ETHICAL / LEGAL ISSUES

Chapter/Issue	Page	Chapter/Issue	Page
5/Poverty	81	31/Parental Refusal of Immunizations for Child	687
8/Research Studies on Human Subjects	129	32/Delegation of Care to Unlicensed Personnel	723
10/Confidentiality of Assessment Findings	158	33/Following Orders	766
15/Accuracy of Records	232	34/Withdrawal of Ventilator Support	846
16/Alternative Therapies	264	35/Client's Refusal of Treatment	895
17/Child Abuse	288	36/Decisions Regarding Treatment	928
19/Spousal Abuse	312	37/Ending Tube Feeding	957
20/Refusal of Treatment Based on Prejudice	332	38/Judgment of Client's Self-Care	1004
21/Respecting Client Confidentiality	349	39/Reaction to HIV/AIDS	1045
22/Literacy	368	40/Possible Neglect of a Client	1074
23/Caregiver Involvement in Home Care	386	41/Family Conflict Over Healthcare	1117
24/Health Assessment	397	42/Impact of Night Shift on Healthcare Workers	1153
25/Delegating Vital Signs	469	43/Possible Dependence on Pain Medication	1191
26/Needlesticks	487	44/Client Decision Making	1205
27/Client's Refusal of Medications	523	45/Mistreatment of Client by Staff	1230
27/Possible Substance Abuse by a Healthcare Worker	523	46/Anorexia	1263
28/IV Hydration in the Terminally Ill	599	47/Placement of an Elder in a Nursing Home	1294
29/Informed Consent	630	48/Durable Power of Attorney for Healthcare and Advance Directives	1308
30/Ability of Older Adults to Remain Independent Despite Declining Health Status	660	49/Transferring a Client	1333
		50/Abortion	1365

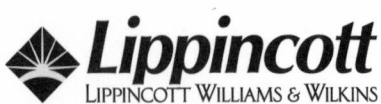

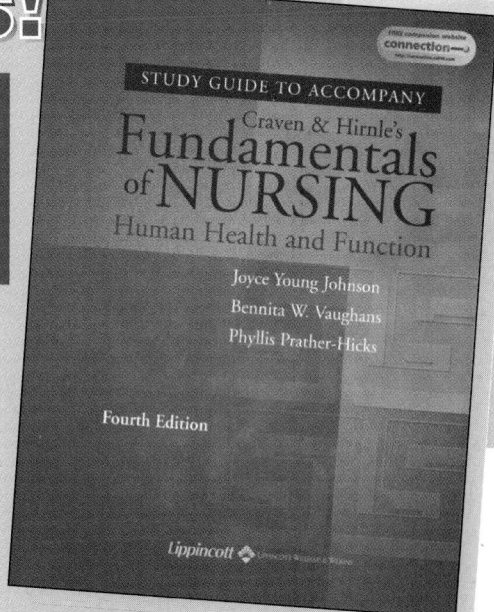
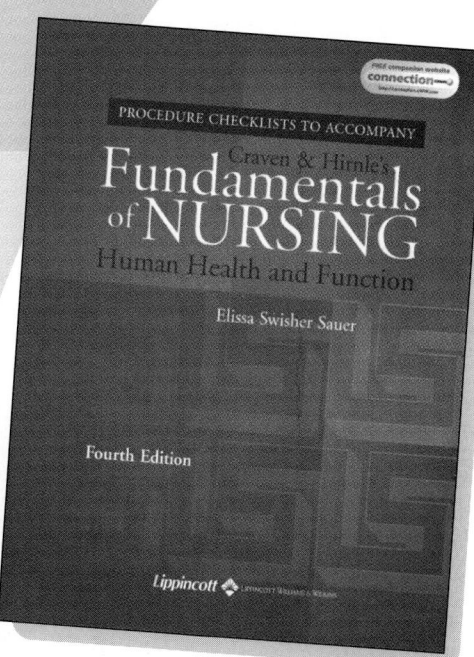
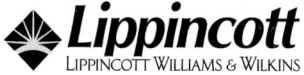

Fundamentals of NURSING
Human Health and Function

Fourth Edition

Ruth F. Craven, EdD, RN, BC, FAAN

Professor
Department of Biobehavioral Nursing
and Health Systems

Associate Dean
Educational Outreach and Community Relations
University of Washington School of Nursing
Seattle, Washington

Constance J. Hirnle, MN, RN

Nursing Development Specialist
Virginia Mason Medical Center
Seattle, Washington

Lecturer, Biobehavioral Nursing and Health Systems
University of Washington School of Nursing
Seattle, Washington

37 Contributors

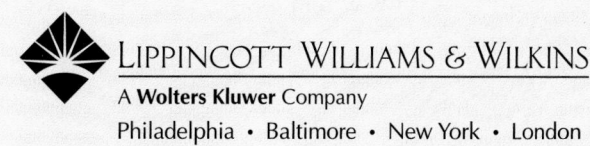

LIPPINCOTT WILLIAMS & WILKINS
A **Wolters Kluwer** Company
Philadelphia · Baltimore · New York · London
Buenos Aires · Hong Kong · Sydney · Tokyo

Executive Editor: Ilze Rader
Managing Editor: Lisa Popeck
Developmental Editor: Renée Gagliardi
Editorial Assistant: Sharon Nowak
Senior Project Editor: Rosanne Hallowell
Senior Production Manager: Helen Ewan

Managing Editor / Production: Erika Kors
Art Director: Carolyn O'Brien
Manufacturing Manager: William Alberti
Indexer: Maria Coughlin
Compositor: Circle Graphics
Printer: Quebecor-Versailles

Fourth Edition

9 8 7 6 5 4

Library of Congress Cataloging-in-Publication Data

Fundamentals of nursing : human health and function / [edited by] Ruth F. Craven,
Constance J. Hirnle.—4th ed.
       p. ; cm.
   Includes bibliographical references and index.
   ISBN 0-7817-3581-5
    1. Nursing. I. Craven, Ruth F. II. Hirnle, Constance J.
   [DNLM: 1. Nursing. 2. Nursing Diagnosis. 3. Nursing Process. WY 100 F97988 2002]
   RT41 .C86 2002
   610.73—dc21

                                                    2002017861

Care has been taken to confirm the accuracy of the information presented and to describe generally accepted practices. However, the authors, editors, and publisher are not responsible for errors or omissions or for any consequences from application of the information in this book and make no warranty, express or implied, with respect to the content of the publication.

The authors, editors, and publisher have exerted every effort to ensure that drug selection and dosage set forth in this text are in accordance with the current recommendations and practice at the time of publication. However, in view of ongoing research, changes in government regulations, and the constant flow of information relating to drug therapy and drug reactions, the reader is urged to check the package insert for each drug for any change in indications and dosage and for added warnings and precautions This is particularly important when the recommended agent is a new or infrequently employed drug.

Some drugs and medical devices presented in this publication have Food and Drug Administration (FDA) clearance for limited use in restricted research settings. It is the responsibility of the health care provider to ascertain the FDA status of each drug or device planned for use in his or her clinical practice.

LWW.com

To Scott, John, and Sarah Hirnle, Nancy
Cassick, and Kathy Schaffer

Bill, Brent, Judy, Shanyce, and Kyle
and Sarah Craven

For their love, support, sacrifice, and
encouragement that allowed us to make this
book a reality

Gail E. Armstrong, ND, RN
Assistant Professor
University of Colorado
Denver, Colorado
   33 – Mobility and Body Mechanics (Chest Tube Procedure)

Debra Beauchaine, MN, ARNP
Adult/Geriatric Nurse Practitioner
Virginia Mason Medical Center
Seattle, Washington
   27 – Medication Administration
   40 – Urinary Elimination

Margaret Auld Bruya, DNSc, RN, CS
Professor
Intercollegiate Center for Nursing Education
Washington State University College of Nursing
Spokane, Washington
   8 – Nursing Research: Evidence-Based Care

James P. Bush, EdD, RN
Associate Professor Emeritus
Department of Biobehavioral Nursing and Health Systems
University of Washington
Seattle, Washington
   44 – Sensory Perception

Terry Cicero, MN, RN, CCRN
Instructor
School of Nursing
Seattle University
Seattle, Washington
   28 – Intravenous Therapy

B. Jane Cornman, PhD, RN
Senior Lecturer
Department of Family and Child Nursing
University of Washington
Seattle, Washington
   16 – Health and Wellness

Susanna Cunningham, PhD, RN, FAAN
Professor
Department of Biobehavioral Nursing and Health Systems
University of Washington
Seattle, Washington
   36 – Fluid, Electrolyte, and Acid-Base Balance

Alice S. Demi, DNS, RN, FAAN
Professor and Acting Director
School of Nursing
Georgia State University
Atlanta, Georgia
   48 – Loss and Grieving

Kathleen Shannon Dorcy, BSN, MN, RN
Research Coordinator
Fred Hutchinson Cancer Research Center
Seattle, Washington
   1 – The Changing Face of Nursing

Kathryn Van Dyke Hayes, DNSc, RN,C
Associate Professor and Associate Chair for Academics
Division of Nursing and Respiratory Care
Shenandoah University
Winchester, Virginia
   9 – Nursing Process: Foundation for Practice
   10 – Nursing Assessment
   11 – Nursing Diagnosis
   12 – Outcome Identification and Planning
   13 – Implementation and Evaluation

Emily Wurster Hitchens, EdD, RN
Professor and Associate Dean
School of Health Sciences
Seattle Pacific University
Seattle, Washington
   5 – Values
   51 – Spiritual Health

Sharon Jensen, MN, RN
Instructor
School of Nursing
Seattle University
Seattle, Washington
   14 – Critical Thinking
   24 – Health Assessment of Human Function
   35 – Oxygenation: Cardiovascular Function

Christina Joy, DNSc, RN
Director of Nursing
Whitman-Walker Clinic
Washington, DC
   26 – Asepsis and Infection Control
   39 – The Body's Defense Against Infection

Lucille Kindely Kelley, EdD, RN
Professor and Dean
School of Health Sciences
Seattle Pacific University
Seattle, Washington
  46 – Self-Concept

Michael Kennedy, PhD, RN
Research Assistant Professor
University of Washington
Seattle, Washington
  21 – Communication: The Nurse–Client Relationship

Carol Landis, DNSc, RN
Professor
Department of Biobehavioral Nursing and Health Systems
University of Washington
Seattle, Washington
  49 – Stress, Coping, and Adaptation

Lisa Lesneski, PhD(c), MS, RN
Assistant Professor, Nursing
University of Scranton
Scranton, Pennsylvania
  3 – The Profession of Nursing
  4 – Nursing Theory and Conceptual Frameworks

Barbara S. Levine, PhD, ARNP, CS
Gerontological Nurse Practitioner
Holy Redeemer Health System
Philadelphia, Pennsylvania
  45 – Cognitive Processes

Louise Martell, PhD, RN
Associate Professor
University of Washington
Seattle, Washington
  17 – Lifespan Development

Katherine E. Matas, PhD, RN
Visiting Assistant Professor
Northern Arizona University
Flagstaff, Arizona
  2 – Community-Based Nursing and Continuity of Care
  23 – Care Management

Karen L. Moe, MEd, RN
Staff Development Specialist
University of Washington Medical Center
Clinical Faculty, School of Nursing
University of Washington
Seattle, Washington
  29 – Perioperative Nursing

Donna Moniz, MN, RN, JD
Attorney
Seattle, Washington
  6 – Ethical and Legal Concerns

Marjorie A. Muecke, PhD, RN, FAAN
Professor, Psychosocial and Community Health
University of Washington
Seattle, Washington
  20 – Culture and Ethnicity

Georgia L. Roberts Narsavage, PhD, RN, CS
Associate Professor and Director of MSN Program
Francis Payne Bolton School of Nursing
Case Western Reserve University
Cleveland, Ohio
  47 – Families and Their Relationships

Ellen F. Olshansky, DNSc, RN,C
Professor
Associate Dean, Graduate Programs
School of Nursing
Duquesne University
Pittsburgh, Pennsylvania
  50 – Human Sexuality

Jane W. Peterson, PhD, RN
Professor
School of Nursing
Seattle University
Seattle, Washington
  19 – Individual, Family, and Community

Marlene Reimer, PhD, RN, CNN(C)
Professor of Nursing
Associate Dean, Research
The University of Calgary
Calgary, Alberta
Canada
  42 – Sleep and Rest

Ginger Salvadalena, MN, RN, CWOCN
Clinical Education Specialist
Enterostomal Therapy Nurse
Hollister Incorporated
Libertyville, Illinois
  38 – Skin Integrity and Wound Healing

Jennifer M. Schaller-Ayers, PhD, RN,C
Associate Professor
College of Nursing
East Tennessee State University
Johnson City, Tennessee
  31 – Health Maintenance

Sarah Shannon, PhD, RN
Associate Professor
Department of Biobehavioral Nursing and Health Systems
University of Washington
Seattle, Washington
  6 – Ethical and Legal Concerns

Mary Shellkey, PhC, RN
Assistant Professor
School of Nursing
Seattle University
Seattle, Washington
  18 – The Older Adult

Andreana Siu, RN, DNSc
Nurse Practitioner
Department of Cardiology
VA Palo Alto Health Care System
Palo Alto, California
  Connections Web Site

Sheila M. Sparks, DNSc, RN, CS
Director and Associate Professor
Division of Nursing and Respiratory Care
Shenandoah University
Winchester, Virginia
  9 – Nursing Process: Foundation for Practice
  10 – Nursing Assessment
  11 – Nursing Diagnosis
  12 – Outcome Identification and Planning
  13 – Implementation and Evaluation

Jessica Thomas, MN, RN
Former Director, Women's Services
General Hospital Medical Center
Everett, Washington
  7 – Nurse Leader and Manager

Unabeth Westfall, PhD, RN
Professor
School of Nursing
Oregon Health Sciences University
Portland, Oregon
  37 – Nutrition

Diana Wilkie, PhD, RN
Professor
Department of Biobehavioral Nursing and Health Systems
University of Washington
Seattle, Washington
  43 – Pain Perception and Management

Weihua Zhang, MS, RN
Clinical Associate
Emory University
Atlanta, Georgia
  48 – Loss and Grieving

Joan M. Baker, MS, RN, CS

Connie Bellin, PhD(C), RN

Diane Britt, MN, RN

Catherine Broom, ARNP, CS

Karen K. Carlson, MN, RN, CCRN

Dona Rinaldi Carpenter, EdD, RN, CS

Ann Tyler Chadwick, MN, RN, CRRN (deceased)

Teresa A. Delarose, EdD, RN, CNOR

Barbara Dikty, BSN, RN

Mary P. Farley, MN, RN, CCRN

Mary Kay Flynn, MA, RN, CCRN

Elaine A. Furst, MA, RN

Polly E. Gardner, MN, RN

Laina M. Gerace, PhD, RN

Mikell Goe, MN, RN, CCRN

Joanne Woodhull Goepfert, MN, PHC, RN

Mary Sue Gorski, MN, RNC

Celia L. Hartley, MN, RN

Judy A. Hartmann, MSN, RN

Robert W. Hirnle, MS, RRT

L. Michele Issel, PhD, RN

Joan M. Jenks, MSN, RN

Don Johnson, PhD, RN

Ann E. Kelly, MSN, RN, CS

Joy Miller Knopp, MN, RN, OCN

Kathleen Kovarik, MN, RN

Claudia Kroll, MSEd, MSN, ARNP

Valerie G. Larson, MN, ARNP, CS

Alice Lind, BSN, RN

Mary McGregor, MN, RN, CDE

Beverly S. McKenna, MN, RN

Kristine Iwersen Moore, MN, RN, CDE

Connie Nakao, PhD, RN

Cheryl M. Prandoni, MSN, RNC

Bonnie Reinert, PhD, RN

Gaie Rubenfeld, MS, RN

Barbara J. Ruff, MN, RN

Jill Salisbury, MSN, RN, CS

Barbara Scheffer, MS, RN

Anita Shoup, MN, RN

Margaret L. Snyder, MN, RN, CCRN

Michelle Thobaben, MS, PHN, RN, FNP

Karen A, Thomas, PhD, RN

Wendy L. Walker, MN, RN

Lorraine A. Watson, PhD, RN

Sharon Weinstein, MS, RN, CRNI

Karen S. Wulff, MN, EdD, RN

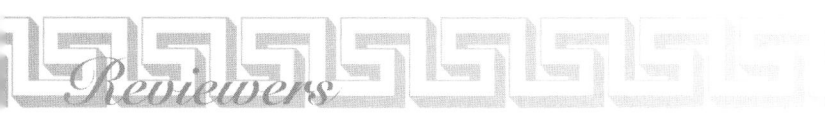
Reviewers

JoAnn Abegglen, PNP, APRN, MS
Assistant Professor
Brigham Young University
Provo, Utah

Valerie Benedix
Clovis Community College
Clovis, New Mexico

Tracy Call-Schmidt, MSN, RN, FNP-C
Nurse Practitioner/Clinical Instructor
Alpine Pain and Stress
University of Utah, College of Nursing
Salt Lake City, Utah

Donna Cartwright, MS, APRN
Dean, Professional and Applied Technology Education
College of Eastern Utah
Price, Utah

Margaret Colyar, DSN, APRN, C-FNP/C-PN
Assistant Professor (Clinical)/Co-director, Nursing Program
University of Utah, College of Nursing
Salt Lake City, Utah

Linda Carman Copel, PhD, RN, CS, DAPA
Associate Professor
Villanova University
Villanova, Pennsylvania

Marianne Craven, RN, MN
Assistant Professor
Utah Valley State College
Salt Lake City, Utah

Emily Donato, RN, BScN, Med
Lecturer
Laurentian University School of Nursing
Sudbury, Ontario
Canada

Kathleen Walsh Free, C-ANP MSN RN-C
Assistant Clinical Professor
Indiana University Southeast
New Albany, Indiana

Donna Funk, RN, MN/E, ONC
Professor of Nursing
Brigham Young University—Idaho
Rexburg, Idaho

Penelope Heaslip, BScN, MEd, RN
Chairperson, Nursing
University College of the Cariboo
Kamloops, British Columbia
Canada

Jennifer Heuberger, RN
Graduate student
Seattle University
Seattle, Washington

Judith Ann Hughes, EdD, RN
Associate Degree Nursing Coordinator
Southwestern Community College
Franklin, North Carolina

Betty Ayotte Jensen, PhD, RN
Associate Professor of Nursing
Humboldt State University
Arcata, California

David C. Keller, MS, APRN
Assistant Teaching Professor
Brigham Young University, College of Nursing
Provo, Utah

Michalene King, RN, BSN, MSEd, MSN
Associate Professor of Nursing
West Liberty State College
West Liberty, West Virginia

Pauline Ladebauche, RNC, MS
Director, Nursing Laboratories
University of Massachusetts Lowell
Lowell, Massachusetts

Carol Lavender, MSN, RN-C
Assistant Professor
Brigham Young University
Provo, Utah

Gayle Lee, PhP, RN, CCRN
Faculty
Brigham Young University—Idaho
Rexburg, Idaho

Geeta Maharaj, MSN, CPNP
Clinical Instructor
University of Utah College of Nursing
Salt Lake City, Utah

Gary Measom, RN, PhD
Department of Nursing
Utah Valley State College
Orem, Utah

Barbara Nubile, RN, MSN
Nursing Department Chair
Northern Marianas College
Saipan, MP

Ann Pinner, RN, BSN, MS
Instructor
Georgia Perimeter College
Clarkston, Georgia

LouAnn Provost, MSN, RN
Associate Professor
Utah Valley State College
Orem, Utah

Catherine B. Talley
Greenville, South Carolina

Iris Woodard, RN-CS, BSN, ANP
Nurse Practitioner
Kaiser Permanente
Springfield, Virginia

Kathleen Zajic, RN, MSN
Associate Professor of Nursing
College of St. Mary
Omaha, Nebraska

As the 21st century begins, nursing's focus has not changed. Promotion and maintenance of individual, family, and community health; management of a healthy environment; and care of the ill remain at the center of nursing. Two basic premises of this fourth edition of *Fundamentals of Nursing: Human Health and Function* relate to these issues.

The first premise is that the art and science of professional nursing practice focus on the health, function, and wellness of the person. The goals are maintaining, supporting, and restoring health and function in various settings. Achieving these goals requires nurses to promptly identify potential alterations in function and their effects on clients' activities of daily living. The second premise is that contemporary nursing practice is based on the appropriate selection and use of nursing interventions. In nursing practice, these activities involve the "diagnosis and treatment of human responses to potential or actual health problems" (American Nurses Association, 1980).

Through the incorporation of both premises, we have attempted to create an innovative text that helps nursing faculty prepare beginning nursing students for the challenging and dynamic nursing practice of the new millennium. Our intent is to provide students with the knowledge base to assess a client's ability to function independently, evaluate the client's ability to cope with altered function, help the client identify realistic outcomes, and intervene as appropriate to maximize the client's function. These nursing responsibilities are critical as health care delivery occurs in various community-based settings and focuses on promoting the client's responsibility for self-care.

ORGANIZATION OF THE TEXT

The text is organized in two main sections: **Section I, Conceptual Foundations of Nursing,** and **Section II, Human Function and Clinical Nursing Therapeutics.**

Section I presents the professional and clinical concepts essential to nursing today. This section contains six units.

- **Unit 1, The Delivery of Nursing Care,** discusses the current health care delivery system. *Chapter 1, The Changing Face of Nursing,* is an innovative approach to presenting issues in current nursing practice. It introduces students to the "reality" of nursing by presenting the stories of several actual nurses. Reflection questions following the stories encourage students to tie together related themes and to explore how the experiences of others may apply to their own careers. *Chapter 2, Community-Based Nursing and Continuity of Care,* shows how health care and nursing are now community-focused, rather than solely hospital-focused. Continuity of care, important to ensuring that clients are not lost in the increasingly complex health care system, is also part of chapter 2.
- **Unit 2, Concepts Essential for Professional Nursing,** introduces students to concepts essential for nursing practice. *Chapter 3, The Profession of Nursing,* presents nursing's

history, current standards, and other issues. Chapter 4 summarizes theories and conceptual frameworks basic to nursing. The remaining chapters discuss topics that underscore nursing's vital roles and key issues: values, ethical and legal concerns, leadership and management, and nursing research.

- **Unit 3, The Nursing Process: Framework for Clinical Nursing Therapeutics,** explains the nursing process to beginning students and explores each component in detail. The unit provides the framework for the application of the nursing process throughout the text. First is an overview of the nursing process and how the steps are related. The unit continues with the skills and activities needed to assess a client's health, analyze and cluster data to formulate nursing diagnoses, identify realistic outcomes, formulate plans of care, select nursing interventions, and evaluate the effectiveness of those interventions, including outcome criteria. Next is *Chapter 14, Critical Thinking.* This revised chapter shows students how to combine the components of the nursing process with critical thinking to provide the most effective care possible. It also reinforces the strong critical thinking component of the entire textbook. The final chapter discusses forms of documents and reporting—the communication aspect of the nursing process—with a focus on technology, including computerized systems.
- **Unit 4, Concepts Essential for Human Functioning and Nursing Management,** provides foundational concepts and knowledge about clients essential for providing safe, effective nursing care. It begins with *Chapter 16, Health and Wellness. Chapter 17, Lifespan Development,* presents the concepts of human growth and development. The information in Chapter 17 sets the stage for the "Lifespan Considerations" sections in each chapter in Section II. *Chapter 18, The Older Adult,* is a brand new chapter that explores issues related to care of the burgeoning older adult population. Chapters 19 and 20 explore the individual as part of a family and community, and in terms of culture and ethnicity. Chapter 21 focuses on the communication skills nurses need to establish therapeutic relationships with clients; Chapter 22 follows this idea by exploring teaching skills nurses need to maximize their clients' learning. Chapter 23 explores the important components of discharge planning and home care, vital to ensuring that clients can manage their health care needs independently.
- **Unit 5, Essential Assessment Components,** explores the fundamental skills in each component of health assessment. *Chapter 24, Health Assessment of Human Function,* details an overall health assessment. *Chapter 25, Vital Sign Assessment,* covers the assessment of body temperature, pulse, respirations, and blood pressure.
- **Unit 6, Selected Clinical Nursing Therapeutics,** focuses on nursing responsibilities associated with common

clinical situations that provide the basis for many aspects of nursing care. Topics include asepsis and infection control, medication administration, intravenous therapy, and perioperative care.

Section II, Human Function and Clinical Nursing Therapeutics, is organized by areas of human function. Each chapter contains a consistent nursing process format that presents health care concepts and nursing responsibilities for each functional area. This format focuses on assessment and diagnosis of altered function and human responses, and identification of outcome criteria, followed by implementation of appropriate nursing care strategies, and evaluation of those interventions.

Each clinical nursing care chapter in the 11 units in this section first presents "normal" function, so that students can fully understand the expected function before proceeding to changes or alterations in those areas. Next are factors that may affect the specific function, followed by possible alterations. Understanding of both normal and altered function sets the framework for the assessment of subjective and objective data and for implementation of interventions for both health promotion and altered function. Each chapter in this section emphasizes the latest North American Nursing Diagnosis Association (NANDA) nursing diagnoses, outcome identification, and possible outcome criteria. Additionally, Section II contains many step-by-step, illustrated procedures that cover purpose, assessment, equipment, and steps with rationales. "Lifespan Considerations" and "Home Care Modifications" assist the student with modifying a procedure or making adjustments while caring for all types of clients across different health care settings. "Collaboration and Delegation" assists students to know how to work most effectively with other members of the health care team when performing these common procedures.

KEY FEATURES

Fundamentals of Nursing: Human Health and Function presents the essential concepts, processes, and skills that help students build a solid foundation for professional nursing practice. To achieve this goal, the text

- **Emphasizes human health, function, and wellness.** Building on the foundational sciences helps students fully understand normal function, which provides a solid background for understanding the scientific rationales for basic nursing care.
- **Emphasizes critical thinking.** The student learns to apply critical thinking to a growing knowledge base of nursing care. The book contains a separate, fully revised critical thinking chapter that helps students integrate the concept with the components of the nursing process. Each chapter begins with a vignette and related critical thinking considerations to enhance thinking related to the chapter topic. The pedagogical features throughout the book contain critical thinking exercises that ask students to further explore the issues discussed.
- **Stresses how normal function and dysfunction vary throughout the life cycle.** This emphasis encourages

students to view people and their differing needs within the context of their developmental stage.
- **Discusses the effects of dysfunction on activities of daily living.** Understanding how dysfunction affects a person's daily life enables students to better assist clients to maintain optimal wellness.
- **Reinforces nursing responsibility for promoting optimal function in wellness and illness.** This thread runs throughout the text and helps students to understand the effects of health and illness on human responses and to implement nursing care strategies for people across the health–illness continuum.
- **Emphasizes holistic care across the life cycle.** This emphasis helps students to see clients as having equally important physiologic, psychosocial, and spiritual needs.
- **Provides a strong nursing process and nursing diagnosis framework.** The nursing process is fundamental to nursing care. This organizing structure creates a strong theoretical underpinning, which assists students to understand how to use the nursing process and nursing diagnoses in clinical practice.
- **Emphasizes client goals and outcome criteria.** Nursing interventions relate to outcomes, and measurable client behaviors help students evaluate the effectiveness of interventions performed.
- **Explores community-based nursing.** Discharge planning and home care have been expanded to meet the changing environments for care in the health care system and to help students understand the importance of continuity of care.
- **Emphasizes collaborative care.** An integral part of community-based care is collaboration among various health care professionals. The nurse is part of this team and, in fact, often manages the team. To help the student understand collaborative care, displays entitled "Collaborative Care Plan: Critical Pathway," appear in the text.
- **Features a family focus.** This perspective encourages students to view clients in light of their family relationships and roles, and to view families as critical members of the team that helps clients meet their needs.
- **Emphasizes communication.** Communication is an essential component of all human relationships. This text helps students become effective listeners and reliable communicators on the health care team. Boxed displays called "Therapeutic Dialogues" compare less effective and more effective ways for nurses to communicate with clients and colleagues. These dialogues serve as excellent learning tools.
- **Emphasizes nursing research.** By introducing research early, beginning students learn to be discriminating consumers of nursing research, understand its relevance to clinical practice, and value its importance in the advancement of professional nursing.
- **Considers the client as an individual.** The student learns that at the center of all the applied knowledge and care is an individual with human needs. The text avoids gender bias and emphasizes ethnic and cultural needs without resorting to stereotypes.

FEATURES FOR STUDENT LEARNING

To reinforce and enhance learning and involve the student in the learning process, numerous features summarize or highlight text information.

- **Learning Objectives, Key Terms, and Key Concepts** alert students about what to expect in the chapter, provide important terms that are defined within the chapter, and help students focus on and review chapter content.
- **Critical Thinking Challenge.** Clinical "vignettes" related to the chapter's content open each chapter and emphasize the real world of nursing practice. Related photos and critical thinking questions accompany the vignettes.
- **Outcome-Based Teaching Plans.** This feature contains client-focused methods for teaching, geared toward health promotion and the underlying concepts of fundamentals. The plans present brief scenarios and the related desired outcomes. They then explain targeted strategies for helping clients achieve their goals.
- **Nursing Research and Critical Thinking.** These displays focus on nursing-related topics that groups of experts have examined along with their conclusions. They present studies and their overall implications for nursing practice and related critical thinking.
- **Clinical Research.** These displays target strategies for specific client problems based on guidelines established by governmental agencies.
- **Therapeutic Dialogues.** These displays provide examples of "less effective" and "more effective" communication with clients and colleagues. Critical Thinking Challenges appear at the end of each Therapeutic Dialogue display.
- **Planning: Examples of NIC/NOC Interventions.** These updated boxes list specific interventions based on NIC/NOC nomenclatures.
- **Safety Alerts.** These small boxes appear close to related text issues and address specific safety concerns for nurses.
- **Ethical/Legal Issues.** These displays present scenarios related to the chapter topic, focusing on an ethical or legal dilemma. Reflection questions make the student ponder implications for themselves personally and professionally.
- **Apply Your Knowledge.** These features ask students to answer questions based on knowledge they have gained from the chapter and previous chapters. These questions have clear and definite answers, found in Appendix A.
- **Nursing Plans of Care.** These revised displays are found in all chapters in Section II. These sample plans are linked with nursing diagnoses used in the chapters to enrich the student's understanding.

- **References and Bibliographies** provide students with classic readings, current nursing resources, and a broad base of substantive reading material.
- **Boxed displays and tables** throughout the text, in addition to the recurring features listed above, emphasize and summarize essential material.
- **Color photos and art** clarify the text, illustrate procedures, and enhance understanding.

NEW TO THIS EDITION

The following elements to guide student learning are new to this edition:

- A brand new chapter: *Chapter 18, The Older Adult*
- A fully revised *Chapter 14, Critical Thinking*
- New content on care of the dying person in *Chapter 48, Loss and Grieving*
- Expanded coverage of alternative and complementary therapies in *Chapter 16, Health and Wellness*
- Updated NANDA Nursing Diagnoses throughout the book
- Updated NIC/NOC displays
- New, illustrated nursing procedures:
  - Denture Care
  - Performing a Surgical Hand Scrub
  - Donning Surgical Gown and Gloves
  - Setting Up a Sterile Field
  - Using a Mechanical Lift
  - Transferring a Client to a Stretcher
  - Care of a Client with a Chest Drainage Tube
  - Removing Contact Lenses
  - Assisting an Adult with Inserting a Hearing Aid
  - Drawing Up Two Medications in a Syringe
- More than 30 new photos and line drawings

TEACHING–LEARNING PACKAGE

Fundamentals of Nursing: Human Health and Function has an extensive ancillary package, designed with both the student and instructor in mind. A *Study Guide* augments the text and provides a means of student self-evaluation. *Procedures Checklists* provide guidelines for student practice and evaluation tools for faculty. The *Instructor's Resource CD-ROM* includes teaching-learning plans. The Connections web site (*www.connections/lww.com*) provides much supplemental material for both instructors and students.

Ruth F. Craven, EdD, RN, BC, FAAN
Constance J. Hirnle, MN, RN

Fundamentals of Nursing: Human Health and Function, Fourth Edition

34 Oxygenation: Respiratory Function

Key Terms
alveoli
apnea
atelectasis
bronchioles
bronchospasm
diffusion
dyspnea
hyperventilation

hypoventilation
hypoxemia
hypoxia
oxygen saturation
pulse oximetry
respiration
tracheostomy
ventilation

Learning Objectives
Upon completion of this chapter, the student will be able to do the following:
1. Identify factors that can interfere with effective oxygenation of body tissues.
2. Describe common manifestations of altered respiratory function.
3. Discuss lifespan-related changes and problems in respiratory function.
4. Describe important elements in the respiratory assessment.
5. List three appropriate nursing diagnoses and outcomes for the client with altered respiratory function.
6. Describe nursing measures to ensure a patent airway.
7. Discuss safe administration of oxygen using different modes of delivery.
8. Describe the impact of respiratory dysfunction on activities of daily living.
9. Identify home care considerations for the respiratory client.

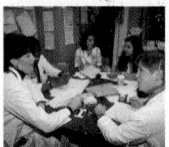

Critical Thinking Challenge
You are a nurse working in an intermediate care facility. In the past, your facility has served primarily geriatric clients. Recently the facility has begun to care for stable, ventilator-dependent clients. Although staff respiratory therapists regularly monitor the ventilator-dependent clients, the clients' arrival has caused considerable anxiety among the nurses. You have volunteered to serve on a committee to address their concerns.

After you have completed this chapter, return to the above scenario and reflect on the following areas of Critical Thinking:
1. Identify the nurses' concerns about the clients and about themselves that may contribute to their feelings of anxiety.
2. Compare and contrast special needs of these ventilator-dependent clients with those of the average geriatric client.
3. Describe how nursing personnel may collaborate with respiratory care personnel to optimize care for these clients.
4. Identify and plan strategies that may make the nursing staff feel more comfortable caring for the new clients.

Chapter Openers include Key Terms, Learning Objectives, and Critical Thinking Challenges. *Key Terms* highlight important terms found in the chapter. *Learning Objectives* help you review the most important points of the content. *Critical Thinking Challenges* emphasize the real world of nursing practice through scenarios for your consideration and response. Related photos and questions to accompany these everyday examples will help you integrate your learning as you prepare for practice.

Nursing Research and Critical Thinking
Does the Medicare Hospice Nursing Home Benefit Supplement, Not Duplicate, Care Already Provided in Nursing Homes?

Grief and bereavement are common to families of clients with end-stage Alzheimer's disease. Many clients with end-stage dementia reside in the nursing home setting, where clients with dementia may comprise up to 70% of the client population. Many people do not understand the unique aspects of hospice care in the nursing home and imagine these services to duplicate care that is already given. Hospice providers designed this study to determine the prevalence of grief and bereavement services in nursing homes. The researchers performed a telephone survey of 121 nursing homes regarding their on-site grief and bereavement services. A structured telephone survey was administered to nursing home staff, either the social worker or director of nursing. A total of 111 nursing homes responded to the survey, a response rate of 91%. An estimation of prop... interval (CI) wa... The results of t... sent sympathy... 99% did not pro... mary caregiver... after death, 99%...

From Murphy, K.,...
The importance...
Journal of the An...

able bereavement support groups, 76% did not offer referral for counseling when bereavement intervention was deemed appropriate, 54% sent a representative from the nursing home to the funeral home or the funeral of a client who died at their facility, 99% had no contact with family members after the death of their clients.

Critical Thinking Considerations. The subjects for this study were limited to nursing homes in one small area of the United States. However, the researchers point out several issues that are important to nurses who provide care for end-stage dementia clients in other settings:

• Nursing home staff and families of clients are unaware of the unique service hospice provides in the nursing home for clients with end-stage Alzheimer's disease.

Nursing Research and Critical Thinking boxes focus on nursing-related topics and conclusions arrived at by groups of experts. They present the relevance of such findings for nursing practice.

OUTCOME-BASED TEACHING PLAN

George Porter, a 54-year-old executive, is being discharged from the telemetry unit following a r... infarction. He and his wife have both express... that an emergency could arise when they retu... They want to be prepared to handle such an e...

OUTCOME: Mr. and Mrs. Porter can verba... recognize and treat anginal pain.
Strategies
• Provide handout explaining angina and its t...
• Review medications (names, dosages, when special considerations) for each new medica... has been ordered.
• Provide above information about medicatio... ing and have client restate it.
• Stress the necessity for rest when Mr. Porter... pain or pressure to see if it subsides.
• Instruct Mr. Porter to space oxygen-consum... ties (e.g., don't exercise right after eating).
• Review specifics regarding PRN nitroglyceride. Have Mr. and Mrs. Porter reverbalize.

OUTCOME: Mrs. Porter can verbalize when to call 911 and develop a plan to become proficient in CPR.
Strategies
• Discuss with Mr. and Mrs. Porter their plan for handling a cardiac emergency (unrelieved chest pain and cardiac arrest).
• Explore Mrs. Porter's comfort with performing CPR on her husband if needed.
• Assess Mrs. Porter's specific plans for taking a community course to learn CPR.
• Provide a written list of when to call 911 (unrelieved chest pain; new onset of rapid, irregular, or very slow heart rate, especially if accompanied by severe fatigue or dizziness; fainting or loss of consciousness).
• Provide a sticker with emergency numbers for the Porters to keep on the phone.

Outcome-Based Teaching Plans direct strategies for client and family education toward specific goals. They focus on health promotion and interventions for altered function.

THERAPEUTIC DIALOGUE
Cardiac Surgery

Scene for Thought
Jean Norman is a 77-year-old woman lying in her bed in the ICU with tubes and beeping monitors around her. She turns to the nurse, who approaches with an extra blanket that she had requested.

Less Effective	More Effective
Client: Thank you for the blanket, dear. I'm so cold here. *(Speaks softly and weakly.)*	**Client:** Thank you for the blanket, dear. I'm so cold here. *(Speaks softly and weakly.)*
Nurse: How are you feeling otherwise, Ms. Norman? *(Arranges the blanket over her.)*	**Nurse:** How are you feeling otherwise, Ms. Norman? *(Arranges the blanket over her.)*
Client: Very tired and sore. I guess a bypass operation takes a lot out of you. *(Smiles weakly.)* But I'm sure it will turn out fine. *(Doesn't maintain eye contact.)*	**Client:** Very tired and sore. I guess a bypass operation takes a lot out of you. *(Smiles weakly.)* But I'm sure it will turn out fine. *(Doesn't maintain eye contact.)*
Nurse: You seem to be doing just great—your vital signs are normal, your incisions are healing well, and everything else looks good. I don't think I've seen too many people recover from surgery this fast, honestly. Are you in much pain right now? *(Stands quietly by the bed and holds the client's hand.)*	**Nurse:** Tell me more about that. *(Stands at the bedside, looking at her.)*
Client: A little. If you have some time perhaps you could get me something? *(Still smiling.)*	**Client:** What do you mean, dear?
Nurse: Right away, Ms. Norman. You only have to let me know. *(Smiles and gives her hand a warm squeeze.)*	**Nurse:** You sound a little worried.
...k you, dear. I appreciate it. *(Squeezes back.)*	**Client:** *(Her eyes fill with tears, and she looks toward the hallway where her husband is sitting.)* Yes. I'm really worried if I'll be able to be as active as I was. *(Cries.)*
	Nurse: *(Holds her hand, stands quietly by the bed.)*
	Client: I know I'm being silly. People go through this operation all the time. *(Dries her eyes.)*
	Nurse: It's usual for people to be worried. I'm glad you decided to share that worry with me.
	Client: Do you think so? You don't think I'm being neurotic about this?
	Nurse: I'm not sure what you mean by neurotic, but I know that you seem fearful, and sometimes talking about fears helps them become more manageable.
	Client: That's true. *(She begins to talk about her fear of becoming an invalid and not being able to golf with her husband.)*

Therapeutic Dialogues compare "less effective" and "more effective" communication to help direct typical interactions between nurses and clients, families, and colleagues.

...inking Challenge
...s cared for Ms. Norman's needs. Compare and contrast the dialogues.
...the first dialogue less effective?
...ow the nursing assessment, diagnoses, and interventions differ between the first and second
• Discuss which nursing outcome would be most effective in Ms. Norman's care.

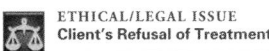

ETHICAL/LEGAL ISSUE
Client's Refusal of Treatment

Mrs. Chow, a competent 74-year-old client, li[...]
tirement center. She has had congestive heart [...]
the past 12 years. Her feet are swollen and pa[...]
she walks on them. Difficult breathing from th[...]
failure limits her activity tolerance. When you[...]
room to give her the "water pill," Lasix, she s[...]
don't want to take it any more." You explain [...]
water pill is necessary to help her kidneys exc[...]
excess fluid. Her response is, "When I take it,[...]
myself. I would rather have my dignity than h[...]
happen." Over the course of several days, her [...]
worsens to the point where she needs the Lasix to live.
She continues to state that she would rather die with
dignity than take the Lasix.

Reflection
- Identify the important issues in this case.
- Explore how your own feelings, values, and beliefs are
  the same or different from Mrs. Chow's.
- Consider your position. What is your role as a nurse in
  this situation?
- Target ways to work with the client to help her make
  choices about her healthcare and the outcomes.

Ethical/Legal Issue boxes focus on an ethical
or legal dilemma related to the chapter topic. Reflection questions ask you to ponder the implications
for yourself as a student and as a practicing nurse.

Apply Your Knowledge boxes help
ensure that you understand the clinical relevance
of what you have learned. You can check your
responses against those found in Appendix A.

APPLY YOUR KNOWLEDGE

Stan Myer, 76, lives in an assisted living faci[...]
occasionally has some confusion. He has bee[...]
you that his new glasses are worthless. The g[...]
seemed to work at first, but now he says he s[...]
thing wavy or distorted in the center of his vision. He
keeps asking you to clean the glasses and get rid of
whatever is making it difficult for him to see. You have
cleaned his glasses several times and they look clear to
you, yet you have noticed that Mr. Myer no longer
reads the paper and his signature has changed.
  What assessment data do you need to collect at this
point? Discuss how you will help to clarify Mr. Myers'
sensory perception.
  Check your answers in Appendix A.

500 *Unit 6* Selected Clinical Nursing Therapeutics

PROCEDURE 26-2

SURGICAL HAND SCRUB

Purpose
1. Remove as many microorganisms from the
   hands as possible before a sterile procedure.
2. Decrease the risk of infection for high-risk groups
   (e.g., newborns, transplant recipients).

Assessment
- Assess agency policy regarding surgical hand scrub.
- Assess hands for cuts, abrasions, or traumatized
  skin that can harbor microorganisms.
- Assess length and conditions of nails and cuticles.
  Long nails, artificial nails, and nail polish should be
  avoided.

Equipment
Deep sink with knee or foot controls for soap and water.
Agency-approved antimicrobial soap.
Surgical scrub brush
Plastic nail stick or sterile nail cleaner
Sterile towel for drying

Procedure
1. Remove rings. Apply surgical attire (scrubs, shoe
   cover, cap or hood, face mask and protective eye
   wear)
   *Rationale: Rings can harbor microorganisms.
   Applying attire after handwashing would
   contaminate hands.*
2. Wash and rinse hands for the initial wash.
   *Rationale: To remove gross contamination and
   transient microorganisms.*
3. Open disposable brush impregnated with antimicrobial soap and adjust water temperature to
   warm using water control lever.
   *Rationale: Antimicrobial soap is more effective at
   reducing microorganisms. Use of warm water
   decreases drying of the hands. This is especially important in areas where surgical hand
   scrubs are performed frequently.*
4. Wet hands and arms. Keep elbows bent so that
   hands remain higher than elbows. Water will
   flow down hands and off elbows.
   *Rationale: Movement of water and dirt will flow
   from hands to less clean areas, thus not contaminating hands during the scrub.*
5. Use nail stick or cleaner to clean under nails of
   both hands.
   *Rationale: The nails can harbor significant bacte-
   ria and need to be cleaned thoroughly.*
6. Wet scrub brush or apply antibacterial soap if not
   already impregnated in the brush.

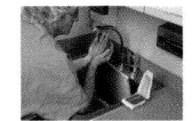

Step 4 When wetting arms and hands, elbows are
bent and hands remain higher than the elbows.

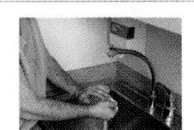

Step 5 Use the nail stick to clean under the nails.

*Rationale: Antibacterial soap assists in removing
transient and resident microorganisms.*
7. *Anatomic Timed Scrub.* Starting with the fingertips, scrub each anatomic area (nails, fingers
   each side and web space, palmar surface, dorsal
   surface, and forearm) for the designated amount
   of time according to agency policy (total usually
   around 5 minutes). Scrub vigorously using vertical strokes. Repeat with other hand.

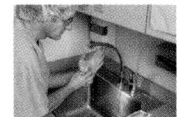

Step 7 Use the scrub brush with vertical strokes.

80 Detailed Procedures include many
illustrations, along with carefully spelled out steps
and their rationales. They also include *Lifespan
Considerations, Home Care Modifications,* and
Collaboration and Delegation guidelines to assist
with modifying procedures based on age, setting,
or acting in a supervisory capacity.

Chapter 38 Skin Integrity and Wound Healing 1013

PROCEDURE 38-3 (Continued)

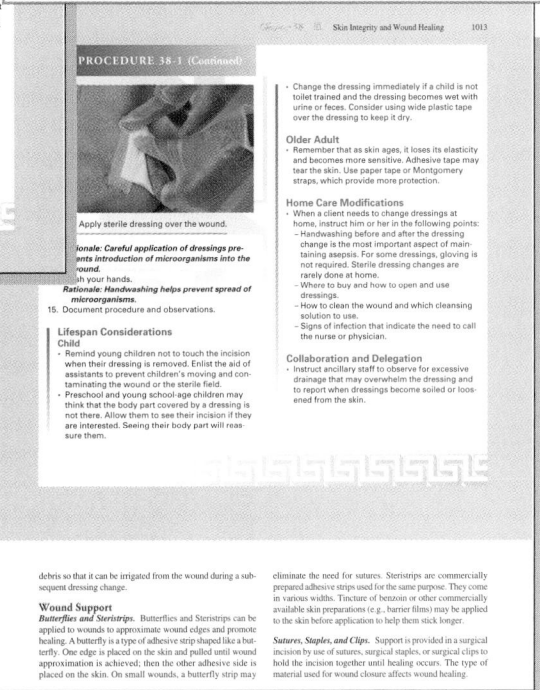

Apply sterile dressing over the wound.

*Rationale: Careful application of dressings pre-
[ve]nts introduction of microorganisms into the
[w]ound.*
[Wa]sh your hands.
   *Rationale: Handwashing helps prevent spread of
   microorganisms.*
15. Document procedure and observations.

Lifespan Considerations
Child
- Remind young children not to touch the incision
  when their dressing is removed. Enlist the aid of
  assistants to prevent children's moving and contaminating the wound or the sterile field.
- Preschool and young school-age children may
  think that the body part covered by a dressing is
  not there. Allow them to see their incision if they
  are interested. Seeing their body part will reassure them.

- Change the dressing immediately if a child is not
  toilet trained and the dressing becomes wet with
  urine or feces. Consider using wide plastic tape
  over the dressing to keep it dry.

Older Adult
- Remember that as skin ages, it loses its elasticity
  and becomes more sensitive. Adhesive tape may
  tear the skin. Use paper tape or Montgomery
  straps, which provide more protection.

Home Care Modifications
- When a client needs to change dressings at
  home, instruct him or her in the following points:
  - Handwashing before and after the dressing
    change is the most important aspect of main-
    taining asepsis. For some dressings, gloving is
    not required. Sterile dressing changes are
    rarely done at home.
  - Where to buy and how to open and use
    dressings.
  - How to clean the wound and which cleansing
    solution to use.
  - Signs of infection that indicate the need to call
    the nurse or physician.

Collaboration and Delegation
- Instruct ancillary staff to observe for excessive
  drainage that may overwhelm the dressing and
  to report when dressings become soiled or loosened from the skin.

debris so that it can be irrigated from the wound during a subsequent dressing change.

Wound Support
Butterflies and Steristrips. Butterflies and Steristrips can be
applied to wounds to approximate wound edges and promote
healing. A butterfly is a type of adhesive strip shaped like a butterfly. One edge is placed on the skin and pulled until wound
approximation is achieved; then the other adhesive side is
placed on the skin. On small wounds, a butterfly strip may

eliminate the need for sutures. Steristrips are commercially
prepared adhesive strips used for the same purpose. They come
in various widths. Tincture of benzoin or other commercially
available skin preparations (e.g., barrier films) may be applied
to the skin before application to help them stick longer.

Sutures, Staples, and Clips. Support is provided in a surgical
incision by use of sutures, surgical staples, or surgical clips to
hold the incision together until healing occurs. The type of
material used for wound closure affects wound healing.

THE CLIENT WITH INEFFECTIVE AIRWAY CLEARANCE

Nursing Diagnosis

Ineffective Airway Clearance related to tracheobronchial infection as manifested by weak cough, adventi-
sounds, and copious green sputum production.

Client Goal

Client will mobilize pulmonary secretions.

Client Outcome Criteria

• After teaching session, client demonstrates proper coughing techniques.
• Client drinks at least six glasses of water per day while in hospital.
• Client demonstrates correct self-suctioning technique before discharge.

Nursing Interventions	Scientific Rationale
1. Provide and teach the client the importance of ade-quate hydration. Encourage fluids (2,000–3,000 mL per 24 hours). Monitor intake and output. Avoid milk and milk products. Ultrasonic nebulizer treatment.	1. Adequate hydration thins secretions, which prevents mucus from plugging airways. Evaluate hydration status of client. Milk products tend to thicken secretions. Moisten and aid mobility of respiratory secretions.
2. Position and encourage client to cough to promote mobilization of secretions. Deep breathing every 2 hours. Huff coughing. Have client assume sitting position if possible.	2. Open alveoli and prevent further atelectasis. Prevent airway collapse. Permit deep inspiration and forceful abdominal con-tractions necessary for coughing.
3. Administer analgesic before cough session if pain limits coughing effectiveness.	3. If client fears pain, he or she hesitates to breathe deeply and cough effectively.
4. Provide or teach client tracheal suctioning if he or she is unable to remove secretions with effective coughing. Hyperoxygenate with 100% O₂ before and after suc-tioning procedure. Suction for no longer than 10 seconds per suctioning attempt. Provide opportunities for client to practice and demonstrate suctioning technique if self-suctioning is necessary.	4. A weak, nonproductive cough causes secretions to be retained in airways and interfere with gas exchange. Hypoxemia, which can occur during the suctioning procedure, is prevented. Longer periods of suction can contribute to tissue trauma and hypoxemia. Suctioning is a complex motor skill that requires practice for skill acquisition and comfort.
5. Provide or teach postural chest physiotherapy as or-dered. Have client or family members demonstrate when comfortable with skill mastery.	5. Secretions drain from major airways using the force of gravity.

Nursing Plans of Care, found in all chapters in Section II, are linked with nursing diagnoses
to enrich your understanding of the content.

PLANNING   Examples of NIC/NOC Interventions

**Accepted Loss and Grieving Nursing Interventions
Classification (NIC)**
Grief Work Facilitation

**Accepted Loss and Grieving Nursing Outcomes
Classification (NOC)**
Coping
Grief Resolution
Psychological Adjustment Life Change

Refer to the following for specifics regarding NIC/NOC:
   McCloskey, J., & Bulechek, G. (2000). *Iowa Intervention
   Project: Nursing Interventions Classification (NIC)* (3rd ed.).
   St. Louis, MO: C. V. Mosby.
Johnson, M., & Maas, M. (2000). *Iowa Outcomes P
   Nursing Outcomes Classification (NOC)* (2nd ed.).
   MO: C. V. Mosby.

Planning: Examples of NIC/NOC Interventions

list specific interventions based on the increasingly important NIC/NOC nomenclatures.

Acknowledgments

Sincere appreciation and warmest thanks are extended to the many people who contributed to the production of this book.

- The contributors, who worked diligently to provide up-to-date information in their specialty areas and were patient with our never-ending requests that were always needed yesterday.
- Our students, who have taught us much and continue to keep our feet planted in the real world.
- The Lippincott Williams & Wilkins editorial team who ensured that the fourth edition meets the market's demands and remains the highest quality possible: Renée Gagliardi, Developmental Editor; Lisa Popeck, Managing Editor; and Ilze Rader, Executive Editor.
- Freelance developmental editors who helped ensure the book published on time: Sarah Kyle, Michael Porter, and Hilarie Surrena.
- Lippincott Williams & Wilkins Production team who kept us on schedule and saw the project through with patience and professionalism: Tom Gibbons, Rosanne Hallowell, and Mike Carcel, as well as freelance copyeditors Beverly Braunlich and Charlotte Kidd.
- Helen Miske, MN, RN, Director of the Learning Resources Center at Seattle University; Debra Beauchaine, MN, ARNP, CA, Adult/Geriatric Nurse Practitioner; Robin Thomas, MN, RN, Providence Medical Center; and Daniel Hallett, Photographer, for their assistance with photographs used in the third edition that were carried over to this text.
- Danielle DiPalma, Maryann Foley, Brett MacNaughton, Joe Morita, and Barbara Proud, who assisted with photographs new to this edition.
- Seattle University, Bessie Burton Sullivan Skilled Nursing Residence, Providence Medical Center, Meydenbauer Medical and Rehabilitation Center, University of Washington, friends, colleagues, and others who contributed photos for use in this text.
- Maureen Niland, PhD, RN, and Jessica Thomas, MN, RN, for consultation and advice on botanicals and financial changes in the health care delivery systems, respectively.

Finally, but most importantly, we acknowledge with love and gratitude the constant support and encouragement of family, friends, students, and colleagues throughout this revision.

Contents

Section I
Conceptual Foundations of Nursing

Unit 1   The Delivery of Nursing Care
1   The Changing Face of Nursing, 5
2   Community-Based Nursing and Continuity of Care, 19

Unit 2   Concepts Essential for Professional Nursing
3   The Profession of Nursing, 39
4   Nursing Theory and Conceptual Frameworks, 55
5   Values, 69
6   Ethical and Legal Concerns, 85
7   Nurse Leader and Manager, 109
8   Nursing Research: Evidence-Based Care, 121

Unit 3   The Nursing Process: Framework for Clinical Nursing Therapeutics
9   Nursing Process: Foundation for Practice, 137
10   Nursing Assessment, 149
11   Nursing Diagnosis, 163
12   Outcome Identification and Planning, 185
13   Implementation and Evaluation, 201
14   Critical Thinking, 215
15   Communication of the Nursing Process: Documenting and Reporting, 229

Unit 4   Concepts Essential for Human Functioning and Nursing Management
16   Health and Wellness, 255
17   Lifespan Development, 267
18   The Older Adult, 295
19   Individual, Family, and Community, 309
20   Culture and Ethnicity, 325
21   Communication: The Nurse-Client Relationship, 343
22   Client Education, 361
23   Care Management, 379

Unit 5   Essential Assessment Components
24   Health Assessment of Human Function, 393
25   Vital Sign Assessment, 443

Unit 6   Selected Clinical Nursing Therapeutics
26   Asepsis and Infection Control, 479
27   Medication Administration, 513
28   Intravenous Therapy, 575
29   Perioperative Nursing, 611

Section II
Human Function and Clinical Nursing Therapeutics

Unit 7   Health Perception and Health Management
30   Safety, 649
31   Health Maintenance, 679

Unit 8   Activity and Exercise
32   Self-Care and Hygiene, 703
33   Mobility and Body Mechanics, 753
34   Oxygenation: Respiratory Function, 809
35   Oxygenation: Cardiovascular Function, 865

Unit 9   Nutrition and Metabolism
36   Fluid, Electrolyte, and Acid-Base Balance, 909
37   Nutrition, 941
38   Skin Integrity and Wound Healing, 983
39   The Body's Defense Against Infection, 1027

Unit 10   Elimination
40   Urinary Elimination, 1063
41   Bowel Elimination, 1101

Unit 11   Sleep and Rest
42   Sleep and Rest, 1143

Unit 12   Cognition and Perception
43   Pain Perception and Management, 1167
44   Sensory Perception, 1199
45   Cognitive Processes, 1219

Unit 13   Self-Perception and Self-Concept
46   Self-Concept, 1253

Unit 14   Roles and Relationships
47   Families and Their Relationships, 1275
48   Loss and Grieving, 1299

Unit 15   Coping and Stress Management
49   Stress, Coping, and Adaptation, 1325

Unit 16   Sexuality and Reproduction
50   Human Sexuality, 1351

Unit 17   Values and Beliefs
51   Spiritual Health, 1381

Appendix A: Answers to "Apply Your Knowledge," 1405
Appendix B: Diagnostic Studies and Interpretation, 1411
Appendix C: Medical Terminology: Prefixes, Roots, and Suffixes, 1451
Appendix D: Selected Information Resources for Nursing Practice, 1459
Appendix E: Herbal Preparations Used As Health Remedies, 1471
Glossary, 1481
Index, 1491

Section **I**
Conceptual Foundations of Nursing

Unit 1   The Delivery of Nursing Care
1   The Changing Face of Nursing, 5
   • Issues and Trends in Current Nursing, 8
   Influence of Today's Healthcare Settings, 8
   Rising Consumerism, 10
   Technologic Advances, 11
   Access to Healthcare and Financial Resources, 12
   Today's Nurse, 13
   • Conclusion, 16
2   Community-Based Nursing and Continuity
   of Care, 19
   • Levels of Healthcare, 20
   Community-Based Healthcare Trends and the
      Determinants of Health, 20
   Community-Based Healthcare, 21
   Community-Based Nursing, 22
   • Community-Based Healthcare Issues, 27
   Fragmentation of Service, 27
   Quality of Care, 27
   Complementary and Alternative Healthcare Services, 27
   Self-Care, 28
   Continuity of Care and Entrance and Exit Within
      the System, 28

Unit 2   Concepts Essential for Professional Nursing
3   The Profession of Nursing, 39
   • Highlights of the Historical Evolution of
   Professional Nursing, 40
   Ancient History, 43
   Contributions of the Greeks, 43
   Early Christian Era, 43
   The Middle Ages, 43
   The Renaissance, 43
   The Reformation, 43
   Nursing in the 18th Century, 44
   Nursing in the 19th Century, 44
   Nursing in the 20th Century, 44
   Nursing in the 21st Century, 45
   • Socialization to Professional Nursing, 45
   Nursing and Professionalism Defined, 45
   Educational Preparation and Career Opportunities, 46
   • Nursing Responsibilities, 49
   Caregiver, 49
   Decision Maker, 49
   Client Advocate, 49
   Manager and Coordinator, 50
   Communicator, 50
   Educator, 50
   • Career Development and Expanded
   Nursing Roles, 50
   Nurse Practitioner, 50

   Clinical Nurse Specialist, 50
   Nurse Midwife, 50
   Nurse Anesthetist, 50
   Nurse Researcher, 51
   Nurse Administrator, 51
   Nurse Educator, 51
   • Professional Nursing Practice, 51
   Standards of Practice, 51
   Nurse Practice Acts, 51
   Nursing Organizations, 51
   • Current and Future Trends in Nursing Practice, 53
4   Nursing Theory and Conceptual Frameworks, 55
   • Nursing Theory, 56
   Development of Nursing Theory, 56
   Four Major Concepts, 57
   • Non-nursing Theories Used in Nursing, 57
   General Systems Theory, 57
   Human Needs Theory: Maslow's Hierarchy of
      Human Needs, 62
   Change Theory, 64
   • Functional Health Patterns as a Framework
   for Nursing, 65
   Health Perception and Health Management, 65
   Activity and Exercise, 65
   Nutrition and Metabolism, 65
   Elimination, 66
   Sleep and Rest, 66
   Cognition and Perception, 66
   Other Patterns, 66
5   Values, 69
   • Value and Belief Patterns, 70
   Professional Values in Nursing, 70
   • Sources of Values, 73
   Cultural Influences, 73
   Socializing Influences, 73
   Lifespan Considerations, 75
   • Effects of Values on Functional Health, 76
   Health Perception and Health Management, 77
   Activity and Exercise, 77
   Nutrition and Metabolism, 77
   Elimination, 77
   Sleep and Rest, 77
   Cognition and Perception, 77
   Self-Perception and Self-Concept, 77
   Roles and Relationships, 79
   Coping and Stress Management, 79
   Sexuality and Reproduction, 79
   Values and Beliefs, 79
   • Manifestations of Nurses' Values, 79
   • Value Conflicts, 80
   Client and Family Conflicts, 80
   Client and Healthcare Conflicts, 80
   Resolving Value Conflicts in the Healthcare System, 80
   Nursing Values Challenged by Managed Care, 81

6   Ethical and Legal Concerns, 85
      • Ethics in Nursing, 86
        Theoretical Frameworks in Ethics, 88
        Principles of Healthcare Ethics, 89
        Ethical Principles of Professional–
           Patient Relationships, 93
        Model for Case Analysis, 94
        Resolving Ethical Dilemmas, 96
      • The Law and Nursing, 98
        Sources of Laws, 98
        Licensure, 98
        Standards of Care, 98
        Torts and Crimes, 99
        Legally Sensitive Areas of Nursing Practice, 102
        Protecting Yourself Legally, 104
7   Nurse Leader and Manager, 109
      • Leadership, 110
        Styles of Leadership, 110
      • Management, 111
        Resource Management, 111
        Skills for Effective Management, 112
      • Applying Leadership and Management
        to Nursing Roles, 114
        Clinical Practice Roles, 114
        Advanced Clinical Practice Roles, 117
        Nursing Management Roles, 118
8   Nursing Research: Evidence-Based Care, 121
      • Research and Nursing, 122
        Scientific Process and Nursing Research, 123
        Historical Appreciation of Nursing Research, 123
        Characteristics of Nursing Research, 124
        Methods of Nursing Research, 125
      • The Research Process, 125
        Problem Area Identification, 125
        Formulation of a Problem Statement, 126
        Proposed Research Questions or Hypotheses, 127
        Data Management, 127
        Analysis of Results, 127
        Dissemination of Results, 127
      • Ethical and Legal Issues, 128
        Institutional Review Boards, 128
        Subject Rights, 129
      • Research and the Professional Nurse, 129
        Levels of Nursing Participation, 129
        Clinical Nursing Practice, 129

**Unit 3   The Nursing Process: Framework
for Clinical Nursing Therapeutics**
9   Nursing Process: Foundation for Practice, 137
      • Historical Development of the Nursing Process, 138
      • Components of the Nursing Process, 138
        Definition, 138
        Phases, 139
        Interactive Nature of Each Phase, 141
      • Theoretical Foundations for Use of the
        Nursing Process, 142
        Systems Theory, 142

Problem-Solving Process, 142
Decision-Making Process, 142
Information-Processing Theory, 143
Diagnostic Reasoning Process, 144
      • Skill Requirements, 144
        Sound Knowledge Base, 144
        Ability to Communicate in Writing, 144
        Ability to Listen, 144
      • Nursing Practice and the Nursing Process, 144
        Professional Relevance, 144
        Functional Health Approach, 145
        Nursing Process Trends, 146
10 Nursing Assessment, 149
      • Preparing for Assessment, 150
        Types of Assessment, 150
        Setting and Environment, 151
      • Assessment Skills, 151
        Observation, 152
        Interviewing, 153
        Physical Examination Techniques, 154
      • Assessment Activities, 155
        Collect Data, 155
        Validate Data, 158
        Organize Data, 160
11 Nursing Diagnosis, 163
      • Historical Development, 164
      • Nursing Diagnosis Taxonomy, 164
        Definition, 165
        Nursing Diagnosis Taxonomy Development, 165
        Nursing Diagnosis Extension and
           Classification Project, 167
        Nursing Diagnoses and Other Healthcare Problems, 168
      • Components of a Nursing Diagnosis, 169
        Diagnostic Label, 169
        Descriptors, 169
        Definition, 175
        Defining Characteristics, 175
        Risk Factors, 175
        Related Factors, 175
      • Diagnosis Activities, 175
        Identify Pattern, 175
        Validate Diagnosis, 177
        Formulate the Diagnostic Statement, 177
      • Nursing Practice and Nursing Diagnoses, 179
        Significance of Nursing Diagnosis, 179
        Functional Approach to Nursing Diagnosis, 182
12 Outcome Identification and Planning, 185
      • Outcome Identification, 186
        Nurse-Sensitive Client Outcomes, 186
      • Outcome Identification Activities, 186
        Establish Priorities, 186
        Establish Client Goals and Outcome Criteria, 188
      • Planning, 188
        Nursing Intervention Classification, 189
        Planning Activities, 189
        Functional Approach to Planning, 198

13 Implementation and Evaluation, 201
  • Implementation, 202
    Implementation Skills, 202
    Implementation Activities, 202
    Types of Nursing Interventions, 203
    Functional Approach to Implementation, 206
  • Evaluation, 206
    Evaluation Skills, 207
    Types of Evaluation, 207
    Evaluation Activities, 207
    Functional Approach to Evaluation, 210
  • Quality Improvement Programs, 210
    American Nurses Association, 211
    *Joint Commission on Accreditation of
      Healthcare Organizations, 211*
    Peer Review, 211

14 Critical Thinking, 215
  • Importance of Critical Thinking in Nursing, 216
  • Conceptual Development of Critical Thinking, 216
  • Factors Affecting Critical Thinking, 217
    Anxiety, 217
    Attitude, 217
    Level of Preparation, 217
    Learning Styles, 218
    Gender Issues, 219
  • The Links Between Knowledge, Critical Thinking,
    Reflection, and Clinical Reasoning, 220
    Development of Critical Thinking Skills, 220
    Diagnostic Reasoning, 222
    Nursing Judgment, 224
    Reflection, 224
    Developing Expertise, 226
  • Applying Critical Thinking to Learning Activities, 227

15 Communication of the Nursing Process:
    Documenting and Reporting, 229
  • Written Communication: The Client Record, 230
    Purpose, 230
    Principles of Data Entry and Management, 231
    Computers in Documentation, 233
    Nursing Entries on the Client Record, 237
  • Oral Communication: Reporting, 245
    Nurse to Nurse, 247
    Report to Primary Care Provider, 247
    Interdisciplinary Team, 248
  • Ethical Concerns in Documentation
    and Reporting, 249
    Confidentiality, 249
    Access to Records, 249

Unit 4 Concepts Essential for Human Functioning
and Nursing Management
16 Health and Wellness, 255
  • Health and Wellness, 256
  • Health Models, 256
    Clinical Model, 256
    Host–Agent–Environment Model, 256
    Health Belief Model, 256

    High-Level Wellness Model, 257
    Holistic Health Model, 258
  • Wellness and Holistic Healthcare, 258
    Holistic Practice, 258
    Meaning of Disease, Illness, and Dysfunction, 259
    Effect of Stress, 261
  • Nursing in Wellness and Holistic Healthcare, 261
    Nursing as a Therapeutic Partnership, 262
    Nursing Diagnoses for Wellness, 262
    Examples of Holistic Healthcare Modalities, 263

17 Lifespan Development, 267
  • Genetics and Environment, 268
    Change, 268
    Reorganization and Integration, 269
  • Concepts of Development, 269
    Principles of Growth and Development, 269
    Growth and Development Theories, 269
  • Growth and Development Through
    the Lifespan, 272
    Intrauterine Development, 272
    Newborn (Birth to 1 Month), 274
    Infant (1 Month to 1 Year), 275
    Toddler (1 to 3 Years), 275
    Preschooler (3 to 6 Years), 276
    School-Age Child (6 to 11 Years), 276
    Adolescent (11 to 22 Years), 277
    Young Adult (21 to 40 Years), 278
    Middle Adult (40 to 60 Years), 279
    Older Adult (60 Years and Older), 279
  • Functional Health and Anticipatory Guidance
    Across the Lifespan, 281
    Health Perception and Health Management, 281
    Activity and Exercise, 282
    Nutrition and Metabolism, 283
    Elimination, 284
    Sleep and Rest, 285
    Cognition and Perception, 286
    Self-Perception and Self-Concept, 287
    Roles and Relationships, 287
    Coping and Stress Tolerance, 288
    Sexuality and Reproduction, 289
    Values and Beliefs, 291

18 The Older Adult, 295
  • Demographics, 296
  • Cognition and Communication, Mood,
    and Self-Care, 297
    Cognition and Communication, 297
    Mood, 298
    Self-Care, 298
  • Mobility, Elimination, and Skin Integrity, 298
    Mobility, 298
    Elimination, 299
    Skin Integrity, 300
  • Nutrition and Health Maintenance, 300
  • Chronic Illness, Infections, and Immunity, 301
    Chronic Illness, 301
    Infections and Immunity, 303

xxiii

- Sleep and Rest, 303
- Pain Management, 304
- Loss and Grief, Loneliness, Coping and Stress, 304
  Loss and Grief, 304
  Loneliness, 304
  Coping and Stress, 305
- Sexuality, Roles and Relationships, and Self-Perception, 305
  Sexuality, 305
  Roles and Relationships, 305
  Self-Perception, 306
- Values, Beliefs, and Spirituality, 306

19 Individual, Family, and Community, 309
- Individual, 310
  Individual Responsibility for Healthy Function, 310
- Family, 310
  Family Conceptual Frameworks, 310
  Family Assessment, 313
  Family Responsibility for Healthy Function, 314
- Community, 314
  Definition of Community, 315
  Community Assessment, 317
  Community Responsibility for Healthy Function, 317
  Advanced Community Concepts, 318
- Functional Approach to Individual, Family, and Community, 320
  Health Perception and Health Maintenance, 321
  Nutrition and Metabolism, 321
  Elimination , 321
  Activity and Exercise, 321
  Sleep and Rest, 321
  Cognition and Perception, 321
  Self-Perception and Self-Concept, 321
  Roles and Relationships , 321
  Sexuality and Reproduction, 321
  Coping and Stress Tolerance, 321
  Values and Beliefs, 321

20 Culture and Ethnicity, 325
- What is Culture?, 326
  Characteristics of Culture, 327
  Concepts Related to Culture, 330
- Concepts of Culture and Nursing Care, 332
  Culturally Sensitive Nursing Care, 333
  Biocultural Variation, 334
  Nursing Assessment Based on the Client's Perspective, 334
  Language Differences Between the Client and the Nurse, 337
  Increased Effectiveness of Client Education, 337

21 Communication: The Nurse–Client Relationship, 343
- The Communication Process, 344
  Types of Communication, 344
  Elements of the Communication Process, 345
  Importance of Language and Experience, 345
- The Nurse–Client Relationship: A Helping Relationship, 347

Phases, 347
Contract Setting, 347
Advocacy, 348
Circle of Confidentiality, 349
- Ingredients of Therapeutic Communication, 349
  Empathy, 349
  Positive Regard, 350
  Comfortable Sense of Self, 350
- Communication and Nursing Process, 350
  Assessment, 350
  Implementation, 351

22 Client Education, 361
- Teaching–Learning Process, 362
  Approaches to Learning, 362
  Information Processing, 362
  Domains of Knowledge, 363
  Qualities of a Teaching–Learning Relationship, 364
- Purposes of Client Education, 364
  Wellness Promotion, 364
  Disease Prevention, 364
  Restoration of Health or Function, 364
  Promotion of Coping, 365
- Assessment For Learning, 365
  Assessing Learning Needs, 365
  Assessing Learning Readiness, 367
- Nursing Diagnoses, 368
  Diagnostic Statement: Deficient Knowledge, 368
- Outcome Identification and Planning, 368
  Outcome Identification, 368
  Planning Teaching Strategies, 368
  Teaching Aids and Resources, 369
  Use of Translators, 371
  Timing and Amount of Information, 372
  Appropriate Family and Friend Involvement, 372
  Written Teaching Plan, 372
- Implementation of Client Teaching, 372
  Meeting Priority Needs First, 372
  Comfortable Environment, 372
  Individualized Teaching Sessions, 373
  Communication, 373
  Repetition, 373
  Teaching Methods, 373
- Evaluation of Learning, 374
  Written Tests, 374
  Oral Tests, 374
  Return Demonstration, 374
  Simulation, 374
- Documentation of Learning, 374
- Lifespan Considerations, 375
  Newborn and Infant, 375
  Toddler and Preschooler, 375
  School-Age Child and Adolescent, 375
  Adult and Older Adult, 375

23 Care Management, 379
- Home Healthcare, 380
  Trends Affecting Home Healthcare, 380
  Tele-Home Health, 381
  Home as Healthcare Setting, 381

Home Care Versus Acute Care, 381
Role of Family and Community: A Systems View, 381
Factors Affecting Home Healthcare Management, 381
The Nurse and Home Healthcare, 383
- Hospice, 389

Unit 5   Essential Assessment Components
24   Health Assessment of Human Function, 393
- Purpose of the Health Assessment, 394
- Frameworks for Health Assessment, 394
   Functional Health Framework, 394
   Head-to-Toe Framework, 394
   Body Systems Framework, 394
- Conducting a Health Assessment, 396
   Reviewing General Information, 396
   Considering Culture, 396
   Preparing the Client and Environment, 396
- Obtaining Subjective Data: The Interview, 397
   Reason for Seeking Healthcare, 398
   Health History, 398
   Pain Assessment, 398
   *Assessment of Health Perception and
      Health Management, 398*
   Assessment of Activity and Exercise, 399
   Assessment of Nutrition and Metabolism, 400
   Assessment of Elimination, 401
   Assessment of Sleep and Rest, 401
   Assessment of Cognition and Perception, 401
   Assessment of Self-Perception and Self-Concept, 404
   Assessment of Roles and Relationships, 404
   Assessment of Coping and Stress Tolerance, 405
   Assessment of Sexuality and Reproduction, 405
   Assessment of Values and Beliefs, 406
- Obtaining Objective Data: The Physical
   Examination, 406
   Positioning and Draping, 407
   Inspection, 407
   Palpation, 407
   Percussion, 408
   Auscultation, 409
- Head-to-Toe Physical Assessment of Function, 410
   Assessment of Head, Face, and Neck, 410
   Assessment of Skin, Hair, and Nails, 419
   Cardiac Assessment, 421
   Respiratory Assessment, 422
   Assessment of Breasts, 427
   Abdominal Assessment, 427
   Assessment of Extremities, 427
- Concluding the Assessment, 437
- Lifespan Considerations, 437
   Newborn and Infant, 437
   Toddler and Preschooler, 437
   School-Age Child and Adolescent, 439
   Adult and Older Adult, 439
25   Vital Sign Assessment, 443
- Body Temperature, 444

Regulation of Body Temperature, 444
Factors Affecting Body Temperature, 445
Factors Affecting Body Temperature Measurement, 446
Assessing Body Temperature, 446
- Pulse, 449
   Characteristics, 449
   Factors Affecting Pulse Rate, 449
   Assessing the Pulse, 449
- Respirations, 459
   Factors Affecting Respirations, 459
   Assessing Respirations, 459
   Methods, 460
- Blood Pressure, 460
   Physiologic Factors Determining Blood Pressure, 461
   Factors Affecting Blood Pressure, 463
   Assessing Blood Pressure, 464
   Methods, 468
   Abnormalities, 471
- Documenting Vital Signs, 473
- Lifespan Considerations, 473
   Newborn and Infant, 474
   Toddler and Preschooler, 474
   School-Age Child and Adolescent, 475
   Adult and Older Adult, 475

Unit 6   Selected Clinical Nursing Therapeutics
26   Asepsis and Infection Control, 479
- Role of Microorganisms in Infection, 480
   Agents Causing Infection, 480
   Chain of Infection, 481
   Nosocomial Infections, 483
- Infection Control, 484
   Regulatory Agencies, 484
   Employee Health, 484
   Waste Disposal, 486
- Aseptic Practices, 486
   Handwashing, 488
   Cleaning, Disinfection, and Sterilization, 491
   Use of Barriers, 492
   Isolation Systems, 494
   Surgical Asepsis, 496
- Lifespan Considerations, 501
   Newborn and Infant, 501
   Toddler and Preschooler, 505
   Child and Adolescent, 505
   Adult and Older Adult, 505
27   Medication Administration, 513
- Drugs and Medications, 513
   Medication Standards, 513
   Types and Forms of Drugs, 513
   Sources of Information About Medications, 513
   Systems of Medication Distribution, 515
   Nonprescription and Prescription Medications, 517
   Medication Order, 518
- Legal Aspects of Medication Administration, 521
   Food and Drug Administration (FDA), 521
   Controlled Substances, 521

Nurse Practice Acts, 522
Institutional Medication Policies, 522
Client's Rights, 522
Substance Abuse, 523
- Principles of Drug Action, 523
Pharmacokinetics, 523
Pharmacodynamics, 524
- Medication Assessment, 526
Information Collected During Initial Assessment, 526
Assessment Before Medication Administration, 527
Assessment of Knowledge and Compliance, 528
- Safe Medication Administration, 529
Interpretation of the Order, 530
Calculating Adult Medication Dosages, 530
Calculating Children's Medication Dosages, 530
Administering Medications According to the
   "Five Rights," 530
Documentation of Medication Administration, 532
Medication Errors, 532
Medication Administration in the Home, 533
Oral Medications, 533
Topical Medications, 537
Inhaled Medications, 540
Parenteral Medications, 540
Healthcare Planning and Home/Community-
   Based Care, 562
Evaluation, 564
- Lifespan Considerations, 564
Newborn and Infant, 564
Toddler and Preschooler, 570
Child and Adolescent, 571
Adult and Older Adult, 572

28 Intravenous Therapy, 575
- Intravenous Therapy, 576
Types of Intravenous Solutions, 576
Equipment for Intravenous Infusion, 577
Intravenous Flow Rates, 582
- Role of the Nurse in Intravenous Therapy, 586
Initiating Intravenous Therapy, 586
Maintaining Intravenous Infusions, 588
Assessing for Complications, 588
Discontinuing an Intravenous Infusion, 598
Lifespan Considerations, 598
- Parenteral Nutrition, 599
Total Parenteral Nutrition (TPN), 600
- Blood Transfusion, 603
Blood Components, 603
Blood Compatibility, 603
Selection of Blood Donors, 604
Transfusion Technique, 604
- Community-Based Nursing, 607
Client Teaching, 607
Monitoring, 608

29 Perioperative Nursing, 611
- Surgical Intervention, 612
Phases of Perioperative Nursing, 612
Classification of Surgery, 612

Surgical Facilities, 612
Impact of Surgery on Health and Function, 613
Lifespan Considerations, 621
- Preoperative Nursing, 622
Nursing Assessment, 622
Nursing Diagnoses and Outcome Identification, 623
Nursing Interventions, 624
Evaluation, 632
- Intraoperative Nursing, 632
Nursing Assessment, 632
Nursing Diagnoses and Outcome Identification, 632
Nursing Interventions, 632
Evaluation, 638
- Postoperative Nursing, 638
Nursing Assessment, 638
Nursing Diagnoses and Outcome Identification, 639
Nursing Interventions in the Recovery Facility, 639
Nursing Interventions on the Surgical Unit, 641
Community-Based Nursing, 643
Evaluation, 643

Section II
Human Function and Clinical Nursing Therapeutics

Unit 7 Health Perception and Health Management
30 Safety, 649
- Normal Safety, 650
Characteristics of Safety, 650
Lifespan Considerations, 650
- Factors Affecting Safety, 652
Physiologic Factors, 652
Coping and Stress Tolerance, 653
Environmental Factors, 653
Disease, 655
Disregard for Safety, 656
- Altered Safety, 656
Manifestations of Altered Safety, 656
Impact on Activities of Daily Living, 659
- Assessment, 660
Subjective Data, 660
Objective Data, 661
- Nursing Diagnoses, 663
Diagnostic Statement: Risk for Injury, 663
Related Nursing Diagnoses, 663
- Outcome Identification and Planning, 663
- Implementation, 664
Health Promotion, 664
Nursing Interventions for Altered Safety, 673
Healthcare Planning and Home/Community-
   Based Nursing, 673
- Evaluation, 675

31 Health Maintenance, 679
- Normal Health Maintenance, 680
Characteristics of Normal Health Maintenance, 680
Normal Health-Maintenance Patterns, 681

Lifespan Considerations, 683
• Factors Affecting Health Maintenance, 685
Cognition and Perception, 685
Age and Developmental Level, 685
Previous Experiences, 685
Lifestyle and Habits, 685
Environment, 685
Economic Resources, 686
Culture, Values, and Beliefs, 687
Roles and Relationships, 687
Coping and Stress Tolerance, 687
• Altered Health Maintenance, 687
Manifestations of Altered Function, 687
Impact on Activities of Daily Living, 688
• Assessment, 688
Subjective Data, 688
Objective Data, 690
• Nursing Diagnoses, 691
Diagnostic Statement—Ineffective Health
  Maintenance, 691
Diagnostic Statement—Health-Seeking Behaviors, 693
Diagnostic Statement—Therapeutic Regimen
  Management: Effective and Ineffective—Focus:
  Individual, Family, and Community, 694
Related Nursing Diagnoses, 694
• Outcome Identification and Planning, 694
• Implementation, 694
Health Promotion, 694
Nursing Interventions for Altered Function, 697
Healthcare Planning and Home- or Community-
  Based Nursing, 697
• Evaluation, 698

Unit 8 Activity and Exercise
32 Self-Care and Hygiene, 703
• Normal Self-Care, 704
Characteristics of Normal Self-Care, 704
Normal Self-Care Patterns, 705
Lifespan Considerations, 705
• Factors Affecting Self-Care, 706
Culture, Values, and Beliefs, 706
Environment, 706
Motivation, 707
Emotional Disturbance and Depression, 707
Cognitive Abilities, 707
Energy, 707
Acute Illness and Surgery, 707
Pain, 707
Neuromuscular Function, 708
Sensorimotor Deficits, 708
• Altered Self-Care, 708
Manifestations of Altered Self-Care, 708
Impact on Activities of Daily Living, 708
• Assessment, 710
Subjective Data, 710
Objective Data, 711
• Nursing Diagnoses, 711

Diagnostic Statement: Bathing/Hygiene
  Self-Care Deficit, 712
Diagnostic Statement: Feeding Self-Care Deficit, 712
Diagnostic Statement: Toileting Self-Care Deficit, 713
Diagnostic Statement: Dressing/Grooming
  Self-Care Deficit, 713
Related Nursing Diagnoses, 713
• Outcome Identification and Planning, 713
• Implementation, 713
Health Promotion, 713
Nursing Interventions for Altered Self-Care, 714
Healthcare Planning and Home/Community-
  Based Nursing, 742
• Evaluation, 749
33 Mobility and Body Mechanics, 753
• Normal Mobility, 754
Structures of the Musculoskeletal System, 754
Normal Physiologic Function, 755
Characteristics of Normal Movement, 760
Lifespan Considerations, 760
• Factors Affecting Mobility, 763
Lifestyle and Habits, 763
Intact Musculoskeletal System, 763
Nervous System Control, 764
Circulation and Oxygenation, 764
Energy, 765
Congenital Problems, 765
Affective Disorders, 765
Therapeutic Modalities, 765
• Altered Mobility, 765
Manifestations of Altered Mobility, 765
Impact of Immobility on Function, 766
Impact on Activities of Daily Living, 771
• Assessment, 771
Subjective Data, 771
Objective Data, 776
• Nursing Diagnoses, 778
Diagnostic Statement: Impaired Physical Mobility, 778
Diagnostic Statement: Impaired Walking, 779
Diagnostic Statement: Impaired
  Wheelchair Mobility, 779
Diagnostic Statement: Impaired Transfer Ability, 779
Diagnostic Statement: Impaired Bed Mobility, 779
Diagnostic Statement: Activity Intolerance, 779
Diagnostic Statement: Risk for Disuse Syndrome, 779
Related Nursing Diagnoses, 779
• Outcome Identification and Planning, 780
• Implementation, 780
Health Promotion, 780
Nursing Interventions for Altered Mobility, 781
Healthcare Planning and Home/Community-
  Based Nursing, 801
• Evaluation, 804
34 Oxygenation: Respiratory Function, 809
• Normal Respiratory Function, 810
Structure of the Respiratory System, 810
Function of the Respiratory System, 810

Normal Breathing Pattern, 812
Lifespan Considerations, 812
- Factors Affecting Respiratory Function, 813
Body Position, 813
Environment, 813
Lifestyle and Habits, 813
Increased Work of Breathing, 814
- Altered Respiratory Function, 815
Manifestations of Altered Respiratory Function, 815
Impact on Activities of Daily Living, 816
- Assessment, 818
Subjective Data, 818
Objective Data, 819
- Nursing Diagnoses, 821
Diagnostic Statement: Ineffective Breathing Pattern, 821
Diagnostic Statement: Ineffective Airway Clearance, 824
Diagnostic Statement: Impaired Gas Exchange, 824
Related Nursing Diagnoses, 824
- Outcome Identification and Planning, 824
- Implementation, 824
Health Promotion, 824
Nursing Interventions for Altered Respiratory Function, 828
Healthcare Planning and Home Care/Community-Based Nursing, 858
- Evaluation, 860

35 Oxygenation: Cardiovascular Function, 865
- Normal Cardiovascular Function, 866
Structure of the Cardiovascular System, 866
Function of the Cardiovascular System, 867
Lifespan Considerations, 870
- Factors Affecting Cardiovascular Function, 870
Cigarette Smoking, 871
High Blood Pressure, 871
Nutrition, 871
Lack of Exercise, 872
Diabetes, 872
Obesity, 876
Medical and Family History, 872
Medications and Drug Use, 872
Stress, 872
Aging, 873
- Altered Cardiovascular Function, 873
Manifestations of Altered Cardiovascular Function, 873
Impact on Activities of Daily Living, 879
- Assessment, 879
Subjective Data, 879
Objective Data, 880
- Nursing Diagnoses, 884
Diagnostic Statement: Decreased Cardiac Output, 884
Diagnostic Statement: Ineffective Tissue Perfusion (Renal, Cerebral, Cardiopulmonary, Gastrointestinal, Peripheral), 884
Diagnostic Statement: Activity Intolerance, 884
Related Nursing Diagnoses, 884
- Outcome Identification and Planning, 884

- Implementation, 885
Health Promotion, 885
Nursing Interventions for Altered Cardiovascular Function, 889
Healthcare Planning and Home Community-Based Nursing, 901
- Evaluation, 902

Unit 9 Nutrition and Metabolism

36 Fluid, Electrolyte, and Acid-Base Balance, 909
- Normal Fluid and Electrolyte Balance, 910
Fluid Compartments, 910
Electrolytes, 912
Fluid and Electrolyte Distribution, 913
Lifespan Considerations, 914
- Normal Acid–Base Balance, 916

37 Nutrition, 941
- Normal Nutrition, 942
- Nutrients, 942
Nutrient Guidelines, 942
Carbohydrates, 943
Proteins, 943
Fats, 943
Vitamins, 944
Minerals, 947
Water, 950
The Food Guide Pyramid, 950
- The Digestive System, 951
Structure of the Digestive System, 951
Function of the Digestive System, 952
- Characteristics of Normal Nutrition, 953
Nutrient Density, 953
Dietary Guidelines for Americans, 953
Energy Balance, 953
Nutritional Status, 954
Lifespan Considerations, 954
- Factors Affecting Nutrition, 957
Physiologic Factors, 957
Lifestyle and Habits, 958
Culture and Beliefs, 961
Economic Resources, 961
Drug and Nutrient Interactions, 961
Gender, 961
Surgery, 961
Cancer and Cancer Treatment, 961
Alcohol and Drug Abuse, 961
Psychological State, 961
- Altered Nutritional Function, 962
Manifestations of Altered Function, 962
Impact on Activities of Daily Living, 963
- Assessment, 963
Subjective Data, 963
Objective Date, 964
- Nursing Diagnoses, 965
Diagnostic Statement—Imbalanced Nutrition: Less Than Body Requirements, 966
Diagnostic Statement—Imbalanced Nutrition: More Than Body Requirements, 966

*Diagnostic Statement—Imbalanced Nutrition:
 Risk for More Than Body Requirements, 966*
Diagnostic Statement—Impaired Swallowing, 966
- Outcome Identification and Planning, 967
- Implementation, 967
Health Promotion, 967
*Nursing Interventions for Altered Nutritional
 Function, 968*
*Healthcare Planning and Home- or Community-
 Based Care, 977*
- Evaluation, 977

38 Skin Integrity and Wound Healing, 983
- Normal Integumentary Function, 984
Structure of the Skin, 985
Function of the Skin, 985
Characteristics of Normal Skin, 985
Lifespan Considerations, 985
- Factors Affecting Integumentary Function, 986
Circulation, 986
Nutrition, 989
Lifestyle and Habits, 989
Condition of the Epidermis, 989
Allergy, 989
Infections, 989
Abnormal Growth Rate, 990
Systemic Diseases, 990
Trauma, 990
Excessive Exposure, 991
- Altered Integumentary Function, 991
Manifestations of Altered Integumentary Function, 991
Wound Healing, 991
Impact on Activities of Daily Living, 997
- Assessment, 997
Subjective Data, 997
Objective Data, 998
- Nursing Diagnoses, 1001
Impaired Skin Integrity, 1001
Impaired Tissue Integrity, 1002
Risk for Impaired Skin Integrity, 1002
Related Nursing Diagnoses, 1002
- Outcome Identification and Planning, 1002
- Implementation, 1003
Health Promotion, 1003
Nursing Interventions for Skin Impairment, 1005
*Healthcare Planning and Home/Community-
 Based Nursing, 1021*
- Evaluation, 1022

39 The Body's Defense Against Infection, 1027
- Normal Resistance to Infection, 1028
*Characteristics of Normal Resistance to Infection,
 1028*
Lifespan Considerations, 1031
- Factors Affecting Normal Resistance to Infection,
 1032
Presence of Infectious Agents, 1032
Compromised Host, 1039
- Altered Resistance to Infection, 1041

Type of Infection, 1041
Progress of an Infection, 1041
Manifestations of Infection, 1043
Impact on Activities of Daily Living, 1044
- Assessment, 1044
Subjective Data, 1044
Objective Data, 1045
- Nursing Diagnoses, 1051
Risk for Infection, 1051
Related Nursing Diagnoses, 1051
- Outcome Identification and Planning , 1051
- Implementation, 1052
Health Promotion, 1052
Nursing Interventions for Altered Function, 1054
*Healthcare Planning and Home- or Community-
 Based Nursing, 1057*
- Evaluation, 1058

Unit 10 Elimination
40 Urinary Elimination, 1063
- Normal Urinary Function, 1064
Structures of the Urinary Tract, 1064
Function of the Urinary System, 1065
Characteristics of Normal Urine, 1066
Normal Pattern of Urinary Elimination, 1066
Lifespan Considerations, 1066
- Factors Affecting Urinary Elimination, 1068
Fluid Intake, 1068
Loss of Body Fluid, 1068
Nutrition, 1068
Body Position, 1068
Psychological Factors, 1068
Obstruction of Urine Flow, 1069
Infections of the Urinary Tract, 1069
Hypotension, 1069
Neurologic Injury, 1069
Decreased Muscle Tone, 1069
Pregnancy, 1070
Surgery, 1070
Medications, 1070
Urinary Diversion, 1070
- Altered Urinary Function, 1070
Manifestations of Altered Urinary Function, 1070
Impact on Activities of Daily Living, 1073
- Assessment, 1073
Subjective Data, 1073
Objective Data, 1074
- Nursing Diagnoses, 1081
*Diagnostic Statement: Stress Urinary Incontinence,
 1082*
*Diagnostic Statement: Urge Urinary Incontinence,
 1082*
*Diagnostic Statement: Reflex Urinary Incontinence,
 1082*
*Diagnostic Statement: Functional Urinary Inconti-
 nence, 1082*
*Diagnostic Statement: Total Urinary
 Incontinence, 1082*

Diagnostic Statement: Urinary Retention, 1082
Related Nursing Diagnoses, 1083
- Outcome Identification and Planning, 1083
- Implementation, 1083
Health Promotion, 1083
Nursing Interventions for Altered Function, 1084
*Healthcare Planning and Home or Community-
   Based Nursing, 1097*
- Evaluation, 1098

41   Bowel Elimination, 1101
- Normal Bowel Function, 1102
Structures of the Gastrointestinal Tract, 1102
Function of the Intestine, 1103
Characteristics of Normal Feces, 1103
Normal Bowel Pattern, 1103
Lifespan Considerations, 1103
- Factors Affecting Bowel Elimination, 1105
Nutrition, 1105
Fluid Intake, 1105
Activity and Exercise, 1105
Body Position, 1105
Ignoring the Urge to Defecate, 1106
Lifestyle, 1106
Pregnancy, 1106
Medications, 1106
Diagnostic Procedures, 1107
Surgery, 1107
Fecal Diversion, 1107
- Altered Bowel Function, 1108
Manifestations of Altered Bowel Function, 1108
Impact on Activities of Daily Living, 1110
- Assessment, 1110
Subjective Data, 1111
Objective Data, 1111
- Nursing Diagnoses, 1116
Diagnostic Statement: Constipation, 1116
Diagnostic Statement: Perceived Constipation, 1116
Diagnostic Statement: Diarrhea, 1116
Diagnostic Statement: Bowel Incontinence, 1117
Related Nursing Diagnoses, 1117
- Outcome Identification and Planning, 1117
- Implementation, 1117
Health Promotion, 1117
*Nursing Interventions for Altered Bowel Function,
   1120*
*Healthcare Planning and Home/Community-
   Based Care, 1137*
- Evaluation, 1137

Unit 11   Sleep and Rest
42   Sleep and Rest, 1143
- Normal Sleep and Rest, 1144
Physiologic Function, 1144
Psychological Function, 1145
Characteristics of Normal Sleep and Rest, 1146
Normal Sleep and Rest Patterns, 1146
Lifespan Considerations, 1148

- Factors Affecting Sleep and Rest, 1150
Need, 1150
Environment, 1150
Relationships, 1151
Shift Work, 1151
Nutrition and Metabolism, 1151
Elimination Patterns, 1151
Exercise and Thermoregulation, 1151
Vigilance, 1151
Lifestyle and Habits, 1151
Illness, 1152
Medications and Chemicals, 1154
Mood States, 1154
- Altered Sleep and Rest, 1154
Manifestations of Altered Sleep, 1154
Impact on Activities of Daily Living, 1156
- Assessment, 1156
Subjective Data, 1156
Objective Data, 1157
- Nursing Diagnoses, 1157
Diagnostic Statement: Disturbed Sleep Pattern, 1157
Diagnostic Statement: Sleep Deprivation, 1158
Related Nursing Diagnoses, 1158
- Outcome Identification and Planning, 1158
- Implementation, 1158
Health Promotion, 1158
Nursing Interventions for Altered Function, 1159
*Healthcare Planning and Home/Community-
   Based Care, 1160*
- Evaluation, 1160

Unit 12   Cognition and Perception
43   Pain Perception and Management, 1167
- Pain Perception, 1168
Structures Related to the Pain Process, 1168
Pain Modulation, 1169
Pain Theories, 1169
Characteristics of Pain, 1169
Lifespan Considerations, 1171
- Factors Affecting Pain Perception and
   Pain Response, 1172
Physiologic Factors, 1172
Affective Factors, 1174
Behavioral Factors, 1174
Cognitive Factors, 1174
- Altered Function Resulting in Pain, 1174
Manifestations of Pain, 1174
Impact on Activities of Daily Living, 1176
- Assessment, 1176
Subjective Data, 1176
Objective Data, 1180
- Nursing Diagnoses, 1181
Diagnostic Statement: Acute Pain, 1181
Diagnostic Statement: Chronic Pain, 1181
Related Nursing Diagnoses, 1181
- Outcome Identification and Planning, 1182
- Implementation, 1182

Health Promotion, 1182
Nursing Interventions for the Client
Experiencing Pain, 1183
Healthcare Planning and Home/Community-
Based Nursing, 1194
- Evaluation, 1194

44   Sensory Perception, 1199
- Normal Sensory Perception, 1200
Structure and Function of Sensory Perception, 1200
Characteristics of Normal Sensory Perception, 1200
Normal Sensory Pattern, 1200
Lifespan Considerations, 1201
- Factors Affecting Sensory Perception, 1201
Environment, 1201
Previous Experience, 1201
Lifestyle and Habits, 1201
Illness, 1201
Medications, 1202
Variations in Stimulation, 1202
- Altered Sensory Perception Function, 1204
Manifestations of Altered Sensory
Perception Function, 1204
Impact on Activities of Daily Living, 1205
- Assessment, 1206
Subjective Data, 1206
Objective Data, 1207
- Nursing Diagnoses, 1207
Diagnostic Statement: Disturbed Sensory
Perception, 1207
Related Nursing Diagnoses, 1208
- Outcome Identification and Planning, 1208
- Implementation, 1209
Health Promotion, 1209
Nursing Interventions for Altered Sensory
Perception Function, 1210
Healthcare Planning and Home/Community-
Based Nursing, 1211
- Evaluation, 1214

45   Cognitive Processes, 1219
- Normal Cognitive Processes, 1220
Anatomic Structures Involved in Cognition, 1220
Normal Cognitive Function, 1220
Characteristics of Normal Cognition, 1223
Normal Cognitive Patterns, 1224
Lifespan Considerations, 1225
- Factors Affecting Cognitive Function, 1226
Personal Factors, 1226
Environmental Factors, 1229
Culture, Values, and Beliefs, 1229
- Altered Cognitive Function, 1230
Manifestations of Altered Cognitive Function, 1230
Impact on Activities of Daily Living, 1232
- Assessment, 1233
Subjective Data, 1233
Objective Data, 1236
- Nursing Diagnoses, 1237
Diagnostic Statement: Acute Confusion, 1237

Diagnostic Statement: Chronic Confusion, 1238
Diagnostic Statement: Impaired Memory, 1239
Diagnostic Statement: Disturbed Thought Processes,
1239
Diagnostic Statement: Impaired Verbal Communica-
tion, 1239
Related Nursing Diagnoses, 1239
- Outcome Identification and Planning, 1240
- Implementation, 1240
Health Promotion, 1240
Nursing Interventions for Impaired Cognitive Func-
tion, 1241
Healthcare Planning and Home/Community-Based
Nursing, 1246
- Evaluation, 1247

Unit 13   Self-Perception and Self-Concept
46   Self-Concept, 1253
- Normal Function of Self, 1254
Characteristics of Self-Concept, 1254
Normal Self-Concept Patterns, 1254
Lifespan Considerations, 1254
- Factors Affecting Self-Concept, 1259
Biologic Makeup, 1259
Culture, Values, and Beliefs, 1259
Coping and Stress Tolerance, 1261
Self-Efficacy, 1261
Previous Experience, 1261
Developmental Level, 1262
Role Transition, 1262
Illness, Trauma, and Surgery, 1263
- Altered Self-Concept, 1263
Manifestations of Altered Function, 1263
Impact on Activities of Daily Living, 1264
- Assessment, 1264
Subjective Data, 1264
Objective Data, 1265
- Nursing Diagnoses, 1265
Diagnostic Statement: Body Image Disturbance, 1265
Diagnostic Statement: Self-Esteem Disturbance, 1265
Diagnostic Statement: Chronic Low
Self-Esteem, 1265
Diagnostic Statement: Situational Low
Self-Esteem, 1265
Diagnostic Statement: Altered Role Performance, 1266
Related Nursing Diagnoses, 1266
- Outcome Identification and Planning, 1266
- Implementation, 1266
Health Promotion, 1266
Nursing Interventions for Altered Self-Concept, 1269
Healthcare Planning and Home/Community-
Based Nursing, 1270
- Evaluation, 1270

Unit 14   Roles and Relationships
47   Families and Their Relationships, 1275
- Normal Family Relationships, 1276

Family Structure, 1276
Family Function, 1277
Normal Functional Family Pattern, 1278
Lifespan Considerations, 1278
• Factors Affecting Family Function, 1280
Culture, Values, and Beliefs, 1280
Economic Resources, 1280
Lifestyle, 1281
Previous Life Experience, 1281
Coping and Stress Tolerance, 1281
Acute Illness, 1281
Chronic Illness, 1282
Traumatic Experiences, 1282
Substance Abuse, 1282
• Altered Family Relationships, 1282
Manifestations of Altered Family Function, 1282
Impact on Activities of Daily Living, 1285
• Assessment, 1286
Subjective Assessment, 1286
Objective Data, 1286
• Nursing Diagnoses, 1287
Diagnostic Statement: Caregiver Role Strain, 1287
Diagnostic Statement: Risk for Caregiver Role
    Strain, 1288
Diagnostic Statement: Interrupted Family
    Processes, 1288
Diagnostic Statement: Dysfunctional Family
    Processes: Alcoholism, 1288
Diagnostic Statement: Compromised Family
    Coping, 1289
Diagnostic Statement: Disabled Family Coping, 1289
Diagnostic Statement: Readiness for Enhanced
    Family Coping, 1290
Diagnostic Statement: Ineffective Family Therapeutic
    Regimen Management, 1290
Diagnostic Statement: Impaired Parenting, 1290
Diagnostic Statement: Risk for Impaired
    Parenting, 1290
Diagnostic Statement: Parental Role Conflict, 1291
Diagnostic Statement: Risk for Impaired Parent/
    Infant/Child Attachment, 1291
Related Nursing Diagnoses, 1291
• Outcome Identification and Planning, 1291
• Implementation, 1292
Health Promotion, 1292
Nursing Interventions for Altered Family
    Function, 1292
Healthcare Planning and Home/Community-
    Based Nursing, 1293
• Evaluation, 1294
48 Loss and Grieving, 1299
• Normal Grieving, 1300
Characteristics of Normal Loss and Grieving, 1300
Lifespan Considerations, 1302
• Factors Affecting Grieving, 1304
Meaning of the Loss, 1304
Circumstances of the Loss, 1304

Religious Beliefs and Cultural Practices, 1305
Personal Resources and Stressors, 1305
Sociocultural Resources and Stressors, 1305
• Altered Grieving, 1305
Manifestations of Altered Grieving, 1305
Impact on Activities of Daily Living, 1305
• Assessment, 1306
Subjective Data, 1306
Objective Data, 1307
• Nursing Diagnoses, 1307
Diagnostic Statement: Anticipatory Grieving, 1307
Diagnostic Statement: Dysfunctional Grieving, 1307
Related Nursing Diagnoses, 1308
• Outcome Identification and Planning, 1308
• Implementation, 1308
Health Promotion, 1308
Nursing Interventions for Altered Grieving, 1311
Healthcare Planning and Home/Community-
    Based Nursing, 1311
• Evaluation, 1312
• Caring for the Dying Patient, 1313
Definition of Death, 1313
Response to Dying and Death, 1313
Physical Signs of Dying, 1314
Hospice Care, 1314
Nursing Diagnoses and Nursing Implementation, 1314
Caring for the Deceased, 1315

Unit 15 Coping and Stress Management
49 Stress, Coping, and Adaptation, 1325
• Normal Coping and Adaptation to Stress, 1326
Physiologic Function Related to Stress, Coping,
    and Adaptation, 1326
Characteristics of Stress, Coping, and Adaptation, 1328
Normal Coping Patterns, 1330
Lifespan Considerations, 1331
• Factors Affecting Coping Patterns, 1332
Lifestyle Considerations, 1332
Previous Experience, 1333
Involuntary Relocation, 1333
Social Interaction, 1334
Sensory Deficits, 1334
• Altered Coping Patterns, 1334
Manifestations of Altered Coping, 1334
Impact on Activities of Daily Living, 1336
• Assessment, 1336
Subjective Data, 1336
Objective Data, 1337
• Nursing Diagnoses, 1338
Diagnostic Statement: Ineffective Coping, 1338
Related Nursing Diagnoses, 1339
• Outcome Identification and Planning, 1339
• Implementation, 1339
Health Promotion, 1339
Nursing Interventions for Altered Function, 1342
Healthcare Planning and Home/Community-
    Based Nursing, 1343
• Evaluation, 1344

Unit 16 Sexuality and Reproduction

50 Human Sexuality, 1351

- Normal Human Sexuality, 1352

  Structure of the Reproductive Systems, 1352

  Function of Sexuality and the Reproductive Systems, 1354

  Characteristics of Normal Sexuality, 1356

  Normal Sexual Patterns, 1356

  Lifespan Considerations, 1357

- Factors Affecting Sexuality, 1359

  Relationships, 1359

  Cognition and Perception, 1359

  Culture, Values, and Beliefs, 1359

  Self-Concept, 1359

  Previous Experience, 1359

  Pregnancy, 1359

  Environment, 1360

  Illness, 1360

  Medication, 1360

  Surgery, 1362

- Altered Human Sexuality, 1362

  Manifestations of Altered Sexuality, 1362

  Impact on Activities of Daily Living, 1363

- Assessment, 1363

  Subjective Data, 1363

  Objective Data, 1366

- Nursing Diagnoses, 1366

  Diagnostic Statement: Sexual Dysfunction, 1366

  Diagnostic Statement: Ineffective Sexuality Patterns, 1367

  Related Nursing Diagnoses, 1367

- Outcome Identification and Planning, 1368

- Implementation, 1368

  Health Promotion, 1368

  Nursing Interventions for Altered Function, 1373

  Healthcare Planning and Home/Community-Based Nursing, 1374

- Evaluation, 1375

Unit 17 Values and Beliefs

51 Spiritual Health, 1381

- Normal Spiritual Function, 1382

  Characteristics of Spirituality, 1382

  Normal Spiritual Pattern, 1383

  Lifespan Considerations, 1384

- Factors Affecting Spiritual Health, 1384

  Culture, 1386

  Gender, 1386

  Previous Experience, 1386

  Crisis and Change, 1386

  Separation From Spiritual Ties, 1386

  Moral Issues Regarding Therapy, 1386

  Inadequate or Inappropriate Care, 1386

- Altered Spiritual Function, 1388

  Manifestations of Altered Spiritual Function, 1388

  Impact on Activities of Daily Living, 1388

- Assessment, 1388

  Subjective Data, 1388

  Objective Data, 1391

- Nursing Diagnoses, 1391

  Spiritual Distress (Distress of the Human Spirit), 1392

  Readiness for Enhanced Spiritual Well-Being, 1392

  Risk for Spiritual Distress, 1392

  Decisional Conflict (Specify), 1392

  Noncompliance (Specify), 1393

  Related Nursing Diagnoses, 1393

- Outcome Identification and Planning, 1393

- Implementation, 1394

  Health Promotion, 1394

  Nursing Interventions for Altered Spiritual Function, 1395

  Healthcare Planning and Home/Community-Based Nursing, 1395

- Evaluation, 1395

Appendix A: Answers to "Apply Your Knowledge," 1405

Appendix B: Diagnostic Studies and Interpretation, 1411

Appendix C: Medical Terminology: Prefixes, Roots, and Suffixes, 1451

Appendix D: Selected Information Resources for Nursing Practice, 1459

Appendix E: Herbal Preparations Used As Health Remedies, 1471

Glossary, 1481

Index, 1491

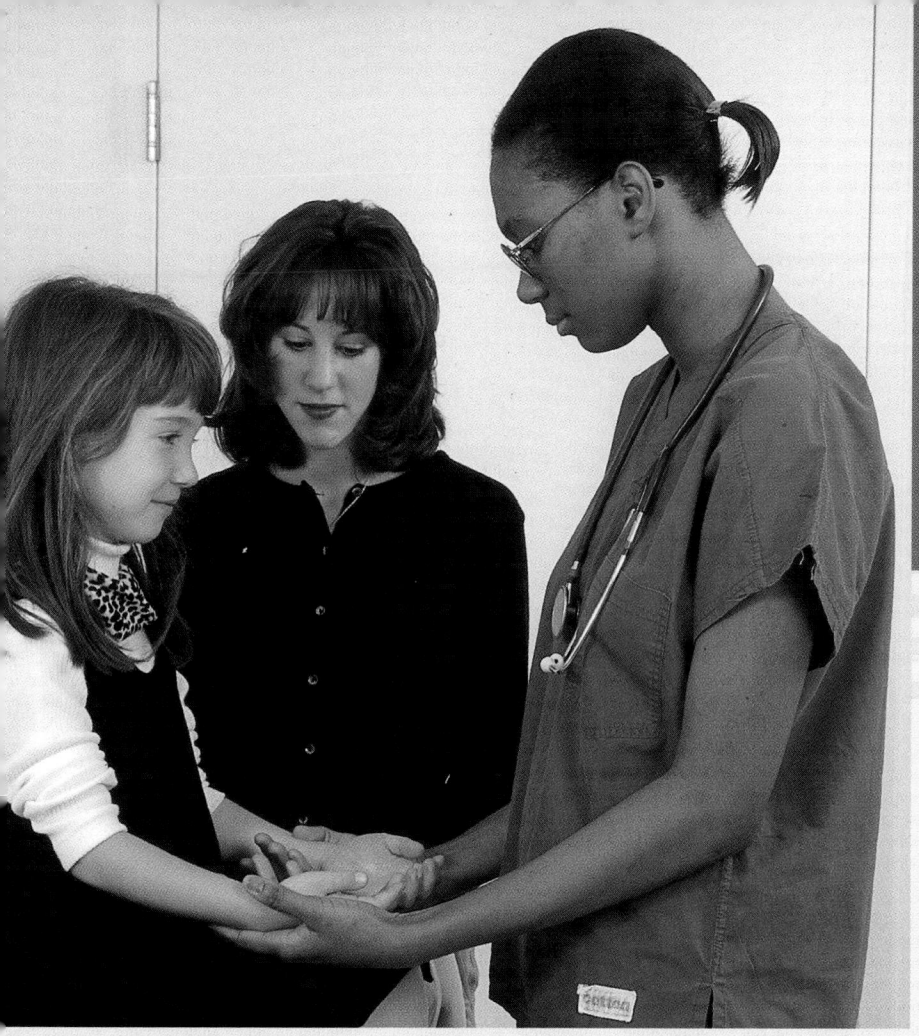

Conceptual Foundations of Nursing

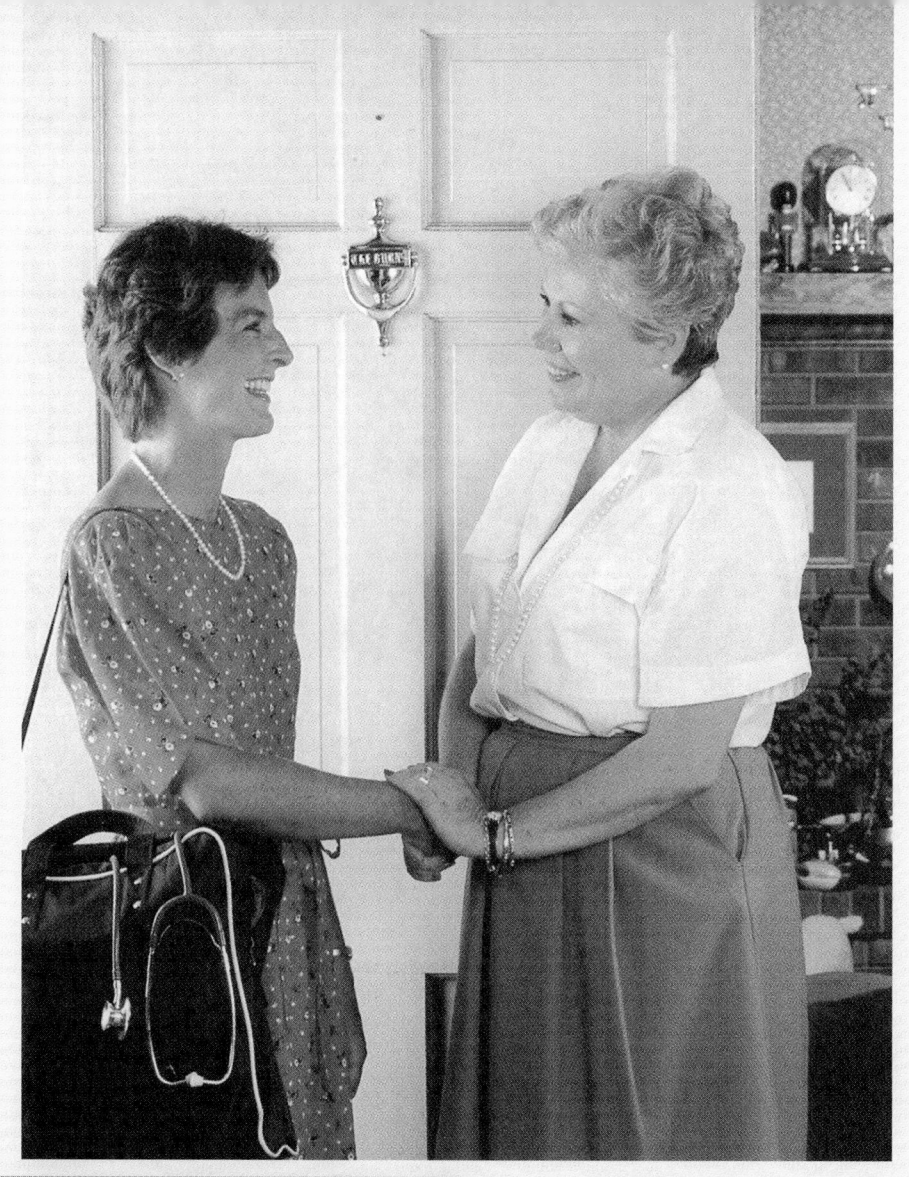

The Delivery of Nursing Care

1 The Changing Face of Nursing

Key Terms

case management
triage

Learning Objectives

Upon completion of this chapter, the student will be able to do the following:

1. Describe how nursing practice has shifted from an institution-based to a community-based paradigm.
2. Discuss how nurses have developed more independent practice over the last 50 years.
3. Explain how nurses must collaborate with other disciplines to care for clients.
4. Articulate how socioeconomic trends influence care delivery.
5. Describe how personal views and experiences influence nursing practice.
6. Identify how critical thinking is integral to nursing education and practice.

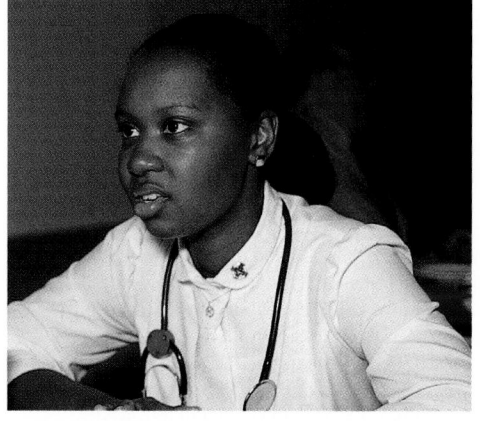

Critical Thinking Challenge

You are a student beginning your nursing program. As you complete your first week of classes, you notice that your instructors have focused on several consistent themes. They are stressing such concepts as community-based care, the need for consumer participation in healthcare, and the influence of technologic advances. They are asking for your opinions on financial, ethical, and legal concerns. Many of your fellow classmates are returning to school after several years away. They mention to you how many responsibilities they are juggling and the hopes that they have for success. You feel both excited and slightly scared but are eager to understand better the many ideas you and your fellow students are encountering.

Once you have completed this chapter, return to the above scenario and reflect on the following areas of Critical Thinking:

1. Describe how you anticipate that current trends in nursing will affect the way you practice, your relationships with clients, and your relationships with coworkers.
2. Identify ways that nurses can promote and uphold the wishes of their clients in terms of healthcare choices and decisions.
3. Explore possibilities for learning more about community-based healthcare delivery, technologic developments, and financial considerations.
4. Based on the information in this chapter, how would you expect nurses to practice 50 years from now?

As you turn the pages of this textbook, you are preparing for a career in nursing. In this journey, you will master many scientific, physiologic, psychosocial, and fundamental facts. You will learn many things: how to touch people, assess for health, and observe for pain. You will learn to see physical clues that a person is suffering from inadequate oxygenation or cardiac insufficiency. You will learn to hear how the heart sounds and how to listen for changes in the breathing of one who is dying. You will see the power of the human body as you witness the processes of labor and birth. You will experience the incredible abilities of technology to extend and improve human life.

In the midst of such experiences, you will develop critical thinking skills that will enable you to place multiple factors into complex equations and arrive at appropriate conclusions. You will learn the importance of knowing yourself, your values, and how you arrive at decisions. You will need to consider the problems of today's society and issues involving healthcare allocation, the extent and use of technology, the treatment of disease, and the promotion of health.

This chapter specifically introduces you to the "changing face of nursing." Throughout, you will read the stories of several nurses who are working in various settings. They represent a broad spectrum of educational preparation as well as diversity in their chosen areas of clinical practice. Political, economic, and social realities have influenced their work. They have agreed to share their experiences to relate how the nursing profession has responded to these realities. In the next section, Ruth Craven and Constance Hirnle, the editors of this textbook, discuss how nursing has shaped their lives, their purpose in writing this textbook, and their advice to you as beginning students. After their discussions you will find a letter of advice written specifically for you from a group of nurses who are in their first weeks of returning to school to earn their baccalaureate in nursing. Their words are carefully chosen, looking back to their first time in nursing school and wanting to share with you some words of wisdom as you embark on the path they took, anywhere from 25 to 4 years ago.

I knew I wanted to be a nurse ever since I was in high school and volunteered at my local hospital. The nurses there encouraged me to go to a diploma school to really learn about bedside nursing. I took their advice. I received a very good education, but as I learned more it became evident that I needed more academic education. Over the next few years, I worked full time and went to the university part time, earning my bachelor of science in nursing (BSN) degree. I moved to the West Coast and completed my master's program. With each level of education, I realized how much there was to learn and how I needed to organize that knowledge into some form that would be useful to me. Working with students, seeing them grow in their confidence and competence, and conveying that knowledge to others were sources of great satisfaction.

During my nursing career, I have had several other careers. I have been a bedside nurse, an educator, a writer, and an administrator, and I have had a family life with a husband and three children. I have worked with interesting clients, dedicated students, creative colleagues, and talented staff who have taught me much about the quality of nursing. I am more involved now in nursing practice than at any point in

my career and more than I ever envisioned when I entered that diploma school.

Connie Hirnle and I met during her graduate studies. We found we shared mutual values and interests. Our association continued over the years and ultimately led to collaboration on this textbook. As we considered how to introduce students to the nursing field, we looked at what had been done in the past, where nursing was moving, and what scholarship and data were available to write a book applying evidence-based practice. As we considered what it is that nursing does, we appreciated the concept of health as related to function and the idea that nurses work with clients to assist them in moving from dysfunction back to healthy function or to whatever outcomes are appropriate.

The organization and content of this textbook have been created to convey our abiding passion for professional nursing and all the components that it includes. Our hope and desire are that students will learn and grow in the profession and have the same commitment to nursing and as exciting careers as we are experiencing.

—Ruth Craven

I have always wanted to become a nurse, a choice that may seem odd to some readers. In the early 1960s, teaching and nursing were the professions that society, family, and young women themselves deemed acceptable. I have never regretted my decision. I entered a 4-year BSN program right out of high school. I was so very young. I can vividly remember my first anatomy laboratory course, seeing and working with a cadaver. It was a shock! My first client, whom I was assigned to bathe, was a homeless woman. I will never forget her popping out her glass eye and calmly handing it to me! Lesson #1—Always be ready for the unexpected!

During the subsequent school years, I learned a lot about myself and about life. I felt the support of my classmates who struggled and rejoiced as we learned the art of nursing together. Lesson #2—Develop a strong, supportive peer group to help you make it through nursing school.

My first job as a registered nurse (RN) was on a busy surgical unit. I loved my clients and their families and learned something new every day. I would go home very tired, but I always thought that what I did mattered. Lesson #3—Nursing is very hard work, but it is work that truly makes a difference.

Fairly early in my career, I decided to go to graduate school, which I found to be easier than my undergraduate program. I became more knowledgeable, but mainly I grew as a person as I learned from fellow students who had diverse nursing experiences. Lesson #4—Always be open to new ways to grow, as a person and as a professional.

After graduate school, I started to teach and to raise my family. I needed the weekends and summers off to keep up with my wonderful children, Scott, John, and Sarah. Teaching taught me a great deal—most importantly, how much I didn't know! I especially enjoyed clinical instruction. Every day, every student, and every client would teach me something new. They asked such wonderful questions. Lesson #5—Be open to all that you can learn from others.

Writing this textbook has been another unexpected adventure. If anyone had told me I might someday write a book, I would have told them they were crazy! I think the reason I really agreed to write this book was that nursing and teaching have meant so much to me. Writing and collaborating with others have helped me broaden my perspective of what nursing is all about. I have seen many changes in healthcare delivery and in the nursing profession. Change is occurring very rapidly and can at times be stressful. How we as individuals, and we as a profession, cope with change will affect the healthcare system of the future. Lesson #6—Learn good coping skills; they are a necessity in life and in your profession.

—Connie Hirnle

An Open Letter to Nursing Students

We are writing from our perspectives and our life experiences to share a little bit of insight that could help to inspire you as you begin your education in nursing. This advice may seem a bit biased; that is because all of us writing to you are dedicated to nursing and greatly enjoy our profession. We want you to feel this energy and vitality as you start out, and we hope that it will sustain you in some of the days when things are less than positive. Here are our words:

Nursing can provide wonderful opportunities to experience new people and new cultures. Whether you travel across the state, across the country, or across the world (as I have done traveling from my home land of New Zealand), the people you meet and care for all have something unique to share with you.

—Bridgette J.

Meet people where they are in their life at the moment you talk with them; clean your mental blackboard of judgments and stereotypes . . . just be with them.

—Pam K.

As you enter the field of nursing I wish you well and hope you remember after a few years of practice why you do this. There is a great deal of stress in caring for others, dealing with peers, doctors, and the whole gamut of healthcare. Try your best but be willing to forgive yourself—for you will make mistakes. Support your peers and they will support you. Learn to laugh when times are awful. Nursing is hard work, but it is extremely fulfilling.

—Pam M.

Stay positive and keep an open mind! Nursing school is truly worth it in the end!! I truly believe that motivation and hard work pay off, especially in nursing school. There are so many opportunities for nurses. You do not just have to work in the hospital. Talk with counselors or professors at a university about the many options there are for nurses. You will be scared to death on your first nursing job. Everyone is! Be patient and ask lots of questions. You will care for so many different people; remember to treat each person as an individual. Everyone is unique and everyone deserves good nursing care regardless of race, age, or personal financial status. One last thing: LISTEN to your patients. Try not to be focused on the tasks you have to do. Focus on the people; they will appreciate it, and you will do a much better job. Good luck!!

—Kristine F.

As you begin your journey as a nurse, the most important skill you will ever use (besides handwashing) is to smile. Your smile will help patients feel better, and it has the ability to heal wounds no surgeon or medication could ever touch.

—Amy F.

My advice is to take each day one at a time and never lose sight of who you are. Always set aside a few hours a week to enjoy life. You will be more rested, more productive, and more enthusiastic about school if you allow yourself to relax and enjoy life. If you begin to feel overwhelmed, take a moment and prioritize. Do not focus on everything, just on one

assignment at a time. Then, before you know it you will be finished with your first class, your first school term, and your first year . . . and then you will be walking down the aisle to graduate!! Good luck!!

—Mary F.

There are many roads to take in nursing. My advice to you as nursing students is to leave your options open. You will be amazed at where you will end up ten years from now. Have fun and good luck!!

—Erin H.

Do not get competitive about grades. Look around at your fellow students and realize that you will be friends with these people by the end of the program. In the working world no one will ask you what your grade point average was.

—Debra H.

My advice to you as new nurses:

1. Know your limits.
2. Know your nurse practice act (the law as related to nursing practice in each state).
3. Be tolerant of others; enjoy and embrace diversity.
4. Remember the practice of mind, body, spirit, and always give compassionate care to the whole person.
5. Keep an open mind.

—Joyce B.

Nursing is a career that should not be limited to the medical-surgical unit, or the operating room, or the labor and delivery unit, or the intensive care unit (ICU), or the emergency department. When entering nursing, look beyond the known clinical areas where traditionally many of us started our careers. Look instead to areas such as the cardiac catheterization laboratory, forensic nursing, or nurse practitioner in primary care. Nursing is an avenue of continued learning. Nursing involves extensive critical thinking skills that we all learn and continue to develop in our daily practice. Enjoy nursing; it is full of joy as well as sadness. You can always find new avenues of personal growth within the profession of nursing.

—Patty J.

Do not be discouraged, because there will be more than one way to do things and you will have to find what is comfortable for you. Always ask questions, no matter how small, if you are not sure about something.

—Mona B.

Nursing is like a relationship: You will receive as much as you give.

—Oksana P.

My words of wisdom to new nursing students:
Be open to change.
Stay excited about nursing as the years go by. Do so by challenging yourself and by trying different fields of nursing.

—Kristy M.

Do not lose your sense of humor; you will need it. Peroxide takes blood out of clothing. Never lose sight of your dreams; they will sustain you.

—Marie E.

ISSUES AND TRENDS IN CURRENT NURSING

Over the past 50 years, nursing has undergone dynamic changes in its scope of practice. Nurses have moved from simply observing and giving prescribed medications to coordinating clinical information for the entire healthcare team. This coordination allows the design of the best possible plans of care. In many instances, nurses are the healthcare professionals who physically assess clients, consult with various team members (e.g., physicians, physical therapists, social workers, pharmacists), design plans of care, and implement plans with clients.

Many changes in the healthcare industry have led to the broadening scope of nursing practice. Settings for healthcare have shifted from hospitals and other institution-based settings to community-based settings. Community-based settings for healthcare are discussed here and in detail in Chapter 2. The shift to community-based care is related to "rising consumerism," or the public's desire to participate more actively in healthcare decisions, issues, and choices. Technologic advances have greatly broadened the possibilities of what healthcare can do for people. Related to all these issues are concerns about healthcare costs and the need for all people to be able to access the healthcare resources they need.

Influence of Today's Healthcare Settings

A person seeking healthcare today faces a tremendous array of settings in which care is provided. Some suggest that this maze is so complex that the average person needs an advocate to help him or her move through it. Services vary: some concentrate on health promotion and disease prevention; others focus on diagnosis and treatment, rehabilitation, or supportive care. Because of the recent increases in the number and variety of agencies that provide healthcare, any attempt to categorize them would be incomplete.

Until recently, hospitals and medical centers were the largest and most organized of healthcare agencies. Because of rising costs, more procedures and treatments are being performed on an ambulatory basis. Clients come to an ambulatory care facility and usually do not stay overnight. A hallmark of good ambulatory care is thorough family and client education. The role of nurses in an ambulatory center can vary considerably, depending on their education and the center's management.

Community healthcare agencies offer care to a neighborhood or community. Many care facilities, such as day care centers and ambulatory care centers, also are community based. Many have come into existence as a result of federal legislation. Because hospital stays are shorter, care provided in the

---

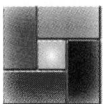 ## Nursing Research and Critical Thinking
Do Current Educational Materials Meet Clients' Needs for Self-Study in Preparation for Procedures?

Changes in healthcare delivery have led to the expectation that clients can learn about many diagnostic procedures that they will undergo by using books and videotapes given to them before such procedures. Two clinical nurse specialists working with clients scheduled for cardiac catheterization realized the need to evaluate the appropriateness and effectiveness of these educational materials. They designed a systematic study to assess the suitability of materials used to prepare clients for cardiac catheterization. They identified materials in common use through a survey of four hospital laboratories and three cardiologists' offices that performed cardiac catheterizations. They evaluated three videotapes and four booklets using the Suitability Assessment of Materials (SAM) instrument. They also evaluated concrete objective information (COI, procedural and sensation information). The SAM assesses six criteria for client education materials: content, literacy demand, graphics, presentation and appearance, learning stimulation, and cultural appropriateness. On two separate occasions, the first author used the SAM and the COI to

rate each videotape and booklet. The second review and rating occurred 6 weeks after the first and was perfectly consistent with the first rating (inter-rater reliability, $r = 1.0$). Only one videotape achieved a rating that supported its use for client education. Two booklets were rated as adequate, and two were rated as unsuitable.

Critical Thinking Considerations. The researchers stated that the study's purpose was to evaluate the suitability of materials without regard to the client's culture. They therefore excluded cultural appropriateness criterion. Because culture can have a great impact on the way people understand what they are told or what they read, the exclusion of this information may have affected the study's results. Implications of this study are as follows:

- Effective and appropriate educational materials that empower clients are essential to professional practice.
- Booklets are frequently used as educational material, yet their reading level and scope of content are often too difficult for clients to understand.

From Smith, P. T., & Cason, C. L. (1998). Suitability of patient education materials for cardiac catheterization. *Clinical Nurse Specialist, 12*(4), 140–146.

community has expanded. Chapter 2 discusses issues surrounding the shift to community-based care in detail. The following stories illustrate how this shift has influenced nursing practice.

Virginia's Story

Virginia entered a diploma nursing program in 1949. Her first nursing job was working on a pediatric unit in a small, rural hospital. She then worked on the other units of the hospital (medical-surgical and obstetrics). RNs administered all medications and treatments, while nursing aides managed personal care. The client population varied from 40 to 10. (Such wide swings in hospital census happen less frequently in today's hospitals, because there are fewer admissions for observation and most beds are filled with acutely ill clients.) Team nursing was the model used to provide care: two RNs supervised the work of many aides. Although she remembers being very busy, Virginia also remembers how wonderful it felt to work with clients and their families, both in hard and in happy times.

From 1961 to 1979, Virginia served as an administrator at two different hospitals. Her nursing background was a great benefit, because she understood the needs of clients and staff, which positively affected institutional growth and development. Virginia was often called on to work in the emergency and delivery rooms. She loved being able to remain active in bedside clinical practice while also facing the challenges of nursing administration. During these years, Virginia witnessed the beginning of Medicare and other federal government programs. As these programs became chief payers of care in hospitals, many new regulatory directives emerged. Changes were most evident in procedures that involved medical records, documentation, and financial systems.

From 1980 to 1986, Virginia worked in nursing administration in Alaska, which coincided with a shift from the team nursing model to the primary nursing model. In primary nursing, RNs provide most care for clients. This meant that Virginia had to find new ways to recruit RNs to her staff. This shift was difficult because the area was isolated and staff somewhat limited. During this time, technologic advancements in client care exploded. By this time, licensed practical nurses (LPNs) were practicing at the level that used to be common only for RNs. Administrators like Virginia focused on creating budgets and educational opportunities that would allow for expansion of the clinical practice and acquisition of the necessary equipment for technologic support of clients within the hospital.

Virginia has since left administration and is now working in home care. Using case management as the model for care delivery, she is able to make decisions specific to each individual client to promote his or her independence for as long as possible. **Case management** means that Virginia coordinates many resources to maximize the opportunity for people to manage their own healthcare at home (see Chapter 25). She says of her current position, "I think I have learned a whole lot in life skills and in my nursing experience on how to view the various unique aspects of people and then how to pull

them together in a community-building endeavor. This establishment of 'community' makes this the best job I have had so far. It is truly the most personally rewarding."

Liz's Story

After graduation from a BSN program, Liz worked on telemetry, medical, and pediatrics units in a large hospital. She went on to graduate school and worked as a nurse specialist in transfusion services. She was responsible for reviewing and analyzing blood counts and ordering blood, platelets, and other blood products. Liz earned her master's degree in 1996, having completed research on health education for preschool children. After the birth of her third child, Liz decided that she would like to be home more during the day and work during the evenings.

Her job search took her down many paths. She finally decided that she could best use her clinical experience and graduate education by working with a consulting nurse services unit. Such units have increased dramatically with the shift to community-based nursing. In her current position, Liz works 6 to 8 hours a day, answering questions from callers in the community. Examples of calls that Liz receives include, "My doctor told me that I will be having a CT-guided rib biopsy; what does that mean, and what might they be looking for with this test?" "On TV, I saw the *E. coli* warnings on cold cereal; what should we do?" The Centers for Disease Control and Prevention (CDC) and the local health department work in conjunction with the staff to keep employees informed about public health issues and concerns. Staff then provide relevant information to callers who express interest in such topical health concerns.

Liz's county is currently exploring options to improve use of emergency medical services (EMS) in conjunction with such consulting services. The study's results may allow more efficient use of staff and resources and increased customer satisfaction. Many people who call 911 may require only a verbal discussion with a nurse to adequately address their healthcare concerns. Consulting nurses may be able to **triage** specific calls, or prioritize them in order of importance. For example, flu, minor injuries, and stuffy noses would be handled after life-threatening or traumatic experiences.

Liz's work illustrates how public policy and procedure evolve with economic concerns, the public's needs, and the resources available to a community. Liz states, "This work exemplifies what nurses do best: education, evaluation, personal reassurance, and community-accessed and -integrated care—people in their own homes calling and attempting to understand how best they can meet their needs in the real-life situation."

Reflection

- What benefits do you see in the transition toward community-based healthcare? How do you perceive these changes will affect the nursing field as a whole? Do you believe the changes strengthen or weaken nursing's role in client care?
- How do you suppose a nurse with a strong background in institution-based care (such as Virginia) would

approach this transition? As a new nurse, how would you prepare to work in community-based settings?

- Do you agree with Liz's comment that her work exemplifies what nurses do best? Why or why not?

Rising Consumerism

Consumerism is the public's expectation that it will have a voice in determining the type, quality, and cost of healthcare it receives. Today's consumers are informed and are asserting their rights in the area of healthcare delivery. The consumer movement was fostered by the advent of managed care organizations (MCOs), which promote the prevention and treatment of illness (see Chapter 2). Legislation that required facilities to obtain informed consent from clients before beginning certain treatments further encouraged this movement. Previously, the healthcare system operated on the assumption that physicians knew what was best for clients and should make decisions for them. Now clients expect—and demand—to be involved in healthcare decisions.

The right to healthcare also has became a consumer issue. Historically, the poor either had to be satisfied with a decreased quality of care or do without healthcare entirely. Today, many citizens view equal access to healthcare as everyone's right. An ongoing debate centers on who should pay for this care.

Jenny's Story

Jenny graduated in 1984 with her BSN degree. She speaks warmly of people she met as she pursued her education. The sense of community and support from those in her nursing cohort allowed her to develop friendships that continue to be a strong presence in her life.

After working for 3 years on a medical unit, she transferred to pediatrics and worked there for almost 7 years. She learned to care for infants born prematurely who required intensive monitoring of their breathing and heart rate as they "grew and gained" sufficiently to be discharged. She taught parents how to monitor their newborns for signs of respiratory distress and how to allow time for babies to learn to nipple feed after having had gavage feeds (i.e., feedings of fortified formula administered via a feeding tube placed down the baby's throat).

In pediatrics, Jenny also cared for children with terminal illnesses (Fig. 1-1). One client, Josh, arrived full of bravado and with a definite view as to how all things were to be done for him. One day, Josh decided that he wanted to go out on pass to dinner with his family. At the time, some staff members resisted this request. Power struggles erupted over just who would make decisions regarding his daily care.

As Josh's primary nurse, Jenny called a conference for staff to discuss the problems with the situation and to identify possible solutions. This approach did much to resolve tension. So it was that Josh exerted power over his own daily existence. He went out on a pass and had a "night out" with his family.

Within a few days after this "night out," Josh moved into an isolation room to begin chemotherapy for his transplantation. He died a few weeks later. Jenny had never lost sight of

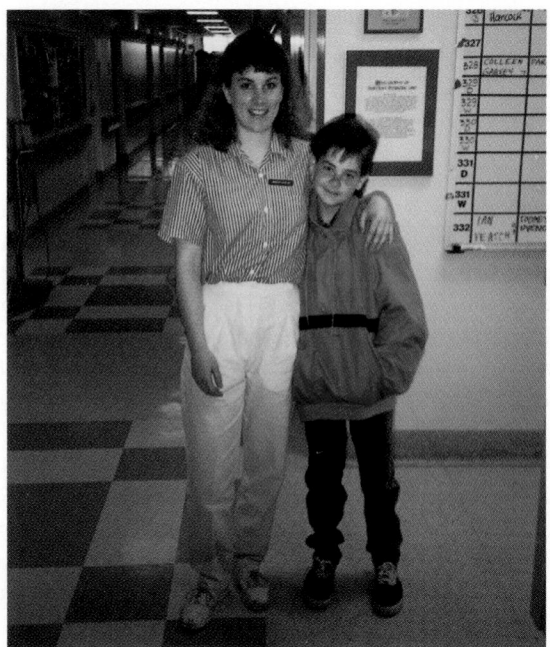

FIGURE 1-1   Jenny with a young client.

the importance of allowing Josh as a person—not his disease or his prognosis—to be her first and foremost concern.

Now, Jenny works in a treatment center, assisting with chemotherapy and antibiotic therapy. There she works with clients, referred by many physicians, who 10 years ago would have been hospitalized for the therapies they are now receiving in the community. Care in this setting is governed by a system called pathways, and nurses act as case managers. This shift is an example of how nursing practices change with influences from healthcare economics and the needs of people in the healthcare setting.

Bill's Story

Bill chose nursing as a second career. He had spent much time in Africa as a missionary pastoral worker. He oversaw a program that imported food from the United States and was responsible for distributing food to the villages. He worked with individual villages to create committees that reviewed and evaluated needs for food delivery. He also worked with nurses who provided maternal and child care to decrease the infant mortality rate. After his missionary work, Bill sought a career that would continue to best maximize his talents. He built houses for a few years before returning to school. He married and enrolled in an associate degree in nursing (ADN) program, graduating in 1992.

Bill's first choice had been to work in a hospital, where he believed he could gain wide exposure and learn a great many clinical skills. But the market was tight at graduation, and he took a job at a nearby nursing home. He found that he was exposed to a wide range of clinical scenarios and was surprised that he actually enjoyed seeing the same faces over a long period. He was able to develop relationships with these clients. Bill's interest in their stories and lives helped his clients "step outside" themselves and create new lives.

Bill felt an immense respect and admiration for the people with whom he worked. He never met any client in the home who initially wanted to be there. Because people needed to adjust to the new environment, Bill helped them to cultivate a sense of dignity. He chose to support what people saw as good and sacred, not to change them or to convert them to a different way of being.

Now, Bill is working in home health hospice. Here, he has an opportunity to help people maintain their ability to remain at home and deal holistically with their health and family needs at the end of their lives. Bill finds his current experience similar to his missionary work in Africa: meeting people on their own ground, honoring their lives and their choices, and supporting them in their decisions about health and death. Bill holds a deep reverence for this final stage, and he understands the desire to greet death on one's own terms without the assistance of high technology involvement. He works to ensure that death and dying do not diminish a person but rather conclude each person's unique life journey.

Reflection

- What ethical issues are involved in healthcare decision making?
- How has the consumer's role changed the way healthcare is administered?
- Whom do you believe should be involved in client care decisions?
- If you had been faced with Jenny's situation, how would you have handled it? Do you believe she made the right decision?
- How does Bill approach client decisions?
- In what way are Jenny's and Bill's situations similar? In what ways are they different?

Technologic Advances

Advances in technology have drastically changed healthcare and significantly altered the profile of the hospitalized client. Less invasive diagnostic tools can assist in identifying conditions at an early stage, while they are still treatable. People with cancer can receive high doses of chemotherapy that destroy the malignant cells. Damaged immune systems can be replaced with transplantations of bone marrow from other people. Premature newborns can be saved with the use of hi-tech computerized monitoring systems and critical care interventions. Nurses translate the newest findings of research, science, and technology into care for their clients.

Many previously incurable diseases can now be treated. Life can now be maintained mechanically long after biologic systems have stopped functioning. Heart, lung, and liver transplantations, unheard of three decades ago, are common. New technology, however, is expensive, and some advances raise formidable questions. For example, should insurance plans cover expensive transplantations? How do we decide when to remove a person from life-support equipment? Who decides to whom the organs should be given?

Linda's Story

Linda graduated in 1982 and started her career in a small, rural hospital, working on an oncology unit. Eventually she worked in a large, urban hospital on a pediatric bone marrow transplantation unit. It was there that she met 6-year-old Mitch (Fig. 1-2), who had a diagnosis of myelodysplastic syndrome, a malignant, life-threatening condition. Mitch had a rather uncomplicated first transplantation and returned to his home and school. He returned for his 1-year checkup and was given a clean bill of health. One month later, unfortunately, his disease had recurred. Mitch returned to Linda's unit for his second bone marrow transplantation. Unlike the first transplantation, this one proved to have a complicated course; he developed severe graft-versus-host disease. It soon became clear that Mitch would not survive. Linda worked with his family in anticipation of his death. A deeply religious family, they were able to be present with Mitch and view every moment together as a gift.

In the midst of physical manifestations of disease, Mitch was still a little boy and given to ways of any other child his age. One day, he was angry with Linda and said things that were quite unkind. The next day, knowing that he had hurt her feelings, Mitch made her a picture. To this day, 8 years after his death, the picture is still on her refrigerator. The paper is almost pure white with most of the color having faded, yet it stays in place.

The faded picture on her refrigerator is a testament to Mitch and the short but vital life he shared with Linda and all that knew him. Mitch is one of the faces Linda holds in her mind's eye as she currently oversees the research and development of new anticancer drugs in a pharmaceutical company. She coordinates a large staff, manages an annual budget, and shares responsibility with other company executives

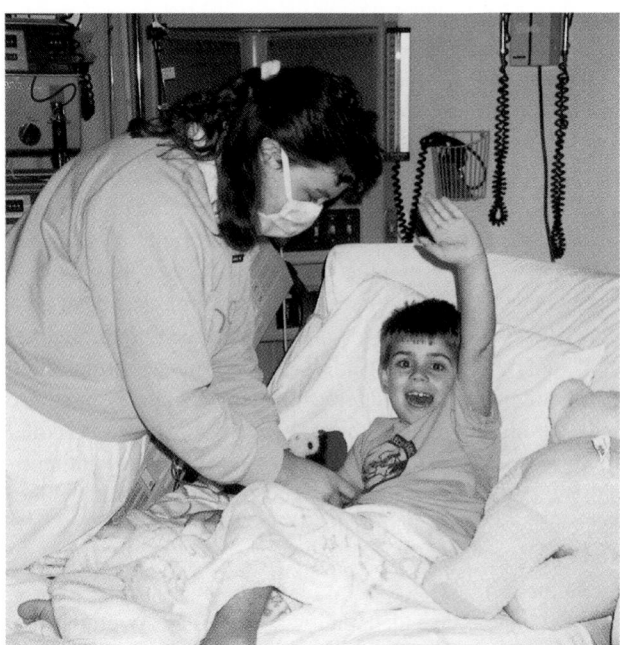

FIGURE 1-2 Linda still keeps the picture that Mitch drew for her on her refrigerator.

to guide the course of evaluating the safety and efficacy of new drugs. Her nursing skills, developed first in her educational program, and her clinical expertise, developed during years of practice, are integral to this job. Linda's professional practice has been able to move to exciting new horizons given the technology and research happening in the area of healthcare.

Denise's Story

Denise had originally pursued her nursing education in a hospital-based program, earning her diploma in 1975. She worked for several years before moving to Colorado, where she married and enrolled in graduate school, completing her master's degree in 1988. She moved to Arizona and worked in a clinic providing family care. It was in this setting that Denise began to ask questions about who received care, who made these decisions, who should provide the care, and where it should be delivered. The people served by the clinic taught Denise much about what it means to "be healthy" and what it means to "have healthcare."

While studying for her master of science in nursing (MSN) degree, Denise had, in her words, "fallen in love with learning." She wanted to continue her education and therefore enrolled in a doctoral program. Denise also worked part-time in postanesthesia recovery room care. She valued the balance of clinical practice with her academic understanding of nursing. Denise earned her doctorate in 1996 and is currently teaching undergraduate and graduate nursing courses. She finds the time spent with nursing students invigorating and inspiring and believes she is helping to create new paradigms of thinking that relate to the profession.

Denise views education as integral preparation for nurses to work in a field that is ever-changing yet also built on a rich history of tradition and scientific research (see Chapters 3 and 8). In 2001, Denise was awarded a grant to pursue a collaborative research project with a colleague on the faculty in the School of Social Work. The research will examine the experiences of women enrolled in welfare programs. Denise, in her doctoral studies, delved into social issues in society, and she has integrated a career in teaching with research that has social justice at its foundation. Social justice in the arena of public health takes into account the most vulnerable of populations and addresses how we as a society can respond with respect to the unmet needs of people. Nurses work with the most vulnerable people in society, sometimes meeting them at their most intimate and painful moments. The relationship between nurses and those with whom they work is most therapeutic when it is rooted in mutual respect. Mutuality allows nurses to deal authentically with the course of care specific to the individual client or population with whom the nurse is working.

Reflection

- Do you believe technologic advances are, overall, for the client's good?
- Compare and contrast the advances in healthcare that have occurred over the past 50 years.

- How has science changed the role that nurses play in the administration of healthcare and their responsibilities for educating the client?
- How would you characterize the roles of biotechnology firms in the advancement of new treatment therapies? How does nursing input relate to these routes of technologic advancement?
- In what way does Linda's nursing background interact with her role in the pharmaceutical company?
- Denise views education as a vital part of the nursing role. How does this relate to technology?

Access to Healthcare and Financial Resources

Healthcare costs in the United States are an ongoing concern. The government and the healthcare industry have adopted several measures to offset some costs. For example, healthcare delivery through organizations such as MCOs has expanded, and the government has established prospective payment for Medicare. As the availability of resources has decreased, however, a number of issues have emerged. With limited resources, the question of healthcare rationing must be addressed. The change to lower-cost providers by hospitals and clinics has created job security concerns for many nurses. All healthcare providers are being asked to put a dollar value on their services and to relate these costs to client outcomes. Finally, quality- versus quantity-of-life questions are being debated at all levels.

Access to healthcare services refers to a person's ability to find and to receive care from a healthcare provider. Access has been a public health issue for many years. Although more people are involved in the healthcare system than ever before, some areas of the United States still lack adequate healthcare resources. Research has suggested that access varies depending on an individual's income, race, and geographic location. Numerous plans have been attempted to solve the access issue. The need for solutions is a continuing concern.

Betty's Story

Betty's first clinical job was at a large teaching hospital. Afterward, she spent 4 years in Papua New Guinea. She volunteered at a school, teaching and preparing local nurses. The school's faculty consisted of nine people who emphasized community health, obstetrics, and medical-surgical care. Papua New Guinea is rich in natural resources such as gold and copper, yet most people there live in poverty. This developing country has pressing social, educational, and health needs, but only a small portion of society benefits from the rich natural resources and commerce.

Teaching medical-surgical nursing meant focusing on infectious diseases such as malaria, leprosy, and tuberculosis. HIV/AIDS education also became a pressing need. Accessing resources such as books, articles, and current research was an ongoing challenge. Betty made it her personal mission to create a library and to establish resources for the school's continued benefit. She worked with contacts from the United

States and Australia, asking them to send books and supplies. The government provided a subsidy, but many needs and supplies were given by various churches.

After leaving Papua New Guinea, Betty traveled in China and Europe. She faced many instances in which she had to triage injuries and illnesses. In one such case, she came upon a car crash in which a woman had been severely injured. Betty performed cardiopulmonary resuscitation and revived the woman; however, the woman died in Betty's arms while on the way to the hospital. This incident and her experience in Papua caused Betty to reflect on how people take healthcare in the United States for granted. When nurses perform cardiopulmonary resuscitation, they assume that an EMS team will transport the victim quickly for needed care in an appropriate ICU. The lack of EMS and ICUs in other countries highlights the reality of different priorities in different areas.

Returning to the United States, Betty assumed a position as a field nurse, working with pregnant teens and young mothers in a public health department. After 3 years, Betty decided to go to graduate school to understand healthcare at the level of research. She obtained an MSN and a master of public health (MPH) degree.

Betty took a job as a nurse epidemiologist, working in community assessment. In this occupation, Betty analyzed small geographic populations using qualitative and survey data to describe and understand unique communities. Betty worked with an entire team of environmental specialists, nurses, community development specialists, volunteers from the community, youth, university students, and other agency members. The team's very composition mirrored that found in the larger community. Recently, Betty took a new opportunity in public health administration and management. Her goal is to develop leadership skills for herself and within her team. Betty says of her new job, "In some respects the work is more satisfying, because I am not putting Band-Aids on wounds. I am helping to create a situation where injury and illness are less of a threat to people and where a standard of healthiness can be made manifest for whole populations, as opposed to treating a single client at a time."

Sharon's Story

Sharon is a woman with a broad spectrum of interests. She took classes in history, French, art, philosophy, and theology in addition to those required for her BSN program. After graduation, Sharon worked in a small rural hospital, regularly serving in the surgery, recovery, and emergency departments; on holidays, she covered obstetric care. Sharon needed the skills to master any clinical scenario as it unfolded, because she was often the only nurse on the shift. From this rural setting, Sharon transferred to a university-affiliated hospital as a member of the surgical unit. Here, she worked with some of the earliest recipients of kidney transplantations and open heart surgery.

Sharon worked for 5 years as a visiting nurse, which allowed her to use physical assessment skills, make critical analyses, and apply theory to arrive at differential diagnoses for her clients. In this fairly autonomous position, Sharon had

responsibility for approximately 50 clients at a time, most of whom were elderly and fragile. During these years, Sharon frequently witnessed her clients' having to choose between food and medicine. Fixed incomes mandated such difficult decisions; more often than not, older adults chose medicine over food. Resulting malnutrition and other health complications left fewer choices for independent living and decision making. Such dilemmas inspired Sharon to examine how she could influence institutional structures that rendered her clients vulnerable to the ravages of poverty and ill health. She believed that she could more completely address the principle of distributive justice and human rights at the policy formation level than at the bedside. She chose to move from home care into advocacy work, focusing on the issue of senior citizens and healthcare.

An example of Sharon's advocacy work was the passage of the Senior Citizen's Service Act, in which the state government appropriated funds for Area Agencies on Aging to evaluate the needs of seniors and then establish programs to address these needs. Such needs ranged from transportation, to access to healthcare clinics, to the provision of nutrition sites. While active in advocacy work, Sharon also attended graduate school and earned a degree in theology with a concentration in biomedical ethics. For 20 years, she has been working on end-of-life issues with lawmakers and national leaders. The combination of experience as a legislative advocate and nursing experience has given Sharon wonderful opportunities to serve people. She summarizes her nursing career by saying, "I am grateful that I have had the chance to practice nursing and to work at the policy formation and implementation level. Nursing encompasses a wonderful body of knowledge, and it can be used every day. It tells us about ourselves and all those with whom we work and have our being."

Reflection

- Why is economics an issue in healthcare? How would you suggest healthcare be made more accessible?
- Why do you think there are areas in the United States with inadequate healthcare?
- How must the healthcare community adapt to maintain the vision of healthcare access for all without compromising quality?
- In what ways has the role of nursing changed in order to provide healthcare access to those in need?
- How would a nurse with Betty's or Sharon's background react to the statement, "I'm sorry, but your healthcare insurance does not cover these services."
- How would Betty and Sharon characterize the current condition of the United States healthcare system as compared with systems in underdeveloped nations?

Today's Nurse

Fifty years ago, most nurses were young women who entered hospital-based programs right after graduation from high school. Their nursing education involved a strict academic program and a strong clinical component of mandatory time spent working at the hospital with which the school was affiliated. Nursing students had to adhere to dress codes and curfews. They could not be married and had to observe all rules of their programs.

Today's students reflect a much more diverse population. Some still enter their programs immediately after high school, but many more have pursued other paths before choosing nursing as a career. Consequently, nursing students must find ways to balance the demands of being an adult learner with the responsibilities of adult life. Many have children, partners, and other employment demands. These learners must balance family, finances, and career development.

Roberta's Story

Roberta, a 58-year-old nurse, currently works on a medical isolation floor in a large urban hospital. Roberta received her associate of arts degree from a community college as an adult learner while raising four young children alone. Her time in school was difficult because she had to juggle academic and clinical work along with her family's care and support. "Sometimes I doubted that I would complete it all. It seemed all my time belonged to everyone else, and I never had a moment to call my own," she recalls.

Her hard work and determination paid off. After graduation, Roberta began working night shift on a medical isolation floor. The job was fast-paced with many demands. She was responsible for monitoring all intravenous (IV) fluids and administering all medications. Roberta needed to juggle the tasks of physical assessment, decision making, and coordination of care for 12 clients with documenting in each client's chart all that had transpired during the night shift.

Several years after her entry into nursing, Roberta's hospital changed from the team model to the primary nurse model for care delivery. Coincident with the shift to the primary care model, the level of care required for clients in hospitals increased. Such clients were sicker and had a greater need for Roberta's clinical expertise and time. Although caring for fewer clients gave her more time to get to know each person better, the clinical demands of their increasingly complex conditions meant that Roberta still had an enormous amount of work to accomplish during each shift. She recalls that one gentleman who was about to be discharged from the hospital told her, "I really appreciated the gentle little tap you gave my toe every time you came by to see me." This exchange made Roberta realize just how much little things meant to those entrusted to her care.

Over time, the population of people admitted to Roberta's hospital unit changed primarily from older adults to young people, particularly with the emergence of acquired immunodeficiency syndrome (AIDS). Roberta found herself working with people who were dying at the height of their personal and professional lives. Her experiences with these people led Roberta to begin volunteering in hospice care. She also became a member of the hospital's nursing educa-

tion committee, presenting a workshop twice a year to facilitate her colleagues' professional ability to deal with death and dying.

In 1988, Roberta's stepson, Richie, was lost in a mountain climbing accident. His death was one of those moments in which the support of other nurses, her colleagues on night shift, and the nursing education committee were most important. The experience of her professional practice and her personal loss were closely interrelated. Her work with grieving clients and their families had given her expertise in encountering death, yet the death of her stepson pushed her to realms of understanding she could never before have imagined. The people with whom Roberta worked proved to have a significant role in supporting her during her time of rebuilding and coping.

Kathy's Story

Kathy provides another perspective. Kathy is one of the four young children Roberta was raising while attending nursing school in the 1970s (Fig. 1-3). Kathy was born in Seattle, married a military man, and moved to Alabama. She describes how she came to pursue nursing as a career: "I had dropped out of school in the 10th grade because I could not deal with school. Instead, I just got my general education document (GED) in 1982. For 13 years, I ran a home day care center, and then I realized I needed to do something else with my life and nursing came to me as the option."

As she made this decision to pursue a nursing career, she had family responsibilities to consider, as had Roberta years before. It was her mother's love for nursing that made an impression on Kathy and inspired her to be a nurse.

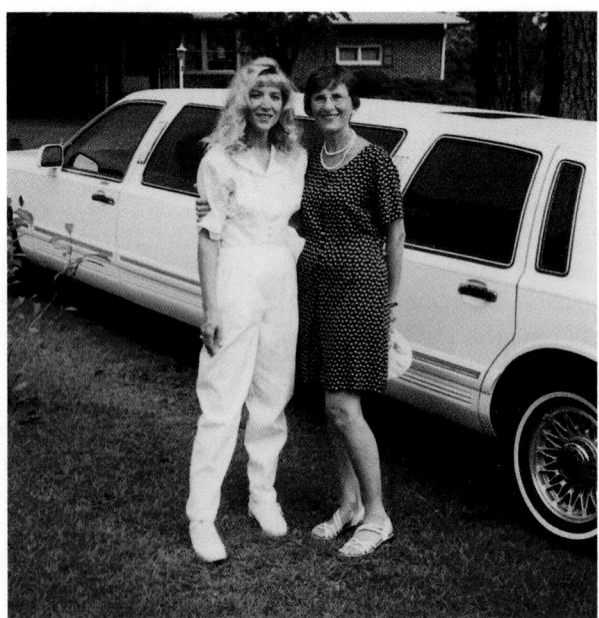

FIGURE 1-3   Kathy and Roberta, mother and daughter nurses, reflect the changes in nursing practice and its future development.

As she recalls the time she spent in school, she mentions the challenges that touched her heart and made her question whether she would succeed in her decision to be a nurse. She remembers moments of learning, like the first time she had to give medications. When someone needed an IV line started in order to receive the appropriate medication, the instructor told Kathy to do it. She did the procedure correctly but did not get the line placed. Then the clinical instructor attempted to start the line and she too was unsuccessful. It was reassuring to realize that even experts have trouble always performing procedures perfectly.

On another occasion, Kathy was working in the labor and delivery unit when she faced an experience with death. A woman came into the facility expecting to give birth and go home with her baby. But the ultrasound and fetal monitoring were unable to locate heart sounds. Hope quickly transformed into loss and grief. This lesson was painful but important about expectations surrounding healthcare.

Kathy, 28 years old, graduated in 1998. During her job search, Kathy noted with pride, "It is time to start working in this field in which I am now qualified to practice. These years of school have prepared me so that clients can be entrusted to my care. This makes it all worthwhile." Kathy proceeded to get a job in a labor and delivery/postpartum unit and has found her work most rewarding. In 2000 she gave birth to a baby girl, Katie Rose. As Kathy balances the demands of being a wife, a mother to two teenagers and a new baby, and a professional nurse, she sees her career in nursing as an opportunity to pursue many new and challenging horizons.

Gayle's Story

Gayle attended Seattle Central Community College and has had her ADN since 1986. She began her career as an agency nurse and explored various agencies in her area. At the time of her graduation, hospitals were requiring 6 months of clinical experience before coming to work. In her agency, she found a nursing home she liked and applied for a position there. Gayle worked in the nursing home as a charge nurse and as a medication nurse. She was working with elderly people and saw many unmet needs within the group for which she was caring. This inspired her to look into other career options. She then went to work at Providence Hospital in a medical unit. From there she developed many professional skills, including the teaching of CPR classes and precepting of new employees, eventually becoming charge nurse of the medical unit. After 8 years in that unit Gayle transferred to the ICU, and this is where she has been most recently.

During the course of her career in nursing, Gayle contemplated returning to school for her degree but found it problematic with the competing demands of family, two children, and work. Her mother-in-law, though, was a constant source of encouragement to return.

In 2000, Gayle took the plunge and began the BSN completion program at the university. She began taking some course electives, including effective writing and the physical assessment class. She found it very exciting to be in school.

Now Gayle has determined that as she completes her BSN degree in 2002 she wants to pursue a career as a nurse practitioner in women's health. "Women are the key to families. If women can maintain physical and mental health, I believe they can and will promote wellness in their families." Women are, in Gayle's' view, extremely important to the functioning of a family. In her experience, some women often pay little attention to their own self-growth and health needs; however, she sees how much more powerful women could be if both self-growth and healthcare needs were attended to. She is also very interested in the health issues related to the human immunodeficiency virus (HIV), so she sees her future tied to clinical practice as well as research. She sees herself addressing the concerns of women, their bodies, their sexuality, their health, and their emotional balance. HIV has become a bigger issue in the African American community as the incidence of infection among African women has increased. Gayle views prevention and teaching of women to care for themselves as pivotal to decreasing the risks of HIV for African American women.

Gayle reports that school is truly wonderful. She encourages students to have a goal, to hold tight to that goal, and not to give up on their dreams.

Joyce's Story

Joyce began her nursing career as an LPN, graduating from her initial educational program in 1978. She worked as an LPN while she and her husband were raising a family. In the ensuing years she attained her ADN and continued working in a hospital setting. As her youngest child graduated from high school, Joyce decided to return to school for her BSN degree. She continued to work full time and earned her BSN over 2 years. While enrolled in the BSN completion program, she discovered that there were many dimensions to nursing and advanced practice that she had never even contemplated. Her work had always been very important to Joyce, and she practiced with integrity and commitment. Indeed, her clinical excellence and expertise were acknowledged in 2001, when she was chosen by her peers at her hospital as Nurse of the Year. Joyce's energy for learning and desire for increasing her abilities as a practitioner inspired her to reflect on the choices she had before her in the next 20 years of her career. How could she continue to expand her role in nursing and remain vital in her capacity as a nurse? She made a monumental decision: she would attend graduate school!

It was a very important step in Joyce's life to consider applying for graduate school. Before attending the BSN program, Joyce had never viewed herself as a scholar, yet while enrolled at the university for her BSN she discovered that she greatly enjoyed school and that she was quite adept at learning. Still, the thought of taking on the challenge of graduate education was somewhat daunting. After doing some quiet soul searching and taking the Graduate Record Examination,

Joyce summoned up her courage and applied to the graduate program. Her acceptance letter came quickly, and as she graduated in 2001 with her BSN she looked forward to 2002 and the beginning of her graduate classes. In her years as a nurse, Joyce never wavered in her high expectations of herself. In continuing her education, she has amplified her abilities to provide excellent care to clients and leadership within the profession of nursing.

Reflection

- Both Roberta and Kathy earned their nursing degrees as adult learners. How does your nursing education experience compare with theirs?
- Gayle identified women and their healthcare as pivotal to improving the general health of the family and thus of the community. Can you think of other groups of people or culturally diverse populations whose healthcare issues are in need of acknowledgment?
- How can the healthcare industry best prepare nurses today for the next millennium?
- How will you balance the demands of your education with your work, your family, and your other responsibilities?
- Both Gayle and Joyce took the opportunity to plan to attend graduate school. Do you see potential areas where you might one day wish to have further study and attain a graduate degree?

CONCLUSION

The glimpses into the lives of working nurses give you a broad view of nursing practice in today's healthcare industry. As you read the vignettes, reflect on the intricate relationship that links the needs of clients, the healthcare system, and scientific and technologic resources. Notice how needs and resources combine to give nurses an opportunity to hold a unique place within the healthcare system. The dynamic nursing profession encourages people to use individual gifts that enhance clinical responsibilities and practice.

Clients, their families, and other members of the healthcare team rely on nurses for informed, critically analyzed judgments. The future of professional nursing is evolving with the arenas of medicine, science, research, and political and economic policy. Within this milieu, you will have the opportunity to influence and shape the profession's future.

KEY CONCEPTS

- Awareness of one's capabilities and own biases is important.
- Nursing has become an autonomous profession, in which nurses collaborate with professionals of multiple disciplines in the care of clients.
- Over the years, nursing practice has evolved from an institution-based model toward a community-based model.
- Nurses must be aware of the political and socioeconomic trends that influence nursing and healthcare.
- Cultural diversity and awareness are necessary for advancing nurse practice and creating a healthy community.

- Hospital care has changed over the years. These changes have allowed for more skill specialization and development of the nurse's role as an expert within the healthcare system.
- Because of advances in technology and science, the population requiring healthcare is now more complex with regard to injury and disease acuteness, mandating more critical evaluation and intervention.
- Critical thinking is a key skill in nursing; it is the tool that enables development of one's own concept of nursing.
- Effective nursing is characterized by the ability not only to administer quality care but also to evaluate situations critically and adapt as necessary.
- Nursing operates within a complex matrix of client needs and resources.
- Nursing education can serve to provide a foundation upon which many new opportunities for creative practice can emerge.
- Nursing opportunities have evolved to new levels, including data analysis, research-based therapies, client and community education, and policy formation in the international as well as local and national arenas.

BIBLIOGRAPHY

Allen, D. (1998). Record-keeping and routine nursing practice: The view from the wards. *Journal of Advanced Nursing, 27*(6), 1223–1230.

Allen, D. I., & Kahn, N. B., Jr. (1998). Educational guidelines for women's health are available from AAFP [letter; comment]. *Family Medicine, 30*(6), 400.

Allen, D. W. (1998). How nurses become leaders. Perceptions and beliefs about leadership development. *Journal of Nursing Administration, 28*(9), 15–20.

Amyot, D., Gray, P., Demong, C., Wilson, W., Murphy, D., Watson, J., & Duff, J. (1996). The nurse's role in clinical trials. *Canadian Nurse, 92*(10), 30–32.

Benner, P. (1996). A response by P. Benner to K. Cash, "Benner and expertise in nursing: A critique" [comment]. *International Journal of Nursing Studies, 33*(6), 669–674.

Bozzo, J., Carlson, B., & Diers, D. (1998). Using hospital data systems to find target populations: New tools for clinical nurse specialists. *Clinical Nurse Specialist, 12*(2), 86–91.

Chinn, P. L. (1996). Editorial 3: Publication, collaboration and clarity. An editorial view with Peggy Chinn [interview by Annette Street]. *Contemporary Nurse, 5*(3), 96–100.

Diers, D., Bozzo, J., Blatt, L., & Roussel, M. (1998). Understanding nursing resources in intensive care: A case study. *American Journal of Critical Care, 7*(2), 143–148.

Dow, K. H. (1996). The quality of lives: 1,525 voices of cancer. Betty R. Ferrell, PhD, FAAN, 1996 Oncology Nursing Society Distinguished Researcher. *Oncology Nursing Forum, 23*(6), 907–908.

Drevdahl, D. (1999). Sailing beyond: Nursing theory and the person. *Advances in Nursing Science, 21*(4), 1–13.

Ersek, M., Ferrell, R. B., Dow, K. H., & Melancon, C. H. (1997). Quality of life in women with ovarian cancer. *Western Journal of Nursing Research, 19*(3), 334–350.

Fagin, L., Carson, J., Leary, J., DeVilliers, N., Bartlett, H., O'Malley, P., & West, M. (1996). Stress, coping and burnout in mental health nurses: Findings from three research studies. *International Journal of Social Psychiatry, 42*(2), 102–111.

Kang, D. H., Coe, C. L., Karaszewski, J., McCarthy, D.O. (1998). Relationship of social support to stress responses and immune function in healthy and asthmatic adolescents. *Research in Nursing & Health, 21*(2), 117–128.

Lewis, C. K. (1996). The clinical nurse specialist's role as coach in a clinical practice development model [editorial]. *Journal of Vascular Nursing, 14*(2), 48–52.

McHugh, M., Duprat, L. J., & Clifford, J. C. (1996). Enhancing support for the graduate nurse. *American Journal of Nursing, 96*(6), 57–62.

McKane, C. L., & Schumacher, L. (1997). Professional advancement model for critical care orientation. *Journal of Nursing Staff Development, 13*(2), 88–91.

Nicol, M. J., Fox-Hiley, A., Bavin, C. J., & Sheng, R. (1996). Assessment of clinical and communication skills: Operationalizing Benner's model. *Nurse Education Today, 16*(3), 175–179.

Richardson, S. L. (1996). The historical relationship of nursing program accreditation and public policy in Canada. *Nursing History Review, 4*, 19–41.

Salvage, J. (1998). Opportunities to reshape health policy. *Nursing Times, 94*(17), 20.

Simpson, J. (1996). Public health policy and the nursing profession. *Journal of the Royal Society of Health, 116*(2), 118–120.

Watson, J. (1996). The wait, the wonder, the watch: Caring in a transplant unit. *Journal of Clinical Nursing, 5*(3), 199–200.

Watson, L. J. (1996). A national profile of nursing centers: Arenas for advanced practice. *Nurse Practitioner, 21*(3), 72–74.

Watson, M. F. (1997). Transitions in nursing education: A model for designing practical/vocational nursing curriculum. *Journal of Practical Nursing, 47*(4), 18–24.

Whitman, M. (1998). Nurses can influence public health policy. *Advanced Practice Nursing Quarterly, 3*(4), 67–71.

Zerwekh, J. V. (1997). The practice of presencing. *Seminars in Oncology Nursing, 13*(4), 260–262.

Zerwekh, J. V. (1997). Do dying patients really need I.V. fluids? *American Journal of Nursing, 97*(3), 26–31.

2 Community-Based Nursing and Continuity of Care

Key Terms

community-based
  healthcare
community-based nursing
  care
continuity of care
discharge planning

healthy communities/
  healthy cities
health determinants
levels of healthcare
nursing competencies for
  community-based care

Learning Objectives

Upon completion of this chapter, the student will be able to do the following:
1. Discuss what is meant by community-based healthcare.
2. Identify three levels of healthcare and the services under each level.
3. Identify the role of various settings for community-based healthcare.
4. Explain how social, professional, and financial considerations have influenced the growth of community-based healthcare.
5. Determine the focus of nursing care in all settings and situations.
6. Discuss forms of community-based nursing practice, both traditional and more recent.
7. Identify the importance of continuity of care and discharge planning.

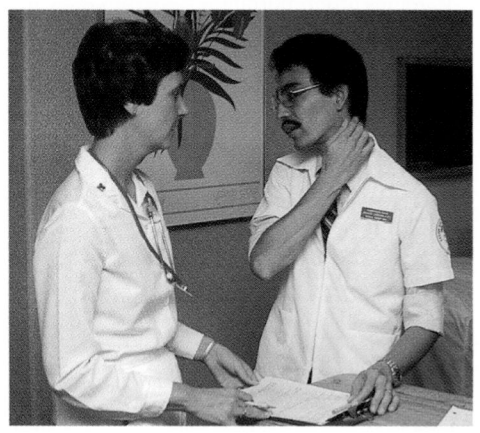

Critical Thinking Challenge

You are employed as a clinic nurse at an Indian Health Service (IHS) facility serving a population of 4300 tribal members on a reservation. You note that there is a high rate of missed appointments in the diabetes clinic. You find it difficult to reach people because many have no phones. Clients tell you that some of their difficulties are due to lack of reliable transportation to the clinic (many have to travel a long distance). Some clients say they don't feel they are respected when they come to the clinic. In addition, grandparents and great-grandparents may be unable to leave home because of child care responsibilities for extended family members. You wonder why the incidence and severity of diabetes problems is escalating quite dramatically for tribal members. The nearest hospital and dialysis facility is over 100 miles away at another IHS unit. You decide to consult with the community health nurses who work for the Tribal Health Department to assist you in developing a plan that will lead to more effectively meeting the health needs of the people you serve with the resources available regionally.

Once you have completed this chapter and incorporated the community-based healthcare delivery system into your knowledge base, review the above scenario and reflect on the following areas of Critical Thinking:

1. Describe the work skills and knowledge base you will need to function effectively in community-based nursing practice.
2. Explain the importance of continuity of care and discharge planning in the emerging healthcare system.
3. Propose how nurses will work with various sectors of the community and healthcare professionals.
4. Predict the opportunities for the nursing profession within the changing healthcare system.
5. Calculate what will happen to hospitals in the future.

The United States healthcare system has been in a state of crisis and tumultuous change for two decades (American Nurses Association [ANA], 1991; Brook, Kamberg, & McGlynn, 1997; Donley, 1996; Iglehart, 2001). The pivotal problem is how to deliver cost-effective, quality healthcare that is accessible and results in positive health outcomes for everyone. The crisis, however, presents opportunity. Healthcare policymakers are eager to find solutions that will work. Healthcare professionals are seeking creative ways to decrease both provider and consumer frustrations. So far, efforts to reform the healthcare system have not contained costs; meanwhile concerns continue about quality of care (Heffler, Levit, Smith, Smith, Cowan, Lazenby, & Freeland, 2001; Kohn, Corrigan, & Donaldson, 2000).

Most legislative discussions about national healthcare share two key strategies: primary healthcare measures and health promotion/disease prevention services. The World Health Organization (WHO) (1978), a United Nations agency that promotes worldwide health, includes the components of universality, essentiality, community empowerment, community participation, and community development in its definition of primary healthcare.

Because hospital stays are shorter, care provided in the community has expanded. Community-based care is becoming more significant than institution-based care as emphasis moves to primary healthcare, health promotion, and disease prevention. Studies predict that in the future more nurses will work in community-based settings than in institution-based settings.

To provide an understanding of current and future trends in healthcare delivery and nursing care, this chapter presents background information related to industry changes, emerging models of community-based nursing practice, and the critical role nurses play in the continuity of care. Although everything in this textbook is related to community-based nursing (because the hospital is, after all, a part of the community), the clinical chapters in Section II use community-based nursing as an integral part of their "Implementation" sections.

LEVELS OF HEALTHCARE

The U.S. Department of Health and Human Services Division of Nursing has analyzed current nursing practice and education in relation to population healthcare needs. **Levels of healthcare** are categorized as primary, secondary, and tertiary (Fig. 2-1). Most current resources, services, nursing practice, and nursing education exist within the category of secondary healthcare: emergency care, acute and critical care, diagnosis, and treatment. The population's needs, however, fall mostly within the categories of primary healthcare (health promotion, education, protection, and screening) and tertiary healthcare (rehabilitation, long-term care, support services, and hospice care). Most primary and tertiary services are best delivered in community-based settings. As the twenty-first century begins, the healthcare industry must work to better align these levels of need with actual provision of care.

Community-Based Healthcare Trends and the Determinants of Health

According to the Healthcare Forum (1994, p. 3), "Americans are moving away from a narrow concept of health as the absence of disease to a broader definition that encompasses quality of life issues." In a random survey to determine what the public considers vital to individual and community health, results revealed that Americans are moving toward an approach that emphasizes actively "creating" health. Survey participants shared the following values:

- Individuals can influence their own health through behavior and lifestyle changes.
- Prevention strategies are important.
- Health and well-being include quality-of-life issues.

A significant finding is that people believe "quality of life" to be synonymous with a healthy community. The public believes that decreasing crime rates, strengthening families and

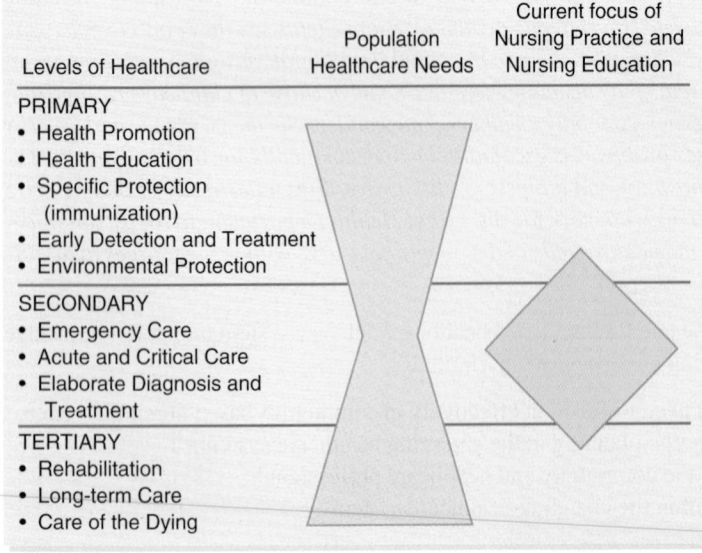

Levels of Healthcare	Population Healthcare Needs	Current focus of Nursing Practice and Nursing Education
PRIMARY • Health Promotion • Health Education • Specific Protection (immunization) • Early Detection and Treatment • Environmental Protection		
SECONDARY • Emergency Care • Acute and Critical Care • Elaborate Diagnosis and Treatment		
TERTIARY • Rehabilitation • Long-term Care • Care of the Dying		

FIGURE 2-1 Levels of healthcare need. Whereas the population's needs are clustered at the primary and tertiary levels, nursing practice and education concentrate at the secondary level. (Developed by the Nursing Practice Branch, Department of Health and Human Services.)

their lifestyles, improving environmental quality, and providing behavioral or mental healthcare are critical elements to creating healthy communities. In relation to healthcare within the community, the Healthcare Forum (1994) found that desire for high-quality healthcare, affordable healthcare, and good access to healthcare were almost equal (Fig. 2-2). There is growing recognition that to achieve the goals of *Healthy People 2010: Understanding and Improving Health* (U.S. Department of Health and Human Services, 2000), a model inclusive of multiple **health determinants** is needed. Healthcare services, per se, make a relatively small contribution (10% to 20%) to the overall health status of individuals and communities (Durch, Bailey, & Stoto, 1997; Evans, Barer, & Marmor, 1994; Keating & Hertzman, 1999; Lee & Estes, 1997; Marmot & Wilkinson, 1999; McGinnis & Foerge, 1993; Tarlov & St. Peter, 2000). To impact social, economic, political and educational health determinants, effective health initiatives are community-based by necessity. Behavior and lifestyle account for an estimated 50% of individual health (McGinnis & Foerge, 1993).

The above information reinforces the importance of predictions the National League for Nursing (NLN) made in 1992. The NLN predictions included the following:

- Nurses will emerge as community leaders.
- Community nursing centers and health programs to assist in preventing disease and promoting health will expand and become more available to the consumer.
- Home care will become the center of healthcare.
- Health will become a value with moral force for the public, thereby creating a demand for consumer-driven services (Executive Wire, 1992).

In addition, the NLN (1994) has identified community-based nursing to include the following concepts:

- The individual and the family have primary responsibility for healthcare decisions.
- Health and social issues are acknowledged as interactive.
- Treatment effectiveness, rather than technologic imperative, drives decisions.

As a result, the trend in healthcare delivery is in the direction of community-based care with consumers leading

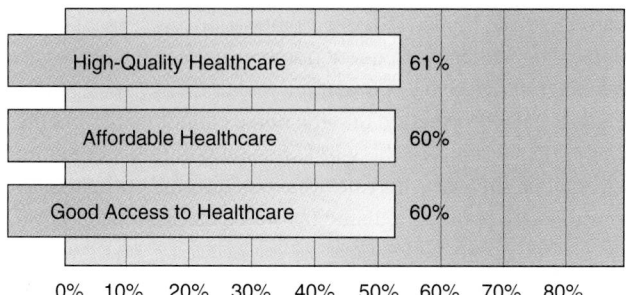

FIGURE 2-2   In a healthcare survey, respondents deemed quality, affordability, and access to healthcare as equally important. (Data from Healthcare Forum [1994]. *What creates health?* San Francisco: Author.)

the way (Kretzmann & McKnight, 1993; McKnight, 1995; Ray & Anderson, 2000; Rosenbaum, 2001; Rothschild & Leape, 2000).

Community-Based Healthcare

Community-based healthcare is the design, delivery, and evaluation of healthcare services developed in partnership with communities. "Community" is broadly defined and may be a work place, school district attendance area, enrollees of a managed care insurance provider, a geographically defined area, or a group or place identified by a categorical or medical need. Community-based healthcare is found where people are—where they work, recreate, go to school and church, etc.—and is developed within the context of a given community, i.e., its unique needs and strengths. Partnerships assume equity in contributions, participation, commitment to common interests, and close association. Respect, appreciation, and cooperation characterize successful partnerships. The nature of the cures–client relationship in community-based care is one of partnership.

Experts believe that future integrated models of care will supply a broad range of services, from in-house to ambulatory care, within their own system (vertically integrated) or arrange for other systems to provide the services (horizontally integrated) through contracts (Riley, 1994). Primary care providers, hospitals, retirement communities, pharmacies, rehabilitation centers, and other types of providers from a large geographic area will be connected formally.

Formal integration of services is expected to restructure the economic activity of the healthcare delivery system (Buerhaus, 1999). Networks are expected to compete for clients by becoming more efficient, charging lower prices, and providing quality services. They will guarantee quality care for a fixed price for the individual's life and maintain a central database to ensure comprehensive care as the client moves within the system.

Nursing's Agenda for Health Care Reform (ANA, 1991; *www.nursingworld.org/readroom/rnagenda.htm*) is the nursing community's proactive position on how, where, and by whom healthcare should be delivered. It promotes an approach in which healthcare is taken to the consumer who, in turn, will be an increasingly informed participant in decisions affecting his or her care. Healthcare services will be delivered in such places as the place of employment or school-based clinics. Hospitals and other institutions will remain significant components of the healthcare system, but they will no longer be the central focus or dominant influence. The consumer will assume a more dominant position (NLN, 1994).

Healthcare delivery will increase where people spend their time: home, schools, work, shelters, church parishes, senior citizen centers, ambulatory settings, long-term care facilities, and hospitals. Common to all programs will be the need for greater individual authority, accountability, and responsibility with a lesser reliability on institutional authority and policies (NLN, 1994).

Community-Based Nursing

Changes in the healthcare system result in changes in the delivery of nursing care. Nursing education is evolving and redirecting its emphasis to meet society's changing needs. Nursing began its focus of care in the community in the 1800s, was redirected to acute care for much of the twentieth century, and now is returning to the community. Nurses have a critical role to play in the evolving models of community-based care. It behooves us to review lessons from our history and from great role models such as Lillian Wald (Keeling, 2001; Stanhope & Lancaster, 2000).

Community-based nursing care can be defined as nursing care directed toward a specific group or population within the community and may be provided for individuals and groups as described above. The level of care can be primary, secondary, or tertiary. In community-based nursing, nurses have more authority, are more accountable for their actions, and are responsible to consumers rather than institutions. The emphasis is on a "flowing" kind of care that does not necessarily take place in one setting. Community-based nursing presents a special opportunity for nurses to apply their knowledge, perhaps more than ever before.

Nursing scholars differentiate between community-based nursing and community health nursing; the main difference is that community health nursing focuses on client and populations as community, while community-based nursing focuses on individuals and families within the community (Naylor & Buhler-Wilkerson, 1999; Stanhope & Lancaster, 2000; Zotti, Brown & Stotts, 1996).

Focus of Nursing Care

Although the setting for care and the type of intervention may change, the nursing focus is always the same. Wherever he or she practices, the nurse's concern is for health of the whole person (not only physiologic needs but also psychosocial and spiritual needs) in relation to the person's environment (ANA, 1995).

In nursing practice in the hospital, physical and mental stabilization is a primary goal for most clients. Needs include physiologic monitoring, complete or partial personal care, exercise, nutritional support, pain management, treatment and medication administration, anticipatory guidance, counseling, and teaching. Care needs are complex. Because of the trend toward shorter lengths of stay, the client may be discharged before counseling and teaching are finished.

In settings outside the hospital, the nurse's activities change. If nursing care is directed toward an individual, as, for example in home healthcare, the physiologic crisis is resolving but care needs may remain intense. Assessment of the home and involvement of family/significant others in direct care are essential. Planning and intervention focus on using individual, family, and community resources to assist in restoring a client's health to maximum possible functioning, while continuing to monitor for possible side effects to treatment or complications.

If community-based nursing is directed toward a population, the needs of that population, as determined by epidemiologic and demographic data and input from the population, help to set priorities. For example, work site healthcare services are individualized to the industry involved (factory workers versus white-collar workers).

Community-Based Nursing Practice in Transition

For most of the twentieth century, community settings for nursing practice primarily included county and state health departments. These departments carried out the traditional functions of public health: assessing community health status, ensuring health, and developing health policy. The focus of community health nursing is the health of a population. As a result of funding reductions in recent years, national, state, and county health departments continue to attempt to perform their mission with limited resources. Although public health/community health nurses still conduct home visits, nursing practice in many state health departments now focuses on client contact during clinic visits for maternity and child services, infectious diseases, and primary care.

Other common community-based settings for nursing practice include schools (school nursing), the workplace (occupational health nursing), and homes (hospice and home healthcare nursing). School nurses focus on the health of children attending their schools. Health screening, education, and counseling, crisis intervention, and first aid or chronic care management are some functions within school nursing practice. Occupational health nurses focus on worker populations; they stress the promotion, protection, and restoration of workers' health within the context of a safe and healthy work environment. Hospice nurses focus on the dying. Palliative care within a multidisciplinary team and family support are essential elements of hospice practice.

Nurses have delivered nursing care in the home setting since the late 1800s, although the focus of that care has changed over time. Currently the focus of nursing care in home healthcare is on complex chronic health situations (e.g., multiple medications, client confusion, or poor social support) and/or acute care assistance (e.g., fetal monitoring or home intravenous antibiotic therapy). This focus is largely determined by care covered by the healthcare system and may not meet all client needs. Home care nursing is discussed in detail in Chapter 23.

All nurses working in community settings should be prepared to make home visits. The school or occupational health nurse may make less frequent home visits than the nurse case manager or health department nurse, but many times a home visit reveals information that the nurse cannot gather in other ways. By focusing on the whole person within his or her environment, the nurse may be able to determine optimal interventions not apparent outside the home environment.

Newer Community-Based Nursing Settings

Community Nursing Centers. Newer forms of community-based nursing practice include community nursing centers that may be located in schools, workplaces, or other sites within the community. Nurse-managed centers deliver primary health-

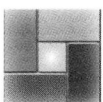
Nursing Research and Critical Thinking
Would Inner-City Minority Children With Chronic Asthma Benefit From a School-Based Management Program?

Nurses working in the community noted that inner-city minority children appear to have a high incidence of asthma and relatively poor management of the disease. They designed this study to examine the efficacy of a school-based program to prevent exacerbation of asthma symptoms and to manage asthma using measured doses of an inhaled anti-inflammatory medication. The researchers reviewed health records from an inner-city school and identified 40 students as having been previously diagnosed with asthma. They sent letters to the parents of each child, informing them of the study. The parents of 25 children attended the initial information session. After a detailed explanation of the study, all 25 families agreed to participate. Each child's diagnosis of asthma was confirmed by pre- and post-inhaled bronchodilator spirometry, or a methacholine challenge test, with demonstration of symptoms such as wheeze or cough. Three children were excluded from participation when they failed to demonstrate symptoms of asthma. Therefore, the purposive sample was comprised of 22 children (N = 22) with a confirmed diagnosis of asthma. For 3 months, each child came to the school clinic two times per day for medication administration and measurement of respiratory peak flow rates. Data were collected for a number of variables including bronchodilator use, school absences, self-reports of asthma symptoms, and number of visits to the physician. During the study, mean peak flow rates improved approximately 15% ($P = .0029$), and bronchodilator use decreased 66% ($P = .0015$).

Critical Thinking Considerations. This study had a small sample size and used a nonprobability sampling design, which did not allow use of a control group. Thus, it is unknown if improvements were due to the interventions or to other factors. Implications for nurses from this study are as follows:

• The use of regular inhaled anti-inflammatory medication significantly reduced the need for inhaled bronchodilators and helped improve peak flow readings.
• The consistent use of inhaled anti-inflammatory medication through school-based management led to a substantial reduction in complaints of nocturnal asthma symptoms.

From McEwen, M., Johnson, P., Neatherlin, J., Millard, M. W., & Lawrence, G. (1998). School-based management of chronic asthma among inner-city African-American schoolchildren in Dallas, Texas. *Journal of School Health, 68*(5), 196–201.

---

care to specific populations. Nurse Practitioners (NPs) and community health nurses staff these centers with backup from physicians as needed. The NLN defines a community nursing center as follows:

• A nurse occupies the chief management position.
• The nursing staff is accountable and responsible for client care and professional practice.
• Nurses are the primary providers that clients see when visiting the center (Murphy, 1995, p. 3).

Nursing centers, however, are not only sites that clients visit. They also are a concept that shapes broader services that nurses offer in practice arrangements within the community (Sharp, 1992). A nursing center must "also support nurse-managed services to clients in their home, community, hospital, nursing home, or a site across the healthcare continuum" (Murphy, 1995, p. 3). A further description of types of centers is given in Display 2-1.

Employee Assistance and Wellness Programs. Employee assistance programs (EAPs) and wellness programs represent additional settings for community-based nursing practice (Masi, 1992; Oss & Clary, 1998). Traditionally, EAPs focused on assistance with behavioral health and substance abuse problems. Today, EAPs incorporate wellness programs into their services. One example is the Arizona State University

(ASU) EAP and Wellness Program. Community health graduate nursing students were involved in the program planning and development of a campus-wide coalition for 3 years (Fig. 2-3 and Fig. 2-4). The resulting program model and evaluation plan (Matas & Mermis, 1993; 1994) have strong

DISPLAY 2-1

🔲 CATEGORIES OF COMMUNITY NURSING CENTERS

Community outreach: Free-standing clinics similar to traditional community public health clinics
Institution-based: Derive their mission from a large parent organization such as a hospital, university, or corporation
Wellness/health-promotion models: Provide triage, screening, education, counseling, and health maintenance services
Independent practice nurses: Faculty, nurse entrepreneurs

The first three categories are described in Riesch, S. K. (1992). Nursing centers: an analysis of the anecdotal literature. *Journal of Professional Nursing, 8*(1), 16–25. The fourth category is described in Aydelotte, M. K., Hardy, M. A., & Hope, K. P. (1988). *Nurses in private practice.* Kansas City, MO: American Nurses Association.

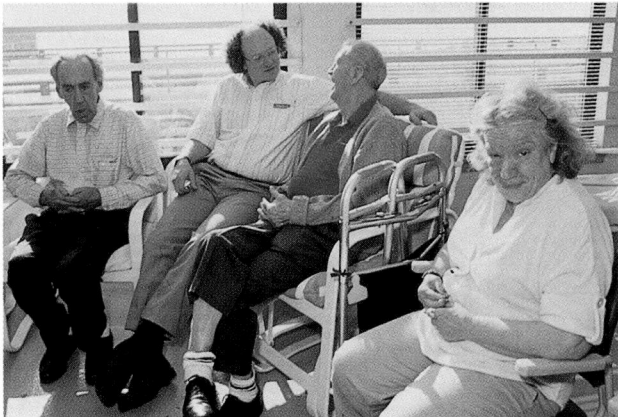

FIGURE 2-3   Nurses provide mental health counseling within community groups.

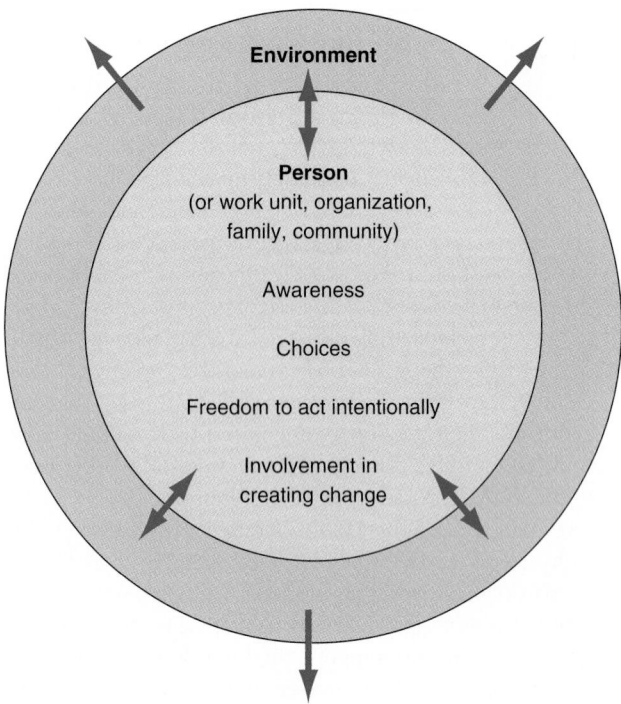

FIGURE 2-5   The Arizona State University Well-Being Model shows the dynamic process of knowing participation in change. Well-being is defined as actualizing choices based on awareness of intentional action and involvement in a changing environment. Power is defined as the capacity to knowingly participate in change. Well-being enhances the powers of the individual, organization, and community. (© K. Matas, 1994.)

support from ASU administration, faculty, and staff. Nursing theory and practice form the model's core (Fig. 2-5). The program, implemented in 1995, received the Governor's Award for Excellence in 1997.

Wellness programs can be found in various settings, and nurses often manage and staff them. These programs exist in integrated healthcare systems and other places such as a component of healthy cities projects (Matas, 1994). Other wellness programs have been established in the workplace and schools. Nursing theory and current research literature on wellness programs (Murdaugh & Vanderboom, 1997; Pelletier, 1991; 1993; Watt, Verma, & Flynn, 1998) suggest that, to be effective, a wellness program must be comprehensive and oriented to the whole person within the context of community and family needs. Additional outcome studies are needed.

Other Forms of Practice.   Other emerging forms of community-based nursing practice include parish or block nursing (Jamieson, 1996), lay health worker networks (McFarlane, Kelly, Rodriguez, & Fehir, 1994), case management, independent nursing practice, and work with community coalitions

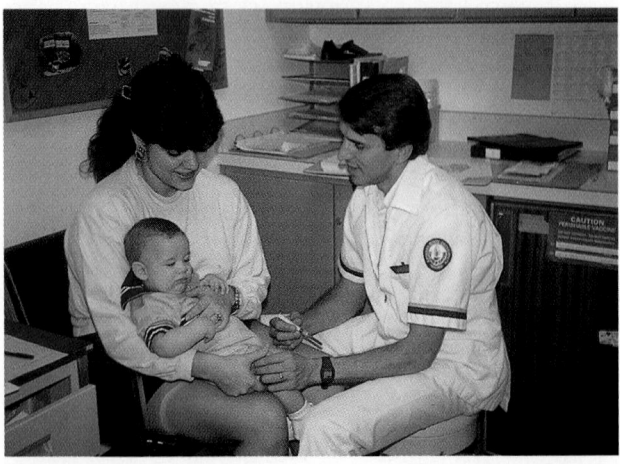

FIGURE 2-4   This student nurse from Arizona State College, Tempe, AZ, interviews a woman and her infant.

such as the healthy cities projects (Butterfoss, Goodman, & Wandersman, 1993; Flynn, 1998). Nurses have been active in parish nursing in the Midwest for some time. Many churches have full-time nurses on their staffs; others hire nurses part-time as consultants. Some plan health fairs for the congregation. As the population ages, churches may find that adding a nurse to the staff will assist in meeting their senior citizens' needs. President George W. Bush's White House Office of Faith-Based and Community Initiatives may also provide opportunities for nurses to partner with faith communities for health programs (*http://www.faithbased communityinitiatives.org*).

In some communities, lay health workers are critical links between underserved or high-risk populations and the formal healthcare system. Nurses have collaborated with community members to identify, support, and provide training and consultation to lay health workers. Lay health workers are community members committed to assisting themselves and their neighbors through outreach networks. In this way, nurses can significantly eliminate barriers to healthcare, increase accessibility of needed services, and thus improve the community's health status.

Case management involves healthcare provided through the direction of a case manager, usually a nurse, who plans, coordinates, and tracks client care through a variety of settings. Case management provides continuity of care. This type of care is useful when the client is high risk, and the care is more complex. Nurses involved in case management are primary care nurses or skilled clinicians.

Some advanced practice nurses and NPs work independently by setting up their own offices for private or group practice. Some state laws require that the independent NP be linked to a medical backup. "Success depends on the possession of specific resources, such as adequate skills, finances, emotional support, and the desire to be one's own boss" (Calmelat, 1993). An advanced practice nurse in private practice is accountable to professional standards and the clients served. An example of this type of practice is described by Matas (1997) as the Health Patterning Clinic. Matas developed a nursing theory-based practice model for an ambulatory adult population; the model demonstrates improved client health and well-being across all types of presenting problems.

According to Butterfoss, Goodman, & Wandersman (1994, p. 316), "community coalitions unite individuals and groups in a shared purpose." Recently many efforts have focused on building community coalitions to improve communities' health. These efforts usually take a multifaceted approach such as developing gang prevention programs or substance abuse programs along with more traditional public health measures (e.g., community assessment). Nurses are key participants and contributors in community coalitions and are well prepared to assume leadership positions.

One example of such an effort is the Building a Healthy Mesa project under the sponsorship of the Mesa United Way in Arizona. Several faculty members, undergraduate community health nursing students, and graduate community health students contributed significantly to this coalition. The undergraduate students conducted community assessments in several neighborhoods over 2 years. The graduate students worked in a neighborhood, assessing, planning, implementing, and evaluating an immunization program for an ethnically diverse and economically vulnerable high-risk group. They also developed a lay health worker outreach program. The effort has received funding from the city of Mesa to develop a community resource center in a neighborhood school. Faculty have contributed not only by guiding the students but also by serving in leadership positions on various committees (Matas, 1994). They provide consultation for writing grants and proposals and advise on program planning and development.

In Battle Creek, Michigan, a coalition of churches was formed to study and plan how to promote, maintain, or improve the community health in and through faith communities. Nurses, pastors, other health professionals, the county health department, and community members collaborated to form the Faith Health Network, which is currently funded by a local foundation. Its formation and development has been nurse-lead. The coalition aims to impact significant health disparities in the larger Battle Creek community through the participation of 10 faith communities in developing and completing a spirituality and health survey used as a tool for community empowerment (Matas, 2001; Matas & Davies, 2001).

Global Initiatives

As nurses become valued and recognized for their contributions to health promotion, they will become sought-after members of global networks. Globalized practice is a new form of community-based nursing. A non-local network of individuals and/or organizations defines the community. Computer communication skills become critically important as linkages form worldwide. Global networks are both interdisciplinary and discipline specific.

Interdisciplinary. Blue Sky Associates is an interdisciplinary organization dedicated to educational transformation. In 1996, members held a conference at St. Olaf's College in Northfield, Minnesota, entitled "The Spirit in Education." From this conference, an effort was begun to create a worldwide "wisdom project." A gathering held in Honolulu in January 2001 provided a forum for a worldwide dialogue about self-care wisdom. Members of the nursing field assisted in developing this project (*http://worldwisdomproject.org*).

Global Good Services, Inc. (*http://www.globalgoodservices. org*) expresses a vision for healthy communities on a global level, beginning with Native American communities. Due to lack of funding, this organization was unable to implement its first community partnership effort in building the Viable Village. The group's experience is a good case study exemplifying the difficulties involved in moving beyond the current system's status quo to develop innovative ways for communities to realize their true potentials. The Viable Village model encompasses assisting communities toward not only innovative healthcare delivery and services but also toward healthy economies and educational systems that will ensure the well being of future generations. Again, nurses were involved in defining and articulating the Viable Village model.

Kenzer (2000) has summarized healthy cities literature from around the world, and Fawcett and colleagues (2000) provide excellent information on web-based resources for building healthier communities.

Discipline (Nursing) Specific. In 1986, under the auspice of St. Mary's Hospital in Tucson, Arizona, a group began meeting in Mexico to focus on nursing case management. The group invited nurses from around the country to share their experiences and concerns related to nursing case management. The group's evolution is reflected in its name change from the Nursing Case Management Exchange to the Global Nursing Exchange. In 1999 the group gathered at the International Council of Nursing meeting in London. The Global Nursing Exchange includes administrators, basic and advanced practice clinicians, educators, researchers, authors, editors, and consultants. This international community of nurses supports and collaborates together to sustain and encourage personal self-care. Its larger purpose is promoting worldwide access to quality nursing and primary healthcare (Matas & Brown, 1997).

It will be important to remember to think broadly and "outside the box" as nursing moves more and more into community-based settings. Many times you may find you are the first (and only) nurse on the scene. With no one to mentor or guide you on-site, being connected to virtual or local nursing support systems will be essential. Remind yourself of the unique contribution nursing can make and take the lead in advocating for meeting needs that consumers are becoming more sophisticated about expressing. Visit the Nursing Manifesto web site at *www.nursemanifest.com* to learn about one virtual support network for nurses. Table 2-1 lists web sites for community-based initiatives.

Competencies Needed for Community-Based Nursing Care

As mentioned previously, educational programs are restructuring to prepare nurses for community-based practice. The Pew Health Professions Commission (O'Neil & the Pew Commission, 1998) issued the *Recreating Professional Practice for a New Century* report. The Pew Commission's "agenda for action" identifies 21 competencies that future health professionals must possess. These competencies, listed in Display 2-2, emphasize community and public health principles. Nursing practice in community-based, integrated healthcare systems will require basic competencies in community health nursing including primary, secondary, and tertiary prevention; community health assessment; knowledge and use of epidemiologic principles; community planning and coalition building; population health interventions (such as screening and educational programs); case management; and evaluating community- or population-focused care (Association of Community Health Nurse Educators, 1990).

Koerner (2000) identifies four capacities as the hallmarks of nursing leaders practicing in the community:

1. Capacity to create negotiated partnerships. Negotiation skills and the capacity to be authentic are basic to this skill.

2. Capacity to create new order. In this time of chaos, creating new order involves the capacity to see relationships and synthesize new systems.
3. Capacity for fluency and numeracy. Fluency and numeracy refer to the capacity of creative flow with ideas, words, images and metaphors in both quantification and qualitative capture of those things critically important in nursing practice.
4. Capacity for moral courage and integrity. The leader's character and courage determine the act's intention, thus the quality of outcomes that may affect many people.

Familiarity with current national, state, and local documents concerning health is critical to community-based nursing. An example of a national document is *Healthy People 2010* (*http://web.health.gov/healthypeople*). An example of a state document is *Arizona 2000: Plan for a Healthy Tomorrow* (Arizona Department of Health Services, 1993). Examples of local documents are the *Kalamazoo County Healthier Community Assessment* (Public Sector Consultants, 1995) and *Kalamazoo Community Indicators* (Healthy Futures, 1998). At the national, state, and local levels, all these documents identify health priorities for communities and at-risk groups. Other important recent documents providing direction for the future of community-based healthcare include the Pew Health Professions Commission report (O'Neil et al., 1998), the Institute of Medicine's report, *The Future of Public Health* (1988), and *Nursing's Agenda for Healthcare Reform* (ANA, 1991), the *U.S. Preventive Services Task Force* report (1998) and *Implementing Community-Based Education in the Undergraduate Nursing Curriculum* (American Association of Colleges of Nursing, 2000).

TABLE 2-1

Web Sites for Community-Based Initiatives	
Web Site Address	**Web Site Name/Description**
http://www.ncl.org	National Civic League, Healthy Communities program
http://www.healthycommunities.org	Coalition for Healthier Cities and Communities
http://www.bphc.hrsa.dhhs.gov/hshc	Healthy Schools, Healthy Communities
http://www.hmhb.org	National Healthy Mothers, Healthy Babies
http://www.sustainable.org	Sustainable Communities Network
http://www.paho.org	Pan American Health Organization
http://electronicvalley.org/hv2000	Health Valley 2000
http://www.globalhealthaction.org	Global Health Action
http://globalgoodservices.org	Native American Viable Village HealthCare Reform
http://worldwisdomproject.org	Blue Sky Associates, Community Wisdom
http://www.fetzer.org/rcc/	Relationship-Centered Care
http://www.nursemanifest.com/manifesto.htm	Community Formation for Nurses
http://www.futurehealth.ucsf.edu/ccph/html	Campus-Community Partnerships for Health
http://www.compact.org	Coalition of campuses to support students and faulty in community partnership efforts
http://www.faithbasedcommunityinitiatives.org	White House Office of Faith and Community-based initiatives

DISPLAY 2-2

⬚ **PEW COMMISSION 21 COMPETENCIES FOR THE 21ST CENTURY**

1. Embrace a personal ethic of social responsibility and service.
2. Exhibit ethical behavior in all professional activities.
3. Provide evidence-based, clinically competent care.
4. Incorporate the multiple determinants of health in clinical care.
5. Apply knowledge of the new sciences.
6. Demonstrate critical thinking, reflection, and problem-solving skills.
7. Understand the role of primary care.
8. Rigorously practice preventive health care.
9. Integrate population-based care and services into practice.
10. Improve access to health care for those with unmet health needs.
11. Practice relationship-centered care with individuals and families.
12. Provide culturally sensitive care to a diverse society.
13. Partner with communities in health care decisions.
14. Use communication and information technology effectively and appropriately.
15. Work in interdisciplinary teams.
16. Ensure care that balances individual, professional, system, and societal needs.
17. Practice leadership.
18. Take responsibility for quality of care and health outcomes at all levels.
19. Contribute to continuous improvement of the health care system.
20. Advocate for public policy that promotes and protects the public health.
21. Continue to learn and help others learn.

O'Neil, E. H. and the Pew Commission for the Health Professions. (1998). *Recreating professional practice for a new century.* San Francisco: Pew Health Professions Commission.

COMMUNITY-BASED HEALTHCARE ISSUES

Fragmentation of Service

The explosive growth of knowledge has led to specialization throughout the healthcare system.

The price for this specialization is fragmented care. For example, a surgical client who suffers from diabetes receives care from a surgeon and an endocrinologist or internist. If that same client has heart problems during surgery, a cardiologist is called. The client may spend time in surgery, the recovery room, the intensive or coronary care unit, a step-down unit, and/or a medical or surgical unit. After discharge, this fragmentation may continue as different specialists prescribe dif-

ferent medications and require follow-up visits. This can confuse and upset the client and family. It can also compound the client's health problems.

Of equal importance is the fragmentation that often results as clients move from one system of care to the next or when a government agency or program is not able to address communities' needs because the issues are so complex. For example, to address a community issue such as domestic violence, professionals in law enforcement, the judicial system, social services, and health services may be required to work together where no such collaborations have been established. Without systematic partnership building and coordination of services and communication, the individuals, families and communities continue to suffer and problems go unaddressed. In addition, all services must be evaluated to determine outcomes of care (Holt, 2000; Rowell, 2001; VanOrt & Townsend, 2000).

Quality of Care

Changes in the healthcare industry have led to concerns over the quality of care clients are receiving. Licensing, accreditation, and certification are examples of attempts to guarantee that people and places in the healthcare system are prepared to do what the public expects. Both people and institutions may be licensed. Mechanisms, often tests, are established to recognize minimum competence in a profession. One example is the National Council Learning Extension NCLEX-RN®, an examination that all states use to license registered nurses (see Chap. 3). Practicing without a license is a criminal offense. Institutions are licensed based on their ability to meet established criteria. Typical factors considered are physical structure, administration, personnel qualifications, and practice standards. Hospitals, nursing homes, and pharmacies are licensed in all states; licensing of other facilities and nonhospital services varies from state to state.

Accreditation, a popular approach to quality measurement, is a voluntary system that healthcare organizations use. Groups with mutual interests establish standards of quality and inspect themselves accordingly. Although not legally required, strong incentives exist to attain and maintain accreditation. In many instances, accreditation is necessary to secure federal funding for care. For hospitals, the accrediting body is the Joint Commission of Accreditation of Healthcare Organizations (JCAHO); for HMOs, it is the National Committee for Quality Assurance (NCQA).

Certification, the third approach to quality control, combines features of licensing and accreditation. Boards use standards for education, experience, and performance on examinations to determine a person's competence. Although certification is usually voluntary, incentives exist for people to become certified. Certification is often used to designate a person's professional specialty (e.g., certified nurse midwife).

Complementary and Alternative Healthcare Services

Complementary and alternative healthcare is care composed of treatments outside Western medicine. These treatments may include acupuncture, acupressure, therapeutic touch, herbal treatments, hypnosis, imagery, homeopathy, and chiropractic. Alternative health treatments are under study to see how they can support standard plans of care. Congress established the Office of Alternative Medicine as a part of the National Institutes of Health (NIH) in 1992 to examine these treatments and their effects on client outcomes. Reflecting the increasing significance and impact of these practices, the office was recently upgraded to an NIH "Center" with the subsequent name change to the National Center for Complementary and Alternative Medicine (*www.nccam.nih.gov*).

In response to consumer pressure, some insurers are beginning to pay for alternative treatments. Based on a 1993 random telephone sample of American adults, Eisenberg and colleagues reported that 34% of respondents used at least one unconventional therapy in the last year (Eisenberg, Kessler, Foster, Norlock, Calkins, & Dellono, 1993). Most respondents (72%) did not inform their physicians of these actions. Extrapolating these results to the U.S. population in 1990, Eisenberg and colleagues found that citizens made an estimated 425 million visits to providers of unconventional therapy. This number exceeds the total visits to all U.S. primary healthcare physicians (388 million). In 1998, Eisenberg and coworkers replicated and extended their earlier study that examined consumer actions during 1997 (Eisenberg, Davis, Etter, Appel, Wilkey, Van Rompay, & Kessler, 1998). The prevalence and expenditures associated with alternative medical therapies in the United States increased substantively. Overall prevalence of use increased 25%. Visits to alternative practitioners rose by 47%, and expenditures on services increased by 45%.

Self-Care

Self-care is a concept whose time has come as evidenced by several trends. As of 1997, more than 38 million Americans are without health insurance (Centers for Disease Control and Prevention, 1999). This number is projected to rise to 46 million by 2005. By necessity, self-care becomes important and highly valued. Consumers are no longer passive regarding their health; they understand the relationships of lifestyle, attitudes, and behaviors to health and well-being. In addition, many healthcare providers and services are promoting self-care as a strategy to reduce consumption of expensive medical services. Providers in capitated care systems benefit financially, and consumers benefit through personal empowerment and active partnership.

Herbert Benson, MD, president of the Mind/Body Institute associated with Harvard Medical School, predicts that self-care will be one of the three main influences in the healthcare system of the twenty-first century (1996). Self-care is a strong nursing disciplinary value and knowledge base. Nurses are in a significant position to encourage individuals, families, communities, and organizations to build on inherent strengths, capacities, and self-care abilities (Grandinetti, 1996; Lipson & Steiger, 1996; Payor & Provider News, 1996; Vernarec, 1997).

Continuity of Care and Entrance and Exit Within the System

Continuity of care is provision of health services without disruption, regardless of movement between settings. Continuity of care is a concern across the healthcare continuum. All models of community-based nursing address it. An organizational structure must be in place to ensure continuity of care from one healthcare setting to the next and among health professionals and community systems.

Admission to the Healthcare System

During admission to the healthcare system, clients generally experience some apprehension. Because they are placing themselves in the hands of healthcare professionals, they may fear becoming dependent and losing control over their lives or their decisions. The admission process is significant to the client's well-being; nursing confidence and competence can exert positive influence on the course of care. To decrease the client's fear or anxiety, nurses can assist in the following ways:

- Establishing rapport and showing a willingness to listen
- Clearly defining the purpose and expectations of the admission
- Assisting the client to understand how to participate as fully as possible in care-related decisions
- Clarifying the nursing role in relation to the client's healthcare needs
- Documenting the procedure

Whether the visit is a short emergency or an extended stay, the client receives an identification bracelet at the same time that required paperwork (e.g., admissions questions, insurance coverage, consent forms) is completed. The identification bracelet contains the client's name, healthcare provider's name, unit and room number, and possibly allergies. For the client's safety, check the identification bracelet before carrying out any diagnostic test, medication, or other treatment.

When working with a client who enters a unit or room, welcome the client and address him or her by name. Introduce yourself, and give the client full attention. Although the admission may be routine to a nurse, no healthcare admission is routine for the client. Convey empathy and concern to put the client at ease. Consider the client's cultural and spiritual needs: e.g., the need for an interpreter, awareness of what this admission means culturally, and respect for spiritual beliefs. Chapters 22 and 51 provide more in-depth discussion on these subjects.

Whether the client is admitted to a unit within an emergency or outpatient setting, hospital, or long-term care facility, the client and family need to know the following:

- How to access assistance (call bell signal, telephone number, or other electronic alerting)
- The physical environment and healthcare arrangements (unit or room arrangement)
- Basic care equipment
- Frequency of contact with care provider

Table 2-2 lists possible admission procedures that nurses perform at admission.

When admitting clients to a setting other than home, nurses need to orient them to the facility's organization, the care-giving supplies in the unit, and safety equipment in the unit and facility. Teaching clients and families about safe operation of the bed, side rails, overbed table, and lighting system and controls gives them power over some aspects of care and makes the unit less intimidating.

Support the family by familiarizing them with the location of waiting rooms, restrooms, public telephones, the nurses' station or desk, and other areas. This information helps to decrease anxiety. It gives the family an opportunity to contact other family members or spiritual leaders.

Client units also have other equipment for use in caregiving: e.g., the sphygmomanometer, outlets for oxygen and suction, personal care materials in the bedside stand such as bath basin, bedpan, urinal, emesis basin, and personal articles such as soap, toothpaste, toothbrush, and extra linen. Explain the location and purpose of such equipment. If the client is expected to stay overnight in a unit, usually there will be a telephone and television or radio.

Be sure to take complete admission information. The approach depends on the purpose of care. For example, in an emergency department, nurses conduct a focused admission that emphasizes the purpose of the current visit, symptoms, and information pertaining to the current problem. For a hospital admission, nurses complete a more in-depth admission form.

In some hospitals, this form runs to 12 pages. The assessment focuses on the current problem but covers other aspects of the client's health and lifestyle. In a community-related facility or if the client's condition is not life threatening, nurses may perform an even more detailed admission assessment that includes problems and information about the family or the client's environment.

During the assessment phase, help the client understand how he or she can participate in decisions and planning. For instance, the nurse may say, "After the physical examination, your physician will talk to you in his office." Leaving the client alone in the room without any information increases his or her anxiety. Give the client as much information as is appropriate. For example, the nurse may say, "Your laboratory results will arrive before lunch," "Some technicians will be here shortly to take an x-ray and take some blood for tests," or "I will bring you a pill for the pain as soon as your physician prescribes it."

Discharge Planning

Discharge planning prepares a client to move from one level of care to another within or outside the current healthcare facility. Traditionally, this process involved discharge from the hospital to the home. In the current healthcare system, discharge planning occurs from all settings including ambulatory surgical centers, rehabilitation units, drug treatment centers, and childbirth centers. Discharge can also occur within a facility as a client moves from one unit to another (e.g., a

TABLE 2-2

Overview of Admission to Various Healthcare Facilities	
Facility	**Possible Admission Procedures**
Hospital	Introduction; orientation to room and equipment; complete nursing history, vital signs, and other physical assessment
Emergency room	Introduction; ABCs (airway, breathing, and circulation); vital signs; focused assessment for acute problems; orientation to surroundings
Clinic or physician's office	Introduction; explore reason for seeking medical care and focused assessment of that problem; vital signs
Nursing home	Introduction; review of written or verbal report from transferring agency; nursing history and assessment focusing on functional abilities; orientation to new surroundings
Hospice	Introduction; review of referral; nursing history and assessment focusing on pain control, functional abilities, coping, and support; wishes concerning terminal care and death (e.g., living will); orientation to procedures and care
Psychiatric facility	Introduction; mental health evaluation including history, mood state, suicide risk, use of drugs, support system
Home visit	Introduction; review of referral and client's medical and nursing problems; home environment, caretaker and family support, community resources

client with a cerebral vascular accident moves from a medical-surgical unit to the rehabilitation unit). Discharge planning is also important with home care when for various reasons clients no longer require services.

As a collaborative function, discharge planning is done with, not for, the client and family. The discharge planner is the health or social services professional who is responsible for coordinating the transition and serving as a link between the discharging facility and the community. Often the discharge planner is a nurse who cares for the client. Frequently, the discharge planner may be a specialized role filled by a nurse or social worker who works collaboratively with the healthcare team, client, and family to assist with more complex needs. Discharge planning does not solve all problems but it can reduce readmissions, minimize residual effects of the health condition through continuity of care, and improve client and family satisfaction with the healthcare system.

Blaylock Risk Assessment Screen. Blaylock developed a discharge planning screening tool to help quantify the risk and amount of discharge planning that different people would require (Blaylock & Cason, 1992). The tool presents ten categories of risk factors for scoring: age, living situation/social supports, functional status, cognition, behavior pattern, mobility, sensory deficits, number of previous hospital/emergency room visits, number of medical problems, and number of medications. The higher the score, the greater the client's risk and the greater the need for discharge planning. The score helps identify people who might require home care resources, extended discharge planning, or placement in a retirement or nursing home (Display 2-3).

Discharge Planning Elements for the Client

Goal Setting. The nurse should develop goal setting in the areas of education, advocacy, and case management in collaboration with the client and family/caregiver. Outcomes for each identified health goal should be stated in realistic, clear, measurable, and time-oriented terms. Factors to consider in setting goals should include the following:

- Client's level of functioning and independence to achieve or maintain goals
- Extent of family/caregiver involvement
- Availability of community resources and the client's and family/caregiver's motivation to use those resources

An example of a goal is "Mr. Jones will be able to walk 15 to 20 steps with his walker in his home within 7 days of discharge from the hospital."

Transition. When people undergo transitions, their assumptions about themselves change and they develop new assumptions that allow them to adapt. Issues involving transition are particularly obvious when a client moves between settings such as from the hospital to home or from home to a long-term care facility. The physical move is only one type of transition the client makes. Other related changes may involve self-concept, role performance, mobility, self-care,

or communication with family members. For example, a mother with terminal cancer may experience the transition from her role as caregiver for her children to the role of care recipient.

Continuity of Care. Continuity of care is both an ideal and a necessity. Continuity of care is the provision of health services without disruption, regardless of the client's movement between settings. From the client's perspective, it involves having a home health nurse visit within 24 hours of hospital discharge or having the physician's office contact the local pharmacy about the client's medication needs. When health services are disrupted, the client may experience a relapse and require additional healthcare or hospitalization. Thus, continuity of care helps to maintain the client's health status and reduces healthcare costs.

Organizational policy and financial realities can work against continuity. Communication between health professionals about a client's needs may not occur. Starting discharge plans at admission can help ensure continuity of care by identifying needs early on; planning ahead allows for expedient referrals to community services and agencies.

Discharge Planning Elements for the Nurse. The nurse is responsible for ensuring that the client is prepared for discharge and that the family or caregiver has received necessary information and assistance. Safety is a key factor in planning for the client to return home. For the nurse, the key elements of discharge planning are coordination, facilitation, and negotiation.

Coordination. Coordination is the act of assembling and directing activities to provide services harmoniously. The result of coordination is a team working together with a unified purpose (Fig. 2-6). Payment based on diagnosis-related groups has led to shorter hospital stays; as a result, nurses must coordinate health and social services for clients' needs after discharge (Kee & Borchers, 1998). One way to coordinate services is to initiate and conduct team and family conferences, preferably before the client is discharged. Otherwise the client's problems may become unnecessarily complex. At a team conference, the discussion should focus on individualizing the client's care. For example, as the client's advocate, the nurse can bring to the team's awareness any special considerations regarding the client's home setting or other circumstances. At a family conference, professionals and the family gather to discuss family issues related to the client. For example, concern may exist about the availability of family members to assist with care, their understanding of care required, and/or other issues. Both types of conferences provide an opportunity for clients, family, and healthcare professionals to plan care and set goals. If clients require special equipment (e.g., oxygen, ventilation equipment, walking aids) to receive care in the home, the nurse may be responsible for securing the appropriate orders or authorizations, contacting the vendor, and arranging for delivery to the client's home.

Facilitation. Facilitation means making something easier and smoother, eliminating problems and barriers. To facilitate the client's transition, the discharge planner must anticipate needs

DISPLAY 2-3

BLAYLOCK RISK ASSESSMENT SCREEN (BRASS)

Circle all that apply and total. Refer to the Risk Factor Index.*

Age
- 0 = 55 years or less
- 1 = 56 to 64 years
- 2 = 65 to 79 years
- 3 = 80+ years

Living Situation/Social Support
- 0 = Lives only with spouse
- 1 = Lives with family
- 2 = Lives alone with family support
- 3 = Lives alone with friends' support
- 4 = Lives alone with no support
- 5 = Nursing home or residential care

Functional Status
- 0 = Independent in activities of daily living and instrumental activities of daily living

Dependent in:
- 1 = Eating/feeding
- 1 = Bathing/grooming
- 1 = Toileting
- 1 = Transferring
- 1 = Incontinent of bowel function
- 1 = Incontinent of bladder function
- 1 = Meal preparation
- 1 = Responsible for own medication administration
- 1 = Handling own finances
- 1 = Grocery shopping
- 1 = Transportation

Cognition
- 0 = Oriented
- 1 = Disoriented to some spheres† some of the time
- 2 = Disoriented to some spheres all of the time
- 3 = Disoriented to all spheres some of the time
- 4 = Disoriented to all spheres all of the time
- 5 = Comatose

Behavior Pattern
- 0 = Appropriate
- 1 = Wandering
- 1 = Agitated
- 1 = Confused
- 1 = Other

Mobility
- 0 = Ambulatory
- 1 = Ambulatory with mechanical assistance
- 2 = Ambulatory with human assistance
- 3 = Nonambulatory

Sensory Deficits
- 0 = None
- 1 = Visual or hearing deficits
- 2 = Visual and hearing deficits

Number of Previous Admissions/Emergency Room Visits
- 0 = None in the last 3 months
- 1 = One in the last 3 months
- 2 = Two in the last 3 months
- 3 = More than two in the last 3 months

Number of Active Medical Problems
- 0 = Three medical problems
- 1 = Three to five medical problems
- 2 = More than five medical problems

Number of Drugs
- 0 = Fewer than three drugs
- 1 = Three to five drugs
- 2 = More than five drugs

Total Score

* Risk Factor Index: Score of 10 = at risk for home care resources; score of 11 to 19 = at risk for extended discharge planning; score greater than 20 = at risk for placement other than home. If the patient's score is 10 or greater, refer the patient to the discharge planning coordinator or discharge planning team.
† Spheres = person, place, time, and self.
© Copyright 1991, Ann Blaylock.

and plan ahead. For example, the client may be overwhelmed by just thinking about going home, let alone planning for transportation from hospital to home. The nurse may be able to reduce the client's anxiety by anticipating and planning for transportation. Anticipation of discharge needs begins at admission and continues through the client's stay. The nurse must consider the different settings, the client's needs, and available resources.

A family conference helps to determine the most comprehensive service delivery. Coordination of care within the home includes assessing the family's capability to provide needed services and arranging services from other healthcare providers (e.g., physical therapy, occupational therapy, home health aides) and volunteers. For example, if a client needs home care and the spouse works full-time outside the home, plans need to be formulated so that the client has the help and assistance he

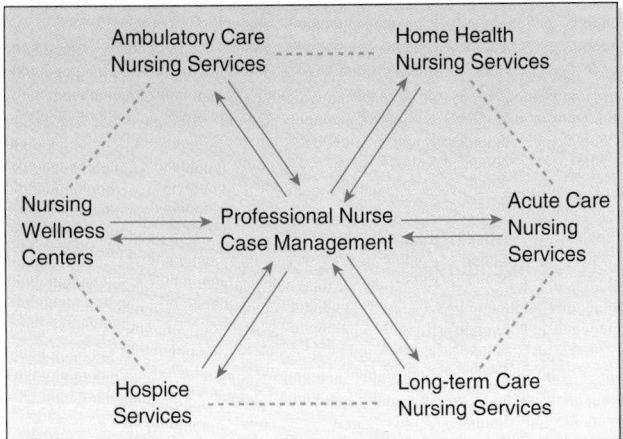

FIGURE 2-6   Coordination among healthcare team members is vital to the success of a client's discharge planning.

or she needs during those times alone. The home environment (e.g., the presence of stairs or the bathroom's location) may need modification based on the client's needs.

Negotiation. Negotiation is the process by which the client, nurse, and family determine goals. The most elaborate plan of care is doomed if the client, family, or healthcare professional hampers attempts to achieve the goals. Negotiation may be formal or informal; it must involve dialogue with the client and family to help articulate desires, values, and feelings about their views of a realistic plan of care. For example, the home care priorities of a young mother with a respirator-dependent infant may differ from those of the nurse. Negotiating with the mother over which goals and objectives take priority has two effects: the mother will be more willing to work with the nurse to attain goals and the mother will feel more in control of the situation.

At times clarification is a priority so a more formal process involving contracts is necessary. A contract is a written agreement between the nurse and client that delineates each person's roles and responsibilities. A contract regarding care clarifies expectations of the nurse, client, and family members. It provides a concrete reference for all parties to access should issues arise. Contracts help to limit the helplessness, stress, or disempowerment that clients and families may feel. The sense of control and empowerment achieved through the contract enhances the client's internal resources—specifically, motivation

and commitment. The nurse and the client or caregiver discuss who will be responsible for what and all participants reach a consensus. The consensus on responsibilities is written, then each person receives a copy so every participant can see clearly who is accountable for which responsibilities.

Levels of Discharge Planning. Discharge plans vary depending on the client's needs and the nursing interventions required to assist the client after discharge. All client goals and nursing interventions should be developed from the perspective that human responses to health and illness occur regardless of setting. Discharge planning is needed when a child is discharged from a day surgery center after a tonsillectomy, an older woman leaves a clinic requiring additional diagnostic tests to rule out a diagnosis of cancer, or a young man with a long history of substance abuse is discharged from a drug rehabilitation center. The level of discharge planning increases depending on the complexity of healthcare required and the complexity of the client's transition. The three levels of discharge planning are summarized in Table 2-3.

Basic Discharge Plan. The least complicated and most common discharge plan is teaching the client about self-care. Client teaching may include instruction about medications, treatments, community resources, or energy conservation techniques. The teaching should anticipate problems that the client may experience at home. For instance, when discharging a newborn with an apnea monitor to a home with three other small children, the nurse should teach the parents to check the monitor frequently to ensure that the other children have not inadvertently changed the monitor's parameters.

Simple Referral. The second type of discharge plan involves referring the client to community resources (e.g., a smoker to a smoking cessation clinic, a high-risk mother to the local health department, a caregiver to a respite service). A referral is a request for a service outside the referring professional's scope. The nurse acts as the discharge planner and must know both the community resources and the client's ability to reach those resources. Knowledge of the community resources is based on the community assessment and on personal knowledge.

Complex Referral. The third and most complex type of discharge plan involves referring the client to the discharge planner. The nurse may choose to involve the discharge planner because the client's situation is complex, so planning and

TABLE 2-3

Levels of Discharge Planning		
Discharge Plan Level	**Nursing Interventions**	**People Involved**
Basic, universal	Self-care and illness teaching	Nurse, client, caregiver
Simple referral	Refer to community resources	Nurse, client, caregiver
Complex referral	Refer to discharge planner	Nurse, discharge planner, family

TABLE 2-4

Healthcare Providers Used in Discharge Referrals	
Healthcare Provider	**Role**
Home health nurse	Provides assessments; directs care, client teaching and support; coordinates services; evaluates outcomes
Home health aide	Provides hygiene care, cooking, supervision, and companionship
Social worker	Assists in finding and connecting with community resources or financial resources, provides counseling and support
Physical therapist	Assists with restoring mobility, strengthens muscle groups, teaches ambulation with new devices
Occupational therapist	Helps clients adjust to limitations by teaching new vocational skills and better ways to perform activities of daily living
Nutritionist	Teaches clients about meal planning and diet restrictions
Speech therapist	Assists clients to communicate better and works with clients who have swallowing problems
Respiratory therapist	Provides home follow-up for clients with respiratory problems including assessment, oxygen administration, and home ventilator care

making referrals to appropriate community resources would be too time consuming or beyond the nurse's knowledge level or ability. This type of discharge planning is particularly appropriate for clients who are considered high risk.

This level of discharge plan involves interdisciplinary collaboration and coordination. The discharge planner takes responsibility for coordinating the activities necessary to transfer the client from one setting to another. Referring the client to a discharge planner, however, does not absolve the nurse of responsibility. The nurse must follow up to ensure that the discharge planner has acted and must evaluate to learn if the client is satisfied with the discharge plan. The nurse may need to reinforce plans.

A referral to the discharge planner is appropriate for coordinating placement of the client in a skilled nursing facility or a long-term care facility. The discharge planner can also coordinate and initiate services the client will need if discharged to home (e.g., a visiting nurse). Table 2-4 provides a list of healthcare providers often used as referrals during discharge planning.

KEY CONCEPTS

- The central issue of today's healthcare industry is how to deliver cost-effective and quality healthcare that is accessible to and results in positive health outcomes for everyone.
- Levels of healthcare are categorized as primary, secondary, and tertiary. Most current sources and services are in secondary healthcare, but the population's needs fall within the categories of primary and tertiary healthcare.

- Care once considered safe only within the hospital now is delivered routinely in community-based settings.
- Common to all community-based programs is the need for nurses to have greater individual authority, accountability, responsibility, and allegiance to clients while relying less on institutional authority and policies. At the same time, nurses have a greater need to collaborate effectively as members of interdisciplinary teams.
- Although the site and circumstances of nursing care may change, the focus is always the nurse's concern for health of the whole person in relation to that person's environment.
- Community nursing centers deliver primary healthcare to a specific population, are managed and staffed by nurses, and have physician backup and consultation as needed.
- An organizational structure must be in place to ensure continuity of care from one healthcare setting to another and among healthcare professionals.

REFERENCES

American Association of Colleges of Nursing. (2000). *Implementing community-based education in the undergraduate nursing curriculum.* Washington, DC: Author.

American Nurses Association. (1991). *Nursing's agenda for health care reform.* Kansas City, MO: Author.

American Nurses Association. (1995). *Nursing's social policy statement.* Washington, DC: Author.

Arizona Department of Health Services. (1993). *Arizona 2009: Plan for a healthy tomorrow.* Phoenix, AZ: Author.

Association of Community Health Nurse Educators. (1990). *Essentials of baccalaureate nursing education for entry level practice in community health nursing.* Louisville, KY: Author.

Benson, H. (1996). *Healing words, healing practices* [Videotape]. Harvard Medical School, Department of Continuing Education. Boston, MA: Reunion Productions.

Blaylock, A., & Cason, C. L. (1992). Discharge planning: Predicting patient's needs. *Journal of Gerontological Nursing, 18*(7), 5–10.

Brook, R. H., Kamberg, C. J., & McGlynn, E. A. (1997). Health system reform and quality. In P. R. Lee & C. L. Estes (Eds.), *The nation's health* (pp. 381–394). Boston, MA: Jones and Bartlett Publishers.

Buerhaus, P. (1999). Is a nursing shortage on the way? *Nursing Management, 30*(2), 54–55.

Butterfoss, F. D., Goodman, R. M., & Wandersman, A. (1993). Community coalitions for prevention and health promotion. *Health Education Research, 8*(3), 315–330.

Calmelat, A. (1993). Tips for starting your own nurse practitioner practice. *Nurse Practitioner, 18*(4), 58.

Centers for Disease Control and Prevention. (1999). *Health insurance coverage.* Washington, DC: Author. [Online] Available: *http://www.cdc.gov/ncswww/fastats/hinsure.htm*

Donley, R. (1996). Ethics in the age of health care reform. *Nursing Economics, 11*(1), 19–24, 51.

Durch, J. S., Bailey, L. A., & Stoto, M. A. (1997). *Improving health in the community.* Washington, DC: National Academy Press.

Eisenberg, D. M., Davis, R. B., Etter, S. L., Appel, S., Wilkey, S., Van Rompay, M., & Kessler, R. C. (1998). Trends in alternative medicine use in the United States, 1990–1997. *Journal of the American Medical Association, 280*(18), 1569–1575.

Eisenberg, D. M., Kessler, R. C., Foster, C., Norlock, F. E., Calkins, I. R., & Dellono, T. L. (1993). Unconventional medicine in the United States. *New England Journal of Medicine, 328*(4), 246–252.

Evans, R. G., Barer, M. L., & Marmor, T. R. (1994). *Why are some people healthy and others not?* New York: Aldine De Gruyter.

Executive Wire. (1992). *Trends to watch for in '92: Health highest on American agenda.* New York, NY: National League for Nursing.

Fawcett, S. B., Francisco, V. T., Schultz, J. A., Berkowitz, B., Wolff, T. J., & Nagy, G. (2000). The community tool box: A web-based resource for building healthier communities. *Public Health Reports, 115,* 274–278.

Flynn, B. C. (1998). Communicating with the public: Community-based nursing research and practice. *Public Health Nursing, 15*(3), 165–170.

Grandinetti, D. (1996). Teaching patients to take care of themselves. *Medical Economics, 22*(73), 83–86.

Healthcare Forum. (1994). *What creates health?* San Francisco, CA: Author.

Healthy Futures. (1998). *Kalamazoo community indicators.* Kalamazoo, MI: Author.

Heffler, S., Levit, K., Smith, S., Smith, C., Cowan, C., Lazenby, H., & Freeland, M. (2001). Health spending growth up in 1999; Faster growth expected in the future. *Health Affairs, 20*(2), 193–203.

Holt, F. M. (2000). Challenges of community-based practice. *Clinical Nurse Specialist, 14*(1), 39.

Iglehart, J. K. (2001). U.S. health care: Taking the long view. *Health Affairs, 20*(7), 6–7.

Institute of Medicine (1988). *The future of public health.* Washington, DC: National Academy Press.

Jamieson, M. (1996). Grass roots efforts: Nurses involved in the political process. In E. Cohen (Ed.), *Nurse case management in the 21st century* (pp. 21–27). St. Louis, MO: Mosby.

Keating, D. P., & Hertzman, C. (1999). *Developmental health and the wealth of nations.* New York: The Guilford Press.

Kee, C. C., & Borchers, L. (1998). Reducing readmission rates through discharge interventions. *Clinical Nurse Specialist, 12*(5), 206–209.

Keeling, A. W. (2001). Professional nursing comes of age: 1859–2000. In K. K. Chitty, *Professional nursing: Concepts and challenges* (3rd ed.) (pp. 1–32). Philadelphia: W. B. Saunders.

Kenzer, M. (2000). Healthy cities: A guide to the literature. *Public Health Reports, 115,* 279–289.

Koerner, J. G. (2000). Nightingale II: Nursing leaders remembering community. *Nursing Administration Quarterly, 24*(2), 13–18.

Kohn, L. T., Corrigan, J. M., & Donaldson, M. S. (Eds.). (2000). *To err is human: Building a safer health system.* Washington, D.C.: National Academy Press.

Kretzmann, J. P., & McKnight, J. L. (1993). *Building communities from the inside out.* Evanston, IL: Northwestern University, Institute for Policy Research.

Lee, P., & Estes, C. (1994). *The nation's health.* (4th ed.). Boston: Jones & Bartlett.

Lipson, J. G., & Steiger, N. J. (1996). *Self care nursing in a multicultural context.* Thousand Oaks, CA: Sage Publications.

Marmot, M. G., & Wilkinson, R. G. (1999). *Social determinants of health.* New York: Oxford University Press.

Masi, D. (Ed.). (1992). *Handbook for developing employee assistance and counseling programs.* New York, NY: American Management Association.

Matas, K. E. (1994). *Health theme team framework: Building a healthy Mesa.* Unpublished manuscript, Mesa, AZ: United Way.

Matas, K. E. (1997). Therapeutic touch: A model for community-based health promotion. In M. Madrid (Ed.), *Patterns of Rogerian knowing.* New York, NY: National League for Nursing.

Matas, K. E. (2001). *Faith Health Network annual program evaluation report.* Report submitted to the Battle Creek Community Foundation, Battle Creek, MI: In One Accord.

Matas, K. E., & Brown, C. F. (1997). *Cochise community self care project: Annual report.* Unpublished manuscript, Tucson, AZ: Community Nursing Services, Carondelet Health Systems.

Matas, K. E., & Davies, G. R. (2001). *Congregational survey final summary report.* Report submitted to the Faith Health Network of In One Accord, Battle Creek, MI: In One Accord.

Matas, K. E., & Mermis, W. L. (1993). *Campus wellness project.* Report submitted to the Department of Human Resources, Tempe, AZ: Arizona State University.

Matas, K. E., & Mermis, W. L. (1994). *Campus wellness project year 2.* Report submitted to the Department of Human Resources, Tempe, AZ: Arizona State University.

McFarlane, J., Kelly, E., Rodriguez, R., & Fehir, J. (1994). De madres a madres: Women building community coalition for health. *Health Care for Women International, 15*(5), 46–76.

McGinnis, J. M., & Foerge, W. H. (1993). Actual causes of death in the United States. *Journal of the American Medical Association, 270*(18), 2207–2212.

McKnight, J. L. (1995). *The careless society.* New York: Basic Books.

Murdaugh, C. L., & Vanderboom, C. (1997). Individual and community models of promoting wellness. *Journal of Cardiovascular Nursing, 3*(11), 1–7.

Murphy, B. (Ed.). (1995). *Nursing centers: The time is now.* New York, NY: National League for Nursing Press.

National League for Nursing. (1994). *A vision for the future.* New York, NY: Author.

Naylor, M. D., & Buhler-Wilkerson, K. (1999). Creating community-based care for the new millennium. *Nursing Outlook, 47,* 120–127.

O'Neil, E. H. and the Pew Commission for the Health Professions. (1998). *Recreating professional practice for a new century.* San Francisco: Pew Health Professions Commission.

Oss, M., & Clary, J. (1998). The evolving world of employee assistants. *Behavioral Health Management, 4*(18), 20–26.

Payor & Provider News. (1996, November 26). Self-care shown to produce happier healthier patients. *Medical Industry Today.*

Pelletier, K. R. (1991). A review and analysis of the health and cost-effective outcome studies of comprehensive health promotion and disease prevention programs. *American Journal of Health Promotion, 5*(4), 311–315.

Pelletier, K. R. (1993). A review and analysis of the health and cost-effective outcome studies of comprehensive health promotion and disease prevention programs at the work-site: 1991–1993. *American Journal of Health Promotion, 8*(1), 50–62.

Public Sector Consultants. (1995). *Kalamazoo County healthier community assessment.* Kalamazoo, MI: HealthConnect.

Ray, P., & Anderson, S. R. (2000). *The cultural creatives: How 50 million people are changing the world.* New York: Harmony Books.

Riley, D. (1994). Integrated health care systems: Emerging models. *Nursing Economics, 12*(4), 201–206.

Rosenbaum, S. (2001). *An overview of managed care liability: Implications for patient rights and federal and state reform.* Washington, DC: American Association of Retired Persons, Public Policy Institute.

Rothschild, J. M., & Leape, L. L. (2000). *The nature and extent of medical injury in older patients.* Washington, DC: American Association of Retired Persons, Public Policy Institute.

Rowell, P. (2001). Beyond the acute care setting: Community-based nonacute care nursing sensitive indicators. *Outcomes Management for Nursing Practice, 5*(1), 24–27.

Sharp, N. (1992). Community nursing centers: Coming of age. *Nursing Management, 23*(8), 1–20.

Stanhope, M., & Lancaster, J. (2000). *Community and public health nursing* (5th ed.). St. Louis: Mosby.

Tarlov, A. R., & St. Peter, R. F. (2000). *The society and population health reader* (Vol. II.). New York: The New Press.

U.S. Department of Health and Human Services. (2000). *Healthy people 2010: Understanding and improving health* (2nd ed.). Washington, DC: GPO.

U.S. Preventive Services Task Force (1998). *Guide to clinical preventive services* (3rd ed.). Baltimore, MD: Williams and Wilkins.

VanOrt, S., & Townsend, J. (2000). Community-based nursing education and nursing accreditation by the Commission on Collegiate Nursing Education. *Journal of Professional Nursing, 16*(6), 330–335.

Vernarec, E. (1997). The consumer as health care manager. *Business and Health, 15*(5A), 51–55.

Watt, D., Verma, S., & Flynn, L. (1998). Wellness programs: A review of the evidence. *Canadian Medical Association Journal, 158,* 224–230.

World Health Organization. (1978). *Primary health care: Report of the International Conference on Primary Health Care.* Geneva, Switzerland: Author.

Zotti, M. E., Brown, P., & Stotts, R. C. (1996). Community-based nursing versus community health nursing: What does it all mean? *Nursing Outlook, 44,* 211–217.

BIBLIOGRAPHY

American Nurses Association. (1994). *Clinician's handbook of preventive services.* Waldorf, MD: American Nurses Publishing.

Burge, B. J. (1994). Occupational health: Nursing in the workplace. *Nursing Clinics of North America, 29*(3), 431–441.

Burgel, C. J. (1993). *Innovation at the work site.* Washington, DC: American Nurses Publishing.

Burner, S. T., Waldo, D. R., & McKusick, D. R. (1992). National health expenditures projections through 2030. *Health Care Financing Review, 14*(1), 14.

Castro, J. (1994). *The American way of health.* Boston: Little, Brown.

Coffey, R. J., Fenner, K. M., & Stogis, S. L. (1997). *Virtually integrated health systems.* San Francisco, CA: Jossey-Bass.

Cohen, E. L., & DeBack, V. (1999). *The outcome mandate: Case management in health care today.* St. Louis, MO: Mosby.

DeTornyay, R. (1992). Reconsidering nursing education: The report of the Pew Health Professions Commission. *Journal of Nursing Education, 31*(7), 296–301.

Elliott, B. (1993). *Vision 2010: Families and health care.* Minneapolis, MN: National Council on Family Relations.

Ellis, J. R., & Hartley, C. L. (1995). *Nursing in today's world: Challenges, issues, and trends* (5th ed.). Philadelphia: J. B. Lippincott.

Flarey, D. L. (1995). *Redesigning nursing care delivery: Transforming our future.* Philadelphia: J. B. Lippincott.

Global Nursing Exchange. (1997). *A special presentation* [videotape]. Tucson, AZ: Digivideo.

Green, K. (1998). *Home care survival guide.* Philadelphia: Lippincott-Raven.

Gruman, F. (1995). An expanded view of health: Implications for how healthcare works. *Healing, 3*(2), 2–26.

Harrington, C., Estes, C., & Davis, S. (1997). The medical-industrial complex. In C. Harrington & C. Estes (Eds.), *Health policy and nursing.* Boston: Jones & Bartlett.

Hayward, C. (1998). Market memo: What are we going to do with all our surplus capacity? *Health Care Strategic Management, 16*(3), 1, 20–23.

Hunt, R., & Zurek, E. L. (1997). *Introduction to community based nursing.* Philadelphia: Lippincott-Raven.

Johns, C., & Freshwater, D. (1998). *Transforming nursing through reflective practice.* Malden, MA: Blackwell Science.

Kritek, P. B. (1994). *Negotiating at an uneven table.* San Francisco, CA: Jossey-Bass.

Lamb, G., & Huggins, D. (1990). The professional nursing work. In G. M. Mayer, M. J. Madden, & E. Lowrenz (Eds.), *Patient care delivery models.* Rockville, MD: Aspen.

Longest, B. B. (1996). *Health professionals in management.* Stanford, CT: Appleton-Lange.

McEwen, M. (1998). *Community-based nursing: An introduction.* Philadelphia: W. B. Saunders.

Mundt, M. H., & Cohen, E. L. (1999). Emerging competencies for nurse case managers. In E. L. Cohen & V. DeBack (Eds.), *The outcomes mandate: Case management in health care today.* St. Louis, MO: Mosby.

Pew Health Professions Commission. (1991). *Healthy America: Practitioners for 2005.* Durham, NC: Author.

Pollock, A. J., & Biester, D. J. (1994). Community nursing center: An approach to caring for the underserved. *Journal of Pediatric Nursing, 9*(5), 330–334.

Porter-O'Grady, T. (1996). Nurses as advanced practitioners and primary care providers. In E. L. Cohen, (Ed.), *Nurse case management in the 21st century* (pp. 10–20). St. Louis, MO: Mosby.

Porter-O'Grady, T., Hawkins, M. A., & Parker, M. L. (1997). *Whole-systems shared governance.* Gaithersburg, MD: Aspen.

Raffel, M. W., & Raffel, N. K. (1989). *The U.S. health system: Origins and functions* (3rd ed.). New York: John Wiley & Sons.

Rogers, B. (1994). *Occupational health nursing: Concepts and practice.* Philadelphia: W. B. Saunders.

Samuelson, R. J. (1998, September 28). Having it all. *Newsweek.*

Shorr, L. B. (1997). *Common purpose: Strengthening families and neighborhoods to rebuild America.* New York, NY: Anchor Books.

Smith, L. (1993). The coming health care shakeout. *Fortune, 127*(10), 7–75.

Stackhouse, J. C. (1998). *Into the community: Nursing in ambulatory and home care.* Philadelphia: Lippincott-Raven.

Touros, A. O. (1990). *World Health Organization healthy cities project: A project becomes a movement.* Copenhagen, Denmark: FADL Publishers.

U.S. Senate Special Committee Report on Aging. (1991). *Aging America: Trends and projections* (1991 ed.). Washington, DC: Public Health Service, Department of Health and Human Services.

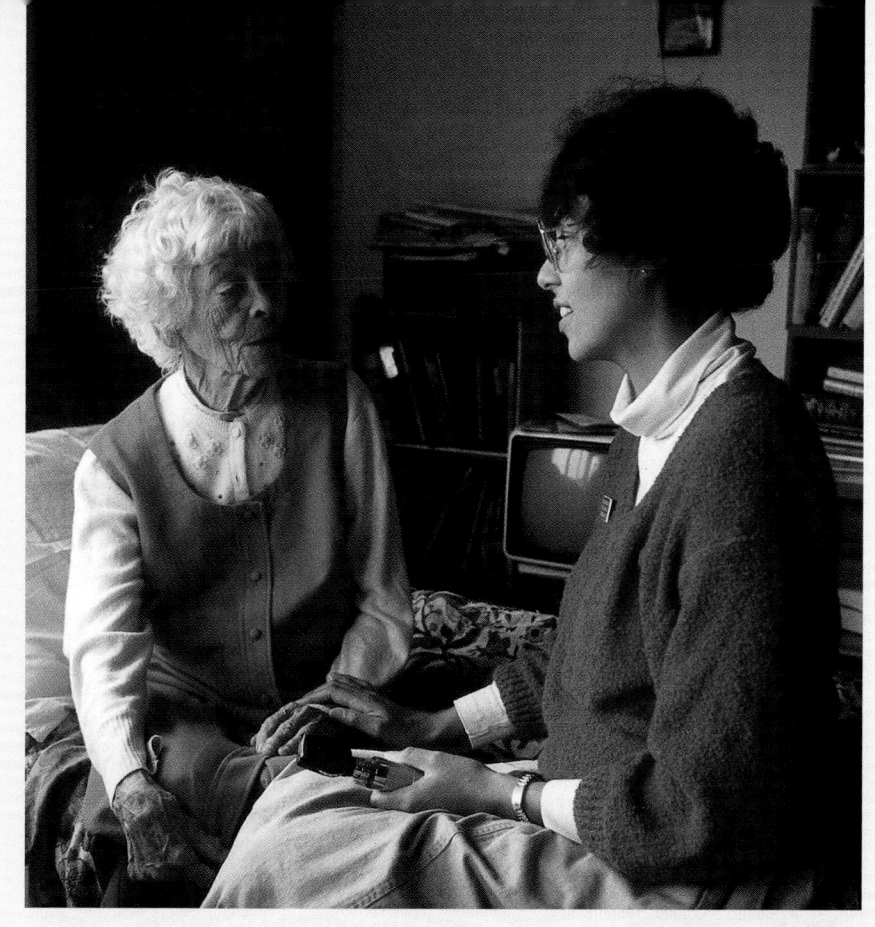

Concepts Essential for Professional Nursing

3 The Profession of Nursing

⑤ Key Terms

advanced practice nursing
American Nurses
  Association
associate nurse
clinical nurse specialist
International Council
  of Nurses
licensed practical nurse
National League for Nursing

nurse administrator
nurse anesthetist
nurse educator
nurse midwife
nurse practice acts
nurse practitioner
nurse researcher
professional nurse
socialization

⑤ Learning Objectives

Upon completion of this chapter, the student will be able to do the following:

1. Describe the evolution of professional nursing.
2. Discuss the influence of nursing's historical development on contemporary views of professional nursing.
3. Identify distinct pathways for entrance into professional nursing practice.
4. Explain types of graduate educational programs in nursing.
5. Identify roles and responsibilities of professional nursing within the healthcare delivery system.
6. Describe career development opportunities and expanded nursing roles.
7. Describe the purpose and function of professional nursing organizations.
8. Discuss the impact of current and future social trends on professional nursing practice.

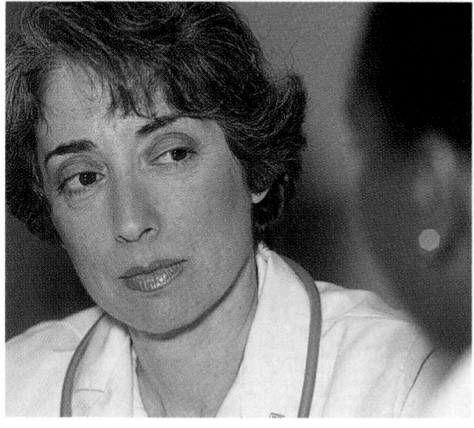

⑤ Critical Thinking Challenge

You are a nursing student beginning your first clinical rotation on a medical-surgical unit. This is your first experience caring for clients in a hospital setting. When you arrive on the unit to review your assignment, a member of the nursing staff pulls you aside and asks, "Why are you entering the nursing profession? Do you know what it entails? Are you sure that you can handle all that it requires?"

Once you have completed this chapter and have added its concepts to your knowledge base, review the above scenario and reflect on the following areas of Critical Thinking:

1. Describe your immediate reaction to this situation, and reflect on your choice of nursing as a career.
2. Examine the rationales or conclusions that led to your decision to become a nurse.
3. Analyze what you think the other nurse may be experiencing that resulted in the questions asked in the situation.
4. List all the pros and cons of a career in nursing. Prioritize the list, and discuss your rationales for choosing or not choosing nursing as a career.

The word *nursing* calls to mind many ideas and images. For some, these images are from traditional and perhaps outdated sources, including white uniforms, nursing caps, needles, and bedpans. For others, images of nursing include kindness, skill, compassion, and intelligence. Modern nursing practice involves many such images and also encompasses new and perhaps unique perspectives on what the profession involves.

Many factors have affected the way the public, nursing professionals and their colleagues, and those beginning their nursing careers perceive nursing. History, especially the social, political, and cultural events of the 20th century, has influenced today's practice. Evolving roles of women, portrayals of nursing in the media, and issues involving educational preparation have had a considerable impact on the image of nursing today. Nurse historians have examined past contributions and their influences on contemporary practice (Came, Gregory, English, & VenKatesh, 1996; Lusk, 1997; MacKintosh, 1997; Egenes, 1998; Griffon, 1998). The roles and responsibilities of nurses are changing along with the evolving healthcare environment, and the profession must be prepared to face the challenges of the new millennium.

Nursing is caring, commitment, and dedication to meeting the functional health needs of all people. Within a functional health pattern framework, nurses direct care to promote, maintain, and restore health in various settings. Nurses are prepared to identify and to assist with the healthcare needs of individuals, families, communities, and groups. As technology advances, society's healthcare needs increase in complexity, and the demands of the healthcare system change. The need for educated nurses who are committed to maintaining expertise in the theory and practice of professional nursing will continue to grow in response to such developments.

Providing nursing care in settings outside hospitals, such as in the homes of clients or in ambulatory clinics, is now very common. The assumption that nurses will care for most clients in acute care environments is no longer valid. Changes in reimbursement for healthcare services and cost-containment measures have moved nursing practice to areas beyond such settings. Nursing means caring for communities and groups of people, such as the homeless, and addressing issues with far-reaching social implications, such as human rights and acquired immunodeficiency syndrome (AIDS). Nursing means being socially responsible, involved, and committed to the health of all people.

Nursing offers many challenging and exciting career opportunities. Students embarking on professional nursing careers accept responsibility for society's healthcare needs and for the advancement of nursing as a profession. Never in nursing's history has there been a more opportune time to move the profession forward and to make a difference in the healthcare of all people. This chapter provides a starting point for understanding where nursing has been, where it is now, and where it is headed.

HIGHLIGHTS OF THE HISTORICAL EVOLUTION OF PROFESSIONAL NURSING

Although nursing in some form has probably existed throughout history, documentation of the profession is available only for the last 150 years. Nursing probably began as women intuitively identified and provided for their families' healthcare needs. As certain individuals emerged with the desire and ability to nurture others and provide care for them, the profession of nursing began. This section highlights critical events that have shaped nursing's history and that have influenced issues affecting today's profession. An overview of this historical evolution provides the background necessary to understanding current nursing practice (Fig. 3-1). Table 3-1 highlights events in nursing's history. For more in-depth discussions of nursing's historical evolution, the reader should examine textbooks dedicated solely to this topic.

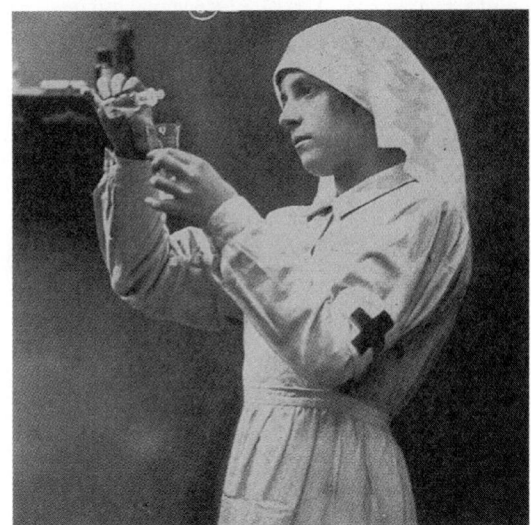

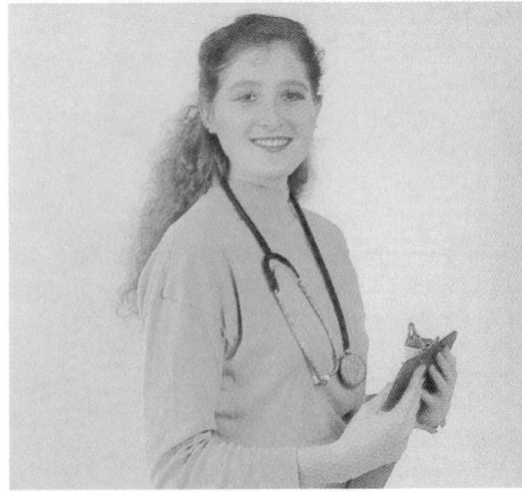

FIGURE 3-1   Comparison of the nurse at the beginning of the 20th century and a professional nurse today.

TABLE 3-1

Then and Now—A Selection of Significant Events in the History of Nursing		
Date	**Then**	**Now**
1–500 AD (approximately)	Nursing care primarily involves meeting the hygiene and comfort needs of individuals and families. Christians working in close association with an organized church primarily provide care.	Nursing care today involves a high degree of technical skill and includes responsibilities above and beyond hygiene and comfort measures, although these components of care continue to be important. Today's nurse must be highly skilled and up to date with technologic advances, must be computer literate, and have a strong foundation in the sciences and humanities. Responsibilities are complex and require critical thinking skills. Nursing is no longer tied to the church, and nurses are educated in colleges and universities.
1836	Theodor Fliedner opens a small hospital and training school in Kaiserworth, Germany, where Florence Nightingale, "the founder of modern nursing," receives her nursing education.	Hospital-based schools of nursing continue to exist, but these programs have been declining in number as the profession moves forward and requires education in academic settings.
1854–1860	Florence Nightingale makes major contributions to modern nursing, is named Superintendent of Nursing, cares for soldiers in the Crimean War, opens a training school at St. Thomas Hospital in London, and publishes *Notes on Nursing, What It Is, What It Is Not.*	Nightingale's many contributions to nursing continue to influence the profession. The components of her theory apply even today, and nurses around the world recognize the courage, dedication, and work of this early professional leader.
1861–1865	Dorothea Dix establishes the Nurse Corps of the United States Army. Dix was not a nurse but an advocate for the mentally ill.	Nurses continue to choose careers in the armed services where opportunities for exciting and rewarding careers are offered.
1872	America's first trained nurse, Linda Richards, graduates from the New England Hospital for Women in Boston.	Nursing continues to prepare educated, competent individuals to provide nursing care in institutions of higher education.
1873	Three nursing schools patterned after the Nightingale plan develop in the United States: Bellevue Training School, Connecticut Training School, and Boston Training School. In 1874, the first "Nightingale model" school of Nursing in Canada is set up in St. Catherines, Ontario.	New nursing programs continue to develop. The profession now offers several routes to a career in nursing, including diploma, associate degree, baccalaureate degree, the generic master's, and doctoral degree.
1882	Clara Barton organizes the American National Red Cross.	The Red Cross continues to exist today, offering care to victims of disasters, maintaining the nation's blood supply, and educating about AIDS.
1893	Lillian Wald and Mary Brewster found the Henry Street Settlement, the first home visiting nurse organization in the United States. The Henry Street Settlement can still be visited in New York City.	Visiting nurse associations have grown and become essential healthcare components in society. Cost containment and healthcare reform concerns have moved nursing from the hospital setting to the community once again.
1897	The American Society of Superintendents of Training Schools of the United States and Canada is organized. It is renamed the American Nurses Association in 1911 and the Canadian Nurses Association in 1907.	The ANA and the CNA continue to function as nursing's professional organizations.

(continues)

TABLE 3-1 (Continued)

Then and Now—A Selection of Significant Events in the History of Nursing		
Date	**Then**	**Now**
1899	International Council of Nurses is established.	ICN continues to represent and speak to international nursing concerns.
1900	*American Journal of Nursing*—first nursing journal to be owned, operated, and published by nurses—is developed.	*American Journal of Nursing* and *The Canadian Nurse* continue to be major references for clinical nursing practice.
1923	Goldmark report of the Rockefeller Foundation is published, advocating financial support of university-based schools of nursing. A similar report, the Weir report, is published in Canada in 1932.	There is a decline in available financial support to incoming students of nursing. However, nursing organizations and leaders are working to improve financial assistance to students.
1940	World War II results in another nursing shortage. Esther Lucille Brown completes the Brown report on nursing education, advocating that education for nursing belongs in colleges and universities, not in hospitals.	Although hospital-based schools of nursing continue to exist, they are declining in number, and students are more frequently choosing college and university educations.
1953	National Student Nurses' Association (NSNA) is established.	NSNA continues today to encourage students of nursing to become involved in professional issues. Students are given opportunities to hold leadership positions at state and national levels. The equivalent organization in Canada is known as the Canadian University Nursing Students Association.
1965	ANA issues its first "position paper on nursing education," calling for all nursing education to take place in institutions of higher education and stipulating the baccalaureate as minimum preparation for professional nursing and the associate degree for technical nursing practice.	The entry level debate has not been completely resolved. Preparation of nurses for the future continues to be one of professional nursing's concerns.
1985	National Center for Nursing Research is established at the National Institutes of Health in Bethesda, Maryland.	1993—The National Center for Nursing Research is upgraded by President Clinton to Institute status.
1994	Healthcare reform is a discussion that permeates professional circles. Cost-containment measures, access to health care, and the need for health promotion are integral components of the issues.	Healthcare reform will continue to be an integral issue to the nursing profession. Nurses will continue to explore options for advanced practice nurses to maintain nursing's role and move it forward in this environment of change.
1999		Managed care, cost, reimbursement issues, and complex technologic advances continue to affect healthcare. Advanced practice roles for nurses are increasing as issues related to access to healthcare and the need for health promotion programs become central.
2001		Redesigning and downsizing of the workforce and the changes in patient profiles have numerous effects on nursing. Healthcare is facing the implications of the supply and demand of nurses.

Ancient History

Ancient history makes few references to nursing as its own discipline; any discussions of nursing are blurred with those of medicine. Brief accounts of men and women engaging in practices that may be associated with nursing have been found. For example, in ancient Egypt, maternal–child nursing was the responsibility of midwives, and wet nurses were hired to breast-feed infants. Priests were primarily responsible for healing practices, and the people's security was directly related to keeping the gods appeased. Israelites practiced principles of sanitation by using boiled or filtered water and carefully inspecting meat for spoilage. Today, Orthodox Jews continue to practice purification rites, such as bathing and isolation, that they practiced in ancient times (Mitchell & Grippando, 1993).

In ancient Babylonia, Egypt, and Sumeria, rich families were the primary recipients of nursing care. If and when nursing care was available outside wealthy homes, nurses were primarily servants. In Egypt, the treatment of disease and care of the sick were left to those in the priesthood (Kalisch & Kalisch, 1995). Subservient roles for women and nurses were rooted in sexual discrimination and overall devaluation of human life reflective of this era. Women's low status combined with society's negative attitudes toward the sick provided major obstacles to nursing's development (Dolan, Fitzpatrick, & Herrmann, 1983).

Contributions of the Greeks

The Greeks made significant contributions to the care of the sick and, to an extent, to the nursing profession. Hippocrates, the "father of medicine," made a major advance in medicine by rejecting the belief that diseases had supernatural causes. He also is credited with developing assessment standards for clients, establishing overall medical standards, and recognizing a need for nurses (Kalisch & Kalisch, 1995; Doheny, Cook, & Stopper, 1997; Kelly & Joel, 1999).

Early Christian Era

Evidence of nursing roles became more apparent in the early Christian era. Women performed duties that reflected components of today's nursing practice: care related to nutrition, mobility, medication administration, personal counseling, hygiene, and comfort measures was paramount (Dolan et al., 1983). Men and women committed to the church spread the philosophy of Christianity while providing nursing care to the ill.

Religion's influence raised the social position of nursing by placing more value on human life. Compassion, charity, and willingness to serve were qualities associated with nurses. Deacons and deaconesses (individuals working for the church ministry) were designated to perform services for the sick (Doheny et al., 1997; Kelly & Joel, 1999).

Deaconesses functioned as visiting nurses, dedicating their lives to charity work. This role allowed widowed and un-married women to hold respectable places in society. Phoebe (55 AD) is the most noted deaconess in nursing's history. The early deaconesses identified a need for hospitals to care for the sick, resulting in the emergence of several Christian hospitals. Fabiola established the first general hospital in Rome at about 380 AD (Mitchell & Grippando, 1993).

The Middle Ages

Poverty was a critical problem during the Middle Ages. Nursing continued to shape the purpose and direction of healthcare and to provide leadership in the field. These advancements were enhanced by the continuing spread of Christianity, which had positive effects on cultural values and institutions. Christianity's influence also improved the status of nursing by attracting intelligent individuals from respected families (Dolan et al., 1983). During the Middle Ages, society also faced epidemics of leprosy, typhus, and bubonic plague (Kalisch & Kalisch, 1995).

The Crusades resulted in the establishment of military nursing orders and the recruitment of men into nursing, which was well organized at this time (Mitchell & Grippando, 1993). The Church dictated the scope of nursing practice and viewed the spiritual needs of clients as the priority for care. Obedience and devotion were maintained with rigid discipline and remained central to organized nursing for centuries (Mitchell & Grippando, 1993).

Clearly, however, nursing roles that are relevant today were beginning to emerge. The nurse's role as midwife from early civilization into the present day was evident, as was the importance of community and public health nursing.

The Renaissance

"The revival of learning during the Renaissance spurred the advance of medicine" (Kalisch & Kalisch, 1995, p. 13). This revival contributed to recognition of the need for sound educational preparation in nursing and contributed to the profession's further advancement. Unfortunately, the continuing lack of effective sanitation and increasing poverty resulted in serious healthcare problems. The need for healthcare providers to respond immediately to these problems further delayed the move toward improved nursing education.

The Reformation

Nursing encountered another setback during the Reformation. The dispersion of religious orders, which had been the primary source of healthcare, resulted in a serious deterioration in hospital conditions and nursing care. Attempts to improve nursing education and the image of nurses were abandoned. The role of women changed dramatically during this time. Women were viewed as subordinate to men and were expected to remain at home caring for children; this decreased the number of qualified women practicing nursing (Mitchell & Grippando, 1993).

Nursing in the 18th Century

Revolutions and epidemics resulted in the expansion of nursing roles in the 18th century. Continuing problems related to healthcare needs included poor sanitation and low standards of living. By the end of the century, nursing was present in hospitals, but working conditions were poor, resulting in a loss of social status for members of the profession. As nursing's social status deteriorated, few qualified individuals chose to enter the profession. According to Kalisch and Kalisch (1995):

> Nursing was considered an inferior, undesirable occupation. During the previous century religious attendants had been largely replaced by lay people who were employed without any attention given to their selection. Often drawn from the criminal class and lacking a spirit of self-sacrifice, they exploited and abused the patients (pp. 37–38).

Nursing in the 19th Century

Society's attitudes about nursing during this time were reflected in Charles Dickens' *Martin Chuzzlewit* (1844), in which criminals and women of low moral standards provided care. One character, Sarah Gamp, was a nurse who abused alcohol and treated her clients cruelly. Such negative portrayals of nursing seriously damaged the profession's image. Fragments of such images are still found in some media portrayals today.

New problems and social changes affected the profession and the nurse's role in the 19th century. The Industrial Revolution initiated political, economic, and social expansion throughout North America and Europe. Poverty; long workdays for men, women, and children; and the prevalence of disease increased the need for nurses to address community health problems. Continued emphasis was placed on the need for proper preparation of nurses. Religion once again was influential; the caring image of the nurse was believed to be based on a spiritual calling to the profession. Poverty, innocence, and submissiveness were qualities associated with potential nursing candidates (Dolan et al., 1983).

Florence Nightingale

Florence Nightingale has been called the founder of modern nursing. Stubborn and unyielding, Nightingale improved health laws, reformed hospitals, reorganized military medical services, and established nursing as a profession with two missions: sick nursing and health nursing. Nightingale viewed "sick nursing" as helping clients use their own reparative processes to get well and "health nursing" as preventing illness (Kalisch & Kalisch, 1995; Kelly & Joel, 1999).

Nightingale was born May 12, 1820, in Florence, Italy, to a wealthy English family. She was educated in languages, philosophy, and the liberal arts. She entered the nursing profession against the wishes of her parents. Her hope was to replace the "Sarah Gamp" image with one of education, intelligence, and kindness (Kalisch & Kalisch, 1995).

Nightingale was the superintendent of nurses at King's College Hospital until she left to care for soldiers during the Crimean War. Her efforts during this war were credited with decreasing the mortality rate by half, and she soon became known as "the lady with the lamp" because of her midnight rounds to the soldiers. In 1860, Nightingale published *Notes on Nursing* and started the Nightingale Training School for Nurses. Nightingale was gracious and hard working, and her many contributions to nursing continue to influence the profession (Kalisch & Kalisch, 1995; Donahue, 1996).

Nursing During the American Civil War

During the American Civil War (1861–1865), more hospitals and better-prepared nurses were needed. Although she was not a nurse, Dorothea Dix established the Nurse Corps of the United States Army, further expanding nursing's role. Another early nursing leader, Clara Barton, practiced nursing on Civil War battlefields. Barton founded the American Red Cross, an organization that continues to contribute significantly to contemporary healthcare needs (Dolan et al., 1983; Chambers & Subera, 1997).

Nursing Education in the 19th Century

In 1869, the American Medical Association developed the Committee on the Training of Nurses; as a result of this committee's recommendations, hospital-based schools of nursing under medical supervision emerged. In 1874, Linda Richards, America's first trained nurse, graduated from Women's Hospital in Boston.

Public health nursing emerged toward the end of the 19th century. Two early leaders, Lillian Wald and Mary Brewster, established the first public health nursing service for the sick and poor, the Henry Street Settlement on New York City's Lower East Side. This settlement was one of the first community health services to address the needs of poor people living in New York City. The Henry Street Settlement is now a famous center of public health nursing (Dolan et al., 1983).

Nursing in the 20th Century

Military Influences

Military influences on nursing education in the 20th century have been numerous. During the Spanish American War, the Volunteer Nurse Corps (1898) was established and, in 1901, became the Army Nurse Corps. In 1908, Congress authorized the Navy Nurse Corps (Mitchell & Grippando, 1993). During World War I, nurses were transported to war areas in Europe and the Far East to care for the sick and wounded.

The casualties of World War II brought a critical nursing shortage, prompting quick solutions to increase the number of nurses and causing a setback in the move toward university-based nursing education. Nonetheless, Esther Lucille Brown, in her report on nursing education published at that time, wrote that nursing education belonged in colleges and universities, not in hospitals. This report provided further documentation of the need for university-based nursing education programs (Dolan et al., 1983). During World War II, black nurses were first admitted to the nursing service.

During the Korean War, Congress authorized the creation of the Air Force Nurse Corps (1949), and, by 1950, Air Force nurses were evacuating wounded soldiers from Korea. In 1956, the Army Student Nurse Program was established (Mitchell & Grippando, 1993).

The Vietnam War saw many nurses involved in the Army and Navy Nurse Corps caring for the wounded. In addition, Air Force nurses were assigned to Vietnam. In 1970, Anna Mae Hayes, chief of the Army Nurse Corps, was promoted to Brigadier General.

Operation Desert Shield/Desert Storm once again saw the mobilization of nurses to Saudi Arabia (1991). As in other war situations, the nursing shortage in the United States placed pressure on the military to provide nursing and medical care.

Professional Development in the 20th Century

In the early 20th century, professional organizations such as the American Nurses Association (ANA), the Canadian Nurses Association (CNA), the International Council of Nurses (ICN), the National League for Nursing (NLN), and the American Association of Colleges of Nursing (AACN) emerged. Nursing journals were developed, and research was conducted into the need for higher education in nursing. The *American Journal of Nursing,* (AJN), first published in 1900, was the first nursing journal to be owned, operated, and published by nurses (Dolan et al., 1983).

In 1923, a noteworthy milestone in the history of nursing education occurred with the publication of the Goldmark Report, which advocated financial support for university-based schools of nursing. This report's findings eased the transition from hospital-based schools of nursing to university settings, marking a major advance (Dolan et al., 1983).

In 1965, a report by the National Commission on Nursing and Nursing Education addressed several issues, including supply and demand for nurses, clarification of nursing roles and functions, nursing education, and available career opportunities. The report, called the Lysaught report in honor of the study's director, helped clarify the role of professional nursing practice (Dolan et al., 1983).

Rapid scientific advances and increasingly complex technology marked the latter part of the 20th century. Longer lifespans, increased incidence of chronic illness, and new family structures dramatically affected where and how nurses practiced. Despite such changes, nurses continued to focus on delivery of care that is safe, comprehensive, and effective.

Nursing in the 21st Century

Nursing's history has influenced today's educational requirements, practice settings, and roles. Likewise, when, how, and why the profession evolves will directly relate to the contributions of present and future nursing professionals. Social forces can be expected to influence future definitions of nursing, just as these forces have shaped nursing practice to date.

SOCIALIZATION TO PROFESSIONAL NURSING

Socialization is a process that involves learning theory and skills and internalizing an identity appropriate to a specific role. Internalizing a specific role allows one to participate as a member of a group.

Many students enter nursing with the perception that their professional identity will center on providing service to people who are ill or who require care in regaining health. Although this initial perception may be true, it is only a small part of the professional identity that students must internalize when they join the profession. Socialization to nursing involves changes that ultimately affect a student's knowledge base, attitudes, and values regarding professional nursing practice. This socialization continues as the individual grows personally and professionally. As the student becomes socialized to nursing, he or she develops and internalizes an understanding of the profession.

Professions generally have a specific body of knowledge, set of values, and skills that differentiate them from one another. Professional nursing curricula teach foundations of the discipline. Theoretical and clinical instruction facilitates the development of a professional identity and prepares students to function as beginning nurses. Beyond this initial socialization, continuing socialization occurs as nurses gain experience in the workplace and perhaps pursue advanced education.

Patricia Benner, in *From Novice to Expert* (1984), discussed socialization and skill acquisition in nursing using the Dreyfuss model (Table 3-2). According to this model, a nurse passes through five levels of proficiency when acquiring and developing a skill: novice, advanced beginner, competent, proficient, and expert. Differences in each level reflect changes in three areas of skill performance. In the first area, the nurse moves from relying on abstract principles to using concrete experiences. The second area involves a change from seeing situations in parts to seeing them more conceptually, or as a whole. Finally, in the third area, the nurse is no longer outside the situation observing but is directly involved.

Nursing and Professionalism Defined

Because definitions of nursing reflect society's values and influences, the profession is subject to misinterpretation. One common misconception is that nurses are handmaidens to physicians; other misconceptions have been shown in portrayals in the media (e.g., Nurse Ratchett in *One Flew Over the Cuckoo's Nest*). Beginning nursing professionals must develop a clear, accurate understanding of professional practice if other members of the healthcare team and the public are to share this precise interpretation.

Nursing is a multifaceted profession and, as such, has been defined in many ways. Florence Nightingale defined nursing as "the act of utilizing the environment of the client to assist him in his recovery" (Nightingale, 1859/1992). The ANA defined nursing as "the diagnosis and treatment of human responses

TABLE 3-2

Dreyfuss Model of Skill Acquisition Applied to Nursing	
Level of Proficiency	**Summary Description**
Novice	A beginning nursing student or any nurse entering a situation in which he or she has had no previous experience. Behavior is governed by established rules and is limited and inflexible.
Advanced beginner	The advanced beginner can demonstrate marginally acceptable performance. He or she has had enough experience in actual situations to identify meaningful aspects or global characteristics that can be identified only through prior experience.
Competent	Competence is reflected by the nurse who has been on the same job for 2 or 3 years and who consciously and deliberately plans nursing care in terms of long-range goals.
Proficient	The proficient nurse perceives situations as a whole rather than in terms of aspects and manages nursing care rather than performing tasks.
Expert	The expert nurse no longer relies on rules or guidelines to connect understanding of a situation to an appropriate action. The expert nurse, with an enormous background of experience, has an intuitive grasp of the situation and zeroes in on the problem.

The five levels of proficiency listed in the left column were developed by Stuart Dreyfuss and Hubert Dreyfuss. The second column reflects the author's summary of a discussion by Patricia Benner in *From novice to expert: Excellence and power in clinical nursing practice.* San Francisco: Addison-Wesley, 1984.

to actual or potential health problems" (American Nurses Association, 1980, p. 1). The CNA (1987, p. 3) published the following definition:

The nursing profession exists in response to a need of society and holds ideals related to human health throughout the life span. Nurses direct their energies toward the promotion, maintenance, and restoration of health; the prevention of illness; the alleviation of suffering and the ensurance of a peaceful death when life can no longer be sustained. Nurses value a holistic view and regard an individual as a biopsychosocial being who has the capacity to set goals and make decisions and who has the right and responsibility to make informed choices congruent with personal beliefs and values. Nursing, a dynamic and supportive profession guided by its code of ethics, is rooted in caring, a concept evident throughout its four fields of activity: practice, education, administration, and research.

Despite the many definitions, common themes are evident. Holism, caring, teaching, advocacy, and supporting, promoting, maintaining, and restoring health are all components of nursing practice. Nursing care involves creativity, sensitivity, and applications based on scientific rationales. All of these components are essential to the practice, but nurses should not limit themselves to these themes.

The question of whether nursing is a profession has been an ongoing debate. To answer this question, it is first helpful to examine the established criteria for a profession. Several criteria to evaluate nursing's professional status have been proposed, including the need for higher education, a specific body of knowledge, public interest and responsibility, and internal organization. Flexner (1915) published criteria that can serve as a benchmark for determining professional status. Table 3-3 compares Flexner's criteria of patterns identified in developing professions with characteristics specific to nursing. Higher and more specialized education and increased autonomy in

practice have contributed to the growth of professionalism in nursing. Increased levels of research activity, accountability, and responsibility have enhanced nursing's status. As more nurses obtain master's and doctoral degrees and as research contributions grow, the profession's specific body of knowledge becomes clearer and more accurately defined.

Educational Preparation and Career Opportunities

Three distinct pathways exist for entrance into professional nursing practice, and new approaches emerge continually. Basic preparation and selected examples of new approaches are presented here. Career opportunities in nursing depend on the person's educational preparation and area of clinical expertise.

Accelerated changes in healthcare with an emphasis on primary care have intensified interest in **advanced practice nursing.**

Regulation of advanced practice nursing is done by statute or by certification. Regulation by statute involves modification of the state nurse practice act to regulate advanced nursing practice and involves issuance of a second license. Regulation by certification involves a process whereby professional boards validate an individual nurse's advanced qualifications in a particular area of nursing (Ziemer, 1994, p. 7).

An example of an advanced practice nurse is the nurse practitioner.

The issue of educational preparation for entry into practice has been debated since the 1930s and 1940s, when the Brown and Goldmark reports recommended two levels of nursing preparation. In 1965, the ANA adopted a resolution proposing that minimum preparation for beginning professional

TABLE 3-3

Flexner's Professional Development Patterns Compared With Nursing	
Patterns of Developing Professions	**Nursing Profession**
Professions are basically intellectual.	Nurses are educated in institutions of higher learning and function in a responsible and accountable manner. Critical thinking is now being emphasized to a great extent at all levels of nursing education.
Professions are based on a specific body of knowledge that can be learned.	Nursing has identified and continues to develop its own specific body of knowledge from which nursing practice emerges. Application of theory derived from research provides the rationales for action.
Professions are practical as well as theoretical.	Nursing professionals accept great responsibility for providing for people's healthcare needs. The profession evolved in response to needs identified by society and is guided by an ethical code.
Professional work can be taught through professional education.	Nurses are educated primarily in associate degree and baccalaureate degree programs.
Professions have strong internal organization.	The American Nurses Association and other bodies provide internal organization.
Practitioners are motivated by altruism.	Many nurses enter the profession out of a desire to help others.

practice should be a baccalaureate degree in nursing, and that minimum preparation for technical practice should be an associate degree in nursing. The ANA's 1965 resolution also prompted the 1985 ANA statement adopting the titles of **associate nurse** (a nurse prepared in an associate degree program) and **professional nurse** (a nurse possessing the baccalaureate degree in nursing) for these two levels. Canada has one level of nursing practice: the professional level. Although nurses are educated at the diploma and university levels, all are considered to be professional nurses. The

---

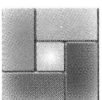

Nursing Research and Critical Thinking

Is It Possible to Measure the Effects of Educational or Clinical Experiences on a Nurse's Professional Self-Concept?

Many nurse educators believe that factors such as the evolving role of women in society, changing patterns of professional education and socialization, and escalating demands within the nursing workplace are creating significant challenges to a positive professional self-concept for nurses. They believe that one of nursing's greatest sources for future development is the potential to improve the collective professional self-concept of nurses. Before educators can design and evaluate educational programs to enhance the development of professional self-concept in nursing students, they must develop standardized instruments or techniques of measurement from which to draw conclusions. Two nurses designed a study to evaluate The Professional Self-Concept of Nurses Instrument (PSCNI). A sample of 127 students enrolled in four strata of nursing education at a Canadian university completed the PSCNI. The researchers used confirmation factor analysis to investigate the notion of multidimensionality of the concept. Items on the PSCNI clustered into three subscales and Cronbach's alpha were used to estimate scale reliability:

professional practice (.89); satisfaction (.86); and communication (.40). This suggests that the information is reliable, particularly in terms of the first two scales. Furthermore, there was a statistically significant ($P < .05$) difference between scale scores based on educational preparation.

Critical Thinking Considerations. The PSCNI was developed to study professional self-concept in a population of Australian nursing students. The scale was grounded within two central assumptions: that professional self-concept can be measured and that the attitudes nurses have about themselves as professionals can be usefully detected using a measurement instrument. Implications from this study are as follows:

- The instrument may be flexible across cultures and sensitive among distinct groups of nursing students.
- Further testing of the PSCNI will develop a deeper understanding of the professional self-concept of nursing students and graduates as they evolve professionally.

From Arthur, D., & Thorne, S. (1998). Professional self-concept of nurses: A comparative study of four strata of nursing students in a Canadian university. *Nurse Education Today, 18*(5), 380–388.

CNA endorsed the baccalaureate standard for entry to practice in 1982, although several provinces had adopted this standard earlier.

The debate over entry-level preparation continues to influence many critical issues. Included in this debate are the competencies of new nursing graduates, the public view of nursing roles, the need for professional status within the healthcare community, the organization of nursing education, and the supply and demand for nursing professionals. Finally, the variety of programs available for entry into nursing practice is confusing to students, employers, and the public. Professional nursing must resolve the problems of entry-level requirements.

Nursing in the United States continues to have three major routes leading to the registered nurse licensure. Educational preparation may be the diploma, associate, or baccalaureate degree. Now emerging are programs that have the master's degree and nursing doctorate as entry-level preparation.

All nursing programs require a minimum of state or provincial approval. In addition to state approval, the NLN and Commission on Collegiate Nursing Education (CCNE) provide accreditation standards for all types of nursing programs in the United States. Such accreditation signifies excellence in nursing education. Accreditation from the Canadian Association of University Schools of Nursing signifies excellence in Canada.

Types of Educational Programs
Would-be nurses may enter licensed practical nursing programs or may pursue diploma, associate, baccalaureate, master's, or doctoral degrees. Students may choose the educational route that best suits their needs and goals.

Practical Nursing Program. People interested in a practical nursing career attend 1-year programs that prepare them to perform technical skills under the supervision of registered nurses (RNs). In the United States, students successfully completing the program requirements may sit for the licensure examination given by the state board of nursing to become a **licensed practical nurse** (LPN) or licensed vocational nurse. A similar process controlled by the provincial association is in place in Canada. LPNs are employed in hospitals, long-term care facilities, and rehabilitation centers and by healthcare providers such as physicians. LPNs differ from RNs in two areas: educational preparation and scope of practice. Practical nursing was established to prepare healthcare providers for client care and to assist professional nurses with routine technical procedures.

Diploma Nursing Program. Diploma nursing schools were the first type of educational preparation available for RNs. In the United States, diploma programs usually require 3 years of study. Students earn some college credit, but college credit is not awarded for nursing courses. Clinical experience is extensive, which is an advantage of this route. In Canada, diploma programs can be at the hospital (3-year) level or at the college (2-year) level. College credit is awarded for all courses at the college level.

Students successfully completing diploma programs take the state or provincial board of nursing examination for reg-

istered nurse licensure. Graduates of diploma programs work as beginning practitioners in acute, intermediate, long-term, and ambulatory healthcare facilities. Graduates must demonstrate competency in the assessment, planning, implementation, and evaluation phases of the nursing process (National League for Nursing, 1978b).

The number of diploma programs has declined as nursing education moves into institutions of higher learning. This decline is also related to efforts to achieve professional status and control over nursing practice.

Associate Degree Nursing Program. Associate degree nursing (ADN) began in 1952 in the Division of Nursing Education of Teachers College, Columbia University, under the direction of Mildred Montag. Initially developed in response to a nursing shortage, ADN education continues to thrive today. Students pursuing this degree attend a junior college for 2 years, receiving college credit for all courses and clinical experience in nursing. The goal of this program is to prepare technical nurses who are capable of functioning as quality practitioners under the supervision of professional nurses. Students successfully completing the requirements of an ADN program also take the state board of nursing examination for registered nurse licensure. Canada does not have an ADN program.

As providers of nursing care, ADNs use the nursing process to formulate and maintain individualized nursing plans of care. They also teach clients who need information or support to maintain health. As managers, ADNs provide care for a group of clients with common, well-defined health problems in structured settings (National League for Nursing, 1978c).

Baccalaureate Degree Nursing Program. The baccalaureate degree in nursing offers students a full college or university education with a background in liberal arts. The programs are rigorous and provide students with credits for nursing courses and clinical experience in all areas of nursing practice. Baccalaureate degree programs in nursing emphasize community health, research, leadership, and management. They are offered in college or university settings.

Students successfully completing the baccalaureate degree in nursing take the state board of nursing examination for registered nurse licensure. In Canada, students take a provincial board examination for registration; there is no licensure. Nurses are prepared as generalists at the baccalaureate level and provide comprehensive services that assess, promote, and maintain the health of individuals, families, communities, and groups (National League for Nursing, 1978a).

Advanced Nursing Education Opportunities
Master's Degree Nursing Program. Master's level education in nursing began in the last quarter of the 19th century in response to a need for better-educated faculty and supervisory staff (Mitchell & Grippando, 1993). Nurses interested in attaining advanced education in specialties may complete graduate programs in their specific area of interest. Graduate education prepares nurses for advanced, independent practice with continued emphasis on research. Graduate education

requires independent critical thinking, and nurses pursuing graduate education must have solid scholastic abilities.

Accelerated tracks are also available for RNs seeking graduate degrees who do not possess baccalaureate degrees in nursing. Usually, these students enter baccalaureate programs after completing diploma or associate degree requirements. Senior-level nursing courses are replaced with similar-level coursework for exceptional students. These accelerated options can save both time and money for qualified students.

In an innovative movement, several colleges in the United States offer a generic Master of Science degree in nursing in preparation for professional nursing practice. Usually, students begin the programs with baccalaureate degrees in fields of study other than nursing. Students completing generic master's programs have advanced research capabilities and some opportunity for clinical concentration in a nursing specialty.

Doctoral Degree Program. In the United States, the first four doctoral degree programs were offered at Boston University, New York University, Teachers College at Columbia University, and the University of Pittsburgh. In Canada, the first doctoral degree programs were at McGill University, the University of Alberta, the University of British Columbia, and the University of Toronto. Students may earn a Doctor of Philosophy (PhD), Doctor of Education (EdD), or Doctor of Nursing Science (DNS) degree. People interested in careers as nurse researchers or nurse educators usually must obtain doctoral degrees. Doctoral education has become more available to nurses, and the number of nurses earning doctoral degrees continues to increase. Nurses usually obtain doctoral education after completing master's programs. Many PhD programs incorporate the master's degree for students who enter from Bachelor of Science in nursing programs.

An innovative program combines entrance into professional nursing practice with a professional nurse doctorate program. Case Western Reserve University began the first program in 1985, and the University of Colorado has a similar program. Advanced preparation in clinical research is a major component.

NURSING RESPONSIBILITIES

Historically, the nurse's sole duty was to provide care and comfort to the sick. Advances in technology, knowledge, health promotion, and prevention have expanded the functions of today's nurses. Nursing functions include activities that nurses perform independently or collaboratively. For instance, nurses may initiate activities, such as turning or positioning bed clients every 2 hours, that are nurse-prescribed interventions (Carpenito, 2002). On the other hand, when physicians delegate actions (physician-prescribed interventions) that require nurses to use their own judgment, nurses are addressing collaborative problems. For example, although physicians must prescribe medications, they rely on the judgment of nurses for proper administration. Nurses must thoroughly understand medications, observe for side effects, and teach clients about medications. Nurse- and physician-prescribed interventions are discussed further in Unit 3.

In addition to these roles, the profession has many other requirements, including assertiveness; a sound knowledge base in the sciences, humanities, and arts; the ability to make safe judgments; the ability to communicate the healthcare needs of clients in written and oral form; and a spirit of collegiality with other members of the healthcare team. Professional nurses are autonomous and assume the responsibilities of caregivers, decision makers, client advocates, managers and coordinators of healthcare needs, educators, and communicators.

Caregiver

As providers of care, nurses assume responsibility for helping clients promote, restore, and maintain health and wellness (Fig. 3-2). Nurses view each client as unique and consider the "whole" person in the caring process. Nurses address not only physiologic concerns but also spiritual, emotional, and social needs. They must set priorities for care and assist clients in meeting all needs in the most timely and cost-effective manner possible, while ensuring excellence.

Decision Maker

Nurses are continually identifying obstacles or difficulties in the promotion, restoration, and maintenance of health. Problem resolution requires the ability to make sound judgments and decisions. Nurses must choose the best approaches to client care, help clients participate in this decision making, and use safe and effective judgments when providing care. They are also responsible for involving other members of the healthcare team and the families of clients in decision making to ensure that sound choices are made (Fig. 3-3).

Client Advocate

One of the nurse's most important functions is to protect clients. Nurses act as client advocates in many situations; examples include communicating the needs and concerns of clients and ensuring that clients understand their treatments.

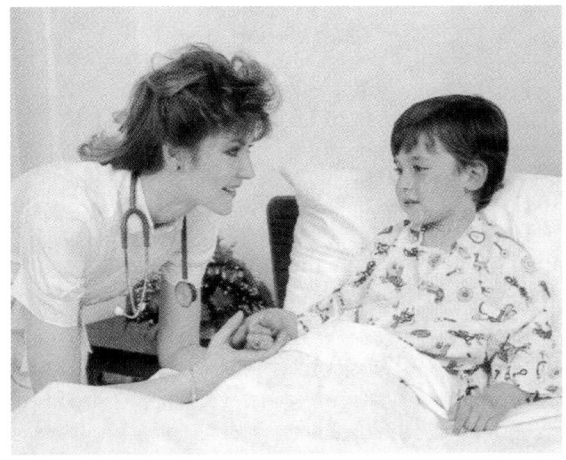

FIGURE 3-2 Nurses provide care to clients from across the lifespan.

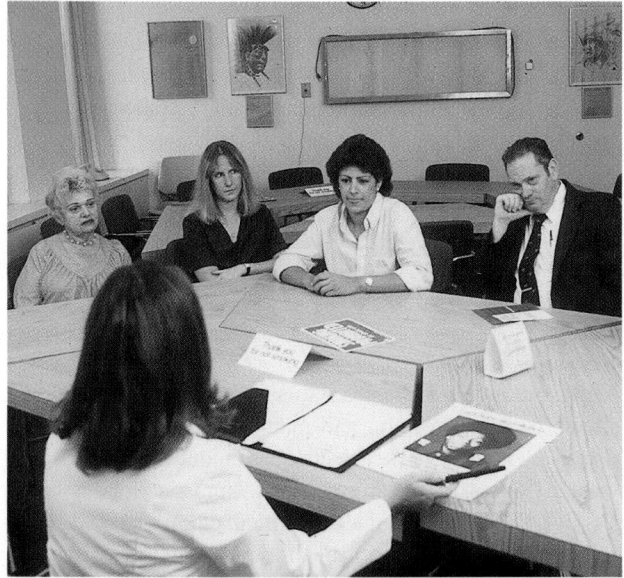

FIGURE 3-3   Nurses are responsible for involving other members of the healthcare team in decision making.

Nurses must promote safe environments that facilitate the restoration of health. They are responsible for thoroughly understanding their clients' health problems, histories, and potential problems. They consistently take responsibility for protecting clients and helping them assert their legal rights.

Manager and Coordinator

Promoting, restoring, and maintaining health involve coordinating the services that a variety of healthcare professionals offer. In addition to managing their own time, nurses also must coordinate all activities or treatments that involve clients. The goal of their role as manager and coordinator is to complete client care effectively, efficiently, and in a manner that benefits the client.

Communicator

Central to all other roles is the role of communicator. Because nurses usually are the healthcare professionals who spend the most time with clients, they have the best opportunity for observing, communicating, and identifying problems or improvements in the plan of care. Nurses are responsible for communicating findings to the healthcare team in oral and written form. The quality of this communication is critical to helping clients meet their healthcare needs; nurses must be knowledgeable, articulate, and capable of effective written and verbal expression.

Educator

Health promotion and disease prevention are a growing concern and focus of the healthcare delivery system. Educating clients about diseases, prevention, nutrition, and healthy behaviors is essential. Nurses must explain treatments and pro-

cedures for which they are responsible, answer any questions clients have, and evaluate the progress of clients toward health. Education is involved in all nursing activities.

CAREER DEVELOPMENT AND EXPANDED NURSING ROLES

Many additional opportunities for career development and advancement are available in nursing. These opportunities, some of which require advanced education, lead to new and varied roles and exciting challenges. Some expanded nursing roles include nurse practitioner, clinical nurse specialist, nurse midwife, nurse anesthetist, nurse researcher, nurse administrator, and nurse educator.

Nurse Practitioner

A **nurse practitioner** has advanced education (at least a master's degree in nursing) and is a graduate of a nurse practitioner program. Nurse practitioners function with more independence and autonomy than other nurses and are highly skilled at doing nursing assessments, performing physical examinations, counseling, teaching, and treating minor health problems. Nurse practitioners have a specialty, such as obstetrics, pediatrics, or family care.

Clinical Nurse Specialist

A **clinical nurse specialist** has a master's degree in nursing and may have advanced experience and expertise in a specialized area of practice (e.g., gerontology, pediatrics, critical care, oncology, endocrinology, cardiovascular disease, or pulmonary disease). Clinical nurse specialists work in various settings, depending on their specialty. Roles of clinical nurse specialists include clinician, educator, manager, consultant, and researcher.

Nurse Midwife

A **nurse midwife** is educated in nursing and midwifery and, in the United States, is certified by the American College of Nurse Midwives. Nurse midwives provide independent care for women during normal pregnancy, labor, and delivery. They practice in conjunction with specific healthcare agencies from which medical services are available should a client develop complications. Nurse midwives also may perform routine Papanicolaou (Pap) smears and breast examinations and assist clients with family planning. In Canada, midwives are trained as autonomous professionals and may or may not be nurses. Provincial colleges of midwives (similar to state boards of nursing) set and enforce standards of education.

Nurse Anesthetist

A **nurse anesthetist** provides general anesthesia for clients undergoing surgery under the supervision of a physician prepared in anesthesiology. Nurse anesthetists are RNs with advanced education in anesthesiology. They work in hospitals. There are no nurse anesthetists in Canada.

Nurse Researcher

A **nurse researcher** is responsible for the continued development and refinement of nursing knowledge and practice through the investigation of nursing problems. Nurse researchers have advanced education, usually at the doctoral level. They work in large teaching hospitals and research centers, such as the National Institute for Nursing Research in Bethesda, Maryland. Many nurse researchers also are employed in academic settings. All nurses have a responsibility to do research to improve nursing care and to practice from a research basis. Even nurses without advanced preparation in research can work with individuals who have such training.

Nurse Administrator

A **nurse administrator** manages and controls client care. Nurse administrators are responsible for specific nursing units and serve as liaisons between staff members and directors of nursing. Educational preparation for nurse administrators requires at least a baccalaureate degree in nursing and, in some cases, a master's or doctoral degree.

Nurse Educator

The **nurse educator** role can be developed in many settings, including schools of nursing and hospital staff development departments. Advanced education in nursing is required, usually a master's degree. Teaching at the baccalaureate, master's, or doctoral level in nursing usually requires a doctoral degree. Nurse educators generally have specific clinical specialties and advanced clinical experience. People in this career role must continue to maintain expertise in the practice setting, develop expert knowledge of theory, perfect classroom presentation style, and have in-depth knowledge of curriculum development and higher education.

PROFESSIONAL NURSING PRACTICE

Standards of Practice

As nursing became an independent profession, it began to develop its own standards of practice. Standards of practice are essential because they serve as guidelines for providing and evaluating nursing care. They help to ensure high-quality care and serve as criteria in legal questions of whether adequate care was provided. Standards of practice for the United States and Canada appear in Display 3-1.

The ANA's standards include two lists: standards of care and standards of professional performance. Measurement criteria are printed in the ANA booklet, *Standards of Clinical Nursing Practice*, 2nd edition (1998). The standards of care list designates professional nursing responsibilities as assessment, diagnosis, outcome identification, planning, implementation, and evaluation. These responsibilities are inherent in the nursing process and are discussed throughout this text. Standards of professional performance include quality of care, performance appraisal, education, collegiality, ethics, collaboration, research, and use of resources. All of these performance standards are integrated into this text under related discussions.

The CNA has set similar standards of practice. Its four central standards of nursing practice are use of a conceptual model for nursing, effective use of the nursing process, initiation of a helping relationship between the client and the nurse, and fulfillment of professional responsibilities. In addition, each province has written standards of nursing practice for which nurses are accountable.

Nurse Practice Acts

The **nurse practice act** of each state or province defines the practice of nursing within that area. In the United States, each state's licensing board sets requirements for licensure in conjunction with the board of nursing. In Canada, the provincial nursing association sets requirements for registration. New graduates must take and pass the nursing licensure examination to qualify for a nursing license or registration. With the emergence of more autonomous and expanded roles for nurses, many states have started to revise their nurse practice acts to reflect the greater responsibilities associated with current nursing practice.

Nursing Organizations

As the nursing profession has developed and advanced, organizations that have become integral to the profession have increased. The number of associations continues to grow at local, state, and national levels. Nursing organizations may be related to a specialty, or they may encompass all areas of nursing.

The organizations that involve most nurses or student nurses are the ANA, the CNA, the NLN, the CCNE, the National Student Nurses' Association (NSNA), and the Canadian University Nursing Students Association. The ICN includes nurses throughout the world and addresses international healthcare concerns in nursing. See Display 3-2 for a list of specialty nursing organizations.

American Nurses Association
The **American Nurses Association** is nursing's professional organization in the United States. Membership in state constituents of the ANA is open only to registered professional nurses. The ANA is important because it makes decisions about the functions, activities, and goals of the nursing profession. The ANA is a voice for nurses because it acts on issues and wishes expressed by its membership (Kelly & Joel, 1999).

The ANA's functions and activities have been adapted or expanded in accordance with the changing needs of the profession and public. Its goals, as stated in the current bylaws, are to work for the improvement of health standards and the availability of healthcare services for all, to foster high standards

DISPLAY 3-1

⬜ STANDARDS OF PRACTICE

American Nurses Association Standards of Clinical Nursing Practice Standards of Care

Standards of Care

Standard I. Assessment

The nurse collects patient health data.

Standard II. Diagnosis

The nurse analyzes the assessment data in determining diagnoses.

Standard III. Outcome identification

The nurse identifies expected outcomes individualized to the patient.

Standard IV. Planning

The nurse develops a plan of care that prescribes interventions to attain expected outcomes.

Standard V. Implementation

The nurse implements the interventions identified in the plan of care.

Standard VI. Evaluation

The nurse evaluates the patient's progress toward attainment of outcomes.

Standards of Professional Performance

Standard I. Quality of care

The nurse systematically evaluates the quality and effectiveness of nursing practice.

Standard II. Performance appraisal

The nurse evaluates his or her own nursing practice in relation to professional practice standards and relevant statutes and regulations.

Standard III. Education

The nurse acquires and maintains current knowledge and competency in nursing practice.

Standard IV. Collegiality

The nurse interacts with, and contributes to the professional development of, peers and other healthcare providers as colleagues.

Standard V. Ethics

The nurse's decisions and actions on behalf of patients are determined in an ethical manner.

Standard VI. Collaboration

The nurse collaborates with the patient, family, and other healthcare providers in providing patient care.

Standard VII. Research

The nurse uses research findings in practice.

Standard VIII. Resource utilization

The nurse considers factors related to safety, effectiveness, and cost in planning and delivering patient care.

Canadian Nurses Association Standards for Nursing Practice

Standard I.

Nursing practice requires that a conceptual model or models for nursing be the basis for that practice.

Standard II.

Nursing practice requires the effective use of the nursing process.

Standard III.

Nursing practice requires that the helping relationship be the nature of client–nurse interaction.

Standard IV.

Nursing practice requires nurses to fulfill professional responsibilities.

From American Nurses Association. (1998). *Standards of clinical nursing practice* (2nd ed.) Kansas City, MO: Author. (Measurement criteria for these standards are listed in their publication); Canadian Nurses Association. (1987). *A definition of nursing practice: Standards for nursing practice.* Ottawa: Author. (Sets of related behaviors are included with their standards.)

of nursing, and to stimulate and promote the professional development of nurses and advance their economic and general welfare (Kelly & Joel, 1999).

Canadian Nurses Association

The CNA, Canada's professional nursing organization, promotes high standards of practice and professional development for Canadian nursing. Its functions are similar to those of the ANA.

National League for Nursing

The main purpose of the **National League for Nursing** is to ensure that the public need for nursing is met. Members of the NLN include nurses and other members of the health team, lay people, and agencies concerned with nursing education

and service. The NLN works within the community and in association with individuals and groups outside nursing.

Commission on Collegiate Nursing Education

The CCNE is an autonomous accrediting agency that contributes to the improvement of public health by ensuring the quality and integrity of baccalaureate and graduate education programs. CCNE was established by the AACN and by representatives of nursing's community of interest. As with the NLN, accreditation by the CCNE is a nongovernmental peer review process that uses nationally recognized standards to evaluate the integrity of nursing programs and to foster continued improvement in nursing education programs and therefore in professional practice.

DISPLAY 3-2

⬚ SPECIALTY NURSING ORGANIZATIONS

Academy of Medical Surgical Nursing
American Association of Critical-Care Nurses
American Association of Colleges of Nursing
American Association for the History of Nursing, Inc.
American Association of Neuroscience Nurses
American Association of Nurse Anesthetists
American Association of Nurse Attorneys
American Association of Occupational Health Nurses
American Assembly for Men in Nursing
American College of Nurse-Midwives
American Nephrology Nurses' Association
American Organization of Nurse Executives
American Society of Post Anesthesia Nursing
Association of Operating Room Nurses
Association of Rehabilitation Nurses
Canadian Association of Critical Care Nurses
Canadian Intravenous Nurses Association
Emergency Nurses Association
Intravenous Nurses Society
National Association of Pediatric Nurse Practitioners
National Black Nurses Association, Inc.
Oncology Nursing Society

National Student Nurses' Association

The NSNA, established in 1953, is the national organization for nursing students in the United States. Its goals are to contribute to nursing education to provide for the highest quality healthcare; to provide programs representative of fundamental and current professional interests and concerns; and to aid in the development of the whole person, his or her professional role, and his or her responsibility for the healthcare of people in all walks of life. The NSNA is autonomous, student financed, and student run. It serves as the voice of nursing students, speaking out on issues of concern to the entire profession (Kelly & Joel, 1999).

International Council of Nurses

The oldest international association of professional women is the **International Council of Nurses.** This nonpolitical group brings together people from many countries who have a common interest in nursing and a common purpose of developing nursing throughout the world (Kelly & Joel, 1999).

CURRENT AND FUTURE TRENDS IN NURSING PRACTICE

Professional nursing changes to reflect society's values. Examples of issues that are affecting today's profession include healthcare cost containment, scientific and technologic advances, and the women's movement. Current trends in nurs-

ing practice include the development of nursing centers, wellness promotion programs, care of older adults, birthing centers, and home and community healthcare. As nursing practice changes, so too must the preparation of its practitioners.

Given the limits on resources, cost containment has become imperative. Clients enter the healthcare system acutely ill and leave much sooner than they did in the past, increasing the demand on nurses to ensure high-quality, comprehensive care before discharge. The healthcare system must place increasing emphasis on such areas as illness prevention, nutrition, and healthy lifestyles.

Science and technology continue to affect the nursing profession. In the past, nurses relied on their experience, observation, and intuition to make decisions. Today, the profession has defined a specific body of knowledge that continues to develop through research and practice. Contemporary nurses work in a more technical and more controversial healthcare delivery system that demands a high degree of skill. New ethical dilemmas and questions continue to arise in the process of providing healthcare.

The women's movement has brought attention to the need for equality and the recognition of universal human rights; as a result, nurses have become more assertive as professionals and are demanding more autonomy in client care. Some believe, however, that the movement has hurt nursing by encouraging women to enter nontraditional careers, thus diminishing the pool of capable women from which nursing has traditionally drawn. In contrast, more men are pursuing nursing as a professional career. The profession must continue to address the need for more nurses from nonwhite population groups, both to enhance the profession's diversity and to better reflect today's society.

Social issues and concerns are intimately linked to the provision of healthcare. Just as past issues have affected today's nursing practice, those of today will influence what happens in the future. The profession must remain dynamic in its attempts to meet society's healthcare needs.

KEY CONCEPTS

- The nursing profession has evolved over hundreds of years and continues to grow in response to society's needs.
- Nursing's history has shaped the profession's educational requirements, roles, and practice settings.
- Educational preparation and career opportunities in nursing are numerous. Diploma, associate, baccalaureate, master's, and doctoral degrees are available to those seeking a career in nursing.
- Nursing roles have expanded as the profession has developed more autonomy and gained status.
- Nurses function as caregivers, decision makers, client advocates, managers/coordinators, communicators, and educators.
- Individual state nurse practice acts govern and define the scope of nursing practice within each state.
- The ANA's standards of practice guide and direct the practice of nursing in the United States, designating nursing responsibilities that include collecting data, making nursing diagnoses, planning and implementing care, and evaluating outcomes of client care.

- Nursing organizations have emerged to represent both nurses in general and nurses involved in specialties.
- The ANA is the professional organization for American nurses.
- Trends in nursing practice develop in response to changes in society. Trends affecting modern nursing practice include financial concerns, advances in technology, and the women's movement.

REFERENCES

American Nurses Association. (1998). *Standards of clinical nursing practice* (2nd ed.). Washington, DC: American Nurses Publishing.

American Nurses Association. (1980). *Nursing: A social policy statement.* Kansas City, MO: Author.

Benner, P. (1984). *From novice to expert: Excellence and power in clinical nursing practice.* San Francisco: Addison-Wesley.

Came, D., Gregory, D., English, J., & VenKatesh, P. (1996). A struggle for equality: Resistance to commissioning of male nurses in the Canadian military, 1952–1967. *Canadian Journal of Nursing Research, 28*(1), 103–117.

Canadian Nurses Association. (1987). *A definition of nursing practice: Standards for nursing practice.* Ottawa: Author.

Carpenito, L. (2002). *Nursing diagnosis: Application to clinical practice* (9th ed.). Philadelphia: Lippincott Williams & Wilkins.

Chambers, L. E., & Subera, P. A. (1997). Nursing history as a tool for development of a professional identity within nursing students. *Journal of Nursing Education, 36*(9), 432–433.

Doheny, M. O., Cook, C. B., & Stopper, M. C. (1997). *The discipline of nursing: An introduction* (4th ed.). Stamford, CT: Appleton & Lange.

Dolan, A. J., Fitzpatrick, M. L., & Herrmann, E. K. (1983). *Nursing in society: A historical perspective* (15th ed.). Philadelphia: W. B. Saunders.

Donahue, M. P. (1996). *Nursing: The finest art, an illustrated history* (2nd ed.). St. Louis, MO: Mosby.

Egenes, K. J. (1998). An experiment in leadership: The rise of student government at Philadelphia General Hospital Training School, 1920–1930. *Nursing History Review, 6,* 71–84.

Flexner, A. (1915). Is social work a profession? *School Society, 1*(26), 901.

Griffon, D. P. (1998). "A somewhat duskier skin": Mary Seacole in the Crimea. *Nursing History Review, 6,* 115–127.

Kalisch, P. A., & Kalisch, B. J. (1995). *The advance of American nursing* (3rd ed.). Philadelphia: J. B. Lippincott.

Kelly, L. Y., & Joel, L. A. (1999). *Dimensions of professional nursing* (8th ed.). New York: McGraw-Hill.

Lusk, B. (1997). Professional classifications of American nurses, 1910 to 1935. *Western Journal of Nursing Research, 19*(2), 227–242.

MacKintosh, C. (1997). A historical study of men in nursing. *Journal of Advanced Nursing, 26,* 232–236.

Mitchell, P. R., & Grippando, G. M. (1993). *Nursing perspectives and issues* (5th ed.). New York: Delmar Publishers.

National League for Nursing. (1978a). *Characteristics of baccalaureate education in nursing.* Pub. No. 15-1758. New York: Author.

National League for Nursing. (1978b). *Roles and competencies of graduates of diploma programs in nursing.* Pub. No. 16-1735. New York: Author.

National League for Nursing. (1978c). *Roles and competencies of the associate degree nurse on entry into practice.* Pub. No. 23-17211. New York: Author.

Nightingale, F. N. (1992). *Notes on nursing: What it is and what it is not.* Philadelphia: J. B. Lippincott. (Original work published 1859).

Ziemer, M. (1994, August). Advanced practice nursing. *The Pennsylvania Nurse, 7.*

BIBLIOGRAPHY

Ashley, J. (1976). *Hospitals, paternalism, and the role of the nurse.* New York: Teachers College Press.

Cunningham, M. P. (2000). Breaking the mold. *American Journal of Nursing, 100*(10), 125–133.

Dossey, B. M. (2000). *Florence Nightingale.* Springhouse, PA: Springhouse Corporation.

Fairman, J. (1992). Watchful vigilance: Nursing care, technology, and the development of intensive care units. *Nursing Research, 41*(1), 56–60.

Kelly, L. Y., & Joel, L. A. (1996). *The nursing experience: trends, challenges, and transitions.* New York: McGraw-Hill.

Lewenson, S. B. (1993). *Taking charge: Nursing, suffrage and feminism, 1873–1920.* New York: Garland Press.

Lewenson, S. B. (1990). The women's nursing and suffrage movement, 1893–1920. In V. Bullough, B. Bullough, & M. Stanton (Eds.). *Florence Nightingale and her era: A collection of new scholarship* (pp. 117–118). New York: Garland Publishing.

O'Brian, P. A. (1987). All a woman's life can bring: The domestic roots of nursing in Philadelphia, 1830–1885. *Nursing Research, 36*(1), 12–17.

Pokorney, M. E. (1992). An historical perspective of Confederate nursing during the Civil War, 1861–1865. *Nursing Research, 41*(1) 28–32.

Reverby, S. (1987). A caring dilemma: Womanhood and nursing in historical perspective. *Nursing Research, 36*(10), 5–11.

Schorr, T. M., & Kennedy, M. S. (1999). *100 years of American nursing: Celebrating a century of caring.* Philadelphia: Lippincott Williams & Wilkins.

Thibodeau, J. A., & Hawkins, J. W. (1994). Moving toward a nursing model in advanced practice. *Western Journal of Nursing Research, 16*(2), 205–218.

Widerquist, J. G. (1992). The spirituality of Florence Nightingale. *Nursing Research, 41*(1), 49–55.

4 Nursing Theory and Conceptual Frameworks

📗 Key Terms

conceptual framework
environment
functional health patterns
general systems theory
health
human needs
Maslow's hierarchy of
   human needs

movement
nursing
nursing theory
person
refreezing
self-actualization
theory
unfreezing

📗 Learning Objectives

Upon completion of this chapter, the student will be able to do the
following:
1. Define *nursing theory* and *conceptual framework*.
2. Recognize major nursing theories and their relevance to nursing
   practice.
3. Identify the four major concepts of nursing theories.
4. Discuss the relationship between nursing theories and non-
   nursing theories.
5. Summarize non-nursing theories and their use in nursing.
6. Explain the relationship of functional health pattern typology
   to nursing.

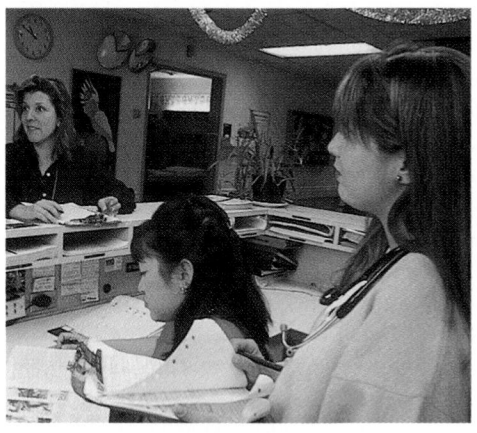

📗 Critical Thinking Challenge

*You are a nursing major completing your clinical laboratory in a local hospi-
tal. You are assigned to a unit that cares primarily for clients who have diabetes mellitus and cardiovascular diseases. The unit is large, usually holding
40 clients. Each client's room is private. Nurses care for five to six clients as
part of their regular assignments. In a meeting, nursing administration and
staff members decided to use a nursing framework to develop the unit's organizational structure and the provision of all subsequent nursing care.*

Once you have completed this chapter and have incorporated nursing theories
and conceptual frameworks into your knowledge base, review the above scenario and reflect on the following areas of Critical Thinking:

1. Explore how the hospital might go about accomplishing this task.
2. Select a nursing theory you believe would best apply to this type of unit, and state your rationale.
3. Illustrate how the four concepts of the selected theory might be addressed on this unit.
4. Compare arguments for and against using your chosen theory in this practice setting.
5. Formulate a plan for how you might convince your colleagues that this theory applies to the practice setting.

"As a practice discipline and profession, nursing is often described as both an 'art' and a 'science'" (Schultz & Meleis, 1988, p. 217). Although many people view nursing as primarily a practice discipline, the art of practice is grounded in scientific principles. The science and practice of nursing are recognized as the profession's two major dimensions. Without nursing science, nursing practice could not exist (Rogers, 1970). Development of the science and practice of nursing is an essential component of the discipline; it generates knowledge that supports and advances healthcare. The contemporary move to use, refine, and develop theoretical models for nursing practice and education has received increased attention throughout nursing's history, thus reinforcing the profession's emphasis on theory-based practice.

The science of nursing incorporates the study of relationships among nurses, clients, and their environments within the context of health. Conceptual and theoretical nursing models generate knowledge that improves nursing practice, guides nursing research, and facilitates the organization of curricula for all levels of nursing education (Fawcett, 1995; Marriner-Tomey & Alligood, 1998). From nursing science, conceptual models and nursing theories evolve. As the profession continues to expand its own body of knowledge, concepts and theories develop to support nursing's practice component. Development and clarification of theoretical frameworks applied to the practice of professional nursing facilitate the description of what nurses do, why, and how. Theoretical frameworks are important to the advancement of nursing knowledge and professional practice.

Over the years, nursing has incorporated theories from nonnursing sources, including theories of systems, human needs, change, problem solving, and decision making. More recently, a functional health approach to nursing has become popular. Functional health patterns provide an organizing framework for nursing practice grounded in the discipline of nursing. This framework is clear and appropriate and provides a way to organize information that is important to nursing's unique body of knowledge. Functional health patterns are discussed in more detail toward the end of this chapter, and they provide the organizational framework for this textbook.

NURSING THEORY

A **conceptual framework** or model is defined as a set of concepts and the propositions that integrate them into a meaningful configuration (Marriner-Tomey & Alligood, 1998). Conceptual frameworks are composed of concepts or *constructs* that describe ideas about individuals, groups, situations, and events of particular interest to a discipline (e.g., nursing). The concepts and propositions of a conceptual framework are highly abstract and general. Conceptual frameworks have the "basic purpose of focusing, ruling some things in as relevant, and ruling others out due to their lesser importance" (Williams, 1979, p. 96).

Barnum (1998, p. 1) defines **theory** as "a construct (the way to put together the 'parts' of something) that accounts for or organizes some phenomenon. A nursing theory, then, de-

scribes or explains nursing." Theories contain concepts that provide meanings for terms and propositions and clarify how these concepts are related, similar to conceptual frameworks. Theories, however, go a step beyond conceptual frameworks. A theory is a way to relate concepts by using definitions that state significant relationships between them. The concepts and propositions of a theory are much more specific than those of a conceptual framework. In nursing, concepts include how the theorist describes person, environment, health, and nursing. Propositions within the theory show the relationship of these four concepts.

Nursing theory provides the foundation for nursing knowledge and gives direction to nursing practice. Nursing theory should guide the development and future direction of nursing research. Barnum (1998) offers this vivid analogy to describe nursing theory:

> A theory is like a map of a territory as opposed to an aerial photograph. The map does not display the full terrain (buildings, moving vehicles, or grazing livestock); instead, it picks out those parts that are important for its purpose. If its aim is to guide travelers, the map will highlight roads; if its purpose is to describe the physical terrain, it will show mountains, plains, and rivers. But no map (or theory) reflects all that is contained within a phenomenon. Such a map would defeat its purpose: giving one a handle on the phenomenon. The handle is created by making the essential parts stand out in relief (p. 1).

Development of Nursing Theory

The development of nursing theory has provided direction for the structure of professional nursing practice, education, and research. Chinn (1994) emphasized the importance of nursing theory to students and practicing professionals, stating that "nursing theory ought to guide research and practice, generate new ideas, and differentiate the focus of nursing from other professions" (p. 145).

The introduction of nursing theory historically began with Florence Nightingale (1860), who, in *Notes on Nursing,* was the first nurse to discuss a framework for nursing. She conceptualized the nurse's role as manipulating the environment to facilitate and encourage the reparative process by attending to ventilation, warmth, light, diet, cleanliness, and noise. Her framework for nursing can be seen in today's nursing practice in terms of monitoring clients' nutritional status and following standard precautions.

Since Nightingale, nursing theories have become increasingly sophisticated. Some theories and frameworks are easily adapted to practice settings, whereas others are better suited for research. Nurse theorists continue to contribute to nursing's body of knowledge. An excellent example was presented by Eakes, Burke, and Hainsworth (1998) in their article, "Middle-Range Theory of Chronic Sorrow." They presented the nursing theory related to chronic sorrow "as a normal response to ongoing disparity due to loss . . . [and] chronic sorrow as the periodic recurrence of permanent, pervasive sadness or other grief-related feelings associated with a significant loss. The theory provides a framework for understanding and working with people following a single or ongoing loss" (p. 179). Often, in professional nursing practice, nurses must address the needs of clients who are experiencing loss and sorrow. This article provides an excellent example of theory development. In another example, Jaarsma, Halfens, Senten, Saad, and Dracup (1998) described the development of a supportive-educative program for clients with advanced heart failure using Orem's nursing theory (1971).

Four Major Concepts

Nurses have developed various theories that provide different explanations of the nursing discipline. All theories, however, share four central concepts: person, environment, health, and nursing. Each theory defines, relates, and emphasizes these concepts differently.

In a broad sense, the concept of **person** refers to all human beings. People are the recipients of nursing care; they include individuals, families, communities, and groups. **Environment** includes factors that affect individuals internally and externally. It means not only everyday surroundings but also settings where nursing care is provided. **Health** generally addresses the person's state of well-being. The concept of **nursing** is central to all nursing theories. Definitions of nursing describe what nursing is, what nurses do, and how nurses interact with clients. Most nursing theories address each of the four central concepts implicitly or explicitly. Table 4-1 lists each major nursing theorist, the central purpose of each theory, and each theorist's definitions of the four major concepts.

NON-NURSING THEORIES USED IN NURSING

General Systems Theory

The general systems theory, or a systems framework, provides another approach for studying individuals in their environments and is used by many disciplines. **General systems theory** includes purpose, content, and process, breaking down the "whole" and analyzing the parts. The relationships between the parts of the whole are examined to learn how they work together.

Von Bertalanffy (1969, 1976) developed general systems theory, which assumes the following:

- All systems must be goal directed.
- A system is more than the sum of its parts.
- A system is ever changing, and any change in one part affects the whole.
- Boundaries are implicit, and human systems are open and dynamic.

(text continues on page 62)

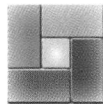

Nursing Research and Critical Thinking
Is It Possible to Measure Client Satisfaction Based on a Nursing Model of Care?

For nurses to be able to compete successfully in today's consumer-oriented healthcare market, they must be able to evaluate the outcomes of their services, including client satisfaction with the nursing care they receive. Nurses designed this descriptive, correlational study to investigate the validity and reliability of the Client Satisfaction Tool (CST). The CST is based on Cox's Interactional Model of Client Health Behavior and is explicitly developed to measure client satisfaction with a nurse practitioner model of care. The nurses used a nursing framework to develop the CST to conceptualize validly the nurse practitioner model of care. This model integrates the physical and psychosocial aspects of client health and includes therapeutic listening, client education, goal setting, and technical aspects of primary care. A convenience sample of 38 clients who had received care at a nurse-managed primary care clinic completed the questionnaire. Responses to the CST indicated that people receiving care at the clinic were satisfied with the care they received. Reliability testing of the instrument showed that the tool has high internal consistency (Cronbach's alpha was .956) and high stability ($r = .974$). Construct validity testing with measures of perceived health changes showed that the tool has both convergent ($r = .599$, $P > .01$) and divergent ($r = .194$, $P < .10$) validity.

Critical Thinking Considerations. Subjects for this study had received care at this clinic at least 2 weeks before data collection and were interviewed by people who were not directly involved with care delivery at the clinic. Rationales for this method of subject selection and data collection and implications of the study are as follows:

- Responses are likely to be biased due to gratitude for services rendered, the wish to reward staff, and/or the fear of repercussions for negative care appraisal.
- The CST is a methodologically sound measure of client satisfaction that can be used in future research to examine client satisfaction with nurse practitioner care.
- The study supported the idea that healthcare consumers value the integration of the physical and psychosocial aspects of healthcare.

From Bear, M., & Bowers, C. (1998). Using a nursing framework to measure client satisfaction at a nurse-managed clinic. *Public Health Nursing, 15*(1), 50–59.

TABLE 4-1

Overview of Major Nursing Theorists		
Theorist	**Purpose**	**Views of Components**
Florence Nightingale (1860), *Notes on Nursing: What It Is, What It Is Not*	To help individuals responsible for caring for the sick to "think how to nurse." Theory addresses fundamental needs of the sick and basic principles of good healthcare.	Person: An individual with vital reparative processes to deal with disease. Environment: External conditions that affect life and the individual's development. Focus is on ventilation, warmth, odors, and light. Health: Focus is on the reparative process of getting well. Nursing: Goal is to place the individual in the best condition for good healthcare.
Hildegard E. Peplau (1952), *Interpersonal Relations in Nursing*	To develop an interpersonal interaction between client and nurse	Person: An organism striving to reduce tension generated by needs. Environment: Implicitly defined; the interpersonal process is always included, and the psychodynamic milieu receives attention, with emphasis on the client's culture and mores. Health: Ongoing human process that implies forward movement of personality and other ongoing human processes in the direction of creative, constructive, productive, personal, and community living. Nursing: Interpersonal therapeutic process that "functions cooperatively with other human processes that make health possible for individuals in communities. Nursing is an educative instrument, a maturing force that aims to promote forward movement of personality."
Virginia Henderson (1955), *The Nature of Nursing*	To assist the client in gaining independence as rapidly as possible	Person: Individual requiring assistance to achieve health and independence or a peaceful death. Mind and body are inseparable. Environment: All external conditions and influences that affect life and development. Health: Equated with independence, viewed in terms of the client's ability to perform 14 components of nursing care unaided: breathing, eating, drinking, maintaining comfort, sleeping, resting, clothing, maintaining body temperature, ensuring safety, communicating, worshiping, working, recreation, and continuing development. Nursing: Assists and supports the individual in life activities and the attainment of independence.
Faye Glenn Abdellah (1960), *Patient-Centered Approaches to Nursing*	To deliver nursing care for the whole individual	Person: The recipient of nursing care having physical, emotional, and sociologic needs that may be overt or covert.

TABLE 4-1 (Continued)

Overview of Major Nursing Theorists		
Theorist	**Purpose**	**Views of Components**
		Environment: Not clearly defined. Some discussion indicates that clients interact with their environment, of which the nurse is a part.
		Health: Implicitly defined as a state when the individual has no unmet needs and no anticipated or actual impairments.
		Nursing: Broadly grouped in "21 nursing problems," which center around needs for hygiene, comfort, activity, rest, safety, oxygen, nutrition, elimination, hydration, physical and emotional health promotion, interpersonal relationships, and development of self-awareness. Nursing care is doing something for an individual.
Ida Jean Orlando (1961), *The Dynamic Nurse-Patient Relationship*	To interact with clients to meet immediate needs by identifying client behaviors, nurse's reactions, and nursing actions to take	Person: Unique individual behaving verbally and nonverbally. Assumption is that individuals are at times able to meet their own needs and at other times unable to do so.
		Environment: Not defined.
		Health: Not defined. Assumption is that being without emotional or physical discomfort and having a sense of well-being contribute to a healthy state.
		Nursing: Professional nursing is conceptualized as finding out and meeting the client's immediate need for help. Medicine and nursing are viewed as distinctly different.
Lydia E. Hall (1964), *Nursing: What Is It?*	To provide professional nursing care to people past the acute stage of illness	Person: Client is composed of body, pathology, and person. People set their own goals and are capable of learning and growing.
		Environment: Should facilitate achievement of the client's personal goals.
		Health: Development of a mature self-identity that assists in the conscious selection of actions that facilitate growth.
		Nursing: Caring is the nurse's primary function. Professional nursing is most important during the recuperative period.
Ernestine Wiedenbach (1964), *Clinical Nursing— A Helping Art*	To assist individuals in overcoming obstacles that prevent meeting healthcare needs	Person: Any individual who is receiving help (care, instruction, or advice) from a member of the health profession or from a worker in the field of health.
		Environment: Not specifically addressed.
		Health: Not defined. Concepts of nursing, client, and need for help and their relationships imply health-related concerns in the nurse–client relationship (Marriner-Tomey & Alligood, 1998, p. 245).

(continues)

TABLE 4-1 (Continued)

Overview of Major Nursing Theorists		
Theorist	Purpose	Views of Components
Myra Estrin Levin (1973), *Conservation Model*	To use conservation activities aimed at optimal use of client's resources	Nursing: The nurse is a functioning human being who acts, thinks, and feels. All actions, thoughts, and feelings underlie what the nurse does. Person: A holistic being. Environment: Broadly, includes all the individual's experiences. Health: The maintenance of the client's unity and integrity.
Dorothy E. Johnson (1980), *The Behavioral System Model for Nursing*	To reduce stress so the client can recover as quickly as possible	Nursing: A discipline rooted in the organic dependency of the individual human being on his or her relationships with others. Person: A system of interdependent parts with patterned, repetitive, and purposeful ways of behaving. Environment: All forces that affect the person and that influence the behavioral system. Health: Focus on person, not illness. Health is a dynamic state influenced by biologic, psychological, and social factors. Nursing: Promotion of behavioral system, balance, and stability. An art and a science providing external assistance before and during system balance disturbances.
Martha E. Rogers (1970), *The Science of Unitary Man*	To assist the client in achieving a maximum level of wellness	Person: Unitary man, a four-dimensional energy field. Environment: Encompasses all that is outside any given human field. Person exchanging matter and energy. Health: Not specifically addressed, but emerges out of interaction between human and environment, moves forward, and maximizes human potential. Nursing: A learned profession that is both science and art. The professional practice of nursing is creative and imaginative and exists to serve people.
Dorothea E. Orem (1971), *Nursing: Concepts of Practice*	To provide care and to assist the client to attain self-care	Person: Biopsychosocial being capable of self-care. Includes physical, psychological, interpersonal, and social aspects of human functioning. Environment: Internal and external stimuli. Requisites for self-care have their origins in human beings and the environment. Health: State of wholeness or integrity of human beings, including physical, mental, and social well-being. Nursing: A creative effort of one human being to help another human being. Consists of three nursing systems: wholly compensatory, partially compensatory, and supportive/educative.

TABLE 4-1 (Continued)

Overview of Major Nursing Theorists		
Theorist	**Purpose**	**Views of Components**
Imogene M. King (1971), *Open Systems Model*	To use communication to help the client reestablish a positive adaptation to his or her environment	Person: Biopsychosocial being. Environment: Internal and external environment continually interact to assist in adjustments to change. Health: A dynamic life experience with continued goal attainment and adjustment to stressors. Nursing: Perceiving, thinking, relating, judging, and acting with an individual who comes to a nursing situation.
Joyce Travelbee (1966, 1971), *Interpersonal Aspects of Nursing*	To assist individuals, families, communities, and groups to prevent or cope with illness and regain health	Person: A unique, irreplaceable individual who is in a continuous process of becoming, evolving, and changing. Environment: Not explicitly defined. Health: Health includes the individual's perceptions of health and the absence of disease. Nursing: An interpersonal process whereby the professional nurse practitioner assists an individual, family, or community to prevent or to cope with the experience of illness and suffering and, if necessary, to find meaning in these experiences.
Betty Neuman (1972), *The Neuman Systems Model*	To address the effects of stress and reactions to it on the development and maintenance of health	Person: A client system that is composed of physiologic, psychological, sociocultural, and environmental variables. Environment: Internal and external forces surrounding humans at any time. Health: Health or wellness exists if all parts and subparts are in harmony with the whole person. Nursing: A unique profession concerned with all variables affecting an individual's response to stressors.
Sister Callista Roy (1979)	To identify the types of demands placed on a client and the client's adaptation to the demands	Person: A biopsychosocial being and the recipient of nursing care. Environment: All conditions, circumstances, and influences surrounding and affecting the development of an organism or groups of organisms. Health: The person encounters adaptation problems in changing environments. Nursing: A theoretical system of knowledge that prescribes a process of analysis and action related to the care of the ill or potentially ill person.

(continues)

TABLE 4-1 (Continued)

Overview of Major Nursing Theorists

Theorist	Purpose	Views of Components
Jean Watson (1979), *Nursing: Human Science and Human Care*	To focus on curative factors derived from a humanistic perspective and from scientific knowledge	Person: A valued being to be cared for, respected, nurtured, understood, and assisted; a fully functional, integrated self. Environment: Social environment, caring, and the culture of caring affect health. Health: Physical, mental, and social well-being. Nursing: A human science of people and human health; illness experiences that are mediated by professional, personal, scientific, aesthetic, and ethical human care transactions.
Rosemarie Rizzo Parse (1981), *Man–Living–Health: Theory of Nursing*	To focus on humans as living unity and humans' qualitative participation with health experience	Person: A major reason for nursing's existence, evidenced by a "pattern of patterns of relating" (p. 26). Environment: "Man and environment interchange energy to create what is in the world, and man chooses the meaning given to the situations he creates" (p. 27). Health: A lived experience that is a process of being and becoming. Nursing: "Nursing practice is directed toward illuminating and mobilizing family interrelationships in light of the meaning assigned to health and its possibilities as language in the cocreated patterns of relating" (p. 82).

Nursing Theorists' Use of General Systems Theory

Examples of nursing theories that have used the systems approach to client care include Roy's adaptation model (1980), Hall's philosophy of nursing (1964), Neuman's healthcare systems model (1972), Johnson's behavioral model (1980), and Parse's theory for nursing (1981).

Human Needs Theory: Maslow's Hierarchy of Human Needs

Human needs are any physiologic or psychological factors necessary for a healthy existence. The most prominent theorist to focus on human needs has been Abraham Maslow. **Maslow's hierarchy of human needs** (1970) states that all humans are born with instinctive needs. These needs, grouped into five categories, are arranged in order of importance from those essential for physical survival to those necessary to develop a person's fullest potential. Maslow's hierarchy provides a framework for recognizing and prioritizing basic human needs. This hierarchy is constructed as a pyramid (Fig. 4-1). From the pyramid's base to its apex, people must meet lower-level needs to some degree before they can address higher-level needs. A person is not motivated by all five categories of human needs at the same time. The category most relevant to the person's circumstances at a particular time is the primary motivator. Meeting needs is a dynamic process that involves continual resolution of, progression beyond, and return to any given category of needs.

Human needs are motivational forces (Yura & Walsh, 1988). Culture, socioeconomic factors, personal values, and health influence the motivational strength for and manner of expression of these needs. All people develop behaviors that help them meet their needs. They can learn to delay meeting their needs and modify the specific behaviors that satisfy needs, depending on each need's motivational strength. If a need goes unmet, physical illness, psychological disequilibrium, or death can occur.

Physiologic Needs

Physiologic needs are fundamental motivating forces and provide the base for Maslow's pyramid. Oxygen, food, water, elimination, activity, rest, temperature maintenance, and sexuality are essential for existence. Nurses assess each client's ability to meet his or her physiologic needs and identify the nature and degree of nursing interventions necessary to enable the person to satisfy these needs.

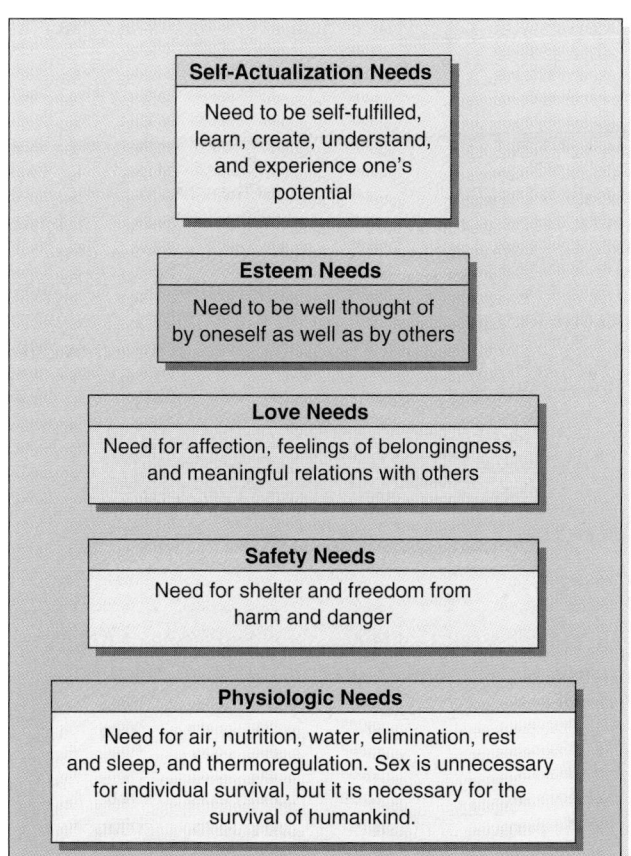

FIGURE 4-1 A pyramid represents Maslow's hierarchy of human needs. According to Maslow, basic physiologic needs, such as nutrition and water, must be met before the person can move on to higher-level needs. Nursing helps people meet needs they cannot meet by themselves.

Air. Oxygen is essential for the body's metabolic processes. Satisfying this need requires properly functioning respiratory and cardiovascular systems (see Chapters 34 and 35).

Nutrition. Proper nutrition is essential for energy production and the body's metabolic processes. Satisfying this need requires adequate food and a properly functioning gastrointestinal tract (see Chapters 37 and 41).

Water. Fluids are necessary for metabolic processes. Proper fluid balance is critical for life (see Chapter 36).

Elimination. Elimination is a crucial part of the metabolic process. It enables the body to dispose of waste products and to maintain fluid and electrolyte balances (see Chapters 36, 40, and 41).

Sleep and Rest. Sleep and rest are necessary for the body to revitalize itself. People vary considerably in the total amount, frequency, and duration of sleep and rest they require. These requirements also vary throughout each person's lifespan. Failure to meet needs for sleep and rest leads to fatigue, irri-

tability, behavioral changes, difficulty concentrating, and eventual exhaustion (see Chapter 42).

Thermoregulation. Temperature maintenance is necessary for life. Extremes in either direction can lead to death. The body monitors and maintains its temperature through sensors in the skin, the hypothalamus, and the effector system. Any alteration in these structures can affect temperature regulation. The body can adapt to environmental temperatures within broad limits, but age and health status greatly affect this capacity (see Chapter 25).

Sex. Sexual relations are not essential for a person's survival but are necessary for the continuation of the species. The importance of this need varies widely among individuals. Meeting this need can affect how the person deals with higher-order needs, such as love, belonging, and self-esteem (see Chapter 50).

Safety Needs

After meeting basic physiologic needs, the person must address safety needs. Humans need to be physically safe and free from the fear and anxiety that result from a lack of security and protection. Safety is often a dominant motivator. For example, in a country at war, safety becomes a primary force as long as physiologic needs are minimally satisfied. The same is true during natural disasters, such as floods or tornadoes. Such events cause major disruptions in personal, family, and societal routines and can lead to chaos. According to Maslow (1970), an essential aspect of safety is the need for predictability and routine (see Chapter 30).

Love Needs

The need for love and belonging is the next tier on Maslow's pyramid. After a sense of safety is achieved, people need to feel that they belong and are loved to avoid loneliness and isolation. To meet this need, a person must give and receive love (see Chapter 47).

Esteem Needs

According to Maslow (1970), there are two types of esteem needs: esteem derived from others and self-esteem. People need to know that others think well of, admire, and respect them. Self-esteem is a person's sense of his or her own adequacy and worth. To be genuine, it must be firmly grounded in a realistic appraisal of one's strengths and weaknesses. If esteem needs go unmet, the person faces a life characterized by self-doubt and feelings of helplessness and worthlessness. What others value in a person and what that person values in himself or herself may differ, and these evaluations are influenced by cultural, social, and psychological variables (see Chapter 46).

Self-Actualization Needs

According to Maslow (1970), the need for **self-actualization** is the innate need to realize fully all of one's abilities and qualities, that is, to maximize one's potential. Maslow sees this process as never-ending. Although early life experiences affect self-actualization, people have the capacity to change and to reach a state of optimal psychological health as they strive for it.

Nursing Theorists' Perceptions of Human Needs

Through the years, nursing theories have incorporated ideas from human needs theory. Typically, nurses identify a client's needs, using them as a basis for planning and implementing care. Human needs theory has led to the development of nursing models and frameworks for holistic nursing. Nurse theorists who have used human needs theory are listed in Table 4-2.

Change Theory

People grow and change throughout their lives. This growth and change are evident in the dynamic nature of basic human needs and how they are met. Change happens daily. It is subtle, continuous, and manifested in both everyday occurrences and more disruptive life events. Reactions to change are grounded in the basic human needs for self-esteem, safety, and security.

TABLE 4-2

Nurse Theorists and Human Needs	
Nurse Theorist	Integration of Human Needs
Florence Nightingale	In *Notes on Nursing* (1860/1946), Nightingale wrote that nurses should create an environment in which healing could take place; the need for a positive environment, free from filth and vermin, is paramount to the client's recovery.
Virginia Henderson	Henderson (1966) described 14 principles of nursing that focus on physiologic, social, psychological, and spiritual needs.
Ida Jean Orlando	The concept of need is central to Orlando's theory, which focuses on clients and their unmet needs. Orlando believed that the purpose of nursing is to provide the assistance that a client requires to meet his or her needs.
Dorothea Orem	Orem placed human needs into three categories: universal self-care requisites, developmental self-care requisites, and health deviations. *Universal healthcare requisites* include the need for air, food, water, elimination, and safety. *Developmental requisites* address human needs throughout the lifespan. Finally, *health deviations* address needs that develop as a result of an illness.
Imogene M. King	King viewed nursing as a process that involves action, reaction, interaction, and transaction. The nurse operates on the belief that each person is an open system who interacts with interpersonal and societal systems. The client and nurse establish a relationship to cope with or improve a health state.
Sister Callista Roy	Roy's adaptation model identifies five essential elements: *person, goal of nursing, nursing activities, health,* and *environment.* Each person constantly interacts with the environment. Roy includes four modes of adaptation: physiologic needs (adaptation to satisfy basic needs), self-concept (adaptation to maintain psychological integrity), role function (adaptation to society's roles and duties), and interdependence (adaptation to enable need fulfillment; support systems).
Martha E. Rogers	Rogers (1970) described nursing as a humanistic science dedicated to compassionate concern for maintaining and promoting health. Preventing illness and rehabilitating the sick and disabled are primary goals.
Lydia E. Hall	Hall saw nursing as having different functions in three interlocking circles: *care circle* (client's body), *cure circle* (disease), and *core circle* (client's inner feelings and motivations). The nurse helps the client become aware of his or her needs, feelings, and motivations. It then becomes the client's task to set goals and priorities. This learning process encourages maximum growth. The client freely expresses ideas regarding the disease process and his or her own needs, and through this expression the client gains self-identity.
Jean Watson	Watson believed that caring is central to nursing. Watson's hierarchy of *10 carative factors* is similar to Maslow's: Clients must satisfy lower-order needs before attaining higher ones.
Faye Glenn Abdellah	Abdellah described nursing as a service to people, families, and society. The nurse helps people, sick or well, to cope with their health needs. In Abdellah's model, nursing care means providing information to the client or doing something to the client with the goal of meeting needs or alleviating an impairment.

Change involves a modification or alteration. It may be planned or unplanned. Although a variety of change theories exist, Kurt Lewin (1962) developed the classic theory of change, which identifies the following six components:

1. Recognition of the area where change is needed
2. Analysis of a situation to determine what forces exist to maintain the situation and what forces are working to change it
3. Identification of methods by which change can occur
4. Recognition of the influence of group mores or customs on change
5. Identification of the methods that the reference group uses to bring about change
6. The actual process of change

Lewin identified three states of change: unfreezing, movement, and refreezing. **Unfreezing** is the recognition of the need for change and the dissolution of previously held patterns of behavior. **Movement** is the shift of behavior toward a new and more healthful pattern. Movement marks the initiation of change. **Refreezing** is the long-term solidification of the new pattern of behavior.

The healthcare delivery system and the practice of professional nursing continually evolve. Nurses must recognize the dynamic nature of change and assist individuals and groups to adapt (Lutjens & Tiffany, 1994; Tiffany, 1994). The impact of change on basic human needs is constant and should be recognized to best use this framework to organize nursing care.

Nursing Theorists' Use of Change Theory

Change theory offers insight into expected behaviors when significant change occurs within an environment. Nurse theorists have incorporated various aspects of change theory. For example, Peplau's (1952) use of the nursing process applies aspects of change theory as client needs are assessed and necessary alterations in specific patterns of behavior are determined.

FUNCTIONAL HEALTH PATTERNS AS A FRAMEWORK FOR NURSING

Nurses deal with the "whole" person, examining the physical, psychological, interpersonal, and spiritual aspects of each client's life. The "whole" person concept emphasizes a holistic approach to professional nursing (see Chapter 16). Holistic practice also considers the client's family and community, which is especially important now that the community is a common location for healthcare delivery.

Nursing faculty and clinicians have struggled to organize information in a way that is more nursing focused. In addition to using specific nursing theories, another way to organize nursing information in a holistic way is to use Marjory Gordon's concept of **functional health patterns.** These patterns delineate the human needs of the person, family, community, and group. The patterns, which focus on behaviors that occur with time, present a total picture of the client, rather than just a small part of his or her life. Functional health patterns represent basic

health needs that develop as people strive to meet those needs. These patterns are unique because they are interrelated: One pattern often provides answers to another. No pattern can be studied as a separate category.

Gordon's patterns, which are consistent with the human needs philosophy and general systems theory, can provide a framework for holistic nursing assessment (Fig. 4-2). Gordon provides a comprehensive discussion of client needs; Maslow's hierarchy offers a rationale for determining the order in which to address those needs; and systems theory requires an analysis of relationships, purposes, reasons, and tasks.

Health Perception and Health Management

The health perception–health management pattern is the first in a series of 11 patterns that Gordon addressed (1994). This pattern focuses on health values and beliefs and the resources in the community that are available to meet health needs. It is based on the awareness that, although promoting health is a primary nursing function, clients actually manage their own health. Success in meeting human needs in this pattern relies heavily on culture, societal beliefs, personal expectations, and one's own health. The client's family may play an important part in this function because one family member may make major health decisions for the entire group.

Activity and Exercise

Energy required to meet human needs is examined in the activity and exercise pattern. Clients must be evaluated for their ability to engage in self-care activities to meet basic physiologic needs. Another aspect involves determining how much energy is available to ensure the safety of their environment. For example, energy requirements for an older person who lives alone differ vastly from those of a young adult who lives in an intact family. The relationship of activity–exercise to health perception–health management is evident because the nurse must learn the importance the client places on the person, family, or community. The community may not have adequate transportation for its members to engage in exercise or activity. Problems meeting needs in this category may affect other needs, such as human companionship and nutritional concerns.

Nutrition and Metabolism

Life cannot be sustained without meeting human needs in the category of nutrition and metabolism. People establish patterns for meeting these needs early in life, and many such behaviors are learned in the family. This pattern does not deal simply with "eating." It encompasses food knowledge, food preparation, financial resources and limits, and cultural ideas and beliefs. The community is important here because of the resources it can offer.

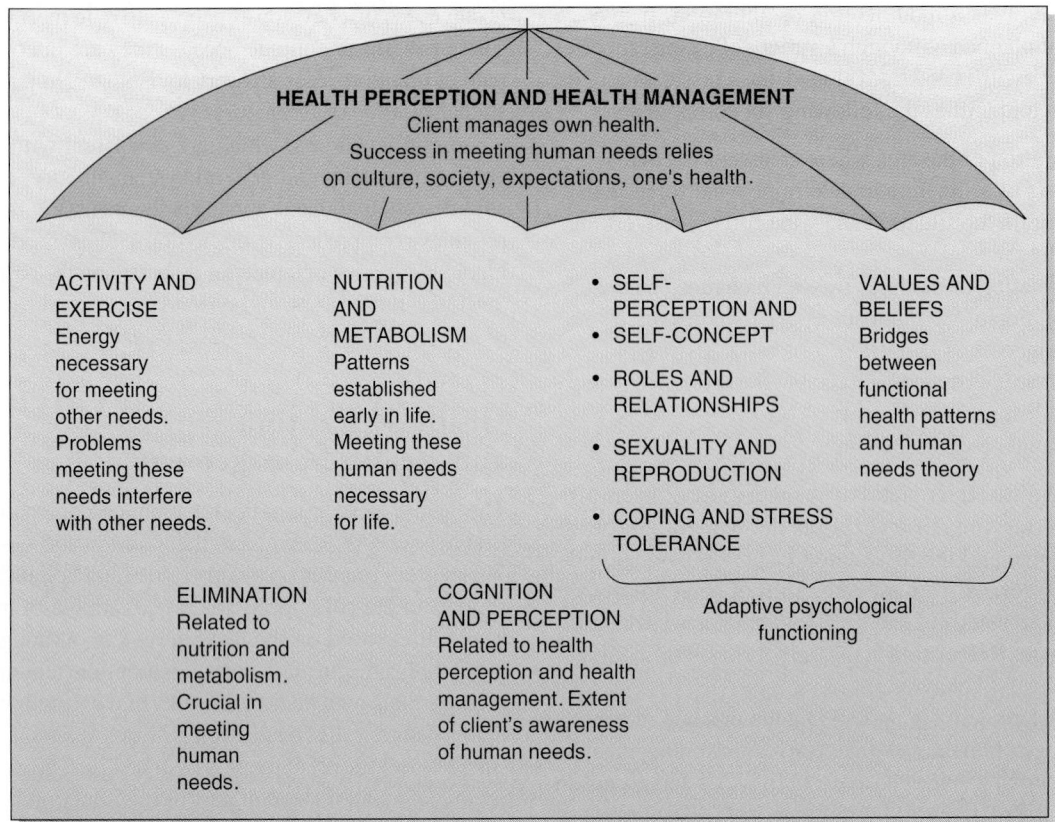

FIGURE 4-2   Relationship of functional health patterns, human needs theory, and delivery of nursing care. The first function, health perception and health management, forms an umbrella for the remaining ten patterns.

Elimination

Elimination is closely related to nutrition and metabolism. Often, these areas can be assessed simultaneously. Both are crucial to understanding the client's needs.

Sleep and Rest

Sleep and rest are primary human needs. Patterns begin to develop at birth and change throughout life. Newborns, for example, spend much time sleeping. Parents can reveal the amount of time and how an infant sleeps, thus showing a pattern. The person's environment may help or hinder this category of needs.

Cognition and Perception

The cognitive–perceptual pattern examines the extent of the client's awareness of human needs, which ties in with the first pattern, health perception–health management. Lifespan considerations are important when evaluating this pattern.

Other Patterns

The remaining patterns—self-perception and self-concept, roles and relationships, coping and stress tolerance, sexuality and reproduction, and values and beliefs—involve a complex

group of needs that are intimately related to the person's level of adaptive psychological functioning. Adequate examination of these patterns requires assessment of the client's intrapsychic and interpersonal functioning, which means looking at the client in relation to self, family, significant others, and community.

Values and beliefs provide the bridge to connect functional health patterns, human needs, and other theories. Understanding the client's value and belief system is crucial to learning about the importance of each human need as a motivating factor in the client's life, as a community member, and in relationships in his or her family.

KEY CONCEPTS

- Conceptual frameworks are a set of concepts that describe ideas about individuals, groups, situations, and events that are of special interest to nursing.
- Nursing theories use definitions of significant relationships between concepts to describe nursing. Common to all nursing theories are four major concepts: person, environment, health, and nursing.
- General systems theory requires analysis of the parts of a system, the relationships among these parts, and the purposes, reasons, and tasks of the system.
- Human needs (including any physiologic or psychological factor in life that is necessary for a healthy existence) are

motivational forces influenced by culture, socioeconomic factors, personal values, and health status.

- Maslow's theory of human needs presents a hierarchical ordering of human needs: physiologic needs, safety needs, belonging and love needs, esteem needs, and self-actualization needs.
- Change theory recognizes the dynamic nature of growth and the need for constant reevaluation of nursing practice.
- Use of functional health patterns offers a holistic approach to nursing. Patterns delineate the human needs of the client, family, and community. Functional health patterns provide for a comprehensive discussion of client needs by incorporating other nursing and non-nursing theories into a pattern design and description.

REFERENCES

Abdellah, F. G. (1960). *Patient-centered approaches to nursing.* New York: Macmillan.

Barnum, B. J. S. (1998). *Nursing theory: Analysis, application, evaluation* (5th ed.). Philadelphia: Lippincott Williams & Wilkins.

Chinn, P. L. (1994). *Theory and nursing. A systematic approach* (4th ed.). St. Louis, MO: Mosby.

Eakes, G. G., Burke, M. L., & Hainsworth, M. A. (1998). Middle-range theory of chronic sorrow. *Image: Journal of Nursing Scholarship, 30*(2), 179–184.

Fawcett, J. (1995). *Analysis and evaluation of conceptual models of nursing* (3rd ed.). Philadelphia: F. A. Davis.

Gordon, M. (1994). *Nursing diagnosis, process and application* (3rd ed.). St. Louis, MO: Mosby.

Hall, L. E. (1964). Nursing: What is it? *Canadian Nurse, 60,* 150–154.

Henderson, V. (1955). *The nature of nursing.* New York: Macmillan.

Jaarsma, T., Halfens, R., Senten, M., Saad, H. H. A., & Dracup, K. (1998). Developing a supportive-educative program for patients with advanced heart failure within Orem's general theory of nursing. *Nursing Science Quarterly, 11*(2), 79–85.

Johnson, D. E. (1980). The behavioral system model for nursing. In J. P. Riehl & C. Roy (Eds.), *Conceptual models for nursing practice* (3rd. ed.). New York: Appleton-Century-Crofts.

Lewin, K. (1962). Quasi-stationary social equilibria and the problem of permanent changes. In G. W. Bennis, K. D. Bennee, & R. Chin (Eds.), *The planning of change.* New York: Holt, Rinehart and Winston.

Lutjens, L. R., & Tiffany, C. R. (1994). Evaluating planned change theories. *Nursing Management, 25*(3), 54–57.

Marriner-Tomey, A., & Alligood, M. R. (1998). *Nursing theorists and their work* (4th ed.). St. Louis, MO: Mosby.

Maslow, A. H. (1970). *Motivation and personality* (2nd ed.). New York: Harper & Row.

Neuman, B. (1972). *The Neuman systems model: Application to nursing education and practice.* New York: Appleton-Century-Crofts.

Nightingale, F. (1860). *Notes on nursing: What it is and what it is not.* London: Harrison & Sons.

Orem, D. E. (1971). *Nursing: Concepts of practice* (3rd ed.). New York: McGraw-Hill.

Orlando, I. J. (1961). *The dynamic nurse–patient relationship: Function, process, and principles.* New York: Putnam.

Parse, R. R. (1981). *Man–living–health: Theory of nursing.* New York: John Wiley and Sons.

Peplau, H. E. (1952). *Interpersonal relations in nursing.* New York: Putnam.

Rogers, M. E. (1970). *An introduction to the theoretical basis of nursing.* Philadelphia: F. A. Davis.

Roy, C. (1980). The Roy adaptation model. In J. P. Riehl & C. Roy (Eds.), *Conceptual models for nursing practice.* New York: Appleton-Century Crofts.

Schultz, P. R., & Meleis, A. I. (1988). Nursing epistemology: Traditions, insights, questions. *Image: Journal of Nursing Scholarship, 20*(4), 217–221.

Tiffany, C. R. (1994). Analysis of planned change theories. *Nursing Management, 25*(2), 60–62.

Travelbee, J. (1971). *Interpersonal aspects of nursing.* Philadelphia: F. A. Davis.

von Bertalanffy, L. (1969). *General system theory.* New York: George Braziller.

von Bertalanffy, L. (1976). *Perspectives on general system theory: Scientific-philosophical studies.* New York: George Braziller.

Williams, C. A. (1979). The nature and development of conceptual frameworks. In F. S. Downs & J. W. Fleming (Eds.), *Issues in nursing research.* New York: Appleton-Century-Crofts.

Yura, H., & Walsh, M. (1988). *The nursing process: Assessing, planning, implementing, and evaluating* (5th ed.). Norwalk, CT: Appleton & Lange.

BIBLIOGRAPHY

Barrett, E. A. (1994). *Rogerian scientists, artists, revolutionaries* (NLN Publication 15-2610). (pp. 61–87). New York: National League for Nursing.

Benner, P. (2000). Links between philosophy, theory, practice, and research. *The Canadian Journal of Nursing Research, 32*(2), 7–13.

Bunting, S. (1993). *Rosemarie Parse: Theory of human becoming.* Newbury Park: Sage.

Carper, B. A. (1978). Fundamental patterns of knowing in nursing. *Advances in Nursing Science, 1*(11), 12–23.

Conway, J. (1994). Reflection: The art and science of nursing and the theory–practice gap. *British Journal of Nursing, 3*(3), 114–118.

Dixon, E. L. (1999). Community health nursing practice and the Roy Adaptation Model. *Public Health Nursing, 16*(4), 290–300.

Elkan, R., & Robinson, J. (1993). Project 2000: The gap between theory and practice. *Nurse Education Today, 13*(4), 295–298.

Evans, C. L. S. (1993). *Imogene King: A conceptual framework for nursing.* Newbury Park: Sage.

Forchuk, C. (1993). *Hildegard E. Peplau: Interpersonal nursing theory.* Newbury Park: Sage.

Hagerman, Z. J., & Tiffany, C. R. (1994). Evaluation of two planned change theories. *Nursing Management, 25*(4), 57–60, 62.

Hartweg, D. L. (1993). *Dorothea Orem: Self-care deficit theory.* Newbury Park: Sage.

Ireland, M. (2000). Martha Roger's odyssey. *The American Journal of Nursing, 100*(10), 59.

King, I. M. (1971). *Toward a theory of nursing.* New York: Wiley.

Laurent, C. L. (2000). A nursing theory for nursing leadership. *Journal of Nursing Management, 8*(2), 83–87.

Levesque, L., Ricard, N., Ducharme, F., Duquette, A., & Bonin, J. P. (1998). Empirical verification of a theoretical model derived from the Roy adaptation model: Findings from five studies. *Nursing Science Quarterly, 11*(1), 31–39.

Levine, M. C. (1973). *An introduction to clinical nursing* (2nd ed.). Philadelphia: F. A. Davis.

Lutjens, L. R. J. (1993). *Martha Rogers: The science of unitary human beings.* Newbury Park: Sage.

Lutjens, L. R. J. (1993). *Callista Roy: An adaptation model.* Newbury Park: Sage.

Marchione, J. (1993). *Margaret Newman: Health as expanding consciousness.* Newbury Park: Sage.

Montague, A. (1970). *The direction of human development.* New York: Hawthorne.

Newman, M. A. (1994). Theory for nursing practice. *Nursing Science Quarterly, 7*(4), 153–157.

Nursing Theories Conference Group. (1980). *Nursing theories: The base for professional nursing practice.* Englewood Cliffs, NJ: Prentice-Hall.

O'Connor, N. (1993). *Paterson and Zderad: Humanistic nursing theory.* Newbury Park: Sage.

O'Connor, N. (1990). *Nursing: Concepts of practice* (3rd ed.). St. Louis, MO: Mosby–Year Book.

Reed, S. (1993). *Betty Neuman: The systems model.* Newbury Park: Sage.

Reynolds, C. L., & Leininger, M. M. (1993). *Madeleine Leininger: Cultural care diversity and universality theory.* Newbury Park: Sage.

Rogers, M. E. (1994). *Nursing science evolves* (NLN Publication 15-2610). (pp. 3–9). New York: National League for Nursing.

Scammell, J. & Miller, S. (1999). Back to basics: Exploring the conceptual basis of nursing. *Nurse Education Today, 19*(7), 570–577.

Schmieding, N. J. (1993). *Ida Jean Orlando: A nursing process theory.* Newbury Park: Sage.

Selanders, L. C. (1993). *Florence Nightingale: An environmental adaptation theory.* Newbury Park: Sage.

Vander, A. J., Sherman, J. H., & Luciano, D. S. (1993). *Human physiology: The mechanisms of body function* (6th ed.). San Francisco: McGraw-Hill.

Watson, J. (1985). *Nursing: The philosophy and science of caring.* Boulder, CO: University Press.

Wright, P. S., Piazza, D., Holcombe, J., & Foote, A. (1994). A comparison of three theories of nursing used as a guide for the nursing care of an 8-year-old child with leukemia. *Journal of Pediatric Oncology Nursing, 11*(1), 14–19.

5 Values

Key Terms

attitudes
behaviors
beliefs
cultural value orientation
focus value
foundation value
future values
hierarchy of skills

imaginal skills
instrumental skills
interpersonal skills
moral values
systems skills
values
value system
world view

Learning Objectives

Upon completion of this chapter, the student will be able to do the following:
1. Define values.
2. Explain how behaviors relate to values.
3. Identify sources of professional nursing values.
4. Apply cultural and developmental perspectives when identifying values.
5. Relate values to functional health patterns.
6. Examine values conflict and resolution in nursing care situations.

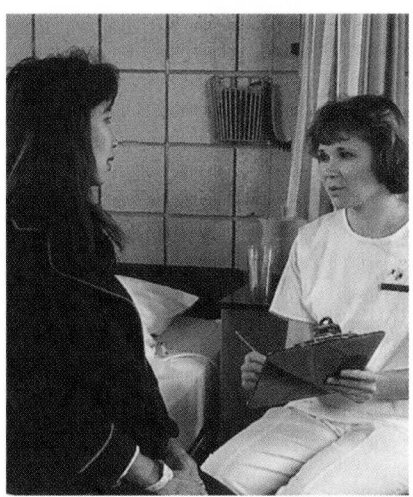

Critical Thinking Challenge

You are a nurse who is teaching health promotion measures to pregnant women. One woman with whom you have talked before approaches you after class. She asks you to look at her abdomen. Although she is in the early stages of pregnancy, her abdomen is the size of a soccer ball, and she complains of severe abdominal cramping. The woman is afraid to approach her regular healthcare provider because she is afraid that she will lose the pregnancy or will need to undergo a procedure that will compromise her ability to have children. She describes her family of origin as very child-focused, and she says she will not agree to any surgery that would make having children impossible.

Once you have completed this chapter and added values to your knowledge base, review the above scenario and reflect on the following areas of Critical Thinking:

1. Describe your initial thoughts and feelings concerning this woman and her situation.
2. Compare your responses with what the woman appears to be telling you about her values.
3. As you explore this situation, identify your values, and determine their origin.
4. As you imagine working with this woman, list sources for potential agreement and potential conflict.
5. Name some values that might be key in building a common ground and working relationship with this client.

What is really important in your life? How do you decide what actions to take? On what do you base your decisions? By thinking about the factors that influence your decision making, you find cues as to the critical values that have an impact on your life choices. By reflecting on your values, you become clearer about your purpose in life. Understanding these values assists you in decision making because you can more effectively articulate and defend your position. Evaluating your values also helps you develop a stronger sense of self.

Consciously or unconsciously, values have an impact on most of your decisions. These values reflect your needs, responses to situations, and relationships to significant others, culture, religion, and society at large. Values are not stable but vary among individuals and change according to life experiences and level of maturity. For example, what may be of value to you at age 20 may no longer matter to you at age 60.

As a beginning student of nursing, you have decided that you want to work with people and help them improve their health. If you examine your thoughts and feelings connected with this decision, you may find that you have a positive attitude toward people and that you like to be with others. You also probably like the study of biology and social sciences. A variety of other factors may have influenced your choice to become a nurse, such as your family, community, and religion. Perhaps you understood the critical need for caring nurses in a world of pain and suffering. Your decision to become a professional nurse reflects your values that will ultimately emerge in the way you care for clients and their families.

Just as you have core values, so do the clients, families, and healthcare organizations with whom you will work. Conflicts that arise usually relate to values. These value conflicts represent a variety of preferences and levels of development, and they can lead to ethical dilemmas for those involved. Whatever the conflict, nurses must understand their own values and be sensitive to those of others to be effective healthcare providers.

VALUE AND BELIEF PATTERNS

Values are standards for decision making that endure for a significant time in one's life (Hall, Kalven, Rosen, & Taylor, 1982). They are abstract ideas that have four parts: thinking, choosing, feeling, and behaving (King, 1984). Consider the values of "truth" and "honesty." These words mean little until a person has thought about them, makes a choice about being honest based on his or her feelings, and consequently behaves truthfully.

A **value system** is an enduring set of principles and rules organized into a hierarchy (Rokeach, 1973). When choosing between alternatives and making decisions, value systems help people decide which values are most important. Suppose a nurse is confronted with the following situation:

A client undergoes a series of diagnostic tests that reveal the early stages of a particular cancer. His doctor explains that this cancer typically progresses rapidly but has an excellent prognosis if treated aggressively with radiation and surgery. Later that day, the client informs you that he intends to try self-treatment with herbal and other natural remedies for a few months before progressing with the doctor's recommendations.

The nurse may be unsure how to respond to the client's decision. Values that the nurse will need to balance include truth, caring, harmony, duty, and responsibility. The situation might be further complicated if the nurse knows that the client's family or other healthcare team members have different preferences.

Attitudes, beliefs, and behaviors are often linked with values but are not the same as values (Hall et al., 1982). An **attitude** is one's disposition toward an object or a situation; it can be a mental or emotional mindset, and it can be positive or negative. **Beliefs** are ideas that one accepts as true; they may be expressed by such things as decisions, opinions, and creeds.

Behaviors are observable actions. Attitudes can be seen in behaviors and opinions. To continue with the above example of the client with cancer, the nurse's attitudes and beliefs about the client's condition would influence the valuing process. The nurse's ultimate behaviors, however, would demonstrate the values that held priority. Attitudes, beliefs, and behaviors are value indicators; if nurses take time to reflect on them, they will be able to realize and articulate their values and value systems.

Moral values involve correct behavior, such as having some sense of right and wrong or "oughtness" (Rokeach, 1973). They are moral because they deal with human interactions that involve the integrity of life or health.

Professional Values in Nursing

Professional nursing values can be traced in the discipline's history and traditions. As described in Chapter 3, nursing's Judeo-Christian heritage promoted care for the sick and poor. This heritage contributed many of the foundational values on which professional nursing was established. Florence Nightingale reflected these values when she described a personal "call to service" and showed commitment to this calling at a time when nursing was looked on as a service provided by the lowest members of society. From the Nightingale Pledge in 1893 (Display 5-1) to documents such as the current Code for Nurses of the American Nurses Association (ANA, 1985), nurses have endeavored to identify and define standards of practice. These standards are based on universal moral principles or values, the central one being respect for people, or human dignity. Other values based on human dignity include promoting self-determination, doing good, avoiding harm, telling the truth, respecting privileged information, keeping promises, and treating people fairly. When one enters nursing, however, one also "inherits a measure of both the responsibility and the trust that have accrued to nursing over the years" (American Association of Colleges of Nursing, 1998); thus, one becomes a part of the nursing tradition of service.

A second statement of values, advanced by the American Association of Colleges of Nursing (AACN) in *Essentials of Baccalaureate Education for Professional Nursing Practice* (American Association of Colleges of Nursing, 1998), identifies five core values for nurses: altruism, autonomy, human

DISPLAY 5-1

⬚ **NIGHTINGALE PLEDGE**

"I solemnly pledge myself before God and in the presence of this assembly to pass my life in purity and to practice my profession faithfully. I will abstain from whatever is deleterious and mischievous, and will not take or knowingly administer any harmful drug. I will do all in my power to maintain and elevate the standard of my profession, and will hold in confidence all personal matters committed to my keeping and all family affairs coming to my knowledge in the practice of my calling. With loyalty will I endeavor to aid the physician in his work, and devote myself to the welfare of those committed to my care."

dignity, integrity, and social justice. The AACN stresses that nurses need to adopt these essential values to have a sense of commitment and social responsibility, a sensitivity and responsiveness to the needs of others, and responsibility for themselves and their actions.

Although both the ANA and the AACN have provided statements on the importance of values (Table 5-1), how do nursing students develop these values? Three important ways of doing so are through socialization, classroom study, and clinical study.

Socialization

Initial learning of values begins in childhood as part of ongoing socialization in the family, school, religion, ethnicity, and social groups. People may not begin to question why they hold certain values until they face experiences apart from those shared with important socializing groups. Essentially, socialization happens by the process of living and experiencing in family and society. If the student comes from a family

TABLE 5-1

Values in Professional Nursing	
ANA Code of Ethics	**AACN Essentials**
Human dignity	Altruism
Autonomy	Autonomy
Doing good	Integrity
Avoiding harm	Human dignity
Truth-telling	Social justice
Confidentiality	
Keeping promises	
Justice	

From: American Nurses Association. (1985). *Code for nurses with interpretive statements.* Kansas City, MO: Author; American Association of Colleges of Nursing. (1998). *Essentials of baccalaureate education for professional nursing.* Washington, DC: Author.

of healthcare professionals, this too is part of the socialization process.

Classroom Study

Values Clarification. Values clarification is "a method of self-discovery by which people identify their personal values and their value rankings" (King, 1984, p. 25). This process does not evaluate values as such but helps people identify their own values. According to Raths, Harmin, and Simon (1978), there are three phases to this process (choosing, prizing, and acting) and seven steps (Display 5-2).

People can use values clarification in several ways:

- To examine past situations and decisions
- To conduct general case studies
- To explore how they spend their time by listing activities in a typical 24-hour period

Whatever the vehicle for examination of values, certain assumptions underlie the process. First, for people freely to choose beliefs and behaviors, they must have a sense of who they are, or a sense of self (King, 1984). Sense of self generally begins to develop in late childhood, and individuation is well established by young adulthood. If individuation has not occurred to some degree, a person's chosen values will reflect those of others and be externalized rather than internalized. Second, people need to have basic self-esteem to be confident in relying on their feelings, beliefs, and behaviors as guides for decision making (King, 1984).

The prizing and cherishing of one's beliefs and behaviors tend to affirm self-worth and contribute to a sense of inner harmony, purpose, and meaning (King, 1984). These feelings are rewarding and enable one to act more easily on indicated choices. As a person acts on his or her beliefs repeatedly and consistently in various situations, a mature, self-conscious, personal value system begins to emerge.

Values Inquiry. Whereas values clarification is a method of self-discovery of personal values, values inquiry (King, 1984) is a method of examining social issues and the values that motivate human choices. Case studies and issue-laden incidents provide ways to facilitate the inquiry process. A predetermined series of questions aids in discussing the issues. One set of questions follows:

- What are the facts?
- What can be inferred from the facts?
- What can be inferred from the person's value system?
- What evidence supports these inferences?

Another set of questions useful in assisting with values inquiry is based on problem solving:

- What is the problem?
- What other alternatives are options?
- What are the possible consequences of each alternative?
- What is the evidence that these consequences might occur?
- What are the advantages and disadvantages of each consequence and why?

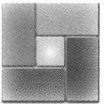

Nursing Research and Critical Thinking
Does Forgiveness Reduce Tension as a Result of a Reprioritizing of Values Frequently Caused by a Diagnosis of Cancer?

A significant goal for nursing is improving or maintaining the quality of life of patients with cancer. Terminally ill patients frequently find that an inability to forgive hurtful events from their pasts often causes severe negative emotional responses that stay with them over time. Recent research into the concept of forgiveness has shown that becoming able to forgive the hurts experienced in one's life leads to the general benefits of psychological and spiritual growth; reduced negative emotions such as sadness, anger, and anxiety; ability to let go of the past and get on with life; cessation of hurtful behaviors; increased ability to reestablish or build new relationships; and transcendence. Furthermore, there are indications that forgiveness may lead to a more accepting and peaceful death, help solidify a sense of meaning in life, help restore healthy relationships, and promote serenity in the dying process.

Nurse researchers designed a study to generate a grounded substantive theory of the process of forgiveness in patients with cancer. Employing a qualitative approach—grounded theory—the researchers used a sample of 25 adult patients with cancer between ages 35 and 88 years (mean = 62.4 years): 13 men and 12 women receiving active, palliative, or terminal treatment. The researchers used open-ended interviews that they transcribed verbatim and analyzed using constant comparative analysis, and expert and participant validation. The main research variable was forgiveness as reflected in the participants' past and current experiences.

The researchers found that a cancer diagnosis promotes a rethinking of life priorities. They found that each participant could describe hurtful events that initially caused severe negative emotional responses. However, the participants also described a desire to focus on living out priority values that was prompted by their cancer diagnosis. It was found that an escalating tension developed for the participants between their maintenance of negative emotions and being able to act on their personal values. Forgiveness was used to relieve this tension. To gain perspective, the participants used several methods that allowed them to resolve negative emotions and learn to live out their priority values. The participants used forgiveness to help clarify their personal values as well as to eliminate the negative emotions that remained from an inflicted hurt.

Critical Thinking Considerations. When grounded theory methodology is used, data are simultaneously collected, analyzed, and interpreted from the time of the initial encounters with the research participants. All of the data are compared with each other, and the theory evolves into categories that are compared constantly with each other and with new data as it is collected. Possible implications include the following:

- A cancer diagnosis often promotes reprioritizing values that involve forgiveness.
- Tension often results between harboring anger or bitterness and wanting to achieve reprioritized goals.
- Patients may use forgiveness to help resolve this tension.
- Nurses can facilitate the healing process by helping patients to identify and clarify priority values.

From Mickley, J. R. & Cowles, K. (2001). Ameliorating the tension: Use of forgiveness for healing. *Oncology Nursing Forum, 28(1), 31–37.*

DISPLAY 5-2

PHASES AND STEPS IN VALUES CLARIFICATION

Choosing One's Beliefs and Behaviors
1. Choosing freely
2. Choosing from among alternatives
3. Choosing after consideration of the consequences

Prizing One's Beliefs and Behaviors
4. Prizing and cherishing
5. Affirming

Acting on One's Beliefs
6. Acting on choices
7. Repeating

Adapted from Raths, L. E., Harmin, M., & Simon, S. B. (1966). *Values and teaching* (2nd ed.). Columbus, OH: Charles E. Merrill.

- What would you do if you were in this situation and why?

Unlike values clarification, which can be an individual or a group experience, values inquiry lends itself more exclusively to group discussion (Fig. 5-1). The process increases understanding, enhances empathy within a broader social context, and increases communication skills and the ability to verbalize one's position.

Applied Ethics. Nurses must acknowledge and be aware of their personal and professional values when they confront ethical dilemmas. Of particular importance are moral values, or those that deal with right and wrong behavior toward other human beings. Analyzing and critiquing case studies assists in applying certain ethical principles or values, such as respect for people, honesty, and justice. Consideration of case studies also aids in developing moral reasoning skills and, if done in a group discussion, communication skills (King, 1984).

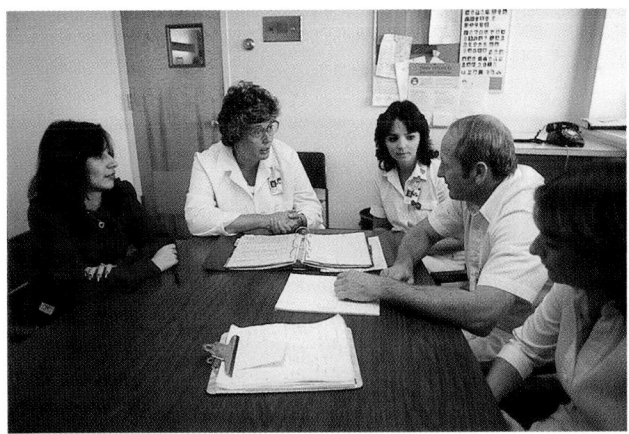

FIGURE 5-1 Values inquiry uses group discussion to examine social issues and values that motivate human choice.

Clinical Study

The major learning experience in clinical study is client care. After nurses become proficient in giving basic client care, they usually examine whether the care was effective, what made it effective, and whether it was acceptable to the client. When answering these questions, what is important to the client and to the nurse becomes apparent. The whole care-planning process is a value-rich situation. The questions asked during the nursing assessment, the prioritizing of nursing diagnoses, and the establishment of client goals all reflect values.

If the care-planning process is mutual and the nurse takes the client's values into account, the nursing care will support the client's unique qualities; "if a person's values are ignored or replaced with the values of others, the person ceases to exist as a singular human being" (Curtin & Flaherty, 1981, p. 90). If the nurse affirms the client's values during the caring process, he or she also affirms the client as a worthwhile person. Therefore, the study of client care includes a consciousness of the client's values and the nurse's values and how these interact in the care-giving process.

SOURCES OF VALUES

Values come from many sources. Some authors, such as Fromm and Maslow, believe that values are rooted in the conditions of human existence, which are intrinsic in the structure of human nature, both genetically and culturally (Fromm, 1959). Kidder (1994), a long-time columnist for the *Christian Science Monitor,* explored the proposition that some values are so fundamental to humans that they transcend cultural boundaries. He interviewed 24 articulate, thoughtful people from all over the world to discover their core values and whether commonalities existed. His goal was to explore the possibility of a global code of values. Through an analysis and synthesis process, he identified eight core, universal values: love, truthfulness, fairness, freedom, unity, tolerance, responsibility, and respect for life. These values were elicited from visionary people and demonstrate that humans share a basic understanding of how to live together.

Cultural Influences

If some values appear universal, why do cultures seem so different from one another? Daily living is expressed in so many different traditions and customs that it is hard to discern universal qualities. Two ideas are important to understanding why this is; one is world view, and the other is cultural value orientation.

World view (Walsh & Middleton, 1984) is an unquestioned framework or predominant set of assumptions through which people view life; it is a perspective, an outlook, or an image of reality. A world view also guides actions and determines values. For example, one culture's world view may be more easily captured in a story or a myth that explains how the people came to be and how they ought to live. The "American dream" encompasses a whole range of values, such as individualism, equality, freedom, privacy, change, progress, achievement, and materialism.

Cultural value orientation, a theory originated by Kluckhohn in the 1950s and applied to nursing by Brink (1984), can be seen as a subset of world view. There are four general orientations: nature, time, activity, and relationships. Each orientation has three types of responses. Consider the nature orientation and its three responses: mastery, subjugation, and harmony. If one believes that humans are masters of nature, then one values problem solving and intervention. If one believes that humans are subjugated to nature, then one values wonder, awe, or fate and focuses more on safety and survival. If one believes that humans should act in harmony with nature, then one values balance with it. Table 5-2 outlines the four general orientations and their different responses.

By understanding the premise of universal values identified by Kidder (1994), along with the concepts of world view and cultural values orientation, one can better appreciate the variation in meanings of behavior across cultures.

Socializing Influences

In addition, values are codified in such social institutions as the family, school, and religion. Children learn values in several ways. Parents and family caregivers, teachers, and other authority figures reward and punish behavior; language colors thinking and perception; significant others model behavior; the media produce a variety of images that influence behavior; and unspoken expectations direct behavior (Hall et al., 1982). During adolescence and young adulthood, people are likely to encounter a variety of values and become more aware of differences. The process of value refinement continues throughout life. It may be a result of a planned, self-conscious discovery process, or it may be a matter of living and dealing with life situations as they arise. Two more phenomena that make it possible to become more conscious of values manifest themselves in adolescence: social perspective taking and formal reasoning. Both abilities enable a person to understand and have empathy for another's thoughts, feelings, and points of view.

TABLE 5-2

Cultural Value Orientations with Associated Values from Hall			
Orientations		**Associated Values**	
Person–nature	**Mastery**	**Subjugation**	**Harmony**
	Control	Fate	Equilibrium
	Order	Awe	Balance
	Planning	Survival	Integration
Time	**Future**	**Present**	**Past**
	Management	Wonder	Tradition
	Achievement	Flexibility	Ritual
	Research	Sensory pleasure	Obligation
Relational	**Individual**	**Collateral**	**Linear**
	Independence	Mutual accountability	Authority
	Competition	Belonging	Discipline
	Success		Hierarchy
Activity	**Doing**	**Being**	**Being-in-Becoming**
	Productivity	Being self	Self-actualization
	Efficiency	Expressiveness	Wholeness
	Profits	Celebration	Search/meaning

From: Brink, P. J. (1984). Values orientations as an assessment tool in cultural diversity. *Nursing Research, 33,* 198–203; Hall, B. (1980). *The personal discernment inventory.* New York: Paulist Press.

Community

An institution (e.g., college, workplace) forms a sense of community by fostering values and goals that it consistently integrates into its various activities. The institution further enhances these values when it treats people with consideration, according to its stated values. The experience of community also provides a supportive environment in which one can experiment more freely with various attitudes, beliefs, and behaviors.

Peer Culture

The attitudes, beliefs, and behaviors that grow out of peer group relationships are powerful (Fig. 5-2). Peer groups define themselves by common interests, needs, and problems. Out of these similar interests and bonds, the group clarifies its values.

Role Models

Effective role models demonstrate the values that they believe and promote. Affirming values in this manner has a more powerful impact than "preaching." Young adults, especially quick to recognize incongruities between talking and doing, respond to mature adults who make an effort to live by what they say. Unfortunately, many role models fail to reflect on their own values and as a result model conflict and confusion.

Experiences That Challenge a Way of Thinking

All of life's experiences can challenge a person's values, but it is the discerning person who actually reflects on these experiences and articulates and integrates them into practice.

One theorist, Brian Hall (1980), considers life experiences and potential growth by recognizing phases of values development. People using his tools can assess where their core values lie and make plans to develop them through exposing themselves to a variety of life experiences in a planned way.

As discussed previously, values are reflected through a person's attitudes, beliefs, and behaviors. Behavior, however, demonstrates whether a person truly holds and lives out a value. Brian Hall (1991) identified three levels of valuing: foundation, focus, and future (Fig. 5-3).

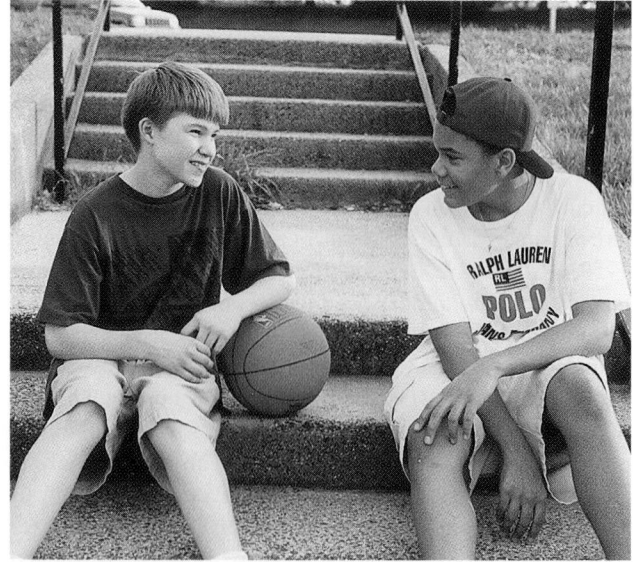

FIGURE 5-2 Peer relationships can have a significant influence on an individual's values.

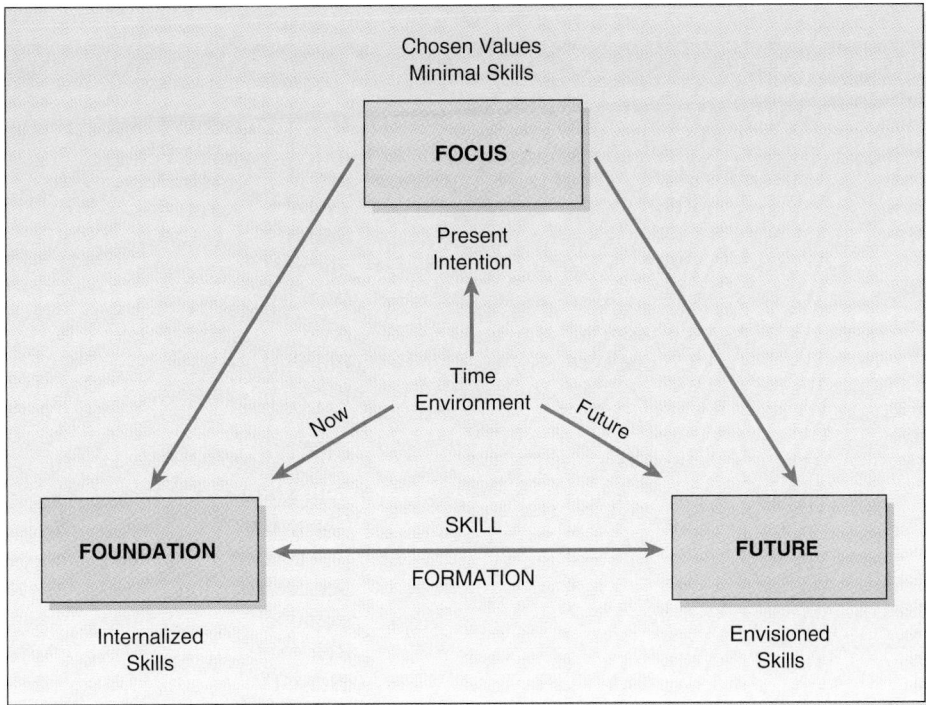

FIGURE 5-3   Three levels of valuing: Focus, Foundation, and Future. (From Hall, B. [1980]. *The personal discernment inventory* (p. 36). New York: Paulist Press.)

In this schema, two kinds of behavior indicate a held value. One kind is habitual; the person does not have to think about it. For example, such health practices as brushing and flossing teeth can become a routine part of morning care; maintaining these habits would indicate a **foundation value.** Another type of behavior relies on choice; the person does this behavior only when he or she sets it as a goal. For example, a dentist also recommends the use of a water-spray oral hygiene device. To add this procedure to the morning routine, the person would need to purchase the equipment and allow additional time for using it. He or she might also need to set the alarm to get up earlier. Until these additional behaviors become habits, the extra dental care would remain a choice or **focus value.** On the other hand, if the person only thought about buying a water-spray device, telling the dentist that he or she thought it was a good idea, the value of additional dental care would remain a vision or **future value;** it would not become "real" until the person acted on it. Future values are those that people ultimately would like to hold but that they momentarily lack the knowledge or skills necessary to integrate into their lives.

Lifespan Considerations

Values can reflect a person's age and stage of development. Although not everyone automatically develops all values, most people's values change or are refined by their various life experiences. Table 5-3 illustrates key values during dif-

ferent stages of life, combining Erikson's (1982) and Hall's theories of development.

Newborn and Infant

At the most basic level, infants begin value development with the establishment of trust and autonomy. Moral development and cognitive ability are closely related during these life stages.

Toddler and Preschooler

As children progress to toddlerhood, moral and values development begins as they identify behaviors that elicit reward or punishment. Kohlberg (1964) refers to this process as the first-level preconventional stage; children learn to distinguish right from wrong and understand the choice between obedience and punishment.

Preschoolers learn that rules are unchanging and are imposed by parents and other adults. In this later stage of development, children recognize and accept fairness and cooperation, although their self-interest and self-will limit the capacity to do so. Children are concerned when the situation seems "unfair" to them, yet do not have enough maturity to project that same sense of fairness to their peers.

Child and Adolescent

School-age children are industrious, recognizing the need for moral codes and social rules. Younger children in this age group maintain a strict understanding and application of the rules, seeing things in clearly dichotomous ways (i.e., right or wrong). As children grow into preadolescence, they become

TABLE 5-3

Values and Life Stages		
Developmental Stage	**Erikson's Values**	**Hall's Phases of Consciousness and Associated Values**
Infant	Hope	**Phase I**
		Security
Toddler	Will	Survival
		Wonder
Preschool	Purpose	Awe
School age	Competence	**Phase II**
		Belonging
		Work
Adolescence	Loyalty	Self-competence
		Self-worth
Young adulthood	Love	**Phase III**
		Independence
		Service/vocation
Middle adulthood	Care	Creation
		Being self
Older adulthood	Wisdom	**Phase IV**
		Harmony
		Interdependence
		Intimacy
		Esthetics

From: Erikson, E. (1982). *The life cycle completed.* New York: W. W. Norton; Hall, B. (1980). *The personal discernment inventory.* New York: Paulist Press.

more flexible. The threat of discipline becomes less important than social expectations. Kohlberg (1964) refers to this as the second-level or conventional stage, characterized by conformity to expectations and behaviors of others.

For adolescents, the influence of peer identification reaches its greatest persuasiveness. Although this period of development is often characterized by rebellion, adolescents have a high level of moral judgment with a law-and-order orientation. Adolescents understand that morality derives from principles of conscience and that rules are cooperative agreements that can be modified. As people reach late adolescence, they begin to move away from strong peer influence according to their individual principles, and peer group values decrease in importance.

Adult and Older Adult

Adults focus on intimacy and generativity as they form careers and families. Primary moral concerns are now directed toward meeting the expectations of employers, family, and adult social groups. Values that adults learned and developed in childhood usually evolve into what they will accept as guiding principles for life.

Older adults focus on personal integrity and the wisdom that they have accumulated over a lifetime. Values are firmly ingrained, yet older adults are often more accepting of values of others that may differ from their own.

EFFECT OF VALUES ON FUNCTIONAL HEALTH

When assessing values related to functional health, the nurse needs to be aware of three levels of information: general human needs, social and culture-specific needs, and individual or personal needs. These needs are discussed in detail in Chapters 4, 19, and 20. These levels determine client behaviors and indicate the values that influence health status.

The nursing profession has identified 11 functional health patterns that represent general, basic human needs. For example, the preceding discussion about values and dental care falls under the second pattern, nutrition and metabolism.

Functional health patterns of clients, whether individuals, families, or communities, evolve for client-centered interactions. Each pattern is an expression of biopsychosocial integration. No one pattern can be understood without knowledge of other patterns (Gordon, 1997). In assessing these functional health patterns, nurses need to consider the individual's baseline health status; established norms for specific age groups; and cultural, social, or other norms.

The culture or social group also defines how the client views health. The culture may promote specific beliefs about health, the body, and the cause and cure of illness that, in turn, dictate certain behaviors and indicate values. For example, in a Southeast Asian culture, the top of a person's head is sacred; if something covers this area, the person's spirit is harmed. For people from this culture, certain diagnostic procedures, medical treatments, or surgeries are frightening and cause conflicts between values of spiritual well-being and medical care.

Finally, each client is unique, expressing personal preferences and values. For example, some clients like touch, whereas others do not.

Understanding includes being sensitive to clients' values and their perceptions of the functional health patterns. Nurses should move from the perspective of general human needs to cultural or social needs and finally to unique individual needs to avoid stereotyping. The following sections briefly review the 11 health patterns, relating values issues to each. The values identified with each pattern are taken from the list of 120 values (Display 5-3) identified by Hall (1980).

Health Perception and Health Management

Personal health is a value. The basis of this value resides in people's value to themselves, usually expressed as self-esteem or self-acceptance. Health values also reflect beliefs about the nature of health and health practices; most of these beliefs and practices are culturally or socially defined. For example, a culture may view good health as an indicator of balance in life or of being a good person. To maintain health as a value, additional values are necessary to carry out health practices; these might include discipline, planning, responsibility, education, and cooperation. When working with specific people, nurses need to assess how the clients experience health and what they do to maintain health, all within their cultural and social environment. A client's level of self-esteem, which also is a value, reflects the ability to incorporate new health behaviors into his or her lifestyle.

Activity and Exercise

The activity and exercise pattern deals with a person's energy level. Values associated with this pattern include sensory pleasure, competition, image, play, leisure, relaxation, and recreation. People give different levels of value to exercise. Some people give priority to other values or do not have the time management skills to incorporate exercise programs into their schedules.

Nutrition and Metabolism

The essential value represented by the nutrition and metabolism pattern is survival; however, various attitudes and beliefs about nutrition represent cultural and personal preferences. Food presentation may reflect esthetic values, such as art and beauty, and meal times may reflect socialization values, such as family, work, service, or ritual. For example, some cultures emphasize the color, texture, and design of food; others emphasize social interaction at meal times. An example of values involving food preparation is expressed in the book *Like Water for Chocolate* (Esquivel, 1992).

Elimination

Values associated with excretory functions may include sensory pleasure, control, discipline, and self-competence. Practices associated with these functions are learned within cultural and family frameworks. For example, one can observe the various body care products (e.g., cleansers, deodorants, perfumes) that are advertised and available in a culture or society to ascertain that group's perception of the body.

Sleep and Rest

Survival is the value basic to the sleep and rest pattern, but culture and family also support practices related to sleep and rest; siestas and coffee breaks are examples. Also, the manner of sleeping varies across cultures and families; family members might sleep in separate beds and bedrooms or in a large family room on mats on the floor. Generally, all people need 6 to 8 hours of sleep per day, but much variability relates to age, occupation, and individual needs.

Cognition and Perception

The cognition and perception pattern involves the five senses, language, memory, and decision making. Values associated with this area include sensory pleasure, expressiveness, communication, rationality, evaluation, and intuition. Language is probably the most important of these aspects, because it reflects cultural patterns of thinking in such areas as time, space, and world view. Within that culture, a person's sentence structure indicates his or her thinking process, reality orientation, and sensory preference.

The four value orientations (human nature, time, activity, and relationships) have numerous implications for thinking and perceiving. They affect a person's understanding of the illness process, interventions in the process, the decision as to which people are to be involved in the process, and acceptable treatments. One way to understand this pattern is to read Tony Hillerman's detective novels, which are set in the Navajo culture of the southwestern United States (e.g., Hillerman, 1999). Hillerman successfully captures the value orientations of "present," harmony with nature, collateral or tribal relationships, and "doing" as the investigation unfolds. Because a murder is usually involved, the reader should pay particular attention to the author's understanding of the body and the spirit.

Self-Perception and Self-Concept

Values underlying this pattern are self-preservation, self-delight, self-worth, self-competency, self-assertion, self-actualization, integration, and being oneself. Initially, the family and larger society prescribe how one should think and feel about oneself. In a culture that values individuality and independence, the emphasis is on a unique sense of self apart from the group.

DISPLAY 5-3

⌐ **HALL'S VALUE LIST WITH SKILLS**

Values	Skills	Values	Skills
1. Accountability/mutual	IS	50. Family belonging	IP
2. Achievement/success	I_2	51. Fantasy/play	IM
3. Adaptability/flexibility	IP	52. Food/warmth/shelter	I_2
4. Administration/control	I_2	53. Friendship/belonging	IP
5. Affection/physical	IP	54. Function	I_2
6. Art/beauty as pure value	IM	55. Generosity/service	IP
7. (Self) assertion	IP	56. Growth/expansion	IS
8. Being liked	IP	57. Harmony/system	IS
9. Being self	IS	58. Health/personal	IS
10. Care/nurture	IP	59. Hierarchy/property/order	IS
11. (Self) centeredness	IP	60. Honor	IS
12. Communications	I_2	61. Human dignity	IS
13. Community/personalist	IS	62. Independence	IP
14. Community/supportive	IS	63. Instrumentality	I_2
15. Competition	I_2	64. Integration/wholeness	IP
16. (Self) competence/confidence	I_2	65. Interdependence	IS
17. Congruence	IP	66. Intimacy	IP
18. Construction/new order	IS	67. Intimacy and solitude as unitive	IP
19. Contemplation/asceticism	I_2	68. Justice	IS
20. (Self) control	IP	69. Knowledge/discovery/insight	I_2
21. Control/order/discipline	I_2	70. Law/guide	IS
22. Convivial tool/intermediate	IS	71. Law/rule	I_2
23. Cooperation	IS	72. Life/self-actualization	IP
24. Corporation/construction/new order	IS	73. Limitation/celebration	IP
25. Courtesy/respect	IP	74. Loyalty/respect	IP
26. Creativity/ideation	IM	75. Macroeconomics	IS
27. Criteria/rationality	I_2	76. Management	I_2
28. (Self) delight	IM	77. Membership	I_2
29. Decision/initiation	IP	78. Mission/goals	IS
30. Design/pattern/order	I_2	79. Obedience/duty	IP
31. Detachment/solitude	IS	80. Obedience/mutual accountability	IS
32. (Self) directedness	IP	81. Objectivity	I_2
33. Discernment/communal	IM	82. Ownership	IP
34. Discovery/delight	IS	83. Patriotism/esteem	IP
35. Duty/obligation	IP	84. Pioneerism/innovation/progress	IS
36. Economics/profit	I_2	85. Play/leisure	IP
37. Economics/success	I_2	86. Poverty/simplicity	IS
38. Ecority/beauty/aesthetics	IM	87. Pluriformity	IS
39. Education/certification	I_2	88. Power/authority/honesty	IP
40. Education/knowledge/insight	I_2	89. Presence/dwelling	IP
41. Efficiency/planning	I_2	90. (Self) preservation	IP
42. Empathy	IP	91. Prestige/image	IP
43. Equality/liberation	IP	92. Productivity	I_2
44. Equilibrium	IS	93. Property/control	I_2
45. Equity/rights	IP	94. Recreation/freesence	IM
46. Ethics/accountability/values	I_2	95. Relaxation	IS
47. Evaluation/skill self system	IP	96. Research/originality/knowledge	IM
48. Expressiveness/freedom	IM	97. Responsibility	IP
49. Faith/risk	IP	98. Ritual/meaning	IS

(continued)

DISPLAY 5-3 (Continued)

🔳 HALL'S VALUE LIST WITH SKILLS

Values	Skills	Values	Skills
99. Rule/accountability	I_2	110. Tradition	IS
100. Safety/survival	I_2	111. Transcendence/global confluence	IS
101. Search/meaning	IM	112. Truth/wisdom/intuitive insight	IM
102. Security	IP	113. Unity/solidarity	IP
103. Sensory pleasure/sex	IP	114. Wonder/awe/fate	IM
104. Service/vocation	IS	115. Wonder/curiosity	IM
105. Sharing/listening/trust	IP	116. Word	IS
106. Simplicity/play	I_2	117. Work/labor	I_2
107. Social affirmation	IS	118. Workmanship/craft	I_2
108. Support peer	IP	119. Worship/duty/creed	I_2
109. Synergy	IS	120. (Self) worth	IP

I_2, instrumental skills; IP, interpersonal skills; IM, imaginal skills; IS, system skills.
Adapted from Hall, B. (1980). *The personal discernment inventory.* New York: Paulist Press.

Roles and Relationships

How people relate to others is often defined by their function or role. Some values associated with the many possible role relationships include belonging, social affiliation, support, work, duty, ownership, membership, education, service, power, authority, cooperation, and intimacy. The major roles in our society are family roles, student or work roles, and social roles.

Coping and Stress Management

Although people respond to stress in many ways, the basic values underlying this pattern are self-preservation, safety, and survival. Other values related to this pattern reflect various coping styles; such values include support, competition, equilibrium, control, planning, management, flexibility, assertion, relaxation, sharing, listening, education, creativity, detachment, cooperation, and insight.

Sexuality and Reproduction

The pattern of sexuality and reproduction is closely associated with self-concept and role relationships. Self-delight, self-control, belonging, sharing, wholeness, being oneself, and intimacy are values associated with this pattern. Participation and levels of satisfaction are usually defined within the society and culture. For example, the focus of sexuality may be primarily on reproduction, or it may be on intimacy and pleasure.

Values and Beliefs

The values and beliefs pattern reflects a person's overall attitude or feeling about life and is associated with hope, meaning, and purpose. It may involve spiritual and religious issues that support the person's world view and attitudes about the importance of life and the meaning of death. Values typical of this pattern include wonder, duty, loyalty, tradition, worship, design, law, unity, service, search, human dignity, intimacy, justice, mission, faith, truth, and transcendence.

MANIFESTATIONS OF NURSES' VALUES

Nurses demonstrate their professional and personal values in their attitudes and behaviors. For example, a nurse may say that he or she values family and belonging. Observation of the nurse's interaction with families can either conform to these values or indicate a discrepancy between what the nurse says and what he or she does. When a nurse claims to value family and belonging but does not demonstrate this through behavior when caring for clients, the nurse might be deficient in communication skills or might not understand family dynamics. Therefore, this value would be a future value or an ideal not yet incorporated into the nurse's behavior.

In Hall's schema, values also can be organized in a **hierarchy of skills** (Hall, 1980). These skills are instrumental, interpersonal, imaginal, and systems. **Instrumental skills,** the first level, are associated with basic physical and intellectual competencies that enable one to shape ideas and the external environment. Nursing examples of instrumental skills are the knowledge and clinical application necessary to provide basic client care (e.g., skin care, wound care, range of motion, vital signs). **Interpersonal skills** determine a person's ability to relate happily and productively with others. Communication skills, such as listening and sharing; problem-solving skills; teaching; and counseling are some of the interpersonal skills that are necessary in nursing (Fig. 5-4). **Imaginal skills** bring imagination and creativity into play, enabling the nurse to en-

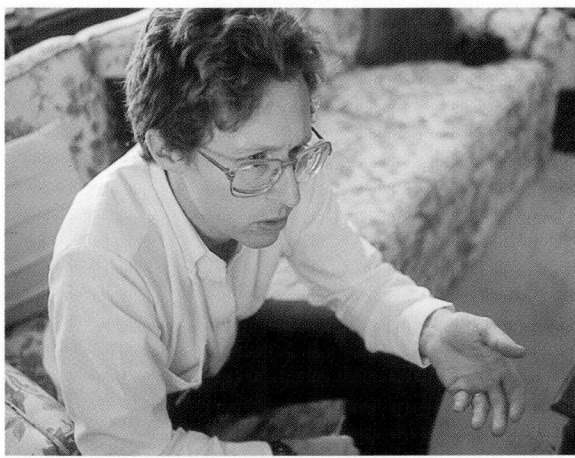

FIGURE 5-4   Effective communication is an example of an interpersonal skill necessary in nursing.

vision a plan for adapting and personalizing client care. The values that support imaginal skills are esthetic; esthetics also was an essential value of nursing, as identified by the AACN (1985). **Systems skills** are those that help a person see the whole picture and how various parts relate. As nurses initiate changes in one aspect of client care, they need to be aware of how these changes may affect other institutions in the community, such as home health or hospice, family group homes, senior citizens centers, multiservice agencies, community health departments, schools, and churches.

Returning to the example of the nurse whose future values are family and belonging, knowledge of family dynamics and communication are instrumental skills. Understanding the process of the nurse–client relationship and being able to form relationships built on trust are interpersonal skills. For the value of family and belonging to become a behavioral reality, the nurse sets goals to use family dynamics knowledge and to practice communication. That is, this value is a choice (focus) value until the nurse does the behaviors automatically. An essential value of the nursing profession is human dignity. Knowledge of family dynamics and communication are values that support the higher value of human dignity. In Hall's schema, human dignity is a systems skill, the most complex of all the skills. It requires incorporation not only of instrumental and interpersonal skills but also of imaginal skills. When these skills are integrated, the nurse can move beyond a particular family and begin to think of family health programs in the larger healthcare system. At this level, human dignity for all families becomes an action (foundation) value.

VALUE CONFLICTS

Whenever there is human interaction, value conflicts are likely to occur. These conflicts can be resolved if nurses are aware of their own values and the values of others. Resolving such conflicts may entail a values clarification and an appreciation

and acceptance of differences. Because value conflicts may affect a client's compliance with nursing care, the nurse's appreciation and acceptance of value differences can be the basis of negotiation and compromise.

Client and Family Conflicts

Value conflicts between family members arise from differences in developmental stages, experiences, and personal preferences. One fairly common example is when one spouse refuses to take the time to have a health checkup. Depending on how a person experienced the healthcare system in early life, the person refusing care may hold the values of tradition, self-control, competition, self-directedness, independence, fate, and risk in higher regard than the value of regular preventive healthcare. These values may reflect an underlying struggle with the values of the other spouse, such as security, self-competence, or self-worth. The nurse's role might be to help the spouses explore their personal health history and needs rather than continuing the argument about the health checkup. Ideally, the nurse could assist each spouse in setting some attainable personal health goals, helping both realize the values of sharing, listening, trust, accountability, and responsibility.

Client and Healthcare Conflicts

Areas of conflict between clients and healthcare providers can center on values related to knowledge, cultural differences, developmental differences, and personal preferences. For example, in the case of a family in which the grandmother has died, parents may prefer that young children not attend the funeral, believing that children do not understand death and that it might be difficult for them. Realizing that death is a traumatic event for the survivors and that the parents' protection of the children is really a protection of their own feelings, the nurse might explore ways in which to meet the children's grief and loss needs (see Chapter 48). Depending on the children's ages, possibilities other than attending the funeral might include telling stories, drawing, or playing with a dollhouse family that includes a grandmother. A good example of a book for a child about 8 years of age is *Annie and the Old One* (Miles, 1971).

Resolving Value Conflicts in the Healthcare System

Three main issues that arise regarding resolution of value conflicts are the perception of conflict, the meaning of resolution, and the values underlying the resolution process. Nurses who face value conflicts need to examine their own values regarding conflict. A nurse who views conflict as negative might feel threatened, because his or her own values of self-competence, duty, success, authority, and esteem may be questioned. However, a nurse who views conflict as positive

ETHICAL/LEGAL ISSUE
Poverty

You are working as a home care nurse and have been assigned to Pearl Jones, a 74-year-old widow. Pearl has no living relatives and lives in a run-down home in an old section of town. Her house is cold as you enter. A strong odor is in the air, spoiled food is in the sink and refrigerator, dirt and dust are everywhere, and cockroaches scurry about. The bathroom has not been cleaned in a long time, and the toilet has not been flushed recently. It is obvious that Mrs. Jones also has not bathed in a long time. Her hair is unwashed, and her clothes are soiled. You talk with Mrs. Jones about her situation and offer to contact agencies to help with the home and with assisted living services, or to help her find a better living situation. Mrs. Jones makes it clear that she is quite comfortable with her lifestyle and does not want help from anyone. She just wants you to help with her dressing on her leg ulcer and leave her alone. She tells you that she owns this home and doesn't plan to leave it until she goes to her grave by her husband.

Reflection
- Reflect on your feelings about this situation and identify them.
- Identify the concerns you may have about this home visit and this client. What possible conflicts might stem from differences in values?
- Identify possible approaches to seeking additional information about this situation.
- Recognizing the client's right to make choices, define what you see as your ethically appropriate behavior.

might find the values of respect, communication, care, equilibrium, harmony, service, and creativity enhanced. These two views of conflict are based on the nurse's life experience and level of values development.

Several definitions of the word *resolution* apply to resolving value conflicts. One definition is that it is a clarifying or explanatory process. For example, many people do not take the time to reflect on their values, so, when conflicts occur, they are unable to articulate their position. Therefore, one of the first goals for the nurse is to assist the client in exploring and defining the relevant issues, attitudes, and beliefs. This clarification or explanation may be the resolution, or it may be the first step in a resolution process.

A second definition of resolution is that it occurs by answering questions. Clients have many questions related to their care. What nurses take for granted as routine care may be strange to clients. Encouraging questions by saying something like, "I have asked you a lot of questions; now do you have some that you would like to ask?" can be helpful. For example, an adolescent woman is admitted for a suicide ges-

ture; she cut her wrist. After a lengthy assessment, the nurse asks the client whether she has any questions. Her question is, "How is the food here?" Although a suicide attempt indicates that the client is dealing with survival issues, this question also is a concrete demonstration that the client is focusing on food and shelter. She is not able to focus on setting goals related to communication skills, assertiveness, or dealing with loss and grief. The first nursing intervention would be getting the client something to eat. If the nurse insisted on focusing on the counseling goals of communication or assertiveness in the ensuing 24 hours, a values conflict would occur.

Another definition of resolution involves coming to a decision or a determination for future action. For example, a client may have several treatment options. Even after examining all the facts and getting a second opinion, the client decides to take a course of action that the nurse does not like. If the nurse were to impose his or her decision on the client at this point, it is highly likely that a value conflict would arise, and the client might not comply with any treatment measures.

A fourth definition of resolution involves breaking up the issue or problem into its elements. Perhaps the nurse and client can agree on some elements of the situation, thus facilitating care. Arriving at areas of common ground is especially important when nurses work with clients from sociocultural backgrounds different than their own. A client often has a different belief system concerning the cause of illness, resulting in different values regarding prevention and cure. For example, a male refugee from Africa becomes psychotic because of major losses and culture shock. He is hospitalized for several months, discharged, and then rehospitalized because he did not take the prescribed psychotropic medications. Exploring the client's belief system reveals that he believes that his problems are a result of displeasing his family and being a coward. He views his mental illness as a punishment. Rather than focusing on the scientific explanation supported by Western values of knowledge, the nurse assists the client in learning about the community by taking him to various activities and facilities. The client likes this approach, finding that a prayer meeting held at a church of his ethnic group is especially helpful.

Nursing's Values Challenged by Managed Care

The ways in which healthcare and nursing care are delivered are changing. *Managed care* is the current term used for describing systems of care that focus on groups or populations of persons who are enrolled, most often through their employment, in a health benefit plan. The plans represent a variety of organizational structures, such as preferred provider, health maintenance organization, or integrated service network. Each of these systems has different values underlying the delivery of care; however, all reflect the values of the business model, efficiency and effectiveness. These values

THERAPEUTIC DIALOGUE
Values

Scene for Thought

Mrs. Haverford, 42 years old, is in the hospital with an acute episode of her chronic rheumatoid arthritis. Her husband of 20 years has come to visit. He asks to speak to his wife's primary nurse because he has some questions. He meets the nurse in the hallway.

Less Effective

Nurse: Hi, Mr. Haverford. I'm Vicki Driessen, your wife's primary nurse. You wanted to speak to me?

Husband: Yes, my wife is looking awfully sick this time around. I wondered what's going on. I've seen her through a lot of flare-ups of the arthritis, but . . . (Vicki interrupts).

Nurse: I understand that you're worried about your wife's condition. You know we're doing everything we can for her. When she's home, you work hard to care for her, but now it's time for you to relax and let us take over. I'll be down to her room in a little while to see how she's doing. We can talk more then.

More Effective

Nurse: Hello, Mr. Haverford. I'm Darla Jessup, your wife's primary nurse. You wanted to talk to me?

Husband: Yes, my wife is looking awfully sick this time around. I wondered what's going on. I've seen her through a lot of flare-ups. I wanted to ask you some questions about the care my wife is getting. (Looks serious.)

Nurse: How can I help? (Offers self.)

Husband: Well, I don't know if you can. I don't remember her ever being this sick before. I'm thinking it might be the new medicine her doctor put her on. What do you think? (Continues to look worried.)

Nurse: I can see that you are troubled. What have you been told about why she's in the hospital? (Observing and seeking information.)

Husband: Not much, but I want to know more. She's a very independent woman, and I don't want her to get so sick that she won't be as independent as she was. That would bother her a lot.

Nurse: It sounds as though you would like some information and that your wife might like it, too. How about setting up a time when we can talk together? (Offers information.)

Husband: Fine. Millie will be pleased, but let me ask her. She's still not feeling too good yet.

Nurse: Okay. I'll be coming to her room soon to give her some medication and see to her comfort. I'll see you then.

Critical Thinking Challenge

- From Hall's Value List (see Display 5-3), record the values that the husband exhibits while talking to the nurses about his wife.
- Make a similar list for each nurse.
- Compare the difference between Ms. Driessen's and Ms. Jessup's list of values.
- Examine what kind of effect this difference might have on the client and her husband.

---

are reflected in the decision making and policy development of two organizations, the employer and the healthcare plan. If these values dominate both environments, then nurses may find that they have value conflicts when serving individual clients. These conflicts fall into three areas: (1) caring for vulnerable persons, including children, the elderly, and the poor; (2) balancing cost-effectiveness with respectful care that enhances human dignity; and (3) being mindful of caring for both the individual and his or her right to healthcare and the needs of the represented group. For example, you are an adult nurse practitioner and prescribe a newer cardiac medication for a midlife client. The client goes to the pharmacy and is told that his health benefit does not cover this medication. You know from your assessment of the client, the pharmacologic literature, and research that this medication

is the best practice and that its use potentially prevents additional health problems from developing. What do you do? Whom do you serve, the employer who buys the health benefit, the health benefit plan that limits prescriptions, or your client? What values will direct your decisions? You are concerned about giving the best possible care to your client, and in the larger picture you are also concerned about all potential clients represented by this employer and this plan.

The Coalition for Accountable Managed Care (1997) has suggested that managed care can facilitate high-quality healthcare if healthcare providers and the public support a more socially-oriented ethic of care that balances individual rights with community needs. Some of the principles include

- Promotion of access to services without discrimination in enrollment
- Provision of quality care through clinical excellence
- Identification and response to the needs of communities through community accountability and commitment to community service, including provision of care to persons who are unable to pay, the community's underserved members, and high-risk patients
- Health system improvement and participation in community public health initiatives
- Provision of consumer information, education, and choice
- Governance of plans that are representative of the interests and needs of populations and the community as well as the enrolled population
- Financial responsibility that includes budgeting of adequate resources to carry out the previously described principles

Nurses who are now working in a managed healthcare system are beginning to express value conflicts as they broaden their focus from the client to the healthcare plan. They are particularly reflecting on the value of social justice as they deal with limited resources (Wurzbach, 1998). In addition to being challenged by different values, they are being challenged to become more reasoned and articulate when defending their own values. This is particularly true when the nurse acts as an advocate for client care.

Nurses in the 21st century will be confronted more and more with conflicts arising from differences in organizational versus service value priorities, individual versus community focus, and access to care for all, whether well served or underserved. So nurses will need to own and balance the values of mutual accountability and efficiency with equity and service, all the while maintaining an ethic of care and respect. Nurses are challenged to maintain integrity as they become accountable to both the consumer and society (Raines, 1997).

KEY CONCEPTS

- All human interactions are value based.
- Nurses must clarify and respect the values of others and examine their own values.
- Values are enhanced and refined by experiences that cultivate values development, such as interactions with people of differing values and viewpoints and experiences that challenge one's way of thinking.
- The ANA Code for Nurses is a set of standards based on universal moral principles or values.
- The AACN identifies five core values for nurses: altruism, autonomy, human dignity, integrity, and social justice.
- Values in nursing are developed through classroom study and clinical study.
- Values clarification is a method of self-discovery by which people identify their personal values without evaluating the values.

- An understanding of values and their influence on the nurse–client–family interaction is vital for acceptance of healthcare and the integration of the value of personal health into the lives of the client and family.

REFERENCES

American Association of Colleges of Nursing. (1998). *Essentials of baccalaureate education for professional nursing practice.* Washington, DC: Author.

American Nurses Association. (1985). *Code for nurses with interpretive statements.* Kansas City, MO: Author.

Brink, P. J. (1984). Values orientation as an assessment tool in cultural diversity. *Nursing Research, 33,* 198–203.

Coalition for Accountable Managed Care. 1997. *Principles for accountable managed care.* Washington, DC: Author.

Curtin, L., & Flaherty, M. J. (1981). *Nursing ethics: Theories and pragmatics.* New York: Appleton-Lange.

Erikson, E. (1982). *The life cycle completed.* New York: W. W. Norton & Co.

Esquivel, L. (1992). *Like water for chocolate: A novel in monthly installments, with recipes, romances, and home remedies.* New York: Doubleday.

Fromm, E. (1959). Values, psychology and human existence. In A. Maslow (Ed.), *New knowledge in human values.* New York: Harper & Row.

Gordon, M. (1997). *Manual of nursing diagnosis 1997–1998.* St. Louis, MO: Mosby–Year Book.

Hall, B. (1980). *The personal discernment inventory.* New York: Paulist Press.

Hall, B. (1991). *Spiritual connections: The journey of discipleship and Christian values.* Dayton, OH: Values Technology Inc.

Hall, B., Kalven, J., Rosen, L., & Taylor, B. (1982). *Readings in value development.* Ramsey, NJ: Paulist Press.

Hillerman, T. (1999). *Hunting Badger.* New York: Harper & Row.

Kidder, R. M. (1994). *Shared values for a troubled world.* San Francisco, CA: Jossey-Bass.

King, E. C. (1984). *Affective education in nursing.* Rockville, MD: Aspen.

Kohlberg, L. (1964). Development of moral character and moral ideology. In M. L. Hoffman & L. N. W. Hoffman (Eds.), *Review of child development research* (Vol. 1.) New York: Russell Sage Foundation.

Miles, M. (1971). *Annie and the old one.* Boston: The Atlantic Monthly PressBook.

Nursing World/Nursing Trends and Issues. (1998, January). Nursing's values challenged by managed care. Available at: http://www.nursingworld.org/readroom/nti/980lnti.htm.

Raines, D. A. (1997). From covenant to contract: How managed care is changing provider/patient relationships. *Association of Women's Health, Obstetrics, and Neonatal Nurses Lifelines, 1*(4), 41–45.

Raths, L. E., Harmin, M., & Simon, S. B. (1978). *Values and teaching* (2nd ed.). Columbus, OH: Charles E. Merrill.

Rokeach, M. (1973). *The nature of human values.* New York: The Free Press.

Walsh, B. J., & Middleton, J. R. (1984). *The transforming vision, shaping a Christian world view.* Downers Grove, IL: InterVarsity Press.

Wurzbach, M. E. (1998). Managed care: Moral conflicts for primary health care nurses. *Nursing Outlook, 46*(2), 62–66.

BIBLIOGRAPHY

Fagermoen, M. S. (1997). Professional identity: Values embedded in meaningful nursing practice. *Journal of Advanced Nursing, 25,* 434–441.

Felton, G. M., Parsons, M. A., & Bartoces, M. G. (1997). Demographic factors: Interaction effects on health-promoting behavior and health related factors. *Public Health Nursing, 14*(6), 361–367.

Felton, G. M., Parsons, M. A., Misener, T. R., & Oldaker, S. (1997). Health-promoting behaviors of black and white college women. *Western Journal of Nursing Research, 19*(5), 654–666.

Flynn, L. (1997). The health practices of homeless women: A causal model. *Nursing Research, 42*(2), 72–77.

Hall, B. (1986). *The genesis effect.* New York: Paulist Press.

Krach, P., DeVaney, S., DeTurk, C., & Zink, M. H. (1998). Functional status of the oldest-old in a home setting. *Journal of Advanced Nursing, 24,* 456–464.

Williams, A. M. (1998). The delivery of quality nursing care: A grounded theory study of the nurse's perspective. *Journal of Advanced Nursing, 27,* 808–816.

Yarcheski, A., Mahon, N., & Yarcheski, T. J. (1997). Alternate models of positive health practices in adolescents. *Nursing Research, 46*(2), 85–92.

6 Ethical and Legal Concerns

Key Terms

advance directives
assault
autonomy
battery
beneficence
community-based no
    code order
confidentiality
crime
double effect
durable power of attorney
    for healthcare decisions
ethics
fidelity
futility
informed consent
justice

laws
liability
libel
living will
malpractice
morals
negligence
nonmaleficence
privacy
proxy directive
res ipsa loquitur
respondeat superior
resuscitation
slander
tort
veracity

Learning Objectives

Upon completion of this chapter, the student will be able to do the following:

1. Define the chapter's key terms.
2. Differentiate personal values and morality from professional values.
3. Explain ethical philosophy.
4. Discuss the eight principles of healthcare ethics.
5. Describe a systematic approach for resolving ethical dilemmas.
6. Analyze an ethical dilemma, citing ethical principles.
7. Explain licensure.
8. Describe standard of care.
9. Compare and contrast crimes and torts; cite appropriate examples.
10. Define four elements of negligence.
11. Describe legal protections for nurses and cite measures to take.

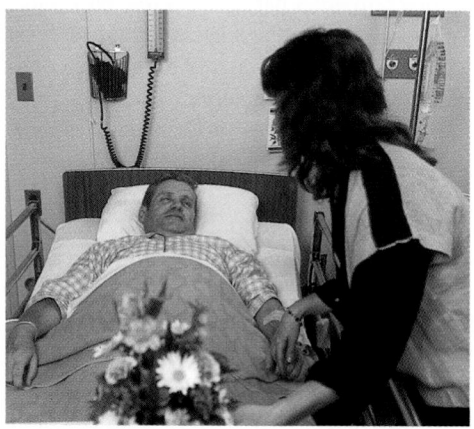

Critical Thinking Challenge

You are a home health nurse. One of your clients is a 59-year-old man with chronic restrictive pulmonary disease. He lives alone but has two adult children who live nearby and take turns transporting him to clinic appointments. In recent visits, your client seemed weak and fatigued; he struggled with shortness of breath and had lost approximately 10 lb. in the last month. Recently he needed to be hospitalized. His daughter mentions her concern about her father's worsening respiratory condition and the increasing amount of care he needs. You know that clients with this disease deteriorate over time and usually require ventilator support when they no longer have the strength to breathe on their own.

Once you have completed this chapter and have incorporated ethical and legal concerns into your knowledge base, review the above scenario and reflect on the following areas of Critical Thinking:

1. Develop a plan for gathering information about the client's and the family's comprehension and expectations of the client's health.
2. Based on the information collected, identify appropriate strategies that you believe are needed.
3. Propose additional information you need to supply the family to assist them in planning realistic possibilities for the future.
4. Describe the ethical dilemmas that may be part of the planning decisions.
5. Examine the legal concerns you see as inherent in this situation.

Healthcare delivery has undergone notable changes during the last decade including increased client participation in decision making, shorter hospital stays, and restructuring services to provide care in settings such as outpatient clinics, short-stay units, long-term care, and in-home care. Emphasis on multidisciplinary collaboration and care coordination attempts to ensure that clients' needs are met across the health and illness continuum. For nurses, these changes have contributed to development of new clinical environments and expanded practice. Nurses today frequently encounter difficult situations involving decisions about the best course of action. Changes in healthcare delivery can result in fragmented care for patients. The nurse plays an important role in assisting patients to identify and access the services they need.

Nurses are obligated to provide ethical and legal client care that demonstrates respect for others. Both fundamental principles of healthcare ethics and laws governing the scope of nursing guide nursing practice in all situations. Applying ethical thinking and moral reasoning to the decisions and actions inherent in client care promotes ethical nursing practice. Legal nursing practice is based on standards of care and the applicable nurse practice act.

Addressing ethical problems in clinical practice is a moral obligation that fosters empowerment for all nurses. It increases nurses' satisfaction about what they can achieve for the clients to whom they provide care. Nurses achieve personal and professional success by identifying ethical problems and legal responsibilities in clinical practice then using their knowledge and skills to bring about resolution.

ETHICS IN NURSING

Ethics is a branch of philosophy dealing with standards of conduct and moral judgment. Healthcare ethics pertain to how professionals fulfill their responsibilities and provide care to clients. While no set of absolute guidelines provides answers for all problems, the fundamental principles of ethics serve as a basis for interpreting and analyzing clinical situations in decision making. To understand ethics as it pertains to nurses or other clinicians, it is important to distinguish professional ethics from personal morality, personal values, institutional policies, or legal obligations (Kipnis, 1990).

Personal morality is the set of beliefs about the standards of right and wrong that help a person determine the correct or permissible action in a given situation. *Personal values* are ideas or beliefs a person considers important and feels strongly about. As discussed in Chapter 5, values, rooted in each person's unique experience, develop through family relationships, religious affiliations, education, and associations with friends and professionals. America, like many countries, is comprised of citizens from different cultural, religious, and ethnic backgrounds. In a pluralistic society, people have diverse ways of thinking about what is important and right. Life choices and healthcare decisions vary according to what each person values and believes to be morally right or wrong. Nurses must distinguish between their own personal values and shared professional ethics.

Institutional policies are guidelines developed by healthcare institutions to direct professional practice. Hospitals, nursing homes, and other organizations that employ nurses may have policies concerning issues such as do-not-resuscitate orders and withdrawal of tube feedings. Institutional policies are often developed by consulting legal guidelines and professional standards but also may reflect an institution's religious affiliation. For example, some nursing homes do not permit artificially provided nutrition and hydration to be withdrawn due to religious teachings even though stopping this medical therapy is legally permissible in appropriate situations. Nurses need to be aware of institutional policies but these policies are not the same as professional values. In some cases, nurses need to work actively to ensure that institutional policies reflect professional ethics.

Legal guidelines are drawn from state and federal laws. The laws pertinent to healthcare are discussed later in this chapter. Nurses should be aware of the legal guidelines that govern their particular area of practice; they should also recognize that myths abound particularly around withholding and withdrawing life support (Meisel, 1991; Meisel, Snyder, & Quill, 2000; Quill, Lo, & Brock, 1997). Also, legal guidelines are not synonymous with professional ethics. In many cases, the law establishes a minimum code of conduct while professional ethics suggest an ideal.

Professional ethics involve principles and values with universal application and standards of conduct to be upheld in all situations. Personal values and personal morality are what each person holds as significant and true for himself or herself. These personal convictions apply only to situations and decisions pertaining to that individual. In ethical practice, nurses avoid allowing personal judgments to bias their treatment of clients. For example, a particular nurse may value candor in family relationships, but as a nurse should abide by the professional ethics obligation to maintain patient confidentiality. Decision making can be very challenging when professional ethics conflict with institutional policies, personal morality or values. For example, Jehovah's Witnesses often refuse blood products in their treatment, a decision that affects how or if surgery will be conducted. Although conflicting values are inherent in such a situation, respectful client treatment is still essential.

The ANA recently revised the Code of Ethics for Nurses (ANA, 2001) that delineates the conduct and responsibilities expected of all nurses in their nursing practices. Nurses' ethical obligations include acting in the best interest of their clients not only as individual practitioners but also as members of the nursing profession, the healthcare team, and the community at large. Nurses are responsible to know and comply with the standards of ethical practice and to ensure that other nurses also comply. Interpretive statements have been developed that explain how each item in the code is manifested in nursing practice. The complete document can be obtained from the American Nurses Association (ANA). The Canadian Nurses Association and the International Council of Nurses also have published codes of ethics that reflect the basic tenets of nursing practice (Display 6-1).

DISPLAY 6-1

🖅 PROFESSIONAL CODES OF ETHICS FOR NURSES

American Nurses Association Code for Nurses*

The American Nurses Association (ANA) House of Delegates approved these nine provisions of the new Code of Ethics for Nurses at its June 30, 2001 meeting in Washington, DC. In July 2001, the Congress of Nursing Practice and Economics voted to accept the new language of the interpretive statements resulting in a fully approved revised Code of Ethics for Nurses With Interpretive Statements.

1. The nurse, in all professional relationships, practices with compassion and respect for the inherent dignity, worth and uniqueness of every individual, unrestricted by considerations of social or economic status, personal attributes, or the nature of health problems.
2. The nurse's primary commitment is to the patient, whether an individual, family, group, or community.
3. The nurse promotes, advocates for, and strives to protect the health, safety, and rights of the patient.
4. The nurse is responsible and accountable for individual nursing practice and determines the appropriate delegation of tasks consistent with the nurse's obligation to provide optimum patient care.
5. The nurse owes the same duties to self as to others, including the responsibility to preserve integrity and safety, to maintain competence, and to continue personal and professional growth.
6. The nurse participates in establishing, maintaining, and improving healthcare environments and conditions of employment conducive to the provision of quality health care and consistent with the values of the profession through individual and collective action.
7. The nurse participates in the advancement of the profession through contributions to practice, education, administration, and knowledge development.
8. The nurse collaborates with other health professionals and the public in promoting community, national, and international efforts to meet health needs.

The profession of nursing, as represented by associations and their members, is responsible for articulating nursing values, for maintaining the integrity of the profession and its practice, and for shaping social policy.

Canadian Nurses Association Code of Ethics for Nursing†

  I. A nurse treats clients with respect for their individual needs and values.
 II. Based on respect for clients and regard for their right to control their own care, nursing care reflects respect for the right of choice held by clients.
III. The nurse holds confidential all information about a client learned in the healthcare setting.

 IV. The nurse is guided by consideration for the dignity of clients.
  V. The nurse provides competent care to clients.
 VI. The nurse maintains trust in nurses and nursing.
VII. The nurse recognizes the contribution and expertise of colleagues from nursing and other disciplines as essential to excellent healthcare.
VIII. The nurse takes steps to ensure that the client receives competent and ethical care.
 IX. Conditions of employment should contribute in a positive way to client care and the professional satisfaction of nurses.
  X. Job action by nurses is directed toward securing conditions of employment that enable safe and appropriate care for clients and contribute to the professional satisfaction of nurses.
 XI. The nurse advocates the interests of clients.
XII. The nurse represents the values and ethics of nursing before colleagues and others.
XIII. Professional nurses' organizations are responsible for clarifying, securing, and sustaining ethical nursing conduct. The fulfillment of these tasks requires that professional nurses' organizations remain responsive to the rights, needs, and legitimate interests of clients and nurses.

International Council of Nurses Code for Nurses‡

An international code of ethics for nurses was first adopted by the International Council of Nurses (ICN) in 1953. It has been revised and reaffirmed at various times since, most recently with this review and revision completed in 2000.

Preamble

Nurses have four fundamental responsibilities: to promote health, to prevent illness, to restore health and to alleviate suffering. The need for nursing is universal.

Inherent in nursing is respect for human rights, including the right to life, to dignity and to be treated with respect. Nursing care is unrestricted by considerations of age, colour, creed, culture, disability or illness, gender, nationality, politics, race or social status.

Nurses render health services to the individual, the family and the community and co-ordinate their services with those of related groups.

The Code

The ICN Code of Ethics for Nurses has four principal elements that outline the standards of ethical conduct.

Elements of the Code

1. Nurses and people

The nurse's primary professional responsibility is to people requiring nursing care.

(continued)

DISPLAY 6-1 (Continued)

🔲 **PROFESSIONAL CODES OF ETHICS FOR NURSES**

In providing care, the nurse promotes an environment in which the human rights, values, customs and spiritual beliefs of the individual, family and community are respected.

The nurse ensures that the individual receives sufficient information on which to base consent for care and related treatment.

The nurse holds in confidence personal information and uses judgement in sharing this information.

The nurse shares with society the responsibility for initiating and supporting action to meet the health and social needs of the public, in particular those of vulnerable populations.

The nurse also shares responsibility to sustain and protect the natural environment from depletion, pollution, degradation and destruction.

2. Nurses and practice

The nurse carries personal responsibility and accountability for nursing practice, and for maintaining competence by continual learning.

The nurse maintains a standard of personal health such that the ability to provide care is not compromised.

The nurse uses judgement regarding individual competence when accepting and delegating responsibility.

The nurse at all times maintains standards of personal conduct which reflect well on the profession and enhance public confidence.

The nurse, in providing care, ensures that use of technology and scientific advances are compatible with the safety, dignity and rights of people.

3. Nurses and the profession

The nurse assumes the major role in determining and implementing acceptable standards of clinical nursing practice, management, research and education.

The nurse is active in developing a core of research-based professional knowledge.

The nurse, acting through the professional organisation, participates in creating and maintaining equitable social and economic working conditions in nursing.

4. Nurses and co-workers

The nurse sustains a co-operative relationship with co-workers in nursing and other fields.

The nurse takes appropriate action to safeguard individuals when their care is endangered by a co-worker or any other person.

* From American Nurses Association. (2001). *Code for nurses.* Kansas City, MO: Author. [Online] Available at: *http://www.nursingworld.org/ethics/chcode.htm*

† From Canadian Nurses Association. (1997). *Code of ethics for nursing.* Ottawa, Ontario: Author. [Online] Available at: *http://www.cna-nurses.ca/pages/ethics/ethicsframe.htm*

‡ From International Council of Nurses. (2000). *ICN code of ethics for nurses.* ICN-International Council of Nurses, 3, place Jean-Marteau, CH-1201 Geneva, Switzerland. [Online] Available at: *http://www.icn.ch/ethics.htm*

Theoretical Frameworks in Ethics

Frameworks in ethics provide a systematic way of organizing reasons that serve as a basis for deciding the right and best action to take. Major theoretical frameworks in ethics are differentiated based on which values are emphasized as most important. Goals, duties, and rights are central considerations to all ethics theories, but each framework varies in how it assigns priority to goals, duties, and rights (Beauchamp & Childress, 2001; Benjamin & Curtis, 1992). Conceptualization of a particular situation within each framework yields different conclusions.

In frameworks that emphasize goals, actions are judged to be right based on whether or not they contribute to the achievement of identified outcomes. In the utilitarian framework, actions are right when they contribute to the greatest good and are wrong when they detract from the greatest good (Beauchamp & Childress, 2001). In some utilitarian frameworks, the greatest good refers to the greatest happiness for an individual. For clients with cancer, this type of framework would evaluate alternatives such as radical surgery, chemotherapy, or radiation according to which choice will give the client the greatest comfort and chance for survival. Some utilitarian theories define "good consequences" according to whether or not an action results in the greatest good for the greatest number. In this type of framework, funding very expensive or experimental treatments beneficial to only a few clients might be refused to preserve dollars for wellness and prevention services that benefit more people.

Deontologic frameworks emphasize roles or responsibilities that one is morally obligated to fulfill. These frameworks expect the individual to remain faithful to a certain set of duties that take precedence over other considerations (Beauchamp & Childress, 2001). Decisions about the right action to take are based on which action is in keeping with these duties regardless of consequences. For example, a nurse is obligated to protect a client's confidentiality. When rights are identified as the primary consideration, the focus is on the claims or entitlements of each person (Beauchamp & Childress, 2001; Benjamin & Curtis, 1992). Actions are judged according to whether or not they uphold each person's rights. The Right to Life campaign is an example of an ethical position based on rights. The central element is the unborn child's entitlement to life. Judgments about actions are based on whether or not the actions support this right.

Principles of Healthcare Ethics

Principles are basic ideas that serve as starting points for both understanding and working through problems (Jonsen, 1994). The major principles of healthcare ethics important to uphold in all situations include beneficence, nonmaleficence, respect for autonomy, and justice. These principles serve as the basis for rules that govern the relationships between healthcare providers and clients.

Beneficence and Nonmaleficence

Beneficence means doing or promoting good. This principle is the basis for all healthcare. Nurses, physicians, and all other healthcare practitioners work to accomplish good for clients by promoting their best interests and striving to achieve optimal outcomes. People may differ in how they define what is 'good' or 'best.' In these cases, healthcare providers should promote good as defined by the patient. Nurses take beneficent actions when they administer pain medication, perform dressing changes to promote wound healing, and provide emotional support to clients who are anxious or depressed.

Nonmaleficence is often viewed as an extension of beneficence. The principle of **nonmaleficence** means to avoid doing harm, to remove from harm, and to prevent harm. When working with clients, nurses must not cause injury or suffering; they accomplish this by maintaining competency in clinical practice. Upholding the principle of nonmaleficence is evidenced by providing medication to prevent clients from further suffering, protecting clients from a chemically impaired practitioner, or reporting suspected child abuse to prevent further victimization.

Doing good and avoiding harm seem fairly simple but in many cases are complex and difficult to discern. For example, bone marrow transplantation often saves lives; however, clients undergoing the procedure experience a great deal of pain and suffering to benefit from the intervention. Saving the life of an expectant mother with a cardiac problem who is unlikely to survive childbirth may necessitate death to the fetus through abortion. Confronting a colleague's substance abuse may lead that person to obtain therapeutic help but may also result in that person being temporarily suspended from employment, which could cause embarrassment or hostility.

Respect for Autonomy

Autonomy essentially means independence and the ability to be self-directed. In healthcare, respect for autonomy is the basis for the client's right to self-determination. That is, clients are entitled to make decisions about what will happen to them and their bodies. Adult clients with the capacity to make decisions have the right to consent to or to refuse treatment. Even if healthcare providers do not agree with a client's decision, they must respect the client's wishes (Beauchamp & Childress, 2001).

Infants, young children, persons who are mentally handicapped or incapacitated, and people in a persistent vegetative state or coma do not have the capacity to participate in decision making about their healthcare. For such a person, a surrogate decision maker must be identified to act on the client's behalf. Through nursing assessment and therapeutic relationships, nurses gain in-depth understanding of what clients need and want from their healthcare. Nurses promote client autonomy by integrating clients' wishes into the treatment plan. Clients communicate their wishes to healthcare providers by verbally participating in healthcare decision making and through written documents called **advance directives,** which specify what interventions the client would or would not want if he or she became terminally ill or sustained an injury or illness that impeded the ability to make or communicate decisions (Fig. 6-1). A **living will** is a type of advance directive that specifies the types of medical treatment a client does and does not want to receive should they be unable to speak for themselves and in a terminal condition. Often included are instructions about resuscitation, drugs, blood transfusions, tube feedings, and mechanical ventilation. A second type of advance directive is a **proxy directive,** sometimes referred to as **a durable power of attorney for healthcare decisions.** This type of advance directive allows an individual to designate another person to make decisions if the client becomes incapacitated and unable to make decisions independently. This "surrogate decision maker" would then act on the client's behalf. The legal aspects of these documents are discussed later in this chapter. Clients are entitled to rescind or to change their directives at any time. Nurses are often the first to learn about changes a client is contemplating. The nurse must then document the client's wishes and notify the client's physician and other involved professionals so the plan of care is altered to reflect these changes.

A Patient's Bill of Rights, published by the American Hospital Association (AHA, 1990), identifies key elements of clients' rights and responsibilities in their relationships with healthcare providers (Display 6-2). A client is entitled to considerate and respectful care, which includes assurances of confidentiality, complete information, continuity of care, and access to treatment providers. The bill also identifies the client's right to information about costs and financial liabilities and to know if the organization has rules and regulations by which the client must abide.

Cultural diversity has implications for upholding client autonomy. Providers must modify care to reflect respect for values and beliefs of different ethnic or social groups. Some cultures prefer to withhold information about severe or terminal illness from a client. Religious beliefs and allegiance to tradition affect how much information clients will share and how receptive they are to the recommendations of healthcare providers.

Justice

Justice, the principle of fairness, is the basis for the obligation to treat all clients equally and fairly. Justice is the foundation for decisions about resource allocation throughout a society or group. While there are many ways to judge justice,

(text continues on page 92)

DECLARATION

I, *Mildred Jones*, being of sound mind, willfully and voluntarily make this declaration to be followed if I become incapacitated. This declaration reflects my firm and settled commitment to refuse life-sustaining treatment under the circumstances indicated below.

I direct my attending physician to withhold or withdraw life-sustaining treatment that serves only to prolong the process of my dying, if I should be in a terminal condition or in a state of permanent unconsciousness.

I direct that treatment be limited to measures to keep me comfortable and to relieve pain, including any pain that might occur by withholding or withdrawing life-sustaining treatment.

In addition, if I am in the condition described above, I feel especially strongly about the following forms of treatment. **I realize that if I do not specifically indicate my preference regarding any of the forms of treatment listed below, I may receive that form of treatment.**

• Cardiac resuscitation:	I do want (x)	I do not want( )
• Mechanical respiration:	I do want ( )	I do not want (x)
• Tube feeding or any other artificial or invasive form of nutrition (food):	I do want ( )	I do not want (x)
• Any artificial or invasive form of hydration (water):	I do want ( )	I do not want (x)
• Blood or blood products:	I do want ( )	I do not want (x)
• Any invasive diagnostic tests:	I do want ( )	I do not want (x)
• Any form of surgery:	I do want ( )	I do not want (x)
• Kidney dialysis:	I do want ( )	I do not want (x)
• Antibiotics:	I do want (x)	I do not want ( )

Other instructions:

I(x) do ( ) do not want to designate another person as my surrogate to make medical treatment decisions for me if I should be incapacitated and in a terminal condition or in a state of permanent unconciousness.

Name and address of surrogate (if applicable):

Jonathan Jones
423 Main Street
Crossroads SC

Name and address of substitute surrogate (if surrogate designated above is unable to serve):

Trudy Conover
619 Wyoming Drive
Crossroads SC

I made this declaration on the *21* day of *10/95* (month, year).

Declarant's signature: *Mildred Jones*
Declarant's address: *423 Main Street*
                           Crossroads SC

The declarant or the person on behalf of and at the direction of the declarant knowingly and voluntarily signed this writing by signature or mark in my presence.

1. Witness's signature: *Mary Martin*
   Witness's address: *818 Hill Drive*
                          Bayside GA

2. Witness's signature: *Rosa Diaz*
   Witness's address: *1043 River Road*
                          Summit SC

FIGURE 6-1   Sample of an advance directive.

DISPLAY 6-2

☐ A PATIENT'S BILL OF RIGHTS

A Patient's Bill of Rights was first adopted by the American Hospital Association in 1973. This revision was approved by the AHA Board of Trustees on October 21, 1992.

Introduction
Effective health care requires collaboration between patients and physicians and other health care professionals. Open and honest communication, respect for personal and professional values, and sensitivity to differences are integral to optimal patient care. As the setting for the provision of health services, hospitals must provide a foundation for understanding and respecting the rights and responsibilities of patients, their families, physicians, and other caregivers. Hospitals must ensure a health care ethic that respects the role of patients in decision making about treatment choices and other aspects of their care. Hospitals must be sensitive to cultural, racial, linguistic, religious, age, gender, and other differences as well as the needs of persons with disabilities.

The American Hospital Association presents A Patient's Bill of Rights with the expectation that it will contribute to more effective patient care and be supported by the hospital on behalf of the institution, its medical staff, employees, and patients. The American Hospital Association encourages health care institutions to tailor this bill of rights to their patient community by translating and/or simplifying the language of this bill of rights as may be necessary to ensure that patients and their families understand their rights and responsibilities.

Bill of Rights*
1. The patient has the right to considerate and respectful care.
2. The patient has the right to and is encouraged to obtain from physicians and other direct caregivers relevant, current, and understandable information concerning diagnosis, treatment, and prognosis.

   Except in emergencies when the patient lacks decision-making capacity and the need for treatment is urgent, the patient is entitled to the opportunity to discuss and request information related to the specific procedures and/or treatments, the risks involved, the possible length of recuperation, and the medically reasonable alternatives and their accompanying risks and benefits.

   Patients have the right to know the identity of physicians, nurses, and others involved in their care, as well as when those involved are students, residents, or other trainees. The patient also has the right to know the immediate and long-term financial implications of treatment choices, insofar as they are known.

3. The patient has the right to make decisions about the plan of care prior to and during the course of treatment and to refuse a recommended treatment or plan of care to the extent permitted by law and hospital policy and to be informed of the medical consequences of this action. In case of such refusal, the patient is entitled to other appropriate care and services that the hospital provides or transfer to another hospital. The hospital should notify patients of any policy that might affect patient choice within the institution.
4. The patient has the right to have an advance directive (such as a living will, health care proxy, or durable power of attorney for health care) concerning treatment or designating a surrogate decision maker with the expectation that the hospital will honor the intent of that directive to the extent permitted by law and hospital policy.

   Health care institutions must advise patients of their rights under state law and hospital policy to make informed medical choices, ask if the patient has an advance directive, and include that information in patient records. The patient has the right to timely information about hospital policy that may limit its ability to implement fully a legally valid advance directive.
5. The patient has the right to every consideration of privacy. Case discussion, consultation, examination, and treatment should be conducted so as to protect each patient's privacy.
6. The patient has the right to expect that all communications and records pertaining to his/her care will be treated as confidential by the hospital, except in cases such as suspected abuse and public health hazards when reporting is permitted or required by law. The patient has the right to expect that the hospital will emphasize the confidentiality of this information when it releases it to any other parties entitled to review information in these records.
7. The patient has the right to review the records pertaining to his/her medical care and to have the information explained or interpreted as necessary, except when restricted by law.
8. The patient has the right to expect that, within its capacity and policies, a hospital will make reasonable response to the request of a patient for appropriate and medically indicated care and services. The hospital must provide evaluation, service, and/or referral as indicated by the urgency of the case. When medically appropriate and legally permissible, or when a patient has so requested, a patient may be transferred to another facility. The institution to which the patient is to

(continued)

DISPLAY 6-2 (Continued)

A PATIENT'S BILL OF RIGHTS

be transferred must first have accepted the patient for transfer. The patient must also have the benefit of complete information and explanation concerning the need for, risks, benefits, and alternatives to such a transfer.

9. The patient has the right to ask and be informed of the existence of business relationships among the hospital, educational institutions, other health care providers, or payers that may influence the patient's treatment and care.

10. The patient has the right to consent to or decline to participate in proposed research studies or human experimentation affecting care and treatment or requiring direct patient involvement, and to have those studies fully explained prior to consent. A patient who declines to participate in research or experimentation is entitled to the most effective care that the hospital can otherwise provide.

11. The patient has the right to expect reasonable continuity of care when appropriate and to be informed by physicians and other caregivers of available and realistic patient care options when hospital care is no longer appropriate.

12. The patient has the right to be informed of hospital policies and practices that relate to patient care, treatment, and responsibilities. The patient has the right to be informed of available resources for resolving disputes, grievances, and conflicts, such as ethics committees, patient representatives, or other mechanisms available in the institution. The patient has the right to be informed of the hospital's charges for services and available payment methods.

The collaborative nature of health care requires that patients, or their families/surrogates, participate in their care. The effectiveness of care and patient satisfaction with the course of treatment depend, in part, on the patient fulfill-

ing certain responsibilities. Patients are responsible for providing information about past illnesses, hospitalizations, medications, and other matters related to health status. To participate effectively in decision making, patients must be encouraged to take responsibility for requesting additional information or clarification about their health status or treatment when they do not fully understand information and instructions. Patients are also responsible for ensuring that the health care institution has a copy of their written advance directive if they have one. Patients are responsible for informing their physicians and other caregivers if they anticipate problems in following prescribed treatment.

Patients should also be aware of the hospital's obligation to be reasonably efficient and equitable in providing care to other patients and the community. The hospital's rules and regulations are designed to help the hospital meet this obligation. Patients and their families are responsible for making reasonable accommodations to the needs of the hospital, other patients, medical staff, and hospital employees. Patients are responsible for providing necessary information for insurance claims and for working with the hospital to make payment arrangements, when necessary.

A person's health depends on much more than health care services. Patients are responsible for recognizing the impact of their life-style on their personal health.

Conclusion
Hospitals have many functions to perform, including the enhancement of health status, health promotion, and the prevention and treatment of injury and disease; the immediate and ongoing care and rehabilitation of patients; the education of health professionals, patients, and the community; and research. All these activities must be conducted with an overriding concern for the values and dignity of patients.

* These rights can be exercised on the patient's behalf by a legally designated surrogate or proxy decision maker if
  the patient lacks decision-making capacity, is legally incompetent, or is a minor.
Reprinted with permission of the American Hospital Association. © 1992.

most agree that a just healthcare system provides care on the basis of medical need rather than by ability to pay, social status, race, or gender.

Nurses commonly face issues of justice in their clinical practice. When organizing care for a group of clients, nurses must decide how much time to spend with each client. A just decision is based on client need and a fair distribution of resources rather than on how much a nurse likes each client (Liaschenko, 1999). Nurses also encounter justice issues in working with clients who have different healthcare insurance. For example, basic Medicare coverage does not cover

prescriptions or extended care in a nursing home. Nurses work with patients and families who are forced to make hard decisions for their elderly family members due to these financial constraints. In these situations, it is helpful for nurses to identify governmental and community resources to assist patients. It is also important for nurses to work at a policy level to help alleviate healthcare disparities (Caplan, Light, & Daniels, 1999; Kopelman & Mouradian, 2001; Weiner, 2001). This can be done by providing information to policy makers and the general public about client needs and healthcare system injustices (Curtin, 2000).

Ethical Principles of Professional-Patient Relationships

In addition to the principles of respect for autonomy, beneficence, nonmaleficence, and justice that guide healthcare decision making, there are principles that guide the behavior of healthcare professionals toward patients and their families. These principles include veracity, fidelity, privacy, and confidentiality (Beauchamp and Childress, 2001). Although some circumstances create exceptions to the rules, for the most part nurses are required to adhere to these obligations.

Veracity

Veracity means telling the truth, which is essential to the integrity of the client-provider relationship. Healthcare professionals are obliged to be honest with clients. The right to self-determination becomes meaningless if the client does not receive accurate, unbiased, and understandable information (President's Commission, 1982).

Clients and families frequently disclose their questions and concerns to nurses. Nurses assist them to obtain information and understand how it applies to their situation by arranging discussions between client, family, and physician, and by providing emotional support to those adjusting to illness.

Telling a client about serious health problems can be distressing for both the client and the healthcare professional. Several studies reveal that clients prefer to receive accurate information about their condition and prognosis even when the outlook is bleak (Woodard & Parmies, 1992; Sardell & Trierweiler, 1993). Candid discussions about their condition and treatment reassure some clients (Sell et al., 1993). A study of clients with cancer showed a large percentage wanted more information than their physicians were inclined to reveal and that informed clients were less anxious and more cooperative (Espinosa, Gonzales-Baron, Poveda, Ordonez, & Zamora, 1993).

Fidelity

Fidelity means being faithful to one's commitments and promises. Nurses' commitments to clients include providing safe care and maintaining competence in nursing practice. In some instances, nurses make promises to clients in an overt way. For example, in psychiatric day treatment programs, detailed client care contracts are made between client and team. If a nurse agrees to be the resource to a client during crisis, the nurse must fulfill this commitment. If the nurse cannot be available, the ethical action is to discuss this with the client and to arrange a substitute when needed.

Making promises to clients requires good judgment. Being responsive to a client's request is important, but the nurse must evaluate whether or not he or she can uphold agreements. Consider this example:

Dave Meyers, registered nurse (RN), admitted a client with a history of alcohol abuse. The client asked for assurance that leather restraints would not be used under any circumstances. In an attempt to calm the client, Dave agreed to this request. After surgery, the client grew agitated, delirious, and combative. Although restraints were indicated to pre-

serve the client's safety, Dave opposed using them because of the promise he made.

This promise was not safe. Ethical practice in this case would have incorporated the client's concerns and an explanation of circumstances in which restraints would be applied.

Privacy

Privacy is important to most people. A loss of privacy occurs if others inappropriately use their access to a person. Nurses protect patient privacy by ensuring that the patient's body is appropriately covered, by not discussing medically irrelevant physical features, and by not engaging in discussion of intimate details about the patient unless necessary for the provision of good care.

Ms. Baglia, a 38-year-old nurse, had a breast biopsy done for a suspicious lump by a physician within the facility where she is employed. Her co-worker is worried for her and accesses the computerized record to learn the biopsy results.

Ms. Baglia's co-worker has violated her privacy by accessing her medical record unnecessarily. While nurses have the authority to access medical records, this access is limited to patient care related reasons. Nurses need to establish a culture of privacy to ensure that personal information of patients is kept as private as possible.

Confidentiality

The principle of **confidentiality** requires that information about a client be kept private. What is documented in the client's record is accessible only to those providing care to that client. No one else is entitled to that information unless the client has signed a Consent for Release of Information that identifies with whom information may be shared and for what purpose. Discussing clients outside the clinical setting, telling friends or family about clients, or even discussing clients in the elevator with other workers violates client confidentiality and must be avoided (Pinch, 2000).

Bill Fry, a 72-year-old man, has been hospitalized for nearly a month following an acute myocardial infarction and subsequent coronary artery bypass surgery. Mr. Fry's recovery was complicated by compromised pulmonary function caused by a 50-year history of smoking cigarettes. Once transferred out of the intensive care unit, Mr. Fry requested an escort to the smoking area of the hospital so he could have a cigarette. He also directed the nursing staff to not inform his wife and three adult children that he had resumed smoking.

In this situation, the nurse is obligated to protect the client's confidentiality and not to give the family information about the patient. One approach the nurse can take is to talk with Mr. Fry about the resources available to help him stop smoking, his reasons for choosing to continue smoking, and strategies for discussing his decision with his family. Recently, medications have been found to assist patients with the experience of craving that is a part of addiction (Covey et al., 2000; Hughes, 1999). If asked directly by the family, the nurse should explain that patient confidentiality requires the nurse to not reveal patient information.

Breaking confidentiality may be ethically justified if there is a well-defined reason to share information. Information can only be shared if doing so would substantially benefit someone else and that benefit would outweigh or override harm that would come from a breach of confidentiality (Walters, 1988). In situations where the nurse is tempted to break confidentiality for these reasons, he or she should consult with a supervisor, ethics consultant, and possibly legal counsel to confirm that the breach in confidentiality is indeed justified.

Model for Case Analysis

Clinical judgment is comprised of three questions: What is wrong with this patient? What can be done? And what should be done for this patient? (Pellegrino, 1979). For example, a nurse, caring for a 72-year-old woman 12 hours after surgery for a hip replacement, notes that the patient is slightly febrile. After listening to the patient's lungs, the nurse concludes that the patient's elevated temperature is due to inadequate ventilation. She treats the patient by assisting with deep breathing and coughing. An hour later the patient's temperature is normal. In this situation, the question of what should be done is clear. Imagine, however, that the patient has end-stage cancer, has a no-code order, and is becoming increasingly obtunded. The question of what should be done for an elevated temperature becomes more complex. If the woman is actively dying, it may be more appropriate to provide acetaminophen for comfort rather than to promote pulmonary hygiene.

The ability to analyze clinical situations and to integrate ethical considerations with relevant clinical data and surrounding issues is an essential skill for ethical clinical practice. Jonsen, Siegler, and Winslade (1998) have developed a model for case analysis that aids organizing the salient features of a clinical situation to promote problem solving and decision making. This model divides information about each case into four categories: Indications for Medical Intervention, Patient Preferences, Quality of Life, and Contextual Features (Display 6-3). Using the model assists the nurse to sort through the case facts to identify what is known, what is not known, and where conflicts exist.

Indications for Medical Intervention

For each person entering the healthcare system as a client, questions must be answered about whether or not that individual is in need of treatment and, if so, what intervention will be used. Indications for medical treatment include consideration of the client's diagnosis and condition. Treatment alternatives, including medical and nursing therapeutics, are then evaluated according to whether or not they are indicated and what they can accomplish for that particular client.

Beneficence and nonmaleficence are relevant in this category. A clinical judgment must be made about whether or not a treatment alternative will produce a benefit and what action or nonaction will achieve the greatest good for the client. The distinction between available treatment and that which is truly indicated is important. The criterion for this distinction rests on whether or not the intervention can achieve a therapeutic or desired benefit for the client. Nurses participate in determining if interventions are indicated by continually as-

---

DISPLAY 6-3

🔲 **MODEL FOR CASE ANALYSIS**

Indications for Medical Intervention
- What is the health problem? Diagnosis? Prognosis?
- What is the range of treatment options from aggressive to palliative? Which are legally forbidden? Which are morally/ethically repugnant?
- What is the goal of each treatment option?
- Common problem: Who judges futility?

Patient Preference
- What are the patient's preferences regarding the treatment options identified above?
- If the patient is unable to communicate preferences at this time, is there verbal or written evidence of what his/her preferences might have been (e.g., living will or conversations with others)?
- If no written or verbal evidence of the patient's preferences exist a.) have all potential sources been exhausted, and b.) is there "relational" evidence based on how the patient lived his/her life and prior health care choices?
- With minors, patient preferences are "held in trust."
- Suggestion: Be creative in considering potential sources of information.
- Common problem: Do we "believe" this patient (surrogate)?

Quality of Life
- If possible, the patient's view of his/her quality of life is respected. If the patient's view is unknowable, whose standards do we use to judge quality of life?
- What are the clinical facts devoid of judgments of worth?
- Suggestion: Compare quality of life for each treatment option outlined in step one based on clinical facts.

Contextual Features
- Who is the primary beneficiary of treatment?
- What is the impact on the family; are the costs unduly burdensome to the patient/family?
- Is the public at risk?

Adapted from Jonsen, A. R., Siegler, M., & Winslade, W. (1998). *Clinical ethics* (4th ed.). New York: McGraw-Hill.

---

sessing the client's condition and response to treatment, then integrating this information into the plan of care.

The concept of double effect stems from Catholic theology and arises when considering possible treatments. **Double effect** means that an action can produce two outcomes that can be helpful and harmful at the same time. Usually one outcome is desired, whereas the other is not intended but is foreseen. The reason for taking an action must be sufficiently compelling to justify the negative consequences. Providing adequate pain management to dying persons, while recognizing that this may hasten their death, can be justified by the concept of double effect. It is important to note however that adequate pain management rarely hastens death in these situations. The fear is that respiratory depression will result from high doses of opioids. However, in a patient who has been on opioids, this side effect is unlikely to occur unless the dose is increased significantly.

A determination of medical **futility** results when interventions are unlikely to preserve life, restore health, or relieve suffering (Schneiderman, Jecker, & Jonsen, 1990). Determinations of futility are made in reference to goals. Therefore, a treatment course is best designed around outcomes on which the client and healthcare provider mutually agree. Consider this example:

Paula Hastings, 30 years old, had cancer for several years. After surgical tumor resections, chemotherapy, and radiation, she was found to have several tumors including lung metastases. Her condition was considered terminal. The physician discussed with Paula that no further aggressive interventions would be used and care would be directed toward making her as comfortable as possible. Paula agreed.

Weeks later, Paula presented in the emergency room with bleeding through an enterocutaneous fistula near her colostomy. The resident on call admitted Paula and ordered blood products to be given. The assistant head nurse on the unit where Paula was admitted was familiar with her case. He recalled the "Do Not Resuscitate" order for this client. He was concerned that resuscitating this terminally ill client would be providing futile treatment. The nurse identified that the goals of treatment needed to be reviewed and that interventions should be discussed in light of these goals.

Client Preference

A client's choice about what is done is essential to healthcare decision making. Each person is uniquely qualified to make decisions about his or her own best interest. After a clinical judgment has been made about the client's condition and indicated interventions have been determined, this information is discussed with the client who may then accept or refuse the treatment alternatives. The wishes of an informed client with the capacity for decision making must always be respected and incorporated into the plan of care. Consider this example:

Grace Hall, 73, was diagnosed with cancer 10 years ago. Over the years, she has undergone several forms of treatment. She has suffered many negative side effects of these treatments such as nausea and vomiting, hair loss, fatigue, and pain. When another mass was discovered, her physician presented the treatment options to her and informed her that, without treatment, chances of surviving for more than 6 months were very poor. The physician indicated that he would be scheduling her for radiation treatment. Mrs. Hall told the nurse that she did not want treatment. She was worried that, if she told the doctor this, he would not see her as a client any more. Because she was in a great deal of pain and needed medication, this concern of abandonment frightened her.

A nurse's primary ethical responsibility in this case is to advocate for the client, ensuring that her wishes be respected by informing the physician of the client's statement, and supporting the client to talk with the physician. Although the physician believes treatment would provide a substantial therapeutic gain, he must respect the client's preference to forego further intervention. Ethical care in this case would also include assessing the preservation of the client's function and prevention of suffering to whatever degree possible.

The principle of **informed consent** protects the client's right to self-determination in healthcare decision making. To determine preferences, clients must have information about their condition, about proposed treatment, about risks and benefits of the specified treatment, and about existing alternatives including not having the proposed interventions (Meisel & Kuczewski, 1996). Ethically valid consent is meant to be a process of shared decision making with mutual respect and participation.

Clients frequently disclose their concerns and fears to nurses. When this happens, nurses must listen carefully to identify if clients need further information, clarification, or reassurance. Ethical nursing action involves advocating for clients by answering questions, arranging for more information, and/or accommodating the need for time to adjust to the implications of the information. All these actions help to insure that clients' preferences will be known, respected, and incorporated into decisions about care.

Quality of Life

Quality of life, in the context of healthcare decision making, focuses on a person's physical and neurological functioning. Yet an evaluation of quality of life is inherently subjective. One person might value physical mobility and independence above other qualities while another might judge the ability to communicate with others as critical. Whenever possible, quality of life should be judged by the person to whom it applies. However, sometimes this is not possible either because the person is acutely ill or has suffered a neurological insult. When the patient is unable to judge his or her own quality of life, others must weigh the facts.

It is important to be aware of the perspectives on quality of life of different stakeholders including the family, doctors, and nurses. To effectively weigh quality of life, the stakeholders should discuss the clinical facts without attaching judgment to these facts. For example, what is the patient's current and expected ability to communicate with the external world verbally or through touch? What pleasures can the patient enjoy such as taste, feeling the sun on one's face, or listening to music? Is the patient in pain and can that pain be effectively ameliorated? What is the patient's ability to do the activities of daily living? Once the clinical facts have been discussed, the patient's possible judgment of those facts can be considered based on the patient's prior history.

Contextual Features

Contextual features are benefits and burdens that affect individuals or groups in addition to the client but have compelling influence on the situation. Factors in this category include matters of finance, family situations, availability and use of resources, pressures from family or friends, and organizational or public policy.

The significance of these issues can be illustrated by comparing the perspectives that these features lend to a case. A man has a stroke resulting in severe brain injury. If he survives, he will require total care including tube feeding and nursing home placement. His only insurance is Medicare, which does not cover nursing home placement for extended periods. His wife has a chronic illness causing pain and loss of mobility that is alleviated by expensive medications, also not covered by Medicare. The three adult children consider whether their parents' savings would best be spent on nursing home care for their father who lacks awareness or on medication for their mother. They approach the medical team to request that treatment be withdrawn from their father.

Resolving Ethical Dilemmas

Responsibilities for ethical nursing practice encompass managing oneself as a moral being, functioning as a member of the healthcare team, acting as an accountable employee in an organization, and participating in the community. Taking

action in any of these spheres promotes ethical client care (Broom, 1990).

A dilemma is a situation in which:

- Two or more choices are available.
- It is difficult to determine which choice is best.
- Available alternatives cannot solve the needs of all those involved.
- Each alternative in a dilemma may have both favorable and unfavorable features.

Ethical dilemmas in healthcare involve issues surrounding professional actions and client care decisions. They can lead to discomfort and conflict among the members of the healthcare team, between providers and the client and family, or between the provider, nurses, and healthcare organization (Shannon, 1997). Several strategies may be used to prevent and resolve ethical dilemmas (Broom, 1990).

Strategies

Validate Feelings and Values. Emotions affect how people think and act in any situation. Healthcare providers have strong feelings and values about their work with clients. When clients are dying despite extensive treatment efforts, it is normal for professionals to grieve. When clients do not adhere to treatment, thereby compromising their own safety,

---

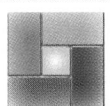

Nursing Research and Critical Thinking
Do Hospice Agencies Have More Experience Addressing the Ethical/Legal Dimensions of Care Than Nonhospice Agencies?

The researchers in this study define hospice as an interdisciplinary program of palliative care and supportive services that address the physical, spiritual, social, and economic needs of terminally ill clients and their families. Historically, hospice has been viewed as an alternative to an institutionalized and medicalized death. More high-tech services, however, are being used to aid in the delivery of palliative care. Home care providers can expect that greater numbers of these new procedures and devices will be found in any given client's home. The researchers designed a survey to collect data from executive directors of a national sample of home healthcare agencies in the United States. A 5% stratified, systematic random sample of agencies (n = 650) was drawn. Executive directors of each of the 650 sampled agencies received a six-page, structured questionnaire containing 45 open-ended and closed-ended questions. The response rate was well below 30%. Personal requests by telephone to all nonresponding agency directors were carried out and resulted in a final response rate of 33%. As a part of the survey, a Legal-Ethical Index (LEI) was developed that measured the extent to which home healthcare agencies have dealt with a range

of ethical and legal issues pertaining to the provision of technology-enhanced care in the home. Factor analysis of index items resulted in the identification of three dimensions of ethical-legal practice: "right to die" issues, "delegation of authority" issues, and "clients' rights" issues. Hospice providers reported significantly more involvement in ethical and legal issues generally and in "right to die" issues specifically ($t = -2.5$; $P < .05$).

Critical Thinking Considerations. The response rate for this study was only 33%. When only a small subsample of respondents complete a survey, researchers are faced with the possibility that those who did not complete the survey would have answered the questions differently from those who did. Implications of this study are as follows:

- Ethical and legal dimensions of care are surfacing with increased frequency in all categories of home healthcare, whether or not high-tech services are offered.
- The law imposes obligations that are enforceable in a court of law, whereas ethical norms tend to be enforced within the context of a particular profession's code of ethics.

Kaye, L. W., & Davitt, J. K. (1998). Comparison of the high-tech service delivery experiences of hospice and non-hospice home health providers. *The Hospice Journal, 13*(3), 1–20.

physicians and nurses may experience frustration and anger. Sometimes team members blame each other when things go wrong; this reaction can cause conflict.

Validation is a way of acknowledging and identifying feelings as credible. When a person is validated, he or she feels accepted. Acceptance promotes communication necessary for well-coordinated healthcare. Because conflict may erupt in situations involving ethical dilemmas, conflict resolution strategies such as clarifying misunderstanding, validating, consensus building, and collaborating also contribute to resolution of the ethical dilemmas.

Conduct a Case Analysis. Analyzing the case according to the model previously presented organizes the facts and elucidates the ethical issues to consider. Using the model also prompts consideration of areas that might be overlooked. A case analysis can be done by those directly involved in the case. Assistance also may be requested from a member of the organizational ethics committee or ethics consultation service.

The people involved in a case fulfill different roles with the client and family and contribute different data to the case analysis and management (Shannon, 1997). For example, the physician contributes facts about the client's medical condition and prognosis. Nurses describe the client's adaptation to illness and response to treatment. A physical therapist describes how physical capabilities will affect quality of life. Social workers provide information about community resources.

Compiling all the information about the case helps clarify problems and issues. Significant factors become more apparent and ethical conflicts become more evident. Alternatives are weighed in light of both ethical considerations and the specifics of that case.

Identify Outcomes. Planning care according to outcomes provides focus and consistency to a treatment plan. Many times ethical conflicts arise because the parties involved hold different ideas about the goals of intervention. Once information in all the categories has been considered, realistic outcomes can be formulated.

Identify Short- and Long-Term Goals. Outcomes for the care and treatment of a terminally ill client may include such goals as planning for pain relief, setting up hospice care, identifying a surrogate decision maker, and determining whether or not the client will be resuscitated if cardiac arrest occurs. Clarifying what will be done with each of these concerns promotes the client's sense of well-being.

For healthcare team members, answers to such questions prevent confusion about what care is meant to achieve. Crisis management is avoided. Cost savings result from working toward realistic and desirable goals rather than allowing a situation to linger or to grow more complex without a clear plan.

Clarify Accountabilities. Different people may be accountable for carrying out actions identified as part of the plan. For instance, if the team has received information that an incompetent client had completed a living will, a nurse or social worker can take responsibility for contacting the family and requesting that they bring in a copy of this document for review and consideration of the client's wishes. If questions remain about whether or not a medical condition would respond to treatment, the physicians may need to pursue further tests or request consultation. If client preference is unclear, a psychosocial clinical nurse specialist may be designated to work with the client to assess what he or she wants or hopes from treatment. In cases when a decision is made to withhold medically futile care, the physician is accountable to communicate this to the family.

Follow Through. Once a plan has been established, participants are ethically bound to uphold their accountabilities and professional responsibilities by following through with their part of what is to be done. Failing to do so breaks the implicit contract between nurse and client, possibly jeopardizing the client's health, safety, or well-being. It also undermines the integrity of the nursing profession and healthcare system, violating the confidence and trust that the public can have in the professionals from whom they seek care.

Resolve Reactions. Healthcare decisions are complex and can have dramatic consequences. The existence of an ethical dilemma can make a situation more vexing, which adds to the emotional reactions of those involved. Working through the reactions to a particularly significant event is an important step for learning from the experience and preventing residual feelings from hampering one's ability to work through similar situations in the future. Discussing feelings and reactions among the team, with peers, or a supervisor is an important step to promote resolution. This type of discussion can lead to planning care for future clients in a way that avoids repeating the same problems.

Ethics Committees

Organizational Ethics Committees required by the Joint Commission on Accreditation of Healthcare Organizations (JCAHO) are important vehicles for working through ethical issues in practice. The AHA encourages the development of these committees as interdisciplinary vehicles for identifying and addressing ethical issues. These committees have three primary functions: policy development, education, and consultation (Fost & Cranford, 1985). As part of the education and consultative functions, regular case reviews can promote ethical practice by assisting staff to recognize the ethical implications in practice and to develop strategies for resolution (Otto, 2000; Walker, 1993).

Additional Actions

Beyond case-by-case intervention, nurses contribute to identification and resolution of ethical problems by participating within their organizations and communities and helping to identify what contributes to ethical dilemmas and suggesting ways to minimize these dilemmas. Nurses also can contribute to the development of a healthcare system that respects all people and abides by the fundamentals of ethical practice.

Ways to do so include being an educated voter, participating in public forums in which decisions are made about health-care, and informing public officials of how the decisions they make affect healthcare.

THE LAW AND NURSING

Laws are rules or standards of human conduct established by government through legislative bodies and interpreted by courts to protect the rights of citizens. As a society changes its moral standards, laws generally evolve to correspond with current thinking about morality and ethics. At any time, different views about morality or ethics may not conform to law.

In healthcare and other areas of society where technology has a major impact, moral and legal standards lag behind technologic advances. As a result, the law alone may not provide specific answers to difficult healthcare dilemmas. Nurses have a responsibility to understand the current legal and ethical guidelines that govern client care.

Sources of Laws

Three kinds of law have the potential to affect nursing practice:

- Civil law generally governs actions by one individual or corporation against another.
- Criminal law involves actions by the state against an individual for violations of criminal statutes.
- Administrative law involves actions by state administrative agencies against individuals or organizations.

Malpractice cases are generally the kind of civil cases that involve nurses. A client or family member sues the nurse or the nurse's employer for malpractice because of a claim of client injury caused by nursing care. Fortunately, criminal prosecution of nurses is rare. Examples of criminal law violations include drug diversion, client assault, failure to report child abuse, and mercy killing. Administrative agencies govern the practice of nursing through boards or commissions of nursing in each state.

Laws come from three major sources: statutes passed by state and federal legislatures; specific details of statutory implementation governed by regulations adopted by state or federal agencies; and court decisions about individual cases that develop precedents for the interpretation of statutes. In addition, courts will interpret federal and state constitutions.

Licensure

The major type of administrative law that governs nursing is licensing law. Each state has a nurse practice act, although the language of each state act is different. Generally, nurse practice acts define nursing, address the scope and expectations of practice, describe how the profession will be governed, and provide criteria for nursing education. Licensure is mandatory (i.e., to practice nursing, one must be licensed as a nurse). In all states, there are exceptions for those who provide uncompensated nursing care to ill friends or family

members (Creighton, 1986). Almost all states recognize advanced registered nurse practitioners, most of whom have prescriptive authority.

Three current challenges to state boards of nursing include the development of multistate licensure, telemedicine, and the use of unlicensed assistive personnel (Health Professions Regulatory Issues, 1997; Telehealth Legislation, 1997). Liability for licensing arises in several areas. Care given below nursing standards can result in liability to the Board of Nursing for malpractice. In addition, the Board of Nursing is concerned with nurses practicing beyond the scope of their license even when the practice meets quality standards. For example, a nurse without an advanced practice license who decides to suture wounds or prescribe medicine may be liable for practice beyond his or her scope in accordance with the Nurse Practice Act. Drug diversion or abuse gives rise to a number of licensing actions, although many states provide an alternative program that promotes treatment and rehabilitation rather than discipline.

Unfortunately, client abuse and sexual contact with clients constitute an increasing area of liability in licensing cases. Sex with a current patient or client is almost never acceptable. Particularly in psychiatric nursing, sexual contact with former clients will probably violate disciplinary standards. Violation of other statutes or regulations may give rise to licensing action.

Standards of Care

Standards of care, which comprise the expected level of performance or practice as established by guidelines, authority, or custom, are important in malpractice and licensing cases. Each state's nurse practice act provides one set of guidelines for the standard that nursing care should meet. These guidelines vary as to how specifically they govern practice. The ANA and other specialty organizations define standards of care on the national level. JCAHO accredits healthcare facilities and sets nursing standards for some aspects of care such as documentation.

Institutions or agencies usually have their own policies and procedures that define their standards for nursing care. Standardized nursing plans of care or protocols also may reflect the care expected for a specific client group. Healthcare reform efforts continue to raise new issues for nursing boards or commissions (Moniz, 1992; Porter-O'Grady, 1998). The care provided by each nurse also is measured against the expected behavior of a nurse with a similar level of expertise and experience. Nurses involved in setting standards should be certain that standards are realistic in light of available resources. Standards that an agency sets should be updated frequently to reflect technologic changes. Nurses must familiarize themselves with the standards. Standards of practice are discussed in Chapter 3. When circumstances prevent compliance with standards, nurses should document the reasons for deviation.

Informed Consent

Healthcare providers are legally required to involve clients in healthcare decisions. Nurses have a moral obligation to ensure that clients give informed consent, which is voluntary permission for specific procedures based on information and knowledge. The law has evolved from first demanding that physicians simply obtain permission for experimental treatment and surgery to the current concept of giving clients full information regarding all therapeutic and diagnostic procedures. For consent to be "informed," the following elements must be addressed:

- The client's current medical status and the general course of the illness
- The proposed treatment and its rationale
- Risks and benefits of the proposed treatment
- Risks of not consenting to the treatment
- Alternatives to the proposed treatment, including non-treatment, and their associated risks and benefits

The healthcare provider who performs a procedure is charged with obtaining informed consent. Generally, however, nurses are responsible for obtaining the client's signature and verifying that the client was informed about a proposed treatment. JCAHO stipulates that an agency's policy must specify the procedures requiring signed consent. Once a consent form is signed, the burden of proof falls to the plaintiff in a legal action against the hospital or nurse. A sample informed consent form is shown in Chapter 29. Each state defines the criteria for informed consent, the need for the client's legal competency, and who is authorized to give consent for an incapacitated client. In all states, healthcare personnel may administer emergency treatment without consent if necessary. Because not all clients can read and many do not understand the complex terms contained in informed consent documents, healthcare personnel must ensure that consent is truly informed by providing whatever assistance is appropriate.

Torts and Crimes

Torts and crimes are legal wrongs committed against a person or property. A **tort** is subject to action in a civil court; a **crime** is a violation punishable by the state. Types of torts and crimes and their differences are listed in Display 6-4.

Tort actions compensate for damages. Successful tort actions result in money damages paid to the victim. Torts may be intentional or unintentional (discussed below).

A crime is any wrong punishable by the state. Two elements are necessary: evil intent and a criminal act. Crimes may exist, however, in which intent is not absolutely clear (e.g., reckless driving). Crimes are prosecuted in the criminal justice system and classified as felonies (e.g., rape, murder) or misdemeanors.

Intentional Torts

Assault and Battery. **Assault** is the threat of touching another person without his or her consent. **Battery** is the actual carrying out of such a threat (i.e., the unlawful touching of a person's body). A nurse can be sued for battery any time he or she fails to obtain consent for a procedure. For example, a hospital was sued for battery after a coronary care nurse re-

---

DISPLAY 6-4

⅃ DIFFERENCES BETWEEN CRIMES AND TORTS

Crime
Results in prison term or fine or short jail sentence to punish offender.
Felony
Pre-meditated killing (first-degree murder)
Impulsive or unintentional killing (second-degree murder; manslaughter)
Misdemeanor
An offense punishable by imprisonment of less than 1 year or a fine of less than $1,000. Does not amount to a felony.

Tort
Results in civil trial to assess compensation for plaintiff
Intentional
Assault and battery
Defamation of character
Fraud
Invasion of privacy
False imprisonment
Unintentional
Negligence—mistake or failure to be prudent
Malpractice—negligence in the practice of a profession (e.g., failure to assess a significant change in condition, failure to act appropriately in treating a patient, error in sponge counts, causing a burn, failure to use aseptic technique, falls, medical errors, misadministration of blood)

---

suscitated a client who had expressed wishes not to be resuscitated (*Anderson v. St. Francis-St. George Hospital,* 1996).

Defamation of Character. Defamation of character includes false communication that results in injury to a person's reputation by means of print (**libel**) or spoken word (**slander**). The nurse is permitted to make statements about clients only as part of his or her nursing practice and only within the limits provided by law. For example, disclosure of a false AIDS diagnosis may constitute defamation of character.

Fraud. Fraud is the willful, purposeful misrepresentation of self or an act that may cause harm to a person or property. A nurse who misrepresents his or her qualifications or bills for care not given may be committing a fraud.

Invasion of Privacy. The nurse is bound to limit discussion about a client to appropriate parties. Disclosing confidential information to an inappropriate third party subjects the nurse to liability for invasion of privacy, even if the information is true. The nurse should discuss the client with others only when the discussion is necessary for treatment and care or when the client consents to disclosure. For example, a nurse who discloses that a client is HIV positive may be liable for invasion of privacy. There is a new federal law, the Health Insurance Portability and Accountability Act (HIPAA) which passed in 1996. The Department of Health and Human Services promulgated the final privacy rule in late 2000. Agencies will need to study this lengthy regulation carefully to meet strict provisions regarding the handling of medical records and healthcare information. Violations may lead to criminal as well as civil liability.

False Imprisonment. Prevention of movement or unjustified retention of a person without consent may be false imprisonment. Nurses must use restraints only in accordance with agency policies and usually with a physician's order. A client cannot be forced to remain in the healthcare facility against his or her will (assuming that the client is mentally alert, oriented, and capable of participating in care decisions). If the client refuses to remain in the facility, the agency will have him or her sign a release stating that he or she left without medical approval. Those with mental impairments may be committed involuntarily in accordance with court proceedings if they are dangerous to themselves or others.

Unintentional Torts

Negligence. **Negligence** may be an act of omission (neglecting to do something that a reasonably prudent person would do) or commission (doing something that a reasonably prudent person would not do). **Malpractice** is negligence on the professional's part. Intent to harm is not an element of a malpractice suit. To prove nursing malpractice, a lawyer must prove that a deviation from the standard of care occurred that resulted in damage to a client. In a malpractice case, violations of the standard of care are generally proved or disproved by expert testimony. A nurse expert in a given field of nursing will be called to testify about the standard of practice as it relates to the particular case.

To prove malpractice, four elements are necessary:

- A duty to the plaintiff
- A failure to meet the standard of care, or a breach of duty, which may be an act of omission
- Causation (i.e., that the breach of duty produced the injury in a natural and continuous sequence)
- Damages, which require a physical, emotional, financial or other injury to the client

Duty. Duty describes the relationship between the plaintiff (the person bringing suit) and the defendant (the person being sued). Nurses have a duty to care for their clients. The existence of a duty is rarely an issue in a malpractice suit. Recently, however, cases have arisen in the managed care setting in which an organization may be liable for damage to a client who was not seen but should have been.

Breach of Duty. Breach of duty is the failure to conform to the standard of practice, thus creating a risk for a person that a reasonable person would have foreseen. Breach of duty may be charged when a nurse fails to meet published standards of any

relevant professional organization or the agency in which the nurse is employed. The nurse may be accused of breach of duty whenever reasonably accepted standards of nursing care are not met. Failure to observe and monitor a client's condition and behavior is a breach of duty (Cavico & Cavico, 1995). Failure to make a proper nursing assessment or nursing diagnosis is a breach of the standard of care. As nurses assume more responsibility for client care, the amount of independent client diagnosis judgment afforded nurses surely will increase. Failure to communicate relevant information about the client to the physician or other healthcare provider is a breach of duty (*Iacano v. St. Peter's Medical Center,* 2000). Failure to follow doctors' orders is a breach of duty unless the nurse knows or should know that executing an order would pose a clear risk of harm to the client. In those cases, the nurse is obliged to clarify the order or to use independent judgment in calling on others to intervene. Increasingly, the law sets specific standards. In California, legislation even governs patient care ratios in acute care settings (Perla, 2001).

Proximate Cause. Causation must be proven for the courts to find negligence. A nurse's carelessness might not result in injury. Or injury may occur without the nurse's carelessness as its proximate cause. For example, a nurse was found to have failed to be alert to signs of infections at intravenous needle sites, but no liability would adhere because there was no evidence of causation (*Simmons v. U.S.,* 1993).

A nurse or hospital may not be liable for damage to a client, even if the nurse is negligent, when the negligence does not cause the plaintiff's injury. In one case, a plaintiff alleged that the discharge nurse's failure to relate the plaintiff's complaint of chest pain to an attending physician was negligent. An expert testified that if the nurse had reported to the physician, the result would not have been different because there was no evidence the doctor would have reexamined the plaintiff. The doctor already knew of the pain and had misdiagnosed it (*Gill v. Foster,* 1992).

Courts frequently use foreseeability as a criterion for determining whether or not a cause is considered proximate. The question becomes whether or not a reasonable person should have foreseen that injury would result from a failure to conform to the standard of care (Cavico & Cavico, 1995). More commonly, plaintiffs are able to establish proximate cause between a breach of duty and damages. For example, there was proximate cause between improper monitoring by a recovery room nurse and failure to ascertain drugs administered and the client's respiratory arrest in *Eyoma v. Falco,* 1991; and between failure to properly stock the code cart leading to delayed intubation and brain death in *Dixon v. Taylor,* 1993. In *Conerly v. State* (1997), the court found that the nurses failed to detect fetal distress and continued to administer oxytocin (Pitocin) to a client in labor, causing asphyxia-related brain damage and eventual death of the baby.

When it is obvious that the client's injury resulted from someone's negligence but it is impossible to prove who was at fault, the doctrine of **res ipsa loquitur** ("the thing speaks for itself") may be invoked. Three elements must be proven (Cavico & Cavico, 1995):

- The injury could not have occurred if negligence were not present.
- The defendant or defendants (e.g., nurse, doctor, or hospital) were in complete control of the instrument causing the injury.
- The plaintiff (client) did not voluntarily create the injury.

Damages. For a plaintiff to prevail in a malpractice suit, the plaintiff must have suffered damages. The purpose of the suit is to compensate for these damages. General damages include pain and suffering, disfigurement, and disability. Special damages are for losses and expenses related to the injury such as medical expenses and lost wages. Punitive damages, rarely seen in nursing cases, are imposed when there is reckless, indifferent, or malicious conduct (Cavico & Cavico, 1995).

Manning v. Twin Falls Clinic and Hospital (1992) involved a lawsuit by the family of a deceased client against a nurse and hospital. The client was 67 years old when he was admitted to the hospital with a lengthy history of respiratory problems including chronic obstructive pulmonary disease and carbon dioxide retention. He had been on oxygen for several years. He was on no code status and on oxygen in the hospital. However, the client was to be moved to a private room because he was already near death. The nurse elected to move him without using portable oxygen for transport. The client's family protested, claiming he could not survive without his oxygen and requested a portable oxygen unit. The nurse refused. The court affirmed punitive damages against the nurse personally because the care given was found to be such an extreme deviation from the community standard of nursing care (830 P.2d 1191).

Trends in Nursing Malpractice. In the past, nurses generally were not named in malpractice suits because it was considered better to sue the person or institution with the most money or insurance. Today, however, nurses are increasingly named in malpractice litigation because of higher income or insurance and because of their increasing autonomy. Clients still sue nurses for medication errors, falls, and retained sponges. In *Bailey v. Cooper Green Hospital, et al.* (2000), the patient complained of pain following abdominal surgery; she sued the surgical nurses and was awarded $78,000.

During the past few decades, medical care has seen dramatic advances in knowledge about disease processes and technology for diagnosis and treatment of illnesses. The number of malpractice suits has increased as a result of these highly complex and advanced methods of delivering healthcare. The result has been higher standards of care for nurses, with a corresponding increase in liability (Erlen & Sereika, 1997). Managed care systems have given rise to liability in varied circumstances. A health system was found liable for $45 million in the case of a call by the mother of a 6-month-old child with a fever. The telephone triage nurse instructed the parents to take the child to a hospital 42 miles away that gave discounts to the managed care system. On the way, the baby arrested. He required amputation of both hands and feet due to impaired

perfusion. The nurse was found to have breached standards in not making a reasonable assessment of respiratory distress (Sullivan, 1997).

The nurse may experience pressure to delegate professional functions. In *Singleton v. AAA Home Health, Inc.* (2000), a home health client sued the agency when a nurse allegedly delegated wound care to an unqualified aide without direct supervision. They left the original deep packing in the hip wound, changing only the outer dressing. The court awarded more than $100,000 for delayed healing of over a year.

Nurses rushing to perform technical tasks correctly may forget to really listen to their patients. In one case, nurses who were giving chemotherapy apparently did not listen to a client's reports of burning on administration nor did they communicate with the physician about the client's continuing problems. A court awarded half a million dollars for damages that included multiple surgeries and skin grafting (*Iacano v. St. Peter's Medical Center, 2000*).

Financial constraints have led some institutions to reduce nurse-patient ratios. California has passed legislation mandating hospital nurse-to-patient ratios to safeguard patients. The law specifies the minimum requirements by type of license (Perla, 2001).

Liability

Liability denotes legal responsibility to pay damages. When the four elements of negligence are proven (i.e., when the nurse's breach of a duty owed to the client was the proximate cause of injury to the client), the nurse can be found liable. The hospital, clinic, or community nurse service may be held responsible for a nurse's negligence under the doctrine of **respondeat superior** ("let the master answer"). This notion of vicarious liability, or liability assigned to an employer by way of the terms of employment, can be applied whenever the nurse is acting within the scope of employment. Rarely, the employer may attempt to prove that the nurse was not acting within the scope of employment when the negligent act occurred. This is one reason why individual liability insurance is important. Nurses are generally covered by vicarious liability when they are acting under their employer's control. It is important to remember that this means both the employer and the nurse are responsible. The employer cannot make the nurse immune from liability. General areas of liability are summarized in Table 6-1.

Hospitals have a legal duty to treat clients who come to their emergency rooms; nurses as hospital employees have a duty to treat clients that the hospital admits (42 USC 1395 dd). In some cases, clients were denied emergency treatment because they could not pay hospital fees. A nurse who refuses care to a client can be held liable for injuries resulting from such refusal. In addition, the federal government may impose a fine on the hospital for such refusal.

Crimes

Criminal proceedings arise when the state brings charges against a defendant who has violated a criminal statute (e.g., robbery, rape, or manslaughter). The state seeks punishment

TABLE 6-1

General Areas of Liability			
	To Whom Is Healthcare Provider Responsible?	Client Injury Necessary?	Result if Successful
Malpractice or Negligence	Client	Yes	Money paid to client by healthcare provider
Administrative/ Licensing	Board of nursing	No	Loss of license or keeping license on certain conditions; fine
Criminal	State represented by prosecutors	No	Jail or fine

for that wrongdoing. Negligence that leads to a client's death is tried as a civil tort, a lawsuit filed by the client's family. Only rarely will the state file a criminal action. In a criminal procedure, the prosecution must prove guilt beyond a reasonable doubt. In a civil case, the plaintiff need only prove the case on a "more likely than not" basis.

Assault and battery (described previously) also may be criminally tried. Other examples of crimes for which nurses have been tried include robbery, narcotics laws violations, and murder. In one notorious case, a nurse who wanted to prove the need for a pediatric intensive care unit administered succinylcholine to several children in a pediatrician's office. The first five children experienced respiratory arrest and survived. When the sixth child died, the nurse was tried and convicted for murder (Tammelleo, 1986).

In another case, criminal charges resulted when a nurse forcefully searched a client whom she suspected of stealing money from another client. When the client objected to being searched, a guard held the client's arms so the nurse could search the pockets. Finding no money, they left the client, who subsequently suffered a cardiac arrest and died. Criminal intent was shown because the nurse should have been aware that her search was illegal (Tammelleo, 1985).

Legally Sensitive Areas of Nursing Practice

Controlled Substances

In 1970, the Comprehensive Drug Abuse Prevention and Control Act was passed in the United States. In most states, nurses may administer controlled substances (narcotics, depressants, stimulants, and hallucinogens) only under the direction of a physician or other authorized provider. Misuse can lead to criminal penalties unless the substances are authorized under advanced practice licenses. In institutions, most controlled substances must be kept secure and monitored closely in accordance with institutional policies and state regulations. Failure to do so may lead to disciplinary action against the nurse's license.

Death and Dying

Death occurs when there is an absence of brain function despite the function of other body organs. It is the nurse's duty to recognize legal death. In some states, the nurse may pronounce death at the bedside. In most states, however, the physician has the legal responsibility of pronouncing the person dead.

Euthanasia. Physician- or nurse-caused death (active euthanasia) is controversial. Many healthcare providers believe that actively causing a client's death violates professional ethics. *Active euthanasia, deliberately hastening a person's death, is considered murder in all states and almost all other countries.* Despite these concerns, there is growing support for physician-assisted suicide and related measures to reduce suffering at the end of life (Gostin, 1997). Passive euthanasia measures are those that withhold or withdraw treatment to allow death to occur naturally over time.

Advance Directives. In 1990, the federal legislature passed the Patient Self-Determination Act, which requires that each hospital, nursing home, visiting nurse agency, hospice, or health maintenance organization admitting clients to their services inform clients about their rights regarding end-of-life decisions. The agency is required to inform clients of state law, local policy, and agency policies, if any, regarding end-of-life decisions. The statute has been successful only to a limited degree in that most Americans have not executed any kind of advance directive (Hite, 1995; Rich, 1998).

Nurses must become familiar with statutes in their states regarding the execution of living wills or directives to physicians (ANA, 1991). These statutes list specific procedures to follow while granting civil and criminal immunity to those following the guidelines. The living will should be prepared before people become incapacitated. Be aware of the requirements for witnessing a living will. Usually, the state's Natural Death Act prohibits an employee of the healthcare provider caring for the client to be a witness. Also, be familiar with the ANA standards for these areas. These practice requirements are absolute. Thus, each nurse is accountable for providing care congruent with these standards.

Resuscitation. Nurses must always know the code status of their clients regarding **resuscitation,** verify the code status on the client's order sheet, and follow agency policy. When nurses are unaware and encounter a client in cardiac arrest, they should resuscitate the client pending confirmation that there is a no code order. If there is a no code order, resuscitation may be stopped once initiated. And if there is not a code order and the client's wishes for end-of-life care are not followed because of this lack of order, then the nurse is responsible for ensuring that an order is obtained.

Issues have occurred around do not resuscitate orders for home care clients. A **community-based no code order** can be obtained in many states and have various names including EMS-No CPR orders, portable no code orders, or community-based DNR orders. These documents generally require the signatures of the physician and the patient or their legal surrogate. Unlike advance directives, these orders must be obtained through a healthcare provider. A community-based no code order allows emergency medical personnel, if called, to provide care and support to the patient and family without attempting resuscitation.

Death Certificate. Laws are specific in each of the states regarding who may sign death certificates. Determine that information for your state.

Care of the Body. After the physician pronounces death, the nurse is responsible for preparing the body for the morgue or mortuary. Be familiar with the facility's instructions for care and the wishes of the deceased and family. Always treat the body with dignity.

Organ Donation. Always check to see if the deceased wished to donate organs to a transplant program. If the death was accidental and no donor card is available, the nurse may discuss with the family the possibility of donating the deceased person's organs. Figure 6-2 shows a sample organ donor card. A section of the living will also may provide this information. If functional organs are to be donated, the hospital should have specific care instructions for the body. The Uniform Anatomical Gift Act is in effect in all 50 states and the District of Columbia with some variation. State law governs the procurement process while safeguarding donor intentions and designates procedures for use and distribution of organs. Some states use the driver's license to identify those persons who agree to organ donation in the event of their untimely death.

Autopsy. An *autopsy* is a postmortem examination of the body's organs and tissues to determine the cause of or pathologic conditions contributing to death. Except in certain circumstances, consent for an autopsy is required. The patient

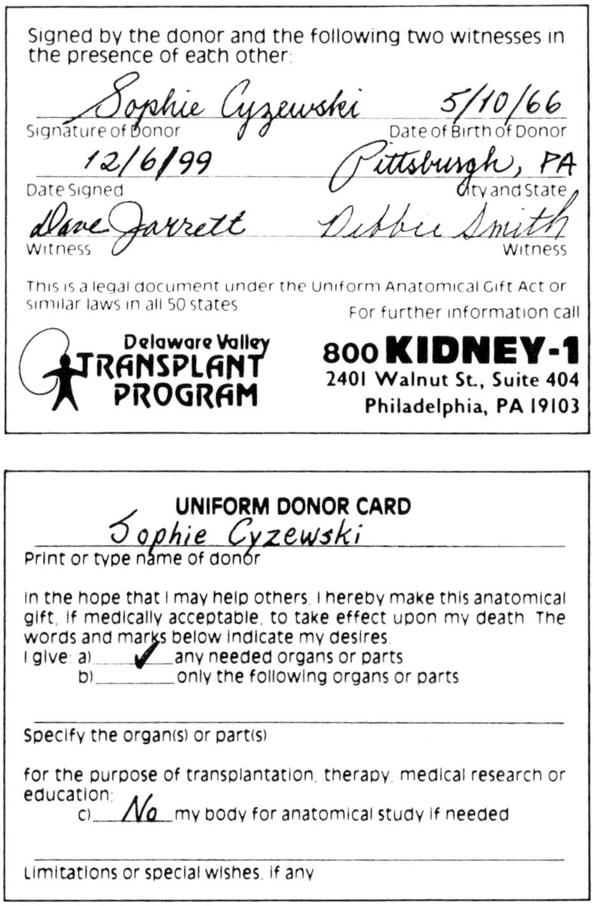
Signed by the donor and the following two witnesses in the presence of each other:

Sophie Cyzewski — Signature of Donor; 5/10/66 — Date of Birth of Donor

12/6/99 — Date Signed; Pittsburgh, PA — City and State

Dave Jarrett — Witness; Debbie Smith — Witness

This is a legal document under the Uniform Anatomical Gift Act or similar laws in all 50 states

For further information call

Delaware Valley TRANSPLANT PROGRAM

800 KIDNEY-1
2401 Walnut St., Suite 404
Philadelphia, PA 19103

UNIFORM DONOR CARD

Sophie Cyzewski
Print or type name of donor

In the hope that I may help others, I hereby make this anatomical gift, if medically acceptable, to take effect upon my death. The words and marks below indicate my desires.
I give: a) ✓ any needed organs or parts
b) ______ only the following organs or parts

Specify the organ(s) or part(s)

for the purpose of transplantation, therapy, medical research or education;
c) No my body for anatomical study if needed

Limitations or special wishes, if any

FIGURE 6-2 Sample of an organ donor card.

may consent to an autopsy before death or a close family member may consent after death. State laws require an autopsy regardless of consent if the death meets certain state criteria such as suspected murder or suicide.

Wills. The nurse may be asked to witness a will, which is a person's declaration regarding how his or her property is to be handled after death. Many institutions have policies about nurses witnessing legal documents. If a nurse does witness a will, he or she makes a note on the client's chart about the client's mental and physical condition at the time of the signing and of the nurse's role in the proceedings. A nurse cannot be a beneficiary to any will he or she witnesses.

Good Samaritan Law

The Good Samaritan Law offers legal immunity for healthcare professionals who assist in an emergency and render reasonable care under such circumstances. Because most states do not require nurses or citizens to aid the distressed, such assistance becomes an ethical, rather than a legal, duty. Although this law limits liability for the nurse, he or she may be liable for gross negligence. A nurse who stops to help is obligated to remain until additional assistance is obtained. The nurse should then

THERAPEUTIC DIALOGUE
Ethical Issues

Scene for Thought

Mrs. Miller, who has been unconscious since major abdominal surgery for metastatic cancer, has been in the intensive care unit for 3 weeks. Her 23-year-old daughter, Melanie, is meeting with the physician and the nurse. The purpose of this meeting is to re-explain the plan for Mrs. Miller and its rationale. Melanie seems to be confused about her mother's prognosis.

Less Effective

Physician: We need to talk again about why we're decreasing your mom's IVs and oxygen.

Melanie: I thought you were taking her oxygen and IVs away because she's getting better! I don't understand what you're doing. *(Cries and looks angry.)*

Nurse: I thought you understood, Miss Miller, that your mother isn't getting any better and that, in fact, she probably won't come out of her coma at all. *(Said softly but firmly.)*

Melanie: No, I didn't get that! My mother is still a young woman, and she's never been sick like this. How can she be dying? How can you take away the things she needs to live?

Nurse: I know it's hard for you to understand. I think it would be a good thing if you called your minister and the rest of your family so you can talk it over and decide what to do.

Melanie: I think I'll call our family lawyer too. There's something funny going on here! *(Cries as she strides purposefully away to the phone.)*

More Effective

Physician: We need to talk again about why we're decreasing your mom's IVs and oxygen.

Melanie: I thought you were taking her oxygen and IVs away because she's getting better! I don't understand what you're doing. *(Cries and looks angry.)*

Physician: I really thought you understood, Melanie. I'm sorry you're upset about this.

Nurse: Could you tell us what you see when you go in to visit your mother, Melanie? *(Assesses her viewpoint before making any assumptions.)*

Melanie: I see that she's lying there, resting quietly, looking like she's asleep. *(Still cries quietly, face set in a stiff frown.)*

Nurse: We've all noticed some changes in her over the last few weeks. Have you? *(Assesses her perceptions.)*

Melanie: Well . . . I've noticed that her color is getting paler and that she doesn't move around at all anymore, even when you do something to her. I suppose you think that means something! *(Looks frightened and angry at the same time.)*

Nurse: Yes, we think it means that your mom is going deeper into her coma and that there is very little chance that she'll come out. *(Nurse and physician further explain coma and its relationship to the cancer.)*

Melanie: *(Puts her head in her hands and cries quietly. The room is quiet. She looks up.)* I knew this. The doctor said that before. I didn't want to believe it.

Nurse: We know it's difficult to "give up" on someone you love. It might be helpful to talk some more about what to expect over the next few days and how you can help us with your mother's care. Would that be good for you?

Melanie: Yes, that would be helpful. I hope you don't mind if I cry, though. I thought she would get better.

Nurse: That's very understandable. We won't mind. *(Discussion with Melanie continues. Nurse and family suggest support from clergy, father, and siblings. Family meeting is arranged the next day to include all.)*

Critical Thinking Challenges

- Determine which of the 11 items of the ANA Code of Ethics that the second nurse reflected in her care of the Miller family.
- After studying the Patient's Bill of Rights, propose those rights that are particularly relevant to the Miller family's situation.
- Explain who is the client: Mrs. Miller, Melanie, or the family.
- Critique the first nurse's failure to meet Melanie's needs.

relinquish care to official rescue personnel unless asked to remain. Because emergency assistance is generally outside the scope of the nurse's employment, the employer's malpractice insurance will not provide coverage. This is another reason for nurses to carry their own insurance.

Protecting Yourself Legally

Nurses may minimize the risk of legal problems, including malpractice, in a number of ways. First, nurses should keep current with advances in practice. Continuing education is absolutely essential to stay knowledgeable about general and specialized care. Likewise, nurses should be familiar with state regulations governing nursing and with standards of professional organizations.

Professional Practice

Nurses involved in the development of policies, procedures, protocols, or standardized nursing plans of care should be sure to make them realistic for their own practices and/or for an agency. Such standards should be practicable with the resources available. Staffing and equipment to conform to these guidelines must be available at all times. Those who develop standards to apply to various practice settings should keep in mind the differences in resources and facilities of different sizes, acuity, and geographic area. Those involved in policy making need to continue to update policies in a timely and sensible manner in accordance with nursing's demands. New knowledge must be applied. Policies, procedures, and protocols must be followed. Propounding unrealistic policies and procedures then not following them is an invitation to malpractice suits.

The client's condition must be monitored, and observations must be documented. Whether the client is in a hospital recovering from surgery, in home care coping with a chronic illness, or in a setting where direct observation is impossible (e.g., as a telephone triage nurse), assessment of the client must be recorded. Significant changes in the client's condition need to be reported to a physician or other professional in a timely manner. The report to the physician also must be documented. When physicians do not follow up with assessment intervention, the nurse needs to challenge the physician's care. Hospitals and nurses may be liable when nurses do not challenge physicians in the face of obvious negligence. In *Reinen v. Northern Arizona Orthopedics, LTD* (2000), the nurse allegedly failed to follow the chain of command when a diabetic patient deteriorated following trauma surgery. The appellate court held that the nurse could be found negligent when she did not get a physician to follow up on abnormal laboratory values and to treat his critical condition. She did not seek the assistance of her supervisor, which the court clearly expected.

Professional Liability Insurance

With increasing numbers of malpractice claims involving nurses, nurses will find it prudent to have professional liability insurance. Although nurses are generally covered under their employers' insurance, there may be conflicts of interest with other employees. Increasingly, nurses are being named specifically in lawsuits, so having their own insurance ensures the best representation. Because a nurse may be sued for some act related to nursing but outside the limits of her or his employment, every nurse also should have her or his own insurance. Nursing students are generally covered for their student clinical experiences as long as they are registered students and are practicing under appropriate supervision.

Documentation

Documentation should be accurate, complete, and contemporaneous with care given (Wisser, 1998). Documentation should include normal findings in the form of a flowsheet, checklist, or narrative. Assess and record vital signs in accordance with the agency's policy and the client's condition. When critical events occur, note the precise time and event in the records. Documentation should be objective. Criticism of other providers has no place in the medical record. Do not include negative comments about the client or family unless they constitute objective documentation of behavior or accurate quotations of statements made. Never obliterate an entry by erasing it or using correction fluid. The presumption will be that the matter erased or covered up is more damaging than whatever was actually written. Correct charting errors by marking a line through the error and recording the nurse's initials. If a specific incident, such as a fall or medication error, occurs, follow these principles:

- Maintain rapport with the client. Do not avoid communication with the client who is experiencing stress and uncertainty. Offer simple explanations if you can do so honestly, calmly, and without blaming anyone.
- Document the incident in the progress notes and on the appropriate forms of your institution. Incident reports are useful to remind you of the events surrounding the incident. They are useful to enhance continuous quality improvement.

Nursing students must perform only duties within the scope of their professional training to date. These acts are performed with the same degree of competence that an RN would exhibit. Under the auspices of a clinical supervisor, nursing students may carry out assignments. Nursing students assume liability for their negligent or wrong acts. The clinical supervisor or school may be held liable as well.

KEY CONCEPTS

- **Morals** are standards of right and wrong. Values are ideas and beliefs that a person holds to be important.
- The ANA code of ethics is the nurses' value statement to the public and should be acted upon by all nurses.
- Principles of healthcare ethics include beneficence, nonmaleficence, autonomy, and justice. Principles of professional ethics include confidentiality, privacy, veracity, and fidelity.
- An ethical dilemma involves choosing between conflicting values. Resolution of a dilemma involves the application of structured analysis based on moral principles.
- Licensing law, a type of administrative law, governs nursing practice through the Nurse Practice Act of each state.
- Individual state nurse practice acts provide some guidance for standards of nursing. Following the current standard of nursing care as evidenced in state statutes and regulations, standards of professional organizations, and current literature helps to minimize the risk for legal problems.
- The four elements of negligence are duty, breach of duty, proximate cause, and damage.
- The nurse has legal responsibilities regarding the dying client and the deceased (e.g., euthanasia, living wills, resuscitation,

the death certificate, care of the body, organ donations, the autopsy, and wills).
- Although the Good Samaritan Law provides immunity for professionals under specific circumstances, nurses should carry personal liability insurance.
- Nurses need to obtain professional liability insurance to protect their best interests should their practice be called into question through legal action.
- Clear, accurate documentation will substantiate care provided to the client.

REFERENCES

American Hospital Association. (1992). *A patient's bill of rights.* Chicago, IL: Author.

American Nurses Association. (1991). *Position statement—Nursing the patient self-determination acts.* http://nursingworld.org/readroom/position/ethics/etsdet.htm

American Nurses Association. (2001). *Ethics code for nurses with interpretive statements.* Kansas City, MO: Author. [Online] *http://www.nursingworld.org/ethics/chcode.htm*

Beauchamp, T. L., & Childress, J. F. (2001). *Principles of biomedical ethics* (5th ed.). New York, NY: Oxford University Press.

Benjamin, M., & Curtis, J. (1992). *Ethics in nursing.* New York, NY: Oxford University Press.

Broom, C. (1990). Conflict resolutions strategies for ethical dilemmas: When ethical dilemmas evolve to conflict. *Dimensions of Critical Care Nursing, 10*(6), 354–363.

Caplan, R. L., Light, D. W., & Daniels, N. (1999). Benchmarks of fairness: A moral framework for assessing equity. *International Journal of Health Services, 29*(4), 853–869.

Cavico, F. J., & Cavico, N. M. (1995). The nursing profession in the 1990s: Negligence and malpractice liability. *Cleveland State Law Review, 43,* 557–626.

Covey, L. S., Sullivan, M. A., Johnston, J. A., Glassman, A. H., Robinson, M. D., & Adams, D. P. (2000). Advances in non-nicotine pharmacotherapy for smoking cessation. *Drugs, 59*(1):17–31.

Creighton, H. (1986). *Law every nurse should know* (5th ed.). Philadelphia: W. B. Saunders.

Curtin, L. (2000). On being a person of integrity . . . or ethics and other liabilities. *Journal of Continuing Education in Nursing, 31*(2), 55–58.

Erlen, J. A., & Sereika, S. M. (1997). Critical care nurses: Ethical decision-making and stress. *Journal of Advanced Nursing, 26*(5), 953–961.

Espinosa, E., Gonzales-Baron, M., Poveda, J., Ordonez, A., & Zamora, P. (1993). The information given to the terminal patient with cancer. *European Journal of Cancer, 29*(12), 1795–1796.

Fost, N., & Cranford, R. E. (1985). Hospital ethics committees: administrative aspects. *Journal of the American Medical Association, 253*(18), 2687–2692.

Gostin, L. O. (1997). Deciding life and death in the courtroom: From Quinlan to Cruzan, Glucksberg, and Vacco—a brief history and analysis of constitutional protection of the "right to die." *Journal of the American Medical Association, 278*(18).

Health Professions Regulatory Issues. (1997). [Online] Available at: *www.nursingworld.org/gova/hod97/regulate.htm*

Hite, C. (1995). Advance directives & end-of-life decisions. [Online] Available at: *http://www.euthanasia.org/hite.html*

Hughes, J. R. (1999). Four beliefs that may impede progress in the treatment of smoking. *Tobacco Control, 8*(3), 323–326.

Jonsen, A. R. (1994). Clinical ethics and the four principles. In R. Gillon & A. Lloyd (Eds.), *Principles of health care ethics.* Chichester: John Wiley and Sons Ltd.

Jonsen, A. R., Siegler, M., & Winslade, W. J. (1998). *Clinical ethics: A practical approach to ethical decisions in clinical medicine* (4th ed.) New York: McGraw Hill.

Kipnis, K. (1990). Professional ethics in health care: An introduction. *Hawaii Medical Journal, 49*(8), 292–294.

Kopelman, L. M., & Mouradian, W. E. (2001). Do children get their fair share of health and dental care? *Journal of Medicine and Philosophy, 26*(2), 127–136.

Liaschenko, J. (1999). Can justice coexist with the supremacy of personal values in nursing practice? *Western Journal of Nursing Research, 21*(1), 35–50.

Meisel A. (1991). Legal myths about terminating life support. *Archives of Internal Medicine, 151*(8), 1497–1502.

Meisel A., & Kuczewski M. (1996). Legal and ethical myths about informed consent. *Archives of Internal Medicine, 156*(22), 2521–2526.

Meisel, A., Snyder, L., & Quill, T. (2000). Seven legal barriers to end-of-life care: Myths, realities, and grains of truth. *Journal of the American Medical Association, 284*(19), 2495–2501.

Moniz, D. M. (1992). The legal danger of written protocols and standards of practice. The nurse practitioner. *The American Journal of Primary Health Care, 17*(9), 58–60.

Otto, S. (2000). A nurse's lifeline. A nursing ethics committee offers the chance to review and learn from ethical dilemmas. *American Journal of Nursing, 100*(12), 57–59.

Pellegrino, E. (1979). The anatomy of clinical judgments. In H. T. Engelhardt, Jr., S. F. Spicker, & B. Towers (Eds.), *Clinical judgment: A critical appraisal.* (pp. 169–194). Dordrecht, Holland: D. Reidel.

Perla, L. (2001). AB 394: Changes in Patient Care and Nurse Staff Ratios. *Journal of Nursing Law, 8,* 27–32.

Pinch, W. J. (2000). Confidentiality: concept analysis and clinical application. *Nursing Forum, 35*(2), 5–16.

Porter-O'Grady, T. (1998). Signposts for the next century. *Nursing Management, 29*(12), 5.

President's Commission for the Study of Ethical Problems in Medicine and Biomedical and Behavioral Research. (1982). *Making health care decisions* (Vol. I.). Washington, DC: U.S. Government Printing Office.

Quill T. E., Lo, B., & Brock, D. W. (1997). Palliative options of last resort: A comparison of voluntarily stopping eating and drinking, terminal sedation, physician-assisted suicide, and voluntary active euthanasia. *Journal of the American Medical Association, 278*(23), 2099–2104.

Rich, B. A. (1998). Advance directives: The next generation. *Journal of Legal Medicine, 19,* 63–97.

Sardell, A. N., & Trierweiler, S. J. (1993). Disclosing the cancer diagnosis. *Cancer, 72*(11), 3355–3365.

Schneiderman, L. J., Jecker, N. S., & Jonsen, A. R. (1990). Medical futility: Its meaning and ethical implications. *Annals of Internal Medicine, 112*(12), 949–954.

Sell, L., Devlin, B., Bourke, S. J., Munro, N. C., Corris, P. A., & Gibson, G. J. (1993). Communicating the diagnosis of lung cancer. *Respiratory Medicine, 87,* 61–63.

Shannon, S. E. (1997). The roots of interdisciplinary conflict around ethical issues. *Critical Care Nursing Clinics of North America, 9,* 13–28.

Sullivan, G. (1997). Advice or diagnosis? A legal perspective. *Business and Health, 12*(5), 40.

Tammelleo, A. D. (Ed.). (1985). Chaos in the O.R. *The Regan Report on Nursing Law, 26,* 4.

Tammelleo, A. D. (Ed.). (1986). Nurse murders pediatric patient. *The Regan Report on Nursing Law, 27,* 6.

Telehealth Legislation. (1997). [Online] Available at: *http://www.nursingworld.org*

Uniform Anatomical Gift Act, Amend. 1987. 18A U.L.A. 2 (1987).

Walker, M. U. (1993). Keeping moral space open: New images of ethics consulting. *Hastings Center Report, 23*(2), 33–40.

Walters, L. (1988). Ethical issues in the prevention and treatment of HIV infection and AIDS. *Science, 239,* 597–603.

Weiner, S. (2001). "I can't afford that!": Dilemmas in the care of the uninsured and underinsured. *Journal of General Internal Medicine, 16*(6), 412–418.

Wisser, S. H. (1998). Chart documentation: For reading concerns. *Journal of Neuroscience Nursing, 30*(5), 326–329.

Woodard, L. J., & Parmies, R. J. (1992). The disclosure of the diagnosis of cancer. *Primary Care, 19*(4), 657–663.

Legal Case References

Anderson v. St. Francis-St. George Hospital, 671 N.E.2d 225 (Ohio 1996).

Bailey v. Cooper Green Hospital, et al., Ala. S. Ct., 2000 Ala. LEXIS 550 (2000).

Conerly v. State, 690 So.2d 980 (La. 1997).

Dixon v. Taylor, 431 S.E.2d 778, 781–82 (N.C. App. Ct. 1993).

Eyoma v. Falco, 589 A.2d 653, 655–56 (N.J. Super. Ct. 1991).

Gill v. Foster, 232 Ill. App.3d 768, 173 Ill. Dec. 802, 597 N.E.2d 776 (4th Dist.1992).

Iacano v. St. Peter's Medical Center, 760 A.2d 348 N.J. Super. Ct. App. Div. (2000).

Manning v. Twin Falls Clinic and Hospital, 830 P.2d 1185 (1992).

Reinen v. Northern Arizona Orthopedics, LTD, 991 P. 2d 242, 2000 Ariz. LEXIS 1(2000).

Simmons v. U.S., 841 F. Supp. 748, 750 (W.D. La. 1993).

Singleton v. AAA Home Health, Inc., 772 So. 2d 346 (La. App. 2000).

BIBLIOGRAPHY

Astrom, G., Jansson, L., Norberg, A., & Hallberg, I. R. (1993). Experienced nurses' narratives of their being in ethically difficult care situations. The problem to act in accordance with one's ethical reasoning and feelings. *Cancer Nursing, 16*(3), 179–187.

Bandman, E., & Bandman, B. (2002). *Nursing ethics through the life span* (4th ed.). New Jersey: Prentice-Hall.

Barnard, A., & Sandelowski, M. (2001). Technology and humane nursing care: (Ir)reconcilable or invented difference? *Journal of Advanced Nursing, 34*(3), 367–375.

Brent, N. J. (1997). *Nurses and the law: A guide to principles and application.* Philadelphia: W. B. Saunders.

Broom, C. (1992). Administering pain medications for a terminal patient: Part 2: Case analysis. *Dimensions of Critical Care Nursing, 11*(3), 158–161.

Broom, C. (1994). Patient–family conflicting issues: Part 2: Case analysis. *Dimensions of Critical Care Nursing, 13*(1), 44–50.

Burns, J. P., Mitchell, C., Griffith, J. L., & Truog, R. D. (2001). End-of-life care in the pediatric intensive care unit: attitudes and practices of pediatric critical care physicians and nurses. *Critical Care Medicine, 29*(3), 658–664.

Cameron, M. E. (1997). Legal and ethical issues. Professional boundaries in nursing. *Journal of Professional Nursing, 13*(3), 142.

Cameron, M. E., Crisham, P., & Lewis, D. E. (1993). The basic nature of ethical problems experienced by persons with acquired immunodeficiency syndrome: Implications for nursing

ethics education and practice. *Journal of Professional Nursing, 9*(6), 327–335.

Canadian Nurses Association. (1997). *Code of ethics for nursing.* Ottawa: Author. [Online] Available at: *http://www.cna-nurses.ca/pages/ethics/ethicsframe.htm*

Cochran, M. (1999). The real meaning of patient-nurse confidentiality. *Critical Care Nursing Quarterly, 22*(1), 42–51.

Curtin, L. (2001). The ICN code of ethics for nurses: Shared values in a troubled world. International Nursing Review, 48(1), 1–2.

Guido, G. W. (2001). *Legal and ethical issues in nursing* (3rd ed.). New Jersey: Prentice-Hall.

International Council of Nurses. (2000). *The ICN code of ethics for nurses.* ICN-International Council of Nurses, 3, place Jean-Marteau, CH-1201 Geneva, Switzerland. [Online] Available at: *http://www.icn.ch/ethics.htm*

International Council of Nurses. (1973). *ICN Code for Nurses: Ethical concepts applied to nursing.* Geneva, Switzerland: Imprimeries Polpularies.

Leipert, B. D. (2001). Feminism and public health nursing: partners for health. *Scholarly Inquiry Nursing Practice, 15*(1), 49–61.

Ludwick, R., & Sedlak, C. A. (1998). Ethical issues and critical thinking: Students' stories. *Nursing Connections, 11*(3), 12–18.

Martin, J. (1993). Lying to patients: Can it ever be justified? *Nursing Standards, 7*(18), 29–31.

Matzo, M. L., & Schwarz, J. K. (2001). In their own words: Oncology nurses respond to patient requests for assisted suicide and euthanasia. *Applied Nursing Research, 14*(2), 64–71.

Patient Self-Determination Act, 42 U.S.C. 1396a(a); 42 U.S.C. 1396m(1)(a); 42 U.S.C. 1396n(c)(2). (1990).

Pellegrino, E. D. (1992). Is truth telling to the patient a cultural artifact? *Journal of the American Medical Association, 268*(13), 1734–1735.

Porter-O'Grady, T. (1998). Ethics in health care: Are nurses at the table? *Advanced Practice Nursing Quarterly, 4*(2), 83–84.

Shannon, S. E. (2001). Helping families prepare for and cope with a death in the ICU. In J. R. Curtis & G. D. Rubenfeld (Eds.), *The transition from cure to comfort: Managing death in the intensive care unit* (pp. 165–182). New York: Oxford University Press.

Streiner, D. L., Saigal, S., Burrows, E., Stoskopf, B., & Rosenbaum, P. (2001). Attitudes of parents and health care professionals toward active treatment of extremely premature infants. *Pediatrics, 108*(1), 152–157.

Trott, M. C. (1998). Legal issues for nurse managers. *Nurse Manager, 29*(6), 38–41.

Uhlman, R. F., & Pearlman, R. A. (1991). Perceived quality of life and preferences for life-sustaining treatment in older adults. *Archives of Internal Medicine, 151*(3), 495–498.

Watson, C. (1993). The role of the nurse in ethical decision making in intensive care units. *Intensive Critical Care Nursing, 9*(3), 191–194.

Werner, P., & Mendelsson, G. (2001). Nursing staff members' intentions to use physical restraints with older people: testing the theory of reasoned action. *Journal of Advanced Nursing, 35*(5), 784–791.

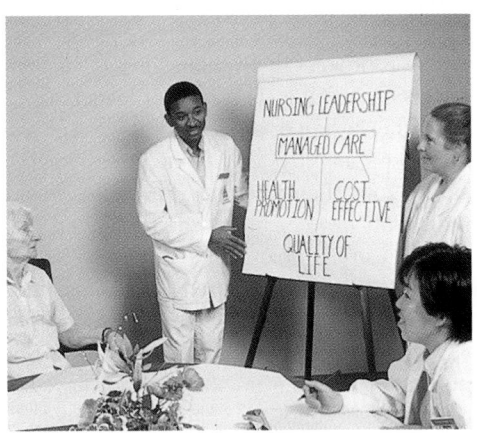

7 Nurse Leader and Manager

Key Terms

charge nurse
clinical nurse specialist
delegation
directive leadership
financial resources
human resource
   management
information resources
leadership
managed care
management

nurse anesthetist
nurse executive
nurse midwife
nurse practitioner
participative leadership
planning
primary nursing
problem solving
resource management
team leader
team nursing

Learning Objectives

Upon completion of this chapter, the student will be able to do the following:

1. Explain the differences between leadership and management.
2. Describe the three areas of resource management focus.
3. Identify three skills required for effective management.
4. List interventions that can control perceptions and reactions to change.
5. Describe common clinical practice, management, and education roles in nursing.
6. Characterize leadership and management functions of common nursing roles.
7. Describe the three most popular models of nursing care delivery.
8. Explain why problem solving, management, and nursing processes are similar.

Critical Thinking Challenge

Your nurse manager wants to change the practice model on your unit from primary care nursing to modular nursing (care partners). You have been working on the unit for 3 years. You are pleased with the current system and wonder how the new changes will affect you.

Once you have completed this chapter and have incorporated information about the nurse as leader and manager into your knowledge base, review the above scenario and reflect on the following areas of Critical Thinking:

1. Compare and contrast the advantages of primary nursing and modular nursing (care pairs) for clients. Do the same for nurses in the two situations.
2. Examine possible reasons that the manager might want to change the current model.
3. Analyze how you have adjusted to big changes in your life. Identify those factors that were helpful and those factors that were counterproductive.
4. Identify ways to decrease your own stress (professionally and personally) during a significant change at work.

The environment for delivery of nursing care has become increasingly complex and fluid. Nurses practice in a variety of settings, assuming greater independence and responsibility than ever before. As the various organizations that provide healthcare become more business oriented, nurses are challenged to be highly skilled resource managers as well as providers of "the diagnosis and treatment of human responses to actual or potential health problems" (American Nurses Association, 1995). The American Organization of Nurse Executives (AONE) defines three essential role components of nursing: "(1) a contingent component which requires medical authorization for treatment, (2) an independent component of practice, and (3) a role as integrator and coordinator of care, across the lifespan of individuals, as well as across settings and among disciplines" (American Organization of Nurse Executives, 1993). For nursing professionals to meet the service responsibilities to society and fulfill the accountabilities of these three component roles, the profession needs internal organization and leadership.

At the institutional level, leadership abilities and management skills are required of all nurses so as to use dwindling resources to achieve the best outcomes for clients and to support the success and survival of the organization. As those who pay for healthcare become more concerned about increasing costs, nurses must know how to select the most effective methods for solving client problems. At the individual nurse–client level, leadership and good management skills are necessary to determine plans of nursing care, to collaborate effectively with other healthcare professionals, and to coordinate interdisciplinary treatment plans for clients. At the management level, individual nurses must be provided with appropriate resources to allow for the implementation of plans of care.

LEADERSHIP

Leadership is the ability to influence others to strive for a vision or goal or to change. Leadership results from the effective practice of behaviors that are selected to meet the needs of the situation. Leadership behaviors can be learned.

No one best way (or one best set of behaviors) exists for effective leadership. Research on leaders and leadership has shown that different leaders have different inherent traits and abilities (Bass, 1990; Porter-O'Grady, 1997). Although certain personality traits are more common in leaders than in followers, no single set of traits is found in every leader. Although many leaders are courageous, optimistic, assertive, decisive, logical, thorough, and innovative, some followers also have these traits. A leader's effectiveness depends not only on his or her traits, skills, and behaviors, but also on characteristics of the followers, the relationship between the leader and followers, and factors in the situation, such as shared purpose and desire for change (Rost, 1993; Bass & Avolio, 1994; Irurita, 1994; Swanson, 2000).

Just as knowledge of pathophysiology enables nurses to make appropriate decisions regarding client care priorities, knowledge of economics provides a foundation for effective decision making. Briefly stated, economics is concerned with the causes and consequences of scarcity. To obtain one thing of value, we must give up another. To make good choices, people must consider not only the intended consequences of a choice, but also the unintended or secondary effects. The most well-intentioned program or intervention can become ineffective as a result of unforeseen "costs" or secondary effects. Successful leaders have sufficient depth of knowledge of the economics of healthcare so that their decisions consider a broad range of consequences (Millman, 1996; Finkler & Kovner, 2000).

Styles of Leadership

Effective leadership occurs when a person with the right combination of personality traits and abilities uses behaviors appropriate for the circumstance. A leader who is effective in one situation may be ineffective in another. Leaders are often described by the style of leadership that they predominantly use. Leadership style describes how a leader interacts with followers; leadership style is reflective of the leader's traits, values, abilities, and behaviors.

In a classic article that has been the basis for many subsequent leadership theories, Tannenbaum and Schmidt (1973) describe leadership styles along a continuum from directive to participative (Fig. 7-1):

- **Directive leadership** describes a leader who makes all the decisions and tells followers what to do. The leader is in complete control. The directive leader does not involve followers in problem solving, discussion, or decision making. This type of leadership is also called authoritarian or autocratic. It was formerly used in hospitals. Physicians told nurses what to do, and nurses told clients what to do. As the roles of nurses and clients have changed, the leadership style in hospitals also has changed.
- **Participative leadership,** also referred to as democratic, is at the opposite end of the continuum. The participative leader involves followers in goal setting, problem solving, and decision making. This involvement acknowledges the importance of followers in goal achievement and effective organization and promotes a sense of control over individual situations. Participative leadership also tends to involve those most familiar with the details of the situation in the decision. To be effective, a participative leader also must provide overall direction to the group process.

Under most circumstances, some degree of participation is appropriate to promote job satisfaction and commitment, but in a crisis or emergency no time is available for group discussion and decision making, so directive leadership is most appropriate. A more directive style also may be appropriate when the leader is sharing new skills or knowledge with immature, insecure, or unskilled followers. Effective leaders

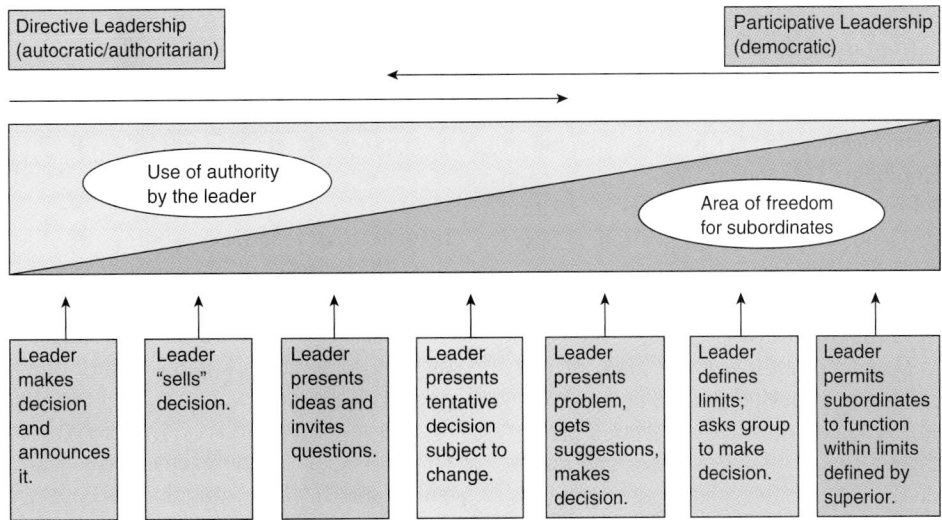

FIGURE 7-1   Leadership style has been described along a continuum from directive to participative. Directive leadership is sometimes called autocratic, authoritative, or boss-centered. Participative leadership is also called democratic or subordinate-centered leadership. (Adapted by permission of *Harvard Business Review*. An exhibit from "How to choose a leadership pattern" by R. Tannenbaum & W. H. Schmidt, [May/June 1973]. Copyright © 1973 by the Presidents and Fellows of Harvard College; all rights reserved.)

learn how to vary their style to match the circumstances appropriately (Trott & Windsor, 1999).

Today's postindustrial information age has seen rapid change and major transitions. For example, much of healthcare has moved from the hospital to the home, and the focus of nursing has changed from tasks and treatments to coordination of interdisciplinary treatment plans. Therefore, certain leadership competencies and actions are more effective today. Effective leaders are driven by their own values and sense of purpose. They communicate a vision and coach, facilitate, and empower others to master change and work toward that vision (Senge, 1990; Cover, 1991; McDaniel & Wolf, 1992; Noer, 1993; Bass & Avolio, 1994).

MANAGEMENT

Management involves getting a job done or accomplishing a goal. In today's complex healthcare environment, effective nurse managers must manage human, financial, and information resources to accomplish goals (Fig. 7-2). The process they use is similar to the problem-solving process, which is based on the scientific or research method.

Resource Management

In modern healthcare organizations, managers usually are responsible for accomplishing the work of the unit within the constraints of available resources. This process is called **resource management.** Managers must be able to organize people, things, and activities and to direct them toward overall objectives. They must manage human, financial, and information resources.

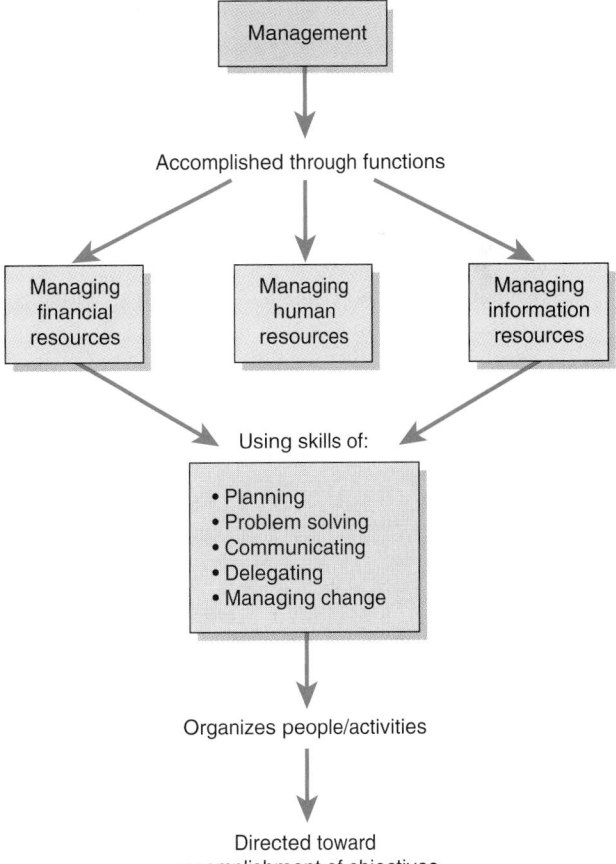

FIGURE 7-2   Effective management includes managing human, financial, and informational resources by using the skills of planning, problem solving, communicating, delegating, and managing change.

Human Resources

Human resource management is concerned with maximizing the value of the people who do the work of the organization. Activities associated with human resource management include staff selection, performance appraisal, reward, and development. They occur in a cyclic fashion (Devanna, 1994). First, the manager identifies a position that must be filled. The description of the position is based on the manager's analysis of what needs to be done—at present and in the future. A participative manager will seek input from the staff in creating the description, because staff members have a deep understanding of the work. Usually with the help of human resources personnel, qualified candidates are sought and screened. After a selection process that includes interviews by the manager, peers, and others, a selection is made. During the orientation period, performance appraisal must be continuous. With feedback, the new team member forms work habits appropriate to the organization and rapidly becoming a productive member of the staff. Informal feedback is far more effective in shaping daily behavior than a formal evaluation process, although both are important.

Performance appraisal is continuous throughout employment. Each organization determines a reward structure to define and to acknowledge success. Rewards include increased pay, expansion of responsibility and power, recognition, and job security. The manager is also responsible for the ongoing development of employees. Especially in a highly technical area such as nursing, there is a constant need to upgrade skills. To produce high-quality care, the manager must constantly be developing the staff to meet new challenges.

With the addition of unlicensed assistive personnel to the care team, staff nurses must increase their own human resource management skills (Flanagan, 1997). Along with their managers, they engage in delegation, problem solving, and conflict resolution as well as teaching, critical thinking, and prioritization. Staff nurses must be able to give excellent feedback to assist unlicensed assistive personnel to provide client care safely and appropriately.

If, during a thorough process of feedback and development, an employee cannot work to the standards that the organization has set, the employee is removed from the position and the selection process begins again. More commonly, employees leave voluntarily for new opportunities.

Financial Resources

At one time, nurses did not need to be concerned with the management of **financial resources** (allocation and expenditure of money). Nurses provided skilled care, and payors paid bills without scrutiny. As pressure to control skyrocketing healthcare costs increased, healthcare organizations first simply decreased the budgets of nursing units without input from the nursing profession. This method proved unworkable. For nurse managers to provide useful input into financial planning and management, knowledge of business skills in addition to client care is necessary. Nurse managers must be able

to develop budgets that provide sufficient resources to accomplish unit goals. Once developed, budgets must be monitored in a timely fashion so that behavior can be changed to achieve budget compliance or the budget can be adjusted to account for unforeseen changes.

Information Resources

Information resources, sources of all types of data, are available to managers in various forms (e.g., clinical information about clients, budget compliance data, productivity ratios, client satisfaction surveys). The ability to use this information to make decisions is becoming increasingly important to the success of a manager and his or her unit. Information about trends is necessary to project human and financial resource needs and to create plans and budgets. Accurate and timely information is necessary to monitor budgets and to make adjustments. Specific information about clients and their care must be available to provide a context for medical and nursing decision making. Computers are able to process huge amounts of data in an array of formats. The manager, however, must be able to formulate questions that data analysis can answer and to interpret the results of inquiries. Only then can computerized data be useful to make correct decisions. The data must also be accurate, complete, and presented in a usable format. A fully computerized client record has the possibility of being the source for billing, management data, productivity information, and statistics. Technologic and confidentiality issues are yet to be solved, however, and nurse managers must be involved in such discussions in their organizations.

Skills for Effective Management

Planning

Planning is deciding what to do, when, where, how, by whom, and with what resources. Planning is an ongoing process that involves assessing, setting goals, establishing priorities, developing action plans, and evaluating whether the actions are meeting the objectives. Planning provides direction for the people involved and meaning for the work activities. It also provides a scheme for efficient use of people, space, and equipment.

In the nursing department, the top-level manager, or nurse executive, devotes a great deal of time to planning. The nurse executive plans the department's goals and services and determines the numbers and types of nurses and other personnel required to provide those services. In contrast, the department's lowest-level manager, the staff nurse, devotes less time to planning. The staff nurse assesses each client and determines needs, sets priorities, and develops a plan for nursing care. The plan of care answers the questions of what to do, when, where, and how.

For all employees, planning requires an ability to look into the future and to predict accurately any changes in the work of the day or the unit. Change in the healthcare environment is too rapid to allow today's plan to be a copy of the plan used yesterday.

Problem Solving

Problem solving is a systematic process that involves the following steps:

1. Identifying and analyzing the problem
2. Determining possible solutions to the problem
3. Considering the consequences of each possible solution and choosing a solution
4. Implementing the solution
5. Evaluating the results

Identifying and analyzing the problem involves collecting information about the issue to clarify the problem and its circumstances. Gathering information helps to clarify the problem and also offers clues to possible solutions and their consequences. After speculating on the possible consequences of each proposed solution, the manager chooses the solution that is expected to result in the most positive outcome. After the solution has been implemented, another assessment determines whether the desired results were obtained.

Communicating

Communication, a prerequisite to problem solving, is one of the fundamental skills of management. Managers spend a significant amount of time communicating in one form or another with others. Staff nurses spend a large amount of their time communicating with clients, families, other nurses, physicians, other healthcare professionals, and support staff.

For implementation to be successful, managers must have effective writing, speaking, and listening skills. For effective communication, the sender must be able to translate what he or she means into what he or she says or writes, and the receiver must be able to receive and objectively interpret that message. Factors such as differences in the sender's and receiver's skills, background experiences, education, trust, values, semantics, and emotional states can influence the interpretation of the message. The status difference between the leader and followers also may have an impact on the effectiveness of communication.

The nonverbal cues that accompany the message are essential aspects of verbal communication. If the sender's tone, speed, inflection of voice, facial expression, or other nonverbal behaviors are consistent with the verbal message, communication will be enhanced. If any of these variables is inconsistent with the verbal message, the receiver will believe the nonverbal message instead of the verbal one.

Listening is an important part of effective verbal communication. Listening can be hampered by the listener's lack of interest in the topic, premature interpretation of the message, or preoccupation with preparing a response. Good listening is a choice of actions that can be improved with practice. To be more effective, the listener should do the following:

- Give full attention to what the speaker is saying.
- Listen to the facts and feelings.
- Avoid formulating a response or judging the meaning until the speaker has finished.
- Use questions to clarify meanings.

Communication skills are necessary for successful implementation of the management process. Managers depend on communication to stay informed, to assist with planning and decision making, and to convey decisions to others. Effective leaders inspire followers by successfully communicating a shared meaning of goals, direction, and vision. Staff nurses rely on communication to care for clients and families, to relate to coworkers, and to function as effective interdisciplinary team members.

Delegating

"**Delegation** is transferring to a competent individual the authority to perform a selected nursing task in a selected situation" (National Council of State Boards of Nursing, 1995). Delegation is an essential activity for all levels of nurses. Executives and managers cannot actually perform all the activities required of them; delegating to others becomes an important time management tool. In addition, because successful completion of delegated activities helps staff members to grow and to become more committed to the organization, delegation is an important development method (Marelli, 1997).

With the changes in care delivery systems discussed later in this chapter, nurses must delegate to non-nursing personnel aspects of client care that they once performed themselves. Delegating is a new skill for some nurses, especially for those who have practiced within a primary nursing model. Some nurses find delegation difficult to learn. Safe and effective delegation is based on knowledge of the laws governing nursing practice and familiarity with job descriptions and training of unlicensed assistive personnel (Display 7-1). Once a task is identified as

DISPLAY 7-1

回 PRINCIPLES OF SAFE DELEGATION AND SUPERVISION

Right Task
Be sure the task that you are assigning is within the delegate's scope of practice. The task must also be within the delegate's job description.

Right Person
Competency to perform a delegated task is determined by the following measures:
- Certification/licensure
- Job description
- Skills checklist
- Demonstrated skill

Right Communication
Be sure to give directions that are clear, concise, correct, and complete.

Right Feedback
Work collaboratively with the delegate:
- Ask for the delegate's input first.
- Recognize his or her efforts.
- Learn the delegate's solution to the problem.

Adapted from Hansten, R. I., & Washburn, M. J. (1998). *Clinical delegation skills* (2nd ed.). Gaithersburg, MD: Aspen.

being appropriate for delegation, the nurse must make sure that the assistant is competent to do the task. The nurse must provide clear directions, set parameters, and resolve any conflict or confusion. Once the task is completed, the nurse must evaluate the work of the assistant and provide feedback (Hansten & Washburn, 1998). In this way, high-quality, cost-effective client care is achieved.

Managing Change

Change is sometimes defined as growth or learning. To be effective, managers must be masters of the change process. They must be able to assess situations and anticipate future needs in order to determine when change is needed and implement the needed change. Managers must also be able to manage change that others impose.

Managers need to know how to overcome resistance to change in themselves, their followers, and the overall organization (Fig. 7-3). Lack of knowledge, inaccurate information, fear of the unknown, threats to status or position, and threats to economic benefits can cause resistance to change. Education and enhanced communication are the best ways to reduce resistance caused by a lack of information or inaccurate information. Participation and involvement are effective approaches when the initiators of the change do not have all the information they need to design the change and when others have the power to resist the change. When people are resisting change because of emotional adjustment problems, the best interventions are facilitation and support. Negotiation and agreement may be appropriate when the change adversely affects the person's position or economic status.

People can control their perceptions and reactions to change by being aware of emotional reactions associated with change and by actively seeking information, increasing communication, and getting involved in the change process. For those who perceive it as an opportunity for learning and personal growth, change is a positive force that requires little resistance. For others who obtain comfort from things remaining the same, change can be very stressful. To implement change effectively, managers must assess the implications of any change for themselves and their followers and must intervene by providing needed communication, information, support, and involvement.

APPLYING LEADERSHIP AND MANAGEMENT TO NURSING ROLES

A subtle difference exists between leadership and management. Leadership focuses on people and inspires them to perform or to change. Management focuses on getting the job done by planning, organizing, directing, and controlling people and activities. To be effective, managers must also have leadership abilities. To be effective, nurses use both leadership and management skills in their various professional roles (Marquis & Huston, 1996; Huber, 2000).

Clinical Practice Roles

Nursing delivers its service to society through clinical practice roles. Teaching and administrative roles within the profession exist to support and to represent the clinical practice roles. Circumstances such as the availability of nurses, changing client populations, changes in technology, variations in the healthcare delivery system, and altered financial conditions lead to the development of new models of care delivery or variations in current models.

Confronted with the need to cut costs and increase productivity, organizations across the country are reengineering or restructuring. A great deal of uncertainty and turmoil exists because of these changes. With new care systems continuing to emerge, nurse managers must retain the position and power necessary to be involved in these changes (Marelli, 1997). Nurses use their knowledge of systems, current circumstances, and priorities of care to adjust to the current model of care delivery or to create a new one.

Staff Nurse

The core role of nursing is that of staff nurse. Most nurses are staff nurses who deliver most nursing care directly to clients, whether in hospitals, the community, clinics, long-term care facilities, or homes. Staff nurses fulfill many functions in the delivery of client care: provider of care, decision maker, client advocate, team member, communicator, and

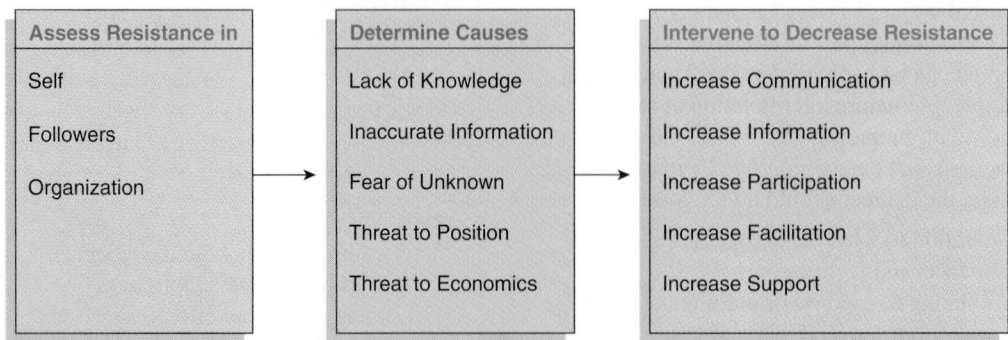

FIGURE 7-3   To be effective, managers must be masters of the change process. They need to know how to intervene to overcome resistance to change in themselves, their followers, and the overall organization.

THERAPEUTIC DIALOGUE
Leadership and Management

Scene for Thought

Two nurse managers (Edith and Emily) want to change the current way that staff on their units schedule their work hours. They both call staff meetings to discuss the proposed change.

Less Effective

Edith: The way it works now is that you give me your requests by a certain time and then I figure out how to fit everyone in a grid. I try to give everyone the days off they want and still ensure that enough people are on the unit so clients are safe and cared for. There have been problems with this system. I've come up with a better plan. I was thinking that all of you could schedule yourselves each month. That way you could plan ahead what days off you want to have and work it out among yourselves if you needed to change something.

Mabel: That sounds really interesting, Edith, but what happens if you need more people on a given day?

Roland: Yeah, and what if we want to work an extra shift or whatever?

Jordan: I can only work very specific times because of my school schedule, Edith. (Begins to look panicked.)

Edith: I guess I'll have to go back to the drawing board. We'll keep things as they are for now, and if anyone has any ideas, please let me know. (Begins to gather up her things as the staff looks at each other discouragedly.)

More Effective

Emily: The way it works now is that you give me your requests by a certain time and then I figure out how to fit everyone in a grid. I try to give everyone the days off they want and still ensure that enough people are on the unit so clients are safe and cared for. I think there have been problems with this system and that we can come up with a better plan. What do you think?

Joanne: There have been definite problems, especially when something unexpected has come up, like a flood of admissions or discharges.

Richard: Or many new people on the unit are on the same shift. They don't quite know what's going on and really can't be counted on to fill in the gaps until they are better oriented.

Emily: James, you haven't said anything. What do you think?

James: Well, I like the system as it is, but I have a set schedule because of school. A new system might not work as well for me.

Emily: I was thinking of a schedule that all of you would fill in yourselves each month. That way you could plan ahead what days off you wanted and work it out with one another if you needed to change something.

Maureen: That sounds really interesting, Emily, but what happens if you need more people on a given day?

Richard: Yeah, and what if we want to work an extra shift or whatever?

Emily: I have a certain number of nursing hours per client day that I have to keep to according to the budget. When the census goes up we can have more staff. When it goes down, we'll use fewer people, but still have enough staff for effective client care. We could build flexibility into the system. I have some examples of schedules from two other units whose staff schedule themselves. Let's look and see how they do it. (The staff members lean forward eagerly.)

Critical Thinking Challenge

- Based on the descriptions of leadership style in this chapter, what style does Emily use?
- Which (one or all) of the four management functions does she demonstrate?
- Give examples of how she is going about problem solving, communicating, and managing change.
- Both Edith and Emily had the same idea for scheduling, but arrived at very different conclusions with their staff.
- How did their leadership and management abilities contribute to these differences? What could Edith do to be more productive and effective?

---

educator. Regardless of the setting, staff nurses use the nursing process: assessing clients and families, determining nursing diagnoses, establishing plans of care, and evaluating outcomes of care. In addition, staff nurses consult with other healthcare professionals, report the most current client status, and coordinate the care given by other professionals. They use management skills to integrate nursing plans of care with the therapy plans of other healthcare professionals. They use leadership skills to coordinate interdisciplinary

care for clients (American Organization of Nurse Executives, 1998).

Nurses use various models of care delivery to provide client care. The most popular models of care delivery are team nursing, total client care, primary nursing, modular nursing, case management, and client-centered care.

Team Nursing. In **team nursing,** a specific group of caregivers works with a group of clients, and team members are as-

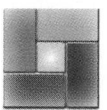

Nursing Research and Critical Thinking

What are the Influences of Nurses' Attributes, Unit Characteristics, and Elements of the Work Environment on the Job Satisfaction of Nurses Working in Pediatric Critical Care Units?

Nursing researchers have shown that frequent turnover of nursing staff occurs because of high levels of stress and the challenges of meeting the complex needs of critically ill patients. Nurses working with critically ill children and their families experience this stress every day in their work. The difficulty or working under such stressful conditions poses a threat to job satisfaction and leads to the loss of experienced nurses from critical care areas. Nurse researchers designed a study to explore the influences of nurses' attributes, unit characteristics, and elements of the work environment on the job satisfaction of nurses working in pediatric critical care units. They also sought to determine stressors that are unique to nurses working in pediatric critical care. The researchers used a cross-sectional survey design to sample 1973 staff nurses in pediatric critical care units in 65 institutions in the United States and Canada. The nurses designed the survey to measure the following variables: nurses' perceptions of group cohesion, job stress, nurse–physician collaboration, nursing leadership, professional job satisfaction, and organizational work satisfaction. Significant associations ($r = 0.37$ to $r = 0.56$) were found between job stress and group cohesion, professional job satisfaction, nurse–physician collaboration, nursing leadership behaviors, and organizational work satisfaction. Organizational work satisfaction was positively correlated ($r = 0.35$ to $r = 0.56$) with group cohesion, professional job satisfaction, nurse–physician collaboration, and nursing leadership behaviors. Furthermore, job stress, group cohesion, job satisfaction, nurse–physician collaboration, and nursing leadership behaviors explained 52% of the variance in organizational work satisfaction. Nurses participating in the study cited dealing with patients' families as the most frequently experienced job stressor.

Critical Thinking Considerations. Conducting such a large study across many diverse institutions required that the project coordinator carefully manage the study and maintain communication across institutions. This was achieved by designating a site coordinator at each institution who was responsible for obtaining approval from the appropriate institutional review board and for implementing the study at that site. Implications of this study are as follows:

- Job stress and nursing leadership are the most influential variables in the explanation of job satisfaction for nurses working in pediatric intensive care units.
- Retention efforts need to be targeted toward management strategies that empower staff to provide quality care along with focal interventions related to the diminishment of stress caused by nurse–family interactions.
- Because of the pivotal role of stress in job satisfaction, research efforts should focus on testing interventions targeted to areas of most concern to PICU nurses, namely family concerns and care of dying children.

From Bratt, M. M., Broome, M., Kelber, S. & Lostocco, L. (2000). Influence of stress and nursing leadership on job satisfaction of pediatric intensive care unit nurses. *American Journal of Critical Care, 9*(5), 307-317.

signed specific care functions or procedures to perform for all the clients. Members of the team usually include registered nurses (RNs), licensed practical nurses (LPNs), and unlicensed assistive personnel. The **team leader** is the nurse who manages the team by using management techniques.

An advantage of team nursing is the collaboration it provides in decision making about the plan of care for each client. Team nursing in inpatient settings also provides an easy mechanism for more experienced nurses to supervise and to teach less experienced nurses. A disadvantage is that more staff members deliver care to each client, potentially leading to fragmented care. This fragmentation may result in decreased accountability for the overall plan and delivery of care, which can result in decreased quality of client outcomes. Clients and families are less likely to receive consistent care and to develop rapport with nursing staff.

Total Client Care. With this model of care delivery, each nurse is given the full responsibility for a client or group of clients, depending on the acuteness of the setting. Assignments are often based on each nurse's skill and experience. For example, experienced nurses may be assigned clients who are unstable or require complex care. The assigned nurse performs all of the client's care. Therefore, fewer caregivers interact with the client and family, ultimately facilitating communication and continuity of care. Because the nurse is fully responsible for all aspects of care, his or her knowledge of that client is enhanced. A main disadvantage is the increased cost of RN salaries. If the primary nurse is an LPN, an RN must do assessment. In agencies that hire many part-time nurses, continuity of care may be lost.

Primary Nursing. In **primary nursing,** an RN assumes responsibility for developing a 24-hour nursing plan of care and for integrating that plan with the therapy plans of other healthcare professionals. The primary nurse accepts total responsibility for the quality of nursing care for a client. The nurse uses management skills in planning and coordinating client care. He or she also uses leadership abilities to ensure that the prescribed plan is implemented and that nursing care is integrated with care delivered by others.

Primary nursing results in increased continuity of care, improved interdisciplinary communication, and enhanced coordination of the total therapy plan. Primary nursing provides improved quality and consistency of nursing care for clients. The primary nursing model can result in increased job satisfaction for nurses because it provides increased autonomy in practice, close working relationships with clients and families, enhanced collaboration with other healthcare professionals, and increased focus of the nurse's role on planning and delivering client care. However, primary nursing requires enough RNs so that all clients have a nurse responsible for their plan of care, while allowing a reasonable caseload for each RN. It may not be possible to have a staff of all RNs because of availability and cost. The professional nurse must have enough direct contact with the client to make critical judgments about the client's diagnoses, required care, response to therapy, and ongoing disease process. Other potential disadvantages of the primary nursing model are the lack of a built-in system for experienced nurses to supervise and teach less experienced nurses and the lack of a natural nurse-to-nurse consultation. The busy routine in the work setting detracts from nurse-to-nurse consultation and joint decision making. With economic changes in healthcare delivery, primary nursing may be viewed as economically inefficient.

Modular Nursing or Care Partners. In this model, an RN is assigned responsibility for a group of clients in partnership with another caregiver, who may be licensed or unlicensed. Essentially, this model is a form of team nursing with a smaller team and caseload. The RN assigns tasks to the care partner based on principles of delegation. This model has the advantages and disadvantages of team nursing, although it is more flexible than team nursing.

Case Management. In some healthcare agencies, primary nursing has evolved into a managed care delivery model. In the **managed care** model, the facility uses a predetermined critical pathway to establish and monitor the extent and timing of care within an anticipated length of stay. (Critical pathways are discussed and an example is given in Chapter 12.) For common conditions, an interdisciplinary team develops a standard plan of care that includes time frames. Key elements that are slotted at specific times in the plan include diagnostic tests, consultations, treatments, activities, procedures, discharge planning, and teaching.

As the client moves through the critical pathway, variances (any deviation from outcomes indicated in the critical pathway) are noted and dealt with appropriately. Variances may be caused by the system, the client's condition, or the caregiver. Data collected in the process are analyzed to improve the quality and cost-effectiveness of care.

Clients with complex and multiple healthcare needs or inadequate support may require more individualized plans of care. Case management is used in such situations to ensure optimum, high-quality care in the most efficient and economical manner.

Client-Centered Care. In client-centered care models, all work of the organization that is related to the customer or client is analyzed. Then the care model is redesigned so that a multidisciplinary care team performs all client activities in the same location. Examples include admission, general care, laboratory, and radiology services.

The advantage of this model is that it brings the care to the client and promotes interdisciplinary collaboration and communication. Although it is not less expensive, the efficiency that results from taking care to clients and working as a team has been shown to decrease overall costs and increase client satisfaction.

Advanced Clinical Practice Roles

Nurses with advanced clinical practice roles provide direct client care and consultation to staff nurses. Some provide direct nursing care through group or independent practice. To be effective, these advanced practitioners must use good management techniques when planning and implementing client care, consultations, and educational programs. Others in the nursing profession also expect these advanced practitioners to be leaders in the profession through delivery of advanced care, consultation on complex care issues, development of new nursing practices, and participation in nursing research and publication. Often through their pioneering efforts, nursing is clarified, refined, and, in some instances, redefined.

Clinical Nurse Specialists. **Clinical nurse specialists** are RNs who hold a master's degree and advanced preparation in a specialty area of nursing (e.g., cardiovascular, neuroscience, critical care, psychosocial, rehabilitation). Clinical nurse specialists usually practice in hospitals, hospital clinics, community home health agencies, or private practice. They provide direct client care, consult with staff nurses, offer advanced education for nurses in specialty areas, evaluate nursing care outcomes, and develop new nursing practices to support new therapies or new technology.

Advanced Registered Nurse Practitioners. Nurse practitioners are RNs with advanced nursing degrees and preparation in health assessment and treatment. Their advanced preparation is usually concentrated in a specialty area, such as pediatrics, geriatrics, women's health, or adult health. These nurses also hold either certification or advanced licensing that allows them to practice independently in a specialty area. They usually work in community clinics or offices as independent practitioners or as members of a group practice. In some states, nurse practitioners can prescribe medications with some limitations.

Other Roles. Nurse midwives and nurse anesthetists are two other advanced specialty roles within the nursing profession. A **nurse midwife** is an RN with advanced education and certification in the care of women during uncomplicated pregnancy and delivery. The **nurse anesthetist** is an RN with additional education in anesthesiology. The nurse anesthetist administers anesthesia to surgical clients under the supervision of an anesthesiologist.

Nursing Management Roles

First-Line Managers

Through experience, staff nurses gain increasing abilities to manage care for a group of clients, to assist team members, and to serve as resources for new nurses. These enhanced abilities indicate to supervisors that staff nurses are ready to assume beginning management functions. Two such first-line management roles are team leader and charge nurse (Fig. 7-4).

When team leading is the model of nursing care delivery, the team leader manages a team of nurses, LPNs, and nursing assistants to provide nursing care for a group of clients. The team leader is responsible for the performance of team members and the quality of nursing care delivered.

The **charge nurse** is responsible for the functioning of a nursing unit for a particular work shift. The charge nurse makes management decisions and supervises the unit's staff as needed to provide quality client care on that shift. The charge nurse is a resource person for other staff members and may be pulled into issues that require interdepartmental or interdisciplinary problem solving. During the shift, the charge nurse determines staff work assignments and evaluates whether the numbers and skills of the staff on the next shift are adequate to meet current client needs safely.

Although the staff supervision and decision-making functions of the team leader and the charge nurse are similar, the scope of responsibility is different. The charge nurse has responsibility for the entire unit, which may have more than one team. The charge nurse supervises the team leaders (or, if primary nursing, case management, or another model of care delivery is used, the total unit staff) and facilitates communication and work among the teams (or staff members).

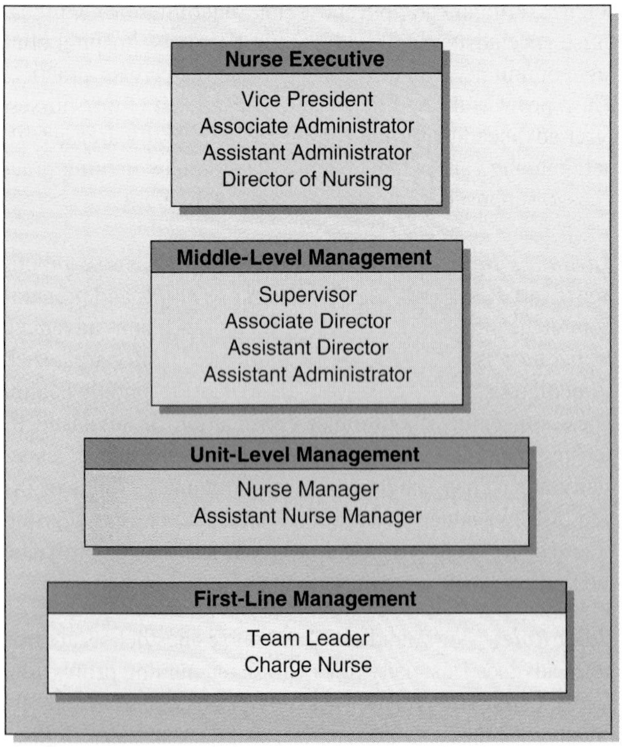

Unit Level Managers

Permanent management roles at some healthcare agencies include nurse manager and assistant nurse manager. In many agencies, nurse managers are recognized as department heads and are held accountable for 24-hour operations of nursing units, including such functions as staff scheduling and supervision, budget management, staff education, and quality client care. Nurse managers provide vital communication links among clients, direct caregivers, and administrative personnel. Nurse managers alert administrators to changing client needs, care preferences, and staff characteristics. They also represent the administration to staff members and clients by communicating changes in the organization that may affect them.

Assistant nurse managers help with overall management of nursing units by performing functions delegated by the nurse managers (e.g., hiring, evaluating, and counseling staff; preparing work schedules; preparing and monitoring unit budgets). In addition to performing delegated management functions, assistant nurse managers often serve as unit-based clinical resources and educators or permanent charge nurses.

Middle Managers

Depending on the size and complexity of the healthcare agency, there may be several levels of middle management. Between the nurse manager or coordinator and the nurse executive may be managers with titles of supervisor, director, or assistant administrator. These middle managers are usually responsible for the activities of several departments and programs. They spend more time planning for the department and focusing on interdepartmental or interdisciplinary problem solving than nurse managers do, but less time dealing with management of day-to-day client care. As organizations follow the trend of fewer layers of management, middle managers are often eliminated.

Nurse Executive
Vice President
Associate Administrator
Assistant Administrator
Director of Nursing

Middle-Level Management
Supervisor
Associate Director
Assistant Director
Assistant Administrator

Unit-Level Management
Nurse Manager
Assistant Nurse Manager

First-Line Management
Team Leader
Charge Nurse

FIGURE 7-4   Depending on the size and complexity of the healthcare agency, there may be several levels and roles in management. These management roles exist to support and to represent the clinical practice roles in nursing.

🖫 **APPLY YOUR KNOWLEDGE**

One RN, one LPN, and two nursing assistants comprise the team that will deliver care to 28 nursing home residents. You are the RN and designated team leader. One of the nursing assistants is still becoming oriented to the facility, having been on the job for only a few days. The other nursing assistant calls in sick. In trying to readjust work assignments to provide quality care for all the residents, you ask the new nursing assistant to perform the blood glucose monitoring for the three residents who need it. He responds that he cannot do that in addition to his other assigned work. Besides, he hasn't been properly instructed in this procedure. What are your options in this situation? How can you and the rest of the team provide care in the most efficient, safe manner?

Check your answer in Appendix A.

Nurse Executives

The **nurse executive** has a variety of titles and duties, depending on the type and complexity of the institution or healthcare agency. Some titles are vice president, associate administrator, assistant administrator, or chief nurse executive (CNE). Nurse executives are administrators and leaders of professionals. Because they are involved in strategic planning and decision making for institutions, nurse executives must effectively negotiate with nonclinical administrators, medical directors, and other top-level clinical administrators. They also must be able to lead, influence, and represent nursing professionals.

Implications for Nurses

To be effective in any management role, nurses must be skilled in the techniques of business management. The proportion of time they spend on specific activities will vary with each role. Beginning managers, nurse managers, and assistant nurse managers focus primarily on current operations and client care management. Nurse executives focus primarily on strategic planning involving issues within the agency that affect nursing practice or issues with the community or other agencies.

A manager's success depends on effective management strategies and effective leadership practices. The higher the level of management, the more essential it is that the nurse be an effective leader. Nurse executives are expected to be leaders within their agency and in the nursing profession. Effective nurse executives establish circumstances that allow nurses to function as professionals while providing quality client care.

KEY CONCEPTS

- Nurses are professionals who are responsible for providing a service to society through effective leadership behaviors and management skills.
- Leadership is the ability to influence others to strive for a goal or vision or to change. Management is getting the job done or accomplishing the goal through managing resources.
- As managers, nurses need to be skilled in planning, problem solving, communicating, delegating, and managing change.
- The five steps of the problem-solving process are identifying and analyzing the problem, determining possible solutions, considering the consequences of each possible solution and choosing a solution, implementing the solution, and evaluating the results.
- Effective communication involves transferring the meaning of information between people, using good verbal and nonverbal communication, and listening effectively.
- Change is inevitable. People can influence their own perceptions and reactions to change by being aware of the emotions associated with them and by actively seeking information, increasing communication, and getting involved in the change process.
- Effective leadership behaviors and management skills contribute to the success of nurses in their many clinical, management, and teaching roles.

REFERENCES

American Nurses Association. (1995). *Nursing's social policy statement.* Washington, DC: ANA Publishing.

American Organization of Nurse Executives. (1993). *Nursing's contribution to the health of the American people.* Chicago, IL: Author.

American Organization of Nurse Executives. (1998). *Nursing and the continuum of care (Leadership series).* Chicago, IL: American Hospital Publishing.

Bass, B. M. (1990). *Bass and Stogdill's handbook of leadership: Theory, research, and managerial applications.* New York: Free Press.

Bass, B. M., & Avolio, B. J. (1994). *Improving organizational effectiveness through transformational leadership.* Thousand Oaks, CA: Sage.

Covey, S. R. (1991). *Principle-centered leadership.* New York: Summit.

Devanna, M. A. (1994). Human resource management: Competitive advantage through people. In E. G. C. Collins & M. A. Devanna (Eds.). *The new portable MBA.* New York: John Wiley and Sons.

Finkler, S. A. & Kovner, C. T. (2000). *Financial management for nurse-managers and executives* (2nd ed.). Philadelphia: W. B. Saunders.

Flanagan, L. (1997). Staff nurses: Who are they, what do they do, and what challenges do they face? In J. C. McCloskey & H. K. Grace (Eds.). *Current issues in nursing* (5th ed.). St. Louis, MO: Mosby.

Hansten, R. I., & Washburn, M. J. (1998). *Clinical delegation skills* (2nd ed.). Gaithersburg, MD: Aspen.

Huber, D. (2000). *Leadership and nursing care management* (2nd ed.). Philadelphia: W. B. Saunders.

Irurita, V. (1994). Optimism, values and commitment as forces in nursing leadership. *J Nurs Admin, 24*(9), 61–71.

Marelli, T. M. (1997). *The nurse manager's survival guide* (2nd ed.). St. Louis, MO: Mosby.

Marquis, B. L., & Huston, C. J. (1996). *Management decision making for nurses* (2nd ed.). Philadelphia: Lippincott-Raven.

McDaniel, C., & Wolf, G. (1992). Transformational leadership in nursing service: A test of a theory. *Journal of Nursing Administration, 22*(2), 60–65.

Millman, D. (1996). *Economics: Making good choices.* Cincinnati, OH: Southwestern College Publishing.

National Council of State Boards of Nursing. (1995, December). Delegation: Concepts and decision making process. *Issues,* 1–2.

Noer, D. M. (1993). *Healing the wounds: Overcoming the trauma of layoffs and revitalizing downsized organizations.* San Francisco, CA: Jossey-Bass.

Porter-O'Grady, T. (1997). Process leadership and the death of management. *Nursing Economics, 15*(6), 286–293.

Rost, J. C. (1993). *Leadership for the twenty-first century.* Westport, CT: Praeger.

Senge, P. M. (1990). *The fifth discipline: The art and practice of the learning organization.* New York: Doubleday Current.

Swanson, J. W. (2000). Zen leadership: Balancing energy for mind, body, and spirit harmony. *Nursing Administration Quarterly, 24*(2), 29–33.

Tannenbaum, R., & Schmidt, W. H. (1973). How to choose a leadership pattern. *Harvard Business Review, 51,* 164–173.

Trott, M. C. & Windsor, K. (1999). Leadership effectiveness: How do you measure up? *Nursing Economics, 17*(3), 127–130.

BIBLIOGRAPHY

Barnum, B. S. (1994). Realities in nursing practice: A strategic view. *Nursing and Health Care, 15*(8), 400–405.

Curtin, L. (2000). The first ten principles for the ethical administration of nursing services. *Nursing Administration Quarterly, 25*(1), 7–13.

Douglass, L. M. (1996). *The effective nurse leader and manager* (5th ed.). St. Louis, MO: Mosby.

Forbes, B. A. (1993). *Profile of the leader of the future: Origin, premises, values, and characteristics of the Theory of Transformational Leadership Model.* Unpublished monograph, Seattle, WA.

Gillies, D. A. (1994). *Nursing management: A systems approach* (3rd ed.). Philadelphia: W. B. Saunders.

Jaco, P. R., Price, S. A., & Davidson, A. M. (1994). The nurse executive in the public sector: Responsibilities, activities, and characteristics. *Journal of Nursing Administration, 24*(3), 55–62.

Kerfoot, K. M. (1994). Leaders: Yesterday, today, and tomorrow. In R. Spitzer-Lehmann (Ed.), *Nursing management desk reference: Concepts, skills, & strategies.* Philadelphia: W. B. Saunders.

Mark, B. A. (1994). The emerging role of the nurse manager: Implications for educational preparation. *Journal of Nursing Administration, 24*(1), 48–55.

Napolitano, C. S. & Henderson, L. J. (1998). *The leadership odyssey: A self-development guide to new skills for new times.* San Francisco: Jossey-Bass.

Porter-O'Grady, T., & Wilson, C. K. (1998). *The health care team book.* St. Louis, MO: Mosby–Year Book.

Pritchett, P., & Pound, R. (1998). *Business as UnUsual.* Dallas, TX: Pritchett and Associates, Inc.

Senge, P. (1998). *The dance of change.* New York: Doubleday.

Simmons, G. F., Vasquez, C., & Harris, P. R. (1993). *Transcultural leadership: Empowering the diverse workforce.* Houston, TX: Gulf.

Sullivan, E. J., & Decker, P. J. (1997). *Effective management in nursing* (4th ed.). Menlo Park, CA: Addison-Wesley.

Tappan, R. M. (2001). *Nursing leadership and management* (4th ed.). Philadelphia: F. A. Davis.

Wheatley, M. J. (1994). *Leadership and the new science.* San Francisco, CA: Bennett-Koehler.

Wilson, C. K. (1992). *Building new organizations: Visions and realities.* Gaithersburg, MD: Aspen.

Zander, K. (1994). Nurses and case management: To control or to collaborate. In J. C. McCloskey & H. K. Grace (Eds.), Current issues in nursing (4th ed., p. 257). St. Louis, MO: Mosby.

8 Nursing Research
Evidence-Based Care

🔲 Key Terms

anonymity	networking
confidentiality	nursing research
dependent variable	problem statement
evidence-based care	qualitative research
hypothesis	quantitative research
independent variable	research design
literature review	theory
methods	variables

🔲 Learning Objectives

Upon completion of this chapter, the student will be able to do the following:
1. Trace the historical appreciation of nursing research.
2. Explain the contributions of evidence-based research to nursing practice.
3. Discuss the role of evidence-based research in nursing.
4. Review the research process for the beginning professional nursing student.
5. Summarize legal and ethical issues related to nursing research.

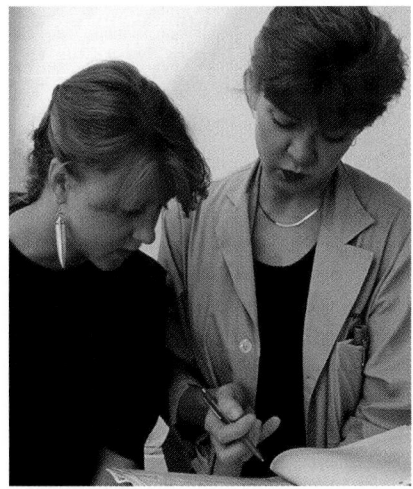

🔲 Critical Thinking Challenge

You are a nurse working in a rehabilitation unit of a large medical center. As you enter a client's room to conduct a follow-up assessment, you find the client engrossed in a conversation with a woman in a lab coat, who introduces herself as a graduate nursing student from the university affiliated with the medical center. The student says that she is conducting research for her master's thesis. You know that no arrangements have been made for this client to be a participant in a research study to evaluate nursing care, and you had no knowledge that this student might collect data in this setting. You reviewed the client's records at the beginning of your shift and know that the client did not sign a consent form to participate in any study. The student states that she was only interviewing the client, not providing any treatment, and was not putting the client at any risk. Therefore, she does not think that she needed to obtain consent.

Once you have completed this chapter and have incorporated nursing research into your knowledge base, review the above scenario and reflect on the following areas of Critical Thinking:

1. Critique the graduate student's actions in light of how you understand the protection of client rights in research.
2. Critique the actions of the faculty members in charge of this student in light of your understanding of the client's rights in research.
3. Based on your understanding of client rights, describe your reaction to the graduate student's response.
4. Now that you have clarified your understanding and considered the graduate student's response, identify how you will proceed.

Biomedical, environmental, psychological, and sociologic research has resulted in monumental advances in modern healthcare. Research into the complexities of the human immune system has led to the ability to transplant body organs and other parts and has provided essential information about the care and treatment of people with acquired immunodeficiency syndrome (AIDS). Other research efforts have led to improvements in psychiatric care through the understanding of neurotransmitters, challenging previously held beliefs about mental disorders while improving quality of life for clients and their families. One major reason for conducting research is to expand a profession's knowledge base. Second and most currently, research focusing on outcomes, or evidence-based research, has molded clinicians' practice in the hope of improving health outcomes for recipients.

One of the goals of this textbook is to emphasize the pivotal role of research in everyday nursing practice. Throughout the text, there are "research displays" that highlight the focus of each chapter. Take an opportunity to read, contemplate, and perhaps apply the research display as you learn about the concepts in that chapter.

Nursing practice and probably client outcomes are enhanced when professional nurses choose to use treatment methods that are based on research. Untested treatments may seemingly improve or alter the outcome a client experiences, but no confirmation exists that choosing the same treatment a second time would similarly improve outcome. Research-based nursing practice leads to improved care. The science of nursing draws heavily on other sciences, in particular the biopsychosocial fields, such as physiology, pharmacology, psychology, and sociology. Nurses must be able to discriminate "good" research from "poor" research to know what to use in clinical practice. Therefore, they must have a working knowledge of research methods and a beginning ability to read for application and to critique research. This chapter helps nursing students understand the research process and, in particular, the application of research to the practice of nursing. Research utilization forms the underpinnings of all nursing practice, continuing throughout the nurse's career and altering outcomes for clients.

RESEARCH AND NURSING

For the purposes of this chapter, *research* is defined as a formalized process of systematic investigation designed to test a research question or **hypothesis** and draw conclusions from collected data. Many similarities are found between the formalized research process and the nursing process format that is an integral part of nursing education.

Nursing research is defined as a "systematic inquiry into the problems encountered in nursing practice and into the modalities of client care, such as support and comfort, prevention of trauma, promotion of recovery, health education, health appraisal and coordination of health care" (Gortner, 1975). Waltz and Bausell (1991, p. 1) included in addition the precision of the research process to "gain solutions to problems and/or discover and interpret new facts and relationships." "Nursing research concerns nursing and things

nurses do that are different from the actions of other disciplines" (Neiswiadomy, 1997, p. 4). **Evidence-based care** is an approach to healthcare that realizes that pathophysiologic reasoning and personal experience are necessary but not sufficient for making decisions. This technique emphasizes decision making based on the best available evidence and the use of outcome studies to guide decisions.

Nursing research is identical to that of any other discipline in which practitioners are interested in seeking the truth. Nurses interested in the underpinnings of nursing practice attempt to describe events and phenomena, define and interpret the relationships among the phenomena, and eventually control and predict the phenomena studied (Munhall & Boyd, 1993; Kearney, 2001). The patterns exposed through research can predict future nursing outcomes. Knowledge is essential for healthcare practice (Brown, 1999).

Research affects the clinical practice of nurses in all areas, particularly in relation to the goals of nursing (Fig. 8-1). Historically, nursing has valued research that "develops knowledge about health and the promotion of health over the full lifespan, care of persons with health problems and disabilities, and nursing actions to enhance the ability of individuals to respond to actual or potential health problems" (American Nurses Association, 1981). Nurses working in critical care might be interested in a study on oral temperature accuracy (Fallis, Gupton & Kassum, 1994) or in one about sternal wounds (Hussy, Leeper & Hynan, 1998). Nurses working with older clients might be more interested in Bader's (1993) work on physical health impairment and depression, or Kleinpell and Ferrans' work with older intensive care clients (1998). Specialists become familiar with research related to their disciplines by paying attention to reviews of research or through the use of expert or consensus panels relevant to their areas. The change in focus from pure research to outcomes research is changing the way practitioners view their profession.

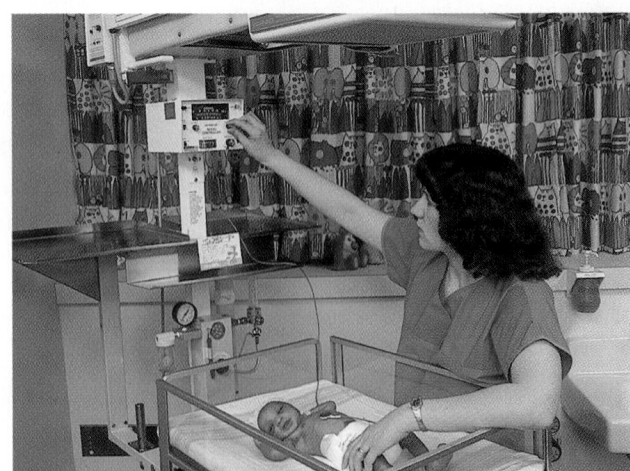

FIGURE 8-1   Clinical research defines nursing practice and raises the standards of nursing care. Research findings about newborn thermoregulation help promote evidence-based nursing care during the newborn period.

Although many problems that nurses encounter in clinical practice affect people of all ages, some problems are age- or person-specific. One nurse may be interested in the health benefits of aerobic exercise for a healthy geriatric population; another may be interested in the effect of positioning on the oxygen saturation of clients who have undergone coronary artery bypass surgery. A community initiative, the Fifth Vital Sign Task Force of the Missoula Demonstration Project, focused on improving the assessment and treatment of pain in Missoula, Montana. Using surveys, community education, and continuous quality-improvement teams, the group of community and university faculty from several disciplines, including nursing, set a goal for the entire community of healthcare providers, from emergency medical technicians on the ambulances to the critical care and home nursing staff, to use the same pain scale. Such research led to a community-wide commitment to pain relief (Mayer, Torma, Byock & Norris, 2001). Every nurse needs to be interested in prevention in the cost-conscious healthcare arena (Griffith, 1993). Each researcher contributes to the body of nursing knowledge in a specific way. All nurses should contribute in some fashion to expanding nursing knowledge.

The focus of nursing research must be on generating fundamental knowledge to guide nursing practice (Barnard, 1980; LoBiondo-Wood & Haber, 1994; Brown, 1999). Progress in nursing education, practice, or administration requires systematic analyses of research applicable to a nurse's area of expertise (Mason & Leavitt, 1993). With the widespread use of the World Wide Web, nurses, like all others, have widespread ability to seek, find, and apply information about healthcare. One of the thousands of sites available is the Cochrane Collaboration and Library. This international, nonprofit organization aims to help people make well-informed decisions about healthcare. Through its web site, www.cochrane.org, healthcare workers and others can access systematic reviews of relevant randomized controlled trials regarding healthcare interventions. The availability of electronic media information alters the depth and breadth of information available to all, thereby changing the way in which fundamental knowledge is disseminated and used.

Scientific Process and Nursing Research

In general, research means the search for a valid answer to a question. How the question is raised and by whom often are key to solving the problem. The scientific method, the problem-solving method, and the nursing process all use research methods. The problem-solving method and the nursing process are compared in Chapter 9. In this section, the scientific process is compared with nursing practice.

Ways of seeking and finding answers and acquiring knowledge in any field include formal and informal classes, clinical experiences, discussions with classmates or expert panels, scientific problem solving, continuing education courses, and research studies relevant to the area of interest. These methods of seeking knowledge have the following common characteristics:

- Identifying what one needs to know
- Deciding the approach to seeking the answer
- Devising a plan
- Implementing the plan
- Assessing the evidence

The first step for the practicing nurse is to assess a problem; for the researcher, the first step is to recognize the general problem area. The next step for the practicing nurse is to make a nursing diagnosis, and defining the specific problem is the second step in the research process. The clinical nurse then proceeds with planning and intervention, whereas the researcher proposes hypotheses and manages data. In the final step, the clinician evaluates outcomes; the researcher analyzes results and disseminates the findings in relation to the patterns uncovered.

Nurses can become involved in research and research utilization in several ways. Staff nurses can use the nursing process framework to begin to formulate and answer questions they encounter in clinical settings. Such behavior encourages self and others to improve the nursing care delivered. The presumed outcome should be improved client care. Another way to become involved in research is to be a research subject or a data collector for another person's research project (Glass, 1991). Of course, nurses can conduct research in their practice area, with guidance from others skilled in research methods.

Historical Appreciation of Nursing Research

Appreciation of the place of research in professional nursing has grown significantly. Nursing research has been an integral part of the profession since Florence Nightingale documented the care of soldiers in the Crimean War. Nightingale's careful statistical records are a model for nurses and social scientists alike (Cohen, 1984).

LoBiondo-Wood and Haber (1994), Neiswiadomy (1997), and Polit and Hungler (1999) identified several historical events that have been key to developments in nursing research. Between 1900 and 1940, research in nursing centered on education, methods of teaching, and methods of evaluating how nurses learned. During and after World War II, research interest turned to supply and demand for nurses as the need for nurses to serve in both the military and civilian sectors increased.

More master's programs in nursing emerged in the 1950s. True to the emerging scientific focus, most programs included courses on research methods. Increased federal funding enabled nurses to continue these studies. Publications of nursing research became more common. The journal *Nursing Research* began publishing the results of studies by individuals and schools of nursing. At about the same time, a 5-year research project sponsored by the American Nurses Association (ANA) focused on nurses' activities and functions.

Federal funding for graduate study and research expanded in the 1960s. Many baccalaureate-prepared nurses were able to continue with graduate education. The nursing profession was strengthened with the development of conceptual frameworks (an early stage of theory development wherein interrelated concepts help shape the proposed research) and the use of the scientific method in nursing practice. Nursing organizations established priorities for research investigations. Such research endeavors led to improvements in the quality and specificity of nursing care.

With the base of nurses prepared at the master's level, rapid growth in nursing research continued during the 1970s and 1980s. Three more journals of nursing research were born in the 1970s: *Advances in Nursing Science, Research in Nursing and Health,* and *Western Journal of Nursing Research.* In 1980, the ANA Commission on Nursing Research recommended further research in areas of health promotion, illness prevention, cost-effective healthcare, and nursing care for high-risk clients. Researchers also examined the conceptual frameworks that were offered in the 1960s and 1970s.

In a 1983 study, the Institute of Medicine urged the federal government to increase the level of funding for nursing research. As a result, the National Center for Nursing Research was established under the National Institutes of Health. The center's purpose was to place nursing securely in the sphere of scientific investigation and to support research and training into client care, health promotion, disease prevention, and the mitigation of effects of acute and chronic disabilities (Merritt, 1986). This center, now the National Institute for Nursing Research (established in 1985), has continued to fund and support nursing research and is key in the support and dissemination of seminal work in nursing.

Groups began to establish priorities in nursing research during the 1980s (Polit & Hungler, 1999). In 1985, the ANA Cabinet on Nursing Research identified 11 priorities for nursing research (Display 8-1). *Applied Nursing Research,* a journal with studies related to the practice of nursing, was established. The recommendation for essential knowledge for healthcare practice continues unabated into the 1990s (Brown, 1999).

Question areas of interest to nurse researchers vary with the types of positions that nurses hold, the settings for healthcare practice, and each individual. Polit and Hungler (1999) identified promotion of positive health practices, the nursing process of clinical judgments, groups at risk for specific health problems, description of holistic nursing situations, issues of minority/racial groups, and compliance with prescribed programs of treatment as current topics of research interest.

Characteristics of Nursing Research

Traditionally, nursing has been concerned with the whole person, not just the individual "parts." This style has its proponents and detractors. When nurses conduct research, they tend to focus on the physiologic, psychological, sociologic, cultural, and economic factors that affect a person. They view

DISPLAY 8-1

🔄 THE 11 PRIORITIES FOR NURSING RESEARCH

1. Promote health, well-being, and ability to care for oneself among all age, social, and cultural groups.
2. Minimize or prevent behaviorally and environmentally induced health problems that compromise the quality of life and reduce productivity.
3. Minimize the negative effects of new health technologies on the adaptive abilities of individuals and families experiencing acute or chronic health problems.
4. Ensure that the care needs of particularly vulnerable groups, such as the elderly, children with congenital health problems, individuals from diverse cultures, mentally ill people, and the poor, are met in effective and acceptable ways.
5. Classify nursing practice phenomena.
6. Ensure that principles of ethics guide nursing research.
7. Develop instruments to measure nursing outcomes.
8. Develop integrative methodologies for the holistic study of human beings as they relate to their families and lifestyles.
9. Design and evaluate alternative models for delivering healthcare and for administering healthcare systems so that nurses will be able to balance high quality and cost-effectiveness when meeting the nursing needs of identified populations.
10. Evaluate the effectiveness of alternative approaches to nursing education for the kind of practice that requires broad knowledge and a wide repertoire of skills and for the kind of practice that requires specialized knowledge and a focused set of skills.
11. Identify and analyze historical and contemporary factors that influence the shaping of nursing professionals' involvement in national health policy development.

From: American Nurses' Association Cabinet on Nursing Research. (1985). *Directions for nursing research: Toward the twenty-first century.* Kansas City, MO: ANA, with permission.

the situation from a nursing perspective and ask questions about what they see. Diers (1979) listed four properties of nursing research and how to maintain a holistic perspective:

1. The focus of nursing research must be on a variance that makes a difference in improving client care.
2. Nursing research has the potential for contributing to the development of theory and the body of scientific nursing knowledge.

3. A research problem is a nursing research problem when nurses have access to and control over the phenomena being studied.
4. A nurse interested in research must have an inquisitive, curious, and questioning mind.

Methods of Nursing Research

Just as subjects of studies are diverse, so are methods. Two broad approaches to research are quantitative and qualitative research. **Quantitative research** involves the systematic collection of numeric information, usually under conditions of considerable control, and the analysis of that information using statistical procedures. **Qualitative research** involves the systematic collection and analysis of more subjective narrative materials, using procedures in which there tends to be a minimum of researcher-imposed control (Polit & Hungler, 1999). Furthermore, quantitative researchers tend to use deductive reasoning, logic, and measurable attributes of human experience, whereas qualitative researchers tend to use dynamic, individual aspects of the human experience in a holistic approach (Table 8-1). Both methods have strengths and weaknesses and specific applications.

THE RESEARCH PROCESS

An understanding of the process that researchers use is essential for beginning practitioners and users of nursing or evidence-based research. Understanding the process helps nurses judge the appropriateness of the research presented and allows them to apply the findings to clinical situations. The process of research forms the underpinnings of the nursing profession and will be used throughout one's professional career. The steps

summarized here are universal for all professions who use research as their base.

Problem Area Identification

Practical experience, scientific literature, and untested theories or theories with limited testing influence the development of a research idea. Clinical practice can provide numerous opportunities to piece together observations that may lead to a problem for research. For example, nurses working in the recovery room observe that temperatures taken with an aural (in the ear) device appear to be more quickly determined and just as accurate as more traditional oral or rectal methods. The nurses note the differences in methods and speculate about other factors that might contribute to the ultimate adoption of the aural rather than the traditional methods. Every day, the practical experience and puzzlement of nurses can lead to questions that need solving. Evidence-based studies of "how we think, feel and behave profoundly influence the onset of some diseases, the progression of many and the management of nearly all" (Health and Health Care 2010, 2000, p. 194). Taking the opportunity to question and investigate can lead to problem identification and research-based practice. Following a hunch, Pratt et al. (1996) reported that depressed and socially isolated persons were four times more likely to have a heart attack than those who were not depressed and isolated. Similarly, Oxman, Freeman, and Manheimer (1996) reported that 232 elderly patients undergoing elective heart surgery who did not have any group of strength or comfort from religion had three times the risk of dying as those who did. Nurses can work together to design and implement different methods for investigating such problems (Dilorio, Hockenberry-Eaton, Maibach & Rivero, 1994). Every day

TABLE 8-1

Comparison of Quantitative and Qualitative Research		
	Quantitative Research	**Qualitative Research**
Focus	Focuses on a relatively small number of specific concepts	Attempts to understand entirety of some phenomena rather than focusing on specific concepts
Initial concept	Begins with preconceived ideas about how concepts are interrelated	Has few preconceived ideas: stresses importance of people's interpretations of events and circumstances rather than researcher's interpretation
Method	Uses structured procedures and formal instruments to collect information	Collects information without formal, structured instruments
Controls	Collects information under conditions of control	Does not attempt to control the context of the research, but attempts to capture that context in its entirety
Objectivity versus subjectivity	Emphasizes objectivity in collection and analysis of information	Attempts to capitalize on subjective data as a means for understanding and interpreting human experiences
Analysis	Analyzes numeric information through statistical procedures	Analyzes narrative information in an organized, but intuitive, fashion

Adapted from Polit, D. F., and Hungler, B. P. (1997). *Essentials of nursing research: Methods, appraisal, and utilization* (4th ed.). Philadelphia: Lippincott-Raven.

can be a revelation of problem area identification if the nurse is constantly questioning and linking events and observations.

Review of Scientific Literature

Literature review is the process of selecting published materials. These materials can be research- or evidence-based, or they may be anecdotal (short, written experiences and impressions that convey a greater understanding of a problem but are not considered research literature). Such materials contribute to and substantiate a summary of the concepts to be studied.

Scientific literature can be a valuable source for research ideas. For example, articles on a family's adaptation to a child's head injury (Baker, 1990), the expectations of obese persons in their weight loss programs (Foster, Wadden, Vogt & Brewer, 1997), the health problems that abound among women who are living in transitional shelters (Hatton, 1997), or the effects of prepared childbirth classes on obstetric outcomes (Hetherington, 1990) may be valuable for your clinical practice area.

Untested theories are good starts for nursing research. For example, Haase (1987) studied critically ill adolescents using a "courage" theory. The study gave insight into this special population and served to further develop a knowledge base surrounding adolescent care. Research interviews can help researchers understand people's responses to illness or particular situations (Hutchinson, Wilson, & Wilson, 1994). The work of Johnson, Wicks, Milstead, Hartwig, and Hathaway (1998) on racial and gender differences in kidney transplantation could lead transplantation nurses to examine their own practice.

Critical appraisal of the scientific literature may lead nurses to speculate about a problem area, particularly if the literature is in conflict or is inconsistent with their own practice. For example, a nurse working in coronary care may read two articles on postoperative pain management after cardiac surgery that suggest two different protocols. The nurse may wonder which of the protocols is more valid. Because of the conflict in the literature, an evaluation of this area may provide the answer.

Literature review must be systematic and exhaustive. Researchers must take a critical, almost dubious, approach to the available material. Research builds on previous work; hence, an extensive literature review, properly executed, allows researchers to place current ideas in the context of previous work. A complete review also helps develop the conceptual frame of reference for the study. It gives clues on how to study the problem (the **methods**) and suggests instruments that might help.

The literature search can seem overwhelming. An indispensable skill is the ability to identify and locate pertinent documentation on a particular topic. To do so, students must know which library sources to use. Books and indexes of journals, reports, the Internet, and abstracts are places to start. Books provide overviews of topics or deal with a specific detailed topic, although they become dated almost as soon as they are published. Bibliographies in books are valuable because they provide sources for original articles. Indexes are the gateway to the enormous volume of literature in the health sciences. Indexes such as the *Cumulative Index to Nursing and Allied Health Literature* (CINAHL), *International Nursing Index, Index Medicus, Nursing Studies Index, MedLine,* and *Nursing Research Index* are valuable. Such references are available in print and electronically, such as on CD-ROM databases; consult a librarian for details.

Continually growing as a resource for nursing research is the Internet, a global directory of commercial, educational, and governmental agencies. The Internet has developed into a sophisticated tool in information retrieval and research, both for the public and for nursing and health professionals. Literally hundreds of nursing sites are available to researchers through the World Wide Web. Researchers can seek and find information from online databases such as CINAHL.

Theoretical Framework

Nursing science and theory development are being refined. As discussed in Chapter 4, a **theory** is a set of interrelated constructs or propositions that attempts to present or explain some phenomenon systematically. Several nursing theorists have developed models and theories that remain incompletely tested. This incomplete testing and the evolving nature of models and theories give researchers an opportunity to use the work of a nursing theorist to test concepts from that theory for practice application. An example might be a nurse who wants to study Orem's self-care model for clients undergoing ambulatory surgical procedures. The nurse might design a study to investigate factors influencing self-care abilities before and after surgery, or self-care practices of homeless children (Norton & Ridenour, 1995).

The nursing model or theory should be a guide to identify and study systematically the logical relationships between variables. Each nursing model depends on the individual researcher's philosophy of human behavior and how that philosophy meshes with other ways of looking at science (Fawcett & Downs, 1992).

Often, a theoretical framework is likened to an architectural blueprint. These renderings, although not exact models of vision, help the user move from vision to reality. They help nurses further construct theories and distinguish nursing from other disciplines.

Formulation of a Problem Statement

The **problem statement,** a key step in the research process, identifies the direction that a research project will take. As beginning consumers of research literature, nursing students are in a position to evaluate whether the study is a logical extension of the problem. Sometimes, the problem area is not clearly stated, and the reader is unsure of the study's direction. The problem statement should be clear and unambiguous, express a relationship between two or more variables, identify the population to be studied, and encourage empiric testing. The problem statement is introduced early in the research and should reflect a well-defined, specific focus.

Stating the problem requires specifying the population to be studied. In the problem statement, the researcher states who will be the focus. For instance, the problem statement, "Is there a relationship between fathers who have been abused as children and their school-aged sons' emergency room records for suspicious injury?" suggests that the populations to be studied are fathers and sons.

The focus is best viewed when the problem has significance for nursing, either directly as with evidence-based research, or as a foundation for the development of further research. Research applicable to nursing practice, education, or administration is highly useful to a practice-based profession. That is, the outcomes have the potential for altering nursing practice or protocol and benefiting clients, other nurses, or students. Research that is theoretically relevant is also more useful.

Questions about judgments, ethics, morals, or values are not as amenable to a scientific research process without changing the question. For example, the question, "Is it better to tell clients about their diagnosis of terminal cancer or let them discover it themselves?" is impossible to answer. What is meant by "better"? Whose value system is being considered? The study of values has no right answer. If the question were framed differently, it could be researched through clinical inquiry. For instance, a nurse interested in determining how often each method is used could investigate attitudes toward each method.

Proposed Research Questions or Hypotheses

In the problem statement, the relationship is expressed between two or more variables or operationalized concepts. **Variables,** or properties that vary from each other, are the focus of the study. For example, a researcher studying postoperative clients might be interested in preoperative preparation in relation to the outcome of respiratory function.

Variables can be dependent or independent, according to their role in a particular study. An **independent variable** has the presumed effect on the dependent variable. It may be manipulated if the researcher is doing an experimental study; in a nonexperimental study, it is assumed to have occurred naturally before or during the study. The **dependent variable** is the consequence or presumed effect that varies as changes occur in the independent variable. The dependent variable is the one that the researcher is interested in understanding and explaining. For example, a nurse may study the problem that cardiac output measurement (the dependent variable) varies with the temperature of the injectate solution (the independent variable). In this case, the researcher would try to explain the effects of temperature on the measurements.

The final consideration when evaluating a research problem is testability. The problem must be measurable by qualitative or quantitative methods. If the question is posed in such a way that there is a relationship between an independent and a dependent variable and that relationship can be measured, probably the question can be researched.

Data Management

Research Design

Research design is the overall plan for the collection and analysis of the data. The study's design is crucial. If the design can limit the number of research problems before the study, the outcome may be more useful. If an instrument is to be used in a study or a new instrument needs to be developed, a consultant in methods (methodologist) can alleviate some reliability and validity problems by helping the novice researcher select or develop the instrument.

Because most nursing research occurs outside laboratory settings, the institution's policies, parameters, and constraints must be considered. Researchers must consider the costs of the facility, equipment, and personnel time (Fig. 8-2). Sometimes a study cannot be conducted because the costs outweigh the benefits.

Analysis of Results

Data are not the final results. They are a raw form of the answer. Reviewers put the data through various types of analysis and interpretation and manage them in an orderly, planned manner. Researchers look for patterns of information. They may analyze this information objectively or subjectively (see Table 8-1) by quantitative or qualitative analysis.

The results must make sense and be consistent with the data; this is part of the responsibility of researchers in interpretation. The implications are examined. The following question is asked: "How do these implications apply in the broader context?" Researchers return to their original question or problem statement and should be able to answer it with the analysis and interpretation of the results.

Dissemination of Results

Once the results of a study are determined, the findings must be disseminated so that clinical application or research replication by other nurses can occur. Conclusions

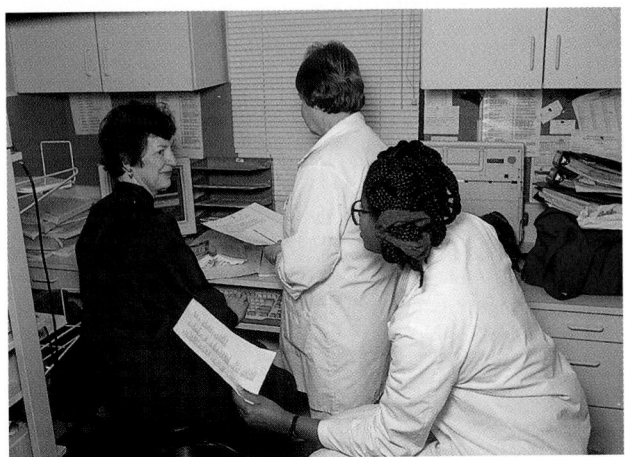

FIGURE 8-2 Nursing research can be time consuming for personnel, and the value of research must be weighed against the cost.

are strengthened and validated by similar findings in more than one research study.

Communication of Findings

Findings can be disseminated by oral and poster presentations at research meetings or in print through research and clinical journals. Presentations and publication of the results of studies allow other nurses interested in improving nursing practice to act on the findings. Nurses may adopt the findings for their clinical practice. A nurse acquainted with the original research may choose to do the same study but with a different group of study subjects or subjects in another clinical area. Others may extend the same study or stop using a clinical procedure or therapy that has shown little or no merit. A bonus of presenting the results at meetings or publishing them may be that the researcher will meet other nurses with similar interests. This practice is called **networking,** and it is a good way to disseminate and to expand one's knowledge, as well as to meet with other professional nurses.

Adoption of Findings

When a research report is being considered for use in clinical practice, preparation for change is made. Sister Callista Roy, a venerated nursing theorist, offers her guidance for dissemination and utilization of nursing literature in practice through a state-of-the-art review (Roy, 1999). All those professionals who may be affected should be brought together if the change is to be made smoothly. For example, nurses in one unit may read a study concluding that selective decontamination of the digestive tract of mechanically ventilated clients may reduce the incidence of nosocomial infections (Meijer, Van Saene, & Hill, 1990) and decide they want to implement the findings. To make such a change, nurses would collaborate with physicians, microbiologists, pharmacists, and respiratory therapists to consider how this change would influence client care.

ETHICAL AND LEGAL ISSUES

Ethical and legal issues related to the research process continually arise. The primary issue is that of human rights or subject rights. In the past, research has been conducted without proper consent or any consent from the participants. There has been an evolution of ethical principles in nursing as in all research projects. The five rights outlined in 1985 by the ANA guidelines—self-determinism, privacy and dignity, anonymity and confidentiality, fair treatment, and protection from discomfort and harm—apply to all people involved in research projects.

Institutional Review Boards

In 1974, the National Research Act was passed, requiring any agency applying for funding for any project involving biomedical or behavioral research on humans to submit assurances that it had an institutional review board (IRB) to review the research and protect the rights of human subjects. It resulted from the Senate hearings on the Tuskegee Syphilis Study (Jones, 1993). At agencies where no federal money has been awarded, usually a review mechanism is present similar to the IRB.

Why are IRBs necessary? After World War II, the Nuremberg military tribunal was charged with prosecuting Nazis who had done biomedical research on concentration camp prisoners. Because the tribunal had no measures against which to test the defendants, a set of basic principles of ethical, moral, and legal concepts for the conduct of acceptable experiments had to be written. The Articles of the Nuremberg Tribunal are listed in Display 8-2.

DISPLAY 8-2

ARTICLES OF THE NUREMBERG TRIBUNAL RELATED TO ETHICAL, MORAL, AND LEGAL CONCEPTS FOR THE CONDUCT OF EXPERIMENTS

- The voluntary consent of the human subject is absolutely essential.
- The experiment should be such as to yield fruitful results for the good of society, unprocurable by other means of study, and not random and unnecessary in nature.
- The experiment should be so designed and based on the results of animal experimentation and knowledge of the natural history of the disease or other problems under study that the anticipated results will justify the performance of the experiment.
- The experiment should be conducted to avoid all unnecessary physical and mental suffering and injury.
- No experiment should be conducted where there is a prior reason to believe that death or disabling injury will occur.

- The degree of risk to be taken should never exceed that determined by the humanitarian importance of the problem to be solved by the experiment.
- Proper preparations should be made and adequate facilities provided to protect the subject against injury, disability, or death.
- The experiment should be conducted only by scientifically qualified persons.
- The human subject should be at liberty to bring the experiment to an end.
- During the experiment, the scientist, if he has probable cause to believe that a continuation of the experiment is likely to result in injury, disability, or death to the experiment subject, will bring it to a close.

From: Katz, J. et al. (1972). *Experimentation with human beings* (pp. 289–290). Copyright 1972 Russell Sage Foundation.

Subject Rights

The first statement of the Nuremberg code, developed in 1949, addresses the rights of research subjects. Voluntary consent; the right to withdraw from investigations at any time without penalty; protection from physical and mental suffering, injury, disability, and death; and a balance between benefits and risks are paramount (Levine, 1981; McMahon & O'Carroll, 2000). Nursing researchers must provide the following information to human subjects (Commission on Nursing Research, 1981):

- An explanation of the study
- The procedures to be followed and their purposes
- A clear description of physical and mental discomforts, any invasion of privacy, and any threat to dignity
- The methods used to protect anonymity and ensure confidentiality

These provisions may seem obvious, but before 1974 several human research studies were conducted in the United States that probably would not be allowed today. Subjects in these studies underwent unethical experimental procedures, including sterilization, euthanasia, injection with live cancer cells, and the withholding of treatment for syphilis (Diers, 1979; Faulder, 1985; Tetting, 1990; LoBiondo-Wood & Haber, 1994). The ethical principles of autonomy, beneficence, and justice remain as guides for research gauging the goals of research, while maintaining the rights of research participants (Orb, Eisenhauer, & Wynaden, 2001).

Clients involved in research must be assured that their privacy is being protected. Privacy is protected in two general ways. **Anonymity** is the protection of the subject so that not even the researcher can link the subject with the information provided. **Confidentiality** ensures that the subjects' identities will not be linked with the information they provide and will not be publicly divulged.

Although students may have few opportunities to seek or to obtain informed consent from people selected as potential subjects for research, students may have a role in data collection or may provide medications or treatments in a research study. The role that nurses or students are to play in research studies must be clarified with involved faculty members. Any educational institution will have an IRB for their faculty and student projects involving human subjects. Ask about your school's IRB.

RESEARCH AND THE PROFESSIONAL NURSE

Levels of Nursing Participation

Some nurses may think mistakenly that they have little to contribute to research. Nurses actually have a great deal to contribute by observing client responses to treatments and techniques. A nurse with several years of clinical experience in a particular unit may generate many unanswered questions. He or she would be in a position to initiate research with a skilled researcher or would value assisting with client management or data collection in someone else's research project.

ETHICAL/LEGAL ISSUE
Research Studies on Human Subjects

Michael Thomas, 29, an accountant, was diagnosed 3 years ago with human immunodeficiency virus (HIV) infection. Over the past few months, his diagnosis has progressed into acquired immunodeficiency syndrome (AIDS) with the appearance of some related cancers. He has been admitted to the hospital to participate in a research program that is studying new drugs to treat AIDS-related cancers. His partner is trying to talk him out of participating, knowing that this type of drug trial is a "double-blind" study, in which Michael may receive a placebo rather than the drug. The research team is encouraging Michael to participate in the study. When you enter the room to check on Michael, he appears distraught and upset. He says to you, "I don't know what to do. I know this drug trial may be my best chance of living, but I don't want to upset my partner. Can you help me be sure that I get selected for the trial drug and not the placebo?"

Reflection

- Review Chapter 6 about informed consent and information in this chapter about the protection of human subjects. What information might apply to the above scenario?
- Reflect on your feelings in this situation and identify them.
- Articulate your role as a nurse providing care and as a nurse assisting in a research project.
- Think about the ways in which you might respond to this situation. Identify possible approaches.

The education of nurses who are clinical specialists usually emphasizes clinically relevant research. In the practice arena, they can do their own research, act as consultants to novice researchers, and collaborate with other healthcare professionals on more complex client situations. For example, a clinical specialist in oncology may collaborate with a clinical psychologist to study stressors of pain or side effects related to therapy.

The ANA's Commission on Nursing Education has developed guidelines for the investigative function of nurses (Display 8-3). These standards give information about how different educational levels may enhance the research contributions that nurses can make.

Clinical Nursing Practice

Clinical Research

The problem-solving methods that nurses use can help practicing nurses translate clinical problems into research projects. Nurses in clinical areas regularly raise questions that

DISPLAY 8-3

🔲 GUIDELINES FOR INVESTIGATIVE FUNCTION OF NURSES

Associate Degree in Nursing
- Demonstrates awareness of the value or relevance of research in nursing
- Assists in identifying problem areas in nursing practice
- Assists in collection of data within an established, structured format

Baccalaureate Degree in Nursing
- Reads, interprets, and evaluates research for applicability to nursing practice
- Identifies nursing problems that need to be investigated, and participates in implementation of scientific studies
- Uses nursing practice as a means of gathering data for refining and extending practice
- Applies established findings of nursing and other health-related research to nursing practice
- Shares research finding with colleagues

Master's Degree in Nursing
- Analyzes and reformulates nursing practice problems so that scientific knowledge and scientific methods can be used to find solutions
- Enhances the quality and clinical relevance of nursing research by providing expertise in clinical problems and by providing knowledge about the way in which these clinical services are delivered
- Facilitates investigation of problems in clinical settings through such activities as contributing to a climate

supportive of investigative activities, collaborating with others in investigations, and enhancing nursing's access to clients and data
- Conducts investigations for the purpose of monitoring the quality of the practice of nursing in a clinical setting
- Assists others to apply scientific knowledge in nursing practice

Doctoral Degree in Nursing or Related Discipline
- Graduate of a practice-oriented doctoral program
- Provides leadership for the integration of scientific knowledge with other sources of knowledge for the advancement of practice
- Conducts investigations to evaluate the contribution of nursing activities to the well-being of clients
- Develops methods to monitor the quality of the practice of nursing in a clinical setting and to evaluate contributions of nursing activities to the well-being of clients
- Graduate of a research-oriented doctoral program
- Develops theoretical explanations of phenomena relevant to nursing by empirical research and analytical processes
- Uses analytic and empirical methods to discover ways to modify or extend existing scientific knowledge so it is relevant to nursing
- Develops methods for scientific inquiry of phenomena relevant to nursing

This language was developed as a part of the work of the ANA Commission on Nursing Education and was included in the report of that commission to the 1980 ANA House of Delegates. *From:* Commission on Nursing Research. (1981). *Guidelines for the investigative function of nurses.* Kansas City, MO: Author.

---

could be considered researchable. Because of daily interactions with clients, nurses have the opportunity to solve problems but, in the strict sense, do not research nursing questions.

Nurses interested in research, especially in the clinical area, use the resources at hand: clients and the clinical setting in which the nurse works. Client care allows nurses to define and to seek solutions to various problems. Using observation skills, discussions with colleagues, and personal clinical experience, nurses can learn to organize priorities and offer clients the most efficient and timely care.

Nurse researchers use techniques similar to those they developed first as students and then refined as skilled clinicians. Nurse researchers broaden the area of study and try to discover various conditions (variables) that affect the situation. For example, a nurse in the neonatal unit might be concerned with the temperature balance of newborns receiving phototherapy for physiologic jaundice. The researcher recognizes that to study this problem the related fields of physical

thermodynamics and developmental physiology must be investigated. The researcher also needs to investigate the placement of temperature probes, site selection, nurse technique, and the soundness of previous research.

Nurse researchers recognize the need to consult other experts and to consider other organizational patterns. Recruitment of those skilled in particular areas ensures that the results will be more useful and gives the design and statistical analysis more merit. Often, for example, the skills of a statistician are needed.

Multidisciplinary Clinical Research
No one discipline can provide the breadth of evidence needed for evidence-based practice. The Agency for Health Care Policy and Research (AHCPR) was established in December, 1989, under Public Law 101-239 (Omnibus Budget Reconciliation Act of 1989). AHCPR, a part of the U.S. Department of Health and Human Services, is the lead agency charged

with supporting research designed to improve the quality of healthcare, reduce its cost, and broaden access to essential services. AHCPR's broad programs of research, including nursing research, bring practical, science-based information to healthcare practitioners and to consumers and other healthcare purchasers. The findings of studies across disciplines are combined to provide guidelines for clinical care, including guidelines for therapies for practitioners as well as education guides for clients.

Providers, health plans, and public payers around the country report that adoption of AHCPR recommendations has brought real cost savings (Display 8-4). Even very conservative projections indicate that national cost savings from past AHCPR research range up to $175 million per condition, re-

inforcing the importance of careful research. The adoption of AHCPR recommendations has enabled the public and private sectors to improve quality and reduce costs, demonstrating that solid scientific research can identify how to target and design cost-reduction efforts without jeopardizing quality, and how to improve quality without increasing costs. Facilities and providers want to deliver high-quality, cost-effective care and are eager audiences for information that will help them do so (Agency for Health Care Policy and Research, 1995).

Applying Research to Practice

Student nurses and beginning practicing nurses are not usually involved in direct research, except in the role of data collection or administration of medications and treatments as a protocol in a research project. Even with limited direct participation in research, beginning nurses should be consumers of research. They can read research literature applicable to the practice setting and attempt to evaluate it or use it in clinical practice after collaboration with more expert practitioners. For beginning nurses, the ability to read articles carefully and critically is important. Rasmussen, O'Connor, Shinkle, and Thomas (2000) offer a checklist designed to help nurses with varying skills critique reported qualitative and quantitative research studies.

Through the teaching and learning process in basic nursing education, new nurses can be exposed to evidenced-based nursing care practice (Rambur, 1999). Analysis of the material learned does not necessarily mean finding flaws and faults. It is the conscious decision to undertake an objective and careful evaluation of the research project in light of how practicing nurses, working directly with clients or a client population, would be able to use this knowledge. Knowing that the "answers" are not always known, the nurse is wise to keep learning and being aware that every day new practices could be employed with knowledge gained through research and new evidence. The thrust to use more evidence-based practice should lead to better outcomes for all consumers (Friedland et al., 1998). Practitioners need skills and resources to appraise, synthesize, and use the best evidence for nursing care (Rosswurn & Larrabee, 1999).

After a study or research project has been evaluated, the findings might be used in clinical practice. However, nurses should not assume that, just because something has been published, it is appropriate for clinical practice. On the contrary, because something is published, nurses should view the contents with some degree of skepticism before adopting them to the clinical setting.

Applying research findings to clinical practice has utility. Nurses need to narrow the gap between research and application by selecting useful studies to put into place. The expanding use of community-based nursing and family-centered care offers a completely new area of research. Collaboration between researchers and practitioners will enhance diffusion of evidenced-based practice (Rosswurn & Larrabee, 1999).

In the meantime, while research continues, a planned program of evaluation and implementation will help nurses find appropriate approaches to client care situations. For example,

DISPLAY 8-4

COST SAVINGS EXAMPLES

Even if the Agency for Health Care Policy and Research recommendations affect only one client in five, the implications for cost and quality could be substantial. For example:

- Employers and other private sector payers could save $370 million in treatments and tests for low-back pain among the working-age population, according to Medstat, Inc., a private research and consulting firm.
- Stroke prevention therapies could save $132 million a year.
- Reduced use of acetaminophen could limit kidney damage and save $100 to $140 million a year for Medicare's end-stage renal disease program.
- Optimal antibiotic treatment before surgery could reduce the risk of postsurgical infections and save $22.5 million in hospital costs each year.
- Movement of appropriate cardiac catheterizations to an outpatient setting could save at least $13 million a year. Urinary incontinence therapies could save $7.2 million a year in hospital costs for the under-65 population alone.
- On-call medical care to terminally ill clients living at home could reduce hospitalization rates and save up to $27 million a year.
- Following acute pain management protocols could shorten hospital stays and save as much as $81 million a year in hospital costs for hip replacement patients alone.
- Reducing unnecessary interventions for otitis media in children under the age of 2 could save up to $170 million a year in medical and indirect costs.
- Preconception care and enhanced prenatal care for pregnant diabetic women would net savings of $8.5 million a year.

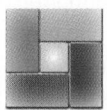

Nursing Research and Critical Thinking
How Does Nursing Research Rate When Considered in Relation to Other Types of Research Conducted at the University Level?

Formal assessment of university research in Britain began in 1985. Assessments are carried out by the Higher Education Funding Council, usually every 4 years. Various subject panels examine pieces of research that departments submit on a voluntary basis. Research funding received and the coherence and scale of research programs are also considered. Nurses concerned about the poor showing that nursing research had in the assessments during the past two rating periods (in 1992 and 1996, nursing as a discipline came in last) developed a survey to examine and improve nursing's contribution to research. The survey asked heads of nursing departments in universities about their entries, or nonentries, to the assessments and about the research culture in their departments. Sixty-eight responses to the survey were received from 107 questionnaires (64%). The survey discovered both diversity and consensus.

Many departments had no established links with other researchers or research networks, whereas a few had well-developed links. This difference did not appear to be related to length of time in higher education. A strong theme that emerged was that of a tension between a desire for academic credibility in higher education and a desire for clinical or professional credibility with other providers. Main nursing research areas identified in the survey data were care of the elderly; rehabilitation; primary/secondary care interface; nursing informatics; practice development; specialized and advanced nursing roles; nursing outcomes and their evaluation; dissemination of research findings; lay participation and views of users and caregivers; and nurses' career patterns.

Critical Thinking Considerations. This study was specific to university-based nursing research in Britain. The findings are not generalizable internationally. Further research would be useful in other university systems around the world. The researchers and respondents discuss the fact that nursing research is a recent arrival in higher education. Implications of this study are as follows:

- Many respondents wrote about a need for an improved research capacity for nursing.
- Established researchers were overburdened, and teaching commitments imposed restraints on research time.

From Traynor, M. (1998). Survey looks at problems in university nursing research. *Nursing Times, 94*(29), 66–67.

---

the journal *Focus on Critical Care* has a column, "Research Review," that helps critical care nurses apply relevant research to their practice. Other journals provide similar information.

KEY CONCEPTS

- Expanding nursing's knowledge base is an important goal of nursing research.
- Nursing research is the systematic inquiry into clinical practice problems, modes of client care, nursing education, and nursing administration.
- The scientific method of research and the nursing process are similar.
- Research is a step-by-step process of defining ideas, reviewing literature, developing a theoretical framework, formulating a problem statement, proceeding with the study, and disseminating findings.
- Nursing research results must be disseminated so that the profession can evaluate and apply the findings.
- Legal and ethical considerations, including the rights of human subjects, anonymity, and confidentiality, are central to any research study.
- Practicing nurses encounter many questions that may be bases for research studies.

REFERENCES

Agency for Health Care Policy and Research. (1995). *Better quality can cost less: The evolving role of AHCPR.* Highlights of a September 1995 interim report to the National Advisory Council for Health Care Policy, Research, and Evaluation. Rockville, MD: Agency for Health Care Policy and Research. Available at: http://www.ahcpr.gov/about/quality.htm.

American Nurses Association. (1981). *Research priorities for the 1980s: Generating a scientific base for nursing practice* (Publication #D-68). Kansas City, MO: Author.

American Nurses Association. (1985). *Human rights guidelines for nurses in clinical and other research* (Document No. O-465M). Kansas City, MO: Author.

American Nurses Association Cabinet on Nursing Research. (1985). *Directions for nursing research: Toward the twenty-first century.* Kansas City, MO: American Nurses Association.

Bader, A. (1993). Physical health impairment and depression among older adults. *Image: Journal of Nursing Scholarship, 25*(4), 326–330.

Baker, J. L. (1990). Family adaptation when one member has a head injury. *Journal of Neuroscience Nursing, 22,* 232–237.

Barnard, K. E. (1980). Knowledge for practice: Directions for the future. *Nursing Research, 29,* 208–212.

Brown, S. J. (1999). *Knowledge for health care practice: A guide to using research evidence.* Philadelphia: W. B. Saunders.

Cohen, I. B. (1984). Florence Nightingale. *Scientific American, 250*(3), 128–137.

Commission on Nursing Research. (1981). *Guidelines for the investigative function of nurses.* Kansas City, MO: Author.

Diers, D. (1979). *Research in nursing practice.* Philadelphia: J. B. Lippincott.

Dilorio, C., Hockenberry-Eaton, M., Maibach, E., & Rivero, T. (1994). Focus groups: An interview method for nursing research. *Journal of Neuroscience Nursing, 26*(3), 175–180.

Fallis, W. M., Gupton, A., & Kassum, D. (1994). Determination of oral temperature accuracy in adult critical care patients who are orally intubated. *Heart and Lung, 23*(4), 300–307.

Faulder, C. (1985). *Whose body is it?* London: Virago.

Fawcett, J., & Downs, F. S. (1992). *The relationship of theory and research* (2nd ed.). Philadelphia: F. A. Davis.

Foster, G. D., Wadden, T. A., Vogt, R. A., & Brewer, G. (1997). What is reasonable weight loss? Patient's expectations and evaluations of obesity treatment outcomes. *Journal of Consulting and Clinical Psychology, 65*(2), 79–85.

Friedland, D. J., Go, A. S., Davoren, J. B., Shlipak, M. G., Bent, S. W., Subak, L. L., & Mendelson, T. (1998). *Evidence-based medicine.* Stamford, CT: Appleton & Lange.

Glass, E. C. (1991). Importance of research to practice. In M. A. Mateo & K. T. Kirchhoff (Eds.), *Conducting and using nursing research in the clinical setting.* Baltimore, MD: Williams & Wilkins.

Gortner, S. (1975). Research for a practice profession. *Nursing Research, 24*(6), 193–197.

Griffith, H. M. (1993). Needed—a strong nursing position on preventive service. *Image: Journal of Nursing Scholarship, 25*(4), 272.

Haase, J. E. (1987). Components of courage in critically ill adolescents: A phenomenological study. *Advances in Nursing Science, 19*(2), 64–80.

Hatton, D. C. (1997). Managing health problems among homeless women with children in a transitional shelter. *Image: Journal of Nursing Scholarship, 29*(1), 33–37.

Hetherington, S. L. (1990). A controlled study of the effects of prepared childbirth classes on obstetric outcome. *Birth, 17*(2), 86–89.

Hussy, L. C., Leeper, B., & Hynan, L. S. (1998). Development of the sternal wound infection prediction scale. *Heart and Lung, 27*(5), 326–336.

Hutchinson, S. A., Wilson, M. E., & Wilson, H. S. (1994). Benefits of participating in research interviews. *Image: Journal of Nursing Scholarship, 26*(2), 161–164.

Institute for the Future. (2000). *Health and health care 2010: The forecast, the challenge.* Menlo Park, CA: Author.

Johnson, C. D., Wicks, M. N., Milstead, J., Hartwig, M., & Hathaway, D. K. (1998). Racial and gender differences in quality of life following kidney transplantation. *Image: Journal of Nursing Scholarship, 30*(2), 125–130.

Jones, J. H. (1993). *Bad blood: Tuskegee syphilis experiment.* New York: The Free Press.

Kearney, M. H. (2001). Levels and applications of qualitative research evidence. *Research in Nursing and Health, 24*(2):145–153.

Kleinpell, R. M., & Ferrans, C. E. (1998). Factors influencing intensive care until survival for critically ill elderly patients. *Heart and Lung, 27*(5), 337–343.

Levine, R. J. (1981). *Ethics and regulation of clinical research.* Baltimore, MD: Urban & Schwarzenberg.

LoBiondo-Wood, G., & Haber, J. (1994). *Nursing research: Critical appraisal and utilization* (3rd ed.). St. Louis, MO: Mosby.

Mason, D. J., & Leavitt, J. K. (1993). Policy and politics: A framework for action. In D. J. Mason, S. W. Talbott, & J. K. Leavitt (Eds.), *Policy and politics for nurses* (2nd ed.). Philadelphia: W. B. Saunders.

Mayer, D. M., Torma, L., Byock, I., & Norris, K. (2001). Speaking the language of pain. *American Journal of Nursing, 101*(2), 44–50.

McMahon, A., O'Carroll, D. (2000, February 23–29). Research ethics. *Nursing Standards, 14*(23), 31.

Meijer, K., Van Saene, R., & Hill, J. (1990). Infection control in patients undergoing mechanical ventilation: Traditional approach versus a new development—Selective decontamination of the digestive tract. *Heart and Lung, 19*(10), 11–20.

Merritt, D. H. (1986). The National Center for Nursing Research. *Image: Journal of Nursing Scholarship, 18*(2), 84.

Munhall, P. L., & Boyd, C. O. (1993). *Nursing research: A qualitative perspective* (Publication #19-2535). New York: National League for Nursing Press.

Neiswiadomy, R. M. (1997). *Foundations of nursing research* (3rd ed.). Norwalk, CT: Appleton & Lange.

Norton, D., & Ridenour, N. (1995). Children from homeless families describe what is special in their lives. *Nurse Practitioner Forum, 6*(1), 29–33.

Orb, A., Eisenhauer, L., & Wynaden, D. (2001). Ethics in qualitative research. *Journal of Nursing Scholarship 33*(1), 93–96.

Oxman, T. E., Freeman, D. H., & Manheimer, E. D. (1996). Lack of social participation or religious strength and comfort as risk factors for death after cardiac surgery in the elderly. *Psychosomatic Medicine, 57*, 5–15.

Pratt, L. A., et al. (1996). Depression, psychotropic medication and risk of myocardial infarction. *Circulation, 94*, 3123–3129.

Polit, D. F., & Hungler, B. P. (1999). *Nursing research: Principles and methods* (6th ed.). Philadelphia: Lippincott Williams & Wilkins.

Rambur, B. (1999). Fostering evidenced-based practice in nursing education. *Journal of Professional Nursing, 15*(5), 270–274.

Rasmussen, L., O'Connor, M., Shinkle, S., & Thomas, M. K. (2000). The basic research review checklist. *Journal of Continuing Education in Nursing, 31*(1), 13–17.

Rosswurn, M. A., & Larrabee, J. H. (1999). Clinical scholarship: A model for change to evidenced-based practice. *Image: Journal of Nursing Scholarship 31*(4), 317–322.

Roy, C. (1999). State of the art: Dissemination and utilization of nursing literature in practice. *Biological Research for Nursing, 1*(2), 147–155.

Tetting, D. W. (1990). Preparing for human subjects review. *Critical Care Nursing Quarterly, 12*(4), 10–16.

Waltz, C., & Bausell, R. P. (1991). *Nursing research: Design, statistics and computer analysis.* Philadelphia: F. A. Davis.

BIBLIOGRAPHY

Brent, N. J. (1990). Legal issues in research: Informed consent. *Journal of Neuroscience Nursing, 22*(3), 189–191.

Briones, T., & Bruya, M. A. (1990). The professional imperative: Research utilization in the search for scientifically based nursing practice. *Focus on Critical Care, 17*(1), 78–81.

Dempsey, P. A., & Dempsey, A. D. (1996). *Nursing research: Text and workbook.* Boston: Little, Brown.

Elliott, D. (2000). Making research connections to improve clinical practice. *Australian Critical Care, 13*(1), 2–3.

Fitzpatrick, J. J., Stevenson, J. S., & Polis, N. S. (1994). *Nursing research and its utilization.* New York: Springer.

Fonteyn, M. E. (1990). The need for nurse involvement in critical care research. *Critical Care Quarterly, 12*(4), 1–4.

Home Box Office (Producer). (1997). *Ms. Ever's boys.* New York: HBO.

Holloway, I., & Wheeler, S. (1996). *Qualitative research for nurses.* London: Blackwell Science.

Hunt, J. (2001). Research into practice: the foundation for evidence-based care. *Cancer Nursing, 24*(2), 78–87.

Johnson, B. (2000). Evidence-based nursing for older people. *Nursing Times, 96*(16):45.

Kingry, M. J., Tiedje, L. B., & Friedman, L. L. (1990). Focus groups: A research technique for nursing. *Nursing Research, 39*(2), 124–125.

Leininger, M. (1990). Ethnomethods: The philosophic and epistemic bases to explicate transcultural nursing knowledge. *Journal of Transcultural Nursing, 1*(2), 40–51.

Maerker, M., Lisper, H., & Rickberg, S. (1990). Role-playing as a method in nursing research. *Journal of Advanced Nursing, 15*(2), 180–186.

Morrison-Beedy, D., Beeber, L., & Hahn, E. (2000). Progressive involvement of baccalaureate nursing students in research. *Nurse Educator, 25*(4), 155–156.

Nativo, D. G. (2000). Advanced practice: Guidelines for evidenced-based clinical practice. *Nursing Outlook, 48*(2), 58–59.

Neidich, B. (1990). A method to facilitate student interest in research: Chart review. *Nurse Educator, 29*(3), 139–140.

Ray, L. (1999). Evidence and outcomes: Agendas, presuppositions and power. *Journal of Advanced Nursing, 30*(5), 1017–1026.

Rempusheski, V. F. (1990). Ask an expert: Formulating research questions. *Applied Nursing Research, 3*(1), 44–46.

Resnick, B. (2000). Incorporating outcomes research into clinical practice: The four-step approach. *AACN Clinical Issues, 11*(3), 453–462.

Spross, J. A., & Heaney, C. A. (2000). Shaping advanced practice in the new millennium. *Seminars in Oncology Nursing, 16*(1), 12–24.

Streubert, H. J., & Carpenter, D. R. (1999). *Qualitative research in nursing.* Philadelphia: Lippincott Williams & Wilkins.

Wood, M. J. (2000). Influencing health policy through research. *Clinical Nursing Research, 9*(3), 213–216.

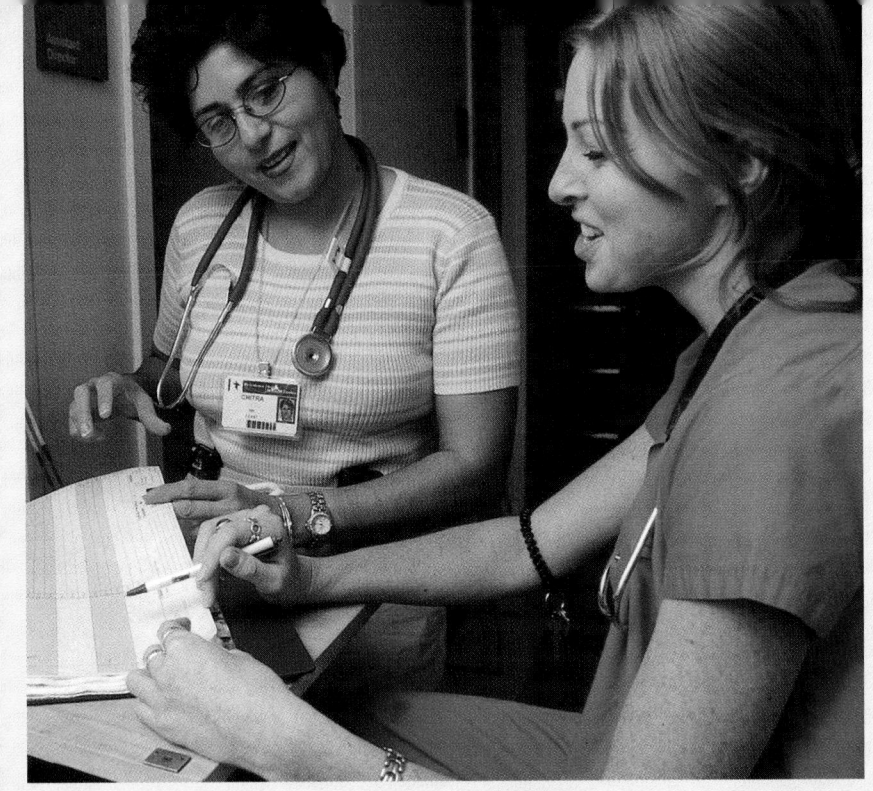

The Nursing Process
Framework for Clinical Nursing Therapeutics

9 Nursing Process
Foundation for Practice

Key Terms

decision making
diagnostic reasoning process
functional health pattern
information-processing
   theory
input
nursing process

output
primary source
problem-solving process
secondary source
systems theory
throughput

Learning Objectives

Upon completion of this chapter, the student will be able to do the following:
1. Identify the components of the nursing process.
2. Describe significant historical developments in the evolution of the nursing process.
3. Discuss the requirements for effective use of the nursing process.
4. Explain the major theoretical foundations on which the nursing process is based.
5. Describe the functional health approach to the nursing process.
6. Appraise future trends that will influence the nursing process.

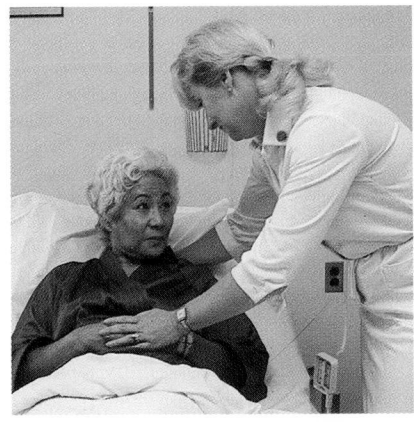

Critical Thinking Challenge

You are assigned to care for a client who had a total hip replacement 3 days ago. As you enter the room, the client is awake and greets you cheerfully. You introduce yourself and ask how she is feeling. The client replies, "I'm doing as well as can be expected." Your morning assessment reveals the following:

- *Vital signs: blood pressure 148/84, pulse 86, respirations 18, temperature 36.5°C*
- *Pain controlled adequately while in bed, but verbalizes pain when ambulating with PT*
- *Eating soft diet; no BM since surgery; bowel sounds present*
- *Repositioned client to maintain proper hip alignment*
- *Incision dry with no signs of inflammation*
- *Teaching initiated about signs and symptoms of wound infection in preparation for discharge*
- *Ambulated twice yesterday with PT; complained of dizziness and pain; states she does not know how she will manage walking at home because she lives alone, and her house is large, with steps*
- *Referral to social services for discharge planning*

Once you have completed this chapter and have incorporated the nursing process into your knowledge base, review the above scenario and reflect on the following areas of critical thinking:

1. Reflect on the assessment findings. Consider what you think are the client's problems. State whether they are actual or potential problems.
2. Determine the information-processing methods (inductive and deductive) that you used to arrive at these conclusions, and validate your findings.
3. Explain how a sound knowledge base, ability to listen, and ability to communicate in writing are important in developing and implementing an individualized and effective plan of care for this client.

The foundation of the nursing profession is nursing process. Skill in using the nursing process is necessary for the clinical application of knowledge and theory in nursing practice. Concepts related to nursing process continue to evolve. For instance, what was previously a five-phase process has now become a six-phase process. This textbook uses the six-step nursing process of assessment, diagnosis, outcome identification, planning, implementation, and evaluation.

This chapter discusses the historical development of nursing process, summarizes each phase, and gives a brief review of the theoretical foundations of the nursing process. This chapter also describes the requirements for effective use and professional relevance of the nursing process. The chapter concludes with a discussion of a functional health approach to the nursing process and future nursing process trends.

HISTORICAL DEVELOPMENT OF THE NURSING PROCESS

The term *nursing process* is synonymous with the problem-solving approach for discovering the healthcare and nursing care needs of clients. Before the widespread use of the term *nursing process* in the late 1960s, nurses cared for clients using a loosely structured framework based on the medical model. Since then, several nursing leaders have been instrumental in developing today's nursing process, and many models of the nursing process have been created.

Lydia Hall is credited with originally introducing the term *nursing process* in 1955 (George, 1995), but nursing publications did not use the term extensively until the 1960s. A few years later, Dorothy Johnson (1959), Ida Jean Orlando (1961), and Ernestine Wiedenbach (1963) described a three-step nursing process. In 1967, Lois Knowles published a five-step nursing process using "the five D's:" discover, delve, decide, do, and discriminate. The discover and delve steps are synonymous with the assessment phase; decide is the planning stage; do is the implementation phase; and discriminate is the evaluation of client responses to nursing interventions.

In 1967, several publications defined the nursing process and delineated the steps. The Western Interstate Commission for Higher Education (WICHE) and the faculty at the Catholic University of America were instrumental in moving the nursing process forward. WICHE published this definition: "The nursing process is that which goes on between a client and a nurse in a given setting; it records the behaviors of client and nurse and the resulting interaction. The steps of the process are perception, communication, interpretation, and evaluation" (Western Interstate Commission for Higher Education, 1967, p. 6). Although this definition was never widely accepted, it was an impetus to the development of the nursing process.

Helen Yura and Mary Walsh (1973), along with the nursing faculty at the Catholic University of America, identified the steps of the nursing process as assessing, planning, implementing, and evaluating. Since 1967, Yura and Walsh

have continued to develop and refine the nursing process concept.

In 1973, the American Nurses Association (ANA) distinguished diagnosis as a separate step of the nursing process in their *Standards of Nursing Practice*. The standards were arranged according to the five steps of the nursing process (see Chapter 4). The use of the five-step nursing process model by nursing educators and practitioners began at about this time.

In the 1980s, further support was gained for making diagnosis a distinct nursing function and a separate step of the nursing process. In *Nursing: A Social Policy Statement,* the ANA (1980, 1995) again identified diagnosis of actual and potential health problems as an integral part of nursing practice.

The newest development in nursing process is the six-step nursing process model, which the ANA introduced in its revised *Standards of Clinical Nursing Practice* (1991). In this six-step model, the ANA distinguished outcome identification as the third step of the nursing process. The six steps of the ANA model are used throughout this text. Table 9-1 summarizes selected contributions of people and organizations to the development and evolution of the nursing process.

COMPONENTS OF THE NURSING PROCESS

Definition

The **nursing process** generally is defined as a systematic problem-solving approach toward giving individualized nursing care. A number of authors have defined it in various ways. Display 9-1 includes a few definitions for your consideration. Note the similarities among the definitions. Regardless of the specific definition, nurses use the nursing process as a problem-solving method in all settings with clients of all ages to identify and treat human responses to potential or actual health problems. By incorporating each client's unique aspects, the nursing process facilitates the development of individualized care. The nursing process is also used to identify and treat potential or actual health problems of families and communities. In the chapters on nursing process in this book, the term *client* refers to an individual, family, or community.

The nursing process complements the current role of consumers in healthcare. That is, clients play an active role in decisions affecting their health, no longer passively accepting the decisions that healthcare professionals make.

The nursing process serves as a guide for professional nursing practice. It has the following characteristics:

- It is a framework for providing nursing care to individuals, families, and communities.
- It is orderly and systematic.
- It is interdependent.
- It provides specific care for individuals, families, and communities.
- It is client centered, using the client's strengths.
- It is appropriate for use throughout the lifespan.
- It can be used in all settings.

TABLE 9-1

Contributions of Selected Individuals and Organizations to the Development and Evolution of the Nursing Process		
Decade	**Individual/Organization**	**Contribution**
1950s	L. Hall (1955)	Originally used the term *nursing process*.
		Identified three aspects of nursing care as care, cure, and core.
		Three steps of nursing process: note observations, ministration of care, validation.
	D. Johnson (1959)	Nursing seen as fostering the behavioral functioning of the client.
		Three steps of nursing process: assessment, decision, nursing action.
1960s	I. J. Orlando (1961)	Nursing process set into motion by client behavior.
		Three steps of nursing process: client's behavior, nurse's reaction, nurse's actions.
	Western Interstate Commission for Higher Education (1967)	Nursing defined as an interactive process between client and nurse.
		Four steps of nursing process: perception, communication, interpretation, evaluation.
	H. Yura & M. Walsh (1967)	Four components of nursing process: assessing, planning, implementing, evaluating.
	L. Knowles (1967)	Described nursing practice as discover, delve, decide, do, discriminate.
1970s	American Nurses Association (1973)	Published *Standards of Nursing Practice*.
		Diagnosis distinguished as separate step of nursing process.
1980s	American Nurses Association (1980)	Published *Nursing: A Social Policy Statement*.
		Diagnosis of actual and potential health problems delineated as integral part of nursing practice.
1990s	American Nurses Association (1991)	Published *Standards of Clinical Nursing Practice*.
		Outcome identification differentiated as a distinct step of the nursing process.
		Six steps of nursing process: assessment, diagnosis, outcome identification, planning, implementation, evaluation.

Phases

The six phases of the nursing process are assessment, diagnosis, outcome identification, planning, implementation, and evaluation. Figure 9-1 illustrates these phases.

Assessment

Assessment commonly refers to evaluation or appraisal. In nursing, assessment is the systematic collection of subjective and objective data with the goal of making a clinical nursing judgment about an individual, family, or community. During assessment, the nurse appraises the client's total situation by considering the physical, psychological, emotional, sociocultural, and spiritual factors that may affect the client's health status.

The nurse must gather all relevant information about a client's present, past, or potential problems to develop a complete database. Data collection takes place during every nurse–client interaction and from many other available sources (Gordon, 1987, 1994). The client is the **primary source** of information for assessment. **Secondary sources** include family members, significant others, other healthcare professionals, health records, and literature review.

Gathering of assessment data takes place through observing, interviewing, and examining the client and interpreting laboratory data. Observation begins with the first client encounter and is ongoing. The nursing interview allows for the systematic assessment of functional health, including the client's perception and interpretation of problems (Gordon, 1982, 1987, 1994). During the physical examination, nurses use techniques of inspection, percussion, palpation, and auscultation to obtain further data. Objective information from health records, including laboratory and diagnostic data, completes the database (see Chapters 10 and 24).

An in-depth nursing history and physical assessment are usually required at admission to a hospital or long-term care facility, or during the first visit by a community or home health nurse. This initial database becomes the reference point for all further nursing assessments. Thorough assessment data provide the foundation for nursing diagnoses (Yura & Walsh, 1988).

Diagnosis

Diagnosing human responses to actual or potential health problems is the second phase of the nursing process. Diagnosis is the clinical act of identifying problems. It also is the term given

DISPLAY 9-1

DEFINITIONS OF NURSING PROCESS BY SEVERAL AUTHORS

"The nursing process is an orderly, systematic manner of determining the client's health status, specifying problems defined as alterations in human need fulfillment, making plans to solve them, initiating and implementing the plan, and evaluating the extent to which the plan was effective in promoting optimum wellness and resolving the problems identified" (Yura & Walsh, 1988, p. 1).

"Nursing process is a method of problem identification and problem solving. Although derived from the supposedly objective scientific method, nursing process is not applied in an objective, value-free way. Human values influence both problem identification and problem solving. The components of nursing process discussed in textbooks vary but generally include assessment and diagnosis. These are the problem-identification components. Outcome projection, intervention, and outcome evaluation are the problem-solving components" (Gordon, 1994, pp. 9–10).

"After a client has sought healthcare in his or her home, office, clinic, hospital, or institution, the nurse uses systematic assessment and problem-solving techniques to evaluate the client's functional status: Is it positive or altered, or is the client at risk for altered functioning? Does the client identify a problem with his or her health status? The nurse and client collaborate on planning and implementing appropriate interventions and on evaluating the effectiveness of these interventions. The nursing process describes this method, for through its five components—assessment, diagnosis, planning, intervention, and evaluation—it sets the practice of nursing in motion" (Carpenito, 1997, p. 45).

"The nursing process, which consists of five interrelated steps—Assessment, Diagnosis, Planning, Implementation, and Evaluation—is a systematic, dynamic way of giving nursing care. Central to all nursing approaches, the nursing process promotes humanistic, outcome-focused (results-focused), cost-effective care. . . . It's based on the belief that as we plan and deliver care, we must consider the unique values, interests, and desires of the consumer (person, family, community)." (Alfaro-LeFevre, 2002, p. 4).

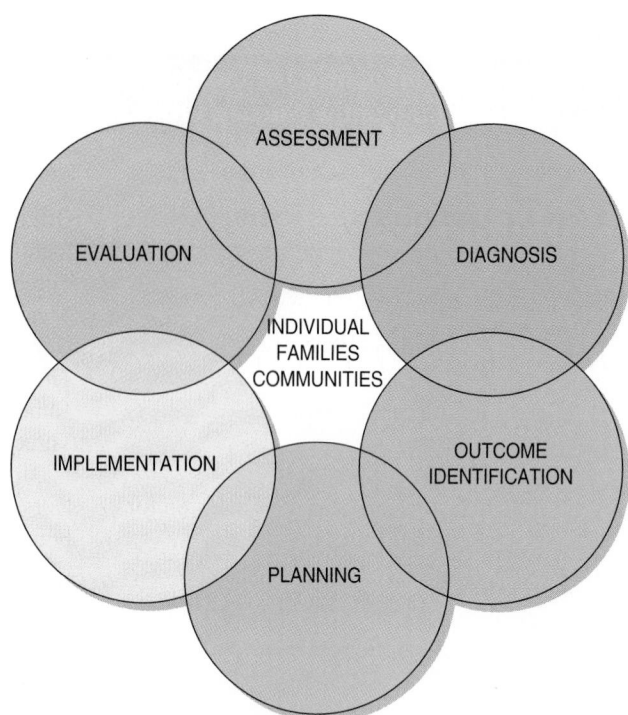

FIGURE 9-1   Six phases of the nursing process.

ment based on them. The North American Nursing Diagnosis Association (NANDA) defines *nursing diagnosis* as "a clinical judgment about individual, family, or community responses to actual or potential health problems/life processes. Nursing diagnoses provide the basis for selecting nursing interventions to achieve outcomes for which the nurse is accountable" (North American Nursing Diagnosis Association, 2001, p. 245). Registered nurses are responsible for identifying nursing diagnoses for clients under their care.

The clinical skills that nurses use to make nursing diagnoses are the nursing diagnostic process and the formulation of a nursing diagnostic statement. The nursing diagnostic process uses cue clustering, cluster interpretation, and diagnostic validation to ensure accuracy in the selection of the correct diagnoses. Formulating the diagnostic statement requires knowledge of the differences among actual, risk, possible, and wellness nursing diagnoses.

Outcome Identification

According to the ANA's *Standards of Clinical Nursing Practice* (1991), outcome identification refers to formulating and documenting measurable, realistic, client-focused goals. Identification of outcomes, including client goals and outcome criteria, is an integral part of the nursing process.

Planning

After determining nursing diagnoses, establishing priorities, and writing expected outcomes, nurses begin the planning phase. Nurses work together with clients to identify goals and intervention strategies that will reduce identified problems. The planning phase involves preparing a nursing plan of care,

to the client's problem. To diagnose means to analyze assessment information and derive meaning from this analysis.

Registered nurses are educated and licensed to make nursing diagnoses. They are responsible for identifying nursing diagnoses for their clients and for planning client manage-

which directs the activities of the nursing staff in the provision of client care.

The nursing plan of care is a written summary of the care that a client is to receive. The Joint Commission on Accreditation of Healthcare Organizations (JCAHO) requires a written plan of care for each client. The plans of care may be handwritten notes, electronic records, preprinted forms, care paths or maps, individualized preprinted plans of care, or standards of practice (Joint Commission on Accreditation of Healthcare Organizations, 1996). Although many institutions have developed standardized plans of care, all plans must be individualized. Chapter 12 discusses nursing plans of care further. The skills involved in planning include establishing client goals and outcome criteria and determining nursing interventions.

Writing the plan of care on the client record formally recognizes what the nurse planned and accomplished to assist the client. Because the plan of care remains a permanent part of the record, the beginning practitioner sometimes feels intimidated in writing information that another nurse may criticize or change. As nurses develop their skill in writing plans and begin to recognize their responsibility to carry out other nurses' plans of care, this fear should be reduced. Once the plan of care is written, it must be implemented on the client's behalf.

Implementation

Implementation is the action phase of the nursing process. It is the actual initiation of the plan, evaluation of response to the plan, and recording of nursing actions and client response to these actions. To implement means to carry out, to perform, to intervene, or to do something. Implementation may include delegating or coordinating interventions within the plan of care. This phase also may include designating the client, significant others, or healthcare providers to implement the pre-established plan of care (American Nurses Association, 1991). Nursing actions are goal directed, assisting the client to reach maximum functional health. Because nursing care is provided to assist in meeting client goals, nurses must focus on their actions, making sure that each action they undertake is necessary and required.

The components of implementation include reassessment, initiation of the plan, evaluation of the response, and recording of actions taken. Nursing actions focus on resolving or improving a client's functional health status problems.

Implementation requires the use of intellectual, interpersonal, and technical skills. Developing expertise in each of these areas is required for professional nursing practice. Once nurses have provided the care, they evaluate it.

Evaluation

Evaluation commonly refers to rating, grading, and judging. In the evaluation phase, nurses discover why the nursing plan of care was a success or failure (Alfaro-LeFevre, 2001). They determine the client's reaction to nursing interventions and judge whether the goals of the plan of care were achieved. The plan of care provides the basis for evaluation. Reassessing clients provides new information for changing or eliminating nursing diagnoses, goals, or interventions. Determining goal achievement is a joint decision between the client and the nurse (Yura & Walsh, 1988).

Evaluation focuses on individual clients and groups of clients. Quality assurance monitors provide input for development and refinement of standards of care for groups of similar clients.

Although evaluation is a separate and distinct phase, it also is an ongoing and continuous process performed throughout all phases of the nursing process. Judgments in previous phases of the nursing process result in prompt reassessment, rediagnosing, and replanning. The evaluation phase involves a detailed reassessment of the entire plan of care. An in-depth, comprehensive judgment about client goal attainment and fulfillment of outcome criteria takes place in this phase (Yura & Walsh, 1988).

The process of evaluation requires a variety of skills. These skills include knowledge of standards of care, normal client responses, and conceptual models of nursing; the ability to monitor the effectiveness of nursing interventions; and awareness of clinical research.

Interactive Nature of Each Phase

Each phase of the nursing process interacts with and is influenced by the other phases (Fig. 9-2). For example, a nurse collecting assessment information may implement some aspects of care at the same time. In a similar manner, as the nurse evaluates nursing care, he or she makes and implements new plans. During an emergency, a nurse may carry out all phases of the nursing process with no apparent divisions among them.

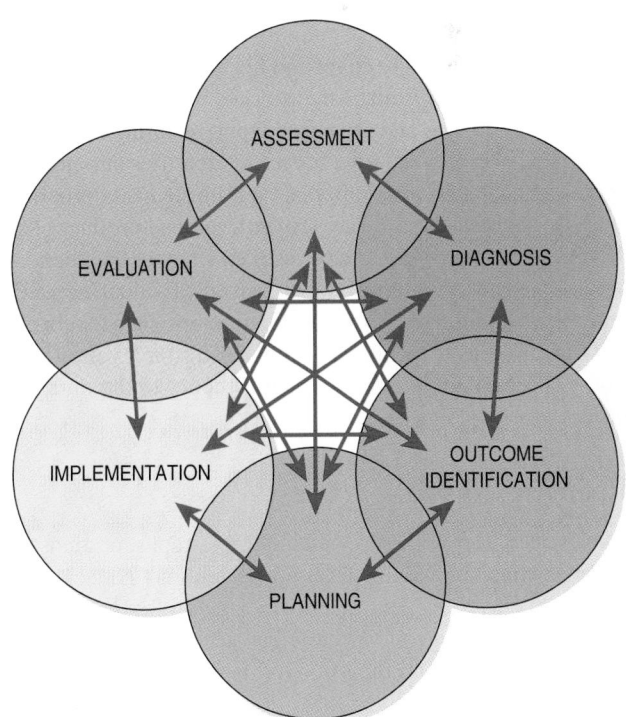

FIGURE 9-2   Interactive nature of the nursing process.

As the client's condition changes, the nurse gathers and incorporates new data into the plan of care. When care is provided, evaluation of the client's response may indicate a need for immediate revision of the plan or for the identification of new nursing diagnoses.

THEORETICAL FOUNDATIONS FOR USE OF THE NURSING PROCESS

An understanding of the theoretical foundations of the nursing process is necessary to apply it effectively. Systems theory, problem-solving process, decision-making process, information-processing theory, and diagnostic reasoning process are the basic structural units of the nursing process.

Systems Theory

Systems theory, one conceptual foundation on which nursing process is built, illustrates how the steps of the nursing process interact with each other, forming a unique blend that is greater than the sum of its parts. Systems terminology provides a common language for the members of the healthcare team (Fawcett, 2000).

A system is composed of a set of subsystems, and each higher level is made up of systems of the lower levels. All systems, including the nursing process, have cyclical patterns. The nursing process has six subsystems—assessment, diagnosis, outcome identification, planning, implementation, and evaluation—which overlap and influence subsequent subsystems.

Input, the information that enters a system, is the data collected during the assessment step (observation, nursing interview, and physical examination). Input includes assessment data about the client and his or her immediate environment. **Throughput** is the process by which a system transforms, creates, and organizes input, resulting in a reorganization of the input. After the nurse identifies nursing diagnoses and outcomes and plans and implements nursing care, throughput takes place. **Output,** the end product of a system, is the client's health status (i.e., whether the client's health has been maintained or improved). Evaluating goal attainment and the need for modification provides feedback for revising the plan, thereby completing the cycle. (See Fig. 9-3 for a comparison of systems theory to the nursing process.)

Problem-Solving Process

Nurses encounter problems, ranging from simple questions to complex clinical situations, that require solutions. Nurses confront problems with clients, family members, other healthcare team members, and equipment. Approaches to problem solving vary depending on the nature of the problem (e.g., complex or simple); the problem solver's experience, knowledge, and mental ability; and the alternative or option chosen to solve the problem.

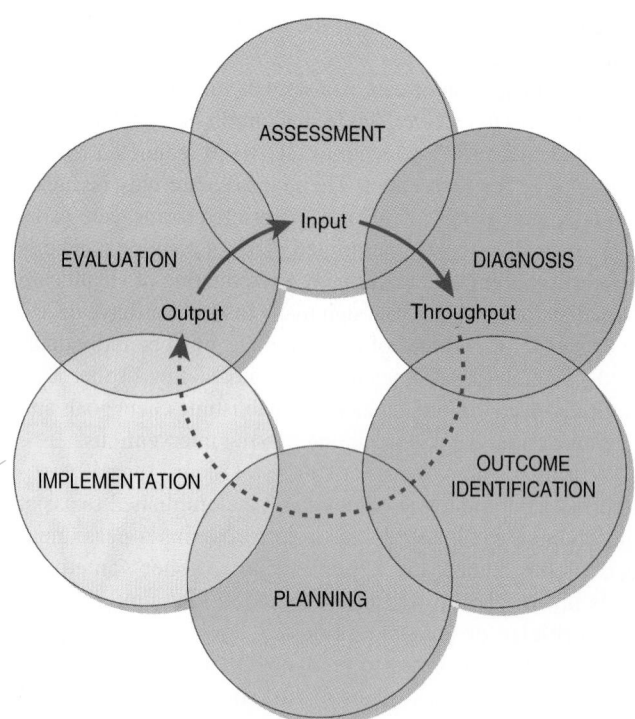

FIGURE 9-3   Systems theory in comparison to the nursing process.

Problem solving is the basis for the nursing process. The **problem-solving process** is a modified version of the scientific problem-solving method. The scientific method focuses on one problem, is carried out in a laboratory, has an extended time element, and controls as many variables or factors as possible. In contrast, the problem-solving process takes place in a clinical setting and involves clients with multiple problems. It occurs under shorter time constraints, and unforeseeable factors and events frequently intervene. The problem-solving process allows for the flexibility needed in the "real world" of clinical nursing practice.

Problem solving does not occur in isolation. Nurses solve problems by interacting and working with clients, family members, and other healthcare team members. It is an interpersonal approach that may involve two or more people. The client, whenever possible, is involved in solving problems.

The problem-solving process is composed of six steps. The phases of the nursing process are similar to the steps of the problem-solving process. Table 9-2 illustrates the similarities of the scientific problem-solving method, the problem-solving process, and the nursing process.

Decision-Making Process

Making decisions about client care is the essence of nursing practice. Decision making is integral to every step of the nursing process. In its simplest form, **decision making** consists of three phases: identifying the problem, determining the alternatives, and selecting the most appropriate alternative. People make decisions constantly, such as what to wear, what

TABLE 9-2

Similarities and Differences Among the Scientific Problem-Solving Method, the Problem-Solving Process, and the Nursing Process		
Scientific Problem-Solving Method	**Problem-Solving Process**	**Nursing Process**
Define problem	Recognize existence of problem	Assessment
Collect data	Collect data	Assessment
Formulate a hypothesis	Analyze data; specify problem	Diagnosis
Select method to test hypothesis	Determine ways to achieve solution to problem	Outcome identification, planning
Test hypothesis	Execute the planned actions	Implementation
Formulate conclusion; evaluate hypothesis	Judge the effectiveness of selected actions	Evaluation

to eat, and when to study. Past experiences and exposure to different life events influence all these decisions.

In clinical situations, nurses must decide which client should receive care first, when care may be delegated to other healthcare team members, and which client care activities are needed. Each decision is carried out or changed depending on the immediate circumstances. On some days, decisions made early in the day present no problems, but usually priorities change to meet emergency needs. Nurses must deal with uncertainty and must be adept at making astute clinical decisions.

The steps used in this process can be compared with the phases of the nursing process. Gathering information is analogous to assessment; identifying the problem area is similar to diagnosing; considering alternative courses of action and selecting a course may be likened to the planning phase. Evaluating information and the course of action is implied in this process.

Information-Processing Theory

After completing the interview, reviewing the chart, and examining the client, nurses must synthesize the data. In this complex task (Benner & Tanner, 1987; Benner, Tanner, & Chelsea, 1996), the processing of information requires the cognitive skills of logical and inductive–deductive thinking and the decision-making and diagnostic processes.

Nurses can use **information-processing theory** (Fig. 9-4) to help cluster data to arrive at a diagnosis (Newell & Simon, 1972; Simon, 1979). Because the brain can process only five to seven pieces of information at once, data need to be organized in a framework or outline. The framework model used in this textbook is functional health. In this way, nurses can see how each piece fits into the whole. Studies have shown that experienced nurses need fewer cues to make accurate diagnoses (Benner, 1984; Benner et al., 1996; Benner, 2000).

Gathering and processing information can proceed inductively or deductively. Nurses use both approaches to identify and resolve problems. *Induction* is a reasoning process that proceeds from the specific to the general:

A rose has petals.
A daisy has petals.
A petunia has petals.
Therefore, all flowers have petals.

Deduction proceeds from the general to the specific:

All flowers have petals.
A rose has petals.
Therefore, a rose is a flower.

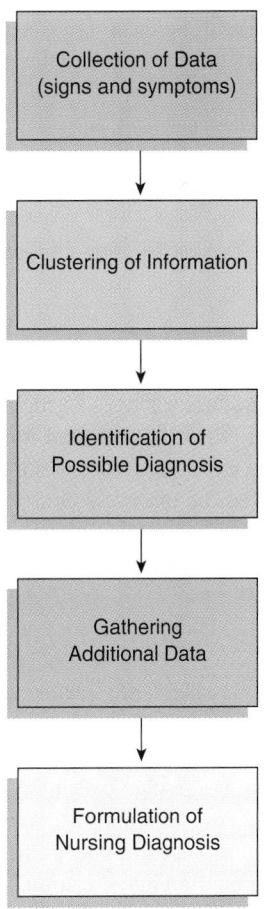

FIGURE 9-4 Information processing model.

Diagnostic Reasoning Process

The **diagnostic reasoning process** is used to make accurate clinical diagnoses about client problems. It is a complex process that is composed of several interrelated steps and is affected by variables such as the background of the diagnostician and the client. The diagnosis requires that the practitioners should (1) acquire a good working knowledge of the relevant structures and their function, (2) be able to comprehend the meaning of that knowledge, (3) know when and how to apply the knowledge, (4) be able to analyze the relationships among different pieces of information, (5) be able to synthesize pieces of information and their relationships into a meaningful whole, and (6) cross-check the processing of the entire information to evaluate whether their conclusions are defensible (Nkanginieme, 1997). Although the steps are discussed sequentially, in practice there is much overlap until the diagnosis is made and confirmed (Carnevali & Thomas, 1993). The steps include the following:

- Considering the backgrounds of the diagnostician and client
- Collecting pre-encounter data about the client
- Entering into the assessment situation
- Collecting the database
- Gathering and coalescing cues and cue clusters
- Selecting priority cue clusters
- Identifying possible diagnoses
- Confirming or refuting the diagnosis
- Selecting the diagnosis or making the clinical judgment

SKILL REQUIREMENTS

Sound Knowledge Base

To use the nursing process successfully, nurses must have a general understanding of the basic sciences and humanities. Nurses use this scientific knowledge during assessment, planning, implementing, and evaluating client care. For example, for a client with chronic obstructive pulmonary disease, several factors may produce changes in the physiology of the lungs. Culture and ethnic background may affect how the client adapts. Also, exposure to pollutants acquired at work may have influenced the disease's course. Drawing all the pieces together to plan care requires a broad knowledge base.

Nurses need a working knowledge of computers. Increasing numbers of institutions and agencies use computerized records. Keyboarding is necessary for entering client data at a computer terminal or on a notebook (laptop) computer. Also, word processing skills are needed for entering client data and for writing professional reports. Internet access is becoming increasingly important to obtain healthcare information for developing the plan of care. Nurses may e-mail peers for information or use computer databases for research.

Nurses add to their basic knowledge formally and informally by attending continuing education programs, reading professional journals, learning about related fields, and having discussions with peers and others. Incorporating new re- search findings into practice is necessary to achieve better client outcomes, develop new standards for practice, and provide cost-effective care.

Ability to Communicate in Writing

Writing skills are necessary to communicate information on the client's health record and other agency forms. Writing enables others to develop a picture of the client at the time of the assessment. Often written records are the only way to discover historical information about the progression of a disease and the client's response to it. Writing skillfully requires the ability to summarize information while maintaining comprehensiveness and accuracy. Succinct descriptive terms are useful for providing an accurate, detailed written report.

Ability to Listen

One way to obtain information for written reports is by listening. Active listening implies that nurses are responsive to the cues that clients are sending. Clients who are anxious or preoccupied may respond to questions with short or inappropriate answers. Astute nurses listen to what the client says to follow up on misconceptions and misunderstandings or to correct misinformation.

Being an active listener involves paying attention to nonverbal cues and spoken responses. Clients may hesitate to give certain information. Although respecting clients and not prying are important, nurses need to gather information that is essential for good client care. As interviewing skills develop, nurses learn how to phrase certain questions and approach personal matters. Often, the way in which questions are asked can make the difference between complete and superficial responses.

NURSING PRACTICE AND THE NURSING PROCESS

Professional Relevance

The nursing process is a systematic, organized way of providing nursing care for any client in any situation. Its adaptability and practicality contribute to high-quality nursing care. Because a concise nursing plan of care is written, continuity of care is facilitated and communication among nurses is enhanced.

The nursing process focuses on the client's unique problems. The client or family members are involved in setting priorities, developing goals and outcome criteria, and selecting nursing interventions. Because of this involvement, they play an important role in decisions that directly affect client care. The client's responses to nursing interventions are continually assessed and evaluated, which fosters individualized nursing care.

Legally, the nursing process is recognized as the standard for nursing practice. Nurses are held accountable to practice according to legal statutes and the nurse practice act of the state. Most states use the term *nursing process* when describing the act of nursing.

THERAPEUTIC DIALOGUE
Nursing Process

Scene for Thought
Linda Castro, a 34-year-old mother of two, is scheduled for a course of chemotherapy for leukemia. She has been in the oncology outpatient clinic for this treatment twice before and is known to the staff. She is sitting in the treatment chair.

Less Effective	More Effective
Nurse: Hi, Ms. Castro. I'm Carol Keegan; do you remember me from last time?	**Nurse:** Hi, Ms. Castro, I'm Lesley Jory; do you remember me from last time?
Client: Yes. Hi. I'm glad you're still here. (Looks tired and pale.)	**Client:** Yes. Hi. I'm glad you're still here. (Looks tired and pale.)
Nurse: Is it good to see a familiar face? (Checking out the client's perception.)	**Nurse:** Is it good to see a familiar face? (Checking out the client's perception.)
Client: Yes. I was worried that there would be a lot of changes since I was here last.	**Client:** Yes. I was worried that there would be a lot of changes since I was here last.
Nurse: We're all still here. How have you been since we last saw each other? (Assessment of coping outside the hospital.)	**Nurse:** We're all still here. How have you been since we last saw each other? (Assessment of coping outside the hospital.)
Client: Not too bad. The kids are a handful, but my husband helps most of the time, and I manage. Then I get so tired I can't do anything. The bruising is back again, too. (Shows several large bruises on her arms and legs.)	**Client:** Not too bad. The kids are a handful, but my husband helps most of the time, and I manage. Then I get so tired I can't do anything. The bruising is back again, too. (Shows several large bruises on her arms and legs.)
Nurse: Yes, I see. Well, that's to be expected. (Turns away from client to get chart.)	**Nurse:** I see. They look painful. You look tired. Is there something I can help you with or get you? (Assessment of immediate needs.)
Client: When do the treatments start, Carol?	**Client:** I'd love it if you could adjust the foot rest for me. I can't seem to move today.
Nurse: (Looks at client's chart; hears phone ring. Looks away, and doesn't hear client's question.)	**Nurse:** Sure. Is that okay? (Evaluation of intervention.)
Client: Carol, can you tell me when the treatments start?	**Client:** That's good. When do the treatments start, Lesley?
Nurse: In about an hour, I think. The lab results have to come up yet. Then we can get started.	**Nurse:** In about an hour, I think. The lab results have to come up. Then we can get started. Are you concerned? (Assessment.)
Client: I'm wondering if I'll have the same problem with my veins as the last time. (Looks worried)	**Client:** Well, I'm wondering if I'll have the same problem with my veins as the last time. (Looks worried.)
Nurse: I doubt it. Don't worry. We'll take care of it.	**Nurse:** Let me check your old chart. I think we did some magic with warm compresses that seemed to work last time; remember? (Evaluation of prior intervention.)
	Client: Oh yeah. That worked great. I'm glad you remembered.
	Nurse: Anything else you need before I see to those labs?
	Client: Yes. Could you get me a laxative order? I've been too tired to eat or drink much, so I guess I'm all out of whack right now. (Laughs, a little embarrassed.)
	Nurse: Not a problem. Perhaps we could talk about foods that will keep you regular. I'll bring in some ice water. We'll work on it together. (Planning with the client.)

Critical Thinking Challenge
- Identify all the phases of the nursing process you could see Lesley using.
- Analyze whether it was an orderly progression or whether she skipped phases and then returned to them.
- Describe how the less effective interaction by Carol affected the interaction. Discuss alternative responses Carol may have stated.
- Determine what you would need to assess Ms. Castro's functional health and make further diagnoses.

Professionally, the nursing process is recognized as the method of practicing nursing. It is the model on which professional nursing standards are based. Although it sometimes is criticized for not being adaptable to the changing healthcare environment, the nursing process remains the almost universally accepted method for providing nursing care.

Functional Health Approach

Gordon (1982, 1987, 1994) developed a method for organizing nursing assessment data that involves the appraisal of 11 **functional health patterns.** These functional health patterns provide a framework for the collection of assessment data.

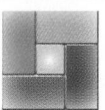

Nursing Research and Critical Thinking

Do Perceived Self-Efficacy and Functional Ability Affect the Level of Depression That Older Adults Experience After Major Elective Surgery?

Many nurses have witnessed that decline in functional ability as a consequence of medical illness or surgery often leads to the development of depressive symptoms in older clients. In this study, the nurse wanted to learn the relationship between postoperative functional ability and depressive symptoms in older adults. She designed a longitudinal study to test a theoretical path model of the effects of perceived self-efficacy and functional ability on depressive symptoms in older adults after major elective surgery. A correlational, prospective, single-cohort design was used to test the proposed theoretical model. Seventy-six older adult inpatients (60% women; mean age, 72.3 years; SD, 5.16) who had undergone elective total hip replacement surgery participated in a face-to-face interview 4 to 5 days after surgery (Time 1) and a telephone interview 6 weeks after surgery (Time 2). Perceived self-efficacy was measured by the Self-Efficacy Expectation Scale, functional ability by the Functional Status Index, and depressive symptoms by the Geriatric Depression Scale. The data were analyzed by path analysis. The results of the study revealed that Time 1 perceived self-efficacy had a direct, negative effect on Time 2 depressive symptoms. Time 1 perceived self-efficacy also had an indirect effect on Time 2 depressive symptoms through its positive effect on Time 2 functional ability. Time 1 perceived self-efficacy together with Time 2 functional ability explained 29% of the variance in depressive symptoms ($F \{2, 73\} = 4.78$, $P < .0001$).

Critical Thinking Considerations. Although the generalizability of the study findings is limited by the choice to control for a number of potentially confounding variables by exclusion, the researcher discussed several issues that are applicable to nursing practice. Possible implications include the following:

- Interventions to enhance the perceived self-efficacy of older clients while hospitalized after elective total hip replacement surgery may enhance functional ability, which, in turn, may decrease the likelihood of postoperative depressive symptoms.
- The short length of hospital stays reinforces the importance of identifying and strengthening personal resources in older clients that foster recovery, such as perceived self-efficacy.

Kurlowicz, L. H. (1998). Perceived self-efficacy, functional ability, and depressive symptoms in older elective surgery patients. *Nursing Research, 45*(4), 219–226.

Gordon originally developed the functional health pattern typology (systematic classification) in 1974 while teaching nursing assessment and diagnosis to nursing students at Boston College. Comments from nurse scholars, nurse educators, clinical nurse specialists, and students who used the categories in their practice resulted in some modification of her original health pattern categories.

Functional health patterns help the nurse ascertain the client's strengths and any dysfunctional or potentially dysfunctional pattern that exists. All 11 patterns are considered a composite of the client–environment situation and are examined collectively. Display 9-2 lists the typology of the 11 patterns. The patterns are built on the data collected during the interview and physical examination and are relevant for the individual, family, or community (Gordon, 1982, 1987, 1994).

Functional health patterns are the blueprint for the rest of the nursing process. Although functional health patterns guide the collection of assessment data, they also serve as a guide for the identification of nursing diagnoses, development of the plan of care, implementation of the plan, and the organization of evaluative data for revision of the plan. Figure 9-5 diagrams the relationships between functional health and the nursing process.

Nursing Process Trends

Although the steps of the nursing process are likely to remain the same, the way the nursing process is used will change. Many institutions have computerized their data-collection methods and nursing plans of care. Written documentation is often minimal. Instead, nurses systematically enter data into computer terminals, often at the bedsides of clients, providing easy access to all types of information necessary for quality client care. For example, a client's laboratory test results may be available for rapid interpretation and possible changes in the nursing plan of care.

Computerization, not to be equated with a lack of personalized care, aims to provide a larger, more comprehensive database to improve client care and outcomes. Frequently, clients require complex medical treatment and nursing care. Often, the treatment involves the use of sophisticated technologic devices. In this technologic environment, remember the client's need for a human touch.

As nursing diagnoses are researched and the taxonomy is scientifically validated, approaches to nursing care delivery can be standardized and evaluated. Use of national health databases will assist in evaluating and modifying nursing care. The Nursing Diagnosis Extension Classification (NDEC) research team is focusing on improving and refining the clin-

DISPLAY 9-2

TYPOLOGY OF 11 FUNCTIONAL HEALTH PATTERNS

Health perception–health management: Describes client's perceived pattern of health and well-being and how health is managed

Activity–exercise: Describes pattern of exercise, activity, leisure, and recreation

Nutritional–metabolic: Describes pattern of food and fluid consumption relative to metabolic need and pattern indicators of local nutrient supply

Elimination: Describes patterns of excretory function (bowel, bladder, skin)

Sleep–rest: Describes patterns of sleep, rest, and relaxation

Cognitive–perceptual: Describes sensory-perceptual and cognitive pattern

Self-perception–self-concept: Describes self-concept pattern and perceptions of self (e.g., body comfort, body image, feeling state)

Role–relationship: Describes pattern of role-engagements and relationships

Coping–stress tolerance: Describes general coping pattern and effectiveness of the pattern in terms of stress tolerance

Sexuality–reproductive: Describes client's patterns of satisfaction and dissatisfaction with sexuality pattern; describes reproductive patterns

Value–belief: Describes patterns of values, beliefs (including spiritual), or goals that guide choices or decisions.

From Gordon, M. (1994). *Nursing diagnosis: Process and application* (3rd ed). St. Louis, MO: Mosby.

ical usefulness of the current list of NANDA nursing diagnoses (Craft-Rosenberg & Delaney, 1997). The Nursing Intervention Classification (NIC) research team is concentrating on the development of a nursing intervention taxonomy, and the Nursing-sensitive Outcomes Classification (NOC) research team is focusing on a client outcome taxonomy (Iowa Intervention Project, 1997; Johnson & Maas, 1997; Johnson, Maas, & Moorehead, 2000; McCloskey & Bulechek, 1996; 2000). The work of NANDA, NIC, and NOC will have a significant impact on the future development of nursing knowledge and nursing science. See Chapters 10 and 11 for more information.

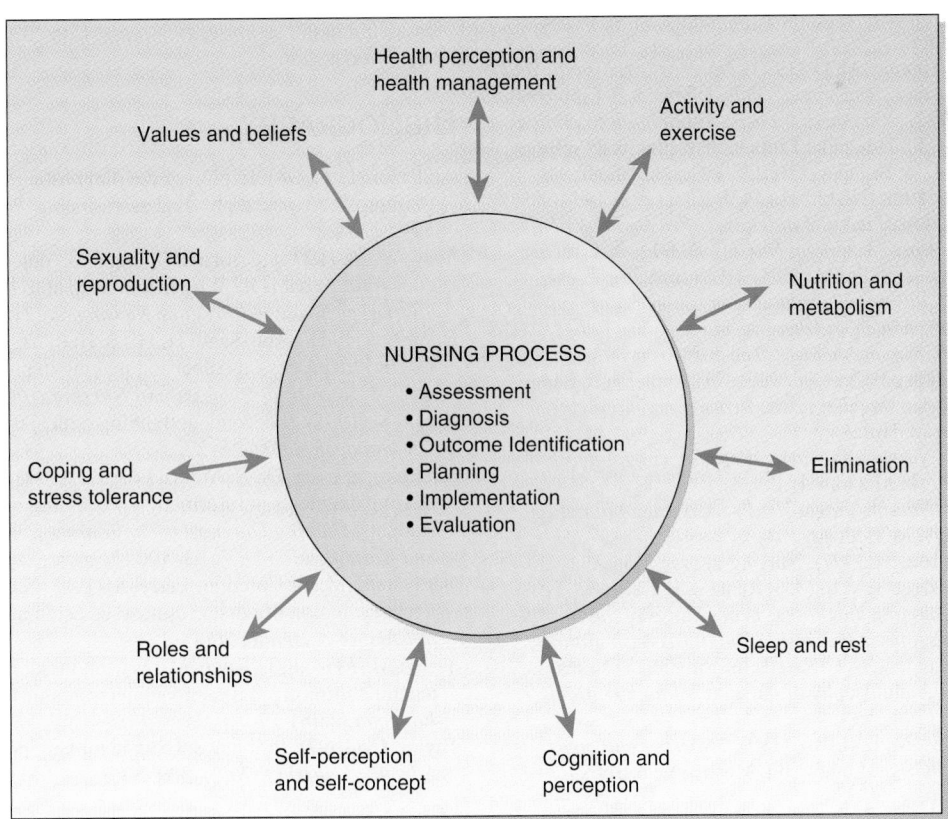

FIGURE 9-5 Functional health permeates every phase of the nursing process.

KEY CONCEPTS

- The nursing process is the systematic, problem-solving approach to providing nursing care to individuals, families, and communities.
- The nursing process has evolved over the last 40 years to consist of six phases: assessment, diagnosis, outcome identification, planning, implementation, and evaluation.
- The nursing process is used in all settings with clients of all ages to identify actual and potential health problems and design strategies to resolve them.
- Systems theory, the problem-solving process, decision-making process, information-processing theory, and diagnostic reasoning process are the theoretical foundations for the nursing process.

REFERENCES

Alfaro-LeFevre, R. (2002). *Applying nursing process: A step-by-step guide* (5th ed.). Philadelphia: Lippincott-Raven.

American Nurses Association. (1973). *Standards of nursing practice.* Kansas City, MO: Author.

American Nurses Association. (1980). *Nursing: A social policy statement.* Kansas City, MO: Author.

American Nurses Association. (1991). *Standards of clinical nursing practice.* Kansas City, MO: Author.

American Nurses Association. (1995). *Nursing: A social policy statement.* Washington, D.C.: Author.

Benner, P. (1984). *From novice to expert.* Menlo Park, CA: Addison-Wesley.

Benner, P. (2000). *From novice to expert: Excellence and power in clinical nursing practice,* [Commemorative ed.]. Englewood Cliffs, NJ: Prentice-Hall.

Benner, P., & Tanner, C. (1987). Clinical judgment: How expert nurses use intuition. *American Journal of Nursing, 87,* 23–31.

Benner, P., Tanner, C., & Chelsea, C. (1996). *Expertise in nursing practice: Caring, clinical judgement and ethics.* New York: Springer Publishing.

Carnevali, D. L., & Thomas, M. D. (1993). *Diagnostic reasoning and treatment decision making in nursing.* Philadelphia: J. B. Lippincott.

Carpenito, L. J. (1997). *Nursing diagnosis: Application to clinical practice* (7th ed.). Philadelphia: Lippincott Williams & Wilkins.

Craft-Rosenberg, M., & Delaney, C. (1997). Nursing diagnosis extension classification (NDEC). In M. J. Rantz & P. LeMone (Eds.), *Classification of nursing diagnoses: Proceedings of the 12th conference, North American Nursing Diagnosis Association* (pp. 26–31). Glendale, CA: CINAHL Information Systems.

Fawcett, J. (2000). *Analysis and evaluation of contemporary nursing knowledge: Nursing models and theories.* Philadelphia: F. A. Davis.

George, J. B. (1995). *Nursing theories: The base for professional nursing practice* (4th ed). East Norwalk, CT: Appleton & Lange.

Gordon, M. (1982). *Nursing diagnosis: Process and application.* New York: McGraw-Hill.

Gordon, M. (1987). *Nursing diagnosis: Process and application* (2nd ed.). New York: McGraw-Hill.

Gordon, M. (1994). *Nursing diagnosis: Process and application* (3rd ed.). St. Louis, MO: Mosby.

Iowa Intervention Project. (1997). Nursing interventions classification (NIC): An overview. In M. J. Rantz & P. LeMone (Eds.), *Classification of nursing diagnoses: Proceedings of the twelfth conference, North American Nursing Diagnosis Association* (pp. 32–39). Glendale, CA: CINAHL Information Systems.

Johnson, D. (1959). A philosophy of nursing. *Nursing Outlook, 7,* 198–200.

Johnson, M., & Maas, M. L. (Eds.). (1997). *Nursing outcomes classification (NOC).* St. Louis, MO: Mosby–Year Book.

Johnson, M., Maas, M. L., & Moorhead, S. (Eds.). (2000). *Nursing outcomes classification (NOC)* (2nd ed.). St. Louis, MO: Mosby–Year Book.

Joint Commission on Accreditation of Healthcare Organizations. (1996). *Comprehensive accreditation manual for hospitals: The official handbook.* Oakbrook Terrace, IL: Author.

Knowles, L. (1967). *Decision-making in nursing: A necessity for doing.* New York: Appleton-Century-Crofts.

McCloskey, J. C., & Bulechek, G. M. (Eds.). (1996). *Nursing interventions classification (NIC)* (2nd ed.). St. Louis, MO: Mosby–Year Book.

McCloskey, J. C., & Bulechek, G. M., (Eds.) (2000). *Nursing interventions: Effective nursing treatments* (3rd ed.). Philadelphia: W. B. Saunders.

Newell, A., & Simon, H. A. (1972). *Human problem-solving.* Englewood Cliffs, NJ: Prentice-Hall.

Nkanginieme, K.E.O. (1997). Clinical diagnosis as a dynamic cognitive process: Application of Bloom's taxonomy for educational objectives in the cognitive domain. *Medical Education Online, 2(1).* URL: http://www.med-ed-online.org.

North American Nursing Diagnosis Association. (2001). *NANDA nursing diagnoses: Definitions and classifications 2001–2002.* Philadelphia: Author.

Orlando, I. J. (1961). *The dynamic nurse–patient relationship.* New York: G. P. Putnam.

Simon, H. A. (1979). *Models of thought.* New Haven: Yale University Press.

Western Interstate Commission for Higher Education. (1967). *Defining clinical content, graduate nursing programs, medical and surgical nursing.* Boulder, CO: Author.

Wiedenbach, E. (1963). The helping art of nursing. *American Journal of Nursing, 63*(11), 54–57.

Yura, H., & Walsh, M. B. (1973). *The nursing process: Assessing, planning, implementing, evaluating.* Norwalk, CT: Appleton-Century-Crofts.

Yura, H., & Walsh, M. B. (1988). *The nursing process: Assessing, planning, implementing, evaluating* (5th ed.). Norwalk, CT: Appleton & Lange.

BIBLIOGRAPHY

Anderson, L. (1998). Exploring the diagnostic reasoning process to improve advanced physical assessments. *Perspectives, 22*(1), 17–22.

Daly, W. M. (1998). Critical thinking as an outcome of nursing education. What is it? Why is it important to nursing practice? *Journal of Advanced Practice Nursing, 28*(2), 323–331.

Hamers, J. P. H., Abu-Saad, H. H., & Halfens, R. J. G. (1994). Diagnostic process and decision making in nursing: A literature review. *Journal of Professional Nursing, 10*(3), 154–163.

Klann, S. (1997). Independent thinking critical to decision making. *OR Manager, 13*(7), 26–27.

Monteiro da Cruz, D., & Arcuri, E. A. M. (1998). The influence of nursing diagnosis in information processing on undergraduate students. *Nursing Diagnosis: The Journal of Nursing Language and Classification, 9*(3), 93–100.

Narayan, S. M., & Corcoran-Perry, S. (1997). Line of reasoning as a representation of nurses' clinical decision making. *Research in Nursing & Health, 20*(4), 353–364.

Su, W. M., Masodi, J., Kopp, M., & Klonowski, E. (1998). Infusing teaching thinking skills into subject-area instruction. *Nurse Educator, 23*(4), 27–30.

Taylor, C. (1997). Problem solving in nursing practice. *Journal of Advanced Nursing, 26*(2), 329–336.

10 Nursing Assessment

Key Terms

assessment
auscultation
cue
inspection
interviewing
intuition
objective data

observation
palpation
percussion
physical examination
subjective data
validation

Learning Objectives

Upon completion of this chapter, the student will be able to do the following:
1. Describe the assessment phase of the nursing process.
2. Discuss the purpose of assessment in nursing practice.
3. Identify the skills required for nursing assessment.
4. Differentiate the three major activities involved in nursing assessment.
5. Describe the process of data collection.
6. Explain the rationale for data validation.
7. Discuss the frameworks used to organize assessment data.

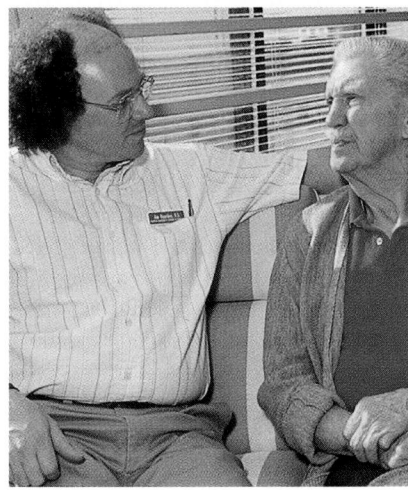

Critical Thinking Challenge

You are a nurse working in a busy medical clinic attached to a large medical center. An older man comes alone to the health clinic. You are asked to make an initial health assessment. His major complaint is generalized abdominal pain and decreased appetite. His wife of 51 years died 2 months ago. He moves slowly but appears steady on his feet. He is able to answer questions but does not look directly at you and mumbles his responses. You have 15 minutes to complete your health assessment.

Once you have completed this chapter and have incorporated nursing assessment into your knowledge base, review the above scenario and reflect on the following areas of Critical Thinking.

1. Measure the importance of rapport in this assessment. Propose methods you would use to establish rapport.
2. From the limited information provided, detect possibilities of what might be wrong with this client, supporting these informed guesses with data from the situation.
3. Summarize subjective and objective data collection and plan techniques or questions you will use to obtain data.
4. Given your limited time for assessment, determine how you will prioritize collection of essential information.

The first phase of the nursing process, called **assessment,** is the collection of data for nursing purposes. Information is collected using the skills of observation, interviewing, physical examination, and intuition and from many sources, including clients, their family members or significant others, health records, other health team members, and literature review. Figure 10-1 shows the assessment phase in relation to the other phases in the nursing process. Interpretation or analysis of the data takes place in the diagnosis phase of the nursing process. Assessment is the phase of the nursing process during which data are gathered for the purpose of identifying actual or potential health problems. Accurate assessment information is essential for the provision of high-quality nursing care.

Although overlap in the collection of some data by other members of the healthcare team may occur, the specific way in which the data are used differs from one profession to another. Nursing assessment focuses on the gathering of data about a client's state of wellness, functional ability, physical status, strengths, and responses to actual and potential health problems (Gordon, 1994).

The purpose of nursing assessment is to gather data about the client (individual, family, or community) that can be used in diagnosing, identifying outcomes, planning, and implementing care. Assessment is done for the following reasons:

- To establish baseline information on the client
- To determine the client's normal function
- To determine the client's risk for dysfunction
- To determine the presence or absence of dysfunction
- To determine the client's strengths
- To provide data for the diagnosis phase

The activities that make up the assessment phase are the following:

- Collect data.
- Validate data.
- Organize data.

PREPARING FOR ASSESSMENT

Types of Assessment

Assessment takes many forms depending on the clinical situation, client status, time available, and purpose of data collection. The types of assessment are the initial assessment, focus assessment, time-lapsed reassessment, and emergency assessment (Table 10-1).

Initial Assessment

An initial assessment, also called an admission assessment, is performed when the client enters a healthcare facility, receives care from a home health agency, or is seen for the first time in an outpatient clinic. The purposes are to evaluate the client's health status, to identify functional health patterns that are problematic, and to provide an in-depth, comprehensive database, which is critical for evaluating changes in the client's health status in subsequent assessments (Gordon, 1994).

Professional registered nurses (RNs) usually perform initial assessments. If a thorough assessment cannot be completed because of the client's health status or the urgency of specific health problems, it is finished at a later time. Frequently, experienced nurses delegate parts of the admission assessment to nonprofessional staff members. However, the professional RN is ultimately responsible for the completeness and accuracy of the information. The Joint Commission on the Accreditation of Healthcare Organizations (1996) has mandated that each client have a documented nursing admission assessment that follows institutional policies. Home health agencies, long-term care facilities, and other healthcare settings have established policies for the collection of admission data.

Focus Assessment

A focus assessment collects data about a problem that has already been identified. This type of assessment has a narrower scope and a shorter time frame than the initial assessment. In focus assessments, nurses determine whether the problem still exists and whether the status of the problem has changed (i.e., improved, worsened, or resolved). This assessment also includes the appraisal of any new, overlooked, or misdiagnosed problems. In intensive care units, nurses may perform focus assessments every few minutes.

Often, nurses assess clients for specific problems and provide nursing care at the same time. For example, while bathing a client with weakness in the lower extremities, the nurse can assess the client's skin, muscular strength, and ability to perform self-care activities (Gordon, 1994).

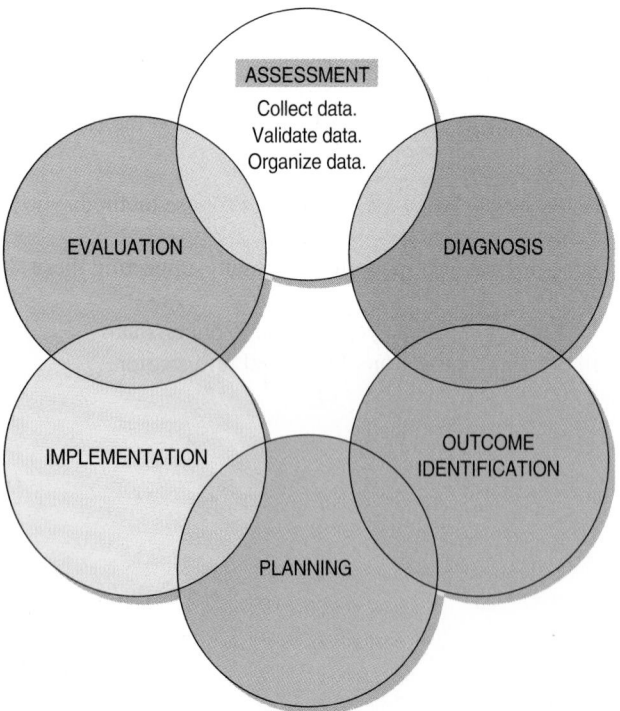

FIGURE 10-1   ANA Standard I states: The nurse collects client health data. This illustration shows activities used in the Assessment phase and also the relationship of Assessment to the other phases of the nursing process.

TABLE 10-1

Types, Aims, and Time Frame for Assessment		
Type	**Aim**	**Time Frame**
Initial assessment	Initial identification of normal function, functional status, and collection of data concerning actual or potential dysfunction Baseline for reference and future comparison	Within the specified time frame after admission to a hospital, nursing home, ambulatory healthcare center, or home healthcare setting
Focus assessment	Status determination of a specific problem identified during previous assessment	Ongoing process; integrated with nursing care; a few minutes to a few hours between assessments
Time-lapsed reassessment	Comparison of client's current status to baseline obtained previously; detection of changes in all functional health patterns after an extended period of time has passed	Several months (3, 6, or 9 months or more) between assessments
Emergency assessment	Identification of life-threatening situation	Anytime a physiologic, psychological, or emotional crisis occurs

Time-Lapsed Reassessment

Time-lapsed reassessment, another type of assessment, takes place after the initial assessment to evaluate any changes in the client's functional health. Nurses perform time-lapsed reassessments when substantial periods of time have elapsed between assessments (e.g., periodic outpatient clinic visits, home health visits, health and developmental screenings). Like the focus assessment, the time-lapsed reassessment determines the status of problems already identified. Because of the varying time interval between reassessments (e.g., 3 to 12 months), a complete review of all functional health patterns is carried out. For example, several weeks or months may elapse between reassessments of a client in an ambulatory setting. Time-lapsed reassessment is usually less comprehensive than the initial assessment (Gordon, 1994).

Emergency Assessment

Emergency assessment takes place in life-threatening situations in which the preservation of life is the top priority. Time is of the essence for rapid identification of and intervention for the client's health problems. Often the client's difficulties involve airway, breathing, and circulatory problems (the ABCs). Abrupt changes in self-concept (suicidal thoughts) or roles or relationships (social conflict leading to violent acts) can also initiate an emergency (Gordon, 1994). Emergency assessment focuses on a few essential health patterns and is not comprehensive.

Setting and Environment

Assessment can take place in any setting where nurses care for clients and their family members: in the client's home, at a clinic, in a hospital room, at a health fair, or at the client's workplace. The client's physical comfort helps facilitate data collection. Therefore, the assessment should be scheduled at an appropriate time of day so that the client is not tired, hungry, or in pain.

Nurses must be aware of environmental factors conducive to the collection of accurate and complete assessment data. An assessment is best performed in a quiet, private setting that lends itself to the discussion of sensitive, personal, and confidential information. The setting must be restricted or secluded to prevent undue embarrassment of the client during the interview and physical examination. Visitors and family members may need to leave the room temporarily. Distractions such as a television or radio, announcements over the intercom, and interruptions by other healthcare personnel should be minimized. Closing the door, pulling the curtains, turning down the heat, or moving the client to another place may be necessary if the environment cannot be modified.

ASSESSMENT SKILLS

To obtain comprehensive data, nurses use a variety of skills as they assess clients and their family members. Reading about various skills is helpful, but actual clinical experience and repeated use of these skills develop proficiency in nursing assessment.

Assessment involves recognizing and collecting **cues,** pieces of information about a client's health status. Cues may be overt (objective) or covert (subjective). Examples of overt cues are a description of an incision site ("reddened, small amount bloody drainage on dressing") or a blood pressure measurement ("180/110"). An example of a covert clue is the client's statement, "I have a sharp pain in my shoulder." In the diagnosis phase, these cues are interpreted, clustered, and analyzed.

Nurses use the clinical skills of observation, interviewing, physical examination, and intuition to assess clients across the lifespan in a variety of settings. Nurses use these skills simultaneously when assessing clients. For example, during the client interview, the nurse asks questions, observes the client, listens to the client's answers, and mentally stores information for further exploration during the physical examination. Table 10-2 summarizes the clinical skills used in assessment.

Nurses come in contact with clients of all ages, so assessment techniques may need to be modified according to each client's age and developmental stage. For example, the assessment of a child often involves parental assistance. The parent or other caregiver may hold the child on his or her lap to facilitate examination. Distraction techniques, such as flashing a light or moving an object, are helpful to divert an infant's attention during assessment, for example, when examining the ear (Bates, Bickley, & Hoekelman, 1998). When assessing an obese client, a larger blood pressure cuff may be needed. Speaking more slowly and distinctly may be required when examining an older adult with degenerative hearing loss. A client with joint problems or muscular weakness may require additional time to change positions during the physical examination.

Observation

Observation lays the groundwork for collecting other kinds of assessment data. As assessment proceeds, nurses anticipate the type of information that will be necessary or appropriate to obtain for a particular client. **Observation** comprises more than the nurse's ability to "see" the client; nurses also use the senses of smell, hearing, touch, and, rarely, the sense of taste (Yura & Walsh, 1988; Gordon, 1994).

Observation begins the moment the nurse meets the client. As the client walks into the room, gets out of the wheelchair, or is assisted into bed, the nurse is constantly observing, using all the appropriate sensory modalities. Observation includes looking, watching, examining, scrutinizing, surveying, scanning, and appraising. Using knowledge of nursing care, physical assessment, basic sciences, social sciences, and pathophysiology, nurses observe clients in a sophisticated manner. Intellectual skills also come into play as nurses decide what data they need to complete the assessment.

Vision

The sense of vision is used in a specialized manner. The nurse's ability to survey how the client "looks" is key. Does the client show signs of distress or discomfort, such as grimacing, scowling, or frowning, and guarding or holding a body part? Is the client sitting upright in a chair with arms resting comfortably at the sides, or curled up in bed? What is the client's body size and nutritional status? Is the client overweight, obese, normal weight, or undernourished and emaciated? What is the client's preferred posture? Can he or she walk? Are there any abnormal movements?

How is the client groomed and dressed? Is the client's clothing clean, excessively worn, or inappropriate for the season or weather? If a client's appearance and clothing are disheveled, further information is needed to determine possible contributing factors to self-neglect. Comparing the client's appearance to the probable norm for the client and taking into account the client's lifestyle, occupation, age, and socioeconomic group are key components of this specialized vision (Yura & Walsh, 1988; Bates et al., 1998).

Nonverbal behavior is noted during every interaction with the client. The client's nonverbal demeanor yields information about feelings toward the nurse, staff, and family (Sundeen, et al., 1997). Does the client show any signs of anger, suspicion, anxiety, or hostility? For example, the client may deny any anxiety or apprehension about health problems but may have an anxious facial expression or tear-filled eyes. The client may be argumentative and hostile with family members but cooperative and friendly with staff.

Smell

A keen sense of smell is used when observing the client. Any body or breath odors may indicate an underlying physical condition. For example, foul-smelling breath may signify an oral or pulmonary infection. A fruity breath odor may indicate a metabolic disorder such as ketosis in diabetes mellitus. Alcohol on the client's breath can mean that alcohol intake is one explanation for mental and physical findings (Bates et al., 1998). Body odors indicate sweat and sebaceous gland function and the client's overall cleanliness. A homeless person may have body odors related to lifestyle circumstances and the inability to bathe.

Hearing

Observation includes the nurse's ability to listen to and hear what the client says. The client's level of consciousness and awareness of surroundings are noted. The client's ability to state his or her name, location, and date accurately is determined when asking questions and observing how the client answers. The ability to initiate conversation or to respond

TABLE 10-2

Clinical Skills Used in Assessment	
Type	**Definition**
Observation	The act of noticing client cues
Interviewing	Interaction and communication process for gathering data by questioning and information exchange
Physical examination	Analysis of bodily functioning using the techniques of inspection, palpation, percussion, and auscultation
Intuition	Use of insights, instincts, or clinical experience to make judgments about client care

only when spoken to provides clues about the client's mental and physical condition. If the client is confused, the validity of the information obtained should be questioned. Family members or significant others, if available, can provide information for a client who is confused or incapacitated.

Touch

General observations continue through the use of touch. Touch is used to greet the client (a handshake), to provide nonverbal communication and reassurance, and to perform a preliminary appraisal of skin temperature and moisture. Observe for perspiration, warmth or coldness, and strength of the client's handshake. A gentle touch on the arm or hand may reassure the client and, at the same time, reveal dry, scaly skin indicative of dehydration or a thyroid problem. A specialized kind of touching called palpation is performed during the physical examination.

Always consider the client's sociocultural background when using touch. In some cultures, the use of touch must be modified to minimize the client's sense that privacy has been invaded. For example, with Chinese-American clients minimizing touching is a means of maintaining a formal distance and is considered a form of respect (Matocha, 1998). Clients from some cultures may interpret touching as a hostile action. Chinese-American clients may believe that drawing blood for laboratory tests depletes the body's energy, which cannot be regenerated (Barkauskas, Stoltenberg-Allen, Baumann, & Darling-Fisher, 1997). Other cultural groups use touch in other ways. For example, Cuban-American clients may hug or kiss a healthcare provider to show gratitude and appreciation (Grossman, 1998).

Interviewing

To conduct a successful interview, nurses must be effective communicators. Among the factors affecting an interview's quality and comprehensiveness are the nurse's skill and experience and the client's willingness to share information.

Several techniques facilitate communication between nurses and clients. These techniques establish rapport, help nurses elicit thoughts and feelings of clients, encourage conversation, and ensure mutual understanding (Sundeen et al., 1997). Barriers that hinder interaction have the opposite effect on communication (Carpenito, 2002; Sundeen et al., 1997). Table 10-3 summarizes the facilitators and barriers to effective communication. Chapter 21 discusses communication techniques further.

Interviewing, an essential skill for obtaining information for the nursing history, consists of asking questions designed to elicit subjective data from the client or family members. The nursing history focuses on the client's account of the actual or potential health problems and their impact on his or her health status. The nursing history helps the nurse

- Clarify and verify the client's perception of his or her health status
- Compare the client's present and past health status, lifestyle behaviors, and coping abilities
- Identify actual and potential nursing diagnoses
- Develop the nursing plan of care
- Implement nursing interventions to support the client's adaptive responses

Healthcare institutions usually have a form for the systematic collection and documentation of the nursing history. Such documentation improves communication among nursing staff and other health team members.

A nursing history can take 30 to 60 minutes to perform. Although it is usually completed in one session, several sessions may be required. If the client's condition (e.g., severe pain, breathing difficulties) or the setting (e.g., excessive noise, lack of privacy) makes data collection difficult, information about urgent problems should be collected and other questions deferred until a more suitable time.

An interview can be divided into four phases: preparatory, introductory, maintenance, and concluding.

TABLE 10-3

Techniques that Facilitate and Block Communication During an Interview	
Facilitators of Communication	**Barriers to Communication**
Use broad opening statements	Make stereotyped comments
Give general leads	Give advice or state your opinion
Listen	Agree with the client
Acknowledge the client's feelings	Defend
Use silence	Give approval
Give information	Use reassuring clichés
Reflect or repeat the client's words	Request an explanation
Share observations	Express disapproval
Clarify	Belittle the client's feelings
Summarize	Change the subject
Validate	Disagree with the client
Verbalize implied thoughts or feelings	

Preparatory Phase

The preparatory or preinteraction phase occurs before the nurse meets the client. Actions taken in this phase help ensure that the interview will be as productive as possible. The nurse's attention is directed toward preparing for the first nurse–client interaction. During this phase, do the following (Sundeen et al., 1997):

- Review as much information as possible about the client.
- Decide what data are needed and what type of data collection form will be used.
- Review the literature pertinent to the client's developmental age, psychosocial aspects, and pathophysiologic considerations, if needed.
- Assess your own feelings or reactions to previous clients that might interfere with the nurse–client relationship.
- Seek assistance from more experienced nurses, mentors, or supervisors if concerned about how to carry out the interview.
- Plan for a private, quiet setting for the interview; schedule a mutually convenient time of day; and determine the length of time needed for data collection.
- Modify the environment to facilitate the interview.

Introductory Phase

The second phase of an interview is called the introductory phase. Also known as the orientation phase, it begins when the nurse and client meet. Actions in this phase assist in establishing rapport, clarifying roles, and alleviating anxiety. The nurse and client are actively involved in asking questions, getting acquainted, and exchanging their expectations for the interview and health assessment. During this phase, do the following (Sundeen et al., 1997):

- Introduce yourself by name and position and explain the purpose and content of the interview.
- Begin to establish rapport with the client by conveying a caring, interested attitude; rapport is essential for a trusting, helpful nurse–client relationship.
- Observe the client's behavior, and listen attentively to determine the client's self-perceptions and the how the client views his or her health problems; validate the client's perceptions as the interview progresses.
- Let the client know how long the nurse–client relationship is expected to last.
- Inform the client how the information collected will be used and that confidentiality will be maintained.
- Start with nonthreatening, specific questions and proceed to open-ended questions.
- Establish a verbal contract with the client, incorporating the goals of the interview.

Maintenance Phase

The maintenance phase, or working phase, is the third phase of an interview. The nurse and client work toward achieving the specific task or goal agreed on in the introductory phase. Both participants maintain the interaction for the purpose of

getting the "work" done, but it is the nurse's responsibility to ensure that the goals are met. The goals may be mutually revised by the client and nurse. In this phase, do the following (Sundeen et al., 1997):

- Keep focused on the tasks or goals to ensure that needed data are obtained and goals are achieved.
- Encourage the client to express his or her feelings, concerns, and questions.
- Use techniques that facilitate communication between the nurse and client (e.g., silence, general leads, validation).
- Observe the nonverbal behavior that accompanies verbal responses (e.g., a client may say she is not nervous, worried, or anxious while biting her fingernails, moving constantly, and smoking throughout the interview).
- Assess the client's ability to continue the interview (e.g., grimace of pain, shortness of breath, fatigue).
- Facilitate goal attainment by moving to the next topic of discussion after needed data are collected.

Concluding Phase

In the concluding or termination phase, the nurse–client relationship is completed. Actions taken in this phase can help ensure that the termination will be a positive experience for both participants. The focus is on reviewing goals or tasks attained and expressing concerns related to this phase. In this phase, do the following (Sundeen et al., 1997):

- Review goal or task attainment; such a review can foster a sense of achievement in the client and nurse.
- Summarize the highlights of the interview and its meaning to the nurse and the client.
- Encourage the client to express and share his or her feelings regarding the termination of the nurse–client relationship.
- Use language congruent with the client's cultural background and local custom (e.g., "goodbye" may mean a final farewell in some cultures; promises to contact the client in the future may be taken literally).

Physical Examination Techniques

The **physical examination** is a systematic data collection method that uses the senses of sight, hearing, smell, and touch to detect health problems. Four techniques are used: inspection, palpation, percussion, and auscultation. Usually, the nursing interview is completed before the physical examination is performed. The physical examination is used to verify and expand the data gathered during the nursing interview (Gordon, 1994).

Inspection

Inspection is a visual examination of the client that is done in a methodical and deliberate manner. Beginning with the first client contact, it is conducted intentionally and continuously to avoid omitting data. Not haphazard or passive, inspection is an important first step in the physical examination process. During inspection, the client's anatomic structures are considered and any abnormalities that may be present are identified. Factors such as color, shape, symmetry, movement, pulsations, and texture of the involved body part are noted (Bates et al., 1998; Fuller & Schaller-Ayers, 1999).

Inspection is carried out during the interview and subsequent physical examination. For example, an enlarged thyroid or growth in the neck may be visible during the interview with the client. Detailed inspection of the neck would take place after the interview.

Palpation

Palpation is the specialized use of touch for data collection that augments the inspection process. The nurse uses the fingertips and palms of the hand to determine the size, shape, and configuration of underlying body structures. The pulsations of blood vessels; the outlines of organs such as the thyroid, spleen, or liver; the size, shape, and mobility of masses; the temperature of the skin; vibration or movement of blood in a blood vessel; and tenderness or sensitivity of a body part are detected.

Percussion

Percussion is a technique in which one or both hands are used to strike the body surface to produce a sound called a percussion note. Underlying body structures have characteristic percussion notes that indicate their denseness or hollowness. Percussion is used to discover the location and level of organs (liver, heart, diaphragm); the consistency of body structures (fluid-filled, air-filled, or solid); the presence of tenderness (over the kidneys or near the spine); and the identification of masses or tumors.

Auscultation

Auscultation is the technique of listening to body sounds with a stethoscope placed on the body surface to amplify normal and abnormal sounds. It yields information by amplifying the movement of air or fluid in the body. Mastery of auscultation lies in practice and the ability to interpret the findings. A novice nurse may consult with a more experienced nurse to verify auscultation findings, often to verify and confirm the presence of abnormal sounds.

Various body systems, including the respiratory, cardiovascular, and gastrointestinal systems, may be auscultated for characteristic sounds. Bowel sounds, breath sounds, heart sounds, and the sound of blood moving through a narrowed or twisted blood vessel (known as a bruit) are heard through auscultation.

Intuition

Only recently acknowledged as a legitimate part of nursing practice, **intuition** is defined as the use of insight, instinct, and clinical experience to make clinical judgments about the client. Intuition is a specialized type of knowing (also called common sense, gut feelings, or a sixth sense) that triggers nursing actions and/or reflection and directly influences the nurse's ability to analyze client cues (Cioffi, 1997; King & Appleton, 1997). "Although not validated or valued in traditional ways, intuitive knowledge appears to be used by nurses, particularly expert nurses, in many aspects of clinical practice" (Beckett, 1990).

Intuition plays a role in the nurse's ability to analyze cues rapidly, make clinical decisions, and implement nursing actions even though assessment data may be incomplete or ambiguous (Rew, 1988). In the past, the concept of intuition appeared infrequently in nursing literature, but nurse researchers and scholars are continuing to examine its role in the various phases of the nursing process. Research results imply that the nursing process addresses only part of the problem-solving process used by nurses (Rew & Barrow, 1987; King & Appleton, 1997). Rew (1988) found that most experienced nurses used intuition during the assessment and implementation phases of the nursing process. Research on intuition in nursing suggests that recognition and use of intuition are necessary in nursing practice, education, and administration (King & Appleton, 1997).

Intuition comes into play when assessment data are incomplete, sketchy, or vague, or when the client looks all right on the surface but the nurse senses that something is not quite right. For example, before obtaining complete assessment data, a nurse may enter a client's room and get a strong "feel" about the client's condition without performing a physical examination or reading the chart, or a nurse may sense that a client with normal vital signs, skin color, and neurologic status is going to have a cardiac or respiratory arrest (Rew, 1988). In the two situations described, the nurse uses intuitive knowledge to analyze cues, make clinical decisions, and implement nursing interventions on behalf of the client. Intuition results in decisions that might not have been made had the nurse used the nursing process alone.

Previous studies on intuition in nursing have involved primarily nurses in critical care units. Additional research studies in both acute care and community settings are needed to verify the exact role that intuition plays in clinical nursing practice (King & Appleton, 1997).

ASSESSMENT ACTIVITIES

During the assessment phase, nurses collect, validate, and organize data. Because these activities are so closely related, shifting from one to another often occurs. For example, collecting and organizing of data may occur at the same time. Nurses may choose to validate information as they collect it rather than at the completion of data collection. As they organize data, they may discover ambiguous cues that require further clarification and validation.

Collect Data

Data collection, the process of compiling information about the client, begins with the first client contact. Nurses use observation, interviewing, and physical examination. Usu-

Nursing Research and Critical Thinking
What Practical Knowledge Do Expert Nurses Use When They Assess Clients at Risk for Impaired Swallowing?

When a group of nurses found that little nursing research had been done to guide practice for clients with impaired swallowing, they undertook a study to identify and describe the knowledge embedded in everyday nursing practice. They designed a descriptive, exploratory study using purposive sampling. The framework for the study was derived from the Dreyfus model of skill acquisition, which states that practitioners move through definable stages, from novice to expert, as they increasingly rely on concrete experience rather than formal rules and procedures. They identified 12 nurses in one teaching hospital who were considered by their peers to be experts in the care of clients at risk for impaired swallowing. They collected data from this sample ($N = 12$) of expert nurses, using written narratives by each participant; group interviews, in which nurses discussed the written narrative; nonparticipant observations and individual interviews of the expert nurses; and reviews of clients' charts. Data were analyzed using interpretive phenomenology. The researchers found that the themes in the nursing care of clients with impaired swallowing included assessment of swallowing; clinical management; the importance of knowing the client; quality of life; and eating as a form of family caring and as a social and aesthetic need.

Critical Thinking Considerations. The researchers state that the sample was drawn from nurses practicing on the units of the hospital that most often have clients with impaired swallowing. Despite the prevalence of this problem and the existence of a clinical advancement program that recognizes nursing expertise, identifying nurses who were expert in caring for clients with impaired swallowing was difficult. Implications are as follows:

- The study suggests that although some nurses have much experiential knowledge of how to assess clients' swallowing ability and how to feed clients, they have difficulty clearly articulating these processes.
- The need for skilled nursing assessment of swallowing ability is critical when feeding is delegated to nonprofessionals. Informed guidance and direction needs to be provided.

From McHale, J. M., Phipps, M. A., Hovarth, K., & Schmelz, J. (1998). Expert nursing knowledge in the care of patients at risk of impaired swallowing. *Image: Journal of Nursing Scholarship, 30*(2), 137–141.

ally, they collect data using a systematic format that ensures comprehensive, accurate information.

Types of Data
Subjective and objective data, both integral parts of assessment, are obtained during data collection. Table 10-4 shows the differences in the methods of obtaining subjective and objective data and provides examples of each type.

Subjective data, also known as symptoms or covert cues, include the client's feelings and statements about his or her health problems. Clients supply subjective data. Often, attempts to validate, confirm, or substantiate subjective data through other sources are not feasible. Subjective data are obtained through the interview and are best recorded as direct quotations from the client, such as

> "I haven't felt good for the last couple of months."
> "I get a sharp pain in my stomach after I eat."
> "Every time I move, I feel nauseated."

Objective data, also known as signs or overt cues, are observable, perceptible, and measurable. Others can validate or verify objective data. Examples include bowel sounds, temperature readings, peripheral pulses, distended neck vessels, and skin rashes. Objective data may be obtained by the senses (e.g., vision, touch, smell) or by measuring devices or equip-

ment (e.g., thermometer, sphygmomanometer), laboratory studies (e.g., complete blood count), or diagnostic procedures (e.g., colonoscopy).

Sources of Data
Two major sources of data exist for the collection of information about the client. The client is considered the primary source of data because only he or she can give a first-hand description of the health problem and its effects on his or her lifestyle. All other sources, including family members, significant others, other members of the healthcare team, laboratory tests, and literature review, are considered secondary sources.

Primary Source. The client is the primary source of data, and the information collected from the client is considered to be the most reliable, unless circumstances such as altered level of consciousness, severe pain, impending surgery, acute illness, or age make data collection impossible. The client is deemed unreliable if he or she is confused or suffering from physical or mental conditions that alter thinking, judgment, or memory. In these situations, secondary sources help provide the necessary assessment information.

Secondary Sources. Secondary sources provide data that supplement, clarify, and validate information obtained from

TABLE 10-4

Comparison of Subjective and Objective Data		
	Subjective Data (Covert Cues)	Objective Data (Overt Cues)
Method of obtaining data	Interview	Techniques of inspection, palpation, percussion, and auscultation Measurement devices Health record Laboratory studies, radiologic tests, diagnostic procedures
Examples	Symptoms Values Perceptions Feelings Attitudes Sensations Beliefs	Physical examination findings: heart sounds, palpable tumor, discolored skin Blood pressure, temperature, intracranial pressure Written reports of other healthcare team members on health record Complete blood count results, chest radiography results

the client. These sources include family members or significant others, the health record, laboratory tests and diagnostic procedures, health team members, and literature review.

Family members or significant others supplement and verify information obtained from the client, often providing information that the client forgets to mention or is unwilling to reveal. They may be the only source of data for children or for confused, unresponsive, or severely ill clients. Data provided by family members and significant others include a description of how the client reacts to illness, the client's perceptions of changes in health status, the client's ability to cope with life stressors, and information about the client's home situation.

Usually, the client's permission is obtained before information is sought from family members or significant others. All people involved must understand the confidential nature of the information they provide. The client's permission must also be obtained to divulge any information (e.g., diagnosis of cancer, positive human immunodeficiency virus status, pregnancy) to family members or significant others.

Past and current health records (e.g., consultation reports, medical and nursing histories, physical examination findings) contain a wealth of information about the client and are helpful in completing assessment data. Facts about the client's previous illnesses, hospitalizations, function, and dysfunction are obtained. The health record may also reveal data not expressed by the client or picked up by the nurse. Reviewing health records can also reduce the number of times a client is asked the same questions by various health team members.

Laboratory tests and diagnostic procedures, another secondary source of data for completing the database, supplement and verify findings from the interview and physical examination. Laboratory test results are always interpreted in relation to the client's underlying health problems and treatment modalities. These results can also identify actual or potential health problems not disclosed by the client or explored by the nurse. Sometimes, laboratory tests and diagnostic procedures are used to judge the effectiveness of nursing interventions.

Written and verbal reports from other health team members are another source of assessment data. Health team members include professional staff such as nurses, social workers, physical therapists, physicians, clergy, respiratory therapists, and nonprofessional personnel such as certified nursing assistants. Take advantage of the expertise of other colleagues who are caring for the client. All of them are valuable sources of information about the client's current and past health status. Consulting other health team members helps verify and supplement the assessment data.

Reviewing the literature helps complete the client's database. Pertinent literature includes textbooks, journals, dissertation abstracts, and unpublished monographs presented at professional meetings. The client's health patterns must be viewed in relation to current knowledge and theory. A thorough review of the literature provides information on recent developments in nursing and medical practice.

Recording Data

Using a framework or outline, assessment data are systematically recorded and become a permanent part of the medical record. Institutions usually have a specific form for recording data and facilitating its use by other nurses who are caring for the client. Baseline assessment data are referred to periodically to reaffirm assessment findings and to compare the client's current status with his or her initial condition. Two methods can be used: the traditional written assessment record and the computerized assessment record. Chapter 15 discusses documentation of client assessment in detail.

ETHICAL/LEGAL ISSUE
Confidentiality of Assessment Findings

Mr. Jones, a 51-year-old client, was recently diagnosed with advanced colon cancer with metastasis. Due to a large bowel obstruction, Mr. Jones had a bowel resection with reanastomosis 6 days ago and is recovering at home. Your assessment reveals that the client lives alone and has been estranged from his wife for the past 2 years. He states, "We really don't talk much." During your home visit. Mr. Jones' wife arrives and asks you to tell her what is wrong with her husband. How would you handle this situation? What information would you give Mrs. Jones?

Reflection
- Consider your responsibilities to the client. Consider your responsibilities to his wife.
- Identify additional information you would need to assess before proceeding.
- Propose possible strategies for handling this situation.

Validate Data

Validation, commonly referred to as double-checking the information at hand, is the process of confirming the accuracy of assessment data collected. As data are collected, multiple cues are identified. Inferences are made about the cues (i.e., a

APPLY YOUR KNOWLEDGE

You have collected the following data for your assigned client:

- Complete blood count (CBC)
- Client's health history: "I haven't felt good for the last 2 weeks. I think it's the flu." History of diabetes for 5 years; no complaints of pain.
- Physical examination: Afebrile; pulse–72; respirations–22; blood pressure–112/64. Abdomen soft and nontender. Bowel sounds present in all four quadrants.
- Family member's description of how the client has reacted to his or her illness
- Client's perception of ability to cope with life stressors
- Chest radiology results
- Consultation report from physical therapy

Which data are considered primary sources and which are considered secondary sources?

Check your answer in Appendix A.

meaning or interpretation is attached to the cue). One or more inferences can be made about a particular cue or group of cues (Alfaro-LeFevre, 2001), as seen in the examples provided in Display 10-1.

Validation assists in verifying and clarifying cues and inferences, thus increasing the likelihood that cues and inferences are accurate, free from bias, and interpreted correctly (Alfaro-LeFevre, 2001). Incorrect cues and inferences lead to the development of inappropriate nursing diagnoses and nursing plans of care. Figure 10-2 illustrates the connection between cues and inferences and methods for data validation.

Identification of relevant cues and correct inferences depends on the nurse's clinical nursing knowledge, assessment skills, personal values, and past experience (Alfaro-LeFevre, 2001). Inferences must be validated before cues are clustered and analyzed for identification of nursing diagnoses.

Methods of validating data include (Alfaro-LeFevre, 2001):

- *Comparing cues to normal function.* For example, Mr. Jones is a professional athlete and has a resting pulse of 50 beats per minute; the nurse knows that physiologic heart changes in physically fit people can result in a slower pulse rate (bradycardia).
- *Referring to textbooks, journals, and research reports.* For example, the nurse may consider the presence of brown macules or "liver spots" on the hands and forearms of an elderly client to be abnormal. After checking a textbook on physical changes that occur with aging, the nurse learns that they are common in older adults.
- *Checking consistency of cues.* Data can be checked, for example, by retaking the client's temperature or blood pressure or by using another piece of equipment. Subjective and objective data can be compared. For example, the client may state, "I feel hot," but his or her temperature is 98.6°F, or the client may state, "I can't get my breath," but respirations are 20 and lung sounds are clear.
- *Clarifying the client's statements.* Ask specific, closed-ended questions; share observations with the client and family members; clarify ambiguous or vague statements; and verify inferences. For example, a client who is asked whether he of she has any allergies to foods, medicines, or pollutants may respond, "I am allergic to antibiotics." If questioned further about the medication bottle labeled "penicillin" the client brought from home, he or she may state, "Oh, I'm not allergic to all antibiotics, just erythromycin." A client may be of normal weight but very fatigued. Further questioning would be needed to determine the client's perspective regarding dietary intake, weight, and other factors. The family member's perspective is also needed. It is possible that the client has a history of bingeing and purging, although his or her weight is within a normal range.
- *Seeking consensus with colleagues about inferences.* This is usually done after the data have been validated using the methods already described. If peers or colleagues independently reach the same conclusion as the

DISPLAY 10-1

⑤ **EXAMPLES OF CUES AND INFERENCES**

Example 1
Group of Cues Client has
- Blurry vision or visual defect
- Headache
- Tingling and numbness in extremities
- Dizziness

Possible Inferences
- Client has a brain tumor.
- Client is having warning signals of a stroke.
- Client may be diabetic.
- Client is anxious.

Example 2
Cue
Mr. Spencer has dry, flaky skin.

Possible Inferences
1. Mr. Spencer may be dehydrated.
2. Mr. Spencer has hypothyroidism.
3. Mr. Spencer has some type of dermatitis.

Example 3
Cue
Client has frequency and burning on urination.

Inference
Client has a urinary tract infection.

Example 4
Cue
Mrs. Smith's blood sugar is 55 mg/dL.

Inference
Mrs. Smith is having a hypoglycemic reaction.

Example 5
Cue
Client states, "I just can't seem to shake this pain in my joints."

Inference
Client has inadequate pain management.

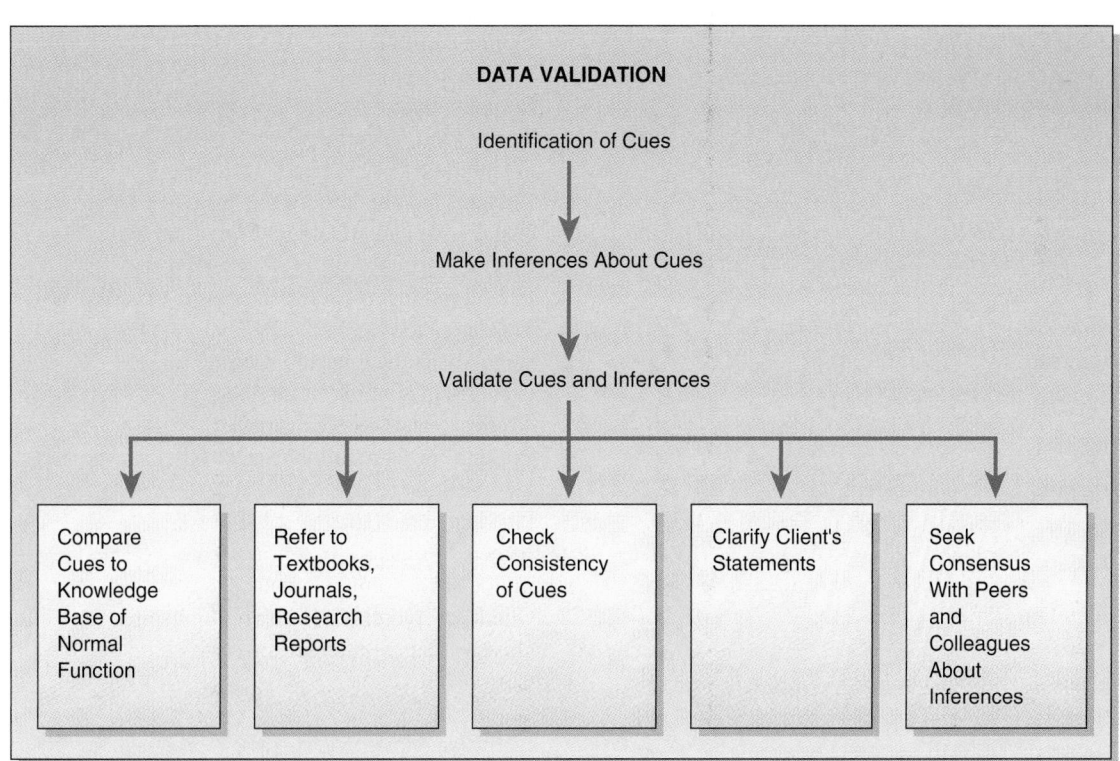

FIGURE 10-2   Methods for the validation of cues and inferences.

nurse did, and if that conclusion is based on valid data, the nurse's inferences are supported. If colleagues present an alternative view, it assists the nurse in questioning the validity of his or her own inferences.

Organize Data

A variety of frameworks exist for the orderly collection and recording of assessment data. Frameworks serve as guides during the nursing interview and physical examination, help prevent the omission of pertinent information, and foster data analysis in the diagnosis phase. Frameworks may be modified based on the client's physical status and the nurse's personal preference (Fuller & Schaller-Ayers, 1999).

Nursing conceptual models provide one such framework. Institutions, nursing schools, and individual nurses use one or

more of these frameworks to guide their nursing practice. Each conceptual framework has a frame of reference for carrying out nursing care. Some examples are Orem's self-care model, Roy's adaptation model, Neuman's systems model, and Johnson's behavioral model (Fawcett, 2000). When using one of these frameworks, refer to specific texts that describe these models in detail. See also Chapter 4 for more information.

Functional Health Patterns Model

The client's strengths, talents, and functional health patterns are an integral part of the assessment data. This information occasionally is obscured or forgotten in some assessment frameworks. An assessment of functional health focuses on the client's normal function and his or her altered function or risk for altered function. Because the information gathered using the 11 functional health patterns is basic to nursing, it is ap-

TABLE 10-5

Functional Health Patterns and Assessment Parameters

Functional Health Pattern	Assessment Parameters
Health perception and health management	General survey of the client's health status Usual health behaviors
Activity and exercise	Mobility status Exercise routine Leisure activities
Nutrition and metabolism	Eating habits Appraisal of appetite Weight loss or gain Changes in skin, hair, or nails
Elimination—excretory function (bowel, bladder, and skin)	Usual bowel and bladder elimination habits Laxative use Excretory function of the skin (e.g., excessive perspiration)
Sleep and rest	Regular sleep habits and routine
Cognition and perception	Changes in cognitive function Ability to hear, see, and speak Presence of pain, numbness, or other sensations
Self-perception and self-concept	Descriptions of self Physical appearance Effects of illness Major life accomplishments
Role and relationships	Client's perceptions of key relationships Observations of interactions with others
Coping and stress tolerance	Current stress level Coping ability Ability to endure life stressors Physiologic responses to stress (e.g., blood pressure, heart rate)
Sexuality and reproduction	Client's appraisal of his or her sexual role and sexual health
Values and beliefs	Identification of valued people and possessions Sources of support Religious practices

plicable to all conceptual models of nursing practice (Gordon, 1994). Functional health assessment can be used for clients of all ages and in all specialty areas, and it is relevant for the assessment of the person, family, or community (Bechtel, 1995; Carlson-Catalano, 1998; Courtens & Abu-Saad, 1998).

Some nurses collect physical assessment data using the body systems model or the head-to-toe model but use a functional health framework to organize and document assessment data. The advantages of a functional health framework include the following:

- Client strengths and assets (not merely deficits, problems, or limitations) can be identified.
- The focus is on nursing diagnoses, not medical diagnoses.
- Clustering is easier to do because of the simple categories and concise typology.
- It may contribute to the delineation of basic assessment areas relevant for all clients.

The components of functional health assessment include the pattern label, assessment parameters for each pattern, and recording of assessment data.

The pattern label is the name given to a category of assessment data. Gordon (1994) identified 11 categories of assessment data, called functional health patterns. Pattern labels indicate whether the client has a functional (asset, strength) or dysfunctional (nursing diagnosis) health pattern.

Assessment parameters help nurses gather specific information about each functional health pattern. Assessment parameters have been identified for each functional health pattern. Specific interview questions, physical examination techniques, and other information such as laboratory data or health records help nurses identify health problems within each pattern.

There are various forms for recording assessment parameters and identifying the client's functional or dysfunctional health patterns (Gordon, 1994). Nurses use the approved institutional form from their place of employment or school of nursing. Data may be recorded by hand on a form or by entering the information into a computer.

Chapter 9 presents the 11 functional health patterns. In-depth information about the assessment parameters for each functional health pattern is described in Chapter 24 and highlighted in Table 10-5.

Head-to-Toe Model

Using the head-to-toe framework for assessment, nurses systematically examine every part of the body starting from the head and progressing down to the toes. Similar to most assessment models, the head-to-toe method first assesses the client's general state of health. Vital signs may be taken before the physical examination begins. Chapter 24 presents the order of physical assessment. Modifications of the head-to-toe framework can be used for young children to ensure that invasive techniques, such as examining the ears with an otoscope, are done last.

Body Systems Model

The body systems model (also called the medical model or review of systems) focuses on the client's major anatomic systems. This framework allows nurses to collect data about the past and present condition of each organ or body system and to examine thoroughly all body systems for actual and potential problems. This review often reveals information that the client did not consider important or neglected to mention. It starts with an assessment of the client's general state of health, followed by systematic assessment of each body system (neurologic, cardiovascular, respiratory, gastrointestinal, and so on) until all systems have been assessed. Chapter 24 describes the order of the physical assessment as performed by the staff nurse using a body systems framework.

KEY CONCEPTS

- Assessment is the collection of subjective and objective data from the client and other sources for the purpose of describing health problems.
- Types of assessment vary depending on the clinical situation, the client's health status, the time available, and the purpose of data collection.
- An in-depth, comprehensive appraisal of a client's functional health patterns at the time of entry into a healthcare facility or at the time of the first home health visit or outpatient clinic visit is called an admission assessment.
- Environmental factors can facilitate or hinder collection of assessment data.
- Observation helps the nurse anticipate appropriate data to be collected during the nursing interview and physical examination.
- Proficient interviewing skills are necessary for obtaining comprehensive assessment data.
- The physical examination is a systematic analysis in which inspection, palpation, percussion, and auscultation are used.
- Intuition, a legitimate aspect of nursing practice, involves the nurse's use of insight, instinct, and clinical experience.
- The client, family and significant others, health team members, and health records are sources of assessment data.
- Assessment data are recorded and become a permanent part of the health record.
- The functional health pattern assessment provides a framework for collecting and organizing client data, providing a foundation for the development of nursing diagnoses.

REFERENCES

Alfaro-LeFevre, R. (2001). *Applying nursing process: A step-by-step guide* (5th ed.). Philadelphia: Lippincott Williams & Wilkins.

Barkauskas, V. H., Stoltenberg-Allen, K., Baumann, L. C., & Darling-Fisher, C. (1997). *Health and physical assessment* (2nd ed.). St. Louis, MO: Mosby–Year Book.

Bates, B., Bickley, L. S., & Hoekelman, R. A. M. (1998). *A guide to physical examination and history taking* (7th ed.). Philadelphia: J. B. Lippincott.

Bechtel, G. A. (1995). Enhancing functional health patterns among homebound elderly. *Journal of Nursing Science, 1*(1/2), 33–39.

Beckett, J. E. (1991). Intuition in clinical nursing. *Research Review: Studies in Nursing Practice, 6*(3), 2.

Carlson-Catalano, J. (1998). Nursing diagnoses and interventions for post-acute phase battered women. *Nursing Diagnosis: The Journal of Nursing Language and Classification, 9*(3), 101–110.

Carpenito, L. J. (2002). *Nursing diagnosis: Application to clinical practice* (9th ed.). Philadelphia: Lippincott Williams & Wilkins.

Cioffi, J. (2001). Heuristics, servants to intuition, in clinical decision-making. *Journal of Advanced Nursing, 26,* 203–208.

Courtens, A. M., & Abu-Saad, H. H. (1998). Nursing diagnoses in patients with leukemia. *Nursing Diagnosis: The Journal of Nursing Language and Classification, 9*(2), 49–61.

Fawcett, J. (2000). *Analysis and evaluation of contemporary nursing knowledge: Nursing models and theories.* Philadelphia: F. A. Davis.

Fuller, J., & Schaller-Ayers, J. (1999). *Health assessment: A nursing approach* (3rd ed.). Philadelphia: J. B. Lippincott.

Gordon, M. (1994). *Nursing diagnosis: Process and application* (3rd ed.). St. Louis, MO: Mosby.

Grossman, D. (1998). Cuban-Americans. In L. D. Purnell & B. J. Paulanka (Eds.), *Transcultural health care: A culturally competent approach* (pp. 189–215). Philadelphia: F. A. Davis.

Joint Commission on Accreditation of Healthcare Organizations. (1996). *Comprehensive accreditation manual for hospitals: The official handbook.* Oakbrook Terrace, IL: Author.

King, L., & Appleton, J. V. (1997). Intuition: A critical review of the research and rhetoric. *Journal of Advanced Nursing, 26,* 194–202.

Matocha, L. K. (1998). Chinese-Americans. In L. D. Purnell & B. J. Paulanka (Eds.), *Transcultural health care: A culturally competent approach* (pp. 163–188). Philadelphia: F. A. Davis.

Rew, L. (1988). Intuition in decision-making. *Image: Journal of Nursing Scholarship, 20,* 150–154.

Rew, L., & Barrow, E. M. (1987). Intuition: A neglected hallmark of nursing knowledge. *Advances in Nursing Science, 10*(1), 49–62.

Smeltzer, S. C., & Bare, B. G. (2000). *Brunner and Suddarth's textbook of medical-surgical nursing* (9th ed.). Philadelphia: J. B. Lippincott.

Sundeen, S. J., Desalvo, E. A., & Rankin, E. D., et al. (1997). *Nurse–client interaction: Implementing the nursing process* (6th ed.). St. Louis, MO: Mosby.

Yura, H., & Walsh, M. B. (1988). *The nursing process: Assessing, planning, implementing, evaluating* (5th ed.). Norwalk, CT: Appleton & Lange.

BIBLIOGRAPHY

Baldwin, D. R. (1998). Implementation of computerized clinical documentation. *Home Health Care Management and Practice, 10*(2), 43–51.

Hinshaw, A. S. (2000). Nursing knowledge for the 21st century: Opportunities and challenges. *Journal of Nursing Scholarship, 32*(2), 117–123.

Jones, D. A. (1994). Alternative conceptualizations of assessment. In R. M. Carroll-Johnson & M. Paquette (Eds.), *Classification of nursing diagnoses: Proceedings of the tenth conference, North American Nursing Diagnosis Association* (pp. 105–112). Philadelphia: J. B. Lippincott.

McHale, J. M., Phipps, M. A., Horvath, K., & Schmelz, J. (1998). Expert nursing knowledge in the care of patients at risk of impaired swallowing. *Image: Journal of Nursing Scholarship, 30*(2), 137–141.

Moran, M., Kosmahl, E., & Brimer, M. (1997). Computer use in documentation and clinical practice. *Topics in Geriatric Rehabilitation, 13*(1), 72–78.

Parke, B. (1998). Gerontological nurses' way of knowing: Realizing the presence of pain in cognitively impaired older adults. *Journal of Gerontological Nursing, 24*(6), 21–28, 48–49.

Sarna, L. (1998). Effectiveness of structured nursing assessment of symptom distress in advanced lung cancer. *Oncology Nursing Forum, 25*(6), 1041–1048.

Staggers, N., & Mills, M. E. (1994). Nurse computer interaction: Staff performance outcomes. *Nursing Research, 43,* 144–150.

11 Nursing Diagnosis

⌐ Key Terms

actual nursing diagnosis	possible nursing diagnosis
cluster	premature closure
collaborative health problem	risk nursing diagnosis
cue	taxonomy
medical diagnosis	validation
nursing diagnosis	wellness nursing diagnosis

⌐ Learning Objectives

Upon completion of this chapter, the student will be able to do the following:

1. Define *diagnosis* in relation to the nursing process.
2. State the meaning of *nursing diagnosis*.
3. Describe the components of a nursing diagnosis.
4. Discuss the significance of nursing diagnosis for nursing practice.
5. Discuss the Nursing Diagnosis Extension and Classification (NDEC) project.
6. Differentiate between a nursing diagnosis and other healthcare problems.
7. Identify the clinical skills needed to make nursing diagnoses.
8. Formulate nursing diagnoses for a client situation.
9. Discuss the categorization of nursing diagnoses by functional health patterns.

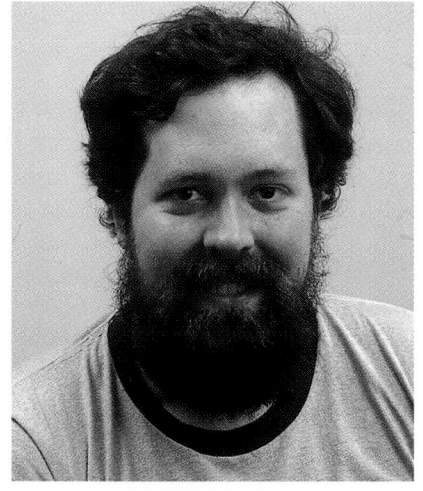

⌐ Critical Thinking Challenge

Jake Mason, a middle-aged former carpenter, comes to the health clinic with a temperature of 101°F. He has paralysis of all four extremities and has been wheelchair dependent for 6 months since he was injured in a construction accident. He is not working but still considers himself to be the provider for his wife and two children. He displays anger that his wife has to work to pay the bills and that she also has the responsibility of disciplining the children. You are the nurse caring for him.

Once you have completed this chapter and have incorporated nursing diagnosis into your knowledge base, review the above scenario and reflect on the following areas of Critical Thinking:

1. Cluster the data provided in this situation under various nursing diagnoses, and provide justification for your decisions regarding placement. (*Note:* Some data may fit under several diagnoses.)
2. Evaluate patterns in data clustering that indicate adequate support for identifying a nursing diagnosis.
3. Construct a list of additional data you need to validate each diagnostic statement, and propose a plan for obtaining this information.
4. Reflect on factors that could bias your interpretation of these data.
5. Create a three-part nursing diagnostic statement based on your assessment.

Diagnosing human responses to actual or potential health problems is the second phase of the nursing process. After collecting relevant information about clients, nurses need to analyze and interpret the data. The result of this interpretation is the nursing diagnosis. Registered nurses are educated and licensed to make nursing diagnoses. As such, they have a duty to identify and plan care for clients based on them.

The North American Nursing Diagnosis Association (NANDA, 2001) defines **nursing diagnosis** as follows:

> A clinical judgment about individual, family, or community responses to actual or potential health/life processes. A nursing diagnosis provides the basis for selection of nursing interventions to achieve outcomes for which the nurse is accountable (p. 245).

The term *nursing diagnosis* serves as both the label and the action of describing a client's functional problems. Its purpose is to identify problems and synthesize the information gathered during the nursing assessment by

- Analyzing collected data
- Identifying the client's strengths
- Identifying the client's normal functional level and indicators of actual or potential dysfunction
- Formulating a diagnostic statement in relation to this synthesis

In the diagnosis phase, the nurse does the following:

- Identifies patterns.
- Validates the diagnosis.
- Formulates the nursing diagnosis statement.

Figure 11-1 shows the diagnosis phase in relation to the other phases of the nursing process.

HISTORICAL DEVELOPMENT

As early as 1926, Harmer suggested that nurses should include problem statements when documenting client care. In 1947, Lesnich and Anderson argued that diagnosis was within the scope of nursing practice. Fry (1953) is generally credited with the first use of the term *nursing diagnosis* in the nursing literature. During the 1960s, a series of research studies focused on the nurse's ability to make clinical judgments using client cues (Hammond, 1966). These studies revealed that knowledge and interpretation varied widely and that the terms used to describe client problems were not standardized. In 1972, Gordon (1987) completed her dissertation on diagnostic reasoning in nursing. The formal development of the identification and classification of nursing diagnoses began with the first National Conference on the Classification of Nursing Diagnoses, convened by Gebbie and Lavin in 1973.

Although implied in the assessment phase of the nursing process (Yura & Walsh, 1973, 1988), nursing diagnosis emerged as a separate phase in the early 1970s. The act of diagnosing was recognized by the American Nurses Association (ANA) in *Standards of Nursing Practice* (ANA, 1973) and reaffirmed by the publication of revised standards in

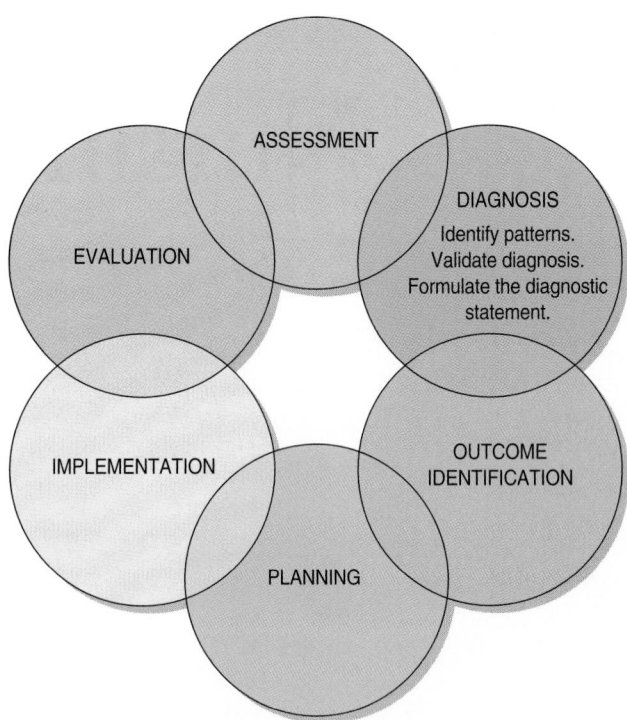

FIGURE 11-1   American Nurses Association Standard II states: The nurse analyzes the assessment data in determining diagnoses. This illustration shows activities used in the nursing diagnosis phase and also the relationship of nursing diagnosis to the other phases of the nursing process.

1991 (ANA, 1991). It gained further support when the ANA included diagnosis as a separate activity in *Nursing: A Social Policy Statement* (1995). Since that time, most state nurse practice acts have included diagnosis as part of the domain of nursing practice for which the nurse is held accountable. Standards developed by the Joint Commission on the Accreditation of Healthcare Organizations (JCAHO) mandate that each client's nursing care be based on identified nursing diagnoses or client care needs (JCAHO, 1996).

Interest in the nursing diagnosis movement has been stimulated by the "contribution that nursing vocabularies can make in (a) documenting care, (b) linking nursing contributions to quality outcomes, and (c) costing out nursing care services" (Jones, 2001, p. 379). Nurses continue to develop new nursing diagnoses, refine existing diagnoses, and organize them into a classification system useful to practicing nurses. NANDA has been the leader in nursing diagnosis classification and has been endorsed by the ANA as having the responsibility to do so. To date, 14 conferences have been held to refine the classification system for nursing diagnoses.

NURSING DIAGNOSIS TAXONOMY

Professions require a sound scientific base; the nursing process is nursing's scientific base. To achieve this scientific foundation, nursing requires a **taxonomy,** or classification system, to provide a structure for nursing practice. "The purposes of a taxonomy are to provide vocabulary for classifying phenomena in a discipline, provide new ways of looking at the discipline, and play a part in concept derivation" (NANDA, 1999, p. 173). A classification system for nursing diagnoses involves a knowledge of nursing practice, theoretical frameworks, and the characteristics of taxonomies.

Definition

A taxonomy is a method for ordering complex information. Each classification system is based on a single principle or set of principles (criteria) that establish the ground rules for selecting and placing individual elements in the system. A simple example of an ordering system is an outline:

    I.
        A.
        B.
            1.
            2.
                a.
                b.
    II.
    III.

The *set* (in this case, I, II, III) is a well-defined collection. The *subset* is a smaller unit or category of the set (in this case, A, B). Such elements, or subsets, can be further subdivided into smaller units (1, 2 or a, b). The further down the classification, the more concrete the unit becomes. It may name a real thing and may be observable and measurable. An example of a simple classification system is the dictionary: Words are grouped under each letter of the alphabet, which simplifies finding them.

The goal of a taxonomy is to produce a workable classification system. If the system is too complex, confusion occurs. If the system is too simple, the categories may be vague and duplicated. "In every system the component classes must have something different. Without the sameness there is no identifiable class; without the differences there are no discrete entities to group" (Gebbie & Lavin, 1975, p. 34).

The classification of diseases has been evolving since the 1770s. Today, the International Council of Nursing is sponsoring the development of the International Classification of Nursing Practice (ICNP), and NANDA is a contributor to this effort (Warren, 1996).

The most widely accepted classification system of diseases is the *International Classification of Diseases,* 10th edition, Clinical Modification (ICD-10-CM). The ICD-10-CM codes diseases by cause or manifestation. Other classification systems include the *Systemized Nomenclature of Medicine* (SNOMED®), published by the College of American Pathologists; *Current Procedural Terminology,* published by the College of American Pathologists; and *Current Procedural Terminology,* published by the American Medical Association. In psychiatry, the *Diagnostic and Statistical Manual of Mental Disorders* (DSM-IV; American Psychiatric Association, 2000) is used to classify mental health disorders. All these systems respond to changes in epidemiology and practice to maintain accuracy.

Nursing Diagnosis Taxonomy Development

NANDA's goal has been to develop a nursing diagnosis taxonomy. At the first conference in 1973, eighty-six nursing diagnoses were listed alphabetically and published for use and development by all registered nurses (RNs) (Gebbie & Lavin, 1975). There was no claim as to the validity of the diagnoses, nor was the list considered final. No classification system was selected.

Through the first six conferences, the listing of nursing diagnoses remained alphabetical, but attention was focusing on selecting a classification system. Involved with the classification from the outset, nursing theorists in 1977 were formally asked to participate in the development of the classification system.

As of 2000, NANDA has accepted 155 nursing diagnoses for clinical use and testing. NANDA is reviewing and staging additional diagnoses. Psychiatric nurses requested inclusion of their nursing diagnoses at the 11th biennial conference, and their labels were accepted for development (NANDA, 1999).

A summary of the activities of each conference is presented in Table 11-1. To illustrate the development of taxonomy, one nursing diagnosis, Grieving, has been selected to highlight changes made throughout the 14 conferences. The numbers indicate its placement in the classification system.

NANDA Process for Review and Staging of Nursing Diagnoses

New or revised nursing diagnoses may be submitted to NANDA for review and staging. To obtain new guidelines for submission and an abstract form, write NANDA, 1211 Locust Street, Philadelphia, PA, 19107 (1-800-647-9002) or visit the NANDA website at http://www.nanda.org.

After a diagnosis is submitted, the diagnostic review committee completes a review and the diagnosis is staged using the following criteria (NANDA, 2001, pp. 242–243):

2.0   Accepted for Clinical Development (Authentication/ Substantiation)

2.1   Label, Definition, Defining Characteristics or Risk Factors, References, and Literature Review

At stage 2.1, the label is forwarded to the Taxonomy Committee for classification. A narrative review of relevant literature is required to demonstrate the existence of a substantive body of knowledge underlying the diagnosis. The literature review is consistent with the label and definition. Literature should include discussion and support of the defining characteristics or risk factors (for risk diagnoses) and related factors (for actual diagnoses).

2.2   Case Study

The criteria in 2.1 are met. The narrative includes description of an actual case that exhibits the nursing diagnosis and includes defining characteristics or risk factors. Related factors, interventions, and outcomes are optional.

TABLE 11-1

Summary of the Classification of Nursing Diagnosis Conferences		
Year/#	Accomplishments	Chronological Development of the Nursing Diagnosis: Grieving
1973 1st National Conference	86 nursing diagnoses identified, listed alphabetically Established clearinghouse for nursing diagnoses	11.73 Grieving 11.74 Normal Grieving 11.75 Normal Grieving, Potential 11.76 11.77 Arrested Grieving 11.78 Arrested Grieving, Potential 11.79 Delayed Onset of Grieving 11.80 Delayed Onset of Grieving, Potential
1975 2nd National Conference	Further identification of nursing diagnoses, listed alphabetically	11.73 Grieving, Acute 11.76 Grieving, Anticipatory 11.77 Grieving, Delayed
1978 3rd National Conference	Diagnoses listed alphabetically "Unitary man" schema introduced as classification	11.73 Grieving
1980 4th National Conference	Patterns of nursing diagnoses discussed; no definite recommendations Diagnoses listed alphabetically	11.73 Grieving, Dysfunctional 11.74 Delete 11.75 Delete 11.76 Grieving, Anticipatory 11.77 Delete 11.78 Delete 11.79 Delete 11.80 Delete
1982 5th National Conference	Patterns of unitary man described Diagnoses listed alphabetically Vote to become NANDA	Grieving, Anticipatory Grieving, Dysfunctional
1984 6th Conference	First conference open to nursing public Further refinement to patterns of unitary man Diagnoses listed alphabetically	Grieving, Anticipatory Grieving, Dysfunctional
1986 7th Conference	Endorsement of NANDA taxonomy I Human response patterns replaced patterns of unitary man Development of rules for submission of new diagnoses	9.2.2 Grieving 9.2.2.1 Dysfunctional 9.2.2.2 Anticipatory 9.2.2.3
1988 8th Conference	Endorsement of NANDA taxonomy I (rev.)	9.2.1.1 Dysfunctional Grieving 9.2.1.2 Anticipatory Grieving
1990 9th Conference	NANDA taxonomy II proposed Definition of nursing diagnosis approved	Same as 1988
1992 10th Conference	New nursing diagnoses added	Same as 1988
1994 11th Conference	18 "to be developed" nursing diagnoses Psychiatric nursing diagnoses proposed Revised submission guidelines for nursing diagnoses	Same as 1988

TABLE 11-1 (Continued)

Summary of the Classification of Nursing Diagnosis Conferences		
Year/#	Accomplishments	Chronological Development of the Nursing Diagnosis: Grieving
1996 12th Conference	Two levels of acceptance for diagnoses; changes approved and added to nursing diagnosis Liaison with International Classification of Definitions and Classification of Nursing Practice (ICNP)	Defining characteristics updated
1998 13th Conference	Diagnoses revised by NDEC 21 new diagnoses submitted by Association of Rehabilitation Nurses (ARN), Association of Perioperative Registered Nurses (AORN)	Defining characteristics updated
2000 14th Conference	7 new diagnoses, significant label changes, taxonomy # format approved	Domain 9 Coping/Stress Tolerance Class 2 Coping Responses Diagnostic Concept: Denial Approved Diagnoses: 00136 Anticipatory Grieving, 00135 Dysfunctional Grieving

2.3 Clinical Case Studies

The criteria in 2.1 and 2.2 are met. The narrative includes the description of a series of at least ten cases that exhibit the diagnosis and include defining characteristics or risk factors, related factors, interventions, and outcomes.

2.4 Consensus Studies Related to Diagnosis Using Nurse Experts

The previous criteria are met. Studies include opinionnaire, Delphi, and similar studies of diagnostic components (e.g., diagnostic content validity) in which nurses are the subjects.

3.0 Clinically Supported (Validation and Testing)

3.1 Clinical Studies Related to Diagnosis, But Not Generalizable to the Population

3.2 Well-Designed Clinical Studies with Small Sample Sizes

3.3 Well-Designed Clinical Studies with Random Sample of Sufficient Size to Allow for Generalizability to the Overall Population

In 2000, NANDA approved seven new nursing diagnoses and placed them on the taxonomy for clinical use and testing. They also modified labels for many diagnoses. The most significant changes were deletion of the modifier "altered," listing of diagnoses by concept label, and new modifiers for several diagnoses (NANDA, 2001).

Taxonomy II

The complete NANDA Taxonomy II (2000) is presented in Display 11-1. Taxonomy II was approved at the 14th Biennial NANDA Conference. It uses a multiaxial format to aid in adding new diagnoses or modifying existing ones. The seven axes are as follows:

Axis 1: The diagnostic concept

Axis 2: Time (acute to chronic, short-term, long-term)

Axis 3: Unit of care (individual, family, community, target group)

Axis 4: Age (fetus to elder)

Axis 5: Health status (actual, risk for, opportunity or potential for growth/enhancement)

Axis 6: Descriptor (limits or specifies the meaning of the diagnostic concept)

Axis 7: Topology (parts/regions of the body)

In addition to changes in the format, Taxonomy II has a code structure that can be used in computer database systems. These changes help "clinicians to see where there are gaps/or potentially useful new diagnoses" (NANDA, 2001, p. 232).

Nursing Diagnosis Extension and Classification Project

Under a collaborative agreement between a team of researchers at the University of Iowa College of Nursing and NANDA, the Nursing Diagnosis Extension and Classification (NDEC) project began in 1993. The major purposes of NDEC are to evaluate and revise existing NANDA nursing diagnoses, develop new diagnostic terms, and organize the NANDA diagnoses into a classification structure (Craft-Rosenberg & Delaney, 1997). The NDEC team of nurse researchers are using concept analyses, expert validation, hierarchical clustering, multidimensional scaling, and other research methodologies to complete these activities. Reports from the NDEC research team are given at NANDA board meetings and presented to the membership at biennial conferences. Information about the work of NDEC can be obtained through the NDEC Research Dissemination Coordinator, Janice Denehy, RN, PhD, The University of Iowa College of Nursing, Iowa City, IA 52242.

Nursing Diagnoses and Other Healthcare Problems

Nursing diagnoses must be distinguished from medical diagnoses. A **medical diagnosis** describes a disease or pathology of specific organs or body systems. Medical diagnoses convey information about the signs and symptoms of disease processes and provide a convenient means for communicating treatment requirements. The physician focuses on treating the underlying pathology.

In contrast, a nursing diagnosis describes an actual, risk, or wellness human response to a health problem that nurses are responsible for treating independently. Nursing diagnoses describe the client's response to the disease process, developmental stage, or life process and provide a convenient way to communicate nursing therapies or interventions.

Nursing diagnoses carry legal ramifications. Only healthcare problems within the scope of nursing practice can be identified as nursing diagnoses. A nurse cannot diagnose a medical disease and is not licensed to treat such a problem. Registered nurses must take care to identify client problems within their scope, practice abilities, and education.

When identifying problems from assessment data, nurses determine whether they can address such problems legally and independently. If so, the problems can receive nursing diagnoses. If such problems require physician-prescribed and nurse-prescribed actions, however, they are **collaborative health problems.** Collaborative problems refer to actual or potential physiologic complications that can result from disease, trauma, treatment, or diagnostic studies for which nurses intervene in collaboration with personnel of other disciplines (Carpenito, 2002). Table 11-2 compares nursing diagnoses with collaborative and medical diagnoses, and Figure 11-2 shows how a nurse makes these determinations. Procedures, medical terminology, symptoms, client needs, and treatments are often confused with nursing diagnoses. For example, if the nurse writes "Foley catheter," this is a treatment, not the response the client may have to the treatment. Other examples include "Need for oxygen" or "Dyspnea," terms that describe symptoms and do not provide enough information to validate the presence of a nursing diagnosis. Another common mistake is to write "Lack of adequate nutrition" as the nursing diagnosis. This phrase describes a client need, but it is not a nursing diagnosis. The nursing diagnosis, in this case, would be Imbalanced Nutrition: Less than Body Requirements.

The following list shows the proper use of a variety of terms for a client with a specific breathing problem. These terms are often confused:

- *Medical diagnosis:* Pneumonia
- *Nursing diagnosis:* Ineffective Airway Clearance related to tracheobronchial secretions
- *Client need:* Oxygenation
- *Procedure:* Bronchoscopy
- *Treatment:* Oxygen therapy

TABLE 11-2

Comparison of Nursing Diagnoses With Collaborative Problems and Medical Diagnoses		
	Nursing Diagnoses	**Collaborative Problems and Medical Diagnoses**
Focus of assessment activities	Main focus is on monitoring human responses to actual and potential health problems.	Main focus is on monitoring for pathophysiologic response of body organs or systems.
Problem identification	Nurse identifies and validates independently that problem exists and can be treated legally by nursing staff.	Nurse may identify problem but is required to refer to physician for validation that problem exists (may require additional diagnostic studies to label the problem). Nurse may not be qualified to diagnose exact nature of problem but refers abnormal data to physician.
Treatment	Nurse legally initiates actions for treatment.	Nurse collaborates with physician to initiate interventions for treatment. Nurse may have standing orders from physician or institution (delegated authority) to initiate diagnostic studies or treatment interventions for the problem without physician's orders.

From Alfaro-LeFevre, R. (2001). *Applying nursing diagnosis and nursing process: A step-by-step guide* (5th ed.). Philadelphia: Lippincott-Raven.

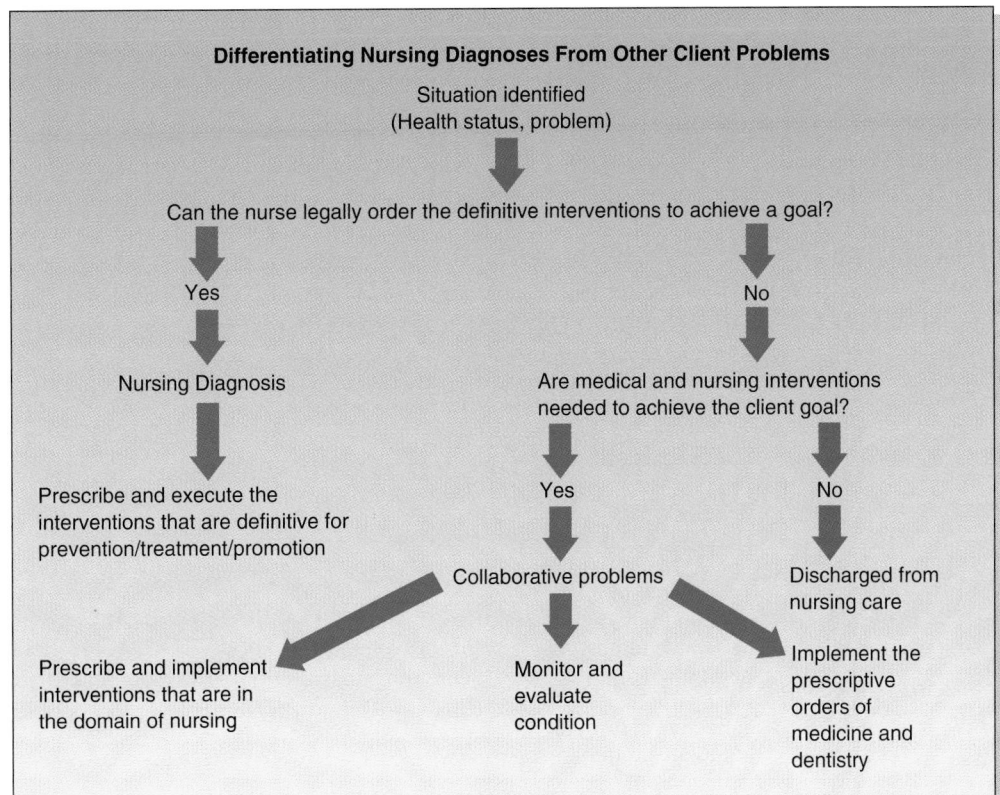

FIGURE 11-2 Differentiating a nursing diagnosis from other client problems. (From Carpenito, L. [2002]. *Nursing diagnosis: Application to clinical practice* [9th ed.]. Philadelphia: Lippincott.)

Formulating an accurate nursing diagnosis is a clinical judgment, but nursing diagnoses should not be written judgmentally. For example, it is incorrect to write "Failure to carry out medical regimen related to drug use." The reasons for the client's noncompliance with the regimen should be explored and analyzed to avoid labeling or stereotyping a client's behavior based on insufficient evidence.

COMPONENTS OF A NURSING DIAGNOSIS

Diagnostic Label

The diagnostic label is the name of the nursing diagnosis as listed in the taxonomy. It describes the essence of the problem using as few words as possible. Some examples include Stress Urinary Incontinence, Anxiety, and Feeding Self-Care Deficit. Each nursing diagnosis represents a pattern of related client cues.

Descriptors

Descriptors are words used to give additional meaning to a nursing diagnosis. They describe changes in condition, state of the client, or some qualification of the specific nursing diagnosis. They accompany the labels in Display 11-1. Examples of descriptors used by NANDA (2001) include the following:

- *Ability:* Capacity to do or act
- *Anticipatory:* To realize beforehand, foresee
- *Balance:* State of equilibrium
- *Compromised:* To make vulnerable to threat
- *Decreased:* Lessened; lesser in size, amount, or degree
- *Deficient:* Inadequate in amount, quality, or degree; not sufficient; incomplete
- *Delayed:* To postpone, impede, and retard
- *Depleted:* Emptied wholly or in part, exhausted of
- *Disproportionate:* Not consistent with a standard
- *Disabling:* To make unable or unfit, to incapacitate
- *Disorganized:* To destroy the systematic arrangement
- *Disturbed:* Agitated or interrupted, interfered with
- *Dysfunctional:* Abnormal, incomplete functioning
- *Effective:* Producing the intended or expected effect
- *Excessive:* Characterized by an amount or quantity that is greater than that necessary, desirable, or useful
- *Functional:* Normal complete functioning
- *Imbalanced:* State of disequilibrium
- *Impaired:* Made worse, weakened, damaged, reduced, deteriorated
- *Inability:* Incapacity to do or act
- *Increased:* Greater in size, amount, or degree
- *Ineffective:* Not producing the desired effect
- *Interrupted:* To break the continuity or uniformity
- *Organized:* To form as into a systematic arrangement

(text continues on page 175)

DISPLAY 11-1

 NANDA TAXONOMY II (2001)

Domain 1—Health Promotion

The awareness of well-being or normality of function and the strategies used to maintain control of and enhance that well-being or normality of function

Class 1—Health Awareness: Recognition of normal function and well-being

Class 2—Health Management: Identifying, controlling, performing, and integrating activities to maintain health and well being

Diagnostic Concepts	Approved Diagnoses
Therapeutic regimen	00082 Effective therapeutic regimen management
Management	00078 Ineffective therapeutic regimen management
	00080 Ineffective family therapeutic regimen management
	00081 Ineffective community therapeutic regimen management
Health-seeking behaviors	00084 Health-seeking behaviors (specify)
Health maintenance	00099 Ineffective health maintenance
Home maintenance	00098 Impaired home maintenance

Domain 2—Nutrition

The activities of taking in, assimilating, and using nutrients for the purposes of tissue maintenance, tissue repair, and the production of energy

Class 1—Ingestion: Taking food or nutrients into the body

Diagnostic Concepts	Approved Diagnoses
Infant feeding pattern	00107 Ineffective infant feeding pattern
Swallowing	00103 Impaired swallowing
Nutrition	00002 Imbalanced nutrition: Less than body requirements
	00001 Imbalanced nutrition: More than body requirements
	00003 Risk for imbalanced nutrition: More than body requirements

Class 2—Digestion: The physical and chemical activities that convert foodstuffs into substances suitable for absorption and assimilation

Class 3—Absorption: The act of taking up nutrients through body tissues

Class 4—Metabolism: The chemical and physical processes occurring in living organisms and cells for the development and use of protoplasm, production of waste and energy, release of energy for all vital processes

Class 5—Hydration: The taking in and absorption of fluids and electrolytes

Diagnostic Concepts	Approved Diagnoses
Fluid volume	00027 Deficient fluid volume
	00028 Risk for deficient fluid volume
	00026 Excess fluid volume
	00025 Risk for fluid volume imbalance

Domain 3—Elimination

Secretion and excretion of waste products from the body

Class 1—Urinary System: The process of secretion and excretion of urine

Diagnostic Concepts	Approved Diagnoses
Urinary elimination	00016 Impaired urinary elimination
Urinary retention	00023 Urinary retention
Urinary incontinence	00021 Total urinary incontinence
	00020 Functional urinary incontinence
	00017 Stress urinary incontinence
	00019 Urge urinary incontinence
	00018 Reflex urinary incontinence
	00022 Risk for urge urinary incontinence

Class 2—Gastrointestinal System: Excretion and expulsion of waste products from the bowel

Diagnostic Concepts	Approved Diagnoses
Bowel incontinence	00014 Bowel incontinence
Diarrhea	00013 Diarrhea
Constipation	00011 Constipation
	00015 Risk for constipation
	00012 Perceived constipation

Class 3—Integumentary System: Process of secretion and excretion through the skin

Class 4—Pulmonary System: Removal of byproducts of metabolic products, secretions, and foreign material from the lung or bronchi

DISPLAY 11-1 (Continued)

⑤ NANDA TAXONOMY II (2001)

Diagnostic Concepts	Approved Diagnoses
Gas exchange	00030 Impaired gas exchange

Domain 4—Activity/Rest
The production, conservation, expenditure, or balance of energy resources
Class 1—Sleep/Rest: Slumber, repose, ease, or inactivity

Diagnostic Concepts	Approved Diagnoses
Sleep pattern	00095 Disturbed sleep pattern
	00096 Sleep deprivation

Class 2—Activity/Exercise: Moving parts of the body (mobility), doing work, or performing actions often (but not always) against resistance

Diagnostic Concepts	Approved Diagnoses
Disuse syndrome	00040 Risk for disuse syndrome
Mobility	00085 Impaired physical mobility
	00091 Impaired bed mobility
	00089 Impaired wheelchair mobility
Transfer ability	00090 Impaired transfer ability
Walking	00088 Impaired walking
Diversional activity	00097 Deficient diversional activity
Wandering	00154 Wandering
Self-care deficit	00109 Dressing/grooming deficit
	00108 Bathing/hygiene self-care deficit
	00102 Feeding self-care deficit
	00110 Toileting self-care deficit
Surgical recovery	00100 Delayed surgical recovery

Class 3—Energy Balance: A dynamic state of harmony between intake and expenditure of resources

Diagnostic Concepts	Approved Diagnoses
Cardiac output	00029 Decreased cardiac output
Spontaneous ventilation	00033 Impaired spontaneous ventilation
Breathing pattern	00032 Ineffective breathing pattern

Activity tolerance	00092 Activity intolerance
	00094 Risk for activity intolerance
Ventilatory weaning	00034 Dysfunctional ventilatory weaning response
Tissue perfusion	00024 Ineffective tissue perfusion (specify type: renal, cerebral, cardiopulmonary, gastrointestinal, peripheral)

Domain 5—Perception/Cognition
The human information processing system including attention, orientation, sensation, perception, cognition, and communication
Class 1—Attention: Mental readiness to notice or observe

Diagnostic Concepts	Approved Diagnoses
Unilateral neglect	00123 Unilateral neglect

Class 2—Orientation: Awareness of time, place, and person

Diagnostic Concepts	Approved Diagnoses
Environmental interpretation	00127 Impaired environmental interpretation syndrome

Class 3—Sensation/Perception: Receiving information through the senses of touch, taste, smell, vision, hearing, and kinesthesia and the comprehension of sense data resulting in naming, associating, and/or pattern recognition

Diagnostic Concepts	Approved Diagnoses
Sensory perception	00122 Disturbed sensory perception (specify: visual, auditory, kinesthetic, gustatory, tactile, olfactory)

Class 4—Cognition: Use of memory, learning, thinking, problem solving, abstraction, judgment, insight, intellectual capacity, calculation, and language

Diagnostic Concepts	Approved Diagnoses
Knowledge	00126 Deficient knowledge (specify)

(continued)

DISPLAY 11-1 (Continued)

NANDA TAXONOMY II (2001)

Confusion	00128 Acute confusion
	00129 Chronic confusion
Memory	00131 Impaired memory
Thought processes	00130 Disturbed thought processes

Class 5—Communication: Sending and receiving verbal and nonverbal information

Diagnostic Concepts	Approved Diagnoses
Verbal communication	00051 Impaired verbal communication

Domain 6—Self-perception
Awareness about the self
Class 1—Self-Concept: The perception(s) about the total self

Diagnostic Concepts	Approved Diagnoses
Identify	00121 Disturbed personal identity
	00125 Powerlessness
	00152 Risk for powerlessness
	00124 Hopelessness
Loneliness	00054 Risk for loneliness

Class 2—Self-esteem: Assessment of one's own worth, capability, significance, and success

Diagnostic Concepts	Approved Diagnoses
Self-esteem	00119 Chronic low self-esteem
	00120 Situational low self-esteem
	00153 Risk for situational low self-esteem

Class 3—Body Image: A mental image of one's own body

Diagnostic Concepts	Approved Diagnoses
Body image	00118 Disturbed body image

Domain 7—Role Relationships
The positive and negative connections or associations between persons or groups of persons and the means by which those connections are demonstrated
Class 1—Caregiving Roles: Socially expected behavior patterns by persons providing care who are not health care professionals

Diagnostic Concepts	Approved Diagnoses
Caregiver role strain	00061 Caregiver role strain
	00062 Risk for caregiver role strain
Parenting	00056 Impaired parenting
	00057 Risk for impaired parenting

Class 2—Family Relationships: Associations of people who are biologically related or related by choice

Diagnostic Concepts	Approved Diagnoses
Family processes	00060 Interrupted family processes
	00063 Dysfunctional family processes: Alcoholism
Attachment	00058 Risk for impaired parent/infant/child attachment

Class 3—Role Performance: Quality of functioning in socially expected behavior patterns

Diagnostic Concepts	Approved Diagnoses
Breastfeeding	00106 Effective breast-feeding
	00104 Ineffective breast-feeding
	00105 Interrupted breast-feeding
Role performance	00055 Ineffective role performance
	00064 Parental role conflict
Social interaction	00052 Impaired social inter-action

Domain 8—Sexuality
Sexual identity, sexual function, and reproduction
Class 1—Sexual Identity: The state of being a specific person in regard to sexually and/or gender
Class 2—Sexual Function: The capacity or ability to participate in sexual activities

Diagnostic Concepts	Approved Diagnoses
Sexual function	00059 Sexual dysfunction
Sexual patterns	00065 Ineffective sexuality patterns

Class 3—Reproduction: Any process by which new individuals (people) are produced

DISPLAY 11-1 (Continued)

NANDA TAXONOMY II (2001)

Domain 9—Coping/Stress Tolerance
Contending with life events/life processes
Class 1—Post-Trauma Responses: Reactions occurring after physical or psychological trauma

Diagnostic Concepts	Approved Diagnoses
Relocation stress	00114 Relocation syndrome
	00149 Risk for relocation stress syndrome
Rape-trauma	00142 Rape-trauma syndrome
	00144 Rape-trauma syndrome: Silent reaction
	00143 Rape-trauma syndrome: Compound reaction
Post-trauma response	00141 Post-trauma syndrome
	00145 Risk for post-trauma syndrome

Class 2—Coping Responses: The process of managing environmental stress

Diagnostic Concepts	Approved Diagnoses
Fear	00148 Fear
Anxiety	00146 Anxiety
	00147 Death anxiety
Sorrow	00137 Chronic sorrow
Denial	00072 Ineffective denial
	00136 Anticipatory grieving
	00135 Dysfunctional grieving
Adjustment	00070 Impaired adjustment
Coping	00069 Ineffective coping
	00073 Disabled family coping
	00074 Compromised family coping
	00071 Defensive coping
	00077 Ineffective community coping
	00075 Readiness for enhanced family coping
	00076 Readiness for enhanced community coping

Class 3—Neurobehavioral Stress: Behavioral responses reflecting nerve and brain function

Diagnostic Concepts	Approved Diagnoses
Dysreflexia	00009 Autonomic dysreflexia
	00010 Risk for autonomic dysreflexia
Infant behavior	00116 Disorganized infant behavior
	00115 Risk for disorganized infant behavior
	00117 Readiness for enhanced organized infant behavior
Adaptive capacity	00049 Decreased intracranial adaptive capacity

Domain 10—Life Principles
Principles underlying conduct, thought, and behavior about acts, customs, or institutions viewed as being true or having intrinsic worth
Class 1—Values: The identification and ranking of preferred modes of conduct or end states
Class 2—Beliefs: Opinions, expectations, or judgments about acts, customs, or institutions viewed as being true or having intrinsic worth

Diagnostic Concepts	Approved Diagnoses
Spiritual well-being	00068 Readiness for enhanced spiritual well-being

Class 3—Value/Belief/Action Congruence: The correspondence or balance achieved between values, beliefs, and actions

Diagnostic Concepts	Approved Diagnoses
Spiritual distress	00066 Spiritual distress
	00067 Risk for spiritual distress
Decisional conflict	00083 Decisional conflict (specify)
Noncompliance	00079 Noncompliance (specify)

Domain 11—Safety/Protection
Freedom from danger, physical injury or immune system damage, preservation from loss, and protection of safety and security
Class 1—Infection: Host responses following pathogenic invasion

Diagnostic Concepts	Approved Diagnoses
Infection	00004 Risk for infection

Class 2—Physical Injury: Bodily harm or hurt

(continued)

DISPLAY 11-1 (Continued)

🖫 **NANDA TAXONOMY II (2001)**

Diagnostic Concepts	Approved Diagnoses	
Oral mucous membrane	00045	Impaired oral mucous membrane
Injury	00035	Risk for injury
	00087	Risk for perioperative positioning injury
	00155	Risk for falls
Trauma	00038	Risk for trauma
Skin integrity	00046	Impaired skin integrity
	00047	Risk for impaired skin integrity
Tissue integrity	00044	Impaired tissue integrity
Dentition	00048	Impaired dentition
Suffocation	00036	Risk for suffocation
Aspiration	00039	Risk for aspiration
Airway clearance	00031	Ineffective airway clearance
Neurovascular function	00086	Risk for peripheral neurovascular dysfunction
Protection	00043	Ineffective protection

Class 3—Violence: The exertion of excessive force or power so as to cause injury or abuse

Diagnostic Concepts	Approved Diagnoses	
Self-mutilation	00139	Risk for self-mutilation
	00151	Self-mutilation
Violence	00138	Risk for other-directed violence
	00140	Risk for self-directed violence
	00150	Risk for suicide

Class 4—Environmental Hazards: Sources of danger in the surroundings

Diagnostic Concepts	Approved Diagnoses	
Poisoning	00037	Risk for poisoning

Class 5—Defensive Processes: The processes by which the self protects itself from the nonself

Diagnostic Concepts	Approved Diagnoses	
Latex allergy response	00041	Latex allergy response
	00042	Risk for latex allergy response

Class 6—Thermoregulation: The physiologic process of regulating heat and energy within the body for the purposes of protecting the organism

Diagnostic Concepts	Approved Diagnoses	
Body temperature	00005	Risk for imbalanced body temperature
Thermoregulation	00008	Ineffective thermo-regulation
	00006	Hypothermia
	00007	Hyperthermia

Domain 12—Comfort
Sense of mental, physical, or social well-being or ease
Class 1—Physical Comfort: Sense of well-being or ease

Diagnostic Concepts	Approved Diagnoses	
Pain	00132	Acute pain
	00133	Chronic pain
Nausea	00134	Nausea

Class 2—Environmental Comfort: Sense of well-being or ease in/with one's environment
Class 3—Social Comfort: Sense of well-being or ease with one's social situations

Diagnostic Concepts	Approved Diagnoses	
Social Isolation	00053	Social isolation

Domain 13—Growth/Development
Age-appropriate increases in physical dimensions, organ systems, and/or attainment of developmental milestones
Class 1—Growth: Increases in physical dimensions or maturity of organ systems

Diagnostic Concepts	Approved Diagnoses	
Growth	00113	Risk for dispro-portionate growth
Failure to thrive	00101	Adult failure to thrive

Class 2—Development: Attainment, lack of attainment, or loss of developmental milestones

Diagnostic Concepts	Approved Diagnoses	
Development	00111	Delayed growth and development
	00112	Risk for delayed development

North American Nursing Diagnosis Association. (2001). *NANDA nursing diagnoses: Definitions and Classification 2001–2002.* Philadelphia: Author.

- *Perceived:* To become aware of by means of the senses; assignment of meaning
- *Readiness for enhanced* (for use with wellness diagnoses): To make greater, to increase in quality; to attain the more desired

Definition

Each nursing diagnosis that NANDA approves for clinical use and testing has a definition that describes the characteristics of the human response under consideration. For example, the definition of the diagnostic label Hypothermia is "body temperature below normal range" (NANDA, 2001, p. 96).

Defining Characteristics

Defining characteristics are the "observable cues/inferences that cluster as manifestations of an actual or wellness nursing diagnosis" (NANDA, 2001, p. 245). Each piece of client information is considered a clinical cue; a set of clinical cues forms a cluster that is present if the diagnosis is accurate.

Risk Factors

The term *risk factors* is used to describe clinical cues in risk nursing diagnoses. They are "environmental factors and physiological, psychological, genetic, or chemical elements that increase the vulnerability of an individual, family, or community to an unhealthful event" (NANDA, 2001, p. 245–246). Examples of risk factors for the nursing diagnosis Risk for Deficient Fluid Volume include extremes of age, physical immobility, and medication (e.g., diuretics). If the risk factors are not addressed, a potential problem may become an actual problem.

Related Factors

Related factors describe the conditions, circumstances, or etiologies that contribute to the problem. Although there is usually not a direct causal relationship between the nursing diagnosis and the cause, some relationships can be described. Terms that can be used are *associated with, related to,* or *contributing to.* Identifying related factors helps nurses to develop specific interventions to resolve the health problem. For example, nurses would use different nursing interventions when caring for a client with Stress Incontinence related to high intra-abdominal pressure than for a client with Stress Incontinence related to overdistention between voidings.

DIAGNOSIS ACTIVITIES

Identify Pattern

After completing the client assessment, nurses analyze the data they obtained to identify specific client problems. The data, both subjective symptoms and objective signs, form **cues,** or pieces of information collected during the nursing assessment. But not all data examined will be grouped to identify problems. Significant cues to be clustered involve subjec-

tive and objective data that deviate from standards or from what is considered normal. Several cues form a **cluster,** which is then interpreted and validated. The result is a nursing diagnostic label that accurately reflects the specific client problem. Because clustering, interpreting, and validating client cues are integral to nursing practice, each step is described separately. However, this process is cyclical. That is, as new information is obtained, new cue patterns may emerge and cue clusters may change. As nurses develop skill in making clinical judgments, they evaluate individual pieces of data, examine trends, and view the client as a whole (Chase, 1994).

Cue Clustering

As cues are collected, some data organization takes place. Typically, nurses use a standardized assessment form (see Chapter 24) that automatically puts information into categories or systems. Clustering goes beyond systems. Cue clustering brings together cues that, if viewed separately, would not convey the same meaning. The purpose of cue clustering is to take individual cues and group them to derive meaning.

Cue clustering can be compared with piecing together a puzzle. All the puzzle pieces form one picture (the client problem), and each piece is a cue. Figure 11-3 illustrates the puzzle concept. The puzzle shows a circle and two triangles. All the pieces of the puzzle with the circle form a cluster, as do all the pieces for the triangles. Placing the circle pieces into a cluster helps identify the pattern of the puzzle (the diagnosis). A separate and distinct cue cluster forms each nursing diagnosis.

During cue clustering, critical thinking is used to analyze and synthesize the cues. Each cue is analyzed for its fit into a particular problem. The cues are then put together to form meaningful clusters that describe specific client problems.

To see how this process works, refer to the client in the situation at the beginning of the chapter. Review the situation of the former carpenter and then see which cues belong together when describing a particular problem.

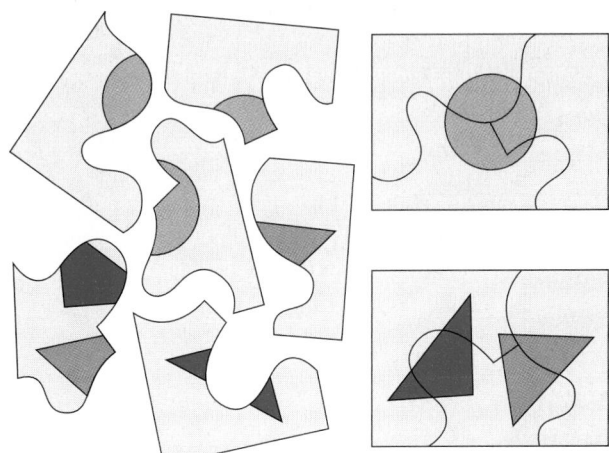

FIGURE 11-3 Collecting the puzzle pieces is assessment. Pieces that are similar form a cluster. Identifying the pattern and putting the puzzle together is nursing diagnosis. Other parts of the puzzle (e.g., a star) would form another diagnosis.

Although the first tendency is to identify Hyperthermia as a nursing diagnosis, look at other cues the client has given. For the purpose of illustration, one nursing diagnosis has been selected here, but the reader is encouraged to select other cues and describe additional nursing diagnoses that may be present. The relevant cues follow:

- Not currently working
- Recent change from active, mobile individual to wheelchair-dependent, quadriplegic person
- Considers self to be provider
- Angry at wife for carrying out role of breadwinner

Taken together, these cues fit the defining characteristics of a specific nursing diagnosis. Recognizing this cue cluster leads to the next step, cluster interpretation. First, however, some problems that can occur in cue clustering must be described.

Problems in Cue Clustering. The major problems in cue clustering are insufficient, inaccurate, and inconsistent cues. Skill in cue clustering comes with experience and practice. Expect to use a variety of reference materials to develop these skills.

Having insufficient cues is a problem. Nurses cannot plan effective care because the problem cannot be determined with confidence. Using the example from the beginning of the chapter, a nurse might select the cue temperature of 101°F and write this nursing diagnosis: Hyperthermia. However, he or she has not gathered enough information to lead to this conclusion. This lack of adequate cues also can be called **premature closure:** selecting a diagnosis before analyzing pertinent information. Additional cues needed to identify Hyperthermia include flushed skin, warm to touch, increased respiratory rate, tachycardia, or seizures/convulsions (NANDA, 2001).

Inaccurate clustering of cues is a problem because nurses may be clustering unrelated information, thus making judgments based on incorrect clusters. Inaccuracy in clustering occurs when nurses are unfamiliar with diagnoses or when the cues for various diagnoses overlap. If, for example, the cues (wheelchair-dependent quadriplegic, not working, and anger) are clustered and the nursing diagnosis of Impaired Physical Mobility related to dependency is made, nursing interventions will be geared toward resolving the dependency, not the problem of impaired mobility.

Inconsistent cues are a problem because the meaning attached to one cue may be altered based on another cue. For example, one client may say that she cannot eat a regular diet, but later she is seen eating a steak and potatoes. Because the cues do not match, further information is needed to validate the problem and the cues.

Cluster Interpretation

Cluster interpretation means synthesizing the cue clusters. This intellectual activity requires nurses to see the whole picture and to attach meaning to the cluster, looking at the pattern the cluster suggests. It is the ability to derive the meaning and implications of the human response for a client.

A specific cue cluster was presented in the critical thinking challenge. Review it now, and think of possible nursing diagnoses. The following nursing diagnoses are listed as possible choices:

- Ineffective Coping related to dependency. Cues: anger, wheelchair-dependent quadriplegic.
- Impaired Adjustment related to disability requiring change in lifestyle. Cues: wheelchair-dependent quadriplegic for 6 months, not working.
- Ineffective Role Performance related to recent change. Cues: not working; angry at wife for carrying out breadwinner role; perceives self as provider; recent change from active, mobile person to wheelchair-dependent quadriplegic.

Analyzing these suggested nursing diagnostic statements would involve reviewing each definition and associated defining characteristics.

The first two possible nursing diagnoses cannot be supported by clinical cues. Ineffective Coping relies on two cues that are not defining characteristics of this diagnosis. This diagnosis requires evidence of a client's verbalization of the inability to cope or to ask for help or the inability to solve problems. More information is needed to support the use of this diagnosis. The diagnosis of Impaired Adjustment may or may not describe this client. The nurse has assumed that, by becoming a wheelchair-dependent quadriplegic, this client has not made a satisfactory adjustment to his new lifestyle. Additional defining characteristics are needed to evaluate the presence of this problem.

In the third diagnosis, Ineffective Role Performance, all the cues supporting the defining characteristics for the diagnosis are present. The client had a change in the perception of his role, in his physical capacity to resume a previous role, and in his usual patterns of responsibility. There is evidence of conflict, as shown by his anger toward his wife. The nurse can make this diagnosis with confidence and plan nursing interventions to assist the client in resolving this problem.

Problems in Cluster Interpretation. Analysis of cue clusters can be impeded by incorrect clustering of data and misinterpretation of cue clusters. If the cues are not clustered correctly, nurses cannot make accurate clinical judgments. For example, if the cues (malnourished, feeds self, and dependent in mobility) are clustered, the nurse may arrive at the erroneous diagnosis of Feeding Self-Care Deficit related to inadequate intake. However, there is no information here about the daily intake of food. The fact that the client feeds himself does not explain the cue of dependent in mobility. Does the client use assistive devices? What is the state of malnourishment? Are supplemental feedings being given? By forming this particular cue cluster, the nurse has neglected other important areas for analysis. In this example, these include defining characteristics for the nursing diagnoses of Imbalanced Nutrition: Less than Body Requirements and Impaired Physical Mobility.

Misinterpretation of cue clusters occurs when the nurse fails to recognize the correct pattern. This can happen if the nurse is unfamiliar with the nursing diagnosis or is inexperienced in relating how these particular cues fit together. If the defining characteristics for the diagnosis under consideration are complex and require extensive analysis for correct interpretation, ask the experienced clinician to assist with interpreting the cues.

Validate Diagnosis

After selecting a nursing diagnosis (Ineffective Role Performance, in the clinical example), the nurse should validate it with the client. **Validation** legitimizes the diagnosis and helps to discover its significance for the client. The client may deny that a problem exists, may not want to deal with it, or may acknowledge it but want to deal with it later. These are acceptable reasons for not dealing with an identified diagnosis, but the presence of the problem and its status should be documented. For most problems, the client will agree that there is a problem that can be resolved with nursing assistance.

Diagnostic validation occurs in two stages. In the first stage, the cue clusters that have been interpreted are compared with norms for the client and for clients in general. In the second stage, the specific nursing diagnosis is evaluated for its nursing research base. This research base is different for each diagnosis.

In the clinical example, these diagnoses may be made if additional data collection identifies cues to support them:

- Ineffective Coping
- Impaired Adjustment
- Hyperthermia

For each diagnosis, the nurse should discuss with the client the significance of the problem, determine the client's perception of the reason for the problem, and ask whether the client desires help to resolve or to diminish the problem. Some clients are not ready or motivated to seek help even when a problem clearly exists.

Problems in Diagnostic Validation. Problems can occur in diagnostic validation because of a nurse's limited experience, lack of a knowledge base about the nursing diagnosis, or insufficient characteristics of a diagnosis.

If the nurse has limited clinical experience, exposure to a variety of clients under the guidance of an instructor, mentor, or expert practitioner can provide an opportunity to practice these skills. Each nursing diagnosis and defining characteristic should be discussed and errors corrected. A nonthreatening environment, patience, and understanding are required for both parties. It is helpful to trace the steps taken to arrive at a particular problem; errors in logic or missing steps in the process can sometimes be identified and suggestions made for avoiding them.

Nurses who are not knowledgeable about specific nursing diagnoses should refer to articles, books, and other materials that discuss the identification of the problem and its management. For example, the proceedings of the NANDA conferences on the classification of nursing diagnosis and *Nursing Diagnosis Reference Manual* (Sparks & Taylor, 2001) can be used to learn about individual nursing diagnoses.

The problem of insufficient research about specific nursing diagnoses can be corrected by participating in clinical research studies sponsored by institutions, organizations, and individual researchers. RNs have an obligation to contribute to the profession's scientific development. Current research on nursing diagnoses can be found in nursing journals and the previously mentioned proceedings of the NANDA conferences. The term *nursing diagnosis* is listed as a subject heading in the *Cumulative Index for Nursing and Allied Health Literature,* enabling nurses to find nursing diagnosis information quickly.

Formulate the Diagnostic Statement

Formulating the nursing diagnostic statement involves writing the label of the actual, risk, wellness, or possible nursing diagnosis that has been made through the nursing diagnostic process. The correct way of stating these diagnoses is described in the following section and illustrated in Table 11-3 and Figure 11-4. Accurate and inaccurate examples also are given in the text and in Table 11-4.

TABLE 11-3

Types of Diagnostic Statements		
Type	**Construction**	**Example**
Actual nursing diagnosis	Three part statement includes diagnostic label, related factors, defining characteristics	Acute Pain related to surgical trauma and inflammation, as evidenced by grimacing and verbal reports of pain
Risk nursing diagnosis	Two-part statement includes diagnostic label, risk factors	Risk for Infection related to surgery and immunosuppression
Possible nursing diagnosis	Two-part statement includes diagnostic label, related factors (unknown)	Possible Self-Esteem Disturbance related to unknown etiology
Wellness diagnosis	One-part statement includes diagnostic label	Readiness for Enhanced Spiritual Well-Being

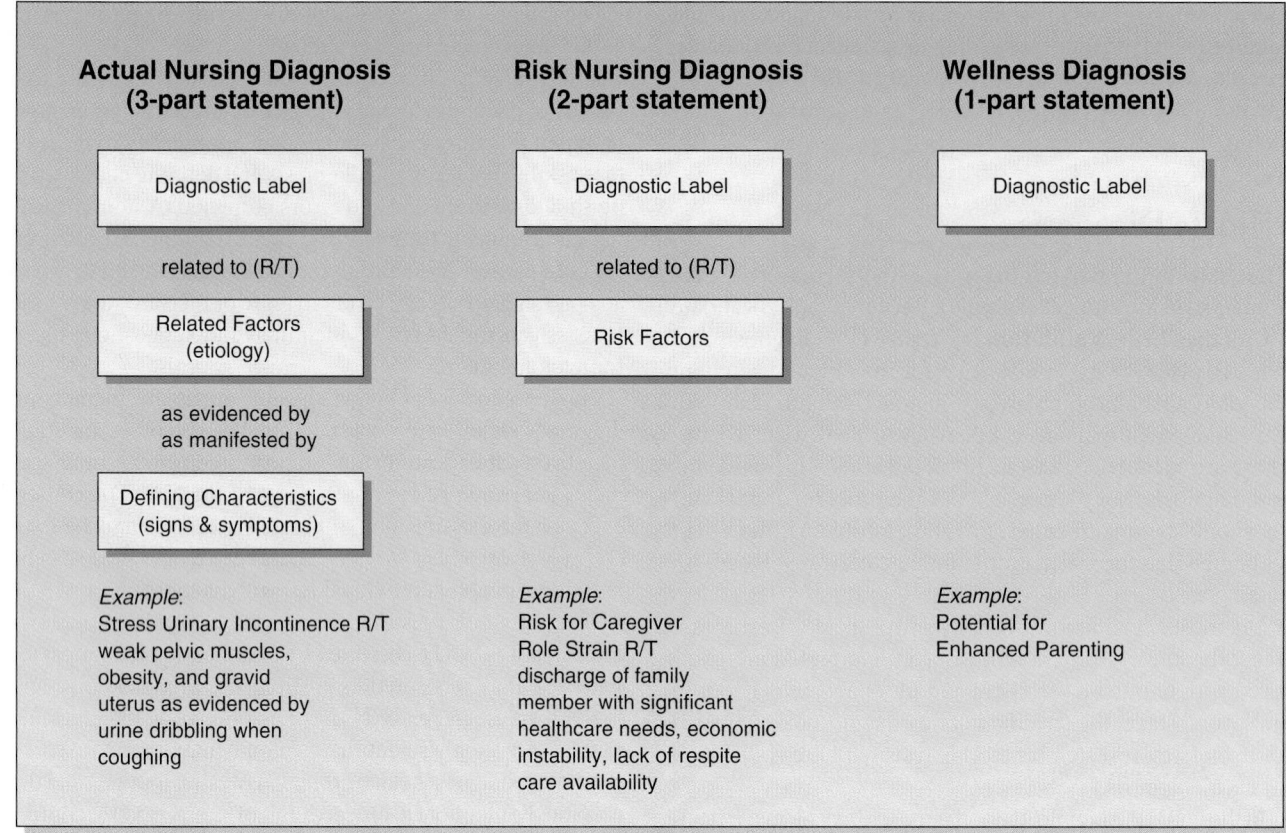

FIGURE 11-4   Examples of a three-part actual nursing diagnostic statement, a two-part risk nursing diagnostic statement, and a one-part wellness nursing diagnostic statement.

Actual Nursing Diagnoses

Actual nursing diagnoses describe a human response to a health problem that is being manifested. They are written as three-part statements: diagnostic label, defining characteristics, and related factors. Client cues supporting the existence of the problem can be found in the documented assessment data. In the nursing diagnosis statement, cues are identified by "as manifested by" or "as evidenced by." Problems sometimes occur when nurses invert the label and the "related to" phrase. To avoid this problem, determine the main focus of the problem (the diagnostic label) and the factor that is contributing to the client's inability to resolve it (related factor).

> *Accurate:* Impaired Physical Mobility related to pain
> *Inaccurate:* Ineffective Movement related to arthritis, which causes pain when moving. (The nurse has selected an incorrect descriptor, has not used an approved diagnostic label, has repeated the problem in the "related to" phrase, and has used a medical diagnosis in the statement.)

Risk Nursing Diagnoses

NANDA replaced the term *potential* with the term *risk* because it was believed that the latter term is more descriptive of some clients' particular vulnerability to health problems. For example, all clients admitted to a hospital are at risk for infection,

but some people, such as those with compromised immune systems, are at higher risk than others. This terminology also could assist in third-party reimbursement for nursing care and is the term used in the ICD-10 list of nursing diagnoses. A **risk nursing diagnosis,** as defined by NANDA, "describes human responses to health conditions/life processes that may develop in a vulnerable individual, family, or community. It is supported by risk factors that contribute to increased vulnerability" (NANDA, 2001, p. 245). Problems in identifying risk nursing diagnoses include lack of knowledge of a client's risk factor profile and the particular risks involved in care and treatment of the underlying health problem. Risk nursing diagnoses are two-part statements because they do not include defining characteristics.

> *Accurate:* Risk for Aspiration related to reduced level of consciousness
> *Inaccurate:* Risk for Secretions entering the airway from impaired swallowing. (The nurse has listed part of the definition and one of the at-risk factors in the label.)

Wellness Nursing Diagnoses

A **wellness nursing diagnosis** is a diagnostic statement that describes the human response to levels of wellness in an individual, family, or community that have a potential for enhancement to a higher state (NANDA, 2001). Readiness for

TABLE 11-4

Examples of Accurate Versus Inaccurate Statement of Nursing Diagnoses

Type	Accurate Statement	Rationale	Inaccurate Statement	Rationale
Actual nursing diagnosis	Constipation related to decreased activity and fluids as manifested by small, hard, formed stool every 4 days	Properly stated using three-part statement, including diagnostic label (constipation), related factors (decreased activity), and defining characteristics (small, hard, formed stool every 4 days)	Altered Bowel Function related to production of hard stool	Incorrect diagnostic label; altered bowel function is nonspecific and not accepted by NANDA. Only a two-part statement; related factors are omitted, and defining characteristics (hard stool) are substituted.
Risk nursing diagnosis	Risk for Activity Intolerance related to prolonged bedrest	"Risk" is used rather than "potential." Risk diagnoses use risk factors. Defining characteristics should not be included.	Activity Intolerance, Potential	"Potential" rather than "risk" used; diagnostic label is reversed, and no risk factors are provided.
Possible nursing diagnosis	Possible Impaired Adjustment related to unknown etiology	Unknown etiology used until more data can be collected to validate diagnosis.	Adjustment impaired, possibly due to recent car accident that resulted in quadriplegia	Diagnostic label is reversed, and cues are included in "related to" without validation.
Wellness nursing diagnosis	Readiness for Enhanced Family Coping	Wellness diagnoses are one-part statements without risk factors or defining characteristics.	Family coping potential due to desire for better health.	Diagnostic statement reversed, and more information than just the diagnostic label is provided.

Enhanced Spiritual Well-Being is an example of a wellness nursing diagnosis.

Possible Nursing Diagnoses

A **possible nursing diagnosis** is made when not enough evidence supports the presence of the problem but the nurse thinks that it is highly probable and wants to collect more information. The statement is phrased in the same way as an actual problem, except the "related to" phrase is "unknown cause." An example of a possible nursing diagnosis statement follows:

Accurate: Possible Impaired Adjustment related to unknown etiology. (One of the first interventions will be to collect additional assessment data.)

Inaccurate: Adjustment Impaired, Possibly due to recent car accident that resulted in quadriplegia. (The nurse has reversed the diagnostic label and included cues in the "related to" phrase.)

NURSING PRACTICE AND NURSING DIAGNOSES

Significance of Nursing Diagnosis

Nursing diagnoses provide a means of communicating nursing requirements for client care to other nurses, the healthcare team, and the public. "Developing our standards and guidelines; our nursing diagnoses, outcomes, and interventions; and fitting these into a unified nursing language system to be incorporated into patient care databases will make nursing visible" (Hoskins, 1997, p. v). Nursing diagnostic labels can serve as shorthand for specific client problems.

Although many nursing diagnoses need further research to be clinically useful, all have suggested lists of defining characteristics or risk factors that validate the existence of the problem. Making accurate nursing diagnoses helps to ensure that clients receive quality nursing care.

DISPLAY 11-2

NURSING DIAGNOSES ORGANIZED BY FUNCTIONAL HEALTH PATTERNS

Health Perception–Health Management
Development, Risk for Delayed
Energy Field, Disturbed
Growth and Development, Delayed
Growth, Risk for Disproportionate
Health Maintenance, Ineffective
Health-Seeking Behaviors
Injury, Risk for
Latex Allergy Response
Risk for Latex Allergy
Risk for Suffocation
Risk for Poisoning
Risk for Trauma
Risk for Falls
Injury, Risk for Perioperative Positioning
Management of Therapeutic Regimen, Effective
Management of Therapeutic Regimen, Ineffective
Management of Therapeutic Regimen, Ineffective Family
Management of Therapeutic Regimen, Ineffective
    Community
Noncompliance

Activity–Exercise
Adult Failure to Thrive
Activity Intolerance
Activity Intolerance, Risk for
Decreased Cardiac Output
Delayed Surgical Recovery
Disuse Syndrome, Risk for
Diversional Activity, Deficient
Impaired Home Maintenance
Impaired Walking
Impaired Wheelchair Mobility
Impaired Transfer Ability
Impaired Bed Mobility
Infant Behavior, Disorganized
Infant Behavior, Risk for Disorganized
Infant Behavior, Readiness for Enhanced Organized
Mobility, Impaired Physical
Mobility, Impaired Bed
Peripheral Neurovascular Dysfunction, Risk for
Dysfunctional Ventilatory Weaning Response
Ineffective Airway Clearance
Ineffective Breathing Pattern
Impaired Gas Exchange
Impaired Spontaneous Ventilation
Feeding, Self-care Deficit
Bathing/Hygiene, Self-care Deficit
Dressing/Grooming, Self-care Deficit
Tissue Perfusion, Ineffective: (Specify) (Cerebral,
    Cardiopulmonary, Renal, Gastrointestinal, Peripheral)
Wandering

Nutritional–Metabolic
Impaired Dentition
Adaptive Capacity, Intracranial: Decreased
Body Temperature, Risk for Imbalanced
Hypothermia
Hyperthermia
Thermoregulation, Ineffective
Fluid Volume, Deficient
Fluid Volume, Risk for Deficient
Fluid Volume Excess
Risk for Fluid Volume Imbalance
Infection, Risk for
Nutrition, Imbalanced: Less Than Body Requirements
Nutrition, Imbalanced: More Than Body Requirements
Nutrition, Imbalanced: Risk for More Than Body
    Requirements
Breast-feeding, Effective
Breast-feeding, Ineffective
Breast-feeding, Interrupted
Feeding Pattern, Ineffective Infant
Swallowing, Impaired
Protection, Ineffective
Tissue Integrity, Impaired
Oral Mucous Membrane, Impaired
Skin Integrity, Impaired
Skin Integrity, Risk for Impaired

Elimination
Bowel Incontinence
Constipation
Risk for Constipation
Constipation, Perceived
Diarrhea
Urinary Elimination, Impaired
Urinary Retention
Total Incontinence
Functional Incontinence
Reflex Incontinence
Urge Incontinence
Stress Incontinence
Risk for Urinary Urge Incontinence

Sleep–Rest
Sleep deprivation
Sleep Pattern, Disturbed

Cognitive–Perceptual
Aspiration, Risk for
Pain, Acute
Pain, Chronic
Confusion, Acute
Confusion, Chronic

DISPLAY 11-2 (Continued)

NURSING DIAGNOSES ORGANIZED BY FUNCTIONAL HEALTH PATTERNS

Decisional Conflict
Dysreflexia, Autonomic
Dysreflexia, Autonomic, Risk for
Environmental Interpretation Syndrome, Impaired
Knowledge Deficit
Memory, Impaired
Nausea
Sensory Perception, Disturbed: (Specify) (Visual, Auditory, Kinesthetic, Gustatory, Tactile, Olfactory)
Thought Processes, Disturbed
Unilateral Neglect

Self–Perception
Anxiety
Body Image Disturbed
Chronic Sorrow
Death Anxiety
Fatigue
Fear
Hopelessness
Personal Identity, Disturbed
Powerlessness
Chronic Low Self-esteem
Situational Low Self-esteem
Situational Low Self-esteem, Risk for

Role–Relationship
Communication, Impaired Verbal
Family Processes, Interrupted
Family Process: Alcoholism, Dysfunctional
Grieving, Anticipatory
Grieving, Dysfunctional
Loneliness, Risk for
Parent/Infant/Child Attachment, Risk for Impaired
Parental Role Conflict
Parenting, Impaired
Parenting, Impaired, Risk for

Role Performance, Ineffective
Social Interaction, Impaired
Social Isolation

Coping–Stress Tolerance
Adjustment, Impaired
Caregiver Role Strain
Caregiver Role Strain, Risk for
Coping, Ineffective
Defensive Coping
Ineffective Denial
Coping, Disabled Family
Coping, Compromised Family
Coping, Readiness for Enhanced Family
Coping, Ineffective Community
Coping, Readiness for Enhanced Community
Post-Trauma Syndrome
Post-Trauma Syndrome, Risk for
Rape-Trauma Syndrome
Rape-Trauma Syndrome, Compound Reaction
Rape-Trauma Syndrome, Silent Reaction
Relocation Stress Syndrome
Relocation Stress Syndrome, Risk for
Self-Mutilation
Self-Mutilation, Risk for
Suicide, Risk for
Violence, Risk for Self-Directed
Violence, Risk for Directed at Others

Sexuality–Reproductive
Sexual Dysfunction
Sexuality Patterns, Ineffective

Value–Belief
Spiritual Distress
Risk for Spiritual Distress
Spiritual Well Being, Readiness for Enhanced

By focusing attention on the actual or potential health needs of clients, nursing diagnoses increase the specificity of nursing interventions for each client. This specificity can be measured and monitored to make sure that effective interventions are acknowledged for their contribution to resolving healthcare problems. Coding of nursing diagnoses in computerized systems allows direct reimbursement for nurses. Acknowledging nursing's specific contribution in resolving health problems advances professional nursing practice.

Studies of specific nursing diagnoses improve understanding of the nursing diagnostic process and contribute to examination of the nurse's role in healthcare. As research supports nursing diagnoses, a clear description of the scope of nursing practice will emerge. The development and publica-

tion of a taxonomy of nursing diagnoses should significantly affect practice, education, research, legislation, and nursing as a profession. A nursing diagnosis taxonomy will help to bridge the gap between knowledge and practice and will articulate the scope of nursing practice, essential to developing nursing's professional role in healthcare.

Each nurse will decide the usefulness of the nursing diagnosis taxonomy. As the profession develops, the taxonomy will be critically reviewed, revised, and tested. For today's practitioner, the taxonomy meets the need for organization of nursing diagnoses.

The limitations of NANDA Taxonomy II do not mean that it cannot or should not be used in clinical practice. Nursing process and nursing diagnosis taxonomy continue to evolve

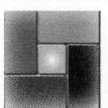

Nursing Research and Critical Thinking
Is it Possible to Validate the Nursing Diagnosis of Relocation Stress Syndrome by Studying Elders Being Relocated En Masse to a New Facility?

The North American Nursing Diagnosis Association accepted the nursing diagnosis of relocation stress syndrome (RSS) in 1992. This syndrome is defined as physiologic and/or psychosocial disturbances that result from the transfer from one environment to another. Increased confusion in the elderly, depression, anxiety, apprehension, and loneliness are the major defining characteristics of this syndrome. These nurses became aware of the fact that many nursing diagnostic labels are used as though they have been generated by rigorous research. However, often they are not. Although RSS appears to be accepted as a basis for nursing intervention, these nurses could find no validation studies of this diagnosis. They designed a study to validate the presence of some defining characteristics of RSS in a group of long-term care residents ($N = 106$) relocated en masse to a new facility. The study population comprised people who had lived at the facility at least 90 days before the move and at least 45 days after the move. The residents ranged in age from 27 to 101 years. Most of the population were women. The presence of five characteristics defining the nursing diagnosis of RSS (dependency, confusion, anxiety, depression, and withdrawal) was measured with the Multidimensional Observation Scale for Elderly Subjects (MOSES) scale. Measures were taken twice before and twice after the move to examine changes in these characteristics over time. During the time of the move, no extraordinary efforts were made to alleviate RSS. The researchers used a repeated measures analysis of variance to analyze the data. There were no differences in the mean scores ($P = <.5$) on the measured factors overall or from one measurement period to another.

Critical Thinking Considerations. The following techniques have been used to validate other nursing diagnoses: (a) establishing content validity by quantifying interrater reliability of expert practitioners, (b) determining the frequency of use of accepted nursing diagnoses in nursing practice, and (c) developing tools to operationalize the measurement of diagnostic characteristics. Such studies are affected by biases inherent in research designed to verify the presence of diagnoses already accepted. Implications for nursing are as follows:

• None of the findings is consistent with the proposition that dependency, confusion, depression, and withdrawal are associated with large-scale relocations.
• Accessibility to the patient advocate may have provided the sense of control that is believed to be a mitigating factor in relocation effects.
• Minimizing staff reassignments and roommate separations may have provided a social support system sufficient to offset the stress associated with the move.

Mallick, M. J. & Whipple, T. W. (2000). Validity of the nursing diagnosis of relocation stress syndrome. *Nursing Research, 49*(2), 97–100.

with the addition of new nursing diagnoses and revisions of existing diagnoses. All nurses have the opportunity and responsibility to use the taxonomy in practice. The challenge for each practitioner is to learn the concepts and skills required to assist clients by accurately diagnosing, planning, and implementing nursing care.

Functional Approach to Nursing Diagnosis

Gordon (1994) suggested a framework for organizing nursing diagnoses based on functional health, thus offering a convenient way to cluster similar diagnoses. Because this book focuses on function, and data collected during assessment are discussed and organized in this fashion, it is useful to organize nursing diagnoses in the same manner. The complete list of nursing diagnoses organized by function is shown in Display 11-2.

Reviewing function and nursing diagnoses for each pattern ensures that nurses have considered all actual, possible, or risk nursing diagnoses, therefore ensuring that physiologic problems do not overshadow the client's emotional, social, or spiritual needs.

KEY CONCEPTS

• Collection of assessment data provides the basis for identifying nursing diagnoses.
• RNs are educated and licensed to make nursing diagnoses.
• A nursing diagnosis is a clinical judgment about individual, family, or community responses to actual or potential health problems and life processes.
• Activities of nursing diagnoses include pattern identification, diagnostic validation, and formulation of the nursing diagnosis statement.
• NANDA-accepted nursing diagnoses are organized according to human response patterns.
• A nursing diagnosis must address a problem within the scope and education of RNs, and RNs must be able to intervene legally and independent of physician-prescribed actions.
• The nurse is responsible and accountable to identify and treat collaborative problems, which focus on pathophysiologic responses, in cooperation with the physician.

- A nursing diagnosis consists of the diagnostic label, definition, defining characteristics, risk factors, related factors, and descriptors.
- A cue is a piece of information (subjective or objective) collected during the nursing assessment.
- Cluster interpretation involves synthesis of the cue clusters. It is an intellectual activity requiring the ability to see the whole picture, attach meaning to the cluster, and discern the pattern the cluster suggests.
- Diagnostic validation occurs in two stages: comparing the clusters with norms and evaluating the specific nursing diagnosis for its particular nursing research base.
- Formulating the nursing diagnostic statement involves writing the actual, risk, wellness, or possible nursing diagnoses.

REFERENCES

American Nurses Association. (1973). *Standards of nursing practice.* Kansas City, MO: Author.

American Nurses Association. (1991). *Standards of clinical nursing practice.* Kansas City, MO: Author.

American Nurses Association (1995). *Nursing: A social policy statement.* Kansas City, MO: Author.

American Psychiatric Association. (2000). *Diagnostic and statistical manual of mental disorders* (4th ed.), text revision. Washington, DC: Author.

Carpenito, L. J. (2002). *Nursing diagnosis: Application to clinical practice* (9th ed.). Philadelphia: Lippincott Williams & Wilkins.

Chase, S. K. (1994). Clinical judgment by critical care nurses: An ethnographic study. In R. M. Carroll-Johnson & M. Paquette (Eds.), *Classification of nursing diagnoses: Proceedings of the tenth conference.* Philadelphia: J. B. Lippincott.

Craft-Rosenberg, M., & Delaney, C. (1997). Nursing diagnosis extension and classification (NDEC). In M. J. Rantz & P. LeMone (Eds.), *Classification of nursing diagnoses: Proceedings of the twelfth conference* (pp. 26–31). Glendale, CA: CINAHL Information Systems.

Fry, V. (1953). The creative approach to nursing. *American Journal of Nursing, 3,* 301–302.

Gebbie, K., & Lavin, M. (1975). *Classification of nursing diagnoses: Proceedings from the first national conference.* St. Louis, MO: C. V. Mosby.

Gordon, M. (1987). *Nursing diagnosis: Process and application* (2nd ed.). New York: McGraw-Hill.

Gordon, M. (1994). *Manual of nursing diagnosis, 1995–1996.* St. Louis, MO: Mosby–Year Book.

Hammond, K. R. (1966). Clinical inference in nursing: A psychologist's viewpoint. *Nursing Research, 15,* 27–38.

Hoskins, L. (1997). Foreword. In M. J. Rantz & P. LeMone (Eds.), *Classification of nursing diagnoses: Proceedings of the twelfth conference* (pp. v–vi). Glendale, CA: CINAHL Information Systems.

Joint Commission on Accreditation of Healthcare Organizations. (1996). *Comprehensive accreditation manual for hospitals: The official handbook.* Oak Brook Terrace, IL: Author.

Jones, D. (2001). Linking nursing language and knowledge development. In N. L. Chaska (Ed.), *The Nursing Profession: Tomorrow and Beyond* (pp. 373–386). Thousand Oaks, CA: Sage Publications.

North American Nursing Diagnosis Association. (1999). *NANDA nursing diagnoses: Definitions and classification.* Philadelphia: Author.

North American Nursing Diagnosis Association. (2001). *NANDA nursing diagnoses: Definitions and classification 2001–2002.* Philadelphia: Author.

Sparks, S. M., & Taylor, C. M. (2001). *Nursing Diagnosis Reference Manual* (5th ed.). Springhouse, PA: Springhouse Corporation.

Warren, J. J. (1996). Introduction to classification of nursing diagnoses. In *NANDA, nursing diagnoses: Definitions, classification 1997–1998.* Philadelphia: NANDA.

Yura, H., & Walsh, M. B. (1973). *The nursing process.* Norwalk, CT: Appleton-Century-Croft.

Yura, H., & Walsh, M. B. (1988). *The nursing process* (5th ed.). Norwalk, CT: Appleton & Lange.

BIBLIOGRAPHY

Barnett-Damewood, H., & Carlson-Catalano, J. (2000). Physical activity deficit: A proposed nursing diagnosis. *Nursing Diagnosis, 11*(1), 24–31.

Correa, C. G., & da Cruz, D. (2000). Pain: A clinical validation with postoperative heart surgery patients. *Nursing Diagnosis, 11*(1), 5–14.

Creason, N., & Sparks, D. (2000). Fecal impaction: A review. *Nursing Diagnosis, 11*(1), 15–23.

Cutler, L. (2000). The diagnostic domain of nursing. *Nursing Critical Care, 5*(2), 59–61.

Mallick, M. J., & Whipple, T. W. (2000). Validity of nursing diagnosis of relocation stress syndrome. *Nursing Research, 49*(2), 97–100.

Wake, M., & Coenen, A. (1998). Nursing diagnosis in the International Classification for Nursing Practice. *Nursing Diagnosis, 9*(3), 111–118.

12 Outcome Identification and Planning

Key Terms

goal
nursing interventions
outcome criteria
outcome identification
planning

priority
qualifier
scientific rationale
variance

Learning Objectives

Upon completion of this chapter, the student will be able to do the following:
1. Define *outcome identification* and *planning*.
2. Explain the purposes of outcome identification and planning.
3. Discuss the Nursing Outcome Classification and the Nursing Intervention Classification projects.
4. Describe the components of the nursing plan of care.
5. Formulate a nursing plan of care for a client given a nursing assessment database.
6. Use a functional health approach to plan client care.

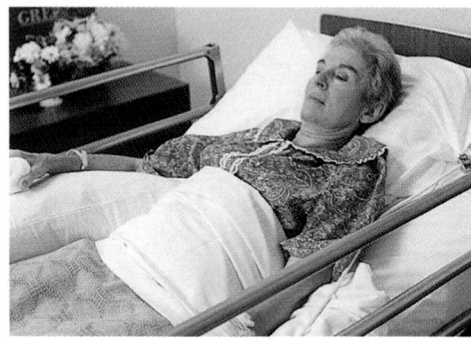

Critical Thinking Challenge

You are working as a nurse in an extended-care facility. You admit a client from the community hospital who had a total hip replacement 1 week ago. Your admission assessment reveals the following:

- *Client states, "They sent me here until I could walk better because my daughter isn't willing to take me like this! I can't even get up to go to the bathroom by myself."*
- *Medical history includes arthritis controlled with nonsteroidal anti-inflammatory drugs and irregular heart rhythm controlled with digoxin; vital signs stable (VSS), incision healing well; fair appetite, no swallowing difficulties; BM every 2 or 3 days (often needs laxative); physical therapy twice a day to work on ambulating with a walker and increasing muscle strength and endurance*

From these data, you identify the following nursing diagnoses:

- *Impaired Physical Mobility related to inability to ambulate or transfer independently and decreased muscle strength and endurance*
- *Constipation related to decreased physical mobility and inability to perform toileting tasks*

Once you have completed this chapter and have incorporated outcome identification and planning into your knowledge base, review the above scenario and reflect on the following areas of Critical Thinking:

1. Analyze how you would prioritize the nursing diagnoses for this client, and suggest additional information you may need to collect.
2. State possible outcomes for each diagnosis that should be met before the client's discharge to the home.
3. Construct possible methods to work with the client to individualize the plan of care and develop realistic outcomes.
4. Develop a hypothetical written plan of care for one of the above nursing diagnoses, indicating what additional information is needed.

Afterhcollecting and analyzing assessment data and identifying and validating nursing diagnoses, nurses are ready to begin planning care with clients. Nursing is a practice discipline involving application of theoretical knowledge to actual client situations. Nurses and clients set realistic goals in what the nursing process calls "outcome identification." A plan specifies interventions to meet client goals.

OUTCOME IDENTIFICATION

Outcome identification is the formulation of goals and measurable outcomes that provide the basis for evaluating nursing diagnoses. Outcome identification is the most recent addition to the nursing process, as described in the current American Nurses Association (ANA) *Standards of Clinical Nursing Practice* (1991). The ANA describes seven measurement criteria for outcome identification, which include specifying intermediate and long-term outcomes that focus on health promotion, health maintenance, or health restoration.

Outcome identification serves the following purposes:

- Providing individualized care
- Promoting client participation
- Planning care that is realistic and measurable
- Allowing for involvement of support people

The following are activities performed in this phase:

- Establish priorities.
- Establish client goals and outcome criteria.

Outcome identification in relation to other phases of the nursing process is shown in Figure 12-1. A classification system for outcomes is described in the next section.

Nursing-Sensitive Client Outcomes

Nurses must demonstrate to the public how they achieve client outcomes. To meet this need, a research team at the University of Iowa College of Nursing is conducting Nursing-Sensitive Patient Outcomes research (Johnson & Maas, 1997; Johnson, Maas, & Moorhead, 2000). The research is aimed at identifying, validating, and classifying nursing-sensitive client outcomes and indicators; field testing the outcomes; and testing measurement procedures for the outcomes and indicators.

Nursing Outcomes Classification

The Nursing-Sensitive Outcomes Classification (NOC) system is organized according to categories, classes, labels, outcome indicators, and measurement activities for outcomes. "The NOC can be used in a manual or computerized clinical information system. The outcomes can be used in critical paths and care plans and can be used to set expected patient goals" (Johnson et al., 2000, p. 72). Each nursing-sensitive outcome has a definition, a measurement scale, and associated indicators and measures. A taxonomy of nursing-sensitive patient outcomes is available from the research team at the

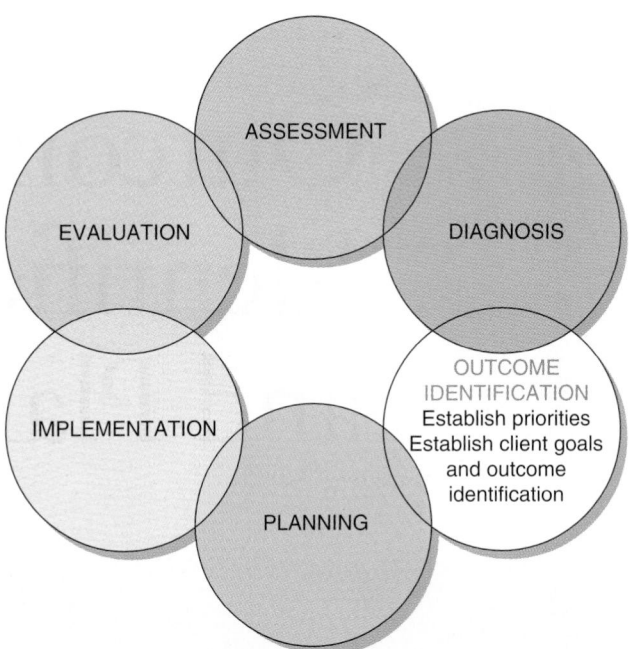

FIGURE 12-1   ANA Standard III states: The nurse identifies expected outcomes individualized to the client. This illustration shows activities used in the outcome identification phase and also the relationship of outcome identification to the other phases of the nursing process.

University of Iowa. The current classification consists of 260 outcomes for individuals, families, communities, or caregivers (Display 12-1).

OUTCOME IDENTIFICATION ACTIVITIES

Establish Priorities

A **priority** is something that takes precedence in position, deemed the most important among several items. Priority setting is a decision-making process that ranks the order of nursing diagnoses in terms of importance to the client. Priorities constantly change as the client's situation and condition change. Nurses use experience, clinical expertise, practice, knowledge, and assessment data collected from clients to determine priorities. High priorities for clients usually involve the following:

- A life-threatening situation (e.g., difficulty breathing, hemorrhage)
- Something that needs immediate attention (e.g., preparation for a test, discharge from the facility that will occur shortly)
- Something that is very important to the client (e.g., pain, anxiety)

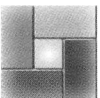

Nursing Research and Critical Thinking
Can Advanced Practice Nurses Demonstrate the Value of Their Role and the Impact of Their Practice on Client Outcomes?

Advanced practice nurses (APNs) need to demonstrate the value of their practice to those who benefit from their care and to those who pay. Nurses designed this study to create and to demonstrate an evaluation model to assess comprehensively the value of the APN role. Outcomes result from structure and process factors. Nursing outcomes are the result of interventions (processes) based on the nurse's clinical judgment and theoretic, practical, and scientific knowledge. It is critical for researchers to track APN-sensitive measures during outcome studies. The researchers demonstrated the usefulness of their evaluation model on a sample of outcome measures from an aggregate neonatal population. The data were based on an average per case for 6 months compared with baseline data. Categories for assessment were developed to measure indicators for resource utilization, satisfaction, long-term functional outcomes, costs, and revenue. Indicators for desired outcomes were compared with actual outcome data. The evaluation model showed that the average length of stay and number of readmissions were reduced when APNs were available to provide care. The study further showed that families were more likely to attend follow-up appointments (85% versus 92%) and were more satisfied with the care received (90% versus 96%). Cost of care was reduced by 18.1%, and loss of revenue was reduced by 43.2%. The model was able to demonstrate an ability to evaluate the impact of APN practice both individually and aggregatively on the issues relevant to today's healthcare system regarding quality, cost, and satisfaction.

Critical Thinking Considerations. This model was developed to enable nurses to evaluate the impact of the APN role in a way that allows them to prove that their presence has a positive impact on the quality and financial outcomes of care for individual clients and entire populations of clients. Implications for further research are as follows:

- The correlations among the structure, strategies of care (process), and their objectives (outcome) are key to the assessment of the quality of care and the impact of the APN role on client care.
- Using the model will give credibility and validity to the positive impact of APNs on care.

From Byers, J. F., & Brunell, M. L. (1998). Demonstrating the value of the advanced practice nurse: An evaluation model. *AACN Clinical Issues: Advanced Practice in Acute and Critical Care, 9*(2), 296–305.

Life-threatening problems always take precedence over routine care. For instance, maintaining an airway when a client is having respiratory difficulty always takes precedence over client teaching. Often, the client's physical condition is more stable and determining priorities is more subtle. For example, if the client is receiving care in the home, establishing priorities might include determining what to teach a newly diagnosed diabetic client during a 60-minute home visit.

DISPLAY 12-1

NURSING OUTCOMES CLASSIFICATION SYSTEM EXAMPLE

MOBILITY LEVEL. Domain Functional Health (I) Class-Mobility (c) Definition: Ability to move purposely. Mobility Level: 1 Dependent, 2 Requires assistive person and device, 3 Requires assistive person, 4 Independent with assistive device, 5 Completely independent. Indicators: Ambulation: walking 1 2 3 4 5.

From Johnson, M., Maas, M., & Moorhead, A. (Eds.). (2000). *Nursing outcomes classification (NOC)* (2nd ed.). St. Louis, MO: Mosby–Year Book.

High-priority nursing diagnoses are those that are potentially life-threatening and require immediate action. Examples include Impaired Gas Exchange, Dysreflexia (a condition in which a spinal cord–injured client experiences life-threatening inhibited sympathetic responses due to noxious stimuli), and Self-Directed Risk for Violence. In each of these situations, the person could die if appropriate intervention is not initiated.

Medium-priority nursing diagnoses involve problems that could result in unhealthy consequences, such as physical or emotional impairment, but are not likely to threaten life. Examples include Fatigue, Stress Incontinence, or Dysfunctional Grieving. Assessment data obtained from the client determine how significant each nursing diagnosis is and what priority it is assigned.

Low-priority nursing diagnoses involve problems that usually can be resolved easily with minimal interventions and have little potential to cause significant dysfunction. Often, the low-priority status is based on the significance for the client and the high likelihood that the problem will be easily resolved. For example, Pain might be a nursing diagnosis for a client after minor surgery, but because the pain is moderate and probably will last only a short time, the diagnosis is of low priority.

Sometimes clients and nurses disagree on the priority given to problems. For example, a postoperative client may view pain as the most important problem and try to avoid moving or ambulating so that pain will decrease. The nurse might view Ineffective Breathing Pattern as much more significant. Through dialogue, the nurse and client are able to share their opinions, experiences, and values so that they can determine an agreeable plan. After listening to the client, the nurse may say, "I understand that you are in pain, but it is important to walk so that you do not develop respiratory complications. How about planning to get you up 30 minutes after you get your pain medication, so your pain is well controlled by then?" During shift changes, client goals and progress can be shared with other staff to promote continuity of care.

Nurses use priorities to plan care and determine the order in which interventions are carried out. Sometimes availability limits whether all desirable interventions can actually be carried out. For example, a nurse may want to wash a client's hair to promote self-esteem, but time may not allow this intervention if the client is scheduled for a diagnostic test or two other clients are scheduled for surgery.

Establish Client Goals and Outcome Criteria

Often, the terms *goals, objectives,* and *outcomes* are used interchangeably because they are statements of expectations. For this reason, nurses should be familiar with the specific use of terms in the clinical setting in which they work. A distinction is made in this textbook: client goals and outcome criteria are not interchangeable. Their definitions and use are described in the following sections.

Client Goals

A client **goal** is an educated guess, made as a broad statement, about what the client's state will be after the nursing intervention is carried out. It directly addresses the problem stated in the nursing diagnosis. Using clinical knowledge and experience, the nurse, in collaboration with the client, determines appropriate goals.

Behavioral goals are written to indicate a desired state. They contain an action verb and a qualifier that indicate the level of performance that needs to be achieved. Some commonly used behavioral verbs are presented in Display 12-2. The **qualifier**

DISPLAY 12-2

🔲 **BEHAVIORAL VERBS USED IN CLIENT GOALS**		
Calculate	Distinguish	Practice
Classify	Draw	Recall
Communicate	Explain	Recite
Compare	Express	Record
Construct	Identify	Stand
Contrast	List	State
Define	Maintain	Use
Demonstrate	Name	Verbalize
Describe	Participate	Walk
Discuss	Perform	

is a description of the parameter for achieving the goal. For instance, "Walks" would not be a specific client goal. Restating this client goal as "Ambulates safely with one-person assistance" clarifies this goal statement.

Goals may be short term or long term. A short-term goal can be met in a relatively short period (within days or less than 1 week). A long-term goal requires more time, perhaps several weeks or months. A long-term goal also may indicate ongoing activity. Long-term goals are usually stated by using the phrase "every day" or "will maintain" (Alfaro-LeFevre, 2001).

Goals need to be revised if the client's situation or medical condition changes. For example, you are working in the home with a client who has mobility deficits from multiple sclerosis. During the home visit, you and the client decide that a goal is, "Ambulates safely with a quad cane." Two weeks later, during another home visit, you notice increased mobility problems due to an exacerbation of multiple sclerosis. This change in the client's medical condition was unexpected and not within your control. An appropriate revision of a goal might be, "Transfers safely to a chair, with one-person assistance." As this client's mobility status improves or deteriorates, mobility goals will need to be revised.

Outcome Criteria

Outcome criteria are specific, measurable, realistic statements of goal attainment. They may restate the goal, but they also present information that will guide the evaluation phase of the nursing process. To be specific and measurable, certain requirements must be met when writing outcome criteria. Outcome criteria answer the questions who, what actions, under what circumstances, how well, and when. According to Alfaro-LeFevre (2001), requirements include the following:

- *Subject:* Who is the person expected to achieve the goal?
- *Verb:* What actions must the person do to achieve the goal?
- *Condition:* Under what circumstances is the person to perform the action?
- *Criteria:* How well is the person to perform the action?
- *Specific time:* When is the person expected to perform the action?

An example of an outcome criterion would be, "The client [who] verbalizes [what action] three dietary modifications of a low-salt diet to his wife [under what circumstances] accurately [how well] after the teaching session [when]."

PLANNING

Planning, the fourth phase of the nursing process, refers to the development of nursing strategies designed to ameliorate client problems. A plan of care is developed to direct nursing care activities related to the person for whom the goals and outcome criteria were developed. A written plan of care directs the activities of the nursing staff in the provision of client care.

Purposes of planning include the following:

- Direct client care activities.
- Promote continuity of care.
- Focus charting requirements.
- Allow for delegation of specific activities.

Activities of the planning phase involve the following:

- Planning nursing interventions
- Writing the nursing plan of care

Planning in relation to other phases of the nursing process is illustrated in Figure 12-2.

Nursing Intervention Classification

Since 1987, a research team at the University of Iowa College of Nursing has been engaged in constructing, validating, and implementing nursing interventions (McCloskey & Bulechek, 2000). The interventions are organized in a three-level taxonomy consisting of domains, classes, and interventions. Interventions can be direct or indirect care activities; they include nurse-initiated interventions as well as treatments initiated by the physician or other provider.

At the most abstract level, the taxonomy includes seven domains:

- Physiologic: Basic
- Physiologic: Complex
- Behavioral

- Safety
- Family
- Health system
- Community

Each domain group contains classes, which are groups of interventions that are then broken down into individual interventions. The domains, classes, and interventions are coded numerically to permit computerization. Each intervention consists of a definition and a list of activities that describe the nursing actions that need to be performed. There are 486 interventions included in the Nursing Interventions Classification (McCloskey & Bulechek, 2000) (Display 12-3).

Planning Activities

Planning Nursing Interventions

Selecting appropriate nursing interventions directs activities to be carried out in the implementation phase. **Nursing interventions** are "any treatment, based upon clinical judgment and knowledge, that a nurse performs to enhance patient/client outcomes" (McCloskey & Bulechek, 2000, p. xix). Alfaro-LeFevre (2001) states that nursing interventions are used to monitor health status; prevent, resolve, or control a problem; assist with activities of daily living (ADLs); or promote optimum health and independence. Interventions are written as specific activities on the plan of care.

Determining appropriate nursing interventions for a specific client requires clinical knowledge and practice. In general, interventions can be grouped to describe the activity being suggested. Types of interventions include the following:

- Psychomotor (positioning, inserting, applying)
- Psychosocial (supporting, exploring, encouraging)
- Educational (demonstrating, teaching, observing return demonstrations)
- Maintenance (skin care, hygiene)
- Surveillance (detecting changes)
- Supervisory (other healthcare providers)
- Sociocultural (spending time, incorporating cultural differences into care regimen)

DISPLAY 12-3

⑤ **NURSING INTERVENTION CLASSIFICATION SYSTEM EXAMPLE**

DOMAIN 1. Physiological: Basic CLASS A. Activity and Exercise Management INTERVENTION 0140 Body Mechanics Promotion

From McCloskey, J. C., & Bulechek, G. M. (Eds.). (2000). *Nursing interventions classification* (3rd ed.). St. Louis, MO: Mosby–Year Book.

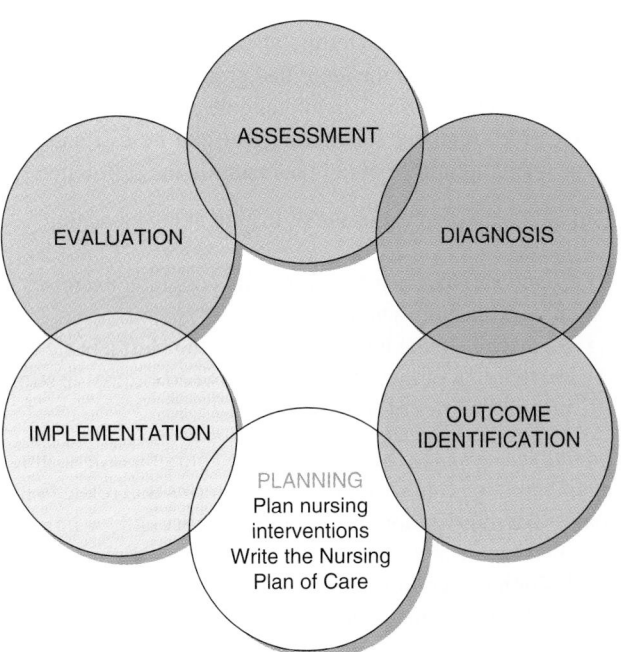

FIGURE 12-2 ANA Standard IV states: The nurse develops a plan of care that prescribes interventions to attain expected outcomes. This illustration shows activities used in the planning phase and also the relationship of planning to the other phases of the nursing process.

Writing a Nursing Plan of Care

A nursing plan of care documents the problem-solving process. The ability to create the nursing plan of care has become a standard expected of every nurse. The plan is a critical element in focusing nursing activity. To serve as evaluation criteria and meet the standards of the Joint Commission for Accreditation of Healthcare Organizations (JCAHO; 1996), the plan must be developed by a registered nurse, it must be documented in the client's health record, and it must reflect the standards of care established by the institution and the profession. Medicare and Medicaid standards and some third-party reimbursement plans require nursing plans of care for each client.

Two important concepts guide a nursing plan of care:

- The plan of care is nursing centered.
- The plan of care is a step-by-step process.

Keeping the plan of care nursing centered is essential to identify the scope and depth of nursing practice. By focusing on the treatment of human responses to actual or potential health problems, the nurse remains in the nursing practice domain.

A step-by-step process is evidenced by the following:

- Sufficient data are collected to substantiate nursing diagnoses.
- At least one goal must be stated for each nursing diagnosis.
- Outcome criteria must be identified for each goal.
- Nursing interventions must be specifically designed to meet the identified goal.
- Each intervention should be supported by a scientific rationale.
- Evaluation must address whether each goal was completely met, partially met, or completely unmet.

Types of Nursing Plans of Care

The nursing plan of care can be written in various ways. Institutions may use a portable metal card file format, a notebook, or a computerized care plan design. Despite these design differences, the plan of care usually contains three key elements: the nursing diagnosis (client problem), client goals, and nursing interventions (nursing orders, nursing actions). The plan of care can be written for the individual client, standardized for a client population, generic for a specific problem, or computer-generated from assessment data. Students learning to write plans use the instructional nursing plan of care format. In practice settings, nurses use the clinical nursing plan of care format.

Instructional Nursing Plans of Care. Instructional nursing plans of care allow students to learn a variety of client problems and the processes nurses use to solve them. Scientific rationales from nursing literature are given as references for the information and to illustrate the nurse's decision-making process. Specific recommendations for completing this type of plan of care are given using each step of the nursing process.

These guidelines also apply to writing a clinical nursing plan of care as a practicing nurse.

Usually, student nurses are required to complete some form of an instructional nursing plan of care to demonstrate in a written format an understanding of the problem-solving process used in assisting clients to maintain or regain a higher level of function. Once assessment data have been collected, organized, and synthesized, one or more nursing diagnoses are identified to develop the plan of care.

Components of instructional nursing plans of care usually include nursing diagnoses, client goals, outcome criteria, nursing interventions, scientific rationale, and evaluation.

The nursing plans of care used in later chapters of this text illustrate this format and include one nursing diagnosis, one or more client goals, several client outcome criteria, nursing interventions, and scientific rationale. These plans are based on the sample format given in the Sample Nursing Plan of Care shown here, along with what to include in each section of the plan. For assistance in learning how to state nursing diagnoses, client goals, outcome criteria, nursing interventions, scientific rationale, and evaluation correctly, refer to Table 12-1.

Nursing Diagnosis. The nursing diagnostic statement is recorded in the space labeled "Nursing Diagnosis," using North American Nursing Diagnosis Association (NANDA) terminology if possible. All identified nursing diagnoses for a client should be listed in order of priority for client care. Use of a functional approach helps nurses to focus on real or potential functional problems rather than on disease pathology.

Client Goals. One or more client goals are established for each nursing diagnosis. Each goal must be measurable, realistic, or observable. Some examples of goal statements are, "Maintains present weight," "Demonstrates no evidence of infection," and "Administers insulin correctly." The goal describes a client outcome in broad terms. The client goal reflects resolution or correction of the identified problem.

Client Outcome Criteria. Client outcome criteria are specific, measurable, realistic statements that can be evaluated to judge goal attainment. Examples include the following:

- Draws up correct dosage of insulin at next teaching session
- Demonstrates deep-breathing and coughing exercises at next teaching session
- Verbalizes to the nurse during evening shift a basic understanding of the relationship between excessive stimuli and feelings of loss of control

Nursing Interventions. Sometimes called nursing orders, nursing interventions are written in specific terms that relate to the goals. "An intervention may be either direct care or indirect care. Direct care interventions include both physiological and psychological nursing actions . . . indirect care interventions include nursing actions aimed at management of the patient care environment and interdisciplinary collaboration" (McCloskey & Bulechek, 2000, p. xix). The statements should be comprehensive but brief; nurses may refer to procedures, protocols, or standing policies for further information. In some cases, nursing interventions include specific measures

---

SAMPLE NURSING PLAN OF CARE

Nursing Diagnosis
(Use the NANDA-accepted list of nursing diagnoses. List in priority order. Use the diagnostic label and "related to" [related factor], followed by "manifested by" [supporting defining characteristics].)

Client Goal
(One or more client goals established from nursing diagnosis. A broadly stated objective that indicates an overall picture of the state of the client if the problem is resolved.)

Client Outcome Criteria
(Specific, measurable, realistic statements that can be evaluated to judge goal attainment. Stated as behavioral objectives, they include a verb, a short phrase describing the specific measure to be accomplished, and a time reference.)

Nursing Intervention	Scientific Rationale
(Write interventions [nursing orders] that are specific and relate to the goal. The "related to" phrase of the nursing diagnostic statement directs choice of nursing interventions. Interventions include who, what, when, and how the order is to be carried out.)	(Gives justification for carrying out the intervention. Demonstrates synthesis of physiologic, psychological, and pathophysiologic concepts.)

---

needed to carry out the medical regimen and are not directed at a nursing diagnosis. Examples are shown in Table 12-2.

Scientific Rationale. The **scientific rationale** is the justification or reason for carrying out the intervention. It often synthesizes psychological and pathophysiologic concepts. The rationale—the "why" of the intervention—describes a research-based reason for performing the intervention. Usually, student nurses are required to supply scientific rationales to show understanding of the basic reasons for carrying out specific nursing interventions. In clinical practice settings, nurses may use rationales to illustrate new research findings or support controversial approaches to problems. A reference for each scientific rationale must be given, citing the author, year, title, and page of the article or book used. Sometimes, nurses think that interventions are based on common sense, but this is not so: many nursing interventions previously thought to be sensible have turned out to be unsafe, impractical, or unnecessary. For example, massaging bony prominences was once thought to promote skin integrity, but research has shown that this practice may cause tissue damage and should *not* be performed (Maklebust & Sieggreen, 1996). Asking why certain nursing interventions are performed aids in the scientific development of nursing practice.

Evaluation. The evaluation of a nursing intervention is a written statement that determines the client's status in relation to the outcome criteria at a particular time. The evaluation stage answers the question: Was the goal achieved? It provides the necessary feedback to guide revision of the plan of care or resolution of the problem. Changes may be needed in the time frame for goal achievement or to facilitate new skill development in the client. In some cases, the student will state what would have been evaluated if nursing care had been provided during additional clinical experiences.

Evaluation of care usually is recorded in the narrative nursing note and includes the client's response to the intervention and the objective clinical findings. Each intervention is evaluated for effectiveness, modified if needed, and deleted if not necessary.

Clinical Nursing Plans of Care. The clinical plan of care used in practice is different from the required instructional plan of care done by students. The nursing process is used, but the plan is organized in a practical, concise format for daily use. Usually, there is less specific detail, and rationales are not documented. The focus is to individualize the plan of care for each client using findings from the nursing assessment and identified nursing diagnoses. The various forms of clinical nursing plans of care are highlighted in Display 12-4.

Nurses continually refine the process of writing plans of care and actively using them in implementing daily care as they gain experience. A well-written, continually updated nursing plan of care is an invaluable tool. The steps of a clinical plan of care follow.

Assessment and Data Collection. The history and physical assessment are guidelines for the initial plan. Data are gathered in each subsequent meeting with the client to revise the plan.

Nursing Diagnosis. The nursing diagnosis in a working plan of care is written using the guidelines in Chapter 11. The clinical plan of care focuses on individual client needs and priority nursing problems.

TABLE 12-1

Correct and Incorrect Plan of Care Entries	
Entry	**Rationale**
Nursing Diagnoses *Correct* Feeding Self-care Deficit (Level 3) related to right-sided weakness manifested by inability to pick up spoon, lack of attention to food on tray, and inability to open containers	Correct statement of actual nursing diagnosis using three-part statement, including diagnostic label, related factors, and defining characteristics.
Incorrect Self-care Deficit, Feeding: due to left cerebrovascular accident, manifested by not eating	Incorrect statement of actual diagnosis. Diagnostic label is inverted, a medical diagnosis is used for the causative agent, and defining characteristics are not provided for validation of the diagnosis.
Client Goal *Correct* Client demonstrates correct skin care regimen	Correctly stated client goal: general statement of overall picture of client if problem is resolved; measurable, realistic, and observable.
Incorrect Client's skin is free of eczema	Incorrect statement of client goal. The goal is not achievable through nursing interventions and may be unrealistic even with medical treatment.
Client Outcome Criteria *Correct* Ambulates 30 feet with walker before discharge	Correctly stated client outcome: specific, measurable, and realistic.
Incorrect Walks in the hall	Incorrectly stated outcome criterion because it is not specific and does not include qualifiers for the outcome.
Nursing Interventions *Correct* Staff will perform passive range-of-motion exercises to all extremities during morning care and evening care	Correctly stated nursing intervention, including who, what, when, and how nursing order will be carried out.
Incorrect Encourage joint mobility	Incorrectly stated nursing intervention because time frame, type of exercise, and who will perform the exercise are not specified.
Scientific Rationale *Correct* Small shifts in body weight promote circulation and help to prevent skin breakdown (Craven & Hirnle, 2000)	Correctly stated rationale: tells scientific basis for nursing action and correctly cites source.
Incorrect Changes position every 2 hours	Incorrectly stated scientific rationale: restates a nursing intervention without documenting why it is an appropriate nursing intervention, and no source is cited.

TABLE 12-1 (Continued)

Correct and Incorrect Plan of Care Entries	
Entry	Rationale
Evaluation	
Correct	
Unable to complete passive range of motion to right upper extremity after morning care because of reported pain when arm is elevated above shoulder level. Physician notified, and patient instructed to rest arm.	Correctly stated evaluation because it indicates that goal was not met, with specific documentation providing the data for revision.
Incorrect	
Range of motion discontinued due to pain	Incorrect evaluation statement: statement does not contain client's response or follow up on the problem.

Outcome Identification. Client goals and outcome criteria are often seen in the same statement. The goals are specific to meeting the client problems identified in the nursing diagnoses. *Interventions.* Nursing actions specific to each client's needs are documented. The healthcare person responsible for performing the nursing action is identified. The action may be most appropriately completed by the nurse. In some instances, it is delegated to auxiliary nursing personnel. This leads to better communication and use of plans for daily assignments. *Rationale.* Although the scientific rationale is not documented in the clinical plan, it is no less important than in the instructional plan. Nurses must know the rationale behind the nursing action or must question and review the rationale before performing the action. This professional responsibility is expected of every practicing nurse. *Evaluation.* Evaluation is ongoing from initial care through resolution of the problem. Evaluation in the clinical plan is based on the specific observations made of client progress toward the outcome criteria. The plan is updated and changed—minute by minute in critical and acute care, weekly or monthly in long-term or home healthcare.

TABLE 12-2

Examples of Nursing Interventions to Include the Medical Regimen	
Medical Order	Nursing Intervention
Weight qd, report loss > 5#	Bedscale weight every day at 6 AM; report weight > (specify #) to team leader and physician.
Increase caloric intake	Provide between-meal snack at 10 AM, 2 PM, and 10 PM. Request consultation with dietitian (done 10/19). Transfer client to chair for each meal and snack.

Collaborative Care Plan: Critical Pathways

Critical pathways (paths) are becoming the current standard guideline for nursing care in many hospitals. The focus on outcome management, controlling costs, and continuous quality improvement has been the driving force for most organizations as they convert to critical paths and case management as a system for care delivery (Johnson, Maas, & Moorhead, 2000). Various terms for critical paths are used: clinical paths, collaborative care plans, CareMaps, multidisciplinary care plan, and case management plans. A standardized plan or critical path is acceptable to the JCAHO (Kobs, 1997).

The critical path is a cause-and-effect grid that describes a client's problems with intermediate outcomes and multidisciplinary staff actions along a timeline. The critical path tool can be designed for clients with a particular illness, diagnostic-related grouping (DRG), procedure, or condition. Timelines can be developed for a continuum of care in the hospital in terms of hours, days, and months; across geographic care units (e.g., emergency room, critical care unit, telemetry); or for a continuum of care in the community. Because the format may vary with the agency, a generic form is included here. In this case, blanks are filled in with generic information. Sample critical paths are provided in selected chapters.

Information on the critical path is based on the most cost-efficient practice patterns for a particular diagnosis or procedure. This method addresses key events in the treatment process that must be accomplished to achieve predetermined outcomes at a minimal cost. The staff nurse is responsible for initiating, maintaining, and completing the critical path, including documentation of variances. A variance is a deviation from expected outcomes. Many hospitals are developing a version of the critical path for clients and families to help increase their understanding of and participation in the plan of care. In addition, continuity of care is being addressed by the use of care maps that cross multiple sites and demonstrate collaboration among healthcare providers (Doran, Sampson, Staus, Ahern & Schiro, 1997; Raiwet, Halliwell, Andruski & Wilson, 1997) and by different organizations

DISPLAY 12-4

🔲 CLINICAL NURSING PLANS OF CARE

Individual Plan of Care

Individual plans of care are written for each client by an RN. The nursing diagnoses are listed, along with specific goals and interventions to resolve the problem. This method is ideal, but it is time consuming.

Standardized Plan of Care

Standardized plans of care are written by a group of nurses who are experts in a given area of practice (e.g., obstetrics, rehabilitation, or orthopedics). The plans are written for a client population with a specific medical diagnosis (e.g., total hip replacement, pressure ulcer, vaginal delivery, coronary artery bypass surgery). These experts identify the most common nursing diagnoses for this client population and write the goals and interventions usually necessary to resolve the problem. Each time a standardized plan of care is used, it must be individualized for a specific client. This method assures the nurse that the plan is correct for the client. The danger of a standardized plan of care lies in the fact that it may not fit a specific client. Nurses must make judgments as to the degree to which standardized plans should be modified or whether they should not be used in individual cases.

Generic Plan of Care

Generalized plans of care usually are written for a specific nursing diagnosis. They contain the goals and interventions most commonly seen when that particular nursing diagnosis is identified. Again, the generic plan of care must be individualized for a specific client. Because generic plans are written by experts in a particular diagnostic area, they may serve as a learning tool for the inexperienced nurse who is unfamiliar with the content.

Computerized Plan of Care

Computerized plans of care are generated from assessment data entered into a computer about a specific client. The plan is written by experts in the area, and the content is similar to that of the standardized or generic plan of care. Once the plan is on the computer screen, the nurse has an opportunity to customize it for the client. Because these plans are linked to assessment data, it is critical that all pertinent information be collected and entered into the system. The generated plan of care is only as good as the data on which it is based.

established criteria. The paths reflect the criteria of the Health Care Financing Administration. Clients who do not meet the discharge criteria and are discharged must be monitored for readmissions and premature discharges.

The impetus for critical paths was the prospective payment system (DRGs) established by the federal government in the early 1980s, which was aimed at controlling costs for Medicare and Medicaid clients. The reduction in healthcare costs was believed to result from shortening the length of stay (LOS) for hospitalized clients. However, hospitals needed to increase the quality and efficiency of healthcare delivery to achieve the predetermined LOS specified by the DRGs. Consequently, critical paths were specifically written to incorporate the DRG-determined LOS into the timeline. If critical paths were followed and clients were discharged within the predetermined LOS, hospitals were reimbursed the predicted cost.

Critical paths became an ideal tool to help clients achieve the predicted LOS, improve quality, and control costs.

A key to the success of critical paths is that they are collaboratively developed by the multidisciplinary team involved in care of a given client population. The collaboration helps ensure that the tool is relevant and will be followed by all members of the health team.

The New England Medical Center Hospital in Boston is credited as being the first hospital to develop critical paths, now called CareMaps. Their case management and critical path/CareMap system has evolved to include a comprehensive tool. Although the critical path was developed primarily as a case management tool, it is being used alone or with case management to guide client care activities in healthcare institutions (Zander, 1993). In some hospitals, critical paths are used as a guideline for client care in as much as 80% of the hospital's population. Clinical pathways can be used by care managers to coordinate care for clients with complex health problems, complications, or need for follow-up or referral (Goehner, 1997).

A criterion for success of the critical path is consistency in healthcare delivery. Lack of consistency in care delivery usually results in a variance from the critical path. **Variances** result when a deviation occurs in the path that alters an expected outcome or the date of discharge. Client, staff, and system variances can occur. Some hospitals also include variances in the community. Variances are monitored concurrently and retrospectively for continuous quality improvement. The use of new computer technology (e.g., optical scanner) can aid in collecting and reporting critical path variance data (Strassner, 1997). Variance measurement has the potential for identifying client problems and complications early in hospitalization, variations in practice patterns, and system problems.

A recent development in the critical path movement has been to include documentation as a permanent part of the client's health record. Incorporating documentation in the design of the critical path eliminates much of the redundancy in charting. Critical path documentation consists of writing the

working together (Hainsworth, Lockwood-Cook, Pond & Lagoe, 1997).

Most critical paths incorporate quality indicators and discharge criteria to measure the quality of care provided. The client's progress at the time of discharge is measured against

(text continues on page 198)

GENERIC COLLABORATIVE CARE PLAN

Critical Pathway (and types of information included in such a plan)

Illness, DRG, Procedure, or Condition

Client Name: _____

Case Type: _____	Admit Date: _____	Expected LOS: _____
DRG: _____	Date Path Initiated: _____	Physician: _____ Actual LOS: _____
ICD-9: _____	Discharge Date: _____	Case Manager: _____

Outcome Criteria

(Timeline)	(Date) Day 1 (may be expressed in hours, days, or events)	D	E	N	Day 2	D	E	N	Day 3 (may extend for more days or expected length of stay)	D	E	N
Client Problems (May be stated as nursing diagnoses or client problems for individualized care. Usually includes 3–5 problems)	(Site of Care)				(Intermediate or expected outcome for each problem)				(Rather than Day, Evening, Night, may be 12-hour shifts with two columns)			
(May include more than one space)												
Interventions					(May be stated as nurse, physician, or client actions or actions of any health-care members)							
Consult/Referral					(List appropriate referrals to specific health-care providers)							

GENERIC COLLABORATIVE CARE PLAN

Critical Pathway (and types of information included in such a plan), *Continued*

(Timeline)	*(Date) Day 1* *(may be expressed* *in hours, days,* *or events)*	Day 2						Day 3 *(may extend for* *more days or expected* *length of stay)*		
	(Site of Care)	*D*	*E*	*N*	*D*	*E*	*N*	*D*	*E*	*N*
Interventions										
Diagnostic Tests										
(Diagnostic or laboratory tests needed for this particular client)										
Assessment										
(Routine or specific assessments required)										
Treatments										
(Multidisciplinary procedures such as antiembolic stockings, oxygen administration, dressing changes, Foley catheter)										
Activity										
(Includes mobility prescriptions or limitations)										

Diet
(Prescribed diet, supplement, or restrictions)

Meds
(Regularly scheduled & prn meds. IV may be included)

Teaching
(Routine teaching expected for client/family—when and by whom)

Discharge/Transfer Planning
(Coordination of services and referrals for transition to home or other healthcare facility. May indicate follow-up services or appointment)

Initials/Signatures:

Write "V" for variance in box if expected outcome not met or intervention not performed as stated. Client variances need to be explained in progress notes.

provider's initials next to the outcome and intervention or indicating whether a variance occurred. Some hospitals place a "V" next to the outcome or intervention if a variance occurs. Documentation of client variance is written in the progress or nurse's notes. Staff and system variances are documented on a separate variance sheet so that the data can be monitored for continuous quality improvement.

Nurses must have a thorough understanding of the nursing process, not only because it is the basis for nursing care but also because it is the underlying framework for the critical path. However, the nursing process is a problem-solving process and a mental function, whereas the critical path is a tool that operationalizes that process. Healthcare facilities that are developing critical paths without listing the client problems (or nursing diagnoses) and intermediate or discharge outcomes have fragmented the nursing process. When outcome is separated from process, outcomes based on that process cannot be evaluated. Nurses and other health team members cannot determine whether a particular outcome was a result of a specific intervention if they are not linked accordingly. Critical paths that function as comprehensive multidisciplinary care plans allow for the evaluation of the nursing process, documentation of that process, and monitoring for continuous quality improvement. Integration of the nursing process within the critical path framework is essential to ensure an outcome-based, accountability-driven system. By including a documentation section next to each outcome and intervention, evaluation of the nursing process is possible, ensuring accountability for the critical path.

Nurses in hospital and community settings will be expected to function as case managers and to develop and use critical paths in their case management role. Care managers approve exceptions to standardized plans to maximize client outcomes, thus ensuring quality care (Kelly & Joel, 1996).

Functional Approach to Planning

Nurses must meet high standards to satisfy professional mandates, including legal, social, and institutional expectations of professional practice. Use of a functional approach facilitates professional nursing practice.

Some clients have good function in many areas but require nursing care for dysfunction in other areas. Understanding the concepts of function and dysfunction allows nurses to see each client's strengths and limitations. Because function is useful for organizing assessment data and identifying nursing diagnoses, it provides a forceful focus for identifying outcomes and planning nursing interventions.

KEY CONCEPTS

- Outcome identification is crucial for selecting and evaluating nursing interventions.
- Client goals are stated as behavioral objectives and indicate the desired state of the client if the problem has been resolved.
- Outcome criteria are specific, measurable, realistic statements of goal attainment.

- The nursing plan of care is designed to direct client care activities, promote continuity of care, focus charting requirements, and specify who is to carry out the nursing actions.
- The key elements of the nursing plan of care are the nursing diagnosis, client goals and outcome criteria, and nursing interventions.
- Nursing interventions are independent, dependent, and interdependent activities that nurses carry out to provide client care.
- The use of critical pathways (paths) is on the rise in many areas. They provide a collaborative plan of care.

REFERENCES

Alfaro-LeFevre, R. (2001). *Applying nursing process: A step-by-step guide* (5th ed.). Philadelphia: Lippincott Williams & Wilkins.

American Nurses Association. (1991). *Standards of clinical nursing practice.* Kansas City, MO: Author.

Doran, K., Sampson, B., Staus, R., Ahern, C., & Schiro, D. (1997). Clinical pathway across tertiary and community care after an interventional cardiology procedure. *Journal of Cardiovascular Nursing, 11*(2), 1–14.

Goehner, E. D. (1997). Integrating nursing diagnoses into clinical pathways. In M. J. Rantz & P. LeMone (Eds.), *Classification of nursing diagnoses: Proceedings of the twelfth conference, North American Nursing Diagnosis Association* (pp. 285–297). Glendale, CA: Cumulative Index to Nursing and Allied Health Literature (CINAHL) Information Systems.

Hainsworth, D. S., Lockwood-Cook, E., Pond, M., & Lagoe, R. J. (1997). Development and implementation of clinical pathways for stroke on a multihospital basis. *Journal of Neuroscience Nursing, 29*(3), 156–162.

Iowa Intervention Project. (1997). Nursing interventions classification (NIC): An overview. In M. J. Rantz & P. LeMone (Eds.), *Classification of nursing diagnoses: Proceedings of the twelfth conference, North American Nursing Diagnosis Association* (pp. 32–40). Glendale, CA: CINAHL Information Systems.

Johnson, M., & Maas, M. (1997). *Nursing outcomes classification (NOC).* St. Louis, MO: Mosby–Year Book.

Johnson, M., Maas, M., & Moorhead, S. (Eds.). (2000). *Nursing Outcomes classification (NOC),* (2nd ed.). St. Louis, MO: Mosby.

Joint Commission on the Accreditation of Healthcare Organizations. (1996). *Comprehensive accreditation manual for hospitals: The official handbook.* Oak Brook Terrace, IL: Author.

Kelly, L. Y., & Joel, L. A. (1996). *The nursing experience: Trends, challenges, and transitions* (3rd ed.). New York: McGraw-Hill.

Kobs, A. (1997). Nursing care plans: Are they required? *Nursing Management, 28*(5), 30, 32.

Maas, M. (1997). Nursing-sensitive outcomes classification (NOC): Completing the essential comprehensive languages for nursing. In M. J. Rantz & P. LeMone (Eds.), *Classification of nursing diagnoses: Proceedings of the twelfth conference, North American Nursing Diagnosis Association* (pp. 40–47). Glendale, CA: CINAHL Information Systems.

Maklebust, J., & Sieggreen, M. (1996). *Pressure ulcers: Guidelines for prevention and nursing management* (2nd ed.). Springhouse, PA: Springhouse Corporation.

McCloskey, J. C., & Bulechek, G. M. (Eds.). (2000). *Nursing interventions classification (NIC)* (3rd ed.). St. Louis, MO: Mosby–Year Book.

Raiwet, C., Halliwell, G., Andruski, L., & Wilson, D. (1997). Care maps across the continuum. *Canadian Nurse, 93*(1), 26–30.

Strassner, L. (1997). Tips, tools, and techniques. Scanner technology to manage critical path variance analysis. *Nursing Case Management, 2*(4), 141–147.

Zander, K. (1994). Case management update. *Seminars in Perioperative Nursing 3*(1), 55–58.

BIBLIOGRAPHY

Chase, S. K. (1997). Teaching baccalaureate nursing students to project outcomes to nursing interventions. In M. J. Rantz & P. LeMone (Eds.). *Classification of nursing diagnoses: Proceedings of the twelfth conference, North American Nursing Diagnosis Association* (pp. 117–125). Glendale, CA: CINAHL Information Systems.

Cruz, D. M., Gutierrez, B. A. O., Lopez, A. L., de Souza, T. T., & Assami. S. (2000). Congruence of terms between lists of problems and the ICNP—Alpha Version. *International nursing review, 47*(2), 89–96.

Delaney, C., Reed D., & Clarke M. (2000). Describing patient problems and nursing treatment patterns using nursing minimum data sets (NMDS and NMMDS) and UHDDS repositories. *Proceedings AMIA Symposium,* 176–179.

Holzemer, W. L., & Henry, S. B. (1999). Therapeutic outcomes sensitive to nursing. In A. S. Hinshaw, S. L. Feetham, & J. L. F. Shaver (Eds.), *Handbook of clinical nursing research* (pp. 185–195). Thousand Oaks, CA: Sage.

The Iowa Intervention Project. (1997). Defining nursing's effectiveness: Diagnoses, interventions, and outcomes. In M. J. Rantz & P. LeMone (Eds.). *Classification of nursing diagnoses: Proceedings of the twelfth conference, North American Nursing Diagnosis Association* (pp. 293–303). Glendale, CA: CINAHL Information Systems.

Johnson, M. (1999). Overview of the Nursing Outcomes Classification (NOC). In M. J. Rantz, *Classification of nursing diagnoses: proceedings of the thirteenth conference, North American Nursing Diagnosis Association* (pp. 267–272). Glendale, CA: CINAHL Information Systems.

13 Implementation and Evaluation

🔳 Key Terms

evaluation
implementation
nursing monitors
peer review

quality improvement
  programs
standards

🔳 Learning Objectives

Upon completion of this chapter, the student will be able to do the following:
1. Define implementation and evaluation.
2. Discuss the purposes of implementation and evaluation.
3. Describe clinical skills needed to implement the nursing plan of care.
4. Explain methods for revising or modifying the nursing plan of care.
5. Describe activities the nurse carries out during the evaluation phase of the nursing process.
6. Discuss quality assurance monitors used in nursing settings.
7. Use a functional approach to implement and evaluate client care.

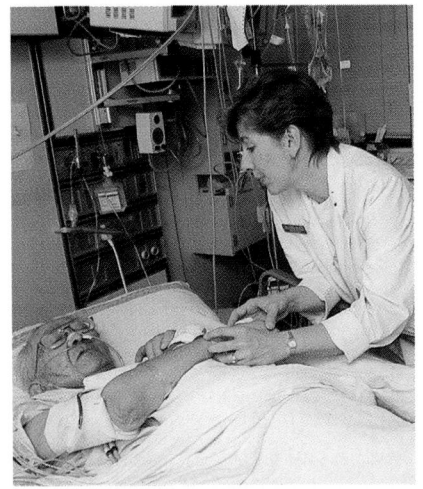

🔳 Critical Thinking Challenge

You are assigned to care for a 68-year-old client who has just returned to your nursing unit after abdominal surgery with general anesthesia. He has a history of arthritis for which he takes nonsteroidal anti-inflammatory agents (NSAIDs) and uses a cane to ambulate. He lives alone in a large two-story home. His postoperative assessment reveals the following: skin pale, warm, and dry; abdominal dressing dry and intact; vital signs-temperature–97.2°F, pulse–78 and regular, respirations–16, blood pressure–136/74; responsive but sleepy; reluctant to cough, deep breathe, and turn because of complaints of pain.

The plan of care identifies the following nursing diagnoses and goals for this client:

- *Risk for Aspiration related to effects of anesthesia and decreased level of consciousness; client will maintain a patent airway and remain free of signs and symptoms of aspiration.*
- *Pain related to surgical trauma; client will report that postoperative pain is well controlled.*
- *Impaired Physical Mobility related to pain and underlying arthritis; client will maintain optimal state of mobility, progressively increasing activities daily.*
- *Risk for Disuse Syndrome related to effects of anesthesia and surgery and underlying arthritis; client will remain free of complications of immobility, achieving optimal level of functioning.*

Once you have completed this chapter and have incorporated implementation and evaluation into your knowledge base, review the above scenario and reflect on the following areas of Critical Thinking:

1. Analyze how you would prioritize your care for this client. Suggest additional data you would need to collect, and propose possible additional nursing diagnoses and goals that might be appropriate.
2. Reflect on the intellectual, interpersonal, and technical skills you would need to care for this client.
3. Propose possible interventions to carry out for this client. Classify each action proposed as cognitive, interpersonal, or technical.
4. Explore how you would evaluate this client's goal achievement. Suggest possible factors that might facilitate or interfere with his goal attainment.

After the nurse and client identify problems and strengths, they plan together methods of helping the client maintain or return to healthy function. Outcome criteria are set for goals, and a plan of care is developed. Now, they are ready for the implementation phase of the nursing process, the activity that provides planned care, and the evaluation phase, in which the client's status is measured in response to the nursing care provided.

IMPLEMENTATION

Implementation refers to the action phase of the nursing process in which nursing care is provided. It is the actual initiation of the plan and recording of nursing actions. Its purpose is to provide technical and therapeutic nursing care required to help the client achieve an optimal level of health.

Competence in intellectual, interpersonal, and technical skills is required to carry out the implementation phase. Nurses can delegate parts of the plan of care to other members of the healthcare team, but the registered nurse maintains accountability for the supervision and evaluation of these people. Figure 13-1 illustrates the activities of implementation, which include the following:

- Reassessing
- Setting priorities
- Performing nursing interventions
- Recording nursing actions

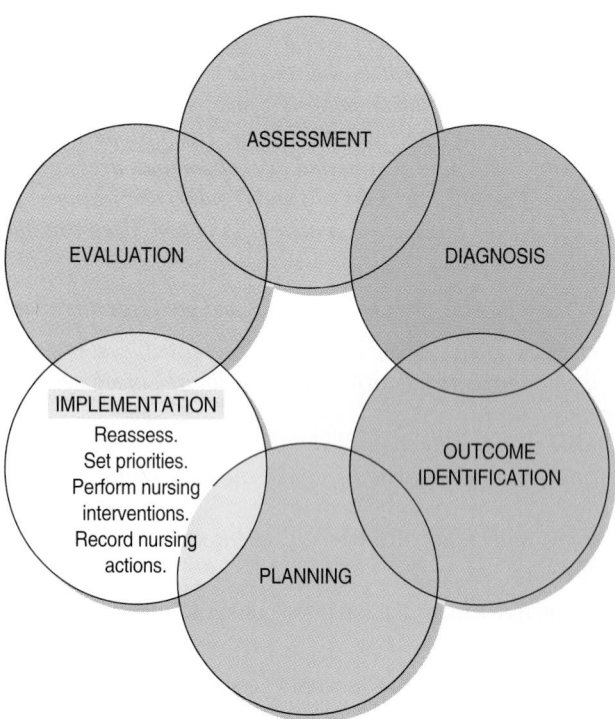

FIGURE 13-1   ANA Standard V states: The nurse implements the interventions identified in the plan of care. This illustration shows activities nurses use in the implementation phase and the relationship of implementation to the other phases of the nursing process.

Implementation Skills

Intellectual Skills

The intellectual skills used in implementation include problem solving, decision making, and teaching. To solve problems, nurses ask clients pertinent questions, discuss alternatives, and are open to new ideas. To enrich the decision-making abilities of clients, nurses give them opportunities to choose which treatments are performed, when, and in what sequence. Teaching requires knowledge about teaching–learning principles and information to convey.

Interpersonal Skills

The ability to work with others to accomplish goals is critical to nursing. Nurses use communication skills to carry out planned nursing interventions. Skill at verbal and nonverbal communication is refined through practice. Chapter 21 gives more details on communication.

Technical Skills

Technical skills are used to carry out treatments and procedures. Nurses learn the specific skills through clinical practice. Technical competence means being able to use equipment, machines, and supplies in a particular specialty. For example, nurses working in delivery rooms must be familiar with fetal monitoring, positioning on the delivery-room table, and neonatal resuscitation devices. On the other hand, nurses working on medical units may need technical competence in using hypothermia blankets, therapeutic beds, or feeding pumps. Home health nurses must be familiar with adaptive equipment, client-controlled analgesia pumps, and wound dressing supplies. Nurses also use technical skills to retrieve and record client information on a computer.

Implementation Activities

Reassess

During each encounter with clients, nurses assess function, ensuring prompt attention to emerging problems. Because a client's condition can change quickly and dramatically, astute nurses remain alert to subtle cues and inferences. For example, the client who is experiencing pain may become quiet and withdraw from external stimuli. Recognizing such a change, nurses can intervene, validate, and assist the client to become more comfortable. A client who is demanding and irritable may be masking anxiety about a surgical procedure or fear about the results of a diagnostic test. As they initiate the nursing plan of care, nurses must ensure that the planned interventions are still relevant.

Set Priorities

Because a person's condition changes, priorities also may change. Priorities are based on information collected during reassessment. When setting priorities, nurses rank nursing problems in order of importance based on several factors (Fig. 13-2):

- The client's condition
- New information from reassessment

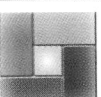

Nursing Research and Critical Thinking
How Does the Use of a Decision Tree Affect the Accuracy of Decision Making for Chronic Wound Care?

Nurses working with chronic wound care implement a nursing intervention that requires complex decision making. The decision–analysis process can be broken down into its component parts and the parts recombined to formulate a logical, temporal, and tangible sequence reflective of the whole. The result is often represented as a flowchart or decision tree that captures key points where a choice must be made from a number of available options. Two nurses designed a descriptive, comparative, replication study to examine the use of a decision tree and its impact on the accuracy of decision making for chronic wound care. Data were collected from two groups of home care nurses in two large, urban settings. One group was measured after initial contact with the decision tree, and the other group was measured 2 years after implementation of the decision tree. The evaluation instrument consisted of the Chronic Wound Management Decision Tree (CWMDT) in combination with pictorial case studies. The main outcome measure of interest was the accuracy and confidence of decision making in wound-care staging and treatment. The researchers found that the accuracy of decision making with the use of the CWMDT improved over time, as did accuracy of decision making after initial contact with the decision tree. Age, experience in nursing and home care, number of in-service sessions attended, and number of chronic wounds treated were not found to correlate with accuracy of decision making.

Critical Thinking Considerations. The reliability of the CWMDT may have an impact on the accuracy of decision making. Content validity has been established for the instrument; interuser and intrauser reliability have not been tested. Implications of this study are as follows:

- Although the use of the CWMDT increased the accuracy of decision making when managing clients with chronic wounds, the instrument did not lead to error-free decision making.
- Further investigation is needed to determine which decision tree, under what conditions and by whom, should be used in clinical practice.

From Letourneau, S. & Jensen, L. (1998). Impact of a decision tree on chronic wound care. *Journal of the Wound, Ostomy, and Continence Nurses Society, 25*(5), 240–247.

- Time and resources available for nursing interventions
- Feedback from the client, family, and healthcare staff
- The nurse's experience in assessing situations and setting priorities

A priority problem requires a nursing intervention before another problem is addressed, but setting priorities does not entail skipping any interventions. Setting priorities affects only the order in which nursing interventions are carried out.

Priorities can be set every few minutes, hourly, daily, weekly, or for longer periods. For example, in the critical care unit, priorities may need to be set every few minutes for an unstable client with multiple trauma. Usually maintaining a patent airway, breathing, and circulation (the ABCs) are top priorities for these clients. Priorities for home care clients may be set for much longer periods. For example, a priority over time may be fostering independent transferring from bed to chair or independent ambulation to the bathroom.

Perform Nursing Interventions

Nurses (or designees) carry out the nursing interventions listed on the nursing plan of care. If a nurse is caring for several clients, he or she develops a schedule so that all clients are cared for in a timely fashion.

Intervention for Collaborative Problems. Nurses manage collaborative problems using both nurse- and physician-prescribed interventions to reduce risk of complications (Carpenito, 2002). Nursing diagnoses are determined, in part, when nurses ask, "Is this a problem that a nurse can legally treat without an order from a physician?" Interventions based on such diagnoses are nurse-prescribed actions. When nurses cannot legally make treatment decisions but have to follow physician's orders, the action is physician prescribed. Both types of interventions involve nursing judgment, because both require legal mandates. The problem is a collaborative problem (Alfaro-LeFevre, 2001) when nurses use both nurse-prescribed and physician-prescribed interventions to give nursing care. For instance, the physician prescribes pain medication, but the nurse sometimes makes decisions as to when the medication is given. The nurse also may use alternative methods for pain relief.

Record Actions

After carrying out nursing interventions, nurses record them in the client's health record. Each institution determines the specific requirements for documentation and should prepare written guidelines for the use of all forms. Chapter 15 discusses the recording of information.

Types of Nursing Interventions

The nursing interventions classification (NIC) assists in defining the role of the professional nurse by listing direct and indirect treatments performed within the nursing role. Similar to

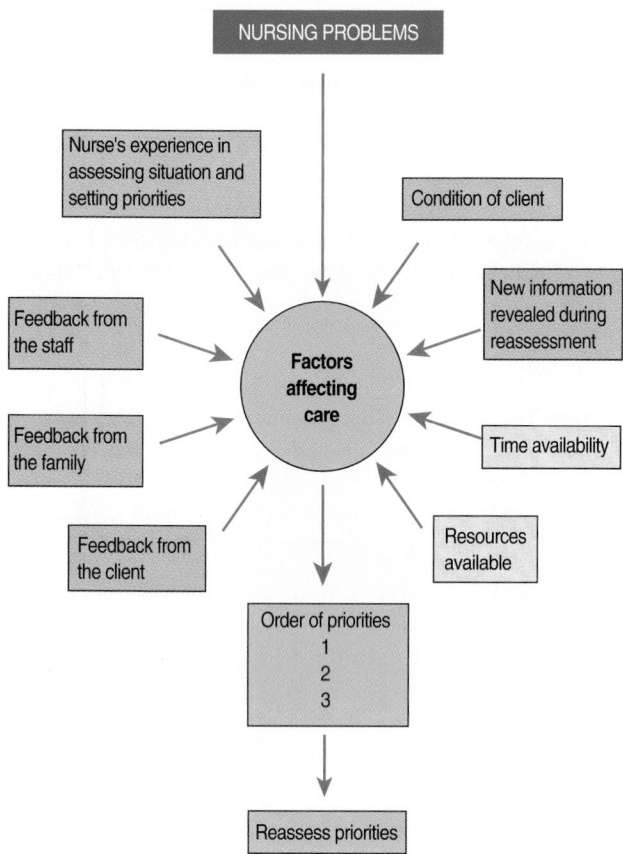

FIGURE 13-2   Nurses set priorities (position of prominence) by considering factors that affect care.

the nursing diagnoses taxonomy of the North American Nursing Diagnosis Association (NANDA), the NIC provides a label or name for each intervention, a definition of the intervention, and a set of defining activities or actions that a nurse performs to implement the intervention (McCloskey & Bulechek, 1996, 2000). The NIC is in its early stages, and interventions will continue to be added and refined.

Possible advantages of the NIC include the following (McCloskey & Bulechek, 1992, 1996, 2000):

- Creation of a standardized language that promotes better understanding and communication of nursing interventions
- Expansion of knowledge about similarities and differences across nursing diagnoses
- Exploration of nursing care information systems
- Assistance in determining cost of services that nurses provide
- Demonstration of the impact nurses have within the healthcare system

Nursing interventions fall within three major categories: those using cognitive skills, those using interpersonal skills, and those using technical skills (Table 13-1). Selection of the type of nursing intervention to be used in client situations depends on the client's dysfunction and functional requirements.

Cognitive Interventions

Educational Interventions.   Nurses carry out educational nursing interventions by applying general principles about the teaching and learning process. They develop teaching plans and provide instruction about health promotion or specific healthcare problems and their management. The ability to teach clients requires knowledge of normal anatomy and physiology, usual patterns of client response to health changes, and pathophysiology of the disease process. A careful assessment of the client yields information about his or her level of motivation, level of knowledge, willingness to follow the health regimen, and physical and psychological abilities to carry out the plan. See Chapter 22 for more information on client education.

Once a nurse is aware of the client's readiness for learning, he or she can implement outcome-based teaching plans, using instruction methods that optimize successful outcomes.

Supervisory Interventions.   The term *supervisory interventions* is applied in the context of overseeing a client's overall care (American Nurses Association, 1996). Supervisory nursing interventions include ensuring that other members of the nursing team carry out specified aspects of the plan of care, and that those involved with the client or family show return demonstration of skills. Supervision of nursing team members requires in-depth knowledge of the job descriptions and capabilities of each person on the team. Nurses may delegate specific aspects of care to nonprofessional staff, but registered nurses are held accountable for selecting appropriate nursing care measures for these personnel to perform. Registered nurses cannot delegate "nursing activities that include the core of the nursing process (assessment, diagnosis, planning, and evaluation) and require specialized knowledge, judgment, and/or skill" to unlicensed assistive personnel (UAP) (ANA, 1996). Nurses also maintain responsibility to ensure that nursing care measures have been carried out correctly. Important information about the client's response to the care is communicated verbally and in written form to the nurse responsible for the client.

Supervising the client or family in skill performance is essential to provide encouragement, give feedback about correct and incorrect performance, and facilitate introduction of new skills to be learned. Clients and their families often are unfamiliar with nursing care regimens, equipment, and supplies. They need ample opportunity to carry out interventions under supervision. Nurses include clients and family members in planning and implementing initial care. They help clients and families begin to assume responsibility for self-management. Skills are built with practice. Doing an activity once usually is not sufficient for a client or family member to achieve proficiency.

Interpersonal Interventions

Coordinating Interventions.   Coordinating client activities serves many purposes. Coordination involves acting as a client advocate, making referrals for follow-up care, collaborating with other healthcare team members, and ensuring that the client's schedule is therapeutic.

TABLE 13-1

Types of Nursing Interventions		
Cognitive	**Interpersonal**	**Technical**
Teach/educate.	Coordinate activities.	Provide basic hygiene, skin care.
Relate knowledge to activities of daily living (ADLs).	Provide caregiving.	Perform routine nursing activities.
Provide feedback.	Use therapeutic communication.	Detect change from baseline data.
Create strategies for clients with dysfunctional communication.	Provide a personal presence.	Reorganize abnormal responses.
Supervise nursing team.	Set limits.	Provide independent and dependent treatment.
Supervise client in performance.	Provide opportunity to examine values and attitudes.	Assist with ADLs.
Supervise family in performance.	Explore and legitimize feelings.	Provide appropriate sensory stimulation.
Alter the environment as needed.	Provide spiritual support.	Mobilize equipment.
	Use humor.	Maintain equipment.
	Provide individual therapy.	Use special abilities or talents.
	Provide group therapy.	
	Become client's advocate.	
	Support client and family plans.	
	Make referrals for follow-up.	
	Serve as a role model.	

For some clients, speaking for the client or encouraging the client to ask questions fulfills the advocacy role. For example, a client may need help in refusing a suggested treatment or requesting a second opinion about surgery. In the advocacy role, the nurse presents the client's point of view and suggests ways in which the client's requests can be met.

Nurses are in a position to know what type of nursing follow-up clients need. They make referrals to home health agencies, visiting nurse associations, or other healthcare providers to facilitate return of optimal function. Many self-help groups and community services are available to provide assistance to clients with health-related problems; creativity in matching clients with these services can help ensure continued monitoring of the client's health status, minimizing the risk for relapses.

Supportive Interventions. Supportive nursing interventions emphasize use of communication skills, relief of spiritual distress, and caring behaviors. A combination of good communication and caring provides comfort and promotes a healthy response to health problems. Being supportive means recognizing the need for encouragement, unconditional acceptance of behaviors, and the positive effects of "being there" for clients during stress or crises. For example, the nurse may sit with a client who is anxious, listen to a client's experience grieving for the loss of a loved one, or touch the forehead of a client with a spinal-cord injury. Such interventions are called "therapeutic use of self."

Nurses provide spiritual support by giving clients time to carry out religious practices, meditate, or read. Respecting the client's privacy during these times conveys acceptance and understanding. If the client wants to talk, the nurse listens to assess spiritual distress without being judgmental. If the

client asks for a spiritual support person, the nurse contacts the client's minister, rabbi, or priest or the hospital chaplain.

Psychosocial Interventions. Psychosocial nursing interventions focus on resolving emotional, psychological, or social problems. Humor, individual or group therapy, role-modeling social skills, and exploring feelings are all ways of carrying out psychosocial nursing interventions.

Some clients and families respond to stress by joking, teasing, or laughing about it. They may use humor as a way to relieve stress and to give clients examples of difficult situations and ways to resolve them. Always use humor judiciously, recognizing underlying themes or deeper problems. A client may say jokingly, "Gee, my arm must be target practice for everyone learning how to draw blood." Pick up on this cue and find out how many times the client has been "stuck," determine why there was such a problem, and instruct the client to speak up and request special consideration for future blood-drawing attempts.

Providing individual and group therapy is the nurse's responsibility in various settings. Individual therapy, used as a means of resolving psychological problems, usually requires additional training or certification. Group therapy is often used to provide support and guidance for clients and their support people with similar needs or problems. Recognizing the need for individual or group therapy, nurses make referrals to healthcare providers with the required expertise. In some settings, nurses hold group meetings with families of Alzheimer's clients or families of children with cancer. Most group therapy sessions have a stated purpose and schedule of activities. Group members rely on their own experiences and gain new ways of dealing with problems from others who have experienced the same problems. The nurse therapist serves as the group facilitator and assists group members to share feelings, advice, and helpful hints with one another.

Sometimes a group member can offer a suggestion that would be unacceptable to the person if made by a healthcare professional. For example, in a group for spouses of Alzheimer's clients, one wife reports that her husband continues to drive even though he admits that he often gets lost and cannot remember the way home. Another group member simply says, "Take the keys away! I don't want to be on the street with him." The wife accepts this blunt advice and follows it. She had previously refused this advice from the therapist because she said driving was her husband's only pleasure; she did not want to rob him of this last piece of independence.

The role-modeling of social skills is used for clients who have not acquired them because of lack of exposure or lengthy illness. In some long-term care settings, clients have grown to depend on the staff to make all their decisions. In other cases, clients have never practiced acceptable social behaviors. Treating clients with respect and using appropriate language and social behaviors (e.g., saying "please" and "thank you" and not interrupting) can help such clients to become socially adept.

Exploring feelings is a way to provide psychosocial intervention. Many clients with chronic or life-threatening illnesses need an opportunity to express their feelings in a nonjudgmental setting. Nurses are in a prime position to help these clients ventilate their feelings and relieve fears and anxiety.

Technical Interventions

Maintenance Interventions. Maintenance nursing interventions help clients retain a certain state of health, preventing deterioration of physical or psychological functioning and preserving independence. Maintenance interventions include basic hygiene, skin care, and other routine nursing activities. Maintenance nursing interventions are sometimes undervalued or considered insignificant, but they allow clients to preserve function and reduce the chance of developing complications.

Surveillance Interventions. Surveillance nursing interventions include detecting changes from baseline data and recognizing abnormal responses. This activity also can be categorized as observation, inspection, or vigilance. Nurses rely on the senses to detect changes: observing the appearance and characteristics of clients; hearing by auscultation, pitch, and tone; detecting odors and comparing them with past experience and knowledge of specific problems; and using touch to assess body temperature, skin condition, clamminess, or diaphoresis. Nurses use all these surveillance activities to determine the current status of clients and changes from previous states. Nurses often detect subtle changes in a client's condition and communicate them to the physician to minimize problems. Expert nurse clinicians develop skill in detecting and preventing complications and usually receive positive feedback for their accurate and

timely interventions based on this "sense" of "something being wrong."

Psychomotor Intervention. Psychomotor nursing interventions—those requiring technical expertise—include inserting, removing, changing, applying, administering, cleansing, or any other activity that requires a psychomotor action. The management and care of equipment, supplies, treatments, and procedures also falls into this category of nursing interventions. Nurses gain technical competence through practice.

Functional Approach to Implementation

When thinking about implementation, consider the overall perspective of nursing. With a functional approach, nursing tries to maximize a client's functional status and resolve dysfunction. With each client encounter, nurses reassess function, revise care when needed, and evaluate the client's response. By focusing on areas of strength or healthy functioning, nurses can optimize interventions to help clients reach their healthiest states.

EVALUATION

Evaluation, the sixth phase of the nursing process, follows implementation of the nursing plan of care. **Evaluation** is defined as the judgment of the effectiveness of nursing care to meet client goals based on the client's behavioral responses. This phase involves a thorough, systematic review of the effectiveness of nursing interventions and a determination of client goal achievement. Nurses use a variety of skills to judge the effectiveness of nursing care. These skills include knowledge of standards of care, normal client responses, and conceptual models and theories of nursing; ability to monitor the effectiveness of nursing interventions; and awareness of clinical research. Critical appraisal of goal attainment is determined jointly by the nurse and client.

Although a separate and distinct phase, evaluation also is ongoing throughout the nursing process (Alfaro-LeFevre, 2001). Judgments made in previous phases usually result in prompt reassessment, rediagnosis, and replanning (Yura & Walsh, 1988). Nurses continually assess responses of clients to particular nursing interventions, establish different priorities for nursing diagnoses, and alter nursing plans of care as necessary. An in-depth, comprehensive judgment about goal attainment is performed only during the evaluation phase of the nursing process (Yura & Walsh, 1988).

The nursing plan of care is the foundation for evaluation. The identified nursing diagnoses, client goals, outcome criteria, and nursing interventions are the guides. Through this process, nurses determine the appropriateness, accuracy, and relevance of these nursing care components. Evaluation also helps nurses discover any errors that may have occurred in previous steps of the nursing process. Nurses always consider evaluation in light of how the client responded or reacted to the planned course of action (Yura & Walsh, 1988). Figure 13-3 illustrates the relationship of the activities of the evaluation phase to the other phases of the nursing process.

There are several purposes for carrying out evaluation:

- To collect subjective and objective data to make judgments about nursing care delivered
- To examine the client's behavioral responses to nursing interventions
- To compare the client's behavioral responses with predetermined outcome criteria
- To appraise the extent to which client goals were attained or problems resolved
- To appraise involvement and collaboration of the client, family members, nurses, and healthcare team members in healthcare decisions
- To provide a basis for the revision of the nursing plan of care evaluation
- To monitor the quality of nursing care and its effect on the client's health status (Yura & Walsh, 1988; Alfaro-LeFevre, 2001; Carpenito, 2002)

Specific activities during this phase include the following:

- Reviewing client goals and outcome criteria
- Collecting data
- Measuring goal attainment
- Recording judgments or measurements of goal attainment
- Revising or modifying the nursing plan of care

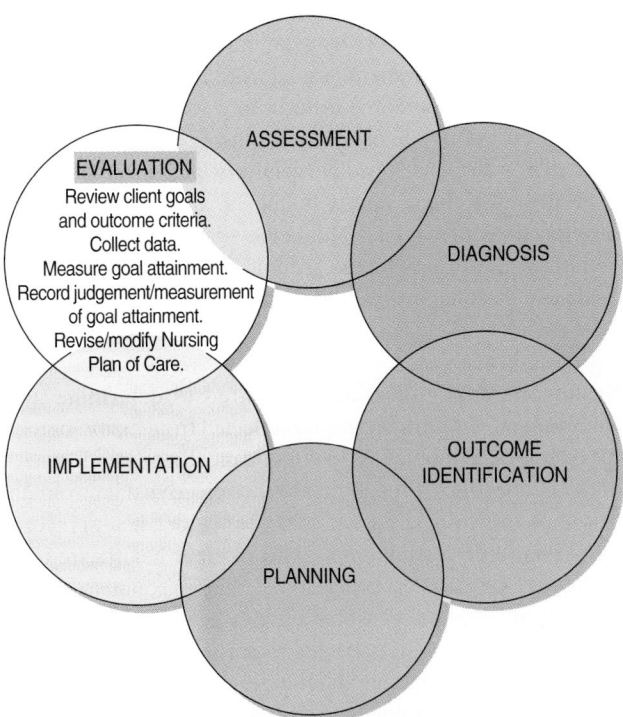

FIGURE 13-3 ANA Standard VI states: The nurse evaluates the client's progress toward attainment of outcomes. This illustration shows activities used in the evaluation phase and also the relationship of evaluation to the other phases of the nursing process.

Evaluation Skills

Knowledge of Standards of Care

Standards of care are authoritative statements made by nursing organizations (e.g., American Association of Neuroscience Nurses), external review boards (e.g., Joint Commission on the Accreditation of Healthcare Organizations [JCAHO], 1996), or healthcare institutions (e.g., your employer) that describe the responsibilities of the nursing profession, against which its practitioners are held accountable (American Nurses Association, 1998). Knowledge about the current standards of care proposed by nursing organizations, external review boards, and one's own healthcare institution (e.g., policies and procedures) is necessary to evaluate nursing care. Standards of care guide professional practice and serve as the framework for the evaluation of practice (American Nurses Association, 1998). See the section in this chapter on quality improvement programs for a discussion of these standards.

Knowledge of Normal Client Response

The nurse's knowledge of many subjects, such as physiology, pathophysiology, biochemistry, psychology, sociology, and pharmacology, comes into play when evaluating normal client responses. Nurses obtain a tremendous knowledge base about client responses during their basic nursing education. They acquire additional knowledge and updating of information through formal and informal continuing education. Obtaining college credits in nursing is an example of formal continuing education. Attendance at nursing conferences and seminars is an example of informal continuing education. Nurses also sharpen skills and update knowledge about client responses through clinical experience, guidance and assistance from mentors, and reading textbooks and journal articles.

Knowledge of Conceptual Models and Theories

Conceptual models and theories of nursing provide information that facilitates evaluation of the nursing plan of care. Every conceptual model or theory describes specific goals of action and consequences of those actions that assist in the evaluation of care. Because the conceptual model or theory guides development of client goals and outcome criteria, the goal of action or desired result of a particular conceptual model or theory is revealed in these components of the plan (Meleis, 1997; Fawcett, 2000). If a client's behavioral responses match the client goal statements and client outcome criteria, the conceptual model or theory's goal has been reached. For example, the goal of the Roy Adaptation Model of Nursing is to promote the client's adaptive behavior (Phillips, 2001; Phillips et al., 2001). The consequences of nursing actions lead to effective coping mechanisms, maximal level of functioning, and adaptive responses. For a client undergoing upper abdominal surgery, physiologic adaptive needs may include oxygenation (coughing and deep breathing), protection (preventing wound infection and pneumonia), and activity and exercise (assisting with activities of daily living and ambulation).

Ability to Monitor the Effectiveness of Nursing Interventions

Many intellectual and technical skills are necessary to monitor the effectiveness of nursing interventions. Nurses need interviewing techniques and physical assessment skills to obtain subjective and objective data from clients and their family members. Knowledge of interviewing techniques, such as types of questions, interview phases, and the appropriate environment for interviewing, facilitates the collection of subjective data for evaluation of the nursing plan of care.

Physical and functional assessment skills are necessary to monitor the effectiveness of nursing interventions. The ability to inspect, palpate, percuss, and auscultate proficiently provides objective data about the effectiveness of nursing interventions. For example, if a client has Impaired Gas Exchange related to altered oxygen supply, auscultation of breath sounds will yield information about the effectiveness of nursing interventions.

Knowledge and skill when using measurement devices yield further information about the effectiveness of nursing interventions. Many technologic advances in medicine and nursing make it mandatory for nurses to have knowledge and skill in the use of multiple measurement devices. Nurses use devices such as blood pressure cuffs, thermometers, arterial lines, intracranial pressure monitors, and intravenous pumps frequently, depending on the practice setting. Measurement devices provide objective information for the evaluation of nursing strategies.

Nursing also requires knowledge and skill in interpreting laboratory data. Laboratory studies, such as complete blood counts, arterial blood gas determinations, and routine urinalysis tests, provide data for evaluation of nursing interventions. For example, in the same client with Impaired Gas Exchange related to altered oxygen supply, arterial blood gas measurements help nurses determine oxygenation, respiratory status, metabolic status, and the necessity for suctioning.

Awareness of Clinical Research

The nursing profession uses research findings to develop innovative methods to sharpen assessment and diagnostic skills; establish future standards for developing client goals, client outcomes, and nursing interventions in the planning stage; and provide the latest knowledge to enhance nursing practice. Journal clubs are a way to integrate current research findings into clinical practice; including nurse scientists in these meetings facilitates interaction between clinicians and researchers (Avant, 1994).

Types of Evaluation

Structure Evaluation

Structure evaluation focuses on the attributes of the setting or surroundings where healthcare is provided. It deals with the environmental aspects that directly or indirectly influence the quality of care provided. Availability of equipment, layout of physical facilities, nurse–client ratios, administrative support, and maintenance of nursing staff competence are some areas

of concern for structure evaluation (Ziegler, Vaughan-Wrobel, & Erlen, 1986; Miller, 1989).

Process Evaluation

Process evaluation focuses on the nurse's performance and whether the nursing care provided was appropriate and competent (Ziegler et al., 1986). The phases of the nursing process are used as the framework for the evaluation of nursing care. Areas of concern for this type of evaluation include the type of information obtained by interview and physical assessment, the validity of the nursing diagnostic statements, and the nurse's technical competence.

Outcome Evaluation

Outcome evaluation, which focuses on the client and the client's function, is currently receiving a great deal of emphasis. Outcome evaluation determines the extent to which the client's behavioral response to nursing intervention reflects the desired client goal and outcome criteria (Ziegler et al., 1986). Outcome evaluation can take place only after standards have been developed. An example of an outcome evaluation is to establish standards of care for a specific diagnosis and then compare actual client outcomes with that standard.

Evaluation Activities

Review Client Goals and Outcome Criteria

Measuring goal attainment starts by reviewing the client goals and outcome criteria, written in measurable terms, that were developed for each nursing diagnosis. Nurses review expected client behaviors by examining the time frames and methods for measurement of goal fulfillment. They evaluate client goals and outcome criteria in a variety of ways, including observing client behaviors, using documentation of the client's responses to interventions, and receiving feedback from the client, family members, and other healthcare providers, if appropriate. This review helps nurses focus on data they need to assess the accuracy and realistic nature of the goals and outcome criteria (Alfaro-LeFevre, 2001).

Collect Data

Systematic data collection is required to determine goal achievement. Subjective data are collected from many sources: the client, family members or significant others, nursing staff, and other healthcare team members. Objective data from observation (e.g., posture, skin color, behavior), health records (e.g., laboratory results, reports from other healthcare team members), physical assessment (e.g., breath sounds, strength of extremities), and measurement devices (e.g., blood pressure, temperature) are collected to judge the client's behavioral responses to nursing interventions.

Nurses also use subjective data to evaluate the effectiveness of nursing care provided. For example, a client with a nursing diagnosis of Acute Pain related to a recent surgical procedure may have as a goal, "Client will state that pain is relieved within 10 minutes after repositioning." The client's subjective statement would be needed to judge whether this goal has been achieved. Chapter 24 provides more information on subjective and objective data.

Measure Goal/Outcome Achievement

After collecting data, nurses form a comprehensive picture of the client's behavioral responses to nursing interventions. The next activity is to make a judgment about goal attainment by comparing the client's actual behavioral responses to the predicted responses or predetermined outcome criteria developed in the planning phase. When possible, the client is involved.

The four possible judgments that may be made are as follows (Alfaro-LeFevre, 2001):

- The goal was completely met.
- The goal was partially met.
- The goal was completely unmet.
- New problems or nursing diagnoses have developed.

The fourth judgment can exist simultaneously with any of the first three. Table 13-2 provides some examples of a com-

pletely met goal, a partially met goal, and a completely unmet goal. Once the judgment about the attainment or lack of attainment of the outcome criteria is made, the plan of care is revised. See the section in this chapter on revision and modification of the nursing plan of care.

Assess Facilitators of Goal Attainment. Clients, family members, significant others, and other healthcare team members are invaluable in facilitating or helping with goal attainment. Occasionally, only those closest to the client can identify the subtle or elusive factors that helped (or hindered) goal achievement. Examples of facilitators include audiovisual materials, written handouts, repetition of material, and easily accessible and interested nursing staff.

Assess Barriers to Goal Attainment. Several barriers to goal attainment have been identified. Barriers may involve the client, family members or significant others, and the nurse or other healthcare team members. Examples of how goal attainment may be blocked include providing incorrect information, withholding information, having an unexpected

TABLE 13-2

Clinical Examples of Evaluation of Goal Attainment				
Nursing Diagnosis	**Client Goal**	**Subjective Data Collected**	**Objective Data Collected**	**Goal Judgment**
Impaired Swallowing related to neuromuscular impairment	Client will demonstrate correct eating techniques to maximize swallowing.	Client states, "I sit up in a chair for a half hour after I eat."	Client wears dentures when eating; performs return demonstration of facial exercises; bends head forward when eating; checks mouth for any remaining food particles; remains in Fowler's position for at least 30 minutes after eating; lies on side while lying in bed.	Goal completely met.
Chronic Low Self-Esteem	Client interacts verbally in group therapy session.	Client states, "I feel uncomfortable when speaking in front of others."	Client observed sitting in group session, looking at floor, and participating minimally.	Goal partially met.
Impaired Physical Mobility related to neuromuscular impairment	Client will carry out prescribed mobility regimen.	Client states, "I can't do anything by myself. I need a lot of help with everything."	Client unable to perform active range-of-motion exercises independently; unable to transfer from bed to wheelchair; unable to dress and groom independently.	Goal completely unmet.

reaction to treatment (e.g., allergic response to therapy), possessing inadequate coping ability, and experiencing a worsened underlying pathologic condition.

Family members also may act as barriers to goal achievement in many ways. For example, their lack of understanding of the plan of care, lack of interest in the client, or failure to realize that the client actually has a problem can impede movement toward a goal. The cultural heritage, moral values, and religious influences of a family also can be barriers (Yura & Walsh, 1988).

Nurses may unwittingly block goal achievement, for instance, by neglecting to collect pertinent assessment data, assigning an inappropriate priority rating to nursing diagnoses, or delegating nursing care to inappropriate nursing staff members. Nurses may fail to include clients in the planning step, neglect to incorporate facets of the medical regimen when developing the nursing plan of care, or forget to share critical information with other members of the healthcare team (Yura & Walsh, 1988).

Other healthcare team members also may be barriers. They may lack communication among themselves, be unable to work together as a team, or fail to coordinate the activities of all healthcare team members (Yura & Walsh, 1988). When healthcare team members do not share information among themselves, continuity in the planning and implementation of care is hampered. The evaluation phase identifies the barriers that are interfering with the client's advancement toward goal achievement.

Record Judgment or Measurement of Goal Attainment

Written documentation of the subjective and objective data gathered and the judgment made about goal attainment is required on the client's health record. Judgments about goal attainment are written clearly and concisely. Avoid ambiguous terms, such as "inadequate," "good," or "extremely well," which can be interpreted differently by different people (Ziegler et al., 1986).

Revise or Modify the Nursing Plan of Care

Revision or modification of the nursing plan of care is part of the evaluation phase. It provides a feedback mechanism that starts the entire chain of events again. Figure 13-4 illustrates the feedback mechanism and the cyclic nature of the nursing process, starting with a complete reassessment of the client.

Nursing diagnoses that are resolved require no further nursing intervention and may be removed from the nursing plan of care. To maintain the client's "problem-free status," a nursing plan of care is developed that incorporates potential for wellness and other health-promoting nursing diagnoses and focuses nursing actions toward maximal functioning. The level of functioning and health status changes are periodically reassessed to determine whether new problems or nursing diagnoses have developed.

Some client goals are partially met or completely unmet. Modification begins with a complete client reassessment. Changes in client goals, client outcome criteria, and nursing in-

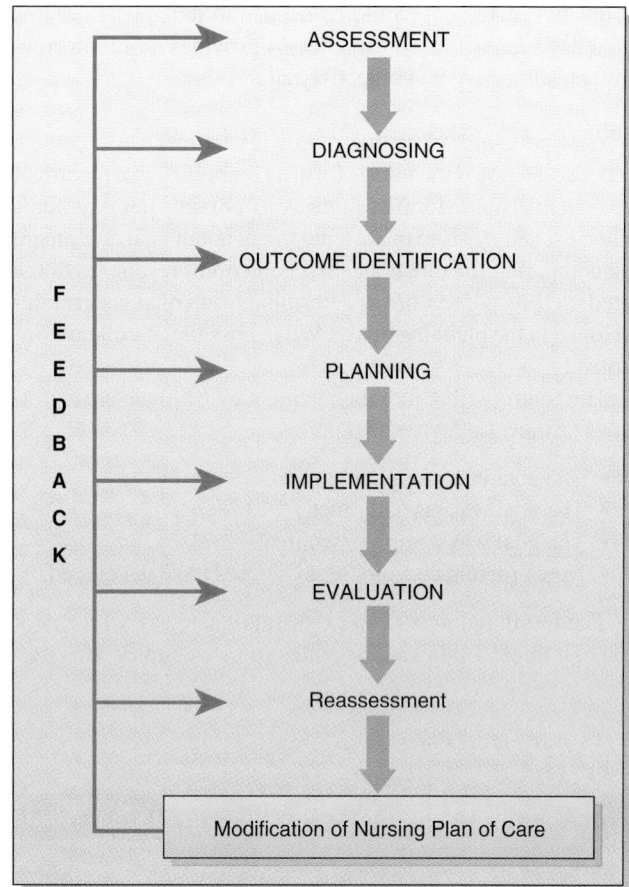

FIGURE 13-4   Feedback mechanism and cyclic nature of the nursing process.

terventions are required. If new problems have arisen, new nursing diagnoses must be identified and a nursing plan of care written. Figure 13-5 illustrates the steps taken after judging goal attainment and needed revisions of the nursing plan of care.

Functional Approach to Evaluation

Evaluation using the functional health approach requires a specific perspective. In addition to measuring attainment of client goals, the client's functional status for each health pattern is established. After implementing the nursing plan of care, the nurse ascertains the client's functional status based on data from the evaluation phase. Subjective and objective data are used to determine the client's movement toward improved function. Evaluation using the functional health approach provides a framework for organizing and evaluating data for revision or modification of the nursing plan of care.

QUALITY IMPROVEMENT PROGRAMS

Evaluation can also focus on the quality of nursing care provided to groups of clients with similar problems or nursing diagnoses. **Quality improvement programs** are mechanisms

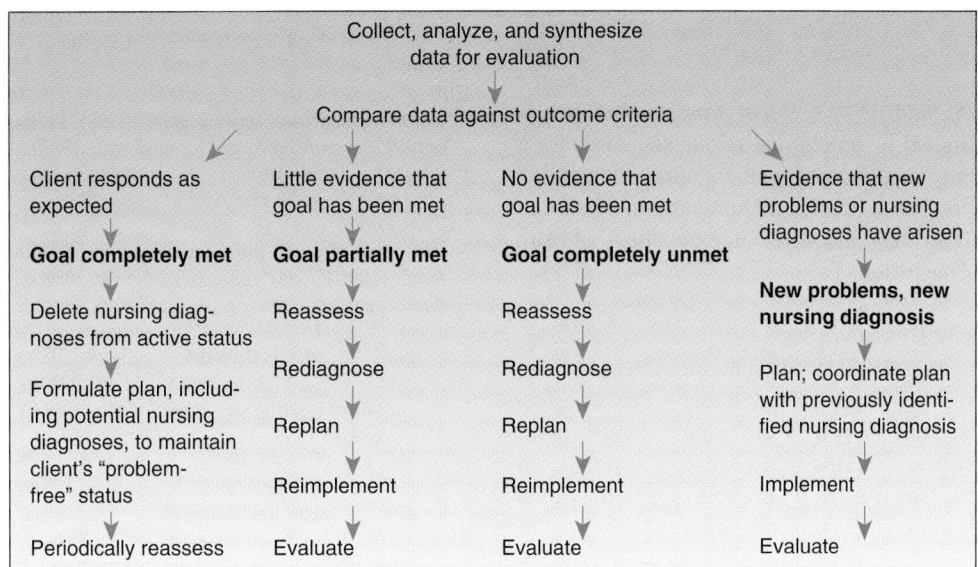

FIGURE 13-5   Flowchart to identify actions taken after judgment of goal achievement.

for healthcare organizations to assess and improve care (Ellis & Hartley, 2000). Formerly called quality assurance monitors, total quality management (TQM), total quality improvement (TQI), or continuous quality improvement (CQI), these programs ensure that quality client care is provided and standards are upheld. They provide input for the development and refinement of standards of care for groups of similar clients. Standards provide the basis for quality monitors "because they are statements of accountability and define requirements for quality nursing care" (Moriconi, 1989, p. 176).

Quality improvement involves measuring the extent to which standards have been achieved. Focus on quality improvement is the combined result of consumers' demands for high-caliber health services and soaring healthcare costs. Also, governmental agencies, accreditation groups, and regulatory bodies have pressured the nursing profession to respond to quality improvement issues. Standards of care have been proposed by ANA, JCAHO, specialty nursing organizations (e.g., Association of Rehabilitation Nurses, American Association of Spinal Cord Injury Nurses), and individual healthcare institutions.

American Nurses Association

The ANA first established the *Standards of Nursing Practice* in 1973; these were updated in 1998 with the second edition of *Standards of Clinical Nursing Practice,* which included "standards of care" and "standards of professional performance." Based on a nursing process framework, "standards of care" are composed of seven nursing standards for providing nursing care to all clients. The behaviors and roles of professional nurses are described in the eight "standards of professional performance." Both sets of standards include measurement criteria for evaluating nursing care and performance.

Some specialty nursing groups, in conjunction with the ANA, have developed processes and outcome criteria for a number of nursing diagnoses. For example, the Association of Rehabilitation Nurses and the American Association of Neuroscience Nurses have set standards based on nursing diagnoses applied to their specialty.

Joint Commission on Accreditation of Healthcare Organizations

The JCAHO (1996) is an external review board that establishes standards for institutions to ensure that the institution functions within specified guidelines. The hospital standards for nursing care are applicable to all clients in every setting where nursing care is provided. Recent changes in the JCAHO guidelines require the continuous monitoring and evaluation of the quality of nursing care provided by the department of nursing. The guidelines are general, and each institution develops a specific quality improvement program suited to its organizational structure.

Peer Review

Peer review is the evaluation and judgment of a nurse's performance by other nurses. It is another mechanism for evaluating and monitoring the nursing care that is provided. The two types of peer review are nursing monitors and individual peer review.

Nursing Monitors

The **nursing monitor,** previously called a nursing audit, is "a review, by a nurse, of the client's care or records to determine the extent to which that care or records meet established standards" (Yura & Walsh, 1988, p. 177). Nursing monitoring committees usually establish the "standards against which their observations will be measured" (Yura & Walsh, 1988, p. 178). Although nursing departments develop their own standards for particular nursing care settings, the ANA's (1998) *Standards of Clinical Nursing Practice* is often used as a model in generating unique standards for a particular setting or institution. Members of the monitoring committee may review a nurse's documentation of care in the health record, or they may determine the client's health status through observation.

Individual Peer Review

The second type of peer review is individual peer review, which focuses on the nurse. An individual nurse's performance is evaluated and judged by other nurses with similar education and experience. This type of review also is based on preestablished standards (Kelly & Joel, 1999). Individual peer review adds to nurse monitoring data.

KEY CONCEPTS

- Nurse-prescribed actions are based on client interventions that nurses can legally perform without a physician's order. Collaborative problems are those in which nurses use both physician-prescribed and nurse-prescribed interventions to give care.
- Implementing the nursing plan of care requires intellectual, interpersonal, and technical skills.
- Evaluation is a judgmental process for determining the effectiveness of nursing interventions to meet client goals. It occurs throughout all steps of the nursing process but also is a distinct, separate step.
- An in-depth, comprehensive judgment about client goal attainment and fulfillment is performed during the evaluation step of the nursing process.
- The nursing plan of care forms the foundation for evaluation. The nurse and client determine goal attainment.
- The nurse, client, family members, significant others, and other healthcare team members may help or hinder goal attainment.
- Revising the nursing plan of care involves reassessment, rediagnosis, and replanning.
- Evaluation determines the reasons why the nursing plan of care was a success or failure.
- Quality improvement involves the monitoring and evaluating of nursing care against standards of nursing practice.

REFERENCES

Alfaro-LeFevre, R. (2001). *Applying nursing process: A step-by-step guide* (5th ed.). Philadelphia: Lippincott Williams & Wilkins.

American Nurses Association. (1973). *Standards of nursing practice.* Kansas City, MO: Author.

American Nurses Association. (1996). *Registered professional nurses and unlicensed assistive personnel.* Washington, DC: Author.

American Nurses Association. (1998). *Standards of clinical nursing practice* (2nd ed.). Washington, DC: Author.

Avant, K. C. (1994). The link of theory to practice. In R. M. Carroll-Johnson & M. Paquette (Eds.), *Classification of nursing diagnoses: Proceedings of the tenth conference* (pp. 11–16). Philadelphia: J. B. Lippincott.

Carpenito, L. J. (2002). *Nursing diagnosis: Application to clinical practice* (10th ed.). Philadelphia: Lippincott Williams & Wilkins.

Ellis, J. R., & Hartley, C. L. (2000). *Nursing in today's world: Challenges, issues, and trends* (7th ed.). Philadelphia: Lippincott Williams & Wilkins.

Fawcett, J. (2000). *Analysis and evaluation of contemporary nursing knowledge: Nursing models and theories.* Philadelphia: F. A. Davis.

Joint Commission on the Accreditation of Healthcare Organizations. (1996). *Comprehensive accreditation manual for hospitals: The official handbook.* Oakbrook Terrace, IL: Author.

Kelly, L. Y., & Joel, L. A. (1999). *Dimensions of professional nursing* (8th ed.). New York: McGraw-Hill.

McCloskey, J. C., & Bulechek, G. M. (1992). *Iowa Interventions Project nursing interventions classification (NIC).* St. Louis, MO: Mosby.

McCloskey, J. C., & Bulechek, G. M. (Eds.) (1996). *Nursing interventions classification (NIC)* (2nd ed.). St. Louis, MO: Mosby–Year Book.

McCloskey, J. C., & Bulechek, G. M. (2000). *Nursing interventions: Effective nursing treatments* (3rd ed.). Philadelphia: W. B. Saunders.

Meleis, A. I. (1997). *Theoretical nursing: Development and progress* (3rd ed.). Philadelphia: Lippincott-Raven.

Miller, E. (1989). *How to make nursing diagnosis work: Administrative and clinical strategies.* Norwalk, CT: Appleton & Lange.

Moriconi, D. (1989). Quality assurance in diagnosis-based nursing practice. In E. Miller (Ed.), *How to make nursing diagnosis work: Administrative and clinical strategies.* Norwalk, CT: Appleton & Lange.

Phillips, K. D. (2001). Roy's adaptation model in nursing practice. In M. R. Alligood & A. Marriner-Tomey (Eds.), *Nursing theory: Utilization and application* (2nd ed.). St. Louis, MO: Mosby–Year Book.

Phillips, K. D., Blue, C. L., Brubaker, K. M., Fine, J. M. B., Kirsch, M. J., Papazian, K. R., Reister, C. M., & Sobiech, M. A. (2001). Sister Callista Roy: Adaptation model. In A. M. Tomey & M. R. Alligood (Eds.), *Nursing theorists and their work* (5th ed.). St. Louis, MO: Mosby–Year Book.

Yura, H., & Walsh, M. B. (1988). *The nursing process: Assessing, planning, implementing, evaluating* (5th ed.). Norwalk, CT: Appleton & Lange.

Ziegler, S. M., Vaughan-Wrobel, B. C., & Erlen, J. A. (1986). *Nursing process, nursing diagnosis, nursing knowledge: Avenues to autonomy.* Norwalk, CT: Appleton-Century Crofts.

BIBLIOGRAPHY

Braunstein, M. S. (1998). Evaluation of nursing practice: Process and critique. *Nursing Science Quarterly, 11*(2), 64–68.

Chance, K. S. (1997). The quest for quality: An exploration of attempts to define and measure quality nursing care [original article condensed for republication, including commentary by Hempsall, K. L., Hughes, L., Woodruff, D., & Maas, M. L.]. *Image: Journal of Nursing Scholarship, 29,* 326–331.

Gordon, M., Murphy, C. P., Candee, D., & Hiltunen, E. (1994). Clinical judgment: An integrated model. *ANS Advances in Nursing Science 16*(4), 55–70.

Johnson, M., & Maas, M. L. (Eds.). (1997). *Nursing outcomes classification (NOC).* St. Louis, MO: Mosby–Year Book.

Johnson, M., Maas, M. L., & Moorhead, S. (2000). *Nursing outcomes classification* (2nd ed.). St. Louis, MO: Mosby.

Maas, M. L. (1997). Nursing-sensitive outcomes classification (NOC): Completing the essential comprehensive languages for nursing. In M. J. Rantz and P. LeMone (Eds.), *Classification of nursing diagnoses: Proceedings of the twelfth conference, North American Nursing Diagnosis Association* (pp. 40–47). Glendale, CA: Cumulative Index to Nursing and Allied Health Literature (CINAHL) Information Systems.

McCloskey, J. C., & Bulechek, G. M. (1994). Standardizing the language for nursing treatments: An overview of the issues. *Nursing Outlook, 42,* 56–63.

Micek, W. T., Berry, L., Gilski, D., Kallenbach, A., Link, D., & Scharer, K. (1996). Patient outcomes: The link between nursing diagnoses and interventions. *Journal of Nursing Administration, 26*(11), 29–35.

Mitchell, P. H., Ferketich, S., Jennings, B. M., American Academy of Nursing Expert Panel on Quality Health Care. (1998).

Quality health outcomes model. *Image: Journal of Nursing Scholarship, 30,* 43–46.

Prowse, M. A., & Lyne, P. A. (2000). Revealing the contribution of bioscience-based nursing knowledge to clinically effective patient care. *Clinical Effectiveness in Nursing, 4*(2), 67–74.

Prowse, M. A., & Lyne, P. A. (2000). Clinical effectiveness in the post-anaesthesia care unit: How nursing knowledge contributes to achieving intended patient outcomes. *Journal of Advanced Nursing, 31*(5), 1115–1124.

Tripp-Reiner, T. (1999). Cultural interventions for ethnic groups of color. In A. S. Hinshaw, S. L. Feetham, & J. L. F. Shaver (Eds.), *Handbook of clinical nursing research* (pp. 107–120). Thousand Oaks, CA: Sage.

14 Critical Thinking

Key Terms

advanced beginner
clinical experience
clinical reasoning
commitment
competence
connected knowing
critical thinking
diagnostic reasoning
dualism
expert
intellectual development
knowledge base

learning styles
multiplicity
novice
nursing judgment
procedural knowledge
proficient
received knowledge
reflection
relativism
search for meaning
silence

Learning Objectives

Upon completion of this chapter, the student will be able to do the following:
1. Identify major factors that affect learning.
2. Explain how critical thinking is used in nursing.
3. Enhance awareness of definitions, behaviors, and standards used in critical thinking.
4. Understand the relationships between knowledge, experience, critical thinking, reflection, clinical reasoning, and nursing judgment.
5. Explore ways to enhance and develop critical thinking skills, especially as they apply to nursing.

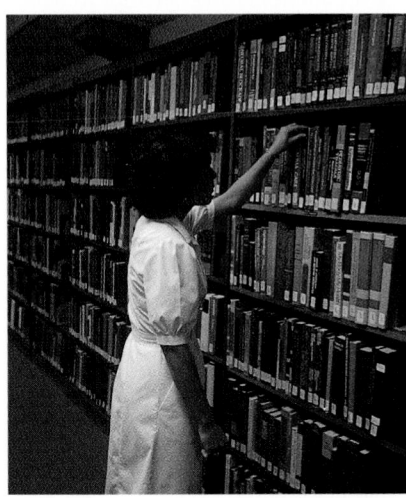

Critical Thinking Challenge

You are a nursing student beginning your clinical nursing program. The nursing courses are different than those you have taken previously, and you are finding it difficult to know how to study. This week will be your first time taking care of a client at a nursing home. You receive your assignment and find you will be caring for an older man who has heart disease. He has five other medical problems and takes 10 medications. His care plan includes 12 nursing diagnoses. Your previous experience with nursing homes is limited, and most of what you have heard and read about them is negative.

This situation is one that nursing students commonly encounter. Although some details may differ, most beginning students worry about being capable of handling clinical situations with a limited knowledge base and little experience. This chapter, other courses you are taking, your life experiences, and later chapters in this text will help you build a solid foundation for learning.

Once you have completed this chapter, review this scenario and reflect on the following:

1. What factors influence your ability to think critically about this client?
2. How do your existing knowledge base and experience influence your ability to make nursing judgments?
3. How can you use critical thinking as you prepare for his care?
4. How do you use critical thinking and clinical reasoning to make nursing judgments as you care for him in the nursing home?
5. What role does reflection have about this client's care in the nursing home?

Beginning students may believe that "nurse-thinking" is a totally new skill to learn. Approached as a new skill, critical thinking may appear overwhelming. Viewing it this way though ignores a person's existing thinking skills. In reality, people save time and energy by building on their existing skills.

This chapter defines and explains critical thinking concepts within the nursing context. A conceptual model illustrates how critical thinking, reflection, and clinical reasoning lead to nursing judgment. The chapter provides an opportunity for learning how to develop further critical thinking skills. Students can take the critical thinking information in this chapter and integrate it with what they already know.

IMPORTANCE OF CRITICAL THINKING IN NURSING

The enormous amount of information available in healthcare changes continually. Simple memorization-style thinking is insufficient to complement the nurse's tasks of sorting, organizing, and identifying relevant information for efficient, effective use. The growing complexity of healthcare demands the use of critical thinking for effective, creative, and efficient nursing care.

Critical thinking helps nurses to choose solutions or identify options for client care situations. The focus of nursing care may be on individuals, families, or communities as the client. Nurses are required to think critically in all settings including home, school, ambulatory care, critical care units, and community centers. Nurses must work from a broad knowledge base then individualize care for each client and setting. A nurse's ability to think critically will be one of his or her most important skills.

CONCEPTUAL DEVELOPMENT OF CRITICAL THINKING

Dictionaries describe *thinking* as a mental activity in which a person forms thoughts in the mind, forms intentions, determines by reflection, or attains clear ideas (*American Heritage College Dictionary,* 1993). *Critical* is defined as a turning point or an especially important juncture (*American Heritage College Dictionary,* 1993). It is the point at which a definite change is made. Critical thinking, then, assumes a turning point because of a thought process.

The term *critical thinking* is not new. It has been prominent in the general educational literature since the early 1980s. The definitions of critical thinking are summarized in Display 14-1. From this review, it is easy to see that a critical thinker has many characteristics. Common explanations are discussed below.

Facione (1990) made a comprehensive attempt to define critical thinking in general. After surveying 46 experts across the United States from the disciplines of philosophy, education, social science, and physical science, Facione developed a consensus addressing both critical thinking and the ideal

DISPLAY 14-1

🔄 SELECTED DEFINITIONS OF CRITICAL THINKING

Alfaro-LeFevre (2000, p. 9)
Purposeful thinking that aims to make judgments based on evidence

American Association of Colleges of Nursing (1998)
"Critical thinking underlies independent and interdependent decision making. Critical thinking includes questioning, analysis, synthesis, interpretation, inference, inductive and deductive reasoning, intuition, application, and creativity."

Deming, W. E. (1993)
"Critical thinking is a process for surfacing, exploring and validating assumptions through reflection and inquiry." (cited in Ulsenhemier, Bailery, Thornton, McCullough, Warden, 1995).

Ennis (1985)
Critical thinking is "reflective and reasonable thinking that is focused on deciding what to believe or do."

Facione (1990)
"We understand critical thinking to be purposeful, self-regulatory judgement which results in interpretation,

analysis, evaluation, and inference as well as explanation . . . upon which judgement is based. Critical thinking is essential as a tool of inquiry. . . . Critical thinking is a pervasive and self-rectifying human phenomenon. . . ."

National League of Nursing (2000)
"Critical thinking in nursing is a logical, context-sensitive, reflective, reasoning process that guides the nurse in generating, implementing and evaluating effective approaches to client care and professional concerns."

Paul (2001, p. 1)
"Critical thinking is the intellectually disciplined process of actively and skillfully conceptualizing, applying, analyzing, synthesizing, and/or evaluating information gathered from, or generated by, observation, experience, reflection, reasoning, or communication, as a guide to belief and action."

Rubenfeld and Scheffer (1995)
Critical thinking is a "blend of five modes of thinking: Total Recall, Habits, Inquiry, New Ideas and Creativity, and Knowing How You Think."

critical thinker. The survey targeted seven characteristics of an ideal critical thinker: inquisitive, open-minded, analytical, systematic, confident, truth seeking, and mature. Facione (1990, p. 2) states, "We understand critical thinking to be purposeful, self-regulatory judgment which results in interpretation, analysis, evaluation, and inference as well as explanation . . . upon which judgment is based. Critical thinking is essential as a tool of inquiry. Critical thinking is a pervasive and self-rectifying human phenomenon."

Richard Paul, the founder of the Foundation for Critical Thinking, offered several definitions for critical thinking. One definition is: "Critical thinking is the art of thinking about your thinking while you are thinking in order to make your thinking better: more clear, more accurate, or more defensible" (Paul, 1993, p. 91). Part of what he described was metacognition, which is thinking about thinking. In another definition, Paul (1993, p. 110) states: "Critical thinking is the intellectually disciplined process of actively and skillfully conceptualizing, applying, analyzing, synthesizing, or evaluating information gathered from, or generated by, observation, experience, reflection, reasoning, or communication, as a guide to belief and action."

FACTORS AFFECTING CRITICAL THINKING

Many factors influence thinking: e.g., cognitive function, physical state, amount of sleep or rest, nutrition, and fluid and electrolyte balances. The person's age, gender, developmental level, learning style, anxiety, attitude, and preparation level also affect thinking. Although not the only factors, these are particularly important for beginning-level nursing students to address to increase awareness of their own thinking skills.

Anxiety

High workload, test-taking, grading, and performance issues can cause stress for students. Additionally, the nursing profession is filled with life-and-death, health-and-illness situations that produce anxiety. Too little anxiety limits thinking, while some anxiety often stimulates thinking. Too much anxiety, however, can paralyze higher-order thinking skills (Angelo & Cross, 1993). Thus a proper balance of anxiety is the key to high-level thinking. To maintain an effective balance, a person needs to determine ways to stay motivated yet reduce excessive anxiety.

Attitude

Nursing classes may differ from other classroom experiences in which the teacher provides the student with all information needed to meet the course requirements. Taking the initiative in the learning process may feel uncomfortable at first. Nursing students, though, will find that learning this new way develops skills for lifelong learning, an essential quality in a nurse.

Critical thinking in nursing requires active participation. Nurses must assume the responsibility for learning. The de-

sire to ask why, to develop inquisitiveness, and to question promotes lifelong learning. Paul (2001) has listed positive attitudes that a person can develop to promote skills in learning (Table 14-1).

When progressing through nursing school, students must set attitudinal goals related to their development. With adaptive attitudes, nurses will find mastering content is much easier.

Level of Preparation

By the time a person enters college, he or she should have mastered basic skills in reading, writing, listening, studying, and thinking. These basic literacy skills provide a foundation for effective learning (Nist, 1993). College reading demands, however, may be higher than a student has previously encountered. It is essential for a nursing student to be able to read for meaning and understanding and be actively involved with the text rather than for memorization. When reading, the following sequence may be helpful:

1. Establish the purpose for the reading.
2. Determine what is expected from the reading.
3. Estimate how much time it will take.
4. Skim and outline based on the purpose and main points.
5. Build a glossary of new words.
6. Read and question during the reading.
7. Assess progress and reread to clarify.
8. Integrate new knowledge with what is already known (Krumseig & Baehr, 2000).

Writing is a tool that can assist in learning. Writing can help a person refine, synthesize, and organize knowledge. Students should spend considerable time thinking and exploring during the pre-writing stage. Students will experience significant progress through forming an outline and shaping the draft. Encourage the flow of ideas during the initial process; focus on spelling and punctuation later in the editing stage. The process and technique for writing as thinking is described below:

1. Pre-write: Think; brainstorm; puzzle; question; talk with others; gather ideas through research, reading, and interviewing; take notes.
2. Produce scrambled first draft: Discover ideas through writing.
3. Shape draft: Settle on thesis statement; identify precise purpose of discourse; decide on audience; arrange paragraphs; develop coherent paragraphs; write transitions.
4. Redraft.
5. Redraft.
6. Edit: Check variety and flow of sentence structure; check grammar, usage, spelling, punctuation, bibliography (Bean, 1996).

When listening, students need to evaluate for the meaning of what is said. They must listen for themes, concepts that link sentences together, and for the basic premises of what is unsaid. Through active listening, students can put the original sounds and words into the appropriate context.

TABLE 14-1

Critical Thinking Attitudes	
Attribute	**Description**
Confidence	Feeling certain in one's ability to accomplish a goal
Thinking independently	Considering a wide range of ideas before making own conclusion
Fairness	Avoiding bias or prejudice and dealing with situations in a just manner
Responsibility and accountability	Acting on sound knowledge and acknowledging actions as one's own
Risk taking	Being willing to try out new ideas
Discipline	Following orderly thinking to do what is best
Perseverance	Staying determined to keep trying until the goal is achieved
Creativity	Formulating new ideas and alternative approaches
Curiosity	Being motivated to achieve and asking "why"
Integrity	Being honest and willing to adhere to principles in the face of adversity
Humility	Admitting one's own limitations

From Paul, R. (1993). Critical thinking: *How to prepare students for a rapidly changing world.* Santa Rosa, CA: Foundation for Critical Thinking.

Developing strong study strategies helps students to study effectively and efficiently. One most important task to learn is how to manage time efficiently. Time management significantly affects how well a person accomplishes his or her goals. Helpful measures include taking time at the beginning of the quarter to plan assignments, identifying study time before tests, and completing class preparation. As students consider time management in their classroom and personal lives, here is a guideline to follow: For every hour a student spends in class, she or he should spend 2 hours studying. Other recommendations are: Avoid procrastination by making a calendar then following it; identify how productive you are with your study time; make sure that study time is free from distractions; and plan ways to study that fit with your personal schedule and how you learn best (learning style).

Learning Styles

People learn in many different ways. It is most important that the learner acknowledges how he or she learns best. **Learning styles** are preferences, not abilities. Students can learn different ways to learn, then use various styles of learning depending upon the situation.

Some learners are people-oriented; others are task-oriented (Anderson & Adams, 1992). People-oriented learners are social: They prefer to study in groups rather than alone and they enjoy the process more than focusing on the task at hand. They find it easier to learn materials within a social context. This preferred style may conflict within that of the traditional classroom where students sitting in rows listen quietly to the instructor. Task-oriented learners focus on the goal at hand and are less easily influenced by the opinions of others.

Another dimension of learning is based on the five senses. Auditory learners receive information through hearing. They do well in classes that are primarily lecture-based. Visual learners like to see written material and prefer to have important points in writing. They like overhead slides, models, and pictures. Kinesthetic learners are tactile so they like to be actively involved. They learn by doing things, e.g., changing dressings and administering medications.

Yet another approach to learning discriminates between lumpers and splitters (Gregorc & Ward, 1977). Some learners (lumpers) need to see the big picture first; others (splitters) want to look at each piece at a time. The lumpers see the concepts, the big picture, but may have difficulty grasping the details. They may understand all the concepts of medication administration but forget to note the dose, route, or time of each medication. Splitters, who process each piece individually, may get lost in details. For example, splitters might be so focused on the "five rights" of medication administration (see Chap. 27) that they forget why the client needs the medication in the first place. Learners at either end of the spectrum are at a disadvantage; a balance of both styles is best.

Abstract thinkers see the big overarching concepts but may have difficulty dealing with day-to-day activities. They may enjoy nursing theory and be able to view the advantages and disadvantages of one theory over another. Concrete thinkers are more focused on knowledge and skills; they like things that fit into a framework. Random thinkers move from topic to topic, connecting ideas as they come to mind. Sequential thinkers like outlines and want to know the direction of thought. They enjoy class outlines and want instructors to follow those guidelines.

In beginning nursing courses, some students will be active experimenters and others will be reflective observers. Active experimenters are the first to try things; they will be excited to perform the first injection. Reflective students may speak little in a communications course; however, when talking they usually have insightful comments based on listening carefully. While active experimenters enjoy clinical rotations and laboratories, reflective students like logs, journals, and thought-provoking questions.

Some learners are competitive; they want to know other classmates' grades. In contrast, collaborative learners enjoy working together and sharing ideas and knowledge. In group work, learning-oriented students often differ with their grade-oriented colleagues. Learning-oriented students view the teacher as a guide but they test knowledge on their own scales. Grade-oriented students try to figure out what the instructor wants and put effort into courses that are based on the grade distribution. Grade-oriented students may put minimal effort into pass/fail courses; learning-oriented students will learn as much as they can from such classes.

Some people are liberal thinkers; others are conservative. Liberal thinkers like to go beyond the guidelines and recommendations; conservative thinkers prefer familiar situations and adhere to rules. Being able to listen to and adapt to both sides is most important.

Students who come to nursing bring many different learning styles. Most people use several of the learning styles discussed above. The nursing student who knows how to use a style appropriate to a particular situation is at an advantage. Students will benefit from attempting to understand and use other learning styles so that they can learn more effectively. They'll also better understand how their clients and colleagues learn and think.

Gender Issues

Intellectual development, as described by Perry (1970), explains how people perceive and function in their worlds. Perry examined intellectual development of college-aged men. He found that those who practice **dualism** in their thinking assume that one right answer exists for every question,

authorities have all the answers, and the best way to learn is to memorize the information. The belief at the next stage, called **multiplicity,** is that no opinion is wrong and all opinions are equally valid. Those at this stage believe that there is no point in arguing for one side or another because one moral principle is as right as another is. **Relativism** is the stage at which a person recognizes that not all approaches are equally valid and that context affects the way of knowing. By analyzing the processes, examining the use of evidence, and using logical reasoning, an individual can test the benefits of one approach. The **commitment** stage is when an individual makes choices and decisions. He or she bases the choices on examining the issue and sometimes considering difficult moral or ethical grounds. The person makes a decision after considering the issue's complexity (Perry, 1981). Operating at the higher levels of intellectual development is desirable for more complex situations.

Belenky, Clinchy, Goldberger, and Tarule (1986) studied the moral and intellectual development of college-aged women. They constructed five perspectives that shift over time. **Silence** was the perspective by which people felt "mindless and voiceless and subject to the whims of external authority" (Belenky et al., 1986, p. 15). These women mostly had grown up in isolation and were subjugated by an authority figure. **Received knowledge** is similar to the dualistic thinking described by Perry. Women with this perspective believed in right and wrong but based their judgments on what others told them. A common belief among these women is "I just listen to inside of me and I know what to do" (Belenky et al., 1986, p. 69). Women who relied on procedures, criteria, and reasoned judgment had the perspective of **procedural knowledge.** They found that being objective gave them a sense of empowerment and control that seemed like independent thinking. Belenky et al. discovered that some women wanted to connect with the knowledge of another person. This process is described as connected versus separate knowing. **Connected knowing** is based on empathy, which is attempting to experience a situation from another's point of view. These women tended to avoid the debating common in college classes. They preferred to postpone judgment and to learn and to explore collaboratively. The highest value is placed on knowledge gained from the perspective of **search for meaning,** which emphasizes the context and the relative and uncertain nature of truth.

Women may be less comfortable than men in the academic environment because women place more emphasis on examining different points of view rather than finding the right answer. Belenky et al. also described the order of women's intellectual growth as one based on a shifting perspective rather than a linear development.

As learners, students should consider which perspective or stage they find comfortable and how they may move to a more developed stage. They also should consider gender issues in learning and what types of academic situations best promote their learning.

THE LINKS BETWEEN KNOWLEDGE, CRITICAL THINKING, REFLECTION, AND CLINICAL REASONING

Critical thinking occurs within an existing knowledge base and is paralleled by **clinical experience.** Models are used often to explain links between concepts. A model for the development of **nursing judgment** (Fowler, 1998) shows how knowledge, experience, critical thinking, clinical reasoning, and nursing judgment are related (Figure 14-1).

In nursing school, students may take many classes that prepare them to work with clients. Thus they build a **knowledge base** before entering into clinical experience. This firm foundation of knowledge gives students a rudimentary understanding of the client.

When nurses encounter health and illness in individuals, families, and communities, they experience rich opportunities for critical thinking and reflection. It is important that students learn, review, and remember knowledge gained from previous courses to apply in clinical settings. When encountering real clients, nurses need to integrate that academic knowledge into a complete view. Using critical thinking, they can see how all preexisting knowledge and current information fit together to create new, higher-level thinking.

For example, consider the client in the nursing home at the beginning of this chapter. One of his medical diagnoses is congestive heart failure. To deal with the client's problem appropriately, the nurse will need to use his or her knowledge base from previous classes. From an assessment course, the nurse will know to auscultate the client's lungs for fluid and the heart for extra sounds. He or she will use knowledge from anatomy, physiology, and pathophysiology courses while examining the client for right-sided versus left-sided heart failure. As the nurse reviews the medication list, he or she will know the purpose, side effects, and nursing care related to digoxin, furosemide (Lasix), and potassium from pharmacology classes. From nutrition classes, the nurse will understand the rationale for a low-salt diet and be able to teach the client about foods to avoid or eat in small quantities. The nurse will be able to communicate and develop a relationship with the client, as well as provide help with bathing, transfers, and ambulation, based on knowledge from foundational nursing courses. In this way the nurse will apply critical thinking, which integrates knowledge that until this point had been theoretical, to an actual client scenario.

As beginning nurses, students will have many opportunities to strengthen and expand their knowledge bases. They can develop mechanisms to build this knowledge. An expanding knowledge base is essential for excellent nursing practice. By thinking about concepts and their relationships to each other, students broaden and deepen their knowledge bases. Continuing with the above example, the nurse will remember that heart failure can cause fluid to accumulate in the lungs. To expand his or her knowledge base, the nurse may review notes or books, ask his or her instructors, or read the chart about breath sounds. The nurse can note that the client has edema but, if he or she has forgotten how edema is scaled, can reinforce the knowledge base by looking up the information in a textbook. He or she can record the findings in a notebook so that the next time a client has edema, the nurse has the information handy as a ready reference.

The clinical experience also provides opportunities for **clinical reasoning.** Students must become actively involved in their learning by taking advantage of every opportunity to learn more. When students think that they have all the answers, they should ask themselves more questions. It is often said that it is better to have the right question than the right answer. Nursing practice highly values the pattern of inquisitiveness. This habit will assist students to become expert nurses more quickly.

Consider again the example of the client with heart failure. The nurse might expect to see clear or frothy sputum from fluid in the lungs. This client, however, is coughing up thick yellow sputum. The nurse could decide to accept this finding and simply chart it. If he or she uses critical thinking, however, the nurse might ask why the client has yellow sputum. Based on previous knowledge, he or she would know that yellow sputum is a characteristic of infection. Thus the nurse uses critical thinking to question why the client has a finding different than expected. Critical thinking helps to solve problems.

Development of Critical Thinking Skills

As students develop within their nursing roles, they will build critical thinking skills and apply them to real healthcare situations. A commitment to think critically often and at a high level will benefit a nurse's ability to care for clients most effectively. Critical thinking requires conscious, deliberate effort. Critical thinking has many facets to analyze and examine. Some aspects of thinking may be well developed, while others have

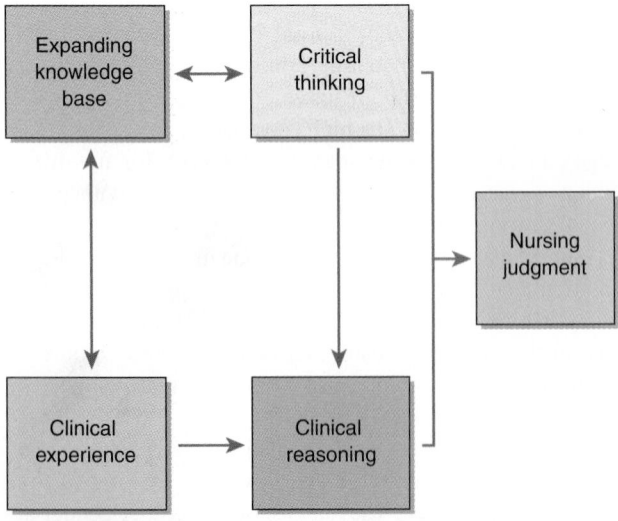

FIGURE 14-1   Model for development of nursing judgment. (Redrawn from Fowler, L. P. (1998). Improving critical thinking in nursing practice. *Journal for Nurses in Staff Development,* 14(4), 185.)

room for improvement. By looking at the parts of critical thinking, the nurse can see skills that he or she needs to develop. The parts of thinking are summarized in Display 14-2 (Paul, 2001). Eventually critical thinking will become a habit, and students will become expert nurses.

Clinical reasoning means using critical thinking in healthcare (Pesut, Herman, & Fowler, 1997). All parts of the nursing process require clinical reasoning: assessment, diagnosis, outcome identification, planning, implementation, and evaluation (Figure 14-2). The National League for Nursing (NLN) (2000) describes behaviors that show critical thinking use at each stage of the nursing process (Table 14-2). As students think about assessment, they should ask relevant questions and validate data. During analysis, they should consider other viewpoints and recognize assumptions. To increase skills in critical reasoning, students must consider how well they are using the described behaviors. They also need to take time to develop their less-used skills.

When caring for clients, nurses must take time to *think through their main purpose* (Paul, 2001). They must differentiate the main purpose from other less important purposes. For example, if a client complains of constipation and shortness of breath, the nurse might want to consider those problems separately. When the main problem is shortness of breath, the nurse should gather more data related to that finding. He or she should examine physical assessment data related to breathing. For example, the nurse should be concerned about the client's pulmonary status. That alerts the nurse to listen more carefully to the lungs to differentiate coarse crackles from the sputum instead of fine crackles from the fluid and to carefully check for dyspnea and oxygenation status. The nurse may decide to obtain an oxygen saturation level in addition to vital signs.

Consider the case in which the client with heart failure was coughing up yellow sputum. If the nurse suspects that the client is short of breath from infection, he or she will evaluate other indicators of infection. The nurse will take the client's

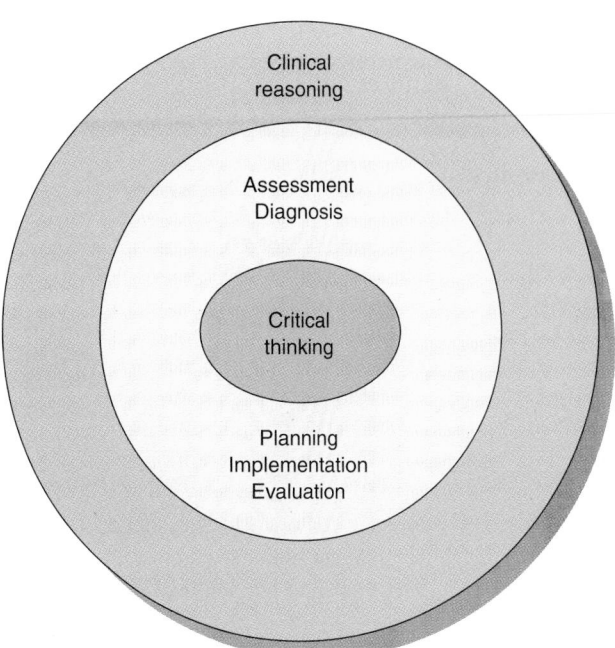

FIGURE 14-2 Role of critical thinking and nursing process in clinical reasoning.

temperature to see if it is elevated and will assess the last white blood cell count in the chart to see if it is elevated. He or she also will consider factors that may place the client at risk for infection such as immobility or immune suppression.

All reasoning has a purpose; by clarifying the purpose, the nurse can better direct thinking to productive nursing care. *Thus, all reasoning is an attempt to figure something out* (Paul, 2001). What is the question you are trying to answer? Students must take the time to clearly and precisely examine the question at issue. To challenge themselves, they should word the question in several ways, changing it to make several questions with slightly different meanings. They should then decide which question is most important. In the client with heart failure and yellow sputum, the nurse could ask questions related to subjective assessment information in different ways. One question might be, "Are you short of breath?" The nurse could ask also, "Are you more short of breath than yesterday?" The client's answer could indicate a change. Another way to phrase it is, "Do you wake suddenly with shortness of breath at night?" That question elicits information about shortness of breath that is common with heart failure.

Another example might be related to coughing. The nurse could ask what type of cough the client has and get information about a dry or productive cough. Breaking the question into subquestions can help elicit more specific information (Paul, 2001). Some subquestions the nurse could ask are, "Where does the cough come from—your chest or your throat?" Responses can provide information that might differentiate a chest problem from a sinus problem. Another question would be "What makes your cough better or worse?" As the nurse gains knowledge, he or she will learn to ask questions that provide quality information.

DISPLAY 14-2

🖫 **PARTS OF THINKING (PAUL, 2001)**

All reasoning

1. Has a purpose
2. Is an attempt to figure something out, to settle some question, to solve some problem
3. Is based on assumptions
4. Is done from some point of view
5. Is based on data, information, and evidence
6. Is expressed through, and shaped by, concepts and ideas
7. Contains inferences or interpretations by which we give meaning to data
8. Leads somewhere or has implications and consequences

TABLE 14-2

Critical Thinking Behaviors from the National League for Nursing (NLN)

Assessment	Ask relevant questions
	Explore ideas
	Validate data
	Recognize issues and concerns
Analysis	Interpret evidence
	Consider viewpoints
	Recognize assumptions
	Identify missing information
	Use reflective skepticism
	Examine alternatives
	Evaluate worth of evidence
	Detect bias
	Consider legal/ethical standards
Planning	Validate/generate hypotheses
	Predict consequences
	Use deductive/inductive reasoning
	Support conclusions with evidence
	Set priorities
	Plan approaches
Implementation	Modify/individualize approaches
	Apply research in practice
Evaluation	Determine outcome attainment
	Revise plans
	Determine perception of results

From National League for Nursing (2000). Guidelines for item writing. New York: Author.

Reasoning is based upon data, information, and evidence (Paul, 2001). In the above situation, the nurse gathered objective physical assessment data and subjective data from the client. He or she could gather data from other sources as well. For example, the health history can provide information on other related diagnoses, a history of similar problems, and the client's family history. The nurse may ask other healthcare providers or family members about changes in the client's health status or new findings. By having a more complete database from several sources, including the client, the nurse can arrive at a more accurate conclusion.

Check the data for consistency with one another (Paul, 2001). For example, an inconsistency exists if the client has other signs of infection but his or her temperature is normal. Using critical thinking, students may be able to understand why there is a cluster of data but not all data fit. In the client with a normal temperature, the nurse may find that the client is malnourished. Poor nutrition inhibits the ability to mount an immune response and might prevent temperature from rising normally.

All reasoning contains inferences and interpretations (Paul, 2001). Students should restrict claims to those supported by evidence and avoid jumping to inaccurate conclusions or judgments. Being busy and rushed, understaffed, stressed, insecure in knowledge, or behind commonly contribute to errors in judgment.

Students also must be careful to *separate correlation and causation* (Paul, 2001). If the client with heart failure is an older adult, his increased age might be correlated with an increased risk for infection; however, the age might not necessarily have caused the infection. Not all older adult clients have infection. The nurse would take a moment to question if this case is similar to or different from other clinical cases. Based on an experience of caring for a client with AIDS and *Pneumocystis carinii* pneumonia, how would a student compare and contrast the clinical presentation and treatment of the client with heart failure? Both clients have lung infections but *Pneumocystis* usually causes a dry, nonproductive cough while a bacterial lung infection may produce large amounts of sputum.

Students must ensure that *judgment is based upon a solid pattern or cluster of data* (Paul, 2001). They should ask themselves if enough evidence supports their conclusions. Patterns of data that develop over time are very meaningful. In the case of the client with heart failure, the nurse could check the chart for the normal range of vital signs and see if such findings vary from day to day or week to week. In that analysis, he or she may find that the client has many separate yet related problems.

When nurses care for clients, it is important to *analyze what problems are most important*. Priority setting is an essential nursing skill. To help decide priorities, consider the following: the severity of the problem (e.g., life-threatening would always be first), amount of time spent on the problem (nursing and medical care), which problems are related, and what the client views as most important. As students gain experience, their priority-setting skills will improve. When nurses gather and analyze data, their prioritizing will lead to the development of important diagnoses and issues. In this case, using critical thinking and clinical reasoning lead to identifying top priorities.

Diagnostic Reasoning

Diagnostic reasoning is the process of gathering and clustering data to draw inferences and propose diagnoses. Weber and Kelley (1998) have formulated seven steps of diagnostic reasoning (Table 14-3).

Following this chapter's Critical Thinking Challenge, the nurse has clustered the data, identified the yellow sputum as abnormal, and drawn some inferences that the client may have a lung infection. The next step is to *propose diagnoses*. Nurses have diagnoses designated by the North American Nursing Diagnosis Association (NANDA) that are separate and different from medical diagnoses. These nursing diagnoses provide guidelines for interventions that nurses may practice independently. The above client may be at risk for infection because of poor nutrition, so the nurse might direct

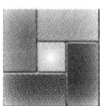

Nursing Research and Critical Thinking
Do Clinical Nursing Teachers Ask Students High-Level Questions in Order to Teach Critical Thinking?

A group of nurse educators believed in the importance of teaching critical thinking, decision making, and problem solving to nursing students. They believed that appropriate use of questioning strategies by clinical teachers would facilitate the development of critical thinking skills and increase the decision-making abilities of nursing students. The nurses designed a study to explore the types and levels of questions that clinical teachers asked of students during postclinical conferences. A comparative–descriptive research design was used for the study. Independent variables were the clinical teachers' academic qualifications, teaching qualifications, years of classroom and clinical teaching experience, and years of nursing experience. The dependent variables were the types and levels of questions asked at postclinical conferences between the clinical teachers and students. Twenty-six clinical teachers from a university school of nursing were recruited as subjects for the study. Each teacher tape recorded one postclinical conference between weeks 2 and 4 of the students' first clinical rotation, and another between weeks 2 and 4 of the students' final clinical rotation. The researchers transcribed and analyzed all the questions asked by the clinical teach-

ers. Two independent raters categorized the 993 questions transcribed for evaluation using a type and level of question-rating scale developed by Craig and Page. The results of the analysis showed that clinical teachers asked more low-level questions (91.2%) than high-level questions (4.4%). There was no significant increase in the number of high-level questions asked as students progressed through the program of study. Furthermore, the qualifications and experience of clinical teachers made no difference in the type of questions they asked.

Critical Thinking Considerations. Although the study used a convenience sample from one university school of nursing, the results demonstrated that these clinical teachers ask few high-level questions. Possible implications of this study are as follows:

• The limited use of high-level questions by clinical teachers may limit the extent to which critical thinking skills in students are facilitated.
• Universities offering higher degrees in nursing need to examine if their courses prepare nurses to be effective teachers in the classroom and clinically.

---

interventions at improving nutrition. The physician may treat the infection with antibiotics. The nurse may address nutrition as part of the nursing care (NANDA, 2001). Thus nurses and physicians both provide interventions but in slightly different ways.

TABLE 14-3

Steps of Diagnostic Reasoning	
Step One	Identify abnormal data and strengths
Step Two	Cluster data
Step Three	Draw inferences
Step Four	Propose possible nursing diagnoses
Step Five	Check for presence of defining characteristics
Step Six	Confirm or rule out
Step Seven	Document conclusions

From Weber, J., & Kelley, J. (1998). *Health assessment in nursing.* Philadelphia: J. B. Lippincott.

The North American Nursing Diagnosis Association (NANDA, 2001) has a list of diagnoses with defining characteristics that nurses use to make the diagnoses. The nurse can make the diagnosis based on assessment data that are present and that cluster together. The nurse should not use a diagnosis if the *defining characteristics* are unmet. A different diagnosis may be better. An example might be diagnosing if the client were at risk for infection because of poor nutrition. Some defining characteristics for Imbalanced Nutrition: Less than Body Requirements are as follows:

• Body weight 20% or more under ideal
• Loss of weight with adequate food intake
• Reported inadequate food intake less than the recommended daily allowance

The client must have the defining characteristics or risk factors for the nursing diagnosis to apply.

The nurse must confirm the diagnosis with the client. He or she can do so by gathering subjective and objective data. For example, the nurse might ask the client about abdominal pain, appetite, and satiety immediately after ingesting food. He or she could gather additional information such as ability to chew or swallow food, food tolerance, nausea, or vomiting. Lastly, the nurse will want to document the data. Usually nurses document assessment information, then think about and analyze the issues. The diagnosis is the nurse's label for the problem.

Using the pattern of collected data, the nurse makes a nursing judgment about what to do next. The outcomes of such judgment are called nursing plans and interventions. Nursing plans and interventions for client care are the products of nursing analysis critical thinking.

Nursing Judgment

Nurses make judgments at each step of the nursing process. Judgments lead to effective care planning, interventions, and intervention revisions based on evaluation of the care. Protocols, care plans, and care maps are ways that nurses use the nursing process to plan care. Nurses base such care on judgments for a common problem; however, every client's care must be individualized. Thus nurses use protocols within the context of critical thinking. They draw upon the individual's assessment and analysis to adapt guidelines to a client.

As beginners, students must realize that they have only small numbers of experiences on which to base their clinical judgment. As they gain experience, they will begin to notice common concepts among situations. Identifying these key concepts and ideas is essential. Thinking critically about each case will help students to *avoid applying inaccurate knowledge* from one situation to another.

Students also must continuously revise ways to *state the concepts that might have slightly different meanings.* For example, a nurse might have cared for clients with infections such as a new mother with a post-Cesarean wound infection, a teen with a sexually transmitted disease, and a client with a urinary tract infection in hospice care. How are the concepts related to infection similar? How do they differ?

Outcomes

Nurses write outcomes for clients so that as they provide care they know if that care is making a difference. In the client with Imbalanced Nutrition (Less than Body Requirements), the nurse may write an outcome such as, "Client will maintain weight at 55 kg within the next week" (Johnson & Moorhead, 2000). The outcomes focus on the client. *The outcomes also must be specific to the client.* This requires critical thinking as the nurse individualizes care. The *outcomes must be realistic and measurable.* Where it may be unreasonable for the client to gain weight, the goal is set for the client to maintain weight. The nurse also must identify a time during which the behavior will be seen, in this case within the next week. Outcomes help nurses know if their interventions actually are working.

Interventions

While outcomes focus on the client, *interventions focus on what the nurse will do* (McCloskey & Bulechek, 2000). For the client with Imbalanced Nutrition, Less than Body Requirements, one intervention includes ascertaining the client's food preferences. Another more specific intervention might be, "Contact client's family to bring in home-cooked meal."

When designing interventions, nurses must be aware not only of positive consequences but also unintended or negative consequences (Paul, 2001). For example, if a home-cooked meal is low in calories or nutrition, the nurse may need to revise the intervention as follows: "Contact dietitian to advise family on highly nutritious food choices that can be brought from home." Clinical reasoning has implications and consequences that nurses can anticipate by using critical thinking. They determine the effectiveness of the care performed when evaluating the nursing process.

Evaluation

When evaluating care, nurses compare the client assessment after the interventions to the client outcomes written earlier. For example, the nurse would weigh the client in the previously discussed example 1 week later to see if he still weighed 55 kg. If the outcomes were met, the nurse may continue the intervention. He or she also may decide to change the outcome. The next client outcome might be "Increase weight to 65 kg by next month." Not all outcomes are met, however. In such cases, the nurse may decide to change the interventions. For example, a new intervention might be, "Encourage 100 cc of nutritional supplement between meals and at bedtime." By *evaluating if the outcomes were met,* the nurse can appropriately continue or revise the interventions, outcomes, or both. He or she uses critical thinking to make these judgments.

Reflection

Paul (2001) has developed a spectrum of universal standards by which to judge thinking (Table 14-4). These standards provide the language by which a student or a nurse can expand his or her abilities. As students write papers, prepare for examinations, and participate in nursing care planning, they may use these standards to improve thinking. Critical thinking and clinical reasoning develop over time if a person makes the effort to improve them (Display 14-3).

TABLE 14-4

Spectrum of Universal Intellectual Standards	
Clear	Unclear
Precise	Imprecise
Relevant	Irrelevant
Accurate	Inaccurate
Deep	Superficial
Significant	Insignificant
Consistent	Inconsistent
Broad	Narrow
Logical	Illogical
Realistic	Unrealistic
Sufficient	Insufficient
Appropriate	Inappropriate
Justifiable	Unjustifiable
Reasonable	Unreasonable
Rational	Irrational
Fair	Unfair
Insightful	Undiscerning

From Paul, R. (2001). *Defining critical thinking. http://www.critical-thinking.org/university/helps.html.*

DISPLAY 14-3

🖫 NURTURING YOUR THINKING SKILLS

1. Make a list of your current thinking skills.
2. Keep a log (diary) of how you use thinking skills on a regular basis.
3. Share your log with a classmate. Learn from and applaud each other.
4. Read an article or book on thinking in nursing and discuss it with a classmate.
5. Draw a picture or write a paragraph that describes how you would like to enhance your thinking and the factors that hinder your thinking. Share it with a classmate.
6. Promise yourself always to consider at least three possible answers (hunches/conclusions) for every question.
7. Remind yourself that the path to responsible nursing care is along the path of critical thinking.
8. Reward yourself for your development of thinking skills.
9. Set goals for further development of your thinking skills.

Reflection is defined as "those intellectual and affective activities in which individuals engage to explore their experiences in order to lead to new understandings and appreciations" (Boud, Keogh, & Walker, 1985). As with the other skills, reflection takes time and attention to develop. Two types of reflection are reflection-in-action, which occurs in clinical practice, and reflection-on-action, which occurs after the event. Since nursing is a practice profession, nurses practice reflection-in-action every clinical day. When practicing reflection-on-action, nurses need deliberate time and effort to think about what has happened.

Mezirow (1981) outlined the levels of critical reflectivity (Table 14-5). Reflection at the most basic level begins with descriptions of events. It is helpful for students to identify a positive or negative situation that they would like to think about further. They should think about the situation, the people, and the environment then recall what happened. Recalling the sequence of events, they can think about both positive and negative feelings and pay attention to those feelings. Students should think about the context of the situation and the relationships involved. What perceptions, judgments, and thoughts occurred? What values were placed on the experience? What assumptions were made that may have been true or false? As they explore the event, students may identify new issues. In reflection, students reevaluate the experience in light of behavior, ideas, feelings, and values surrounding the event.

Learning occurs at the point of critical consciousness. This is similar to Paul's (1993) concept of "thinking about thinking." Higher levels of reflectivity are similar to higher levels of critical thinking. Critical reflectivity is "becoming aware of our awareness and critiquing it" (Mezirow, 1981). It is when a person questions judgments and considers other ways of thinking about the situation. For example, students should ask themselves why an event was important to them. What meaning does it have for them as a person and student or nurse? They should consider values and beliefs different from their own.

All reasoning is based on assumptions and is done from some point of view (Paul, 2001). Nursing values the ability to look at issues from different points of view. Different perspectives allow nurses to recognize more broadly and inclusively the meanings of life experiences. What are some other ways of looking at the issue? How has one's perspective changed? How is a person different because of this experience? Asking these questions helps students prepare to care for clients with different views. Questioning develops skills in understanding, which leads to valuing each person and her or his unique life experience. By avoiding judgments and recognizing assumptions, nurses can provide more competent care to an increasingly diverse group of clients.

The NLN (2000) has outlined critical thinking behaviors that nurses can practice in relation to these issues. One is to *recognize assumptions and consider viewpoints.* This means admitting that a person may take for granted something not based on facts. Television stories about neglect and abuse in long-term care facilities might lead one to assume that these are places to avoid. By gathering facts, a student may learn that the nursing home where he or she has been placed for training has a wide variety of client resources. For example, the home has activities with school children, holds reminiscing sessions, and takes van trips to the countryside. The residents say that they enjoy the environment and the facility delivers high quality care. This example illustrates the importance of taking time to gather facts and be open to new viewpoints.

Students must consider or *understand the position from which something is observed* (National League for Nursing, 2000). As they care for people, nursing students need to think about how they might view the situation differently. A student in long-term care might think about the losses his or her client has experienced. Examples would include the loss of function, loss of independent living, or loss of a spouse. The client's perspective might be different. For example, the client may have struggled through life, working and caring for family with minimal economic resources. The long-term care experience may be the first time the client has had help from others, food prepared for him or her, and activities for enjoyment. Students must take time to talk with clients about their points of view. That process involves asking open-ended, nonjudgmental questions and listening carefully to clients' responses.

The NLN (2000) also describes the use of reflective skepticism. This means *to adopt an attitude of doubt toward supposed truths.* For example, you might assume that a person in a nursing home has a family that doesn't care about her or him. The facts might be that the family cares deeply but does not have the economic or physical resources to care for the elder in the home.

TABLE 14-5

Mezirow's Levels of Reflectivity	
Reflectivity	Becomes aware of a specific perception, meaning, or behavior, and habits of perceiving, thinking, or acting
Affective reflectivity	Becomes aware of how we feel about the specific perceptions, meanings, or behaviors, and habits of perceiving, thinking, or acting
Discriminant reflectivity	Assesses the efficacy of our perceptions, thoughts, actions, and habits of doing things Identifies immediate causes Recognizes reality contexts in which we are functioning Identifies our relationships in reality context situations
Judgmental reflectivity	Makes and becomes aware of our *value judgments* about our perceptions, thoughts, actions, or habits *Critical Consciousness:* Becoming aware of our awareness and critiquing it Applying insights to one's own life
Conceptual reflectivity	Becomes aware of *concepts* used to understand or judge
Psychic reflectivity	Recognizes that interests and anticipations influence the way we perceive, think, or act Becomes aware of the tendency to make precipitant judgments based upon limited information
Theoretical reflectivity	Recognizes that interests and anticipations influence the way we perceive, think, or act Becomes aware of the tendency to make precipitant judgments based upon limited information

From Mezirow, J. (1981). A critical theory of adult learning and education. *Adult Education, 32* (1).

Evaluate the worth of evidence that is present (NLN, 2000). If the nurse works only day shift, recognize that the nurse only knows what happens during the work day. Consider that the family may be making evening visits. When bias is detected, find out if unreasoned judgments have been made. You or the nurse might assume that family members do not participate in care, when in fact they participate but at a different time of day. Take the effort to correct these misperceptions by communicating this information to other shifts.

Paul (2001) describes standards for thought processes (Table 14-6) related to affective issues. These standards can further develop language that helps you to understand the different parts of thinking and reflecting. In analyzing these parts, you can see opportunities to increase your depth of thinking and understanding. Ultimately critical thinking, clinical reasoning, and reflection lead to accurate nursing judgments.

Developing Expertise

As students progress through their nursing careers, they use critical thinking processes to develop skills. Achieving a high level of expertise, however, takes time. As beginners, students need to practice and problem solve. This involves learning to use these processes, finding out what works and what does not, and adapting the processes to themselves as individuals and nurses.

Benner, Tanner, and Chesla (1996) have developed a model of skill acquisition that outlines the stages of increasing expertise. Stage one is the **novice** in which learners use rules to guide practice. Examples of such rules include information and skills that students learn from instructors, practice in laboratory, and read in books. **Advanced beginner** is the next stage. After more experience in clinical situations, students learn to consider more facts and complex rules. If an intervention is unsuccessful, they may question the rule they followed. At **competence,** students devise new rules and reasoning procedures. They feel responsible for the outcomes and may question rules. Students gain competence through more experience. As situations become complex, students assimilate experiences and implement plans. As students become **proficient,** they realize that the events, context, and client situation are as important as the students' individual resources. Based on the evaluation, students develop and implement future actions. The actions become easier. The outcomes become more important than the interventions. Thinking is more flexible and intuitive rather than planned and deliber-

TABLE 14-6

Standards for Valuable Intellectual Traits	
Trait	**Description**
Intellectual Humility	Consciousness of the limits of one's knowledge
Intellectual Courage	True to our own thinking with the need to face and fairly address ideas
Intellectual Empathy	Put oneself in place of others
Intellectual Integrity	True to one's own thinking
Intellectual Perseverance	Struggle with confusion and questions over extended period of time
Faith in Reason	People can learn to persuade each other by reason
Fairmindedness	Consider all viewpoints with reference to one's own

From Paul, R. *Defining critical thinking. http://www.criticalthinking.org/university/helps.html.*

ate. The last stage is **expert.** The expert knows the goal to achieve and how to achieve it. The best of experts think before they act. They intuitively use sound theoretical thinking to reflect on the goal and decide on the seemingly appropriate action. They avoid getting caught in one perspective. The expert can link theory, practice, and intuition. This is the goal. As beginners, students must be patient as this level of expertise takes years after nursing school to develop.

APPLYING CRITICAL THINKING TO LEARNING ACTIVITIES

This textbook will serve as an important tool for students to learn the fundamentals of nursing practice. It presents many critical thinking opportunities. At the beginning of each chapter is a Critical Thinking Challenge that describes a brief situation then asks questions to help students apply what they have learned. As students begin reading, they should consider the guidelines for critical reading. They need to integrate new information into their existing knowledge base. They should ask themselves questions about how things fit together and take the time to apply the information to their own experience. They also should see how critical thinking and clinical reasoning are evident as the text progresses throughout the phases of nursing process: assessment, analysis and diagnosis, planning, implementation, and evaluating.

Students will benefit from reading the highlighted boxes that provide opportunities for critical thinking. The "Apply Your Knowledge" boxes give clinical vignettes related to the chapter's topic. In addition, students can compare their responses against suggested guidelines at the end of the book. The "Outcome-Based Teaching Plans" have situations with outcomes and strategies to meet those outcomes. Students can use clinical reasoning to arrive at nursing judgments

about the best way to approach the situation. The "Ethical and Legal Issue" boxes have situations that ask nurses to synthesize information and arrive at conclusions; many different answers are possible. The boxes provide reflection questions, and nurses can use skills in critical reflection. There is an opportunity for thinking about which answer is best. The "Nursing Research and Critical Thinking" boxes present recent clinical findings. The critical thinking considerations link the research with practice. Key concepts are summarized at the end of each chapter.

Thus students can build their existing knowledge base by reading this book. They can incorporate this knowledge into their clinical experiences in nursing school. Students will have opportunities to use the critical thinking and reflection skills. They will use clinical reasoning as they make nursing judgments. By putting time and effort into developing these skills, they will ultimately provide more individualized and appropriate nursing care.

KEY CONCEPTS

- Many authors have defined critical thinking. Each definition differs slightly but all view critical thinking as a positive process that helps people make decisions and take action.
- Many factors affect thinking: anxiety, attitude, level of preparation, learning style, and gender issues.
- Critical thinking is essential for use in the nursing process and is an important element in effective nursing practice.
- A firm knowledge base and clinical experience provide the base for clinical reasoning to make nursing judgments.
- Critical thinking is important in all nurse–client interactions.
- Students can develop critical thinking skills through self-reflection, building on existing skills, optimizing thinking, expressing thinking verbally and in writing, reading about and discussing critical thinking, listening carefully, and practicing critical thinking.

REFERENCES

Alfaro-LeFevre, R. (2000). Improving your ability to think critically. *Nursing Spectrum Metro Edition,* CE 168B.

American Association of Colleges of Nursing. (1998). *The essential of baccalaureate education for professional nursing practice.* Washington DC: American Association of Colleges of Nursing.

American Heritage College Dictionary. (1993). Boston: Houghton Mifflin.

Anderson, J. A., & Adams, M. (1992). Acknowledging the learning styles of diverse student populations: Implications for instructional design. *New directions for teaching and learning.* San Francisco: Jossey-Bass.

Angelo, T. A., & Cross, K. P. (1993). *Classroom assessment techniques: A handbook for college teachers* (2nd ed.). San Francisco: Jossey-Bass.

Bean, J. C. (1996). *Engaging ideas: The professor's guide to integrating writing, critical thinking, and active learning in the classroom.* San Francisco: Jossey-Bass.

Belenky, M. F., Clinchy, B. V., Goldberger, N. R., & Tarule, J. M. (1986). *Women's ways of knowing: The development of self, voice, and mind.* New York: Basic Books.

Benner, P. Tanner, C. A., & Chesla, C. A. (1996). *Expertise in nursing practice: Caring, clinical judgment, and ethics.* New York: Springer.

Boud, D., Keogh, R., & Walker, D. (1985). Promoting reflection in learning: A model. *In reflection: Turning experience into learning.* London: Kogan Page.

Facione, P. A. (1990). *"The Delphi Report" executive summary critical thinking: A statement of expert consensus for purposes of educational assessment and instruction.* Millbrae, CA: California Academic Press.

Fowler, L. P. (1998). Improving critical thinking in nursing practice. *Journal for Nurses in Staff Development, 14,* (4).

Gregorc, A. R., & Ward, J. B. (1977). Implications for teaching and learning: A new definition for individuals. *Bulletin (National Association of Secondary School Principals [NASSP]), 61,* 20–33.

Johnson, J., & Moorhead, S. (2000). *Nursing outcomes: Classification* (2nd ed.). St. Louis: Mosby.

Krumseig, K., & Baehr, M. (2000). *Foundations of learning* (3rd ed.). Corvalis, OR: Pacific Crest Software.

McCloskey, J. C., & Bulechek, G. M. (2000). *Nursing interventions classification* (3rd ed.). St. Louis: Mosby.

Mezirow, J. (1981). A critical theory of adult learning and education. *Adult Education, 32* (1).

North American Nursing Diagnosis Association (NANDA) (2001). *Nursing Diagnoses: Definitions & Classification 2001–2002.* New York: North American Nursing Diagnosis Association.

National League for Nursing (2000). *Guidelines for item writing.* New York: Author.

Nist, S. A. (1993). What the literature says about academic literacy. *Georgia Journal* of *Reading,* Fall–Winter.

Paul, R. (1993). *Critical thinking: How to prepare students for a rapidly changing world.* Santa Rosa, CA: Foundation for Critical Thinking.

Paul, R. (2001). *Defining critical thinking.* [Online] Available at: *http://www.criticalthinking.org/university/helps.html*

Perry, W. G. (1970). *Forms of intellectual and ethical development in the college years: A scheme.* New York: Holt, Rinehart & Winston.

Perry, W. G. Jr. (1981). Cognitive and ethical growth: The making of meaning. In Arthur Chickering and Associates (Eds.), *The modern American college: Responding to the new realities of diverse students and a changing society.* San Francisco: Jossey-Bass.

Pesut, D. J., Herman, J. A., & Fowler, L. P. (1997). Toward a revolution in thinking: The OPT model of clinical reasoning. In J. McCloskey & H. K. Grace (Eds.), *Current issues in nursing* (5th ed.). St. Louis: Mosby.

Weber, J., & Kelley, J. (1998). *Health Assessment in Nursing.* Philadelphia: Lippincott.

BIBLIOGRAPHY

Benner, P. (1984). *From novice to expert.* Menlo Park, CA: Addison Wesley.

Critical Thinking Foundation (2001). [Online] Available at: *http://www.criticalthinking.org/university*

Deming, W. E. (1993). Critical thinking task team storybook. Winston-Salem, NC: Forsyth Memorial Hospital.

Ennis, R. H. (1985). A logical basis for measuring critical thinking skills. *Educational Leadership, 10,* 44–48.

Facione, P. (1990). Critical thinking: A statement of expert consensus for purposes of educational assessment and instruction. *The Delphi report: Research findings and recommendations prepared for the American Philosophical Association.* (ERIC Doc. No. ED 315-423). Washington, DC: Eric.

Fonteyne, M. E. (1998). *Thinking Strategies for Nursing Practice.* Philadelphia: Lippincott.

Peirce, W. (1998). Understanding students' difficulties in reasoning. Part one: Perspectives from several fields. [Online] Available at: *http://academic.pg.cc.md.us/~wpeirce/MCCCTR/underst.html*

Peirce, W. (2000). Understanding students' difficulties in reasoning. Part two: The perspective from research in learning styles and cognitive styles. [Online] Available at: *http://www.umuc.edu/distance/odell/research/peirce_under2.html*

Rubenfeld, M. G., & Scheffer, B. K. (1999). Critical thinking in nursing: An interactive approach. Philadelphia: Lippincott.

Smith-Stoner, M. (1998). *Critical thinking activities for nursing.* Philadelphia: Lippincott.

Wilkinson, J. M. (2001). *Nursing process and critical thinking* (3rd ed.). Upper Saddle River, NJ: Prentice-Hall.

Winningham, J. L. & Preusser, B. A. (2001). *Critical thinking in medical-surgical settings* (2nd ed.). St. Louis: Mosby.

15 Communication of the Nursing Process
Documenting and Reporting

Key Terms

audit
care plan conferences
change-of-shift report
charting by exception
clinical pathway
computer-based
  personal record
confidentiality
documentation
flowsheets
FOCUS system

incident
Kardex
nursing informatics
nursing plan of care
PIE charting
point of care documentation
quality assurance memo
reporting
SOAP note
variance

Learning Objectives

Upon completion of this chapter, the student will be able to do the following:

1. Describe the purposes of the client record.
2. List the principles of charting.
3. Discuss the relevance of electronic media in documentation.
4. Explain how to use a nursing Kardex.
5. Properly record nursing progress notes by SOAP, PIE, FOCUS, or narrative format.
6. Identify flowsheets and critical pathways used in client records.
7. Identify important data for the change-of-shift report.
8. Describe the procedure for telephone reporting.
9. Discuss the importance of confidentiality in documenting and reporting.

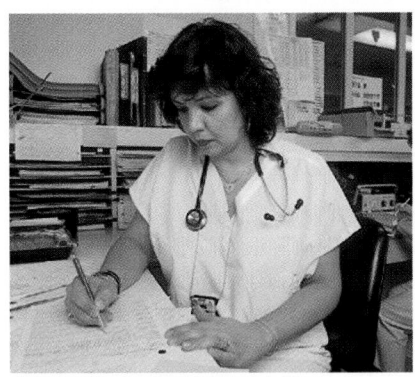

Critical Thinking Challenge

When you come on duty for the morning shift, you check the charts of your clients. You examine the following documentation found on one client's chart from the previous shift:

- *"Client had a terrible night. She was bloated and very nauseated. Bowel sounds present in all quadrants. She complained that her doctor never came in to see her, and when he did, he didn't seem very interested in how she felt."*
- *Vital signs: BP 176/74, P 92, R 18*
- *"Complaining of incisional pain; morphine sulfate given. She was also upset about her family."*

In this chapter, you will integrate information on how to communicate the nursing process both orally and in writing with your coworkers. Correct documentation and reporting of client information are essential to quality client care. After you have completed this chapter and have incorporated written and oral communication (documenting and reporting) into your knowledge base, review the above scenario and reflect on the following areas of Critical Thinking:

1. Formulate any information that you would like to have that was not charted about this client.
2. Rate some positive qualities in the charting. Then, identify at least five weaknesses in this charting and why you see them as problematic.
3. Construct charting for this client using narrative, PIE, and FOCUS formats. Add hypothetical data as necessary to reflect information that would be important to chart. Compare and contrast charting using these different methods.
4. Reflect on possible legal or ethical problems with the chart entries as written originally.

The nursing process is communicated in writing and verbally. Effective communication enhances client care by ensuring comprehensive, coordinated care by a variety of providers. All members of the healthcare team share information through documentation and reporting.

Written communication, or **documentation,** serves as a permanent record of client information and care. The client record or chart provides information during the present visit or admission and may be consulted in the future to review the client's history or for educational, research, and legal purposes. **Reporting** takes place when two or more people share information about client care, either face to face (as in a team meeting or shift report), by audiotape or voice mail, or by telephone (as in reports to a case manager or physician from a nurse making home visits).

Nurses are responsible for accurate, complete, and timely documentation and reporting. As an instrument of continuous client care and as a legal document, the client record should contain all pertinent assessments, planning, interventions, and evaluations for that client.

Documentation and reporting of the client's condition require adherence to the highest standards of **confidentiality.** At all times, nurses must be aware that what is written and spoken about clients is of a personal nature, reflecting consideration for each person's basic human dignity. Clients expect that information about them will be shared only with those who need to know and who will be contributing to their care.

WRITTEN COMMUNICATION: THE CLIENT RECORD

Simply stated, the written record of a client's progress and the care provided is a compilation of health-related data. Management of these data—their organization, input, and retrieval—forms the basis for interdisciplinary communication. The manner in which each member of the healthcare team accesses and contributes to the record may differ. Each piece of data, however, is crucial in forming an actual picture of the client, his or her health status, and the care he or she has received. The client record promotes a coherent plan of care, communication of common and individual goals, and progress of the client toward those goals. An accurate and complete record must be accessible to members of the healthcare team who care for the client. If a client record or portions of it are misplaced, unavailable, or inaccurate, a vital line of communication is blocked.

Documentation of the nursing process within this record provides essential data related to assessment, interventions, and goals. Nurses' entries on the client record are important because they show medical and nursing orders carried out, independent assessments and interventions performed, the exact dates and times of care delivered, and evaluation of care provided. Documented client responses to nursing interventions serve to validate the importance of nursing in promoting health and well-being of clients.

The specific manner in which nursing documentation occurs reflects the philosophy and goals of the agency in which a nurse works. These, in turn, are affected by larger system issues, such as standards of care and documentation established by accrediting bodies, reimbursement requirements, changes in healthcare systems toward multisite and multiagency coordination, and the movement toward a universal computer-based patient record.

Purpose

Communication
Clearly documented information on the client record communicates the plan of care and the client's progress to all members of the healthcare team. Team members who interact with the client at different times and in different ways get a clear picture of what took place in their absence. This communication ensures continuity of care and provides essential data for revision or continuation of care.

Assessment
Nurses and other team members gather assessment data from the client record. By reading about the client's history and initial assessment and comparing these data with additional subjective and objective information that has been obtained, current health status and progress toward goals can be determined. Progressive assessments of lung sounds, for example, might alert the nurse to a developing infection or indicate that fluid is accumulating in the lungs of a postoperative client.

Care Planning
Formulation of a plan of care flows from assessment data in the client record. All data on the client record are considered when nursing diagnoses, goals, outcome criteria, interventions, and evaluation criteria for that client are developed. An individualized nursing plan of care is essential for each client and becomes part of the permanent client record. The exact written form can vary depending on the agency, setting, and specialty in which care is delivered.

Quality Assurance
An **audit** is a review of records. Audits of client records serve a dual purpose: quality assurance and reimbursement. Auditing is done for quality assurance when records are randomly selected to determine whether certain standards of care were met and documented. Results of an audit may then lead to changes in the manner in which care is provided. The goal is to review continually and to improve the quality of nursing care provided. For example, a review of charts in a hospice setting may explain patterns of use of round-the-clock professional care for symptom management. As a result, the agency may provide additional training in symptom management to staff or to family members, or it may establish new policies regarding the use of 24-hour care. The Joint Commission on Accreditation of Healthcare Organizations (JCAHO) audits client records regularly and encourages institutions to set up ongoing quality assurance programs. If deficiencies are detected, educational programs can be designed to improve outcomes in those areas.

Reimbursement

Documentation of client care often provides the basis for decisions regarding care to be provided and subsequent reimbursement to the agency. Medicare, Medicaid, workers' compensation insurance, and third-party insurance companies usually require specific criteria to be met to cover health-related expenses. Documentation may support a diagnostic-related group (DRG) classification or identify interventions that were actually performed for the client.

Several examples illustrate this point. To obtain reimbursement when a wound culture is done, documentation would indicate that appropriate assessment data were gathered and that the test was ordered by a physician and actually carried out by the laboratory; administration of medication or the use of supplies may then be verified with additional documentation. Clients must meet "homebound" eligibility requirements for agencies to receive Medicare reimbursement for home care services; therefore, homebound status becomes an essential documentation component in the admission and ongoing assessment. Hospice beneficiaries generally receive care limited to their admitting diagnosis and must also meet standards for eligibility, such as consent to seek palliative care instead of curative treatments. Nurses must be familiar with the criteria for reimbursement in each setting and knowledgeable about obtaining authorization for care. Their documentation must show that they have adhered to these guidelines in establishing and providing care.

Legal Documentation

The client record serves as a legal document of the client's health status and care received. It may be used in court to prove or disprove injuries a client incurred unintentionally or to implicate or absolve a healthcare professional in regard to improper care. Because nurses and other healthcare team members cannot remember specific assessments or interventions involving a client years after the fact, accurate and complete documentation at the time of care is essential. The care may have been excellent, but the documentation must prove it.

Research

Nursing and healthcare research is often carried out by studying client records. Data may be gathered from groups of records to determine significant similarities in disease presentation, to identify contributing factors, or to determine the effectiveness of therapies. For example, a nurse epidemiologist may review the records of clients who have had tuberculosis to determine patterns of disease in the community. This information might be used to design culturally appropriate education and to plan more effective primary prevention strategies. Examination of nursing care provided may lead to clarification of nursing roles. Research based on documentation of nursing care provided allows the profession to refine the definition of practice.

Education

Members of the healthcare team, including students of nursing, medicine, and other disciplines, use the client record as an educational tool. It contains valuable information about signs and symptoms of disease, diagnostic tests, treatment modalities, and client responses to the disease and to treatment. For example, a nursing student may read the record of a client experiencing a stroke to learn the signs and symptoms that the client initially experienced, the results of the computed axial tomography scan, the effects of medications given to minimize brain injury, and the contribution of physical therapy to help the client reach rehabilitation goals.

Principles of Data Entry and Management

Principles of good documentation are easier to accept and adopt if nurses keep in mind the purposes of the record. Remember that any entry made serves as communication within the healthcare team but also may be scrutinized carefully by students, lawyers, reimbursement agents, and researchers. Client access to records may also be significant, depending on institutional policy and state regulations.

Accuracy

Entries must be accurate. Nurses must write only observations that they have seen, heard, smelled, or felt. An observation made by another health professional must be clearly identified as such. Precise measurements and times must be used whenever possible. For example, a wound should be described as "3 cm by 0.5 cm" rather than "small." If words are not adequate to describe the shape and color of a wound, documentation can also include photographs to depict the actual state of the wound on a given day. Correct spelling and correct use of medical terms are important. Check the spelling of words and grammar used to reduce errors. Proofreading of notes also helps to ensure readability. To avoid confusion, make certain that the names of physicians or other professionals mentioned are correct.

When an error occurs, erasure is not permissible. A notation about the error must be made (Fig. 15-1). Draw a single line through the error, and write the word "Error" and your initials above it. Some institutions require an explanation of the error, such as, "Charted for wrong client."

Accuracy can be enhanced through point of care documentation (see later discussion). This may be as simple as recording data by hand onto the chart during an admission interview with a client, or as sophisticated as using a hand-held electronic device that downloads the information into a system-wide database.

Completeness

Obviously, not every observation is recorded, but information about the nursing process must be complete. Note all relevant data to support an assessment and plan. Without this information, other team members may fail to take appropriate action. For example, if a client's temperature of 100.8°F at 2 PM was not recorded, the nurse arriving at 4 PM might not take the client's temperature. By this time, the temperature may be significantly elevated because of an infection. Complete, pertinent assessment data—such as other vital signs, wound drainage, client complaints, who was notified, and what interventions were carried out—give a complete picture

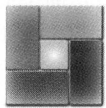

Nursing Research and Critical Thinking
Do Healthcare Professionals Document the Frequency of Abuse, Extent of Injuries, or Follow-Up Referrals for Their Prenatal Clients?

Point prevalence estimates in public and private healthcare settings indicate that 4% to 8% of women experience abuse during pregnancy. Prospective repeated interview assessments of an ethnically stratified cohort of African-American, Hispanic, and Anglo women, however, revealed that 16% were abused during pregnancy. The difference in these rates may stem from a lack of documentation of the abuse in the medical records from which such statistics are usually compiled. These healthcare researchers designed a medical chart audit study to determine the rate of documented assessment of abuse during pregnancy by healthcare providers in public health clinics. The study used a systematic random sample of 540 maternity charts drawn from three health centers over a 15-month period. Each chart was evaluated for presence or absence of designated abuse assessment questions as well as documentation of abuse. All medical and nursing progress notes were reviewed. Among the 540 charts reviewed, no designated abuse assessment questions were asked. Four (0.74%) of the charts documented abuse. On the four charts with documentation of abuse, no referrals, counseling, or follow-up was noted. None of the documentation included frequency of abuse, extent of injuries, or follow-up referrals. Staff ($N = 53$) of the clinics scored an average of 65% (of a possible 100 points) on the knowledge test about abuse to women, and 47% reported asking female clients about partner violence. Furthermore, staff assessing for abuse reported making referrals to shelters, battered women's programs, batterer's treatment programs, legal advocacy, and housing.

Critical Thinking Considerations. The charts reviewed for this study were limited to those from three health centers in an urban public health department. The results of the study should not be generalized to all clinics providing prenatal care. Implications are as follows:

• This research suggests that for abuse of women to be detected, documented, and treated, training of health professionals is needed.
• Because abuse tends to increase over time, designated questions on abuse asked routinely could interrupt the cycle of violence, prevent further trauma, and protect the health and well-being of the pregnant woman and child.

From McFarlane, J., & Wiist, W. H. (1996). Documentation of abuse to pregnant women: A medical chart audit in public health clinics. *Journal of Women's Health, 5*(2), 137–142.

ETHICAL/LEGAL ISSUE
Accuracy of Records

You are working on a busy medical unit where your responsibilities include administering medications to your clients. In preparing morning medications for a client, you notice that an important cardiac medication that should have been given at 6 AM was not signed off as given in the medication record. You consult with another nurse, and she states, "The night nurse probably gave the medication and forgot to sign it off. I will just initial the medication so that she doesn't get in trouble with our charge nurse."

Reflection
• Identify possible consequences of this situation for:
  – The client
  – The nurse signing off the medication
  – The nurse who did not administer the medication
  – You who witnessed the act
• How might you respond if you were witnessing this situation?
• Would your views on the situation differ if the medication was a laxative?

so that nurses on subsequent shifts can make objective evaluations and revise the plan as needed.

Be sure to include the following essential information when charting:

• Any new or changed information
• Signs and symptoms
• Client behaviors
• Nursing interventions
• Medications given
• Physician's orders carried out
• Client teaching
• Client responses

1/17/99	c/o SOB × 15 min. while ambulating.
3:15 pm	Denies chest pain. ~~BP 126/84, P. 64, R. 16~~
	BP 134/90, P. 86 R. 24. Assisted to bed
	with hob elevated. Notified Dr. Smith.
	Sally North RN

FIGURE 15-1 Sample correction of an error in client charting.

Conciseness

Good charting is concise and brief. In narratives, use partial sentences and phrases; drop the client's name and terms referring to the client. Use abbreviations but only those that are commonly accepted and approved by your facility. Table 15-1 lists common abbreviations. Unnecessary elaboration confuses important issues. Being concise also is helpful in time management, because nurses can spend less time charting and more time with clients.

Objectivity

When charting subjective findings, make every effort to identify the source and context for the finding. This point is particularly important when recording information about psychosocial and mental health issues. Directly quoting statements made by the client can help in maintaining objectivity. For example, charting that a client "States he misses the company of friends and is upset that they are no longer visiting" is more objective than charting, "Client lonely and frustrated."

Organization

Each entry must clearly show a logical and systematic grouping of important information by problem or occurrence. For example, assessment is recorded with subjective and objective data, identification of nursing diagnoses, goals, nursing interventions, and the client's response. Information about a routine laboratory test is recorded elsewhere if it does not pertain to this problem.

There must be a chronologic flow of information about client care according to time and procedures completed, with the client's reaction documented. Recording as the events of the day unfold can prevent out-of-sequence or fragmented entries that may cause confusion.

Timeliness

Documentation in a timely manner can help avoid errors. Record all medications at the time they are given and procedures, treatments, and assessments as soon as possible after their completion. When the client's status changes rapidly or frequent assessments are made, document those changes as soon as possible. In inpatient and ambulatory settings, do not leave the unit for breaks or other long periods until important information is recorded. General statements regarding the client's condition may require completion of the shift or visit before their entry into the record to maximize organization and conciseness of the report. Note the time of documentation, and, if an action or significant event takes place at a time earlier than the time of documentation, indicate that time within the note (Carelock & Innerarity, 2001).

Many agencies require documentation using a 24-hour clock (also known as military time) to avoid possible errors (Table 15-2). Initiation of point of care documentation in many settings is another strategy used to maximize accuracy and timeliness of entries. For example, a hospital may maintain assessment records at the bedside, or a home health agency may provide a hand-held computer for nurses who make home visits.

Timeliness also helps avoid forgetting important information. Waiting until the end of the day to record events on several clients may cause a nurse to omit important data or enter inaccurate information. If litigation occurs, lawyers use charted documentation to reconstruct time sequences (Pennels, 2001). Recording events in sequence provides support to demonstrate that appropriate responses were identified and reported. Doing so can be essential for protection from negligence or malpractice claims. See Display 15-1 for a list of high-risk errors in documentation.

Legibility

Writing must be clear and easily read by others. Legibility is especially important when recording numbers and medical terms. For example, a pulse rate of 164 may look similar to 104 but has more serious implications. The term *dysphasia* (difficulty speaking) could be mistaken for *dysphagia* (difficulty swallowing).

Computers in Documentation

With the advance of computer technology, many institutions are transforming the client record to electronic format. The earliest electronic records were a part of the development of hospital information systems in the late 1960s. The first of these systems, at El Camino Hospital in California, was designed to manage all client information accrued throughout the hospital stay (Saba & McCormick, 1996). Nursing care protocols were written, against which nurses could document using a light pen to select appropriate responses. The actual data were then saved in a mainframe computer, which also supported the unit-based terminals. In these systems, nurses would typically return to a standard charting area that contained computer screens, keyboards, and possibly a printer.

Today's electronic records reflect the nature of the computer as a database that is able to record widely diverse types of information in various formats and to provide information specific for the needs of each person retrieving the data. The entire client record or only selected portions of it may be computerized. Multiple people may access portions of the record from different sites at the same time. Depending on individual need, authorization for access may be limited to specific information or may be complete. The record may be linked to a facility-wide information system to assist in ordering supplies and services for a client, store billing and financial data, and maintain nursing and other healthcare data. Typically, the retrieval of information becomes more efficient, making use of the computer's ability to search for specific information requested. Institutions and departments may individualize their reporting formats to address needs specific to their client populations. In contrast, the handwritten chart is generally available to only one person at a time and is maintained in a central location as a single, composite record. With handwritten records, individual disciplines or departments may maintain separate and incomplete records that address their special needs.

(text continues on page 236)

TABLE 15-1

Abbreviations Commonly Used in Documentation

Abbreviation	Meaning	Abbreviation	Meaning
ā	before	os	mouth
abd	abdomen	OOB	out of bed
ac	before meals	oz	ounce
ADLs	activities of daily living	p̄	after
ad lib	as needed	p.c.	after meals
adm.	admitted, admission	post	posterior
amp.	ampule	prep	preparation
ant.	anterior	prn	when necessary
AP	anterior-posterior	q̄, q	every
ax.	axillary	q̄, 2 (3, 4, etc.) hours	every 2 (3, 4, etc.) hours
b.i.d.	twice a day	qd	every day
BP	blood pressure	qh	every hour
BR	bed rest	q.i.d.	four times a day
BRP	bathroom privileges	q.o.d.	every other day
C	Centigrade	q.s.	quantity sufficient
c̄	with	R/O	rule out
caps	capsule	ROM	range of motion
C.C.	chief complaint	s̄	without
cc	cubic centimeter (1 cc = 1 mL)	SBA	stand by assistance
CVP	central venous pressure	SC	subcutaneous
c/o	complains of	SL	sublingual
D/C	discontinue	SOB	shortness of breath
disch; DC	discharge	sol, soln	solution
drsg	dressing	spec	specimen
dr	dram	S/P	status post
elix	elixir	sp. gr.	specific gravity
ext	extract or external	S.S.E.	soapsuds enema
F	Fahrenheit	ss	one half
fx.	fracture, fractional	stat	immediately
gm	gram	tab	tablet
gr	grain	t.i.d.	three times a day
gtt	drop	tinct or tr.	tincture
"H," SC, or sub q	hypodermic or subcutaneous	TKO	to keep open
h	hour	TPN	total parenteral nutrition
HOB	head of bed		hyperalimentation
h.s.	bedtime (hour of sleep)	TPR	temperature, pulse, respiration
hx	history	tsp	teaspoon
I & O	intake & output	TO	telephone order
IM	intramuscular	TWE	tap water enema
IV	intravenous	VO	verbal order
kg	kilogram	VS	vital signs
KVO	keep vein open	VSS	vital signs stable
L	left; liter	W/C	wheelchair
lat	lateral	WNL	within normal limits
MAE	moves all extremities		
mg	milligram	**Selected Abbreviations Used for Specific Descriptions**	
ml, mL	milliliter (1 mL = 1 cc)	AKA	above-knee amputation
NAD	no apparent distress	ASCVD	arteriosclerotic cardiovascular
NG	nasogastric		disease
noc	night	ASHD	arteriosclerotic heart disease
NPO	nothing by mouth		

TABLE 15-1 (Continued)

Abbreviations Commonly Used in Documentation

Abbreviation	Meaning	Abbreviation	Meaning
BKA	below-knee amputation	RLQ	right lower quadrant
ca	cancer	RR, PAR	recovery room, postanesthesia room
chest clear to A & P	chest clear to auscultation & percussion	RUE	right upper extremity
CMS	circulation movement sensation	RUQ	right upper quadrant
CNS	central nervous system	Rx	prescription
DJD	degenerative joint disease	STSG	split-thickness skin graft
DOE	dyspnea on exertion	Surg	surgery, surgical
DTs	delirium tremens	T & A	tonsillectomy & adenoidectomy
D_5W	5% dextrose in water	THR, TJR	total hip replacement; total joint replacement
FUO	fever of unknown origin	URI	upper respiratory infection
GB	gall bladder	UTI	urinary tract infection
GI	gastrointestinal	vag	vaginal
GYN	gynecology	VD	venereal disease
H_2O_2	hydrogen peroxide	WNWD	well-nourished, well-developed
HA	hyperalimentation; headache		
HCVD	hypertensive cardiovascular disease		

Selected Abbreviations Related to Common Diagnostic Tests

Abbreviation	Meaning	Abbreviation	Meaning
HEENT	head, ear, eye, nose, throat	BE	barium enema
HVD	hypertensive vascular disease	B.M.R.	basal metabolism rate
ICU	intensive care unit	CA^{++}	calcium
I & D	incision and drainage	CAT	computed axial tomography
LLE	left lower extremity	CBC	complete blood count
LLQ	left lower quadrant	Cl^-	chloride
LOC	level of consciousness; laxatives of choice	C & S	culture & sensitivity
		Dx	diagnosis
LMP	last menstrual period	ECG, EKG	electrocardiogram
LUE	left upper extremity	EEG	electroencephalogram
LUQ	left upper quadrant	FBS	fasting blood sugar
MI	myocardial infarction	hct	hematocrit
Neuro	neurology; neurosurgery	Hgb	hemoglobin
NS	normal saline	IVP	intravenous pyelogram
Nsy.	nursery	K^+	potassium
NWB	non–weight-bearing	LP	lumbar puncture
O.D.	right eye	MRI	magnetic resonance imaging
O.S.	left eye	Na^+	sodium
O.U.	each eye	RBC	red blood cell
OPD	outpatient department	UGI	upper gastrointestinal x-ray
ORIF	open reduction internal fixation	UA	urinalysis
Ortho	orthopedics	WBC	white blood cell
OT	occupational therapy		
PE	physical examination		

Commonly Used Symbols

Abbreviation	Meaning	Abbreviation	Meaning
PERRLA	pupils equal, round, & react to light and accommodation	>	greater than
PID	pelvic inflammatory disease	<	less than
PI	present illness	=	equal to
PM & R	physical medicine & rehabilitation	≈	approximately equal to
Psych	psychology; psychiatric	≤	equal to or less than
PT	physical therapy	≥	equal to or greater than
RL (or LR)	Ringer's lactate; lactated Ringer's	↑	increased
RLE	right lower extremity	↓	decreased

(continues)

TABLE 15-1 (Continued)

Abbreviations Commonly Used in Documentation			
Abbreviation	**Meaning**	**Abbreviation**	**Meaning**
♀	female	F_1	first filial generation
♂	male	F_2	second filial generation
°	degree	PO_2	partial pressure of oxygen
#	number or pound	PCO_2	partial pressure of carbon dioxide
×	times	:	ratio
@	at	∴	therefore
+	positive	%	percent
−	negative	2°	secondary to
±	positive or negative	Δ	change

Although the principles of documentation remain the same whether the record is handwritten or electronically maintained, the use of the computer can alter the manner in which nurses interact with and record data. To document, nurses must receive instruction in the specific system that their institution uses. A confidential access code is provided to identify the nurse; the access code allows the nurse to sign onto the system and identifies entries as being made by that person, much as a handwritten signature does. The nurse may record information about client progress using separate standard nursing formats, such as a care map and narrative notes (see later discussion). The system may rely on keyboard entry for narrative notes, or it may use mouse-driven commands to access appropriate screens from which interventions may be selected as completed. The nurse may use the computer to review previous nursing interventions, print out a current nursing plan of care, or retrieve data from other disciplines (Fig. 15-2).

Universal Computer-Based Patient Record

In response to a federally initiated goal to have a single record for each citizen, much conversation regarding electronically maintained records now focuses on the **computer-based personal record,** or "CPR" (Staggers, Thompson, & Snyder-Halpern, 2001). Centralization of the client record lends itself to increased accessibility beyond the primary institution. Healthcare practitioners within large and geographically dispersed healthcare organizations can have uniform access to a single client record, allowing greater accuracy and improved care. The goal with the universal CPR is to have these benefits extend beyond specific care providers, allowing clients to share complete health information with any practitioner regardless of institutional affiliation or time and place when care was originally provided. With the CPR, practitioners might, for

TABLE 15-2

24-Hour Time Conversions	
Time	**Conversion to 24-Hour Time**
Midnight	0000
1 AM	0100
2 AM	0200
3 AM	0300
4 AM	0400
5 AM	0500
6 AM	0600
7 AM	0700
8 AM	0800
9 AM	0900
10 AM	1000
11 AM	1100
12 noon	1200
1 PM	1300
2 PM	1400
3 PM	1500
4 PM	1600
5 PM	1700
6 PM	1800
7 PM	1900
8 PM	2000
9 PM	2100
10 PM	2200
11 PM	2300

DISPLAY 15-1

HIGH-RISK ERRORS IN DOCUMENTATION

- Falsifying client records
- Failure to record changes in client's condition
- Failure to document that physician was notified when client's condition changed
- Inadequate admission assessment
- Failure to document completely
- Failure to follow agency's standards or policies on documentation
- Charting in advance

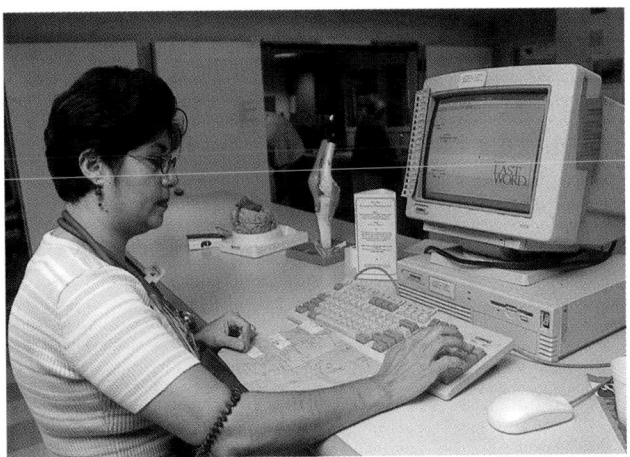

FIGURE 15-2   The nurse may use the computer to document care, print out a nursing plan of care, communicate with other departments, or retrieve data from other disciplines.

example, have access to a listing of the client's current medications and a thorough cardiac history at the time of an emergency. Clients with cancer could share reports between specialists and the primary care team with ease. People who are traveling would know that records of previous illnesses and conditions can be accessed readily. Research shows that lack of an integrated computer system and a standard means of data entry have stalled the process of implementing a CPR system (Staggers, Thompson, & Snyder-Halpern, 2001).

Point of Care Documentation

Documentation that takes place as care occurs is referred to as **point of care (POC) documentation.** With the goal of promoting efficiency, accuracy, and timeliness, POC documentation has become increasingly common. Studies are being performed to measure whether POC documentation has any affect on client satisfaction related to care delivery during hospitalization (Nahm & Poston, 2000). Technology can make this process more efficient than in the past. Nurses may carry hand-held devices or portable computers that allow them to document care as they provide it to clients. In inpatient settings, terminals may be located at clients' bedsides. Information may then be downloaded via secured telecommunication links to the home agency or central computer server. As the field of telehealth develops, POC documentation can become interactive and include multimedia access. For example, homebound clients may be given monitoring equipment that reports vital signs to a remote hook-up and alerts nursing staff to the need for follow-up. The Nightingale Tracker (FITNE Inc., 5 Depot St., Athens, OH 45701), a POC system currently in use in nursing education, allows students, staff, and faculty to access charts, care plans, and electronic mail. It also serves as a speaker phone and can be connected to the Internet for client education.

Standardized Vocabulary

The advent of electronic documentation has given impetus to the use of standardized medical and nursing vocabularies in the client record. The American Nurses Association (ANA) endorses the development of nursing databases to support clinical practice. These databases, using standardized vocabularies, can assist in describing the practice of nursing, supporting research, and identifying the cost and effectiveness of nursing interventions. These can then be incorporated into nursing information systems to facilitate nursing practice and documentation (Coenen, Marin, Park, & Bakken, 2001). The ability to enhance consistency of data through standardization of language also makes retrieval of information easier. The ANA Steering Committee on Data Bases to Support Clinical Nursing Practice approves specific vocabularies as appropriate for nursing practice. At this time, these vocabularies include Omaha, Nursing Intervention Classification (NIC), Nursing Outcome Classification (NOC), Home Health Care Classification (HHCC), North American Nursing Diagnosis Association (NANDA), and Ozbolt's Patient Care Data Set (PCDS).

Nursing Informatics

As technology and sophistication of systems have changed, so too has nursing's contribution to their development. Today, **nursing informatics** is an area of specialization within the profession. The classic definition, provided by Graves and Corcoran (1989, p. 227), defines nursing informatics as "a combination of computer science, information science and nursing science designed to assist in the management and processing of nursing data, information and knowledge to support the practice of nursing and the delivery of nursing care."

In 1990, a national Task Force on Nursing Information Systems was established to address how nursing would interface with healthcare information systems. The organization of nursing information within these systems can vary as greatly among institutions as it has with handwritten records, but the goals remain to promote efficiency, productivity, and effectiveness of care (Zielstorff, Hudgins, Grobe, & the National Commission on Nursing Implementation Project Task Force on Nursing Information Systems, 1993). Nurses specializing in informatics may work within an agency to design and maintain information systems and to provide education and training.

Nursing Entries on the Client Record

Nursing Plan of Care

A **nursing plan of care** should be generated at admission and revised to reflect changes in the client's condition. The nursing plan of care contains nursing diagnoses, goals, outcome criteria, nursing interventions, and evaluation. Standardized plans of care designed for clients with specific medical diagnoses may be used, but they must be individualized. Nursing plans of care are often part of the permanent client record. They may also be incorporated into a multidisciplinary plan of care. (See Chapter 12 for information on nursing plans of care.)

Kardex

The **Kardex** is a series of flip cards usually kept in a portable file (Fig. 15-3). Information entered on the Kardex typically includes the following:

- Pertinent demographic data, such as name, age, occupation, religion, physician, admission date, diagnosis, major procedures, surgery, and emergency contacts
- Basic needs, such as diet, activity, hygiene, how bowel and urinary elimination is accomplished, assistive devices, and safety precautions
- Allergies
- Diagnostic tests
- Daily nursing procedures, such as dressing changes, vital signs, and irrigations
- Medications and intravenous (IV) therapy
- Respiratory therapy, such as use of oxygen, mechanical ventilation, or suctioning

The Kardex is a way to ensure continuity of care from one shift to another and from one day to the next. The Kardex is commonly used in inpatient settings for the change-of-shift report (see later discussion). This most current record of a client's healthcare is updated as the client's condition changes or new physician orders are obtained.

Kardex entries are often in pencil so that they can be changed as the client's condition changes. This means that the Kardex is for planning and communication purposes only. Nursing care and client progress must be documented in the progress notes and appropriate flowsheets. If the Kardex is to become part of the permanent client record, it is written in ink. In either case, nurses are responsible for initiating and updating the Kardex and ensuring that data have been transcribed correctly from the client record.

Nursing Progress Notes

Nursing progress notes are recorded for all clients but vary in format depending on the setting. Narrative notes, SOAP notes, DAR notes, and PIE notes are all descriptive forms of documentation that summarize nursing assessments, interventions, and client responses. They may reflect a specific problem being addressed or the care provided over a specific period. Table 15-3 compares various formats for writing nursing progress notes. Because variations exist within each format, you must be familiar with your agency guidelines to ensure complete documentation of client care.

Narrative Notes. This type of documentation is a method for recording relevant client and nursing activities throughout a shift or during a single visit. It is commonly found in inpatient settings where records are organized according to the discipline charting or have a specially designated area for narrative notes by all disciplines. The note includes the date and time of the entry, identification of the role of the person writing the note, and specific activities accomplished (Fig. 15-4).

In a skilled nursing facility, a typical note might include the type of morning care given (e.g., bath or shower), nutritional intake for the shift, client activity pattern, and comfort mea-

sures provided, along with the client's response. Coordination of services with other disciplines would be noted, such as telephone calls to a physical therapist or home health services, with the time and content of those conversations recorded.

Many settings combine flowsheets with narrative notes to shorten recording time and reduce redundancy. Routine assessments (e.g., vital signs) or routine activities (e.g., IV care, dressing changes, bowel elimination) are recorded on flowsheets. They are then documented as they are completed throughout the day. In some settings, procedures and assessment data are recorded in a separate area of the client record.

Because recording in this method focuses on nursing actions and procedures, specific nursing identification of client problems may not be required. In this case, activities should support information recorded on the nursing plan of care and the nursing Kardex.

A form of the narrative note may also be used in home care settings, but it is distinguished in that case by a limitation of the note to the problem or problems for which the client is being seen. The nurse records assessment data, interventions performed, and responses seen in a narrative format. Each individual visit report may also have a designated area that addresses routine issues covered—such as vital signs, communication with other disciplines, evaluation of care delegated to assisting personnel, or medications reordered.

A disadvantage of narrative notes is that they are time-consuming to write and that much reading can be required to learn about a specific problem. Narrative notes may necessitate checking in a variety of places within the chart to identify all activities that have occurred or to follow assessment data. The narrative form of charting increases the difficulty of performing audits or chart reviews for quality assurance.

SOAP Notes. The **SOAP note** is a progress note that relates to only one health problem. All healthcare team members use the same format. The left-hand column or first line of the SOAP note identifies the problem being addressed from the master problem list. With this method, the client's progress on that particular problem can be assessed without sorting through the whole chart. The team member need only read down the left-hand column of the interdisciplinary progress notes and read the notes of all disciplines that relate to that numbered problem.

After documenting the problem to be addressed, the next step is organizing the information in the SOAP note format. The "S" stands for *subjective* and refers to data or symptoms the client expresses. Quotation marks are often used to document the client's specific statements. Quoting the client allows for different interpretations than the nurse's. If the client cannot give information or gave none relevant to this problem, the "S" may be omitted or noted as "None."

"O" refers to *objective* findings and includes data collected by the nurse that are relevant to the problem. Objective data include what the nurse can see, feel, smell, or hear and relevant laboratory data, diagnostic tests, and vital signs.

"A" stands for *assessment,* which represents a diagnosis, an impression, or a condition change. This assessment is

PLAN		NPO after _____ for OR or tests on _____	PARENTERAL FLUIDS

		GI	*Heplock*

DIET: *2g Na*   ☑ I & O
                ☑ WEIGHT
       1800 cal ADA   ☐ CALORIE COUNT

CONDITION	CODE STATUS
	Full Code

RESPIRATORY

O₂: *4 l/m NC prn*

SUCTION:

ALLERGIES		ENTERAL FLUIDS
Penicillin		DEVICE:

TRACH SIZE/TYPE:

TRACH CARE:

PRECAUTIONS	

CHEST TUBES:

RESIDUALS:

INC. SPIR. *q 1-2° WA*

CDB: *q 1-2° WA*

OTHER:

SURGERIES/MEDICAL HISTORY		ELIMINATION/GI	MONITORING
6/98 Arthroscopy		DEVICE:	VS: *q 4h* POSTURAL ORTHOSTATIC
		BOWEL PLAN:	NEURO CHECKS:
		TESTING:	CMS: *q 4h*

DIAGNOSIS		ELIMINATION/GU	CHEMSTIX: *AC + HS*
PRIMARY	SECONDARY	DEVICE:	OTHER:
1/6/99 Total Knee Replacement Ⓡ	*Diabetes, CHF*		

CALL H.O. IF:

BLADDER PLAN:

TESTING:

T >38.5°	SBP >160< 90
P >120< 50	DBP >100< 40
R >24< 10	UO > < 25 ml/h

346

Bradley, Scott

4/20/25

ROOM	AGE	SERVICE	PHYSICIAN	PRIMARY NURSE
346	69	ORTHO	GREEN	M. CHAVEZ

NURSING KARDEX
HMC 0815   REV MAR 88

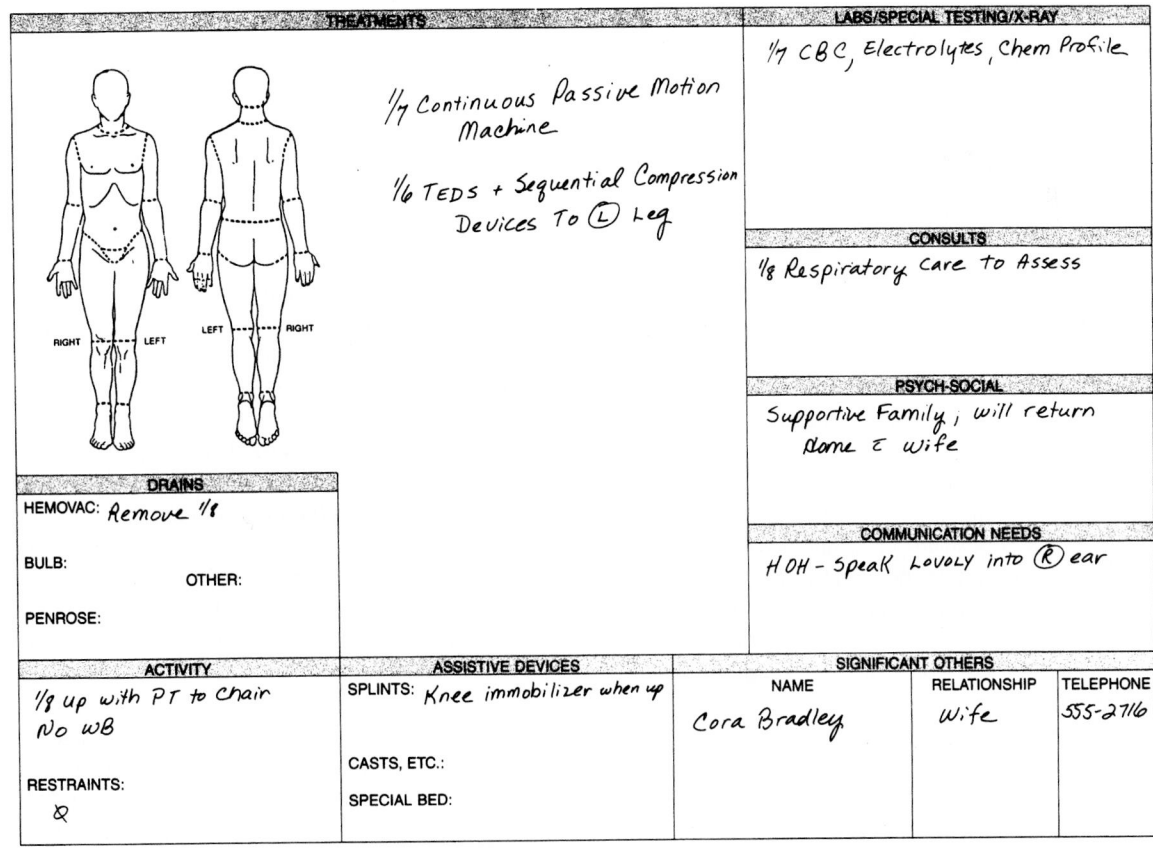

TREATMENTS	LABS/SPECIAL TESTING/X-RAY
	1/7 CBC, Electrolytes, Chem Profile

1/7 Continuous Passive Motion Machine

1/6 TEDS + Sequential Compression Devices To Ⓛ Leg

RIGHT LEFT   LEFT RIGHT

CONSULTS

1/8 Respiratory Care to Assess

PSYCH-SOCIAL

Supportive Family; will return home ē wife

DRAINS	
HEMOVAC: *Remove 1/8*	
BULB: OTHER:	
PENROSE:	

COMMUNICATION NEEDS

HOH - Speak Lovoly into Ⓡ ear

ACTIVITY	ASSISTIVE DEVICES	SIGNIFICANT OTHERS		
1/8 up with PT to chair No WB	SPLINTS: *Knee immobilizer when up*	NAME	RELATIONSHIP	TELEPHONE
	CASTS, ETC.:	*Cora Bradley*	*Wife*	*555-2716*
RESTRAINTS: ⊗	SPECIAL BED:			

FIGURE 15-3   Example of a nursing Kardex.

TABLE 15-3

	Format	**Advantages**	**Disadvantages**
Comparing Documentation Notes			
Narrative	Information provided in written sentences or phrases; usually time sequenced.	Easy to learn; easy to adjust length as needed; can explain in detail.	Time-consuming; difficult to retrieve information; irrelevant information often included; possibly unfocused and disorganized.
SOAP	S subjective data O objective data A assessment P plan	All charting is focused on identified client problems; interdisciplinary—all team members chart on the same progress notes; easy to track progress for identified problem; steps in the nursing process are mirrored.	Difficult to master. Specific focus makes it difficult to chart general information without identifying a problem; lengthy and time-consuming; assessment identification difficult for nurses.
PIE	P problem I interventions E evaluations	Plan of care incorporated into progress notes; outcomes included, which increases quality assurance; daily review to determine progress; less redundancy; easily adapted to automated charting.	Must read progress notes to determine plan of care; if problem has not been identified, difficult to chart; not multidisciplinary.
FOCUS	D data A action R response	Broad view permitting charting on any significant area, not just problems; concise, flexible; works well in long-term care or ambulatory care.	Not multidisciplinary; difficult to identify chronologic order; progress notes may not relate to the care plan.
Charting by Exception (CBE)	Standards met—sign or check off; standards not met—write narrative or SOAP note	Efficient; use of flowsheets permitting rapid detection of changes in condition; outline normal assessments; can take the place of plan of care.	Expensive to institute; inservicing of staff is needed; not prevention focused; not appropriate for long-term or ambulatory care.

made after analyzing the data from the subjective and objective portions and must be supported by those data. If assessment cannot be made from the data gathered, write "Further data gathering necessary" or a statement such as "Abdominal pain, unknown etiology" under the "A" portion of the SOAP note.

"P" stands for *plan.* This portion deals with nursing interventions specifically related to the identified problem. The plan section may simply state, "Continue present regimen," if the assessment shows that the client is progressing adequately using the plan already outlined. The plan also can specify revisions of the present nursing interventions as need is determined. Figure 15-5 provides an example of SOAP nursing progress notes.

Some agencies use the "SOAPIER" format of recording, which adds "I" for *intervention,* "E" for *evaluation,* and "R" for *revision.* This format allows the team member to record interventions, the client's response to the plan, and any revisions needed to the plan. Remember that all information recorded under the SOAP or SOAPIER headings must pertain to the same problem.

In some circumstances, a full SOAP note may be unnecessary. Routine care may be documented on a flowsheet. Routine nursing assessments need not be written as a SOAP note if they are not specifically related to a problem (e.g., routine temperature and blood pressure in a client who has had no problem with fever and has stable blood pressure).

PIE Notes. The **PIE charting** system simplifies documentation by incorporating the plan of care into the progress notes. Documentation is entered for each nursing diagnosis every shift using the acronym "PIE" to structure information according to *problem* (P), *intervention* (I), and *evaluation* (E). Client assessments are not part of the PIE note, because this information is recorded on flowsheets for each shift. Figure 15-6 provides an example of a PIE nursing note. At the end of a 24-hour period, the nurse reviews client documentation to ascertain the client's response to therapeutic intervention and progress. In this way, outdated problems can be eliminated and new problems can be added to the documentation record. This daily review of client progress helps promote continuity of care.

Correct

2/18/98	0730 Client awake, alert, denies com-
	plaints, sitting up in bed watching TV, VS
	taken, lv infusing s̄ difficulty, IV site Ⓡhand
	s̄ redness, Ⓛhip drsg dry and intact. 0830
	100% of full liquid breakfast taken. 0900
	Partial bath at bedside, pt tolerated sitting
	in chair X 30 min without fatigue. 0930
	△Drsg to Ⓛhip approx 50cc pink drng,
	sutures intact, 0 redness or edema at inci-
	sion line, pt tol s̄ pain 1015 1000cc D5 1/2
	NS added to present IV to run at 125cc/hr.
	pt resting. 1100 To x-ray via stretcher. 1145
	Returned from x-ray, back to bed for rest.
	1200 Reg lunch taken 100%
	———————————— MS Gorski RN

Incorrect

2/18/98	0730 Ct fine, states "I like the TV program."
	0830 Took a good breakfast s̄ problems.
	0900 Linen changed with ct up in chair,
	used own toothpaste and hairbrush,
	doesn't like our brand. 0930 Change drsg,
	incision site looks good, new dressing
	applied with cloth tape. 1015 New bag hung.
	1145 Returned to room, tol procedure well.
	1200 Eating lunch.
	————————— MS Gorski RN

FIGURE 15-4 Example of narrative nursing progress notes. Reflect on why the correct nursing note is better.

Correct

Problem	8/18/98	"S" My head hurts right in the back of
#3	0900	my eyes. Client describes pain
		worse bending over, like sinus
		headaches in past.
		"O" Eyes closed, lights dim, hesitant
		to move head when questioned.
		HR80 R20 BP140/90 T98.6
		"A" HA probable 2° sinus pressure.
		"P" 1. Decongestant prn as ordered
		2. Warm wash cloth to eyes
		3. Monitor temp q 4°
		4. Assess pain after med and
		contact physician as indicated
		———————— MS Gorski RN

Incorrect

	8/18/98	"S" Ct states "My head hurts."
#3	0900	"O" History of constipation, ate well
		at breakfast, took shower without
		assist, lungs clear.
		"I hurt all over now."
		"A" Headache
		"P" Contact physician for further
		orders.
		———————— MS Gorski RN

FIGURE 15-5 Example of SOAP nursing progress notes. Reflect on why the correct SOAP nursing note is better.

Variations for the PIE system can be used when appropriate. To designate new problems or abnormal assessments, "A" can be added to the numbered problem (i.e., APIE), allowing the nurse also to provide pertinent assessment data in the documentation. When appropriate, an intervention or an evaluation can be documented without writing the entire PIE statement.

Advantages of the PIE system of documentation include increased efficiency and flexibility; care planning focus; better tracking of client problems, nursing interventions, and client outcomes; and less redundancy. This system easily adapts to automated charting, and client care can easily be audited. A disadvantage of the PIE system is that it is not multidisciplinary; it provides a documentation system only for nursing. Although the PIE system uses a nursing plan of care format, there is no written plan of care, which necessitates review of previous documentation to become knowledgeable about current nursing diagnoses.

Focus Dar Notes. The **FOCUS system** of documentation organizes entries by *data* (D), *action* (A), and *response* (R). This system is broader in its view because a focus can be a problem area (e.g., nursing diagnosis) but does not need to be. An entry can be made on a significant event, positive growth, or learning that occurs during a teaching session. In this way,

9/10/99 0400	Problem #1	Caregiver role strain related to chronically ill spouse, lack of immediate family support, and financial stress.
	Intervention for P(#1)	IP(#1): Acknowledge and talk with caregiver about stress involved with 24-hour care for loved one.
		IP(#1): Allow caregiver to express feelings.
		IP(#1): Help caregiver identify possible supports within the family and community.
	Evaluation for P(#1)	EP(#1): Caregiver discussed the strain of caring for her husband; crying and demonstrating signs of anxiety eg. "I just don't think I will be able to do this for long and then what is going to happen to us all? Sometimes it seems so hopeless." Stated she felt her children were supportive but they lived in another state and could not help with the day-to-day problems. —R. Wolfe, RN
		Note: as additional data are charted for the problem of caregiver role strain, Problem #1 is used to identify the problem.

FIGURE 15-6   Example of a PIE nursing note arranging information by P (problem), I (intervention), and E (evaluation).

client documentation can focus on the client's strengths as well as problem areas.

The data portion of the statement describes subjective and objective data that support the focus of the note. Interventions and treatments are included in the action section of the note, whereas the client's response to therapy is discussed in the response section. Some notes may include all three sections, but flexibility permits the nurse to chart data, actions, and re-

sponses singularly or in combination. An example of a FOCUS nursing note appears in Figure 15-7.

Abbreviated Forms of Documentation

Flowsheets. **Flowsheets** are designed to document routine nursing procedures and to free nurses from writing out continuing procedures repeatedly. One example is a sheet for vital signs that gives a graphic representation of pulse, blood pressure, respirations, and temperature so that trends can be

Date/Time	FOCUS	NOTE
10/2/99	Injection Instruction	**Data:** Referred to injection room for teaching re injection technique as wife will be discharged and need IM injections of Compazine for nausea control. Husband states willingness to learn, yet states anxiety re "sticking wife and causing her pain."
		Action: Demonstrate injection technique including drawing up medication in syringe, locating site, injecting medication, keeping record of medication administered. Have husband verbalize steps and then demonstrate technique.
		Response: Husband able to draw up medication correctly in syringe and verbalize steps to injection technique without cuing. Husband injected model, hands shook, and needed verbal cuing to aspirate. —J. Morales RN
10/3/99	Injection Instruction	**Response:** Husband demonstrated good technique giving wife injection, without cuing. Wife will be discharged in AM with Visiting nurse follow-up. —J. Morales RN

FIGURE 15-7   Example of a FOCUS nursing note arranging information by D (data), A (action), and R (response).

evaluated (see Chapter 25). The intake and output sheet is used to maintain an ongoing record of all fluid intake and output (see Chapter 36). Assessments also can be documented in this manner. Critical care flowsheets are used in intensive care units to document frequently changing data, specific nursing interventions, client responses, and multiple medications and IV fluids administered. In the last decade, flowsheets have evolved in some agencies into charting by exception and clinical pathways.

Flowsheets provide a form on which the nurse can indicate, usually by making a checkmark, that assessment findings and care fall within the agency's standards. Standards require periodic assessments and notations, such as once per shift or weekly, so it is easy to note changes in client status. Documentation is required any time the client's status changes significantly. Additional documentation is required when any deviation from standards is detected. Often, this documentation is a narrative note on the same form to explain the variance, but it can be a SOAP note, PIE note, or DAR note in the progress section of the chart. Flowcharts and critical pathways may require noting "N/A," for not applicable, if an action was not completed. This prevents confusion about what was or was not done (Sullivan, 1996).

Charting by Exception. First developed in 1985 at St. Luke's Hospital in Milwaukee, Wisconsin, **charting by exception** (CBE) permits the nurse to document only those findings that fall outside the standard of care and norms that have been developed by the institution (Barthel, Reichert, Streff, & Twite, 1993). CBE is a shift away from the concept previously held, that "if it hasn't been documented, it hasn't been done." Agencies develop written norms and standards against which client assessments or client care activities can be compared. These standards are made readily available within the nursing site and often are included on the form or in the back of the client's chart for easy reference.

CBE has many advantages:

- It requires less nursing time.
- Guidelines about expected outcomes and normal assessment parameters are clear.
- Changes in client status can readily be detected.
- Information is more readily accessible.

The most significant disadvantage of CBE is the time it takes for each agency to develop and to maintain standards and flowsheets. CBE seems to work best in agencies or with conditions for which routine care can be anticipated.

Clinical Pathways. With increasing interest in outcomes of care, many institutions and agencies have moved to the use of **clinical pathways** as a way to guide the care of clients who have specific and generally predictable conditions. Based on knowledge about best practices and institutional resources, clinical pathways serve as models for ensuring quality of care. The pathway may be for clients who require complex care (e.g., after organ transplantation) or for frequently encountered situations (e.g., home care visits for clients who have

undergone hip replacement surgery). Pathways may look like flowsheets and may use CBE documentation. (See Chapter 12 for a generic clinical pathway.)

Clinical pathways serve as multidisciplinary tools, identifying the expected progression of the client toward discharge. They provide direction about major interventions to be performed: assessments, diagnostic tests, procedures, medications, teaching, activity, diet, and discharge planning. Documentation occurs on the pathway form, and usually the nurse is required to sign his or her initials when a specific intervention has occurred or an outcome has been met. A **variance** occurs when the client does not proceed along the pathway as planned. Any variances are documented in detail, usually with the use of narrative notes.

The physician initiates the clinical pathway for a specific client through standard orders that match those identified in the pathway. Additional orders are written as needed to individualize care. The pathway is then placed in the client's chart, providing orders for care. Institutions may also develop related forms of the pathway for clients to assist in teaching and discharge planning.

The clinical pathway provides a concise means for all members of the healthcare team to view the client's continuing needs and progress toward discharge. Review of variance data can help institutions seek improvements in care and can lead toward changes in pathways themselves.

Admission Entries

When a client enters the healthcare system, a nursing history is completed. Nutrition, activity, sleep, and coping patterns are assessed and documented, as are the pertinent medical history and the history relating to the reason for current care. A complete physical assessment is performed and documented. This information may be entered on the nursing admission history and physical assessment sheet, on another standardized form, or in nursing progress notes. (See Chapter 24 for a full description of nursing history and physical assessment.)

Nursing Discharge Summary

A nursing discharge plan is started at the initiation of care (Fig. 15-8), indicating potential discharge needs and client teaching that will take place. The discharge summary notes the client's condition at discharge and provides specific information about care after discharge. A copy of the discharge summary may be given to the client or sent to a home health nurse or extended care facility.

Nursing discharge summary forms are usually standardized and contain space to write specific instructions for the client. Such information includes medications, diet, activity, follow-up care, and special instructions, such as heat applications and circumstances that require notification of the physician (e.g., signs of wound infection). Sometimes these forms are completed in multiple copies so that a copy can easily be given immediately to the client. More recently, computer-generated discharge forms can be individualized for the client and obtained from software programs installed on the agency

Diagnosis	SELF CARE STATUS LEVEL (Check √ either I - Independent, A - Assistance, U - Unable)		I	A	U
Heart Failure					

Diagnosis: Heart Failure

Procedures/Surgeries (include dates)

SELF CARE STATUS LEVEL (Check √ either I - Independent, A - Assistance, U - Unable)	I	A	U
DRESSES SELF		✓	
SHAVES SELF		✓	
TRANSFERS SELF		✓	
AMBULATES		✓	
FEEDS SELF	✓		
BATHES SELF ☐ TUB ☑ SHOWER		✓	
ORAL HYGIENE		✓	

How Patient Discharged
☐ Ambulatory   ☑ Wheelchair   ☐ Ambulance   ☐ Cabulance

Who Patient Discharged With:
☐ Alone   ☑ M. Hazelet (daughter)
Name and Relationship to Patient

Discharged to:
☐ Nursing Home (name)_____
☐ Own Home or Apt.   ☑ Other (name) Daughter's home

Family/Support System (Name, Relationship, Phone)
May Hazelet (daughter) 698-8650

Sensory Needs
Hearing ☐ within Normal Limits   ☑ Hard of Hearing   ☐ Aids ⊘
Vision ☐ within Normal Limits   ☑ Aids glasses
Speech ☐ within Normal Limits   ☐ Aphasic   ☐ Aids

Languages Spoken: English

Allergies: ☒ None   ☐ Specify

• BLADDER_____

• BOWEL_____

• WOUNDS/DRESSINGS/TUBES
(Type and Location) none

(Supplies/Amt. Provided) _____

• SPECIAL EQUIPMENT/APPLIANCES SENT HOME WITH PATIENT

(If Rental, Obtained from:

YOUR MEDICATIONS

NAME	DOSAGE	WHEN TO TAKE	SPECIAL INSTRUCTIONS	LAST DOSE GIVEN AT
Digoxin	0.125 mg	1 tablet every other day in morning		0900 3-21
Lasix	40 mg	1 tablet every morning		0900 3-21
Potassium	40 mEq	every morning		0900 3-21

PATIENT TEACHING	RETURN DEMONSTRATION	NEEDS PRACTICE	NEEDS MORE INSTRUCTION	SATISFACTORY	REFERRAL AT DISCHARGE
Skills/Topics					Agency Name

FOLLOW-UP CARE

SPECIAL INSTRUCTIONS	CLINIC NAME / PHYSICIAN	DATE	TIME
Diet 2 Gm Na	Lake Beach Clinic	3-29-99	9⁰⁰ am
Activity Up ad lib	Dr. B. Kyle		
Lab Work			
Other			

Address

Phone #   Date Phoned

Referral For:
☐ NURSING CARE
☐ P.T.   ☐ O.T.
☐ MEAL SERVICE
☐ CHORE WORKER
☐ COMPANION
☐ OTHER_____

PHONE NUMBER WHERE YOU CAN BE REACHED
AT UWMC CALL (206) 548-4333 TO MAKE APPOINTMENT(S)
AT HMC CALL _____ TO MAKE APPOINTMENT(S)

Discharge Date/Time 3-21-99   11:30

I have been informed and I understand my home discharge instructions.

Patient Signature or Care-Giver
X Scott Bradley

Primary Nurse Signature
X J. Sidney RN   R.N.

Discharge Unit/Phone Number 689-5342

PT.NO. 029345

NAME Bradley, Scott

D.O.B.

UNIVERSITY OF WASHINGTON MEDICAL CENTERS
HARBORVIEW MEDICAL CENTER - UW MEDICAL CENTER
SEATTLE, WASHINGTON
PATIENT DISCHARGE STATUS REPORT
DIVISION OF NURSING

* U 0 0 2 1 *

WHITE - MEDICAL RECORD
CANARY - PATIENT (BELOW PERFORATION)
PINK - REFERRAL COPY
GOLDEN ROD - CLINIC

UH 0021 REV FEB 94

FIGURE 15-8   Example of a patient discharge summary.

client's current status and any recent changes. Between nurses and other departments, it provides critical current information to enhance client care. Reporting is done face to face, on the telephone, or by taped messages such as shift reports or voice mail. It should be organized, complete, and professional. With increasing computer access in many settings, the sending of electronic messages or e-mail may be used as a written form of reporting to communicate simple messages. In this case, the nurse must become knowledgeable about the institutional policies governing the use and storage of these messages.

Nurse to Nurse

Establishing Continuity between Shifts or Client Visits

In inpatient settings, the **change-of-shift report** serves as the means for the nurse to report to oncoming nursing staff about a client's status and plans of care. This report is a way of ensuring continuity in care from one shift to the next. It may be taped or given face to face (Fig. 15-10). Taping saves time but does not allow for clarification of details. A typical change-of-shift report in an acute care setting includes the following information:

- Name, age, and room number of client
- Medical diagnoses, major procedures or surgery (date)
- Physician name or group
- Significant nursing or medical diagnoses and progress toward goals
- Significant assessment findings, including vital signs
- Diagnostic and laboratory test results
- Specific treatments (e.g., dressing changes, respiratory therapy)
- IV rate and amount of IV fluid remaining

Oral and taped reports may use the nursing Kardex, nursing plan of care, flowsheets, and/or working chart as a basis for the information to be included. The listener also uses the Kardex as a guide to clarify information given by the previous nurse and to fill in the details of routine care.

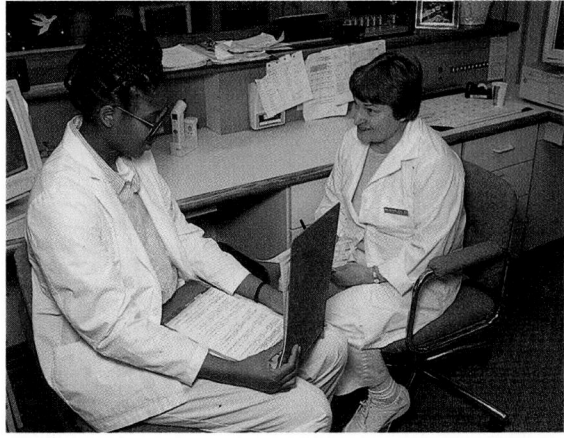

FIGURE 15-10   By reporting to one another, nurses ensure that their clients have continuity of care from one shift to another.

Variations in shift reports occur according to the specialty nursing area. For example, the report in a critical care setting may include an in-depth evaluation of each client's body systems (i.e., respiratory status by assessment and ventilator readings, cardiovascular status by rhythm strips and blood pressure measurements). The report in a long-term care setting might include only those clients with significant status changes and might not address stable clients.

Nursing Rounds

Another method of reporting is nursing rounds (also called walking rounds). Rounds may be used for change-of-shift reports or for care planning. Two or more nurses visit a group of clients, and the nurse assigned to each client summarizes the client's current status and plan of care.

Nursing rounds are advantageous because optimal communication occurs between nurses and client status is confirmed by direct observation. For instance, it may be easier to describe various IV lines and dressing changes when the oncoming nurse is at the client's bedside. However, nursing rounds are time-consuming because other topics may be discussed, and the client may feel excluded or alienated by the medical terms being used. Using understandable language and encouraging the client to participate can facilitate the client's involvement.

Report to Primary Care Provider

A telephone report to a physician is usually prompted by a change in the client's condition. The most important preparation for this type of communication is completion of a focused nursing assessment. The assessment may be focused on the system involved, but all pertinent data should be gathered and communicated as appropriate. It may help to outline on paper the information that needs to be communicated to the physician. Have the client's record handy for reference. Important information to give a physician for status reports or possible medical intervention follows:

- Client name and diagnosis
- Stated symptoms
- Changes in nursing assessment
- Vital signs (compared with baseline)
- Laboratory tests (compared with baseline)
- Nursing treatment initiated and client response

The following is an example of a nurse–physician telephone call:

This is Nancy Newton, RN from Community Home Health. I am calling regarding Mr. Jones, who is now day 8 post CABG [coronary artery bypass graft] surgery. I am calling today because the incision on his left leg is now showing an area of redness extending 3 inches up from the distal end and 1.5 inches on either side. The incision itself remains closed, but the skin is swollen and serous drainage can be expressed. Mr. Jones reported he first noticed the redness yesterday when bathing. He states he has had no other signs of infection, and his temperature today is 98.9°F. He is not taking any medications that would mask a fever at this time.

A telephone report to a physician is often followed by telephone orders that must be documented in the client record and carried out by the nurse. For example, the physician may order a treatment for Mr. Jones that should be started before the client can visit the physician. Write the order in the client record and label it as a telephone or verbal order. Nurses are responsible for correctly identifying the treatment and the physician who ordered it. If it is a medication, accurately record the dose, time, and route. To ensure accuracy, repeat the information and ask the physician to spell the medication and his or her name as necessary. Figure 15-11 is an example of a correctly transcribed telephone order.

Verbal orders need to be cosigned by the ordering physician, usually within a 24-hour period. Make sure this occurs so that the order is validated, thus preventing possible litigation if problems arise (Cirone, 1998). Most home care settings have specific forms for the documentation of verbal phone orders. These are often on carbonless paper so that a copy may be sent for the ordering physician's signature.

Interdisciplinary Team

Client Admission, Transfer, and Discharge

Telephone reports can be used when transferring a client to another unit within a hospital or from one facility or agency to another. Telephone reports also are used extensively to update primary care providers about client status and to communicate between hospital departments. Because telephone reports do not rely on written verification or direct observation, accuracy is vital. Clarify any question. The sender should state the message clearly and concisely, and the receiver should repeat pertinent data for verification.

When a client is transferred to a different facility or unit, the receiving nurse needs to know what to expect. He or she must receive the most current information on the client's status and a summary of the client's progress and general care. The telephone report enables the receiving nurse to prepare for the client before arrival and to clarify any information from written transfer summaries they may have obtained. The following information is generally included in the transfer report:

- Client name and age
- Current diagnosis and medical history
- Reason for transfer
- Most current assessment, particularly abnormalities
- Equipment to be transferred with client (e.g., oxygen, IV infusion, wheelchair)
- Time and method of expected transport

When transferring a client to a different unit within an institution, the client record is transferred with the client.

Reports to and from Other Departments

Nurses often receive telephone reports from other departments, such as radiology centers or laboratories. Information exchanged is crucial to client care, and numbers for laboratory values and complex terminology for diagnostic procedures can easily be misunderstood. When requesting information from another department, be courteous. Identify yourself and the client. Identify any pertinent identification numbers, the client diagnosis, and the attending physician to ensure accuracy in client identification. When you receive a report, repeat the information and speak clearly to verify findings.

Likewise, nurses often give reports to other departments. In the inpatient setting, the client usually is identified by such information as name, room number, date of birth, and diagnosis. This may take place, for instance, when a nurse reports a new client to the dietary department or requests a consultation from physical therapy. The admission of a client to a service such as hospice may necessitate informing a large group of people. In such cases, a standardized script may be used and directed via group voice mail distribution. For example, the nurse may be responsible for notifying the intake department, bereavement program, receptionist, medical records, billing, after-hours staff, volunteer coordinator, and nursing supervisors. A standardized script for all of these people might note the client's name (spelled out as well as spoken), names of case managers, date of admission, payor source, primary care physician, and location of care.

Care Plan Conferences and Team Rounds

Care plan conferences are discussions about client care, involving either several disciplines or just the nursing staff. A conference with other nurses may be held to "brainstorm" ideas about a particular client's care. These conferences are initiated by the nurses who are caring for the client with the goal of enhancing quality and continuity of care.

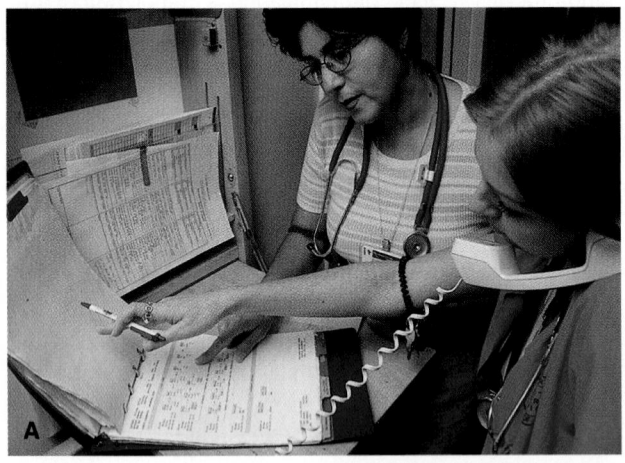

11/6/03	Give rantidine 300 mg. po now and
10 pm	then q6h.
	Telephone order from
	Dr. Lavelle/Ann Smith RN

B

FIGURE 15-11 (A) Nurses may need to communicate with the physician by telephone. (B) Example of documentation of a telephone order from a physician to a nurse.

Interdisciplinary conferences help to coordinate services so that the client's plan of care can be developed and implemented in the most efficient way. Nurses may initiate these conferences and invite members of the healthcare team from other departments (e.g., physical therapy, social services, dietary). Clients who most benefit from such conferences are those with multiple, complex problems. In some settings, routine conferences are held to review client progress and services being provided. For example, in the pediatric oncology setting, such conferences may bring together members from inpatient and ambulatory care teams, allowing for each to anticipate services to be provided.

ETHICAL CONCERNS IN DOCUMENTATION AND REPORTING

Confidentiality

All client care must be confidential. This rule is a basic nursing responsibility and a client expectation and right. In many institutions, the client's privacy is codified in a statement of rights that is signed at the point of entry into care. Nurses must treat the client record as a confidential document entrusted to the healthcare team. They should never leave it in public areas or where it might be read by unauthorized people. Nurses traveling in the community should keep records in a secured filing system. They should not discuss or share the contents of the record with anyone not directly involved in the client's care, including the client's minister, family members, and physicians or nurses who are friends of the family. Strangers, such as new students on a unit, should be asked for identification before they are allowed access to the client's record. The client's right to privacy must be actively guarded.

Discuss clients only in a manner that ensures confidentiality. Do not discuss specific clients in public areas, where family or friends could possibly overhear information. When making telephone reports or engaging in other verbal communication, make sure to speak in a private place and only to those persons who are authorized. In the community, you may need to delay telephone calls to team members until completion of the visit or to coordinate activities in such a way as to group telephone calls after returning to the office.

Carefully follow agency policies regarding transmittal of information via electronic communication such as e-mail and

facsimile transmission. General guidelines for fax transmittal include notifying the recipient that a transmittal is being sent, marking the document clearly on the cover page that it is confidential, and requesting that misdirected fax materials be promptly destroyed or returned (Fiesta, 1996). Legal and professional guidelines regarding electronic messages such as e-mail are currently undergoing definition. Legislation and court decisions in the coming years are likely to affect their status and use among healthcare professionals. Nurses using these methods of communication must remain up to date regarding community and institutional practices. Exercise consistency in adhering to institutional policies regarding use, content, and deletion of messages.

Computers bring a new level of concern to confidentiality in the maintenance of the client record. Securing the transmission of information is of paramount importance. Institutions are responsible for developing policies and procedures that promote security of the electronic record. This stems not only from professional standards but also from external forces. For example, the JCAHO requires a plan to safeguard security and confidentiality whenever hospitals use computers (Joint Commission on Accreditation of Healthcare Organizations, 2001).

Nurses must support these efforts to guard against inadvertent disclosure as well as unauthorized access. Understanding basic principles of security within the system can help the nurse take effective steps to ensure confidentiality and safety of information. Secured access codes must be issued and kept secret, because they constitute the equivalent of a legal signature. Computer programs used for documentation must safeguard the information once it is logged into a client's record, providing strict and clear recording of any subsequent changes to an entry. Computers and any electronic devices that provide access to the record must be safeguarded against theft. Ensure that only authorized people can view the screens when client information is displayed.

Access to Records

Traditionally, the client record has been the property of the healthcare facility, agency, or physician's office. With the advent of the CPR and changing philosophies with respect to personal responsibility for healthcare, ownership of the record itself may also change. At this time, the Federal Privacy Act and other federal laws ensure the right of selected people (e.g., federal government employees; clients receiving care in a Veterans Administration Hospital, Public Health Service facility, or a long-term care facility receiving Medicare or Medicaid payment) to review their health records. Recent federal proposals respond to the need for basic security in the medical records. These proposals deal with ensuring confidentiality and accuracy in the electronic record and its transmission, providing client access to records, and limiting disclosure while maintaining access to information to promote public health. With increasing pressure from advances in telecommunication and heightened consumer awareness, many states are reviewing their legislation with respect to medical records.

|5| APPLY YOUR KNOWLEDGE

You are working in a walk-in medical clinic. You see your cousin's boyfriend sitting in the waiting room. After his appointment, you look through his chart and discover that he was diagnosed and treated for a sexually transmitted disease (STD). You worry about the risk this poses to your cousin. What should you do?

Check your answer in Appendix A.

Ultimately, federal legislation may provide a baseline for security, access, and confidentiality, with state laws providing individually tighter controls. Individual agency policies may provide additional guidance regarding the circumstances and conditions under which records may be accessed. Nurses may be responsible for providing clients with their records and interpreting the information held within them.

KEY CONCEPTS

- The purposes of the client record are communication, assessment, care planning, education, research, auditing, and legal documentation.
- Principles of recording include accuracy, completeness, conciseness, objectivity, organization, timeliness, and legibility.
- The use of computers is increasing in documentation. Either the entire client record or just parts of it (e.g., the nursing plan of care) can be computerized. The universal CPR is designed to bring together all health data on a single client into a readily accessed form.
- The nursing Kardex is a series of cards containing background information, routine care information, and specific treatments for each client. It is used when giving care and for change-of-shift reporting.
- The SOAP format organizes information into subjective (S), objective (O), assessment (A), and plan (P) categories. Chronologic narrative nursing progress notes may be difficult to follow when checking the progress of the client on a specific problem.
- The PIE format incorporates the plan of care into the progress notes. Information is organized according to problem (P), intervention (I), and evaluation (E).
- FOCUS charting permits documentation on any significant topic, not just client problems. Information is organized around data (D), action (A), and response (R).
- Flowsheets for vital signs, intake and output, and routine nursing assessment and care make recording quicker and less redundant.
- CBE enables the nurse to check off normal assessments or treatment administered, writing narrative notes only when deviations from standards or norms are found.
- Clinical pathways allow all members of the team to monitor and to record client progress toward discharge based on care-related norms.
- A nursing discharge summary reports the client's status at discharge and gives instructions for diet, activity, home care, and follow-up.
- Nurse-to-nurse oral reports should be comprehensive but brief, highlighting changes in the past 24 hours or since the last visit.
- In telephone reporting, the sender of the message should speak clearly and the receiver should repeat the message to avoid errors.
- The nurse must maintain the confidentiality of documentation and respect the client's right to privacy in reporting care.

REFERENCES

Barthel, M., Reichert, B., Streff, M., & Twite, K. (1993). Charting by exception eases documentation. *Oncology Nursing Forum, 20*(5), 826.

Carelock, J., & Innerarity, K. (2001). Critical incidents: effective communication and documentation. *Critical Care Nursing Quarterly, 23*(4), 59–66.

Cirone, N. (1998). Does your staff take orders by phone? *Nursing Management, (24)*12, 53.

Coenen, A., Marin, H. F., Park, H., & Bakken, S. (2001). Collaborative efforts for representing nursing concepts in computer based systems: International perspectives. *Journal of the American Medical Information Association, 8*(3), 202–211.

Cordell, B., & Smith-Blair, N. (1994). Streamlined charting for client education. *Nursing '94, 24*(1), 57–59.

Fiesta, J. (1996). Legal issues in the information age: Part 2. *Nursing Management, 27*(9), 12–13.

Graves, J. R., & Corcoran, S. (1989). The study of nursing informatics. *Image: Journal of Nursing Scholarship, 21*(4), 227–231.

Joint Commission on Accreditation of Healthcare Organizations. (2001). Patients rights and organization ethics chapter. In *Comprehensive accreditation manual for hospitals: The official handbook.* Oakwood Terrace, IL: Author.

Nahm, R., & Poston, I. (2000). Measurement of the effects of an integrated point of care computer system on the quality of nursing documentation and patient satisfaction. *Computers in Nursing, 18*(5), 220–229.

Pennels, C. (2001). The art of recording patient care information. *Professional Nurse, 16*(9), 1359–1361.

Saba, V. K., & McCormick, K. A. (1996). *Essentials of computers for nurses.* New York: McGraw-Hill.

Staggers, N., Thompson, C. B., & Snyder-Halpern, R. (2001). History and trends in clinical information systems in the United States. *Journal of Nursing Scholarship, 33*(1), 75–81.

Sullivan, G. H. (1996). Is your documentation all it should be? *RN, 59*(10), 59–61.

Zielstorff, R. D., Hudgins, C. I., Grobe, S. J., & The National Commission on Nursing Implementation Project (NCNIP) Task Force on Nursing Information Systems (1993). *Next-generation nursing information systems: Essential characteristics for professional practice.* Washington, DC: American Nurses Publishing.

BIBLIOGRAPHY

Capone, L. J. (1999). The 12 Cs of clinical documentation. *Home Healthcare Nurse, 17*(6), 382–389.

Clark, J., Christensen, J., Mooney, G., Davies, P., Edwards, J., Fitchett, L., Spowart, B., & Thomas, P. (2001). Professional briefing: New methods of documenting health visiting practice. *Community Practitioner, 74*(3), 108–112.

Cook, A. F., Hoas, H., & Joyner, J. C. (2001). Ethical issues. No secrets on main street: challenges to ethically sound care in rural settings. *AJN 101*(8), 67, 69–71.

Hagland, M. (2001). News and trends. Nursing IS on the leading edge. *Healthcare Informatics, 18*(2), 24–25.

Hardiker, N. R., & Rector, A. L. (2001). Structural validation of nursing terminologies. *Journal of the American Medical Informatics Association, 8*(3), 212–221.

Hebda, T., Czar, P., & Mascara, C. (2001). *Handbook of informatics for nurses and health care professionals.* Upper Saddle River, NJ: Prentice Hall Inc.

Larrabee, J. H., Boldrehini, S., Elder-Sonells, K., Turner, Z. M., Wender, R. G., Hart, J. M., & Lenzi, P. S. (2001). Evaluation of documentation before and after implementation of a nursing information system in an acute care hospital. *Computers in Nursing, 19*(2), 56–68.

Nicoll, L. (1998). *Computers in nursing: Nurses' guide to the Internet.* Philadelphia: Lippincott-Raven.

Raymond, L. (2001). How to chart for peer review. *RN 64*(6), 67–70.

Sardinas, J. L., & Muldoon, J. D. (1998). Securing the transmission and storage of medical information. *Computers in Nursing, 16*(3), 162–168.

Staff, E. J. (1997). Privacy, confidentiality, and security in clinical information systems: Dilemmas and opportunities for the nurse executive. *Nursing Administration Quarterly, 21*(3), 21–28.

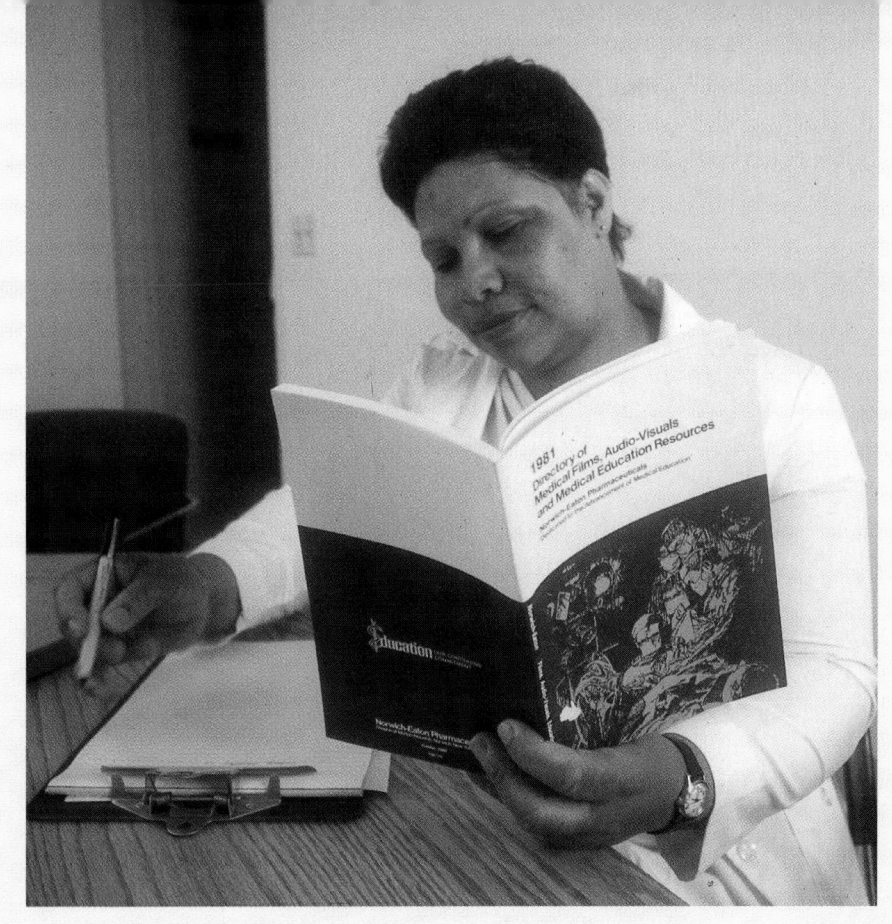

Concepts Essential for Human Functioning and Nursing Management

16 Health and Wellness

Key Terms

agent
disease
dysfunction
environment
health
high-level wellness
holism
homeostasis

host
illness
imagery
meditation
self-awareness
Therapeutic Touch
wellness

Learning Objectives

Upon completion of this chapter, the student will be able to do the following:

1. Define *wellness, holism,* and *holistic care.*
2. Compare and contrast the various models of the concept of health.
3. Identify the connections between mind, body, spirit, and symptoms.
4. Explain the role of the holistic nurse as a colleague with the client.
5. Give examples of some holistic healthcare modalities.
6. During the last half of the twentieth century, healthcare professionals changed their perspectives about health. The concept of holism is at the forefront of current thinking. This chapter will help you understand various definitions of health along with concepts related to wellness. A summary of the practice of holistic healthcare, using Emma Rose's situation for illustration, will help you better understand these concepts.

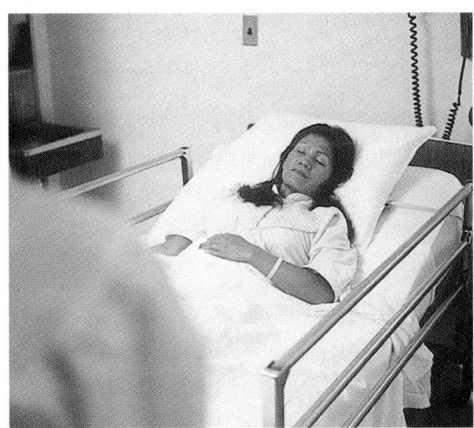

Critical Thinking Challenge

Emma Rose is 25 years old and independent. Yesterday, she had unexpected surgery after a skiing injury that resulted in a compound fracture of her left femur. She has never been in a hospital before. This morning, she overheard the physician on rounds refer to her as "the surgery in Room 304." Being in a hospital bed and overhearing this comment makes Emma Rose feel like a piece of furniture one minute and a child the next. No one seems interested in how this operation has affected her. She has always taken her health for granted. Now, she feels sick and disabled.

As you follow Emma Rose throughout this chapter, you will learn with her more about the concepts of health, wellness, and holistic healthcare. Once you have completed this chapter and have incorporated health and wellness into your knowledge base, review the above scenario and reflect on the following areas of Critical Thinking:

1. Examine Emma Rose's dual feelings of being treated as merely a piece of furniture and as a child. Explain how these feelings may contribute to her feeling disabled or sick.
2. Infer how the connection of mind, body, and spirit accentuated Emma Rose's symptoms.
3. Reflect on the physical, emotional, and spiritual dimensions of Emma Rose's care.
4. Describe health promotion activities that may be appropriate for Emma Rose and how they will help her to feel in control of her own health.

HEALTH AND WELLNESS

The World Health Organization (WHO) defines **health** as "a state of complete physical, mental, and social well-being, not merely the absence of disease or infirmity" (1947, pp. 1–2). This definition is a dramatic departure from the traditional Western view, which considered a person to be healthy if he or she were merely symptom free.

WHO's definition of health is a useful starting point, because it considers all dimensions of the person (functioning physically, psychologically, and socially) as essential to a state of health and wellness. According to Allen (1986), WHO's definition was designed to prevent health from being defined in a Western "disease" orientation. He suggested that, when trying to define health, people should consider historical meanings and implications and understand whose interests were served in each case to better recognize what is necessary for present and future social change.

Health is a dynamic state in which the person constantly adapts to changes in the internal and external environments. Each person has his or her own definition of health. People define health in relation to personal expectations and values. The concept of health must allow for this individual variability. For example, a person may see himself or herself as healthy while experiencing a respiratory infection. Someone who has a temporary disability related to mobility may consider himself or herself "not healthy," but a person with a permanent disability may consider such a condition a "normal" state and define health differently.

The concept of wellness also allows for individual variability. **Wellness** can be thought of as a dynamic balance among the physical, psychological, social, and spiritual aspects of a person's life. As with health, each person also defines wellness in relation to personal expectations. Wellness behaviors promote healthy functioning and help prevent illness. Examples of wellness behaviors include stress management, nutritional awareness, and physical fitness. Chapter 31 discusses wellness behaviors in greater detail.

HEALTH MODELS

Various models of the concept of health exist. Some models are based narrowly on the presence or absence of definable illness. Others are based more conceptually on health beliefs, wellness, and holism.

Clinical Model

The clinical model interprets health narrowly as the absence of signs and symptoms of disease or injury; therefore, the opposite of health is disease. Dunn (1961, p. 2) defines health in this model as "a relatively passive state of freedom from illness . . . a condition of relative homeostasis." Illness, therefore, is something that happens to a person. Many healthcare providers focus on relieving signs and symptoms of disease and conclude that when these findings are no longer present, the person is healthy.

This model may not consider a client's health beliefs or the lifestyle factors that continue to place the client at high risk for disease. Relieving obvious signs and symptoms may not address larger issues in the person's life that affect his or her health. For example, a person who persists in smoking cigarettes and living a sedentary life is likely to develop, eventually, signs and symptoms that relate to these lifestyle patterns, regardless of whether those signs and symptoms are apparent now.

Host–Agent–Environment Model

The host–agent–environment model (Fig. 16-1) was developed to help identify the cause of an illness (Leavell & Clark, 1965). In this model, the following definitions apply:

Host: the person (or group) who may be at risk for or susceptible to an illness
Agent: any factor (internal or external) that can lead to illness by its presence or absence
Environment: factors (physical, social, economic, emotional, spiritual) that may create the likelihood or the predisposition for the person to develop disease

In this model, health and illness depend on the interaction of these three factors. For example, a person (host) may be exposed to the virus for the common cold (agent), but whether a cold develops depends on a variety of conditions (environment). Poor nutrition, inadequate sleep, and unusual stress before the exposure predispose the host to develop a cold. Conversely, a person who is well nourished and physically fit and who is in control of the stresses of life is less likely to develop symptoms.

Health Belief Model

In the health belief model (Rosenstock, 1974), a relation exists between a person's beliefs and actions (Fig. 16-2). Factors that influence those beliefs include the following:

- Personal expectations in relation to health and illness
- Earlier experiences with health and illness
- Sociocultural context
- Age and developmental state

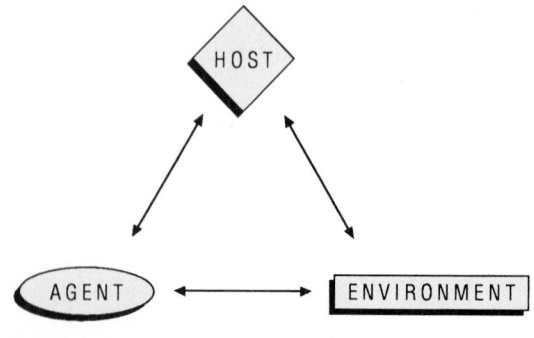

FIGURE 16-1   Host–agent–environment model.

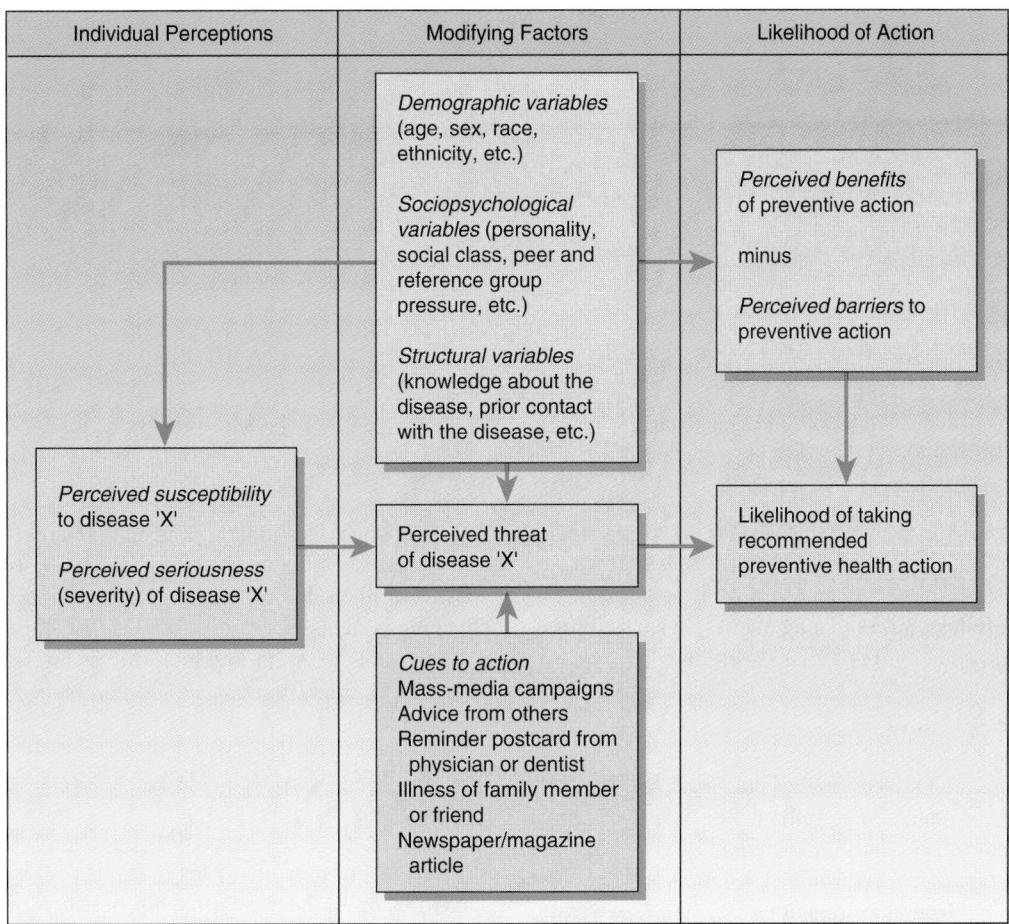

FIGURE 16-2   Health belief model.

According to this model, someone who expects to have a cold at the same time every year may find that those expectations come true. Conversely, positive, health-oriented expectations might keep the person from developing an illness. Previous experience with an illness has a major influence on how the person reacts to subsequent challenges; previous pain experiences, for example, shape future pain experiences.

Peer influence, personality characteristics, ethnicity, and socioeconomic factors may affect a person's response to illness. Someone who gets sick but whose experience is similar to that of his or her peers or socioeconomic group may not consider that he or she is in "poor health." Group values influence the health beliefs of each person.

Age and developmental stage are important considerations in the health belief model. For example, an older adult may be more tolerant of a particular illness or disability than a younger person, because of perceived greater susceptibility to "poor health." Infants and very young children do not differentiate illness from health because they have not developed a conscious memory of one state compared with the other.

The health belief model provides insight into the connection between the way a person sees his or her state of health and that person's response to health, illness, and treatment.

High-Level Wellness Model

Dunn (1961) introduced the term **high-level wellness,** recognizing health as an ongoing process toward a person's highest potential of functioning. This process involves the person, the family, and the community. Dunn describes high-level wellness as "the experience of a person alive with the glow of good health, alive to the tips of their fingers with energy to burn, tingling with vitality—at times like this the world is a glorious place."

The wellness–illness continuum (Travis & Ryan, 1988) is a visual comparison of high-level wellness and traditional medicine's view of wellness (Fig. 16-3). At the neutral point, no signs or symptoms of disease appear. A person moving toward the left experiences a worsening state of health. Someone with wellness-oriented goals wants to move beyond the neutral point (mere absence of disease) to the right (toward high-level wellness). This person evaluates the current conduct of his or her life, learns about available options, and grows toward self-actualization by trying out options in the search for high-level wellness.

High-level wellness, according to Ardell (1977, p. 65) is "a lifestyle-focused approach which you design for the purpose of pursuing the highest-level health within your capability." A

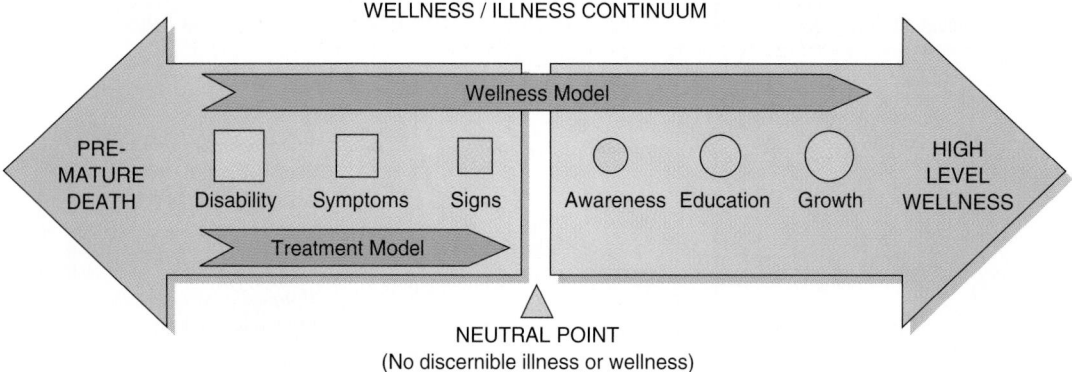

WELLNESS / ILLNESS CONTINUUM

PRE-
MATURE
DEATH

Disability   Symptoms   Signs

Wellness Model

Treatment Model

Awareness   Education   Growth

HIGH
LEVEL
WELLNESS

NEUTRAL POINT
(No discernible illness or wellness)

FIGURE 16-3   Wellness–illness continuum. (From Travis, J. W., & Ryan, R. S. [1988]. *Wellness workbook,* Berkeley, CA: Ten-Speed Press.)

person's lifestyle is a dynamic process that involves beliefs, needs, and values. Choices in life become opportunities to move toward wellness, using methods such as self-responsibility, nutritional awareness, stress management, physical fitness, spiritual growth, and environmental sensitivity.

Holistic Health Model

Holism has been a major theme in the humanities, Western political tradition, and major religions throughout history. Holism acknowledges and respects the interaction of a person's mind, body, and spirit within the environment (Fig. 16-4).

Holism, derived from the Greek *holos* ("whole"), was first used by South African philosopher Jan Christian Smuts (1926) in *Holism and Evolution.* Smuts saw holism as an antidote to the atomistic approach of contemporary science. An atomistic approach takes things apart, examining the person piece by piece in an attempt to understand the larger picture. In the scenario at the beginning of this chapter, the physician on rounds took an atomistic approach, concentrating on the surgery and ignoring other aspects of Emma Rose's life.

Holism is based on the belief that people (or even their parts) cannot be fully understood if examined solely in pieces apart from their environment. Holism sees people as ever-changing systems of energy. As Fig. 16-4 illustrates, the organism and the system in which it lives are seen as greater than and different from the sum of their parts.

WELLNESS AND HOLISTIC HEALTHCARE

Holistic healthcare emphasizes humanism, choices, self-care activities, and a peer relationship between the healthcare provider and the client. A holistic intervention would focus on the interrelated client needs of body, mind, emotions, and spirit.

For centuries, the healthcare community thought of body and mind as distinct entities as Cartesian philosophy reigned. An illness labeled psychosomatic (*psyche,* "mind," and *soma,* "body") was considered a mental health problem, and often the client was referred to a mental health practitioner. Holistic practitioners use the term *psychosomatic* to mean not simply that the mind or emotions cause illness, but that the mind and body are so interrelated that they act on each other in an intimate, direct, inseparable way. Therefore, holistic health practitioners acknowledge the interactive processes of the mind, body, and spirit.

> Emma Rose decides to talk to you about ideas related to holistic care. You give her some questionnaires to complete in order to gather information about her lifestyle, including questions on nutrition, exercise, stress reduction, spirituality, expression of feelings, and environmental awareness. Just answering the questions makes Emma Rose think about lifestyle choices and their role in her desire for wellness. For instance, the questionnaire about nutrition makes her realize that she usually has a doughnut for breakfast but is hungry by midmorning. Her morning coffee really seems to increase her jitters.

Holistic Practice

Holistic health practitioners do not want to abandon the established successes of traditional healthcare. Instead, they try to combine the best of both worlds: the proven success of

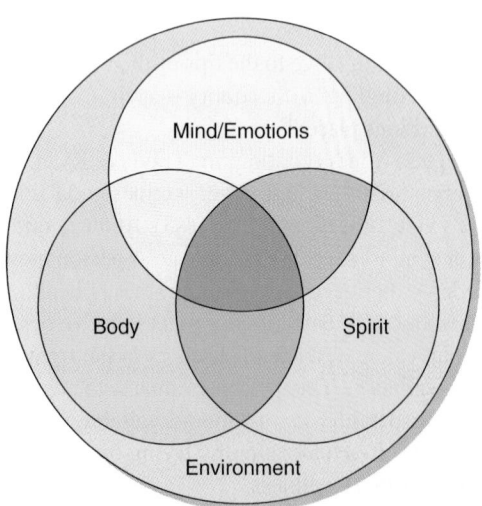

FIGURE 16-4   Schematic representation of holism. The system is greater than and different from the sum of the parts.

Mind/Emotions

Body   Spirit

Environment

Western modern medicine and a wide range of alternative or complementary therapies. The term "complementary" conveys that these therapies are used in conjunction with, rather than in place of, traditional Western biomedicine.

Holistic practitioners recognize the incredible advances that traditional medicine has made, including antibiotics and surgery. They are especially mindful of the risk of iatrogenic illness, or illness that results from treatment and may be traced to overuse and adverse responses to medication, in addition to abuse of prescription medications.

Consumers also are recognizing the need for alternative therapies. In November 1998, the *Journal of the American Medical Association* published a study (Eisenberg et al., 1998) documenting trends in alternative medicine use in the United States between 1990 and 1997. The study's findings showed that Americans spent an estimated $21.2 billion on "unconventional healthcare" in 1997—an increase of 45.2% from 1990. Forty-two percent of the study's respondents (increased from 33.8% in 1990) reported using at least one unconventional therapy during the previous year, with the largest increases in use of herbal medicine, massage, megavitamins, self-help groups, folk remedies, energy healing, and homeopathy. Partly in recognition of the public's demand for healthcare choices and the need for funding of research and resulting publications on alternative modalities of healing, the National Institutes of Health established an Office of Alternative Medicine in 1993. The office was elevated to a center in 1999—the National Center for Complementary and Alternative Medicine (NCCAM)—and now has a web site (http://nccam.nih.gov.).

Self-Responsibility

The first dimension of a wellness lifestyle is self-responsibility, a personal sense of accountability for one's own well-being. As stated in *Healthy People 2010* (U.S. Department of Health and Human Services, 2000), the many roles that each person fulfills in his or her daily life provide numerous opportunities for promoting health and preventing disease. With these opportunities comes responsibility for personal health habits. To make informed choices, the client must first be self-aware. **Self-awareness** means knowing and caring for oneself, recognizing one's strengths and limitations. Holistic health practices add to this self-knowledge on all levels (physical, psychological, social, and spiritual), enabling the person to identify his or her state of being and to decide the priorities of service required. Self-knowing is likely to be the first step toward self-caring.

Informed Choices

Making informed choices, being an active participant rather than a passive recipient, can benefit one's self-concept. As an individual acquires useful self-awareness, this can result in a measure of personal empowerment. Changes in self-concept may facilitate fundamental changes in the person's belief system. The holistic health practitioner can facilitate this decision to change by encouraging the person to examine his or her lifestyle and to consider moving toward high-level wellness.

For example, people learning to use biofeedback to reduce tension headaches must first gather data on their own tension signals and triggers. To initiate relaxation techniques at an early stage, they become aware of the body's symptoms or signals that warn of a tension buildup. By becoming aware of the situations that trigger a stress response, they can learn ways to change those situations, or change their view of the situations, to prevent the stress response before it occurs.

Self-Worth

Psychologist Yetta Bernhard (1975) proposed that self-respect and self-worth are developed in the process of caring for oneself. Participating in self-care gives the client a greater feeling of independence and control. The altered concept of self as an active agent can help the person move toward high-level wellness. The concept of self as an active health agent extends across the wellness–illness continuum and applies to people at all developmental levels.

> After learning signs and symptoms to watch for, Emma Rose begins to monitor her own leg and foot. When she examines her toes, she recognizes that the fact that the toes are pink, warm, and without swelling indicates her leg and foot have healthy circulation. She feels a sense of control that was not present when her other care provider simply pinched the toenail of her great toe, nodded her head, and left without saying a word.

Meaning of Disease, Illness, and Dysfunction

Disease

Because health is a state of harmony, **disease** is a state of disharmony of mind, body, emotions, and spirit. Pelletier, in *Holistic Medicine* (1979), discusses the holistic view of disease as an opportunity to discover meaning. Traditional medicine often equates disease with failure, either of medicine or of the person. Even language, such as "chief complaint," conveys a negative message. When going to see the school nurse, a child is often asked, "What's wrong?"

According to the holistic view, a disease's course and manifestations depend on how the client integrates the experience into his or her life. The school nurse can ask the child, "How are things going for you today?" Disease can be transformed into an experience of personal value and growth.

Illness

Illness is a product of the disharmonious interaction (disease) between mind, body, emotions, and spirit. Claude Bernard, a seventeenth-century French physiologist, developed the concept of **homeostasis,** the organism's attempt to restore balance. With self-regulatory mechanisms, the human body responds to constant challenges from the external environment in an effort to maintain equilibrium or health. Illness is the body's way of signaling that a person has exceeded the natural capacity to mediate between the internal and external environments. Illness can be an opportunity to discover meaning in life and to heal, identifying areas of disharmony and determining how best to move toward a natural state of harmony.

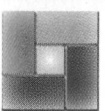

Nursing Research and Critical Thinking

Would a Self-Care Health Promotion Curriculum for African-American Third Grade Students Have a Greater Effect on Their Health and Wellness Than the Traditional Health Curriculum?

A school nurse questioned whether the traditional method of teaching about health was the best way to promote healthy behaviors for inner city, African-American third graders. The nurse developed a self-care health promotion curriculum based on nursing theory for African-American third grade students. The purpose of the research was to assess the effect of the program when compared with the usual way that students learned health at the school. Students in three third grade classes were taught the new curriculum, and three classrooms were taught the traditional curriculum. Pretest and posttest data were collected from all six groups, both treatment and control. Also obtained were several measures of educational performance and demographic information to validate that the groups were similar and homogeneous. The results of the study were that the new self-care curriculum group had higher mean scores on hope and satisfaction with daily living and lower diastolic blood pressure than the traditional group.

Critical Thinking Considerations. This study focused on urban third grade students and is not generalizable to other groups. However, the researcher pointed out the importance of considering culture and community composition in the design of health education curricula in schools. Other implications discussed by the nurse researcher are as follows:

* Teaching self-care and health promotion to younger children may increase positive health outcomes and potential health behaviors in general.
* Schools play a significant role in the lives of urban children of low socioeconomic status by often acting as a link between families and the health profession.
* Educators need to recognize that a shift in thinking about health has occurred from a "rehabilitate and repair" attitude to a "building and strengthening" focus on basic health knowledge to ward off dysfunction.

Baldwin, C. M. (1998). Changing health outcomes for African American children: Utilizing a self-care health promotion curriculum in urban elementary schools. *Journal of Multicultural Nursing and Health, 4*(2), 40–45.

Illness is a product of a complementary interaction between mind and body. Pert, Dreher, and Ruff (1998) refer to the "psychosomatic network," affirmed by psychoneuroimmunologic research, that functions as a living processor of information. Neuropeptides, referred to as the "biochemical substrates of emotion," transmit messages across organs, tissues, cells, and DNA (Pert, Dreher & Ruff, 1998, p. 30). Meek (1977) observed that if a client's mind is fed a daily diet of anger, remorse, revenge, hate, jealousy, suspicion, and envy, the cells of the client's body will reflect this environment. Increased vulnerability to specific diseases seems to correlate with problems expressing certain emotions. For instance, people who deny anxiety seem more prone to cardiac disease. Psychologist Lawrence LeShan (1961) found that cancer clients had a higher than normal incidence of feelings of helplessness and hopelessness before their diagnosis. Cancer also seems to correlate with difficulty expressing feelings, such as anger and depression (Eysenck, 1988).

Feelings do not cause disease, but they do interfere with the immune system and may create an atmosphere in which disease can develop. One study of cancer clients and their families found a powerful relationship between negative images surrounding cancer and treatment outcomes (Simonton, Matthews-Simonton, & Creighton, 1978). The authors counseled clients and people in their support systems about psychological awareness and self-care to achieve the best treatment outcome. Pert et al. (1998) discussed mind–body interventions that facilitate emotional expression and have survival benefits for those with breast cancer or melanoma.

Illness can be a signal that a person's important needs are not being met. It can be an invitation from within to look at the balance between activity and rest or between self- and other-oriented care. *Getting Well Again* (Simonton et al., 1978) suggests a simple exercise to identify the needs being met through illness and ways to find other avenues:

* List the five most important benefits you received from an illness in your life.
* Consider the needs that were met by your illness: relief from stress, love and attention, opportunity to renew energy, and so forth.
* Identify the rules or beliefs that limit you from meeting each of these needs when you are well.

Emma Rose uses this exercise to analyze her situation. Up to this point, she has focused only on the negative aspects of her surgery. She realizes that this event has allowed her to take a break from a project at work she didn't enjoy. She decides to ask her supervisor to assign her to a project she would enjoy more. The cards and telephone calls from her friends show her that they care for her and miss her. She decides to reorganize her calendar so that she can have more contact with caring friends.

Dysfunction

Dysfunction is an action (abnormal, inadequate, or impaired) that does not meet expected norms. The action "generates therapeutic concern on the part of the client, family, or friends, and the nurse" (Gordon, 1994).

Therapeutic interventions for dysfunctional problems are directed at contributing factors. Interventions for potential dysfunction are directed at prevention by reducing risk factors (Gordon, 1994). "An outgrowth of the disease orientation is a disability orientation; an outgrowth of the health orientation is an ability orientation" (Hopkins & Smith, 1993, p. 435). Therefore, the person with altered function is not necessarily disabled but should be able to adapt strengths toward being abled. This transformation is evident in the lives of famous individuals whose illnesses did not limit their potential, such as Helen Keller, Franklin D. Roosevelt, and Stevie Wonder.

> Emma Rose wonders if she will regain her muscle strength and physical activity. She voices her concerns to you. You tell her she will have altered mobility and reduced strength while she recovers and for awhile after she returns to her usual activities. In the meantime, you teach her how to strengthen her quadriceps muscles and wiggle her toes to stimulate the lower leg muscles on the unaffected side. You tell Emma Rose to take short walks and rest periods. You inform her that it is normal to feel tired after exertion. You advise her not to push herself beyond endurance but to move within the limitations of discomfort. "Normal function will return in a few weeks," you say.

Effect of Stress

Holistic practitioners recognize that life stresses affect how and when an illness is manifested. Any change, even a positive one, results in a certain amount of stress. Psychosocial stress, such as the death of a spouse or being diagnosed with a progressively deteriorating illness, can lead to depression, anger, and despair, all of which harm the immune system. A cluster of events that requires life adjustment is associated with the onset of illness. Underlying cardiovascular disease and cancer, the two leading causes of disability and death in the United States, are prolonged states of sympathetic nervous system activity mediated through the hormonal pathways. They are the body's response to prolonged stress reactivity.

Holistic practitioners recognize the impact of stress on health and teach skills to notice and decrease it when possible. See Chapter 49 for more information on stress.

> Emma Rose tells you that she feels uprooted because she is surrounded by unfamiliar objects and is wearing a gown. You suggest that she ask a friend to bring her own pajamas from home and a few things, such as cassette player and tapes, that would make the environment more comfortable. "If you can't be home, you can bring some of your home here," you tell her.

NURSING IN WELLNESS AND HOLISTIC HEALTHCARE

Nursing has traditionally been a holistic profession. Nursing theorists have promoted aspects of holistic care across time. Acknowledging the wisdom of least invasive treatment and the interrelationship of person and environment, Florence Nightingale believed that the purpose of nursing is to put the person in the best condition for nature to restore or to preserve health. Nurses must inquire into all the conditions in which the client lives (Nettina, 2000). Self-responsibility is paramount in Dorothea Orem's nursing theory (Sparks & Taylor, 1998), which focuses on self-care so that the person can maintain life, health, and well-being. According to Martha Rogers (1990), the primary purpose of nursing is to help people achieve their maximum health potential. By promoting high-level wellness and preventing illness whenever possible, the holistic nurse uses an approach that minimizes risk and empowers the client.

In many ways, holistic care mirrors the paradox of the yin-yang symbol, which shows the mutual interdependence of two major forces (Fig. 16-5). Nursing is returning to its historical roots while simultaneously responding to ever-evolving technology, cost containment, and consumer demands. Nurses are challenged to retain the human aspect, including the spiritual aspect of nursing that values the meaning and purpose of life and death. Advances such as cloning and infertility treatments present ethical and legal dilemmas that require nurses to reflect on their own beliefs and values. Many nurses recognize the complementary nature of what Dossey (1991) referred to as "doing" and "being" therapies. "Doing" therapies—such as giving medications, altering diets, and changing dressings—have measurable, linear outcomes. "Being" therapies recognize the less measurable effects of consciousness both within the person and as a bridge between individuals. Meditation, imagery, and prayer are some examples of "being" therapies.

Holistic nurses also recognize a duty to provide the healthiest environment for themselves and generations to come. The American Holistic Nurses Association (AHNA), formed in 1980, states in their *Standards of Holistic Nursing Practice,* "Practicing holistic nursing requires nurses to integrate self-care, self-responsibility, spirituality, and reflection in their lives" (Frisch, 2001, p. 3). These standards reflect the nurse as a member of the global community. Nurses can become nationally certified in the specialty of holistic nursing through the American Holistic Nurses' Certification Corporation. Further information is available at their web site, http://ahna.org/edu/certification.html (accessed November 19, 2001).

There is a range of possible responses on the part of nurses to the popularity of complementary and alternative medicine (CAM) practices. To accurately assess and care for clients,

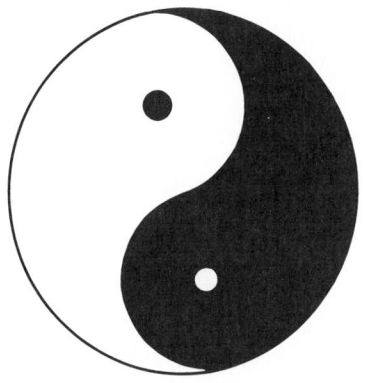

FIGURE 16-5 Tai-chi T'u (yin–yang) symbol.

nurses must include in their intake information whether the individual is currently taking any herbal remedies and/or using any CAM modalities. This helps determine whether there could be any interactive effect between these substances and practices and current recommended medications and treatments. Being familiar with the more popular CAM practices enables nurses to better understand the total healthcare delivery system available to clients. Familiarity with the current research on various modalities gives nurses data to begin to critically evaluate their utility and decide whether a referral is appropriate. Some nurses may choose to become trained in particular CAM modalities and then integrate them into their own practice.

Nursing as a Therapeutic Partnership

The holistic practitioner sees the nurse–client relationship as a therapeutic partnership rather than a dependent relationship. Some nurses believe that the word *patient* connotes a passive, helpless person rather than an individual seeking wellness, which at times includes the support of a healthcare provider; as an alternative, many nurses use the term *client*. The nurse is no longer in a role as a "pill fairy" in a culture that has become accustomed to a quick pharmaceutical fix. Instead, the nurse is an agent for change, helping clients to take responsibility and to take charge of their lives and health. The holistic nurse acts as a "caring colleague" of the client (Blattner, 1981). Holistic nurses offer to help their clients toward high-level wellness while acknowledging that each has the right to choose his or her own path.

> Emma Rose has asked someone for pain medication. She was told it was not time and she would have to wait another 30 minutes. When you stop by her room a few minutes later, she is in pain and anxious. You suggest that using imagery might help her relax and feel more comfortable. You lead her into imagery by suggesting she picture herself on a warm, soft stretch of sand, looking out over a calm, blue-green body of water under a clear blue sky. Before long, Emma Rose realizes she is no longer counting the minutes until her pain medication, and she feels calmer. Later in the day, she again uses the imagery by herself to feel calmer, and she likes feeling that she is in charge.

True helping can occur only when the client wants and needs it. Some helpers become rescuers by entering into what Steiner (1971) called the victim–rescuer–persecutor triangle (Fig. 16-6). In the triangle, the client can be seen as a victim, acting as if he or she wants help. The healthcare provider, as a rescuer, decides to help, but the rescuer neglects to determine whether the help being offered is needed or wanted. The rescuer usually ends up as a victim of the same person he or she was trying to rescue, because the help is ineffective and the effort wasted. The rescuer may feel persecuted by the client and experience resentment ("After all I've done for you!").

People in these roles go around and around the triangle. Rescuing leads to burnout on the part of the healthcare provider, because the great amount of energy expended does

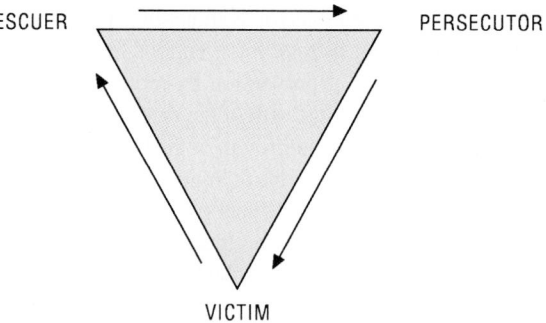

FIGURE 16-6   Victim–rescuer–persecutor triangle.

not result in the desired outcome. Table 16-1 lists characteristics of helpers and rescuers (Travis & Ryan, 1988).

A healthcare provider cannot change or help others unless they want to be changed or helped. Clients cannot be made well unless they want to be well more than they want to be ill (Meek, 1977). Once healed, they will not stay well unless they want to stay well. Clients may be unaware that they want to be well or ill. In these cases, practitioners may help clients clarify and explore their desires in terms of wellness. Is the payoff for becoming well greater than the gains of remaining ill?

Nursing Diagnoses for Wellness

Nursing diagnoses are used to provide organization and clarity when communicating with the healthcare team. The North American Nursing Diagnosis Association (NANDA) has divided nursing diagnoses into the following categories: actual nursing diagnoses, risk nursing diagnoses, wellness nursing diagnoses, and possible nursing diagnoses. Nursing diagnoses

TABLE 16-1

Differences Between Helpers and Rescuers	
Helper	**Rescuer**
Listens for request	Gives when not asked
Presents offer	Neglects to discover if offer is welcome
Gives only what is needed	Gives more help and for longer time than needed
Checks periodically with client	Omits feedback
Checks results that client	Does not check results
Functions better	and feels good when
Meets goals	accepted, bad when
Solves problems independently	turned down by client
Uses suggestions successfully	

From Travis, J. W., & Ryan, R. S. (1988). *Wellness workbook.* Berkeley, CA: Ten-Speed Press.

for wellness serve several purposes. They encourage the nurse and client to examine positive, life-affirming behaviors that contribute to healthy functioning. When written as part of the client's healthcare record, the diagnoses can be used to reinforce continued health promotion. "Assessment of strengths and health-promoting behaviors, shared and supported in collaboration with the recipient of nursing care, encourages the continued use of positive strategies in similar circumstances" (Houldin, Saltstein, & Ganley, 1987, p. 20). Nurses in all settings can use these and other wellness diagnoses to focus on promoting health. Each client should be seen as a whole person with the physical, psychological, and spiritual potential for optimal functioning across the lifespan.

Examples of Holistic Healthcare Modalities.

The NCCAM identifies five major domains of CAM practices: alternative medical systems, mind–body interventions, biologically based therapies, manipulative and body-based methods, and energy therapies. The list of practices keeps changing because those that are considered "mainstream" are not included. The designation of "mainstream" is given to those CAM therapies that have been proven safe and effective. Display 16-1 gives some examples of practices in each of the five domains. Snyder and Lundquist (2001) listed complementary therapies that are commonly used in nursing. Examples of these therapies are starred in Display 16-1, and four of them are discussed in more depth here.

Lifestyle Modification

Holistic practitioners advocate the use of lifestyle modification skills that alleviate stress and promote a state less susceptible to disease. These skills increase an individual's energy level rather than reduce awareness of tension. Programs have been developed to teach the client methods of self-care that include a spiritual component (e.g., meditation, yoga, other relaxation methods), and other approaches include nutrition and cognitive restructuring. Evidence of the paradigm shift from illness care to wellness care and prevention is the coverage by insurance companies of lifestyle modification programs that include mind–body interventions. Notable examples are Benson & Stuart's (1992) Medical Symptoms Reduction Programs through the Mind/Body Medical Institute; Kabat-Zinn's (1990) Stress Reduction and Relaxation Program; and Ornish's (1990, 1998) Program for Reversing Heart Disease. These programs, increasingly considered mainstream, combine a vast array of therapies that some healthcare providers still consider complementary.

Meditation

Meditation, deep personal thought and reflection, may be one of the most basic and powerful self-care activities that can be incorporated into people's lives. It stills the chattering mind and sharpens understanding of the internal and external worlds. Meditation is a way to tune and train the mind, leading to greater efficiency in everyday life. It helps decrease anxiety and helps the individual handle stress with less negative impact. Meditators withstand more life changes with less illness.

Although meditation seems like a simple tool, it can have powerful results. It is considered the cornerstone of the life-

DISPLAY 16-1

DOMAINS OF COMPLEMENTARY AND ALTERNATIVE PRACTICES ACCORDING TO NATIONAL CENTER FOR COMPLEMENTARY AND ALTERNATIVE MEDICINE

1. Alternative Medical Systems: Complete systems of theory and practice that evolved independent of the biomedical approach.
   Examples: Oriental medicine (methods include acupuncture, herbal medicine, oriental massage, and qi gong). Ayurvedic medicine (methods include diet, exercise, meditation, and herbs). Other medical systems developed by Native American, Aboriginal, African, Middle-Eastern, Tibetan, and Central and South American cultures. Homeopathy and naturopathic medicine.
2. Mind–Body Interventions: These interventions utilize a wide variety of techniques to facilitate the positive influence of the mind and body's intimate connections.
   Examples: Meditation*, certain uses of hypnosis, dance, music*, art therapy, prayer*, and imagery*.

3. Biologically Based Therapies: Practices, products, and interventions that are natural and biologically based.
   Examples: Use of herbs*, special diet therapies such as those of Drs. Atkins, Ornish, Pritikin, and Weil*, orthomolecular therapies*, and biological therapies such as the use of laetrile, shark cartilage, or bee pollen.
4. Manipulative and Body-Based Methods: Methods that involve manipulation and/or movement of the body.
   Examples: Chiropractic treatments, osteopathy, and massage*.
5. Energy Therapies: These practices focus on energy originating within or around the body.
   Examples: Qi gong, Reiki*, Therapeutic Touch*, and the use of magnets.

*Complementary therapy commonly used in nursing.
Adapted from the NCAAM; available at http://nccam.nih.gov (accessed November 19, 2001).

style modification programs mentioned previously. It is not a strange and complicated technique requiring great effort and skill; it is merely a way of switching the concentration from the external world to the internal world. Many types of meditation are clearly described in Joel and Michelle Levey's outstanding book, *Simple Meditation and Relaxation* (1999).

Imagery

Imagery is the "internal experience of a perceptual event in the absence of the actual external stimuli" (Achterberg & Lawlis, 1980, p. 27). Use of the term "visualization" can be confusing, because imagery can include qualities from other senses besides sight, including smell, touch, and hearing (Pelletier, 2000). In the Simontons' work with cancer clients (Simonton et al., 1978), they teach their clients to use daily relaxation and mental imagery to enhance their immune system response. The clients are taught to picture cancer cells being destroyed by the current treatment and by their body's white blood cells. The imagery process includes seeing themselves as whole, well, and full of energy. Using these methods, the Simontons report encouraging results: surviving clients in one study lived on average twice as long as clients who received medical treatment alone, and even clients who died lived 1.5 times longer than the control group. In a comprehensive review of studies that examined "psychological interventions," including the use of imagery for oncology clients, Simonton and Sherman (1998) cited numerous studies that reported enhanced quality of life as well as altered immune function and perhaps survival. A certification program called Nurses Certificate Program in Imagery is endorsed by the AHNA and is now available specifically for nurses to incorporate imagery into their professional practice. (For further information, visit the *web site*, *http://www.imageryrn.com/*.)

Therapeutic Touch

Therapeutic Touch is a technique derived from the ancient practice of "laying on of hands." Dora Kunz and Dolores Krieger developed this approach, which nurses have learned worldwide. According to the philosophy of Therapeutic Touch, the client's state of health is reflected in the vital energy field that surrounds him or her. The Therapeutic Touch practitioner learns to attune to this energy field by first centering, or achieving a sense of peace and wholeness within himself or herself. Krieger describes **Therapeutic Touch** as a healing meditation, because the centered state is maintained throughout the process. The practitioner assesses and treats the client's energy field with the goal of restoring harmony. If the practitioner perceives the flow of energy as obstructed, disordered, or depleted, he or she attempts to direct energy to the client to release congestion and balance the areas where flow may be disordered.

Therapeutic Touch relaxes the client, who experiences slower, deeper breathing; decreased muscle tension; and warmer hands and feet. This method has been reported to alleviate discomfort and to speed healing (Horrigan, 1998; MacCrae, 1988; Wirth, 1990). There have been many studies on Therapeutic Touch, but problems have been reported with

ETHICAL/LEGAL ISSUE
Alternative Therapies

Emma Rose has a friend who recommends that when she is discharged home, Emma Rose should consider massage treatments and taking some herbal remedies to enhance her healing. As her primary nurse, you are aware that she will be discharged with a referral to physical therapy as well as a prescription for pain medication to be taken as needed.

Reflection
- Given the ethical obligation of respect for a person's autonomy, what do you consider to be your responsibility, if any, in this case?
- The majority of people who use alternative therapies do not discuss them with their medical doctors and other healthcare practitioners. How would you advise Emma Rose?
- Consider the ethical concept of beneficence—helping your clients to promote health and avoid suffering. How would you see the relationship of beneficence in this situation?
- Should insurance coverage be based on a treatment's efficacy, whether it is traditional or alternative? Give reasons to support your answer.

design and methods in some of these studies (Mulloney & Wells-Federman, 1996). O'Mathuna (2000) urged accurate reporting of research for evidence-based practice of CAM. More research on Therapeutic Touch that will stand the test of scientific rigor is needed. Meanwhile, Therapeutic Touch is a noninvasive process that may decrease clients' need for medication and may enable them to tap into their natural healing potential. The official organization of Therapeutic Touch is the Nurse Healers-Professional Associates International, and its web site is accessible at http://www.therapeutic-touch.org.

KEY CONCEPTS

- Health, as defined by WHO, is a state of complete physical, mental, and social well-being.
- Wellness is a dynamic state that allows for various personal beliefs about health.
- In the clinical model, health is seen as the absence of indications of illness.
- The host–agent–environment model of health seeks a source or cause of illness.
- The health belief model is characterized by the relationship between a person's beliefs and actions.
- In the high-level wellness model, health is an ongoing process toward the person's highest potential.
- The holistic health model recognizes the unique interaction of a person's mind, body, and spirit within the environment.
- Holistic healthcare combines the proven success of modern medicine, participation of the client, and additional activities to complement medical protocol.

- The nursing diagnoses related to health and wellness are important for initiating and reinforcing health promotion.
- Holistic healthcare interventions include many CAM practices, some of which are now considered "mainstream."

REFERENCES

Achterberg, J. A., & Lawlis, G. F. (1980). *Bridges of the bodymind.* Champaign, IL: Institute for Personality and Ability Testing.

Allen, D. G. (1986). Using philosophical and historical methodologies to understand the concept of health. In P. Chinn (Ed.), *Nursing research methodology* (pp. 157–168). Rockville, MD: Aspen.

Ardell, D. B. (1977). *High-level wellness.* Emmaus, PA: Rodale.

Bernhard, Y. (1975). *Self-care.* Millbrae, CA: Celestial Arts.

Benson, H., & Stuart, E. M. (1992). *The wellness book: The comprehensive guide to maintaining health and treating stress-related illness.* New York: Simon & Schuster.

Blattner, B. (1981). *Holistic nursing.* Englewood Cliffs, NJ: Prentice-Hall.

Dossey, L. (1991). *Meaning and medicine: A doctor's tales of breakthrough and healing.* New York: Bantam Books.

Dunn, H. L. (1961). *High-level wellness.* Arlington, VA: R.W. Beatty.

Eisenberg, D. M., Davis, R. B., Ettner, S. L., Appel, S., Wilkey, S., Rompay, M. V., & Kessler, R. C. (1998). Trends in alternative medicine use in the United States. *The Journal of the American Medical Association, 280,* 1569–1575.

Eysenck, H. J. (1988). Personality, stress and cancer prediction and prophylaxis. *British Journal of Medical Psychology, 61,* 57–75.

Frisch, N. C. (2001). Standards for holistic nursing practice: A way to think about our care that includes complementary and alternative modalities. *Online Journal of Issues in Nursing, 6*(2), Manuscript 4. Available at: http://www.nursingworld.org/ojin/topic15/tpc15_4.htm. Accessed November 19, 2001.

Gordon, M. G. (1994). *Nursing diagnosis: Process and application* (3rd ed.). St. Louis, MO: Mosby–Year Book.

Hopkins, H. L., & Smith, H. D. (1993). *Willard and Spackman's occupational therapy* (8th ed.). Philadelphia: J. B. Lippincott.

Horrigan, B. (1998). Dolores Krieger, RN, PhD: Healing with Therapeutic Touch. *Alternative Therapies, 14*(1), 86–92.

Houldin, A., Saltstein, S., & Ganley, K. (1987). *Nursing diagnosis for wellness.* Philadelphia: J. B. Lippincott.

Kabat-Zinn, J. (1990). *Full catastrophe living: Using the wisdom of your body and mind to face stress, pain, and illness.* New York: Delacorte Press.

Kunz, D. (1995). *Spiritual healing.* Wheaton, IL: Quest Books.

Leavell, H. R., & Clark, E. G. (1965). *Preventive medicine for the doctor in his community.* (3rd ed.). New York: McGraw-Hill.

LeShan, L. (1961). A basic psychological orientation apparently associated with malignant disease. *Psychiatric Quarterly, 35,* 314.

Levey, J., & Levey, M. (1999). *Simple meditation and relaxation.* Berkeley, CA: Conari Press.

MacCrae, J. (1988). *Therapeutic Touch: A practical guide.* New York: Alfred A. Knopf.

Meek, G. W. (1977). *Healers and the healing process.* Wheaton, IL: Theosophical Publishing House.

Mulloney, S. S., & Wells-Federman, C. (1996). Therapeutic touch: A healing modality. *Journal of Cardiovascular Nursing, 10*(3), 27–49.

Nettina, S. M. (2000). *The Lippincott manual of nursing practice* (7th ed.). Philadelphia: Lippincott.

O'Mathuna, D. P. (2000). Evidence-based practice and reviews of Therapeutic Touch. *Journal of Nursing Scholarship, 32*(3), 279–285.

Ornish, D. (1990). *Dr. Dean Ornish's program for reversing heart disease.* New York: Random House.

Ornish, D., Scherwitz, L. W., Billing, J. H., Gould, K. L., Merritt, T. A., Sparler, S., Armstrong, W. T., Potts, T. A., Kirkeeide, R. L., Hogeboom, C., & Brand, R. J. (1998). Can intensive lifestyle changes reverse coronary heart disease? Four-year follow-up of the lifestyle heart trial. *Journal of the American Medical Association, 280,* 2001–2007.

Pelletier, K. (1979). *Holistic medicine.* New York: Delacorte.

Pelletier, K. (2000). *The best alternative medicine: what works? what does not?* New York: Simon & Schuster.

Pert, C. B., Dreher, H. E., & Ruff, M. R. (1998). The psychosomatic network: Foundations of mind–body medicine. *Alternative Therapies, 4*(4), 30–41.

Rogers, M. (1990). *An introduction to the theoretical basis of nursing.* Philadelphia: F. A. Davis.

Rosenstock, I. (1974). Historical origin of the health belief model. *Health Education Monographs, 2,* 334.

Simonton, O. C., Matthews-Simonton, S., & Creighton, J. L. (1978). *Getting well again.* New York: Bantam.

Simonton, S. S., & Sherman, A. C. (1998). Psychological aspects of mind-body medicine: Promises and pitfalls from research with cancer patients. *Alternative Therapies, 4*(4), 50–67.

Smuts, J. C. (1926). *Holism and evolution.* New York: Macmillan.

Snyder, M., & Lindquist, R. (2002). Issues in complementary therapies: How we got to where we are. *Online Journal of Issues in Nursing, 6*(2),1–16. http://www.nursingworld.org/ojin/topic15/tpc15_1.htm.

Sparks, S. M., & Taylor, C. M. (1998). *Nursing diagnosis reference manual* (4th ed.). Springhouse, PA: Springhouse.

Steiner, C. (1971). *Transactional analysis made simple.* San Francisco, CA: Transactional Publications.

Travis, J. W., & Ryan, R. S. (1988). *Wellness workbook.* Berkeley, CA: Ten Speed Press.

U.S. Department of Health and Human Services, Public Health Service. (2000). *Healthy people 2010.* Washington, DC: U.S. Government Printing Office.

Wirth, D. P. (1990). The effect of non-contact Therapeutic Touch on the healing rate of full thickness dermal wounds. *Journal of Subtle Energies, 1,* 1–20.

World Health Organization (1947). Constitution of the World Health Organization. *Chronicles of WHO, 1,* 1–2.

BIBLIOGRAPHY

Astin, J. A. (1998). Why patients use alternative medicine. *Journal of the American Medical Association, 279*(19), 1548–1553.

Braden, C. J., Mishel, M. H., & Longman, A. J. (1998). Self-Help Intervention Project (SHIP): Women receiving breast cancer treatment. *Cancer Practice, 6*(2), 87–98.

Cousins, N. (1976). Anatomy of an illness. *New England Journal of Medicine, 12,* 4–51.

Dossey, B. M., Frisch, N. C., Forker, J. E., & Lavin, J. (1998). Evolving a blueprint for certification: Inventory of Professional Activities and Knowledge of a Holistic Nurse (IPAKHN). *Journal of Holistic Nursing, 16*(3), 33–56.

Dossey, B. M., Keegan, L., Guzzetta, C. E. (2000). *Holistic nursing: A handbook for practice* (3rd ed.). Rockville, MD: Aspen.

Geddes, N., & Henry, J. K. (1997). Nursing and alternative medicine: Legal and practice issues. *Journal of Holistic Nursing, 15*(3), 271–281.

Gimbel, M. A. (1998). Yoga, meditation, and imagery: clinical applications. *Nurse Practitioner Forum, 9*(4), 243–255.

Ginzberg, E. (1995). The long view. *Society, 33*(1), 16–21.

Gordon, J. S. (1992, May/June). How America's health care fell ill. *American Heritage,* 49–65.

Jensen, L., & Allen, M. (1993). Wellness: The dialectic of illness. *Image: The Journal of Nursing Scholarship, 25*(3), 220–224.

Jonas, W. B. (1998). Alternative medicine: Learning from the past, examining the present, advancing to the future. *Journal of the American Medical Association, 280*(18), 1616–1617.

Levey, J., & Levey, M. (1998). *Living in balance: A dynamic approach for creating harmony and wholeness in a chaotic world.* Berkeley, CA: Conari Press.

Olshansky, E. (2000). *Integrated women's health: Holistic approaches for comprehensive care.* Gaithersburg, MD: Aspen.

Petit, J. M. (1994). Continuing care retirement communities and the role of the wellness nurse. *Geriatric Nursing, 15*(1), 28–31.

Poplin, C. (1995). The piper's tune. *Society, 33*(1), 8–15.

Sellers, S. C., & Haag, B. A. (1998). Spiritual nursing interventions. *Journal of Holistic Nursing, 16*(3), 338–354.

Stetson, B. (1997). Holistic health stress management program: Nursing student and client health outcomes. *Journal of Holistic Nursing, 15*(2), 143–157.

17 Lifespan Development

⑤ Key Terms

critical period
development
developmental tasks
embryo
environment
fetus

genetics
growth
"nature and nurture"
perception
puberty

⑤ Learning Objectives

Upon completion of this chapter, the student will be able to do the following:
1. Relate genetics and environment to human development.
2. Explain the principles of development.
3. Discuss selected theories of development.
4. Describe physical, psychosocial, and cognitive developmental patterns for different age groups.
5. Identify the major health needs of specific developmental age groups.

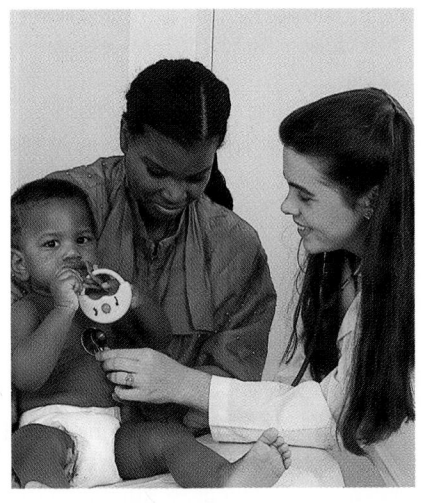

⑤ Critical Thinking Challenge

You are doing a well-child assessment on a 13-month-old boy. You ask the child's mother if anything is of particular concern to her. She seems reluctant to answer but finally says that she is concerned that her son is not yet "potty trained." When you question her further, she tells you that her mother-in-law said that her son (the 13-month-old's father) was completely toilet trained by 12 months, and that either something is wrong with the child or the mother is not working hard enough to accomplish toilet training.

Once you have completed this chapter and added lifespan development to your knowledge base, review the above scenario and reflect on the following areas of Critical Thinking:

1. Determine what the mother may be feeling that she has not expressed verbally.
2. Identify concepts of growth and development that are pertinent to this situation.
3. Relate these components to this child and this situation.
4. Clarify what additional information you will need of the mother and her child.
5. List some appropriate nursing considerations and interventions.

Growth means the physical increase in the body's size and appearance caused by increasing numbers of new cells. **Development** is the process of ongoing change, reorganization, and integration that occurs throughout life. This process includes changes in body structure and physiologic function, psychosocial behaviors, emotional responses, and cognition. As a result of growth and development, a person's competence and capabilities change both quantitatively and qualitatively so that he or she can participate more fully in life.

Traditionally, theorists viewed the process of growth and development as a characteristic of infancy and childhood, giving little attention to the process beyond adolescence. Mounting evidence indicates that predictable patterns of change occur throughout life, and many current researchers (Lynch & Lynch, 1991; Sasser-Coen, 1993; Peterson, 1994; Levenson & Crumpler, 1996) have delineated phases of adult development. Lifespan development is a central and critical issue in attempting to understand human behavior as it relates to health. Beliefs about how people mature across the lifespan influence perceptions of individuals, relationships, and roles. When the word "development" is used in this chapter, "lifespan" is always an assumed qualifier.

GENETICS AND ENVIRONMENT

Two primary factors drive growth and development—genetics and environment. These primary factors are also called **"nature and nurture."** The question of whether genetics or environment has greater impact on developmental outcomes cannot easily be answered because an individual's genetic endowment and environment are, in reality, one indivisible system.

Genetics involves the potential for human function determined by a person's inheritance of 46 single chromosomes, or 23 pairs, that carry information from the birth parents. The code that the chromosomes contain governs the growth, differentiation, and function of all body cells. Current knowledge of the inheritance of physical characteristics (e.g., eye color) is substantial; researchers continue to explore behavioral genetics, or the extent to which behavior is also inherited. Because of the enormous numbers of possible combinations of inherited characteristics, each person possesses a unique genetic makeup, contributing to the wide variety of observed differences among people.

Environment defines the context in which a person exists, including both animate and inanimate surroundings (Bronfenbrenner, 1981). The animate environment comprises specific people (e.g., parents, siblings, spouses, partners, extended family, friends, classmates, workmates, colleagues) and, more broadly, social and cultural groups. The inanimate environment includes all aspects of the physical surroundings. Sensory components of the physical environment include sound and light as well as motion. The inanimate environment at a broader level includes housing, transportation, resources, economics, and other ecologic factors.

Although genetic makeup is stable over generations, surroundings continually change. Two important environmental factors influencing individual development are history and cohort; that is, environment is decidedly different based on a person's year of birth and the experiences of his or her cohort, or generational counterparts. For example, in 1961, schoolchildren across the United States gathered in classrooms and gymnasiums to watch television coverage of Alan Shepherd, the first American astronaut to fly in space. This experience was quite different than the experience of schoolchildren in 1927 who learned from the newspaper or radio of Charles Lindbergh's flight to Europe.

Although the environment can be arbitrarily divided into components, people experience it as a whole. **Perception** is a highly individual, cognitive, neurosensory process that allows each person to experience the environment uniquely. Even when the environments of two people are similar, their individual perceptions differ. Thus, two siblings who share the same family, home, school, and community have different perceptions of their environments, which contribute to the differences in their personalities.

Although all people are different, individuals within specific age groups exhibit similar changes in body structure and function, psychosocial behaviors, and patterns of cognition. Development occurs as a pattern: certain predictable processes follow a time course (e.g., puberty occurs in early adolescence). Patterns provide a way of describing the commonalities of development while preserving the consideration of individual differences. An understanding of change, reorganization, and integration can lead to a better understanding of individual behavior at a point in the lifespan.

Change

Development is a series of changes that start with conception and continue through death. Although ongoing, however, these changes are not consistent across time, nor is development a simple linear process. The school-age child's ability to determine that a set volume of liquid is the same, regardless of the shape of the container, does not demonstrate a gradual but rather a sudden change. Neither does development peak at 18 years of age and plateau until old age. Development includes periods of both relative stability and relative instability. Infancy and adolescence are short in duration but are known for rapid changes in a multitude of functions, including physical maturation, physical coordination, cognition, and social skills.

Although all aspects of human function change with development, not all changes occur on the same time schedule. Body development, cognitive development, and social development are not entirely synchronized. A 3-month-old infant may focus intently on a toy and attempt to reach the toy using a batting motion of the arms. Cognitive development spurs the desire to handle the toy; however, the infant's motor development has not progressed to the level of obtaining it. The young adolescent's social behaviors may indicate an increasing interest in sexuality, even though little physical evidence of puberty may be found.

Reorganization and Integration

Development is also a process of abrupt, dramatic, qualitative shifts in entire behavioral patterns, such as the ability to use tools to solve problems. That is, developmental changes seem to occur in spirals, with periods of relative quiescence, periods of disorganization and seeming regression, and periods of reorganization and integration, in which a person demonstrates new abilities. These newly acquired skills allow the person to view and to interact with the environment in entirely different ways. Despite discontinuity in development, much continuity remains. Experiences during childhood seem to lay the foundations for adulthood.

The question of critical periods in development is another issue related to continuity. A **critical period** is a time during which specific environmental or biologic events must occur for development to proceed normally. Animal studies indicate that such periods exist, but investigations of human development are less conclusive. Nonetheless, studies of the effects of early nutrition (Lucas, 1998) and of language development in children (Newport, 1991) suggest that there are critical periods in the development of the human child.

CONCEPTS OF DEVELOPMENT

Principles of Growth and Development

Knowledge about growth and development is drawn from the biologic and psychosocial sciences and involves certain principles that generally affect all people. These principles express commonalities of the process of growth and development.

- The process of growth and development is continuous and systematic, following a purposeful sequence.
- It is ongoing and complex.
- It is distinctive and predetermined and occurs at a discrete rate for each person.
- It has both quantitative and qualitative aspects.
- It requires experience and practice as well as energy.
- It occurs through adaptation to the conflict of equilibrium versus disequilibrium.
- It produces individuality from the interaction of genetic heredity and environment.
- Its outcome is the attainment of personal potential.

Growth and Development Theories

Theories of development attempt to describe why it occurs as it does and what factors shape outcomes. Some theories stress the impact of "nature," or the biologic aspects of growth and development, while others emphasize "nurture," or the environmental aspects. Four developmental theories, with the broad headings of psychodynamic, cognitive, developmental task, and human needs, are summarized in this section. Most, although not all, theories propose that people progress through universal stages of maturation and that the individual must master each stage before entering subsequent ones.

Psychodynamic Theories

Psychodynamic theories are based on the perspective that humans are essentially emotional, responding to instinctive drives without rationality. By studying childhood events, psychodynamic theorists attempt to explain human behavior throughout the lifespan. Sigmund Freud and Erik Erikson are two well-known psychodynamic theorists. Erikson's theory is more accurately termed *psychosocial*, because he also focused on the connection between the individual and society.

Freud (1856–1939). Freud emphasized the importance of childhood experience on adult personality. His work characterizes psychosexual development as encompassing the oral, anal, phallic, latency, and genital phases (Table 17-1). In Freud's view, the mind consists of the id (concerned with self-gratification), the ego (the mediator between the id and reality), and the superego (the conscience). For the most part, the activities of the mind are subconscious. Freud theorized that all people pass through the five phases, confronting and resolving conflicts of the id–ego–superego in the process. If the person does not resolve these conflicts, his or her movement through succeeding stages may be unsuccessful.

Erikson (1902–1994). Although based on Freud's theory, Erikson's psychosocial theory of development encompassed social and cultural influences as well. Erikson was the first theorist to recognize that development is a lifelong process. The eight stages of his theory progress from birth to death and are presented as developmental crises (e.g., trust versus mistrust) that the person must master before proceeding to the next stage (Table 17-2).

TABLE 17-1

Freud's Psychosexual Theory of Development	
Stage	**Characteristics**
Oral (birth–2 years)	Child seeks pleasure through oral gratification (e.g., sucking, chewing, putting things in mouth).
Anal (2–4 years)	Child delays gratification by learning to control anal sphincter (toilet training).
Phallic (4–6 years)	Child displays curiosity about genitals and gender differences.
Latent (6–12 years)	During this transition period, child focuses on peer relationships and identifies with parent or caregiver of the same sex.
Genital (12–death)	Individual achieves sexual maturity and interest in sex.

TABLE 17-2

Erikson's Psychosocial Stages of Development

Stage	Developmental Conflict	Necessary Accomplishment	Virtues Developed from Successful Resolution
Newborn or infant	Trust vs mistrust	Baby learns to trust caregivers.	Drive and hope
Toddler	Autonomy vs shame and doubt	Toddler gains independence with family's encouragement and learns to cooperate with others.	Self-control and willpower
Preschool	Initiative vs guilt	Preschooler develops confidence in abilities.	Direction and purpose
School-age	Industry vs inferiority	Child derives pleasure from accomplishments.	Method and competence
Adolescence	Identity vs role confusion	Teenager achieves a stable sense of identity.	Devotion and fidelity
Young adult	Intimacy vs isolation	Young adult develops close personal and professional relationships.	Affiliation and love
Middle adult	Generativity vs stagnation	Middle adult finds creativity and productivity in work and relationships.	Production and care
Older adult	Ego integrity vs despair	Older adult understands his or her purpose in life and achieves fulfillment.	Renunciation and wisdom

Adapted from Erikson, E. (1963). *Childhood and society* (2nd ed.). New York: W. W. Norton, and Boyd, M. A., & Nihart, M. A. (1998). *Psychiatric nursing: Contemporary practice.* Philadelphia: Lippincott-Raven.

Cognitive Development Theories

Cognitive development theory, which deals with perception and thinking, focuses on development of intellectual processes. Intellectual growth involves changes in the person's mental operations at various ages. According to this theory, children at various ages respond to cognitive tasks in comparable ways.

Piaget (1896–1980). Jean Piaget based his theory of cognitive development on the assumption that human nature is essentially rational and that the individual's basic goal is to learn to master the environment. The resulting satisfaction the person receives from learning prompts his or her curiosity, problem-solving, imitation, practice, and play activities (Piaget, 1952). Two functions that assist the person in learning and intellectual growth are organization and adaptation. Organization involves the rearranging and structuring of one's knowledge and thoughts. Adaptation means the process of assimilating and accommodating new information. To organize new learning with old and adapt it to expanding environments, the person uses the complementary processes of assimilation and accommodation. Assimilation is the ongoing process of organizing new information into existing knowledge. Accommodation is the process of resolving the disequilibrium resulting from the modifications needed in thought processes to incorporate new data. Piaget's four cognitive developmental stages are the sensorimotor, preoperational, concrete operations, and formal operations (Table 17-3).

Moral reasoning can be defined as judgments people make about what is right and wrong behavior within a social context. Such theorists question how principles of justice, concern for the welfare of others, and altruism affect behavior. As children's cognitive abilities mature and social experiences increase, appropriate behaviors in relation to others within a given culture and society begin to emerge.

Kohlberg (1927–1987). Lawrence Kohlberg (1976, 1984) extended Piaget's work on moral reasoning to develop a theory of moral development. Through a series of short vignettes describing concrete moral dilemmas, Kohlberg assessed children's beliefs about what actions they should take in various situations and why. He identified three major levels of moral development corresponding to Piaget's three later stages of cognitive development. Each level has two stages (Table 17-4).

TABLE 17-3

Piaget's Periods of Intellectual Development			
Age (years)	Period	Cognitive Developmental Characteristics	Description
Birth to 2	Sensorimotor	Divided into six stages, characterized by (a) inborn motor and sensory reflexes, (b) primary circular reaction and first habit, (c) secondary circular reaction, (d) use of familiar means to obtain ends, (e) tertiary circular reaction and discovery through active experimentation, and (f) insight and object permanence	The infant understands the world in terms of overt, physical action on that world. The infant moves from simple reflexes through several steps to an organized set of schemes. Significant concepts are developed including space, time, and causality. Above all, during this period, the child develops the scheme of the permanent object.
2–7	Preoperational	Deferred imitation; symbolic play, graphic imagery (drawing); mental imagery; and language Egocentrism, rigidity of thought, semilogical reasoning, and limited social cognition	Child no longer only makes perceptual and motor adjustment to objects and events. Child can now use symbols (mental images, words, gestures) to represent these objects and events; uses these symbols in an increasingly organized and logical fashion.
7–11	Concrete operations	Conservation of quantity, weight, volume, length, and time based on reversibility by inversion or reciprocity; operations: class inclusion and seriation	Conservation is the understanding of what values remain the same. For example, if liquid is poured from a short, wide glass into a tall, narrow one, the preoperational child thinks that the quantity has changed. For the concrete operation child, the amount stays the same.
11 through end of adolescence	Formal operations	Combination system, whereby variables are isolated and all possible combinations are examined; hypothetical-deductive thinking	Mental operations are applied to objects and events. The child classifies, orders, and reverses them. Hypotheses can be generated from these concrete operations.

From Boyd, M. A., & Nihart, M. A. (1998). *Psychiatric nursing: Contemporary practice.* Philadelphia: Lippincott-Raven.

Developmental Task Theory

Havighurst (1900–1991). Robert Havighurst's theory of development is based on learning and learned behaviors, called **developmental tasks,** which emanate from biologic, psychological, and social origins across the lifespan. Specific developmental tasks are assigned to various life stages (Table 17-5). A person's failure to complete the tasks of each stage may lead to his or her failure at tasks in subsequent stages. According to this theory, success in achieving developmental tasks leads to success with tasks in later stages of life (Havighurst, 1972).

Human Needs Theory

Humanistic theories (also called phenomenologic theories) propose that people are basically good when born and attempt to become all they are capable of becoming throughout their lives. People vary in their experiences, and they have free will and the ability to grow and become what they self-determine.

Maslow (1921–1970). Abraham Maslow is one of the better known humanistic theorists. He organized human needs into a hierarchic framework (discussed in Chapter 4), with a base of physiologic needs and an apex of self-actualization (Fig. 4-2 in

TABLE 17-4

Kohlberg's Stages of Moral Development		
Level and Stage	Characteristics	Example
Level 1: Preconventional		
Stage 1: Punishment/obedience	Decisions are based on avoidance of consequences.	A child obeys his parents to avoid punishment.
Stage 2: Instrumental/relativist	Actions are performed to satisfy needs (trade-offs).	A teenager agrees to mow the lawn if his mother will let him stay out later.
Level II: Conventional		
Stage 3: Approval seeking	Individual behaves to gain approval of significant others.	A child doesn't tattle on her older sister so that her sister will like her.
Stage 4: Law and order	Actions and decisions are based on laws and rules.	A football coach suspends a late player from the game, regardless of the player's excuse.
Level III: Postconventional		
Stage 5: Social contract	Individual rights are of primary importance.	A couple agrees to respect each other's political viewpoints, although they do not share the same view.
Stage 6: Universal-ethical	Relationships are based on mutual trust. The overall "good" is most important, even at the expense of the individual.	A company manager reports illegal environmental practices, although doing so costs him his job.

Chapter 4). To reach the apex of the hierarchy, a person must have met each of the preceding levels of needs. Maslow's theory is often used as a guide for holistic health, focusing on promoting high levels of wellness, preventing illness, and encouraging individual responsibility for health (Murray & Zentner, 2001).

GROWTH AND DEVELOPMENT THROUGH THE LIFESPAN

Normal growth and development are orderly, predictable processes in the human experience. Each person progresses and develops at an individual pace. For example, in the child, a time range exists during which certain developmental phases (e.g., walking, talking) are expected to occur. Progressing through a stage outside the usual time range may have no significant effect on overall development, or it may affect the child's ability to move on to or complete subsequent developmental phases. Usually growth and development are more advanced in the head and upper body than in the lower body. Even though components of growth and development are interrelated, physical, psychosocial, and cognitive development are considered separately in this section.

Intrauterine Development

Growth and development begin at the moment of conception. During the 9 months of the intrauterine stage, development moves from the single cell of the fertilized ovum to a com-

plete human being at the time of birth. Psychosocial and cognitive development also begin during this period, setting the stage for further progress after birth.

Physical Development

The period of intrauterine gestation is divided into three phases or trimesters (Fig. 17-1). The first trimester begins with fertilization of the ovum by the sperm, which unites two sets of chromosomes, creating the genetic program for the new organism. This program determines the child's inherited characteristics, such as eye and hair color. All organ systems are established. Fetal growth and development continue during the second trimester. Organ systems continue maturing in function and size. The third trimester ends with all organs able to support physiologic functioning and life outside the womb.

First Trimester. During the first trimester, all the organ systems of the **embryo** (the stage of development between the 2nd and 8th weeks) develop rapidly. By the 8th week, the embryo possesses a face, legs, arms, a brain and central nervous system, a heartbeat, and a productive digestive system and liver (red blood cell production). The critical development of organ systems during this trimester renders the embryo susceptible to developmental or environmental influences that can cause malformations. When the first bone cells appear in the upper arms, the embryo becomes a **fetus** (child in utero between the 3rd month of gestation and birth). The fetus is approximately 3 inches long and weighs 1 oz.

TABLE 17-5

Havighurst's Age Periods and Developmental Tasks

Infancy and Early Childhood
1. Learning to walk
2. Learning to take solid foods
3. Learning to talk
4. Learning to control the elimination of body wastes
5. Learning sex differences and sexual modesty
6. Achieving psychologic stability
7. Forming simple concepts of social and physical reality
8. Learning to relate emotionally to parents, siblings, and other people
9. Learning to distinguish right from wrong and developing a conscience

Middle Childhood
1. Learning physical skills necessary for ordinary games
2. Building wholesome attitudes toward oneself as a growing organism
3. Learning to get along with age-mates
4. Learning an appropriate masculine or feminine social role
5. Developing fundamental skills in reading, writing, and calculating
6. Developing concepts necessary for everyday living
7. Developing conscience, morality, and a scale of values
8. Achieving personal independence
9. Developing attitudes toward social groups and institutions

Adolescence
1. Achieving new and more mature relations with age-mates of both sexes
2. Achieving a masculine or feminine social role
3. Accepting one's physique and using the body effectively
4. Achieving emotional independence from parents and other adults
5. Achieving assurance of economic independence

6. Selecting and preparing for an occupation
7. Preparing for marriage and family life
8. Developing intellectual skills and concepts necessary for civic competence
9. Desiring and achieving socially responsible behavior
10. Acquiring a set of values and an ethical system as a guide to behavior

Early Adulthood
1. Selecting a mate
2. Learning to live with a partner
3. Starting a family
4. Rearing children
5. Managing a home
6. Getting started in an occupation
7. Taking on civic responsibility
8. Finding a congenial social group

Middle Age
1. Achieving adult civic and social responsibility
2. Establishing and maintaining an economic standard of living
3. Assisting teenage children to become responsible and happy adults
4. Developing adult leisure-time activities
5. Relating oneself to one's spouse as a person
6. Accepting and adjusting to the physiologic changes of middle age
7. Adjusting to aging parents

Later Maturity
1. Adjusting to decreasing physical strength and health
2. Adjusting to retirement and reduced income
3. Adjusting to death of a spouse
4. Establishing an explicit affiliation with one's age group
5. Meeting social and civil obligations
6. Establishing satisfactory physical living arrangements

From Havighurst, R. J. (1972). *Developmental tasks and education* (3rd ed.). New York: David McKay. Copyright © 1972 by Longman Publishers USA. Reprinted with permission.

Second Trimester. A major developmental milestone during this period is that the mother feels fetal movement. Theorists believe fetal activity to be essential for the proper development of the central nervous system (Nathanielsz, 1996). During this growth period, lanugo (downy hair) develops on the fetal arms, legs, and back. Head hair, eyelashes, eyebrows, fingernails, and toenails appear. Skeletal ossification continues. The skin is red and wrinkled. The fetus is nonviable at this point and cannot survive outside the uterine environment. Toward the 20th week, fetal growth slows and the lower limbs are fully formed. The fetus is 11 to 14 inches long and weighs 1 lb 4 oz.

Third Trimester. During the final trimester, fetal features are refined. The hair on the head and the fingernails grow, and lanugo almost disappears. Buds for permanent teeth appear behind the milk teeth buds. The fetus responds to bright lights and internal and external sounds. As the fetus increases in size, his or her activity may diminish because less space is available in the uterus. Arms and legs increase in flexion during the third trimester. The head remains large in comparison to the body. The lungs mature. The fetus receives short-term immunity from the mother because some antibodies pass through the placenta. Chances for survival improve with the approach of the delivery date. The fetus settles into the birth canal.

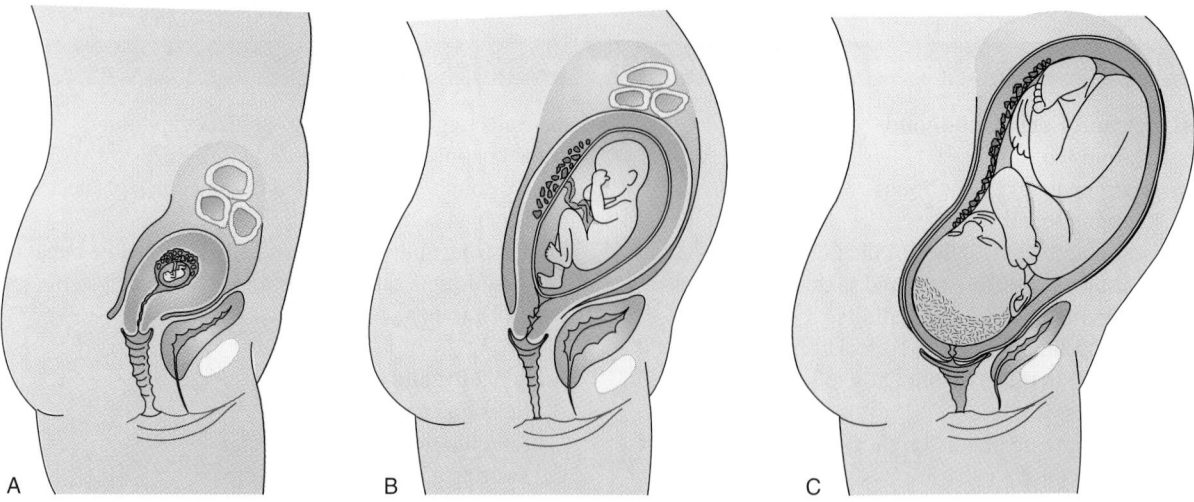

FIGURE 17-1   The period of fetal development is divided into three trimesters. This illustration depicts fetal growth during the first **(A)**, second **(B)**, and third **(C)** trimesters.

Psychosocial Development

Researchers have yet to determine whether events that occur during intrauterine life affect later psychosocial development. Current research methodologies rule out objective study of psychological interactions between fetus and mother. It appears, however, that prebirth events do help to mold cognitive, language, and affective development (Schuster & Ashburn, 1992). Because the pregnant woman's emotional state influences the biochemical environment of the fetus, maternal stress may play a significant, although indirect, role in psychosocial development.

Cognitive Development

Fetal activity represents a form of mother–baby communication that fosters bonding. During the last trimester, the fetus responds to internal and external sounds by changes in heart rate or movement. Researchers believe that stimulation in utero may influence later development. For example, at birth babies are noted, among other things, to respond differentially to their mothers' voices. Furthermore, researchers found that infants changed their rate of sucking on hearing a story that their mothers had read while the infants were in utero (De Casper & Fifer, 1980). Extreme maternal and fetal stressors are thought to affect development adversely (Thompson, 1990; DiPietro, Hodgson, Costigan, Hilton, & Johnson, 1996). Research tends to show that periods of diminished oxygen and severe, long-term prenatal malnutrition adversely affect later developmental functioning (Worthington-Roberts & Williams, 1997).

Newborn (Birth to 1 Month)

Physical Development

During the neonatal period (from birth to 4 weeks), neonates (or newborns) depend on others to meet their physiologic and emotional needs. Newborns must learn new ways of taking in food and oxygen and eliminating waste products, while also learning to adjust to their families' lifestyle. Although all organs are present, they are not all fully mature. Organ maturation continues throughout the neonatal period and into adolescence. At birth, the average newborn weighs 3200 g (7 lb 1 oz), is 49 cm (19.3 inches) long, and has a head circumference of 34 cm (13.5 inches) (Wong, 1999). Arm, leg, and hand movements are reflexive. Movements continue to remain an important means for newborns to communicate with others. Although neonates cannot support their heads while lying on their abdomens, they can lift their heads briefly. When pulled to a sitting position, neonates may hold their heads in line with their backs. They are capable of rolling part way to one side from the back. One-month-old newborns usually keep their hands fisted or slightly open. If their fingers are pried, neonates can grasp the handles of spoons or rattles briefly. Neonates stare at objects, coordinating their eyes; however, they do not reach for objects.

Psychosocial Development

Neonates respond positively to comfort and satisfaction and negatively to pain. They smile back at other faces. Neonates have different temperaments that influence their response to the environment and to caregivers. Usually caregivers can comfort newborns when making direct eye contact with them or talking to them. Through having responsive caregivers, the neonate begins to trust that needs will be met. Attachment or bonding develops at this time (Karen, 1994).

Cognitive Development

Piaget's first period of cognitive development, the sensorimotor stage, begins with the coordination of such activities as grasping objects and displaying basic reflexes. Although neonates were once thought to exhibit reflexive behavior only, current knowledge reveals that, even at birth, neonates are capable of a wide range of behaviors, particularly the ability to provide cues to parents and other caregivers about their needs for interaction.

Infant (1 Month to 1 Year)

Physical Development

Infants progress physically in a sequential pattern. During infancy, weight and height increase at a faster rate than during any other period. At 1 year of age, length has increased by 50% over the birth length, and weight has increased three times over the birth weight. Connections between neurons increase, and more myelin sheaths develop. Myelinization increases the efficiency of neural impulses. Voluntary motor skills begin to replace reflexive behavior (Schuster & Ashburn, 1992). Visual acuity reaches 20/100, facilitating eye–hand coordination. Infants begin holding up their heads for brief periods and advance to supported sitting, independent sitting, creeping, standing with support, and walking while holding on to objects. Infants gain increasing efficiency in energy expenditure while increasing the speed and accuracy of movement. A pincer grasp (picking up objects) replaces the whole-hand carry. Separation of tongue movement from the jaw indicates maturing oral motor development. The refinement of gross, fine, and oral motor skills coupled with the eruption of deciduous teeth allows infants to "munch" on foods and begin self-feeding (Fig. 17-2).

Psychosocial Development

Infants derive primary gratification from sucking and from having caregivers meet their needs. Social responsiveness is evident later on as infants smile in response to familiar faces. Laughing indicates pleasure as they show preferential treatment or responses to caregivers. Infants show fear of strangers or of separation from their primary caregivers. Many theorists consider attachment to be a lifelong process; nonetheless, the ability to trust and to form attachments during this develop-

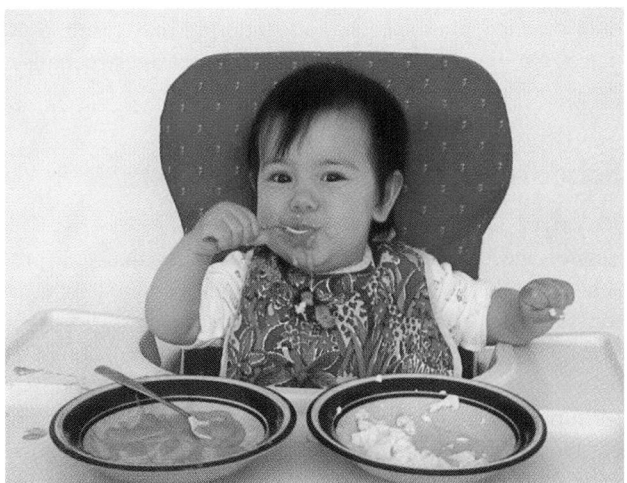

FIGURE 17-2 Although physical development has progressed during infancy to the point where the child can self-feed, neatness is a concept yet to be learned!

mental period is critical to the ability to form meaningful relationships as adults (Karen, 1994). Infants begin to explore the environment while separating briefly from caregivers. They enjoy toys, water and sand play, books, and nursery rhymes. They find human voices and faces particularly fascinating.

Cognitive Development

Infants engage in systematic imitative behavior. They attach meanings to words and, after a period of babbling, utter a few words. They understand language before they are able to talk. Infants are able to solve simple problems by using previously mastered activities or actions. When they discover a pleasurable activity, they repeat it. Through manipulation of objects and motor activities, infants differentiate between self and environment. Infants are fascinated with their own extremities. They achieve personal satisfaction from the ability to direct or control objects. Play remains an important component in self-concept development. Sensory impressions and motor activities provide the groundwork for knowledge of the world. Infants are capable of coordinating one action with another. The "power of association" assists them in understanding cause–effect relationships. The concept of object permanence, or the awareness that an object or person exists even when he or she is not physically seen or heard, develops.

Toddler (1 to 3 Years)

Physical Development

Toddlers possess large heads with relatively long trunks and short, stubby legs. Weak abdominal muscles account for a "pot-bellied" look. At birth, head size is slightly greater than chest size. The head and chest are equal in circumference until about 2 years of age, after which growth in chest size slowly exceeds head size. During the second year, the growth of legs and arms increases. In comparison to the first 12 months of life, growth in height and weight during toddlerhood slows. Toddlers gain approximately 5 lb and 3 to 5 inches per year. At the end of this period, all deciduous teeth have erupted and the mature rotary pattern of chewing allows toddlers to meet nutritional needs by the intake of solid foods. The development of the central nervous, musculoskeletal, cardiopulmonary, gastrointestinal, and urinary systems is almost complete. Gross motor skills rapidly develop. Toddlers learn to use upper muscles of the arms and legs before finger or toe muscles. They kick balls, jump, walk up and down stairs, ride tricycles, and run. Fine motor abilities progress from stacking towers of blocks to drawing stick people. The visual system reaches a more adult level. From 18 to 24 months, visual acuity is 20/40; by 2 to 3 years, it is 20/30. Accommodation is well developed.

Psychosocial Development

The world of toddlers expands to include peers or playmates and other adults. In becoming increasingly autonomous, toddlers see themselves as separate, although emotionally attached to parents or other family caregivers. Separation anxiety is at its peak. Toddlers become aware of the approval or disapproval of others. They express fear, an emotional response to threat against the self (DuPont, 1994). At 2 years, toddlers seem impulsive, inflexible, domineering, defiant, demanding, and always on the go. A major transition occurs in imitation and play behavior. Toddlers are able to imitate behaviors not currently present and to engage in symbolic play. They often exhibit interest in peers in parallel play (i.e., side by side) (Fig. 17-3). Toddlers begin to acquire more language skills and, by the end of this period, respond with more socially responsible behavior and cooperation.

Cognitive Development

Toddlers have definite ideas about how their world should operate, often expressing individual preferences. At the age of 18 months, toddlers respond to requests; "No" is a favorite reply. Self-identity and competency are reflected in common phrases such as "Mine" and "I do it." The egocentric characteristic of this age contributes to sense of self. Young children see the world from their own perspective and attempt to impose order on the environment. Thus, everything has its place, and rituals develop. Piaget's sensorimotor period extends from birth to approximately 2 years. Concepts mastered include causality, spatial relationships, imitation of actions previously observed, and the use of instruments. Between the ages of 2 and 6 years, young children advance to the preoperational stage, in which children assign meaning or identity to an object governed by their own perceptions. Internal and external reality are one. At approximately 18 months of age, use of words seems to increase dramatically. By the time they are 3 years old, toddlers understand well over 2000 words and are able to make short sentences and follow simple commands.

Preschooler (3 to 6 Years)

Physical Development

Physical changes occur at a slow, even, continuous pace. The average 5-year-old child's head circumference is 50 cm (90% of adult size); weight is 39 lb, and height is 40 inches. Arms and legs grow faster during this period; trunk growth follows

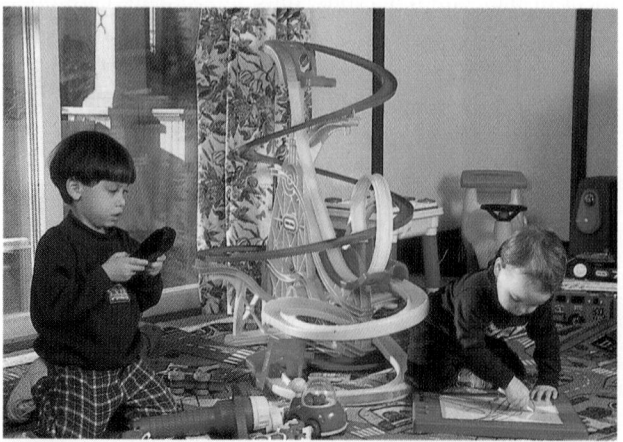

FIGURE 17-3 Toddlers show their growing interest in peers through parallel (side-by-side) play.

later. By 5 years of age, the pot-bellied appearance of the toddler has changed to a more adult appearance. By the end of this period, permanent teeth may appear. Neuromuscular skills are refined. Preschoolers dress themselves, wash their faces and hands, brush their teeth, and attend to their own toilet needs. They are able to copy figures and draw pictures. By 6 years of age, preschoolers should have a visual acuity of 20/20.

Psychosocial Development

Play is critical for early development (Johnsen, 1991; Saracho & Spodek, 1995). A common play style of preschoolers is associative, meaning that these children play together, demonstrating preferences for friends and sharing materials or objects (Parten, 1932). Little organization or goal-oriented behavior is evident. Securely attached preschoolers easily tolerate limited separation from their family caregivers while enjoying the company of other children. Rapid fluctuations between dependence and independence, competence and ineptitude, maturity and infantilism, and growing affection and antisocial destructiveness mark this period. As preschool children strive for individuality, they question and explore their own abilities. They learn to express emotions acceptably along with developing a conscience for moral growth and internalizing control of their actions.

Cognitive Development

In Piaget's preoperational stage, preschoolers can use mental symbols; thinking can include past or future events or events happening elsewhere in the present. Preconceptual thinking (based on concrete perceptions) progresses to intuitive thinking (internally representing events). Magical thinking occurs, in which preschoolers believe that their thinking influences the outside world. Questions from the preschooler begin with "Why," progressing to "Where" and "How." Preschoolers ask meanings of words, talk constantly, count, identify coins, know the days of the week, follow three-step directions in order, and memorize their addresses. During early childhood, the development of receptive language is critical to the development of later expressive abilities. Between 3 and 5 years, children practice adult speech, and stuttering may result. Sentences are grammatically correct and increasingly complex. Preschoolers may attempt to read simple print.

School-Age Child (6 to 11 Years)

Physical Development

School-age children are taller and thinner than are preschoolers. Steady growth continues; on average, height increases 2 to 3 inches per year and weight increases 6.5 lb per year. Baby fat decreases, followed by a reaccumulation of fat between about 7 and 10 years of age. The child's body is forming new bony tissue constantly as bones lengthen and harden and muscle mass increases. Proportions continue to be more adult-like. Lordosis of early childhood disappears. Facial proportions change: the forehead broadens, the nose grows larger, the lips get fuller, and the jaw juts out. Head size continues to increase at a slower rate, about one-half inch every

5 years until puberty. During this period, children lose and gain about four teeth per year (Fig. 17-4). Lymphoid tissues grow rapidly until reaching adult size shortly before adolescence. Advanced motor activities indicate completion of central nervous system myelinization. School-age children engage in large-muscle activities—walking, running, skating, swimming, riding skateboards and horses, and team sports. Small-muscle activities include sewing, printing and script writing, painting, clay modeling, and model building. Vision reaches maximum function, and hearing ability is almost complete but does not reach full maturity until adolescence.

Psychosocial Development

The family and the school are major influences on the development of personality and self-image. School-age children enjoy brief separations from family (overnight). Play is cooperative, with fixed rules and goals. Friendships are an important part of social contacts, usually with children of the same sex. Rivalry for friends is often evident. Although these children quickly form and dissolve relationships, their friendships may be intense while they last. School-age children observe and imitate the attitudes, values, and behaviors of significant people in their environments. In this age of industry (Erikson, 1963), children are determined to master tasks, becoming competent members of their culture.

Cognitive Development

During middle childhood, tremendous growth in the ability to use words occurs. Vocabulary increases, and school-age children follow rules of grammar and syntax. These children have mastered the cognitive operation of concrete thinking, using more logic (Piaget, 1952). They are able to classify and order objects and to mentally conserve their

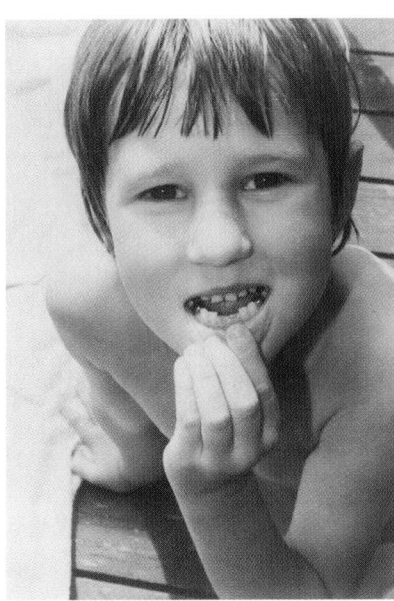

FIGURE 17-4 This school-age child shows the normal developmental pattern of losing his "baby" teeth.

physical properties despite the shapes these objects may take. However, their logic is limited to the "here and now." Comprehension of cause–effect relationships increases, and school-age children better understand the concept of time. Becoming less egocentric, these children begin to appreciate the perspectives of others. They demonstrate public and private selves.

Adolescent (11 to 22 Years)

Physical Development

The early years of adolescence are ones of rapid growth. This period begins with **puberty,** a maturation of the sex organs and reproductive functions along with the appearance of secondary sex characteristics. Girls begin adolescence at approximately 10 years of age, whereas boys enter it 2 years later (Murray & Zentner, 2001). The average age for menarche or onset of menstruation for girls in the United States is approximately 12.5 years (Herman-Giddens, et al., 1997). The end of adolescence varies from ages 18 to 22. Skeletal growth, dependent on the secretion of growth hormones regulated by the pituitary and thyroid glands, occurs through a combination of lengthening of the bones and changes in the ossification centers. Girls (11 to 13 years of age) experience a growth spurt 2 years earlier than boys do, and they plateau in height by 17 years of age. Although girls are initially taller than boys, boys grow rapidly between the ages of 14 to 21 years, eventually surpassing girls in height. Weight gain follows a similar pattern for both sexes. Chronologic age does not always coincide with these changes. One may see a 4-year spread in sexual development among adolescents. These variations may initiate a developmental crisis for some young people. Concern over body normality, sports competition, and social and peer relationships can create major hurdles. Physical growth slows in late adolescence, allowing adaptation to a new body image.

Psychosocial Development

A search for identity and self-discovery characterize adolescent psychosocial development. A changing body challenges the adolescent's sense of identity as he or she integrates physical maturation and sexuality into the self-image. This process occurs within the context of peers. Piaget refers to this stage as adolescent egocentrism, in which adolescents do not distinguish between their own conceptualizations and those of the rest of society. Instability and emotional upheaval characterize early adolescence (11 to 13 years). Increasing independence from family is coupled with increasing time spent with members of the peer group, creating changes that may cause familial tension. Drug abuse, alcoholism, cigarette smoking, and sexual behaviors present challenges to adolescents as they develop personal value systems. Peer contacts and being a part of a group are important (Fig. 17-5). Roles and relationships take on abstract meanings. Initial experiences with dating and early intimate relationships occur in adolescence. Adolescents often attempt their first forays into the working world. Late adolescents

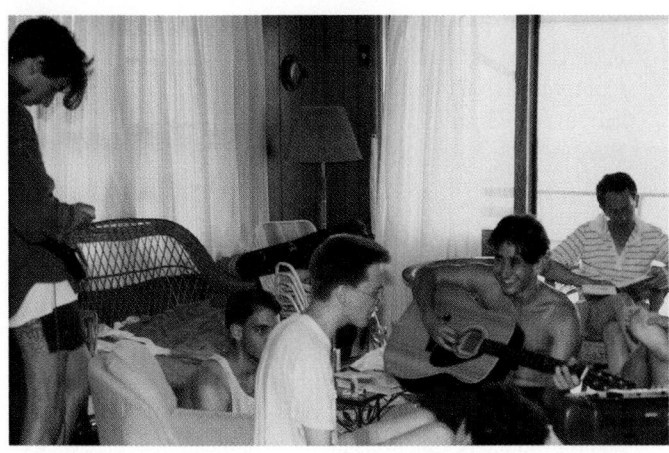

FIGURE 17-5   Throughout adolescence into young adulthood, peer relationships influence psychosocial development.

(18 to 22 years) develop smoother relationships with their parents and other adult authority figures. Older adolescents refine interpersonal skills and gain mastery over drives and emotions as they prepare to enter the world of adults. Late adolescence is often categorized as a period of transition to adulthood, because it often coincides with preparation for a career.

Cognitive Development

Formal thinking begins to emerge around 12 years of age (Piaget, 1952). This level is characterized by the ability to think abstractly; adolescents can express ideas conceptually. The thinking of this age group reflects formal logic. Formal thinking allows people to view situations from multiple perspectives. Formal thinking is not entirely related to chronologic age, and its expression varies among individuals. Adolescents also engage in introspection, self-examination, and personal critique. They develop a more mature morality based on their own judgment.

Young Adult (21 to 40 Years)

Physical Development

The young adult's physical structure stabilizes. Maturational development is complete at this time, with most systems operating at peak efficiency. In early adulthood, individuals often think they are not at risk for health problems. By the end of young adulthood, individuals may realize they are physically vulnerable. Weight and muscle mass may change as the result of the environmental influences of diet and exercise. Dental maturity is evident in the mid-twenties. Sexuality is fully mature, and reproductive function is at a peak.

Psychosocial Development

Early in this stage individuals undergo transition from adolescence to adulthood. The roles of adulthood emerge: work, intimacy, and parenting (Palkovitz, 1996). Adults assume a multitude of responsibilities: civic, parenting, and professional. Social support is important because role conflict often arises as people juggle many roles (e.g., parent, spouse, sibling,

child, friend, worker) while prioritizing to achieve success and happiness.

Young adults face significant decisions, particularly about career and relationships. Establishing intimate relationships and deciding on marriage are priority transitions. The decision whether to have children is another significant transition (Fig. 17-6). Young adults are setting the direction for the remainder of their lives.

Cognitive Development

Having reached Piaget's last stage of cognitive development, abstract thinking comes readily for young adults. Formal educational opportunities along with apprenticeship-type education are common. In some groups, the need to achieve intellectually is strong. Usually, young adults are creative, have effective problem-solving abilities, are realistic, and are less egocentric than they may have been as adolescents. Cognition in adulthood becomes focused on more practical matters than during adolescence (Santrock, 1999).

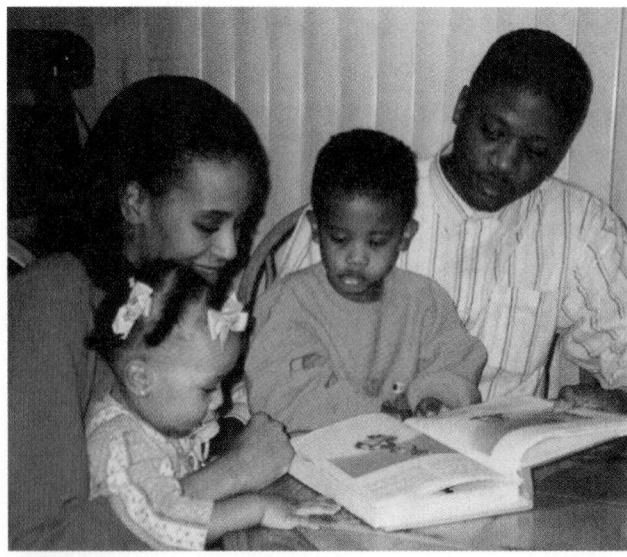

FIGURE 17-6   Starting and shaping a family are significant aspects of the young adult period.

Middle Adult (40 to 60 Years)

Physical Development

The middle adult years are a time of transition between the active, building years of young adulthood and the stabilizing later years of older adulthood. Physiologically, adults in their middle years begin to slow down. Body tissue tends to redistribute, with increased thickening around the trunk's middle portion. Signs of aging become evident. Hair starts to gray, wrinkles begin to show, men may begin to lose hair, and visual acuity for near vision begins to diminish (presbyopia). Decreased function in other body systems is seen, with beginning loss of muscle strength and agility, decreased cardiac output, decreasing hormone production, and increased fatigue.

In the absence of disease or disability, the physical changes of the middle years occur gradually and insidiously and do not interfere with vitality or function. During middle adulthood individuals may confront their physical vulnerability. A healthy lifestyle contributes to continued health in the middle years.

Psychosocial Development

During the middle years, changes in roles occur. Children may leave home, although in recent years many parents have delayed having children until they are well into their thirties or forties (Ventura, Peters, Martin, & Maurer, 1997). If the person is married, role changes may stress or strengthen the spousal relationship. At this time of life, people may be faced with providing support for children who are not totally independent and also for elderly parents who require care. Women, in particular, may feel the burden of both responsibilities (Lynch, 1998). Illness or death of an adult's parents often brings grief and a reminder of one's own mortality. Other major stressors include career changes, divorce and remarriage, or life as a single person or single parent.

Middle-aged adults may view themselves more favorably than they did in younger years, with more time for social and leisure activities. A greater commitment to enjoying relationships may exist. Interpersonal impoverishment or stagnation may develop if mature adults fail to develop generativity (Erikson, 1963). Generativity means a genuine concern for oneself, one's children, community, peers, and society. With generativity, adults feel satisfied with life and that they have contributed to others' development. Inability to accept the physical changes and psychosocial challenges of this time may foster depression, low self-esteem, and feelings of uselessness.

Cognitive Development

Adults in their middle years continue to be interested in learning and show no decrease in ability to learn. They are particularly motivated to learn if the knowledge is relevant and personally applicable. Although the ability to perform may remain unchanged, a reduction in speed of problem-solving or motor skills may interfere with some aspects of functioning (e.g., eye–hand coordination is less keen, leading to a slower reaction time).

Older Adult (60 Years and Older)

Physical Development

The physical changes accompanying old age appear at different times and manifest in different ways. All physiologic systems decline in overall function and efficiency. Chronologic age alone, however, is not a predictor of physical decline. Genetic influence, lifestyle factors, and self-concept combine to determine the course of aging.

Stamina and strength may decrease. Basal metabolic rate decreases, and the gastrointestinal system has decreased digestive juices, less tone, and slower peristalsis. Older adults often find adapting to changing environmental temperatures difficult because they have less subcutaneous fat, diminished circulation to the skin, and decreased core body temperature. Age-related changes in the function of the cardiovascular and respiratory systems contribute to diminished output of the left ventricle, less anaerobic support to muscles, less efficient respiratory ability, and increased time needed for recuperation and healing.

Neurologic changes include increased time required for impulses to travel over multisynaptic pathways, less efficient sleep, and decline in sense of balance. Special senses that began to decline in middle age continue to show decreased function. Vision and hearing changes (presbyopia and presbycusis) become more prominent. Urinary function diminishes because plasma flow to the kidneys may decrease by as much as 50% between 30 and 80 years of age, leading to a comparable decrease in glomerular filtration rate (Robinson, 1997). Decreased urinary bladder tone can contribute to incomplete emptying of the bladder, urinary frequency, and bladder infections. Degenerative changes in connective tissue and cartilage, along with demineralization of the bone, can lead to problems with posture, mobility, and injury from accidents (e.g., falls).

Although older adults experience many physical changes, these changes occur gradually and to varying extents. As a result, in the absence of illness or specific debility, older persons can function adequately in the later years of life.

Psychosocial Development

Older adults must make the transition from working to retirement. Retirement entails loss of the work role and of relationships at work and substantial changes in one's lifestyle (McGoldrick, 1994). Some people welcome retirement, with the increased opportunities it brings for activities such as church, community, and leisure (Fig. 17-7). Other people find that retirement makes them feel useless, and as though they were waiting to die. Retirement planning and a prior devotion to hobbies make the transition easier. Losses are common for elderly people, who experience the deaths of spouses, friends, and possibly children. Women outlive men by an average of 7 years, so many women must face challenges related to newfound independence, finances, and social supports later in life. Physical changes associated with aging may limit social contacts and role performance.

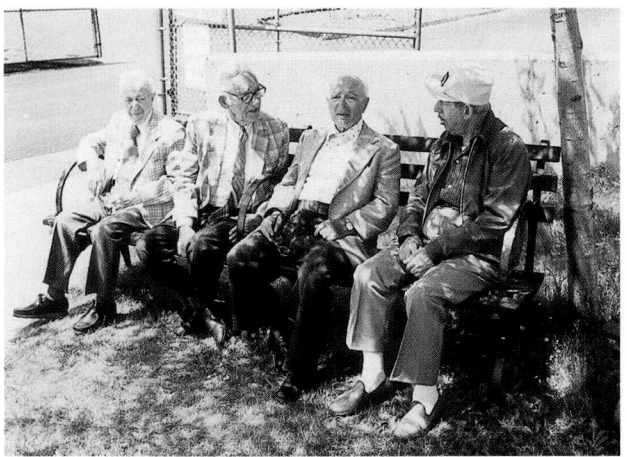

FIGURE 17-7   These retired older adults enjoy opportunities for leisure and discussion.

If older adults successfully accomplish "ego integrity" (Erikson, 1963), they participate in life, feel that their lives have been worthwhile, and do not fear death. Greenberg (1994) offered the concept of family mutuality as a framework for considering the development of elderly adults within

a family context and as a way of fostering empowerment during old age.

Cognitive Development

Although the stereotype of the aging person is one of memory loss and reduced cognitive skills, the actual cognitive changes seen in the latter part of the lifespan do not fit this description (Schulz, 1993; Ackerman, 1996). Aging reduces visual and auditory acuity, potentially affecting function. Changes in cognition more often cause a difference in speed rather than in ability (i.e., learning a new task takes longer and performance time is longer). Increasing experiential knowledge accompanies the aging process.

Most older adults do not experience cognitive impairments. Physical fitness and intellectual stimulation help maintain intellectual functioning in old age. Intellectual loss in later life may reflect interrelated physiologic deficits caused by disease (e.g., atherosclerosis causes blood vessels to narrow). Perfusion to the brain is diminished. Malignancies may metastasize to the brain or other body parts. Cardiovascular disease, emphysema, high blood pressure, poor nutrition, or effects of surgery may temporarily reduce blood supply to the brain, limiting or altering performance. Cognitive dysfunction that results from dementia, delirium, chronic brain disorders, or Alzheimer's disease is not synonymous with old age.

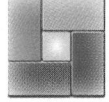

Nursing Research and Critical Thinking

Would Participating in Reminiscence Therapy Sessions Increase Family Coping Strategies of People with Chronic Renal Failure and Their Significant Others?

People diagnosed with chronic renal failure (CRF) and their families are confronted with multiple, complex problems as they attempt to cope with this illness. Reminiscence therapy is a nursing intervention that has been used to help people, especially older adults, adapt to their present life situation. A group of nurses wanted to know what the effects of reminiscence therapy were on family coping for families of clients with CRF. They designed a pretest–posttest experimental study to examine this question. A random sample was obtained from two corporately owned dialysis centers and from one privately owned dialysis center. Seven participants, age 65 years or older and diagnosed with CRF, were obtained from each of these three dialysis centers. Each person was asked to identify a significant family member to also participate in the study. The F-COPES was used to assess family coping. The person with CRF and the significant other were asked to complete the F-COPES in their home before beginning reminiscence therapy. Reminiscence therapy sessions, lasting 45 minutes per session, were held once a week for 6 consecutive weeks. After the sixth session, the F-COPES was admin-

istered as a posttest. Thirty-six participants completed the study. The Student t test was used to examine the difference between participants' pretest and posttest scores. There was a significant increase in family coping scores after reminiscence therapy ($t = 2.94$, $P < .003$).

Critical Thinking Considerations. This study was limited by the small number of older participants obtained from only three dialysis centers. The researchers also discuss the fact that none of the CRF participants could read, so the F-COPES was given verbally, which may have influenced how the participants answered. Possible implications of this study that are relevant to nursing practice are as follows:

• Reminiscence therapy is a useful intervention for helping families with chronically ill older family members.
• This method of capturing the memories of older people and providing insight and information about the past can enrich the lives of those willing to listen and provide a coping mechanism for families adapting to the challenges of chronic illness.

From Comana, M. T., Brown, V. M., & Thomas, J. D. (1998). The effect of reminiscence therapy on family coping. *Journal of Family Nursing, 4*(2), 182–197.

FUNCTIONAL HEALTH AND ANTICIPATORY GUIDANCE ACROSS THE LIFESPAN

Knowledge of lifespan development and an understanding of how humans operate physiologically as well as behaviorally are basic components of nursing. A key to appreciating human function is understanding how development produces qualitative and quantitative differences across the lifespan and how these differences relate to health. The following sections focus on age-related variations in functional health, the ways in which age modifies health needs, and the ways in which nurses can use anticipatory guidance, an educational intervention, to assist with promoting health, maximizing function, and minimizing health problems. Anticipatory guidance focuses on preparing the person or family for unfamiliar or upcoming events. It allows clients to prepare for new roles or experiences.

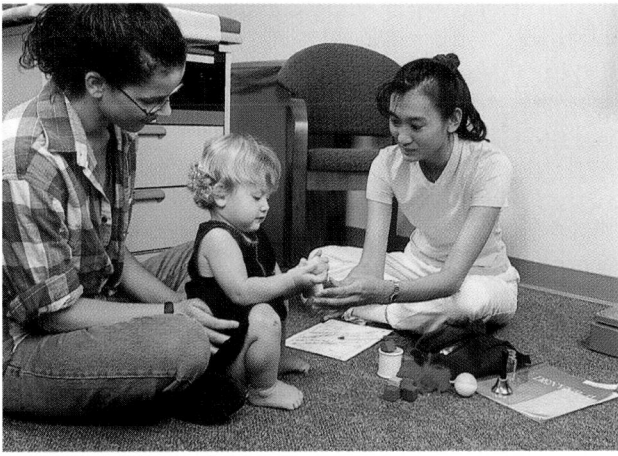

FIGURE 17-8 Regular health monitoring for children of all ages is crucial to their continued well-being. During this well-child assessment, the nurse follows tests outlined in the Denver II Developmental Screening Tool.

Health Perception and Health Management

Fetus, Newborn, and Infant

The earliest effects of health behaviors are seen during the period of fetal development. The intrauterine environment and its effects on the growing fetus have a lifelong impact on health and function. Maternal factors, including the mother's general health and health history, drug and alcohol use, some infectious diseases, smoking, exposure to toxins, diet, and stress are important determinants of fetal outcome. The fetus and the newborn may have malformations or experience dysfunction (e.g., problems affecting the cardiac, musculoskeletal, or nervous systems) as a result of the intrauterine environment.

Optimal care for the fetus is an important means of influencing lifelong health. For this reason, women's health management during the prenatal period is of paramount importance in anticipatory guidance. Encourage pregnant women to seek prenatal care early in pregnancy. They need to avoid exposure to hazards and maintain a lifestyle that will create the optimal fetal environment.

Infants continue to depend on their primary caregivers for health promotion. Encourage families to seek well-child care for regular health monitoring (Fig. 17-8), immunizations, and preventive teaching. Facilitating the transition to the parenting role may help prevent future health and relationship problems for family members.

Neonates and young infants are particularly prone to infections because of immaturity of their immune systems. Certain behaviors, such as mouthing of objects, increase the occurrence of infection. Because day care situations provide more opportunity for exposure to pathogens, it is not surprising that infants in day care have more infections, especially upper respiratory tract infections, than children who are cared for at home (Churchill & Pickering, 1997; Ferson, 1997). The effects of economics and living conditions on infant health are evidenced by a greater incidence of infections among infants from families of low socioeconomic status.

The chief health concern for infants is safety, including safe sleeping conditions and prevention of falls, aspiration, and poisoning. Infants should always be put in approved car seats when riding in automobiles. The increasing mobility involved in rolling over, creeping, crawling, and walking requires modifications in the home to prevent falls and other hazards. In older infants, hand-to-mouth behavior could cause choking or ingestion of harmful substances. Chapter 30 continues a discussion of safety in the home.

Toddler and Preschooler

Toddlers and preschoolers continue to be prone to infections. Because they have more contacts outside their homes, they become prone to many minor illnesses such as colds. Rubella, mumps, rubeola, and varicella (chickenpox) can be prevented through immunization. Immunization (discussed in Chapter 31) is a means of reducing the incidence of certain infections and is a component of normal well-child healthcare.

Safety and accident prevention are the focus of healthcare. Advancing motor and cognitive skills promote exploration, and high levels of energy and activity often lead to injuries. Injuries can range from falls and minor scrapes that occur as part of play, to life-threatening accidents such as drowning, burns, poisonings, or motor vehicle accidents.

Anticipatory guidance for family caregivers of toddlers and preschoolers includes ways to provide a safe environment for exploration—such as storing chemicals, household cleaning products, and medications in safe and protected places. Use of proper restraints (approved car seats or seatbelts with booster seats) in motor vehicles, use of life vests when around water, and close supervision of young children in potentially dangerous situations (e.g., in bathtubs, by swimming pools, at playgrounds) are essential. Children's normal level of curiosity makes them prone to participate in dangerous activities. Adult caregivers need to view the world from children's level and protect against danger at that level (e.g., wall outlets, stove burners and knobs, stairs, space heaters). As children begin to climb, they need protection at higher levels. Dangerous substances (e.g., cleaning products, medications, garden chemicals) should be locked up.

School-Age Child and Adolescent

Minor illnesses and accidents continue to be the most common health problems of school-age children. Exposure to large numbers of other children in school and play environments adds to the kinds and types of infections to which children are susceptible. Daring exploits, imagination, and industriousness of school-age children determine safety needs. Advances in motor skills throughout childhood are associated with the use of bicycles, skateboards, and other riding vehicles; consequently, their related safety concerns become factors. Independent excursions away from home make traffic accidents a possibility, and school-age children need to learn precautions with regard to strangers.

Good hygiene practices are paramount. It is not until children reach 9 years of age that they can physically manipulate a toothbrush and dental floss to clean their teeth adequately without adult supervision. Some adolescents may use over-the-counter products to treat skin problems, but most should be encouraged to keep the skin clean and free of harsh chemicals and to avoid direct exposure to the sun.

Adolescence is a time of trying out different identities and testing limits, coupled with a perception of invulnerability. Although adolescents may have a working knowledge of how the body functions, they have limited abilities to appreciate a cause–effect relationship between health behaviors and outcomes. Increased physical activity in sports and motor vehicle driving place adolescents at risk for serious injuries.

Adolescent health problems are related to lifestyle factors and risk-taking behaviors. Smoking and the use of smokeless tobacco predispose adolescents to changes in the mucosa of the mouth and in the respiratory tract, with the potential for malignant changes in the tissues and vital capacity changes in ventilation. Other health risks include drug use, alcohol consumption, fast driving, drinking and driving, and sexual activity.

In adolescence, the risk of sexually transmitted diseases (STDs) increases and is added to the usual infectious possibilities of youth. Acquired immunodeficiency syndrome (AIDS) is an additional risk, particularly if experimentation with intravenous drugs or unprotected sex occurs. Although the rate is decreasing, teenage pregnancy continues to be of concern to healthcare providers, families, and communities (Ventura et al., 1997). Gang activity is on the rise among adolescents and creates significant concern. Violence within the home, in school, and in the community affects children of all ages; however, it is among adolescents that suicide and homicide have increased dramatically, and the phrase *children killing children* has been coined (Page, 1996; Heide, 1997).

Teach and counsel adolescents regarding safety concerns for sports and driving, sex education, appropriate nutrition, and hygiene. Support and encouragement of positive family relationships are particularly important during these transitional years. Assisting adolescents as they seek personal identity and belonging is crucial. In addition, intense privacy needs may impede adequate healthcare.

Adult and Older Adult

Independence from family of origin, career development, and family establishment characterize young adulthood. Occupation may determine specialized safety concerns. Unhealthy behaviors begun in adolescence, such as smoking, drinking, and promiscuity, may continue into adulthood. The physical effects of such behaviors may become apparent. For example, cigarette smoking results in progressively declining pulmonary function. Health problems common to the middle adulthood group include hypertension, adult-onset diabetes, elevated serum cholesterol concentration, and serious illness (e.g., cancer, cardiac disease).

Acute and chronic illnesses related to lifestyle patterns are manifested late in life. The cumulative effects of smoking, poor nutrition, inadequate exercise, and other health risks become apparent. Common related health problems include chronic pulmonary conditions, cardiovascular problems, and joint degeneration.

Older adults may find that age-related changes impair their ability to manage health independently. Alterations in hearing, vision, and mobility affect practices such as hygiene, diet, and exercise. Changes in sensory and motor abilities intensify safety needs and make falls a major source of injury. Because the immune response is decreased, older people are at increased risk for infection at a time when poor nutrition and other factors may further impede natural defenses.

Anticipatory guidance includes health teaching for behavior modifications, such as following a regular program of exercise, reducing stress, and maintaining an appropriate diet (Caserta, 1995). Encourage adults to have regular physical examinations and to seek referrals as may be warranted for physical or mental health and for relational challenges, such as marital or family relationships, that may benefit from counseling. For more information, see Chapter 31.

Activity and Exercise

Newborn and Infant

Infants explore their world through motor activities. Everyday activity is adequate for developing healthy bodies. Even though developing motor activities can lead to problems related to safety, infants need opportunities to be active. As infants learn to reach and grasp objects and to roll over, they are at risk for injury.

All humans need efficient respiration and circulation for activity. Newborns and infants are prone to respiratory difficulties as a result of the relative immaturity of their airways and lung structures.

Work with adult caregivers to help them understand what factors constitute danger. Close supervision of motor activities and, if needed, of respiratory function is a central teaching element. At the same time, provide families with information about ways to provide a stimulating environment and how to evaluate appropriate toys.

Toddler and Preschooler

The occurrence of respiratory tract infections and the management of congenital problems of the heart or lungs are the leading health problems affecting activity of these age groups. Children of these ages should be given opportunities to be active to the best of their abilities in order to promote a healthy lifestyle.

Anticipatory guidance centers on prevention of respiratory tract infections and early treatment when they occur. Families of children with congenital problems need support and individual teaching.

School-Age Child and Adolescent

School-age children without congenital abnormalities or chronic difficulties have few health problems. Respiratory tract infections continue to occur as a result of contact with classmates. As motor control develops, children become more active, but their bones are not mature and are susceptible to some types of fracture. Because their bones are not completely ossified, children are somewhat more resistant to fractures than are adults. Because their rib cages are not yet rigid, school-age children are vulnerable to injury to the heart and lungs from blows to the chest. School-age children are constantly "on the go." Many school-age children and adolescents participate in organized sports and training of new athletic skills. Sports injuries of all kinds are a major cause of morbidity.

On the other hand, some school-age children and adolescents are becoming less physically active because of increased television watching, video game playing, and work on computers. Such inactivity could impede development of motor skills and an active lifestyle.

Nurses need to be teachers, counselors, and confidants when working with and advising school-age children and adolescents. Helping families understand ways that children of these age groups can minimize health problems and prevent injury is the nursing focus. Children must be provided with and encouraged to wear appropriate protective clothing when riding bicycles, skateboards, or roller blades, and they must be taught to adhere to safe behaviors in all physical activities. Families should encourage their children to spend some of their leisure time in physical activities.

Adult and Older Adult

Changes in motor abilities are noticeable in adulthood. Throughout life, the motor system operates under the "use it or lose it" principle. Exercise is increasingly important in maintenance of muscle function. Mobility is affected not only by muscular changes but also by skeletal changes such as arthritis or loss of bone mineral. Visual and motor changes impair use of means of transportation.

The effects of smoking or other pollution sources on respiration become apparent with aging. When combined with the decline in function that normally occurs with age, resulting health concerns include decreased vital capacity of the lungs, reduced stroke volume and force of heart contraction, and ischemia of tissues that are inadequately perfused. In addition, the vascular system shows accumulation of atherosclerotic plaque and reduced resilience of vessel walls.

Anticipatory guidance includes encouragement to participate in a regular exercise program (Fig. 17-9); to maintain a low-fat, high-fiber diet; and to develop pleasurable leisure activities. Adults are capable of modifying their lifestyles to extend wellness late into life (see Chapter 31).

Nutrition and Metabolism

Newborn and Infant

Infancy is a period of high metabolic rate and high nutritional need. Nutrient intake is particularly important because brain growth occupies a large share of the body's metabolic rate. Breast milk or formula, when breast-feeding is not possible, can meet complex nutritional needs during the first 6 months of life. Health problems related to nutrition focus mainly on an infant's receiving adequate amounts of milk and properly prepared formula. With the eruption of teeth and the introduction of solid foods, nutrient intake is expanded to many types of foods. Even if the infant is eating a variety of foods, breast milk or formula should be continued through at least the first year of life.

Increased metabolic rate and immature renal function lead to high fluid requirements. Breast milk usually provides enough fluid for infants. Errors in formula preparation may result in too high a concentration for newborn kidneys. Or sometimes formula is too dilute, which leads to poor weight gain, fluid overload, and difficulty concentrating urine.

Proper nutrition is important for newborn temperature regulation, which is less well developed during this period, because of less fat storage, increased metabolic rate, and an immature central thermoregulating mechanism. Low blood sugar that results from stressing thermoregulation can lead to acidosis.

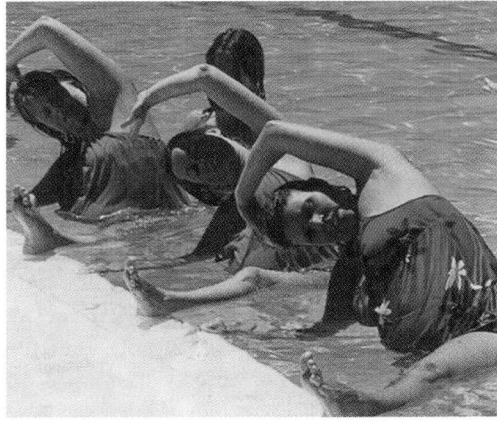

FIGURE 17-9 A regular exercise program is beneficial to health throughout the lifespan, including during pregnancy. Women who are expecting should discuss a program of exercise with their health-care providers before beginning the program.

Early in life children learn that eating can be a time of social interaction and that food can be very enjoyable. Infants before they can sit up on their own should not be left alone to eat or to suck on a bottle. Being left alone to eat or suck on a bottle can lead to choking, ear infections, and inadequate intake.

Teach family caregivers about infant nutrition and feeding, proper preparation of formula, and monitoring of the infant's physical growth. Helping caregivers understand when and how to introduce new foods is supportive. Also, teach caregivers how to use a thermometer and when to call a healthcare provider. Feeding interactions should be enjoyable for both infants and caregivers. Providing nutritious food may be burdensome for low-income families; inform them about food assistance programs in the community.

Toddler and Preschooler

Appetite during toddler and preschool years is extremely variable, but most often toddlers have smaller appetites than infants do. These changes are usually a normal consequence of slowing of growth and change in body composition. Health problems relate to family concerns regarding the adequacy of nutrient intake, because caregivers are beginning to have less control over what children eat. At this age, potential also exists for children to chew food incompletely and possibly choke on pieces of food, especially nuts. Children of these ages are developing skills to feed themselves independently.

Encourage caregivers to provide a variety of easy-to-eat but nutritious food, so that children can select enough for sufficient nutrition. Encourage children to develop good hygiene practices such as washing their hands and brushing and flossing their teeth. Adult caregivers should clean their children's teeth and, at the same time, model appropriate hygiene behaviors and make learning fun. Children should first visit the dentist at about their second birthday.

School-Age Child and Adolescent

As children move beyond the home environment, social influences on food consumption become increasingly important. The food choices of school-age children and adolescents are connected to peer influences and media advertisements. This is an excellent time to involve children in preparing family meals and choosing nutritious snacks.

Adolescence is a period of rapid growth and high nutritional requirements. Adolescents may have difficulty eating sufficient amounts of the right kinds of food to meet requirements for physical growth and physiologic change. Adolescents, in particular, are at risk for less than adequate amounts of iron, calcium, and zinc (Wong, 1999). For some adolescents, the conflict between eating and the desire to be thin is expressed in the health problems of fad dieting, bulimia, and anorexia. Others may respond to stress by overeating, leading to obesity. These health problems may set life-long patterns.

Anticipatory guidance depends on teaching and attempting to influence peer groups in a positive way to encourage good nutrition. Working with adolescents in groups tends to be more effective in changing behaviors. Meeting the nutritional needs of children from low-income families is a challenge and requires the use of community resources to feed all family members adequately.

Adult and Older Adult

Metabolic activity decreases in adults, but the need for adequate nutrition does not. Bone growth, which is accelerated during adolescence, continues in young adulthood. During childbearing years, nutrition is particularly important both for the woman and for the outcome of the pregnancy. People can avoid later health problems by receiving optimal nutrition during the active young adult years. Obesity, bulimia, or anorexia may begin or continue to be a problem. Metabolic disorders, such as diabetes, may be manifested in childhood, adolescence, young adult years, or older adult years.

Health problems related to nutrition are important concerns in the middle and older adult years. Cardiovascular changes make blood cholesterol levels and fat in the diet a concern. The sodium content of food is important for people with renal disorders or high blood pressure. People with diabetes need to regulate total dietary intake. Meeting nutritional needs using fewer calories is a challenge, and many people must monitor excess weight.

During old age, adults may have difficulty in obtaining, storing, and preparing nutritious food. Dental problems and living alone can contribute to poor nutrition in later life.

Anticipatory guidance in the adult years includes providing clients with access to reliable information about nutrition so that they can separate fact from myth. Older adults may benefit from various community-based food programs for both nutritious meals and companionship. Referrals to dietitians, nutrition classes, and support groups may be beneficial. For more information, see Chapter 37.

Elimination

Newborn and Infant

Newborn kidneys are unable to handle high solute levels or concentrate urine. Breast milk usually provides enough fluid for infants. Errors in formula preparation may result in too high a concentration or a high solute load, which can damage tissue. Sometimes formula is too dilute, which leads to fluid overload. Immature kidneys are not efficient in removing drugs or other substances from the body.

Infants are too immature to have control over either bowel or bladder elimination. Health problems relate primarily to skin disorders stemming from diaper use. Monilial infections and diaper rash are common problems.

Teach caregivers of newborns about the importance of correct formula preparation. Direct anticipatory guidance toward teaching adult caregivers proper diapering, disposal of stool and diapers, and skin care. Caregivers will want to learn correct methods of skin hygiene, frequency of diaper changes, and differences in skin rashes and their treatment.

Toddler and Preschooler

Children do not have the neurologic maturation necessary for control over defecation and urination until they can walk independently. Between 2 and 3 years of age, toddlers begin to develop control over elimination. Self-toileting involves recognition of inner signals of the need to eliminate, delaying elimination until at the toilet, handling clothing, and performing proper hygiene. Continence, once achieved, is not guaranteed, and "accidents" are not uncommon. Health problems relate to skin care and delay in progressing toward continence.

Caregivers need to know that children must have a number of skills and a level of maturity for successful toilet training. Toddlers are working toward autonomy and must be praised for their efforts at independence in elimination. Anticipatory guidance can help adult caregivers understand that the attitudes they convey during this time and their reactions to "accidents" influence not only a child's feelings about body function but also feelings about personal mastery and competency. Patience and allowing children to progress at their own pace are necessary during this stage.

School-Age Child and Adolescent

Older school-age children occasionally have difficulty with nocturnal enuresis or "bed-wetting." This problem is often related to levels of maturation of both urinary control mechanisms and sleep but may have emotional or structural causes. Nocturnal enuresis after the age of 6 years is a matter of concern. It is not uncommon to identify a familial pattern of enuresis. The main health problem is related to embarrassment and self-consciousness on the part of the child, who may limit social activities as a result of the enuresis.

Direct anticipatory guidance toward helping family members understand nocturnal enuresis. Encourage a thorough evaluation of the child. Although a physical assessment is essential, psychosocial support also is imperative.

Adult and Older Adult

Continence may be disrupted by "normal" life events, such as pregnancy or childbirth, which result in changes in the pelvic musculature. Decreasing estrogen levels that occur during menopause affect sphincter control, resulting in an increased occurrence of female stress incontinence (Lobo, 1994). Illnesses (e.g., a cerebral vascular accident) or procedures (e.g., prostatic surgery, ureterostomy placement, colostomy) may alter normal elimination patterns and threaten the sense of mastery and personal control at any age.

In older adults, alterations in innervation and changes in muscle tone may produce incontinence or nocturia. Age-related changes in the kidneys may limit adaptability to fluid changes. Decreased glomerular filtration rate can lead to fluid retention and inability to remove drugs or their metabolites. The gastrointestinal tracts of older adults tend to lose tone and motility. Consequently, constipation can develop. Usually increasing fluid and fiber intake helps reduce the risk of constipation.

Shape client teaching to the specific problem related to elimination, teaching either how to manage the alterations or therapies clients can use to regain continence. For more information, see Chapters 40 and 41.

Sleep and Rest

Newborn and Infant

Infants are in the process of organizing sleep and rest. As babies mature, their sleep periods consolidate and become longer. Sleep moves from being free-running to becoming linked to nighttime (Wong, 1999); by about 3 to 4 months of age, many infants sleep through the night. Nighttime sleep relates more to neurologic development than to age or feeding practices. Health problems of sleep in infancy are usually related to problems in the maturation of neurologic integration.

Advise family caregivers that infants normally organize their own sleep patterns. A healthcare provider should assess deviations from orderly progression, however. Remind families that young infants should sleep on their backs on a firm mattress.

Toddler and Preschooler

Toddlers and preschoolers have organized sleep patterns; most sleep occurs at night, with one or two naps during the day. During the second year of life, nightmares often emerge as cognitive development leads to increased memory and the ability to represent experiences mentally, including fearful situations (Wong, 1999). Children of these age groups are not cognitively able to separate reality from "make-believe," especially with regard to television.

Advise caregivers to reassure anxious children in an unhurried manner and to talk in a quiet voice. Caregivers should monitor children's television watching for potentially frightening images.

School-Age Child and Adolescent

Usually school-age children sleep without difficulty. Nighttime bed-wetting, a common problem in young children, may persist and disrupt sleep. As a rule, children outgrow bed-wetting, and adults should understand that scolding and punishment are ineffective. Nightmares continue to occur in children of early school age, producing nighttime awakenings (Stores, 1996). Encourage caregivers to reassure their children regarding nightmares (Fig. 17-10).

Adolescents actually have increased sleep needs as a result of rapid growth and endocrine changes. Sleep deprivation may, in reality, be a health problem for adolescents who are pressured by school, jobs, and multiple activities (Betz, Hunsberger, & Wright, 1994). Counsel adolescents regarding time management and balance of activities, so that they can be active and yet get enough sleep.

Adult and Older Adult

Adult sleep problems are often linked to stress and schedules that lead to sleep deprivation. Sleep patterns in older adults often are within the range of normal. Environmental situations, such as nighttime problems of children in the family, pregnancy, or late-night exercising or eating, may interfere

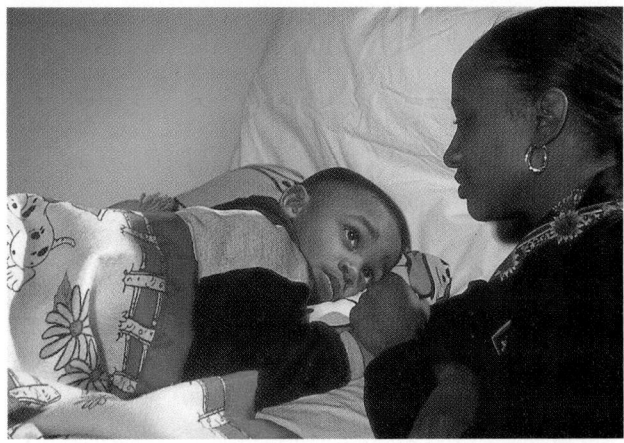

FIGURE 17-10   Children sometimes experience disruptions to their sleep, including nightmares and bed-wetting. Reassurance from a primary caregiver will help the child handle such occurrences.

with sleep as well. Anticipatory guidance includes counseling about activities that foster sleep before bedtime and environments that promote sleep.

Insomnia and sleep apnea are common sleep disorders for adults. Insomnia, a disorder of initiating or maintaining sleep, may become a health problem for which adults may choose to seek evaluation. Sleep apnea is the absence of breathing for 10 seconds or longer that occurs five or more times during an hour and may require thorough assessment and intervention. For more information, see Chapter 42.

Cognition and Perception

Newborn and Infant

Special senses are important components of cognitive-perceptual development in infancy. Sensory stimulation is a basic human need. Studies of sensory deprivation indicate that sensory stimulation is an important requirement for central nervous system development and function (Lobo, Barnard & Coombs, 1992). Although sensory stimulation during early development is extremely important, excess stimulation can overwhelm the central nervous system of neonates and infants.

Even before they can talk, newborns and infants provide caregivers with behavioral cues indicating the appropriateness of stimulation for neurobehavioral development (Barratt, Roach & Leavitt, 1992). During the first year of life, basic language skills, verbal and nonverbal, develop. It is vital that infants hear speech and have contact with others for speech and language development.

Health problems that interfere with the accuracy of sensory input (e.g., hearing) affect cognitive-perceptual development. In connection with immature anatomy and immune response, infants are prone to develop middle ear infections, which, if they become chronic and recurring, may interfere with hearing perception. Infants express ear pain through pulling on or rubbing the ear, disturbances in sleep or eating, or crying or fussiness.

Observation of responses to sounds and expressions of pain is an important form of anticipatory guidance. Help family caregivers understand the need for physical contact and sensory stimulation for adequate cognitive-perceptual development of their child. Holding and cuddling provide physical sensory stimulation, whereas colorful mobiles, pictures, sounds, and toys in the environment stimulate the special senses. Encourage caregivers to talk with the infant and to respond to infant verbal and nonverbal communication.

Toddler and Preschooler

Language and cognitive skills increase dramatically during these ages. Toddlers are still exploring the world through sensorimotor play, and preschool children express themselves through imaginative play and language.

Hearing and vision problems can impede developmental progress and may relate to misperceptions. Careful and informed observation is necessary to identify the subtle pain behaviors in children of this age. Although one might expect to see reduction in activity, children often continue to participate in play despite being in pain. At this age, children are developing cognitive skills, such as language, and are more verbal about indicating the presence of pain. Children as young as 3 years of age can use an objective tool to indicate the level of pain experienced (Beyer, Denyes & Villarruel, 1992; Abu-Saad & Hamers, 1997).

Parents and other caregivers need to be aware that the activity and constant questions of children are part of normal development. They can help children expand their skills by providing stimulating materials and by helping them develop their language skills through reading, conversing, and explaining.

Encourage parents and other caregivers to obtain regular hearing and vision examinations for their children as part of well-child care and to follow up with additional assessment if there are questions about a child's hearing or vision. Assisting caregivers to become observant of subtle behaviors that may be linked to pain or an underlying health problem is part of client teaching.

School-Age Child and Adolescent

Health problems for school-age children and adolescents may be related to previous problems of sensory input. On the other hand, difficulty with schoolwork may be the first indication of a sensory impairment or of attention deficit hyperactivity disorder (ADHD). Physiologic, emotional, and environmental factors may also influence cognitive-perceptual function (see Chapter 45). Use of drugs and alcohol alters cognition. Mental health problems become more prominent during adolescence than at earlier ages, and suicide is a major health concern.

Parents and caregivers need know that high levels of activity do not necessarily mean that a child has ADHD. But if the child's inattention and level of activity interfere with schoolwork and other functions, the child should be evaluated by a specialist. Provide anticipatory guidance at regular well-child examinations at which vision and hearing are examined. Encourage families to be aware of indications of substance use or mental health problems, such as poor academic performance, withdrawal, or changes in personality, and to seek appropriate care.

Adult and Older Adult

In the absence of chronic conditions, the young and middle adult years are associated with few cognitive-related health problems. Hearing and visual acuity diminish with age. Decline in sensory function can contribute to cognitive misperceptions. Pain perception in older adults may vary from the typical pattern seen in younger people and needs careful evaluation. Chapter 45 presents a complete discussion of the various factors that affect cognition in older adults. Reversible confusion and dementia are two major health problems for older adults.

Remind older adults to seek evaluation of pain, sensory deficits, and cognitive changes. They should not accept abnormalities as a "normal" part of aging.

Self-Perception and Self-Concept

Newborn and Infant

The infant's perception of self stems from the relationship with primary caregivers, in which infants learn a sense of worthiness. The infant's successful use of cues in conveying and satisfying needs is early evidence of competency; thus the child learns predictability and trust. Health problems arise when infants are unable to respond to usual interactions or when their needs are not met.

Caregivers and parents need to know that newborns and infants will not be "spoiled" by responding to them immediately. Provide anticipatory guidance by supporting interactions that engender trust.

Toddler and Preschooler

The self-perception of toddlers and preschoolers is related to their developmental tasks of autonomy and initiative. Expressions of anger and regression are common. Health problems exist for children who lack egocentric responses or display exaggerated responses. Excessive fears of injury or altered body image may indicate problems with self-concept. Help families understand the range of normal behaviors, and provide anticipatory guidance about behaviors outside that range that require further evaluation.

School-Age Child and Adolescent

Self-perception in these age groups may be affected by the timing and rapid changes of puberty. At these ages, children's self-concept is tied closely to peers and peer relationships. Peer response and acceptance may challenge a person's self-concept. Poor self-perception may make children in these age groups vulnerable to depression and harmful behaviors. Use of drugs and exposure to STDs and AIDS may indicate the need for peer acceptance to have a positive self-concept. Focus on open communication, interactions with groups that promote development of positive self-concept (e.g., church, Scouts, sports), and health education regarding the consequences of drug use and sexual activity.

Adult and Older Adult

Throughout the lifespan, self-concept and self-perception are reinforced or altered as a consequence of life events, interpersonal relationships, and generativity, the feeling that one has contributed to others (Erikson, 1963; Labouvie-Vief, Chiodo, Goguen, & Diehl, 1995). Changes in self-perception can arise from physical changes such as menopause. In adulthood, this pattern is extremely individual and less predictable, although certain commonalties exist. Older adults may be depressed over life events, or for no definable reason. Evidence of disturbed self-concept that interferes with the ability to carry out activities of daily living necessitates referral for evaluation and treatment. Be supportive of the client and family during periods when self-concept may be altered. Referral to support groups, counselors, or psychiatrists may be appropriate.

Roles and Relationships

Newborn and Infant

The newborn's primary relationship is with the parents or primary caregivers, and attachment is the foundation of development (Goulet, Bell, St. Cyr, Paul, & Lang, 1998). Attachment is a process in which the ongoing interaction between infant and caregiver produces a special bond, offering the infant a safe base from which to launch into the world. Sensitive adults learn to "read" the infant's cues and provide for the infant's needs. Infants, in turn, respond by smiling, sleeping, or not crying. Problems in either party can alter the interaction and interfere with attachment. The change in the relationship produces a sense of loss, which leads to an altered ability for infants to form relationships. Problems in roles and relationships during this time are also thought to contribute to abuse and neglect. The nurse encourages attachment through providing opportunities for positive interaction and by teaching the importance of reciprocal interactions to parents and caregivers.

Toddler and Preschooler

Toddlers and preschoolers are egocentric in their relationships with peers, but they should have opportunities to play with other children to develop social skills. In late infancy and toddlerhood, children express the sense of loss inherent in changes in relationships through separation anxiety and protest. The degree of anxiety and protest, however, is not necessarily direct evidence of the degree of attachment.

Provide anticipatory guidance by assisting families to understand the response of the child to changing relationships and to recognize when it exceeds normal bounds. Parents and caregivers need to recognize that children in these age groups do not have mature social skills (e.g., sharing, playing by rules) in their play.

School-Age Child and Adolescent

Peer relationships are increasingly important in the school-age years. Time spent with friends increases, while time spent with parents and family decreases. During adolescence, peers become very important in the development of

ETHICAL/LEGAL ISSUE
Child Abuse

During a routine home visit to a single mother with two children (ages 2½ years and 8 months), you notice that the mother seems a bit reluctant to talk with you. In an effort to be friendly with the toddler, you observe that the child seems small for her age and that she has no expression on her face (neither smile nor frown). She watches you intently. When you weigh the infant, his weight is significantly below what you had expected for age and length. You also notice that both children seem to have bruise marks on their upper arms. When you ask the mother about these findings, she indicates that the baby just isn't hungry and that both children fall a lot when they play, which is how they got the bruises. You observe no signs of affection among the family, and the mother is anxious to end the visit.

Reflection
- Identify your feelings about this situation.
- Assess the concerns you may have about this home visit.
- Identify possible approaches to seeking additional information.
- Recognizing the client's right to confidentiality as well as legal issues, clarify what you believe to be appropriate actions for you to take.

social and intimate relationship skills. Children who have difficulty relating to peers, leaving home and family, or managing sexuality appropriately may be exhibiting problems in roles and relationships.

Parents and caregivers must be concerned about the risks of poor social skills such as bullying. The nurse can be a safe confidant and counselor for children, a support and encouragement for adult caregivers, and an appraiser and evaluator of the need for further intervention.

Adult and Older Adult

Adults assume many roles, including those related to career, intimacy, marriage, and parenthood. Although these categories help structure thinking, the patterns of resultant roles and relationships are less clear-cut. Patterns of intimacy and parenting are not predictable or set. Although physical intimacy is required for the bearing of biologic offspring, intimacy is not always linked with parenting. Some adults defer parenting in favor of establishing a career. Parenting may be inhibited because of infertility or lack of a mate, or a person may choose not to parent. Conflicts related to the demands of these roles may result in stress.

For middle-aged and older adults, the loss of relationships through relocation, divorce, death, or illness is equally challenging. Middle-aged adults may have elderly parents who require care, and death of parents often occurs in middle age.

Middle age is also a time of evaluation and reflection, which may lead to role conflict and altered relationships. Older adults experience loss of the work role and reduced mobility and activity, which may limit social contacts, as well as changes in family roles and relationships.

Nurses can be helpful by offering support and referring people to community resources. Counsel parents of young children regarding parenting skills and sources for improving and reinforcing them. Reassure middle-aged adults that midlife review is a normal developmental process and that resources are available to assist them in sorting through feelings and conflicts that arise. Preparing for retirement years through development of new interests and activities helps to minimize the adjustment to the various role losses and changed relationships that most older adults experience. See Chapter 47 for further discussion.

Coping and Stress Tolerance

Newborn and Infant

Infants are not immune to stress. Early in life infants develop self-soothing behaviors such as sucking their thumbs and fingers. Thomas and Chess (1977) used the concepts of adaptability and rhythmicity to describe infant behaviors and classified infant temperament styles as easy, slow to warm up, and difficult. Sources of stress in infancy involve satisfaction of basic needs within the context of the caregiving or parental relationship. With the development of object permanence, the major stress of infancy and early childhood is separation, reflecting the impact of attachment (Karen, 1994). A limited understanding of time and absence of the parent or caregiver during this period of trust development are sources of anxiety.

Anticipatory guidance includes counseling families regarding the reason for separation anxiety and the range of normal response. Infants employ self-regulating and soothing behaviors, such as sucking, crying, motor activity, or withdrawal. The responsiveness of caregivers is an important determinant in how infants learn to cope.

Toddler and Preschooler

The stresses of toddlerhood include separation and loss as well as dealing with increasing autonomy. Death, divorce, or illness of a family member can affect toddlers (Behrman, 1994). In addition, sibling rivalry is a common stress, not only during the toddler years but also throughout childhood. With the birth of siblings, older children lose their place as the center of concern. Hospitalization of themselves or of loved ones is especially stressful for toddlers and preschoolers, not only because of the separation but also because they lack the cognitive ability to understand what is happening.

Cognitive development includes changes in memory. The role of memory in coping is twofold. First, children learn from stressful events; this learning can be positive or negative, depending on the coping behaviors the family uses and the outcome. Second, memory sensitizes children to stress. A child who is bitten by a dog may become afraid not only of dogs but of all furry animals. Fears and fantasy, characteristics of preschoolers' thinking, are associated with stress.

Motor development increases the possibilities for coping behaviors. Children can now use mobility to avoid or exit stressful situations, to change such situations directly, or to respond to such situations with aggression. They also are developing the verbal skills to talk about stress. Play is thought to be a major tool in the mastery of stressful events (Henniger, 1995).

Assist families in recognizing the stress their toddlers or preschoolers encounter and in nurturing their children by teaching them coping skills such as how to leave a situation. Successful stress management helps young children manage similar situations in the future.

School-Age Child and Adolescent

Performance expectations, academic pressures, and widening interpersonal contacts are characteristic sources of stress in school-age children. Although performance is a major cause of stress at this age, some of the sources of stress that were problematic during preschool years may continue to some degree. Over the years, school-age children may have developed many coping skills as well as their capacity for learning.

Help children to understand the pressures they are encountering and teach them and their caregivers healthy ways to combat stress. School nurses are in an excellent position to have children confide in them about stress and to teach them effective cognitive coping strategies. Nurses may be instrumental in reducing sources of stress in school settings.

Academic demands, conflicts over issues of independence, threats to identity, and peer pressures dominate adolescent stress. Common signs of stress in adolescents include poor or worsening school performance, changes in behavior, and increased moodiness. Adolescents may turn to dangerous ways to cope with stress and problems. Violence, actual or potential, in school settings is becoming a major source of stress. Some adolescents may react to stressful situations (e.g., being bullied) with violence; this was an element in school shootings in the 1990s and more recently. Substance use and abuse become common means of coping. The increased suicide rate among adolescents reflects the seriousness of the effects of stress on this age group (Centers for Disease Control and Prevention, 1995).

Adolescents need to feel supported and accepted regarding their stress experiences, and nurses are often in the best position to participate in this. Professionals, parents, and caregivers need to be aware of the impact of stress on adolescents and encourage them to use healthy strategies, such as physical activity and effective problem solving, for stress reduction. Guide adult caregivers to observe for signs of excessive stress and dysfunctional coping mechanisms in adolescents. Again, nurses may be instrumental in reducing sources of stress in school settings.

Adult and Older Adult

The various roles of adulthood involve specific types of stress; balancing these roles adds further stress. The underlying features in stressful events are change and loss. Coping is related to the stress or demands posed by the environment as well as the person's or family's capabilities and vulnerabilities (Woods, Haberman & Packard, 1993; Woods & Lewis, 1995). Health problems related to stress include cardiac, nutritional, sleep, and substance use disorders. Chapter 49 presents a complete discussion of stress, coping, and adjustment. Encourage people to learn a variety of methods for managing stress, including exercise, relaxation, imagery, and biofeedback.

Sexuality and Reproduction

Newborn and Infant

Gender is determined at the time of fertilization. In the first weeks of embryonic life, genetic endowment and exposure to hormones determine sexual differentiation. Gender is established at birth based on the baby's physical sexual appearance. Gender identity depends primarily on biologic characteristics, although some theorists believe that environmental factors exert some influence. Difficulty in gender identity and related health problems can occur if gender cannot be established because of ambiguous physical characteristics. Encourage caregivers to provide love, comfort, intimacy, and nurturing, the bases for later sexuality.

Toddler and Preschooler

The exploratory behavior of toddlers includes exploration of the body. Preschoolers recognize physical differences between the sexes, identifying gender based on body parts and appearances. Children of these age groups often engage in exhibitionistic behaviors, such as removing clothing and discussing sexual organs (their own and others'). Masturbation is a common behavior reflecting interest in sexuality.

Anticipatory guidance includes preparing families to expect their children's exploratory behavior and interest in sexuality. Children need to be taught about boundaries of touch by other people so that they can avoid harmful and inappropriate behaviors. Communicate the importance of affection and acceptance of children as a basis for future sexuality and positive self-concept.

School-Age Child and Adolescent

Research suggests that by the time children are 6 or 7 years of age, they have formed a stable concept of themselves as male or female (Cole & Cole, 1993). School-age children have increasing curiosity about sexual function, although peer relationships and friendships are almost exclusively with children of the same gender.

Puberty is the hallmark of adolescence. It prepares the body for reproductive function. Along with these changes, adolescents begin to form intimate relationships, both physical and emotional. Although most sexual activity occurs between heterosexual couples, homosexual experimentation during adolescence is not uncommon. Sometime during adolescence, the identification of oneself as heterosexual or homosexual occurs. The origins of homosexuality are poorly understood, and alternative patterns of sexual development have not been clearly explicated (Chernin & Holden, 1995; Haumann, 1995).

THERAPEUTIC DIALOGUE
Lifespan Development

Scene for Thought

Mr. Rifkin is a 70-year-old man whose wife died 3 years ago. He owns his own home and lives alone. He enjoys the company of a companion, Mrs. Alcott, and she enjoys taking care of him. Mr. Rifkin's only daughter and her family have moved to another state. When he visits his daughter, Mrs. Alcott comes along. Daughter Carol feels that she now has an "intruder" in her relationship with her father and doesn't know what to do. When Carol comes in for her yearly physical, she begins to discuss this situation with her nurse.

Less Effective

Client: I don't know what to do about my Dad's girlfriend. She seems to be taking over a bit too much and getting in the way of our relationship. *(Client looks frustrated and annoyed.)*

Nurse: He's 70 and has a girlfriend? Good for him! I think it's so cute when old folks can get together and take care of each other. Helps them live longer, I hear.

Client: Well, that may be, but I can't get a word in edgewise when she's around. Sure is different from what it used to be. *(Continues to look and sound frustrated.)*

Nurse: Why don't you talk to her about it? I'm sure once you've let her know how you feel she'll be much more sensitive to you.

Client: Sure she will. *(Begins to ask questions about her cholesterol.)*

More Effective

Client: I'd like to tell my Dad that he should leave the woman at home so we can talk together without her butting in all the time.

Nurse: She gets in the way of you and your Dad spending time alone? *(Restating the client's words.)*

Client: Yes, she does. And she can't take a hint, either. I suggested Dad and I take a walk together and she immediately jumped in and came too. *(Client looks frustrated.)*

Nurse: Sounds like she's afraid of being left out. *(Observation of behavior.)*

Client: That's what I'd like to do, leave her out. But I don't want to alienate my Dad or make him choose between her and me or make myself look like a jealous daughter, either. I just want . . . what do I want?

Nurse: Good question. *(Allowing client time to think and come up with her own solution.)*

Client: I want time with my Dad alone. Now I have to figure out how to get it without hurting anyone. *(Client looks determined and a bit more sure of herself.)*

Critical Thinking Challenge

- Based on Erikson's theory of development, analyze what stage Carol is in.
- Determine stages for Mr. Rifkin and Mrs. Alcott.
- Detect the losses Mr. Rifkin has experienced and state how he is coping.
- Consider the losses Carol has experienced and what she is doing about them.
- Appraise the advice given to Carol. Also critique the lack of advice.

For numerous reasons, use of birth control methods is inconsistent among adolescents. Adolescent pregnancy is now regarded as a social problem, especially for young women. Adolescents who become mothers frequently do not complete their education, which contributes to lifelong poverty. Sexual health problems for adolescents are associated with lifestyle activities. STDs and AIDS are significant potential problems for sexually active adolescents, with drug use as a contributory factor.

Adolescents need to have adequate information in order to make effective choices about their sexuality (e.g., abstinence, use of contraceptives). Be supportive of adolescents who are coming to terms with their sexual orientation, and encourage them to be aware of community resources (Fontaine & Hammond, 1996; Radkowsky & Siegel, 1997).

Children of any age are the potential victims of sexual abuse. Indications of abuse in preschoolers include anxiety, fear, sleep disturbances, and holding on to parents or other trusted adults. School-age children exhibit similar clues, plus phobias and a decline in school performance. Adolescents may exhibit

socially unacceptable behavior, sexual promiscuity, running away from home, and failing academic performance. Participate in teaching children of all ages to tell a trustworthy adult when they have been approached or touched in a way that makes them uncomfortable. Encourage families to listen carefully to their children and not to discount what adults might term as "imaginative." Above all, stress that the child is a victim and is not responsible for the abuse.

Adult and Older Adult

Body structure and function, sexual expression, and intimacy are primary aspects of human function throughout adulthood. With the development of intimate relationships, reproduction is a prime concern of early adult years. Most pregnancies and births are healthy life transitions, but reproductive problems may occur (e.g., infertility, STDs, specific sexual dysfunction). During the middle years, women reach menopause and may have health problems related to decreased estrogen production (e.g., hot flashes, osteoporosis). Men may be concerned about waning sexual performance even though most adults can be sexually active throughout their lives. In normal aging, decreased mobility and energy production may limit sexual activity. Health problems are related to interference with sexual expression that may stem from illness (e.g., stroke), death of a spouse, or the environment (e.g., nursing homes). STDs and AIDS remain potential problems throughout adulthood.

Nurses who work with individuals and couples who have sexual and reproductive issues need to be sensitive to their feelings and support their efforts to seek therapies to correct the problem. Encouraging couples to maintain their personal intimacy as well as sexual intimacy is essential throughout life. Preventing STDs and AIDS is important. Nurses can also help older adults to understand that age alone is not a barrier to sexual function and can counsel (or refer to counselors) older people on alternative forms of sexual expression. Sensitivity in anticipating privacy needs for older adults in healthcare settings is a valuable nursing function. For further information, see Chapter 50.

Values and Beliefs

Newborn and Infant

Infants have a limited understanding of right and wrong and do not appreciate cause–effect relationships between their actions and punishments or rewards. Help family caregivers understand that, because infants are not defying them deliberately, punishment is inappropriate.

Toddler and Preschooler

During these ages, children have the cognitive development to comprehend rules imposed on them by adults and the consequences of their actions. These ages are marked by an egocentric approach to right and wrong—children deem whatever they want to be right. Punishment and reward guide behavior.

Toddlers and preschoolers learn religious practices through family activities and imitation. Children of these ages do not have the cognitive functioning to fully comprehend the significance of religious practices; their comprehension reflects the magical thinking typical of these age groups.

The nurse's role is to help families use this stage to enhance positive behaviors through rewarding desired actions. Encouraging adult caregivers to include their children in religious practices fosters spiritual beliefs and development (Cole, 1991).

School-Age Child and Adolescent

Early in the school-age stage, behavior becomes more self-directed and children comprehend the impact of their actions on others. School-age children tend to follow orders to gain the approval of others. Because of the desire for conformity and the wish to fit in, the will to do right guides behavior, with less emphasis on punishment and reward.

Religious beliefs reflect a beginning appreciation of the existence of a deity. Because doing right is associated with reward, school-age children may engage in making "deals" with the deity figure. Being aware of the child's spiritual de-

velopment enhances the parents' ability to further the child's development.

As cognition develops, adolescents move to higher levels of moral thinking. Adolescents learn to make moral judgments that are situation specific, to transfer those judgments across situations, and finally to make autonomous decisions regarding moral issues. The development of moral thinking may differ between boys and girls (Gilligan, 1982). Girls tend to base their judgments in the context of relationships, whereas boys tend to think more in terms of rules. At this time, adolescents question faith and challenge religious beliefs as they develop personal identity and expand their independence from the family.

Behavior problems, or conduct disorders, during these ages have negative effects on children's cognitive, social, and emotional development (Webster-Stratton, 1992). Problems occur when adolescents try out various activities and behaviors, such as substance use and promiscuous sexual behavior.

Nurses can help parents understand that their children's moral and religious values are still developing. If children have behavior problems, nurses should inform the parents and caregivers about resources for parent education and management of behavior problems.

Adult and Older Adult

Values and moral development are at the level of autonomous decisions, in which people apply principles to differing situations. Moral reasoning is bound less by rules, because personal values guide actions to a greater extent. Spiritual beliefs evolve and are applicable across a variety of situations. Health problems occur when disharmony exists between spiritual beliefs and life events (Reed, 1991). Chapter 51 has a complete discussion of spirituality and alterations in spirituality.

KEY CONCEPTS

- Growth and development occur throughout the lifespan.
- Development is the process of ongoing change, reorganization, and integration that occurs throughout a person's life, and it includes body structure and function, psychosocial behaviors, and cognition.
- Genetics and environment are the two primary factors driving development.
- Principles of growth and development are drawn from biologic and psychosocial sciences and express commonalities in the process.
- Theorists have attempted to explain growth and development within various contexts, such as psychodynamics, cognitive development, human needs, and developmental tasks.
- There are progressive, sequenced aspects of development for the various stages of life, on which future development expands.
- The nurse's primary role in growth and development is understanding the person's position in the process, being aware of expectations in terms of functional health, and recognizing functional health problems related to development.

REFERENCES

Abu-Saad, H. H., & Hamers, J. P. H. (1997). Decision-making and paediatric pain: A review. *Journal of Advanced Nursing, 26*(5), 946–952.

Ackerman, P. (1996). A theory of adult intellectual development: Process, personality, interests and knowledge. *Intelligence, 22*(2), 227–258.

Barratt, M. S., Roach, M. A., & Leavitt, L. A. (1992). Early channels of mother–infant communication: Preterm and term infants. *Journal of Child Psychology and Psychiatry and Allied Disciplines, 33*, 1193–1204.

Behrman, R. E. (1994). Children and divorce: Overview and analysis. *Future of Children, 4*, 4–14.

Betz, C., Hunsberger, M., & Wright, S. (1994). *Family-centered nursing care of children* (2nd ed.). Philadelphia: W. B. Saunders.

Beyer, J. E., Denyes, M. J., & Villarruel, A. M. (1992). The creation, validation, and continuing development of the Oucher: A measure of pain intensity in children. *Journal of Pediatric Nursing, 7*, 335–346.

Bronfenbrenner, U. (1981). *The ecology of human development.* Cambridge, MA: Harvard University Press.

Caserta, M. S. (1995). Health promotion and the older population: Expanding our theoretical horizons. *Journal of Community Health, 20*(3), 283–293.

Centers for Disease Control and Prevention. (1995). Suicide among children, adolescents, and young adults—United States, 1980–1992. *MMWR Morb Mortal Wkly Rep, 44*, 289–291.

Chernin, J., & Holden, J. (1995). Toward an understanding of homosexuality: Origins, status, and relationship to individual psychology. *Individual Psychology: Journal of Adlerian Theory, Research and Practice, 51*(2), 90–101.

Churchill, R. B., & Pickering, L. K. (1997). Infection control challenges in child-care centers. *Infectious Disease Clinics of North America, 11*(2), 347–365.

Cole, R. (1991). *The spiritual life of children.* Boston, MA: Houghton Mifflin.

Cole, M., & Cole, S. (1993). *The development of children* (2nd ed.). New York: Scientific American Books.

De Casper, A. J., & Fifer, W. P. (1980). Of human bonding: Newborns prefer their mothers' voices. *Science, 208*, 1174–1176.

DiPietro, J., Hodgson, D., Costigan, K., Hilton, S., & Johnson, T. (1996). Fetal neurobehavioral development. *Child Development, 67*(5), 2553–2568.

DuPont, H. (1994). *Emotional development: Theory and applications.* Westport, CT: Praeger.

Erikson, E. (1963). *Childhood and society* (2nd ed.). New York: W. W. Norton.

Ferson, M. J. (1997). Infection control in child care settings. *Communicable Diseases Intelligence, 21*(22), 333–337.

Fontaine, J., & Hammond, N. (1996). Counseling issues with gay and lesbian adolescents. *Adolescence, 31*(124), 817–830.

Gilligan, C. (1982). *In a different voice.* Cambridge, MA: Harvard University Press.

Goulet, C., Bell, L., St. Cyr, D., Paul, D., & Lang, A. (1998). A concept of analysis of parent–infant attachment. *Journal of Advances in Nursing 28*(5), 1071–1081.

Greenberg, S. (1994). Mutuality in families: A framework for continued growth in late life. *Journal of Geriatric Psychiatry, 27*(1), 79–95.

Haumann, G. (1995). Homosexuality, biology, and ideology. *Journal of Homosexuality, 28*(1–2), 57–77.

Havighurst, R. J. (1972). *Developmental tasks and education* (3rd ed.). New York: David McKay.

Heide, K. (1997). Juvenile homicide in America: How can we stop the killing? *Behavioral Sciences and the Law, 15*(2), 203–220.

Henniger, M. L. (1995). Play: Antidote for childhood stress. *Early Child Development and Care, 105*, 7–12.

Herman-Giddens, M. E., Slora, E. J., Wasserman, R. C., Bourndony, C. J., Bhapkar, M. V., Koch, G. G., & Hasemeier, C. M. (1997). Secondary sexual characteristics and menses in young girls seen in office practice: A study from the Pediatric Research in Office Settings network. *Pediatrics, 99*(4), 505–512.

Johnsen, E. P. (1991). Searching for the social and cognitive outcomes of children's play: A selective second look. *Play and Culture, 4*, 201–213.

Karen, R. (1994). *Becoming attached: Unfolding the mystery of the infant–mother bond and its impact on later life.* New York: Warner Books.

Kohlberg, L. (1976). Moral stages and moralization: The cognitive-developmental approach. In T. Lickona (Ed.), *Moral development and behavior.* New York: Holt, Rinehart & Winston.

Kohlberg, L. (1984). *The psychology of moral development: The nature and validity of moral stages* (vol. 2). New York: Harper & Row.

Labouvie-Vief, G., Chiodo, L., Goguen, L., & Diehl, M. (1995). Representations of self across the life span. *Psychology and Aging, 10*(3), 404–415.

Levenson, M., & Crumpler, C. (1996). Three models of adult development. *Human Development, 39*(3), 135–148.

Lobo, M. L., Barnard, K. E., & Coombs, J. B. (1992). Failure to thrive: A parent–infant interaction perspective. *Journal of Pediatric Nursing, 7*(4), 251–261.

Lobo, R. (Ed.). (1994). *Treatment of the postmenopausal woman: Basic and clinical aspects.* Philadelphia: J. B. Lippincott.

Lucas, A. (1998). Programming by early nutrition: An experimental approach. *The Journal of Nutrition, 128*(2), 401S–407S.

Lynch, M., & Lynch, C. (1991). Self concept development through adult life cycle. *Journal of Research in Education, 1*, 13–17.

Lynch, S. A. (1998). Who supports whom? How age and gender affect the perceived quality of support from family and friends. *The Gerontologist, 38*(2), 231–238.

McGoldrick, A. (1994). The impact of retirement on the individual. *Reviews in Clinical Gerontology, 4*(2), 151–160.

Murray, R., & Zentner, J. (2001). *Nursing assessment and health promotion: Strategies through the life span* (7th ed.). Saddle River, NJ: Prentice Hall.

Nathanielsz, P. (1996). Fetal and neonatal environment has influence on brain development. *Lancet, 347*(8997), 314–315.

Newport, E. (1991). Contrasting concepts of the critical period for language. In S. Carey & R. Gelman (Eds.), *The epigenesis of mind: Essays on biology and cognition.* Hillsdale, NJ: Erlbaum.

Page, R. (1996). Youth suicidal behavior: Completions, attempts and ideations. *High School Journal, 80*(1), 60–65.

Palkovitz, R. (1996). Parenting as a generator of adult development: Conceptual issues and implications. *Journal of Social and Personal Relationships, 13*(4), 571–592.

Parten, M. (1932). Social play among preschool children. *Journal of Abnormal and Social Psychology, 27*, 243–269.

Peterson, M. (1994). Physical aspects of aging: Is there such a thing as "normal?" *Geriatrics, 49*, 45–49.

Piaget, J. (1952). *The origins of intelligence in children.* New York: International Universities Press.

Radkowsky, M., & Siegel, L. (1997). The gay adolescent: Stressors, adaptations, and psychosocial interventions. *Clinical Psychology Review, 17*(2), 191–216.

Reed, P. G. (1991). Spirituality and mental health in older adults: Extant knowledge for nursing. *Family and Community Health, 14*, 14–25.

Robinson, D. (1997). Urinary incontinence in the elderly: A growing problem that needs attention. *Current Opinion in Obstetrical Gynecology, 9*(5), 285–288.

Santrock, J. W. (1999). *Life-span development.* Boston: McGraw-Hill.

Saracho, O., & Spodek, B. (1995). Children's play and early childhood education: Insights from history and theory. *Journal of Education, 177*(3), 129–149.

Sasser-Coen, J. R. (1993). Qualitative changes in creativity in the second half of life: A life-span developmental perspective. *Journal of Creative Behavior, 27*, 18–27.

Schulz, R. (1993). *Adult development and aging: Myths and emerging realities* (2nd ed.). New York: Macmillan.

Schuster, C. S., & Ashburn, S. S. (1992). *The process of human development* (3rd ed.). Philadelphia: J. B. Lippincott.

Stores, G. (1996). Practitioner review: Assessment and treatment of sleep disorders in children and adolescents. *Journal of Child Psychology and Psychiatry, 37*(8), 907–925.

Thomas, A., & Chess, S. (1977). *Temperament and development.* New York: Brunner/Mazel.

Thompson, J. E. (1990). Maternal stress, anxiety, and social support during pregnancy: Possible directions for prenatal intervention. In I. R. Merkatz & J. E. Thompson (Eds.). *New perspectives on prenatal care* (pp. 319–335). New York: Elsevier.

Ventura, S. J., Peters, K. D., Martin, J. A., & Maurer, J. D. (1997). Births and deaths: United States, 1996. *Monthly Vital Statistics Report, 46*(1), (Suppl 2), Sept. 11, 1997.

Webster-Stratton, C. (1992). *The incredible years: A trouble shooting guide for parents of children aged 3–8.* Toronto: Umbrella Press.

Wong, D. (1999). *Whaley & Wong's nursing care of infants and children* (6th ed.). St. Louis: Mosby.

Woods, N. F., Haberman, M. R., & Packard, N. J. (1993). Demands of illness and individual, dyadic, and family adaptation in chronic illness. *Western Journal of Nursing Research, 15,* 25–30.

Woods, N. F., Lewis, F. M. (1995). Women with chronic illness: Their views of their families' adaptation. *Health Care for Women International, 16*(2), 135–148.

Worthington-Roberts, B. S., & Williams, S. R. (1997). *Nutrition in pregnancy and lactation.* Madison, WI: Brown and Benchmark.

BIBLIOGRAPHY

Boyd, M. A., & Nihart, M. A. (1998). *Psychiatric nursing: Contemporary practice.* Philadelphia: Lippincott-Raven.

Bruni, O., Ottaviano, S., Guidetti, V., Romoli, M., Innocenzi, M., Cortesi, F., & Giannotti, F. (1996). The sleep disturbance scale for children. *Journal of Sleep Research, 5*(4), 251–261.

Carman, M. (1997). The psychology of normal aging. *Psychiatric Clinics of North America, 20*(1), 15–24.

Fisher, J. (1993). A framework for describing developmental change among older adults. *Adult Education Quarterly, 43,* 76–89.

Harris, J. R. (1998). *The nurture assumption.* New York: Simon & Schuster.

Herman, S. (1994). Marital satisfaction in the elderly. *Gerontology and Geriatrics Education, 14*(4), 69–79.

Kehn, D. (1995). Predictors of elderly happiness. *Activities, Adaptation & Aging, 19*(3), 11–30.

Kohlberg, L., & Ryncarz, R. (1990). Beyond justice reasoning: Moral development and considerations of a seventh stage. In C. Alexander & E. Langer (Eds.), *Higher stages of human development: Perspectives on adult growth.* New York: Oxford University Press.

Kurtines, W. M., & Gewirtz, J. L. (Eds.). (1991). *Handbook of moral behavior and development. Vol. 1: Theory.* Hillsdale, NJ: Erlbaum.

Reynolds, W., Remer, R., & Johnson, M. (1995). Marital satisfaction in later life: An examination of equity, equality, and reward theories. *International Journal of Aging and Human Development, 40*(2), 155–173.

Schaie, K. W. (1994). The course of adult intellectual development. *American Psychologist, 49,* 304–313.

Santrock, J. W. (1999). *Life-span development* (7th ed.). Boston: McGraw-Hill.

Smotherman, W., & Robinson, S. (1996). The development of behavior before birth. *Developmental Psychology, 32*(3), 425–435.

Van Ausdale, D., & Feagin, J. (1996). Using racial and ethnic concepts: The critical case of very young children. *American Sociological Review, 61*(5), 779–793.

18 The Older Adult

Key Terms

cognition
communication
chronic illness
coping/stress
demographics of aging
elimination
health maintenance
  immunity
infections
loneliness
loss/grief
mobility

mood
nutrition
pain management
rest
roles and relationships
self-care
self-perception
sexuality
skin integrity
sleep
spirituality
values/beliefs

Learning Objectives

Upon completion of this chapter, the student will be able to do the following:
1. Describe the demographics of older adults.
2. Discuss a comprehensive knowledge base that can help nurses display commitment to providing humane and dignified care.
3. Explain physiologic changes and chronic illnesses that place older adults at greater risk for declines in health and quality of life.
4. Identify health promotion and health maintenance strategies that can give older adults advantages in maintaining optimal health.

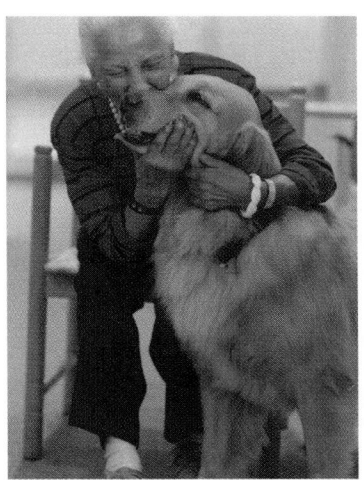

Critical Thinking Challenge

You are a nursing student assigned to do your first clinical rotation in a nearby skilled nursing facility. Many of your classmates comment that they are not looking forward to working with "old people." So far you have had very positive experiences with the older adults in your family; however, you are a little anxious about having to deal with sicker, older frail adults.

When you get to the Alzheimer's unit you see a resident embracing a dog. Although the woman is disoriented (not knowing where she is or the date), she interacts pleasantly with you, smiling and holding your hand, and hugging the dog.

Our previous life experience greatly affects our thoughts, feelings, and behaviors in facing new situations. This tendency prevails in our interactions with specific groups such as the aged. This chapter explores various aspects of aging. It discusses specific characteristics of today's older population and explores misconceptions of aging. After completing this chapter, review the above scenario and reflect on the following areas of critical thinking:

1. Describe your initial reaction to thoughts of caring for older adults.
2. Identify some assumptions that you had about older adults prior to reading this chapter.
3. Identify areas of new information that you will now be able to use in your clinical practice.
4. Construct a care plan that would best fit the specific needs of the woman described in the above scenario.

Older adults are a very heterogeneous group. Myriad differences in lifestyle, experience, and health make it difficult to generalize about this group, especially because their age differences span four decades. As adults age, however, they are more likely to suffer chronic health disorders that impair function and negatively affect their quality of life (Display 18-1). Many older adults suffer multiple health conditions that exacerbate one another. These health conditions interact based on physiology, environment, and the person's unique health profile.

This chapter will examine health conditions that often occur together in older adults. Subsequent chapters will explore these health conditions in more detail. These conditions are not necessarily always found together. In fact, older adults may experience different health conditions in concert at various times. It is critical to remember the principle that as people age, the complex interplay of their health conditions affects function and quality of life.

DEMOGRAPHICS

In the United States and worldwide, the number of persons aged 65 years or older have grown exponentially. Life expectancy has increased for both men and women, mostly because of a substantial decrease in deaths from cardiovascular conditions (primarily heart disease and stroke). In 1900, life expectancy was 47 years. In 1999, life expectancy was 83.6 years for women and 75 years for men. Persons older than age 65 comprise 12.7% of the U.S. population (numbering 34.5 million in 1999) with an expected increase to 20% by the year 2030 (Figure 18-1). Of persons older than 65 years, the fastest growing segment is persons older than 85 years. In 1999, the 65- to 74-year-old age group (18.2 million) was 8 times larger than in 1990; the 75- to 84-year-old age group (12.1 million) was 16 times larger; and the 85 years and older age group (4.2 million) was 34 times larger. The number of centenarians (persons older than age 100 years) is also rapidly increasing; their numbers doubled in the 1980s.

Similar to the total U.S. population, the older U.S. population is becoming more racially diverse. In 1999, 15.7% of persons age 65 or older were minorities (8% Black; 2.1% Asian or Pacific Islander; 1% American Indian or Native Alaskan; 5.1% Hispanic origin) (Figure 18-2). By 2030, minorities are expected to comprise 25.4% of the older adult

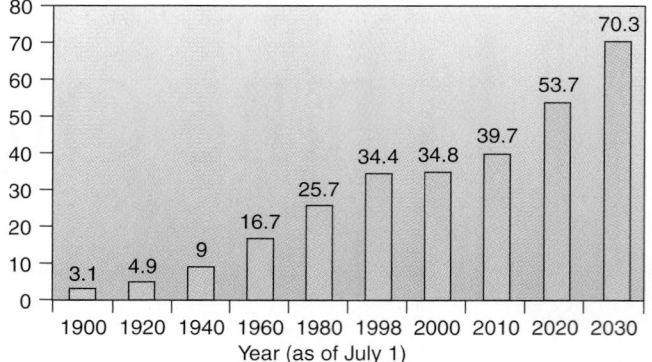

FIGURE 18-1   Number of persons age 65 or older 1900 to 2030.

population. From 1999 to 2030, the white population 65 years or older is expected to increase by 81% compared with 219% for older minorities including Hispanics (328%); African Americans (131%); American Indians, Eskimos, and Aleuts (147%); and Asian and Pacific Islanders (285%).

Living arrangements vary widely based on sex. In 1998, most noninstitutionalized persons older than age 65 years lived in a family setting. The proportion of persons living in a family setting decreased with age; only 45% of those older than age 85 lived in a family setting. In 1998, about 31% (9.9 million) of that age group lived alone (41% of older women and 17% of older men). Among women older than age 85, three of five lived outside a family setting. While only 4.3% (1.4 million) of older adults lived in nursing homes in 1997, the percentage increased with age, ranging from 1.1% of persons aged 65 to 74 years and 4.5% for persons aged 75 to 84 years to 19% for persons older than age 85 years.

Financial situations vary as well. In 1999, the reported median income was $19, 079 for older men compared to $10, 943 for older women. For these persons, 34% reported less than $10, 000 annually; only 23% reported $25,000 or more. The median income was $14,425. One out of 12 (8.3%) white older adults was poor compared to 22.7% of older African Ameri-

DISPLAY 18-1

[5] **MOST COMMONLY REPORTED CHRONIC CONDITIONS (65+)**	
Arthritis	Cataracts
Hypertension	Orthopedic impairments
Heart disease	Sinusitis
Hearing impairments	Diabetes

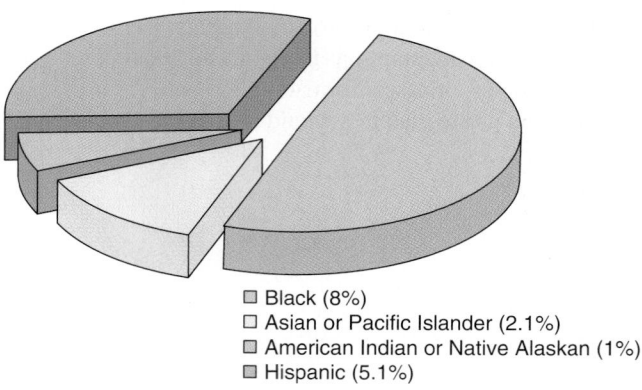

☐ Black (8%)
☐ Asian or Pacific Islander (2.1%)
☐ American Indian or Native Alaskan (1%)
☐ Hispanic (5.1%)

FIGURE 18-2   Estimates of percentages of minority elderly by ethnic origin (1999).

cans and 20.4% of older Hispanics. Older women had higher poverty rates (11.8%) than men (6.9%). Older adults living alone or with nonrelatives had higher poverty rates (20.2%) than those living with family (5.2%). Hispanic women living alone had the highest poverty rate at 58.8%. The U.S. Social Security Administration reported in 1998 that the major income sources for older adults consisted of Social Security (90%), income from other assets (62%), public and private pensions (44%), and earnings (21%) (U.S. Department of Health and Human Services Administration on Aging, 2002).

COGNITION AND COMMUNICATION, MOOD, AND SELF-CARE

Cognition and Communication

Many older adults retain full cognitive (thinking) function into advanced age. As persons enter their 80s and 90s, however, the incidence of dementia (irreversible confusion), such as Alzheimer's disease, increases dramatically. Additionally, older adults experience higher rates of delirium (acute confusion). These conditions disrupt thinking functions in many different ways. Some persons exhibit losses in attention span or short-term memory. Judgment and insight may be impaired. Language deficits may occur. These cognitive and language deficits, in conjunction with any sensory deficits, impair effective communication (exchange of information).

Nurses may use many interventions to facilitate communication and minimize the adverse consequences of confused thinking. Maintaining levels of sensory stimulation that are tolerable for a person with dementia minimizes confusion and fatigue. Appropriate sensory appliances (glasses and hearing aids) assist older adults in interacting appropriately with their environments. An inexpensive hand-held amplifier (e.g., Radio Shack's Optimus Stereo Amplified Listener) serves as an excellent alternative for communicating with clients who are hard of hearing and do not have an available hearing aide. Reality orientation is recommended for orienting persons with reversible confusional states (e.g., delirium). In the latter stages of irreversible confusional states (e.g., Alzheimer's, Parkinson's dementia), reality orientation is less successful and often causes agitated or angry responses. At this latter point, validation therapy (Feil, 1993) is a more effective strategy. Validation therapy is a type of interpersonal interaction in which the health professional attempts to understand and validate the client's current needs (Display 18-2). Environmental modifications, socialization strategies, and family support are other interventions for persons with cognitive disorders and language difficulties (see Chapter 45). Therapies, such as music therapy (Feldt, 2000) and pet therapy (Shelkey, 2000), are also useful in treating dementia.

Antidepressant or antipsychotic medications are commonly used to treat depression or adverse behavioral symptoms (Display 18-3) associated with dementia. Antipsychotics,

DISPLAY 18-2

🔳 VALIDATION THERAPY

Mrs. Leonard is living in a long-term care facility. She encounters one of the nursing caregivers in the hall outside her room. She appears very upset and tearful.

Nurse: Mrs. Leonard, is everything all right? You seem very upset.

Mrs. Leonard: I need to go and get my children who will be getting out of school soon. I don't know where my husband is either.

The nurse knows that Mrs. Leonard's children are adults and that her husband died several years ago. She does not, however, confront Mrs. Leonard with any of these facts, knowing that Mrs. Leonard has had a negative reaction to that approach in the past. The nurse knows that Mrs. Leonard has Alzheimer's disease and that reassurance and distraction will be more successful strategies.

Nurse: It is still a little early to leave and get them. While we're waiting, let's go make some tea and in the meantime you can tell me all about them.

Mrs. Leonard: All right, but I can't be late.

Nurse: I know. I assure you that everything will be fine. Let's go get the tea. I think I even know where there are some delicious cookies.

In this scenario, the nurse is considering that Mrs. Leonard is anxious for any number of reasons. She mentions her family and is worrying about them. The nurse uses distraction (using Mrs. Leonard's short-term memory deficit to her benefit) and a reassuring social interaction to allay Mrs. Leonard's anxieties, while continuing to validate her experience.

DISPLAY 18-3

🔳 ADVERSE DEMENTIA BEHAVIORAL SYMPTOMS

Asking questions repeatedly
Anxiety
Emotional lability (rapid mood fluctuations)
Hoarding
Irritability
Misplacing things
Physically aggressive
Socially/sexually inappropriate
Suspiciousness/paranoia
Undressing in public
Verbally aggressive
Wandering

however, have adverse side effects (including increased confusion and falls) and should be used judiciously with careful monitoring. Their use should be reserved for situations in which behavioral strategies and environmental strategies have failed to be effective (Display 18-4).

Mood

Mood disorders (especially depression) are often unrecognized or misdiagnosed in older adults. Symptoms of depression include poor cognitive performance, sleep problems, and lack of initiative—symptoms commonly seen in persons with dementia. The prevalence of clinically depressive symptoms ranges from 8% to 15% for community-dwelling older adults to 30% in institutionalized older adults (Beers & Berkow, 2000). Suicide is the most serious consequence of depression. Currently, older white men have the highest rate of suicide in the United States. Several assessment tools can screen older clients for depression. Using a standardized screening tool, such as the Yesavage Geriatric Depression Scale (Yesavage & Brink, 1983) (Display 18-5), may help the nurse identify an older person with depression. Many factors place an older adult at risk for depression; factors include recent bereavement, change in environment, alcohol/substance use, and chronic

DISPLAY 18-4

🔄. STRATEGIES FOR PERSONS WITH DEMENTIA

Behavioral

Use a calm, familiar approach; be aware of your non-verbal communication.

Speak slowly and clearly; face the person.

Do not touch the person quickly or without warning.

Use finger foods for persons having problems using eating utensils.

Encourage socialization (music, dancing).

Break tasks down into simple steps; provide verbal cueing.

Do not exceed the person's ability to cope; observe for signs of frustration and redirect client's attention/activity.

Avoid physical restraints.

Environmental

Use clear signage.

Use enclosed bulletin boards.

Reduce the amount of unnecessary noise.

Encourage geriatric-friendly furniture (solid base with arm rests).

Promote life-enhancing art that is conducive to the level of cognitive impairment.

Recommend non-glare flooring.

Ensure ready access to music and snack foods.

Use sound-absorbing wall and ceiling materials.

pain. Knowledge of these risk factors and careful assessment of older adults at risk assist the nurse in providing support, counseling, as well as appropriate and timely referral to a health provider for pharmacologic or psychotherapeutic interventions.

Less common psychiatric disorders, such as delusional disorder, bipolar disorder, anxiety disorder, and schizophrenia, may occur alone or coexist in older clients (Table 18-1). Psychotic symptoms (delusions and hallucinations) may result from delirium, dementia, mood, or psychiatric disorders. These disorders negatively affect the person's function and ability to communicate. Most of these disorders, when recognized and treated, respond to treatment. Antipsychotic medications typically are used to treat delusions (fixed beliefs that contradict reality) and hallucinations (false perceptions such as sounds, smells, visions that have no relation to reality). Nonpharmacologic therapies (e.g., individual therapy, family therapy, peer support groups) are also used in treatment. These psychiatric disorders are severe, persistent, and require treatment throughout the person's lifetime.

Self-Care

Medications or medical conditions may cause or obscure psychotic symptoms. Conditions that mimic dementia or depression present distinct challenges because they impair thinking, mood, and communication. Such conditions also affect the older adult's ability to manage **self-care.** Activities such as shopping, managing finances, and cooking are usually affected first. As the number or severity of impairments increases, the older adult will lose his or her ability to bathe, feed, and ambulate (Chapter 32). The older adult often requires extensive care at this point. Families are the main providers of care to older adults (Archibold & Stewart, 2001). In the absence of family or friends or when the older adult's needs are greater than the family's ability to provide help, institutionalization may be required. When care needs become so extensive as to require institutionalization, the older adult's independence is increasingly compromised. Often, as a result of dementia, decision-making capacity is also lost.

Nurses frequently encounter these older adults and their families in healthcare settings (e.g., emergency rooms, clinics). Numerous community agencies are available to provide necessary assistance (meals, transportation, visiting healthcare providers, home helpers) to the older adult or family. The nurse who is aware of the client's needs and appropriate referral sources may serve as the healthcare provider best situated to link client and families to appropriate services.

MOBILITY, ELIMINATION, AND SKIN INTEGRITY

Mobility

Many chronic conditions of aging negatively affect **mobility** (walking, driving, shopping, exercise). Arthritis, gait and balance disorders (caused by musculoskeletal or neurologic conditions), and cataracts are among the many health conditions

DISPLAY 18-5

🔄 SHORT FORM: GERIATRIC DEPRESSION SCALE

NAME _____ AGE _____ SEX _____ DATE _____
WING _____ ROOM _____ PHYSICIAN _____ ASSESSOR _____

Scoring System
Answers indicating depression are highlighted. Each **Bold faced** answer counts one (1) point.

1. Are you basically satisfied with your life?	YES / **NO**
2. Have you dropped any of your activities and interests?	**YES** / NO
3. Do you feel that your life is empty?	**YES** / NO
4. Do you often get bored?	**YES** / NO
5. Are you in good spirits most of the time?	YES / **NO**
6. Are you afraid that something bad is going to happen to you?	**YES** / NO
7. Do you feel happy most of the time?	YES / **NO**
8. Do you often feel helpless?	**YES** / NO
9. Do you prefer to stay in your room/facility, rather than going out and doing new things?	**YES** / NO
10. Do you feel you have more problems with memory than most?	**YES** / NO
11. Do you think it is wonderful to be alive?	YES / **NO**
12. Do you feel worthless the way you are now?	**YES** / NO
13. Do you feel full of energy?	YES / **NO**
14. Do you feel that your situation is hopeless?	**YES** / NO
15. Do you think that most people are better off than you?	**YES** / NO

Score greater than 5 = Probable Depression   **SCORE** _____

Notes/Current Medications: _____
_____
_____

Instructions for Use:
1. The same CNA caregiver should administer this test each time.
2. Choose a quiet place, preferably the same location each time the test is administered.
3. The administration of this test should not be immediately after some mental trauma or unsteady period.
4. Speak in a soft pleasant tone.
5. Answer all questions by circling the answer (yes or no) to the question.
6. Add the total number of **BOLD FACED** answers circled and record that number in the "SCORE" box.
7. Scores totaling five (5) points or more indicate probable depression.

A 30-item version of the GDS is also available. Address inquiries regarding this scale to: Jerome A. Yesavage, M.D.,
   Director, Psychiatric ICU, Veterans Administration Medical Center, 3801 Miranda Avenue, Palo Alto, CA 94304.

that cause mobility problems. As a result, older adults may experience one or several impairments including hemiparesis (weakness on one side of the body), ataxia (impaired muscular coordination), spasticity (stiff or awkward muscle movements), and coordination or balance problems.

Instituting appropriate interventions relies on a thorough assessment of the person's mobility impairments. Interventions may include muscle strengthening, range of motion exercises, gait and balance training, medication review (especially for medications that cause postural hypotension), and assistive device (canes, walkers) training. Splinting or muscle relaxants help persons with severe spasticity (Cotter & Strumpf, 2002).

As the number and severity of mobility impairment increases, the older adult is increasingly at risk for falls, which are the leading cause of accidental death in older adults. Of fall-related deaths in the United States, 70% occur among older adults (Shelkey, 2001). Elimination problems are among the risk factors for falls (see Chapter 33 for a detailed discussion of mobility).

Elimination

More than 13 million Americans experience urinary incontinence. Both urge incontinence (caused by overactive detrusor muscle causing involuntary bladder contraction) and stress incontinence (caused by pelvic floor muscle weakness or urethral hypermobility) may cause older adults to rush to a toilet, which can contribute to falls. Immobility may cause urinary incontinence if the person cannot toilet independently or does not have sufficient assistance. Overflow incontinence (occurring when bladder muscle distends and urine is forced out) and functional incontinence (occurring when a physical or psychological impairment impedes continence despite a competent urinary system) are other types of urinary incontinence.

Interventions are specific to the type of incontinence. Bladder training, external catheters, medications, and protective pants are the most frequently used strategies (Chapter 40). Careful assessment of the effects of incontinence on the

TABLE 18-1

Psychiatric Disorders	
Disorder	**Characteristics**
Major Depression	Persistent depressed mood (every day for 2 weeks) or loss of interest and other symptoms such as significant change in weight or appetite; problems sleeping; psychomotor retardation or agitation; fatigue; feelings of worthlessness or inappropriate guilt; diminished ability to think or concentrate, or indecisiveness; and recurrent thoughts of death or suicidal ideation. Symptoms cause significant distress or impairment in daily functioning and cannot be the result of medications or medical conditions.
Bipolar Disorder	Mood swings that progress from symptoms of depression to symptoms of mania. Mania is characterized by a distinct period of abnormally and persistently elevated, expansive, or irritable mood lasting at least 1 week. Other symptoms include inflated self-esteem or grandiosity, decreased need for sleep, pressured speech, racing thoughts, distractibility, increase in goal-directed activities, excessive involvement in pleasurable activities with high potential for painful results.
Generalized Anxiety Disorder	Excessive anxiety and worry about several events or activities, occurring more days than not for at least 6 months. Other symptoms include restlessness, being easily fatigued, difficulty concentrating or mind going blank, irritability, muscle tension, sleep disturbance. These symptoms cause significant impairment in functioning, cannot be due to a medication or medical condition, and do not occur exclusively during a mood or psychotic disorder.
Schizophrenia	A psychotic illness characterized by disturbances in many areas of mental functioning. Thinking, perception, behavior, motivation, and emotional life are all affected. The illness impairs functioning in work, relationships, and self-care. Delusions (usually persecutory) are present.
Delusional Disorder	Relatively uncommon disorder characterized by the presence of a persistent, usually well-organized delusion, often persecutory. Hallucinations are not prominent. There is less impairment in the person's functioning as compared with schizophrenia.

person's quality of life is also very important. Unfortunately, some older adults may reduce involvement in social activities because of embarrassment or fear of unexpected incontinence events.

Skin Integrity

Older adults experience many skin changes that put them at risk for disruptions in **skin integrity.** Injuries from falls, problems with repositioning (in bed and chair), and incontinence (bladder and bowel) without proper skin care may result in skin problems. Pressure ulcers are lesions caused by unrelieved pressure that results in damage to underlying tissue (Ayello, 2001). Many factors predispose an individual to have pressure ulcers; factors can be physical (local infections, malnutrition), functional (impaired mobility, incontinence), and psychosocial (poor adherence to treatment, impaired cognition). Several scales have been developed to assess the person's risk (Display 18-6). Using standardized scales, nurses can identify

persons at risk (persons who score in a moderate to severe risk range) and institute preventive strategies (e.g., pressure-relieving mattresses, proper alignment). Initial treatment of pressure ulcers consists of relieving pressure from the area. Based on the stage of the pressure ulcer, various wound treatments (dressings, removal of dead tissue) are initiated. In all age groups, proper skin care (e.g., proper cleansing, lubrication) and maintenance of skin integrity are critical in maintaining optimal health and comfort (see Chapter 38).

NUTRITION AND HEALTH MAINTENANCE

In the United States, an estimated 31% of men and 61% of women aged 65 and older have annual incomes of $10,000 or below, which adversely affects their access to quality food among other things. Among persons aged 75 years or older, an estimated 40% of men and 30% of women are at least 10% underweight. Of men aged 75 years or older, 56.5% could be

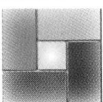

Nursing Research and Critical Thinking
Does Restraining the Elderly Really Prevent Falls?

Since the Omnibus Budget Reconciliation Act (OBRA) of 1987, there has been a significant reduction in the use of physical restraints to prevent falls in older adults who are institutionalized. This decrease in restraint use is due to the developing awareness of the associated physical and psychological problems. This nurse researcher was interested in determining if there were any difference in falls before and after the implementation of a restraint-free policy in a 98-bed southeastern long-term care facility.

An ex post facto (after the fact) descriptive study was used. Data were analyzed from incident reports (one-year pre-implementation and one-year post-implementation) of 97 older adults. Results showed no significant difference in the number of falls before and after the policy change. There were, however, a significantly lower number of falls with injuries and a significantly higher number of falls without injuries.

Critical Thinking Considerations. This study used facility data to compare the rate and severity of falls over

a two-year period (one-year pre-implementation and one-year post-implementation of a restraint-free policy change). Implications of the study are as follows:

- These findings suggest that older adults will continue to fall with or without physical restraints because of changes associated with the aging process and risk factors. However, removing physical restraints and allowing the older adult freedom may decrease the severity of injury sustained in a fall.
- Identifying an older adult at risk for falls involves assessment of intrinsic and extrinsic factors that place them at risk. Extrinsic factors include inadequate lighting, sliding carpets, worn stair treads, lack of arm rests, glare on floors, and ill-fitting walking aids or footwear. Intrinsic factors include altered mobility, sensory impairment, polypharmacy, dizziness, history of falls, pain, and use of alcohol.

From Dunn, K. S. (2001). The effect of physical restraints on the fall rates in older adults who are institutionalized. *Gerontological Nursing, 27* (10), 41–48.

considered overweight (BMI > 25) and 13.2% of those overweight are obese (BMI > 30). Among older women, 52.3% are overweight and 19.2% of those are obese. Body weight is, however, not the only indicator of nutritional health (sufficient intake and utilization of food/nutrients). Nearly 50% of older adults are clinically malnourished on admission to a hospital (based on physical findings and blood work); two-thirds are malnourished at discharge (Amella, 2001).

Consensus is lacking about the optimal nutritional health requirements for older persons as they age. Few research-based findings illuminate the picture; there is a shortage of long-range studies and there are problems with researching older adults with multiple medical disorders. Researchers generally agree, however, that food intake declines with aging (Morley, 2001). Various physiologic processes appear to explain this including decreased thirst and smell, alterations in taste, early satiation (feeling full), and anorexia. Decreased dietary intake is also associated with a decline in physical activity that further limits the intake of essential micronutrients (Wakimoto & Block, 2001).

In recent decades, research exploring the role of nutrition has looked at the role of weight, longevity, and antioxidants in slowing the aging process. Clear evidence is still lacking about the most efficacious strategies for older adults. Good management of chronic illnesses, good nutrition, and health promotion strategies (e.g., immunizations, reduction of stress) have been found to contribute to healthy immune functioning and an increased quality of life (see Chapter 39).

CHRONIC ILLNESS, INFECTIONS, AND IMMUNITY
Chronic Illness

Chronic illness contributes to poor nutrition in many ways. Dental problems (e.g., poorly fitting appliances, broken teeth) may make chewing problematic. Medications may adversely affect appetite or cause a decrease in saliva or a change in taste. Several medical conditions, such as chronic obstructive pulmonary disease, dementia, chronic pain, and depression, contribute to poor appetite. A frail individual may not be able to shop or cook. In addition, psychosocial aspects, such as eating alone after the death of a spouse, also cause problems with maintaining adequate nutrition.

Careful nutritional assessment and client-specific interventions are necessary because nutrition is so critical in maintaining optimal health in older adults. At a basic level, simply eating and digesting food may be difficult for older adults; helpful aids include over-the-counter products that increase saliva so eating is more pleasant for the client and food is easier to digest. Prompt and aggressive treatment of health disorders, such as dental problems, depression or chronic pain, may reverse adverse nutritional consequences. Community agencies are available to deliver meals to homebound elders. Many seniors participate in meals and activities at senior centers; these shared experiences further enhance the psychosocial aspects of nutrition.

DISPLAY 18-6

⑤ BRADEN SCALE FOR PREDICTING PRESSURE ULCER SORE RISK

Sensory Perception: Ability to respond meaningfully to pressure-related discomfort

1. **Completely Limited:** Unresponsive (does not moan, flinch, or grasp) to painful stimuli, due to diminished level of consciousness or sedation, OR limited ability to feel pain over most of body surface.
2. **Very Limited:** Responds only to painful stimuli. Cannot communicate discomfort except by moaning or restlessness, OR has a sensory impairment which limits the ability to feel pain or discomfort over half of body.
3. **Slightly Limited:** Responds to verbal commands but cannot always communicate discomfort or need to be turned, OR has some sensory impairment which limits ability to feel pain or discomfort in 1 or 2 extremities.
4. **No Impairment:** Responds to verbal commands. Has no sensory deficit which would limit ability to feel or voice pain and discomfort.

SCORE

Moisture: Degree to which skin is exposed to moisture

1. **Constantly Moist:** Skin is kept moist almost constantly by perspiration, urine, etc. Dampness is detected every time patient is moved or turned.
2. **Very Moist:** Skin is often but not always moist. Linen must be changed at least once a shift.
3. **Occasionally Moist:** Skin is occasionally moist, requiring an extra linen change approximately once a day.
4. **Rarely Moist:** Skin is usually dry; linen requires changing only at routine intervals.

SCORE

Activity: Degree of physical activity

1. **Bedfast:** Confined to bed
2. **Chairfast:** Ability to walk severely limited or non-existent. Cannot bear own weight and/or must be assisted into chair or wheelchair.
3. **Walks Occasionally:** Walks occasionally during the day, but for very short distances, with or without assistance. Spends majority of each shift in bed or chair.
4. **Walks Frequently:** Walks outside the room at least twice a day and inside room at least once every 2 hours during waking hours.

SCORE

Mobility: Ability to change and control body position

1. **Completely immobile:** Does not make even slight changes in body or extremity position without assistance.
2. **Very Limited:** Makes occasional slight changes in body or extremity position but unable to make frequent or significant changes independently.
3. **Slightly Limited:** Makes frequent though slight changes in body or extremity position independently.
4. **No Limitation:** Makes major and frequent changes in position without assistance.

SCORE

Nutrition: Usual food intake pattern

1. **Very Poor:** Never eats a complete meal. Rarely eats more than $\frac{1}{3}$ of food offered. Eats 2 servings or less of protein (meat or dairy products) per day. Takes fluids poorly. Does not take a liquid dietary supplement, OR is NPO and/or maintained on clear liquids or IV for more than five days.
2. **Probably Inadequate:** Rarely eats a complete meal and generally eats only about half of any food offered. Protein intake includes only 3 servings of meat or dairy products per day. Occasionally will take a dietary supplement, OR receives less than optimum amount of liquid diet or tube feeding.
3. **Adequate:** Eats over half of most meals. Eats a total of 4 servings of protein (meat, dairy products) each day. Occasionally will refuse a meal, but will usually take a supplement if offered, OR is on a tube feeding or TPN regimen, which probably meets most of nutritional needs.

SCORE

DISPLAY 18-6 (Continued)

⌸ **BRADEN SCALE FOR PREDICTING PRESSURE ULCER SORE RISK**

4. **Excellent:** Eats most of every meal. Never refuses a meal. Usually eats a total of 4 or more servings of meat and dairy products. Occasionally eats between meals. Does not require supplementation.

Friction and Shear
1. **Problem:** Requires moderate to maximum assistance in moving. Complete lifting without sliding against sheets is impossible. Frequently slides down in bed or chair, requiring frequent repositioning with maximum assistance. Spasticity, contractures, or agitation leads to almost constant friction.
2. **Potential Problem:** Moves feebly or requires minimum assistance. During a move skin probably slides to some extent against sheets, chair, restraints, or other devices. Maintains relatively good position in chair or bed most of the time but occasionally slides down.
3. **No Apparent Problem:** Moves in bed and in chair independently and has sufficient muscle strength to lift up completely during move. Maintains good position in bed or chair at all times.

SCORE

Braden Scale Scores

1 = Highly Impaired	NPO: Nothing by Mouth
3 or 4 = Moderate to Low Impairment	IV: Intravenously
Total Points Possible: 23	TPN: Total parenteral nutrition
Risk Predicting Score: 16 or Less	

Total Score:

Barbara Braden, PhD, RN, FAAN and Nancy Bergstrom, PhD, RN, FAAN. Copyright © 1987. Used by permission.

Infections and Immunity

As persons become very old and more frail, their immune systems become less efficient. Humoral **immunity** declines result because of changes in T-cell function, and older adults have lower antibody response to the microorganisms that cause influenza and pneumonia (Schelenker, 1998). Inadequate nutrition and the presence of chronic illnesses adversely affect the immune system and the ability to ward off infection. Without the proper nutrients, basic body functions lack the necessary vitamins, minerals, and food substances (proteins, carbohydrates, and fats) to maintain optimal functioning.

Routine health examinations and screening assist in uncovering health problems early and preventing later, more serious complications. Screening needs to encompass the multiple aspects of the person's health including alcohol and substance use, abuse (financial, physical, sexual), and environmental safety (Fulmer, Wallace, & Edelman, 2002). Prevention of health problems and careful monitoring and treatment of co-existing problems are especially important for older adults with compromised immune function (see Chapter 39 for further discussion of immune function and infection).

SLEEP AND REST

Sufficient **rest** and good **sleep** are essential in all age groups for optimal functioning. Normal sleep changes that occur in older persons include an increase in stage one wakefulness and a decrease in deep sleep (Venugopal & Susman, 2000). These changes lead to more frequent nighttime awakenings and less restful sleep. In addition, older persons experience many pathologic processes that further impair good sleep and rest (Chapter 42). Many of these impairments include medications (antipsychotics, beta-blockers, decongestants), restless legs syndrome (uncomfortable sensation in legs relieved by moving or rubbing legs), sleep apnea, pain, cardiovascular, and pulmonary disorders. Sleep disturbances often impair the person's daytime functioning and have a negative effect on health.

Good sleep habits may improve sleep initiation and maintenance (Display 18-7). These strategies, in addition to treatment

DISPLAY 18-7

⌸ **GOOD SLEEP HABITS**

Avoid alcohol, nicotine, and caffeine.
Avoid exercise 3–4 hours before bedtime.
Avoid frequent napping during the day.
Avoid large meals and excitement before bedtime.
Maintain a routine; go to bed at the same time each night.
Sleep in a cool, quiet environment.
Upon awakening, get up and avoid watching the clock.
Use the bed for sleeping (or intimacy or sex) only.

Adapted from M. G. Umlauf & Terri Weaver. (2001). Sleep hygiene measures. In M. D. Mezey (Ed.), *The encyclopedia of elder care* (p. 184). New York: Springer Publications.

of any coexisting medical conditions, may increase the person's effective sleep. Sleep medications may be used but these drugs are most effective when limited to short-term use (7 to 14 days). Persistent, excessive daytime sleepiness may be indicative of a serious sleep disturbance and needs to be evaluated by a sleep specialist.

PAIN MANAGEMENT

Pain is very common in older adults and is a major cause of sleep impairment. The prevalence of chronic pain increases with advancing age. The prevalence of pain in persons over 60 years of age is double of those under 60 years. An estimated 25% to 50% of community-dwelling older persons suffer significant pain, with an estimated 45% to 80% of nursing home residents having substantial, often unrecognized, and undertreated pain. Older persons least likely to receive analgesics include persons 85 years and older, persons of a minority race, and/or persons with low cognitive performance (Coyle, 2001).

Chronic pain is most commonly caused by osteoarthritis. Other conditions causing chronic pain include neuropathic pain, post-stroke central or neuropathic pain, post-herpetic neuralgia, and post-amputation (phantom limb) pain. Cognitive impairments limit an older adult's ability to report pain and may account for sleep disturbances and many of dementia's adverse behavioral symptoms. Barriers to adequate **pain management** in older persons include misconceptions about addiction, lack of knowledge about dose management and tolerance (especially to opioids), belief that older adults suffer less pain, and failure to assess and treat pain in cognitively impaired persons (Martin, Shelkey, & Cranmer, 2000).

Strategies to identify older adults in pain and assist in choosing appropriate therapies include education for healthcare providers, clients, and families; recognition of risk factors (e.g., depression, multiple health problems, immobility); and careful initial assessment and ongoing reassessment (Display 18-8). Inadequate pain management has many negative consequences for older adults; those consequences include decreased quality of life, depression, decreased socialization, suicidal ideation, decreased appetite, increased healthcare utilization, and increased costs. Providing good pain palli-ation is one of the most valuable ways nurses can maximize quality of life for older adults.

LOSS AND GRIEF, LONELINESS, COPING AND STRESS

Loss and Grief

Older adults face myriad potential and immediate **losses** as they continue to age. Typically they face losses related to health, significant others (spouses, family, friends, pets), finances, geography (e.g., moves to assisted living or long-term care facilities), and leisure activities. Loss of a spouse (or significant other) is highly significant and may be a critical threat to self-concept and sense of wholeness. In fact, death, including death from suicide, is most likely to occur during the first year of widowhood. In 1999, almost half of women (45%) were widowed by age 65 compared to 14% of men. Of those women, 70.1% lived alone. Often these older adults are forced to face many losses simultaneously; as a result, their remaining resources are very low.

Persons who suffer losses of any type are expected to grieve. Initial **grief** reactions include shock, disbelief, anger, and/or denial of the loss. The severity and length of the grieving (or bereavement) varies with the individual and the type of loss. Social support, therapy, and religious faith are sources of adaptive coping. Maladaptive coping strategies include using alcohol or drugs to blunt the pain (Siegel & Anderman, 2001). Nursing interventions, which assist the older adult in using adaptive strategies to cope with loss, decrease the risk of prolonged or pathological grief reactions.

Loneliness

Loss of important relationships places an older person at risk for **loneliness.** In addition, loneliness is caused by other extrinsic and intrinsic factors (Ebersole & Hess, 1998). Sensory losses may make it difficult for an older adult to communicate with others. Depression may cause the person to become more socially isolated. Cognitive disorders, such as delirium and dementia, diminish the capacity to interact meaningfully or appropriately in social situations. Cultural differences and language barriers make communication difficult and exacerbate loneliness.

In healthcare settings, nursing staff may focus strongly on tasks while overlooking the older adult's need to maintain her or his integrity and dignity. Often older adults who are dying are isolated further, due in part to the staff's inability to deal with their own feelings and fear of death. Loneliness can predispose a person to poor health outcomes (e.g., increased health utilization, increased medication usage). The nurse, in spending time with the older adult, may uncover reasons for the client's loneliness or even discover ways to decrease loneliness (e.g., pet therapy, reminiscence). Older adults may have musical or art talents to share with others. Many older adults have the occupational and educational skills to serve as mentors or tutors for children and younger adults. Encour-

DISPLAY 18-8

⑤ STRATEGIES FOR TREATING PAIN IN OLDER ADULTS

Acupuncture
Counseling/psychotherapy
Massage
Meditation/imagery
Pharmacological
Psychosocial (socialization, recreational therapies)
Transcutaneous Stimulation (TENS)

aging the older adult to remain active and socially engaged may have many positive physical and psychological effects.

Coping and Stress

Given life's difficulties, it is no surprise that **stress and coping** have been a major nursing interest for decades (Rice, 2000). Older adults are faced with adapting to multiple stressors: i.e., physical/physiological, psychological, sociocultural, and/or environmental stresses. Several theories exist about how individuals manage stress. In one of the most frequently used stress/coping models, Lazarus and Folkman (1984) initially described two major categories of coping strategies: emotion-focused and problem-focused. In emotion-focused coping, the individual attempts to change the way he or she thinks about or appraises a stressful situation rather than changing the situation itself. Problem-focused coping involves attempts to reduce stress by changing the stressful situation.

Victor Frankl (1967), a psychiatrist and Holocaust survivor, described an existential model of managing difficult life events. He observed that many persons who survived the concentration camps did so because they found meaning in their lives or found reasons to live. Later he used these concepts in his therapy (logotherapy) to help his patients find meaning in their suffering. How older adults adapt to stress varies tremendously based on many factors including previous coping styles and current resources (see Chapter 49 for further discussion). Many changes that older adults undergo are permanent (physical changes, employment) in contrast to some temporary changes that younger adults experience. Older adults vary dramatically in their perceptions of as well as their reactions to stressors in their environment. Interventions are most effective when tailored to maximize individual strengths and available resources.

SEXUALITY, ROLES AND RELATIONSHIPS, AND SELF-PERCEPTION

Sexuality

Despite the rapid increase in numbers of older adults, numerous ageist (defined as a process of systematic stereotyping and discrimination against people because of their advanced age; Butler, 2001) myths persist even among older persons. One prevalent myth is that sexual desire or activity diminishes with age. As persons age, the reproductive system loses efficacy; physiologically both men and women experience changes that affect certain aspects of **sexuality** (e.g., arousal and orgasm). Certain medical conditions (e.g., cardiac problems, diabetes, neurological problems, arthritis) and medications (antidepressants, antihypertensives, antipsychotics) make the expression of sexuality difficult (Greenberg, 2001). Despite these changes, research has demonstrated that older persons continue to engage in and enjoy sexual experiences, even into their nineties (Brecher, 1984; Janus & Janus, 1993). Expressions of sexuality extend beyond overt sexual acts and include a yearning for intimacy (psychosocial and physical), security, and belonging. Touch remains an important aspect of sexual expression and integral part of human well-being.

Unfortunately older adults who are alone or institutionalized are often deprived of this important sensory input. Many cultural and social taboos persist (e.g., "dirty old man"). Often older persons lack the privacy necessary to initiate or develop new relationships. In institutional settings, the older person may be subjected to the staff's moral interpretation or restriction of behavior considered to be unacceptable (e.g., same-sex relationships, extramarital relationships). Older gays and lesbians (estimated to be 10% of older adults) experience unique issues. It wasn't until 1973 that the American Psychiatric Association (2000) removed homosexuality from its list of mental illnesses. Currently, eighteen U.S. states still have laws prohibiting lesbians and gay men from consensual intimate relations (Narus & Callen, 2001).

It is important to keep in mind that numerous individual preferences and differences in sexual behavior exist. In one study (Johnson, 1996), men and women expressed differences in describing a satisfying sexual relationship: Older men preferred erotic reading materials/movies, sexual daydreams, physical intimacy, oral sex, and masturbation; older women preferred talking, sitting, making themselves attractive, and saying loving words. For all older adults, however, sexuality is one of the important aspects in which they view their role in society. Sexuality continues to impact their relationships in later life.

To maintain an open, nonjudgmental stance in exploring the older adults' sexuality, nurses need to understand their own cultural and moral belief systems. Nurses are often reluctant to inquire about sexual behavior; their reluctance is based, in part, on the societal norm that considers discussions of sexuality and sexual behavior to be private. Such discussions are crucial, though, in evaluating the older adult's overall health. Older adults surveyed about ways in which healthcare providers may assist them in dealing with sexual questions suggested the following: Spend time with the older adult; use clear, easy-to-understand language; help the client feel more comfortable talking about sex; be open minded and talk openly; listen; encourage discussion; give advice or suggestions as needed; and understand that "sex is not just for the young" (Johnson, 1997).

Currently there is very little accurate, easily accessible information for older adults about their sexuality. As in other healthcare situations, nurses have a unique opportunity to provide support, education, and appropriate referral to their older clients.

Roles and Relationships

Many other factors impact the older adult's roles and relationships throughout aging. Family structures have changed due to increases in lifespan. Older adults divorce or their spouses die. Children divorce and may return to the family home. Four-, even five-generation families have increased. Grandparents and great grandparents play a number of roles depending on a multitude of factors including health, geographic proximity, and cultural expectations. Caregiving often becomes an issue as parents or spouses become very old or ill. Relationships with family, friends, neighbors, and service providers are as unique and complex as the older individuals.

Caregiving for ill children, spouses, or aging parents usually spans several years; sometimes caregiving spans decades. Researchers have found that caregivers (typically women) suffer adverse physical and psychological consequences as a result of caregiving (Ory, Hoffman, Yee, Tennstedt, & Schultz, 1999). Successful nursing strategies include careful assessment of physical and psychological health, referral to appropriate healthcare providers, and assistance in accessing agencies that provide help to caregivers (respite care, day centers, caregiver support groups). For information about services in their community, persons may access the U.S. Administration on Aging web site.

Self-Perception

The older adult's multiple evolving roles define her or his self-concept. The individual's sense of self incorporates many aspects including physical functioning, cognition, social relationships, and life experiences (Whitbourne, 1996; Chapter 45). The older adult attempts to maintain her or his self-esteem despite numerous changes in physiologic and psychological attributes. These changes with aging are a constant challenge to the older adult.

In their interactions with older adults, nurses form part of their clients' social network. Dignified and humane nursing care is essential in positively reinforcing a person's self-esteem and sense of self. In maintaining a high level of quality care, nurses serve as advocates for older adults, especially those who are frail or disadvantaged.

VALUES, BELIEFS, AND SPIRITUALITY

Despite many adverse consequences associated with aging, most older adults retain good function and quality of life into advanced age. **Spirituality** remains a source of health and healing power for most older people. In one survey, 82% of older adults believed in the healing power of personal prayer; 59% to 79% believed spiritual faith did or could help in recovery from illness, injury, or disease; and 75% rated religious belief as a very important means of effectively coping with their illness (Gould, Sherman, Mariano, & Wallace, 2001). Abraham Maslow (1970) described a hierarchy with self-actualization as the highest level. There has been very little appreciation in our society for this aspect of aging. For many older adults, the latter years are ones of creativity as writers, painters, and scholars. Many prominent individuals have continued to contribute to society well into advanced age: e.g., Bertrand Russell, Albert Schweitzer, Frances Scott-Maxwell, Sigmund Freud, Grandma Moses. Scott-Maxwell gives us some insight into her experience of aging: "Age puzzles me. I thought it was a quiet time. My seventies were interesting,

and fairly serene, but my eighties are passionate. I grow more intense as I age" (Fowler & McCutcheon, 1991).

Sometimes the very illnesses and difficulties that older adults experience present an opportunity for higher growth (Dossey, Keegan, Guzzetta, & Kolkmeier, 1995; Vash, 1994). Never before in history has there been a cohort of older people so large in number, creating both great challenges and great opportunities for us all. Having survived world wars and the Great Depression, these older adults are our modern day pioneers; they are helping to pave the path for future generations (Silverman, 1987).

As persons age, they approach death—a stage that has been called the last developmental stage (Murray & Zentner, 2001). Older adults react in numerous and diverse ways to the experience of dying: Some feel fright, anger, resignation; others experience acceptance and equanimity. For many, advancing age provides the opportunity for transcendence or gerotranscendence (a shift in perspective from the material world to the cosmic and an increase in life satisfaction) (Tornstam, 1997). Today most older adults die in a healthcare facility (Fulmer, Foreman, & Walker, 2001). Yet throughout the dying process, persons need to have their physical, psychosocial, and spiritual needs met. Caring for these older adults requires that nurses provide competent palliation and compassionate end-of-life care.

Today, educational opportunities about providing effective palliative care are commonplace. Effective pain management remains an ongoing and primary aspect of care. Hospice provides care for terminally ill older clients and their families. Multiple disciplines (nurses, doctors, clergy, pain specialists, complementary providers, legal/financial advisors) are required to provide the holistic care necessary at this life stage.

Dealing with issues of dying is often very uncomfortable for the older adult, her or his family, and the nurses providing care. For others, death is considered to be a natural part of life's journey. Many nurses who accompany these older adults on their final journeys find the experiences to be some of the most rewarding and meaningful of their professional careers.

KEY CONCEPTS

- Providing excellence in nursing care to older adults depends on a comprehensive knowledge base and a commitment to providing humane and dignified care.
- Older adults, even into advanced age, demonstrate remarkable resilience.
- Physiologic changes and an increased incidence of chronic illnesses place older adults at greater risk for declines in health and quality of life. Health promotion strategies (good lifestyle habits) and health maintenance (disease prevention and treatment) afford even the oldest adult an advantage in maintaining optimal health.
- The U.S. government report, *Healthy People 2010: Understanding and Improving Health* (U.S. Department of Health and Human Services, 2000), and the World Health Organization's *Health for All In the Twenty-First Century* (World Health Organization, 1998), set numerous goals for attaining health for persons around the globe. Their definitions of health encompass the multiple domains (physical, psychosocial, spiritual) of the

The Older Adult

Chapter 18

307

person/family/community necessary to attain and maintain health. Longevity is one of those goals. However, maintaining the quality of the person's life is considered an equally important goal.

- Nursing as a discipline has always been concerned with the multiple domains of the person, family, and community. Nurses are educated to act as providers, advocates, educators, and resource persons for their clients. In caring for older adults, all of those roles are required.

- As the number of persons growing older increases, the task of maintaining excellent nursing care may appear to be daunting. However, our commitment to this task is not entirely selfless. The quality of our nursing care assists not only our older clients. As a result of our efforts, we participate in creating a future for ourselves and for the generations to follow.

REFERENCES

Amella, E. (2001). Nutrition: Eating/meals for older adults. In M. Mezey, T. Fulmer, & C. Mariano (Eds.), *Best nursing practices in care for older adults: Incorporating essential gerontologic content into baccalaureate nursing education* (3rd ed., pp. 8/1–8/20). New York: John A. Hartford Foundation Institute for Geriatric Nursing.

American Psychiatric Association. (2000). *Diagnostic and statistical manual of mental disorders* (4th ed., text revision). Washington, DC: American Psychiatric Association.

Archibold, P. G., & Stewart, B. J. (2001). Family care for frail elders. In M. D. Mezey, (Ed.), *The encyclopedia of elder care* (pp. 257–259). New York: Springer Publishing.

Ayello, E. (2001). Pressure ulcers in older adults. In M. Mezey, T. Fulmer, & C. Mariano (Eds.), *Best nursing practices in care for older adults: Incorporating essential gerontologic content into baccalaureate nursing education* (3rd ed., pp. 7/1–7/16). New York: John A. Hartford Foundation Institute for Geriatric Nursing.

Beers, M. H., & Berkow, R. (2000). *Merck manual of geriatrics* (3rd ed.). Whitehouse Station, NJ: Merck Research Laboratories.

Brecher, E. (1984). *Love, sex, and aging: A Consumer Union report.* Boston: Little, Brown.

Butler, R. N. (2001). Ageism. In M. D. Mezey (Ed.), *The encyclopedia of elder care* (pp. 26–27). New York: Springer Publishing.

Cotter, V. T., & Strumpf, N. E. (2002). *Advanced practice nursing with older adults: Clinical guidelines.* New York: McGraw-Hill.

Coyle, N. (2001). *The who, what, and why of pain.* Paper presentation at Current Controversies in Ethics, Law and Nursing (Sixth Annual Conference). April 11, 2001. Co-sponsored by The John A. Hartford Institute for Geriatric Nursing and The Consortium of New York Geriatric Education Centers and Nursing Spectrum and Partnership for Caring, Inc.

Dossey, B. M., Keegan, L., Guzzetta, C. E., & Kolkmeier, L. G. (1995). *Holistic nursing: A handbook for practice* (2nd ed.). Gaithersburg, MD: Aspen Publishers.

Ebersole, P., & Hess, P. (1998). *Toward healthy aging: Human needs and nursing response* (5th ed.). New York: Mosby.

Feil, N. (1993). *Validation breakthrough: Simple techniques for communicating with people with Alzheimer's Type dementia.* Baltimore: Health Professions Press.

Feldt, K. S. (2000). Aggressive behaviors in cognitively impaired elders. In J. J. Fitzpatrick & T. Fulmer (Eds.), *Geriatric nursing research digest* (pp. 191–195). New York: Springer Publishing.

Fowler, M., & McCutcheon, P. (1991). *Songs of experience: An anthology of literature on growing old.* New York: Ballantine Books.

Frankl, V. (1967). *Man's search for meaning.* New York: Washington Square Press.

Fulmer, T. T., Foreman, M. D., & Walker, M. (Eds.). (2001). *Critical care nursing of the elderly* (2nd ed.). New York: Springer Publishing.

Fulmer, T., Wallace, M., & Edelman, C. L. (2002). In C. L. Edelman & C. L. Mandle (Eds.), *Health promotion throughout the lifespan* (5th ed., pp. 709–743). Philadelphia: Mosby

Gould, E., Sherman, A., Mariano, C., & Wallace, M. (2001). Attitudes about aging. In M. Mezey, T. Fulmer, & C. Mariano (Eds.), *Best nursing practices in care for older adults: Incorporating essential gerontologic content into baccalaureate nursing education* (3rd ed., pp. 1/1–1/24). New York: John A. Hartford Foundation Institute for Geriatric Nursing.

Greenberg, S. A. (2001). Sexual health. In M. D. Mezey (Ed.), *The encyclopedia of elder care* (pp. 589–592). New York: Springer Publishing.

Janus, S. S., & Janus, C. L. (1993). *The Janus report on sexual behavior.* New York: John Wiley & Sons

Johnson, B. K. (1996). Older adults and sexuality: A multidimensional perspective. *Journal of Gerontological Nursing, 22*(2), 6–15.

Johnson, B. K. (1997). Older adults' suggestions for health care providers regarding discussions of sex. *Geriatric Nursing, 18*(2), 65–66.

Lazarus, R. S., & Folkman, S. (1984). *Stress, appraisal, and coping.* New York: Springer Publishing.

Martin, H., Shelkey, M., & Cranmer, K. W. (2000). The team approach to chronic pain management: A multidisciplinary effort in senior care. *Annals of Long-Term Care, June* (Suppl.).

Maslow, A. H. (1970). *Motivation and personality* (2nd ed.). New York: Harper & Row.

Morley, J. E. (2001). Decreased food intake with aging. *Journal of Gerontology, 56A*(Special Issue II), 81–88.

Murray, R. B., & Zentner, J. P. (2001). *Health promotion strategies through the life span* (7th ed.). Upper Saddle River, NJ: Prentice-Hall.

Narus, J. B., & Callen, M. (2001). Gay and lesbian elders. In M. D. Mezey (Ed.), *The encyclopedia of elder care* (pp. 291–294). New York: Springer Publishing.

Ory, M. G., Hoffman, R. R., Yee, J. L., Tennstedt, S., & Schultz, R. (1999). Prevalence and impact of caregiving: A detailed comparison between dementia and nondementia caregiving. *The Gerontologist, 39*(2), 177–185.

Rice, V. H. (Ed.). (2000). *Handbook of stress, coping, and health: Implications for nursing research, theory, and practice.* Thousand Oaks, CA: Sage.

Schlenker, E. D. (1998). *Nutrition in aging* (3rd ed.). New York: McGraw-Hill.

Shelkey, M. (2000). Pet therapy. In J. J. Fitzpatrick & T. Fulmer (Eds.), *Geriatric nursing research digest* (pp. 215–218). New York: Springer Publishing.

Shelkey, M. (2001). Falls of older adults. In M. Mezey, T. Fulmer, & C. Mariano (Eds.), *Best nursing practices in care for older adults: Incorporating essential gerontologic content into baccalaureate nursing education* (3rd ed., pp. 12/1–12/14). New York: John A. Hartford Foundation Institute for Geriatric Nursing.

Siegel, K., & Anderman, S. J. (2001). Bereavement. In M. D. Mezey (Ed.), *The encyclopedia of elder care* (pp. 92–95). New York: Springer Publishing.

Silverman, P. (1987). *The elderly as modern pioneers.* Bloomington: Indiana University Press.

Tornstam, L. (1997). Gerotranscendence: The contemplative dimension of aging. *Journal of Aging Studies, 11*(2), 143–154.

U.S. Department of Health and Human Services, Administration on Aging. (2002). Statistics about Older People. [Online] Available at: *www.aoa.dhhs.gov.*

U.S. Department of Health and Health Services. (2000). *Healthy people 2010: Understanding and improving health.* Washington, DC: U.S. Government Printing Office.

Vash, C. L. (1994). *Personality and adversity: Psychospiritual aspects of rehabilitation.* New York: Springer Publishing.

Venugopal, M., & Susman, J. L. (2000). Insomnia in the elderly: Toward a good night's sleep. *Consultant: Consultations in Primary Care, 40*(7), 1234–1247.

Wakimoto, P., & Block, G. (2001). Dietary intake, dietary patterns, and changes with age: An epidemiological perspective. *Journal of Gerontology, 56A*(Special Issue II), 65–80.

Whitbourne, S. K. (1996). Psychosocial perspectives on emotions: The role of identity in the aging process. In C. Magai & S. H. McFadden (Eds.), *Handbook of emotion, adult development, and aging.* New York: Academic Press.

World Health Organization. (1998). *Health for all in the twenty-first century.* Geneva, Switzerland: The Organization.

Yesavage, J., & Brink, T. L. (1983). Development and validation of the geriatric depression screening scale: A preliminary report. *Journal of Psychiatry Research, 17,* 37–49.

BIBLIOGRAPHY

Abraham, I., Bottrell, M., Fulmer, T., & Mezey, M. (Eds.). (1999). *Geriatric nursing protocols for best practice.* New York: Springer Publishing.

Bergstrom, N., Braden, B., & Boynton, P. (Eds.). (1995). Using a research-based assessment tool in clinical practice. *Nursing Clinics of North America, 30,* 539–551.

Cohen, G. D. (2000). *The creative age.* New York: Avon Books.

Conn, D. K., Herrmann, N., Kaye, A., Rewilak, D., & Schogt, B. (2001). *Practical psychiatry in the long-term care facility: A handbook for staff* (2nd ed.). Seattle: Hogrefe & Huber Publishers.

Fitzpatrick, J. J., & Fulmer, T. (Eds.). (2000). *Geriatric nursing research digest.* New York: Springer Publishing.

Gormly, A. (1997). *Lifespan human development.* (6th ed.). Fort Worth, TX: Harcourt Brace.

Mace, N., & Rabins, P. (1999). *The 36-hour day.* Baltimore: The Johns Hopkins University Press.

Mezey, M., Fulmer, T., & Mariano, C. (Eds.). (2001). *Best nursing practices in care for older adults: Incorporating essential gerontologic content into baccalaureate nursing education* (3rd ed.). New York: John A. Hartford Foundation Institute for Geriatric Nursing.

Mezey, M. D. (2001). *The encyclopedia of elder care.* New York: Springer Publishing.

Papalias, D., & Olds, S. (1998). *Human development* (3rd ed.). Boston: McGraw-Hill.

Rader, J., & Tornquist, E. (1995). *Individualized dementia care: Creative, compassionate approaches.* New York: Springer Publishing.

Rowe, W., & Kahn, L. (1998). *Successful aging.* New York: Pantheon Books.

Strumpf, N. E., Robinson, J., Wagner, J., & Evans, L. K. (1998). *Restraint-free care: Individualized approaches for frail elders.* New York: Springer Publishing.

Chapter

19 Individual, Family, and Community

Key Terms

community
developmental stages
family
feedback loop
systems theory

Learning Objectives

Upon completion of this chapter, the student will be able to do the following:

1. State interactions among individuals, family, and community.
2. Explain two different conceptual frameworks used to study the family.
3. Describe three methods nurses can use to assess a family.
4. Discuss family responsibilities for healthy function of all members.
5. Describe components that could be included in a definition of community.
6. Define *family* and *community*.
7. Compare various types of community.
8. Discuss the implications of different types of communities for nursing care.
9. Discuss community responsibilities for healthy function and the nurse's participation in community.

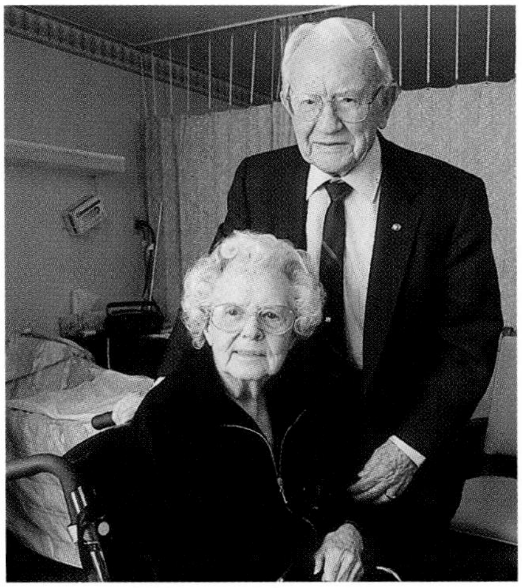

Critical Thinking Challenge

Mrs. Benoli is a 78-year-old Italian-American woman who came to the United States as a young bride. Devoutly Catholic, she and her husband have three grown children, six grandchildren, and two great-grandchildren. Mrs. Benoli enjoys gardening and sewing. She never finished high school. She retired at the mandatory age despite her desire to continue working as a seamstress in a small dress shop in her neighborhood. Before her illness, she went to the dress shop daily to visit friends. Mrs. Benoli states that she has lived in the same neighborhood since her arrival in the United States. She has never had a reason to leave the neighborhood except to visit relatives in Italy.

Mrs. Benoli, who is hospitalized, has passed the acute phase of a cerebrovascular accident. Plans are being made for her discharge. Primary concerns are her support systems and Mrs. Benoli's attitude. She expresses no motivation to walk. She prefers to skip meals to avoid the embarrassment of "eating as babies do." Her speech is slurred, so she prefers not to talk. At present, she cannot continue her hobbies. Her one interest is to continue to go to church whenever possible. Her husband is frail, spends most of his time sitting on the porch, and has never participated in household chores. Mrs. Benoli believes she would be least burdensome to her husband if she remained quietly in bed and ate only when necessary.

Once you have completed this chapter and incorporated the relationship of individual, family, and community into your knowledge base, review the above scenario and reflect on these areas of Critical Thinking:

1. Identify the strengths that could help Mrs. Benoli adjust to her condition.
2. Using your information about Mrs. Benoli, analyze her needs and how her family and community can provide support.
3. Summarize how each member of the healthcare team (e.g., physician, nurse, nutritionist, social worker, physical therapist, speech therapist) can participate in planning for Mrs. Benoli's discharge.

In previous decades, healthcare focused on the client as the sole recipient of care. Many healthcare professionals now believe that care is enhanced when the client is viewed as an individual in the context of family and community. For example, much of Mrs. Benoli's physical and psychosocial support will have to come from sources other than herself. The renewed interest in family and community emerged in the 1970s and was reflected in the American Nurses Association's *Standards: Nursing Practice,* which described nursing practice as "a direct service, goal oriented and adapted to the needs of the individual, the family and the community during health and illness" (American Nurses Association, 1973, p. 2). The Pew Commission report on health professions for the 21st century (1995) includes, among its list of competencies for all care practitioners, clinically competent care for individual clients, involvement of clients and families in the decision-making process, and care for the community's health. *Healthy People 2010* (U.S. Department of Health and Human Services, 2000) also makes clear that the health of an individual is closely linked with the health of the community in which he or she lives.

The beliefs and values that individuals hold and the support that they receive come in large measure from the family and are reinforced by the community. Understanding family dynamics and the community context assists nurses in planning appropriate care for clients.

INDIVIDUAL

Individuals are not isolates. They both influence and are influenced by other people and the environment. Other chapters in this unit address issues related to the individual: lifespan considerations, culture and ethnicity, values, and nurse–client communication. Individuals can meet some basic needs independently, but they require interaction with family and community to meet other needs (Fig. 19-1). Nursing care can be organized around the client's unmet basic needs according to Maslow's hierarchy (Maslow, 1968). Nurses must prioritize these needs, as discussed in Chapter 4, so that clients can sat-

isfactorily meet the lower-level needs first in order to meet the next-level needs fully.

Individual Responsibility for Healthy Function

The ideal goal of healthcare is for individuals to be responsible for their own health. A partnership must develop between healthcare providers, who teach and assist, and healthcare consumers, who ask for specific information or general guidance. A variety of self-help evaluations are available to individuals who want to assess and apply "do-it-yourself" measures. Sample questions appear in Display 19-1.

FAMILY

Traditionally, the family has been considered the basic unit of human society and has played a central role in the organization of social relations. Although debate exists among social scientists about the universality of family functions, the consensus among anthropologists provides a useful perspective on this issue. Most anthropologists agree that the family provides for the following needs: sexual, reproductive, economic, nurturing, educational, socialization, caring, status, and political. Several, if not all, of these seem to be necessary to designate a group as a family. This statement does not mean that other individuals or institutions cannot carry out these functions but that, over time, the family has proved to be a successful social institution in fulfilling these functions. Chapter 47 discusses family functions and structures.

For the purposes of this chapter's discussion of the **family,** the following general definition is offered:

> The family is a social group whose members share common values, occupy specific positions, and interact with each other over time. Adults rear children, engage in economic and political cooperation, and care for elders.

Family Conceptual Frameworks

Conceptual frameworks provide useful guidelines for organizing information about family. Each framework analyzes the family from a different perspective. No one framework is inherently right or wrong, but each requires the nurse to obtain somewhat different pieces of information. It is not the intent of this chapter to acquaint students with all frameworks but rather to show briefly the implications of their use.

A comparison of two frameworks can show how each one guides nursing care. The two frameworks chosen for this chapter are a developmental framework and a systems framework.

Developmental Framework

The developmental framework is popular in the study of families. In the early 1950s, Duvall (1962) directed a group that studied the concept of family developmental tasks. This research focused on developmental tasks and role expectations of parents and children throughout a life cycle. The frame-

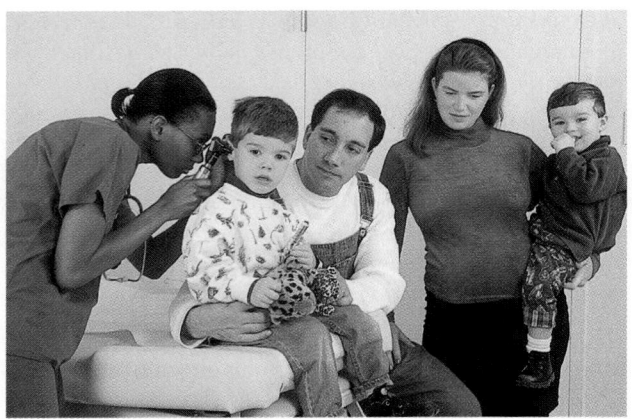

FIGURE 19-1   The nurse assesses individuals and family functions in relation to each individual. Individuals at different developmental levels need different types and amounts of care from the family and nurse.

DISPLAY 19-1

ASSESSMENT QUESTIONS RELATED TO INDIVIDUAL FUNCTION

Health Perception and Health Management
- How would you rate your own health?
- Tell me about the last time you were sick.
- Do you have routine physical examinations? If yes, how often?
- In the past year, how many times have you seen a healthcare provider? For what reasons?

Activity and Exercise
- Are you currently doing any regular exercises? If yes, how often?
- How do you spend your leisure time?
- What hobbies are you engaged in now? Are there others you would like to pursue?

Nutrition and Metabolism
- Describe what you ate last night for dinner. Was that a typical dinner for you?
- What are your favorite foods? How often do you eat them?
- Do you eat between meals? If yes, when and what do you usually eat?
- Who prepares your food, and how is it usually prepared?

Elimination
- Do you have any problems with elimination? If yes, describe them.
- Do you move your bowels regularly? How often?
- Have you ever been taught exercises to strengthen your urinary tract sphincter? If yes, when, and describe the exercises.

Sleep and Rest
- How many hours of sleep do you get a night?
- Do you take naps during the day?
- Do you have a regular bedtime routine?

Cognition and Perception
- How honest can you be with yourself?

- What happens when you set a goal for yourself? Do you usually meet it?
- Have your perceptions of an event ever varied widely from those of others? If yes, what did you think of that?

Self-Perception and Self-Concept
- Have you ever been described in a way you never thought of yourself? How did that make you feel?
- State five adjectives you believe describe you most accurately.
- Finish the following statements:
  My self-concept is most positive when _____.
  My self-concept is most negative when _____.

Roles and Relationships
- Describe your relationship to each of the other members of your family.
- List your various roles at this time in your life.
- How easy is it for you to be the decision maker?

Coping and Stress Tolerance
- Describe a stressful event for you.
- How do you resolve conflicts?
- How satisfied are you with the way you resolve conflicts?

Sexuality and Reproduction
- How do you express tenderness and affection?
- Do you have any questions or concerns about fertility or family planning?
- Do you engage in any high-risk sexual practices?

Values and Beliefs
- How do you define illness?
- Would you rank health at the top, middle, or bottom of what you consider important?
- What do you believe makes a person healthy?

work was meant to allow for biologic and cultural differences as well as differences in values.

Duvall's framework, essentially based on the individual life cycle, demonstrated that families move through a series of eight **developmental stages.** These stages are based on the developmental stage of the oldest child in the family, and they address marriage, childbearing, preschool years, school years, adolescent years, young adulthood, middle-aged parents whose children have left home, and aging parents. The critical family developmental tasks for these stages include, respectively, learning to be a marital partner, adjusting to parenthood, stimulating the curiosity of preschool children, adapting to other school-age families, assisting adolescents

to balance independence and autonomy, launching young adults into the work world, redefining the marital relationship without children, and coping with loss (Duvall, 1977). Tasks that the family does not complete at any one developmental stage can produce chronic difficulties as the family struggles to master tasks at the next stage. Carter and McGoldrick (1999) refined this framework to reflect the changing times and apply it to divorced and remarried families. Visher and Visher (1996) included the stepfamily life cycle.

In 1959, anthropologist Meyer Fortes noted in the introduction to *The Developmental Cycle in Domestic Groups* (1971) that the family life cycle consists of three phases: expansion, dispersion or fusion, and replacement. The papers in

ETHICAL/LEGAL ISSUE
Spousal Abuse

You are observing a public health nurse who works in a blue collar neighborhood. The nurse is making her first visit to the O'Connor family. Mrs. O'Connor delivered a baby boy 4 weeks early; yesterday, the family brought the baby home. Mr. O'Connor works hard as a city bus driver, and he wants peace and quiet when he comes home, especially on hot summer days. As the public health nurse assesses the baby, you notice that Mrs. O'Connor is wearing a long-sleeve blouse buttoned closely around the neck, and long pants. Her hair hides part of her face, but you notice her right eye is puffy, her face swollen, and she does not make eye contact with you or the public health nurse. You ask her about the bruise on her face. She looks away, shrugs her shoulders, and mumbles she bumped into something and will be all right. Then she quickly adds, "You won't tell anyone, will you?"

Reflection
- Reflect on your own feelings in this situation. Try to identify why you might feel the way you do.
- Identify underlying assumptions you have concerning what you think is ethically appropriate behavior.
- What is your obligation regarding confidentiality?
- Think of three different ways you could respond to this situation. Identify a possible approach that might bring about long-term changes in behavior in the O'Connor family.
- Identify possible community resources for this family.

that collection pointed out the universality of the family developmental cycle, analyzing families in Southeast Asia, Africa, and the Western Pacific.

Table 19-1 shows the developmental cycle of the family, combining the work of Duvall, Fortes, and Carter and McGoldrick. At each stage, Duvall and Carter and McGoldrick identified specific tasks for the family to accomplish.

Systems Framework

First described in the social science context by the biologist von Bertalanffy (1968), systems theory has become popular across many disciplines because it takes a holistic approach and tries to encompass all data collected at all levels of abstraction. **Systems theory** looks at the interaction of the parts that make up the whole. There is input to the system, throughput (input from one member in the system to another), and output from the system. When the system is under stress, it tries to regulate itself by use of **feedback loops,** in which the system reroutes some output as input, which in turn affects subsequent output. This response restores the system's balance, or homeostasis. An example can be taken from the opening scenario about Mrs. Benoli:

TABLE 19-1

Developmental Cycle of the Family and Task Accomplishment	
Family Developmental Stage	**Developmental Task**
Preexpansion Unattached adult	Stabilize image Develop independence
Expansion Unit formation	Develop mutual satisfaction Develop independence
Having children (by birth or adoption)	Adjust to child expectation Adjust to birth or adoption of child Establish a home for family
Raising children Newborn through preschool	Nurture growth and development
School-age child	Adjust to less privacy Encourage education of children Develop community socialization
Adolescent	Balance freedom and responsibility Promote adolescent's independence
Dispersion Assist children to move on	Release children with appropriate assistance and stable home base
Readjust unit	Reestablish own interests and careers Readjust the relationships
Replacement Aging Death Children become adults	Maintain connection with other generations Cope with loss of job, significant other, friends, home Adjust to altered living space

Input: The nurse tells the family that Mrs. Benoli has difficulty with fine motor skills and probably will never be able to sew by hand again.

Throughput: Mrs. Benoli tells her family that she is no use to anyone anymore. She can no longer sew, and her identity has been taken from her. Her husband and children each tell her what they valued in her sewing and how she can still be involved in sewing-related activities instead of the sewing itself.

   Output: Mrs. Benoli helps choose patterns and material for her granddaughter's school play.

Because many feedback loops exist, some of which overlap, systems theory describes a circular process, not a deterministic one. When feedback to the system causes the system to move away from homeostasis, it is called "positive feedback"; when the feedback causes the system to maintain homeostasis, it is called "negative feedback." Systems are also considered to be either "open" or "closed." These terms refer to the amount of exchange that takes place between a system and its environment. In a closed system, no exchange occurs, whereas in an open system, exchange occurs readily.

Families are basically open systems; however, the degree to which they are willing to exchange resources with other systems varies greatly. Healthy, functioning families exchange to a greater degree than do dysfunctional families (Fig. 19-2).

Many schools of thought are found within the systems perspective. Systems theorists include Satir (1988), Bowen (1978), Minuchin (1974), Minuchin and Fishman (1981), and Haley (1971). Wright and Leahey (2000) are nurses whose family nursing theory is based on systems theory. Whyte (1992) contends that systems thinking provides the means to develop family nursing practice that will meet contemporary healthcare needs.

Several concepts are important for nurses to understand when viewing a family as a system:

Wholeness—The whole is greater than the sum of its parts. Wholeness includes family values, beliefs,

themes, and the rules by which the family carries out the themes.

Circular interaction—All parts of the system are acting, reacting, and interacting at the same time.

Lack of an identified client—No identified client is found in systems thinking. Individuals are seen as part of family systems. The focus of nursing care is interactional, based on the nurse's behavior (interventions) and the family's response (outcomes). Family members learn positive health habits that they can continually reinforce within their system on their own.

Holistic perspective—All dimensions of the family's life count, including biologic, psychological, social, and cultural aspects.

Family themes—Beliefs and values that are important and reoccur in a family. Examples of themes are religion, health, independence, and travel.

Family rules—Family rules refer to how themes are carried out or operationalized. An easy way to recognize a rule is when the word "should" precedes the activity. Examples of rules for the themes of religion and health are, respectively, "You should go to church every Sunday" and "To stay healthy, you should watch your weight and not eat so much ice cream."

Family Assessment

Once nurses have a framework for understanding the family, they can begin to assess the family. Many nurses (Doherty, 1985; Bomar, 1996; Gillis, 1993; Feetham, Meister, Bell, & Gillis, 1993; McCubbin & McCubbin, 1993; Friedman, 1998; Hanson, 2001) have clinical and research interests in

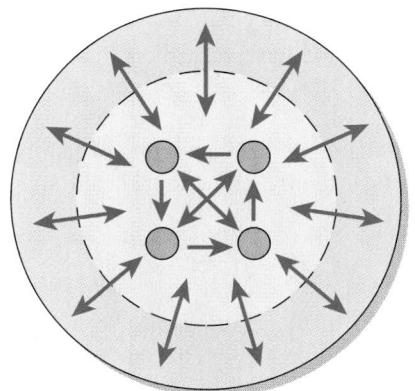 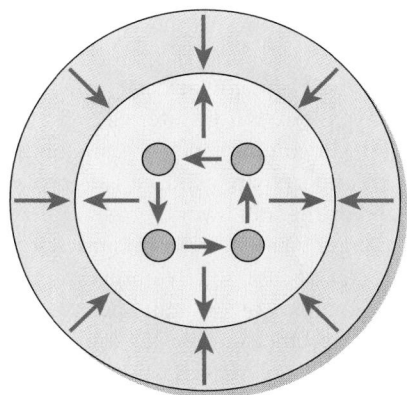

FIGURE 19-2   In a simple systems framework, the family and its members are in the center, and feedback loops interlap. The outer circle is the environment, or, in this chapter, the community: ethnic group, school, church, places of employment, institutions. According to systems theory, the whole is greater than the sum of the parts. In other words, there is no identified person at the center; rather all are equal and inter-related. All systems are acting, reacting, and interacting at the same time. Holistically, everything counts. The functional family (*left*) has interaction among all systems. The boundary between family and community is a broken circle allowing for input and output between family and community. The dysfunctional family (*right*) has limited interaction that goes in only one direction, with a boundary between family and community that does not allow for input and output between those two systems.

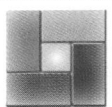

Nursing Research and Critical Thinking
What Factors Promote and Restrain Family Nursing Practice in Finland and in Utah?

The nurses conducting this study wanted to compare the ways that family nursing in public healthcare was conducted in Finland and in Utah. The nurses designed an exploratory study in which they interviewed nurses from each area in focus groups about their practice of family nursing. They were asked about the factors that promote and restrain family nursing practice in the two settings. They also discussed the impact of changes in the way healthcare is delivered on nursing practice. Thirty-six Finnish and 30 Utah nurses participated. T tests were computed to compare age, nursing work experience, and public health nursing work experience of the two groups. Age was not statistically different ($t = -0.924$, $p = .359$), but a significant difference was found for total years working in nursing ($t = 5.76$, $p = .000$) and years working in public health ($t = 3.99$, $p = .000$). Pressure to do more activities with fewer nurses and resources, changes in family problems, and skill level needed by the nurses were common themes in both settings. Differences between the two groups, however, were evident. Finnish public health nurses used emotional support and information to help families empower themselves to use resources and to strengthen their family unit. Utah nurses focused first on individual level goals and then on family cohesion and health. Nurse-initiated referrals and direct physical care were the primary intervention strategies of Utah nurses. Unlike the healthcare system in the United States, access for all in maternal and child healthcare and school health allowed Finnish nurses to develop long-term relationships with families, thus advancing family nursing practice.

Critical Thinking Considerations. Major contributors to the differences between the Finnish and Utah nurses were educational preparation, workplace requirements for nurses, and culture. Such differences between compared groups are confounding variables. Some possible implications for nursing practice found in this study are as follows:

- Both Finnish and Utah public health nurses work primarily in maternal child health, and their emphasis on children is reflected in their definitions of family and family nursing care.
- The child is viewed as a primary client and the entry into the family.
- The family nurse works with the family to place the individual's needs within the context of the family and to improve or strengthen the family.

From Duffy, M. E., Vehvilainen-Julkunen, K., Huber, D., & Varjoranta, P. (1998). Family nursing practice in public health: Finland and Utah. *Public Health Nursing, 15*(4), 281–287.

family nursing and have developed family nursing frameworks. For each framework, nurses collect slightly different data and organize the data according to the framework's focus and principles.

It is beyond the scope of this chapter to discuss various assessment tools; the reader is referred to the references for additional information. At the beginning level, a basic family assessment requires observation, comparison, and interview. The areas to assess depend on the framework; possible areas include developmental stage, wholeness, communication, and support. These areas can be assessed by observation of behavior in the family, by comparison of family behavior to reports in the literature and to other families in similar circumstances, and by interview (Table 19-2). Chapter 47 further discusses the nursing process in relation to the family.

Family Responsibility for Healthy Function

Family members share responsibility with each other for the functional health of all members. Considering the example at the beginning of this chapter, the Benoli family is in the replacement stage of development; they have grown children.

Ways for this family to maintain a healthy lifestyle might include gardening, walking together, or planning simple activities that include some exercise. The Benoli family eats a healthy Mediterranean diet. The younger generations read labels and discuss the nutritional values of the foods they cook. Display 19-2 suggests questions the nurse can ask to elicit information on the interaction of family members as it relates to their family's functional health.

COMMUNITY

Nurses in every setting must be aware of their clients' interactions with and within the community. Beginning nursing students should focus on resources that exist within the community and view clients as individuals within a family within a community. Appropriate nursing care incorporates the interaction of clients with family members and with community institutions (e.g., employer, religious institution, school, other social group). As students progress through the nursing curriculum, they build a foundation that can help them eventually focus appropriate nursing care on any level of need (individual, family, or community) while not losing sight of the relationships among all three levels.

TABLE 19-2

Family Assessment Based on Four Specific Frameworks				
	Developmental Stage	**Wholeness**	**Communication**	**Support**
Observe	Family behavior is consistent with their developmental stage.	Family themes and rules are explicit and implicit.	Family interaction and patterns of communication between members are recognized.	Types of support (e.g., emotional, financial) that family members give each other.
Compare	Family behavior is similar to that of other families at the same stage of development.	Family rules derive from themes and fit a community standard.	Differences and similarities of interaction and communication patterns are noted among different families.	Family members are able to give and receive the amount of support needed for self and each other.
Interview	Tasks and stage of development the family is working on are clear and understood by members.	Members can articulate what is important in their family and what happens if a member breaks a rule.	Members can state functional and dysfunctional communication patterns within the family.	Members can state whether they are receiving sufficient support from others in the family.
References	Duvall (1962, 1977), Wright and Leahey (2000).	Smoyak (1982) uses pictures of the family structure called genograms to display information graphically. This allows the nurse to see patterns of themes and rules repeated over generations. Wright and Leahey (2000) also use an ecomap to depict visually family members' relationships to the larger system.	Satir (1988) describes four dysfunctional patterns. Holman (1983) and Hartman (1978) describe how to depict graphically communication patterns among family members using an ecomap. Minuchin (1974) and Minuchin and Fishman (1981) describe techniques to establish family and communication boundaries. Wright and Leahey (2000) assess emotional, verbal, nonverbal, and circular communication patterns.	Attneave (1975, 1976) and LaFargue (1984) use family network maps to assess family support. Bischoff, Thorburn & Reitmaier (1996) describe neighborhood help to support families.

Definition of Community

Much has been written about community, but there is no agreement on a single definition. Each attempt at a definition has had a particular focus, the one most appropriate to the community in question.

Archer (1985) described three general types of communities: emotional, structural, and functional. These community types are similar to Tucker's view of community "as a spatial unit, as an ethnic group with a common culture, and as an aggregate of people with shared values, interests and goals" (Tucker, 1983, p. 173). Cookfair (1996) added the concept of "aggregates," which may be religious communities, developmental communities, or communities of needs.

Rubin and Rubin (1986) summarized the sociologists' perspective on community as the integration of linkages among

DISPLAY 19-2

ASSESSMENT QUESTIONS RELATED TO FAMILY FUNCTION

Health Perception and Health Management
- What is your perception of your family's state of health?
- Are you able to cope with family health problems?
- Name one thing you do to promote healthy living for yourself and for each member of the family.

Activity and Exercise
- How would you characterize the activity level in this family?
- What types of activities does the family engage in as a group? How often does this occur?
- What are the favorite leisure-time activities of this family?

Nutrition and Metabolism
- Describe your family's eating patterns.
- What are typical meals and when are they served?
- Do you have any special way of preparing family meals?
- Who is the best cook in the house? Why?

Elimination
- Is garbage disposal a problem for your family?
- How is waste and, specifically, human excrement disposed of in this family?
- What hygiene practices are followed by members of this family after using the toilet?

Sleep and Rest
- What is the general sleep pattern in this family?
- What happens when this pattern is disturbed?

Cognition and Perception
- How are decisions made in this family?

- Are your decisions more concrete or more abstract, related more to the past, present, or future?

Self-Perception and Self-Concept
- What does each member like and dislike about being part of this family?
- How would each member describe the family?

Roles and Relationships
- Do you consider the relationship among and between family members to be healthy and supportive? Please explain.

Coping and Stress Tolerance
- Name a stressful event in the family. What was each member's perception of the event? How did each member cope with it?

Sexuality and Reproduction
- Is it acceptable to discuss issues of sexuality openly in this family?
- When, how, and what are children told about sexuality? Are you satisfied with your expression of sexuality within the family?
- Have there been any reproductive problems in the family? Please explain.

Values and Beliefs
- What are important beliefs this family holds? How does each member carry out such beliefs?
- How valued are the activities in which members of the family are engaged?

---

individuals. They placed these characteristics on a continuum, along which eight forms of community emerged. At one end was the "highly affective" or traditional community, such as a rural village, and at the opposite end was the "strictly interest group" or community of interest, such as the American Nurses Association.

Higgs and Gustafson (1985) believed that communities are social units and, like individuals, have a hierarchy of needs. They developed a community typology analogous to Maslow's hierarchy of individual needs. Because they viewed the community as the client, they did not discuss types of communities but rather enumerated functions of a community (Higgs & Gustafson, p. 12):

- Use of space
- Means of livelihood
- Production, distribution, and consumption of goods and services

- Protection of its members
- Education
- Participation
- Linkage with other systems

For the purposes of this chapter, **community** is defined as a social group whose members may or may not share common geographic boundaries, yet who interact because of common interests or shared values to meet their needs within a larger society.

Types of Communities

A list of the types of communities with examples provides awareness of the scope of communities and of the resources that nurses can use for clients.

The early work of Warren (1963) still provides a useful approach to ways of examining communities. His six types of communities (i.e., space, people, institution, interaction, distribution [of power], and social system) are discrete and provide useful guidelines for nursing care. Definitions previously discussed combine several of Warren's types. Warren's list, however, does not address Archer's emotional community (Archer, 1985) or Rubin and Rubin's affective community (Rubin & Rubin, 1986). These can be combined into a seventh category: emotional security. Table 19-3 summarizes the seven types of communities.

Community Assessment

Nurses can take numerous approaches to assessing a community. These have included epidemiologic (Harkness, 1995), ecologic (McFarlane & McFarlane, 1996), systems (Neuman, 1989), and cultural (Leininger, 1991) approaches. When the nurse is able to understand a client's community, he or she can enhance nursing care and discharge planning through the use of appropriate community resources. The case of the Benolis illustrates this point. The nurse might ask Mrs. Benoli to describe her community. Such assessment focuses healthcare planning on two points: a method the client finds acceptable, and a method that maximizes community resources. Table 19-4 summarizes the implications for Mrs. Benoli's nursing care, based on the type of community. This matrix shows possible goals on which the nurse and client could agree. The table is a preliminary way to think of resources based on client and family needs and community types.

Community Responsibility for Healthy Function

The community environment affects the well-being of the individual and the family. Government, educational, recreational, and healthcare services affect all phases of function. One community may have suitable grocery stores with fresh produce and meats at a reasonable price, whereas another neighborhood may sell such products at a higher price. One community may provide free smoke detectors and teach people how to check batteries, while another community ignores the issue of fire safety. Likewise, some communities may be more prone to fires, such as run-down, crowded, inner-city areas with boarded-up houses and litter-strewn areas.

Systems theory suggests that the community has responsibilities toward the family, but the family also is responsible for taking part in community activities and promoting good services. In the same vein, the community is responsible to the healthcare system for providing adequate facilities and resources. Healthcare workers participate in a feedback loop by volunteering in community activities, acting as resources, and assessing community needs and services.

Display 19-3, covering community health, lists questions to be asked of individuals, community representatives, and nurses. The questions apply to the community at large or, on a smaller scale, to institutions such as hospitals, schools, and factories.

TABLE 19-3

Types of Communities: Their Focus and Selected Examples

Type	Focus	Example
1. Space	Geographic boundaries	Town; hospital; unit of a hospital
2. People	Characteristics of people	Cajun population in New Orleans; group adolescent diabetic campers
3. Institution and shared values	Common beliefs and values of a group and their behavior based on those values	American Jesuit universities; support groups for the caretakers of patients with Alzheimer's disease
4. Interaction of people	Usually centered around interest	Parent–teacher association of a specific school; local nurses association
5. Distribution of power	When influence is exerted over others so that, despite resistance, a favorable outcome is obtained	American Association of Retired Persons, American Medical Association
6. Social system	Interaction between systems	Family–school–hospital–church system
7. Emotional security	Emotional ties between people and emphasis on ascribed characteristics	Prenatal classes; ethnic neighbors

Types 1 through 6 are based on Warren (1963). Type 7 is based on Archer (1985) and on Rubin & Rubin (1986).

TABLE 19-4

Implications for Specific Nursing Interventions for Mrs. Benoli by Types of Communities		
	Nursing Needs	
Types of Communities	*Mobility*	*Nutrition*
Space Neighborhood	Set walking criteria within neighborhood boundaries	Eat frequent small meals alone or with one trusted friend
People Friends in dress shop	Walk to dress shop to meet with friends	Eat with friends; allow them to assist periodically
Values Do for self	Walk short distances alone versus longer ones with assistance	Use assistive feeding devices
Interaction Stroke support group	Do what others in same circumstances suggest	Do as suggested by leader of the stroke support group
Power Italian female elders in the neighborhood	Sees very little need to walk because others will come to her; must walk to maintain independence	Eat with family to maintain public image of being in control
Social System Interaction among family, dress shop, neighborhood, church, hospital, elders	Walk outdoors daily to carry out necessary chores	Eat a balanced diet daily with family
Emotional Security Place of birth: Caravaggio, Italy; ethnic group: Italian	Walk as much as possible; would like to visit Caravaggio once again	Eat the foods her grandmother fixed, which she believed had a therapeutic value

Advanced Community Concepts

One way in which communities may improve the health of people within their boundaries is by addressing the healthy people goals proposed for the year 2010 (Office of Disease Prevention and Health Promotion, 1997). The overall goals are (1) to increase quality and years of healthy life and (2) to eliminate health disparities.

Movement toward these goals has started to happen as communities organize themselves, building successful partnerships and obtaining resources (Public Health Service, 1998). One strategy is to organize based on the typology of community as a social system. The Healthy Chico Kids 2000 program in Chico, California, represents such a model. In this case, the community social systems that have come together include various ethnic and socioeconomic popula-

Communication	Interests	Spirituality
Start with face-to-face communication and a one-to-one interaction with a trusted friend	Engage in gross motor activities around light gardening	Allow priest to come to home while planning how to get to church
Communicate first face to face, then in writing, and eventually by phone	Accept suggestions from friends to start new hobbies with them	Allow friends to take to church
Use electric typewriter or computer where no assistance is needed and message is clear	Remain with known hobbies and learn to readjust to limitations	Go to church rather than have priest come to home
Read and keep abreast of what is new for members of the stroke group, try various methods of communication as encouraged within the group	Consider hobbies other members of the stroke support group can do successfully	Use resources of group to get to and from church
Speak within small sphere of other elderly women	Select a hobby that reflects status and can be mastered	Be physically present at church to act as a role model for the younger generation
Contact two people daily: this can be done either face to face, in writing, or by phone	Select one hobby that can be done either alone or in a group	Set aside 1 hour a day for spiritual reflection; allow neighbors to take to church
Speak Italian and English; make contact with relatives in Italy	Select a hobby that centers around "the old days," and "the old country"	Pray, which takes a large part of the day; going to church is not as meaningful as it once was

tions, educational institutions, public health agencies, alternative healthcare centers, businesses, churches, local government, and human service agencies (Public Health Service, 1998).

Organizing and intervening at a community level are advanced concepts that are beyond the level of the beginning nursing student. These concepts require the nurse to conceptualize the community as the unit receiving care. There are several approaches to studying community in this way. Higgs and Gustafson (1985) were among the first nurses to discuss community assessment and diagnosis from four perspectives: epidemiologic, descriptive, systems, and adaptive. The Ottawa Charter for Health Promotion is an example of intervening at a community level. Flynn (1997) described how healthy communities were conceptualized as those in partnerships to develop community leadership and to engage in community

DISPLAY 19-3

 ASSESSMENT QUESTIONS RELATED TO COMMUNITY FUNCTION

Health Perception and Health Management
- Is your community a safe community in which to live? Why?
- What are the major health problems in your community?
- What health problems are on the decline/increase in this community? Why has this decline/increase happened?
- Review morbidity and mortality statistics for the community.

Activity and Exercise
- How efficient is the public transportation system in your community?
- What are the recreational activities in your community? Who plans them?
- Are there parks, and bike and hike paths?
- What are the cultural activities in your community?

Nutrition and Metabolism
- Do residents seem well nourished in your community?
- Are there any specific nutritional programs in your community?
- Observe specific groups in the community such as children, pregnant women, and the elderly. What does their nutritional status appear to be?

Elimination
- How is hazardous waste disposed of in your community?
- Does your community have a recycling plan? How does it work?
- How is household waste disposed of in your community?
- What infectious diseases in your community can be traced to improper waste disposal?

Sleep and Rest
- What is the noise level like in your community at night?
- Do noises in the community interfere with your sleep and rest?

Cognition and Perception
- Are the schools providing a good education?

- How are decisions made in this community? Who participates in decisions that affect all community members?
- Observe the process used by any one group to make their voice heard in the community.

Self-Perception and Self-Concept
- Is there a sense that the community "cares for" its residents?
- Are residents proud of their community? Are they fearful?

Roles and Relationships
- Do community institutions collaborate with each other?
- Can individuals access agencies easily in terms of health-related issues?

Coping and Stress Tolerance
- What are the issues causing stress in your community? (Examples drawn from other communities are racial tension, child molestation, AIDS, and noise pollution.)

Sexuality and Reproduction
- What is the attitude toward sex education in your community? Who should be teaching this material? Are they?
- Review the marriage and birth statistics for the community. Note birth rate, age of mother at pregnancy, abortions, and adoptions.

Values and Beliefs
- How effective are the local media (newspaper, radio, television)? Who makes decisions on programming?
- Do people feel strongly about local government? Do they vote?
- What health-related issues would your community spend money on? What issues would they not?
- How would you complete this sentence related to health issues in your community? We believe that health _____ _____.

assessment, nurse-managed services, research, and policy development.

The concept of a community "at risk" also is useful, because it targets the group most likely to encounter health-related problems. Preventive measures can then be taken to stop these problems either before they occur or in the early stages. Community research and health programs target "at-risk" communities.

FUNCTIONAL APPROACH TO INDIVIDUAL, FAMILY, AND COMMUNITY

Looking again at assessments and care being planned and implemented for Mrs. Benoli at the beginning of the chapter, the team planning for her discharge and care realize that an individual's needs are sometimes met in the family or community. The following section addresses possible plans for care for Mrs. Benoli based on individual, family, and community participation in functional health.

Health Perception and Health Maintenance

Mrs. Benoli considers herself "sick." As a sick person, she believes others should care for her and make her well again. The nurse needs to explore the whole area of chronic illness with Mrs. Benoli, focusing on functions she can control. The local Easter Seal Society has agreed to build a ramp with handrails from the sidewalk to the front door. Mrs. Benoli's oldest son will install grab bars in the bathroom to facilitate her independence.

Nutrition and Metabolism

Mrs. Benoli can no longer shop for groceries, cook, or feed herself. The nurse will assess who among family members and friends can do these chores. For instance, Mr. Benoli can learn to shop for groceries, and Mrs. Benoli's friends can take turns with other family members in preparing food. The nurse will pay special attention to teaching Mrs. Benoli to feed herself. The nurse will also teach Mrs. Benoli to evaluate the nutritional values of food so that she makes wise choices about the foods she eats.

Elimination

Mrs. Benoli is motivated to control this area. Recently, to her delight, she experienced success with her bowel program. The nurse can capitalize on Mrs. Benoli's motivation in this area to praise her and to point out the relationship between input (food and fluids) and output (stool and urine). Mrs. Benoli can limit her fluid intake to morning and afternoon so that she will not have accidents at night.

Activity and Exercise

Mrs. Benoli is hesitant to start walking; she is afraid she will fall and develop more problems. The nurse might build Mrs. Benoli's confidence with exercises to demonstrate to Mrs. Benoli her abilities. Together, the nurse and Mrs. Benoli can set goals and destinations for activities Mrs. Benoli would enjoy. One destination Mrs. Benoli would like to reach is her church, so that she can attend mass.

Sleep and Rest

Mrs. Benoli believes that she gets plenty of rest because she spends so much time in bed. She rests frequently during the day but is fitful at night and hardly ever sleeps more than 2 hours at a time. This is an area of concern, and the nurse must make a careful assessment.

Cognition and Perception

Mrs. Benoli is alert and mentally sharp. As her speech improves, it is easier to understand her. The nurse acts in a manner that is both affirming and empathic by talking "to" the client and not "through" the client. In the meantime, Mrs. Benoli's children and husband speak openly and honestly in front of her. They try to include her in all decisions.

Self-Perception and Self-Concept

Mrs. Benoli sees herself as a burden. She says she has regressed in her abilities, causing others to attend to her needs. Her concept of a positive self is one that does not inconvenience others. The nurse can help build Mrs. Benoli's self-concept with honest praise for her accomplishments. Her family, under Mrs. Benoli's direction, will take care of her garden and encourage her to participate as she is able. The Community Garden Club plans to honor her for a hybrid rose she grew just before becoming ill.

Roles and Relationships

The Benoli children say that their mother has changed since the stroke. She has become a timid, retiring woman who expects her children not only to take over her care but to take care of their father as she did. The nurse can help Mrs. Benoli understand the changes that have taken place and help her find a satisfactory role to play in her family. As Mrs. Benoli's confidence and independence improve, she can become responsible for much of her own care. Her husband will learn to participate in simple household chores. The community will send a housekeeper once a week for heavier chores.

Sexuality and Reproduction

Intimacy has always been an essential part of the Benolis' relationship, which they have managed to maintain throughout Mrs. Benoli's illness. Often, Mr. Benoli sits beside his wife, holding her hand, and singing old Italian love songs to her. She smiles in response. The Benolis function well in this aspect of their lives and do not need help in fulfilling basic needs in these areas.

Coping and Stress Tolerance

In the past, Mrs. Benoli confronted problems head-on. Now, her old coping strategies no longer work. The nurse can help her identify and prioritize her stresses. Mrs. Benoli can develop new coping strategies or adapt old ones to her current abilities.

Values and Beliefs

Mrs. Benoli sees her condition as "old age" and therefore has a resigned attitude toward her present condition. The nurse learns what Mrs. Benoli values and believes before interven-

THERAPEUTIC DIALOGUE
Community Nursing

Scene for Thought
The following conversations are based on the care of Mrs. Benoli, who is discussed throughout this chapter. A community health nurse is making a visit to Mrs. Benoli to see how she is at home. Mrs. Benoli is sitting in a chair on the front porch in the sunshine with her husband.

Less Effective

Nurse: Buon giorno, Signora e Signore. How are you both doing today?

Mrs. Benoli: Hello, Sally. You remembered what we taught you last week. Bene, bene! *(Motions to the nurse to sit down.)*

Nurse: So, how is it going for you?

Mrs. B: Oh, we're okay. It's good to be home from the hospital. *(Looks sideways at her husband.)*

Nurse: Good for you! I wanted to check with you about how you're getting your meals and who's helping you with the housework. *(Takes out notebook to record information.)*

Mrs. B: My daughter comes once a week to clean and then my daughter-in-law brings us our meals or we go over to her house to eat.

Nurse: Sounds like you have it all organized. Are you getting out of the house at all? I remember you liked to go to church as often as you could. *(Continues writing.)*

Mrs. B: Yes, our children take us every Sunday. *(Husband and wife look at each other.)*

Nurse: Terrific! I think you're doing great, Mrs. Benoli. I'll stop in again next week. Hope the week goes well for you. Bye.

More Effective

Nurse: Buon giorno, Signora e Signore Benoli. How are you both today?

Mrs. Benoli: Ah, hello, Susan. You remembered what we taught you last week. Bene, bene! *(Smiles broadly and motions the nurse to sit with them.)*

Nurse: How are you both doing?

Mrs. B: Oh, we're okay. It's good to be home from the hospital. *(Looks sideways at her husband.)*

Nurse: And how are you, Mr. Benoli?

Mrs. B: I'm fine now that my wife is home. I worried so much about her when she had the stroke. And I'm glad to have her here, even though she can't do much around the house. *(Mrs. B. frowns at him.)*

Nurse: You don't look too happy about what your husband said, Mrs. Benoli. What's on your mind?

Mrs. B: Well, I can't help it if I can't do what I used to. He gets his meals and our daughter comes in to clean once a week. *(She looks insulted.)*

Nurse: Perhaps you could talk a little more about what you meant, Mr. Benoli.

Mrs. B: All I meant, Susan, was that she can't get around as much as she used to. This is one busy woman! And I know it bothers her not to do everything she used to. It bothers me, too. We're just getting old, cara mia, we'll just have to face it. *(Pats his wife's hand. She smiles at him, sadly.)*

Nurse: Maybe we three can talk about ways you could continue to do what you want to, Mrs. Benoli. I have some ideas that maybe would work out for you. *(The couple look at each other and then lean forward a little, watching Susan pull pamphlets out of her bag.)*

Critical Thinking Challenge
- Analyze who the client is in the above situation.
- Identify what Susan observed.
- Summarize what Sally missed.
- Determine which nurse had the better eye contact and explain why.
- Critique the questions each nurse asked.

---

ing. The nurse refocuses Mrs. Benoli on her likes, abilities, and accomplishments. The nurse relies on the priest and a nun from the nearby convent as sources of strength for Mrs. Benoli's daily life.

The nurse, after assessing which areas need to be addressed and which do not, helps the team develop a plan of care. For example, intervention is not needed in the area of sexuality. On the other hand, the area of values and beliefs is fundamental to understanding Mrs. Benoli's perceptions of health, and these need to be addressed early in the nurse–client relationship. Strengthening this area will help motivate Mrs. Benoli

to participate in her own care and restructure her image of herself as a burden.

KEY CONCEPTS

- Nursing care for the individual is best developed in the context of the client's family and community. An individual can meet some basic activities of daily living independently but often needs the help of family and community.
- The concept of healthy function is useful at individual, family, and community levels.

- Conceptual frameworks provide useful guidelines for organizing family information.
- Developmental frameworks focus on developmental tasks and role expectations of parents and children throughout the life cycle.
- Family systems frameworks look at the interactions of the parts (individual members) that make up the whole (the family).
- Different types of communities offer different types of resources to their residents.
- The federal government establishes national health goals to be met by communities.

REFERENCES

American Nurses Association. (1973). *Standards: Nursing practice.* Kansas City, MO: Author.

Archer, S. E. (1985). Selected concepts and process for client-centered community health nursing. In S. E. Archer & R. P. Fleshman (Eds.), *Community health nursing* (3rd ed.). (pp. 96–130). Monterey, CA: Wadsworth Health Sciences.

Attneave, C. L. (1975). *Family network map.* Available from The Boston Family Institute, 315 Dartmouth Street, Boston, MA 02116.

Attneave, C. L. (1976). Social network as the unit of intervention. In P. Guerin (Ed.), *Family therapy: Theory and practice* (pp. 220–231). New York: Gardner Press.

Bischoff, R., Thorburn, M. J., & Reitmaier, P. (1996). Neighbourhood support to families with a disabled child: Observations on a coping strategy of caregiving in a Jamaican community-based rehabilitation programme. *Child: Care, Health and Development, 22*(6), 397–410.

Bomar, P. J. (Ed.). (1996). *Nurses and family health promotion: Concepts, assessment, and interventions.* Baltimore: Williams & Wilkins.

Bowen, M. (1978). *Family therapy in clinical practice.* New York: Janson Arson.

Carter, B., & McGoldrick, M. (Eds.). (1999). Overview: The expanded family life cycle: Individual, family and social perspectives. In B. Carter & M. McGoldrick (Eds.): *The expanded family life cycle: Individual, family and social perspectives* (3rd ed.). Boston: Allyn and Bacon, pp 373–380.

Cookfair, J. M. (1996). *Nursing care in the community.* St. Louis: Mosby.

Doherty, W. (1985). Family intervention in health care. *Family Relations, 34,* 129–137.

Duvall, E. M. (1962). *Development* (2nd ed.). Philadelphia: J. B. Lippincott.

Duvall, E. M. (1977). *Marriage and family development* (5th ed.). Philadelphia: J.B. Lippincott.

Feetham, S. L., Meister, S. B., Bell, J. M., & Gillis, C. L. (Eds.). (1993). *The nursing of families: Theory, research, education, practice.* Newbury Park, CA: Sage.

Flynn, B. C. (1997). Partnerships in healthy cities and communities: A social commitment for advanced practice nurses. *Advanced Practice Nursing Quarterly, 2*(4), 1–6.

Fortes, M. (1971). Introduction. In J. Goody (Ed.), *The developmental cycle in domestic groups* [Reprint]. (pp. 1–14). Cambridge: The University Press.

Friedman, M. M. (1998). *Family nursing: Research, theory and practice* (4th ed.). Norwalk, CT: Appleton & Lange.

Gillis, C. L. (1993). Family nursing research: Theory and practice. In G. D. Wegner & R. J. Alexander (Eds.). *Readings in family nursing* (pp. 34–42). Philadelphia: J. B. Lippincott.

Haley, J. (1971). Approaches to family therapy. In J. Haley (Ed.), *Changing families: A family therapy reader* (pp. 227–236). New York: Grune & Stratton.

Hanson, S. M. H. (2001). *Family health care nursing: Theory, practice and research.* Philadelphia: F.A. Davis.

Harkness, G. A. (1995). *Epidemiology in nursing practice.* St. Louis: C. V. Mosby.

Hartman, A. M. (1978). A diagrammatic assessment of family relationships. *Social Casework, 59,* 465–470.

Higgs, Z. R., & Gustafson, D. D. (1985). *Community as a client: Assessment and diagnosis.* Philadelphia: F.A. Davis.

Holman, A. M. (1983). *Family assessment tools for understanding and intervention.* Beverly Hills, CA: Sage Publications.

LaFargue, J. P. (1984). Application of cultural concepts to nursing care: Working with family networks. In J. Uhl (Ed.), *Proceedings of the Ninth Annual Transcultural Nursing Conference* (pp. 14–26). Salt Lake City, UT: The Transcultural Nursing Society.

Leininger, M. (1991). *Culture care and diversity: A theory of nursing.* New York: National League for Nursing.

Maslow, A. H. (1968). *Toward a philosophy of being* (2nd ed.). New York: Van Nostrand Reinhold.

McCubbin, M. A., & McCubbin, H. I. (1993). Families coping with illness: The resiliency model of family stress, adjustment and adaptation. In C. B. Danielson, B. Hamel-Bissell, & P. Winstead-Fry. *Families, health and illness: Perspectives on coping and interventions* (pp. 21–65). St. Louis: Mosby.

McFarlane, R. W., & McFarlane, J. (1996). Ecological connections. In E. T. Anderson & J. M. McFarlane (Eds.), *Community as partner* (2nd ed., pp. 82–122). Philadelphia: Lippincott-Raven.

Minuchin, S. (1974). *Families and family therapy.* Cambridge: Harvard University Press.

Minuchin, S., & Fishman, H. C. (1981). *Family therapy techniques.* Cambridge: Harvard University Press.

Neuman, B. (1989). *The Neuman systems model* (2nd ed.). Norwalk, CT: Appleton & Lange.

Office of Disease Prevention and Health Promotion, U.S. Department of Health and Human Services. (1997). *Developing objectives for healthy people 2010.* Washington, DC: Government Printing Office.

Pew Health Professions Commission. (1995). *Critical challenges: Revitalizing the health professions for the twenty-first century.* San Francisco: UCSF Center for the Health Professions.

Public Health Service, U.S. Department of Health and Human Services. (1998). *Healthy people in healthy communities: A guide for community leaders.* Washington, DC: Government Printing Office.

Rubin, H. J., & Rubin, I. (1986). *Community organizing and development.* Columbus, OH: Merrill.

Satir, V. (1988). *The new peoplemaking.* Mountain View, CA: Science and Behavior Books.

Smoyak, S. (1982). Family systems: Use of genograms as an assessment tool. In I. W. Clements & D. M. Buchanan (Eds.), *Family therapy: A nursing perspective* (pp. 245–250). New York: John Wiley & Sons.

Tucker, W. H. (1983). The nature of a community. In M. J. Fromer (Ed.), *Community health care and the nursing process* (2nd ed., pp. 173–198). St. Louis: C.V. Mosby.

U.S. Department of Health and Human Services. (2000). *Healthy people 2010: Understanding and improving health.* Washington, DC: U.S. Department of Health and Human Services, Government Printing Office.

Visher, E. B., & Visher, J. S. (1996). *Therapy with stepfamilies.* New York: Brunner/Mazel.

von Bertalanffy, L. (1968). *General system theory: Foundations, development, applications.* New York: George Braziller.

Warren, R. L. (1963). *The community in America.* Chicago: Rand McNally.

Whyte, D. A. (1992). A family nursing approach to the care of a child with a chronic illness. *Journal of Advanced Nursing, 17*(3), 317–327.

Wright, L. M., & Leahey, M. (2000). *Nurses and families: A guide to family assessment and intervention* (3rd ed.). Philadelphia: F. A. Davis.

BIBLIOGRAPHY

Bolton, L. B., & Georges, C. A. (1996). National Black Nurses Association community collaboration model. *Journal of National Black Nurses Association, 8*(2), 48–67.

Downs, K., Bernstein, J., & Marchese, T. (1997). Providing culturally competent primary care for immigrant and refugee women: A Cambodian case study. *Journal of Nurse-Midwifery, 42*(6), 499–508.

Gebbie, K. M. (1997). Using the vision of healthy people to build healthier communities. *Nurse Administration Quarterly, 21*(4), 83–90.

Jacobson, S. F., Booton-Hiser, D., Moore, J. H., Edwards, K. A., Pryor, S., & Campbell, J. M. (1998). Diabetes research in an American Indian community. *Image: Journal of Nursing Scholarship, 30*(2), 161–165.

Kantz, B., Wandel, J., Fladger, A., Folcarelli, P., Burger, S., & Clifford, J. C. (1998). Developing patient and family education services: Innovations for the changing healthcare environment. *Journal of Nursing Administration, 28*(2), 11–18.

Keller, L. O., Strohschein, S., Lia-Hoagberg, B., Schaffer, M. (1998). Population-based public health nursing interventions: A model from practice. *Public Health Nursing, 15*(3), 207–215.

Peterson, J. W., Sterling, Y. M., & Weekes, D. P. (1997). Access to health care: Perspectives of African American families with chronically ill children. *Family and Community Health, 19*(4), 64–77.

Shapiro, E. R. (1996). Family bereavement and cultural diversity: A social developmental perspective. *Family Process, 35*(3), 313–332.

Weeks, S. K., & O'Connor, P. C. (1997) The FAMTOOL: Family assessment tool. *Rehabilitation Nursing, 22*(4), 188–191.

20 Culture and Ethnicity

Key Terms

cultural diversity
cultural relativity
culture
culture change
culture shock
cynosure
ethnicity or ethnic identity
ethnocentrism

key informant
minority
race
racism
rituals
stereotypes
subculture
transcultural nursing

Learning Objectives

Upon completion of this chapter, the student will be able to do the following:
1. Discuss characteristics of culture.
2. Define concepts related to culture.
3. Build an understanding of people by viewing human responses in a cultural context.
4. Identify patterns of behavior that reflect cultural and ethnic influences.
5. Communicate effectively with people of diverse orientations.
6. Demonstrate an increased awareness of personal culturation and its influence on nursing practice.
7. Recognize and discuss cultures and ethnic groups, including one's own, that are represented in one's community of practice.

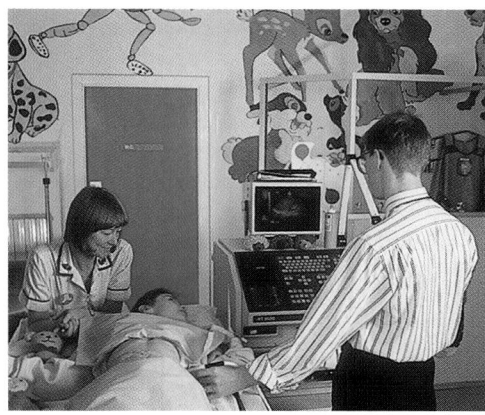

Critical Thinking Challenge

You work in a rehabilitation facility where you are the primary nurse for 6-year-old Spencer. When Spencer was 3 years old, he was in a motor vehicle incident in which his neck was broken at the first cervical vertebra. He is alert and intelligent, but he is immobile from the neck down and requires total care. His parents are Samoan. They have stated that Spencer will come home for future care. Staff members want to send him to another long-term care facility. How will these two different opinions be resolved?

Once you have completed this chapter and have incorporated culture and ethnicity into your knowledge base, review the above scenario and reflect on the following areas of Critical Thinking:

1. Determine the major problems that Spencer's parents would face if they cared for Spencer at home. Propose how the family's cultural beliefs might affect Spencer's care.
2. Considering your own cultural background, analyze how you would feel if you were Spencer's parent and indicate how you would respond in this situation.
3. Analyze how your cultural background affected your thinking (1) when you originally read about the family, and (2) after you studied the chapter.

Nursing is concerned with human responses to actual or potential health problems (American Nurses Association, 1995). In the Critical Thinking Challenge, you are asked to think about how those responses might be affected by the cultural backgrounds of clients, families, and health-care professionals. Understanding culture and ethnicity helps improve the quality of nursing care by doing the following:

- Increasing the diversity of people with whom nurses communicate effectively
- Enabling nurses to attend more accurately to the integrity of the client as a socially and culturally connected person
- Preventing nurses from imposing, however unintentionally, their own culturally shaped presuppositions on clients and peers.

The first part of this chapter examines the theoretical interpretations of culture and related concepts, such as culture change, ethnicity or ethnic identity, minority, race, racism, ritual, subculture, and stereotype. The second part of the chapter discusses the relationship of culture and ethnicity to nursing care. Nursing assessment and intervention are emphasized.

WHAT IS CULTURE?

In nursing, the concept of culture and methods for studying it are derived from anthropology. The anthropologic concept of culture is relatively new; it was first defined in print only in 1871 (Tylor, 1871). Since then, various schools of thought about culture have waxed and waned. Most anthropologists would agree that "culture controls behavior in deep and persisting ways, many of which are outside of awareness and therefore beyond conscious control of the individual" (Hall, 1959). The following definition of culture is used in this chapter:

> **Culture** is a belief system that the members of the culture hold, consciously or unconsciously, as absolute truth. That belief system guides everyday behavior and makes it routine. It provides answers to the unanswerable questions of life, sickness, and death. And it makes the world make sense. In fact, it may explain or comprise common sense. Culture thus enables a person to behave reasonably in contexts that she or he shares with members of the same culture.

Many other definitions of culture exist. Culture can imply qualitative enrichment: the intellectual and aesthetic content of civilizations is called culture, and people become cultured by engaging in the fine arts, such as painting, drama, and opera; bees, fish, and oysters are cultured to increase their supply. Culture is also thought to make humans qualitatively distinct, distinguishing *Homo sapiens* from other orders of being. Both psychological and sociologic characteristics have been found in plants (Goetschs, 1937; Tompkins & Bird, 1972; Rhoades, 1985) and in animals (Darling, 1937; Goodall, 1986). Neither is thought to have and create culture, because other animals and phylogenetically lower forms of life are believed to lack the capacity to communicate in symbols that humans have. Construction and use of symbols as effective and powerful vehicles of human communication reflect the unique human capacity for culture (Douglas, 1973).

Almost anything can carry symbolic meaning. Colors, for example, tend to do so universally, but their meaning varies across cultures and by context (Berlin & Kay, 1969). Black signifies death and mourning among Westerners, but white does the same for Chinese. Westerners color-code sex (pink and blue) and movement (red and green), but not time or social status. The Thai color-code time and social status, but not sex or movement. They designate a specific color as auspicious for each day of the week and reserve blue for royalty and yellow-gold for monks and the king. Christians clothe their priests in black and white; Mahayana Buddhists clothe their monks in gray; Mien* clothe their shamans in red. Traditionally, the white of hospital nurses' uniforms symbolized the cleanliness and purity of nursing. Physicians also wear white jackets or coats that convey the same symbolic meaning, but with dark pants or skirts, the dark color signifying authority.

Nurse anthropologists generally concur that "whatever a person believes to be true or right about any aspect of his [sic] life stems from his culture" (Brink, 1990). Culture patterns ways of perceiving, interpreting and evaluating, and responding to life and the world (Andrews & Boyle, 1999). It provides a blueprint for reacting, feeling, behaving, and interacting socially. People who grow up or live together in the same community of thought and communication share a culture. Their experiences are carved by a shared cultural heritage. That heritage shapes their behavior just as grammar shapes a language, providing rules so well known to a native that he or she follows them automatically.

In most Western societies, for example, spitting in public is considered dirty and aggressive, but exposing the nude body for physical examination by nurses or physicians is a generally accepted protocol. In Muslim societies, in contrast, spitting during ritual ablutions is understood as a religious act of cleansing, whereas exposure of the bare body, particularly to people of the opposite sex, is highly embarrassing and offensive because it violates strong cultural mores associated with intimacy. Such different interpretations of the same behaviors indicate that culture is learned and taught within a society. Culture is the accumulated "common sense" that members of a group share and generate. It provides solutions to common problems of living that have been handed down through generations (Leininger, 1970, p. 49; Leininger, 1997).

In Western societies, spitting was not disparaged for centuries. Spitting became an unattractive behavior in the West only when public health science changed understanding by showing that bacteria cause disease and that sputum carries bacteria. What triggered the reversal of Westerners' attitude toward spitting was the association of spitting with tuberculosis, which in the late 19th century was highly prevalent and feared. This example shows that culture is created by people, often unconsciously, when their old common sense does not

---

* The Mien are a people who live a semi-nomadic lifestyle of agricultural self-subsistence in the hills of Laos and surrounding countries. Some of them fought with the CIA against the Communists in the 1960s and 1970s in the Vietnam War. Upon the 1975 takeover of the Laotian government by the Communists, many Mien fled as refugees, and some have resettled in the United States.

work, as when they attempt to deal with new knowledge, situations, challenges, or threats.

Nurses need to understand how culture affects behavior and what functions it serves, because nurses are accountable for observing and assessing clients' responses, which are influenced by culture. Culture is, consequently, an integral component of nursing's knowledge base. Culture makes communication highly efficient among people who share the same culture, but it can seriously distort and squelch communication between people who do not understand each other's cultures. Culture enables people of similar cultural heritage to understand the meanings of each other's words as part of the particular context in which they are expressed, to "read" each other's nonverbal behavior fairly accurately (usually so well that they are barely aware they are doing so; Hall, 1969), and to communicate through symbols.

At least two thirds of the meaning of a social interaction is estimated to be communicated nonverbally, that is, in gestures, vocalizations (e.g., sighs, throat clearing, laughter, grunts, whistling), and use of space and distance (Birdwhistell, 1970). Even when a nurse and client share the same language, if they do not understand each other's cultures they may misconstrue at least two thirds of each other's messages or information.

Characteristics of Culture

Characteristics of culture are discussed in the following paragraphs. They are also summarized in Display 20-1.

Culture Is Learned

Culture is learned through sustained contact between groups and repeated observations of and participation in a group (Fig. 20-1). It takes time to learn a culture. Some learning is purposeful, and some is absorbed without awareness. When the culture one has learned differs from the culture learned by the people in one's environment, a person can become radically disoriented and stressed. The acute experience of not comprehending the culture in which one is situated is called **culture shock** (Oberg, 1954). Culture shock is a stress syndrome that normally progresses through a series of recognizable stages (honeymoon, disenchantment, beginning resolution, and effective function) to its resolution (Brink & Saunders, 1990). Clients from other cultures or countries where healthcare systems are not as technologically complex as in North America are at risk for culture shock if they are suddenly hospitalized here. Resolution of culture shock requires time, opportunity to observe and participate in the new setting, and careful anticipatory guidance that introduces people, behaviors, and events of the new environment as they affect daily routine.

Culture Is Shared Unequally by Its Members

Not all members of the same culture act and think alike—culture is unequally shared by its members. Knowing a cultural norm does not enable one to predict a person's re-

DISPLAY 20-1

回   CHARACTERISTICS OF CULTURE

Culture Is
- *Learned from other people,* not innate
- *Learned over a period of time*
- *Shared* by people who communicate with each other over time
- *Shared unequally* by its members: some learn and use more of it than others do, and some have and use more access to it or to other cultures than others do
- *Dynamic;* it is always changing at variable rates
- *Diversified;* it increases ideas and opinions
- *Reasonable* from the perspective of the members of the culture; it makes good sense to them
- *Implicit;* it is habit and habituated assumptions
- *Not easily described by its own members*
- *Stabilizing;* it makes human responses generally predictable
- *Ethnocentric;* it uses one's own culture as the correct standard
- *Relative* to socioecologic context
- *Pervasive and holistic*
- *Ritualistic*
- *Recognizable* in patterns at many levels

Culture Is Not
- Predictable at the level of the individual
- Necessarily logical or reasonable to the outside observer
- A set of traits

Culture Functions To
- *Guide behavior* by providing a "blueprint" for action
- *Interpret or give meaning to experience*
- *Explain what is otherwise unknowable:* why we are born; why we are born into the families we are; why we suffer our afflictions, dream our dreams, die our deaths, and have experiences different from others'

sponse. Generalizing about cultural norms in contemporary urban societies is inappropriate because people belong to more than one subcultural group and are influenced uniquely by multiple and diverse reference groups. Exceptions to cultural norms always exist. For example, many people from the United States pride themselves on being generous and altruistic and admire others who are the same. Yet millions of people and families with children are homeless on U.S. streets or do not get basic healthcare because they cannot afford it. Much of American international aid is actually disposal of surplus or obsolete material that otherwise would not be used. Americans also think of themselves as friendly, yet people from other cultures may view this friendliness as

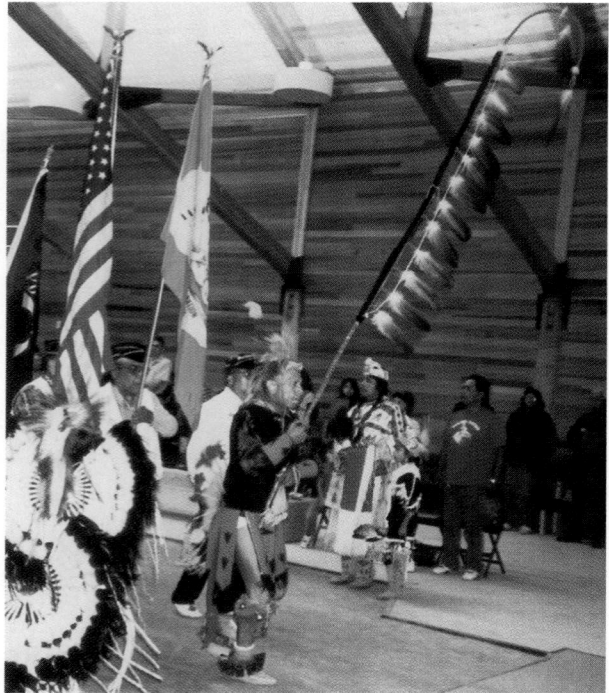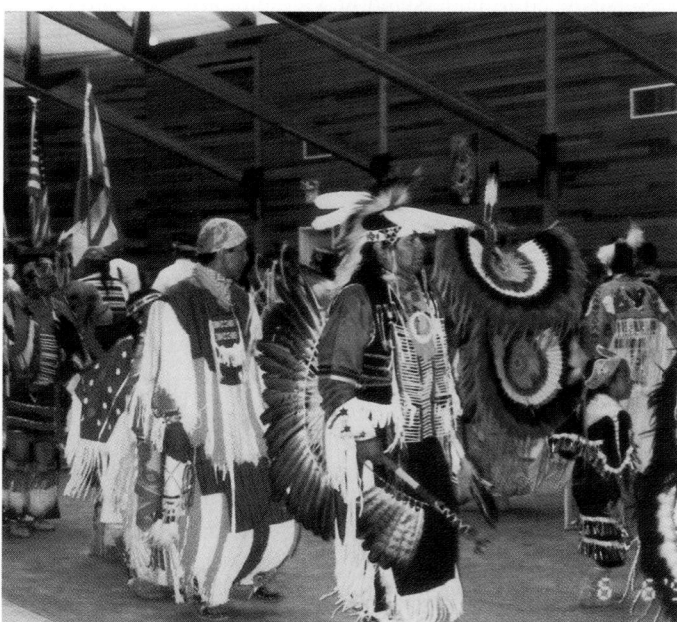

FIGURE 20-1   One of the ways Native Americans pass on their culture and traditions to their children is through costumes and dances.

insensitively intrusive or aggressive; and clients waiting in public hospital and clinic waiting rooms are not likely to find such atmospheres friendly.

People who know certain aspects of their culture better than others do are called **key informants.** Usually, key informants have an especially rich base of cultural knowledge, are reflective, like to talk, and have consciously considered their culture so that they can discuss it. Nurses, for example, often make excellent key informants on hospital culture (Germain, 1979; Muecke, 1993).

Culture Is Dynamic

Culture is dynamic: it changes as people come into contact with new beliefs and ideas. Termed **culture change,** this dynamic is much more rapid than ever before because of the vast reduction in distances between different peoples that the communication and transportation industries have achieved. Immigrants and refugees from developing countries who resettle in North America often change their cultures quickly. Consciously or not, they revise their culture by blending those things from their original culture that seem to work in their new surroundings with new behaviors, attitudes, or beliefs that they find, often by trial and error, work and make life easier for them (Fig. 20-2). Simultaneously, the introduction of cultural ideas from refugees, immigrants, foreign business persons, and media personnel from abroad changes North American society. For example, consumer demand for and use of (Chinese) acupuncture in healthcare have risen. Surges have occurred in the popularity of "ethnic" foods, restaurants, clothes, and music.

Culture Provides Diversity

The **cultural diversity** of a population increases the plurality of ideas and options for behavior to which people are exposed, adding to the texture and complexity of the society's human resources and potential for well-being and achievement. Variety and diversity occur within groups and across groups. Culture provides for diversity only when the playing field is level—when equal opportunity exists for various cultural perspectives. When a dominant culture overpowers the outward, public expressions of other cultures, conflicts and

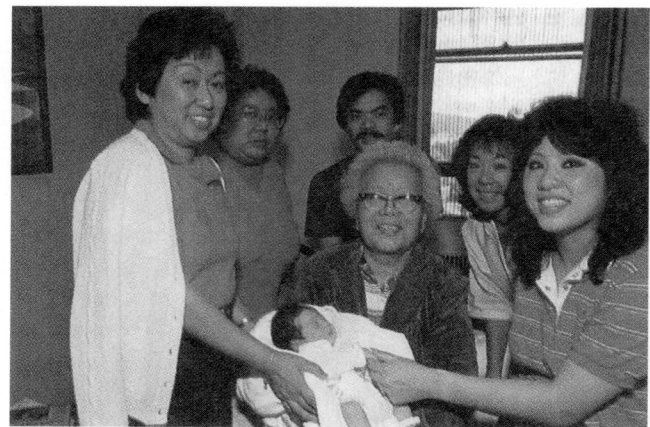

FIGURE 20-2   This family, with immigrant roots, has adapted over time in their cultural exposure and understanding of the dominant culture. Their contributions have also added to and shaped the dominant culture.

suppression may occur in people of differing cultural orientations. Such situations can be highly stressful and, as with slavery and the treatment of Native Americans in the United States, can have lasting disempowering effects.

Culture Is Reasonable From the Perspective of Its Members

Members of the culture in question find their culture reasonable, even though it might seem illogical, counterproductive, or insensitive to outsiders. People such as spouses in cross-cultural marriages, resettling refugees, clients who come from abroad for specialized healthcare, and those who for whatever reasons move quickly from one culture to another tend to act according to the rules of their culture of origin. When those rules do not reasonably fit with cultural rules in their new setting, they are culturally stressed and at risk for culture shock. Ways in which culturally informed nurses can minimize this stress are discussed later in the chapter.

Culture Is Not Easily Described by Its Members

Much of culture is implicit, a combination of habit and habituated assumptions about the world. Habits are enacted without reflection in the daily course of living. Thus, asking clients directly, for example, "What do you believe about prenatal care?" proves a less productive approach than reading about a cultural group or talking with a key informant about it. Cultural dimensions of child-rearing might best be seen by comparing two ethnic groups who are in similar settings, as in DeSantis and Thomas' 1994 study of Cuban and Haitian views of children in Miami, Florida.

Culture Is Habituated Assumptions

Culture is habituated assumptions or the usual way of doing things that people learn through socialization as they mature and become deeply involved in different subcultures. Cultural habituation is advantageous. It reduces the extent to which people must take environmental cues into account—allowing them to respond to routines almost without thinking. This is a key element in expertise. Benner (1984) differentiates the expert nurse from the novice nurse on the basis of being able to take in a large number of cues rapidly; to scan, assess, and prioritize them; and to respond appropriately and effectively in unusually short order. To the extent that culture is shared with others in the community, cultural habituation makes the world familiar and predictable. A predictable environment and being able to perceive the world as coherent are essential for functioning. Without it, people suffer extreme mental stress (Antonovsky, 1980), which can become a chronic form of culture shock.

Culture Is Ethnocentric

Because many aspects of culture are learned from authority figures (e.g., parents, clergy, or celebrities), cultural beliefs usually are held as truths. Viewing one's own culture as the only correct standard by which to view people of other cultures

is **ethnocentrism.** It reflects a fear of difference from one's belief system, and consequent derision or disqualification of people and practices that do not conform to one's own view. Because cultural habituation makes people unaware of many cultural assumptions, they are not always aware of cultural biases. For example, some whites have difficulty accepting the charge of white supremacy that may be leveled against them by blacks. Some men have trouble understanding charges of male chauvinism made by women. Another way of thinking about ethnocentrism is that it can reflect an individual's, group's, or agency's cultural blindness, or lack of capacity to reach out effectively to minorities or culturally stigmatized groups (Giachello, 1995; Murphy and Macleod, 1993).

Culture Is Relative

The earlier example of the variation in the meanings of colors across cultures demonstrates the principle of **cultural relativity,** the way in which cultures relate differently to given situations. Another example is the handshake. Westerners attribute trust and agreement to the handshake and view it as a positive social act. Some Asians avoid shaking hands because the act involves touching a stranger or hands that may be dirty. A cultural interpretation of the difference is that the handshake by itself is meaningless. When carried out by Westerners, it is invested with one meaning. When enacted by Asians, it has another meaning. At the extreme, the principle of cultural relativity would assume that no absolutes exist, nothing has meaning by itself, the meaning or significance of any act or symbol is simply that created and assigned by human groups. Theorists have argued that such an extreme position is untenable because it is amoral. Most nurses accept the principle of cultural relativity only up to a certain (but variable and debatable) degree to preserve moral standards. For example, nursing practice does not condone wife abuse even when a minority group defends it as a culturally appropriate practice. Nurses frequently confront the question, "Where is the line between ethical behavior and cultural integrity?" Issues related to this question require open discussion among staff and with the clients concerned to determine the best among possible decisions. The best decisions would be grounded in ethical principles that are widely used in nursing and medical practice: fairness; respect for persons, families, and communities; and benefit outweighing harm or risk.

Culture Is Pervasive

A culture is a systematic way of interpreting people, behaviors, and events holistically. The holistic nature of culture is congenial with nurses' concern that nursing care be holistic, individualized, and safe. Both the cultural and nursing approaches regard people in their entire humanity, and both direct attention to the total context of a person or group (Leininger, 1970, pp. 21–22; Leininger, 1997). Culture links a wide variety of disparate behaviors and events uniquely. For example, for Western nurses, autopsy is culturally linked to medical beliefs (i.e., that the cause of death can be discovered or validated by examination of the internal organs and tissues, and that by learning the organic cause of death in one person, the deaths of others can be postponed or prevented); to the belief in the separation of the body and soul; and to the Judeo-Christian belief that the body ultimately decomposes into "dust" or generic organic matter. People of other cultural heritages may link autopsy with other belief systems and practices. For example, Hmong* who have not converted to Christianity tend to link autopsy to their recent experience of genocide in Laos and to their beliefs in reincarnation, multiple souls, and the inseparability of body and spirit. They tend to interpret autopsy as preventing the continuation of their society by preventing the union of a person's soul with its body after death, thereby making its rebirth impossible.

Culture Has Common and Observable Rituals

Rituals are common and observable expressions of culture in hospitals, clinics, homes, schools, and work settings. Clients and their families practice rituals that are intimately important to them, particularly during illness and hospitalization. Observance of rituals in times of stress and uncertainty helps restore a sense of control, competence, and familiarity, and to that extent it is a desirable adjunct to nursing care. Nurses' observance of professional rituals helps standardize practice and ensure efficiency. Nurse–client misunderstanding, however, may arise unintentionally when the nurse's rituals are incompatible with the client's. For example, a common home remedy for fever among Southeast Asians is to keep the body well covered with clothes or blankets to keep it warm. This secular ritual of caring conflicts with Western nurses' rituals or procedures of caring for febrile clients, which are designed to cool rather than to warm the body.

Culture Is Recognizable at Many Levels

The easiest level of culture to recognize is material—in artwork, drama, tools, clothes, food, buildings, rituals. Generally, most people think of rituals as events such as Thanksgiving dinner, weddings, funerals, and parades. However, there are also nursing rituals—report, handwashing, gowning, nursing rounds, annual professional meetings, and so forth. Harder to recognize are values and beliefs. Sometimes, they can be accessed by asking about items of material culture. For example, interested, nonjudgmental inquiry about a tattoo on a client's arm could lead to explanations about the person's religious background (from a Coptic Christian), belief in magic (from a Thai), or occupational history (from an American sailor). Sometimes, understanding a people's values and beliefs requires long-term contact, with careful observation and inquiry about patterns in behavior. Although this is the approach of anthropologists, it takes too long for most nurses. Its results are available to nurses in books, journals, documentary movies and videos, lectures, and coursework.

---

* Like the Mien, the Hmong have resettled in Western countries as refugees from the Vietnam War.

Concepts Related to Culture

A number of concepts are so closely related to the concept of culture that each is sometimes used synonymously with culture. Each concept, however, also carries some specific connotation. In North American society, African Americans, American Indians, Chinese, Hmong, Mexican Americans, whites, and other peoples may legitimately be referred to as ethnic groups, minorities, or subcultures, depending on context, but each group may also be misleadingly described or stereotyped.

Ethnicity or Ethnic Identity

Ever since Erik Erikson published his "Reflections on the American Identity" in *Childhood and Society* (1950), ethnicity has implied a culturally informed identity (Petersen, Novak & Gleason, 1980). **Ethnicity** or **ethnic identity** refers to a self-conscious, past-oriented form of identity based on a notion of shared cultural and perhaps ancestral heritage and current position within the larger society. Whites in North America, for example, have an ethnic identity that is grounded in a sense of common European heritage and the associated migrations to the land where they were free to practice their religions, govern themselves, and develop frontiers. The ethnicity of African Americans in North America is linked to a belief in common descent from African peoples and a history of having been brought from Africa against their wills as slaves to a land where white supremacists dominated.

What distinguishes ethnic identity from culture is that ethnic identity is self-conscious about select symbolic elements that are taken as the **cynosure** or emblem of group social identity. In one context, an ethnic group might use native language as its cynosure, as Hmong or Mien do to distinguish themselves from other ethnic groups in North America. In another context, the group might draw on other ethnic indicators, such as style of dress (as when Hmong of one tribe encounter Hmong of another tribe) or religion (as when animist Hmong exclude Christian Hmong from the ranks of "true" Hmong) to stress within-group differences. Ethnicity is a way for people to define themselves and be defined by others. In a society where all cultural groups are not equally respected, these definitions strongly shape what people are able to accomplish (Giachello, 1995).

Ethnicity involves the selection of certain shared cultural characteristics as symbols of a common group origin, history, or descent. That selection may be made by the ethnic group or by the larger society to which it is subordinate. Some European American families have adopted children from a race or ethnic group different from their own. Controversies have arisen regarding raising children in such a home. For instance, will African American children or Korean children lose their roots? Will they have problems assimilating as they enter adolescence if their predominant community is European American?

Margaret Mead (1982, p. 175) documented a history of change in North Americans' images of Native Americans:

> The early explorers in the south painted the portraits of the southeast Indians as royalty and nobles, placing on their impressive physiognomy the mark of European aristocracy and

dressing them in the clothing of the courts. Faced with a need to come to terms with those who possessed the land and knew how to live on it, the settlers elevated them to petty princes before whom it was no shame to ask for help or to admit failure, in the disease-ridden, inexpertly managed colonies of the southeast.

And, after several centuries of subjection, ruthless pillage, and exile into remote reservations, the ethnic emblems of American Indians remained ambiguous status symbols:

> Thus, in the 1930s, the Indians of Oklahoma who were oil rich used to go to New York and buy theatrical Indian costumes for the poorer members of other tribes to wear in local rodeos. In Florida the remnants of different tribes gathered into an artificial synthesis, costumed in European materials, and set themselves up in tourist-oriented Seminole villages.

Ethnic emblems preserve and create a sense of special social identity (e.g., the valuable Indian head nickel), but even such romanticized images as Mead described deny regard for the integrity of ethnically badged groups as human beings.

Minority

Several parameters define the term **minority:** social power, size of the population, and ethnicity. Generally, the term refers to a disadvantaged or less powerful group rather than to a numerical minority (Wirth, 1945). Due to prejudice, discrimination, and sometimes segregation and persecution, a minority does not have the preeminent authority over the society's value system and the allocation of its resources that the dominant segment does (Schermerhorn, 1978, pp. 12–14). Thus, the term emphasizes the political dimension of cultural identity in a pluralistic society such as the United States or Canada, each of which has numerous ethnic groups and ignores the fact that the dominant group is also ethnic and peopled by members with various ethnic ties and identities.

Race

Although the terms *race* and *ethnic group* sometimes refer to the same people, **race** takes biologic characteristics as the markers of separate social status, and ethnic group takes them as markers of cultural identity. Because the biologic features used to differentiate racial groups are easily identifiable only in the extreme or at the level of large population groups (e.g., Asians, blacks, whites), they are highly unreliable. They include blood type, bone length, and size, shape, and number of teeth. Skin color is not biologically linked to ethnic identity. There are no true or readily identifiable physiologic boundaries between races, however, because interracial marriages have made countless people part of more than one racial heritage. In fact, there is more variation in such supposedly "racial" characteristics *within* than across groups. Because the criteria for identifying race are so loose, the U.S. Census Bureau no longer uses standardized criteria to identify racial heritage. Rather, it asks each person to identify his or her own race or racial mix without regard to the criteria for doing so. This practice equates race with ethnic identity.

Racism

Beginning with the Renaissance, European expansion occurred at the expense of peoples whose skin was of darker hue. As a result, skin color became the symbol of both social status or power and cultural difference. **Racism** uses skin color as the primary indicator of social value. In Euro-American society, racism reserves legitimate dominance for those with white skin and penalizes the rest by minimizing their value. This form of racism defines peoples with darker skin as inferior on the basis of accidents of history that denied them resources and privileges of the elite. It is also racist to define people as somehow naturally inferior on the basis of skin color. Racism may be an ideology of the elite who use it to legitimate and perpetuate their dominance and their oppression and exploitation of peoples of different skin color (Schermerhorn, 1978, pp. 73–77), or racism may be any negative belief or action that stereotypes another person on the basis of skin color (American Nurses Association, 1997; U.S. Dept. of Health & Human Services, 1998).

Perhaps the most egregious example of racism in U.S. health care research was the Tuskegee project. The researchers purposefully subjected black prisoners to syphilis without treatment in order to study the natural course of the disease. That is, the researchers consciously caused the study participants, a grossly stigmatized group, decades of increasing suffering leading to their deaths for the sake of medical knowledge (Gamble, 1997). Researchers involved in the Tuskegee project held that medical knowledge was more important than human lives—rather, more important than particular human lives, the lives of black men who as prisoners were powerless against the white researchers.

Subcultures

A **subculture** is a holistic belief system that is marginal and subordinate to the belief system of a culture and that is held most expertly by a recognizable portion of the larger population (Fig. 20-3). The beliefs and standards of a subculture are active only when a person or group acts in a particular social capacity, such as an occupational group or an ethnic group (Harwood, 1981b).

Nursing is considered a middle-class subculture of Western society, particularly of Western medicine, that epitomizes the valued role of nurturers and caregivers. Nurses reflect many values of the dominant group:

- They generally adhere to the work ethic, with work viewed as a reward, independent of other compensation.
- They spend much talent and time on planning for the future.
- They are keenly sensitive to use of time.

Nurses also are recognizable as a subgroup in numerous ways, such as the following:

- Their legally sanctioned authoritative stance vis-à-vis clients and the general public
- Their manner of dress
- Their language ("nurse-ese" includes a large vocabulary of acronyms specific to healthcare professions, as well as its own subcultural lingo)

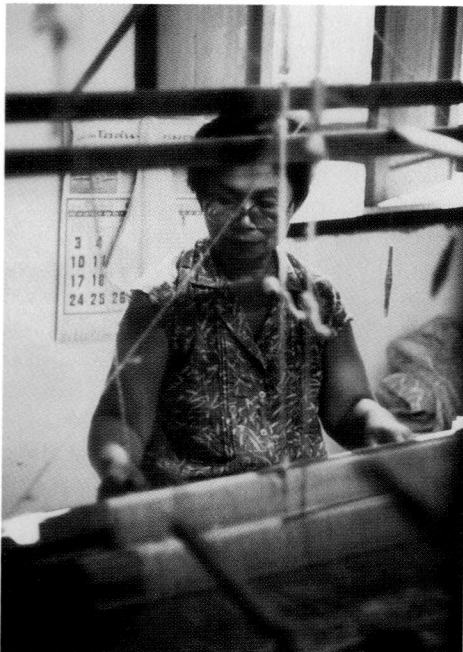

FIGURE 20-3 Cultural traditions are maintained through crafts of members of the cultural group.

- The rituals and ritualized behaviors into which nurses are socialized as nurses

Nurses who are aware of their own subcultural values and behaviors can see how their own cultural makeup might distance, confine, or threaten persons from other cultural backgrounds.

Subcultural identity, like ethnic identity, can be a source of social support, or it can be a target for stigma and exploitation (see Fig. 20-2). For example, in the 1960s the work of Oscar Lewis (1966) spread the misleading notion that poverty is a subculture. He thought that family disorganization made people poor. The theory that culture accounts for poverty blames the poor for being poor, implying that if people were not fatalistic and if they pulled themselves up by their bootstraps, they would not be poor. Critics disproved this theory by demonstrating that societal mechanisms (e.g., the dependency-making welfare system, the lack of adequate day care for children) maintain people in poverty. They noted that many features said to be characteristic of the culture of poverty, such as unemployment and low wages, are characteristic of poverty, not of culture (Valentine, 1968; Stack, 1974). Informed professionals no longer adhere to the notion of a subculture of poverty.

Stereotype

Assigning people to specific categories because of their culture, race, or ethnic emblems is stereotypical thinking. **Stereotypes** are preconceived and untested beliefs about people. They are exaggerated descriptors of character or behavior that are commonly reiterated in mass media, idiomatic expressions, and folklore. They may be demeaning ("People on wel-

fare are lazy, just living off handouts") or idealizing ("Vietnamese are the valedictorians"; "Nurses are client people"; "Physicians are gods on feet"). Either way, they mislead the hearer and deny the individuality of the person.

Use of stereotypes in nursing results in incorrect assessments and, consequently, inappropriate and potentially harmful and unethical interventions or nonaction. For example, acting on the stereotype that "Asians are stoic" could result in a nurse's failure to assess pain and to institute measures to alleviate pain in a client who looks "Oriental." It is imperative that nurses examine their own stereotypes lest they be expressed in unconscious behavior and thereby demean the people they aim to help (Misener, Sowell, Phillips, & Harris, 1997; Allen, Glicken, Beach, & Naylor, 1998; Dootson 2000).

CONCEPTS OF CULTURE AND NURSING CARE

Culture shapes all learned human responses. Clients have the right to receive care that is culturally acceptable to them. Because nursing focuses on human responses to actual or threatened health problems, nurses increase the quality and safety of their care by considering cultural influences on their own responses, as well as those of the individual client, family, or community, to illness. Culture is an integral component of the knowledge base of nursing.

The field of **transcultural nursing,** described as a synthesis of anthropology and nursing, has been gaining ground in

---

ETHICAL/LEGAL ISSUE
Refusal of Treatment Based on Prejudice

As you begin work in the clinic, you overhear the medical assistant and receptionist talking about a client who has come into the waiting room. The client is coughing and appears flushed.

"There he is again. He comes into the clinic over the most minor things and takes up so much of our time. I'm sure he is an illegal alien."

"I know. It isn't right that my tax dollars are spent on noncitizens!"

"Well, just tell him that there are no appointments available."

Reflection
Explore your own feelings about this interaction.
- Identify your personal values and beliefs in this situation.
- Think about ways in which you can respond to this situation.
- Identify a possible approach that might bring about changes in behavior and would improve the quality of client care.

recent years. The focus of transcultural nursing centers on the cultural dimension of care and recognizes that the cultural background of a person influences and determines both health and illness states (Leininger, 1997; Purnell & Paulanka, 1998; Andrews & Boyle, 1999; Meleis 1999). Figure 20-4 illustrates the components of transcultural nursing.

Culturally Sensitive Nursing Care

The culturally sensitive nurse is alert to the possibility of cultural influences on behavior as part of routine assessments of clients, families, and communities. Common cues to subcultural or ethnic identity require assessments including religion, native language or language spoken at home, strong food preferences, characteristic body adornments (e.g., tattoos, amulets, head coverings, cosmetics, jewelry), and communication style (e.g., decision making, relationship to authority figures, relationships with the same sex and the opposite sex). Once such cues are identified, culturally sensitive nurses adapt care to respect each client's subcultural characteristics to the extent that puts the client at greatest ease while ensuring medical safety. They also expect cultural variation in client responses in areas such as pain, hygiene practices, body exposure, food preferences and eating styles, gestures (e.g., eye contact, touch), the sex and age of the healthcare provider,

isolation and quiet, and need for visitors (MacGregor, 1990; Chesla, Skaff, Bartz, Mullan, & Fisher, 2000).

Cultural assessment identifies the client's cultural characteristics to consider for nursing care, and areas of discrepancy between the client's culture and the culture of the nurse and the healthcare setting. Areas of discrepancy indicate the need for providing anticipatory guidance and for clarifying nursing and medical expectations for the client. This clarification might require the assistance of a trained interpreter. Culturally informed case management prevents or minimizes culture shock for the client who is embedded in the subculture of a hospital or healthcare agency. Importantly, it also reinforces the client's sense of competency, thereby promoting learning for self-care.

Exercising cultural sensitivity is becoming increasingly necessary for nurses. Demographic trends, such as increases in the population's average age and ethnic heterogeneity, expand the proportion of clients for whom primary prevention, health education, and long-term care are fundamental intervention strategies. If these interventions are to be effective, an understanding of the client's lifestyle, living environment, and values and beliefs is a must.

Other major but more recent changes in society—the acquired immunodeficiency syndrome (AIDS) pandemic and the practice of early discharge from hospitals—also demand accounting for the client's cultural orientations. The stigma and

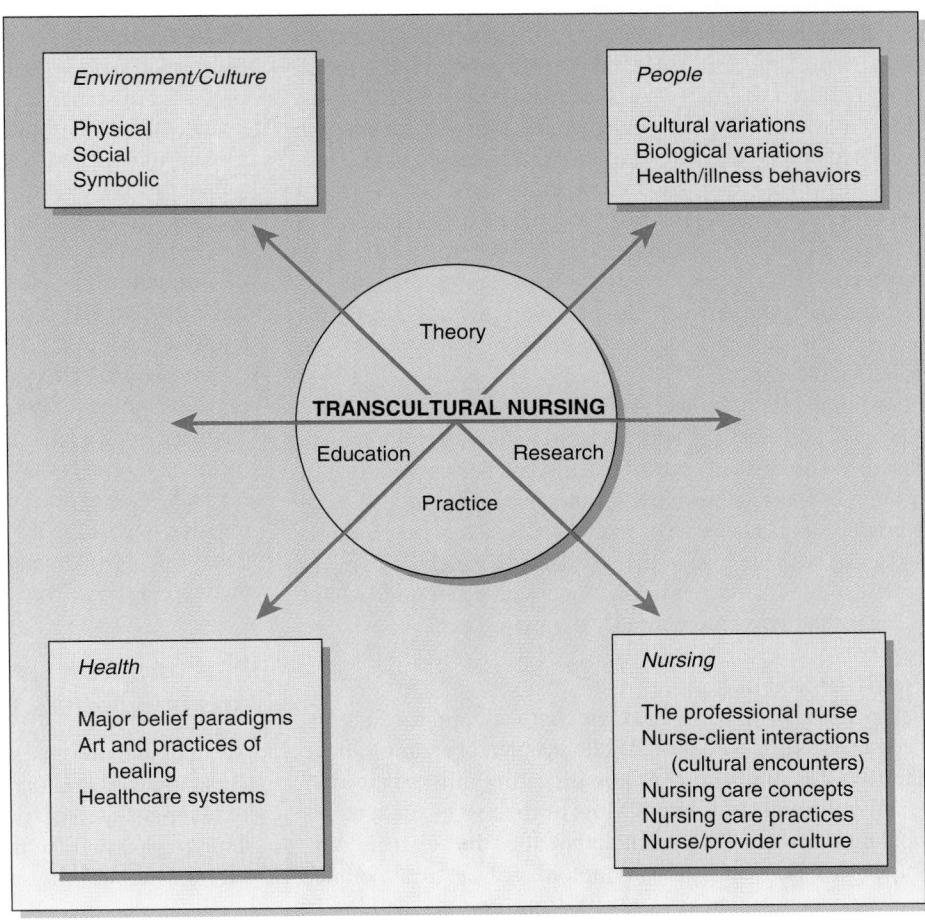

FIGURE 20-4 Model for components in transcultural nursing.

emotional responses attached to human immunodeficiency virus (HIV) infection and AIDS require that nurses be skilled in eliciting what the illness means to the client, the client's support persons, and the public at large when undertaking health education about AIDS prevention and control. The shift in site of nursing care away from hospitals to clients' natural environments (homes, workplaces, schools, ambulatory care settings) has changed the nurse–client power balance in favor of clients. In hospital settings, clients were guests or visitors in the nurse's domain; outside hospitals, nurses are guests of clients. Increasing skill with culturally sensitive assessments and culturally appropriate care is even more crucial.

Biocultural Variation

Together, people's adaptations to their particular econiches over the years, group in-marriage, and the transmission of cultural traditions across generations probably account for much of the genetic variation that occurs among different ethnic and racial groups. Nurses need to consider these variations when assessing clients (Obermeyer, 2000; Graham-Garcia, Raines, Andrews, & Mensah, 2001). The discussion here is limited to noting variations in growth and development, nutritional tolerance, body odor, and skin color.

Growth and Development

Populations differ in their average adult size, tempo of growth, and shape because of complicated interactions between genetic and environmental factors. At the level of population comparisons, there is some racial difference in size, with Asian children distinctly smaller than African or European children, even when comparisons are adjusted for income level. Remember this difference in standing height when evaluating growth curves of children, whether in well-child screening or for pediatric assessment of response to treatment. Asian and African children also have a faster tempo of growth than Europeans do (e.g., on average, girls reach menarche at a younger age), and African children are more advanced than Europeans in skeletal maturity and motor development from birth to adolescence.

Nutritional status strongly influences growth. Although disease may cause some growth retardation among children with inadequate diets, their growth usually catches up with that of children of their age group after the disease is cured. Socioeconomic status also affects growth, most likely because it is associated with the type of diet available to the child. In every society studied, children in the upper socioeconomic sector are larger and grow more rapidly (Crawford et al., 1995).

Nutritional Tolerance

Dietary tolerance is associated with both cultural food preferences and biologic variation. White people, for example, have inherited the ability to continue digesting milk sugar after weaning through adulthood. Most of the rest of the world's population become lactose intolerant after the age of 5 years (Saavedra & Perman, 1989). Symptoms of lactose intolerance are dose dependent and include bloating, cramps, flatulence, and sometimes diarrhea after the ingestion of milk. Because of the associated poor absorption, lactose-intolerant people would do best to avoid milk. Unless they use a lactase enzyme supplement when taking milk and milk products, or follow a diet high in other calcium-rich foods (e.g., nuts, peanut butter, canned fish, cracked roasted meat bones in soups, dark green leafy vegetables), calcium intake may be deficient.

Racial differences are evident in reactions to alcohol and alcoholic beverages (Piette, Baarnett, & Moos, 1998). Enzymatic differences (lower levels of alcohol dehydrogenase and acetaldehyde dehydrogenase) account for the finding that most Asians and Native Americans experience a rapid onset followed by a slow decrease of blood acetaldehyde levels when they consume alcoholic beverages. They consequently experience a long period of exposure to the substance, which is thought to cause many of the symptoms of alcohol intoxication (e.g., facial flushing, other vasomotor symptoms) that are found much less commonly among blacks and whites (Overfield, 1985).

Body Odor

Both body odor and the ways people respond to it vary among populations. Body odor results from deterioration of apocrine sweat, particularly in the axillary area. Populations that have less body odor include Asians and Native Americans (Andrews & Boyle, 1999). In all populations, cultural patterns determine the extent to which people disguise, ignore, or enhance body odor.

Skin Color

Skin color darkens with greater amounts of melanin. Melanin protects the skin from the sun's ultraviolet rays. Its presence accounts for the low prevalence of skin cancers found among blacks and Native Americans. "Mongolian spots," which are clusters of melanocytes, commonly appear (80% to 90% prevalence) in Native American, Asian, and black newborns as poorly circumscribed, macular, blue-black areas of pigmentation, particularly on the lower back around the buttocks. The pigmentation usually disappears by early childhood.

Assessment of oxygenation of the tissues by examination of people with darkly pigmented skin requires practice. Color changes, such as anemic pallor, cyanosis, and jaundice, are most easily observable in areas that are least densely pigmented, such as the sclerae, conjunctivae, nailbeds, buccal mucosa, tongue, palms, and soles. It is normal for some blacks to have bluish pigmentation of the gums and deposits of brown melanin in the sclerae.

Nursing Assessments Based on the Client's Perspective

Accurate nursing assessments require minimizing ethnocentric tendencies and maximizing cultural sensitivity. Cultural assessments identify patterns of behavior over time from the same person and from people of similar background. They are fundamental ways to "locate" culture in carrying out the nursing process.

Subjective data represent the clients' (or the families') views of themselves, their health, their patterns of daily living, demands that are made on them, their usable and unusable resources, and their values and goals. In the subjective data realm, the interviewee is the expert. What is of interest is the client's life, experience, responses, resources, and world as he or she sees them. In the domain of nursing, gathering and recording subjective data without adulterating it is critical.

There are several ways to obtain an understanding of the client's perspective. Usually, combining several methods yields more complete and accurate results than relying on any single one approach. The most effective methods are open-ended interviewing, a variant of which is the ethnographic interview; the use of key informants; and observation over time (Buchwald et al., 1993; Muecke, 1993).

Open-Ended Interviewing

A variety of techniques are used in open-ended interviewing to elicit responses from the interviewee that are as free from influence by the interviewer's comments as possible. Open-ended questions require that the respondent use his or her own words to answer. Silent pauses are sometimes useful because they give the respondent time to think about more things to say. Prompts, such as "Could you tell me more about _____?," encourage the client to elaborate on a point of interest to the nurse.

The Ethnographic Interview

The ethnographic interview is a structured way to elicit the respondent's concepts and understandings (Spradley, 1979). The nurse-interviewer asks questions, the client answers, and the nurse-interviewer asks for repeated clarification of the client's responses. Highly skilled nurse-interviewers conduct ethnographic interviews that sound so much like friendly conversations that respondents do not feel they are being interviewed. In effect, nurse-interviewers guide clients to teach about the subject at hand by expressing interest in the topic, incorporating the clients' own words, and using hypothetical examples. Asking clients to clarify words reveals their individual meaning. Most important is the sense of mutual effort to gain understanding of the client's perspective that the nurse conveys.

There are three parts to an ethnographic interview.

1. It begins with an open-ended, general question such as "How have you been feeling since I saw you yesterday?" or "I'm wondering about your family. . . ."
2. From the client's response, the nurse selects some key terms and asks for clarification. For example, "You felt 'hot in your throat'? I'm not sure what you mean; would you tell me more?" or "You said your 'absent father'—what did you mean by that?" Note the nurse repeats exactly the words and phrases that the client used. The terms are clues to what is important to the client, so the nurse asks the client to talk more about them.
3. The last part of the ethnographic interview is documentation. Information on the client's view of himself

or herself or of the issue discussed should be recorded as soon as possible after the interview so that it can be retained as accurately and completely as possible.

Key Informant Technique

The key informant technique is a method in which the interviewer looks for, locates, and interviews people who have expert or native knowledge about a culture that the interviewer needs to know. A willingness to discuss this knowledge and rapport with the interviewer are critical. The optimal key informant about a client is the client himself, but medically or culturally compromised clients (i.e., those who are unable to function optimally in the culture) might not be able to fill the role. Direct, regular, and ubiquitous contact (in hospital, clinic, home, school, or workplace) of nurses with their clients enables them to observe and assess client behaviors, social support systems, and environmental constraints and resources. But without an understanding of the cultural meaning of what is observed, the nurses' observations have little value.

For most clients with limited English-speaking ability, the most useful key informants in the hospital or clinic situation are bilingual, bicultural, trained interpreters (Putsch, 1985; Carlisle, 1996). Unfortunately, only a small proportion of healthcare agencies have hired such experts. Others who might make useful key informants for nurses include ethnic herbalists or druggists and religious officials (particularly on matters relating to preparation for death, emotional disturbances, social crises, and explanations of illness; Muecke, 1987). The role of religious officials in health is often overlooked. It is important, however, because people usually interpret life–death and health–illness issues in terms of their cultural heritage of religious beliefs.

The following examples indicate the diversity of religious practitioners who might serve as key informants for various ethnic groups in the United States:

- For African Americans, ministers and church mothers can be excellent informants because the church plays a strong central role in many African American communities (Jacques, 1976). Church mothers are particularly well informed about pregnancy, childbirth, and women's health in general.
- For Haitian Americans, a voodoo priest is the expert in the mythology of spirits and the use of plants for home remedies (Laguerre, 1981).
- For Mexican Americans who are Roman Catholic, the priest and the *curandera* (secular folk healer; Kiev, 1968) may be useful informants on people's self-diagnoses and self-care practices.
- For Mexican Americans who are Protestant, a minister of the client's particular sect should be sought because there is a vast difference between the nonpossessional sects (those that do not believe in spirit possession, such as Baptist, Methodist, Seventh-Day Adventist) and the possessional sects (e.g., Pentecostals, who believe in spirit possession and the healing power of prayer and oppose the use of medicines and biomedical services)

THERAPEUTIC DIALOGUE
Culture

Scene for Thought

Spencer, whose situation was described at the beginning of this chapter, is being prepared for discharge. Plans are being made for the next step in Spencer's care. A discharge planner at the hospital is having difficulty discussing Spencer's future care with his parents, who are Samoan. The discharge planner asks the primary nurse to speak with them.

Less Effective

Nurse: Hello again. Thank you for coming in this morning. I wanted to talk to you about where to place Spencer after he gets discharged next month. I understand that you want to care for him at home, is that right?

Mr. Lewis: Yes. *(He looks miserable, and his wife stares straight ahead with her teeth clenched.)*

Nurse: Do you really think that's a good idea? He cannot feed himself, needs to be exercised with the standing board, and turned all the time so his skin stays healthy. Complications can occur at any time. Do you think you can handle that?

Mr. Lewis: Yes. *(His wife is crying quietly beside him and he looks as though he's going to cry, too.)*

Nurse: *(Tries not to act exasperated.)* Okay, if that's your decision, we'll be happy to work with you on that. When do you want to come here to start learning how to take care of him? I think we can do it in a week and then have you practice for a couple of weeks before we send him home with you. *(Mr. and Mrs. Lewis take deep breaths and start to arrange for each of them to come in and learn about Spencer's care.)*

More Effective

Nurse: Hello, Mr. and Mrs. Lewis. I appreciate your coming in today. It seems that there has been some difficulty determining where Spencer will go to be cared for next month after his discharge from here. Could you tell me what you see as the problem with placement?

Mr. Lewis: We can't let him go to another hospital. *(Looks at his hands in his lap. His wife stares straight ahead, her teeth clenched.)*

Nurse: You don't seem very comfortable about that decision. Could you tell me more? *(Uses a relaxed manner, seeks more information.)*

Mr. Lewis: It isn't my decision to make. It doesn't matter what we think. *(He looks ashamed and his wife's eyes fill with tears.)*

Nurse: *(Tries not to look surprised.)* I don't understand. Could you explain that to me?

Mrs. Lewis: *(Breathlessly interrupts.)* We don't want you to think we're bad parents. We think he should go to another hospital. He needs so much care and we don't know how . . . ! *(Cries.)*

Mr. Lewis: It's because my father is in charge of our family and he makes the decisions for all of us. Especially for Spencer, because I was driving the car and my father thinks I was at fault and shouldn't make decisions for him. He thinks we should take care of him at home. *(Looks miserable.)*

Nurse: *(Remains nonjudgmental.)* Thank you for telling me. I understand better now. I have an idea on how we might work this out, but you need to tell me if this will work with your father. *(Shows consideration for both the parents' feelings and the cultural conventions.)* Suppose we ask him to come to a special team meeting with the doctor and me and all the others who care for Spencer and show him what we do with him all day. Perhaps we can then ask his advice about Spencer's placement. What do you think? *(Mr. and Mrs. Lewis talk this over together and decide that Mr. Lewis Senior would feel important and included. They decide it would be a good idea. They look hopeful.)*

Critical Thinking Challenge

- Describe the tone each nurse sets at the beginning of the discussion.
- Determine who did most of the talking in each of the examples.
- Judge if either nurse knew anything about the Samoan culture, and give a reason for your answer.
- Examine the method the first nurse used to determine how this particular family operates.
- Propose places you could learn about the family structure of the various South Pacific cultures.

(Rubel, 1966; Clark, 1970; Kay, 1977; Schreiber & Homiak, 1981).

- For Native Americans, candidates for key informants vary by tribe. Navajo practice a wide diversity of religious practices: on the reservation, a peyote leader would be an important informant on health-related problems and behavior; other informants would be ministers of evangelical groups (e.g., Baptist, Nazarene,

Pentecostal) (Kunitz & Levy, 1981). The Apache and Pueblo of the Southwest rely heavily on medicine men (Joe, Gallerito, & Pino, 1976).

- For Puerto Ricans, both spiritist healers (people who are said to lend their bodies to spirits who communicate through them) and Pentecostal ministers may be helpful informants for conditions not recognized or curable by biomedicine, such as emotional disturbances, incurable chronic or terminal illness, intractable somatic symptoms, and life crisis adjustments (Garrison, 1977; Harwood, 1981a).

Language Differences Between the Client and the Nurse

A deliberate search for the meaning behind client responses enables the nurse to plan and to provide safe and individualized client care. Language differences between the nurse and client compound cultural differences between them and can keep the nurse from understanding the client's point of view. When the client does not speak the same language or does so only to a limited extent, the nurse may decide to act in the client's best interests—without actually knowing what the client believes those interests to be. For example, when a client from an ethnic minority is alert but nontalkative or responds only with affirmatives, healthcare providers might conclude that the client does not understand English. If no interpreter is at hand, the healthcare providers might do what they think is best or necessary for the client even if they do not have the subjective data normally required to guide clinical decision making. The result can be tragic in terms of the client's welfare and loss of trust with a subcultural community.

For example:

A non-Western client with limited English-speaking ability underwent major surgery and recuperated without complications in the intensive care unit (ICU) of a tertiary care hospital. The staff liked him very much. After he was transferred to a regular care unit, his behavior changed dramatically. He exhibited anxious and paranoid behavior. When a psychiatric consultant and interpreter were brought in to handle the problem, they became the first healthcare providers to attempt to access the client's point of view. They found that the transfer from the ICU to a regular unit did not signify recuperation to the client at all. In fact, he interpreted it as meaning the hospital had given up on him because they thought he was so sick that he was no longer worth caring for. In his view, he had been moved from an environment of expert care and the best of technologic assistance into an old part of the hospital that was practically devoid of technologic props and wanting in staff to tend to him. The healthcare team's belief that the transfer was a self-explanatory demonstration of recuperation is a classic example of medical/nursing ethnocentrism, because they neglected to assess the client's perspective.

The client's confusion, fear, and isolation were all preventable. They could be considered *iatrogenic* (i.e., caused by hospitalization). Cases such as this one could be defined as negligent in today's healthcare system because an interpreter should have been obtained to explain to the client the facility's plans for him before he was transferred to another unit. Hospitals are obliged to provide trained language interpreters for "the client who does not speak or understand the predominant language of the community" (Joint Commission on Accreditation of Hospitals, 1996). Furthermore, hospitals that receive Medicare or Medicaid reimbursement are subject to Title VI of the Civil Rights Act, which prohibits recipients

of federal funds from discriminating or denying benefits on the basis of race, color, or national origin: hospitals that fail to provide trained interpreters for people who speak no or only limited English, or for deaf people who use sign language, are in violation of the law (U.S. Department of Health and Human Services, 1982). Nurses who are frustrated in their efforts to communicate with a client owing to language differences or impaired hearing or speech, and who are unable to provide the quality of care deemed appropriate, have the legal recourse to urge the hospital to provide a trained interpreter to resolve the difficulty (U.S. Department of Health and Human Services, 1985).

Obtaining trained interpreters rather than bilingual members of the client's family or friends, however well intentioned or convenient the latter might be, is important because interpretation of behavior goes beyond translation of words. Much medical vocabulary and terminology is difficult to translate into other languages. For example, the phrase, "the lab tech dialed the wrong number," could not be translated into the language of a culture that did not have telephones or scientific laboratories. Furthermore, should the client's condition deteriorate, the emotional burden of responsibility could be overwhelming on someone close to the client.

For example:

A Vietnamese woman was hospitalized with cancer. Her 20-year-old daughter was in a nursing home with leukemia. The husband/father spoke little English. The hospital staff relied on the 12-year-old daughter/sister to act as interpreter. First the sister with leukemia died, then the mother. The 12-year-old, suffering from a sense of complicity in their deaths because of her influence on care owing to her role as translator, suffered an acute psychotic episode for which she needed to be institutionalized. Use of a professional interpreter instead may have prevented this tragic outcome.

Establish a person's need for an interpreter at first contact with the healthcare agency. Provide an interpreter whenever it is requested, and definitely at any time when plans for the client are being made or a change in procedure is being inaugurated. Occasions for involving an interpreter include during admission, for consent for treatment, during treatments, for discharge planning, and for client education. Tips for communicating through an interpreter are given in Display 20-2.

Increased Effectiveness of Client Education

Culturally sensitive nurses look for patterns in the occurrence of unusual behavior in a client from a subculture or ethnic group other than his or her own. An understanding of the principle of cultural relativity suggests an underlying explanation for behavior, particularly for behavior that is repeated by different people of the same culture or ethnic group. When refugees from rural and mountainous areas of Southeast Asia first arrived in the United States, healthcare and social service providers had many stories of the "funny" and "bad" things they did. Analysis of these stories identified clusterings of similar tales, each cluster representing unfamiliarity with

DISPLAY 20-2

COMMUNICATING THROUGH AN INTERPRETER

- Speak to the *client* rather than to the interpreter: this enables the client to "read" your nonverbal language.
- *Watch* the verbal and nonverbal interactions between the interpreter and client: "read" their nonverbal language.
- *Speak slowly.*
- Use *simple* sentences.
- Rephrase a question in different words or ask it indirectly if the answer you received is inappropriate or inconsistent with other indications.
- Avoid using metaphors: they are too hard to translate (e.g., "Have you been feeling down?", "Once in a blue moon," "Does it feel like pins and needles?").
- Expect that it might take an interpreter much longer to say or explain something in another language than in English. This is particularly true when the concept is a medical one for which there is no equivalent in the other language or culture, or when the topic is considered taboo or embarrassing in the other culture.
- When unsure how to bring up a delicate subject, ask the interpreter for advice; *use the interpreter as a key informant* on the culture of the client.
- Try to work consistently with the same interpreter; with practice, you both can learn to communicate better with each other.
- Relate to the interpreter as a professional colleague; your nursing care depends on the interpreter's skill.

Western ways. A culturally sensitive nurse would interpret the unfamiliarity as areas of poor previous communication and, thus, starting points for health education. Some frequent problems in the example just described were the following:

- When women who were taking birth control pills forgot to take a pill, they either took two pills the next day or gave the extra pill to their husbands.
- A large number of newborns in families of non–English-speaking refugees were brought into the emergency room with dehydration.
- Many refugee households with newborns put the heat on in their apartments even during the hot summer, and they swaddled infants and toddlers who had fevers in layers of clothing.

By using the ethnographic interview, observing in clients' homes, and consulting key informants, the nurses discovered the following rationales for the refugee behaviors:

- The women who forgot to take a birth control pill were trying to compensate for its omission. Because they did not know the principles on which the pills work, they

made legitimate guesses about how to overcome their oversight. Also, their cultural heritage had taught them not to ask questions of authority figures, lest they be considered rude and offensive.
- The mothers of dehydrated babies had followed feeding instructions that they had received in the postpartum unit. A hospital nurse who researched the problem discovered that the mothers had learned their lesson well. The problem was that the method they were taught was correct only for the ready-to-use formula for which the hospital gave out free samples. Once those samples were used up, the women began using formula from the Women, Infants, and Children (WIC) Program. The WIC milk was dry powder. Because the women could not read the English language directions on the labels, they guessed how to mix the dry formula. Many guessed wrong, resulting in dehydrated babies.
- The households that turned up the heat and overdressed children with fevers were exercising their belief in the humoral theory of physiology that is prevalent in Southeast Asia (Muecke, 1976). According to this theory, blood is "hot." Because women lose blood during delivery, they lose heat. To keep them from getting sick, their bodies must be kept so warm that they regain the "heat" they have lost. Similarly, children, who tend to have higher fevers than adults, are thought to lose "heat" when they have a fever. Dressing them warmly is thought to prevent "heat" from leaving their bodies.

Culturally sensitive nursing assessments revealed these rationales for untoward self-care practices, providing a highly valid basis for nursing diagnoses and related client education. The health education that resulted from these assessments increased the clients' and their ethnic communities' trust of nurses and of healthcare agencies.

KEY CONCEPTS

- *Culture* is defined as a belief system that the members of the culture hold, consciously or unconsciously, as absolute truth. This belief system guides everyday behavior and makes it routine; provides answers to the unanswerable questions of life, sickness, and death; and makes the world make sense.
- Culture enables a person to behave reasonably in contexts that the person shares with members of the same culture.
- Culture is an integral component of nursing's knowledge base.
- Accurate nursing assessments require that the nurse minimize ethnocentric tendencies and maximize cultural sensitivity.
- Physical assessment skills require knowledge of biocultural variation in such areas as growth, nutritional tolerance and preference, skin color, and body odor.
- Client assessments that consider the client's perspective are most likely to yield diagnoses and interventions appropriate to the client.
- Methods to gain the client's perspective include open-ended interviewing, a variant of which is the ethnographic interview; the use of key informants; observation over time; and use of the client's language.

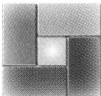

Nursing Research and Critical Thinking
What are the Cultural Variations in Response to the Process of Dying and Grieving Among Four Asian-American Populations?

Asian and Pacific Islander (API) Americans make up the third largest minority group in the United States. Nurses often consider persons identified in this group as coming from the same or similar cultures. These nurse researchers realized that little is known about how the various API American populations respond to the process of dying and grieving or about their traditional beliefs on suicide, euthanasia, advanced directives, and organ donation. Because increased awareness of different cultures can increase the success of nursing interactions with people, they designed an exploratory study to learn more about Asian-American approaches to death and dying through key informant and focus group interviews. In-depth interviews were conducted with people of Chinese, Japanese, Vietnamese, and Filipino descent. The research questions involved asking about the whats, hows, and whys of cultural perceptions and rituals. The questions explored six broad areas: the underlying philosophy or religion influencing death and dying in the culture; burial, memorial services, and bereavement; suicide and euthanasia; advanced directives and organ donation; how beliefs or practices have changed over time;

and advice for healthcare professionals working with dying people from the culture. Results of the study found that, regardless of the religious or philosophical framework of each participant, all had a respect for death and the types of questions it raises. Many differences were found between and among the members of the various ethnic groups.

Critical Thinking Considerations. This study was constrained by a small sample from each ethnic group. All the participants were residents of Hawaii, and their experience differs from that of Asian Americans living on the mainland. Implications of this study are as follows:

* Many factors in addition to cultural heritage influence views and practices related to death and dying: length of time in the United States, educational attainment, occupation, religious upbringing, ethnicity of spouse, and life experience.
* The cultural details provided by the participants in this study are less important than the fact that differences exist and need to be assessed and respected in each nursing encounter.

From Braun, K. L., & Nichols, R. (1997). Death and dying in four Asian American cultures: A descriptive study. *Death Studies, 21*(4), 327–359.

REFERENCES

Allen, L. B., Glicken, A. D., Beach, R. K., & Naylor, K. E. (1998). Adolescent health care experience of gay, lesbian and bisexual young adults. *Journal of Adolescent Health, 23,* 212–220.

American Nurses Association. (1995). *Nursing's social policy statement* (p. 9). Washington, DC: Author.

American Nurses Association. (1997). Position statement: Discrimination and racism in health care [online]. Available at: http://www.nursingworld.org/readroom/position/ethics/etdisrac.htm.

Andrews, M. M., & Boyle, J. S. (1999). *Transcultural concepts in nursing care* (3rd ed.). Philadelphia: Lippincott Williams & Wilkins.

Antonovsky, A. (1980). *Health, stress and coping.* San Francisco: Jossey-Bass.

Benner, P. (1984). *From novice to expert: Excellence and power in clinical nursing practice.* Menlo Park, CA: Addison-Wesley.

Berlin, B., & Kay, P. (1969). *Basic color terms: Their universality and evolution.* Berkeley, CA: University of California Press.

Birdwhistell, R. L. (1970). *Kinesics and context: Essays on body motion communication.* Philadelphia: University of Pennsylvania Press.

Brink, P. J. (Ed.). (1990). *Transcultural nursing: A book of readings* (p. 3). Prospect Heights, IL: Wavel and Press.

Brink, P. J., & Saunders, J. M. (1990). Culture shock: Theoretical and applied. In P. J. Brink (Ed.), *Transcultural nursing: A book of readings* (pp. 126–138). Prospect Heights, IL: Wavel and Press.

Buchwald, D., Caralis, P., Gany, F., et al. (1993). The medical interview across cultures. *Patient Care, 27,* 141–166.

Carlisle, D. (1996). A nurse in any language. *Nursing Times, 92*(39): 26–27.

Chesla, C. A., Skaff, M. M., Bartz, R. J., Mullan, J. T., & Fisher, L. (2000). Differences in personal models among Latinos and European Americans: Implications for clinical care. *Diabetes Care, 23*(12), 1780–1785.

Clark, M. (1970). *Health in the Mexican-American culture* (2nd ed.). Berkeley, CA: University of California Press.

Crawford, P. B., Obarzanek, E., Schreiber, G. B., Barrier, P., Goldman, S., Frederick, M. M., & Sabry, Z. I. (1995, September 5). The effects of race, household income and parental education on nutrient intakes of 9- and 10-year-old girls (NHLBI Growth and Health Study). *Annals of Epidemiology,* 360–368.

Darling, F. F. (1937). *A herd of red deer.* London: Oxford University Press.

DeSantis, L., & Thomas, J. (1994). Childhood independence: Views of Cuban and Haitian immigrant mothers. *Journal of Pediatric Nursing, 9*(4), 258–267.

Dootson, L. G. (2000). Adolescent homosexuality and culturally competent nursing. *Nursing Forum, 35*(3), 13–20.

Douglas, M. (1973). *Natural symbols.* Middlesex, England: Penguin Books.

Erikson, E. H. (1950). *Childhood and society.* New York: W. W. Norton.

Gamble, V. N. (1997). Under the shadow of Tuskegee: African Americans and health care. *American Journal of Public Health, 87,* 1773–1778.

Garrison, V. (1977). Doctor, espiritista or psychiatrist: Health-seeking behavior in a Puerto Rican neighborhood of New York City. *Medical Anthropology, 1*(2), 54–180.

Germain, C. (1979). *The cancer unit: An ethnography.* Wakefield, MA: Nursing Resources.

Giachello, A. (1995). Cultural diversity and institutional inequality. In D. L. Adams (Ed.), *Health issues for women of color: A cultural diversity perspective* (pp. 5–26). Thousand Oaks, CA: Sage Publications.

Goetschs, W. (1937). *The ants.* Ann Arbor, MI: University of Michigan Press.

Goodall, J. (1986). *The chimpanzees of Gombe: Patterns of behavior.* Cambridge, MA: Belknap Press.

Graham-Garcia, J., Raines, T. L., Andrews, J. O., & Mensah, G. A. (2001). Race, ethnicity, and geography: Disparities in heart disease in women of color. *Journal of Transcultural Nursing, 12*(1), 56–67.

Hall, E. T. (1959). *The silent language* (p. 35). Greenwich, CT: Fawcett Premier.

Hall, E. T. (1969). *The hidden dimension.* Garden City, NY: Anchor Press/Doubleday.

Harwood, A. (1981a). Mainland Puerto Ricans. In A. J. Harwood (Ed.), *Ethnicity and medical care* (pp. 397–481). Cambridge, MA: Harvard University Press.

Harwood, A. (Ed.) (1981b). *Ethnicity and medical care* (p. 27). Cambridge, MA: Harvard University Press.

Jacques, G. (1976). Cultural health traditions: A black perspective. In M. F. Branch & P. P. Paxton (Eds.), *Providing safe nursing care for ethnic people of color* (pp. 116–134). New York: Appleton-Century-Crofts.

Joe, J., Gallerito, C., & Pino, J. (1976). Cultural health traditions: American Indian perspectives. In M. F. Branch & P. P. Paxton (Eds.), *Providing safe nursing care for ethnic people of color* (pp. 81–98). New York: Appleton-Century-Crofts.

Joint Commission on Accreditation of Hospitals. (1996). Rights and responsibilities of patients. In *AMH-96 Accreditation manual for hospitals,* (Vol. I). Chicago, IL: Author.

Kay, M. A. (1977). Health and illness in a Mexican-American barrio. In E. Spicer (Ed.), *Ethnic medicine in the Southwest.* Tucson, AZ: University of Arizona Press.

Kiev, A. (1968). *Curanderismo.* New York: The Free Press.

Kunitz, S. J., & Levy, J. E. (1981). Navajos. In A. J. Harwood (Ed.), *Ethnicity and medical care* (pp. 337–396). Cambridge, MA: Harvard University Press.

Laguerre, M. S. (1981). Haitian Americans. In A. J. Harwood (Ed.), *Ethnicity and medical care* (pp. 172–210). Cambridge, MA: Harvard University Press.

Leininger, M. (1997). Transcultural nursing research to transform nursing education and practice: 40 years. *Image: The Journal of Nursing Scholarship, 29*(4), 341–347.

Leininger, M. (1970). *Nursing and anthropology: Two worlds to blend.* New York: John Wiley & Sons.

Lewis, O. (1966). The culture of poverty. *Scientific American, 215*(4), 19–25.

MacGregor, F. C. (1990). Uncooperative patients: Some cultural interpretations. *American Journal of Nursing, 67*(1), 88–91. (Reprinted in Brink, P. J. [Ed.]. [1990]. *Transcultural nursing: A book of readings* [pp. 36–43]. Prospect Heights, IL: Wavel and Press.)

Mead, M. (1982). Ethnicity and anthropology in America. In G. De Vos & L. Romanucci-Ross (Eds.). *Ethnic identity: Cultural continuities and change* (pp. 175–177). Chicago: University of Chicago Press.

Meleis, A. (1999). Culturally competent care. *Journal of Transcultural Nursing, 10*(1), 12.

Misener, T. R., Sowell, R. L., Phillips, K. D., & Harris, C. (1997). Sexual orientation: A cultural diversity issue for nursing. *Nursing Outlook, 45,* 178–181.

Muecke, M. A. (1993). On evaluating ethnographies. In J. Morse, (Ed.), *Critical issues in qualitative research methods.* Newbury Park, CA: Sage.

Muecke, M. A. (1987). Resettled refugees' reconstruction of identity: Lao in Seattle. *Urban Anthropology, 16*(1), 273–290.

Muecke, M. A. (1976). Health care systems as socializing agents: Childbearing the North Thai and Western ways. *Social Science and Medicine, 10,* 377–383.

Murphy, K., Macleod, C. (1993). Nurses' experiences of caring for ethnic-minority clients. *Journal of Advanced Nursing, 18,* 442–450.

Oberg, K. (1954). *Culture shock.* Indianapolis, IN: Bobbs-Merrill.

Obermeyer, C. M. (2000). Menopause across cultures: A review of the evidence. *Menopause, 7*(3), 184–192.

Overfield, T. (1985). *Biologic variation in health and illness: Race, age, and sex differences* (pp. 80–81). Menlo Park, CA: Addison-Wesley.

Petersen, W., Novak, M., & Gleason, P. (1980). *Concepts of ethnicity* (pp. 56, 116). Littleton, MA: Harvard University Press.

Piette, J. D., Baarnett, P. G., & Moos, R. H. (1998). First-time admissions with alcohol-related medical problems: A 10-year follow-up of a national sample of alcoholic patients. *Journal of Studies in Alcohol, 59*(1), 89–96.

Purnell, L., & Paulanka, B. (Eds.) (1998). *Transcultural health care: A culturally competent approach.* Philadelphia, PA: F. A. Davis.

Putsch, R. W., III. (1985). The special case of interpreters in health care. *JAMA, 254,* 3344–3348.

Rhoades, D. F. (1985). Pheromonal communication between plants. In G. A. Cooper-Driver, T. Swain, & E. E. Conn (Eds.), *Chemically mediated interactions between plants and other organisms* (pp. 195–218). New York: Plenum.

Rubel, A. J. (1966). *Across the tracks: Mexican Americans in a Texas city.* Austin, TX: University of Texas Press.

Saavedra, J. M., & Perman, J. A. (1989). Current concepts in lactose malabsorption and intolerance. *Annual Review of Nutrition, 9,* 475–502.

Schermerhorn, R. A. (1978). *Comparative ethnic relations: A framework for theory and research.* Chicago, IL: University of Chicago Press.

Schreiber, J. M., & Homiak, J. P. (1981). Mexican Americans. In A. J. Harwood (Ed.), *Ethnicity and medical care* (pp. 264–336). Cambridge, MA: Harvard University Press.

Spradley, J. P. (1979). *The ethnographic interview.* New York: Holt, Rinehart & Winston.

Stack, C. (1974). *All our kin: Strategies for survival in a black community.* New York: Harper & Row.

Tompkins, P., & Bird, C. (1972). *The secret life of plants.* New York: Avon Books.

Tylor, E. B. (1871). *Primitive culture.* London: Murray.

U. S. Department of Health and Human Services. (1982). *Your rights under Title VI of the Civil Rights Act of 1964 in Health and Human Service Programs, HHS 391.* Washington, DC: Author.

U. S. Department of Health and Human Services. (1998). The initiative to eliminate racial and ethnic disparities in health. Available at: http://www.raceandhealth.hhs.gov. Accessed April, 2001.

U. S. Department of Health and Human Services, Office for Civil Rights. (1985, February). *How to establish effective communication procedures for people with limited English proficiency and for people with impaired hearing, vision, or speech.* USDHHS Region X, Seattle, WA: Author.

Valentine, C. A. (1968). *Culture and poverty: Critique and counterproposals.* Chicago, IL: University of Chicago Press.

Wirth, L. (1945). The problem of minority groups. In R. Linton (Ed.), *The science of man in the world crisis.* New York: Columbia University Press.

BIBLIOGRAPHY

Adams, R., Briones, E., & Rentfro, A. (1992). Cultural consideration: Developing a nursing care delivery system for a Hispanic community. *Nursing Clinics of North America, 27*(1), 107–117.

Andrews, M. M. (1992). Cultural perspectives on nursing in the 21st century. *Journal of Professional Nursing, 9*(1), 1–9.

Campinha-Bacote, J. (1995). The quest for cultural competence in nursing care. *Nursing Forum, 30*(4), 19–25.

Campinha-Bacote, J. (1998). Cultural diversity in nursing education: Issues and concerns. *Journal of Nursing Education, 37*(1), 3–4.

Campinha-Bacote, J., & Ferguson, S. (1991). Cultural considerations in childrearing practices: A transcultural perspective. *Journal of the National Black Nurses Association, 5*(1), 11–17.

Leininger, M. (1998). Transcultural nursing: A scientific and humanistic care discipline. *Journal of Transcultural Nursing, 8*(2), 54–55.

Leininger, M. (1997). Nursing's new paradigm is transcultural nursing. *Advanced Practice Nursing Quarterly, 2*(2), 62–69.

Leininger, M. (1991). *Culture care diversity and universality: A theory of nursing.* New York: National League for Nursing.

Reeb, R. (1992). Granny midwives in Mississippi. *Journal of Transcultural Nursing, 3*(2), 18–27.

Wenger, A. (1992). Transcultural nursing and health care issues in urban and rural contexts. *Journal of Transcultural Nursing, 3*(2), 4–10.

21 Communication:
The Nurse–Client Relationship

🔲 Key Terms

advocacy
circle of confidentiality
communication channel
decode
empathy
encoding
feedback

metacommunication
nonverbal communication
reflection
restatement
therapeutic communication
verbal communication

🔲 Learning Objectives

Upon completion of this chapter, the student will be able to do the following:

1. Define the three major types of communication.
2. Discuss the elements of the communication process and their relevance to nursing.
3. Describe how language and experience affect the communication process.
4. Explain the nature of the nurse–client relationship.
5. Distinguish between a professional and a social relationship.
6. Name the elements of an informal nurse–client contract.
7. Discuss four key ingredients of therapeutic communication.
8. Identify important assessment areas to address when communicating with clients.
9. Give an example for each type of therapeutic communication technique.
10. Identify three key nontherapeutic responses, explaining how each interferes with therapeutic communication.
11. Describe two special situations that affect communication.

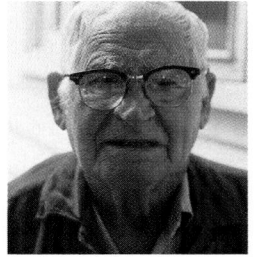

🔲 Critical Thinking Challenge

While you are visiting your client in his retirement apartment, you begin to discuss his recent hospitalization and the fall that occurred during his recovery period. Your concern is for his safety and for preventing further falls. When you ask him why he thinks the fall occurred, you notice that his posture changes. He becomes more erect, and his facial expression is guarded and resolute. He tells you curtly that he simply "lost [his] balance and fell." He goes on to remind you his career has been that of a banker. He continues, "I still advise family and friends, and I am very capable." He does not need "bars" on his bed or little "alarms" to wear like they put on him in the hospital. "Thank you for inquiring, but I understand how to be safe and how to protect myself." You feel that he has no further interest in discussing what you believe is a significant problem.

Once you have completed this chapter and have incorporated therapeutic communication into your knowledge base, review the above scenario, and reflect on the following areas of Critical Thinking:

1. Analyze what might have triggered your client's response to your inquiry and identify how you as the sender of the message might have contributed to his response.
2. Outline the threats that your client may perceive from this interaction.
3. Assess the incongruencies between verbal and nonverbal communication in this visit.
4. Based on your analysis of the above responses, identify the blocks to communication that may be occurring.
5. Construct some options for how you might proceed to improve communication and accomplish your nursing plan of care.

344   *Unit 4*   🔲   Concepts Essential for Human Functioning and Nursing Management

Effective communication within the nurse–client relationship is not so much a natural process as a learned skill. It is a way of being helpful to clients that differs from the way a clerk in a grocery store is helpful or the way friends are helpful to each other. For example, when the grocery clerk gives a courteous answer to a question about a product, the result is a satisfied customer. In a conversation between two friends who are sharing their problems, each friend feels cared for and understood. Although nurse–client communication may include some of the elements in these examples, it differs considerably.

In the nurse–client relationship, the client and his or her experiences and problems are the main subject of communication. The results are directed toward improving coping skills related to the client's health status and well-being. Thus, **therapeutic communication** facilitates interactions focused on the client and the client's concerns. The client expresses and works through feelings and problems related to his or her condition, treatments, and nursing care.

What kind of a process is therapeutic communication, and how does it fit into the context of nursing practice? Because nursing is a practice based on the sciences, nurses master many scientific principles and technical skills. Nursing is an interpersonal process also. Interaction between the nurse and the client has a great deal to do with the outcomes of care. The following things happen during the communication process:

- The nurse and client work together to solve problems centered on the client's healthcare needs.
- The client feels cared for and understood.
- The family or significant others are included in the care.
- Health teaching is conducted.
- Health promotion and preventive care is delivered.

Hildegard Peplau, a psychiatric nurse and nurse theorist, emphasizes that interpersonal competencies of nurses are key to helping clients regain health and well-being (Peplau, 1997). In short, communication is at the heart of all nursing care.

To understand therapeutic communication, an understanding of the communication process and the importance of language and experience is necessary. Specific ingredients and techniques of communication also are important, as is knowledge about the nurse–client relationship, contract setting, advocacy, confidentiality, and developmental issues related to communication.

THE COMMUNICATION PROCESS

Many definitions of communication exist. To communicate means to impart information, to exchange ideas, to express one's self in such a way as to be understood. *Communication* can be defined as a system of sending and receiving messages, forming a connection between the sender and the receiver (Fig. 21-1). It is a process for giving and receiving information, a form of interaction or transaction.

Communication is a continuous human function, much like breathing or cardiac functioning. The process goes on all the time. In many ways, the saying, "You cannot *not* communi-

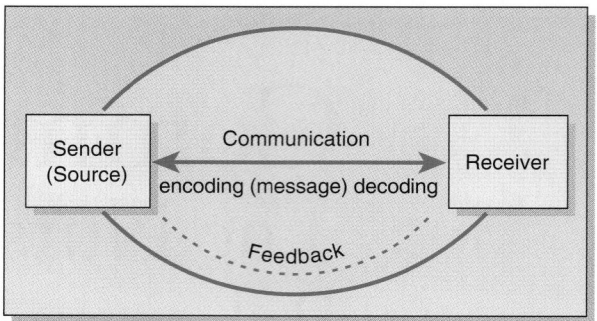

FIGURE 21-1   Communication is a process in which information is sent and received. It is a form of interaction that is continuous and ever-changing.

cate," is true. For example, when a person decides not to share information, or one person stops talking to another person because of hurt or anger, communication has still taken place.

Communication is basic and essential to human life. Through communication, people relate to their environment and to each other. Without it, people would be unable to learn, to direct their lives, or to work together cooperatively in families, organizations, and communities. Communication is basic to human feeling and intellect; without it, the human race could not survive.

Types of Communication

People communicate in a variety of ways. **Verbal communication** involves the spoken or written word. It is an exchange using the elements of language. Equally important is **nonverbal communication.** A person communicates by gestures, facial expressions, posture, body movement, voice tone and volume, rate of speech, and even dress. Silence is a form of nonverbal communication. Display 21-1 lists examples of types of communication.

Another kind of communication, **metacommunication,** is a message about a message. It exists beyond the literal level

DISPLAY 21-1

🔲 EXAMPLES OF TYPES OF COMMUNICATION	
Verbal	**Nonverbal**
Written	Touch
Spoken	Eye contact
Television and radio	Facial expression
Movies	Body posture
Magazines	Gestures
Books	Physical appearance
Computers	Voice tone
Posters	Rate of speech
Brochures	Neatness
	Movement

of communication (i.e., beyond just the words of the message). Metacommunication includes anything that is taken into account when interpreting what is happening, such as the role of the communicator, the nonverbal messages sent, and the context of the communication that is taking place (Crowther, 1991).

Relationships among Types of Communication

The relationships among the different types of communication (verbal, nonverbal, and metacommunication) are important. The way they fit together (are congruent) or do not fit together (are incongruent) reflects just how complex communication is. The following two examples illustrate this concept.

Congruent Relationship. A nurse makes rounds on assigned clients at the beginning of the shift. She explains her role to each client, confers with them about their nursing care needs, and schedules with them the care tasks to be done on that shift. The nurse is dressed in a professional manner and wears a name tag and hospital identification badge. He or she speaks in a well-modulated voice and listens carefully to what each client says.

In this example, each kind of communication conveys messages that are congruent. The messages say, "I am your professional nurse. We will work together to meet your nursing care needs. I respect you." There is a "good fit" between verbal, nonverbal, and metacommunication.

Incongruent Relationship. A client and a nurse have been working together on diabetic teaching. After the teaching session is completed, the client says to the nurse, "Yes, I understand my diabetic diet and how to take my insulin." On the surface, this seems to be a straightforward communication indicating that the client understands the components of care needed to deal successfully with diabetes. If, however, the words of the message are said with an irritated facial expression and a harsh tone of voice, the nonverbal and metacommunication aspects of the message do not "fit" with the verbal message; they are incongruent. The metacommunication in this example may be conveying, "I am tired of being told how to run my life. I am angry about having a chronic illness." Furthermore, if the client is later seen sneaking a candy bar, this nonverbal communication may convey the message that the client has not yet fully accepted his or her condition. In this example, recognizing incongruence between kinds of communication informs the nurse about the client's experience.

Elements of the Communication Process

As shown in Fig. 21-1, communication is a continuous, dynamic, ongoing, and ever-changing operation. Although it is somewhat artificial to break down communication into components, doing so can be useful. Knowing the individual elements of a process can be helpful in identifying where

in the process a problem is occurring. The elements of the model presented here are based on the work of Berlo (1960), a communication theorist.

All communication has a sender (a person or group with a purpose for the communication). The sender's purpose must be translated into a code. This is done with language or nonverbal signals such as gestures, facial expressions, or body cues. The process of getting the purpose translated into the code is called **encoding.** Encoding results in a message.

Another element in the communication process is the **communication channel,** the medium or carrier of the message. For example, television is a channel; the voice or written word is a channel; touch can be a channel.

If the communication process were to stop at this element, no communication would take place because there must be someone at the other end of the channel, the receiver. The receiver is the target of the communication and must be able to understand or **decode** the message. Once messages are decoded and received, feedback occurs. **Feedback** means that the sender and the receiver use one another's reactions to produce further messages.

Understanding the elements of the communication process is useful, because sometimes specific difficulties in communication can be traced to one or more of these elements. A basic example is the client who speaks a different language from the nurse. In this case, the nurse needs to attend to the communication channel. An interpreter may be needed to help carry the message or help the client decode the nurse's messages. Pictures may also be used to convey messages.

Problems in the encoding process also may occur—for example, in clients with thought disorders or certain forms of brain damage. The client has an intent to communicate, but impairment in encoding results in a garbled message. A frightened client whose thoughts are disturbed may say, "The FBI is after me," when he really means, "I am very frightened and out of control." A client who has had a stroke may be able to understand a communication directed at her but not be able to encode a returning message because of brain damage.

Importance of Language and Experience

Language, culture, and experience are crucial to the process of communication. Language, which distinguishes humans from other animals, is used to communicate and develop a person's view of life and the world. Thus, language and experience are closely related. The following discussion is based on the work of Brandler and Grinder (1975).

A person's view of the world is developed through several kinds of filters. One such filter consists of the neurologic receptor systems: sight, hearing, touch, taste, and smell. Stimuli processed through these receptor systems enable the person to experience the outside world. Through language, such experiences can be compared with the experiences of others. Alterations in sensory perceptions can change the person's view of the world. For example, a person with altered hearing or vision may experience the world differently.

Another filter is the particular language system into which the person is socialized. Words and sentences give meaning to things and events. Language allows us to conceptualize the world. For example, a person whose language has only three words for all the possible visible color distinctions would conceptualize colors differently from someone whose language offered more choices. Someone with a limited vocabulary may have more difficulty describing experiences than someone with a rich, diverse vocabulary. In fact, limitations in language skills may actually limit a person's choices in life.

A third filter is the person's unique personal history. Factors such as cultural background, family relationships, place in the sibling ranking, type of parenting received, and genetic makeup all enter into the personal history.

Both the nurse and the client bring their backgrounds into the communication. Some aspects of their background are shared, and some are different. Consider, for example, the image of "a nurse" brought to a nurse–client situation. Some clients may view nursing as a female profession, invoking certain stereotypes about female behaviors and roles. In many societies, women are defined as subservient to men, and their work is devalued. Often, the "caring" image of nursing overshadows the knowledge, decision making abilities, and technical skills of the nurse. Campbell-Heider and Hart

(1993) point out that the language and dress of the nurse reflect not only society's view of the nurse but the nurse's view of self. The professional presentation influences how the client perceives and responds to the nurse.

The nurse–client interaction is productive when communication is aimed toward a common understanding. To communicate effectively, the nurse understands and appreciates his or her own background, while at the same time acknowledging different perspectives held by the client.

In the clinical setting, the extent of successful exchange of information between client and nurse is affected by the degree to which their realities are mutually compatible. The typical nursing work environment, which often involves the use of technical language, produces barriers to communication. Studies have shown that the inability of many clients to understand technical language intimidates them, possibly preventing them from asking questions on their own behalf. Other barriers include talking about the client in front of him or her, withholding information from the client, and being too busy to spend time with the client.

Peplau (1997) stressed that both the nurse and the client tend to have preconceptions and stereotypes about each other. Examples include stereotypes about ethnicity, sexual orientation, social class, age, and psychiatric or medical diagnoses. Examining one's own preconceptions is important to prevent them from interfering with a therapeutic nurse–client relationship.

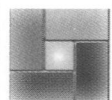

Nursing Research and Critical Thinking
Is There a Difference in the Ways Asian and American Graduate Nursing Students Communicate with the Dying?

Most nurses find it difficult to talk about death with those who are dying. A nurse from Taiwan and a nurse from Illinois designed a study to compare the attitudes toward death and dying in a group of Asian and a group of American graduate nursing students. In this descriptive, comparative study, a questionnaire comprising two instruments, the Collett-Lester Fear of Death Scale and the Health Care Professionals' Experiences With and Attitudes Toward Death and Dying questionnaire, was used to compare the difference in attitudes toward death and dying between the two groups. A convenience sample of Asian and American graduate students was used. Eighteen Asian and 18 American students were sent a questionnaire. Seventeen Asian (94.4%) and 11 American (61.1%) students returned completed questionnaires. The overall response rate was 73.7%. The research showed that Asian students had significantly more fear concerning their own dying process than did the American students ($P < .01$); Asian students were less inclined than the Americans to talk

about death with those who were dying ($P < .05$) and avoided interactions with them more than the Americans did ($P < .05$). However, the Asian students had a significantly more positive attitude than the American students when asked about personal satisfaction gained from caring for the dying ($P < .05$).

Critical Thinking Considerations. The small size of the sample prevented any definitive conclusions being drawn, and the differences in age and religious affiliation between the two groups were confounding variables. However, the researchers discussed several issues that are applicable to nursing practice, including the following:

• If nurses are anxious about death, this anxiety could be manifested as a reluctance to talk about death, think about it, or be with dying people.
• For both Asian and American graduate nursing students, talking about death and dying was the most difficult aspect of caring for the dying.

Kao, S. F., & Lusk, B. (1997). Attitudes of Asian and American graduate nursing students toward death and dying. *International Journal of Nursing Studies, 34*(6), 438–443.

THE NURSE–CLIENT RELATIONSHIP: A HELPING RELATIONSHIP

The nurse–client relationship differs from a social or intimate relationship. Table 21-1 compares the nurse–client relationship with a social relationship. Within the nurse–client relationship, the nurse assumes the roles of a professional and a helper. The client is the one seeking help. The nurse–client relationship focuses on the client, is goal directed, and has defined parameters. In the professional relationship, the nurse also assesses how his or her own role, communication skills, personal history, and values may be affecting the interactions.

Phases

The nurse–client relationship can be thought of in terms of three phases: orientation, working, and termination. The orientation phase consists of introductions and an agreement between nurse and client about their mutual roles and responsibilities. In the psychiatric setting, the orientation phase of the relationship represents the first phase of therapeutic work. The nurse and client get to know each other and develop trust (Forchuk, 1992; Trojan & Yonge, 1993).

With changes in the healthcare delivery system and decreased time for contact between healthcare providers and clients, communication may be less effective than in the past. For clients in acute care settings, the stays are shorter and the clients are more ill, resulting in less time for communication and teaching and less ability to share concerns and absorb knowledge. Additionally, whether in hospitals, long-term care, or home care, the professional nurse is often in the role of supervisor or delegator, needing to deliver nursing care and manage effective communication through licensed and unlicensed assistive personnel. This requires even more skill in communication by the professional nurse.

During the working phase, the nurse and client participate together in nursing care activities. During this period, the client "uses" the nurse's expertise and abilities on his or her behalf. The nurse functions as the client's advocate, caring for the client's physical and emotional healthcare needs. With psychiatric clients, the working phase consists of problem solving around emotional, behavioral, and interpersonal issues.

Termination is the closure of the relationship. The nurse reviews with the client aspects of care and how they have dealt with physical and emotional responses. Discharge planning is a key component in the termination process. Termination can take various forms. For example, the nurse–client relationship can end when the client is discharged or the nurse is reassigned. Be clear about termination. Continued contact beyond professional responsibilities usually is not advisable and may violate professional and ethical codes of conduct.

Contract Setting

The nurse–client relationship is based, in general, on an informal contractual model. In the contractual relationship, clients are seen as having control over the significant decisions that affect their own bodies. Clients are given information necessary for making decisions, and clients choose among options including acceptance, refusal, or termination of treatment. Aspects of care, goals of treatment, and necessary adaptations are discussed with the client. The nurse takes no major action without consulting the client or a family member representing the client. The nurse discusses his or her role, the client's condition, treatment, and nursing care with the client. Decisions about nursing and healthcare are made collaboratively.

TABLE 21-1

Comparison of Professional With Social Relationship		
	Nurse–Client	**Social**
Key Focus	Client	Both participants
Goals	Meeting client's needs. Help client identify feelings and concerns; solve problems, cope, and adapt in relation to healthcare situation.	Meeting own needs. Mutual companionship, enjoyment, and interaction. May lead to intimacy and commitment.
Parameters	Limited primarily to the needs incurred by the healthcare situation. Nurse self-discloses only what is appropriate for the client's benefit. Relationship is terminated when goals are met and service no longer needed.	Sharing of life's events, activities, or other aspects of self. May stay superficial or lead to long-term relationship. Relationship may be terminated when own needs are no longer met.
Self-Assessment	Nurse assesses own role, communication skills, values, and so forth, and how these affect the professional relationship.	Each person assesses how own needs for enjoyment, affection, and sharing, or love and intimacy, are met in the relationship.

The contractual relationship between nurse and client is an informal one that is verbal and is assumed by both parties. Display 21-2 summarizes the elements of an informal contract between nurse and client. In the area of psychiatric nursing practice, contracts usually are more formal, sometimes written. Often, they are used as a therapeutic tool to help a client develop more insight and control over his or her own behavior.

The usual way for a nurse to establish an informal contract with a client is to make a verbal agreement about how they are to work together. A nurse might approach a client as follows: "I will be your nurse while you are a client here. This means I'm responsible for planning your care. I'll be here every day this week but will be off on the weekend and nights. Other nurses will care for you according to the plan we decide on together. Do you have any questions or concerns about your care?"

An important advantage to the informal contractual relationship involves values and rights. The nurse maintains his or her own rights while respecting those of the client. Consider, for instance, a nurse who disagrees with abortion and a client is considering having one. The nurse can contract with the client to provide the information but need not participate in the procedure. The nurse must respect the client's rights. Because abortion is a legal procedure, the nurse cannot restrain the client from having one. Furthermore, the nurse is obligated to provide the client with information so that the client can make an informed decision. However, this does not deny the nurse's personal right to oppose legalized abortion and to choose not to work for an institution that performs abortions.

Advocacy

Advocacy, or taking the client's side, is the basis for communication with clients. Advocacy supports the client's right to the information necessary to make his or her own decisions

DISPLAY 21-2

⌶ **ELEMENTS OF AN INFORMAL NURSE–CLIENT CONTRACT**

- Nurse and client know each other's names.
- Roles and responsibilities are clarified.
- Parameters of the professional relationship are clear.
- Mutual expectations are agreed on.
- Circle of confidentiality is respected.

about treatment options and nursing care. Clients need information about their health status and the course of illness so that they can make the necessary adjustments in their lives. Sharing information reduces anxiety and is an integral aspect of therapeutic communication.

The interaction of increased consumerism and health maintenance organizations has had an effect on nursing advocacy and communication. With advocacy, nurses focus on the knowledge clients need and want to make their own decisions about their health and healthcare. Being an advocate for the client means avoiding an authoritarian approach, which assumes that the professional will make decisions for the client. Inducing guilt or blame is also to be avoided.

An example of inducing guilt is a mother's telling her child, "I cooked this dinner especially for you, and now you aren't going to eat it." The underlying message is, "Because you did not eat the dinner, mother is hurt and you are selfish." Whether it is used in child-rearing situations or in the nurse–client relationship, inducing guilt is inappropriate and manipulative. Table 21-2 compares authoritarian and guilt-inducement approaches with the advocacy approach.

Client advocacy sometimes conflicts with the physician's viewpoint. Physicians tend to see the physician–client relationship as primary and exclusive, with the physician in

TABLE 21-2

Comparison of Authoritarian, Guilt Inducement, and Advocacy Approaches			
Clinical example: Surgery has been recommended, but the client is reluctant to have the operation.			
	Authoritarian	**Guilt Inducement**	**Advocacy**
Approach	No choice	Choice based on consequences of actions	Choice based on information and examination of alternatives
Response	"Surgery is your only choice. You need this operation."	"If you don't have the surgery, you may not live to see your grandchildren. Your family needs you."	"Whether or not you have the surgery is your choice. It is your body. What is your understanding of the situation?"
Underlying Message	The professional knows best and should make the decisions for you.	If you don't do what the professional recommends, you and others will get hurt.	The professional is here to help you make informed choices about your health and well-being.

control of information. To keep the client's best interest in the forefront, the nurse needs to develop a collaborative working relationship with the physician (Fagin, 1992). Helping the client become more assertive with the physician also is a positive approach.

For instance, a client may confide to the nurse that she believes she is not receiving enough information about her condition. The client complains that the physician does not spend enough time with her, and she feels left out of the decisions made about treatment. If the nurse provides the information to the client without conferring with the physician, the nurse has intruded into the physician–client relationship, because the client's perception is that more information is needed from the physician.

In this instance, several options are appropriate. The nurse can discuss the problem with the client and help the client assert herself through such means as writing a list of questions to ask the physician. With the client's permission, the nurse can seek out the physician and share the client's perceptions with him or her. With such actions, the nurse is acting on the client's behalf without interfering in the physician–client relationship, thereby practicing true advocacy.

Circle of Confidentiality

Every client has a right to privacy. However, depending on legal restrictions, certain client information must be shared with other professionals involved in his or her care. This can be thought of as a **circle of confidentiality,** and it includes all the people in a nursing unit who have responsibility for the client. It usually includes the family, unless the client objects.

It is important to clarify with the client that he or she is part of a team. Consider, for example, a nurse who has been caring for a client with a serious prognosis. The client says to the nurse, "If I tell you something, will you promise to keep it in the strictest confidence? Don't tell anyone else, not even my family." The nurse agrees. Then the client says that he plans to kill himself after he is discharged, stating that he has a loaded gun at home.

The nurse in this example failed to adhere to the concept of the circle of confidentiality. The proper response would have been to tell the client that the nurse is part of the healthcare team and that clinically relevant information is shared with the team. This protects both nurse and client and clearly defines the limits of client confidentiality.

Transmission of information beyond the nursing unit is rarely indicated and must be carefully considered. In this day of technical efficiency, client data are readily available (Kreider & Haselton, 1997). The client's right to privacy is important. For example, a client may not want others to know about his or her hospitalization, the nature of his or her illness. This is especially true in cases associated with stigma such as acquired immunodeficiency syndrome (AIDS), substance addiction, and psychiatric illness. Always consider client confidentiality even in such mundane situations as talking at lunch or at home.

 ETHICAL/LEGAL ISSUE
Respecting Client Confidentiality

You are a nursing student and are entering the classroom. You hear your classmates talking about their clients by name and laughing about information related to their clients that your classmates obtained from the clients and their medical records.

Reflection
- Reflect on your feelings in this situation and identify them.
- Identify concerns you may have about ethically appropriate behavior.
- Refer to the Patients' Bill of Rights in Chapter 6. Think about whether this situation demonstrates a violation of this contract.
- Identify possible approaches to your classmates that may alter their behavior yet not impair your communication with them.

INGREDIENTS OF THERAPEUTIC COMMUNICATION

What makes communication therapeutic, and in what ways is it different from other forms of communication? Carl Rogers (1961) studied the process of therapeutic communication, believing that a person cannot be separated from the techniques of communication he or she uses. Based on his research, the characteristics of a therapeutic, "helpful" person were identified. Empathy, positive regard, and a comfortable sense of self were among the key ingredients.

Empathy

Empathy is the ability to enter into another person's experience to perceive it accurately and to understand how the situation is viewed from the client's perspective. Empathy includes the ability to respond receptively to the other person's experience while still maintaining objectivity, and the ability to communicate to the person that he or she is understood (Morse et al., 1992; Williams, 1990). This is done through the process of reflective or "active" listening (see later discussion).

Empathy is a complex process. The nurse must

- Have enough knowledge and experience to perceive the client's perspective accurately
- Feel secure enough not to be intimidated if the client experiences a situation differently
- Feel comfortable enough to be able to imagine what a situation might be like for someone else, while remaining outside that situation to maintain objectivity
- Convey to the client that the nurse perceives the client's feelings, thoughts, and experiences accurately.

Empathy is a strong component in therapeutic relationships. However, the constant exposure to client care can emotionally drain the nurse (Morse et al., 1992). It is not necessarily appropriate to use the entire empathic process (described earlier) in every clinical situation. Simple actions such as touch, kindness, attentiveness, and information sharing also signify empathy.

Positive Regard

Positive regard refers to warmth, caring, interest, and respect for the person, seeing the person unconditionally or non-judgmentally (Fig. 21-2). Respect for the person does not depend on his or her behavior; instead, the person is regarded as worthwhile simply for being human.

How can this work? What if, for example, the nurse is caring for a person who has been convicted of a serious crime? Does positive regard mean that the nurse condones the things this person has done?

Positive regard does not mean that the nurse accepts all aspects of a person's behavior. The nurse does not condone or encourage behavior that is socially inappropriate or abusive. However, the nurse must separate that behavior from the person. The underlying assumption is that the person is worthwhile and has value and dignity.

Positive regard also means that the professional avoids unnecessary labeling of clients. The focus of healthcare professionals on disease tends to label the client as an object (e.g., a diabetic, an amputee, an alcoholic). As a result, the client is seen as someone who is defective. Also, viewing a client as his or her disease rather than as someone who has that disease can interfere with seeing the person behind the label. This viewpoint tends to come through in the communication process. Ignoring the person makes it more difficult to know and understand his or her response to health and illness and to use the client's strengths and potential.

Comfortable Sense of Self

Before a nurse can communicate therapeutically, a comfortable sense of self, such as being aware of one's own personality, values, cultural background, and style of communication, is necessary. A person's sense of self comprises a collection of characteristics. For example, a nurse may be a professional, a

parent, and a sibling, and may be overweight, tall, or athletic. How the nurse experiences these characteristics influences how he or she sees others.

The nurse with a comfortable sense of self can evaluate his or her strengths and weaknesses. For example, one nurse may say, "I work well with postoperative clients, but I have less aptitude for working with rehabilitation clients because I like things to happen more quickly." Another nurse might enjoy working with psychiatric clients because he or she finds working on interpersonal goals rewarding.

Self-evaluation also means taking responsibility for one's actions as a professional. For example, a nurse might think, "I could have said something more supportive," or, "I should have included the family in the planning phase." Through this process, the nurse grows in professional competency.

A person with a comfortable sense of self is open to experiences and is aware of his or her feelings and attitudes. This allows the person to take a more flexible view of life. For example, the nurse may notice that not all clients respond the same way to a similar surgical procedure, and that not all people in a given culture fit the stereotypes of that culture. The differences between the nurse and the client can be seen as interesting or challenging, rather than threatening or "bad."

The professional with a comfortable sense of self feels separate from others, an important aspect of being therapeutic. Because it is easy for a nurse to overidentify with clients, clear interpersonal boundaries need to be maintained. A nurse who becomes too involved in the suffering of clients soon becomes emotionally and physically exhausted, lacking the objectivity it takes to be therapeutic. Also, the ability to separate prevents the nurse from seeking gratification through excessive client dependence. The nurse gives appropriate support and care but has confidence in clients' abilities to make choices about their health and lives.

To maintain professional enthusiasm and job satisfaction, nurses must attend to their own needs as people. Rest, exercise, and a balanced diet are important physical needs. Supportive relationships, interesting activities, and time for relaxation and enjoyment are important emotional needs. Being therapeutic with one's self is necessary before one can be therapeutic with others.

COMMUNICATION AND NURSING PROCESS

The nurse–client relationship and therapeutic communication are instruments used to implement the nursing process. The nursing process can also be applied to the communication that takes place between nurse and client: The nurse assesses the client's communication and uses specific therapeutic communication techniques appropriate for the client's stage of development during nursing interventions.

Assessment

Because therapeutic communication takes place within the nurse–client relationship, the goals of the relationship must be determined. These goals vary depending on the client's

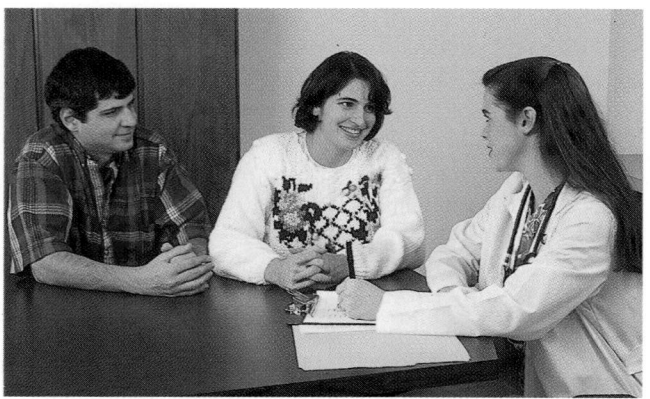

FIGURE 21-2   The nurse communicates positive regard in this interaction with a couple discussing pregnancy.

needs, the area of nursing practice, and the specific role of the nurse in each particular clinical situation. Consider the following two examples.

One nurse works on a postpartum unit where the average length of stay is only 2 days. Each nurse cares for an average of eight clients per shift. The nurse's role is primarily to assist with care of the mother's physical needs, to facilitate mother–infant bonding, and to assess and conduct whatever teaching is necessary to help the family care for and adjust to the newborn. In this situation, the nurse–client relationship is short-term and focused. The nurse renders little direct physical care, working instead as an adviser and health teacher. The nurse and client move through each phase of the nurse–client relationship quickly.

In contrast, another nurse works for a hospice program providing care to terminally ill clients in their homes. The nurse spends 2 hours three times a week with the client and family. Her role is to give direct physical care, to support the client and family, and to teach the family how to care for the client. This relationship is intense and demanding. During the orientation phase, the nurse establishes a working relationship with the family and the client, discussing how the client and family will communicate and work together, thus establishing a verbal contract. In this situation, the nurse works as a direct caregiver, teacher, and therapeutic counselor.

During the initial phase of the relationship, the nurse assesses the client's communication, using the theoretical base presented earlier in this chapter. Some key assessments about communication, summarized in Display 21-3, include the following:

- Are verbal and nonverbal communications congruent?
- What are the feelings and themes conveyed by the client?
- What emotions are expressed?
- What are the client's communication patterns?
- Does the client speak slowly or rapidly?
- Does the client get caught up in minute details?
- Are there long silences?
- Can the client express himself or herself openly and ask the questions he or she needs to ask?
- When the nurse sends messages, does the client return feedback that is precise, pertinent, and directed toward the goals of the nurse–client relationship?

Assessing the environment in which communication takes place is also important. The external environment must be conducive to communication. For example, how are the nurse and client positioned in relation to each other? How far apart are they?

Noise and privacy are other important considerations. Telephones, televisions, radios, and machines such as ventilators, cardiac monitors, and suctioning equipment can be distracting. The presence of other clients and employees can interfere with comfortable communication.

The client's internal environment, made up of his or her cultural background, beliefs, and experiences, also may affect nurse–client communication. For example, do the client's religious beliefs pervade all aspects of his or her life and deci-

sion making? If so, this will affect communication, especially if the nurse has a different belief system. Language and cultural practices also should be assessed.

Many of the same factors assessed in the client pertain to the nurse as well. Consider your own voice tone, quality, and pitch; body language; facial expressions; and verbal fluency; and know how anxiety may affect these factors. Constantly assess your own communication and feedback skills, and also examine how your cultural beliefs and personal history affect your perception of the client (Cravener, 1992; Murphy & Clark, 1993).

Implementation

Once communication has been assessed, how does the nurse use communication as a therapeutic intervention? Table 21-3 summarizes specific techniques to facilitate therapeutic communication. The therapeutic communication skills highlighted in this section are considered basic to any therapeutic relationship. More advanced skills are usually studied in psychiatric nursing, especially at the advanced practice (master's degree) level.

Helping the Client Get Started

Nurses are generally involved in informal therapeutic relationships, which can be important to the client. In the acute care setting, the nurse often combines physical care with a discussion about the client's concerns. The nurse can encourage a client to express concerns by sitting down; often, clients are reluctant to express themselves to someone who is always in a hurry or seems too busy. Draw the curtain between beds, and focus the client's attention away from any roommates and toward the nurse.

Call the client by name, asking whether he or she prefers to be called by the first or last name. Many adults find being called by their first name intrusive or rude. Convey interest and readiness to listen. By leaning toward the client, making eye contact, and assuming a relaxed, open posture, the nurse offers himself or herself to the client. Display 21-4 lists general guidelines for facilitating communication.

Open-Ended Questions. An open-ended question is one that elicits more than a "yes" or "no" answer. Such questions ask how, what, where, or when. Examples of appropriate questions include "How are things going for you at this point?" and "What have your experiences been like?"

Opening Remarks. Other ways to help a client get started include opening remarks based on observations and assessment about the client. For example, assessment-based statements, such as "You've been having a pretty rough time," "I notice you're going through some important changes," or "You seem to be feeling better" provide the client with the opportunity to respond.

These questions and statements must be neutral and tentative, not probing or interrogating. "Why" questions usually are not considered therapeutic because they are too intrusive;

DISPLAY 21-3

🔄 **COMMUNICATION ASSESSMENT TOOL**

Name _____ Age _____ Sex _____ Diagnosis _____

I. Sender or receiver impairments
  A. Structural deficit _____
  B. Sense deficits: hearing, sight, smell, touch, taste
     _____
  C. Loss of functions _____
  D. Disease _____
  E. Drugs _____
  F. Other _____

II. Message variables
  A. Nonverbal communication
     1. Facial expression _____
     2. Gestures _____
     3. Body movements _____
     4. Affect _____
     5. Tone of voice _____
     6. Posture _____
     7. Eye contact _____
     8. Voice volume, quality, pitch _____
  B. Verbal communication
     1. Content of message _____
     2. Communication patterns _____
        a. Blocking _____
        b. Slow _____
        c. Rapid _____
        d. Quiet _____
        e. Halting _____
        f. Aphasic _____
        g. Discontinuous _____
        h. Excessive _____
        i. Detailed _____
        j. Stammering _____
        k. Circumstantial _____
        l. Tangential _____
        m. Long silences _____
        n. Other _____

III. Noise

IV. Communication skills
  A. Openness, spontaneity _____
  B. Use of clarification _____
  C. Request for feedback _____

  D. Tolerance of silence _____
  E. Acceptance of confrontation _____
  F. Other _____

V. Setting
  A. Inpatient unit _____
  B. Community settings _____
  C. Other _____

VI. Media

VII. Feedback
  A. Precise _____
  B. Pertinent _____
  C. Goal directed _____
  D. Informative _____
  E. Solicited _____
  F. Positive _____
  G. Negative _____
  H. Clarified _____
  I. Opportune _____

VIII. Environment
  A. External influences
     1. Temperature _____
     2. Physical arrangement _____
     3. Lighting _____
     4. Noise level _____
     5. Other _____
  B. Internal influences
     1. Beliefs _____
     2. Experiences _____
     3. Thoughts _____
     4. Attitudes _____
     5. Other _____

IX. Cultural influences
  A. Health practices _____
  B. Religious implications _____
  C. Language barriers _____
  D. Food preferences _____
  E. Other _____

Adapted from Johnson, B. S. (1997). *Psychiatric mental-health nursing: Adaptation and growth.* (4th ed.). Philadelphia: J.B. Lippincott.

TABLE 21-3

Therapeutic Communication Techniques	
Technique	**Definition**
Offering self	Making self available to listen to the client
Open-ended questions	Asking neutral questions that encourage the client to express concerns
Opening remarks	Using general statements based on observations and assessments about the client
Restatement	Repeating to the client the main content of his or her communication
Reflection	Identifying the main emotional themes contained in a communication and directing these back to the client
Focusing	Asking goal-directed questions to help the client focus on key concerns
Encouraging elaboration	Helping the client to describe more fully the concerns or problems under discussion
Seeking clarification	Helping the client put into words unclear thoughts or ideas
Giving information	Sharing with the client relevant information for his or her healthcare and well-being
Looking at alternatives	Helping the client see options and participate in the decision-making process related to his or her healthcare and well-being
Silence	Allowing for a pause in communication that permits nurse and client time to think about what has taken place
Summarizing	Highlighting the important points of a conversation by condensing what was said

DISPLAY 21-4

🔄 GUIDELINES FOR FACILITATING COMMUNICATION

- Speak in a normal tone.
- Do not raise your voice or shout.
- Realize that speaking louder does not increase comprehension.
- Speak to the client on an adult level.
- Remember that impaired communication does not indicate impaired intelligence.
- Avoid carrying on more than one conversation at a time.
- Ask simple questions that require simple answers.
- Keep the atmosphere quiet and relaxed.
- Reduce or eliminate environmental noises.
- Make sure you have the client's attention before you speak.
- Maintain eye contact with the client throughout the conversation.
- Assume clients can understand you. Do not discuss their cases or other inappropriate topics in front of them.
- Do not rush the client. Give the client adequate time to respond.
- Do not correct mistakes.
- If you do not understand, ask the client to repeat what he or she said.
- Praise clients for their attempts at speech.

newspaper reporters and schoolteachers ask "why" questions. For example, asking clients why they are upset is more threatening than just noting that they seem to be upset.

Active Listening

Nurses often underestimate the value of listening and the skills needed to listen well (Gibbons, 1993). Listening actively involves the ability to focus on the client and what the client's messages are about, conveying back to the client an accurate picture of what he or she is expressing.

Active listening also involves constant decoding of the content and feeling of the messages sent by the listener. The content part of the message includes thoughts, words, opinions, and ideas. The feeling part refers to the client's emotions. Emotions may be described verbally, but usually they are manifested more accurately through nonverbal means such as facial expression, body posture, laughter, or crying. Note congruence or incongruence among these messages to help understand how clients are experiencing the things they are discussing.

Also observe what is behind the message sent by the client. For example, is the client conveying an attitude of helplessness, rejection, or aggression toward the nurse?

While decoding the conversation, listen actively by using two important techniques: restatement and reflection. These key techniques are used to help a client feel listened to and understood.

Restatement. **Restatement** refers mainly to the content portion of the communication. After listening carefully to the client, repeat the content of the message back to the client, to verify understanding with the client. When the content is restated, the client has the opportunity to hear himself or herself and to gain understanding of his or her own communication.

Reflection. **Reflection** means identifying the main emotional themes contained in a communication and directing them back to the client. The purpose is to verify and check the feelings that are being heard. Listen for the underlying feeling that a client is conveying; then repeat this understanding in a neutral, open manner. With this technique, the client gains a clearer understanding of the feelings he or she is experiencing.

These two techniques do not involve exact repetition of the client's statements. Rather, the nurse picks up on the content or feeling, rephrases it, and then states it back to the client. The following example shows how these techniques might be used in an informal therapeutic relationship:

> *Client:* I can't sleep. It's too hot in here and the noise is bothering me.
> *Nurse:* You can't sleep because it's uncomfortable in here. *(Restatement.)*
> *Client:* That's right. All I can think about is having that operation in the morning. *(Sounds irritable, looks anxious.)*
> *Nurse:* The thought of having surgery is keeping you awake. *(Reflection.)*
> *Client:* Yes. I'm really scared.

In this situation, the nurse listened carefully and found that it was not really the environment but the anxiety about having surgery that was keeping the client awake. By communicating back to the client in a careful way the things being heard, the nurse opened up an opportunity to clarify concerns and misperceptions about the impending surgery.

Exploring

Exploring is a way of communicating therapeutically without giving direct advice. Instead, the nurse helps clients express their concerns and solve their own problems by investigating the situation, how the client feels about it, and what some alternatives might be.

Focusing. Focusing involves asking goal-directed questions to help the client stay on the topic and talk more about it. The questions, still open-ended, are directed toward the client's key concerns. An example of focusing is, "We were talking about how people will respond to your mastectomy. Can you say more about that?"

Asking focused questions helps the client discuss the main issues of concern. It keeps the conversation on target without changing the subject or becoming too generalized, conveying the message that the nurse will stay with the client and help explore concerns.

Sometimes, helping a client express things of importance can be frightening. The nurse encounters a variety of suffering when working with ill and dying clients. To be therapeutic, maturity and a sense of perspective about life, which takes time and experience, are crucial.

Encouraging Elaboration. Encouraging elaboration is a technique used to help the client describe more fully the concerns or problems being discussed. Nodding one's head, using an attentive demeanor, and making comments such as "Go on" or "I see" encourages the client to keep talking and express himself or herself more thoroughly. This provides additional information about the client's emotional state, coping abilities, and view of the situation.

Seeking Clarification. Seeking clarification means helping the client put into words unclear thoughts or ideas. It can also be used to clarify events by putting them in a time sequence. Examples include, "I'm not sure I understand what you mean," "What else happened?" and "What happened then?" Such questions help the client to order his or her thoughts, put events into context, and place things in a more manageable perspective. By clarifying the problem or event being discussed, the client gains new insight into his or her situation.

Giving Information. Giving information involves sharing information about the client's health and well-being in a timely manner and based on what is currently known about the client's condition. Giving information can mean sharing what is known about a client's illness, treatment, and recovery. It can also mean correcting misperceptions.

For example, a young woman is brought to the emergency room after being raped. After medical care has been completed, police reports filled out, and her family notified, the nurse sits with the client for a few minutes while she waits for a family member to come. The client says, "I should have been more careful. I was wearing a short skirt. Maybe that caused the rape." Based on what the nurse knows about rape victims' perceptions, a timely intervention might be for the nurse to say, "When people are raped, it is usual for them to look for the cause within themselves. But the rape is not your fault. You are the victim in this situation." This information is based on research showing that rape victims commonly assume that they provoked the rape. In addition to giving this information, the nurse might also refer the client to a rape counseling center in the community.

Giving information is a skill commonly used in health teaching, often done while giving physical care. Information must be distinguished from suggestions or advice. A typical way to give advice is to start by saying, "Why don't you . . .?" or "You should. . . ." Such advice-giving reinforces the client's dependence on the nurse. A more useful strategy is giving the information the client needs to be able to make a decision.

Looking at Alternatives. Looking at alternatives means exploring options for the client's consideration. When more options are identified, the client's perceived choices are increased (Fig. 21-3). The nurse does not always need to present the alternatives; the client can be asked for them instead. Examples of questions to use are as follows:

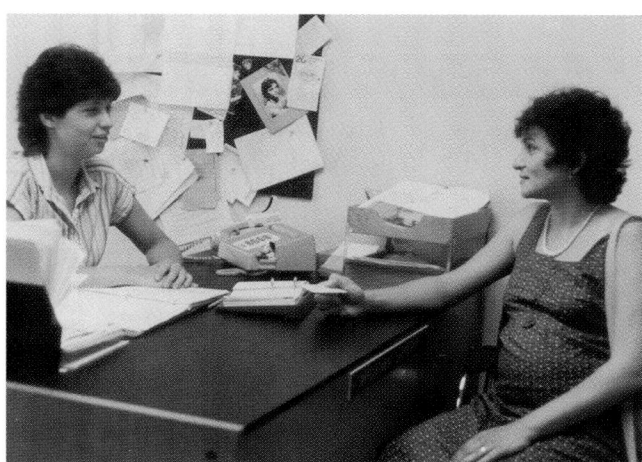

FIGURE 21-3 Assisting the client to examine alternatives increases the client's perceived choices.

- What are some of your ideas about how to handle this?
- Have you thought about [alternative courses of action]?
- What else could you do?
- If you met someone in the same situation as you, what would you advise him or her to do?
- What are some advantages (or disadvantages) of the alternatives we have just discussed?

Alternatives should not be discussed too early or before the client has a clear understanding of the current situation. Sometimes, a client must first express feelings such as grief or anger before he or she can explore how to deal with the situation.

Using Silence. Another useful therapeutic technique is using silence, a pause in communication that allows the nurse and client to reflect on what has taken place. By waiting quietly and attentively, the nurse encourages the client to initiate and maintain conversation. Silence is sometimes difficult for nurses who are used to more active forms of communicating. However, it is important to recognize when silence is appropriate.

Summarizing. Summarizing means highlighting the important points of a conversation by condensing what has been said. This is useful toward the end of a therapeutic conversation. Summarizing helps both nurse and client review the main themes of the conversation and gives a sense of closure. It also enables the nurse and client to think about what else needs to be considered or discussed in the future. It emphasizes the progress made toward self-understanding and problem solving. Examples of summarizing include, "Today, it seems that you've thought about . . ." and "Let's review what we've talked about today."

Developing Communication Skills

Communication between nurse and client in the clinical setting is based on client needs, not on personal or social interests. When the nurse has a professional approach and is client

centered, a focus on the client's health and well-being is maintained.

Time and experience are needed to become skilled at using therapeutic communication. One way to develop this skill is to study one's interactions, either by tape recording a therapeutic conversation (after obtaining the client's permission) or by recreating the conversation from memory. After making a transcript of the conversation, analyze it by reviewing the techniques used, their timing and appropriateness, and how the client responded to the nurse. The nurse's own thoughts and feelings also are noted, because these affect how he or she responds to the client. An example of how to use a process recording to enhance communication skills is shown in Table 21-4.

Nontherapeutic Responses

Nontherapeutic responses interfere with or block therapeutic communication. Often, such responses are the more natural responses that people make in social situations. Nontherapeutic responses may prevent nurses from functioning as professionals and therapeutic agents in the care of clients.

Nurses must meet their own needs outside the therapeutic context. For example, some nurses might become overly involved with clients because they have not developed social lives in ways that meet their needs. Other nurses might be uncomfortable with clients who express feelings because they have never been able to express their own. Engage in self-evaluation to determine your own strengths and weaknesses.

Inexperienced healthcare workers may believe that serious problems can be solved easily. On television, dire problems are solved in half an hour, but in real life this is not always the case. Presenting quick solutions and unwarranted cheerfulness blocks the therapeutic process. Some people have terminal illnesses. Others must adapt to situations for which there are no quick or simple answers. Through experience, nurses learn that they can help but cannot always provide perfect solutions. Maintain a supportive presence and provide competent care while clients struggle with their difficulties.

Rescue Feelings. Rescue feelings occur when a nurse feels essential to the client's welfare. The nurse thinks that he or she has exceptional abilities to help the client, and the nurse's expectations for the client will be high.

Some rescue feelings are useful, because having confidence in one's ability to be helpful is part of being therapeutic. Strong rescue feelings, however, impede the therapeutic process. The nurse may believe that only he or she can meet the client's needs, alienating himself or herself from the healthcare team. The nurse may also raise the client's expectations too high. When these expectations are not met, the client is disappointed.

False Reassurance. False reassurance means giving reassurance that is not based on the real situation. It is a way of minimizing the client's situation. For example, saying, "Don't worry, everything will be fine," minimizes the client's concerns. Other forms of false reassurance include telling a

TABLE 21-4

How to Use a Process Recording to Enhance Communication Skills

The purpose of a process recording is to help the nurse analyze verbal and nonverbal communication with clients with the goal of identifying helpful techniques and areas for improvement. Consider the following situation: *The client is a 35-year-old man who sustained burns on his face and upper body due to a car accident. He was transferred from the burn unit to the rehabilitation unit 2 days ago.*

Verbal and Nonverbal Interaction	Analysis
Less Effective	
Nurse: How are you doing today? *(Standing next to door.)*	Open-ended question invites response, but nonverbal communication (i.e., standing near door) indicates nurse may be busy and needs to move on.
Client: It's been a rough 2 days.	Client makes a general statement.
Nurse: Do you need any pain medication?	Nurse makes assumption that client is referring to physical discomfort. Nurse's question is narrowly focused and limits client's options in responding.
Client: No, I think I'm OK for now. *(Looks down at floor.)*	
Nurse: Well, let me know if you need anything.	Nurse ends interaction without exploring other reasons for client's distress.
Client: OK, thanks.	Client does not feel invited to discuss what is really bothering him.
More Effective	
Nurse: When I left you yesterday things weren't going very well for you.	Opening remark establishes that nurse remembers events from previous day. Indicates working phase of relationship.
How are you doing today? *(Nurse sits down, facing client.)*	Open-ended question helps client get started. Nurse offers self.
Client: It's been a rough 2 days.	Client makes a general statement.
[SILENCE]	Nurse allows silence so client can collect his thoughts.
Client: I've come to the realization that I'm not going to look the same as I did . . .	Client begins to clarify what he means.
Nurse: . . . and . . . ? *(Remains attentive.)*	Encouraging elaboration.
Client: It's hard. *(Becomes tearful.)*	Client showing feelings nonverbally.
Nurse: *(Gently)* It is upsetting to deal with the after-effects of your burns.	Reflection. The nurse reflects the client's feelings so he can own them.
Client: I shouldn't cry. *(Appears embarrassed.)*	Nurse assesses that client's past experiences and personal history have led him to the conclusion that men should not cry.
Nurse: You think men shouldn't cry when they have a really difficult adjustment to make?	Reflection of metacommunication (embarrassment about crying). The nurse shows the client what he feels about his feelings.
Client: *(Laughs slightly.)* I guess it's okay for me to cry. My situation isn't easy to deal with.	The client gains understanding of his feelings and his metacommunication.
[SILENCE]	
Client: *(Looks sad. Remains thoughtful.)*	
Nurse: Some of what you are experiencing is a natural grieving process that people in your situation go through. You have lost part of your former self, and that is a painful experience.	Giving information. The nurse, experienced and well read in the rehabilitation of burn clients, shares this information in a timely manner. The nurse realizes there is no easy solution for this client's problem. She provides support.

Table developed by Laina Gerace, PhD, RN, Associate Professor, University of Illinois at Chicago, College of Nursing.

client not to dwell on his or her problems and saying that an injection will not hurt. Although the intention of such comments is to reassure the client, they actually serve to diminish trust in the professional.

Real reassurance must be based on fact. For example, telling a client that there will be postoperative pain and how it will be controlled is much more reassuring than saying, "There's nothing to this operation. We do it all the time." A procedure may seem routine to the nurse, but to the client it is a major event. The client will feel much more supported if allowed to express anxiety and ask questions.

Giving false reassurance violates the client's trust. If the nurse tells a client not to worry when the client actually is worried, or that something does not hurt when it does hurt, how can the client have confidence in the nurse? Instead, supply any needed information and give reassurances based on actuality.

Giving Advice. Giving advice is another common nontherapeutic response. Giving advice focuses exclusively on the nurse's experiences and opinions. Examples of giving advice include statements that begin, "I think you should . . . ," "Why don't you . . . ," and "The same thing happened to me and I. . . ." Giving advice diminishes the client's responsibilities and choices and tends to be controlling. Clients may believe they must do what the nurse says, even though the advice might not work well for them.

Giving advice is different from giving a suggestion, an alternative idea for the client's consideration. If carefully done, giving a suggestion increases the client's perceived options. Usually, however, it is better if the client comes up with his or her own ideas. A helpful way to give a suggestion is to frame it tentatively, such as, "I wonder if you have thought about [an alternative course of action]."

Changing the Subject. Changing the subject is a nontherapeutic response that usually indicates anxiety on the nurse's part. It is a way of resisting hearing about a client's distress, sadness, and difficulties. Changing the subject might be an attempt to cheer the client up or to distract the client from painful thoughts. However, changing the subject can be a way to avoid listening to what the client has to say.

Being Moralistic. Being moralistic means seeing a situation as good or bad, or right or wrong. It is a judgmental approach. The nurse must become aware of how he or she uses the word "should." Talking to clients in terms of "shoulds" infers a preconceived idea about the "right" thing to do. For instance, saying to an unwed mother, "I think you should keep the baby," is being moralistic. Many factors go into making a decision of this magnitude. What works for one person might not work for another.

Another way of being moralistic is to give approval or disapproval by judging the client's actions as good or bad. Everyone has moral attitudes, and being moral is part of being human. Nurses have a right to their own values. However, in the clinical situation, they must transcend them and view their clients in more objective terms.

Nonprofessional Involvement. Nonprofessional involvement means being overly social or trying to be the client's friend or buddy (Burgess, 1990). Although appropriate at times (e.g., chatting briefly about the weather or a major news event), too much social chit-chat points to a nonprofessional relationship. Nurses who talk too much with clients about themselves and their own goals and problems are being nonprofessional. The purpose of a professional relationship is to meet the client's needs, not the nurse's. Self-disclosure, the act of revealing personal information within the context of a professional relationship, is rarely indicated and should be used judiciously.

Sexual misconduct is another example of nonprofessional involvement. Sexual misconduct occurs when the nurse initiates romantic or sexual interaction with a client or responds to a client in a flirtatious or sexual manner (Smith, Taylor, Keys, & Gornto, 1997). The nurse is responsible for defining and maintaining professional boundaries, even if the client behaves sexually toward the nurse.

Nontherapeutic involvement has pitfalls for both nurse and client. The client is receiving nursing care because of a need for professional services and wants to feel confident that a professional is in charge of nursing care. The nurse must maintain a professional attitude to remain objective in clinical decision making. Becoming a friend to the client abdicates the professional role.

Special Situations

Not all communication techniques are effective with all clients. Certain situations call for particular communication techniques or modifications depending on the client's developmental stage or environment.

Children and Adolescents. Children and adolescents present unique challenges to effective communication. Persons in these age groups are undergoing many changes that make clear communication more difficult.

Children are responsive to nonverbal communication, such as body movements, voice tone, and eye contact. Talking to children at eye level can help to minimize intimidation (Fig. 21-4). Speaking gently and calmly and using quiet body movements engenders greater trust.

When children first learn words, they sometimes have difficulty understanding what they mean. The way words are combined does not always convey the exact meaning intended. Clarify meanings with children until they can understand the message, using restatement and clarification. Consider the following example.

> *Child:* "Baby socks."
> *Nurse:* "You have little socks?"
> *Child: (No response.)*
> *Nurse:* "You have socks?"
> *Child: (Shakes head to indicate "no.")*
> *Nurse:* "You want your socks?"
> *Child: (Smiles and nods head to indicate "yes.")*

Young children are more attentive to simplified speech. Use language that children can understand. When speaking

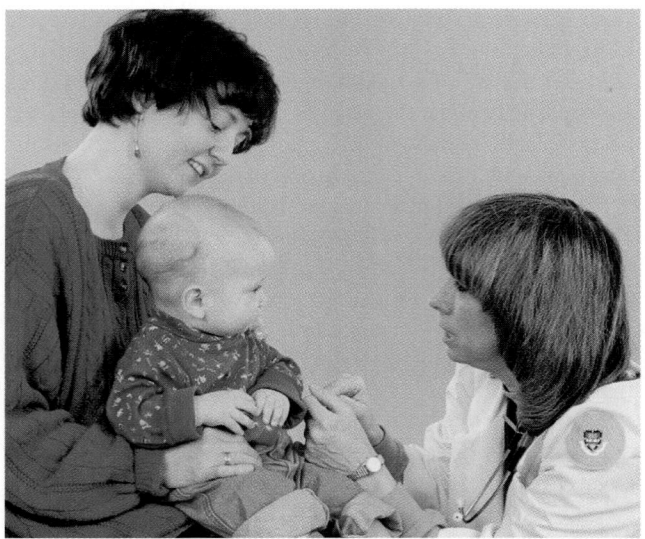

FIGURE 21-4 Communicating at eye level is important for all clients, even infants.

to children who do not respond, rephrase the communication. For example:

> *Nurse:* "It's time for your dinner now."
> *Child: (No response.)*
> *Nurse:* "Time to eat now."
> *Child: (Takes nurse's hand to go to dining area.)*

Use play to help children deal with the stress of hospitalization. For example, having children play with dolls representing physicians and nurses can help them act out their fears appropriately. By participating in such play, children can develop feelings of mastery over the situation. Many hospitals caring for young children provide structured play to help clients deal with their illnesses and treatments. By observing play, nurses can identify children's concerns.

Hospitalization for physical problems in this age group produces anxiety. Children and adolescents often feel embarrassed about their bodies and vulnerable to the control of adults. Therefore, be considerate of personal space, and do not be too intrusive. Use touch judiciously, and maintain modesty. Adolescents are particularly conscious of the need for privacy and modesty in communication situations with health professionals.

Provide information about procedures and treatments in a straightforward manner without giving false reassurance. For example, if a procedure might be painful, it is best to share this information in a matter-of-fact way.

To work effectively with children and adolescents, a sense of give and take is needed. Although the approach may be a little less formal than with adults, some professional distance is still maintained. Limit setting is a key factor in working effectively with children and adolescents. To set limits, the nurse must be seen as authoritative by the young client. Being authoritative means being in charge but permitting freedom within reasonable, closely established behavioral limits that elicit participation in their reinforcement. This is different

from being authoritarian, which means exerting power over another person.

Adults and Older Adults. Specifying communication strategies for any phase of development is difficult, and this is especially true for adulthood. Adulthood is an ongoing developmental period. As people grow and age, they must constantly adapt to many changes. Less is known about adulthood than about any other phase of development.

Hospitalization can create a period of transition in which adults question the progress of their lives, their goals, and even life's meaning. When illness disrupts their responsibilities, feelings of vulnerability may overwhelm them. Active, achieving adults may find it difficult to suddenly need assistance from nurses. Adults may sometimes behave in ways that are difficult to manage.

Nurses also may experience a range of feelings in relation to various adult clients. For example, an older male client may remind the nurse of his or her grandfather. The nurse may then relate to the client as if to the grandfather. Or the nurse may treat the client as if he were helpless and unable to make any decisions. If the client is a physician or a wealthy or well-known person, feelings of intimidation may arise on the nurse's part. Numerous complex situations come into play when communicating therapeutically with adults. Recognizing feelings and sharing them with fellow professionals is important because these feelings affect the way in which communication takes place.

For older adults, normal age-related changes further challenge communication skills. Age-related changes in hearing and vision often add barriers and additional obstacles to effective communication. Decreased hearing and impaired vision diminish the ability of some older adults to participate comfortably in some areas of communication. These clients may require additional communication skills to help them compensate for these changes.

Communication strategies with adults draw on all the concepts discussed in this chapter. The contractual approach provides an opportunity to establish with the client how communication will take place. For example, discuss whether to call an adult by his or her first or last name at the outset. Remember that all human beings, no matter what their job, social status, or income, at some point in their lives are vulnerable and suffer anxiety and worry. Use of therapeutic communication skills will facilitate expression and problem solving with any adult.

Cross-Cultural Communication. The population of the United States is becoming increasingly diverse. Nurses must be prepared to communicate with clients from a variety of cultural and ethnic groups. It is helpful if the nurse is aware of which ethnic groups live in the community and is familiar with common beliefs and practices of those groups related to healthcare, but this may be unrealistic in urban centers with multiple ethnic communities. Fortunately, there are numerous books, journals, and web-based resources to assist healthcare professionals to provide culturally competent care.

When working with clients who have limited English-speaking ability, it is important to remember that the client has a language barrier, not a hearing problem (unless one exists). Speak clearly and distinctly in a normal tone of voice, using hand motions, pictures, and demonstrations when appropriate. Even with the most careful efforts, misunderstandings may occur, and in healthcare it is particularly important to avoid them. Language interpreters should be used whenever possible. Skillful interpreters can provide insight into cultural meanings and nuances of the language and the related culture that may have a bearing on the client's healthcare needs. Family members, particularly children, should not be used as interpreters. Display 21-5 summarizes guidelines for working with language interpreters in health care settings.

The nurse should also be aware of cultural differences in nonverbal communication. For example, direct eye contact in some cultures is considered rude or threatening. Touching a client's head, except when clinically indicated, is prohibited in some cultures, as is touching a person of the opposite gender. Cultural norms may also determine which family members should be addressed and who makes decisions for the family. It is unrealistic to expect nurses to know the cultural beliefs and practices of all of the clients with whom they will work. However, sensitivity and a willingness to learn enhance the nurse's ability to communicate effectively in a variety of cultural contexts.

The Client in the Intensive Care Unit. The intensive care unit (ICU) is an environment designed to help maintain the lives of seriously ill clients. Unfamiliar sounds and noises, artificial lighting, and undefined colors characterize the ICU. Being admitted to the ICU is stressful. The client fears the di-

agnosis and the extent of the injury and may be unable to communicate. Communication is hindered further if the client does not know or understand the severity of the illness, feels a lack of control over what is happening, does not know the reason for therapies, receives care from several different providers, or loses contact with the outside world, including a sense of day and time.

Getting caught up in the complexities and technology of the ICU is easy. As a result, minimal communication may occur with the client. Be constantly aware that the client in this life-threatening situation is a person for whom communication is more important than ever. Even when the client cannot answer (because of decreased level of consciousness, intubation, or other reasons), assume that the client can hear. Talk to the client about what you are doing, just as you would with any other client. Nonverbal communication (e.g., touch, facial expressions) is especially meaningful for ICU clients.

To give cues about day and time, provide clocks and calendars where the client can see them. For clients who can use their hands but cannot speak, notepads or magic slates aid in communication. Call bells within easy reach help clients to communicate their needs.

Once the client has been stabilized, help the client understand the illness and the reason for various therapies. Explanations must be clear, direct, and simply stated. Because of the client's state, expect to repeat the explanations. If the client is able, discussing his or her perceptions and understanding enhances the client's sense of control and decreases stress.

KEY CONCEPTS

- Effective communication within the nurse–client relationship focuses on the client and the client's experiences and results in improved health status and well-being.
- Communication is a system of sending and receiving messages that forms a connection between the sender and the receiver.
- Verbal communication involves language; nonverbal communication includes gestures, facial expressions, body posture, body movement, voice tone, rate of speech, and dress.
- The elements of communication are the source (sender), the message, and the receiver; the processes are encoding, decoding, and feedback.
- The nurse–client relationship is focused on the client and is goal directed with defined parameters.
- The three phases in the nurse–client relationship are orientation, working, and termination.
- Empathy, positive regard, and a comfortable sense of self are among the key ingredients of the nurse–client relationship.
- The nurse–client relationship and therapeutic communication are instruments used to implement the nursing process.
- Skillful use of therapeutic responses is essential for accurate assessment and interventions.
- Nontherapeutic responses, such as rescue feelings, false reassurance, giving advice, changing the subject, being moralistic, and nonprofessional involvement, block communication.
- Communication techniques may need to be modified when dealing with children, adolescents, older adults, persons who speak a foreign language, or persons admitted to the ICU.

DISPLAY 21-5

GUIDELINES FOR INTERPRETER-DEPENDENT COMMUNICATION

- Take time to meet with the interpreter before meeting with the client.
- Allow sufficient time—working with an interpreter may take twice as long as a meeting in which a common language is spoken.
- Speak directly to the client.
- Speak in short sentences and allow the interpreter to interpret.
- Develop alternatives to direct questions.
- Avoid ambiguous language, abstractions, and technical jargon.
- Speak slowly and clearly; use repetition as needed.
- Be aware of nonverbal messages that may require interpretation just as verbal messages.
- Avoid using family members as interpreters.

Adapted from Kennedy, M. G. (1997). Cultural Competency. In N. K. Worley (Ed.). *Mental Health Nursing in the Community.* St. Louis: Mosby

REFERENCES

Berlo, D. K. (1960). *The process of communication: An introduction to therapy and practice.* New York: Holt, Rinehart & Winston.

Brandler, R., & Grinder, J. (1975). *The structure of magic: A book about language and therapy.* Palo Alto, CA: Science & Behavior Books.

Burgess, A. W. (1990). *Psychiatric nursing in the hospital and the community.* Englewood Cliffs, NJ: Appleton & Lange.

Campbell-Heider, N., & Hart, C. A. (1993). Updating the nurse's bedside manner [Comments]. *Image: Journal of Nursing Scholarship, 25*(2), 133–139; 25(4), 362–363.

Cravener, P. (1992). Establishing therapeutic alliance across cultural barriers. *Journal of Psychosocial Nursing and Mental Health Services, 30*(12), 10–14.

Crowther, D. J. (1991). Metacommunications: A missed opportunity? *Journal of Psychosocial Nursing and Mental Health Services, 29*(4), 13–16.

Fagin, C. M. (1992). Collaboration between nurses and physicians: No longer a choice. *Academic Medicine, 67*(5), 295–303.

Forchuk, C. (1992). The orientation phase of the nurse–client relationship: How long does it take? *Perspectives in Psychiatric Care, 28*(4), 7–10.

Gibbons, M. B. (1993). Listening to the lived experience of loss. *Pediatric Nursing, 19*(6), 597–599.

Kreider, N. A., & Haselton, B. J. (1997). *The systems challenge: Getting the clinical information support you need to improve patient care.* Chicago: American Hospital Publishing.

Morse, J. M., Anderson, G., Bottorff, J. L., et al. (1992). Exploring empathy: A conceptual fit for nursing practice? *Image: Journal of Nursing Scholarship, 24*(2), 273–280.

Murphy, K., & Clark, J. M. (1993). Nurses' experiences of caring for ethnic-minority clients. *Journal of Advanced Nursing, 18,* 442–450.

Peplau, H. E. (1997). *Interpersonal relations in nursing.* New York: G.P. Putnam's Sons.

Rogers, C. (1961). *On becoming a person.* Boston: Houghton Mifflin.

Smith, L. L., Taylor, B. B., Keys, A. T., & Gornto, S. B. (1997). Nurse-patient boundaries: Crossing the line. *American Journal of Nursing, 97,* 26–32.

Trojan, L., & Yonge, O. (1993). Developing trusting, caring relationships: Home care nurses and elderly clients. *Journal of Advanced Nursing, 18,* 1903–1910.

Williams, C. A. (1990). Biopsychosocial elements of empathy: A multidimensional model. *Issues in Mental Health Nursing, 11,* 155–174.

BIBLIOGRAPHY

Gallop, R. (1998). Abuse of power in the nurse–client relationship. *Nursing Standard, 12*(37), 43–47.

Loomis, M. (1985). Levels of contracting. *Journal of Psychosocial Nursing and Mental Health Services, 23*(3), 9–14.

Proctor, A., Morse, J. M., & Khonsari, E. S. (1996). Sounds of comfort in the trauma center: How nurses talk to patients in pain. *Social Science and Medicine, 42*(12), 1669–1680.

Reid-Ponte, P. (1992). Distress in cancer patients and primary nurses' empathy skills. *Cancer Nursing, 15*(4), 283–292.

Reisch, S. K., Tosi, C. B., Thurston, C. A., et al. (1993). Effects of communication training on parents and young adolescents. *Nursing Research, 42*(1), 10–16.

Roberto, K. A., Richter, J. M., Bottenberg, D. J., & Campbell, S. (1998). Communication patterns between caregivers and their spouses with Alzheimer's disease: A case study. *Archives of Psychiatric Nursing, 12*(4), 202–208.

Sherrell, K., & Buckwalter, K. C. (1998). Therapeutic approaches with the physically ill elderly: The value of listening, history, and personality. *Journal of Gerontological Nursing, 24*(1), 54–57.

Sundeen, S. J., Stuart, G. W., Rankin, E. A. D., & Cohen, S. A. (1998). *Nurse-Client Interaction: Implementing the Nursing Process.* St. Louis: Mosby.

Stuart, G. W. & Laraia, M. T. (2001). *Principles and practice of psychiatric nursing* (7th ed.). St. Louis: Mosby.

22 Client Education

🔲 Key Terms

affective
andragogy
cognitive
compliance
illiteracy
learning

motivation
noncompliance
pedagogy
psychomotor
return demonstration

🔲 Learning Objectives

Upon completion of this chapter, the student will be able to do the following:
1. Compare and contrast pedagogy with andragogy.
2. Describe important qualities of a teaching–learning relationship.
3. Explain the domains of knowledge and how learning relates to each.
4. Identify four purposes of client education.
5. Define factors that inhibit and facilitate learning.
6. Discuss important assessment data used to individualize client teaching.
7. Describe teaching methods and evaluation strategies.
8. Explain the abilities, needs, and motivations of different age groups as they pertain to learning.

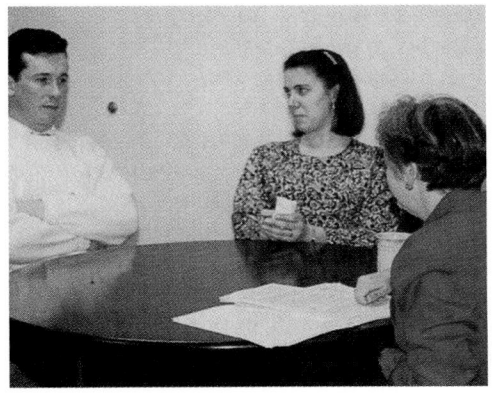

🔲 Critical Thinking Challenge

A woman, accompanied by her husband, comes to the clinic for a blood pressure check. As they enter the office, you hear the husband speaking rapidly in a foreign language. He appears upset. The wife does not respond but looks down and appears to withdraw. Because her blood pressure is elevated for the third consecutive visit, the physician decides to prescribe a blood pressure medication and a low-sodium diet. As the office nurse, you have 15 minutes to teach the couple about these topics.

Once you have completed this chapter and have incorporated client education into your knowledge base, review the above scenario, and reflect on the following areas of Critical Thinking:

1. Prioritize important assessment data to collect from the couple so you can individualize your teaching.
2. Describe factors that might hinder or facilitate the couple's learning.
3. Role play how you might individualize teaching, focusing on three realistic goals.
4. Identify how you will evaluate learning and use your findings to revise future teaching.

The well-known adage, "If you give a man a fish, you feed him for a day, but if you teach a man how to fish, you feed him for a lifetime," illustrates the importance of client education. The teaching–learning process empowers clients and usually enables them to achieve a higher level of wellness or to manage specific healthcare needs. Nurses frequently become primary teachers for clients and coordinate and reinforce information from other healthcare professionals.

Client education is integral to nursing practice. The American Hospital Association's Patient's Bill of Rights (first published in 1975, updated in 1992, and printed in Chapter 6) emphasizes that clients have not only the right to considerate, responsible care but also the right to receive current information on diagnosis, treatment, and prognosis (American Hospital Association, 1992). The American Nurses Association's Standards of Clinical Nursing Practice include "educating clients about their illness, treatment, health promotion, or self-care activities" (American Nurses Association, 1991) as a nursing responsibility for all clients. The Joint Commission on Accreditation of Healthcare Organizations (JCAHO) also has established standards for client education that healthcare agencies must meet to receive accreditation (JCAHO, 1995). Today, as the cost of healthcare is a continuing concern and clients are discharged from facilities more quickly, research has demonstrated the cost-effectiveness of client education.

Client teaching has always been a primary focus for nurses, regardless of the setting. School nurses talk with adolescents about contraception and safe sex practices. Industrial nurses conduct classes on plant safety. Clinic nurses discuss normal childhood development and age-appropriate activities with parents. Ambulatory surgical center nurses discuss postoperative care with clients before discharge. Public health nurses stress the importance of current immunizations to prevent the spread of illness.

Nurses can influence but cannot control their clients through education. Learning and changing behaviors are voluntary actions. Nurses can encourage clients to improve their health status, but no matter how important a nurse believes certain actions and attitudes to be, the choice is the client's.

Client education is seldom the formal process that most people experienced in school. Much client teaching occurs informally during nursing care. During any client care activity, a client or family member may ask questions. This curiosity indicates a degree of motivation that nurses must honor. At such times, client education can be extremely effective.

Client education consists of more than handouts, pamphlets, and videotapes. It requires a therapeutic relationship. Every time a nurse empowers a client toward autonomy and self-care, the client reflects some autonomy and power to the individual nurse and the nursing profession.

TEACHING–LEARNING PROCESS

Learning is the acquisition of a skill or knowledge by practice, study, or instruction. Learning theory has changed over the centuries. According to an early, teacher-centered theory, learning required a disciplined mind, and the goal was to memorize many facts. Later, student-centered theorists believed that learning could be completely intuitive; by encouraging self-direction, an active unfolding of knowledge would occur. Still others claimed that learning must build on prior knowledge and experience, with the teacher actively imparting new ideas and the learner passively associating them with related ideas to grasp principles. Different conceptual models of the learning process also viewed the teacher's role differently, conceptualizing the teacher as director, designer, or programmer.

Nursing students have experienced all these theories at work. For example, to learn anatomy, one must memorize facts. Dealing with people, especially clients, always requires an intuitive component. Pharmacology builds on the student's previous knowledge of pathophysiology, chemistry, anatomy, physiology, and mathematics.

Approaches to Learning

Early research on teaching and learning was conducted in American classrooms, usually studying the learning process of children or adolescents. A more complete understanding of learning evolved as researchers studied how adults learn. The term **pedagogy** is used to describe the approaches and assumptions about teaching as it usually applies to children or adolescent learners. The word **andragogy**, first coined by Knowles (1990), refers to his adult learning theory. Table 22-1 illustrates some differences between pedagogic and andragogic learning.

Pedagogy

The study of traditional classroom instruction of children focuses on the teacher's role in ensuring that learning occurs. The teacher determines what to teach and the methods that will promote learning. The teacher is responsible for motivating students to learn and for directing the process. The student's biologic and academic development also influence the amount of learning that will occur. This conceptual picture of learning is one in which the teacher is in control and the learner passively participates.

Andragogy

Knowles' theory of adult learning (1990) differs significantly from the passive pedagogic approach. Knowles viewed adult learning as based on the individual's need to know something, which is often influenced by a developmental task or a social role. The adult view of self often includes assuming personal responsibility for decision making and valuing independence. Rich life experiences assist in future learning for adults. Andragogy assumes that adults learn better when learning directly relates to their lives or to problems they anticipate. Andragogy focuses teaching on the client's needs and personal goals.

Information Processing

Much research is being conducted to better understand how learning occurs. One such model concludes that learning involves a sophisticated method of information processing.

TABLE 22-1

Pedagogic Versus Andragogic Learning		
Assumptions About Learning	**Pedagogy**	**Andragogy**
Need to know	Teacher establishes what learner needs to know.	Teaching relates to learners' needs.
Self-concept	Learner accepts direction from teacher.	Learner's need for self-direction increases.
Role of experience	Process happens to learner.	Experience is integrally involved with self-concept, which others must acknowledge.
Readiness to learn	Biologic and academic development set learning parameters.	Evolving social and life roles set parameters.
Orientation to learning	Teacher selects logic and system.	Orientation is life-centered or task- and problem-centered.
Motivation	Learner's motivation is external and based on teacher's approval.	Learner's motivation is based on internal drives and life goals.

Adapted from Knowles, M. (1990). *The adult learner: A neglected species.* Houston, TX: Gulf Publishing Co.

This model begins with a sensory register, which determines whether the brain notes or registers an internal or external stimulus. Once registered, this information is stored in short-term memory, which is limited to five to seven thoughts at a time (Babcock & Miller, 1994). Thus, the amount of data that can be processed at any one time is limited.

While an idea is in short-term memory, it is encoded by such factors as meaning, importance, or novelty so that transfer to long-term memory can occur. The human brain is thought to store outlines of encoded information as electrochemical deposits. When these deposits are stimulated, changes occur that can be reconstructed into memories. The more these pathways are accessed, the more stable the connection becomes and the more readily the memory can be retrieved (Babcock & Miller, 1994). Repetition in learning helps ensure that the memory is stored and can be retrieved more easily.

Domains of Knowledge

Knowledge can be acquired in three different domains: cognitive, affective, and psychomotor learning (Bloom, 1956). Frequently, learning does not occur in one domain alone but encompasses all three.

Cognitive

The word **cognitive** refers to rational thought, what one generally considers "thinking." Cognitive learning may involve learning facts, reaching conclusions, making decisions, or inferring. Nurses frequently participate in teaching–learning experiences in which clients assimilate new information to promote optimal wellness. During a cognitive teaching session, moving from the simple to the complex is likely to yield the best results. Ideally, nurses start with basic facts and concepts and then discuss how they are related. Finally, clients learn to apply the material correctly in various situations.

Teaching a new mother the anatomy and physiology of the breast and its role in breast-feeding is an example of cognitive learning. When the mother understands the physiology of her milk supply, the let-down reflex, and the way these two factors work together, the client has demonstrated her cognitive knowledge.

Affective

Affective refers to emotions or feelings. Affective learning changes beliefs, attitudes, or values. Sensitivity and emotional climate influence all types of learning but are especially important in the affective domain. Affective learning is more difficult to measure than cognitive or psychomotor learning because it focuses on thoughts and feelings. An example of affective learning is helping a new mother explore the possible benefits of breast-feeding for the health of her baby.

Psychomotor

Psychomotor refers to the muscular movements that result from some sorts of knowledge. Learning in this domain often means mastering a new task or skill. This type of knowledge is easiest to measure because it can be physically demonstrated. Teaching a new mother to breast-feed is an example of psychomotor learning. When the mother can successfully and independently breast-feed her infant to the physical satisfaction of both, she has demonstrated psychomotor learning.

Nurses are frequently responsible for teaching clients to perform certain skills independently (e.g., effective handwashing, good body mechanics). Nurses teach principles and demonstrate skills; clients practice these skills; nurses answer any questions and identify further resources. In a **return demonstration,** the nurse observes the client performing the new skill; this tool is valuable for evaluating psychomotor learning.

Qualities of a Teaching–Learning Relationship

In nursing, the relationship between teacher and learner is special, characterized by mutual sharing, advocacy, and negotiation. Unlike some traditional views, nurses are not experts who generously bestow knowledge upon clients, nor do nurses barter knowledge for compliance. Both images represent the relationship as a power imbalance in which nurses, because of their knowledge and expertise, control the situation. Effective learning occurs when clients and healthcare professionals are equal participants in the teaching–learning process. At times, teaching must be delayed until clients desire to participate actively. Positive qualities that characterize the teaching relationship include client focus, negotiation, holism, and interaction.

Client Focus
Client education is a therapeutic relationship that should focus on the client's specific needs. Clients are living with whatever health issue necessitated treatment or involvement with the healthcare system. Clients also have unique values, beliefs, cognitive abilities, and learning styles that affect learning. Allowing clients to share enables nurses to better understand this uniqueness and to individualize teaching to the client's needs.

Holism
The teaching–learning relationship should consider the whole person, rather than focusing on the specific content. Assessment data permit nurses to determine the "big picture," which provides broad contextual meaning. Nurses also use their own experiential knowledge. For example, a nurse teaching insulin injections to a client newly diagnosed with diabetes anticipates problems or questions based on those that past clients have had; thus, the nurse anticipates the impact of diabetes on all areas of functioning.

Negotiation
Together, nurses and clients determine what is already known and what is important to learn. They can then develop a plan with input from both parties. Sometimes, negotiation is a more formalized process with a written contract that guides the learning experience. More often, the process is informal and ongoing with continual checking and validating to guide the learning process.

Interactive
The teaching–learning relationship is a dynamic, interactive process that involves active participation from nurse and client. Nurses learn from clients, and clients learn from nurses

as they discuss content, clarify and revisit specific points, or determine new needs. This interactive, nonlinear model differs from the simplistic model that many texts describe: presentation of content, learning, and evaluation of learning.

PURPOSES OF CLIENT EDUCATION

Nurses are involved in client education to promote wellness, prevent illness, restore optimal health and function if illness has occurred, and assist clients and families to cope with alterations in health status. Such teaching encompasses all areas of function, as reflected in Table 22-2.

Wellness Promotion

Focus on health promotion has gained much momentum in recent decades. Nurses, regardless of their practice arena, are involved in client education to promote optimum health and function. Knowledge and values are important when determining choices people make daily. Such things as food, rest, coping abilities, and hygiene and safety practices may influence optimal wellness. People may lack the motivation to change comfortable, unhealthy habits when they are feeling well. Nurses often aim health promotion at young people to prevent bad habits from developing.

The transtheoretical model (or stages of change model) is based on the belief that most people experience similar stages as they attempt to change health behavior over time (Table 22-3). Previously, theorists believed that a person progressed through these stages in a linear fashion, but now they accept that progression is nonlinear and that relapse is expected (McKenzie & Smeltzer, 1997).

Disease Prevention

Client education also focuses on teaching clients the knowledge and skills for early detection or prevention of disease and disability. As research increases, the understanding of risk factors for disease improves. For example, studies have recently improved understanding of the link between some types of cancer and a high-fat diet. This knowledge enables nurses to focus on dietary teaching to help decrease cancer risk. Studies also have proven the importance of early detection and support the teaching of regular testicular or breast self-examination. Research has better identified people at risk for specific illnesses, so resources and teaching programs can be directed at high-risk groups.

Restoration of Health or Function

When illness or dysfunction occurs, client education is important to help limit disability or restore function. In the home, community, and rehabilitation center, much teaching focuses on helping people deal with chronic health problems such as heart disease or diabetes (Fig. 22-1). In the acute care facility, teaching also focuses on restoring health. Clients who are

TABLE 22-2

Examples of Client Teaching for Functional Areas	
Health Pattern	**Example of Possible Teaching**
Health perception/ health management	Breast self-examination, importance of regular physical examinations and immunizations
Activity/exercise	Importance of regular exercise, how to use ambulation devices (e.g., crutches, walker), deep breathing and coughing, leg exercises
Nutrition/metabolic	Healthy diet, dietary restrictions, wound care, how to monitor temperature, total parenteral nutrition at home
Elimination	How to maintain regular bowel function, Kegel exercises to decrease stress incontinence, self-catheterization
Cognitive/perceptual	Pain management (e.g., how to use client-controlled analgesia), how to use memory aids, importance of regular eye and ear examinations
Sleep/rest	Importance of getting adequate rest, aids to promote sleep
Self-concept	Normal body changes, methods of promoting self-esteem
Role/relationship	Assertiveness training, parenting classes
Coping/stress	Biofeedback, relaxation techniques
Sexuality	Prenatal classes, contraception
Values and beliefs	Client's rights, "do not resuscitate" options

admitted for surgery receive instruction during the preoperative and postoperative periods to help prevent complications and to ensure optimal recovery. In the ambulatory care setting, nurses explain medications or diagnostic procedures to clients to reduce anxiety and to assist them in making informed healthcare decisions. Other important client teaching opportunities occur during admission and before discharge (Table 22-4).

Promotion of Coping

Client education is important for individuals and families who must cope with new and frightening procedures or adjust and continue to live with chronic illness or disability. Teaching before surgery or a diagnostic procedure improves coping by minimizing what is unknown and can lessen postoperative anxiety (Brouphy, 2001). Adjusting to loss of function can be difficult for clients and their families. Teaching may assist people to adapt to using new devices (e.g., walker to assist with ambulation) or altering diet or activity. Some teaching assists with changes in body image or role expectations. Teaching may be necessary to prepare caregivers for the technical and psychological challenges of caring for loved ones who have impaired function. Client education also

is important for helping clients and families deal with grief, loss, and eventual death.

ASSESSMENT FOR LEARNING

Assessing Learning Needs

The educational assessment begins with determining what the client needs to know or do to function more independently. New knowledge or skill acquisition may need to occur before a client leaves a clinic or is discharged from the hospital or home care. For example, parents must demonstrate the ability to feed their infant with a new feeding tube before the infant can be discharged to their rural home.

Baseline Knowledge

Many times, clients articulate specifically what learning is important to them and why. Other times, requests for knowledge are less direct. For example, a client may say, "I'm just not sure about all these new medications." Compare the client's knowledge, attitudes, and skills with those necessary for independent functioning. "Tell me what you know about (relevant topic)" is a useful opener. Finding out about previous client-education experiences may give some indication about where to begin.

TABLE 22-3

Stages of Change	
Stages	**Timeframe**
Precontemplation	Not thinking about change in the next 6 months
Contemplation	Seriously thinking about change in the next 6 months
Preparation	Actively planning change
Action	Overtly making changes
Maintenance	Taking steps to sustain change and resist temptation to relapse

TABLE 22-4

Important Teaching Opportunities	
Opportunity	**Possible Learning Need**
Admission	Unit policies, how to work call light and bed, specific treatments that have been ordered and why
New medication	Action of drug, possible side effects, frequency, and any special considerations
Diagnostic procedure	Preparation that is necessary, what will be experienced during procedure, any restrictions or special considerations after procedure
Surgery	Preoperative preparation, postoperative protocols (e.g., deep breathing, leg exercises), pain control, how to get out of bed and turn easily
Discharge	Limitations on activity or diet, procedures such as wound care, when to call the physician

Cultural and Language Needs

Religion, health beliefs, language, and sex-role beliefs are important factors to consider when planning client education. Cultural norms can influence a client's beliefs about what constitutes illness and personal responsibility; it is imperative that the nurse understand this to provide the best care possible (Daddy & Clegg, 2001). Assess the client's beliefs and ability to understand and speak English for effective teaching and learning. Not all groups share certain "mainstream" healthcare norms and values. For instance, Jehovah's Witnesses do not accept blood transfusions, most Islamic sects do not donate or receive organs, and many Native American and Chinese people practice and trust folk medicine beliefs. People who do not speak English require an interpreter.

If a client from a different culture needs to be educated about nutrition, a registered dietitian may be able to help. Registered dietitians often are familiar with cultural food beliefs and can tailor a plan for individual clients' needs. In many cultures, women are the only ones to prepare food or care for the sick. Therefore, identify and include these women in any dietary or health teaching for male clients.

Priorities

Clients usually have many learning needs, so nurses must set priorities to help ensure that teaching will be effective. Priority setting may result in teaching clients basic skills in the hospital and arranging home nursing visits for follow-up teaching. Because time is usually the scarcest resource, assessment and priority setting should start early in the client–nurse interaction, whether in a clinic, a school, or an acute care facility.

Ask clients to identify their learning needs. Clients may perceive learning needs when they wish to learn more to maintain or promote health or to fix a perceived problem that has occurred. For example, a routine physical examination may reveal an elevated cholesterol concentration. This information can increase a client's need and desire to learn about lifestyle changes that can prevent heart disease. Teaching should occur when learning is a high priority for the client. Sometimes, the perceived need for health teaching comes from a client's per-

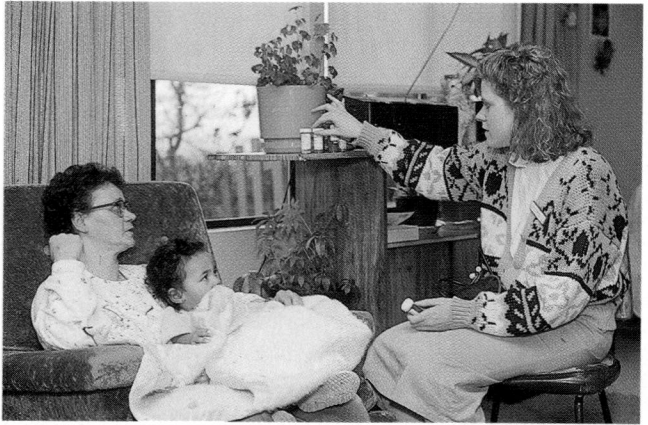

FIGURE 22-1   The nurse teaches the client about medications so that the client can manage many chronic health problems. (Photo courtesy of Seattle University, School of Nursing.)

sonal reflection (e.g., a desire to exercise more and lose weight after the holidays).

In many situations, nurses also share with clients aspects that they believe are important to include in the teaching plan. For example, after listening to a client who comes to the clinic for treatment of a urinary tract infection, the nurse shares that it might be helpful to learn how to prevent future infections and provides information about the medication that was just ordered.

Realistic Approach

Nurses who take a realistic approach set priorities and try not to teach too much in any one teaching session. Consider the following:

* *The client's energy level:* Physical weakness and fatigue can affect attention span and decrease learning.
* *The client's age:* Educational goals for children, adolescents, and adults differ, and clients require different teaching styles at different ages.
* *The client's emotional state:* Clients may be too anxious or depressed to learn. It is not uncommon for those who have received a new diagnosis, suffered a loss, or experienced trauma to have difficulty learning.

Assessing Learning Readiness

Motivation

Motivation provides drive or incentive. This powerful determinant of success in client education is closely related to compliance or adherence to a treatment plan. Motivation for learning starts with the client's recognition of the need to know. Financial problems, inconvenience, denial, lack of social support, nonacceptance of the disease, anxiety, fear, shame, and negative self-concept can affect motivation. Motivation can also change daily. Some clients are less motivated to learn ways to maintain optimum health independently if they derive important secondary gains from the "sick role." Attitudes and beliefs also influence motivation. For instance, a middle-aged man who has started antihypertensive medications to control blood pressure may be less motivated to learn about them if a close friend confides that he became impotent when he took a similar medication.

Motivation is sometimes difficult to assess. There may be verbal cues (e.g., a client who says, "My wife takes care of all that") or nonverbal cues (lack of attention, missed appointments) that point to decreased motivation to learn. When assessing motivation, learn what a client values. Clients who associate healthcare goals with something they already value will probably be more motivated.

Compliance

Assessing the client's history of **compliance** or **noncompliance** (i.e., following or not following the recommended plan) is important. "What have you done in the past for your problem?" may yield different answers from clients and from their family members. Unless a written record is available, past compliance may be hard to assess. "People often find it hard to take blood pressure pills twice a day, every day. Has this ever been a problem for you?" is a useful lead when assessing compliance. Giving clients an agenda can be useful: "As I listen to you, it sounds like we need to talk about wound care and diet. What do you think?" Compliance is not just linked to inadequate knowledge. Many people decide not to follow conventional medical advice for a variety of reasons. This is often frustrating to nurses and other healthcare providers, but the choice to follow advice is the client's and must be respected.

Sensory and Physical State

The client's sensory abilities and physical state affect learning readiness, and the teaching plan must be modified accordingly. For example, clients with poor vision or compromised fine motor skill may be unable to give subcutaneous injections safely. Clients who receive pain medication postoperatively may have difficulty concentrating. A woman who has just given birth may be too tired to participate actively in the learning session.

Literacy Level

Illiteracy (inability to read or write) is found in every walk of life, among all races, and at all socioeconomic levels. A person's appearance and use of spoken language do not indicate his or her literacy. Many people with low literacy levels are of average intelligence and speak articulately. A roughly dressed laborer may be able to read well, but a professionally dressed person may be unable to read at a functional level. Educational level gives only a rough estimate of literacy.

The U.S. Department of Education estimates that as many as 90 million American adults have poor literacy skills and low ability to comprehend and retain information (Wilson, 2000). A correlation does not always exist between literacy and the number of grades completed in school. Many adults read three to five grade levels below the highest grade they completed in school. They may not understand written directions, videotapes, or even some audiotapes. Most client education materials are aimed at people who read at a high school level or above, so this material confuses a huge segment

---

🗉 APPLY YOUR KNOWLEDGE

Mrs. Babbitt, an 84-year-old woman with chronic heart problems, is being discharged with three new heart medications, a stool softener, and a PRN pain medication for her arthritis. She is very compliant, always patting your hand and saying, "Oh, you are so smart. I will try my best to follow all your instructions."

What additional information should you collect to individualize Mrs. Babbitt's teaching?

Describe some principles that might guide your teaching with Mrs. Babbitt.

How might you evaluate Mrs. Babbitt's learning?

Check your answer in Appendix A.

of the population who may be too ashamed to admit their inability to read and understand. Also, the ability to interpret clocks and calendars is not universal, and this can contribute to the inability to follow instructions and keep appointments (Vezeau & Oja, 1996).

Reading tests such as the Wide Range Achievement Test (WRAT) and Rapid Estimate at Adult Literacy in Medicine (REALM), which ask a person to read a passage out loud, can assess literacy. These tests evaluate the person's ability to pronounce words but do not assess comprehension. The Cloze tests may be given to clients who score higher than sixth grade level on the WRAT or REALM reading test. The Cloze test is a written test that measures reading comprehension and the appropriateness of specific educational material (Wilson, 2000).

Direct testing is the most accurate way to assess literacy, but it is often impractical in the clinical setting. Here are some less accurate, but expedient, methods:

- Check the level of the client's pleasure reading.
- Give the client something to read, and later ask for a description of the contents in his or her own words.
- If possible, offer the client several options for learning methods (reading, watching, or listening).

When in doubt, use lower literacy material. When teaching stressed people, it is better to start with simpler material and add complexity later.

NURSING DIAGNOSES

Diagnostic Statement: Deficient Knowledge

Definition. Absence or deficiency of cognitive information related to a specific topic (NANDA, 2001).

ETHICAL/LEGAL ISSUE
Literacy

The physician writes discharge orders for Mrs. Gonzales. They include a complex medication regimen and self-management of an indwelling catheter. Mrs. Gonzales speaks very little English. Her daughter is at work, and when you call for a translator, one is not available until tomorrow. You realize the physician will be upset if Mrs. Gonzales is not discharged today because her insurance coverage will not pay for a longer stay.

Reflection
- Legally, must you provide a translator for Mrs. Gonzales during the teaching session?
- Role play how you might respond to the upset physician in this situation.
- Brainstorm other alternatives to help provide Mrs. Gonzales with the teaching she requires for safe discharge.

Defining Characteristics. Defining characteristics include verbalization of the problem, inaccurate follow-through of instructions, inaccurate performance of tests, and inappropriate or exaggerated behaviors (e.g., hysterical, hostile, agitated, apathetic) (NANDA, 2001).

Related Factors. Many factors can contribute to a knowledge deficit, such as lack of exposure, lack of recall, information misinterpretation, cognitive limitations, lack of interest in learning, and unfamiliarity with information resources (NANDA, 2001).

OUTCOME IDENTIFICATION AND PLANNING

The planning phase of client education involves working with clients to develop a teaching plan, identifying appropriate teaching strategies, and developing a written plan to coordinate teaching among healthcare team members. Factors to consider in planning include the client's assessed learning need and motivation level, learning style preference, literacy level, inclusion of family member or support persons, timing, and the appropriate amount of information to cover.

Outcome Identification

Client-centered, client-involved goals are most effective. Including clients in the planning process helps show clearly what clients are willing or unwilling to do, clarifying goals.

Be brief and realistic when writing goals and outcome criteria. Do not promise overly optimistic outcomes. Create measurable goals with a time frame. A possible form for writing client outcomes is the following:

Who + Does + What + How + When = Goal

For example:

Client + will demonstrate + dressing change + without cueing + before discharge.

Evaluate and revise learning goals as necessary. If learning has been successful, new learning goals may be formulated. If outcomes have not been met, the time frame may be changed, or, based on additional assessment data, the outcomes may be revised.

Planning Teaching Strategies

Availability of resources, learning style preference, and literacy level affect planning of effective teaching strategies. Teaching sessions can be individual, small group, or large group sessions. One-to-one teaching can be individualized, so it is usually most effective, but it also is most expensive in terms of money and time.

Choosing the right strategy for client education can make the experience more enjoyable for both nurse and client. If possible, use a variety of strategies to enhance learning and retention. Combining modalities such as seeing, hearing, and touching promotes better learning than using only one modality.

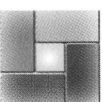

Nursing Research and Critical Thinking
What are the Best Methods of Preparing Clients for Surgery?

Less time for client care has greatly affected nursing practice. Time for preoperative teaching is usually very limited. The nurses in this study questioned, "What is the best method for providing people with the information they need during the limited time nurses have to teach them?" They wanted to examine the effects of a structured education program for clients undergoing ambulatory gynecologic surgery. They designed a relation-searching study with an experimental design. They compared clinical outcomes, length of time in the postanesthesia care unit (PACU), and client satisfaction using two different educational structures. Thirty female subjects who were scheduled for elective laparoscopic tubal ligation over a 9-month period were recruited into the study. The subjects were randomly assigned to a control group ($n = 15$), who received the customary informal unstructured instruction on the day of surgery, and an experimental group ($n = 15$), who received the customary information and a structured presurgical program that modeled adaptive behaviors and described sensations they would experience. On *t*-tests, repeated measures (ANOVA), and sign tests, no significant differences were found between the groups in preadmission and discharge pulse, respiratory rate, and blood pressure readings; incidence of nausea and vomiting and administration of antiemetics; or total length of stay in the PACU between the groups. No significant differences were found in client satisfaction with the education. The control group requested and received significantly more pain medication than did the experimental group ($P < .05$).

Critical Thinking Considerations. The sample size and the fact that all clients came from one medical center were limitations of this study. Generalization of the findings is therefore difficult. Possible implications are as follows:

- The study's clinical significance lies in the identification of a decrease in self-reported pain and requests for analgesics in the group that received the structured educational intervention.
- With positive clinical outcomes being a hallmark of healthcare, nursing interventions that enhance these outcomes need to be encouraged and facilitated.

From Franzen Coslow, B. I., & Eddy, M. E. (1998). Effects of preoperative ambulatory gynecological education: Clinical outcomes and patient satisfaction. *Journal of PeriAnesthesia Nursing 13*(1), 4–10.

Lectures

A lecture is a formal presentation of information by a teacher to a group of learners. This format is most effective when communicating facts (cognitive learning), but it can be used for psychomotor or affective learning. A simple lecture (a one-way communication from teacher to learner) is much more effective when combined with discussion. A lecture may stifle learners who are eager to contribute. Determine whether clients appear bored, anxious, or easily distracted.

Discussion

Discussion is an opportunity for clients to focus learning through exchange of ideas by sharing information, clarifying feelings, or asking questions. It can be useful with individual clients or groups. Discussion involves learners more deeply in the process because it requires participation. This strategy can enhance cognitive and affective learning.

Demonstration

Demonstrations are particularly useful for psychomotor learning. Explaining a skill while slowly demonstrating it leads to talking clients through the procedure for the first few times. Videotapes or audiotapes can be used, but human contact is almost always preferable. Repeated practice can help clients move toward independent functioning. Return demonstrations

help nurses evaluate learning. Praise the client's learning while noting any areas for improvement.

Role Playing

Role playing, or acting out feelings or knowledge, is especially useful for teaching affective behavior to adults or children. It can be used to work through past, present, or anticipated feelings or new situations. Clients react based on their experiences, while nurses offer guidance and feedback. Dolls can be used, especially with children. For example, a child may be asked to demonstrate how his or her mother's illness has affected the family by using dolls to represent each family member.

Teaching Aids and Resources

Teaching aids assist learning but are not substitutes for human contact. They are best used to supplement or reinforce face-to-face teaching.

Pamphlets

Access to written materials can assist nurses in planning teaching–learning sessions. Agencies such as the American Cancer Society, American Heart Association, American Diabetes Association, and other health-related groups frequently prepare written materials. Some are prepared within agencies by clinical nurse specialists or other nurses with a specialized teaching role. Being familiar with available written resources is important. Material should pertain to the client's concern and should be written clearly, with up-to-date information that is consistent with what is taught verbally.

The reading level of any written material must be screened for appropriateness for the individual client. Educational pamphlets should be written at the fifth or sixth grade reading level (Winslow, 1998). The SMOG Readability Formula can be used to assess the reading grade level of printed material (Display 22-1). When evaluating educational material for the person of low literacy, look for materials that contain short sentences and words with few syllables. Large print is important for clients with visual impairment.

Frequently, written materials are provided in advance of a teaching session to give clients time to assimilate information and formulate questions or concerns. Whenever possible, encourage clients to make use of such materials immediately by circling important information or indicating important areas to review before the teaching session. It is best to select a few well-written materials rather than overwhelming clients with dozens of pamphlets (Fig. 22-2).

Audiovisual Aids

Videotapes, slide-tape programs, and even computer-assisted instruction can be useful for subjects that are taught often, such as insulin injections or breast-feeding. Visual

DISPLAY 22-1

🔄 THE SMOG READABILITY FORMULA

To calculate the SMOG reading grade level, begin with the entire written work that is being assessed, and follow these four steps:

1. Count off ten consecutive sentences near the beginning, in the middle, and near the end of the text.
2. From this sample of thirty sentences, circle all of the words containing three or more syllables (polysyllabic), including repetitions of the same word, and total the number of words circled.
3. Estimate the square root of the total number of polysyllabic words counted. This is done by finding the nearest perfect square, and taking its square root.
4. Finally, add a constant of three to the square root. This number gives the SMOG grade, or the reading grade level that a person must have reached if he or she is to fully understand the text being assessed.

A few additional guidelines will help to clarify these directions:

- A sentence is defined as a string of words punctuated with a period (.), an exclamation point (!), or a question mark (?).
- Hyphenated words are considered as one word.
- Numbers that are written out should also be considered, and if in numeric form in the text, they should be pronounced to determine if they are polysyllabic.
- Proper nouns, if polysyllabic, should be counted, too.
- Abbreviations should be read as unabbreviated to determine if they are polysyllabic.

Not all pamphlets, fact sheets, or other printed materials contain 30 sentences. To test a text that has fewer than 30 sentences:

1. Count all of the polysyllabic words in the text.
2. Count the number of sentences.

3. Find the average number of polysyllabic words per sentence as follows:

$$\text{Average} = \frac{\text{Total \# of polysyllabic words}}{\text{Total \# of sentences}}$$

4. Multiply that average by the number of sentences *short of thirty*.
5. Add that figure to the total number of polysyllabic words.
6. Find the square root and add the constant of three.

Perhaps the quickest way to administer the SMOG grading test is by using the SMOG conversion table. Simply count the number of polysyllabic words in your chain of thirty sentences and look up the appropriate grade level on the chart.

SMOG Conversion Table[a]

Total Polysyllabic Word Counts	Approximate Grade Level (±1.5 Grades)
0–2	4
3–6	5
7–12	6
13–20	7
21–30	8
31–42	9
43–56	10
57–72	11
73–90	12
91–110	13
111–132	14
133–156	15
157–182	16
183–210	17
211–240	18

[a] Developed by Harold C. McGraw, Office of Educational Research, Baltimore County Schools, Towson, MD.

From Department of Health and Human Services. (1989). *Making health communication programs work: A planner's guide* (NIH Pub. No. 89-1493). Washington, DC: U.S. Government Printing Office.

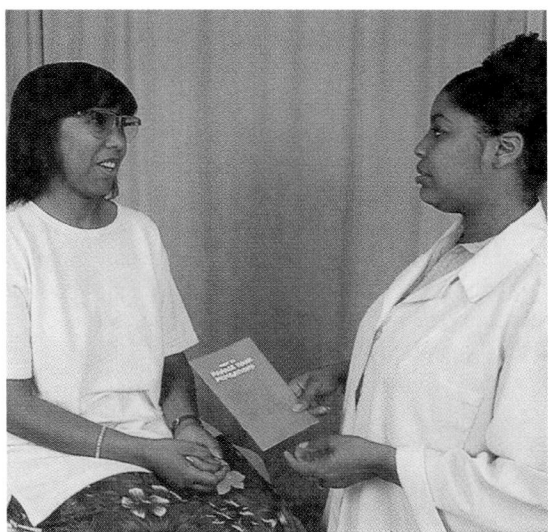

FIGURE 22-2   The nurse provides an instructive, well-written pamphlet to the client to support teaching regarding medication management.

aids often increase learning during a formal lecture presentation. An overhead projector or chalkboard can be used. Some healthcare facilities have a special television channel with programming to provide health education on various topics. Let clients decide which aid might be helpful if more than one form is available. Do not use audiovisual aids in isolation, but combine them with discussion or one-on-one teaching (Fig. 22-3).

Equipment and Models
Seeing and being able to practice on equipment promote learning. Whenever possible, obtain the equipment that a client will actually use for practice. For instance, when teaching glucose monitoring to a client with diabetes, use the type of monitor that the client will use in the future. Models can be used to simulate actual conditions. For example, model breasts have been

developed to assist teaching breast self-examination, permitting clients to palpate what a lump would feel like.

Use of Translators

If a client, family, or caregiver cannot speak English, a translator is necessary during the teaching session. A 2000 law requires all federally run programs to make accommodations for individuals with limited English proficiency. JCAHO and American Hospital Association standards and some state laws also mandate the use of translators for non–English-speaking clients (Gravely, 2001). When an interpreter is needed, the teaching session will take longer, because each message must be repeated twice. In addition to speaking the language, the translator must be aware of the culture and be able to interpret medical information clearly and objectively. Sometimes, doing so is difficult when a family member or friend acts as translator. Better choices are bilingual staff members or professional translators (who may be available in large medical centers) (Fig. 22-4). Female translators may be able to communicate more freely with female clients without encountering cultural prohibitions.

When using a translator, continue to talk to and look at the client. Keep information simple and direct. Instruct the translator to translate word for word as much as possible. Keep the name and number of the translator in a Kardex file or in the client's record. A nod or "Yes" from the client does not always indicate understanding, because some people agree just to avoid "losing face." Be sure to also provide written translated material.

Many telephone companies now offer a Language Line Service whereby the client and healthcare provider talk on the telephone with a bilingual operator who provides translation. This service is cost-effective and provides 24-hour coverage in most languages. It valuable for small agencies and for agencies located in rural or nonurban areas. One disadvantage of this service is the inability to see nonverbal communication.

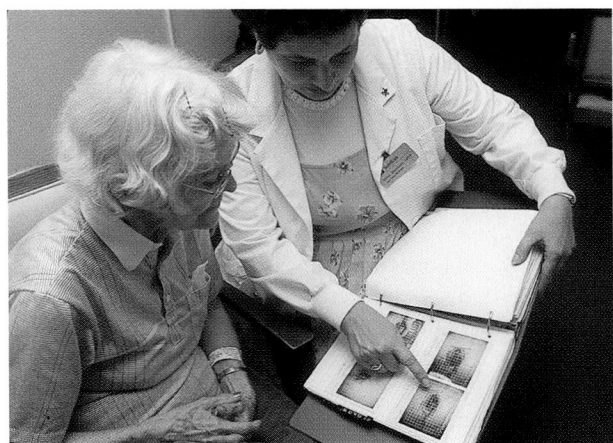

FIGURE 22-3   Combining audiovisual aids with discussion and client participation will lead to more effective learning.

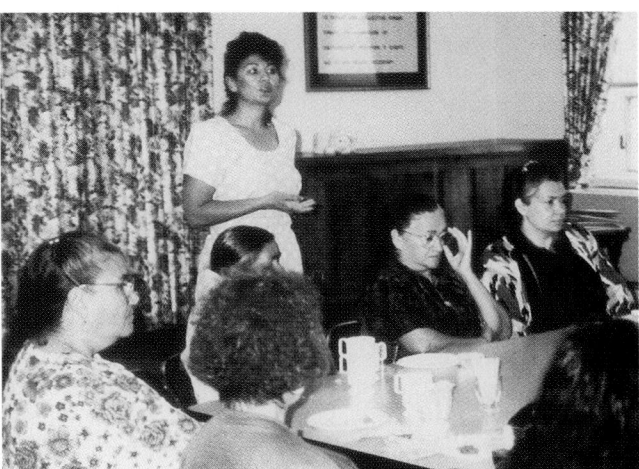

FIGURE 22-4   The bilingual nurse is a valuable resource for clients who need instruction about healthcare in their native language.

Timing and Amount of Information

When planning a teaching session, consider factors such as the amount of time available and the amount of material that needs to be covered. Most teaching sessions are brief and informal. Providing the client with information in a concise format can assist in alleviating treatment-related anxiety and increasing client satisfaction (D'Haese et al., 2000). Sometimes, clients ask questions or seem especially interested in learning. This time when clients are very receptive to teaching is often referred to as a "teachable moment" (Hansen & Fisher, 1998). For example, if the client asks questions when you pass out medications, take a few minutes to explain each newly ordered medication and possible side effects. Reinforce this informal teaching whenever the medication is administered until the client can verbalize this information to you. When a more formal teaching session is necessary, planning the best time can help ensure teaching effectiveness. Consider the following principles when planning a good time to teach:

- The client should not be tired.
- The client should be comfortable.
- Family members or caregivers may be present.
- Uninterrupted time must be available so that meals or necessary treatments do not interrupt the teaching session.
- Teaching should not occur just before an event (e.g., discharge, surgery).

Hospital teaching sessions should be limited to 20 to 30 minutes to avoid tiring clients. Warn clients about any time restraints. Saying "I have 20 minutes to talk" communicates clearly the nurse's time limit, minimizing the chance that clients will feel slighted.

Hospitalization is not the best time for teaching. Plan to cover essential material, but do not expect clients to learn all that is necessary while anxiety or pain is present. Outpatient education is usually more effective than inpatient education for several reasons. Clients are usually less stressed and therefore better able to learn when they are no longer in the hospital. They have lived at home with the change and bring practical, everyday questions to the session. Simply attending an outpatient education session indicates a willingness to learn, and motivation is a strong indicator of educational success.

Appropriate Family and Friend Involvement

Whenever possible, plan to include family members and friends in client education. Their support strongly affects client success. A statement such as, "I'm here because my wife made me come" may indicate denial on the client's part and tells the nurse about the wife's attitudes and influence. Never assume that because someone is a blood relative, he or she automatically wants to participate in client education or care. Friends are often as supportive as family members. When a family member or friend assumes the caregiver role, it may be necessary for that person to attend teaching sessions and demonstrate mastery of important skills and knowledge.

Written Teaching Plan

The written teaching plan guides the teaching process and coordinates teaching among members of the healthcare team. Without a written plan, teaching is likely to be haphazard and ineffective. A written plan clearly stating expected outcomes also serves as a useful reference for evaluation and fosters communication with other professionals so that they may participate. A written teaching plan may be incorporated into critical pathways, indicating at what point specific teaching should occur. Display 22-2 shows the format for an outcome-based teaching plan, examples of which are provided in each clinical chapter in this text.

IMPLEMENTATION OF CLIENT TEACHING

Meeting Priority Needs First

Before any teaching, the client should be comfortable. Easing acute symptoms, such as pain, hunger, thirst, nausea, or dyspnea, allows the client to focus on learning. Give the client a chance to use the toilet. Offer pain medication, and determine whether the client is comfortable.

Anger, fear, anxiety, worry, grief, and guilt block learning. Nurses who are sensitive to distress can modify the plan accordingly. Supportive body language and statements are useful. No matter how thorough planning has been, last-minute changes may be needed.

Comfortable Environment

Anyone who has tried to study in a room that was too hot, cold, dim, bright, noisy, or distracting knows that the environment affects learning. During client education sessions, try to make the environment conducive to learning. If neces-

DISPLAY 22-2

EXAMPLE OF OUTCOME-BASED TEACHING PLAN

Outcome/Deadline
Client will demonstrate blood glucose testing independently by discharge.

Plan/Strategies:
- Assess client's fears and readiness to learn.
- Assess preferred learning style.
- Provide handouts outlining steps in procedure.
- Verbalize steps in procedure as performed by the nurse.
- Ask if client has questions and/or feels comfortable trying procedure.
- Verbally cue client as he or she completes blood glucose testing, including family members in teaching.
- Have client practice blood glucose testing until he or she verbalizes comfort.

sary, send uninvolved visitors away temporarily. Privacy is important; closing the curtains in a semiprivate room, sitting near the client, speaking quietly, and facing the client all contribute to a greater sense of privacy.

Individualized Teaching Sessions

Trying to teach too much at once can block learning. Because people can store only five to seven thoughts in short-term memory at one time (Babcock & Miller, 1994), be selective with information. Lecturing is appropriate only when addressing a group; discussion is much more effective when teaching a small group or one person. Listening to the client's response gives excellent feedback about his or her progress.

People have different learning styles. Some prefer to do, and others prefer to watch. When teaching a psychomotor skill, be sensitive to those who like to do. A demonstration may have been planned, but if the client reaches out to touch the materials, consider talking the client through the skill instead. Children learn through play and are usually energetic and eager "doers." However, if a child prefers to watch, a demonstration instead of instructive play may be best.

Communication

Good communication is necessary for effective client teaching. Chapter 21 discusses communication in the nurse–client relationship in more detail. Active listening requires the nonverbal communication techniques of silence, attending, and observing. If a client is comfortable and believes that he or she has the nurse's undivided attention, learning is greatly enhanced.

Participation is the best measure of involvement. Getting a person to participate can occur by leading—making a pointed, specific statement. The client who rambles may need to be focused.

To clarify understanding, repeat what you hear the client saying and ask whether it is accurate. Reflecting or restating (repeating the client's words) also can be a valuable communication tool.

Repetition

The realities of today's healthcare system—short hospital stays, limited home care opportunities, and very ill clients—provide less time for client teaching. Setting priorities and repeating information are imperative. When cognitive or psychomotor learning is the goal, try repeating the information in various ways. For example, if the client has been learning a therapeutic diet, ask about appropriate food choices in different restaurants, on a picnic, or at a party. Have clients repeat information several times. Ask clients how new learning will affect their daily routines, and check to see whether they are integrating new routines into activities of daily living. Ask clients to practice and demonstrate psychomotor skills several times before discharge. Repetition may point out deficits in learning that would not be evident in a single session.

Because discharge instructions can be overwhelming, clarify important concepts, provide written instructions, review

factual information, and have clients repeat the knowledge and practice the skills. Most healthcare agencies have discharge forms that are printed in duplicate, so nurses can give a copy of the specific discharge teaching to clients as they document it. These forms also help alert nurses to essential information that they must provide before discharge.

Teaching Methods

Methods of teaching differ in the three domains of knowledge. Principal teaching methods are listed in Display 22-3.

Cognitive

Because the cognitive domain of learning involves expanding knowledge, the material must be organized from the simple to the complex. Introduce clients to the basic concepts, and give definitions. Then help clients integrate these concepts into something meaningful and beneficial to health. People do not learn isolated facts well. Learning is enhanced when information builds on previous knowledge. The most common error is trying to teach too much in a single session. It is better to teach some basic ideas well than to overload clients with many hard-to-remember facts.

Affective

When trying to modify an attitude or emotional response, keep a nonjudgmental, nonthreatening attitude. Acknowledging the client's ability to accept or reject the material can empower the client and lead to more healthy decision making. The nurse who states emphatically the rightness of his or her position and the wrongness of the client's position loses all credibility and influence. Listen carefully to what the client values, and work from there.

DISPLAY 22-3

ⓢ PRINCIPAL TEACHING METHODS

Cognitive (knowledge)
1. Lecture
2. Discussion (factual questions and answers)
3. Stimulation (application of knowledge in different contexts)
4. Independent study

Affective (values)
1. Discussion and values clarification
2. Role playing
3. Simulation
4. Discussion

Psychomotor (skill)
1. Skill demonstration
2. Talking the learner through the skill
3. Repeated practice

For example, a nurse is trying to encourage a depressed, noncompliant paraplegic to join a support group. The client is too depressed to be involved in self-care but does seem to have a strong sense of contributing as a family member. The nurse gently approaches the client with the idea that better physical and mental health would enable him to contribute better to his family's well-being. The client may begin to assign a higher value to health when it is tied to better family functioning.

Psychomotor

Psychomotor methods involve the muscular motions needed to learn a skill. Assemble the appropriate equipment (e.g., dressings, syringes); having the necessary supplies at hand can save time and prevent interruptions. Written material, providing a step-by-step guide, acts as a reference during the session and as a reminder to clients the first few times they practice the skill independently. Allow clients to ask questions and make comments. Many adults are intimidated by learning a new skill, so encouragement and praise almost always improve performance. Comments such as, "Lots of people have that same concern" or "I've had many clients with that same problem" help clients feel less isolated.

EVALUATION OF LEARNING

Evaluation of learning is most effective when it is systematic, practical, and ongoing. Measurable, clearly stated outcomes streamline evaluation. When clients actively participate in outcome formation, they are likely to be able to do much of the evaluation.

This final phase depends heavily on what has preceded it. If evaluation becomes unclear, review the outcomes. Were they realistic for the client's abilities, time frame, and resources? Were they clearly stated and measurable?

Evaluation occurs continually as teaching proceeds, rather than after teaching is completed. In this way, the teaching session can be continually adjusted to meet the client's needs. Feedback from nurse to client is most effective when it enhances the client's self-concept and motivates the client to higher learning. Asking clients to repeat or demonstrate what they have learned to family members is one way to accomplish this, especially with children. Remind clients of the progress they have made rather than what still needs to be done. Evaluation can take several forms, including written tests and questionnaires, oral tests, return demonstrations, and simulations.

Written Tests

Written tests are time-consuming, intimidating, and not always specific to the client. They are useful only in the following situations:

- The client is literate (do not take this for granted).
- Clear educational objectives have been mutually decided.
- It is necessary to measure a broad sample of factual information.
- A skilled test writer has prepared the test.

As in the classroom, written tests are most useful for evaluating cognitive learning. Affective learning cannot be tested this way because no answer is right or wrong. Tests may be useful as assessment tools (pretests) or as evaluation tools to check a client's progress. A questionnaire may be used to evaluate how helpful an educational program has been for a group of learners, so positive changes can be made if the program is offered again.

Oral Tests

Oral tests are usually more expedient and less intimidating than written ones. Questions can be informally phrased, and clients usually give immediate, specific, and useful feedback. Stay as casual as possible, because the greater the client's anxiety about being tested, the less likely it is that the evaluation will be accurate. Evaluation of the client's verbal response can be useful in testing cognitive learning, but affective learning in the form of an attitude change is more difficult to measure.

Return Demonstration

The return demonstration is a way of testing skill performance. A client's degree of accuracy and independence in performing a skill is almost always a clear indication of learning. Psychomotor skills can be evaluated with this method. Give feedback about parts done well, along with areas for improvement. Figure 22-5 shows how nurses use return demonstration to evaluate learning breast self-examination techniques.

Simulation

Simulation evaluates whether the client can apply learning in different situations. Offer a scenario to the client, and ask what the best choice or choices would be. For example, the nurse could evaluate dietary learning by asking the client about the best choices in various restaurants, or the nurse could evaluate diabetic sick-day care by posing various sick-day scenarios.

DOCUMENTATION OF LEARNING

Documenting client education is as important as documenting any other aspect of client care. Documentation of client education serves several purposes:

- It communicates the plan and progress to other healthcare professionals.
- It fulfills the nursing job description as delineated by local, state, and national licensing agencies.
- It provides a legal record.

Documentation must contain the subject matter, the client's response, and any necessary break in the process (e.g., if, after evaluation, the nurse found it necessary to return to the planning stage). Well-documented client education is a record of methods that did or did not work, and it can give some indication of client compliance over time.

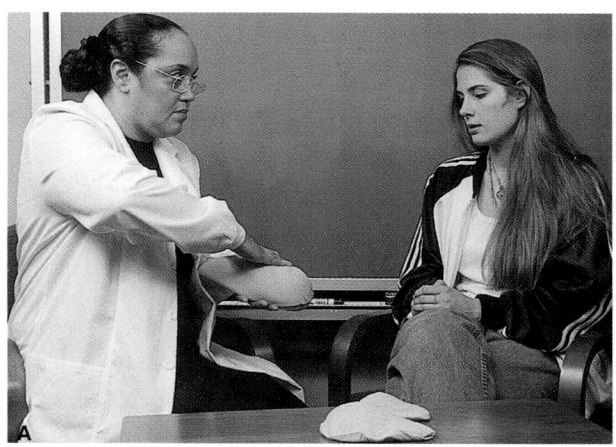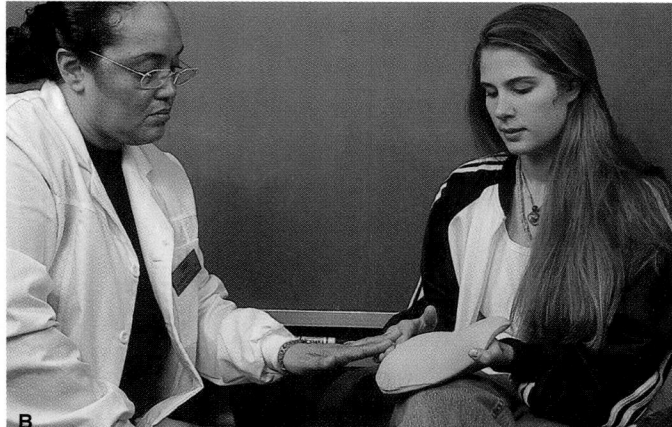

FIGURE 22-5 **(A)** The nurse teaches the client how to conduct a breast self-examination using a prosthetic breast. **(B)** In the return demonstration, the client tests her skill performance in this vital preventive measure.

LIFESPAN CONSIDERATIONS

Newborn and Infant

Newborns and infants learn by interacting with their environment. During this period of rapid development, infants learn a great deal (e.g., how to recognize their mothers, how to follow objects as they move, how to hold toys). Encourage an environment rich in appropriate stimuli to foster normal cognitive development.

During this stage, infants are not ready for formalized teaching; instead, any necessary teaching is directed at parents and caregivers. Teaching about various aspects of child care helps promote positive bonding.

Toddler and Preschooler

Because toddlers and preschoolers are accustomed to learning from and communicating with their parents, the parents are usually the most effective teachers. Children learn through play, so using dolls or toys as models can enhance learning (Fig. 22-6).

Children 2 to 5 years old like to be addressed with their parents listening. Trust is vital. If you tell a preschooler that a procedure will not hurt, but it does, you have lost credibility with the child, and learning is hindered. Children of these ages are likely to have many questions and may ask the same ones many times. Answer their questions immediately, directly, and in language they can understand. Sometimes, this means checking with a parent or caregiver about words that a child uses to describe body functions or important things. Preschoolers are generally energetic and restless, so try to limit the session to 10 minutes. Let children handle machines or supplies as soon as possible. Children of this age can understand some anatomy, so, when possible, use models and correct anatomic names.

Preschoolers, compared with toddlers, have learned to do many more things (e.g., using the toilet, eating, dressing).

They are usually proud of such accomplishments. Relate teaching to children's specific life experiences when possible.

Evaluate learning frequently to ensure that children understand. Preschoolers usually enjoy displaying new knowledge, giving nurses the chance to praise them repeatedly and to offer rewards such as stickers, picture books, or rubber stamps.

School-Age Child and Adolescent

School-age children are usually eager to learn. They can understand cause and effect ("If I don't stay off my leg, it won't heal as quickly, and it'll be longer before I can play outside at recess"). Include children in educational planning, allowing them to help set goals. Being accustomed to a classroom atmosphere, they understand the scheduling of work and play.

Answer all questions quickly and truthfully. Trust is vital to learning and to establishing a relationship in which children feel comfortable enough to express fears and concerns.

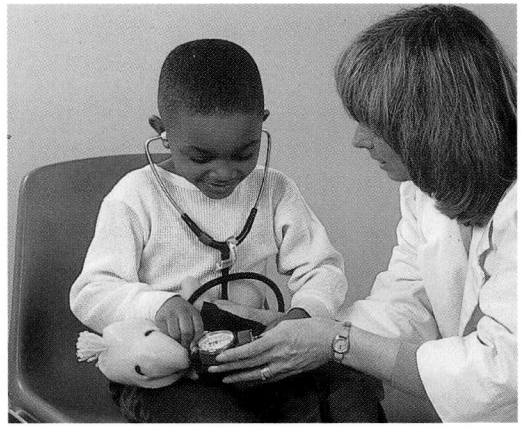

FIGURE 22-6 Allowing the child to participate and using models to demonstrate procedures are two effective methods for educating children about healthcare.

Educational content can be more sophisticated for this group than for preschoolers. Coloring books for teaching anatomy work well. Written material is fine at the proper reading level. Keep in mind that hospitalized children may regress. Explain procedures directly to these children with the parents in the background. Sessions should be no longer than 20 minutes.

"Winning" is important for school-age children, so they usually value success highly. Use of charts with stickers to mark progress is effective with this group.

Adolescents usually appreciate complete, open, and honest explanations to their questions. Their peers are usually more influential than parents, teachers, or nurses. It is fine to include peers in a teaching session; in fact, general healthcare information may be included for the benefit of these visitors. A sensitive, caring attitude is essential to educate adolescents effectively. To maintain the adolescent's trust, keep confidences; if a confidence must be broken, explain to the client whom you must tell and why.

Include adolescents in any educational planning, because their struggle for independence makes them averse to having anything imposed on them. They are more likely to comply when alternatives and consequences are explained. Ask them

THERAPEUTIC DIALOGUE
Client Teaching

Scene for Thought

Jennifer Cohan is 14 years old and has been diagnosed with diabetes mellitus. She wants to learn to give herself her own insulin injections. The diabetes nurse specialist comes to the clinic to talk to her.

Less Effective

Nurse: Hi, Jennifer. I'm Laurel Mandrake, the diabetes nurse. I'm here to teach you to give yourself your shots.
Client: *(Looks doubtfully at the equipment but doesn't say anything.)*
Nurse: I see you're looking at the equipment I brought. It's OK to be nervous. I'll show you how to do it, and then you can ask me questions.
Client: Can I see it first? I know I need this insulin stuff, so I don't get sick like I did at school. That was so embarrassing! But I hate shots so I don't know how good I'll be at this. *(Begins to take out syringes, alcohol swabs, vials, and so forth.)*
Nurse: It will be easier if you just let me show you what to do. I have to cover a lot of information. I'll give you some pamphlets to take home after you are done. I'll go over all this stuff with your mom, too, so she'll be able to help you.
Client: OK. *(Mumbles the word. Bites her lip to keep from crying.)*

More Effective

Nurse: Hi, Jennifer. I'm Lorraine Morris, the diabetes nurse. Your doctor told me you wanted to learn how to give yourself your shots. Is that right? *(Makes sure information is accurate.)*
Client: Yeah, I told him that, but I don't know now. *(Looks doubtfully at the equipment.)*
Nurse: It's okay to be unsure. I see you're looking at the equipment I brought. Do you want to see it or talk about it first? *(Assesses client's learning readiness and gives choices.)*
Client: Can I see it first? I know I need this insulin stuff, so I don't get sick like I did at school. That was so embarrassing! But I hate shots so I don't know how good I'll be at this. *(Begins to take out syringes, alcohol swabs, vials, and so forth.)*
Nurse: *(Sits and watches Jennifer explore.)*
Client: Look at those needles. They're so little!
Nurse: They do look small, don't they?
Client: Do we have to do this today? *(Looks pleadingly.)*
Nurse: I have a suggestion. How about if we go over the equipment today, and I'll give you a few pamphlets to take home and read. We can reschedule the actual teaching next week. How does that sound?
Client: I like that better. Maybe if I read this for a week I'll get more courage. *(Looks relieved.)*
Nurse: That means your Mom will have to give you the insulin until next week. Is that OK with you?
Client: Yeah, if it's OK with Mom. She hates shots, too! *(Laughs.)* *(Lorraine and Jennifer look at the equipment together and make plans for next week. Jennifer's mother comes in and learns how to give insulin as Jennifer watches.)*

Critical Thinking Challenge

* Determine how many of the three domains of learning Jennifer will use to acquire knowledge.
* Evaluate from the above information what kind of learner Jennifer might be.
* Examine how the first nurse approached Jennifer's learning style. What actions contributed to a less effective teaching session?
* Detect what the second nurse did that makes you think she knew the principles of teaching adolescents.
* Develop additional options the nurse might consider for teaching Jennifer.

what they need to know. Find out the value system a teen associates with an illness, and work from his or her point of view. Adolescents are generally sophisticated learners, able to understand broad concepts and assimilate much information. They are oriented to the present, however, and are more in tune with immediate advantages than with long-term results.

This age group is accustomed to teaching sessions of 45 to 50 minutes in school, and this is probably the maximum effective length. It may be better not to include parents in the session, to encourage client autonomy and heighten self-concept; parents can be informed later. Literature to review between sessions can be useful with this group.

Adult and Older Adult

Adults tend to be motivated by activities that enhance or maintain their self-esteem. Self-direction and achievement generally boost self-esteem; dependence and error generally decrease it. Adults tend to take errors personally, thinking poorly of themselves if they believe they are taking too long to grasp a concept.

Adult learners respond well to a straightforward teaching approach and can apply knowledge immediately. Try to provide a comfortable, informal, friendly learning environment where the client can feel appreciated.

Young adults usually have plenty of energy and take good health for granted. Learning must be practical, because these people usually lead busy lives. When setting educational goals with clients from this group, take a practical approach, if possible explaining how the change will improve daily life. Young adults are often motivated by the thought of maintaining their functioning to care for their children.

In general, middle-aged adults are more aware of health problems and do not take good health for granted the way younger adults do. People in this age group sometimes lack the self-confidence to try something new. Middle-aged adults should be involved in all aspects of the teaching plan, because they are usually familiar with the concepts of goal setting and achievement. These people have a broad base of life experience, and teaching goals will more likely be met if they are given time to assimilate new knowledge into old. Approach learning directly, and explain all rationales fully. Try to keep sessions to less than 1 hour, and allow time for clients to practice skills in private.

Middle-aged people also enjoy praise. Evaluate clients in a supportive atmosphere, stressing how much progress they have made. Gently correct misconceptions, and be sensitive to fears and anxieties.

Older adults are the fastest-growing segment of our population. General adult learning principles apply to this group; some special considerations are required, however.

Motivation to learn may be decreased if clients believe life is near its end. Two motivational strategies may be tried:

• Show clients how new knowledge will improve their quality of life, regardless of its length.

• Show how the new knowledge could improve the client's independence.

Physiologic changes that normally occur with aging may hinder learning. Vision may decrease because of cataracts; smaller, less-reactive pupils; or a decrease in color perception. The ability to hear high-pitched sounds usually decreases, although low-pitch hearing may be intact. Rapid speech may become unintelligible because older adults often take longer to process what they hear. Hearing loss can be a source of shame and frustration for the older learner, causing withdrawal and worsening feelings of isolation.

Older adults may suffer from short-term memory loss. Do not assume that memory loss exists, but be sensitive to it. When it does exist, it is usually associated with meaningless learning, complex learning, or new information that has required a reassessment of old learning. If new information conflicts with old, time is needed to reexamine the old learning; this may cause some anxiety and may be a barrier to new learning (Babcock & Miller, 1994). The older learner has large stores of information, so scanning for recall may take longer. Generally, older learners need more time to learn psychomotor skills. Often, they compensate by putting a great deal of effort into accuracy. Display 22-4 lists guidelines for assisting older adults with learning.

DISPLAY 22-4

🖳 TEACHING THE OLDER LEARNER

Teaching Tips
• Use a brightly lit, glare-free room.
• Use visual aids with large, well-spaced letters and primary colors.
• Eliminate extraneous noise.
• Face the learner.
• Speak in low, slow tones.
• Limit sessions to 20 to 30 minutes.
• Watch for cues indicating inadequate hearing, such as leaning forward, cupping an ear, frowning when trying to hear, or starting a separate conversation.
• Relate new material to past experiences in a meaningful way.
• Supply one idea at a time. Use frequent summaries and positive feedback.
• Provide a written or recorded summary of the session.

Medication Teaching
• Be sure the client knows what each medication does, how many pills to take, and when.
• Discuss what to do if the client misses a dose. (Containers that hold a week's worth of medications improve accuracy and consistency.)
• Be sure the client has written medication instructions in appropriate size, form, and language.

KEY CONCEPTS

- Client education is a dynamic process used to empower the client toward autonomy and high-level wellness.
- In client education, the nurse can influence but cannot control. Education must be client centered.
- Determining whether the learning will be primarily psychomotor, cognitive, or affective affects the entire process.
- The nurse, in collaboration with the client, assesses the client's learning needs and readiness to learn; he or she then forms a teaching plan. The plan is implemented, the learning is evaluated, and the process is documented.
- People have varying learning styles, and different age groups require different approaches.

REFERENCES

American Hospital Association. (1992). *A patient's bill of rights.* Chicago, IL: Author.

American Nurses Association. (1991). *Nurse's agenda for healthcare reform (PR—12—91).* Kansas City, MO: Author.

Babcock, D., & Miller, M. (1994). *Client education: Theory and practice.* St. Louis, MO: C. V. Mosby.

Bloom, B. (1956). *Taxonomy of educational objectives: The classification of educational goals.* New York: David McKay.

Brouphy, N. C. (2001 Aug 21). Preoperative education builds a bridge to postoperative care. *Nursing Spectrum, 10*(17), 15.

Daddy, J., & Clegg, A. (2001). Cultural sensitivity: a practical approach to improving services. *Nursing Standard, 15*(33), 19–27.

D'Haese, S., Vinh-Hung, V., Bijdekerke, P., Spinnoy, M., DeBeukeleer, M., Lachie, N., Deroover, P., & Storme, G. (2000). The effect of timing of the provision of information on anxiety and satisfaction of cancer patients receiving radiotherapy. *Journal of Cancer Education, 15*(4), 223–227.

Gravely, S. (2001). When your patient speaks Spanish and you don't. *RN, 64*(5), 65–67.

Joint Commission on Accreditation of Healthcare Organizations (1995). *Accreditation manual of hospitals.* Chicago, IL: Author.

Knowles, M. (1990). *The adult learner: A neglected species* (4th ed.). Houston, TX: Gulf.

McKenzie, J., & Smeltzer, J. (1997). *Planning, implementing, and evaluating health promotion programs* (2nd ed.). Boston, MA: Allyn and Bacon.

North American Nursing Diagnosis Association (NANDA). (2001). *Nursing diagnosis: Definition and classification, 2000–2001.* Philadelphia: Author.

Vezeau, T. M., & Oja, J. (1996). Clock and calendar skills in a client population. *Mother Baby Journal, 1*(3), 19–26.

Winslow, E. (1998). Caring for patients with limited literacy. *American Journal of Nursing, 98*(7), 55–57.

Wilson, F. L. (2000). Measuring patients' ability to read and comprehend: A first step in patient education. *Nursing Connections, 13*(3), 19–27.

BIBLIOGRAPHY

Baker, R. (2001). Child health education for the foreign-born parent. *Issues in Comprehensive Pediatric Nursing, 24*(1), 45–55.

Davidhizar, R., Bechtel, G. A., & Juratovac, A. L. (2000). Responding to the cultural and spiritual needs of clients. *Journal of Practical Nursing, 50*(4), 20–24, 26.

MacDonald, D. (1998). Meeting special learning needs. *RN, 61*(4), 33–34.

Maddox, M. (2001). Teaching spirituality to nurse practitioner students: The importance of the interconnection of mind, body and spirit. *Journal of the American Academy of Nurse Practitioners, 13*(3), 134–139.

Redman, B. (1996). *The process of client education* (8th ed.). St. Louis, MO: C. V. Mosby.

Weissman, M., & Jasovsky, R. (1998). Discharge teaching for today's times. *RN, 61*(6), 38–40.

23 Care Management

⑤ Learning Objectives

Upon completion of this chapter, the student will be able to do the following:
1. Describe the management of healthcare needs in the home from a systems perspective.
2. Identify factors that influence the client's ability to manage healthcare within the home.
3. Explain the major areas requiring assessment by a home care nurse.
4. Describe nursing roles and responsibilities in home care.
5. Identify the importance of community resources in the care of clients receiving home care services.

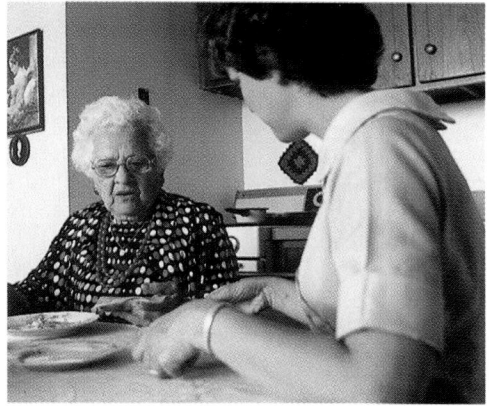

⑤ Critical Thinking Challenge

You are a home care nurse making the first visit to a married couple in their eighties. The husband was recently discharged from the hospital after a stroke. He is paralyzed on his right side and requires assistance with dressing, washing, and eating. Currently, he can tolerate only pureed foods. As you enter, his wife is in the kitchen, finishing her lunch. She has a history of severe degenerative joint disease. She says, "We're managing OK. Our only daughter, who lives about 15 miles away, works full-time. But she said she will drop by every evening to help us out. She has a family, so I hope we can manage during the day without her help." She looks at you with tears in her eyes.

Once you have completed this chapter and have added these topics to your knowledge base, review the above scenario and reflect on the following areas of Critical Thinking:

1. Role play verbal and nonverbal interactions that will help you establish rapport and trust with this couple.
2. Explore additional assessment data you need to collect at this time.
3. Prioritize immediate teaching needs and construct a plan to complete necessary teaching and evaluation during this first visit.
4. Propose additional supports and community resources that might be appropriate for this family.

In this chapter, you will learn the importance of the nurse's collaborating with people to manage their healthcare needs in the home setting and using community resources to support clients in this effort. The management of healthcare needs in the home setting involves not only the client but also family members, friends, and other sources of support. The goals are to allow people to regain or maintain optimal health, to function within their limitations, and to remain in the home environment. A key to successful care management is the quality of the nurse–client (family) relationship. In partnership with clients, the nurse facilitates their abilities to accomplish health and self-care goals.

As discussed in Chapter 2, the last two decades have seen tremendous changes in healthcare delivery. More care management takes place in homes than in hospitals. As the "baby boom" generation ages and the focus of healthcare changes, home care nursing assumes an even greater significance. Home care nursing has expanded from visits to chronically ill people to include care management for individuals and groups with specific healthcare needs and disorders to promote an optimal level of wellness and function. Delivery of advanced technology has also become commonplace in the home setting (Kaye & Davitt, 1999).

People have a perception of themselves in relation to the world and their ability to maintain independence. Independence is often linked to the ability to manage and care for oneself at home. It involves the ability to meet basic needs and to manage the complex activities necessary for self-care and independent functioning in society.

As a client moves or is moved from one environment to another, nurses must consider the client's ability to carry out activities of daily living (ADLs). Understanding the client in relation to the living environment is important in developing plans for care that maximize the person's ability to maintain independence safely.

HOME HEALTHCARE

Home healthcare is characterized by a range of health issues and related services. Such services are delivered to persons at home who are recovering from illness, are disabled, or are chronically or terminally ill and need various services to progress, maintain function, or perform their ADLs (National Association for Home Care, 1996). Services to manage healthcare needs at home can involve a team of interdisciplinary professionals, including social workers; physical, occupational, and speech therapists; and home health aides. Humphrey and Milone-Nuzzo (1996) further defined home care nursing as the provision of nursing care to acute, chronically ill, and well clients of all ages in their homes while integrating community health nursing principles that focus on health promotion and on environmental, psychosocial, economic, cultural, and personal health factors affecting an individual's and family's health status.

Trends Affecting Home Healthcare

One aspect of the changing healthcare system is the increasing role of home management. The federal government has called home care one of the fastest growing areas of the healthcare system (Gonzales, 1997). A major reason for this growth has been earlier discharge of people from the hospital to home since the 1980s. Several other factors have contributed to this growth (Green, 1998). Table 23-1 presents such factors and their implications.

TABLE 23-1

The Impact of National Trends on Home Care	
Trend	**Impact**
Technological advances in medical equipment	Advanced medical technologies have allowed clients previously required to remain in institutional settings to receive necessary healthcare services at home.
Increased demand for cost-effective healthcare options	The relative cost-effectiveness of home care has resulted in an increased demand for services.
Managed care plans	Increased enrollment in managed care plans is driving healthcare services out of institutional settings and into the home.
Graying of America	As the population ages, the incidence of chronic diseases that require home care interventions is expected to increase.
Changes in family status	The number of single-person households is growing, resulting in increased reliance on organizations such as home care agencies to provide care once performed by families.
Increased self-care responsibility	Individuals are taking greater responsibility for making healthcare choices. When possible, the majority of people choose to receive healthcare in their own homes versus an institutional setting.
Increased expectations of lay caregivers	As healthcare shifts to nonclinical settings, the burden of care is shifting to lay caregivers. Home care nurses need to teach sometimes complicated healthcare concepts and procedures to these individuals.

From Green, K. (1998). *Home care survival guide.* Philadelphia: Lippincott-Raven.

In addition, prospective payment has been introduced in home healthcare. Home health agencies are now required by Medicare to collect and report standardized information: the Outcome and Assessment Information Set (OASIS). OASIS provides standardized guidelines for admission and care, as well as a national database for evaluation, reimbursement, and quality improvement (Health Care Financing Administration, 1998; Marrelli, 2001). Current information on home health prospective payment and OASIS can be accessed at http://www.hcfa.gov/medicare/hhmain.htm#billing (accessed 1/14/02).

Tele-Home Health

Harris (2000) advises home health nurses to welcome the increasing use of technology. The use of interactive television and transmittal of data (e.g., cardiac rhythm strips) for selected patients has been implemented by some agencies and has been demonstrated to be well accepted by clients, professionals, and agency administrators (Johnson, Wheeler, Deuser, & Sousa, 2000). More efficient use of professionals' time through use of telephone "visits" to supplement home visits is also a strategy that can be highly effective (Sienkiewicz & Davidson, 2000). In Canada, a telenursing service is available in the Province of Quebec. A widely used service by community dwellers (more than 2 million calls in 1997), the telenursing service is not only cost-effective from a healthcare delivery perspective, but consumers report that using this service saves them time and indirect costs (e.g., childcare, transportation, time away from their jobs). The results of a random survey of callers also revealed that use of this nursing service increased self-reliance and facilitated respondents' self-care practices (Hagan, Morin, & Lepine, 2000).

Home As Healthcare Setting

A person's environment comprises his or her physical, psychological, and social surroundings. An important aspect of this environment is that it is where a person turns for support, intimacy, relaxation, sustenance, and protection from the outside world. For most people, this place is called "home." Home may take many forms, such as a house, apartment, or nursing home. For some it may be a homeless shelter. It may mean living alone or with others. Living in one's own home is usually linked to the ability to manage and care for oneself.

Optimal management in the home occurs when a person can independently maintain a growth-promoting environment (Fig. 23-1). The home is comfortable and safe, and the person performs self-care and hygiene tasks, interacts with others, meets financial obligations, and engages in activities that are satisfying and worthwhile. Although some people may have deficits, they can adjust to their situation through their own resourcefulness or with assistance from others.

Home Care Versus Acute Care

An essential difference in home care versus acute care is that the home care nurse is a "guest" in the client's home and on the client's turf. In the home, clients and families retain the

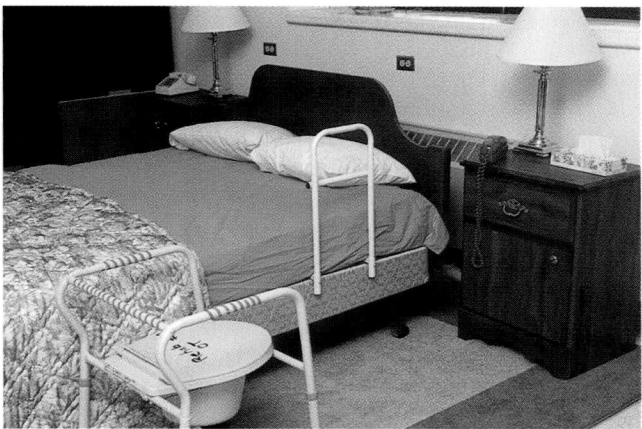

FIGURE 23-1 Safety features such as guardrails and helpful equipment such as a commode can assist clients to manage their healthcare independently.

power and control that they give to providers in other settings. Nurses in the home usually work as members of a therapeutic team. In addition, home care nurses usually have a caseload of clients of varying ages and with a range of health concerns. Therefore, a generalist background and focus are useful. The home management of many healthcare needs also requires broad assessment skills and a knowledge base to provide clients with appropriate teaching to help them remain as independent as possible. Because of the increased independent role in home management, the nurse must know resources within the agency and community to support care at home and must have basic knowledge of payors and their regulations. Support and education of lay caregivers such as family or friends require that the nurse in the home collaborate closely with them (Green, 1998).

Role of Family and Community: A Systems View

The home management of a person's healthcare needs usually occurs within the context of family, friends, and community. A systems view suggests that the individual, family, and community continually interact and influence one another by exchanging information and energy (see Chapter 19). This interaction and influence occur within all environments: physical, social, behavioral, economic, and political. What involves a person can affect his or her family and the community in which they all live. For example, if a person has a communicable disease, this disease may spread to the family as well as friends and neighbors. Community resources such as the local health department may then provide services to the individual and family.

Factors Affecting Home Healthcare Management

Altered ability to manage healthcare needs independently may result from decreased functional abilities, insufficient family or social supports, or insufficient community resources.

Physical deficits or chronic debilitating diseases that decrease the client's ability to perform ADLs can lead to difficulty in maintaining independence. Such factors include the medical diagnosis of a chronic debilitating or limiting condition, the medical prognosis for the condition, and the need for treatments and complex medication regimens (Carpenito, 2000). In addition, deficits in social support and/or community resources may compromise a family's capacity for independence in all ADLs.

The healthcare environment—that is, regulations and the extent of services covered through various insurance programs—also affects home healthcare management. An example is the new home health prospective payment system (HHPPS) and OASIS system of data collection used by Medicare. Agencies receive a set rate for a specific amount of service (by type of visit, or for an entire episode of home healthcare) and are required to collect data demonstrated by research to affect home care service delivery. These changes have been implemented in order to contain costs while keeping the quality of services high (Shaughnessy, Crisler, & Schlenker, 1998).

Functional Abilities

Developmental Stage. The client's developmental stage necessitates specific home care needs. The client requires physical care, but the nurse also needs to address developmental needs. An advanced understanding of the many challenges of various developmental levels is imperative if the nurse is to meet the client's physical and developmental needs.

A high-risk infant may require equipment to monitor breathing or to assist ventilation that is intimidating to parents. That infant, however, still needs closeness and bonding with parents. The nurse supports the parents to meet the infant's physical and emotional needs and encourages them to strengthen the parent–child bond. A school-aged child who requires home care for either an acute or a chronic condition needs support for normal socialization and peer relationships and for continuity in education. The needs that home care nursing can immediately meet are only part of this child's overall needs.

The adolescent who is in need of long-term home care has a unique combination of support needs. In addition to the physical needs that necessitated home care, the adolescent may be struggling with issues related to independence, maintaining peer relationships while unable to participate in activities, and keeping up with educational demands. The home care nurse can assist in coordinating care needs and encouraging family, teachers, schoolmates, and friends to understand the client's struggles and help support his or her needs.

Two more examples illustrate differences in home care needs related to lifespan. A young, single parent with two children lives in a two-bedroom apartment in the suburb of a large midwestern city. Many factors affect her ability to manage her own and her children's health at home. The family requires safe, affordable shelter. Adequate financial resources are necessary to purchase food, clothing, and medical care and to pay for utilities. Household tasks such as cleaning and washing clothes are important in maintaining a healthy environment. The mother must be able to perform ADLs (e.g., hygiene, cooking, dressing, grooming) for herself and for the children. Mobility, or the ability to move freely both within and outside the home, is important for performing many necessary tasks. The cognitive ability to understand how to organize work, manage financial responsibilities, and ensure safety within the home is essential. Transportation is necessary to purchase food, keep appointments within the community, and participate in social activities. Sometimes independence can be maintained with adequate support from the family or the community. Potentially, many issues (economic, physical, cognitive, and social) affect this family's ability to manage at home.

A 68-year-old woman is able to return to her home after having surgery if her daughter stays with her for the first week after discharge. In other situations where there is a lack of financial resources and lay caregivers, many community resources may be needed to support an older person in independent living at home. When management of healthcare needs in the home is no longer feasible, the client may need to be placed in a facility to provide adequate support.

Health Promotion and Safety Deficits. Injury potential, altered health maintenance, and knowledge deficit regarding self-care procedures are important considerations in home management. Injury potential becomes a risk factor if any person's safety is threatened; an example is a stairway without railings, on which children could fall and hurt themselves. Altered health maintenance due to health beliefs, change in financial situation, or lack of supervision can also impair a person's ability to live at home. If a client cannot learn to manage necessary diets or treatments, the ability to promote health at home is impaired. People living alone who have decreased functional abilities may manifest the following:

- Decreased ability for self-care or care of family members
- Decreased maintenance of safe and clean living space
- Decreased maintenance of economic obligations
- Decreased cognitive functioning and ability to respond appropriately to environmental stimuli

Cognitive and Sensory Deficits. Sensory loss, especially blindness, can hinder the ability to manage independently. Loss of sight can decrease independent functioning and increase the risk for injury. Severe pain can also decrease a person's ability to carry out daily activities and functions. An alteration in thought processes, if not responsive to treatment, can profoundly affect the ability to manage at home. Dementia (e.g., Alzheimer's disease) is a progressive condition in which memory loss and confusion greatly affect the client's functional abilities. The severely confused person cannot live independently and may be unable to live safely with the family because of the care demand. Mental illness such as schizophrenia and substance abuse also may impair a person's ability to manage at home with or without significant support from family or community resources.

Decreased Mobility. Many medical problems (e.g., arthritis, neurologic impairments, fractures, respiratory disease, cardiovascular disease, cancer) can impair a client's mobility and alter self-care abilities. Minor mobility problems may make housework or home repairs difficult; limited mobility may also hinder the client's ability to leave the house safely in case of fire or emergency. The inability to do grooming, toileting, and personal hygiene tasks may impair the person's ability to live independently. The inability to maintain home hygiene and cleanliness may pose health and safety risks.

Altered Elimination. Inability to control bowel or bladder function affects the ability to manage independently in a home setting. Often, such impairment occurs with other dysfunction, such as mobility problems after a cerebral vascular accident, neurologic insult, or decreasing cognitive function.

Altered Nutrition. The inability to provide adequate nutrition impairs the client's ability to manage independently. Buying and cooking food and cleaning up require energy. Depression can decrease the desire to eat properly, especially when the person lives alone or a specialized diet is required. Lack of financial resources may also hinder proper nutrition. Physical changes affecting chewing and swallowing also contribute to the potential for impaired home management.

Family and Social Supports

Family and social supports can compensate for functional deficits, and the extent to which family members and friends are interested or able to help is a crucial factor. Their coping abilities and reserves, commitment and ability to be caregivers, and personal health are factors in the balance and fit equation. Busy adults may need their energy for their own home and family; they may not have time to meet the needs of an older person or a person with special needs. Family members of the person with functional health deficits may show signs of not being able to maintain the client or themselves at home. Caregivers responsible for round-the-clock supervision of the client may show signs of stress, reduced ability to cope, alterations in functional abilities, and financial loss. Physical or verbal abuse may signal severe family stress.

People with decreased family, social, or community resources and decreased internal resources may manifest altered or impaired home management in any of the following ways:

- Decreased ability or availability of caregivers to assist with or perform self-care activities
- Decreased assistance in meeting financial obligations
- Inability to reach available resources
- Unavailability of community resources or services specific to the client's needs

Community Resources

Community and service deficits (lack of community agencies that provide supportive health and social services to assist the client) affect a client's ability to manage in the home. Some chronically mentally ill and developmentally disabled people cannot manage their finances or maintain hygienic living conditions without community assistance. Their environmental conditions may be stable, but without daily supervision from professionals or family they would be evicted and could become homeless.

Unhealthy or unsanitary living conditions indicate impaired home management. Unsanitary conditions, rodents, infestation, or environmental hazards are visual cues to an unhealthy environment. Lack of running water, electricity, heat, or proper storage facilities for food also are seen in poor living conditions.

The Nurse and Home Healthcare

A Framework for Home Care: The Rice Model

According to Rice (2001, p. 19), "the purpose of home care is to provide patients (and caregivers) with the understanding, support, treatment, information, and caring they need to successfully manage their health care needs at home." Active self-care management by the client and family in the home can lead to the best level of functioning.

Key components of the Rice model for home care include motivational factors of the client and family (caregiver) and the nurse as **facilitator** of self-determination for self-care in the roles of educator, advocate, spiritual communer, and case manager (Fig. 23-2). The client and family (caregiver) move along a continuum from dependence to interdependence to independence. According to Rice, after an initial assessment, the nurse asks relevant questions to collaboratively identify needs of the client and family (caregiver) for education, advocacy, aesthetic/spiritual communion, and case management. The home care nurse would also ask, first, whether the client or caregiver is willing and able to participate in the plan of care and, second, whether the home environment can support safe delivery of services. An answer of "No" to either of these questions may indicate that the client and caregiver are not candidates for home care. However, the nurse must explore with the family for possible sources of lack of information, misunderstandings, anxieties, and fears to fully assess motivational factors for self-care. The Rice model emphasizes the importance of shared responsibility among the nurse, client, and caregiver to promote the whole person's health and optimal self-care capacities.

Standards of Home Health Nursing Practice

The American Nurses Association (1999) described Standards of Home Health Nursing Practice that have two parts, Standards of Care (following steps of the nursing process) and Standards of Professional Performance, which are shown in Display 23-1. These standards can guide the home care nurse in his or her collaborative role with the client and family (caregiver) to identify the healthcare needs for management in the home setting.

Phases of the Home Nursing Visit

Stanhope and Lancaster (2000) suggested five phases of the home visit. First, the *initiation phase* includes clarifying the source of referral and the purpose of the visit and initial contact

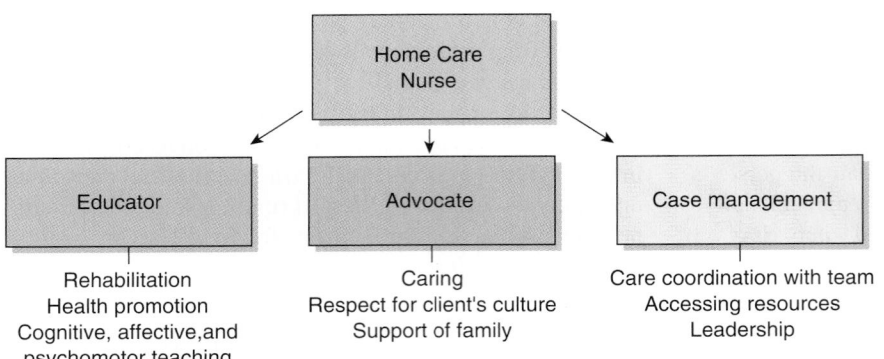

FIGURE 23-2   Components of nursing's role in the Rice model for home care.

with the family. The *previsit phase* includes establishing an understanding with the family for the purpose of the visit, scheduling the visit, and reviewing pertinent records and information. The *in-home phase* involves establishing the professional therapeutic relationship and implementing the nursing process. Social interactions help to establish rapport in this phase of home visiting. In the *termination phase* of the home visit, the nurse and family summarize accomplishments of the visit and make plans for future visits. Finally, the *postvisit phase* includes recording findings and carrying out activities necessary to plan for the next visit.

Assessment

Assessment should encompass the functional abilities, strengths, and assets of the client, family, home, and community. The nurse collects subjective information to assess how the person normally manages at home, what the home is like, and what family and community support is available. The nurse must explore the client's beliefs and culture, competencies, capabilities, concerns, deficits, and limitations to understand how the client manages at home and what he or she desires. Display 23-2 provides key questions that can be used to elicit this information.

DISPLAY 23-1

🖺   STANDARDS OF CARE AND PROFESSIONAL PERFORMANCE

Standards of Care

Standard I—Assessment
The home health nurse collects client health data.

Standard II—Diagnosis
The home health nurse analyzes the assessment data in determining diagnoses.

Standard III—Outcome Identification
The home health nurse identifies expected outcomes customized to the client and the client's environment.

Standard IV—Planning
The home health nurse develops a plan of care that prescribes interventions to attain expected outcomes.

Standard V—Implementation
The home health nurse implements the interventions identified in the plan of care.

Standard VI—Evaluation
The home health nurse evaluates the client's progress toward attainment of outcomes.

Standards of Professional Performance

Standard I—Quality of Care
The home health nurse systematically evaluates the quality and effectiveness of nursing practice.

Standard II—Performance Appraisal
The home health nurse evaluates his or her own nursing practice in relation to professional practice standards, scientific evidence, and relevant statues and regulations.

Standard III—Education
The home health nurse acquires and maintains current knowledge and competency in nursing practice.

Standard IV—Collegiality
The home health nurse interacts with and contributes to the professional development of peers and other health care practitioners as colleagues.

Standard V—Ethics
The home health nurse's decisions and actions on behalf of clients are determined in an ethical manner.

Standard VI—Collaboration
The home health nurse collaborates with the client, family, and other health care practitioners in providing client care.

Standard VII—Research
The home health nurse uses research findings in practice.

Standard VIII—Resource Utilization
The home health nurse assists the client or family in becoming informed consumers about the risks, benefits, and costs in planning and delivering client care.

American Nurses Association. (1999). *The scope and standards of practice for home health nursing.* Washington, DC: Author.

DISPLAY 23-2

KEY QUESTIONS FOR ASSESSING HOME MANAGEMENT

Client

- What goals do you have for yourself?
- What will help you achieve these goals?
- How will you manage at home on a day-to-day basis?
- What treatments will you be doing at home?
- What medications will you be taking at home?
- Is there anything within yourself or your home that you would like to change?
- What do you need to make these changes?
- What do you want it to be like at home?
- What kinds of problems do you think you will have at home?
- How have you dealt with challenges in the past?

Family and Social Support

- Have you ever needed help and support in the past?
- How much can you rely on friends and relatives?
- What kind of help and support do you need now?
- What help will you have at home?
- How much do you think your friends and relatives understand your health and medical problems?
- Whom would you like me to talk to about your health and medical problems?
- How do you think your spouse and friends will handle or cope with your being home?

DISPLAY 23-3

ASSESSMENT OF HOME CONDITIONS

From Client

- Ownership: rent hotel room, apartment, or house; own; live with others
- Access: ground floor, stairs
- Condition
  Utilities: heat, water, telephone, electricity
  Hygiene: housekeeping habits
  Sanitation: rodents, sewer, infestations
  Safety: hand rails

From Home Visit

- Neighborhood: crime potential, located near environmental hazards
- Access: ground floor, condition of stairs and sidewalk, proximity to public transportation
- Utilities: type of utilities available and in service; cooking arrangements
- Hygiene: odors, facilities for cleaning, appropriateness of food storage
- Sanitation: presence or evidence of vermin or rodents
- Safety: short electrical cords, hand rails, fire alarms, stable rugs
- Telephone: private phone, accessibility, answering machine

Assessing the Individual. Interviewing the client provides valuable information about his or her ability to manage at home, risk factors contributing to decreased ability, and identification of actual problems. Assessment starts by asking the client to describe his or her ability to manage self-care tasks such as bathing, dressing, grooming, and eating (see Display 2-3 in Chapter 2). Document the client's ability to carry out household chores independently or with assistance from others. The client can describe how he or she handles functional limitations at home and whether management has been satisfactory. Determine whether the client needs aids such as walkers, oxygen equipment, or a hospital bed. Assess medications and treatments and the client's ability to manage self-care.

Assessing the Family. Assess family support to determine how well a person can function at home. Family assessment can be done with questionnaires covering a broad range of topics. The most significant factors to assess are strengths and barriers to home care within the abilities of family members to provide care. Display 23-2 lists questions that can be used to obtain this information.

Assessing family support focuses on characteristics that show decreased family involvement with or support for the client. To assess family involvement with the client, ask directly how much support family members are willing and able

to provide. Observe for evidence of family visits. Look for evidence of family concern, such as cards and presents. Observe family communication patterns and dynamics. Families differ in their reactions to a member's illness. The prognosis and severity of the illness can affect family interactions and subsequent involvement with the client. Chronic illness can lead to rejection of the client and can impair family dynamics.

Assess the caregivers' ability and willingness to perform, or to help the client perform, any therapeutic treatments. Caregiving often consists of bathing, dressing, toileting, transferring, feeding, housekeeping, shopping, preparing meals, managing finances, and providing transportation. Therefore, assess caregivers for their ability and willingness to carry out these activities and for the emotional and physical strains of providing care or an overload of responsibility. Wound dressing changes, ostomy care, home parenteral therapy, and physical therapy may require additional time and energy. (See also Chapters 21 and 47.)

Assessing Risk. Currently the basis for most reimbursable home healthcare services is acute illness or exacerbations of a chronic problem that require skilled care. Rarely is a single factor the basis for home care. The relationship between functional impairments and available internal and external supports determines the risk for impaired ability to manage at home: the greater the functional impairment, the greater the

ETHICAL/LEGAL ISSUE
Caregiver Involvement in Home Care

You have been assigned to care for Mr. Springs, an 82-year-old man with heart failure and recurrent un-explained falls. His condition is of increasing concern to his wife. Mr. Springs does not want his wife to call their children for help. In her anxiety and exasperation about her husband's situation and her fears related to handling him, Mrs. Springs has been calling her daughter (the only child who lives nearby) at work with increasing frequency. The daughter has become frustrated with her parents' increasing dependency on her when she has her own family to care for and job to maintain. The daughter calls you and appeals to you to "make some decisions" regarding care for her parents.

Reflection
- What is your reaction to this situation? How would you feel if you were Mr. Springs? Mrs. Springs? Their daughter?
- Identify the concerns you may have about this family's situation and the nurse's appropriate role.
- Identify which persons have the legal and ethical authority to make decisions.
- Examine possible approaches to assisting the family in resolving this home care dilemma.
- Recognizing the client's rights and the family's concerns, define what you see as the nurse's ethically appropriate behavior.

From Taylor, C. (1997). Ethical issues in case management. In E. L. Cohen, & T. G. Cesta, *Nursing case management: From concept to evaluation*. St. Louis: Mosby.

risk, and the fewer available supports, the greater the risk. Common risk factors associated with the need for home care include the following:

- Multiple or catastrophic illnesses
- Limited social, mental, or physical functioning
- Repeated hospital admissions within 6 months
- Age older than 80 years, especially for women
- Age older than 70 years with a disability
- Lack of social or family support and living alone
- Complex medical treatment regimen and multiple medications

The presence of these risk factors does not automatically indicate a problem; the importance of the risk factors for each client must be determined. During the entire assessment, be continually aware of cues that would indicate cognitive impairments, such as repeating the same question or giving vague answers that are not consistent. People with cognitive impairments often are unable to manage in the home but rarely are able realistically to identify their own limitations.

Community deficits also can contribute to decreased ability to manage at home. The incidence is greater in the following situations:

- Unsafe neighborhoods
- Inadequate housing for the disabled
- Refusal of agencies to accept difficult clients
- Inadequate home health services
- Lack of volunteer programs
- Long waiting lists for services (especially nursing homes)
- Lack of affordable housing

A dysfunctional pattern can be identified when the client or family verbalizes the inability to perform daily tasks and manage at home. People have a deficit when they cannot perform self-care and hygiene tasks, do not engage in activities and interactions with others, and do not do things from which they would otherwise derive enjoyment and a sense of worth.

Assessing the Home. Although its assessment is often performed at the same time as the client and family assessment, the client's living area is important enough to be considered a separate assessment element. A comprehensive home assessment includes safety, sanitation, mobility, temperature, and personal space. Display 23-3 summarizes home assessment. (See also Chapter 30). Before discharging a client to the home setting, ensure a safe environment:

- Learn whether the house is rented or owned, because this determines whether modifications are feasible.
- Look for smoke or fire alarms, adequate lighting, flat door sills, and adequate security.
- Determine whether the house is clean and free of insect or rodent infestation.
- Ask about sewer and garbage services.
- Determine the source of water and the condition of the plumbing.
- Assess for adequate and safe cooking and food storage equipment, including running water and working electricity. Although rural and urban areas differ in the types of sanitation measures, sanitation should not be a source of disease.
- Assess for easy access throughout the house.
- Look for handrails on tubs and staircases, wide doorways for wheelchair access, and flat, even floors that contribute to easy mobility. There should not be any scatter rugs, and halls should be uncluttered.
- Determine the adequacy of heating and cooling systems. Inadequate temperature control can lead to hypothermia or hyperthermia.

Do not overlook the home's personal aspects. The presence of mementos, pictures, or religious items in a home reflects self-image. A garden, sewing equipment, or a workshop provides additional information on the person's values and avocations. A person may be unable to continue such self-actualizing activities in the face of health challenges. Being aware of the client's past gives the nurse a more complete understanding of the client and how the current health condition has changed his or her way of living. For example, an active 80-year-old man who gardens daily may interpret a broken hip as devastating, but a sedentary man who enjoys watching television and doing crossword puzzles may find the same situation less devastating.

The nurse may recommend changes in the home based on home assessment. Common physical changes include installing ramps and handrails, moving furniture to make room for a rented hospital bed, or installing equipment such as oxygen tanks and suction machines. If a severely disabled client is expected to return home, a home visit should ideally be made before discharge.

Assessing Community Resources. The purpose of community assessment is to identify resources that people needing assistance at home can use. A comprehensive community assessment is not needed to diagnose impairments, but being familiar with **community resources** allows the nurse to develop a more realistic and individualized nursing plan of care for the client. The nurse needs information about the community's economic stability, the client's neighborhood, the social and health resources available in the community, and the community's cultural norms. An overview of community assessment is presented in Chapter 19. The presence of services as recorded in service directories is one way to validate objectively what the client describes. Nurses should be familiar with available emergency care, equipment rental stores, chore and homemaker services, home-delivered meals, visiting nurse services and should know where welfare and Medicare/Medicaid offices are located.

Care Management and Responsibilities in Home Care

Although care management is a nursing responsibility in all settings of practice, home care provides for an exemplary setting within the extant health care system. In the Rice Model of Dynamic Self-Determination for Self-Care (2001), the home care nurse acts a facilitator of the patient/caregiver system through education, advocacy, communion, and case management.

Patient Education. **Patient education** is an interactive, collaborative process between the nurse and client to progress toward the client's goal of assuming responsibility for his or her health and self-care. The education process includes several steps. First, nurses assess. They gather information about the readiness of client and family to learn and target their learning needs and priorities. They interpret their findings to arrive at a nursing diagnosis for education needs.

Second, nurses negotiate the learning objectives and anticipated outcomes with the client and family. Well-written behavioral objectives are characterized as measurable, related to assessment data, developed collaboratively, and oriented to the learner. They contain the elements of performance, conditions, and criteria. Objectives can be classified as cognitive (knowledge-based), affective (values, feelings), or psychomotor (motor skills) (Smith & Mauer, 2000; Stanhope & Lancaster, 2000). (See also Chapter 24.)

Third, nurses and the client and family develop and implement a teaching plan. The teaching plan includes objectives and outcomes, a content outline, teaching format (i.e., group discussion with client and family), teaching tools (i.e., handouts, videos, return demonstration, role playing), and use of a teaching–learning contract with mutually developed objectives to achieve outcomes.

Finally, nurses evaluate client education. Such an evaluation can be done continuously during home visits. In the evaluation, nurses include a measurement of the achievement of the objectives, analyze the barriers and facilitators to learning, summarize the results with the client and family, provide and receive constructive feedback, and continuously reinforce the client's and family's learning (Kraus, 1995).

General areas for teaching to manage healthcare needs at home include information specific to a diagnosis of altered health status (e.g., signs and symptoms, diet, rest, activity, spirituality, self-image, developmental tasks, role transitions, medications, equipment, technical procedure), ways to cope or adapt to limits and restrictions related to the health issue, relevant community resources to support the client and family, and source of payment for healthcare at home (e.g., Medicare). The home care nurse is challenged by the wide range of information needed for client and family education.

Advocacy. Cary (1995, p. 13) defined **advocacy** as "engagement in activities for the purpose of protecting the rights of others while supporting the patient's responsibility for self-determination." A client advocate model suggests that nurses are responsible for promoting client autonomy and self-actualization. Nurses make decisions with clients and caregivers to assist clients to achieve the best possible health outcomes and to access appropriate health services. Advocacy develops from ongoing, caring relationships with clients and families. In a three-step advocacy process, nurses initially explore personal values and beliefs and then begin the informing process (Stanhope & Lancaster, 2000). To inform, nurses engage clients and family about the nature, content, and consequences of their choices. Informing is not merely exchanging information, but viewing information in light of a client's values and understanding. Supporting is the second step of advocacy: that is, nurses uphold the client's right to make and act on a choice and help the client and family to access and communicate with a range of resources and other providers. In the third step in advocacy, affirming, nurses validate with the client and family that choices are consistent with their values and goals. Home care nurses recognize that the needs of clients and their families are dynamic and may vary; therefore, ongoing evaluation of choices is needed to promote self-determination.

At different stages of clients' independent functioning, the nurse's role as advocate may change. Areas in which nurses may act as advocates include helping the client and family to clarify and prioritize their choices, to promote optimal functioning at home, or to communicate with other family members, friends, or professional services (e.g., healthcare providers, third-party payors) to access information or services in the home setting.

Aesthetic/Spiritual Communion. In order to acknowledge the holistic nature of patients (and caregivers), an important aspect of care management within the nurse's role as facilitator is what Rice (2001) terms **aesthetics/spirituality.** Aesthetic/spiritual communion has been described as entering into the "caring moment" (Watson, 1999) with families to accomplish the following:

- Know health through the arts
- Explore alternative and complementary therapies
- Experience self-awareness, faith, hope, and love

For care management to be balanced, the nurse's approach must include strategies that engage the whole person: body, mind, and spirit. Communion of the nature described allows (facilitates) meeting needs within the patient/caregiver in the domain of larger meaning, which can lead to greater self-knowledge, self-reverence, self-healing, and self-care processes. Often this type of relationship is facilitated through aesthetic expression (e.g., drawings, stories, music, poetry) and the use of alternative or complementary health modalities (Eliopoulos, 1999).

Care/Case Management. **Case management** is a term with numerous definitions (Siefker, Garrett, Genderen, & Weis, 1998; Stanhope & Lancaster, 2000). According to Siefker et al., case management focuses on the whole person, not just health-related issues. They suggested that the holistic approach requires the case manager to be a generalist with a range of skills and knowledge. For example, the case manager should have "medical expertise, but he or she also needs counseling skills, a wide knowledge of community resources, possible vocational expertise, mental health expertise, sensitivity to multicultural issues, proficiency in doing research, finesse in working with people with widely differing viewpoints, and a high level of ingenuity and problem-solving ability" (p. 7). The components of the case management process include the following:

- Assessment
- Planning
- Coordinating
- Making referrals
- Monitoring medical progress
- Filing and completing paperwork
- Monitoring outcomes and the plan's effectiveness
- Determining case closure
- Transferring the case at closure

These steps do not necessarily occur in sequence; sometimes, they may seem to happen simultaneously (Siefker et al., 1998).

For home care nurses who may be the client's and family's most direct contact with the healthcare system, these skills are necessary to promote the client's health and function. Hence, nursing care management is integrally related to case management. The complex array of skills has been likened to the nursing process (Stanhope & Lancaster, 2000). See also skills for discharge planning described in Chapter 2.

Coordination of care for a client and family requires development of plans of care that maximize the person's ability to remain in a safe environment, and often that environment is the client's home. Nurses work collaboratively with many healthcare professionals in planning, implementing, and evaluating the client's care, including physicians; social workers; physical, occupational, and speech therapists; and home health aides. Nurses integrate their understanding of community-based nursing with their abilities to collaborate, coordinate, provide, and evaluate care within many settings.

If the client requires special equipment, the home care nurse needs to know how to obtain the equipment and to whom it will be charged. Once such equipment is in the client's home, the nurse needs to know how to operate it, how to handle common malfunctions, and how to assist the client and family with learning to use it.

In the role of coordinating services, the home care nurse may work with a case manager from a managed care system or other third-party payor. Although both persons provide care for the client, they have slightly different concerns. The case manager may focus more on the aspects of reimbursable care to limit the insurer's financial liability. The home care nurse may focus on objective documentation of the client's care needs in order to convince the healthcare provider and the insurer of the need for continued home health services. In this function, the home care nurse acts as the client's advocate.

Accessing Community Resources. As mentioned previously, the home care nurse may need to access and coordinate the procurement of needed equipment for clients. This activity may be as simple as obtaining a prescription from a local pharmacy or as complex as arranging for reimbursement and delivery of large pieces of equipment from a durable medical supply house.

In today's healthcare environment, changes in funding for home services, especially through Medicare and managed care regulations, affect their availability. The challenge for home care nurses is to plan creatively with individuals and families to meet their needs. "As agencies more efficiently prepare patients for discharge, providers may feel as though they are leaving the patients without the assistance for them to remain safely in their homes" (Cochran & Brennan, 1998, p. 219). As a result, home care nurses must stay aware of community resources to assist individuals and families in the home.

Agencies may provide services at no cost or across a range of fees. The United Way funds many types of community services and programs. Churches and social service agencies may also support or provide direct services to individuals and families. For older adults, nurses should contact any agency that has "older," "aging," or "senior" in its title. Local senior centers may be a source of information. Often, a community has an umbrella agency that supports and/or organizes a number of services for particular groups, such as older adults, low-income families, or selected ethnic or racial groups. Local government agencies (city, county, and state) may also

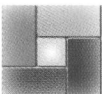

Nursing Research and Critical Thinking
Would Nurse-Led Shared Care of Clients Awaiting Coronary Artery Bypass Surgery Improve Care Management?

These nurses were aware that clients awaiting coronary artery bypass graft (CABG) surgery are usually anxious, suffer pain, and need to prepare for lifestyle changes in order to gain maximum benefit from surgery. They conducted a study to test a number of interventions designed to support clients waiting for surgery. A total of 98 clients waiting for CABG surgery, with an equal distribution between the sexes, were randomly selected. Subjects were randomly assigned to a control group ($n = 49$) and an intervention group ($n = 49$). Clients were assessed within 2 months after being placed on the surgical waiting list and again on admission for their surgery. All primary care team nurses completed a questionnaire at the study's conclusion. The intervention group received a shared care program of family health-centered education and counseling sessions based on their individual needs. The nurse-led interventions were carried out jointly by nurses in the primary care team and those in the cardiac surgery department. The researchers examined client satisfaction, changes in lifestyle, and the prevalence of risk factors for coronary heart disease. They measured anxiety and depression using the Hospital Anxiety and Depression Scale, quality of life using Short Form 36, and symptomatic angina using Likert scales and the level of use of glyceryl trinitrate spray. The study's results showed a significant reduction in the prevalence of risk factors for coronary heart disease and angina in the intervention group. This group also had reduced levels of anxiety and depression and improved quality of life.

Critical Thinking Considerations. This study used a randomized controlled design that enabled the researchers to compare the differences in the variables between the control and intervention groups. These interventions were community based (i.e., not during an episode of acute care) in their delivery. Implications of the study are as follows:

- The nurse-led shared care that provided clients with individualized education and counseling before their admission for surgery led to significant improvements in the client's care management.
- The high level of satisfaction from clients and care providers in the study suggests that there may be a significant demand for this type of service.

From McHugh, F., Lindsay, G., & Wheatley, D. (1998). A study of nurse-led shared care for coronary patients. *Nursing Standard, 12*(45), 33.

---

be sources of information. Some agencies have toll-free numbers. Organizations focusing on health issues also offer information; for example, local chapters of the national heart, lung, diabetes, or Alzheimer's associations often provide support groups, printed materials, and other information. Professional colleagues are frequently excellent resources. With the increased use of technology, on-line sources are more accessible to clients and families.

HOSPICE

Hospices, run by public or private agencies, are designed to care for terminally ill clients and their families by providing supportive, palliative services (Castro, 1994). Many clients receiving these services are suffering from cancer, acquired immunodeficiency syndrome (AIDS), multiple sclerosis, congestive heart failure, or end-stage renal disease. Nurses play a major role in hospice care; a team approach also usually involves physicians, therapists, trained volunteers, and clergy members. Nurses focus on managing pain, treating symptoms, and helping clients live life to the fullest until death. They work with family members to assist in bereavement and reorganizing their lives. Hospice care was initially provided in the home and still is. More recently, hospital- and community-based units have developed hospice programs as well.

KEY CONCEPTS

- The goal of home care is to allow people to regain or maintain optimal health and to function within their limitations in the home environment.
- The home management of a person's healthcare needs usually occurs within the context of family, friends, and community.
- Altered ability to manage healthcare needs independently may result from decreased functional abilities, insufficient family or social supports, or insufficient community resources.
- Key components of the Rice model for home care include motivational factors of the client and family and the nurse as facilitator of home independence in the roles of educator, advocate, aesthetic/spiritual communer, and case manager.

REFERENCES

American Nurses Association. (1999). *The scope and standards of practice for home health nursing.* Washington, DC: Author.

Carpenito, L. J. (2000). *Nursing diagnosis: Application to clinical practice* (8th ed.). Philadelphia: Lippincott.

Cary, A. H. (1995). Role of the nurse as patient advocate. In K. J. Morgan & S. L. McClain (Eds.), *Core curriculum for home health care nursing.* Gaithersburg, MD: Aspen.

Castro, J. (1994). *The American way of health.* Boston: Little, Brown.

Cochran, M., & Brennan, S. J. (1998). Homehealth care nursing in the managed care environment: Part I. *Homehealth Care Nurse, 16*(4), 214–220.

Eliopoulos, C. (1999). *Integrating conventional and alternative therapies: Holistic care for chronic conditions.* St. Louis: Mosby.

Gonzales, T. I. (1997). An empirical study of economics of scope in home healthcare. *Health Services Research, 32*(3), 313–324.

Green, K. (1998). *Home care survival guide.* Philadelphia: Lippincott-Raven.

Hagan, L., Morin. D., & Lepine, R. (2000). Evaluation of tele-nursing outcomes: Satisfaction, self-care practices, and cost savings. *Public Health Nursing, 17*(4), 305–313.

Harris, M. D. (2000). Challenges for home healthcare nurses in the 21st century. *Home Healthcare Nurse, 18*(1), 39–44.

Health Care Financing Administration. (1998). *Outcome and assessment information set: User's manual.* Washington, DC: U.S. Department of Health and Human Services.

Humphrey, C. J., & Milone-Nuzzo, P. (1996). *Orientation to home care nursing.* Gaithersburg, MD: Aspen.

Johnson, B., Wheeler, L., Deuser, J., & Sousa, K. H. (2000). Outcomes of the Kaiser Permanente tele-home health research project. *Archives of Family Medicine, 9*(1), 40–45.

Kaye, L. W., & Davitt, J. K. (1999). *Current practices in high-tech home care.* New York: Springer.

Kraus, M. B. (1995). Role of the nurse as patient educator. In K. J. Morgan & S. L. McClain (Eds.), *Core curriculum for home health care nursing.* Gaithersburg, MD: Aspen.

Marrelli, T. M. (2001). *Handbook of home health standards and documentation guidelines for reimbursement.* St. Louis: Mosby.

National Association for Home Care. (1996). How to choose a home care provider: What is home care? Available at: http://www.nahc.org/consumer/wihc.html. Accessed 1/14/02.

Rice, R. (2001). *Home health nursing practice: Concepts and application.* St. Louis: Mosby Yearbook.

Shaughnessy, P. W., Crisler, K. S., & Schlenker, R. E. (1998). Outcome-based quality improvement in home health care: The OASIS indicators. *Quality Management in Health Care, 7*(1), 58–67.

Siefker, J. M., Garrett, M. B., Genderen, A. V., & Weis, M. J. (1998). *Fundamentals of case management: Guidelines for practicing case managers.* St. Louis, MO: Mosby.

Sienkiewicz, J. I., & Davidson, L. (2000). Using M & E and telephonic case management in PPS. *Home Healthcare Nurse, 18*(8), 541–547.

Smith, C. M., & Mauer, F. A. (2000). Community health nursing: Theory and practice (2nd ed.). Philadelphia: W. B. Saunders.

Stanhope, M., & Lancaster, J. (2000). *Community and public health nursing* (5th ed.). St. Louis, MO: Mosby.

Watson, J. (1999). *Postmodern nursing and beyond.* New York: Churchill Livingstone.

BIBLIOGRAPHY

Bennett, R. L., & Tandy, L. J. (1998). Postpartum home visits: Extending the continuum of care from hospital to home. *Home Healthcare Nurse, 16*(5), 295–303.

Brennan, S. J., & Cochran, M. (1998). Homehealth care nursing in the managed care environment: Part II. *Homehealth Care Nurse, 16*(5), 280–287.

Bond, N., Phillips, P., & Rollins, J. A. (1994). Family centered care at home for families with children who are technologically dependent. *Pediatric Nursing, 20*(2), 123–130.

Chaska, N. L. (Ed.). (2001). *The nursing profession: Tomorrow and beyond.* Thousand Oaks, CA: Sage.

Cohen, E. L., & Cesta, T. G. (1997). Nursing case management: From concept to evaluation (2nd ed.). St. Louis: Mosby.

Cohen, E. L., & De Back, V. (1999). *The outcomes mandate: Case management in health care today.* St. Louis: Mosby.

Daley, B. J., & Miller, M. (1996). Defining home health care nursing: Implications for continuing nursing education. *Journal of Continuing Education in Nursing, 27*(5), 228–237.

Ellenbecker, C. H., & Warren, K. (1998). Nursing practice and patient care in a changing home healthcare environment. *Home Healthcare Nurse, 16*(8), 531–539.

Landry, M. T., Landry, H. T., Beare, P. G., & Roe, C. W. (2001). Guidelines for developing clinical paths in your agency. *Home Healthcare Nurse, 19*(2), 69–74.

Madigan, E. A. (1998). Evidence-based practice in home healthcare: A springboard for discussion. *Home Healthcare Nurse, 16*(6), 411–415.

Matzo, M. P., & Sherman, D. W. (2001). *Palliative care nursing: Quality care at the end of life.* New York: Springer.

Peters, D. A., & McKeon, T. (1998). *Transforming home care: Quality, cost, and data management.* Gaithersburg, MD: Aspen.

Redman, B. K. (2001). *The practice of patient education* (9th ed.). St. Louis: Mosby.

Smith, S. A. (2001). *Hospice concepts: A guide to palliative care in terminal illness.* Champaign, IL: Research Press.

Snowden, F. (Ed.). (2001). *Case manager's desk reference* (2nd ed.). Gaithersburg, MD: Aspen.

Taylor, C. (1997). Ethical issues in case management. In Cohen, E. L., & Cesta, T. G., *Nursing case management: From concept to evaluation.* St. Louis: Mosby.

Weinstein, S. (1993). A coordinated appearance to home infusion care. *Home Healthcare Nurse, 11*(1), 15–20.

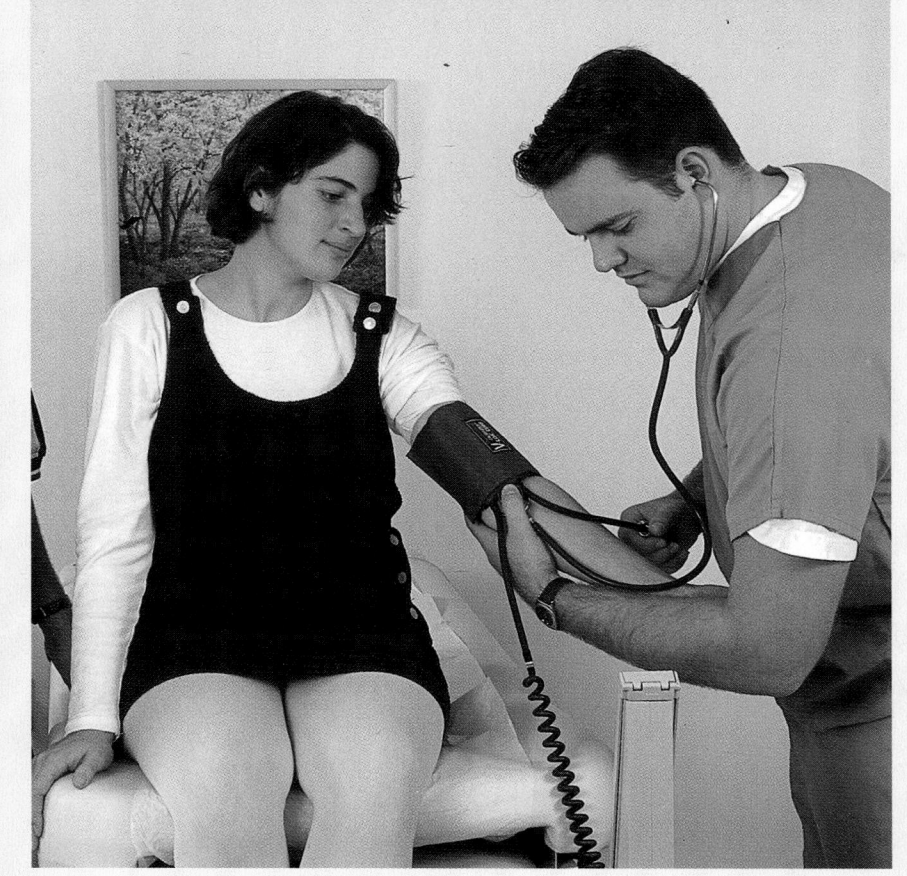

Unit 5

Essential Assessment Components

24 Health Assessment of Human Function

🔲 Key Terms

auscultation
comprehensive health
  assessment
focused health assessment
functional health assessment
health history
inspection
objective data
ophthalmoscope

otoscope
palpation
percussion
physical examination
primary data
secondary data sources
stethoscope
subjective data
tangential lighting

🔲 Learning Objectives

Upon completion of this chapter, the student will be able to do the following:
1. Organize a nursing assessment.
2. Discuss preparation of the client and the environment to foster data collection.
3. Differentiate between subjective and objective data.
4. Discuss methods to obtain subjective information during the client interview.
5. Describe the techniques of inspection, palpation, percussion, and auscultation used in the physical assessment.
6. Describe methods to obtain objective data during the physical examination.
7. Individualize the nursing assessment based on lifespan considerations.

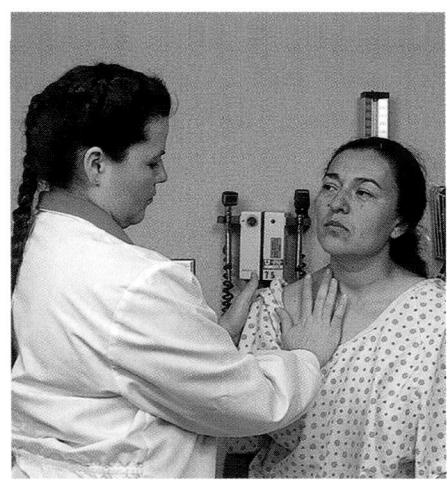

🔲 Critical Thinking Challenge

The chart describes your client as a 38-year-old woman, married, and the mother of two children in the sixth and eighth grades. She works full-time as a paralegal professional. Her past medical history is listed as a tonsillectomy at age 8 and a urinary tract infection at age 14 years (none since then). She has sought health-care at this clinic for the last 2 years, and had a comprehensive assessment when she entered the system. Her husband says that she has been fatigued for the last 2 weeks, and that she gets short of breath on exertion. The client's reason for seeking care is "stabbing chest pain on my right side when I take a deep breath or cough." Her height is 67 inches, weight is 160 lb, and she is alert and oriented. Her vital signs are temperature, 102.2°F; pulse, 120 beats per minute and regular; respirations, 32 per minute and regular; and blood pressure, 152/80 mm Hg. She is coughing up moderate amounts of thick, yellow sputum. A pleural friction rub is present.

Once you have completed this chapter and have incorporated health assessment of human function into your knowledge base, review the above scenario and reflect on the following areas of Critical Thinking:

1. Construct a list of which data presented in the situation were primary data and which were secondary data. Determine which data were subjective and which were objective.
2. Develop the order in which you would collect your assessment information about the client.
3. Using a functional health, head-to-toe, or body systems framework, cluster the data into meaningful groups.
4. Select which data are of priority and which data are irrelevant at this time.
5. Identify gaps in the priority data. List what further data you should gather. Summarize the procedures you would use to obtain these data.
6. Determine if you are able to make a nursing diagnosis at this time. If yes, identify the diagnosis. If not, explain why.

A comprehensive health assessment encompasses the physical, psychological, social, and spiritual dimensions of living. Physical health includes basic functions such as breathing, eating, and walking. Psychological health involves intellect, self-concept, emotions, and behavior. Social dimensions of health encompass relationships and interactions among family, friends, and coworkers. Spiritual health refers to belief in a higher being, personal interpretation of the meaning of life, and attitudes toward moral decisions and personal conduct. In performing a comprehensive health assessment, nurses consider all of these dimensions.

A comprehensive health assessment may be performed as a client makes initial contact within the healthcare system. It should take approximately 45 minutes but can vary in length depending on the specific client.

A comprehensive assessment is complete, but it may not always be practical or feasible. Often, nurses must select the most important interviewing questions or assessment techniques to use and perform a **focused health assessment** based on the client's problems. Components of a focused assessment include performing a general survey, taking vital signs, and assessing specific areas that relate to the problem. Nurses need to use critical thinking to determine which assessment skills to use with each client (Carpenito, 2002).

Assessment includes collecting subjective data through interviewing the client and obtaining objective data by physically examining the client. **Subjective data** are those symptoms, feelings, perceptions, preferences, values, and information that only the client can state and validate. **Objective data** can be directly observed or measured, such as vital signs or appearance (Weber & Kelley, 1998).

PURPOSE OF THE HEALTH ASSESSMENT

The purpose of the health assessment is to establish a database for the client's normal abilities, risk factors that can contribute to dysfunction, and any current alterations in function. A clear description of the client's health status and health-related problems is the desired outcome of a health assessment. From this information, the nurse and the client together can plan strategies to encourage continuation of healthy patterns, prevent potential health problems, and alleviate or manage existing health problems.

The information gathered in health assessment is organized into meaningful groupings to elicit patterns, similarities, and differences. Pieces of information are not used in isolation but rather in combination with other pieces to provide a holistic view of the client. Unclear data are validated, missing information is collected, and connections between patterns are analyzed.

A complete assessment provides an adequate database to help formulate a conclusion or a problem statement, such as a nursing diagnosis. By comparing the client's assessment findings with the defining characteristics for the diagnosis, the nurse can determine whether obtained data has been obtained to meet the diagnosis, whether further data should be gathered, or whether another diagnosis is more appropriate. An accurate assessment provides an essential foundation for the care of the client (Carpenito, 2002).

FRAMEWORKS FOR HEALTH ASSESSMENT

The three major frameworks for organizing assessment data are the functional health framework, the head-to-toe framework, and the body systems framework. Each framework helps nurses to organize the information they collect and to ensure that they do not inadvertently omit important assessment data. Each assessment framework begins with observing the client's general appearance and obtaining vital signs. Developing a consistent, comprehensive method for assessment is more important than which specific framework a nurse decides to use. Table 24-1 compares data collection using the functional health, head-to-toe, and body systems frameworks.

Functional Health Framework

A **functional health assessment** evaluates the effects of the mind, body, and environment in relation to a person's ability to perform the tasks of daily living. The functional health framework for assessment organizes data collection in terms of Gordon's 11 functional health patterns: health perception–health management; nutrition–metabolic; activity–exercise; elimination; sleep–rest; cognitive–perceptual; self-perception–self-concept; roles–relationships; sexuality–reproduction; coping–stress tolerance; and values–beliefs (Gordon, 1994). Often, nurses collect subjective information using functional health patterns but conduct the physical assessment using a head-to-toe approach. Then after all data have been gathered, the nurse may use a functional health framework to organize and analyze the data obtained. This method is used in this chapter.

Head-to-Toe Framework

The head-to-toe framework is a system for collecting data in an organized manner, starting from the head and proceeding systematically downward to the toes. This framework is used to improve efficiency and to expedite the actual physical examination. Display 24-1 outlines the organization for head-to-toe assessment. The interview is conducted separately, usually before the physical examination, to guide and focus data collection. A typical outline of data collection is head (hair, scalp, eyes, ears, oral cavity, and cranial nerves), neck, chest, abdomen, extremities, genitals, and rectum.

Body Systems Framework

Body systems is a framework that medical practitioners commonly use. It focuses on the pathophysiology involved within specific body systems (e.g., cardiovascular, genitourinary). A

TABLE 24-1

Comparison of Functional Health, Head-to-Toe, and Body Systems Frameworks		
Functional Health Pattern	**Head-to-Toe**	**Body Systems**
Health perception and health management		
Activity and exercise	Upper and lower extremities (pulses and circulation); precordium and anterior thorax, posterior thorax	Respiratory Cardiovascular Musculoskeletal
Nutrition and metabolism	Hair and scalp, head, oral cavity, thyroid, nails, abdomen	Gastrointestinal Integumentary Endocrine
Elimination	Abdomen, pelvis, anus, rectum	Genitourinary Gastrointestinal
Sleep and rest	Eyes, ears, cranial nerves	Neurologic
Cognition and perception		Sensory
Self-perception and self-concept		Psychosocial
Roles and relationships		Psychosocial
Coping and stress tolerance		Psychosocial
Sexuality and reproduction	Breasts, testicles, pelvic exam, genitalia	Endocrine Reproductive
Values and beliefs		Psychosocial

DISPLAY 24-1

🔄 PHYSICAL ASSESSMENT COLLECTION USING HEAD-TO-TOE FRAMEWORK

General
General health state
Vital signs and weight
Nutritional status

Mobility and Self-Care
Observe posture
Assess gait and balance
Evaluate mobility
Activities of daily living

Head, Face, and Neck
Evaluate cognition
Level of consciousness
Orientation
Mood
Language and memory
Sensory function
Inspect and examine eyes
Test vision
Inspect and examine ears
Test hearing
Cranial nerves
Inspect oral cavity and teeth
Inspect lymph nodes
Inspect neck veins

Skin, Hair, and Nails
Inspect scalp and hair
Evaluate skin turgor

Observe skin lesions
Assess wounds
Inspect nails

Chest
Inspect and palpate breasts
Inspect and auscultate lungs
Auscultate heart

Abdomen
Inspect, auscultate, palpate four quadrants
Palpate and percuss liver, stomach, bladder
Bowel elimination
Urinary elimination

Genitalia
Inspect female client
Inspect male client

Extremities
Palpate arterial pulses
Observe capillary refill
Evaluate edema
Assess joint mobility
Measure strength
Assess sensory function
Assess circulation, movement, and sensation
Deep tendon reflexes
Inspect skin and nails

body systems approach may be used during the focused assessment of an acutely or critically ill client. It is also commonly used when the purpose of the examination is to determine function of a particular body system. In an unconscious client, it is more important to obtain physical assessment data from all body systems because the client is unable to communicate any difficulties. A focused assessment may be used, for example, after orthopedic surgery; a musculoskeletal assessment may be important to assess the impact of surgery on mobility and activity.

CONDUCTING A HEALTH ASSESSMENT

Reviewing General Information

Usually it is possible to obtain some general information about the client by using secondary data sources before introducing yourself to the client. **Secondary data sources** include sources of data other than the client, such as the chart or other healthcare providers. Such sources help to personalize the interview.

If the chart is available, note the client's name, age, primary language, health history, and current medications or treatment. Doing so promotes efficient communication with the client and prevents repetition of the same questions by several different people. If friends or family are available, they may be able to provide information about the client's symptoms and history.

Primary data are gathered from the client. During the initial stage of the assessment, the nurse takes the client's vital signs to obtain a general overview of the client's status and to detect any conditions that require immediate intervention. The nurse also interviews the client to obtain primary data.

Considering Culture

Cultural sensitivity is important when conducting a health assessment. Often, the client's language, customs, beliefs, and values differ from those of the nurse performing the assessment. A nurse's conscious or unconscious biases can influence his or her interpretation of data. For example, if in the nurse's culture people freely express discomfort and pain, the nurse may misinterpret cues from a stoic client in whose culture it would be weak or embarrassing to verbalize pain. Examination of cultural customs, values, and beliefs helps nurses and clients avoid miscommunication.

When a client who does not speak English is being assessed, an interpreter may be needed. Additional time is required when an interpreter is used. Family members are sometimes helpful, but staff or official translators often provide a more objective translation. For example, information that is emotionally difficult for the family, such as that pertaining to a life-threatening illness, could be traumatic and interfere with the translation process. Recognize that even translators who have a good command of English may need explanations for specific medical terms or may use different terms to describe body functions.

When using an interpreter, speak to the client and use language as if you were speaking directly to the client. Instead of saying, "Ask her if she has pain," say, "Do you have pain?" Look and listen to the client when he or she responds. Observe cues the client expresses with body language, and listen to the tone of voice. This communication can be very important in understanding what the client is saying and underlying emotional messages.

Be sensitive to communication differences across cultures. For example, in some cultures it is comfortable to talk close to another's face, whereas in others additional space is more comfortable. Some cultures find it more comfortable to discuss personal issues (e.g., bowel or bladder elimination) than do others. Additionally, some people regard direct questioning as invasive and are more receptive to a warmer and more casual type of interview. In some cultures, the husband is the family spokesperson and must be present during the health assessment of his wife and children. Knowledge and awareness of these differences between cultures can help prevent inadvertent miscommunication.

Preparing the Client and Environment

Thoughtful preparation of the client and the environment is advantageous for both the client and the nurse. Understanding the process and knowing what to expect ensures the client's physical and emotional comfort. The nurse who is well organized, calm, and efficient reassures the client.

Most clients undergoing a health examination are anxious. Pain, fear, and embarrassment may all contribute to a client's distress. Thoughtfully preparing the client and environment before the assessment can eliminate some controllable sources of anxiety.

Environment

The environment should be comfortable for both nurse and client. A warm, quiet, well-lit room is ideal. Gather all necessary pieces of equipment in advance, making sure they are fully functional. Leaving the client to find equipment is distracting and time-consuming.

Privacy and confidentiality are important concerns for the client who is about to share personal information and submit to a physical examination. The client should feel confident that others will not view or overhear the interview or physical examination. Providing such privacy can be a challenge if the client shares a room with another client. Family members and visitors may leave or stay, depending on the client's preference. Pull the curtains around the bedside, and position yourself so you are away from others in the room.

The client should be as physically comfortable as possible during the assessment. A relaxed client is more attentive and can provide more accurate and complete information. Ask the client if he or she needs to use the bathroom before beginning the assessment, especially if you anticipate an abdominal assessment. Occasionally, you may be unable to provide comfort to the client who is in acute pain or distress until you have accomplished an assessment of the client's condition. When this occurs, acknowledge the distress and promptly begin the assessment, focusing immediately on the client's primary problem. The assessment of the problem usually takes priority when a client is uncomfortable or acutely ill.

Organizing and Documenting
The major portion of the client interview may be conducted either before the physical examination is performed or during dialogue with the client throughout the assessment. Document pertinent information (e.g., quotations, abnormal values) during the interview, and complete the remainder of the form after the conclusion. Practice how and what you will document during the conversation to develop skills in documenting without distracting from the conversation.

During most health assessments, a preprinted form is used to record information. Health assessment forms vary in title and format, depending on the institution, the client population, and the purpose of the assessment. Some common titles for health assessment forms are Nursing History, Nursing Admission Form, Client Database, and Nursing Assessment Form.

The format may be structured, using specific questions and lists of required data, or it may be unstructured, defining broad areas of health. Following a printed form is useful, particularly when you are learning to perform health assessment, because it provides a structure for moving logically from one health area to another. It also helps to prevent the omission of any pertinent information.

Introduction to the Client
Introduce yourself to the client, and explain the nature and purpose of the health assessment. Describe assessment as a series of questions about the client's past and present state of health, followed by a physical examination. During this introductory phase, tell the client approximately how long the assessment will take. Reassure the client that information obtained during the assessment process is confidential and will be shared only with other healthcare professionals participating in provision of care (Girard, 1997).

OBTAINING SUBJECTIVE DATA: THE INTERVIEW

The **health history,** or interview, is a goal-directed conversation between nurse and client. Goals may include the following:

- Obtain the client's history and perceptions of past experiences.
- Identify factors that either positively or negatively influence the client's health status.
- Describe how health status influences the client's abilities.
- Identify what changes the client has made to adapt to the health problems.

The interview component of a health assessment is often the client's first encounter with the nurse and therefore the first step toward establishing a trusting and therapeutic nurse–client re-

ETHICAL/LEGAL ISSUE
Health Assessment

Bob Ellis is the nurse assigned to Mrs. Androni, a 73-year-old widow, who was recently admitted for observation after a fall. Bob introduces himself and explains that he needs to ask the client some questions and to perform a physical examination. Mrs. Androni states, "I just don't feel comfortable having a man examine me. It is against the beliefs and ways of my people. I feel just fine, so you go along and find someone else to practice on."

Reflection
- How would you feel if you were the nurse in this situation?
- Explain factors that might contribute to Mrs. Androni's feelings.
- Can the healthcare facility provide safe care to Mrs. Androni if Bob avoids performing the physical examination?
- Brainstorm advantages and disadvantages to switching the client assignment so that Mrs. Androni receives care from a female nurse.

lationship. Be professional, concerned, and attentive throughout the interview. When the client responds to a question, convey interest by maintaining eye contact, occasionally nodding, or verbally responding to his or her remarks (Arnold & Boggs, 1999).

Nonverbal behavior, particularly body language, can convey a strong message during an interview. The nurse who sits at eye level with the client, appears unhurried and alert, and takes notes conveys to the client that the information being shared is important and deserves attention. In contrast, the nurse who stands over a client during an interview communicates that the nurse's stay will be brief, and the client may feel powerless or conclude that the nurse is in a hurry or has more important tasks to do. The nurse who sits on the bed may invade the client's personal space or appear unprofessional. Throughout the interview, continuously evaluate your verbal and nonverbal messages. These messages can either promote or discourage the client's trust and confidence.

Questioning clients about their health is a skill that requires study and practice to achieve competence. Before the first assessment and interview, prepare questions in each health area. Some questions, such as those about allergies, can be asked with a closed-ended (Yes/No) question. Open-ended questions are preferable in other areas of health concern. For example, the question, "Describe what you eat on a normal day" will yield more valuable information than "How is your appetite?" Ask follow-up or probing questions when a problem area is discovered or suggested. Solicit further detail by statements such as, "Tell me more about that" or "That seems to concern you."

Special techniques may be necessary to control the interview if a client is overly talkative, particularly in regard to unrelated information. Many clients have difficulty staying on a topic or limiting their answers to significant points. A sensitive yet effective method for directing the client might be, "Because our time is limited, we won't be able to discuss that in detail now. I would like to hear more about. . . ." The ability to skillfully, yet sensitively, control the interview is essential for obtaining pertinent information in a timely manner.

Reason for Seeking Healthcare

The first subject usually discussed in a client interview is the client's specific reason for seeking care (Jarvis, 2000). This subject is often called the client's "chief complaint" or "chief concern." Listen carefully to the client's description of the primary problem and document it, quoting the client's exact words. In-depth questioning and discussion of this problem should follow. Information you obtain during the interview helps target areas of pain or probable abnormality so that the examination of the affected areas can be especially careful, thoughtful, and thorough.

Health History

During the interview, obtain information about the client's health history and family health history. Health history information should include known allergies, childhood illnesses, previous surgeries, and chronic health conditions. Ascertain what, if any, medications the client is currently taking. Some clients may have a written list or be able to show you the bottle with the medication's name. Family history includes a review of major illnesses, listing the family member who is affected (e.g., paternal grandfather, sister).

Pain Assessment

Addressing pain early in the health assessment allows the nurse to individualize the rest of the assessment, avoiding positioning and techniques that are especially uncomfortable for the client. If the client is in severe pain, lengthy questioning is best postponed. Acknowledging the client's pain and verbalizing your efforts to limit discomfort during the assessment are important.

Acute illness, chronic disability, surgical intervention, and treatment modalities can all cause the client pain. Pain can limit normal function and affect wellness and quality of life. Accurate assessment of pain is necessary to identify and treat the underlying cause of pain. Assessment permits a better understanding of the client's pain experience (Lawler, 1997).

Because the pain experience is personal and subjective, the client interview is the best way to collect information to assess pain. Such an assessment should include asking the client to describe the location, intensity, quality, onset, and chronology of his or her pain experience. Also determine factors that influence the pain experience and methods of effective pain management. Last, explore the impact the pain experience has

on daily life and other health patterns. Some clients are reluctant to discuss and describe their pain experience because of personal beliefs or values.

Questions helpful in soliciting subjective information concerning the client's pain experience include the following:

- Do you have any pain or discomfort? How long have you had it?
- If yes, tell me how bad it is on a 1 to 10 scale, with 10 being the worst.
- Show me where it is. Does it move or radiate anywhere?
- Describe what it feels like.
- When does it come on? How long does it last?
- What makes it better? What makes it worse?

Objective data are not always available to document the experience of pain. Acute pain stimulates the sympathetic nervous system and produces the following objective symptoms: increased blood pressure, increased pulse, increased respiratory rate, dilated pupils, and diaphoresis. This sympathetic response is not present in chronic pain states, and these parameters may be absent if pain has been present for several days. Observing the client's body position and facial features also gives clues to the presence of pain. Grimacing, guarded positioning, tense body posture, refusal to move a body part, muscle spasms, or rubbing a body part can all indicate the presence of pain despite verbal denial. A "facial mask of pain," in which the client's facial expression is flat or fixed, the eyes appear dull, and fatigue is evident, commonly occurs in chronic pain. Emotional expression such as crying, moaning, or yelling also can occur during severe pain.

Assessment of Health Perception and Health Management

The major focus in health perception–health management is the client's perception of health status, preventive health practices, compliance with medical treatment, and client safety (Gordon, 1994). Discuss the client's health-promotion activities, such as exercise, nutrition, routine preventive examinations (e.g., dental, vision, hearing), immunization history, safety precautions (e.g., child safety seats, bicycle helmets), and stress management. Inquire about the use of nicotine (including chewing tobacco, pipe, cigar, and use of nicotine gum or patches), alcohol (amount, frequency, and type), and drugs (recreational and prescription). Assess the client's overall willingness and ability to follow health-related advice, such as taking medications on schedule or following a prescribed diet. Also elicit other sources of health advice used by the client, such as an acupuncturist, herbalist, or naturopath.

Obtain a detailed allergy history for every client, including medication, food, pollen, insect, and any environmental allergens. Inquire about the specific type of reaction that the client experienced. Some clients may confuse a medication side effect, such as nausea, with an allergic reaction. Document any severe allergic reactions, and communicate them to other members of the healthcare team.

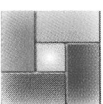

Nursing Research and Critical Thinking

Does Asking Someone, "How Do You Feel?" Provide Any Useful Information?

Self-reported health, as measured by a single question, is rarely used in primary care settings or as a part of health screening programs. A group of researchers wondered whether self-reported health should be routinely used in healthcare settings. They designed a study to explore the relationship between self-reported health and chronic illness and physical disability among older adults living in the community. This study assessed relationships between objective measures of physical and mental health and self-reported health status among a representative sample of 912 older persons. Data were collected through telephone interviews, and augmented with personal interviews in low socioeconomic census tracts (where households were less likely to have working telephones). Questions addressed self-reported health, presence of physical and mental health conditions, health service use, health behaviors, and sociodemographic characteristics. The analysis included the dependent variable, self-reported health, with five response categories ranging from excellent to poor, and objective indicators of physical and mental health. The researchers found that one or more days of poor health in the past month increased the risk of report-

ing poor health 4.4 times. Having one or more days of restricted activity increased reporting of poor health 2.7 times. The study also found that people in good physical health, but who experienced poor mental health, express their mental health problems through self-reports of poor health.

Critical Thinking Considerations. The sample used in this study was taken from an original sample of 5,506 persons who lived in two counties in central New Jersey as a part of a larger health needs assessment project. The participants in this study were limited to persons older than 65 years of age from that original sample. The findings are not generalizable to other age groups or persons living in other communities. According to the researchers, possible implications for nursing practice are as follows:

* Self-reported health can serve as a reliable indicator of a person's physical health status and future morbidity and mortality.
* Among physically healthy older persons, the experience of poor mental health is reflected in self-reports of poor health, and can be helpful in ascertaining the need for further assessment or referral.

Grau, L., West, B., & Gregory, P. (1998). "How do you feel?" Self-reported health as an indicator of current physical and mental health status. *Journal of Psychosocial Nursing, 36*(6), 24–30.

Many people live with chronic diseases, such as heart disease, cancer, or stroke. Control of these health problems depends directly on modification of a person's behavior and habits of living. Prevention necessitates eliminating activities that many people enjoy: overeating, overindulgence in alcohol, and nicotine use. Prevention also implies doing things that require special effort: exercising regularly, eating a healthy diet, seeking regular health examinations, and striving for a harmonious life. Assessment of a person's health perception and health maintenance reveals knowledge, behavior, and attitudes toward preventing disease and living a healthy lifestyle. The following are selected sample interview questions in a health history:

* How would you describe your health?
* When was your last dental, eye, or physical examination?
* Have you ever used tobacco, alcohol, or recreational drugs? What type? How often?
* What safety practices do you follow (e.g., safety belt, bicycle helmet)?

Assessment of Activity and Exercise

Mobility affects independence and self-care abilities. For clients with no deficits, only a brief discussion of mobility and self-care is necessary. Observing the client's posture, gait, and

movement as he or she enters the room provides much information. If you detect deficits, a detailed evaluation is needed.

Posture

Inspect the spine for straight alignment and symmetry. The client's posture should also be straight, without abnormal curving. In kyphosis, the shoulder and upper back tend to curve forward, such as occurs in normal aging. Many schools screen for scoliosis, which is a curvature of a portion of the spine to the side laterally. Scoliosis can be seen better by having the client bend over and evaluating for symmetry. Also observe for lordosis, commonly known as "swayback," in which the lumbar region curves inward and the sacral region curves outward.

Gait and Balance

Gait describes a person's manner of walking. Balance refers to stability and equality between both sides of the body. An evaluation of gait and balance contributes to the assessment of a client's mobility as well as risk for injury due to falling. Gait and balance abnormalities may also indicate dysfunction or disease in other body systems, particularly the brain, spinal cord, muscles, and skeleton. A client may acquire a slowed, cautious, or unnatural gait as an unconscious means of protection from pain, weakness, or loss of balance.

The nurse may observe gait and balance during many activities that naturally occur in the course of a health assessment. Assess the client's balance as he or she walks into the room, moves around in bed, rises from the sitting position, or rolls onto his or her side. To assess gait further, ask the client to walk a distance of about 10 feet down a hallway. A normal gait is quick, springy, and rhythmic, with the arms naturally swinging back and forth. Characteristics of abnormal gait include the following: slow, measured steps; limping; leaning to one side; shuffling the feet; shorter steps taken on one side compared to the other; wide outward swinging of one leg; a wide gait or stance; leaning the trunk forward; lifting the knee higher than normal with each step; and short, hurrying steps.

Decreased Mobility

Foot pain is a common cause of decreased mobility. Inspect the client's feet for the presence of bunions, corns, calluses, ingrown toenails, spurs, and ulcers.

If the client uses any assistive devices for ambulation, such as a cane, crutches, walker, prosthesis, or brace, assess the client's use of the aid, focusing on coordination, stability, comfort, and safety. For additional information on assessing mobility status, refer to Chapter 33.

A program of regular physical activity should be discussed with every client. Participation in sports and recreational activities contributes to not only physical but psychological well-being. Determine whether the client has any pain or discomfort associated with exercise and whether the client is unable to participate in any desirable activities. Energy level also affects the desire and ability to be physically active. Fatigue is frequently associated with cardiac or respiratory disease, anemia, or cancer.

When a client's mobility or self-care functions are compromised, a daily living assessment should be performed. A daily living assessment includes evaluation of the ability to perform self-care skills (bathing, toileting, dressing, grooming, and eating) and simple motor activities (sitting, standing, walking, climbing stairs, and opening doors). Depending on the client's living situation, an assessment of some home maintenance skills may also be appropriate (Halfmann, Keller, & Allison, 1997). These skills include cooking, shopping, housekeeping (making a bed, cleaning, vacuuming, washing dishes), doing the laundry, paying bills, and using the telephone. The architecture of a home, particularly the presence of stairs, can complicate independent activity and should be considered.

A scale is used to rate these self-care abilities (Display 24-2). The daily living assessment provides key information about a person's ability to live independently or the amount of assistance that he or she requires to do so. If major disabilities are present, an occupational therapist may be consulted for further evaluation. More information on daily living assessment is provided in Chapter 32.

Mobility assessment is preventive as well as descriptive. Clients with impaired mobility are at risk for accidents and injury. Older people, particularly those who have fallen in the

DISPLAY 24-2

SELF-CARE ABILITIES SCALE

0—Full self-care, independent
I—Needs to use equipment or device
II—Needs supervision
III—Needs equipment or device and supervision
IV—Unable to perform, dependent

past, are most susceptible. A thorough assessment of risk factors can determine the risk for falling, and appropriate safety precautions may be instituted (Lane, 1999).

Subjective data can be collected concerning adequate peripheral (arm and leg) circulation, evaluating arterial and venous blood flow. Evaluate the client's use of vasoconstricting agents such as nicotine. The following are suggested client interview questions related to mobility:

- Describe your usual activities in a normal day (or week).
- What limitations in ability do you have (eating, toileting, walking, dressing, bathing)?
- Have you recently fallen or consider yourself to be at risk for falling?
- What do you do to keep healthy or prevent disease progression?

Assessment of Nutrition and Metabolism

Assessment of nutrition and metabolism includes dietary habits and metabolic needs. Information reflects how well the client's body is able to ingest, digest, absorb, metabolize, and use food to maintain tissue integrity, maintain fluid and electrolyte balance, and fight infection (Hammond, 1997).

Assessment of nutrition and metabolism requires specific information about the client's normal diet and careful observations of the physical features that reflect nutritional state. The nutrition–metabolism assessment should focus on normal food and fluid intake, alterations in normal eating patterns, how dietary changes have affected daily living, and the development of medical problems secondary to altered nutritional status (Evans-Stoner, 1997).

Interview questions to focus a nutrition–metabolism assessment might include some of the following:

- Tell me what you've eaten in the last 24 hours.
- What is your usual weight? Has it changed in the past 6 months? How much?
- Do you have any problems with tasting, chewing, or swallowing food?
- Do you have any problems with getting groceries or preparing food?

Weight measurement can provide important information regarding nutritional status. Standardized tables have been developed (e.g., Metropolitan Height and Weight Tables for Men and Women, Ages 25 to 59) that recommend ideal body weights for men and women. Standardized tables are also available to evaluate growth in children (McLaren & Green, 1998). Such tables provide a baseline for evaluating the client's weight. Deviations from normal body size, ranging from obese to severely underweight, can influence not only the nutritional state but other areas, such as exercise, activity, and self-concept.

Use of the standardized weight tables to evaluate nutritional status has recently been questioned because the tables fail to consider individual and group (e.g., cultural, ethnic) variances. Determination of the percentage of weight change, which uses the client's usual weight as the standard, may be more meaningful. The following formula can be used to calculate the percentage of weight change:

$$\text{(Current weight} - \text{Usual weight)} / \text{Usual weight} = \text{Percentage of weight change}$$

In general, a change in weight of 10% over the last 6 months is considered to be abnormal (Jarvis, 2000). A dietitian should be consulted for further evaluation.

Weight measurement can also be used to evaluate fluid status or the response of the client to medical treatment (e.g., diuretic therapy to treat congestive heart failure). Rapid weight gain or loss (e.g., 10 lb in 2 weeks) usually results from the gain or loss of body fluid rather than body fat.

Weight measurement can be done on a variety of scales; the choice depends mainly on the client's status. An upright scale is appropriate for clients with normal mobility who can step onto a platform and maintain balance while weight is determined. A chair scale is used for clients who can transfer to a chair but are unable to support the body in a standing position for accurate weight measurement. A bed scale is used for clients who are too weak or immobile to use other scales safely. Special infant scales are used to determine the height and weight of babies.

Scales can be calibrated in terms of pounds or kilograms, with some scales providing both measures of weight. To convert from pounds to kilograms, divide by 2.2; to convert from kilograms to pounds, multiply by 2.2. For most clients, height and weight measurements are obtained on admission to a healthcare agency. When daily or frequent weights are required to evaluate client progress, weight is measured at the same time each day (usually before breakfast), using the same scale. Procedure 24-1 outlines steps in measuring weight.

Height is measured with a measuring stick attached to a standing scale. The client stands erect without shoes on the scale, and the height is determined by lowering the sliding arm until it rests on the client's head. Height can be measured in inches or centimeters. To convert inches to centimeters, multiply by 2.54; to convert centimeters to inches, divide by 2.54.

Assessment of Elimination

Elimination assessment focuses on determining the adequacy of bladder and bowel function, identifying risk factors that may contribute to problems in elimination, assessing the im-

pact of bladder or bowel dysfunction on daily living, and understanding the client's methods of managing and coping with any dysfunction (Bardsley, 1999/2000).

Focus on the client's normal urinary and bowel patterns, noting any recent changes. Questions to elicit such information from the client include the following:

- Describe your normal voiding pattern.
- Have you experienced any changes in your usual voiding pattern?
- Have you had any discomfort, pain, frequency, incontinence, or difficulty starting the urinary stream?
- Tell me your normal bowel pattern.
- What things do you do to stay regular?
- Have you had any changes in your normal bowel pattern?
- Have you had any problems with discomfort or control with bowel movements?
- Do you have problems with nausea, vomiting, constipation, or diarrhea?

Assessment of Sleep and Rest

The assessment of sleep and rest focuses on the client's normal sleep patterns, alterations from the normal pattern, and satisfaction with quality of rest and sleep.

Sleep habits, problems with obtaining adequate rest or sleep, and any aids that the client uses to induce sleep are important areas to consider. The following are suggested questions to elicit this information:

- Tell me when you usually go to sleep. Tell me when you usually wake up. Do you awaken during the night?
- Can you easily fall asleep? What do you do to promote sleep?
- Do you feel rested on awakening?

Most data indicating a dysfunctional sleep pattern are subjective, although a few objective signs may support subjective data (Richardson, 1997). Frequent yawning, decreased attention span, and dark circles or puffiness around the eyes may be related to sleep deprivation. Continual dozing during the day may also occur when the amount or quality of sleep is inadequate. During periods of apparent sleep, note snoring, rapid eye movements, or jerking movements. Observe the client's pattern of breathing while he or she sleeps.

Assessment of Cognition and Perception

Cognitive function refers to a person's ability to think, which is evaluated primarily through written and verbal communication. Factors that contribute to cognition include awareness, thought processes, memory, language, judgment, and attention span. Whereas significant impairment in cognitive abilities is readily noticeable on first interaction, repeated assessments over time are often required to detect
(text continues on page 404)

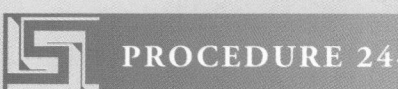

PROCEDURE 24-1

MEASURING WEIGHT

Purpose
1. To provide baseline data from which to assess total fluid balance or nutritional status.
2. To provide baseline data to determine drug dosages or information for diagnostic testing with dye or radioactive injections.

Assessment
- Assess necessity for baseline, daily, or weekly weight measurements.
- Review previous weight measurements, if available.
- Identify time of day previous weights were measured. Weights can vary considerably during a 24-hour period, so serial weights must be done at the same time each day. Most facilities weigh clients in the early morning. Check your facility's current policy.
- Assess client's mental and physical status to determine whether a standing, sitting, or bed scale is appropriate.

Equipment
An appropriate scale. *Note:* Use the same scale each time you weigh the client.
Protector towel or plastic sheet

Procedure
1. Have client void before weighing. *Note:* A full bladder, wet gowns, and saturated dressings affect the measurement.
2. Client should wear same clothing for each weight measurement. He or she should remove slippers or shoes before measurement.
   Rationale: Maintaining consistency increases the accuracy of measurement. Other helpful measures include using the same scale and measuring weight at the same time each day.
3. Place protective paper or cloth on scale.
   Rationale: Help prevent the transfer of microorganisms.
4. Check that scale registers zero. Adjust as necessary.
   Rationale: Ensure accuracy of readings.

Weight With Standing Scale
1. Assist client onto scale. Client must stand in center of platform and not lean or hold onto supports.
   Rationale: Depending on type of equipment, movement may cause inaccurate weight.
2. Read digital display or adjust counterweights to determine client's weight.
3. Assist client from scale and record weight in the client's record.

Rationale: Prompt, accurate recording of data provides information for other members of the healthcare team.

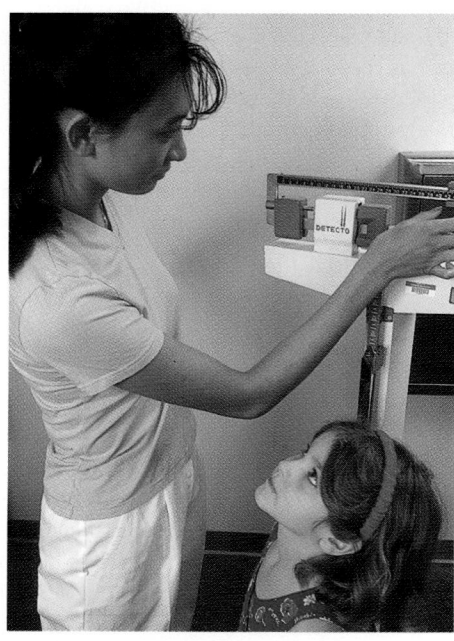

Step 2 Adjust the counterweight to determine the client's weight.

Weight With Chair Scale
1. Place scale beside client and lock wheels.
   Rationale: Safety measures prevent accidental falls.
2. Transfer client onto chair. If arm of chair is removable, unlock and remove before transfer. Lock back into place after transfer.
   Rationale: Provide security and prevent accidental falls. Some scales allow wheelchairs to be wheeled onto scale.
3. Read digital display or adjust counterweights to determine client's weight.
   Rationale: Help ensure accurate weight measurement.
4. Transfer client back to bed or wheelchair.
   Rationale: Provide for the client's safety and comfort.
5. Clean the scale according to agency policy.
   Rationale: A clean scale helps prevent transfer of microorganisms.
   Return to proper location and plug in.
   Rationale: Keep battery charged for next use.

PROCEDURE 24-1 (Continued)

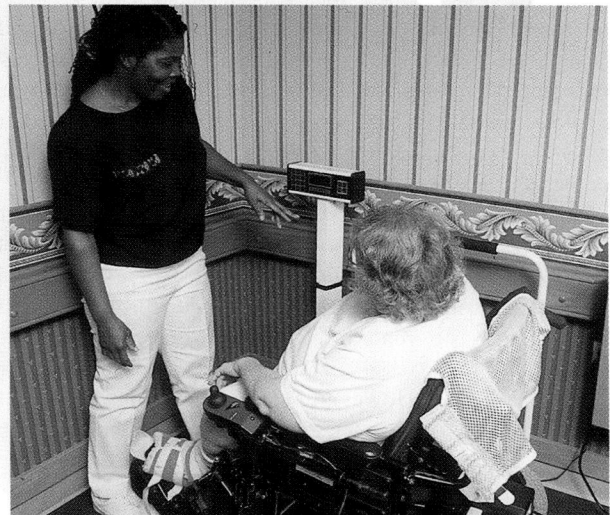

Step 2 The client is able to remain in the wheelchair on this scale.

Weight With Bed Scale

1. Elevate client's bed to level of stretcher scale.
2. With one or two assistants, turn client on the side with back toward the scale.
   Rationale: Prepare for a smooth transfer to the scale.
3. Roll scale toward the bed, lock wheels in place, and lower stretcher onto bed.
   Rationale: Provide for safe transfer of client to bed scale.
4. Position folded stretcher under client. Roll client onto stretcher.
5. Attach stretcher arms to stretcher and gradually elevate stretcher about 2 inches above mattress surface. *Note:* Inform client before elevating. Reassure the client that he or she will not fall but the head may feel lower than the body.
   Rationale: Decrease the client's anxiety and improve cooperation.
6. Determine that the stretcher is not touching any equipment. Lift all drains and tubing away from stretcher.
   Rationale: Equipment alters measurement and affects accuracy.

7. Read digital display for client's weight. *Note:* This is a good time to change client's linen as he or she is elevated off the bed.
8. Gradually lower stretcher to the bed. Remove stretcher arms and transfer client off stretcher. Remove stretcher.
   Rationale: Ensure the client's safe transfer.
9. Unlock bed scale wheels and move away from bed.
10. Assist client to comfortable position.
11. Clean stretcher and scale according to agency policy. Return to proper location and keep plugged in for next use.
    Rationale: Prevent the transfer of microorganisms and keep battery charged for next use.
12. Record weight, and note any extra linen or equipment weighed with the client.

Lifespan Considerations
- Infants are usually weighed nude. Be careful that room temperature is warm because infants' body temperature can fluctuate severely because of their immature thermoregulatory system.
- Infants often roll and kick. The nurse's hand should always be within 1 to 2 inches of the child's body to prevent accidental falls.

Home Care Modifications
- Encourage clients requiring serial weights to keep a written log of their weights.
- Instruct clients to weigh themselves at the same time each day, usually in the morning before breakfast, and to wear similar-weight clothing for each measurement.
- If visual problems restrict the client's ability to read the scale, family members may be able to assist.

Collaboration and Delegation
- Unlicensed nursing personnel (UAP) usually assess clients' weights. Inform UAPs of any client's mobility restrictions and safety precautions that are important. Ask them to notify you of any significant (1 kg) change in a client's daily weight from previous measurement.

subtle changes or minor deficits in cognitive ability (Brackley, 1997).

Subjective data for appraising mental abilities are gathered throughout the health assessment, from the context of a client's conversation and his or her degree of cooperation during the physical examination. Assess whether the client has difficulty understanding or answering questions or following directions. Evaluate the client's responses to questions in terms of clarity and appropriateness. The client should be able to express any health concerns in a coherent and clear manner.

Possible questions to elicit further information concerning a person's cognitive and communication ability include the following:

- Tell me how your memory is. Have you had any recent changes?
- Do you have problems with speaking? reading? writing?
- Describe the last experience you had learning something. How do you believe you learn best?

If deficits in cognition are present, ask:

- Tell me your full name.
- What is today's date?
- Where are you right now?

The purpose of assessing the client's sensory status is to determine functioning of the five senses: vision, hearing, touch, taste, and smell. Assessment should also include the impact sensory deficits have on activities of daily living (ADLs) and any devices the client uses to cope with sensory impairment.

Sensory losses may be congenital but are often associated with the aging process. Assess older clients carefully for sensory deficits, because many adaptive techniques are available to improve the safety, pleasure, and independence of their lives.

Clients are usually aware of sensory loss and can verbalize specific deficits when questioned. During the interview, observe the client for signs of sensory impairment, such as asking questions to be repeated, watching lips closely during speech, squinting to improve vision, or holding reading material at arm's length. Questions concerning sensory status include the following:

- How is your vision? Do you have glasses, contact lenses, or a prosthesis?
- How is your hearing? Do you use a hearing aid?
- Do you notice that it is difficult to feel in your hands or feet?
- Do you have any numbness or tingling in your hands or feet?
- Have you noticed any changes in your taste or smell?

Assessment of Self-Perception and Self-Concept

The self-perception and self-concept pattern focuses on the content and feelings associated with a person's self-evaluation (Gordon, 1994). The components of self-concept include one's self-knowledge, self-expectation, social self, and self-evaluation. The ways in which others evaluate and interact with a person throughout the lifespan influence self-concept (Bohlander, 1995). Body image, the mental picture and feelings about one's body, is an important component of self-concept. Individual beliefs concerning locus of control are also important to explore. Some people believe that life events are self-determined (internal locus of control), whereas others view individual happenings as a matter of fate, luck, or the influence of others (external locus of control).

During a basic health assessment, the goal in assessing self-perception is to describe the client's general view of self and his or her satisfaction with that image. Clients whose primary health problem directly relates to a disturbance in self-concept (such as psychiatric, chemically dependent, abused, or anorectic clients) require an extensive evaluation by a mental health specialist. However, many illnesses alter one's self-concept because of changes related to physical strength, appearance, and loss of control. For this reason, consideration of self-concept should be integrated into the health assessment of every client.

Collect subjective and supporting objective data concerning normal self-concept, recent changes in self-concept, and the presence of conditions (e.g., burns, skin disorders, colostomy, mastectomy, obesity) that could threaten or alter body image.

Possible questions that help the client describe self-perception include the following:

- What are you most concerned about in relation to your health?
- How would you describe yourself?
- How has being sick made you feel differently about yourself?

Eye contact, personal grooming and appearance, posture, body movements, mood, emotions, and voice and speech pattern are nonverbal cues to a client's self-concept. Poor eye contact, inattention to personal grooming, and body language that conveys embarrassment or shame may reflect low self-concept.

Assessment of Roles and Relationships

Most people fill a variety of roles, such as spouse or partner, parent, worker, student, colleague, friend, coach, and adviser. These roles may be rewarding and stimulating, or they may be overwhelming and stressful.

The goal in a basic health assessment is to identify the client's major roles in the family, at work, and in social life and to identify the client's relative satisfaction or dissatisfaction with each role. The assessment should also indicate how health problems or hospitalization may interfere with a person's ability to fulfill role expectations and maintain relationships (Stewart et al., 1997). Although the client normally provides this information, it is often helpful (and sometimes necessary) to consult other members of the family unit to obtain meaningful data.

Information you obtain in the assessment should focus on the client's family configuration and occupation, recent or anticipated changes in the client's roles or relationships, and the client's level of satisfaction with current roles and relationships (Gordon, 1994).

Within the family unit, important information includes who shares the household, what responsibilities or dependencies each member has, and the presence of specific problems, such as issues related to parenting, caring for elderly parents, or marital discord. The illness of a family member may necessitate shifting responsibilities within the family, such as financial support, child care, cooking, and home maintenance. Chronic illnesses often involve the client in long and sometimes permanent dependence on others. Evaluate the specific circumstances of that dependence, the client's attitude, and the client's coping ability.

Roles and relationships related to work are an important area to assess. Factors such as job-related stress, insufficient time for leisure activities, unsafe work environment, job insecurity, inadequate pay, or lack of recognition may negatively affect physical and psychological well-being.

A change in relationships may contribute to the cause or exacerbation of an illness. Explore any areas in which recent change has occurred, such as divorce, death, or illness of a family member, loss of a job, change in job status or pay, increase in job responsibility, or transition from student to worker.

Suggested questions to help obtain this information from the client include the following:

- Are you employed? retired? disabled?
- What do you see as your primary role at work? home?
- Who do you live with?
- Who do you ask for help when you need it?
- Are there any problems at work or home that influence your health?
- Do you have any insurance or financial concerns that you desire help with?

Obtain objective data by watching the interactions of the client with family members and others. Verbal interactions and nonverbal communication can support what the client has discussed in the interview. Observing visitors, cards, and flowers can help to validate that the client has positive relationships with others. Likewise, the absence of visitors and communication from others might suggest a lack of positive relationships.

SAFETY ALERT

Note repeated unexplained injuries, such as bruises, burns, or fractures, as a possible sign of abusive relationships. Frequently, people involved in abusive relationships verbally deny that abuse has occurred.

Assessment of Coping and Stress Tolerance

Stress is an event that disrupts or challenges a person's equilibrium (Gordon, 1994). Although stress is most readily conceptualized as negative, positive life changes also challenge a person and therefore create stress. Examples of positive stressors include marriage, planned pregnancy, job promotion, and a long-awaited vacation. Serious illness, hospitalization, and surgery are universally perceived as stressful events.

Whether something is a stressor depends largely on a person's perception of the event. Each person's response to stress is unique. The way in which a person reacts, and, it is hoped, adapts to stress is called a *coping behavior.*

Coping behaviors can be adaptive, producing relief from stress and even growth. For example, a client who is experiencing work-related stress may cope by exercising more. Coping behaviors can also be maladaptive, leading to further disintegration and disorganization. Elderly persons may be particularly at risk (Ondus et al., 1999). In assessing coping and stress tolerance, the goal is to identify and acknowledge current stressors the client is experiencing, determine how the client has handled stressful events in the past, and identify current methods the client is using to cope.

Subjective data concerning coping and stress tolerance can be obtained through the interview, with the use of open-ended or specific questions. Another technique is to ask the client to describe a stressful event that has occurred in the past and his or her response to it. Such a description can help the nurse identify past stressors and how the client managed the situation. The manner in which a client handled past life crises is often a good predictor of how he or she will manage present or future situations. Suggested questions for interviewing the client regarding coping and stress tolerance include the following:

- Have there been any changes or stress recently in your life? What are they?
- How do you usually handle stress?
- Would you like help to deal with the stress of being sick?

Stress activates the sympathetic nervous system, which produces certain physiologic effects. Sympathetic stimulation may increase the force and rate of the heart beat; increase respiratory rate and depth; decrease blood flow to the skin, resulting in pallor and diaphoresis; and increase blood flow to the muscles. These symptoms may be pronounced in the event of a sudden stressful event. When a person is exposed to chronic stress, the symptoms may be less sudden and less dramatic.

Assessment of Sexuality and Reproduction

Sexuality is the behavioral expression of sexual identity. It may involve, but is not limited to, sexual relationships with a partner. Sexual expression is a complex integration of physiologic, psychological, and social aspects of human nature (LeMone & Jones, 1997). Physical illness and its treatment may influence sexual function. For example, impotence is frequently associated with diabetes mellitus, alcoholism, chronic renal disease, and certain drug therapies. Clients may question their own desirability after such surgeries as mastectomy, radical neck dissection, ostomy, and hysterectomy. Diseases that reduce tolerance, such as heart or lung disease, may limit physical endurance.

Many clients and nurses are hesitant in addressing sexual matters during a health interview. However, sexuality is such an integral aspect of human nature that to ignore it would be neglecting a vital component of health. Including sexuality in the initial client contact conveys to the client that sexual health is an appropriate, legitimate concern. The sexual assessment is not meant to illuminate nonexistent problems. Rather, the client is, in effect, given permission and encouragement to present sexually related questions.

The areas for assessment of sexuality and reproduction include reproductive functioning, sexual role and satisfaction with that role, and potential for alteration in sexual role or function (Gordon, 1994). Discuss the impact of the client's current health status on sexual role and functioning. Examination of the reproductive organs is not usually performed unless the client has problems in that area or as part of a preventive health examination.

The best approach to obtaining a sexual history is to introduce subjects of least sensitivity first. Begin by focusing on chronologic events such as puberty, menstruation, menopause, and reproductive history. Invite the client to elaborate on any problems or expectations in these areas. Also determine the client's knowledge and compliance with preventive health practices such as breast self-examination, regular Papanicolaou (Pap) smear, and testicular and prostate examination.

A sexual assessment is appropriate at every age and should be adapted to correlate with the client's developmental level. Many adolescents are concerned about changes in their bodies and early sexual experience. Use this opportunity to educate, support, and guide the adolescent in matters involving sexuality. Married people may have concerns about their own sexuality and concerns related to parenting and sex education for their children. Many elderly clients enjoy sexual relations throughout their lives and may desire acknowledgment and discussion of their concerns.

Selected questions to elicit information concerning the sexual–reproductive pattern should be individualized for each client and may include the following:

- Are you concerned about pregnancy? What method of contraception do you use? Is this method acceptable to you and your partner?
- Have you ever been diagnosed as having a sexually transmitted disease (gonorrhea, genital herpes, chlamydia, or AIDS)?
- Many men (or women) in your situation have questions about how their illness or surgery will affect the sexual aspects of their lives. What questions do you have?
- Has your illness interfered with your being a mother (or wife, husband, father, partner)?
- Has anything changed your ability to function sexually?
- *For adolescents:* Many boys (or girls) at your age have questions about dating, becoming intimate, contracting a disease, or getting pregnant. What questions do you have?

Assessment of objective data includes the genitalia in men and women and the breasts in a woman; this assessment is described in the physical examination section later in this chapter.

Assessment of Values and Beliefs

Assessment of values and beliefs is also referred to as a spiritual assessment because it focuses on the spiritual dimension of life. Spirituality may be defined as the quality that transcends the physical world, permeates and unifies a person's entire being, and gives life purpose, meaning, and importance. Spirituality usually, but not always, involves a belief and relationship with a higher being. Values and beliefs emerge from one's sense of spirituality and guide one's opinions about what is right, good, proper, and meaningful. Values help determine choices about the conduct of one's life, including health-related decisions concerning personal practices, treatments, and even life or death. The spiritual realm is one aspect of being human that often comes into focus during illness or crisis.

Illness, injury, loss, aging, and disability are spiritual as well as physical and emotional experiences. Serious or life-threatening illness often triggers a person's first encounter with mortality. Crisis often provides the motivation to question one's life, goals, and what is important.

Because body, mind, and spirit are intertwined, distress in any one area affects the health of the whole person. Nurses should include spiritual assessment and care in their daily practice (Brush & Daly, 2000). A nurse who understands a client's spiritual beliefs is better prepared to support coping strategies and provide resources that are spiritually helpful to the client.

Assessment of values and beliefs focuses on the significance of religious affiliation and religious practices; the client's spiritual needs and the resources available to meet those needs; and the relationship between spiritual beliefs and the client's current state of health (Gordon, 1994).

Mention of spiritual beliefs may arise during discussion of the client's coping–stress tolerance pattern. If so, smoothly direct the conversation toward the values–beliefs pattern. The following interview questions may be used to discuss the values–beliefs pattern:

- Are any religious or spiritual practices significant to you?
- Has this illness affected any of these practices or beliefs?
- Is there a religious person or practice that you would like during this illness?

Assessment of the values–beliefs pattern depends primarily on subjective data. However, visible expression of spiritual values is sometimes present. Notice religious articles belonging to clients, such as a Bible, Buddha, Koran, or rosary. You may observe the client in prayer, either alone or with family, friends, or clergy.

OBTAINING OBJECTIVE DATA: THE PHYSICAL EXAMINATION

Physical examination involves the use of one's senses to obtain information about the structure and function of an area being observed or manipulated. The four basic techniques of physical examination are inspection, palpation, percussion, and auscultation. It is often suggested that beginning students practice newly learned physical assessment skills on fellow

You are a clinic nurse seeing Mr. Schorr, who has been experiencing back pain for the last 7 months. He is currently out of work and receiving disability. His vital signs are as follows: temperature 37°C, pulse 78, respirations 18, and blood pressure 128/78. Mr. Schorr sits very quietly, holding himself in one position during most of the interview. His face is nonexpressive as he describes his pain as incapacitating. "All I can do is lay in bed and watch TV and read. The pain pills I have been taking don't seem to be working any more." When you ask him to rate his pain, he says 7 on a scale of 1 to 10.

- Classify subjective and objective data in this pain assessment.
- What data have the most validity in this situation. Why?

Turn to Appendix A to check your answer.

students or willing friends. Doing so can help students to acquire some skill, confidence, and organization before approaching clients. Expertise in the techniques of physical examination can be learned only through practice.

Positioning and Draping

The client may need to assume various positions for the physical examination (see Chapter 33). Clients may need assistance with positioning and, if in pain, should not remain in any position for an extended length of time.

Draping is a method to help ensure privacy. During the examination, cover the client's body parts that are not included in the specific examination taking place, exposing only the part of the body being examined. As you examine another part of the body, redrape the client. Draping also keeps the client warm during examination. Draping materials include paper sheets, linens, or blankets.

Inspection

Inspection is used to make specific observations of physical features and behavior. The nurse's vision is the most valuable tool for this part of the examination. Inspection is the natural beginning to physical examination because it starts immediately on meeting the client. The initial observations provide an overall impression of the client's present state of health and whether immediate interventions are indicated. If the nurse determines that the client is in acute distress, the comprehensive health assessment is deferred. The nurse may obtain assistance and perform a focused assessment instead. General inspection of a client focuses on the following areas:

- Overall appearance of health or illness: Does the client appear weak, frail, or older than the stated age?

- Signs of distress: Is the client grimacing, as if in pain? Is breathing labored? Is the skin color blue or pale?
- Facial expression and mood: Does the client appear anxious, depressed, angry, or uninterested?
- Body size: Does the client appear thin and malnourished or overweight?
- Grooming and personal hygiene: Are the client and his or her clothing clean and neat? Is there an unusual odor?

In addition to the role of inspection in the general survey of a client, inspection is the first method used in examination of a specific area. The chest and abdomen, for example, are inspected before palpation, percussion, or auscultation is performed.

The optimal conditions for effective inspection are full exposure of the area and adequate lighting. Removal of clothing and bed linen is necessary. In respect for the client's modesty and comfort, expose only the specific area you are examining. A well-lit room is essential for good visualization. **Tangential lighting** is provided by indirectly shining light with a lamp or flashlight to create a shadow over the examined area. The shadow brings out subtle differences in contour and movement.

Palpation

Palpation usually follows inspection. **Palpation** is the use of the hands and fingers to gather information through touch. Palpation is used to discriminate position, texture, size, consistency, masses, and fluid. For client comfort, the nurse's hands should be warm and the touch should be gentle and respectful.

During palpation, different parts of the hand are more suitable for different tactile sensations. The fingertips are concentrated with nerve endings and can sense fine differences in texture and consistency. They are used to discriminate raised versus flat skin lesions or to evaluate an arterial pulse. The skin over the dorsum of the hand is sensitive to temperature because it is thin and its nerve density is great. Skin temperature over a specific area may be evaluated by comparing its temperature with that of adjacent areas or the opposite side of the body. The palm of the hand is sensitive to vibration and is useful in locating a vibration associated with a heart murmur.

In addition to this superficial palpation, nurses use light or deep palpation to examine the abdomen. These two latter types of palpation require the client to relax, because tensed muscles block access to underlying tissue. The nurse will enhance the client's ability to relax if actions are explained to the client before touching.

With light palpation, three or four fingers of the dominant hand are used to depress an area of the client's skin approximately 0.5 to 1 inch (Fig. 24-1A). The fingers evaluate the skin temperature and moistness. Move the hand in a gentle, circular motion to detect abnormal masses and locate areas of discomfort. Using a systematic pattern, lightly palpate and then release. Discomfort is best monitored by observing the client's facial expression while palpating. A ticklish client may place his or her hand on top of the nurse's hand to reduce ticklish sensations. This pattern of light palpation always

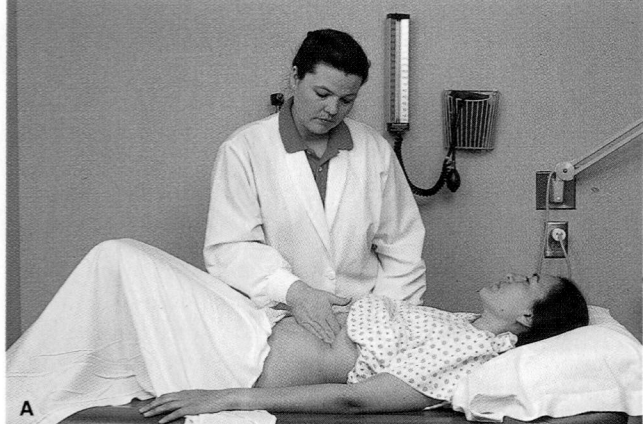

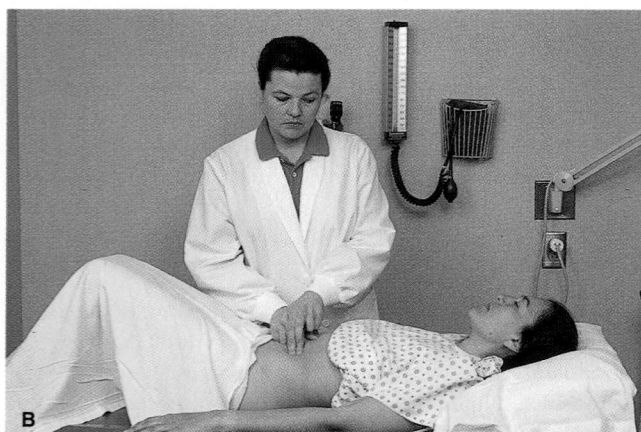

FIGURE 24-1 **(A)** Light palpation. Move the fingertips in a circular motion, depressing the body surface 0.5 to 1 inch. **(B)** Deep palpation. Hold the fingers at a greater angle to the body surface than in light palpation, and depress the skin 1.5 to 2 inches.

precedes deep palpation. If discomfort is elicited in an area, avoid deep palpation there.

Deep palpation involves compression of an area to a depth of 1.5 to 2 inches and requires significantly more pressure than light palpation (Fig. 24-1B). In addition, the fingers are placed at a greater angle to the body than in light palpation. One or both hands may be used, depending on the structure being examined. When using both hands, place the fingers of one hand over the fingers of the other hand. The top hand presses and guides the bottom. The purpose of deep palpation is to locate organs, determine their size, and detect abnormal masses.

Percussion

Percussion, which uses the sense of hearing, involves using the fingers and hands to tap an area on the client to produce sound. The type of percussion tone is determined by the density of the medium through which the sound is traveling. Percussion provides information about the nature of an underlying structure. It is used to outline the size of an organ, such as the bladder or liver. Percussion is also used to determine whether a structure is air-filled, fluid-filled, or solid. Such findings are important during percussion of the lungs and abdomen.

The degree to which sound propagates is called *resonance.* Sound propagates through air; therefore, air-filled spaces are resonant, whereas solid tissue is not. Percussion produces five characteristic tones: tympanic, hyperresonant, resonant, dull, and flat (Table 24-2). Characteristically, percussion of the abdomen is tympanic, hyperinflated lung tissue is hyperresonant, normal lung tissue is resonant, the liver is dull, and bone is flat. The sound is also characterized in terms of intensity, or loudness. The more dense the medium, the quieter the percussion sound. Tympanic tones are the loudest, and flat ones are the quietest.

Percussion may be performed directly or indirectly. Direct percussion is accomplished by tapping an area directly with the fingertip of the middle finger or thumb. Indirect percussion interposes a finger between the area to be percussed and the finger creating the vibrations; indirect percussion usually is used (Fig. 24-2). The steps for indirect percussion are as follows:

1. Rest the nondominant middle finger flatly against the client's skin over the area to be percussed. The remainder of this hand should not touch the client. Identify the interphalangeal joint of this middle finger, because it is the striking area for the opposite hand.
2. Poise the dominant hand about 4 to 5 inches above the striking area, and slightly flex the fingers. Snap this wrist downward, and with the tip of the middle finger, sharply tap the striking area. (The fingernail should be short to facilitate percussing with the tip, not the pad, of the finger.)
3. Deliver several sharp successive blows, rapidly withdrawing.

TABLE 24-2

Characteristics of Percussion Tones				
Tone	Quality	Pitch	Intensity	Location
Flatness	Extreme dullness	High	Soft	Sternum, thigh
Dullness	Thud-like	Medium	Medium	Liver, diaphragm
Resonance	Hollow	Low	Loud	Normal lung
Hyperresonance	Booming	Very low	Very loud	Emphysematous lung
Tympany	Musical, drum-like	High	Loud	Air-filled stomach

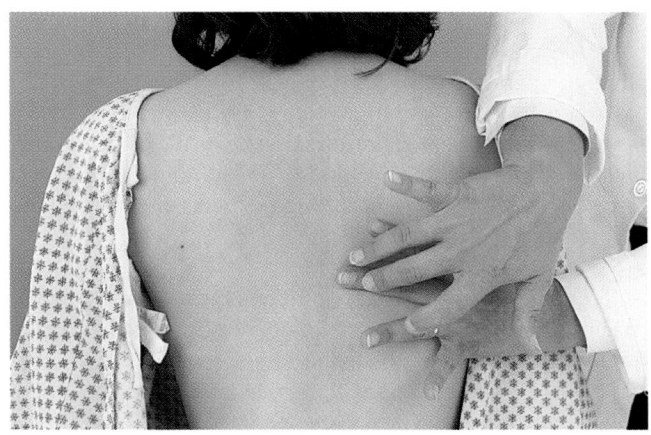

FIGURE 24-2 Perform indirect percussion with two hands, using the finger of one hand to tap on the finger of the other hand.

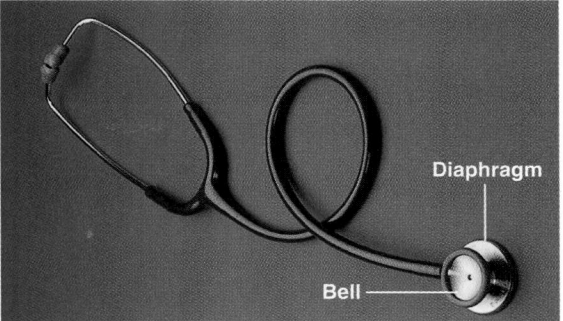

FIGURE 24-3 The diaphragm of the stethoscope is used to auscultate high-frequency sounds, and the bell is used to auscultate low-frequency sounds.

4. Identify the percussion sound (Table 24-2).
5. Proceed to the next area, moving from more resonant to less resonant areas.

Perfecting the percussion technique is often difficult; repetition and practice are essential. Additionally, smaller hands generate less sound. Begin by refining the technique over a tympanic area such as the stomach. Once the percussion sound is clearly audible, move to another area and listen for changes in tone and intensity. Try to label the tone and intensity in this second area. Work from areas of tympany to areas of dullness, and repeat the percussion until the tone and intensity are clear.

Auscultation

Auscultation is listening for sounds of movement within the body. The heart and blood vessels are auscultated for moving blood; the lungs are auscultated for moving air; the abdomen is auscultated for movement of gastrointestinal contents.

The **stethoscope** collects and transmits sound, selects frequencies, and screens out extraneous sound. Although sound transmitted through the stethoscope seems loud, the stethoscope does not amplify the sound. A machine called a Doppler ultrasound device is used to make sound louder if needed.

The head of the stethoscope applied to the skin collects the sound from beneath it. Most stethoscopes have two types of heads, a diaphragm and a bell (Fig. 24-3). The diaphragm is a flat piece that is applied firmly against the skin and responds best to high-frequency sounds. The bell is a funnel- or cup-shaped head that collects low-pitched sounds. The bell should simply be allowed to rest on top of the skin; if too much pressure is applied, the skin is stretched and a diaphragm effect is produced. Some sounds that are very clear with one side may not be audible at all on the other side. Table 24-3 contrasts usage of the diaphragm and bell.

The ability to auscultate clearly also depends on transmission of sound. The tubing should be short (12 to 18 inches) to avoid distortion. The rubber should be thick and heavy to conduct the sound optimally. The head of the stethoscope must be completely sealed by the client's skin over the area of auscultation. Place it on an area that is flat enough to touch the skin surface on all sides. If a client has body hair over the area of auscultation, wetting it with water reduces the crackling sound that hair creates. The earpieces of the stethoscope should fit snugly, occluding the ear canal and screening out environmental noise. Stethoscopes with angled earpieces should be worn so that the angle points toward the nose, thereby directing sound toward the tympanic membrane.

It is essential that the room be as quiet as possible during auscultation. Also, extraneous noise can be generated by rustling bed linen or clothing, rubbing against the stethoscope, bumping the stethoscope tubing, or moving the head of the stethoscope. Attempt to hold the stethoscope and other equipment still to avoid these extraneous noises.

Four properties are used to describe sound: frequency, intensity, duration, and quality. *Frequency* is the measure of

TABLE 24-3

Stethoscope Diaphragm and Bell Usage			
	Technique	Purpose	Example
Diaphragm	Press firmly against the skin	Detects high-pitched sounds	Breath sounds, normal heart sounds, bowel sounds
Bell	Lay lightly on the skin	Detects low-pitched sounds	Abnormal heart sounds, bruits

vibration, expressed in cycles per second, which is heard as pitch. A vibration of many cycles per second (i.e., high frequency) produces a high-pitched sound; one of few cycles per second produces a low-pitched sound. *Intensity* describes the loudness of sound. Breath sounds over the trachea are loud, whereas most heart sounds are soft. *Duration* is the length of the sound. An abnormal heart sound is described according to its duration within the cardiac cycle. Timing of the sound may also be described, such as during inspiration or expiration. *Quality* reflects the musical characteristic of a sound. Blowing, squeaking, and humming are adjectives frequently used in describing the quality of a sound.

HEAD-TO-TOE PHYSICAL ASSESSMENT OF FUNCTION

Assessment of Head, Face, and Neck

Assessment of Cognition

Objective data concerning the client's cognitive abilities are obtained through the neurologic examination. This examination also provides information on sensory function. The neurologic examination is a systematic method of assessing the integration of brain function and motor response. Abnormalities often reflect impairment to the brain or spinal cord. If a client is fully alert and oriented, the nurse may perform a full neurologic assessment to obtain baseline data. In many agencies, comprehensive, detailed neurologic testing is performed by advanced practitioners. See Procedure 24-2 for a detailed description of how to perform a neurologic assessment.

Level of Consciousness. Consciousness is awareness of and responsiveness to the surrounding environment. Impairment in consciousness is evaluated on a continuum. At the highest level of consciousness, a person responds to environmental stimuli with appropriate verbal and motor activity. The person is attentive, cooperative, and completely oriented to self, time, and place. A client may demonstrate impaired consciousness by loss of orientation and inability to follow simple commands. At the lowest level of consciousness, the comatose state, painful stimuli are necessary to induce a verbal or motor response.

The Glasgow Coma Scale (Table 24-4) is a standardized assessment tool that is used when serial assessments are done for high-risk clients (e.g., brain tumor, after brain surgery, after a cerebral vascular accident). Nurses are able to detect subtle changes in a client's consciousness state by reviewing the scale and noticing deviations from baseline. In addition, this tool evaluates the best verbal response and the best motor response so that increased intracranial pressure can be detected and treated quickly. The client's reactions are scored according to the best response he or she gives, and the results are documented appropriately in the client's record.

Orientation. Evaluate orientation by asking simple, direct questions about time, place, and person. Orientation × 1 indicates person orientation, such as knowing one's own name,

knowing the names of significant others, or knowing the nurse. Orientation × 2 indicates person and place, which includes knowing location, city, or state. Orientation × 3 indicates person, place, and time of day, day of week, or date. If the client is not oriented, information he or she provides may not be accurate. Asking the family for additional information or having a family present during the assessment may help verify data the client provides.

Mood. Abnormalities of mood may indicate psychological or neurologic problems. Normal mood is described as happy or pleasant. A client who is unusually overjoyed may be described as elated or euphoric. Depression is being overly sad. Clients who are easily provoked or annoyed are described as irritable. Those with a rapid change of emotions may be described as labile. A client whose affect is clearly out of context with the situation may be described as having an inappropriate affect. Flat affect describes the client who expresses few emotions.

Language and Memory. Communication and memory are specific aspects of cognitive functioning that are important to effective client teaching. Speech deficits may take on a variety of appearances. It is important to differentiate between problems in receiving the communication (receptive aphasia) and problems in expressing communication (expressive aphasia). With receptive aphasia, clients are unable to understand simple directions. With expressive aphasia, the client understands and follows directions but is unable verbally to communicate effectively with the nurse. Mechanical, muscular, or sensory problems may cause difficulties with articulation of words (dysarthria).

If impaired reading ability is suspected, ask the client to read aloud a short passage from the newspaper or from a client education pamphlet and then paraphrase what he or she has read. Some clients are unable to read for reasons other than neurologic deficits, such as illiteracy or understanding a different language. Writing ability involves a complex series of tasks and can simply be evaluated by having the client write his or her name.

Evaluate short-term memory by asking the client to recall events of the day, such as activities, visitors, or meals eaten. Cues to short-term memory loss include losing direction easily and inability to remember a discussion that took place earlier in the same conversation. Intermediate memory might include remembering events that took place earlier in the day. Long-term memory is reflected in the ability to provide historical information about family, health problems, or past hospitalizations.

Assessment of Sensory Function

Physical examination of the senses usually is not performed in a basic health assessment, unless evidence of impaired function is uncovered during the client interview. Physical examination of the senses is a routine part of a health screening examination, such as hearing or vision screening in elementary schools.

(text continues on page 415)

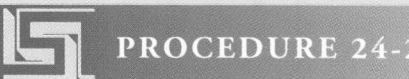

PROCEDURE 24-2

ASSESSING THE NEUROLOGIC SYSTEM

Purpose
1. To obtain baseline information about the client's neurologic status.
2. To assess the client's orientation to his or her environment.
3. To evaluate the client's cognitive function and ability to make judgments.
4. To assess the integrity of motor and sensory pathways and the client's ability to ambulate safely.
5. To detect increased intracranial pressure.

Assessment
- Explain to the client what you plan to do and approximately how long it will take. A complete neurologic assessment can be very lengthy. Decide how extensive the assessment should be, based on the client's diagnosis, level of consciousness, and physical disabilities. An efficient nurse learns how to integrate components of the neurologic assessment with other parts of the client's functional assessment (e.g., assess cranial nerves during head and neck examination, evaluate mental status during nursing history, and test reflexes during musculoskeletal assessment).
- Determine whether any immediate need (e.g., pain, urge to urinate) is distracting the client. Attend to that need first.
- Ask significant others whether they have noted memory loss or changes in the behavior of the client.
- Question the client about the presence of headache, seizures, dizziness, visual changes, or numbness or tingling of any body parts.
- Review medication history for any drugs that can alter level of consciousness or cause behavioral changes (e.g., analgesics, sedatives, antidepressants, antipsychotics, central nervous system stimulants).

Equipment
May need all or part of equipment depending on comprehensiveness of assessment.
Toothpick
Cotton applicator or cotton ball
Vials of hot and cold water
Tongue blade
Penlight
Vials of coffee, vanilla, or clove extracts
Vials of salt, sugar, lemon solutions
Snellen chart
Tuning fork
Reflex hammer

Procedure
Cognitive–Sensory Assessment
1. Assess the client's level of consciousness by asking direct questions that require a verbal response. Note appropriateness of response and emotional state.
   Rationale: Irritability, decreased attention span, inability or unwillingness to cooperate, and an abnormal perception of the environment may be signs of decreased level of consciousness.
2. Evaluate client's speech patterns.
   Rationale: Normally, speech should be clear, well paced, and coherent. Language should seem appropriate for educational level.
3. Observe general appearance: hygiene, appropriateness of clothing to setting and weather.
   Rationale: Unkempt appearance or inappropriate clothing for weather conditions may give clues to client's altered mental status.
4. If client responses are inappropriate, ask direct questions related to person, place, and time (e.g., "What is your name?" "Where are you right now?" "What city do you live in?" "What day is this?").
   Rationale: Measure the client's orientation to immediate environment. As consciousness deteriorates, clients become disoriented to person, place, and time. Note: Be sure a communication or language problem is not causing the client's inappropriate response.
5. If client doesn't respond or inappropriately responds to orientation questions, give simple commands (e.g., "Squeeze my fingers," "Wiggle your toes"). If the client gives no response to verbal commands, test response to painful stimuli by applying firm pressure on client's sternum or finger nailbed with your thumb.
   Rationale: Level of consciousness can vary from fully alert and oriented, to unable to follow commands, to unresponsiveness to external stimuli. Note: Avoid pinching client's skin to elicit a pain response.
6. Document cognitive or sensory assessment objectively by stating specific client responses to verbal or tactile stimulation. Use of Glasgow Coma Scale (see Table 24-4) helps charting of frequent level-of-consciousness testing.
   Rationale: Assessments are more objective and consistent.
7. Assess function of cranial nerves (see Table 24-5).
   Rationale: An increase in intracranial pressure (ICP) puts direct pressure on the optic nerve (C-II). The oculomotor (C-III), the trochlear (C-IV), and the abducens (C-VI) exit the brain

PROCEDURE 24-2 (Continued)

stem at the level of the tentorial notch. When ICP increases and the brain shifts downward, changes in the functions of these nerves are noted.

8. Assess sensory pathways:
   a. Client's eyes are closed during all sensory tests.
      Rationale: Tests are valid only if client doesn't see where stimulus strikes skin.
   b. Apply stimuli to skin in a random, unpredictable order while comparing one side of body with the other.
      Rationale: Client should feel sensations equally on both sides of the body. Random stimuli prevent client from anticipating and correctly guessing where stimulus is.
   c. Client should verbally state when he or she feels a particular stimulus. If you detect an area of altered sensation, note which spinal cord segment is affected by referring to a dermatome chart. *Note:* Boundaries of sensory dysfunction can be found by testing responses about every 2.5 cm in a localized area.

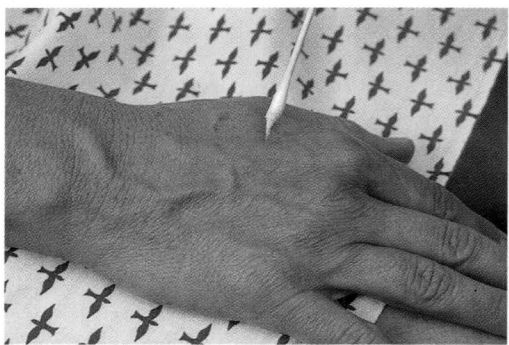

Step 8 Assessing light touch with a cotton applicator.

9. Test pain sensation first by lightly touching pointed, then blunt, end of sterile toothpick to proximal and distal aspects of the arm and legs.
   Rationale: Assess intactness of spinothalamic tract. If pain sensation is intact, nurse may omit tests for temperature.
10. Test temperature sensation by touching skin with vials of hot, then cold, water. *Note:* Client should identify hot versus cold sensation.
11. Lightly stroke proximal and distal aspects of client's arms and legs with a cotton applicator or ball. Ask client to tell you when and where each stroke is felt.

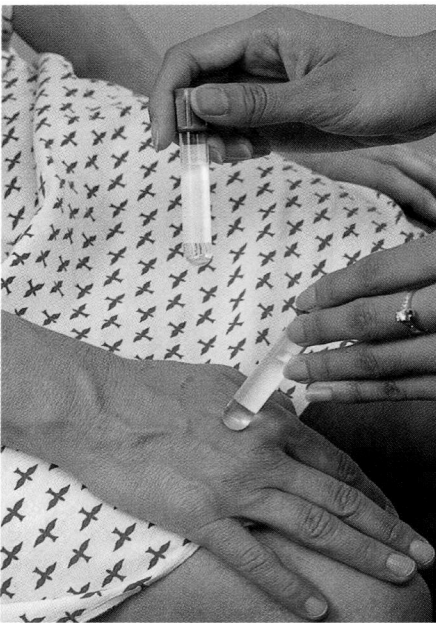

Step 10 Assessing temperature sensation.

Rationale: Testing the client's perception of light touch and the following tests of vibration and position assess intactness of the posterior column. Loss of any of these sensations may indicate a lesion of the posterior column on the same side as the loss.

12. Apply a vibrating tuning fork to the distal interphalangeal joints of fingers and great toe. Ask client to describe what he or she feels and when it stops. *Note:* If client does not feel vibration, move the tuning fork proximally to the next joint until sensation is felt.

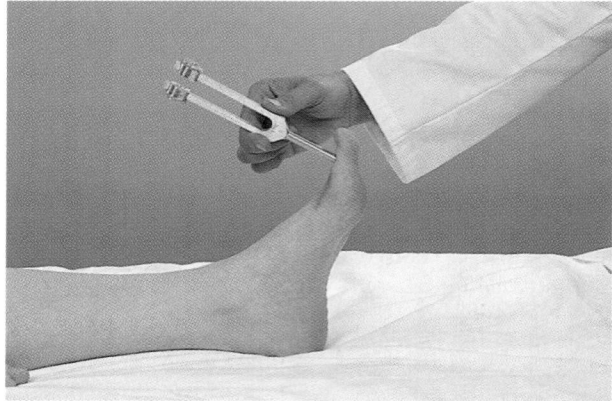

Step 12 Assessing vibratory sensation with a tuning fork.

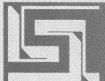

PROCEDURE 24-2 (Continued)

Activity–Mobility Assessment

13. Inspect arm and leg muscles for atrophy, tremors, fasciculations, or other abnormal movements.

14. Assess strength of specific muscle groups by having client extend or flex individual joints against resistance provided by examiner's hands. Test biceps, triceps, wrist, leg muscles, and ankle.
    Rationale: Lack of symmetry of same muscle groups can indicate neurologic impairment.

15. Ask client to close eyes and hold arms in front of body with palms up. Have client hold position for 30 seconds and observe for pronation of hands or drifting of arms. *Note:* Notice weaknesses on one or both sides.
    Rationale: This test detects presence of deformities, reduced mobility of joints, or decreased muscle strength. Upper and lower extremities of dominant side are usually stronger than nondominant side.

16. Evaluate coordination and balance
    a. Perform a series of rapid alternating movements.
       (1) Have client pat upper thigh by rapidly alternating his or her palm and back of the hand.
       (2) With dominant hand, have client touch his or her thumb to each finger on that hand as quickly as possible.
       (3) Have client use his or her dominant forefinger to first touch your forefinger, then his or her nose. Instruct client to repeat this many times as fast as he or she can.
          Rationale: Difficulty performing any of these tests may suggest that further evaluation for cerebellar disease is indicated.
    b. Romberg test: Ask client to stand with feet together, arms at sides. Have client maintain this position for 30 seconds with eyes open, then 30 seconds with eyes closed. Assess for swaying. Stay close to client to assist in case he or she begins to fall.
       Rationale: Clients with cerebellar disease may not maintain balance with eyes open or shut; problems with proprioception cause difficulty only with eyes shut. Stay close to avoid injury.
    c. Ask client to walk across the room. Observe gait for symmetry, rhythm, limping, shuffling, or other abnormalities.

Rationale: Changes in gait may be characteristic of specific neurologic diseases.

17. Assess deep tendon reflexes (see Table 24-8).
    a. Compare symmetry of reflex on each side of body.
    b. Extremity to be tested should be completely relaxed and slightly extended.
    c. Hold the reflex hammer loosely and allow it to swing freely in an arc.

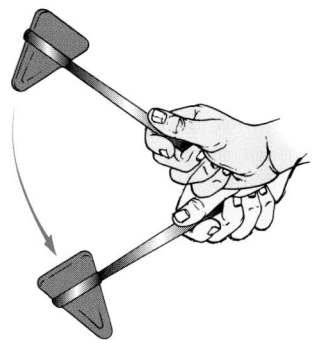

Step 17C Swing reflex hammer in an arc.

    d. Tap tendon briskly.
    e. Document reflexes by grading from 0 to 4+ on stickman, comparing bilaterally.
       Rationale: The quality of a reflex response varies among individuals and by age.

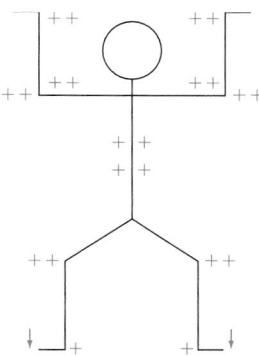

0 —no response
1+—diminished reflex (may be normal)
2+—normal
3+—brisker than normal (may be normal)
4+—hyperactive—upper neuron disorder suspected

Step 17E Document reflexes by grading 0–4 + on a stickman.

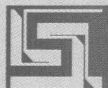

PROCEDURE 24-2 (Continued)

Lifespan Considerations
Newborn and Infant
- The infant at birth has little or no voluntary control over muscular movements. Much of the infant's motor activity is seen as mass responses to stimuli, and the infant has built-in reflexes:
- *Rooting reflex*—Infant turns head toward a warm object placed against his or her cheek; function is to help infant locate the mother's breast when nursing.
- *Sucking reflex*—Swallowing and gagging reflexes are well developed in healthy infants at birth.
- *Moro reflex*—In response to loud noise or sudden movement, infant extends arms in tense, quivering embrace and often cries.
- *Tonic neck reflex*—When relaxed or asleep on back, infant has head turned to one side with arm and leg of that side extended, whereas extremities of opposite side are flexed.

Toddler and Preschooler
- Children are often fearful of strangers and of examining equipment. Spend several minutes becoming acquainted with the child. Allow the child to handle the equipment before the examination. Using a "This is a game" approach often helps allay the fear. Several screening tools are available, such as the Denver Development Test, which is designed to evaluate cognitive and psychomotor skills of infants and children of varying ages.

Older Adult
- A lengthy examination may exhaust the older adult. You may need to complete it in phases.
- Arthritic changes in joints may limit range of motion and physical mobility and should be considered when evaluating assessment data.
- Some reflex responses may become less intense as a person ages. The Achilles reflex and the plantar reflex may be difficult to elicit.
- Short-term memory may be decreased in the older adult; long-term memory is usually unaltered.
- Being in an unfamiliar place or situation can be stressful and promotes confusion.

Collaboration and Delegation
- Report abnormal findings to the physician/neurologist.
- Nurses who do not frequently work with neurologic clients may collaborate with clinical nurse specialists to perform comprehensive neurologic assessment for high-risk clients.

TABLE 24-4

Glasgow Coma Scale

Best Eye-Opening Response		Best Verbal Response		Best Motor Response	
Purposeful and spontaneous	4	Oriented	5	Obeys commands	6
To voice	3	Disoriented	4	Localizes pain	5
To pain	2	Inappropriate words	3	Withdraws to pain	4
No response	1	Incomprehensible sounds	2	Flexion to pain	3
Untestable	U	No response	1	Extension to pain	2
		Untestable	U	No response	1
				Untestable	U

Sensory Aids. Document the use of glasses, contact lenses, hearing aids, and other assistive devices in the client's health assessment. The proper care of such devices should also be solicited and written in the client's record. Doing so helps ensure proper use and care of expensive devices during the client's stay in a healthcare agency.

Visual Acuity. To test the client's near vision, hold newsprint 14 inches from the client's face. If the client is unable to focus well enough to read, experiment with the distance to determine whether improvement occurs when the print is moved closer or farther away. Visual problems with close objects occur more frequently after the age of 40 years. To test far vision, ask the client to read the time on a clock across the room or to read a sign across the hall or room. If problems are detected, refer the client for further testing.

Visual screening is an important part of routine health examinations. The Snellen "E" is used for assessing distant visual acuity. Position the client 20 feet from the Snellen chart, which has been placed at eye level. Test each eye separately and then both eyes together. As the client covers one eye, direct the client to read the smallest line that he or she can see. Young children who do not yet know the letters of the alphabet may be tested with another chart that has pictures. Compare the client's distance from the chart (20 feet) to the number by the smallest line that the client can read. For example, if the client can read the 100-foot line, report visual acuity as 20/100. Refer any person with less than 20/20 acuity to an ophthalmologist or optometrist for evaluation.

Extraocular Movement and Visual Fields. The oculomotor, trochlear, and abducens nerves control the horizontal, vertical, and diagonal movement of the eyes. Assessment of peripheral visual fields and the six ocular movements is important in a comprehensive visual assessment. To evaluate extraocular movements, ask the client to visually follow an object (such as a pencil) through various positions (horizontal, vertical, and diagonal). The client's head remains still as the eyes move to follow the object. At each position, pause to evaluate the presence of nystagmus (involuntary, rhythmic oscillations of the eyes) and evaluate whether the client's eyes can follow the object smoothly.

Peripheral vision can be tested in a similar manner. Have the client look straight ahead and cover one of the client's eyes as you bring your finger or another object within the field of vision. Repeat for each eye from different fields (temporal, upward, downward, and nasal).

Pupils and Pupillary Reflexes. As a beam of light is directed through the pupil and onto the retina, stimulation of the third cranial nerve causes the muscles of the iris to constrict. Evaluate pupils bilaterally for size, shape, accommodation, and reaction to light. Normally, pupils are black and round, and they constrict briskly when exposed to a bright light source. To test pupils, first dim the light in the room. As the client gazes straight ahead, shine a penlight into the pupil from the side of the head. Observe both pupils and estimate initial size and reaction size (Fig. 24-4). The directly illuminated pupil should constrict briskly and the other pupil consensually. Accommodation can be tested by having the client look at a close object (e.g., a finger held approximately 4 inches from the nose) and then look at a distant object (e.g., a picture on the wall). As the client is doing this, observe the client's pupils to see whether they constrict to focus on the close object and dilate to see the distant object. Normal pupil assessment data are recorded as PERRLA: pupils equal, round, reactive to light and accommodation.

Pupils can appear cloudy when cataracts are present. Dilated pupils can occur when glaucoma is treated with drops or neurologic impairment is present. Unilateral changes in pupil reflexes can signify increased intracranial pressure caused by tumor, trauma, or cerebral vascular accident. Report changes in pupillary response to the physician.

Cranial Nerve Assessment. Intact cranial nerve function is important for normal sensory functioning. Vision depends on normal functioning of cranial nerves II, III, IV, and VI. Cranial nerve VIII is important for hearing, and cranial nerve I is important for the sense of smell. Cranial nerves V, VII, IX, and XII are important in the coordination of facial movement or reflex activity. During an initial neurologic assessment, or at specific intervals for high-risk clients, evaluate normal functioning of the cranial nerves. Table 24-5 lists the cranial nerves and techniques used to assess their functioning.

External and Internal Eye Structures. External eye structures should be free of lesions or inflammation. A blink reflex should be present. An **ophthalmoscope** is the instrument used to assess internal eye structures (Fig. 24-5A). Usually, advanced practitioners with additional training and practice perform such examinations. Ophthalmic examination permits visualization of the retina, optic nerve disc, macula, fovea centralis, and retinal vessels. As the fundus is observed through the ophthalmoscope, a round red glow (the red reflex) is noted (Fig. 24-5B). Normal findings include uniform red reflex; round, white, or pink optic nerve disc; reddish retina; and bright red arterioles and dark red veins (Fig. 24-5C).

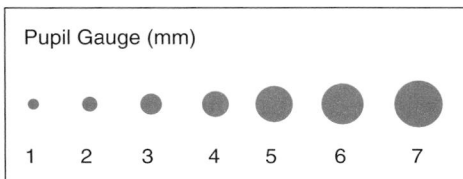

FIGURE 24-4   Pupil size chart. To test the pupil reflex, the nurse shines a penlight from the side into the pupil, observing the rate and amount of pupil constriction. The pupils should constrict briskly and be equal in size after constriction.

TABLE 24-5

Cranial Nerve Function and Assessment			
Number	**Name**	**Function**	**Method of Assessment**
I	Olfactory	Sense of smell	Ask client to identify different mild aromas, such as vanilla, coffee, chocolate, cloves.
II	Optic	Vision	Ask client to read Snellen chart.
III	Oculomotor	Pupillary reflex	Assess pupil reaction to penlight.
		Extraocular eye movement	Assess directions of gaze by holding your finger 18 inches from client's face. Ask client to follow your finger up and down and side to side.
IV	Trochlear	Lateral and downward movement of eyeball	Assess directions of gaze. Test with cranial nerve II.
V	Trigeminal	Sensation to cornea, skin of face, nasal mucosa	Lightly touch cotton swab to lateral sclera of eye to elicit blink.
			Measure sensation of touch and pain on face using cotton wisp.
VI	Abducens	Lateral movement of eyeball	Assess directions of gaze. Test with cranial nerve III.
VII	Facial	Facial expression	Ask client to smile, frown, raise eyebrows.
		Taste—anterior two thirds of tongue	Ask client to identify different tastes on tip and sides of tongue: sugar (sweet), salt, lemon juice (sour).
VIII	Auditory	Hearing	Assess ability to hear spoken word.
IX	Glossopharyngeal	Taste—posterior tongue	Ask client to identify different tastes on back of tongue as above.
		Swallowing	Place a tongue blade on posterior tongue while client says "ah" to elicit a gag response.
		Movement of tongue	Ask client to move tongue up and down, and side to side.
X	Vagus	Swallowing	Assess with cranial nerve IX by observing palate and pharynx move as client says "ah."
		Movement of vocal cords Sensation of pharynx	
XI	Spinal accessory	Head and shoulder movement	Ask client to turn head side to side and shrug shoulders against resistance from examiner's hands.
XII	Hypoglossal	Tongue position	Ask client to stick out tongue to midline, then move it side to side.

Auditory Assessment. Assessment of auditory function can occur simply during normal conversation. During the interview, lower your voice to assess the client's ability to hear. Hearing loss is suggested in a client who turns a particular ear or leans toward the speaker, hears only when able to see the speaker's face (evidence of lip reading), or speaks in a loud or distorted voice. People with hearing loss may avoid social settings because conversation is especially difficult in groups with background noise. Other physical symptoms associated with the ear are tinnitus (ringing in the ears) and vertigo (dizziness).

If hearing loss is suspected, inspect the client's external ear canal for inflammation or cerumen (ear wax). Using an **otoscope** (the instrument for examining the ear), visualize the canal after pulling the pinna up, out, and back to straighten the ear canal (Fig. 24-6A). In an infant, pull the pinna down and back. A buildup of cerumen may prevent visualization of the tympanic membrane. Insects or other foreign objects may

be present in the ear canal. Because these objects can temporarily impede normal hearing, remove them before performing further assessment related to hearing.

Visualization of the inner ear structures usually is performed by an advanced practitioner. To do this, insert the otoscope as far as is comfortable to the client. Support the otoscope by resting a finger against the client's head or cheek and wiggle the auricle until the tympanic membrane is visualized. The normal tympanic membrane is pearly, gray, shiny, translucent, and intact. A cone-shaped reflection of the light from the otoscope is usually seen between the 5 and 7 o'clock positions. The small bones of the ear may also be visualized (Fig. 24-6B).

Health screening may include hearing tests using an audiometer. The client wears headphones that are capable of transmitting sounds of different frequencies. The client indicates when he or she hears a sound by raising the hand. Such tests may also be administered to high-risk clients who are re-

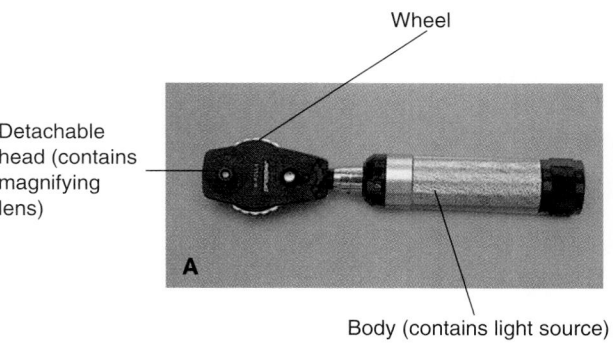

Wheel

Detachable head (contains magnifying lens)

A

Body (contains light source)

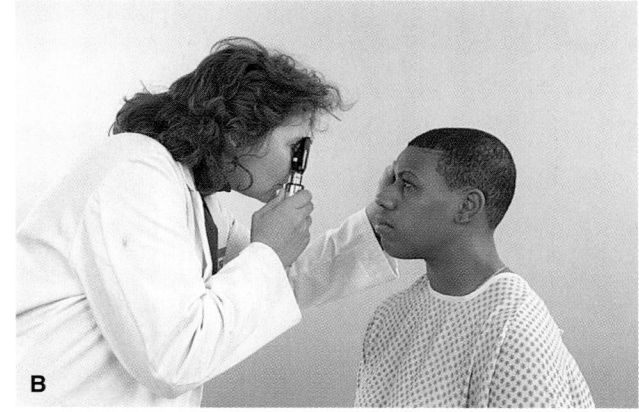

B

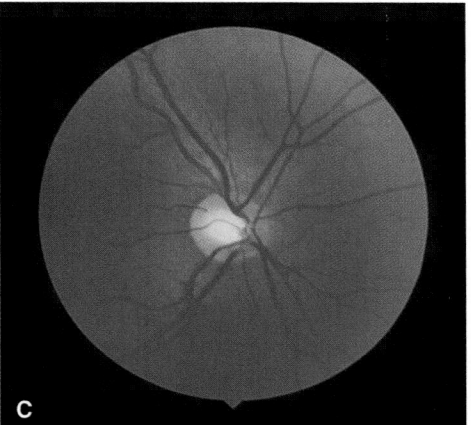

C

FIGURE 24-5 Ophthalmoscopic examination. (**A**) Ophthalmoscope. (**B**) The nurse inspects the red reflex with the ophthalmoscope. (**C**) Fundus of the eye seen through the ophthalmoscope.

ceiving medications (e.g., aminoglycoside antibiotics) that can cause hearing impairment.

The Weber test and the Rinne test, which require a tuning fork, can be used to evaluate hearing loss further. The Weber test can evaluate lateralization of sound (Fig. 24-7A). Acti-vate the tuning fork, and place it at the top of the client's head. Normally, the client will hear vibrations equally in both ears. Clients with conduction deafness will best hear vibrations in the affected ear, whereas in those with sensorineural loss the sound lateralizes to the unaffected ear.

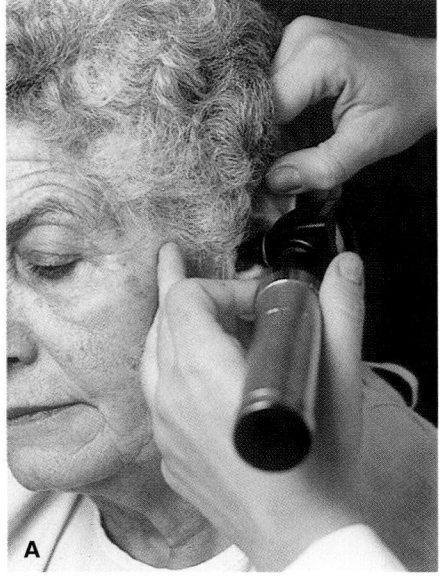

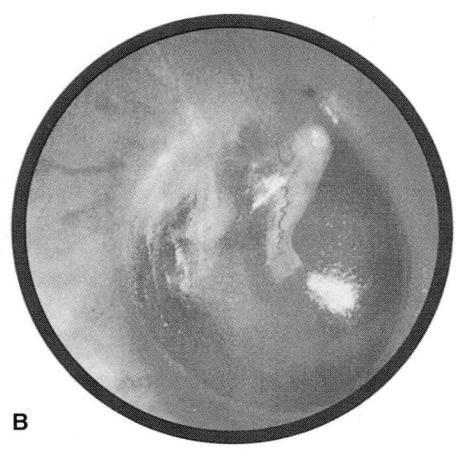

FIGURE 24-6 Internal ear examination. (**A**) Inserting the otoscope into the ear. (**B**) Normal eardrum with cone of light, malleus, and incus visible.

A

B

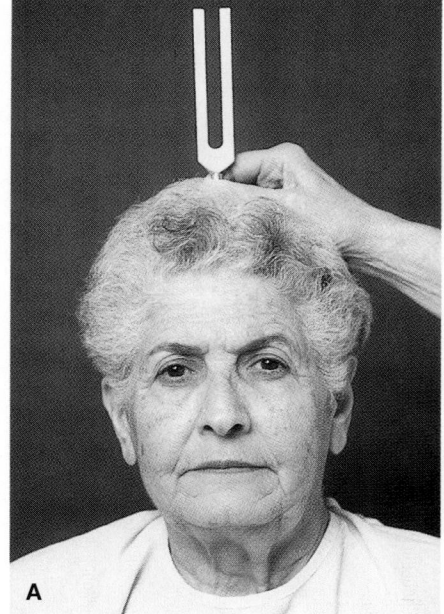
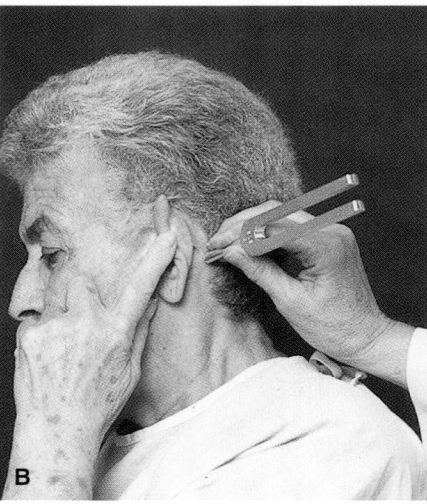

FIGURE 24-7 Evaluating for hearing loss. **(A)** In the Weber test, the base of the lightly vibrating tuning fork is placed on the client's head (or midforehead). **(B)** In the Rinne test, the base of the lightly vibrating tuning fork is placed on the mastoid bone.

The Rinne test discriminates between bone conduction and air conduction of sound. Strike the tuning fork, and place its stem firmly against the mastoid process (Fig 24-7B). When the client can no longer hear the tuning fork, remove it from the bone, and allow sound to conduct through the air near the ear. Normally, the client should hear the sound of the tuning fork when it is placed near the ear, indicating that air conduction of sound is greater than bone conduction. When the client does not detect sound until the tuning fork is placed on the mastoid process, bone conduction of sound is greater than air conduction because of a conductive hearing loss.

Assessment of the Mouth

Examination of the mouth includes the buccal mucosa (cheek), teeth, lips, gums, tongue, tonsils, and uvula (Fig. 24-8). Evaluate the lips for color, moisture, cracks, and lesions. Use a bright light and a tongue blade to inspect the mucous membranes, teeth, and gums. Remove and inspect dental appliances, especially if the client complains of pain or has ill-fitting dentures. Mucous membranes should appear pink and moist. Observe for lesions in the mouth, gums, or tongue. Ask the client to say "Ahh" while the uvula is observed; it should rise symmetrically. The tonsils should be pink, symmetric, and slightly visible. Inspect the teeth for stability and overall hygiene. Evaluate the bite. A major concern when examining the mouth is to detect any abnormalities that might impede the client's ability to taste, chew, swallow, or enjoy food.

Assessment of the Neck

Auscultation is used to detect bruits, which are abnormal arterial sounds, similar to murmurs, caused by increased turbulence of blood flow. Bruits can be detected by placing the

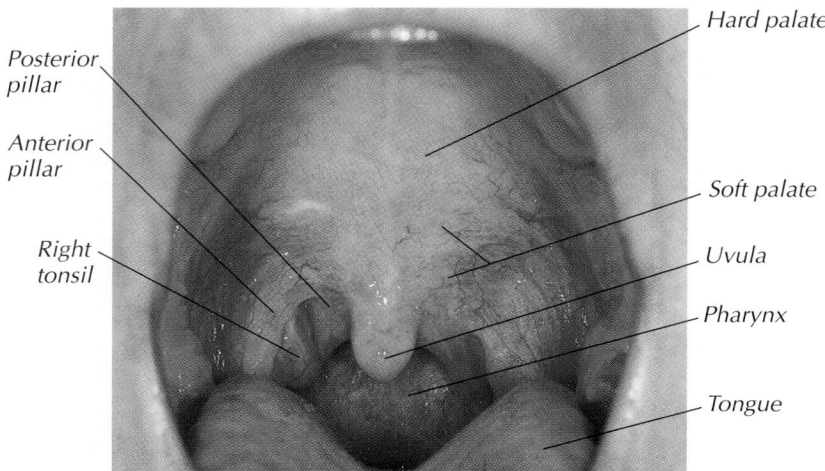

Posterior pillar

Anterior pillar

Right tonsil

Hard palate

Soft palate

Uvula

Pharynx

Tongue

FIGURE 24-8   Structures of the mouth.

stethoscope over major blood vessels, such as the carotid artery, renal artery, iliac artery, femoral artery, or the abdominal aorta. Bruits occur when an artery is partially obstructed or distended, which prevents blood flow from moving straight through the vessel. Palpate the lymph nodes for enlargement, mobility, and tenderness. The lymph nodes may become enlarged or tender with inflammation or infection. Figure 24-9 identifies the location of lymph nodes in the neck. Evaluate the veins in the neck for distention, which often occurs with fluid volume excess. Figure 24-10 identifies the technique for inspection of jugular venous distention.

The trachea is normally in a straight, vertical position. Some lung disorders, such as large masses and pneumothorax, can cause a shift in the trachea from its normal midline position. Stand behind the client and reach across the client's shoulders, placing the index finger on each side of the trachea in the suprasternal notch. The space on either side of the trachea and the ends of the suprasternal notch should be equal. To palpate the thyroid, place the fingers on either side of the trachea below the cricoid cartilage. Using the fingers on the left, push the trachea to the right and ask the client to swallow as you palpate the gland. Do the opposite to palpate the left side of the thyroid (Fig. 24-11).

Evaluate cranial nerve XI by having the client shrug the shoulders and turn the head. Evaluate strength by having the client perform these movements against resistance. Movements should be of equal strength on both sides.

Assessment of Skin, Hair, and Nails

The skin is the largest organ of the body. It protects underlying structures, regulates temperature, and senses stimuli. The epidermis is the outer layer of skin; the dermis below it contains the oil and sweat glands. The subcutaneous tissue is a layer of connective tissue below the epidermis that thins with aging.

Clients may complain of problems with the skin, indicating underlying abnormalities. The skin is a reflection of the body's nutrition and metabolism. Some skin disorders may interfere with the client's body image, especially if present on the face. Examples of questions used in assessment include the following:

- What is your usual daily care routine for skin, hair, and nails?
- Describe any birthmarks, tattoos, moles, or freckles.
- Have you had any hair loss or change?
- What level of protection do you use against sun exposure?

The skin is examined through inspection and palpation. Assess the skin for color, moisture, temperature, texture, and hygiene. Normal skin color may be pink, tan, brown, olive, or yellowish. The color and appearance of the skin and nails may reflect insufficient delivery of oxygenated blood to the tissues because of respiratory dysfunction. With a normal supply of oxygen, the nailbeds, the tongue, and the lips appear pinkish-red in color. Hypoxia (decreased supply of oxygen to the tissues) changes this color to a grayish, bluish, or purplish tone. When this change in color is confined to the nailbeds and lips, it is called *peripheral cyanosis;* when it progresses to the tongue and mucous membranes of the mouth, it is called *central cyanosis.* Central cyanosis indicates a significant problem with oxygenation of body tissues and can result from respiratory, cardiac, or metabolic problems. Chronic bronchitis may also cause the skin to become reddish and leathery, which appears as ruddiness.

The skin is normally dry; either extreme dryness or excessive sweating (diaphoresis) is abnormal. Skin temperature is normally warm; hot may indicate fever, and cool may indicate poor circulation. Skin texture is usually soft, and rough over the elbows, knees, and heels of the feet. Hygiene can be described as well groomed or poor personal hygiene. Observe the skin for past injuries, calluses, stains, scars, needle marks, and insect bites. Note the location of rashes. Frequently, a diagram is helpful in identifying the location of lesions.

Scalp and Hair

Inspect the scalp and hair for color, quantity, distribution, texture, hygiene, nodules, and lesions. Hair color may range from pale blonde to deep black; graying begins normally in the third decade of life. Texture may be straight, curly, kinky, fine, or coarse. Examine the base of the hair follicle for pest infestation and dandruff.

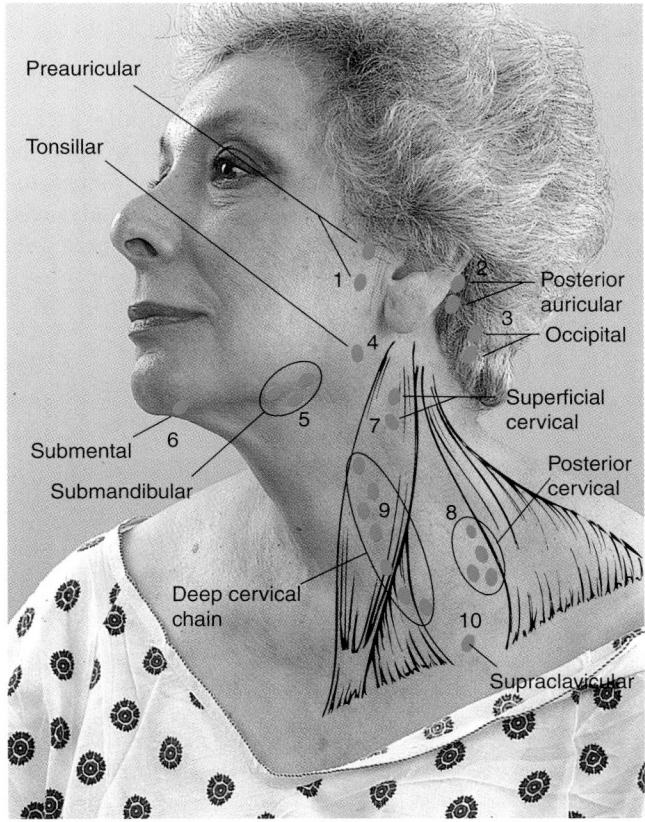

FIGURE 24-9 Lymph nodes in the neck are lightly palpated.

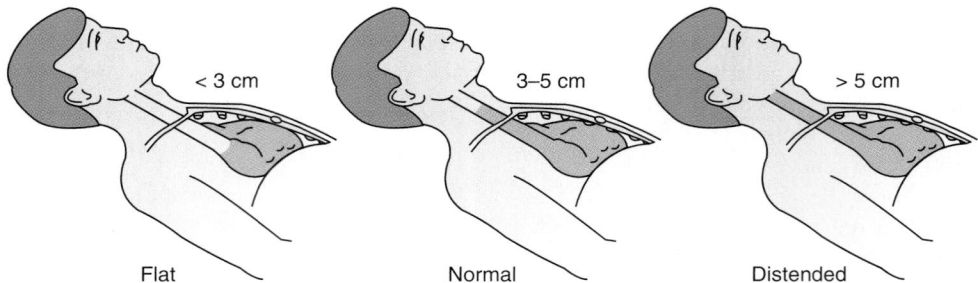

FIGURE 24-10 Height of jugular venous pressure is measured in relation to the sternal angle at the second intercostal space. Normal height is less than 3 cm.

Skin Turgor

Assess the amount of fluid in the tissues by checking skin turgor. Check for skin turgor by pinching a small area of skin on the medial arm or anterior chest and noting how quickly it returns to position when you release it. If skin turgor is poor, the skin remains elevated (tenting) or slowly resumes position. Poor skin turgor may indicate dehydration, but it may also occur with normal aging or with weight loss.

Skin Lesions

A skin lesion is an abnormality in the structure of the skin that results from injury or disease. Describe every lesion in terms of size, color, type, and location. Lesions may be measured with a metric ruler to ensure accurate size determination. Take note of the appearance of the border of the lesion and surrounding skin. It is also important to palpate the lesion to distinguish between flat and raised lesions. Lightly press the lesion to determine whether it blanches with pressure. These steps will assist in labeling the lesion and identifying the cause. A lesion that exhibits asymmetry, irregular borders, uneven color, a raised surface, or a recent change in size may indicate malignancy, and the patient should be referred for evaluation. Refer to Chapter 38 for a complete description and graphic representation of various types of lesions.

Wounds

Accidents, pressure, or surgeries may cause wounds (Hampton, 1997). It is especially important to note a wound's color. Yellow or green coloring may indicate infection. A black, brown, or gray color may indicate necrotic (dead) tissue. Pink is the color of the tissue, and bright pink or red is the color of new granulation tissue. Be sure to note the color, character, and amount of any drainage (exudate) from the wound (Thomas, 1997). Creamy, colored drainage indicates infection. Bright red drainage indicates blood. A watery, clear drainage is serum. Refer to Chapter 38 for a complete description of various characteristics of wounds and exudate.

Nails

Inspect the nails for shape, color, and texture. Clubbing of the nails is a sign of chronic hypoxia. To determine whether clubbing is present, examine the contour of the nail and its adherence to the nailbed. When viewed in profile, normal fingernails present an angle of 160 degrees between the nailbed and the finger. With clubbing, swelling flattens the angle to 180 degrees or less (Fig. 24-12). With advanced clubbing, the nail becomes less adherent to the base of the nail and feels spongy. The nails and fingertips appear large and swollen, and are sometimes described as "drumstick-like."

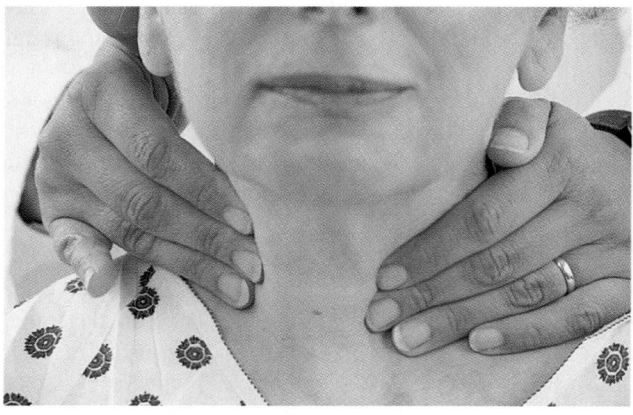

FIGURE 24-11 Palpation of the thyroid below the cricoid cartilage.

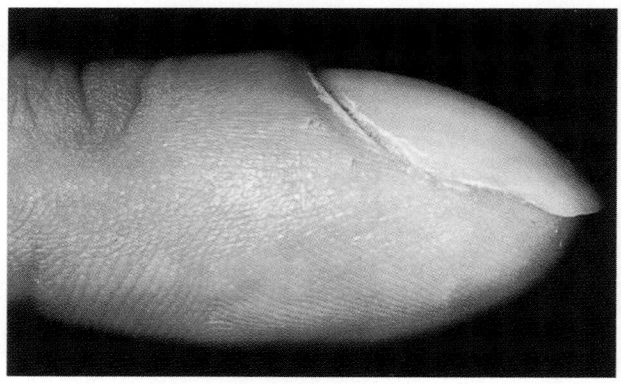

FIGURE 24-12 Clubbing of the nail and fingers.

Cardiac Assessment

Activity and exercise are impeded when the heart cannot work effectively to pump blood or when the vasculature is unable to supply the perfusion of blood that body tissues need. Assessment of cardiac and peripheral vascular status provides clues about circulation and oxygenation to every part of the body.

The major areas for cardiovascular assessment include risk factors for cardiovascular disease (e.g., hypertension, elevated cholesterol concentration, smoking); signs and symptoms of cardiovascular dysfunction (e.g., pain, dizziness, palpitations); the impact of cardiovascular dysfunction on ADLs; and specific adaptations to cardiac or circulatory impairment. Interview questions to help elicit this information might include the following:

- Describe your normal diet or exercise pattern.
- Do you have a history of heart attack, heart rhythm problems, high blood pressure, or high blood cholesterol?
- Have you had any chest pain, shortness of breath, cough, swelling in the legs, calf or leg pain, fluttering in the heart, or fatigue?
- How has this problem limited your activities?

Obtain objective data about the client's cardiovascular status by assessing vital signs, the heart, and arteries and veins. In most cases, assessment of the client's vital signs is the first objective information gathered in a health assessment. Significant deviation from normal heart rate and blood pressure may be the first indicator of a serious problem in circulatory function.

Landmarks for Cardiac Assessment

The precordium is the area on the anterior chest that overlies the heart and its great vessels. Knowledge of the location of structures within the precordium is necessary to perform effective cardiac assessment.

There are four major areas on the precordium for examining the heart (Fig. 24-13). Each area corresponds to one of the heart's four valves sounds.

Aortic area—second intercostal space, right sternal border
Pulmonic area—second intercostal space, left sternal border
Tricuspid area—fifth intercostal space, left sternal border
Mitral (or apical) area—fifth intercostal space, just medial to the midclavicular line

Inspection, palpation, and auscultation are the three basic techniques used to assess the precordium and vasculature. Percussion may be used to estimate the size of the heart, but radiographic examination has generally replaced this method.

Inspection

Inspect the entire precordium for movement. Using tangential light across the chest and observing the heart at eye level can enhance inspection. Normally, the only movement seen is in the mitral valve area. A visible pulsation occurs with ventricular contraction as the left side of the heart strikes the anterior chest wall. This pulsation is called the point of maximal impulse (PMI). Often, the PMI is not visible, especially in clients with thick chest walls or large breasts. Abnormal movements over the precordium include forceful movement around the area of the PMI, called a *heave;* anterior movement of the sternum, called a *lift;* and small areas of pulsation in the intercostal spaces or around the sternum.

Palpation

Palpation follows and complements inspection. Palpate in each of the four precordial areas, noting any vibrations (termed *thrills*) or pulsations. The fingertips are the most sensitive to pulsation, whereas the heel and ulnar surfaces of the hand are most sensitive to vibration. Feel for the PMI in the mitral area, and note its exact location and size. The normal PMI is a light tap, located at the medial to midclavicular line,

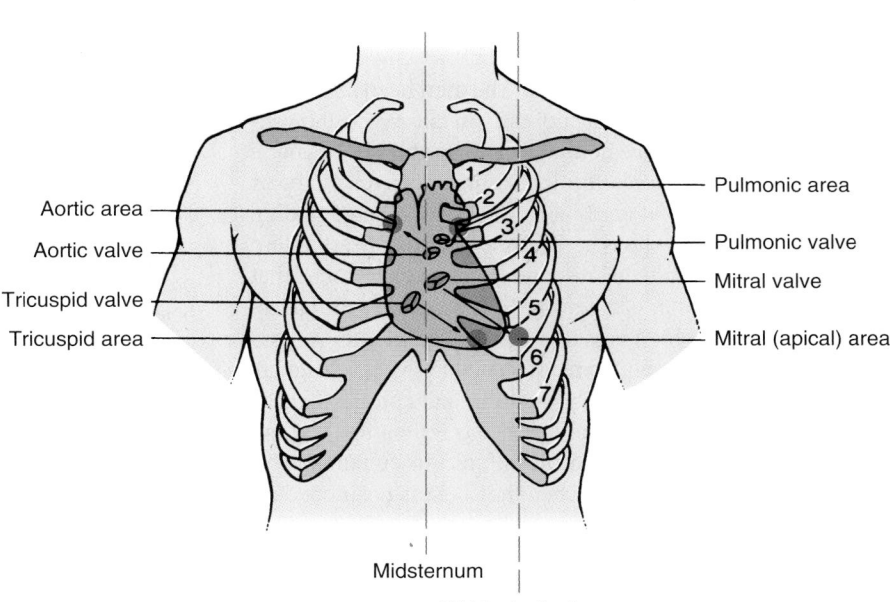

FIGURE 24-13 Heart sounds are referred from valvular points of origin to the auscultatory or precordial landmarks. Sound travels in the direction of blood flow and may be heard some distance from the valve.

Aortic area
Aortic valve
Tricuspid valve
Tricuspid area

Pulmonic area
Pulmonic valve
Mitral valve
Mitral (apical) area

Midsternum
Midclavicular line

confined to the area of one intercostal space. A PMI lateral position to this may indicate an enlarged heart. Pulsations or vibrations over the aortic, pulmonic, or tricuspid areas may indicate problems with those heart valves.

Auscultation

Valuable information can be obtained from listening to heart sounds. Learning the basic techniques of cardiac auscultation is enhanced by using a consistent pattern for auscultating the precordium and by concentrating on one heart sound or phase in the cardiac cycle at a time. Positioning the client in the left lateral position or sitting forward will help to move the heart closer to the chest wall and make the heart sounds easier to hear. Procedure 24-3 details steps in auscultation of heart sounds.

Normal Heart Sounds. Normal heart sounds include the first and second heart sounds (S_1 and S_2, respectively). Systole (ventricular contraction) is the period from the beginning of S_1 to the beginning of S_2. Diastole (ventricular relaxation) is the period from the beginning of S_2 to the beginning of the next ventricular contraction.

S_1 coincides with the beginning of systole, when the mitral and tricuspid valves close. S_1 is louder at the mitral and tricuspid areas. When an audible difference in closure of the two valves is detected, S_1 is said to be split. Because the force generated in the left ventricle is much greater than that in the right ventricle, S_1 is dominated by the mitral valve and is best heard in the mitral (apical) area. S_2 coincides with the beginning of diastole, when the aortic and pulmonic valves close. S_2 is heard more loudly in the aortic and pulmonic areas.

S_1 and S_2 are high-pitched sounds that are best heard with the diaphragm of the stethoscope. When the heart rate is slow, it is easy to differentiate the two sounds. Systole is shorter than diastole, so two "paired" sounds (S_1, then S_2) are heard, followed by a pause. When the heart rate is faster, the pause is less distinctive or even absent. To distinguish S_1 from S_2 in this situation, feel the client's carotid pulse when listening to the heart. The carotid pulse and S_1 occur almost simultaneously.

Extra or Abnormal Heart Sounds. The third heart sound (S_3) is an extra heart sound that occurs early in diastole as the ventricle rapidly fills. It can be normal in healthy children or young adults, but in older people it often signifies congestive heart failure. The presence of an S_3 is an important clinical finding to look for in a client who is at risk for congestive heart failure (Field, 1997). The fourth heart sound (S_4) is an extra sound that occurs late in diastole, just before S_1. It coincides with atrial contraction, when blood is actively propelled into the ventricle. S_4 is thought to result from a stiffened left ventricle and is frequently associated with hypertension and coronary artery disease. The development of an S_4 is not as serious as an S_3 and does not necessarily indicate heart failure. Auscultation of S_3 and S_4 is clearest at the apex when the client is positioned on the left side. Figure 24-14 illustrates where S_3 and S_4, commonly called gallops, occur in the cardiac cycle.

A murmur is vibrating sound that results from turbulent blood flow through the heart, especially across the valves.

The more common causes for a murmur include partially obstructed flow through a valve opening (stenosis), increased blood flow across a normal valve, backward blood flow (regurgitation) caused by a leaky (incompetent) valve, blood flow into a dilated chamber, and blood flow through an abnormal opening between heart chambers. Murmurs resemble blowing or swishing noises and may occur during systole or diastole. They may be low pitched or high pitched, so both the bell and the diaphragm of the stethoscope are appropriate for detecting murmurs. When a murmur is heard, note whether it occurs during systole (between S_1 and S_2) or during diastole (after S_2) and where it is heard on the precordium. Figure 24-15 illustrates where systolic and diastolic murmurs fall in the cardiac cycle. Heart disease almost always causes diastolic murmurs; systolic murmurs may be related to heart disease but frequently are benign.

Respiratory Assessment

Assessment of general respiratory status occurs every time you interact with the client. A survey of skin color, respiratory difficulty, and position the client takes to breathe is important to determine the acuteness of the client's problem. For acute respiratory distress, obtain immediate assistance so that appropriate interventions can begin.

Respiratory assessment should focus on four major areas: risk factors for lung disease (e.g., smoking, occupational exposure to pollutants); signs and symptoms of respiratory dysfunction (e.g., cough, sputum production, dyspnea); impact of respiratory status on ADLs; and adaptive measures for any respiratory dysfunction. Suggested interview questions that can help to elicit this information include the following:

- Have you been exposed to environmental or occupational materials that have affected your breathing? What are they?
- Have you had allergies, asthma, bronchitis, emphysema, tuberculosis, or other lung problems?
- How often do you cough? Describe the sputum.
- Do any breathing difficulties limit your activity? What are they?
- What position do you assume for sleeping?

Anatomic Landmarks of the Chest and Lungs

Nurses use anatomic landmarks and imaginary reference lines during the assessment of structures that lie within the thorax (chest). During lung auscultation and percussion, these lines and landmarks define the specific area of the lung being examined (Fig. 24-16). They also provide a standard vocabulary for use in describing and documenting assessment findings (Fritz, 1997).

Inspection

Inspection related to the respiratory examination focuses on four general areas: configuration of the thorax, breathing patterns, signs of labored breathing, and observation of the skin and nails. The shape of the thorax is best examined by

(text continues on page 425)

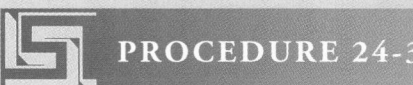

PROCEDURE 24-3

AUSCULTATING HEART SOUNDS

Purpose
1. To assess normal and abnormal functioning of the heart valves.
2. To detect cardiac problems.

Assessment
- Determine whether any immediate need is distracting the client (e.g., pain, urge to urinate). Attend to that problem first.
- Explain to the client what you plan to do and approximately how long it will take.
- Provide for privacy so that the client is not concerned about being viewed or overheard. Visitors and family members may be asked to leave the room.
- Ensure that the room is warm and quiet.

Equipment
Stethoscope with a bell-shaped diaphragm

Procedure
1. Wash hands. *Note:* Moderately warm water increases circulation to warm your hands and decreases discomfort to the client during the examination.
2. Assist the client to the supine position. You may want to re-examine the client in the upright sitting position and a left lateral position. Lift client's gown to expose the chest.
   Rationale: Certain positions accentuate some heart sounds.
3. Warm the diaphragm of the stethoscope by holding it between your hands for a few moments.
   Rationale: A warm stethoscope is more comfortable and will not startle the client, which could alter his or her heart rate.
4. Listen in the mitral area using the diaphragm. Identify the first and second heart sounds (S_1 and S_2). Count the heart rate, noting whether the rhythm is regular or irregular. If the rhythm is irregular, count the heart rate for a full minute. Also note whether the irregularity has a pattern or whether it is totally unpredictable.
   Rationale: Auscultation is best performed systematically, concentrating on one sound at a time in each area.
5. Listen in the aortic area using the diaphragm. Concentrate first on S_1, then S_2, noting whether splitting occurs. Shift your concentration to sys-

tole and then diastole; listen for extra sounds, such as murmurs.
   Rationale: The diaphragm of the stethoscope transmits the high-pitched sounds of S1 and S2. Murmurs are best heard over the valvular areas in the direction in which the blood is flowing through the heart.
6. Listen in the pulmonic area, still using only the diaphragm. Repeat the sequence described in step 5, concentrating on S_1, S_2, systole, and diastole. Compare the loudness of S_2 in the aortic and pulmonic areas.
   Rationale: Loudness of S_2 in the aortic area relates to the systemic arterial blood pressure and can be louder than normal in adults with hypertension. Loudness of S_2 in the pulmonic area relates to the pulmonary artery pressure and may be louder than normal in patients with chronic obstructive pulmonary disease. It is abnormal for the pulmonic S_2 to be louder than the aortic S_2 in adults older than 40 years of age.
7. Move the diaphragm and listen to the tricuspid and mitral areas.
8. Return to the aortic area, this time using the bell of the stethoscope. As before, concentrate individually on S_1, S_2, systole, and diastole.
9. Repeat the same process, using the bell, in the pulmonic, tricuspid, and mitral areas. Especially in the mitral area, concentrate during diastole to detect the presence of a third or fourth heart sound.
   Rationale: The lower-pitched sounds of the mitral and tricuspid valves, as well as an S_3 or S_4, are best transmitted through the bell of the stethoscope. Note: To increase your ability to hear an S_3 or mitral murmur, have the client lie on the left side while you auscultate with the bell. An S_3 often disappears when the client sits up.
10. Replace the client's clothes. Assist the client to a comfortable position.
    Rationale: Provide comfort and warmth before leaving.
11. Record your assessment findings, describing the intensity, quality, and location of the sounds.

Lifespan Considerations
Newborn and Infant
- Newborns have difficulty maintaining body temperature. Uncover only the body area that you are directly assessing.
- Heart rates are normally very rapid, so S_1 and S_2 are often difficult to discern.

PROCEDURE 24-3 (Continued)

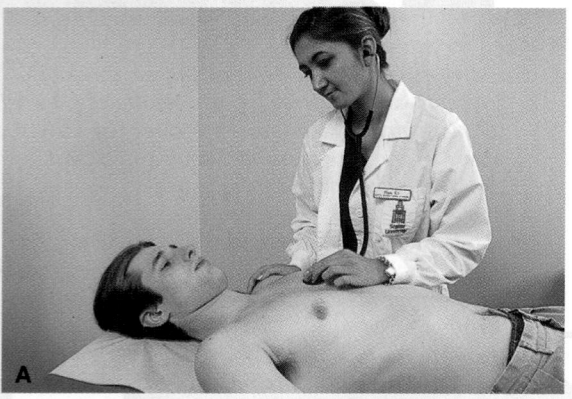

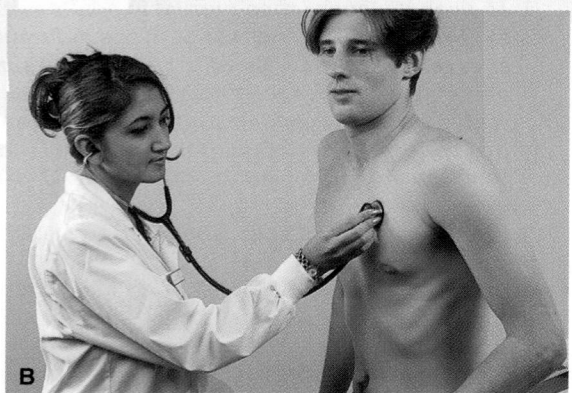

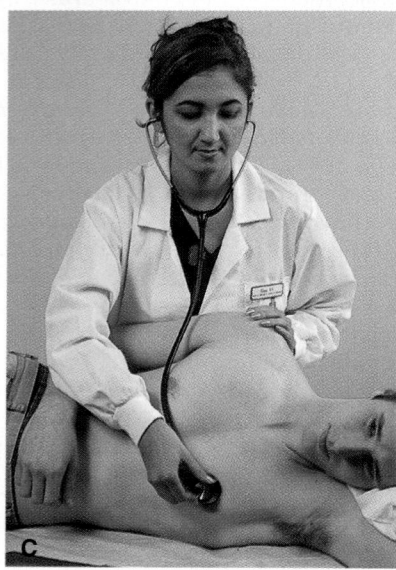

Step 2 (A) Supine, **(B)** forward sitting, and **(C)** left lateral precordial positions for heart auscultation.

- At 8 to 12 months of age, infants become fearful of strangers. Spend several minutes becoming acquainted with the child before proceeding with the examination.

Toddler and Preschooler
- Children 2 to 5 years of age are often afraid of examining equipment. Letting them handle the stethoscope and using a "This is a game" approach often help allay the fear.
- Auscultate heart sounds before performing any invasive examination, which may cause the child to cry.

School-Age Child and Adolescent
- Older children are modest. They may or may not want a parent to be with them during the examination; give the child the choice. Protect modesty through use of gowns or drapes.
- An S_3 is normal in children and young adults.

Older Adult
- An S_3 may indicate heart failure in older adults. An S_4 may be present in patients with coronary artery disease or hypertension.
- A lengthy physical examination may be exhausting for the older adult and may need to be completed in phases.
- Older adults can become easily chilled. Provide warmth through adequate draping or gowning.

Collaboration and Delegation
- Assessing heart sounds takes much practice. Consult with cardiac nurses or cardiologists to compare your assessment findings.
- Notify the physician or cardiologist of new abnormal heart sounds.

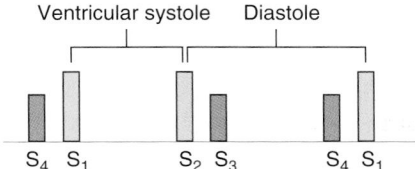

FIGURE 24-14 Occurrence of the third and fourth heart sounds (S₃ and S₄, respectively) in the cardiac cycle.

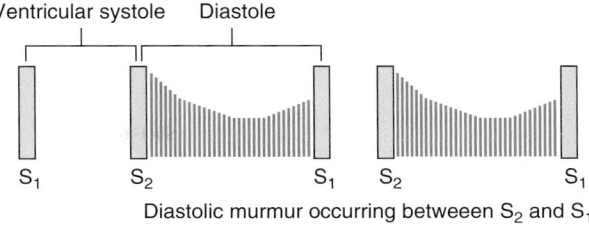

Diastolic murmur occurring between S₂ and S₁

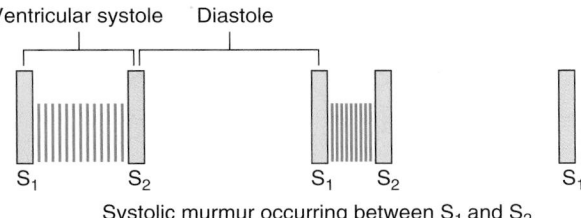

Systolic murmur occurring between S₁ and S₂

FIGURE 24-15 Location of heart murmurs in the cardiac cycle.

having the client sit upright with the chest area unclothed. The *anterior-posterior (AP) diameter* is a term used to describe the distance between the sternum and the vertebral column, drawn as a straight line through the thorax. In the normal adult, the AP diameter is approximately one half of the lateral diameter (width) of the chest.

One of the most common abnormalities of thorax configuration is seen in clients with chronic obstructive pulmonary disease. These clients exhibit a "barrel-shaped" chest in which the AP diameter is enlarged and approximately equal to the lateral diameter. Other thoracic abnormalities include kyphosis, an exaggerated convex curve of the spine; scoliosis, a lateral deviation of the spinal curve; and kyphoscoliosis, a combination of abnormal lateral and convex curvature of the spine. The presence of any of these conditions may deform the rib cage, impede lung expansion, and interfere with breathing.

Normal breathing is silent, effortless, and occurs at a rate of 12 to 20 times per minute in adults. Careful observation of the client's breathing should normally reveal a pattern that is smooth, regular, symmetric, and rhythmic. Conditions to observe for include breathing that is too fast (tachypnea), too slow (bradypnea), too shallow (hypoventilation), too deep (hyperventilation), or irregular (Cheyne–Stokes breathing). Chapter 25 discusses abnormal breathing patterns.

While observing the client's breathing pattern, look for indications of respiratory distress or increased effort in breathing, noting the position that the client has assumed to breathe. Clients with difficulty will be sitting and may be leaning forward or need a pillow for support. Symptoms such as nasal flaring, facial straining, and pursed-lip breathing indicate abnormal respiratory effort. Abnormal effort during inspiration is evidenced by active, visible use of the scalene and sternomastoid muscles of the neck and shoulders. These muscles are called accessory muscles. Contraction of the abdominal muscles, which assists upward movement of the diaphragm, may also be observed. During inspection of the client's breathing, observe the intercostal spaces. Airway obstruction or decreased lung compliance may result in retraction of the intercostal spaces during inspiration, whereas some respiratory diseases (e.g., emphysema) can cause bulging of the intercostal spaces during expiration.

Palpation

Palpation is used in respiratory assessment to evaluate painful or abnormal areas on the chest wall, to test for symmetry of chest expansion, and to detect tracheal deviation. To examine any areas on the chest where the client has complained of

discomfort, or where visible abnormalities are present, lightly palpate the area and surrounding area. Note any tenderness, masses or bulges, or a crackling feeling (crepitus), which may indicate an air leak into the subcutaneous tissue.

Normal chest expansion during inspiration is symmetric, indicating equal expansion of both lungs. To evaluate chest symmetry, stand behind the client, place your thumbs at the level of the tenth rib, and wrap your hands around the lateral rib cage (Fig. 24-17). Ask the client to inhale deeply, and observe your thumbs for equal, outward movement.

Percussion

Percussion of the lung normally reveals a hollow, loud, low-pitched, resonant sound because the lung is filled with air. Percussion that reveals dullness or reduced resonance may indicate masses, fluid, or tissue-filled lung space. Percussion that is hyperresonant indicates hyperinflation of the lung, such as with the air trapping that occurs with emphysema. Diagnostically, examination of the chest radiograph has largely replaced chest percussion.

Auscultation

Lung auscultation involves listening with a stethoscope over the anterior and posterior chest wall for variations in breath sounds. The movement of air in and out of the airways with each inspiration and expiration creates breath sounds. Auscultation of the lungs reveals direct, objective data about the client's ventilatory status. Data gathered through auscultation provide important clues to underlying pathophysiology. Refer to Procedure 24-4 for the steps in pulmonary auscultation.

Normal Breath Sounds. Normal breath sounds are classified as bronchial, bronchovesicular, and vesicular. They are described according to location, ratio of inspiration to expiration, intensity, and pitch, as summarized and illustrated in Table 24-6.

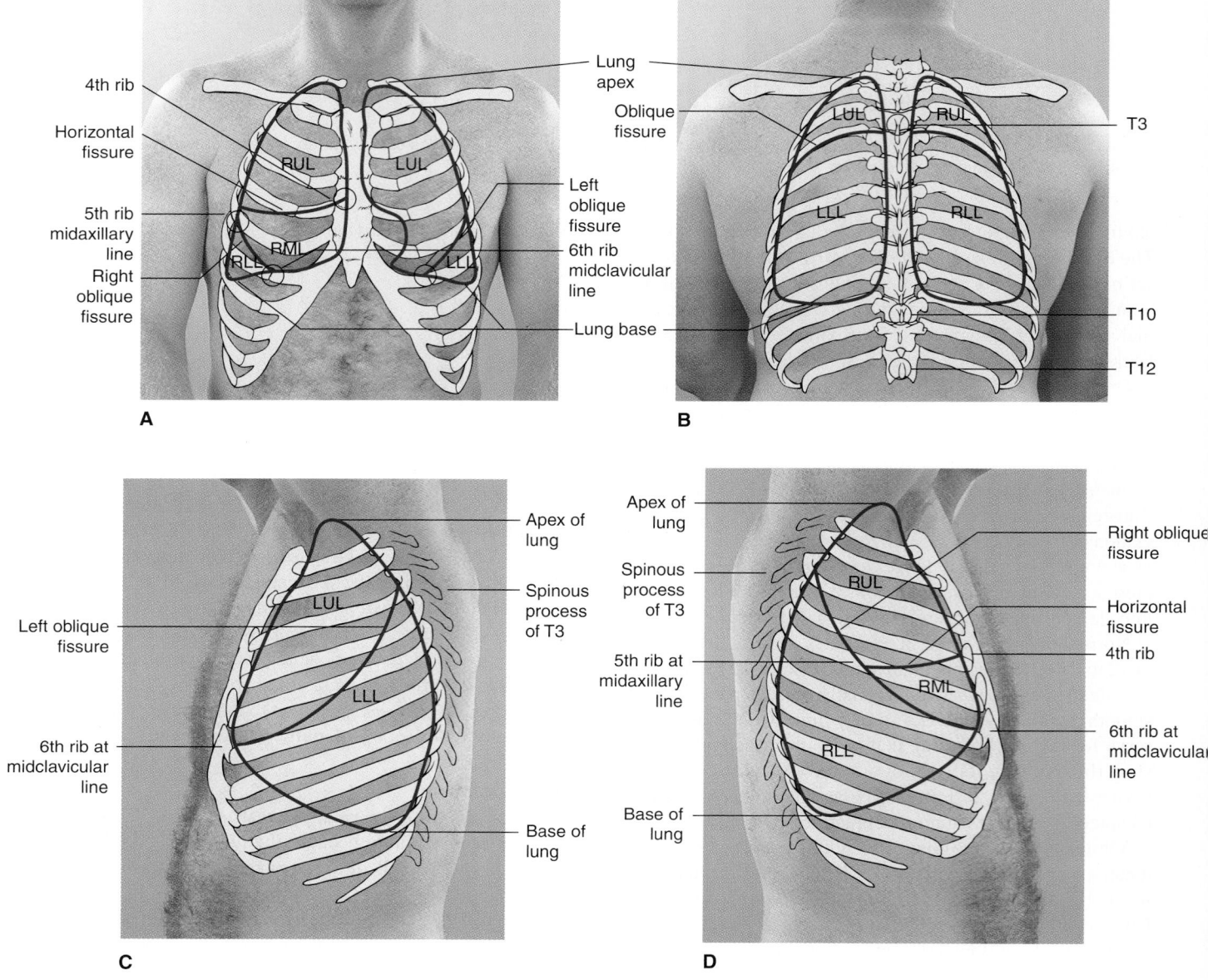

FIGURE 24-16   Landmarks of the anterior and posterior chest wall.

Bronchial breath sounds are loud and high pitched, with a hollow quality often compared to the sound of air blowing through a pipe. Expiration is longer and louder than inspiration with bronchial breath sounds. They are normal when heard over the trachea but indicate a lung abnormality when heard elsewhere. Abnormal bronchial sounds may be associated with pneumonia, pleural effusion, tumor, or atelectasis.

Vesicular breath sounds are normally heard over all areas of the lung except over or near the major airways. Vesicular sounds are described as soft and breezy, with inspiration markedly longer than expiration.

Bronchovesicular breath sounds are intermediate in character between bronchial and vesicular sounds. They are described as breezy but softer and lower pitched than bronchial sounds. Inspiratory and expiratory times are approximately

equal. Bronchovesicular sounds are normally heard in two areas only: on the anterior chest over the bifurcation of the main bronchi in the first or second intercostal spaces, and posteriorly between the scapulae. Like bronchial sounds, bronchovesicular sounds should not be detected elsewhere over the chest.

Adventitious Breath Sounds.   Adventitious breath sounds are abnormal sounds that occur from air passing through narrowed airways or fluid, or from an inflammation of lung pleura. The major adventitious breath sounds are crackles, wheezes, and friction rubs (Fig. 24-18). These sounds are often superimposed over normal breath sounds and take much practiced listening to discern. Chapter 34 describes adventitious breath sounds in detail.

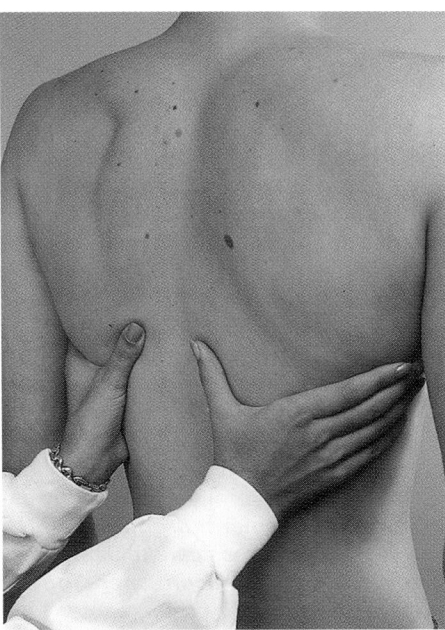

FIGURE 24-17 Palpation of thoracic excursion. In the posterior approach, the nurse's hands are placed at the level of the tenth rib and observed for equal outward movement as the client inhales.

When you detect abnormal breath sounds in a client, continue to listen, requesting the client to say words or sounds. If consolidation or atelectasis is present, the words (such as "ninety-nine") will sound louder and clearer than they usually do. This is known as *bronchophony*. Also, if the client says "ee," the sound will transmit as "ay"; this is called *egophony*.

Assessment of Breasts

Breast examination is important in early detection of breast cancer. This procedure should be conducted as a joint activity of the client and the nurse, with the nurse's primary role as educator. Although breast cancer is rare in men, a brief examination of the male breast is also appropriate. Some questions that you may ask as part of your interview include the following:

- Do you examine your breasts? How often?
- Do you have a family history of breast cancer?

Inspection

Teach the client to do a breast self-examination while you are performing the breast examination (Display 50-2 in Chapter 50). Chapter 50 outlines teaching related to self-examination of breasts. Normal breasts appear rounded and essentially symmetric, although one breast is often slightly larger than the other. The skin should be smooth and intact, with the areola darker in color, round, and symmetric. The nipple should be everted and without discharge or lesions. Abnormal findings with inspection include flattening, bulges or changes in breast size, marked asymmetry, redness, dimpling, and edema.

Palpation

Palpation is done to determine whether masses or lumps are present in the breast. Palpate the breast with the client in the supine position with his or her hands behind the head. Palpate each breast for tenderness, nodules, or masses. Use three or four fingers, pressing the flat part of the fingers in small circles, and moving the circles slowly around the breast. Follow a sequential pattern of palpation so that all breast areas are included. Begin at the outer edge of the breast, gradually working toward the nipple. The tail of the breast extends into the axillary area. Because most breast cancers occur in this upper outer quadrant of the breast, it is especially important to palpate this area carefully. The final step in breast examination is gentle squeezing of the nipple to check for discharge. Again, during the palpation, teach the woman how to perform breast self-palpation.

Abdominal Assessment

The abdomen contains organs for digestion of food, organs for elimination of waste, major arteries and veins, and organs of reproduction in the female. Problems arising from this area may be difficult to diagnose (Wright, 1997). Elimination is the excretion of waste products from the body through the gastrointestinal and urinary systems. Elimination assessment focuses on determining the adequacy of bowel and bladder function, observing characteristics of feces or urine, identifying risk factors that may contribute to problems in elimination, assessing the impact of bowel or bladder dysfunction on daily living, and understanding the client's methods of management and coping for any bowel or bladder problems.

Bowel Elimination

Some clients may consider bowel function to be a private matter, but it is important for nurses to develop ease in asking clients questions regarding their bowel status. Basic abdominal assessment consists of inspection, auscultation, and palpation. Abdominal assessment provides clues to general gastrointestinal function and any related problems.

Landmarks for Abdominal Assessment. For descriptive purposes, the abdomen is divided into four quadrants. An imaginary horizontal line through the umbilicus separates the upper and lower quadrants. An imaginary vertical line between the xiphoid and symphysis pubis separates the right and left quadrants. Table 24-7 lists and illustrates the structures underlying each of the four quadrants.

Inspection. During inspection, note the contour, skin, and movement of the abdomen. Observe the client at eye level from the side, from the foot of the bed, and from directly over the abdomen. Use tangential lighting across the abdomen to accentuate subtle changes. Evaluate the contour of the abdomen by placing the client supine and viewing at eye level from the side. Possible descriptions are flat, rounded, protuberant, or scaphoid (boat shaped or hollowed). Ascites is the

(text continues on page 430)

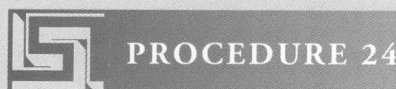

PROCEDURE 24-4

AUSCULTATING BREATH SOUNDS

Purpose
1. To listen for variations in breath sounds that may indicate the presence of airway obstruction or disease process.
2. To assess the effectiveness of medications or therapies in opening or clearing airways.

Assessment/Preparation
- Explain to the client what you plan to do and approximately how long it will take.
- Determine if any immediate need is distracting the client (e.g., pain, need to void). Attend to that need first.
- Provide for privacy so that the client is not concerned about being viewed or overheard. You may ask visitors and family members to leave the room.
- Ensure that the room is warm and quiet.

Equipment
Stethoscope

Procedure
1. Wash hands. *Note:* Moderately warm water increases circulation to warm your hands, decreases discomfort to the client during the examination, and prevents transfer of microorganisms.
2. Assist the client to an upright sitting position. Remove client's gown to expose chest.
   Rationale: Upright position improves chest excursion. Assessing breath sounds through clothing would muffle or distort them.
3. Warm the diaphragm of the stethoscope by holding it between your hands for a short time.
   Rationale: A warm stethoscope is more comfortable for the client and helps put the client at ease.
4. Ask client to breathe deeply through the mouth. Client should breathe slowly.
   Rationale: Mouth breathing enhances volume of breath sounds; nasal breathing decreases volume and can simulate adventitious sounds. A slow breathing rate is necessary to avoid hyperventilation.

Auscultate Anterior Chest
5. Place diaphragm of stethoscope about 1 inch below the middle of the right clavicle, making sure it lies between the ribs. Listen to one full

inspiration and exhalation. Repeat the process at the corresponding site on the left side.
   Rationale: Placement of stethoscope over intercostal space improves sound quality. Representative sounds of right and left upper lobes are audible here.
6. Note normal and adventitious breath sounds at each point on the chest as you proceed.
   Rationale: Movement of air through airways produces characteristic sounds. Abnormal sounds are indicative of airway disturbances.
7. Move stethoscope downward about 1.5 to 2 inches along midclavicular line. Note sounds; move stethoscope laterally to opposite side.
   Rationale: Air movement through other (larger) airways of upper lobes can be heard here. Listening to sounds at corresponding points on opposite sides of sternum allows you to compare similar lung fields.

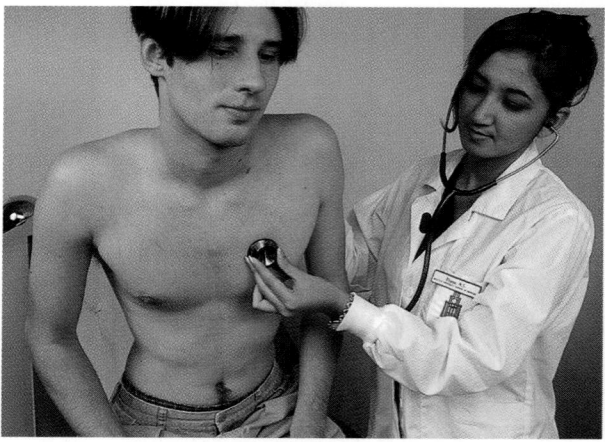

Step 7 Auscultating along the midclavicular line.

8. Move stethoscope downward another inch or two along midclavicular line to fifth intercostal space. (This space lies just below the nipple line on men, approximately across from the head of the xiphoid process of the sternum.) Note sounds, then move to same spot on opposite side.
   Rationale: Right middle lobe and corresponding segments on left can be heard here.

Auscultate Posterior Chest
9. Instruct client to lean forward and cross arms in front.
   Rationale: This position separates scapulae and facilitates listening to posterior breath sounds.

PROCEDURE 24-4 (Continued)

10. Begin by auscultating the area about 2 inches below the shoulders and 2 inches to the right of the spine. Note sounds, then move to corresponding point on left.
    Rationale: These positions allow comparison of breath sounds of posterior segments of the upper lobes.
11. Move stethoscope directly downward 2 or 2.5 inches; note sounds, then move stethoscope laterally and listen on the right.
    Rationale: Superior segments of lower lobes are audible here.
12. Repeat process, moving downward 2 to 2.5 inches; listen to corresponding opposite side.
    Rationale: Each placement of stethoscope allows you to hear sounds of different segments of lung.
13. Move stethoscope downward to area just below scapula. Listen on right and left. Listen also to areas laterally along lower rib cage.
    Rationale: The lower lobes end at the level of the tenth thoracic vertebra (about 1.5 inches below scapulae) and follow the contour of the lower ribs. Their large size and the fact that many clinical problems can affect the lower lobes make lateral assessment essential.

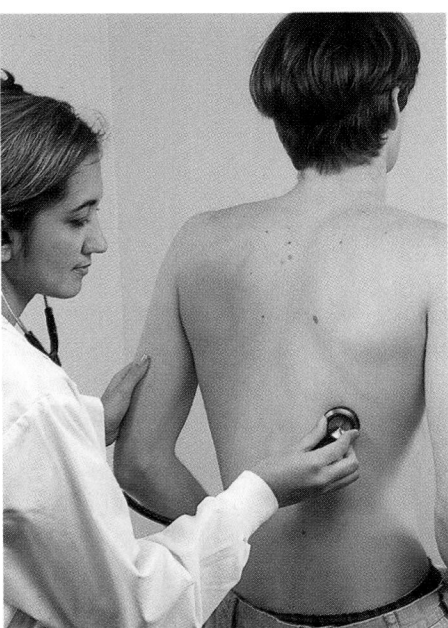

Step 13 Auscultating below the scapula.

14. Replace client's clothes and assist the client to a comfortable position.
15. Discuss your findings with the client.
    Rationale: Discussion provides an opportunity for client feedback on the effectiveness of therapies and provides directions for client teaching if new therapies are to be initiated (e.g., cough, deep breathing, incentive spirometry).
16. Record assessment findings. Be specific as to description and location of adventitious sounds.

Lifespan Considerations
Newborn and Infant
- Newborns have difficulty maintaining body temperature. Uncover only the body area that you are directly assessing.
- At 8 to 12 months of age, infants become fearful of strangers. Spend several minutes becoming acquainted with the child before proceeding with the examination.

Toddler and Preschooler
- Children 2 to 5 years of age are often afraid of examining equipment. Letting them handle the stethoscope and using a "This is a game" approach often help allay the fear.
- Auscultate breath sounds before performing any invasive examination, which may cause the child to cry.

School-Age Child and Adolescent
- Older children are modest. They may or may not want a parent to be with them during the examination; give the child the choice. Protect modesty through the use of gowns or drapes.

Older Adult
- A lengthy physical examination may be exhausting for the older adult and may need to be completed in phases.
- Older adults can become easily chilled. Provide warmth through adequate draping or gowning.

Collaboration and Delegation
- Review your assessment findings with physicians or respiratory therapists (RTs) to improve and refine your skills.
- Collaborate with RT to develop a plan for clients who have adventitious breath sounds.
- Report any significant abnormal findings or respiratory distress to the physician.

TABLE 24-6

Normal Breath Sounds From Anterior Location

Location	Description	Ratio of Inspiration to Expiration	Intensity	Pitch
Bronchial Bronchial breath sounds	Blowing, hollow sounds over the trachea	Inspiration Expiration	Expiration is markedly longer and louder	Expiration is higher
Bronchovesicular Scapula — Intercostal space — Bronchovesicular breath sounds	Intermediate sounds over first and second anterior intercostal spaces and posteriorly between scapula	Inspiration Expiration	Medium and similar	Medium and similar
Vesicular Vesicular breath sounds	Soft and breezy sounds over all lung area except airways	Inspiration Expiration	Inspiration markedly longer and louder	Inspiration is higher

accumulation of serous fluid in the peritoneum. This fluid may cause the shape to become protuberant, or distended and firm. A distended abdomen may also be measured to provide more specific data.

In relation to elimination, observe the abdomen for distention, which can signify decreased peristalsis in the intestines. When distention is present, the abdomen appears larger than usual; in severe distention, the skin appears stretched and taut. The client may be able to verify that the abdomen appears larger than usual or that clothes are tighter.

The abdominal skin should be similar in color and texture to skin on other areas of the body. Note the presence and location of scars, rashes, lesions, petechiae (small, red, hemorrhagic spots), or striae. Striae are streaks caused by rapid or prolonged stretching of the skin. Recent striae are pink or blue; they turn silvery white with age. Pregnancy, ascites, and weight gain or loss are common causes of striae. Fine veins

may normally be visible on the abdomen, especially in the inguinal area. Distended, prominent veins are abnormal and are frequently associated with liver disease. Scars provide clues about previous surgeries.

Visible movement over the abdomen is not uncommon. Wavelike movements of intestinal peristalsis may be seen in thin clients. A normal aortic pulsation is frequently visible in the epigastrium. A rise and fall of the abdomen synchronized with respiration is frequently seen, especially in men.

Auscultation. Always auscultate the abdomen before palpating or percussing, because movement or stimulation can alter motility of the bowel and increase the sounds. Bowel sounds are created as air and fluid mix in the intestine (Kirton, 1997). Procedure 24-5 outlines the method of abdominal auscultation.

(text continues on page 433)

Crackles

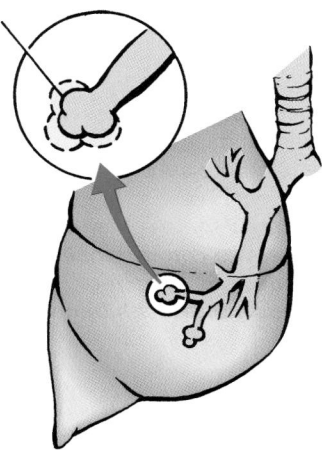

Wheezes

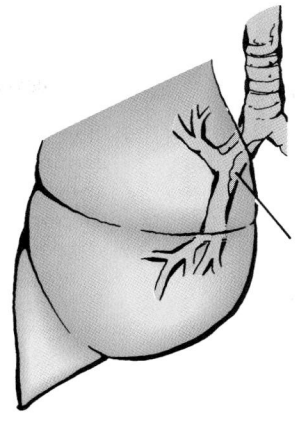

Pleural friction rubs

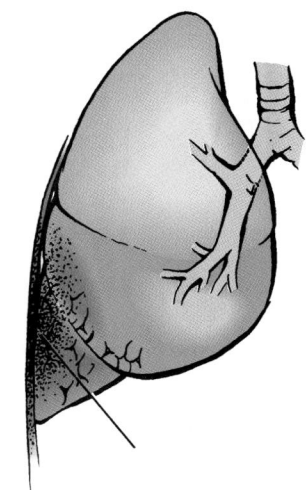

Crackles: high-pitched, discrete, non-continuous crackling sounds heard during the end of inspiration.
Coarse crackles: loud, bubbly noise heard during inspiration; not cleared by a cough

Fine wheeze: musical noise sounding like a squeak; may be heard during inspiration or expiration; usually louder during expiration
Coarse wheeze (rhonchi): loud, low, coarse sounds like a snore heard at any point of inspiration or expiration; coughing may clear sound (usually means mucus accumulation in trachea or large bronchi)

Pleural friction rub: dry, rubbing, or grating sound, usually caused by inflammation of pleural surfaces; heard during inspiration or expiration; loudest over lower lateral anterior surface

FIGURE 24-18   Adventitious breath sounds.

TABLE 24-7

Organs in the Four Abdominal Quadrants[a]		
1—Upper Right Quadrant	**3—Upper Left Quadrant**	
Liver	Left lobe of liver	
Gallbladder	Stomach	
Duodenum	Spleen	
Head of pancreas	Upper lobe of left kidney	
Right adrenal gland	Pancreas	
Upper lobe of right kidney	Left adrenal gland	
Hepatic flexure of colon	Splenic flexure of colon	
Section of ascending colon	Section of transverse colon	
Section of transverse colon	Section of descending colon	
2—Lower Right Quadrant	**4—Lower Left Quadrant**	
Lower lobe of right kidney	Lower lobe of left kidney	
Cecum	Sigmoid colon	
Appendix	Section of descending colon	
Section of ascending colon	Left ovary	
Right ovary	Left fallopian tube	
Right fallopian tube	Left ureter	
Right ureter	Left spermatic cord	
Right spermatic cord	Part of uterus (if enlarged)	
Part of uterus (if enlarged)		

[a]The uterus and urinary bladder fall in the lower midline.

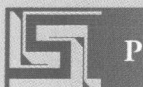

PROCEDURE 24-5

AUSCULTATING BOWEL SOUNDS

Purpose
1. To determine the presence or absence of intestinal peristalsis.

Assessment/Planning
- Explain to the client what you plan to do and how long it will take.
- Determine whether any immediate need is distracting the client (e.g., pain, urge to urinate). Attend to that problem first.
- Plan to auscultate the abdomen before palpating or percussing if performing a complete abdominal examination.
  Rationale: Stimulation of the abdominal wall may alter bowel motility.
- Provide for privacy so that the client is not concerned about being viewed or overheard.
- Ensure that the room is warm and quiet.
- If the client has a nasogastric tube with suction, turn off the suction during auscultation because the sound will confuse your assessment.

Equipment
Stethoscope

Procedure
1. Wash your hands and warm the stethoscope diaphragm.
   Rationale: Cold hands or stethoscope may cause contraction of the abdominal muscles, which you may hear during auscultation.
2. Ask the client when he or she last ate.
   Rationale: Bowel sounds may be increased shortly after eating or if a meal is long overdue.
3. Have the client urinate before the examination.
   Rationale: An empty bladder enhances validity of observations and promotes client comfort.
4. Assist the client to a supine position with abdomen exposed.
   Rationale: Supine position prevents tension in the abdominal muscles.
5. Visually divide the abdomen into four quadrants using the umbilicus as the central crossing landmark (see Table 24-7).
   Rationale: Consistent landmarks facilitate accurate description of assessment findings.
6. Place the stethoscope diaphragm in each of the four quadrants. Listen for pitch, frequency, and duration of bowel sounds at each site.

Rationale: Active bowel sounds are irregular, gurgling noises that occur every 5 to 20 seconds.
7. If you do not hear bowel sounds, listen for 3 to 5 minutes in all quadrants before concluding that they are absent.
   Rationale: Bowel sounds are very irregular and require longer assessment to confirm that they are absent and not hypoactive. Absent or hypoactive bowel sounds indicate inhibited intestinal motility.

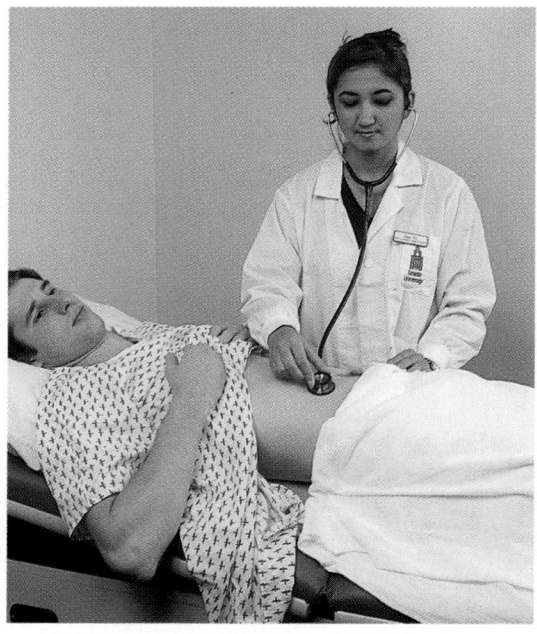

Step 6 Auscultate bowel sounds with diaphragm of stethoscope.

8. Proceed with the rest of the physical examination or cover the client's abdomen and assist him or her to a comfortable position.
9. Document your findings.

Lifespan Considerations
Newborn and Infant
- Newborns have difficulty maintaining body temperature. Uncover only the body area that you are directly assessing.
- At 8 to 12 months of age, infants become fearful of strangers. Spend several minutes becoming acquainted with the child before proceeding with the examination.

PROCEDURE 24-5 (Continued)

Toddler and Preschooler
- Children 2 to 5 years of age are often afraid of the examining equipment. Letting them handle the stethoscope and using a "This is a game" approach often help allay the fear.
- Auscultate bowel sounds before performing any invasive examination, which may cause the child to cry.

School-Age Child and Adolescent
- Older children are modest. They may or may not want a parent to be with them during the exami-

nation; give the child the choice. Protect modesty through use of gowns or drapes.

Older Adult
- Older adults can become easily chilled. Provide warmth through adequate draping or gowning.

Collaboration and Delegation
- Notify the surgeon when the client's bowel sounds return postoperatively, because this development usually warrants a change in diet.

Normal bowel sounds are tinkling, gurgling noises that occurring every 5 to 20 seconds. Bowel sounds of increased frequency and loudness are called borborygmi, or hyperactive bowel sounds. Borborygmus reflects increased intestinal peristalsis, which may be related to diarrhea, laxatives, emotional upset, or intestinal obstruction. Borborygmus heard before a meal is better known as "stomach growling."

Percussion. Percussion is used to detect the location of organs that are not normally palpable and to give clues about the characteristics of the masses underlying the skin. Generalized tympany is present over the intestines, although varying degrees of tympany will be audible depending on the location of food and stool masses. The liver is percussed at the right midclavicular and midsternal lines, and the sound elicited is dull. The gastric bubble in the left lower rib cage is normally very tympanic. The spleen is found at the left tenth rib posterior to the midaxillary line, and is dull (Table 24-7).

Palpation. Light palpation is performed to obtain information about pain or discomfort. Palpate all four quadrants, reserving the area of suspected pain or abnormality until last. Relaxation of the abdominal wall is necessary for an accurate assessment. Promote relaxation by positioning the client with knees slightly flexed and arms at the sides or across the chest. During deep palpation, avoid areas of pain found through light palpation. With deep palpation, masses of stool may normally be palpable in the abdomen. The liver border may be assessed during palpation, although it normally is not palpable at the midclavicular line in adults. Note the location and approximate size of any abnormal masses or enlarged organs.

 SAFETY ALERT
Do not palpate the abdomen of a client complaining of sudden, severe abdominal pain, because doing so could rupture an inflamed appendix, causing peritonitis.

Perirectal Area. Palpation and inspection of the perirectal area should reveal smooth, intact skin without stretching or shininess. To palpate the rectum, insert a lubricated, gloved index finger in the rectum and direct it toward the umbilicus (Fig. 24-19). Document the presence of internal or external hemorrhoids, polyps, or abnormal masses (see Fig. 41-2 in Chapter 41). Frequently, a rectal examination is performed to detect the presence and consistency of stool in the rectum. Hard, dry stool may indicate the presence of a fecal impaction, which may require manual removal.

Urinary Elimination
Inspection. Assessment of the bladder for distention due to urinary retention is warranted if a client complains of lower abdominal (or bladder) discomfort or reports a history of difficulty urinating, or if a prolonged time has elapsed since the last voiding occurred. Inspect the bladder for signs of distention, which appears as a swelling of the lower abdomen, just above the symphysis pubis. Observation of urinary distention may be difficult in the obese person. If the bladder contains less than 500 mL of urine, no bulge is present on inspection.

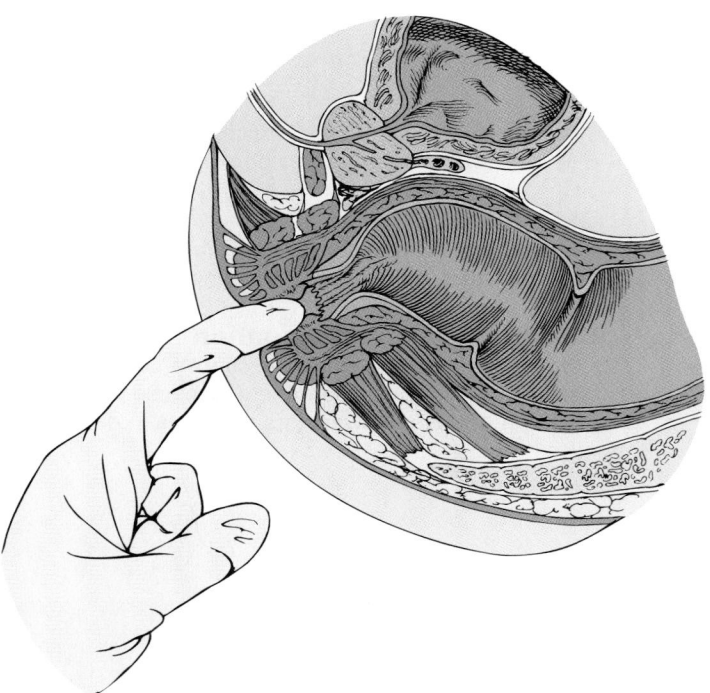

FIGURE 24-19   The nurse inserts a gloved, lubricated index finger into the rectum to detect stool or abnormalities.

Percussion.   Percussion of the lower abdomen follows inspection to determine the presence of a distended bladder. Percussion begins at the umbilicus and proceeds toward the symphysis pubis. If the bladder is empty or contains only a small amount of urine, a tympanic note is heard when the bladder is percussed; percussion over a full bladder produces a duller sound.

Palpation.   Often, the client exhibits signs of sensitivity or discomfort when the full bladder is being palpated. In this case, palpation may be deferred. Light palpation can provide additional data if the client can tolerate it. Palpate from the umbilicus to the symphysis pubis, using the fingertips. With light palpation, you will feel a firm ridge or mass as you locate the bladder. Be aware that palpation can stimulate voiding.

Assessment of the Genitalia

Assessment of a Female Client.   When working with a female client, the following are some questions that you may ask:

- At what age did you begin menstruating?
- How long is your typical menstrual cycle?
- What was the date of your last menstrual cycle?
- Do you have any problems related to menstruation?
- How many times have you been pregnant?
- How many children do you have?

Examination of female internal reproductive organs is not commonly part of the basic health assessment unless the nurse is working in a specialized area such as a gynecology clinic or labor and delivery. Frequently, the nurse is present with the client during a pelvic examination. The following measures can assist relaxation and comfort:

- Assist the client to assume the lithotomy position and drape the client to maintain privacy and warmth.
- Warm the speculum.
- Have a mobile or pictures on the ceiling to focus the client's attention.
- Encourage rhythmic breathing (breathing deeply and slowly through the mouth).
- Ask the client to concentrate on relaxing body muscles with each exhalation.
- Remind client not to hold her breath.

Inspection of the female external reproductive organs includes examining the labia minora, labia majora, clitoris, and vaginal opening. The color of these organs should be pink, with some blue or brown pigments occasionally seen. Bright red color or obvious areas of excoriation are abnormal and often occur in the presence of infection or irritation. Normal vaginal secretions are white, colorless, and odorless. Foul-smelling, purulent drainage is abnormal.

Assessment of a Male Client.   During assessment of the male client, you may ask the following questions:

- Do you examine your testicles? How often?
- Do you have any concerns about sexual function?

Examination of the testicles in men is important for early detection of testicular cancer. As with women, the examination should be undertaken as a joint activity, with the nurse as educator.

Inspection of the external male reproductive organs includes the glans, foreskin, and shaft of the penis, and the scrotum. The man may be circumcised or uncircumcised. If the client is uncircumcised, gently retract the foreskin during the examination to inspect the glans and the urethral opening. Replace the foreskin to the previous position after the inspection. Inspection of the penis should reveal no lesions or abnormal discharge. Smegma is a normal white discharge that may collect around the glans, especially in the uncircumcised man. The scrotal sac is wrinkled in appearance, with the left scrotal sac usually hanging lower than the right.

Perform palpation of the male genitalia to detect the presence of the testicle in each scrotal sac and the absence of pain, swelling, or growths. Palpate one scrotal compartment at a time by grasping the scrotum gently between the thumb and forefinger. Roll the testicle gently to palpate. The testicles should feel round, smooth, and freely movable within the scrotum (Display 50-1 in Chapter 50). Chapter 50 discusses testicular self-examination.

Assessment of Extremities

Inspection

Inspection can be used to assess peripheral circulation. Examine the skin for color and temperature. Poor peripheral circulation may be associated with hair loss and skin discoloration or scaling. Observed varicosities (swollen, twisted veins) can indicate venous problems. Edema, or fluid, may also be detected through inspection. Arterial problems are associated with pallor; dependent rubor; shiny, cool, hairless skin; weak or absent pulses; decreased capillary refill; and sharp pain with increased activity. Venous problems are associated with edema; warmth; bluish discoloration when legs are dependent; brown pigmentation; flaky dermatitis; achy, chronic pain; and ulcers that heal slowly (Vowden, 1998).

Palpation

Palpation is important in peripheral vascular assessment. Skin temperature is best evaluated using the back of the hand. Symmetric coolness or warmth may be normal; unilateral coolness may indicate decreased blood flow; unilateral warmth may indicate local infection. Generalized cool skin accompanied by pallor and moistness may indicate peripheral vasoconstriction due to circulatory shock.

Arterial Pulses. Palpate arterial pulses, noting rate, rhythm, amplitude, and symmetry. Use the brachial, radial, ulnar, femoral, popliteal, posterior tibial, and dorsalis pedis pulses (see Fig. 25-6 in Chapter 25). Comparing pulses between sides is helpful to evaluate for differences in circulation. Also, it can generally be assumed, if a distal pulse is present, that the more medial pulses are also present in the same extremity. A grading scale is used to compare the strength of the pulses (Display 24-3).

Capillary Refill. Palpation is also used to assess capillary refill. Capillary refill time is a simple test of circulatory status that uses the nailbeds. Press down on the nailbed until it turns white, then note how quickly the color returns after you release the pressure. Normal refill time is 3 seconds or less; a prolonged capillary refill time indicates poor circulation.

DISPLAY 24-3

⬚ **GRADING SCALE FOR PULSES**

0 = Absent
1+ = Diminished; thready; easily obliterated
2+ = Normal; not easily obliterated
3+ = Increased; full volume
4+ = Bounding; hyperkinetic

Edema. Edema is evaluated through palpation. Edema is fluid accumulation in the tissues. The degree of edema is estimated by noting how long the tissue remains indented when pressed. Assess edema in dependent areas such as the hands, feet, ankles, and lower legs. Press firmly with the thumb, for at least 5 seconds, behind the medial malleolus, over the dorsum of the foot, and over the shin. If the client is bedridden, the dependent areas are the back and sacrum. A grading system, ranging from +1 to +4, is often used to record edema (see Fig. 35-7 in Chapter 35). Lower limbs may also be measured for circumference to evaluate for changes in edema and symmetry.

Joint Mobility. Joint movement is also important to activity and exercise function. All joints should have appropriate range of motion. Often, range of motion can be observed by watching the extent and ease with which the client moves his or her extremities. If the client complains of stiffness or does not move an area of the body, evaluate joint mobility by moving each joint through its full range of motion and noting any limitations in movement. Generally, greater than 10% reduction in the normal range is abnormal. A physical therapist may be consulted for further evaluation. Refer to Chapter 33 for additional information on assessment of joint mobility.

Muscle Strength. Perform a simple screening of motor function in the arms and legs, because limb movement and strength are essential for many self-care activities. A simple method is to measure hand strength by having the client squeeze your wrists, and foot strength by having the client push the ball of the foot against your hand. Observe muscle strength by evaluating the amount of strength against resistance or gravity. For clients who are able to participate in the examination, have the client move the limb against your resistance. Other clients may be asked to hold a limb in a position, with gravity acting as the resistance. The response is then graded (Display 24-4).

Evaluate symmetry of strength. It is expected that muscle strength is slightly greater in the dominant arm. Notable differences in strength or overall difficulty in performing these tests reveals problems with movement or weakness in the arms. Report any deficits to the physician or to a nurse specialist for a more comprehensive and detailed assessment of muscle function.

DISPLAY 24-4

🖼 GRADING SCALE FOR MUSCLE STRENGTH

0—No detectable muscle contraction
1—Barely detectable contraction
2—Complete range of motion or active body part movement with gravity eliminated
3—Complete range of motion or active movement against gravity
4—Complete range of motion or active movement against gravity and some resistance
5—Complete range of motion or active movement against gravity and full resistance

Sensory Assessment. Loss of tactile sensation may occur with a variety of conditions such as diabetes, peripheral vascular disease, spinal cord injury, brain trauma, tumor, or vascular lesion. Clients with decreased tactile sensations are at risk for injury from heat or cold, prolonged pressure, or shearing force. Sensory function is also evaluated in clients who are recovering from surgery with spinal anesthesia, who are receiving epidural pain medication, or who have spinal cord injuries. Dermatomes are sensory fibers from a single spinal nerve that serve a particular skin surface (Fig. 24-20). Evaluate function in dermatomes around and below (distal to) the suspected problem area. Evaluate sensory perception by observing the client's response to light touch, vibration, and pain. With the client's eyes closed, touch various body areas with a wisp of cotton to assess light touch, with a tuning fork to test vibration, and with a toothpick to test pain. You may use water of different temperatures to assess temperature discrimination. Documentation should include the inability to sense stimuli and the affected location of the body. Report any abnormal sensations such as paresthesias, numbness, or tingling.

Circulation, Movement, and Sensation. When an acute problem with a limb is suspected, circulation, movement, and sensation (CMS) are evaluated. Assess circulation by color, temperature, pulses, and capillary refill. Assess movement by asking the client to voluntarily move the extremity. Assess sensation by asking the client to say when he or she feels the touch. Also, question the client about paresthesias, or sensations of numbness and tingling. CMS is normal if the skin is pink and warm, pulses are present, and capillary refill takes place within 3 seconds. The client should be able to wiggle

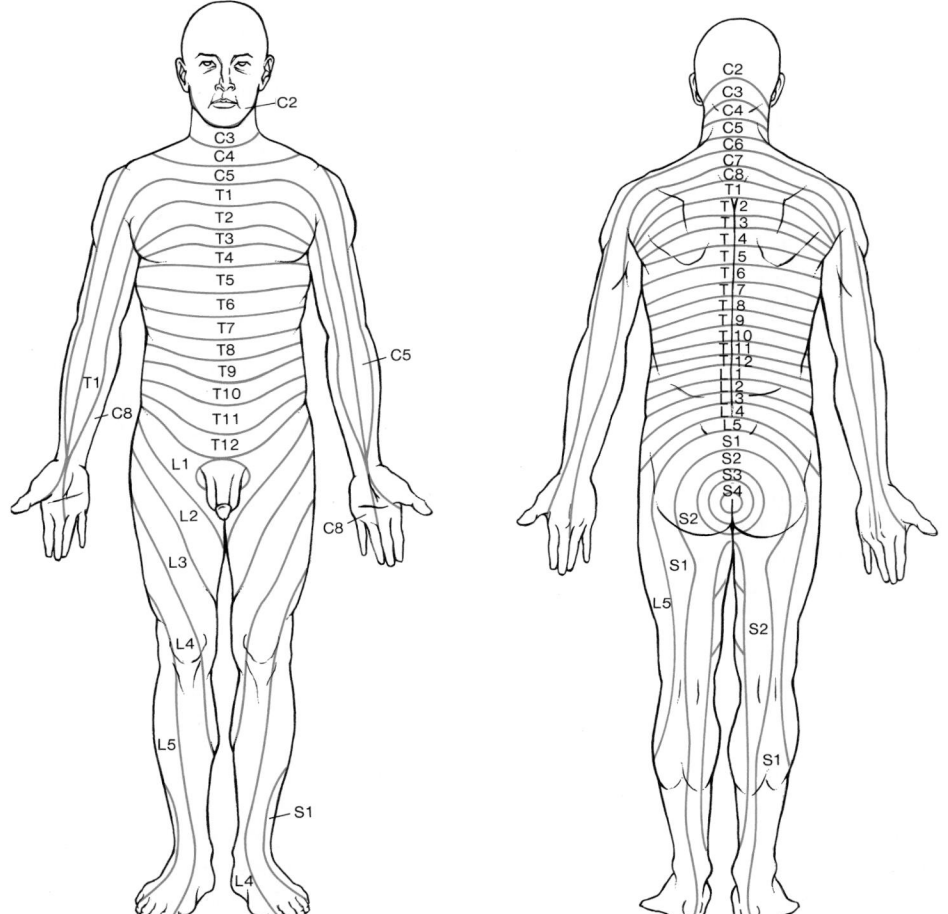

FIGURE 24-20 Dermatomes are sensory fibers from a single spinal nerve that serve a particular skin surface. They are used to evaluate sensory function for high-risk individuals (e.g., after epidural analgesia, spinal anesthesia, spinal cord injury).

the toes or fingers and to report the nurse's touch. No pares-thesias should be present.

Deep Tendon Reflexes. Testing of deep tendon reflexes may be indicated in high-risk clients in specialized practice settings. Use a reflex hammer to tap various tendons in the body to see whether the appropriate reflex arc through the spinal cord is elicited. Normally, a brisk contraction of the muscle occurs. Reflect response can be graded, 0 indicating no reflex activity; +1, minimal activity; +2, normal response; +3, more activity than normal; and +4, hyperactive response. Common reflexes that may be tested include the biceps, the triceps, the patellar, and the Achilles. Table 24-8 illustrates these reflexes and explains the procedure for testing them.

Three significant variations from the normal reflex pattern may be found. First, reflexes on the same side of the body may be different. Second, cortical damage may affect reflexes on one side of the body and not the other. Finally, there can be a difference in the reflex pattern above and below the waist if spinal cord compression has occurred. As a person ages, reflex response may diminish. Bring any abnormal reflex patterns to the physician's attention.

CONCLUDING THE ASSESSMENT

After covering the planned interview questions, ask the client, "Is there anything you would like to discuss that I have not yet mentioned?" This question invites the client to add information that you may have overlooked or did not anticipate. Additionally, you may learn important information if you ask the client for any further information that he or she would like to offer. Before formal closure, you may wish to take a moment to review the assessment to avoid missing or forgetting any information. Doing so can prevent the need to return to collect forgotten information.

In concluding the assessment, summarize your findings and concerns with the client. Sharing this information validates your impressions and clarifies any misunderstandings with the client. The client may want to add to or correct these conclusions. Validate what is the client's most important problem at this time. Explain, particularly to the hospitalized client, that assessment of his or her condition and needs is ongoing. Encourage the client to volunteer additional or new information as changes occur. Document assessment findings in the client's chart in a legible, concise fashion according to agency protocol.

LIFESPAN CONSIDERATIONS

Developmental stage and other age-related factors are important in planning, focusing, and performing a functional health assessment. Nurses should be knowledgeable about common problems of each age group, so that they can include appropriate screening measures that permit early detection of potential or actual problems. Awareness of the client's cognitive development is essential so that questions can be phrased ap-

propriately. Understanding the client's emotional development helps make the examination less traumatic and anxiety provoking. The accompanying Therapeutic Dialogue gives examples of nursing care during assessment and planning.

Newborn and Infant

Nursing assessment is made shortly after birth and at 24 hours of age. If parents are present during the assessment, explain what the examination includes and why it is being performed. Whenever possible, reassure parents about findings that are normal. Permitting parents to see their newborn and participate can help parent bonding and allay fears.

During the first year of life, nurses frequently assess infants during well-baby examinations. These examinations provide an opportunity to educate family caregivers on a variety of infant care topics, reassure them about the wide range of normal growth and development, and allow time for discussion of any concerns they may have about their child.

Keeping the newborn or infant properly covered during the physical examination is important to prevent a drop in body temperature. During the first year of life, head and chest circumference are measured, the infant is weighed, and reflexes are tested. Be sure to finish inspection and auscultation before doing any invasive procedure. Such techniques can frighten the infant or cause pain, which may cause the infant to cry. Encourage the parent or other caregiver to hold the infant during the examination to decrease fear and help the child feel more secure.

🛑 SAFETY ALERT
Never leave an infant on an examining table without being properly guarded. Infants can move quickly and fall. The infant must be properly restrained when you are looking into his or her ears, eyes, nose, or throat, so that quick movements do not result in injury.

Toddler and Preschooler

The young child is often afraid to be examined and may associate physical examination with the discomfort of invasive procedures or getting injections. Encouraging the parent or other caregiver to assist by holding and comforting the child during the examination can be helpful. Explain in simple terms what you plan to do. Demonstrating how equipment works can help alleviate some anxiety in toddlers and preschoolers (Fig. 24-21). Allowing the child to touch the stethoscope or see the shining light of the otoscope can help prepare the child for examination procedures. For some children, it may be helpful to use a puppet or allow the child to role play examining a doll or stuffed animal. Be honest with children. If the child is going to experience pain, it is best to say, "This will hurt for a while, but I'll try and make it quick." Plan uncomfortable procedures toward the end of the examination. Then perform them immediately after the explanation so that anxiety does not escalate.

TABLE 24-8

	Assessment of Deep Tendon Reflexes		
Reflex	**Procedure**		**Normal Response**
Biceps	Flex patient's arm at the elbow with his or her forearm resting on the thigh, palm up. Place your thumb on the base of the biceps tendon in the antecubital fossa. Strike your thumb with the reflex hammer.		Flexion of forearm at the elbow
Triceps	Hold patient's arm across his or her chest, flexing the elbow at a 90-degree angle. Support wrist as patient allows forearm to become limp. Strike the tendon just above the olecranon process.		Extension at the elbow
Patellar	Patient sits upright with legs hanging loosely over side of bed. If patient remains supine, support back of knee while leg is flexed at a 45-degree angle. Strike patellar tendon just below patella.		Extension of lower leg at the knee
Achilles	Patient's knee should be slightly flexed while foot is dorsiflexed. Strike Achilles tendon 1 inch above heel.		Plantar flexion

THERAPEUTIC DIALOGUE
Health Assessment

Scenes for Thought
The nurse practitioner in the pediatrics clinic of a health maintenance organization visits Georgie Stevens, who is 5 years old. Georgie's mother brought him to the clinic because he has a fever of 2 days' duration. He says he is feeling "bad."

Less Effective

Nurse: Hi, Ms. Stevens. How's Georgie doing? I see he's had a fever lately. *(Looking at the chart.)*

Mother: Yes, and coughing all night and sniffles and wheezing. *(She looks weary.)*

Nurse: Let's see what we can find out here. *(Examines Georgie while talking to his mother. Keeps all equipment out of his reach. Doesn't explain what she's doing.)*

Mother: Is it pneumonia? *(Looks worried. Georgie looks worried, too, when he sees his mother's face.)*

Nurse: No, it's just a bad cold. I'll recommend some medications you can buy at the pharmacy. And then give him lots of fluids and get him to wash his hands before he eats and after going to the bathroom so the rest of the family doesn't catch it, too. Okay, Georgie?

Georgie: *(He stopped paying attention when he heard it wasn't pneumonia. He's playing with the paper on the examining table, making little decorative rips in it. He looks up guiltily.)* Uh-huh. Can we go home now, Mommy?

Nurse: Bye, Ms. Stevens. See you next time, Georgie.

More Effective

Nurse: Hi, Georgie, remember me from last time?

Georgie: Yeah, you're Theresa. Can I play with the hearing tube again?

Georgie: Sure you can. You can warm it up before I use it to listen to your breathing. I'm going to talk to your mom now.

Georgie: Okay. *(Plays with stethoscope contentedly.)*

Nurse: How long has he had this fever?

Mother: Two days. And sniffles and coughing all night long and wheezing. I'm worried it might be pneumonia. *(She looks tired.)*

Nurse: I can see it's been a long 2 days. I'm going to examine him and then see what I can recommend so he and you can get some rest. Georgie, here's what my plan is. *(Tells child how she'll proceed with the examination, explaining each step. Georgie is cooperative and "assists" Theresa by holding the tongue depressor, warming the stethoscope, and so forth.)*

Nurse: Okay, Georgie, you've been a great help to me today. You have a cold, my friend, and here's what you need to do. *(Proceeds to tell Georgie and his mother about the importance of fluid intake, getting rest, using cough medicine appropriately, and the like. Includes Georgie in decisions about what kind of fluids he likes and the flavor of the cough syrup they should buy, as well as agreeing to wash his hands before he eats or drinks anything and after going to the bathroom.)*

Georgie: I'll do everything you say, Theresa, because I want to get better and go back to school.

Nurse: Georgie, you're a smart person and I know you'll get better soon. Call me if you have any questions, Ms. Stevens.

Critical Thinking Challenge
- List the subjective data each nurse had at her disposal.
- Based on her behavior toward him, detect what Theresa knew about Georgie that the first nurse did not know.
- Explain the benefits of including Georgie in decisions.
- Judge whether Theresa could treat all her 5-year-old clients this way, and give your reasons.

School-Age Child and Adolescent

As the child ages, nurses can direct more assessment questions specifically to the child. Use vocabulary the child can understand when asking questions or explaining procedures. Encourage the child to ask questions. Whenever possible, give the child simple choices. The child can be distracted during the examination through conversation or playing simple games. Some children are ticklish, especially when the abdomen is examined. Children at this age can be modest, so proper draping and measures to ensure privacy are important.

Adolescence is a period of rapid physical and emotional development. During this time, the youth is often examined alone, unaccompanied by a parent. Sensitive questioning and honest answers to any questions the teen asks help develop good rapport. Because sexual maturation occurs during this period, the examination includes assessment of the sexual organs and appropriate health teaching. Be aware of the sensitivity of adolescents about the body during this time. Discuss any concerns the adolescent has about the maturation process.

Adult and Older Adult

By the time the person has reached adulthood, multiple exposures to physical examinations and assessments have occurred. Some adults still are apprehensive and experience invasion of privacy during assessment procedures. It is important to

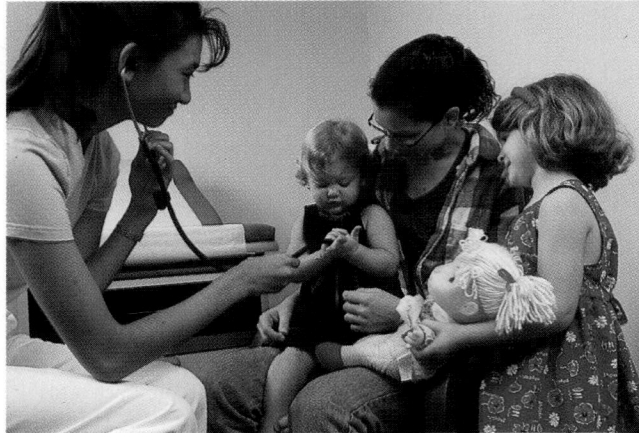

FIGURE 24-21   Physical assessment of the toddler. Allowing the mother to hold her daughter during the examination and permitting the toddler to touch equipment help to reduce the young child's fear of physical examination.

prepare the client for all procedures and to provide for privacy. Include health teaching regarding desirable screening measures, such as breast self-examination, testicular self-examination, and routine gynecologic examinations, in the health examination for the adult.

During later years of adulthood, a person may have chronic health problems that necessitate adaptation of the physical assessment. Arthritic joints or decreased mobility may make getting onto an examination table more difficult. Holding various positions required for examination, especially for long periods, may be tiring. Lengthy examinations may be fatiguing and should be planned for when the client is well rested, if possible. Hearing loss may necessitate speaking more loudly and clearly to facilitate communication. Elderly persons can easily become chilled, so proper draping in a warm examination room is important for client comfort.

Key Concepts

- A health assessment consists of the collection of subjective and objective data about the client's health and health-related problems or concerns.
- The nurse uses interviewing techniques to obtain subjective (client perception) data concerning each functional health pattern.
- The nurse collects objective data through the techniques of inspection, palpation, percussion, and auscultation during the physical examination.
- The focus of a health assessment by the nurse is to determine normal and abnormal aspects, the client's degree of satisfaction, the client's adaptation to dysfunction, and the effect of function on performing ADLs.
- Adequate psychological and physical preparation of the client is important for effective assessment.
- Assessment of health perception and health management should focus on the client's perception of health status, preventive health practices, compliance with medical treatment, and safety.
- Assessment of nutrition and metabolism should focus on food and fluid intake in relation to metabolic demands, skin integrity, and wound healing.

- Assessment of sleep and rest involves eliciting the client's perception of sleep, rest, and relaxation.
- Assessment of self-perception and self-concept focuses on the client's perception of self, such as body image and sense of worth.
- Assessment of roles and relationships describes the quality of a person's family, work, and social roles.
- Assessment of coping and stress tolerance describes current stressors that the client is experiencing, past coping methods, and the effectiveness of current coping methods.
- Assessment of values and beliefs includes the significance of religious affiliation and religious practices, resources available to meet the spiritual health needs of the client, and the relation between spiritual beliefs and the current state of health.
- Assessment of sexuality and reproduction describes reproductive function, sexual role, and the impact of current health status on sexual role function.
- Assessment of the head and neck should focus on cognitive functions such as memory, language, reasoning, problem solving, pain level, and sensory-perceptual capabilities such as vision, hearing, and pain.
- The skin, hair, and nails are assessed throughout the examination as a reflection of processes that occur throughout the body, such as nutrition and oxygenation.
- Respiratory and cardiac function are evaluated through inspection, palpation, percussion, and auscultation using normal landmarks of the thorax and pericardium.
- Assessment of the abdomen should focus on normal excretory function (bowel and bladder) and specific management to assist normal function.
- The breasts and genitalia are examined with an emphasis on health promotion and self-examination.
- The extremities are evaluated for mobility, circulation, sensation, and strength according to ability to move purposefully in the environment.
- Lifespan considerations are important in individualizing assessment techniques to obtain important information from the client.

References

Arnold, E., & Boggs, K. U. (1999). *Interpersonal relationships: Professional communication skills for nurses* (3rd ed.). Philadelphia: W. B. Saunders.

Bardsley, A. (1999/2000). Assessment of incontinence. *Elderly Care, 11*(9), 36–39.

Bohlander, J. R. (1995). Differentiation of self: An examination of the concept. *Issues in Mental Health Nursing, 16*(2), 165–184.

Brackley, M. H. (1997). Mental health assessment/mental status examination. *Nurse Practitioner Forum, 8*(3), 105–113.

Brush, B. L., & Daly, P. R. (2000). Assessing spirituality in primary care practice: Is there time? *Clinical Excellence for Nurse Practitioners, 4*(2), 67–71.

Carpenito, L. J. (2002). *Nursing diagnosis: Application to clinical practice* (9th ed.). Philadelphia: Lippincott.

Engebretson, J. (1996). Considerations in diagnosing in the spiritual domain. *Nursing Diagnosis, 7*(3), 100–107.

Evans-Stoner, N. (1997). Nutritional assessment: A practical approach. *Nursing Clinics of North America, 32*(4), 637–650.

Field, D. (1997). Cardiovascular assessment. *Nursing Times, 93*(35), 45–47.

Fritz, D. J. (1997). Fine tune your physical assessment of the lungs and respiratory system. *Home Care Provider, 2*(6), 299–302.

Girard, N. (1997). Assessment: Part II. *Nurse Practitioner Forum, 8*(4), 131–132.

Gordon, M. (1994). *Nursing diagnosis: Process and application* (3rd ed.). St. Louis: Mosby.

Halfmann, P. L., Keller, C., & Allison, M. (1997). Pragmatic assessment of physical activity. *Nurse Practitioner Forum, 8*(4), 160–165.

Hammond, K. (1997). Physical assessment: A nutritional perspective. *Nursing Clinics of North America, 32*(4), 779–790.

Hampton, S. (1997). Wound assessment. *Professional Nurse, 12,* (12 Suppl), S5–S7.

Jarvis, C. (2000). *Physical examination and health assessment* (3rd ed). Philadelphia: W. B. Saunders.

Kirton, C. A. (1997). Assessing bowel sounds. *Nursing 1997, 27*(3), 64.

Lawler, K. (1997). Pain assessment. *Professional Nurse, 13,* (1 Suppl), S5–S8.

Lane, A. J. (1999). Evaluation of the fall prevention program in an acute care setting. *Orthopaedic Nursing,* Nov/Dec, 37–43.

LeMone, P., & Jones, D. (1997). Nursing assessment of altered sexuality: A review of salient factors and objective measures. *Nursing Diagnosis, 8*(3), 120–128.

McLaren, S., & Green, S. (1998). Nutritional screening and assessment. *Professional Nurse, 13,* (6 Suppl), S9–S15.

Ondus, K. A., Hujer, J. E., Mann, A. E., & Mion, L. C. (1999). Substance abuse and the hospitalized elderly. *Orthopaedic Nursing,* July/Aug.

Richardson, S. J. (1997). A comparison of tools for the assessment of sleep pattern disturbance in critically ill adults. *Dimensions in Critical Care Nursing, 16*(5), 226–239, 240–242.

Stewart, M. J. (1997). Insights from a nursing research program on social support. *Canadian Journal of Nursing Research, 29*(3), 93–110.

Thomas, S. (1997). Assessment and management of wound exudate. *Journal of Wound Care, 6*(7), 327–330.

Vowden, P. (1998). The investigation and assessment of venous disease. *Journal of Wound Care, 7*(3), 143–147.

Weber, J., & Kelley, J. (1998). *Health assessment in nursing.* Philadelphia: Lippincott-Raven.

Wright, J. A. (1997). Seven abdominal assessment signs every emergency nurse should know. *Journal of Emergency Nursing, 23*(5), 446–450.

BIBLIOGRAPHY

Bates, B., Bickley, L. S., & Hoekelman, R. A. (1998). *A guide to physical examination and history taking* (7th ed.). Philadelphia: J. B. Lippincott.

Boughton, K., et al. (1998). Impact of research of pediatric pain assessment and outcomes. *Pediatric Nursing, 24*(10), 31–35, 62.

Colley, W. (1998). Continence assessment. *Nursing Times, 94,* (6 Suppl), 1–2.

Faria, S. H., & Glidden, C. (1997). Assessment of the child: What's different? *Home Care Provider, 2*(6), 282–285.

Flanagan, M. (1997). A practical framework for wound assessment. 1: Physiology. *British Nursing Journal, 5*(22), 1391–1397.

Herrick, C. A., Pearcey, L. G., & Ross, C. (1997). Stigma and ageism: Compounding influences in making an accurate mental health assessment. *Nursing Forum, 32*(3), 21–26.

Heye, M. L. (1997). Pain assessment in elders: Practical tips. *Nurse Practitioner Forum, 8*(4), 133–139.

Kresevic, D. M., & Mezey, M. (1997). Assessment of function: Critically important to acute care of elders. The NICHE Faculty. *Geriatric Nursing, 18*(5), 216–221, 221–222.

Langan, J. C. (1998). Abdominal assessment in the home: From A to Z. *Home Healthcare Nurse, 16*(1), 50–58.

Larsen, P. D., Hazen, S. E., & Martin, J. L. (1997). Assessment and management of sensory loss in elderly patients. *American Operating Room Nursing Journal, 65*(2), 432–437.

Longworth, J. C. (1997). Sexual assessment and counseling in primary care. *Nurse Practitioner Forum, 8*(4), 166–171.

Mannina, J. (1997). Finding an effective hearing testing protocol to identify hearing loss and middle ear disease in school-aged children. *Journal of School Nurses, 13*(5), 23–28.

McCarthy, V. (1997). The first pelvic examination. *Journal of Pediatric Health Care, 11*(5), 247–249.

McLeod, R. P. (1996). Your next patient does not speak English: Translation and interpretation in today's busy office. *Advanced Practice in Nursing Quarterly, 2*(2), 10–14.

Narayan, M. C. (1997). Cultural assessment in home healthcare. *Home Healthcare Nurse, 15*(10), 663–672.

O'Hanlon-Nichols, T. (1998). Basic assessment series: Gastrointestinal system. *American Journal of Nursing, 98*(4), 48–53.

O'Hanlon-Nichols, T. (1998). Basic assessment series: The adult pulmonary system. *American Journal of Nursing, 98*(2), 39–45.

O'Hanlon-Nichols, T. (1997). Basic assessment series: The adult cardiovascular system. *American Journal of Nursing, 97*(12), 34–40.

Owen, A. (1998). Respiratory assessment revisited. *Nursing 98, 28*(4), 48–49.

Pasero, C. L., & McCaffery, M. (1997). Overcoming obstacles to pain assessment in elders. *American Journal of Nursing, 97*(9), 20.

Peters, S. (1997). Constipation: Assessment and treatment in elderly patients. *Advanced Nurse Practitioner, 5*(8), 45–46, 49–50.

Pritchard, P. E., & Dewing, J. (1999). Screening for dementia and depression in older people. *Nursing Standard, 14*(5), 46–53.

Rhodes, V. A. (1997). Criteria for assessment of nausea, vomiting, and retching. *Oncology Nursing Forum, 24,* (7 Suppl), 9–13.

Rogers, A. E. (1997). Nursing management of sleep disorder: Part I—Assessment. *ANNA Journal, 24*(6), 666, 669–671.

Shaw, L. (1997). Protocol for detection and follow-up of hearing loss. *Clinical Nurse Specialist, 11*(6), 240–247.

Thomas, A. J. (1998). Nutrition in practice: 10. Nutrition and the elderly. *Nursing Times, 94,*(8 Suppl), 1–6.

Walker, D. J. (1999). Venous stasis wounds. *Orthopaedic Nursing,* Sept/Oct, 65–74.

Chapter

25 Vital Sign Assessment

Key Terms

apnea
auscultatory gap
blood pressure
bradycardia
bradypnea
core temperature
diastolic blood pressure
dyspnea
hypertension
hypotension

korotkoff sounds
orthostatic hypotension
paradoxical blood pressure
pulse deficit
pulse pressure
stroke volume
systolic blood pressure
tachycardia
tachypnea
tidal volume

Learning Objectives

Upon completion of this chapter, the student will be able to do the following:
1. Describe the procedures used to assess the vital signs: temperature, pulse, respirations, and blood pressure.
2. Describe factors that can influence each vital sign.
3. Identify equipment routinely used to assess vital signs.
4. Identify rationales for using different routes for assessing temperature.
5. Identify the location of commonly assessed pulse sites.
6. Describe how to assess orthostatic hypotension.
7. Recognize normal vital sign values among various age groups.

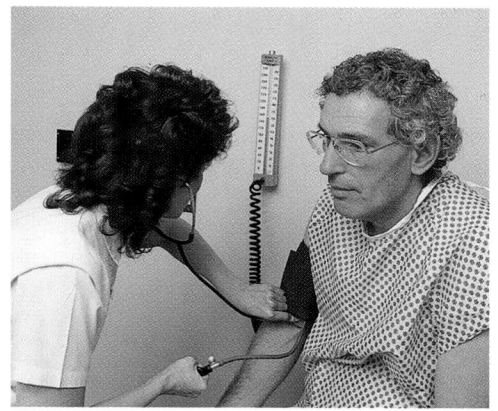

Critical Thinking Challenge

A middle-aged couple is shopping in a mall, where a health fair is set up. You are a nurse participating at a booth for checking blood pressures. After much coaxing, the woman persuades her husband to have his blood pressure taken. You obtain a reading of 168/94. The wife reacts strongly, saying, "I told you that your lack of exercise and overeating would catch up with you one day. How am I going to manage being a widow at such an early age?" The husband responds by saying, "Don't worry about me. I'm just as healthy as ever, and I plan to live until I am 99 years old. I'm sure there is something wrong with that machine." Both of them turn to you. The wife says, "Tell him it's not the machine and that he isn't taking care of himself!"

Once you have completed this chapter and have incorporated vital signs into your knowledge base, review the above scenario and reflect on the following areas of Critical Thinking:

1. Identify possible interpretations of an isolated blood pressure reading of 168/94. List factors that may have affected the reading's accuracy.
2. Analyze the man's reaction to this situation. Indicate health teaching about blood pressure that may be appropriate at this time.
3. Outline possible ways to deal therapeutically with the wife's anxiety, describing possible verbal and nonverbal interactions.

Vital signs—body temperature (T), pulse (P), respirations (R), and blood pressure (BP)—indicate the function of some of the body's homeostatic mechanisms. The blood pressure reading of the man in the opening scenario is more than a number; it can reflect many things about his health status. One important component of assessment involves measuring and interpreting the vital signs. Client teaching concerning the vital signs is an important aspect of health promotion.

Typical or normal values for vital signs have been established for clients of various age groups (Table 25-1). During initial measurement of a client's vital signs, the values are compared with these normal ranges to determine any variation that might indicate illness. When several sets of vital signs have been obtained, this information forms a baseline for comparison of subsequent measurements. Isolated vital sign values are less helpful; nurses should evaluate a series of values and establish trends for the client. Vital sign trends that deviate from normal are much more significant than isolated abnormal values.

The tasks involved in measuring vital signs are simple and easy to learn, but interpreting the measurements and incorporating them into ongoing care and assessment require knowledge, problem-solving skills, critical thinking, and experience. Although vital signs are usually part of routine care, they provide valuable information and should not be taken lightly.

The frequency with which to assess vital signs should be individualized for each client. Healthy people may have vital signs checked only during annual physicals. Very ill, hospitalized clients may have their vital signs monitored more frequently than hospitalized clients who are less ill. Clients seen in ambulatory settings, wellness clinics, or psychiatric institutions may require infrequent vital sign checks. Most inpatient settings have a policy regarding the frequency of vital sign assessment. In addition, physicians order vital signs to be checked at specific intervals based on the client's condition. The nurse caring for the client may decide to monitor vital signs more frequently if the client's condition changes.

BODY TEMPERATURE

Humans are warm-blooded creatures, which means they can maintain internal body temperature independent of the outside environment. The body's tissues and cells are best able to function within a relatively narrow temperature range. The body's surface or skin temperature can vary widely with environmental conditions and physical activity. Despite these fluctuations, the temperature inside the body, the **core temperature,** remains relatively constant, unless the client develops a febrile illness. The body's organs require this constant internal temperature for optimal functioning.

Although normal adult temperature ranges from 36.5° to 37.5°C (97.6° to 99.6°F) when taken orally (Braun, Preston, & Smith, 1998), body temperature can fluctuate with exercise, changes in hormone levels, changes in metabolic rate, and extremes of external temperature. Rectal temperatures are usually 1 degree higher than oral temperatures and axillary temperatures are usually 1 degree lower than oral temperatures. Tympanic temperatures fall about midway between normal oral and rectal temperature measurements (Lee, McKenzie, & Cathcart, 1999). Refer to Table 25-2, which illustrates normal adult temperatures from different body sites.

Regulation of Body Temperature

Regulation of body temperature requires the coordination of many body systems. For the core temperature to remain normal, heat production must equal heat loss. The hypothalamus, located in the pituitary gland in the brain, is the body's built-in thermostat. It can sense small changes in body temperature and stimulates the necessary responses in the nervous system, circulatory system, skin, and sweat glands to maintain homeostasis.

Heat Production
The body continually produces heat as a byproduct of chemical reactions that occur in body cells. This collective process is known as metabolism. The process of thermoregulation

TABLE 25-1

Normal Vital Sign Ranges Across the Lifespan					
	Pulse	**Respirations**	**Temperature (°F)**	**Blood Pressure (mm Hg)**	
				Systolic	*Diastolic*
Newborn (>96 h)	70–190	30–60	96–99.5	60–90	20–60
Infant (>1 mo)	80–160	30–60	99.4–99.7	74–100	50–70
Toddler	80–130	24–40	99–99.7	80–112	50–80
Preschooler	80–120	22–34	98.6–99	82–110	50–78
School-age	75–110	18–30	98–98.6	84–120	54–80
Adolescent	60–90	12–20	97–99	94–140	62–88
Adult	60–100	12–20	97–99	90–140	60–90
Older adult (>70 yr)	60–100	12–20	95–99	90–140	60–90

TABLE 25-2

Normal Adult Temperature Ranges From Different Body Sites			
Oral	Axillary	Rectal	Tympanic
97.6°–99.6°F	96.6°–98.6°F	98.6°–100.6°F	98.2°–100.2°F
36.5°–37.5°C	35.8°–37.0°C	37.0°–38.1°C	36.8°–37.9°C

From Braun, S., Preston, P., & Smith, R. (1998). Getting a better read on thermometry. *RN, 61*(3), 60.

maintains a fairly constant core temperature regardless of where the heat is being produced. The rate of heat production is determined by the person's metabolic rate. The basal metabolic rate (BMR) is the amount of energy the body uses during absolute rest in an awake state. Physical exercise, increased production of thyroid hormones, and stimulation of the sympathetic nervous system can increase heat production.

Heat Loss

Just as the body is continually producing heat, it is also continuously losing heat. Heat is lost through four processes: radiation, conduction, convection, and evaporation.

Exposure to a cold environment increases radiant heat loss. All objects whose temperatures are not at absolute zero constantly lose heat through infrared heat rays. Covering the body with closely woven, dark fabric can reduce radiant heat loss.

Conduction is the transfer of heat from one object to another. The body does lose a considerable amount of heat to the air through conduction. It can also lose heat to water during swimming or during tepid baths. Convection is the loss of heat through air currents such as from a breeze or a fan. Evaporation causes heat loss as water is transformed to a gas. Examples of evaporation include diaphoresis (sweating) during strenuous exercise or when one is febrile.

Factors Affecting Body Temperature

Understanding the factors that can affect body temperature helps nurses accurately assess the significance of body temperature variations.

Age

Newborns have unstable body temperatures because their thermoregulatory mechanisms are immature. It is not uncommon for elderly persons to have body temperatures less than 36.4°C (97.6°F) because normal temperature drops as a person ages (Copstead & Banasik, 2000). When evaluating low-grade temperatures in the elderly or identifying those at risk for hypothermia, remember that older age is associated with lower body temperatures.

Environment

Ordinarily, changes in environmental temperatures do not affect core temperature, but exposure to extremely hot or cold temperatures can alter body temperature. The degree of change relates to the temperature, humidity, and length of exposure. The body's thermoregulatory mechanisms are also influential (e.g., infants and older adults often have diminished control mechanisms). If any person's core temperature drops to 25°C (77°F), death may occur.

Time of Day

Body temperature normally fluctuates throughout the day. Temperature is usually lowest around 3 AM and highest from 5 to 7 PM (Beaudry, VandenBosch, & Anderson, 1996). A person's body temperature can vary by as much as 2°C (1.8°F) from early morning to late afternoon. Theorists attribute this variation to changes in muscle activity and digestive processes, which are usually lowest in the early morning during sleep. Even greater variation in body temperature at various times of the day is found in infants and children.

Although researchers have established no absolute relationship between circadian rhythm and body temperature, 95% of clients have their maximum temperature elevation around 6 PM. A study by Beaudry et al. (1996) suggests once-a-day fever screening of afebrile clients at 6 PM. Reduced routine screening would decrease cost both in terms of staff time and supplies and limit sleep disruption, because clients would not be woken during the night.

Exercise

Body temperature increases with exercise because exercise increases heat production as the body breaks down carbohydrates and fats to provide energy. Strenuous exercise, such as running a marathon, can temporarily raise the temperature as high as 40°C (104°F).

Stress

Emotional or physical stress can elevate body temperature. When stress stimulates the sympathetic nervous system, circulating levels of epinephrine and norepinephrine increase. As a result, the metabolic rate increases, which, in turn, increases heat production. Stressed or anxious clients may have an elevated temperature without underlying pathology.

Hormones

Women usually have greater variations in their temperature than do men. Progesterone, a female hormone secreted at ovulation, increases body temperature 0.3° to 0.6°C (0.5° to 1°F) above baseline. By measuring their temperature daily, women can determine when they ovulate, which is the basis for the rhythm method of birth control. (See Chapter 50.) After menopause, mean temperature norms are the same for men and women (McGann, Marion, Camp, & Spangler, 1993). Thyroxine, epinephrine, and norepinephrine also elevate body temperature by increasing heat production.

Factors Affecting Body Temperature Measurement

Nurses must also consider external factors that can lead to false temperature readings. Small, insignificant alterations in oral temperature readings can occur after smoking or when oxygen is administered by way of mask or cannula. Drinking hot or cold liquids may cause slight variations in oral temperature readings; the most marked variation is found after drinking ice water (20.2° to 21.6°F). Wait 15 minutes after clients have ingested ice water to take their oral temperatures. Many of these factors are less significant now than in the past, because many temperatures are measured tympanically.

Assessing Body Temperature

Temperature measurement establishes a baseline for comparisons as a disease progresses or therapies are instituted. The reliability of a temperature value depends on choosing the correct equipment, selecting the most appropriate site, and using the correct procedure. The nurse must ensure correct placement of the thermometer and must leave it in place for the appropriate length of time.

Sites

Nurses should use their judgment when selecting the route by which to measure temperature. The four sites most commonly used are the mouth, ear, rectum, and axilla. In most clinical situations, any of these sites is satisfactory if the nurse uses proper technique and considers normal variations for the different sites. Additional sites are the esophagus and pulmonary artery, both of which are considered core temperatures. Normal temperature varies within a person, among individuals, and among sites. See Table 25-2.

Oral. The most common site for temperature measurement is the mouth. Advantages of the oral route include easy access and client comfort. Because a client's drinking hot or cold liquids could affect the temperature measurement, wait 15 minutes before placing the thermometer in these situations to allow the client's mouth temperature to return to baseline.

Oral temperature assessment, especially with a glass thermometer, may not be prudent or safe for infants, young children, unconscious or irrational clients, or clients with seizure disorders.

Rectal. The rectal route is believed to be the most reliable, because few factors can artificially influence the reading. Rectal temperatures are recommended infrequently now that

OUTCOME-BASED TEACHING PLAN

Sylvia Yantes, a 16-year-old unwed mother, has just given birth to her first child, a baby boy weighing 5 lb, 10 oz. She stayed in the hospital an extra day because her son had one elevated temperature during his first 24 hours of life. Before Sylvia and her son can go home, she needs to be able to monitor his temperature.

OUTCOME: Before discharge, Sylvia (the mother) will be able to demonstrate accurate assessment of axillary temperature.
Strategies
- Assess the mother's experience monitoring temperature and her ability to read a glass mercury thermometer.
- Encourage the mother to wash her hands first, explaining its importance before handling the baby.
- Have the mother shake down thermometer until it is 95°F and then read temperature by slowly rotating thermometer until she obtains an accurate reading.
- Demonstrate placement of the thermometer in the axilla, explaining the importance of leaving it in place for 5 minutes to obtain an accurate reading.
- Stress the importance of holding the thermometer in place and never leaving the infant unattended while taking the temperature.
- Have the mother demonstrate the procedure until she feels comfortable. Give positive feedback.
- Plan on monitoring temperature once every evening unless the baby becomes febrile.

OUTCOME: During the first postpartum week, the mother will keep a record of daily temperature and bring log to first physician's visit.
Strategies
- Provide the mother with log indicating date and times and a place to fill in the temperatures obtained.
- Provide the mother with written appointment card requesting that she bring the temperature log to that baby visit.
- When you review the log at the first baby visit, give the mother positive feedback.
- Stress that the mother report any temperature elevation above 98.6°, which could indicate infection.

tympanic thermometers are available. Take care to avoid placing the thermometer into fecal material, which may falsely elevate the temperature reading. This route is contraindicated in clients with diarrhea, those who have undergone rectal surgery, those with diseases of the rectum, or those with cancer who are neutropenic. For selected clients (e.g., quadriplegics), rectal temperature measurements may cause vagal stimulation, which can result in bradycardia and syncope. Most clients are uncomfortable having their temperature taken rectally, so avoid this route if possible.

SAFETY ALERT
Rectal thermometers are contraindicated in infants, because they may cause trauma to the rectal mucosa.

Ear. Since the development of the tympanic membrane thermometer, the ear has been added as a site where temperature can be easily and safely measured. This site has many advantages. The tympanic membrane receives its blood supply from the same vasculature that supplies the hypothalamus; thus, tympanic temperature readings reflect core body temperature (Lee, McKenzie, & Cathcart, 1999). Cerumen in the ear canal or the presence of otitis media does not significantly alter temperature readings (Jevon & Jevon, 2001). Smoking, drinking, and eating, which slightly alter oral temperature measurement, do not affect tympanic temperature measurement. The ear is readily accessible and permits rapid temperature readings in very young, confused, or unconscious clients. Because the ear canal has fewer pathogens than the oral or rectal cavities, infection control is less of a concern with the tympanic site. To obtain an accurate reading, snugly fit the probe in the client's ear canal and angle it toward the client's jaw line.

Axillary. The axillary route is considered the least accurate and least reliable site because a number of factors can influence the temperature obtained. For example, if the client has recently bathed, temperature may reflect the temperature of water used. Friction used to dry the skin may influence the temperature. The axillary route is recommended for infants and children and is the route of choice in clients who cannot have their temperatures measured by other routes.

Equipment
Glass Mercury Thermometer. The glass thermometer is still used in some homes, but replacement with tympanic or disposable paper thermometers is recommended due to the risks of mercury exposure to individuals or the environment should the thermometer break. This slender glass tube is sealed at one end and has a bulb of mercury at the other end. It should be handled only at the sealed end because touching the mercury bulb could influence the temperature reading. The tube is calibrated in degrees, using the Celsius or Fahrenheit scale. Exposing the bulb to heat causes the mercury to expand and rise to a point on the scale. The mercury stabilizes at this point and does not fall unless the thermometer is shaken vigorously. The temperature is read by holding the thermometer at eye level and noting the mercury's location on the scale. Figure 25-1 shows the correct way to hold a glass mercury thermometer to obtain an accurate reading.

The tip of the oral glass thermometer is slender and allows for maximal exposure to the oral mucosa. The rectal glass thermometer tip is blunt to decrease the risk of trauma to the rectal mucosa. Often the tips are color-coded (blue for oral and red for rectal) to avoid mixups. The oral thermometer also may be used for axillary temperature measurement.

Electronic Thermometers. The electronic thermometer is widely used in healthcare facilities. Many types are on the market but all have similar characteristics. The thermometer consists of a battery-powered display unit and a temperature-sensitive probe connected to the display unit by a thin cord (Fig. 25-2). When used, a disposable plastic sheath covers the probe to prevent the transmission of infection. These thermometers provide readings in less than 60 seconds and are thought to be most accurate if placed in the sublingual pocket (Braun et al., 1998). The thermometer's display results in Celsius or Fahrenheit; some thermometers can display both scales. The electronic thermometer is ideally suited for use with children because the sheath is unbreakable and the time necessary for accurate measurement is relatively short.

Tympanic Membrane Thermometer. The tympanic membrane thermometer is a portable, hand-held device resembling an otoscope that recharges using a battery pack (Fig. 25-3). It

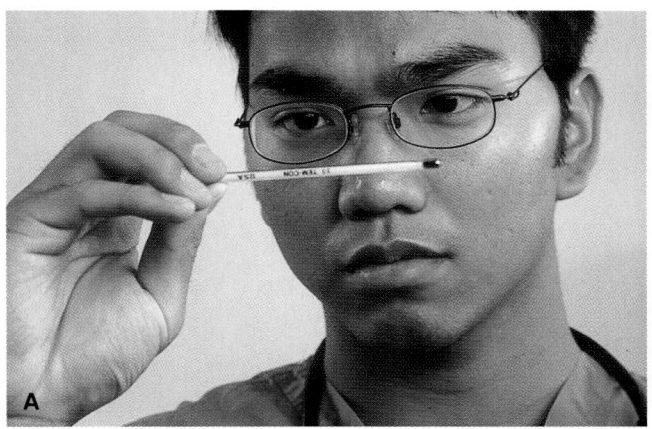
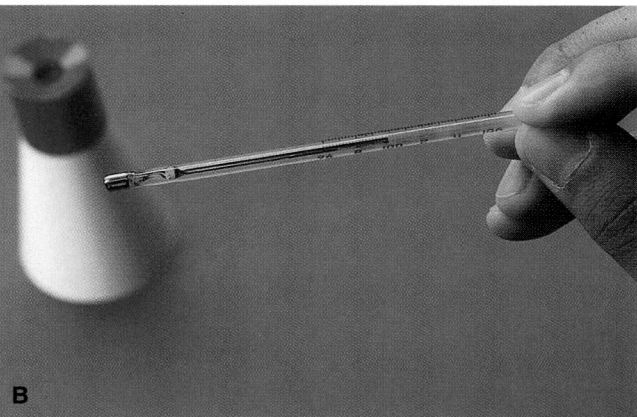

FIGURE 25-1 To read a glass thermometer correctly, hold it at eye level (**A**) and turn it to note the location of mercury on the scale (**B**).

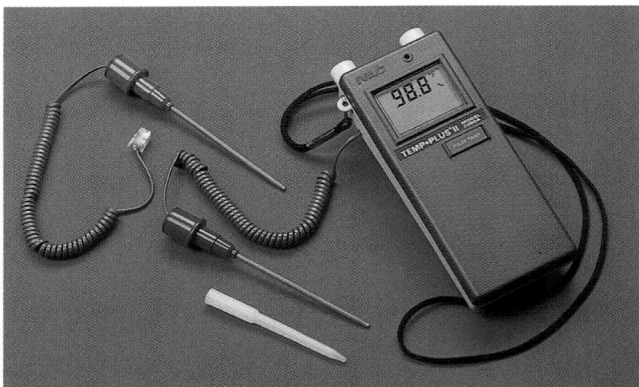

FIGURE 25-2   Electronic thermometer.

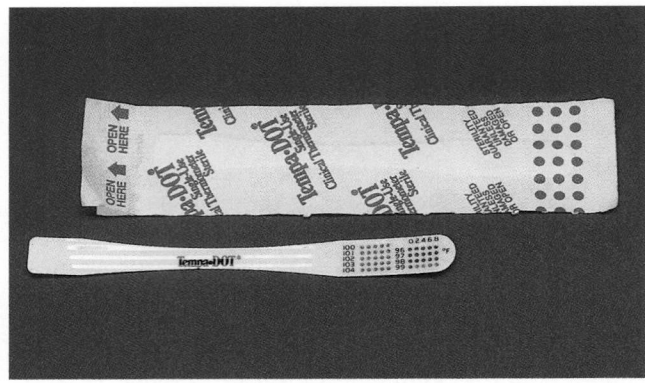

FIGURE 25-4   Disposable paper thermometer. The dots change color to indicate temperature.

records temperature through a sensor probe that is placed in the ear canal to detect infrared radiation from the eardrum. The tympanic membrane thermometer can record temperature in either Fahrenheit or Celsius, with some models providing both readouts. Some studies indicate good correlation between tympanic temperature readings and core body temperature (Baird, White, and Basinger, 1992; Erickson & Meyer, 1994; Kenney & Fortenberry, 1990; Shinozaki et al., 1988), whereas other studies reveal discrepancies (Braun, Preston, & Smith, 1998; Lattavo, Britt, & Dobal, 1995; Winslow, 1997) resulting in both false-positive and false-negative readings. Because discrepancies are usually small, the convenience, safety, and efficiency of tympanic temperature measurement make it useful in monitoring temperature trends and changes.

The tympanic membrane thermometer is especially appropriate for infants over 2 months or very young children who may have difficulty remaining still while temperature is recorded using other methods. Because recordings are obtained in 2 seconds or less, the tympanic membrane thermometer is often preferred in emergency departments or other areas where assessments must be made quickly. Tympanic thermometers should not be used on people who have ear drainage or scarred tympanic membranes (Jevon & Jevon, 2001).

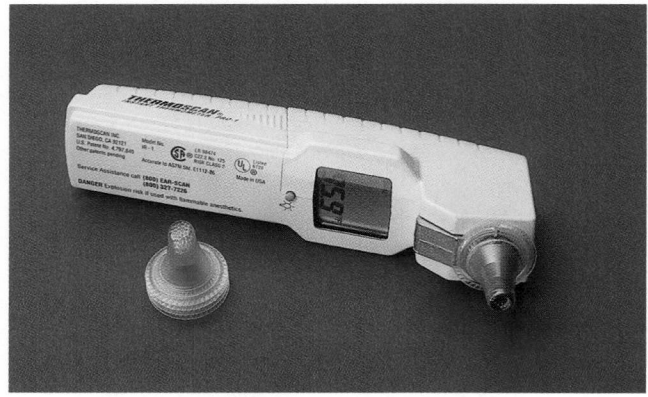

FIGURE 25-3   Tympanic membrane thermometer.

Disposable Paper Thermometers.   Single-use paper thermometers (Fig. 25-4) are thin strips of chemically treated paper with raised dots that change color to reflect the temperature, usually in less than 1 minute. These thermometers are available in Celsius or Fahrenheit scales and are reported to be accurate (Molton, Blacktop & Hall, 2001).

Temperature-Sensitive Strips.   Temperature-sensitive strips can be used to obtain a general indication of body surface temperature. They are usually placed on the forehead or abdomen; the skin under the strip must be dry. After a specified length of time, the strip changes color. On one brand, a green "N" indicates a normal temperature, a brown "N" indicates a transition phase, and a blue-green "F" indicates an elevated temperature. The transition phase reflects the onset of a high temperature in the area where the strip was placed. The strip is removed and discarded after the color change has been noted. This method is particularly useful in the home. Because children younger than 2 years still have immature thermoregulatory systems, any variation from normal should be confirmed using a glass or tympanic thermometer.

Scales

Temperature can be measured on the Celsius or Fahrenheit scale (Fig. 25-5). The scale used varies among agencies. Nurses do not routinely have to convert from one scale to the other; however, if conversion is necessary, they can use simple formulas.

To change Celsius into Fahrenheit, multiply the Celsius reading by 9/5 and add 32 to the result.

$$F = (9/5 \times C°) + 32°$$

For example:

$$F = (9/5 \times 37°) + 32° = (66.6°) + 32° = 98.6°F$$

To change Fahrenheit into Celsius, subtract 32 from the Fahrenheit reading and multiply the result by 5/9.

$$C = (F - 32°) \times 5/9$$

For example:

$$C = (102 - 32°) \times 5/9 = (70) \times 5/9 = 38.8°C$$

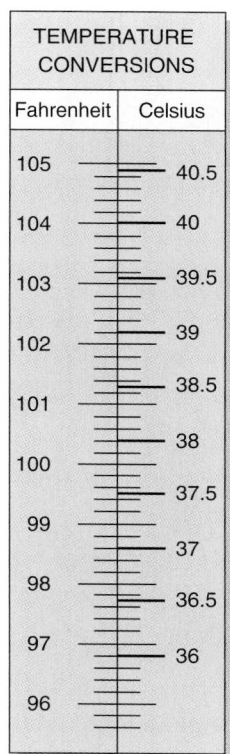

TEMPERATURE CONVERSIONS

Fahrenheit	Celsius
105	40.5
104	40
103	39.5
102	39
	38.5
101	
	38
100	
	37.5
99	
	37
98	
	36.5
97	
	36
96	

FIGURE 25-5 Temperature conversion chart.

Methods

Nurses often delegate temperature taking to unlicensed assistive personnel. Nurses use critical thinking to interpret temperature measurements, document the results, and report abnormal values. Whenever possible, record temperature measurements at the same site so interpretation of fluctuations is easier. See Procedure 25-1 for specific details on how to obtain a temperature measurement using each of the different routes and equipment.

PULSE

Contraction of the ventricles of the heart ejects blood into the arteries. The force of the blood entering the aorta from the left ventricle causes stretching or distention of the elastic aortic wall. As the aorta first expands then contracts, a pulse wave is created that travels along the blood vessels. The pulse wave or pulsation can be felt as a throb or tap where the arteries lie close to the skin surface.

Characteristics

Characteristics of the pulse include rate or frequency, rhythm, and quality. Rate or frequency refers to the number of pulsations per minute. Rhythm refers to the regularity with which pulsation occurs. Quality refers to the strength of the palpated pulsation.

Specialized cells that make up the heart's conduction system establish the rate and rhythm of the pulse. The stimulus for contraction of the heart normally starts as an electrical impulse in the sinoatrial (SA) node of the right atrium. In adults, the SA node initiates the impulse 60 to 100 times per minute. The electrical impulse then spreads quickly through the conduction system to the remainder of the heart so that the heart muscle fibers contract in a synchronous fashion. Irregularities of heart rhythm usually indicate a failure in the conduction system or origination of an impulse in a site other than the SA node.

Several factors determine the quality of the arterial pulse, including the force with which blood is ejected from the ventricles, the amount of blood ejected with each heartbeat (the **stroke volume**), and the patency and compliance or elasticity of the arteries.

Factors Affecting Pulse Rate

Age

The average pulse rate of an infant ranges from 100 to 160 beats per minute. The heart rhythm in infants and children often varies markedly with respiration, increasing during inspiration and decreasing with expiration. The normal range of the pulse in an adult is 60 to 100 beats per minute. Table 25-1 shows the normal pulse ranges for various age groups.

Autonomic Nervous System

Stimulation of the parasympathetic nervous system results in a decrease in the pulse rate. Normally, parasympathetic nervous system input slows pulse rate below 100 beats per minute. Conversely, stimulation of the sympathetic nervous system results in an increased pulse rate. Sympathetic nervous system activation occurs in response to a variety of stimuli including pain, anxiety, exercise, fever, ingestion of caffeinated beverages, and changes in intravascular volume.

Medications

Certain cardiac medications, such as digoxin, decrease heart rate. Medications that decrease intravascular volume, such as diuretics, may cause a reflex increase in pulse rate. Other medications mimic or block the effects of the autonomic nervous system. For example, atropine inhibits impulses to the heart from the parasympathetic nervous system, causing increased pulse rate. Other medications, such as propranolol, block sympathetic nervous system action, resulting in decreased heart rate.

Assessing the Pulse

The pulse is an important part of vital sign measurements. The baseline pulse rate and rhythm are established during the initial nursing assessment and are used for comparison with future measurements.

Sites

The pulse can be assessed in any location where an artery lies close to the skin surface and can be compressed against a firm underlying structure such as muscle or bone. The most commonly assessed pulses are the temporal, carotid, apical,

(*text continues on page 454*)

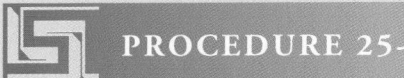

PROCEDURE 25-1

ASSESSING BODY TEMPERATURE

Purpose
1. Obtain baseline temperature data for comparing future measurements.
2. Screen for alterations in temperature.
3. Evaluate temperature response to therapies.

Assessment
- Identify client's baseline temperature.
- Assess for clinical signs and symptoms of temperature alteration.
- Assess for factors that influence body temperature measurement:
- Ingestion of hot or cold foods or liquids in last 15 minutes (oral)
- Smoking within last 15 minutes
- Recent exercise
- Age, hormones, drugs that cause variations in body temperature
- Determine site most appropriate for temperature measurement.

Equipment
Appropriate thermometer
Plastic thermometer sheaths or tissues to wipe thermometer
Water-soluble lubricant and disposable gloves (for rectal temperature)
Pen and vital sign documentation record
Gloves
Assessing Oral Temperature with an Electronic Thermometer

Procedure
1. Wash hands. Identify client and explain the procedure.
   Rationale: Provides for safety and increases client compliance.
2. Remove electronic thermometer from the battery pack, and remove the temperature probe from the unit, noting a digital display of temperature on the screen (usually 34 × C or 94 × F).
   Rationale: The electronic thermometer is stored in a battery pack to ensure that it is always charged and ready for use. Removing the temperature probe prepares the machine to measure and record temperature. The digital display of temperature indicates that it is charged.

3. Securely attach the disposable cover over the temperature probe.
   Rationale: Prevent the transmission of microorganisms.

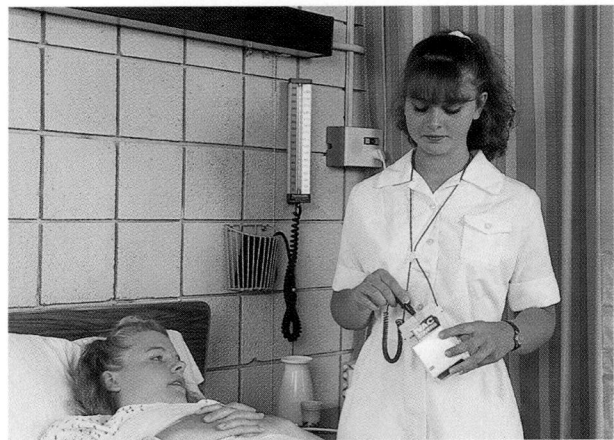

Step 3 Cover temperature probe with disposable cover. (© B. Proud)

4. Hold the probe in the sublingual pocket of the client's mouth.
   Rationale: The sublingual pocket obtains the most accurate temperature. The weight of the probe will displace it from the sublingual pocket if left unsupported.

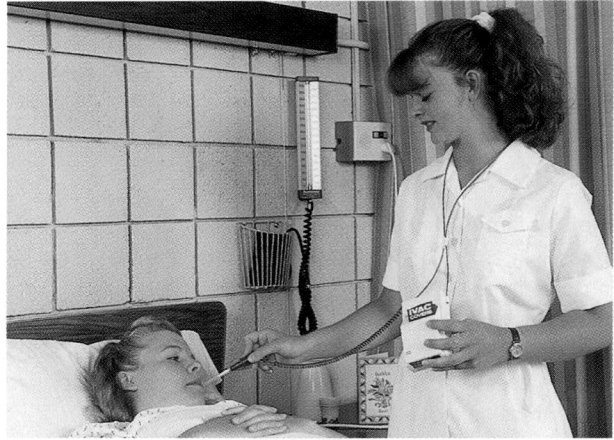

Step 4 Hold probe in sublingual pocket. (© B. Proud)

5. Wait for a beep—usually 10 to 20 seconds—which indicates the estimated temperature. Watch to see if temperature continues to rise. When it stops,

remove the probe from the client's mouth, noting the temperature displayed on the unit.
Rationale: Beep indicates estimated temperature. Usually the final temperature reading is very close to this estimated reading and often this is the temperature recorded if there are time pressures.

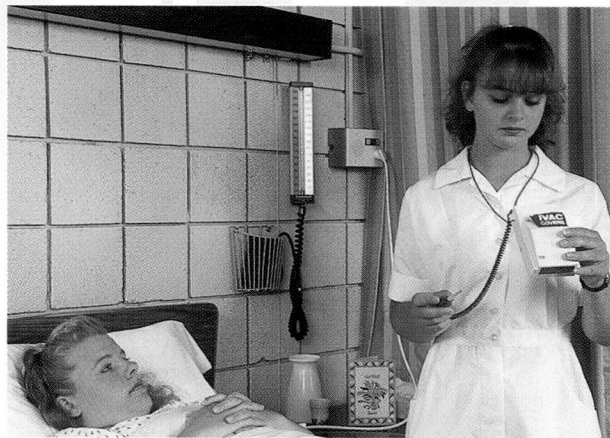

Step 5 After beep, obtain reading. (© B. Proud)

6. Displace the probe cover by pressing the probe release button as you hold the probe over a waste container.
Rationale: The contaminated probe cover can be removed without touching the nurse's hands, thus preventing the transmission of microorganisms.

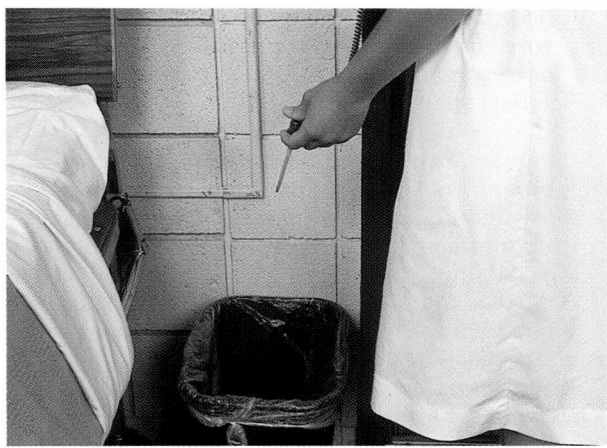

Step 6 Release probe cover into waste receptacle. (© B. Proud)

7. Return the probe to the storage place within the unit and the thermometer to the battery pack.
Rationale: Proper storage prevents damage to the sensitive temperature probe and ensures that the unit will be recharged and ready for use.
8. Record temperature on vital sign documentation record. Discuss findings with client if appropriate.
Rationale: These actions ensure proper documentation and encourage client's understanding of health status.

Assessing Rectal Temperature with an Electronic Thermometer

Procedure

1. Wash hands. Don clean gloves. Identify client and explain procedure.
Rationale: Prevents transmission of microorganisms and increases client compliance.
2. Remove rectal (red) electronic thermometer from battery pack and remove the temperature probe from the unit, noting a digital display of temperature on the screen.
Rationale: Removing the temperature probe prepares the machine to measure and record temperature. Ensure that rectal (red) probe only is used for monitoring rectal temperature to prevent cross contamination of oral probe with rectal bacteria.
3. Securely attach the disposable cover over the temperature probe.
Rationale: Prevent transmission of microorganisms.
4. Close bedroom door or bed curtains. Assist client to Sims' position with upper leg flexed. Expose only anal area.
Rationale: Privacy reduces embarrassment from exposing buttocks. Lateral position exposes anal area for thermometer placement.
5. Apply water-soluble lubricant liberally to thermometer probe tip.
Rationale: Lubricant facilitates insertion of thermometer without irritating or traumatizing the rectum.
6. Separate client's buttocks with one gloved hand.
Rationale: Exposure of anus ensures visualization for accurate placement of probe.
7. Ask client to take a deep, slow breath. Insert thermometer into anus in direction of umbilicus, for an infant ½ inch, for an adult, 1½ inch. Do not force.

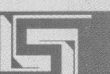

PROCEDURE 25-1 (Continued)

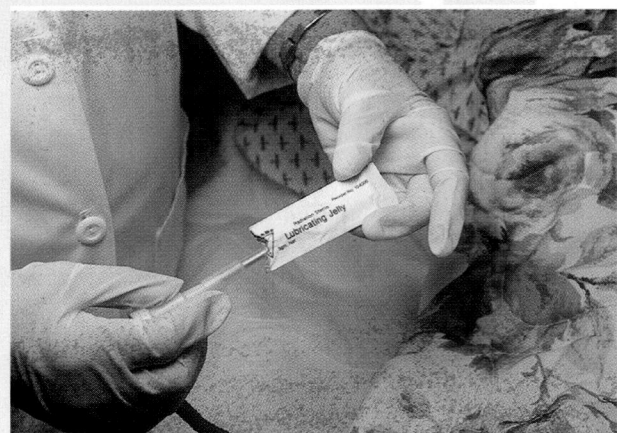

Step 5 Lubricate thermometer probe.

Rationale: Deep, slow breath allows client to relax external sphincter. Insertion depth allows adequate exposure of probe against blood vessels in rectal wall.

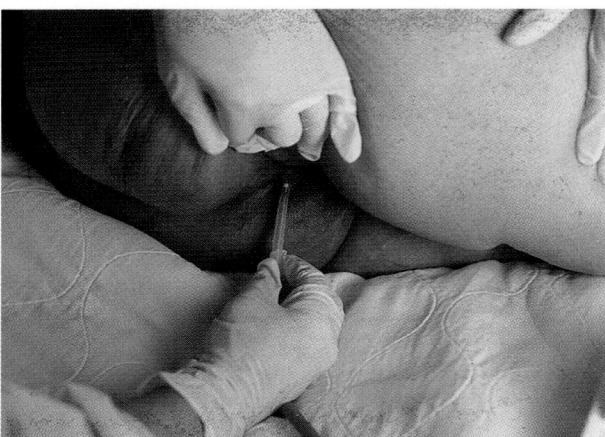

Step 7 Gently insert into anus.

8. Hold in place until beep is heard. Obtain reading.
   Rationale: Holding thermometer prevents rectal damage or perforation from client moving with thermometer in place.
9. Follow steps 6 to 8 in Assessing Oral Temperature With Electronic Thermometer.

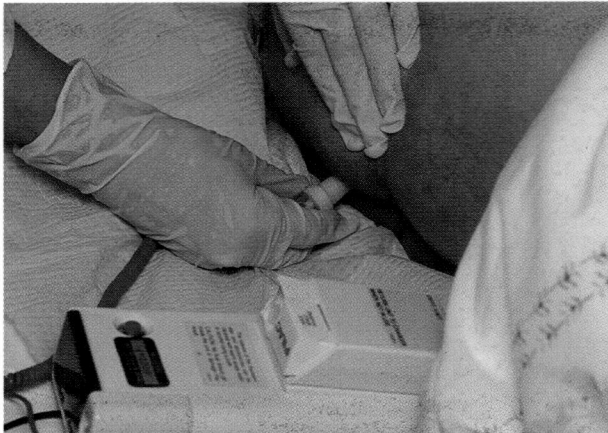

Step 8 Hold thermometer in place.

Assessing Axillary Temperature with an Electronic Thermometer

Procedure
1. Wash hands. Identify client and explain the procedure.
   Rationale: Ensures safety and promotes client compliance.
2. Remove electronic thermometer from the battery pack, and remove the oral temperature probe from the unit, noting a digital display of temperature on the screen (usually 34°C or 94°F).
   Rationale: The electronic thermometer is stored in a battery pack to ensure that it is always charged and ready for use. Removing the temperature probe prepares the machine to measure and record temperature. The digital display of temperature indicates that it is charged.
3. Securely attach the disposable cover over the temperature probe.
   Rationale: Prevent the transmission of microorganisms.
4. Close bedroom door or unit curtains; assist client to comfortable position, and expose axilla removing clothing.
   Rationale: Clothing in the axilla area could interfere with accurate temperature measurement.
5. Insert thermometer into middle of axilla; fold client's arm down, and place across chest.
   Rationale: This position maintains correct position of thermometer against blood vessels in axilla.

PROCEDURE 25-1 (Continued)

6. Wait for a beep that indicates the estimated temperature. Watch to see if temperature continues to rise. When it stops, remove the probe from the client's axilla, noting the temperature displayed on the unit.

   Rationale: Beep indicates estimated temperature. Usually the final temperature reading is very close to this estimated reading and often this is the temperature that is recorded if there are time pressures.

7. Follow steps 6 to 8 in Assessing Oral Temperature With Electronic Thermometer.

Assessing Temperature Using a Tympanic Membrane Thermometer

Procedure

1. Wash hands. Identify client and explain procedure.

   Rationale: Provides for safety and increases client compliance.

2. Remove tympanic thermometer from recharging base, and attach tympanic probe cover to sensor unit.

   Rationale: Probe cover keeps unit clean and prevents the transfer of microorganisms.

3. Insert probe into ear canal, making sure the probe fits snugly. Avoid forcing the probe too deeply into the ear. Pulling on the pinna may help to straighten the ear canal, which permits better exposure of the tympanic membrane. Rotate the probe handle toward the jaw line.

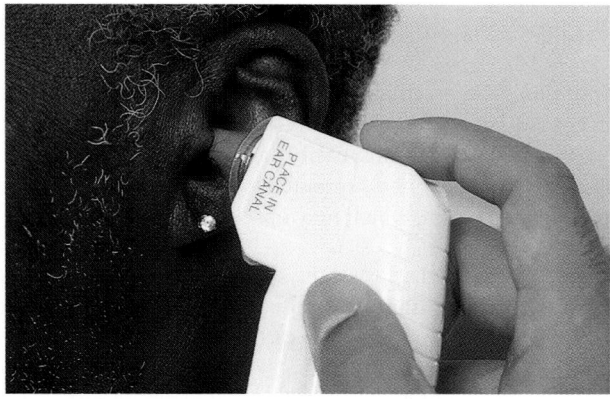

Step 3A Insert probe snugly into ear canal.

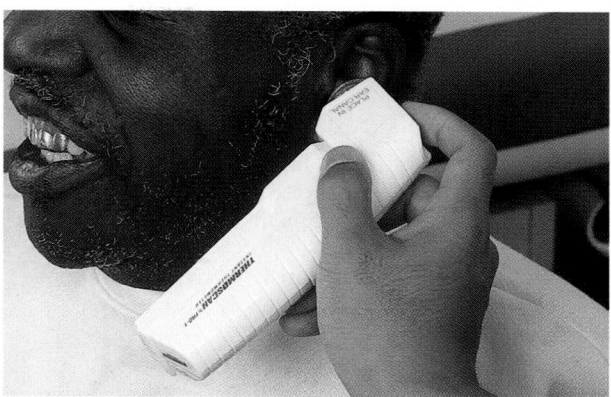

Step 3B Angle probe toward jaw line.

   Rationale: Snug fit into the ear canal is necessary for accurate temperature detection. Forceful deep insertion could result in injury to the eardrum. Angling the probe toward the jaw line ensures an accurate reading.

4. Activate the thermometer, and watch for the temperature readout, which is usually displayed within 2 seconds.

   Rationale: Temperature assessment occurs very quickly with the tympanic membrane thermometer.

5. Eject sensor probe cover directly into waste container, and return tympanic thermometer to base for recharging. Store away from temperature extremes.

   Rationale: Preventing contamination of nurse's hands is important. Recharging tympanic thermometer will prepare thermometer for use. Proper storage will help ensure accurate functioning of the equipment.

6. Record temperature on vital sign documentation record. Discuss findings with client if appropriate.

   Rationale: These actions ensure proper documentation and encourage client's understanding of health status.

Lifespan Considerations
Newborns, Infants, and Children

- Newborns have ineffective and immature thermoregulation. Environmental temperatures greatly affect their body temperatures.
- Tympanic or axillary temperature is the preferred measurement in infants over 2 months and children because it is easily accessible, there is little danger of mercury poisoning from thermometer

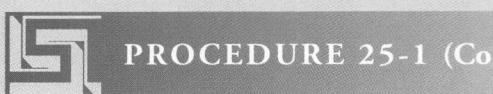

PROCEDURE 25-1 (Continued)

breakage in mouth, and there is no chance of rectal perforation and possible resultant peritonitis.

Older Adults
- Older adults may have difficulty flexing their legs and assuming the left lateral position. Thermometer may be inserted with both legs straight.
- Body temperature drops to an average of 36°C in the older adult.
- Alcoholic clients are at risk for hypothermia because of heat loss from vasodilation.

Home Care Modifications
- Glass thermometers are still sometimes used in the home because they are inexpensive. Caution must be taken if a thermometer breaks, because mercury is harmful if it is swallowed or touched. Tympanic thermometers are becoming less expensive and are frequently given as shower gifts.

- If family members need to assess temperature of clients, they may need to know
- How frequently to monitor temperature
- When to notify home care nurse or physician
- Not to measure temperature orally in children younger than 5 years, or in confused or unconscious clients
- To wash the thermometer in tepid, soapy water, and to store it dry

Collaboration and Delegation
- Unlicensed assistive personnel routinely monitor clients' temperatures. Remind UAPs to promptly report any temperature elevation above 38°C to the RN for follow-up.
- Instruct unlicensed assistive personnel that they must report even low-grade fevers in certain clients (e.g., those who are immunocompromised).
- Usually physicians want to be notified of any temperature over 38.5°C (101°F).

brachial, radial, femoral, popliteal, pedal, and posterior tibial (Fig. 25-6).

Temporal. The temporal artery courses across the temporal bone of the skull. The pulsation of the temporal artery is most easily palpated just in front of the upper part of the ear.

Carotid. The sternomastoid muscles, which stand out when the jaw is forcefully clenched, run from below the ear to the clavicle and sternum. Beneath the sternomastoid muscles lie the carotid arteries. The carotid artery is most easily palpated along the medial border of the sternomastoid muscle in the lower half of the neck. Palpating the carotid artery in the upper part of the neck may result in stimulation of the carotid sinus, which causes a reflex drop in pulse rate. The carotid pulse best represents the quality of pulsation in the aorta because of its proximity to the central circulation.

SAFETY ALERT
Always palpate the carotid artery in the lower half of the neck to avoid stimulating the carotid sinus. Never palpate bilateral carotid pulses simultaneously because this can seriously impair cerebral blood flow.

Apical. The contraction or beating of the heart ventricles also can be palpated with the hand or auscultated with a stethoscope placed over the area of the left ventricle. Normally, this area is at the level of the fifth intercostal space at about the midclavicular line.

Brachial. The brachial artery lies between the groove of the biceps and triceps muscles in the inner aspect of the upper arm. The brachial pulse is most easily palpated with the client's arm flexed at the elbow and supported by the examiner to prevent muscle contraction, which may obscure the pulse.

Radial. The radial artery is the site most commonly assessed in the clinical setting. The radial pulse is palpated on the thumb side of the inner aspect of the wrist.

Femoral. The femoral pulse is palpated in the anterior, medial aspect of the thigh, just below the inguinal ligament, about halfway between the anterior superior iliac spine and the symphysis pubis. Deep palpation may be required to detect the femoral pulse beneath the subcutaneous tissue.

Popliteal. The popliteal pulse is palpable behind the knee in the lateral aspect of the popliteal fossa (the hollow area at the

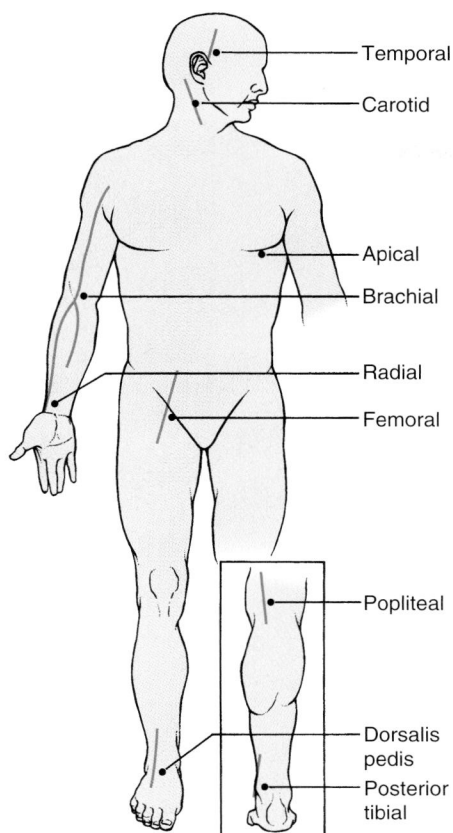

FIGURE 25-6 Pulse sites. The insert shows the left leg. The posterior tibial pulse is on the medial aspect of the ankle.

Temporal
Carotid
Apical
Brachial
Radial
Femoral
Popliteal
Dorsalis pedis
Posterior tibial

back of the knee joint). The pulse is best assessed with the knee flexed and the leg relaxed. The client may be supine or prone.

Pedal. The pedal pulse or dorsalis pedis pulse can be felt on the dorsal aspect of the foot (the area of the foot that is on top in a standing position). The pulse is palpated lateral to the tendon that runs from the great toe toward the ankle. The dorsalis pedis pulse may be congenitally absent in some clients.

Posterior Tibial. The posterior tibial pulse is located behind the malleolus (the rounded protuberance of bone) of the inner ankle. The pulse is palpated by hooking the fingertips behind the bone.

Equipment

Stethoscope. Auscultation of the apical pulse requires a stethoscope. The stethoscope should have snugly fitting ear pieces and thick-walled tubing about 12 inches long for optimal sound transmission. The stethoscope should be equipped with a bell and a diaphragm.

Doppler. Peripheral pulses that cannot be detected by palpation may be assessed with an ultrasonic Doppler device. The transmitter of the device is placed over the artery to be assessed. A conductive gel is first applied to the skin to reduce resistance to sound transmission. High-frequency waves directed at the artery from the transmitter are disturbed by the

pulsating flow of blood and are reflected back to the ultrasound device. The sound disturbances (Doppler shifts) are amplified and heard through ear pieces or a speaker attached to the device (Fig. 25-7).

Doppler assessment of the pulse is generally used to determine the adequacy of blood flow to an area when occlusive vascular disease threatens the blood supply or for postoperative assessment where peripheral circulation can be occluded. The Doppler also may be useful in situations of cardiopulmonary collapse where peripheral vasoconstriction makes pulses difficult to palpate or when obesity or edema makes assessment difficult.

Methods

Palpation. The pulse is palpated using the first and second or second and third fingers of one hand. Use light pressure initially to locate the area of strongest pulsation. You may then use more forceful palpation to count the rate, determine the rhythm, and assess the quality of pulsation. Count the number of pulses for 15, 30, or 60 seconds and multiply as necessary to yield pulses per minute. The time interval used to assess the pulse depends on the client's condition and the agency's norms. Clients with irregular or abnormally slow or fast pulse rates are best assessed for 1 full minute. Clients with regular rhythms and normal rates may be assessed for a shorter time. Intervals of 15 seconds may be used when assessing the pulse frequently, as during recovery from anesthesia.

Regardless of the time interval selected, count the initial pulsation as zero. Do not count pulses at or after completion of the time interval. Counting the first pulse as one or counting pulses after the period of assessment results in overestimation of the pulse. The error is multiplied when intervals of less than 60 seconds are used to assess the rate. Counting even one extra pulsation in a 15-second pulse assessment results in overestimation of the pulse rate by four. Procedure 25-2 gives detailed instructions on taking a pulse.

(*text continues on page 458*)

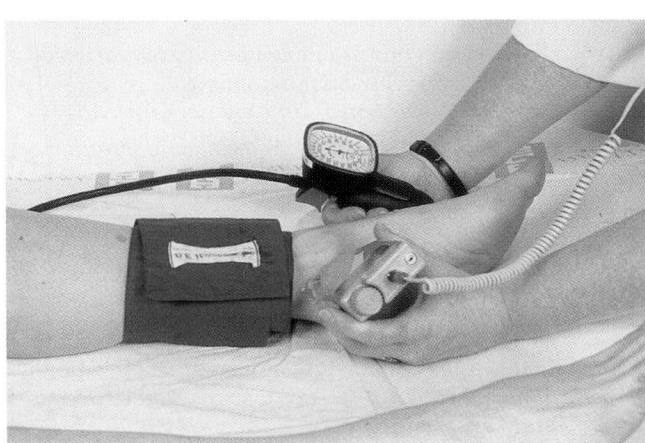

FIGURE 25-7 Doppler devices are used to assess pulse and heart rate in areas that can be difficult to access. (Photo with permission from Cantwell-Gab, K. [1996]. Identifying chronic PAD. *American Journal of Nursing, 96*[7], 40–46.)

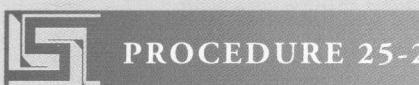

PROCEDURE 25-2

OBTAINING A PULSE

Purpose
1. Obtain a baseline measurement of heart rate and rhythm.
2. Evaluate the heart's response to various therapies and medications.
3. Peripheral pulse may be palpated to assess local blood flow to an extremity.

Assessment
- Review medical history to determine risk factors for alterations in pulse rate (heart disease, fluid or electrolyte imbalances, pain, hemorrhage).
- Assess for physical signs and symptoms of alteration in cardiac or vascular status (dyspnea, chest pain, palpitations, syncope, edema, cyanosis).
- Identify factors that influence pulse (age, medications, fever, exercise).
- Identify site most appropriate for pulse assessment.
- Review previous and baseline pulse assessments, if available.

Equipment
Wristwatch with second hand
Vital sign flowsheet and pen
Doppler and jelly (optional, for difficult-to-palpate pulses)
Stethoscope

Obtaining a Radial Pulse

Procedure
1. Wash hands, identify the client, and explain the procedure.
   Rationale: Provides safety and increases client compliance.
2. Position client comfortably with forearm across chest or at side with wrist extended.
   Rationale: Relaxed position of lower arm with wrist extended allows easier artery palpation.
3. Place fingertips of your first three fingers along the groove at base of thumb, on client's wrist.
   Rationale: Fingertips are the most sensitive part of the hand for palpating pulses. Do not use the thumb to palpate: it has a strong pulse that you may confuse with the client's.
4. Press against radial artery to obliterate pulse, then gradually release pressure until you feel pulsations.
   Rationale: Moderate pressure is needed to accurately assess the pulse's rate and regularity.

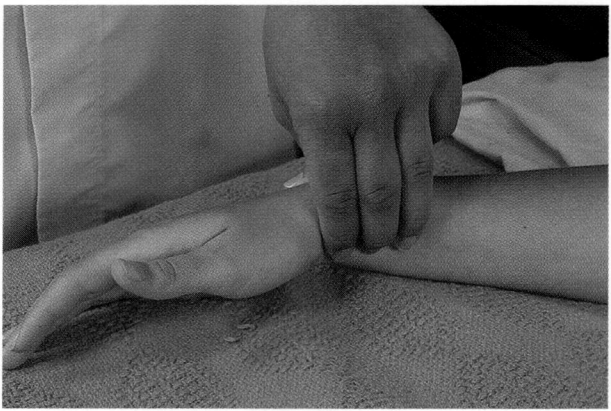

Step 3 Obtaining a radial pulse. (© B. Proud)

5. Assess pulse for regularity and strength.
6. If pulse is not easily palpable, use Doppler (See Fig. 25-7).
   a. Apply conducting gel to end of probe or to radial site.
      Rationale: Doppler works by ultrasound, which transmits sound better with the airtight seal that gel provides.
   b. Press "on" button and place probe against skin on pulse site. Reposition slightly, using firm pressure until you hear pulsating sound.
7. If pulse is regular, count pulse for 30 seconds, and multiply by two. If pulse is irregular, count for 1 full minute. Count the initial pulse as zero.
   Rationale: Prevent overestimation of pulse. If pulse is irregular, a longer counting period ensures a more accurate pulse rate determination.

Obtaining an Apical Pulse

Procedure
1. Wash hands, identify the client, and explain the procedure.
   Rationale: Provides safety and increases client compliance.
2. Position client in supine or sitting position with sternum and left chest exposed.
   Rationale: This position allows easy access for selection of auscultatory site. Rustling from clothing or bed linens will not distract from hearing pulse.

PROCEDURE 25-2 (Continued)

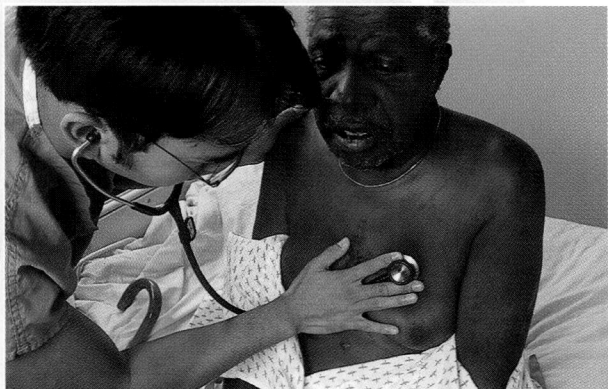

Step 4 Obtaining an apical pulse.

3. Warm diaphragm of stethoscope by holding in the palm of your hand for 5 to 10 seconds.
   Rationale: Cold metal or plastic diaphragm can startle the client when placed directly on the chest. This would possibly alter pulse rate.
4. Insert the ear pieces of stethoscope into your ears and place diaphragm over apex of client's heart.
   Rationale: The heartbeat is usually heard loudest at the fifth intercostal space, near the mid-clavicular line.
5. Assess the heartbeat for regularity and dysrhythmias.
   Rationale: Frequent irregularities within 1 minute may indicate inadequate cardiac perfusion.
6. If rhythm is regular, count the heartbeat for 30 seconds, and multiply by two. Count for 1 full minute if the rhythm is irregular. Count the initial pulse as zero.
   Rationale: Prevent overestimation of pulse. Heart rate is more accurate when counted over a longer period if the rate is irregular.
7. Replace the client's gown and assist the client to return to a comfortable position.
   Rationale: Provide for client comfort.
8. Share results of assessment with client, if appropriate.
   Rationale: Promote the client's understanding of health and response to therapies.

9. Document pulse on vital sign record. Specify in the documentation that you obtained an apical pulse (e.g., AP).
   Rationale: Maintains legal record and communicates with health team members.

Lifespan Considerations
Infants and Children
- Newborns and children younger than age 2 have weak radial pulses. Assess apical pulses for heart rate.
- The apex of the heart on an infant is at the third to fourth intercostal space, to the left of the mid-clavicular line.
- Crying greatly increases the pulse rate. Decrease the child's crying by taking the pulse while the child sits in a parent's or caregiver's lap or by distracting the child with toys.

Older Adults
- If client is taking cardiac medications, such as digitalis preparations or beta blockers, or if he or she has a history of cardiac dysrhythmias, obtain a more accurate assessment of heart rate and rhythm using the apical pulse site.

Home Care Modifications
- Pulse may need to be assessed at home if client is taking various cardiac medications. Teach the caregiver or client how to locate and count the pulse and to keep a diary of daily pulse rate to take to healthcare appointments.
- Digital pulse rate devices are available for home use.

Collaboration and Delegation
- Unlicensed assistive personnel (UAP) often assess pulses. Validate their technique for accuracy. Provide specific information about clients (e.g., if apical pulse is required or if pulse is usually irregular). Indicate what assessment data (e.g., pulse <60 or >110; new irregularity) UAPs need to report promptly for follow-up.
- Report new alterations in rhythm or new episodes of unexplained tachycardia or bradycardia to physician/cardiologist for follow-up.

Auscultation. The apical pulse provides the most accurate assessment of the pulse rate and is the preferred site whenever the peripheral pulses are difficult to assess or the pulse rhythm is irregular.

Assess apical pulse by placing the diaphragm of the stethoscope over the apex of the heart. The sounds heard are due to vibrations caused by the opening and closing of the cardiac valves. Each heartbeat consists of two sounds. The first, S_1, is caused by closure of the mitral and tricuspid valves that separate the atria from the ventricles. The second sound, S_2, is caused by the closure of the pulmonic and aortic valves. The sounds are often described as a muffled "lub-dub." Together, they constitute one heartbeat. To determine the apical pulse, count the heartbeats for 1 full minute.

Assessing Pulse Characteristics

The pulse is assessed for rate, rhythm, and quality. Pulse rate and rhythm are routinely assessed; pulse quality is assessed less often or in exceptional circumstances when abnormalities may be anticipated.

Rate. In adults, the normal rate is 60 to 100 pulsations per minute. Adult pulse rates above 100 beats per minute are called **tachycardia.** Sympathetic nervous system activation may results in tachycardic rates. Tachycardic rates also may occur when the impulse for cardiac contraction comes from an abnormal site in the heart that stimulates the heart to beat faster.

An abnormally slow pulse rate is called *bradycardia.* In adults, a pulse rate below 60 is considered bradycardic. Bradycardia may be the normal resting heart rate in a trained athlete. Disease of the SA node may result in bradycardia due to poor impulse formation. Enhanced parasympathetic nervous system activity may cause bradycardia, as occurs with stimulation of the carotid sinus.

Rhythm. Normally, cardiac contractions occur at evenly spaced intervals, resulting in a regular rhythm. Infants and children often have increased pulse rates during inspiration and decreased rates during expiration; this state is called sinus dysrhythmia.

Heart disease, medications, or electrolyte imbalances may alter the heart's normal rhythmic beating, causing an irregular pulse. An irregular pulse rhythm that still has a consistent pattern of pulsation is called regularly irregular. An example is pulsus bigeminus, in which a normal heartbeat initiated in the SA node is followed by a heartbeat initiated in a different part of the heart. The second beat is early and often weaker than the first, resulting in a regularly irregular pulse.

If the pulse has no pattern, it is called irregularly irregular. Irregularly irregular pulses may be detected in many conditions including a condition known as atrial fibrillation. In atrial fibrillation, the atria do not contract in a synchronous fashion, and the impulse for the heartbeat does not come from the SA node. Consequently, the time interval between successive ventricular contractions varies, and an irregularly irregular pulse is detected.

When you note an abnormal pulse rhythm, consider using the auscultatory method to obtain an apical pulse rate. Also determine if irregularity of the pulse is a new finding for the client.

SAFETY ALERT
Many people have chronically irregular pulse rhythms, but a new finding of pulse irregularity requires immediate investigation to determine the causes and to assess the need for treatment.

Quality. Pulse quality generally refers to the strength of pulsation and may be rated on a numerical scale (Table 25-3). The normal quality of the pulse is described as full or strong and can be easily palpated. Weak pulses are easily obliterated by the examiner's fingers and may be described as thready. A bounding pulse is stronger than normal and difficult to obliterate. Pulse quality reflects the stroke volume, the compliance or elasticity of the arteries, and the adequacy of blood delivery. When stroke volume is decreased, as in severe hemorrhage, the pulse is often thready and may be difficult to palpate in the peripheral arteries. The pulse is usually palpated more easily in the central areas such as the carotid or femoral arteries. With aging, the arteries lose elasticity, and the pulse becomes more bounding. The combination of rapid pulse rate and increased stroke volume with exercise results in a pulse that the client can feel and is sometimes called a pounding heart.

Palpate peripheral pulses bilaterally to compare quality. Equality of pulsation provides information about local blood flow. For example, partial occlusion of a right femoral artery would result in weaker femoral, popliteal, pedal, and posterior tibial pulses on the right than on the left. Bilateral pulse comparison is used to monitor for complications after procedures that are invasive to the arteries, such as arteriography. After an arteriogram, during which a large artery is punctured and injected with radiographic dye, the normal clotting to seal the artery may cause total arterial occlusion. Weakened or absent pulses distal to the puncture site would signal an occlusion.

Pulse Deficits. In some situations, stroke volume may vary from beat to beat during cardiac contraction, resulting in a pulse wave so weak that it cannot be perceived by palpation at a peripheral site. It is important to recognize this situation because it provides information about the heart's ability to per-

TABLE 25-3

Scale to Rate Pulse Quality	
0	No pulse detected
1+	Thready, weak pulse; easily obliterated with pressure; pulse may come and go
2+	Pulse difficult to palpate; may be obliterated with pressure
3+	Normal pulse
4+	Bounding, hyperactive pulse; easily palpated and cannot be obliterated

fuse the body adequately. When some of the ventricular contractions do not perfuse, a difference exists between the apical and peripheral pulses—a pulse deficit. The presence and magnitude of the pulse deficit can be determined by having two nurses simultaneously measure the apical and radial pulses. Both nurses should use the same watch or clock to count the client's pulses for 1 full minute. They then document the difference between the pulses. When a pulse deficit is present, the radial pulse rate is always lower than the apical pulse rate.

RESPIRATIONS

Respiration is a term used to summarize two different but related processes: external respiration and internal respiration. External respiration is the process of taking oxygen into and eliminating carbon dioxide from the body. Internal respiration refers to the use of oxygen, the production of carbon dioxide, and the exchange of these gases between the cells and the blood.

The process of inspiration is active. Inspiratory muscles contract, resulting in increased intrathoracic volume as the lungs are pulled into a more expanded space. The pressure in the airway becomes negative and air flows in. At the end of inspiration, natural lung recoil occurs, the airway pressure becomes slightly positive, and the air flows out as the muscles relax. Expiration is basically a passive process.

Normal breathing is automatic and involuntary. At rest, the normal adult respiratory rate is 12 to 20 breaths per minute. Normal tidal volume (the amount of air moving in and out with each breath) is 500 mL or 6 to 8 L/min (Copstead & Banasik, 2000). In people with healthy respiratory systems, the normal stimulus to breathe is hypercarbia, an increased carbon dioxide level. Chemoreceptors throughout the body sense changes in carbon dioxide levels and stimulate the respiratory center, which increases or decreases respiratory rate and depth accordingly. Chapter 34 provides an in-depth explanation of respiratory control.

Factors Affecting Respirations

Several factors can affect respiratory rate, rhythm, and depth. Familiarity with these factors allows the nurse to determine the significance of alterations.

Age
Normal growth from infancy to adulthood results in a larger lung capacity. As lung capacity increases, lower respiratory rates are sufficient to exchange air. As the adult ages, lung elasticity decreases. With this decrease in lung capacity, the respiratory rate once again increases to allow for adequate air exchange.

Medications
Narcotics decrease respiratory rate and depth. Sympathomimetic drugs (e.g., albuterol) can be used to dilate bronchioles, increasing the person's ability to move air into and out of the lungs.

Stress
Stress or strong emotions can change a person's respiratory pattern, because such conditions stimulate the sympathetic nervous system. Stress increases the rate and depth of respirations.

Exercise
When people exercise, their tissues need more oxygen. Also, exercise produces extra carbon dioxide and heat that the body must eliminate. The body responds to these needs by increasing the rate and depth of respirations.

Altitude
The oxygen content of the air decreases as the altitude increases. To compensate for the decreased oxygen content, the rate and depth of respirations at higher elevations increase to improve the oxygen supply available to the body tissues.

Gender
Because men normally have a larger lung capacity than women, men may have a lower respiratory rate as well.

Body Position
When the body is slumped or stooped, gas exchange can become impaired. As a result, the rate and depth of respiration may increase.

Fever
When a person has a fever, the respiratory system provides an avenue for the release of extra heat. Because heat can be lost from the lungs, the result is an increased respiratory rate.

Assessing Respirations

Respirations should be assessed in every vital sign evaluation. A normal baseline for each client should be established so comparisons can be made. The assessment should include respiratory rate, rhythm, depth, and quality.

The respiratory assessment can provide valuable information, and a thorough assessment of a client's respirations is vital in gathering clues to his or her condition. When assessing a client's respiratory status, keep in mind the client's normal pattern, the influence of any disease conditions, and the influence of any therapies that could affect the client's respiratory status.

Rate
Respiratory rate changes with age. At rest, the normal respiratory rate for an infant is 30 to 60 breaths per minute, decreasing to 12 to 20 breaths per minute for an adult. **Tachypnea** is an abnormally fast respiratory rate (usually above 20 breaths per minute in the adult). **Bradypnea** is an abnormally slow respiratory rate (usually less than 12 breaths per minute in the adult). **Apnea,** the absence of respirations, is often described by the length of time in which no respirations occur (e.g., a 10-second period of apnea). Continuous apnea is synonymous with respiratory arrest and is not compatible with life.

Rhythm and Depth

Respirations should be regular in rhythm and depth. Regularity refers to the pattern of inspiration and expiration. Expiration is normally twice as long as inspiration. Assess depth by observing the movement of the chest wall. Table 25-4 describes abnormal patterns, such as Biot's respirations, Cheyne-Stokes respirations, Kussmaul respirations, and apneustic respirations.

Quality

Respirations are usually automatic, quiet, and effortless. When assessing respirations, be attentive to changes from the normal quality. Abnormalities in quality are usually characterized as problems with effort or noise.

Dyspnea describes respirations that require excessive effort. Respirations can be painful and labored. Clients may report being unable to catch their breath. Dyspnea can occur at rest or with activity; dyspnea that occurs with activity is called exertional dyspnea. Healthy people who are not in good physical condition may experience exertional dyspnea.

Breathing also can be noisy. A number of terms are used to describe the different types of noisy respirations that the nurse can hear without a stethoscope.

Stridor is a harsh inspiratory sound that can sound like crowing. It may indicate an upper airway obstruction. It is commonly heard in children with croup or after aspiration of a foreign object.

Wheezing is a high-pitched musical sound. It is usually heard on expiration but may be heard on inspiration. It is as-sociated with partial obstruction of the bronchi or bronchioles, as in asthma.

Sighs are breaths of deep inspiration and prolonged expiration. Everyone sighs, and sighing aids in the expansion of alveoli. However, more frequent sighing may indicate stress or tension.

Methods

Clients must be unaware that the nurse is doing a respiratory assessment, because if they are conscious of the procedure they may alter their breathing patterns or rate. Often, nurses assess the respiratory rate after taking the radial pulse, while still holding the client's wrist. If respirations are very shallow and difficult to visually detect, count them while observing the sternal notch where respiration is more apparent. If the client is sleeping, rest a hand gently on the client's chest to detect its rise and fall. With an infant or young child, assess respirations before taking the temperature so the child is not crying, which would alter the respiratory status. See Procedure 25-3 for details on assessing respirations.

BLOOD PRESSURE

Blood pressure is the force that blood exerts against the walls of the blood vessels. The pressure in the systemic arteries is most commonly measured in the clinical setting. Blood pressure is stated in millimeters of mercury (mm Hg).

TABLE 25-4

Abnormal Breathing Patterns		
Abnormal Breathing Pattern	**Description**	**Conditions**
Bradypnea	Respiratory rate below 12 beats per minute	Neurologic disturbances, electrolyte disturbances, narcotic or barbiturate overdose, postanesthesia
Tachypnea	Persistent respiratory rate above 20 beats per minute	Trauma, injury, stress, pain; respiratory, cardiac, liver disease
Biot's	Cyclic breathing pattern characterized by shallow breathing alternating with periods of apnea	Neurologic problems (meningitis, encephalitis), head trauma, brain, abscess, heatstroke
Cheyne-Stokes	Cyclic breathing pattern characterized by periods of respirations of increased rate and depth alternating with periods of apnea	Congestive heart failure, drug overdose, increased intracranial pressure
Kussmaul	Increased rate (above 20 beats per minute) and depth of respirations	Metabolic acidosis, diabetic ketoacidosis, renal failure

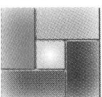

Nursing Research and Critical Thinking

Is It Possible to Identify Clients Who Have an Increased Risk of an Unsuccessful Outcome From Cardiac Arrest Resuscitation in the Hospital?

Critical care nurses wanted to know if there was a way to identify clients with an increased risk of an unsuccessful outcome from cardiac arrest resuscitation in the hospital. Such clients, once identified, could be monitored with heightened vigilance. These nurses designed the first nursing study to examine preexisting variables and outcome of cardiac arrest resuscitation in hospitalized clients. The study design was a retrospective review of medical records on male clients who suffered a cardiac arrest in a hospital setting. The convenience sample for this study consisted of all clients who had a cardiac arrest from 1990 to 1995 while in this hospital. The sample size of 83 was divided into two groups: successful (n = 36) and unsuccessful (n = 47) cardiac arrest resuscitation. A data collection tool was used to collect the data. Analysis of the data revealed no significant differences between successful and unsuccessful cardiac arrest outcomes in relation to clients' preexisting risk factors or prearrest QTc interval. However, the researchers determined a significant difference between the two groups in relation to the clients' vital signs. A significant interaction existed between outcome and res-

piratory rate (F = 3.73, $P < .05$) and between outcome and heart rate (F = 3.36, $P < .05$). The study's major finding is that heart rate and respiratory rate increased 8 hours before the cardiac arrest in the clients with an unsuccessful outcome of resuscitation.

Critical Thinking Considerations. The small convenience sample and the fact that only one institution and only males were studied are study limitations. However, the researchers make the following recommendations for nursing practice in the care of clients at risk for an inhospital cardiac arrest:

- The research suggests that clients who suffer a cardiac arrest within 8 hours following an increase in respiratory rate or heart rate are less likely to be successfully resuscitated, but nurses should not interpret these vital sign changes to mean that resuscitation would be futile.
- Nurses should assess clients for an increase in respiratory rate and/or heart rate and intervene accordingly with heightened vigilance.

From Chaplik, S., & Neafsey, P. J. (1998). Pre-existing variables and outcome of cardiac arrest resuscitation in hospitalized patients. *Dimensions of Critical Care Nursing, 17*(4), 200–208.

Physiologic Factors Determining Blood Pressure

The contractions of the heart result in a pulsating flow of blood into the arteries. The pressure is highest when the ventricles of the heart contract and eject blood into the aorta and pulmonary arteries. The blood pressure measured during ventricular contraction (cardiac systole) is the **systolic blood pressure.** During ventricular relaxation (cardiac diastole), blood pressure is due to elastic recoil of the vessels, and the measured pressure is the **diastolic blood pressure.** The mathematical difference between the measured systolic and diastolic blood pressures is the **pulse pressure.** For instance, a systolic pressure of 120 mm Hg and a diastolic pressure of 80 mm Hg result in a pulse pressure of 40 mm Hg.

Blood pressure is a function of the flow of blood produced by contraction of the heart and the resistance to blood flow through the vessels. The pressure, flow, and resistance relationship is described mathematically as pressure equals flow multiplied by resistance ($P = F \times R$).

Blood Flow

Blood flow is essentially equal to cardiac output. Cardiac output is the product of stroke volume (the amount of blood each ventricle pumps with each heartbeat) and heart rate. A stroke

volume of 70 mL and a heart rate of 72 beats per minute result in a cardiac output of 5,040 mL/min, or about 5 L/min. Average cardiac output in a resting man is 5.5 L/min.

Decreased stroke volume due to poor cardiac pumping (as occurs with a failing heart) or reduced blood volume (as in severe hemorrhage) may result in decreased cardiac output. Bradycardia also may cause decreased cardiac output. Conversely, a rapid heart rate and larger stroke volumes would be expected to increase cardiac output. The magnitude of change in cardiac output created by increases or decreases in one factor (heart rate or stroke volume) is influenced by the other factor's concurrent response. An increase in heart rate in response to a decrease in stroke volume to maintain a normal cardiac output is an example of a compensatory response.

Resistance

Friction among the cells and other blood components and between the blood and the vessel walls causes resistance to blood flow. The friction within the blood components reflects the blood's viscosity and is largely due to the number and shape of the blood cells. Normally, the number and type of blood constituents do not vary greatly, and viscosity is a constant factor.

Friction between the blood and the vessel walls varies with the dimensions of the vessel lumen. Contraction and relaxation

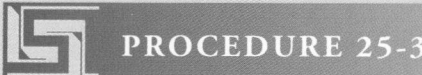

PROCEDURE 25-3

ASSESSING RESPIRATIONS

Purpose
1. Assess respiratory status by evaluating rate and quality.
2. Evaluate the influence of medications and therapies on respiration.

Assessment
- Identify risk factors for altered respiratory status (chest trauma, respiratory disease, smoking history, respiratory depressant medications).
- Assess for physical signs and symptoms of altered respiratory status (cyanosis, clubbed fingers, reduced level of consciousness, pain during inspiration, dyspnea, coughing).
- Review pertinent laboratory studies (arterial blood gases, oxygen saturation, complete blood count).
- Determine baseline respiratory rate.

Equipment
Watch with second hand
Vital signs documentation sheet and a pen

Procedure
1. Wash hands and identify client.
   Rationale: Provides for client safety.
2. After assessment of pulse, keep your fingers resting on client's wrist and observe or feel the rising and falling of chest with respiration. If client is asleep, you may gently place your hand on the client's chest so you can feel chest movement. Do not explain procedure to client.
   Rationale: Explaining procedure may make client self-conscious about respirations and could cause him or her to alter respiratory pattern.
3. When you have observed one complete cycle of inspiration and expiration, look at second hand of watch and count the number of complete cycles. If rate is regular in an adult, count 30 seconds and multiply by two. In children younger than 2 years or in adults with an irregular rate, count for 1 full minute.
   Rationale: Children normally have irregular respiratory patterns. Ensures accuracy of assessment.
4. If respirations are shallow and difficult to count, observe at the sternal notch.
   Rationale: Respirations are more visible at the sternal notch.

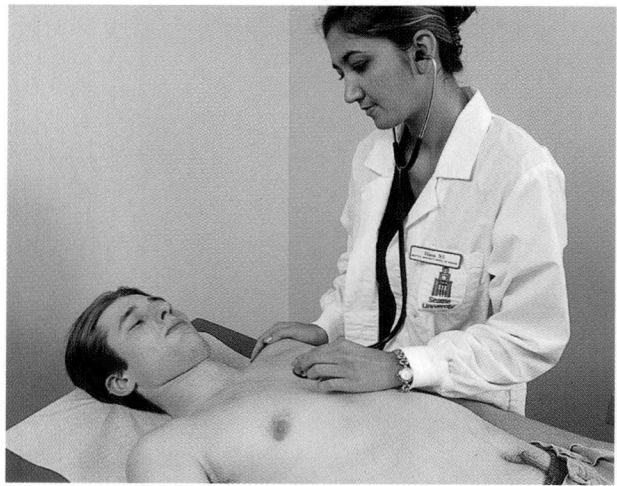

Step 4 Assessing respirations by observing at the sternal notch after taking an apical pulse. Hand on the chest can help detect shallow rise and fall of the chest.

5. Note depth and rhythm of respiratory cycle.
   Rationale: Respiratory characteristics give additional data about alterations in respiratory status.
6. Discuss findings with client and document respiratory rate, depth, rhythm, and character.
   Rationale: Maintains legal record and communicates with health care team.

Lifespan Considerations
Infants and Children
- A crying child's respiratory rate cannot be accurately assessed. Count respirations when the child is sleeping, if possible. If the child is crying, attempt to quiet him or her before assessing respirations. If the child cannot be quieted, write "crying" on the vital signs documentation sheet.

Home Care Modifications
- High-risk infants may be placed on apnea monitors, so that parents can be quickly alerted if respirations dangerously slow or stop.

Collaboration and Delegation
- Unlicensed assistive personnel (UAP) frequently monitor clients' respirations. They must take care to accurately assess rate, especially for clients with shallow breathing patterns. They must report promptly any alterations of rhythm or rate <8 or >24.

of the smooth muscle in the vessel walls control the diameter of the blood vessel. The autonomic nervous system regulates this vascular tone. Constricted vessels offer greater resistance thus increasing blood pressure; dilated vessels offer less resistance thus decreasing blood pressure.

Factors Affecting Blood Pressure

Age

Blood pressure gradually increases throughout childhood and correlates with height, weight, and age. These normal changes make identifying abnormal blood pressure levels for children at various developmental stages difficult. The American Heart Association recommends that a diastolic pressure consistently above the 95th percentile for age indicates a need for diagnostic evaluation.

In adults, the trend is toward gradually increasing systolic and diastolic blood pressure with aging. In part, this trend is due to increased systemic vascular resistance, reflecting arterial narrowing and decreased vessel elasticity due to atherosclerotic vessel disease. The increase in systolic blood pressure is proportionally greater than the increase in diastolic blood pressure; therefore, pulse pressure widens. Table 25-1 shows normal blood pressures for various age groups.

Autonomic Nervous System

The autonomic nervous system influences heart rate, cardiac contractility, systemic vascular resistance, and blood volume. Increased sympathetic nervous system activity results in increased heart rate, stronger contraction of heart muscle, changes in vascular smooth muscle tone, and increased blood volume due to retention of water and sodium. The cumulative effect is increased blood pressure. Therefore, factors that enhance sympathetic nervous system activity (such as pain, anxiety, fear, smoking, and exercise) result in increased blood pressure readings.

Exceptions occur when sympathetic nervous activity cannot keep up with a stressor. An example is a client with severely diminished blood volume resulting from hemorrhage. The sympathetic nervous system is activated to maintain adequate blood pressure, but it may not be enough to compensate for the volume loss. Measured blood pressure may be quite low, although sympathetic nervous system activity is markedly increased.

Circulating Volume

A decrease in circulating volume, either from blood or fluid loss, results in lower blood pressure. Fluid volume deficit can occur with abnormal, unreplaced losses such as diarrhea or diaphoresis. Insufficient oral intake also can cause fluid volume

THERAPEUTIC DIALOGUE
Blood Pressure

Scenes for Thought
Mr. Richards is sitting up in bed with an IV in his left arm and ECG leads attached to his chest. Being careful to use his right arm, the nurse prepares to take his blood pressure.

Less Effective
Nurse: Hi, Mr. Richards. I'm here to take your blood pressure.
Mr. R.: Again? They just took it 20 minutes ago. *(Looks irritated.)*
Nurse: Sure, we have to do that on heart patients. Just let me get this cuff on, and I'll be out of your way in a minute, okay?
Mr. R.: I guess so. Everyone else does. *(Continues to look annoyed.)*
Nurse: There, all done. I'll be back to change your bed and get you up in the chair in a little bit.
Mr. R.: 'Bye. *(Sinks back onto the pillows.)*

More Effective
Nurse: Hi, Mr. Richards. I'm Cheryl Bianco, and I'll be taking care of you today. How's it going?
Mr. R.: Okay, I guess. Are you going to take my blood pressure again? *(Looks irritated.)*
Nurse: Yes, I am. You look irritated about that. Are you? *(Exploring her observation.)*
Mr. R.: Well, yes. I mean, I'm not annoyed at you, but ever since I had the heart attack, people have been taking my pressure every 10 minutes, it seems, and I don't like it. *(Stopping to breathe.)*
Nurse: It feels like the staff is focusing on your pressure. *(Restating.)*
Mr. R.: Are they worried? Am I going to have another heart attack? Should I be worried? I'm confused. *(Looking upset.)*
Nurse: It sounds like you're looking for some information. Let's talk about it. *(Opportunity to provide information and allay his fears.)*

Critical Thinking Challenge
- Analyze the significance of his blood pressure as Mr. Richards sees it.
- Detect his feelings regarding the blood pressure readings.
- Infer what his thinking might do to all of his vital signs if he is upset about frequent blood pressure readings.

deficit. Excess fluid, such as in congestive heart failure or renal failure, can cause elevated blood pressure readings.

Medications

Any medication that alters one or more of the previously described determining factors may cause a change in blood pressure. Examples are diuretics, which decrease blood volume; cardiac medications, which affect the heart's rate or contractile force; narcotic analgesics, which reduce pain and sympathetic nervous system activity; and specific antihypertensive agents.

Normal Fluctuations

Blood pressure fluctuates from minute to minute in response to a variety of stimuli. Increased ambient temperature causes blood vessels near the skin surface to dilate, decreasing resistance and blood pressure. Blood pressure also fluctuates with the respiratory cycle, increasing during expiration and decreasing during inspiration.

In addition to these fluctuations, there is a discernible circadian pattern to blood pressure. Investigators performing direct, continuous monitoring of blood pressure have documented a consistent variation in blood pressure throughout the day.

Assessing Blood Pressure

Blood pressure may be measured directly with a catheter placed into an artery. Direct measurement provides a continuous reading of blood pressure and is used in critical care settings. However, blood pressure is usually measured by indirect methods, using an inflatable cuff to temporarily occlude arterial blood flow through one of the limbs. As the cuff is deflated and flow returns, the blood pressure can be determined by palpation, auscultation, or oscillations. Table 25-5 summarizes potential sources of error in blood pressure measurement. Procedure 25-4 gives detailed instructions for measuring blood pressure.

Sites

Upper Extremity. The blood pressure is usually measured in the arm with a cuff wrapped around the upper part of the limb and the flow auscultated or palpated at the brachial artery. Blood pressure may also be determined by auscultation or palpation of the radial artery in the wrist with an appropriately sized cuff applied to the forearm. Avoid measuring blood pressure in any arm with an internal atriovenous fistula or a peripheral vascular access for hemodialysis. Also, if the client has had a mastectomy, blood pressure monitoring on the same side can further impede circulation, contributing to lymphedema.

Lower Extremity. The cuff may be wrapped around the thigh or above the ankle. Thigh pressure measurement requires a larger, appropriate cuff. Place the client in a flat, prone, or supine position with the cuff centered midthigh over the popliteal artery. Auscultate or palpate blood flow at the popliteal fossa. When an appropriately sized cuff is used,

pressure measurements should vary only slightly (Woods, Froelicher, & Motzer, 2000). Using a cuff that is too small will result in false high readings. To measure blood pressure in the ankle, place the client in a flat, supine position, and place a standard arm cuff just above the malleolus. Auscultate or palpate the posterior tibialis or dorsalis pedis pulse as you deflate the cuff.

Equipment

Sphygmomanometer. A sphygmomanometer consists of an inflatable bladder enclosed in a nondistensible cuff. The bladder is connected to an inflating mechanism such as a bulb or pump, a valve for deflation, and a manometer (Fig. 25-8). The manometer may be a gravity mercury or aneroid type.

Mercury manometers consist of a vertical glass tube marked in 2-mm increments. Cuff pressures are transmitted through the tubing into the manometer and force the mercury to rise in the glass tube. The surface tension of the mercury in the tube causes the top of the mercury column to be curved. The pressure reading is made from the top point of the curved surface (the meniscus) of the mercury. The manometer must be at eye level to ensure an accurate reading. Particulate matter or air bubbles in the glass tube distort readings. Enough mercury must be present in the reservoir to maintain the meniscus at zero with the cuff deflated. The air vent at the top of the glass tube must be clean and allow free passage of air, or the mercury will be unable to rise and fall smoothly in the tube.

Aneroid manometers have a circular gauge marked in 2-mm increments. The pressure transmitted from the cuff causes movement of a metal bellows within the manometer; this movement is indicated by a needle on the gauge. Aneroid manometers require yearly calibration with a properly functioning mercury manometer or other pressure standard. Checks of manometer function should be made throughout the range of pressure measurement to ensure the device's accuracy. Aneroid manometers with a stop peg at the zero point or an external reset are not recommended, because verifying the accuracy of the manometer is impossible.

The tubing and hand bulb must be free of cracks or holes, and connections must be airtight to prevent leaks that cause poor transmission of pressure. The deflation valve must function smoothly to allow the operator to control the rate of deflation.

Stethoscope. A stethoscope is necessary for the auscultatory method of blood pressure measurement. The stethoscope should have snugly fitting ear pieces and thick-walled tubing about 12 in long for optimal sound transmission. The stethoscope should be equipped with a bell and a diaphragm.

Doppler. The Doppler method is useful during low flow states or when the blood pressure is difficult to auscultate by stethoscope. A standard cuff is used to occlude an artery while the ultrasound transducer is placed over the artery distal to the site of occlusion. Systolic blood pressure is the point at which continuous pulsatile flow is heard. Diastolic blood pressure may be difficult to identify reliably with the

TABLE 25-5

Potential Errors in Blood Pressure Measurement

Error	Cause	Recommendation
Falsely low readings	Environmental noise	Turn down TV or radio; stop talking; avoid moving stethoscope or tubing.
	Hearing deficit	Use hearing-amplified stethoscope or hearing aid.
	Ear pieces fitting poorly	Angle ear pieces forward to fit snugly into ear canal.
	Stethoscope tubing too long	Shorten tubing to 30–38 cm (12–15 in).
	Viewing meniscus from above eye level	Place meniscus at eye level.
	Failing to pump cuff up high enough	Palpate systolic pressure to avoid missing auscultatory gap.
	Cuff too wide	Measure arm circumference; bladder should be 80% of arm circumference.
	Arm above heart level	Reposition arm at level of heart, generally fourth intercostal space.
	Releasing valve too rapidly	Practice slow release of 2 mm Hg per second.
	Reading taken at inspiration (in selected high-risk clients, COPD, pulmonary embolus, hypovolemic shock)	Consistently try to record BP at end expiration.
Falsely high readings	Measuring BP when a client has just eaten, is in pain, is anxious, or has a full bladder	Try to assess BP during basal state, or adjust interpretation accordingly.
	Cold hands or stethoscope	Warm hands and stethoscope before measuring BP.
	Viewing meniscus from below eye level	View meniscus from eye level.
	Cuff too narrow	Measure arm circumference; bladder should be 80% of arm circumference.
	Wrapping cuff unevenly or loosely	Rewrap cuff snugly.
	Deflating cuff too slowly	Practice steady deflation of cuff at 2 mm Hg per second.
	Venous congestion	Wait 2 min before reinflating cuff to retake BP; elevate arm to promote redistribution of blood.
	Unsupported arm	Support arm on table to prevent muscle contraction.
	Back unsupported, legs dangling	Provide support for legs and back.
	Arm below heart level	Reposition arm at heart level, usually at the 4th intercostal space.
Inaccurate readings	Meniscus or needle not at zero	Recalibrate or service equipment.
	Faulty valves or leaky tubing	Replace equipment.
	Examiner digit preference	Do not round up or down.
	Forgetting measurement	Record immediately in the room.

Doppler but is considered the point at which continuous flow is heard.

Electronic Devices. Automated devices are frequently used to monitor blood pressure during anesthesia, in the critical care area, postoperatively, or in ambulatory settings when frequent assessments are necessary. The electronic units determine blood pressure by analyzing the sounds of blood flow or measuring oscillations. Although absolute values detected with automatic cuffs may vary slightly, the values are usually within 5 mm Hg of values obtained through direct arterial measurement (Widener, Yang, Costello, & Allen, 1999). Occasionally values can differ by as much as 37 mm Hg, so treatment should not be based on an isolated automated blood pressure reading (Widener et al., 1999). Very irregular heart rates or excessive movement from shivering, transporting the client, or rapid-cycling ventilator can interfere with blood pressure readings. Systolic, diastolic, and mean arterial blood pressure and heart rate are displayed on the monitor (Fig. 25-9). The machine can (*text continues on page 468*)

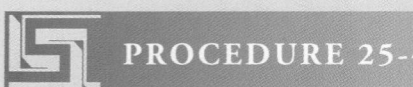

PROCEDURE 25-4

OBTAINING BLOOD PRESSURE

Purpose
1. Evaluate the client's hemodynamic status by obtaining information about cardiac output, blood volume, peripheral vascular resistance, and arterial wall elasticity.
2. Obtain baseline measurement of blood pressure.
3. Monitor the hemodynamic response to various therapies or disease conditions.
4. Screen for hypertension.

Assessment
• Assess blood pressure on initial client examination.
• Identify factors that may alter blood pressure (medications, exercise, age, emotional conditions, smoking, postural changes).
• Assess best site for obtaining blood pressure.
• Review previous blood pressure readings, if available.
• Consider any factors that limit site selection (e.g., mastectomy, dialysis access, PICC line, and so forth).

Equipment
Stethoscope
Sphygmomanometer with bladder and cuff
Documentation record and a pen

Procedure
1. Wash hands; identify client; explain procedure to client; assist client to a comfortable position with forearm supported at heart level and palm up.
   Rationale: Variations in blood pressure can occur with client in different positions. Blood pressure increases when the arm is below heart level and decreases when above heart level. Diastolic blood pressure may increase 10% if arm is unsupported, secondary to isometric exercises used to support arm.
2. Expose the upper arm completely.
   Rationale: Accurate placement of cuff and stethoscope requires complete exposure of upper arm.
3. Wrap deflated cuff snugly around upper arm with center of bladder over brachial artery. Lower border of cuff should be about 2 cm above antecubital space (nearer the antecubital space on an infant).
   Rationale: Placing bladder directly over brachial artery ensures proper compression of artery during cuff inflation. Loose or uneven application can result in falsely high readings.

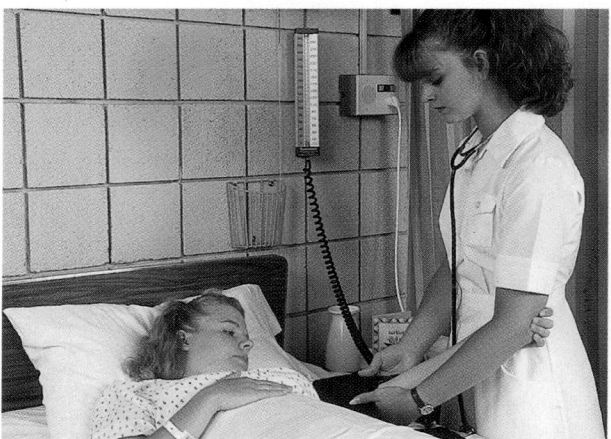

Step 3 Snugly wrap cuff around upper arm. (© B. Proud)

4. If using a mercury manometer, the manometer should be vertical and at eye level.
   Rationale: Prevents distortion and promotes accurate reading of mercury level.
5. Palpate brachial or radial artery with fingertips. Close valve on pressure bulb and inflate cuff until pulse disappears. Inflate cuff 30 mm Hg higher. Slowly release valve and note reading when pulse reappears.
   Rationale: Identify approximate systolic blood pressure reading to prevent underestimating systolic blood pressure should client have an auscultatory gap.

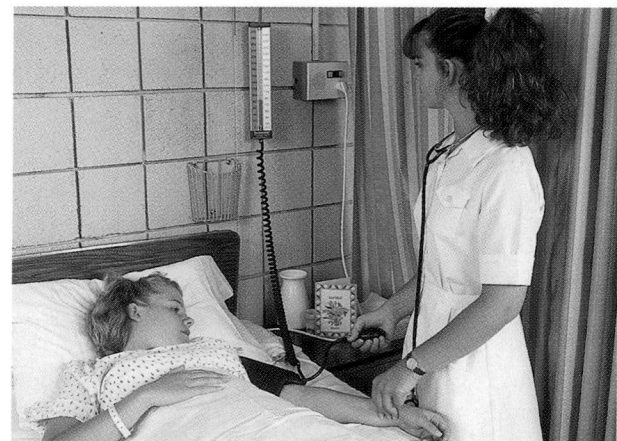

Step 5 Palpate radial pulse to estimate systolic blood pressure. (© B. Proud)

PROCEDURE 25-4 (Continued)

6. Fully deflate cuff, and wait 1 to 2 minutes.
   Rationale: Waiting period prevents falsely high readings by allowing blood trapped in the vein to be recirculated.

7. Place stethoscope ear piece in ears. Repalpate the brachial artery and place stethoscope diaphragm or bell over site.
   Rationale: Blood pressure is a low-frequency sound and is best heard with the stethoscope bell, but the diaphragm is widely used because it is easily placed and more generally available.

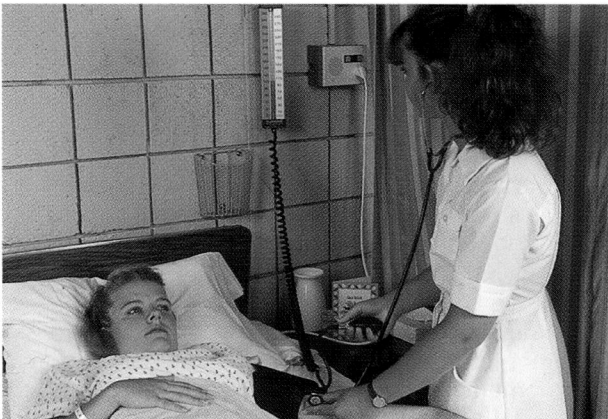

Step 9 Slowly release valve and note systolic and diastolic pressure readings. (© B. Proud)

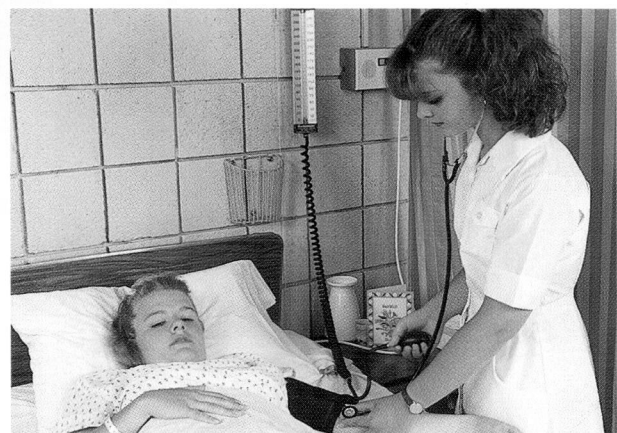

Step 7 Place stethoscope over brachial artery and inflate cuff. (© B. Proud)

8. Close bulb valve by turning clockwise. Inflate cuff to 30 mm Hg above reading where brachial pulse disappeared.
   Rationale: Ensure accurate assessment of systolic blood pressure.

9. Slowly release valve so pressure drops about 2 to 3 mm Hg per second.
   Rationale: Inaccurate measurements may occur if deflation rate is too fast or too slow.

10. Identify manometer reading when first clear Korotkoff sound is heard.
    Rationale: Indicate systolic pressure reading.

11. Continue to deflate, and note reading when sound muffles or dampens (fourth Korotkoff) and when it disappears (fifth Korotkoff).
    Rationale: American Heart Association recommends using the fifth Korotkoff sound as diastolic pressure in adults, fourth Korotkoff in children. In adults, if fourth and fifth Korotkoff are 10 mm Hg or greater apart, note all three readings.

12. Deflate cuff completely and remove from client's arm.

13. Record blood pressure. Record systolic (e.g., 130) and diastolic (e.g., 80) in the form 130/80. *Note:* If three pressures are to be recorded, use the form 130/80/40 (40 is the fifth Korotkoff). Abbreviate RA or LA to indicate right or left arm measurement.
    Rationale: Maintains legal record and communicates with health team members.

14. Assist client to comfortable position and discuss findings with client, if appropriate.
    Rationale: Encourage the client's understanding of health status and promote compliance with therapies.

Lifespan Considerations
Infants and Children

• Selection of proper-sized cuff and bladder is important for obtaining accurate blood pressure measurements in children and adults. The bladder width should be 40% of the circumference of the limb.

• In infants, Korotkoff sounds may be too faint for accurate measurement. Accurate assessment of systolic pressure can be obtained using a Doppler ultrasonic device. Flush method may be used to estimate mean blood pressure.

• When monitoring blood pressure in children, take respirations and pulse rate first because they are less invasive and less likely to cause anxiety.

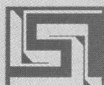

PROCEDURE 25-4 (Continued)

Older Adults

- Adults with hypertension are prone to auscultatory gaps in blood pressure. Estimation of systolic pressure using the brachial artery palpation technique will prevent inaccurate readings secondary to auscultatory gap.
- Diastolic pressure often increases with age as a result of decreased compliance of the arteries.

Home Care Modifications

- You may teach clients with hypertension to monitor their blood pressure at home. A variety of monitors for home use are available. They include digital printouts with time and date for accurate record keeping. Teach the client
- To avoid caffeinated beverages, smoking, and exercise for 30 minutes before measurement

- To use the same arm and body position for each measurement
- At what measurements the client should alert the nurse or physician

Collaboration and Delegation

- Frequently unlicensed assistive personnel (UAP) monitor clients' blood pressures. Validate their techniques for accuracy and provide specific client information (e.g., how frequently to monitor, appropriate size of cuff, site limitations). If client has been experiencing hypertension or hypotension, verbalize what readings they need to promptly report for follow-up.
- Report any cases of significant hypertension or hypotension to the physician. Physicians frequently establish orders for parameters of notification.

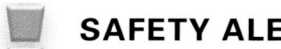

---

be set to record these values automatically at a preset interval (e.g., every 15 minutes). The data obtained are stored in the machine and can be easily retrieved as needed.

🥛 SAFETY ALERT

When using automatic blood pressure devices for serial blood pressure recording, check the cuffed limb frequently to ensure adequate arterial perfusion and venous drainage between measurements.

Methods

Baseline blood pressure ideally is measured with the client in a resting state. Therefore, the client should be in a warm, quiet environment and at least $\frac{1}{2}$ hour should elapse between smoking, exercising, or eating and taking the blood pressure reading. Sometimes blood pressure must be measured when the client is anxious or in pain, but these readings may differ from those made if the client were in a basal state.

Proper Cuff Size. The American Heart Association has made specific recommendations about cuff size and application (Table 25-6). Using an inappropriate size or placement may lead to an erroneous reading. Base cuff size on

the circumference of the limb you are using. The width of the cuff bladder should be 40% of the circumference of the midpoint of the limb. An average adult arm requires a bladder 12 to 14 cm wide. The bladder length should be 80% of the limb circumference, or about twice the bladder width.

Apply the cuff snugly around the limb, with the bladder centered over the artery. Using a cuff that is too small or

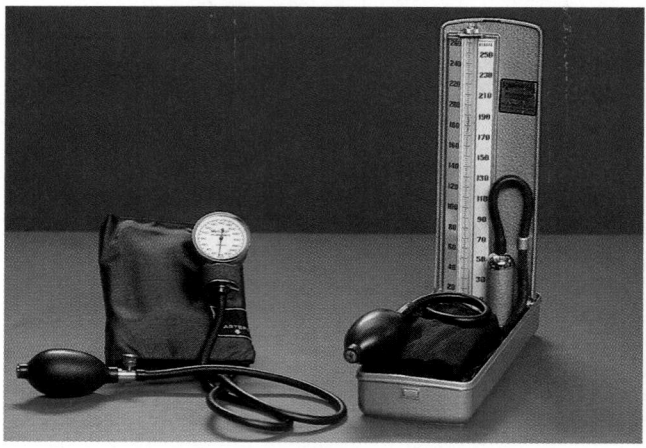

FIGURE 25-8 Sphygmomanometers. *Left,* aneroid; *right,* mercury.

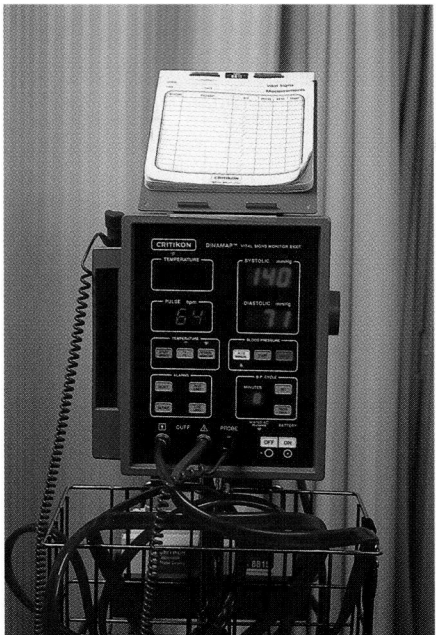

FIGURE 25-9 Automated monitors measure blood pressure and heart rate. They can be set to record these values at certain intervals, and the information is stored for later retrieval.

ETHICAL/LEGAL ISSUE
Delegating Vital Signs

You are working on a busy day surgery center. You delegate to a nursing assistant every-5-minute vital sign assessments for a postoperative client. The nursing assistant is using an automated monitor to obtain blood pressure and pulse readings every 5 minutes. The vital signs she records on the client's record appear stable.

When the client has been back from the operating room about 30 minutes, you notice her hand (distal to the automated cuff) is purple. You quickly release the cuff, but color does not return to the client's hand.

Reflection
- If the client sustains permanent injury due to the malfunction of the automated monitoring system, who might be considered negligent (the hospital, nursing assistant, the RN, the doctor, the manufacturing company)?
- What factors make this client especially vulnerable?
- What could be done to prevent similar situations from occurring?

loosely applied results in spuriously high readings. Using a cuff that is too large results in spuriously low readings.

Proper Positioning. Measure blood pressure with the arm at heart level. Elevating the arm above heart level results in a falsely low measurement; positioning the arm below heart level results in a falsely high reading. When the client is flat, the arm is approximately at heart level. If the client is sitting or standing, support the forearm horizontally at the level of the heart (generally considered the level of the fourth intercostal space, where the ribs join the sternum). Failure to sup-

port the arm causes the client to contract the arm muscles, elevating the blood pressure.

Correlation with the Respiratory Cycle. The intrathoracic pressure changes that occur during a normal respiratory cycle affect the heart and great vessels. Consequently, blood pressure is lower during inspiration than expiration. Exaggerated decreases in systolic blood pressure with inspiration (called pulsus paradoxus or **paradoxical blood pressure**) occur in diseases such as cardiac tamponade, constrictive pericarditis, emphysema, hypovolemic shock, and pulmonary embolus.

TABLE 25-6

Acceptable Bladder Dimensions (in cm) for Arms of Different Sizes*		
Cuff	Bladder Width (cm)	Bladder Length (cm)	Arm Circumference Range at Midpoint (cm)
Newborn	3	6	≤6
Infant	5	15	6–15†
Child	8	21	16–21†
Small adult	10	24	22–26
Adult	13	30	27–34
Large adult	16	38	35–44
Adult thigh	20	42	45–52

* There is some overlapping of the recommended range for arm circumferences in order to limit the number of cuffs; it is recommended that the larger cuff be used when available.
† To approximate the bladder width:arm circumference ratio of 0.40 more closely in infants and children, additional cuffs are available.
From Perloff, D., et al. (1993). Human blood pressure determination by sphygmomanometry. *Circulation, 88*(5), Part 1, p. 2469.

Consistently measuring blood pressure at end expiration eliminates variability of readings due to respiratory changes.

Proper Inflation and Deflation.　An inflated cuff reduces venous blood return to the heart in the extremity. Increased venous pressures are transmitted back to the arterial side of the circuit, and arterial pressures are transiently elevated. Slow, prolonged, or frequent cuff inflation promotes venous congestion. Inflate the cuff rapidly when taking a reading and deflate it completely after measurement. At least 2 minutes should elapse before sequential cuff inflation on any one limb. Elevating the arm above the head between cuff measurements speeds venous return to the heart.

Auscultation.　When determining the blood pressure by the auscultatory method, use an inflatable cuff to occlude flow through a limb temporarily. As you deflate the cuff and blood flow returns, the **Korotkoff sounds** can be heard with a stethoscope placed over the artery. Five distinct phases are identifiable, as shown in Table 25-7. The onset of the Korotkoff sounds of phase I is the recorded systolic pressure. Diastolic pressure is indicated by the onset of phase V sounds in adults and phase IV sounds in children.

Because the Korotkoff sounds are low in frequency, the bell of the stethoscope is best used for auscultation, although most practitioners use the diaphragm because of its larger shape and ease of placement. If the sounds are inaudible with the diaphragm, try the stethoscope bell. Do not press the head of the stethoscope too firmly against the skin because doing so may partially occlude blood flow and alter the reading.

An **auscultatory gap** is the absence of Korotkoff sounds between phases I and II. Failure to identify an auscultatory gap may result in underestimation of the systolic blood pressure or overestimation of the diastolic pressure. An auscultatory gap can be detected by palpating the brachial or radial pulse while inflating the cuff. Inflate the cuff about 30 mm Hg above the number where palpable pulsation disappears. In addition to detecting an auscultatory gap, palpation gives an initial estimate of systolic blood pressure and eliminates the need to inflate the cuff to extremely high pressures in people with normal or low blood pressure. When you detect an auscultatory gap, record the systolic and diastolic pressures as usual, and note the magnitude and range of the auscultatory gap (e.g., 196/90; auscultatory gap from 184 to 150).

Palpation.　When Korotkoff sounds are inaudible, blood pressure may be estimated by palpation. Apply the cuff and inflate as previously described and palpate the brachial or radial artery during cuff deflation. Systolic blood pressure is the point at which pulsation returns. Diastolic blood pressure is difficult to determine reliably with palpation but is indicated by a snap or whipping palpable vibrations. Palpated blood

TABLE 25-7

Korotkoff Sounds			
Phase	**Interpretation**	**Description**	**Recording**
Phase I	← 120 Systolic	Initiated by the onset of faint, clear tapping sounds of gradually increasing intensity	Recorded as systolic pressure
Phase II	← 110	Sound has a swishing quality	
Phase III	← 100	Marked by crisper, more intense sounds; clear intense tapping	
Phase IV	← 90 First diastolic	Characterized by muffled, blowing sounds	Recorded as diastolic pressure in children
Phase V	← 80 Second diastolic	Absence of sound	Recorded as diastolic pressure in adults

BP = 120/90/80

pressure is usually recorded as a systolic reading over "P" for palpated (e.g., 110/P).

Abnormalities

Hypertension. **Hypertension** is the condition in which blood pressure is chronically elevated. Although the natural trend in industrialized societies is for increased blood pressure with aging, hypertension is a dangerous disease associated with increased risk of morbidity and mortality. Therefore, adults of any age with blood pressure above 140/90 mm Hg should be evaluated for hypertension. Hypertension is diagnosed on serial elevated values rather than a single measurement. Studies have shown that some clients demonstrate higher recorded blood pressure in the physician's office than in the home setting. Ambulatory blood pressure measurements refer to blood pressure values obtained away from the clinical setting while the person is engaged in normal activity. Ambulatory blood pressure measurements are helpful to diagnose accurately and treat hypertension. The American Society of Hypertension now recommends ambulatory self-monitoring for all clients except those who are obese or have irregular heart rhythms (Graves, 1999). Chapter 35 covers hypertension in greater detail.

Hypotension. **Hypotension** is blood pressure below 100/60. Low blood pressure readings can be normal for some healthy, young adults and are no cause for concern. A sudden drop in blood pressure, significantly below the normal range for a person, causes hypotension. For example, a hypertensive client who usually has blood pressure readings of 180/94 would be considered hypotensive if the blood pressure fell to 120/80. Once again, a significant change from baseline values is more important than any one specific measurement.

Orthostatic Hypotension. In adults, moving from a flat, horizontal position to a vertical position results in pooling of blood in the lower extremities. People with a healthy, intact autonomic nervous system reflexively compensate for the volume shift by increasing the rate and force of myocardial contraction and vasoconstriction, thus maintaining adequate blood pressure. Even with normal compensation, however, systolic blood pressure usually falls and heart rate increases with a position change.

Inadequate reflex compensation to position change results in **orthostatic hypotension.** Symptoms of orthostatic hypotension are those related to decreased cerebral perfusion such as dizziness, weakness, blurred vision, syncope, and marked changes in blood pressure and heart rate. Orthostatic blood pressure changes may indicate failure of autonomic nervous system protective reflexes or hypovolemia. Hypovolemia or impaired vasoconstriction is signaled by decreased blood pressure and increased heart rate. Autonomic nervous system dysfunction is indicated by decreased blood pressure without marked increases in heart rate (Autonomic Dysfunction Center, Vanderbilt University, 1999). Orthostatic hypotension is a drop in systolic pressure of at least

🔳 APPLY YOUR KNOWLEDGE

Ms. George arrives at the clinic for a blood pressure check and an infusion of IV medications. She appears red in the face and states she hurried over during her lunch hour. Observe the medical assistant taking Ms. George's blood pressure in the accompanying photograph. Identify factors that might result in an inaccurate reading if the assistant uses this technique. It might be helpful to refer to Table 25-5.

Check your answer in Appendix A.

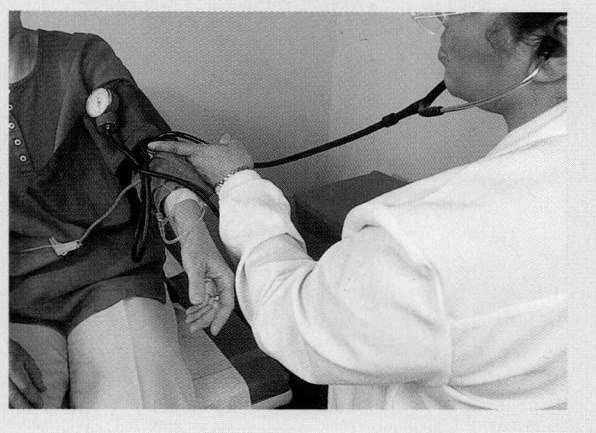

25 mm Hg or a drop in diastolic pressure of at least 10 mm Hg (Jevon, 2001).

🛑 SAFETY ALERT
The person experiencing postural hypotension is at risk for falling. Therefore, checking postural vital signs is one way of screening to ensure client safety.

Instruct clients with chronic orthostatic hypotension to change positions slowly, moving from a lying to a sitting to a standing posture and allowing several minutes to elapse before proceeding to the next position.

Measure orthostatic blood pressure in clients exhibiting symptoms of dizziness, blurred vision, or weakness when changing position; clients taking diuretic medications; and clients with a history of volume loss. Systematic, consistent technique in assessing blood pressure and heart rate response to position change provides the best data for determining and monitoring therapy. Procedure 25-5 gives a step-by-step description for assessing for orthostatic hypotension.

Clients experiencing severe orthostatic hypotension may be unable to tolerate a standing position long enough for you to obtain the blood pressure and heart rate.

🛑 SAFETY ALERT
If the client becomes severely symptomatic while standing, he or she should return to bed without completing the measurements.

⑤ **PROCEDURE 25-5**

ASSESSING FOR ORTHOSTATIC HYPOTENSION

Purpose
1. Assess the compensatory status of the cardio-vascular and autonomic nervous systems to changes in body position.
2. Assess for fluid volume deficit.
3. Assess for the client's safety in getting up and ambulating.

Assessment
- Identify clients at risk for postural drops in blood pressure:
  — Risk of volume depletion
  — Inadequate vasoconstrictor mechanisms secondary to prolonged bed rest
  — Autonomic insufficiency secondary to spinal cord injury or drugs (beta-adrenergic blockers, calcium channel blockers)
- Assess client for complaint of dizziness or light-headedness during position changes.
- Review baseline blood pressure measurements, if available.

Equipment
Stethoscope
Sphygmomanometer
Watch or clock with second hand
Vital sign documentation record and a pen

Procedure
1. Wash hands. Identify client and explain procedure.
   Rationale: Ensures client safety and increases compliance.
2. Position client supine with head of bed flat for 10 minutes.
   Rationale: Allow blood pooled in lower extremities to reenter circulation.
3. Check and record supine blood pressure and pulse. Keep blood pressure cuff attached.
   Rationale: Provide baseline information with which to compare measurements after position changes. Assess pulse rate to help differentiate the cause of postural hypotension. During position changes, if pulse rate rises as blood pressure falls, secondary to sympathetic stimulation, the cause may be volume depletion. If the pulse does not increase when the blood pressure falls, the cause may be related to the lack of sympathetic response.

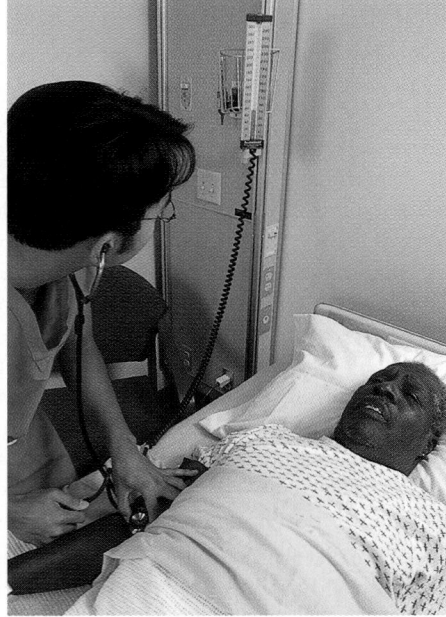

Step 3 Obtain blood pressure and pulse with the client in supine position.

4. Assist client to a sitting position with legs dangling over the edge of the bed. Wait 2 minutes and check blood pressure and pulse rate. *Note:* The waiting period is a convenient time to auscultate the client's lung fields.
   Rationale: Two minutes provides adequate time for the autonomic nervous system to reflexively compensate for volume shifts in the normal person.

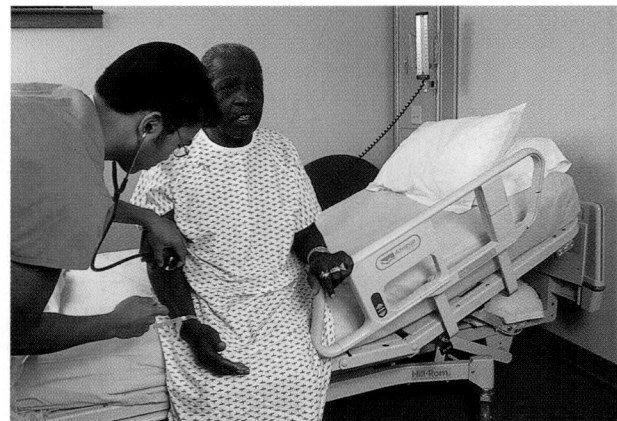

Step 4 Obtain blood pressure and pulse with the client in sitting position with legs dangling over the side of the bed.

PROCEDURE 25-5 (Continued)

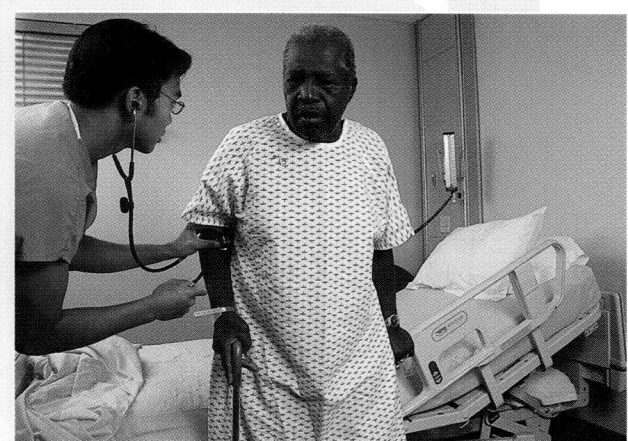

Step 5 Obtain blood pressure and pulse with client in standing position.

5. Assist client to standing position. Wait 2 minutes and check blood pressure and pulse rate. Be alert to signs and symptoms of dizziness.
   Rationale: If blood pressure drops significantly, the client may become lightheaded and may need to be returned to bed before test completion.
6. Assist the client back to a comfortable position.
7. Record measurements and any symptoms that accompanied the postural change. *Note:* Report a drop of 25 mm Hg in systolic pressure or a drop of 10 mm Hg in diastolic pressure.

○—   160/92   82
♀   154/90   82
♀   150/86   84

Rationale: Maintains legal record and communicates with health care team.
8. Discuss findings with client, if appropriate.
   Rationale: If there is a significant postural blood pressure drop, advise the client to sit on the edge of the bed for several minutes before walking to avoid dizziness and possible falls.

Collaboration and Delegation

• Nurses frequently delegate postural blood pressure monitoring to unlicensed assistive personnel. Reinforce to them the order for taking blood pressures: supine first, then sitting, then standing. Caution them that safety is always the most important consideration. If the client becomes dizzy, the assessment must stop and the client should return to bed.
• If other health professionals report that the client complains of dizziness upon rising, validate by obtaining a postural blood pressure.

Record the blood pressure and heart rate values and the position of the client when the values were obtained. Document any symptoms of diminished cerebral perfusion.

DOCUMENTING VITAL SIGNS

Nurses are responsible for assuring that vital signs have been assessed and documented. Frequently vital sign monitoring is delegated to unlicensed assistive personnel. The nurse needs to provide these health team members with guidelines of abnormal readings to be reported promptly. After assessing trends, the nurse may report abnormal findings to the physician. Vital signs are often documented in a graph format, with time as the horizontal axis and the

measured value as the vertical axis (Fig. 25-10). This graph allows trends to be seen easily. Trends may reflect normal variations or a change in response to disease or therapy. For example, the normal trend is toward a decreased body temperature in the early morning. If the graph shows increasing values during the night and early morning, this trend may indicate fever and would require further investigation.

LIFESPAN CONSIDERATIONS

Knowledge of developmental considerations is important for measuring and interpreting vital signs. Table 25-1 summarizes normal ranges for the vital signs across the lifespan.

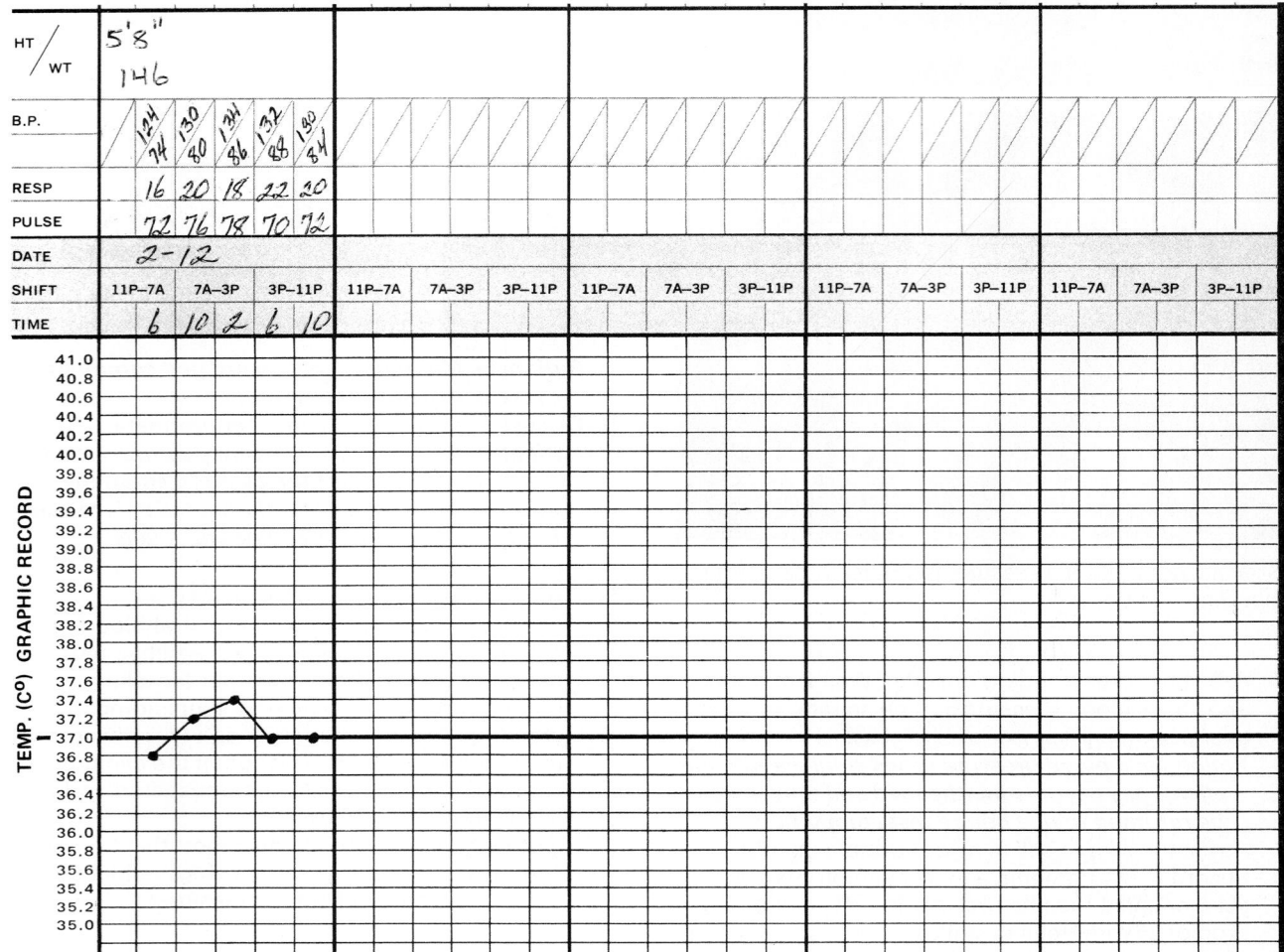

		11P–7A	7A–3P	3P–11P	11P–7A	7A–3P	3P–11P	11P–7A	7A–3P	3P–11P	11P–7A	7A–3P	3P–11P	11P–7A	7A–3P	3P–11P
HT / WT	5'8" 146															
B.P.		124/74	130/80	134/86	132/88	130/84										
RESP		16	20	18	22	20										
PULSE		72	76	78	70	72										
DATE		2-12														
SHIFT		11P–7A	7A–3P	3P–11P	11P–7A	7A–3P	3P–11P	11P–7A	7A–3P	3P–11P	11P–7A	7A–3P	3P–11P	11P–7A	7A–3P	3P–11P
TIME		6	10	2	6	10										

TEMP. (C°) GRAPHIC RECORD

41.0, 40.8, 40.6, 40.4, 40.2, 40.0, 39.8, 39.6, 39.4, 39.2, 39.0, 38.8, 38.6, 38.4, 38.2, 38.0, 37.8, 37.6, 37.4, 37.2, 37.0, 36.8, 36.6, 36.4, 36.2, 36.0, 35.8, 35.6, 35.4, 35.2, 35.0

FIGURE 25-10   Vital signs graphic flow sheet.

Newborn and Infant

Temperature, pulse, and respirations fluctuate widely in newborns. Their thermoregulatory mechanisms are immature, and ambient temperature may markedly affect their body temperature. The inguinal site is an alternative safe site suggested for use in newborns, especially those in superheated environments (Cusson, Madonia, & Taekman, 1997). Pulse and respiration increase rapidly above resting values when a newborn is active, crying, or startled. The apical pulse is the most reliable method of assessing heart rate, because peripheral pulses are faint and difficult to palpate and accurately count. Healthy newborns may exhibit periodic apnea. Blood pressure is not routinely assessed in the newborn or infant because the information obtained is unreliable.

Safety considerations are important when monitoring the vital signs of children of these age groups. Tympanic or axillary temperatures are preferred, because rectal temperature monitoring can cause mucosal tearing or perforation, and infants cannot safely hold oral thermometers in their mouths. Infants move quickly, so protecting them from falling or injury during vital sign monitoring is essential.

Toddler and Preschooler

As a child enters the second year of life, vital signs fluctuate less. The pulse rate decreases to a normal range of 80 to 120 beats per minute, and respirations fall to 22 to 40 breaths per minute. Normal blood pressure ranges from a systolic pressure of 80 to 112 mm Hg over a diastolic pressure of 50 to 80 mm Hg. Blood pressure is routinely monitored after the age of 3 years.

Toddlers and preschoolers may become fearful of procedures involving vital sign measurement, and at this age verbal explanations do little to allay fears. Permitting children to play with stethoscopes or to push the buttons on electronic thermometers may help calm their fears. Having parents or other caregivers hold and talk to frightened children can be comforting.

Safety concerns continue to be important. Monitor temperature using the tympanic or axillary route until the child is 4 or 5 years old and can follow directions about holding the thermometer in the sublingual pocket. It is not safe to use an oral glass mercury thermometer in children in this age group because inadvertently biting down on the thermometer could cause breakage, lacerations, and possibly mercury poisoning.

School-Age Child and Adolescent

The broad range of normal values for children reflects the wide variability in their vital signs. In general, temperature, pulse, and respirations gradually decrease through childhood, but blood pressure increases and correlates with height and weight.

Children in this age group are familiar with vital sign assessment and seldom exhibit fear during monitoring. Health teaching about normal values and the reason for taking vital signs helps to educate them. A child may try to experiment by putting the thermometer under hot water or near a light source, so validate any unlikely temperature readings.

Adult and Older Adult

Vital signs usually stabilize during young adulthood. As adults age, the effects of lifestyle and chronic diseases become evident in the vital signs. Chronic respiratory disease and exposure to pollutants, such as cigarette smoke, can influence respiratory rate and pattern. Cardiovascular diseases may cause changes in the heart rate and rhythm. The incidence of hypertension is increasing in the United States with an estimated one in five Americans and one in four adult Americans—many of whom go undiagnosed and untreated every year—having clinically significant high blood pressure (American Heart Association, 2000). Conversely, orthostatic hypotension is common in older adults although the actual incidence is unclear. It is also uncertain whether orthostatic hypotension is a result of normal aging or is seen only in elderly people with existing disease states. Older adults also have lower normal ranges for body temperature. Often adults ask nurses about the values obtained during monitoring. This discussion is an excellent opportunity for client education.

KEY CONCEPTS

- Temperature, pulse, respirations, and blood pressure are considered the vital signs because significant deviations from normal ranges are not compatible with life.
- Vital sign assessment is an important nursing function that permits the nurse to detect alterations from normal and to evaluate the client's progress.
- Body temperature can be monitored easily in four sites: oral cavity, ear, rectum, and axilla.
- Factors that can affect body temperature include age, environmental conditions, time of day, exercise, stress, and hormone level.
- Equipment to monitor body temperature includes glass mercury thermometers, electronic thermometers, tympanic membrane thermometers, chemically treated paper thermometers, and temperature-sensitive strips.
- As the heart contracts and ejects blood into the circulation, pulsations can be palpated at various arterial sites in the body.
- Evaluation of the pulse should include rate, rhythm, and quality.
- Factors such as age, autonomic nervous system stimulation, and medications can affect the pulse.
- An irregular pulse should be counted for 1 full minute, preferably at the apical site.

- A pulse deficit occurs when a cardiac contraction creates a pulse wave that is weak and not palpable at peripheral sites.
- Age, medications, stress, exercise, altitude, gender, body position, and the presence of a fever can influence respiratory rate, rhythm, and depth.
- Abnormal breathing rates include tachypnea (more than 20 breaths per minute), bradypnea (less than 12 breaths per minute), and apnea (interval of absent respirations).
- Abnormal breathing patterns include Biot's respirations, Kussmaul respirations, and apneustic respirations.
- Blood pressure is a function of the flow of blood produced by the heart and the resistance to blood flow through the vessels.
- Systolic pressure occurs during ventricular contraction, and diastolic pressure occurs during ventricular relaxation. Pulse pressure is the difference between systolic and diastolic pressure.
- Factors that can affect blood pressure include age, autonomic nervous system input, circulating volume, medications, and circadian rhythms.
- Blood pressure is usually measured indirectly using a sphygmomanometer and a stethoscope.
- Auscultation of blood pressure reveals five different phases known as Korotkoff sounds. The first Korotkoff sound corresponds to systolic pressure and the fifth (fourth in children) to diastolic pressure.
- Selecting proper cuff size, keeping the arm at heart level, avoiding venous congestion, and detecting the presence of an auscultatory gap are important steps in obtaining accurate blood pressure readings.
- Orthostatic hypotension occurs when a person experiences a decrease in blood pressure when changing from a supine to an upright position.
- Normal variations in vital signs occur throughout the lifespan.

REFERENCES

American Heart Association (2000). One in five Americans and one in four adults has high blood pressure. [On-line] Available at: http//www.americanheart.org/ hbp/phys_stats.html

Baird, S., White, N., & Basinger, M. (1992). Can you rely on tympanic thermometers? *RN, 55*(8), 48–51.

Beaudry, M., VandenBosch, T., & Anderson, J. (1996). Research utilization: Once-a-day temperatures for afebrile patients. *Clinical Nurse Specialist, 10*(1), 21–24.

Beckstrand, R., Wilshaw, R., Moran, S., & Schaalje, G. (1996). Supralingual temperatures compared to tympanic and rectal temperatures. *Pediatric Nursing, 22*(5), 436–438.

Braun, S., Preston, P., & Smith, R. (1998). Getting a better read on thermometry. *RN, 61*(3), 57–60.

Chamberlain, J. M., Grandner, J., Rubinoff, J. L., Klein, B. L., Waisman, Y, & Huey, M. (1991). Comparison of a tympanic thermometer to rectal and oral thermometers in pediatric emergency department. *Clinical Pediatrics, 30*(4), 24–29.

Copstead, L. C., & Banasik, J. L. (2000). *Pathophysiology: Biological and behavioral perspectives* (2nd ed.). Philadelphia: W.B. Saunders Company.

Cusson, R., Madonia, J., & Taekman, J. (1997). The effects of environment on body site temperatures in full-term neonates. *Nursing Research, 46*(4), 202–206.

Dobbin, K. (1998). Noninvasive blood pressure monitoring. *Critical Care Nurse, 18*(2), 101–102.

Erickson, R., & Meyer, L. (1994). Accuracy of infrared ear thermometry and other temperature methods in adults. *American Journal of Critical Care, (3)*1, 40–54.

Graves, J. W. (1999, November). The clinical utility of out of office self-measurement of blood pressure. *Home Health Consultant, 6*(11), 26–29.

Jevon, P., & Jevon, M. (2001, March 1–7). Practical procedures for nurses: Using a tympanic thermometer no 56.1. *Nursing Times, 97*(9), 43–4.

Jevon, P. (2001, January 18–24). Orthostatic hypotension. *Nursing Times, 97*(3), 39–40.

Kenney, R., & Fortenberry, J. (1990). Evaluation of an infrared tympanic membrane thermometer in pediatric patients. *Pediatrics, 85*(5), 856.

Lattavo, K., Britt, J., & Dobal, M. (1995). Agreement between measures of pulmonary artery and tympanic temperatures. *Research in Nursing and Health, 18*(4), 365–370.

Lee, V. K., McKenzie, N. E., & Cathcart, M. (1999, June). Ear and oral temperatures under usual practice conditions. *Research for Nursing Practice, 1*(1), 8.

Levine B. S. & Underhill-Motzer, S. L. (2000). History-taking and physical examination. In S. L. Woods, E. S. Sivarajan-Froelicher, & S. U. Motzer (Eds.), *Cardiac nursing* (4th ed.). Philadelphia: Lippincott Williams & Wilkins.

McGann, K., Marion, G., Camp, L., & Spangler, J. (1993). The influence of gender and race on mean body temperature in a population of older adults. *Archives of Family Medicine, 2*(12), 1265–1267.

Molton, A. H., Blacktop, J. & Hall, C. M. (2001, Spring). Largest difference in mean temperature values from oral to tympanic thermometers is < .2° C. *Journal of Child Health Care, 5*(1), 5–10.

Molton, A. H., Blacktop, J. & Hall, C. M. (1999). Orthostatic intolerance. *Autonomic Dysfunction Center at Vanderbilt University.* [On-line]. Available at: http//www.mc.Vanderbilt.edu/gcrc/adc/index.html.

Perloff, D., Grim, C., Flack, J., Frohlich, E., Hill, M., McDonald, M., & Morgenstern, B. (1993). Human blood pressure determination by sphygmomanometry. *Circulation, (88)*5, 2460–2470.

Pickering, T. (1996). Recommendations for the use of home (self) and ambulatory blood pressure monitoring. *American Journal of Hypertension, 9*(1), 1.

Pontious, S., Kennedy, A., Chung, K., Burroughs, T., Libby, L., & Vogel, D. (1994). Accuracy and reliability of temperature measurement in the emergency department by instrument and site in children. *Pediatric Nursing, (20)*1, 58–63.

Porth, C. (1998). *Pathophysiology: Concepts of altered health states* (5th ed.). Philadelphia: Lippincott-Raven.

Pransky, S. (1991). The impact of technique and condition of tympanic membrane upon infrared tympanic thermometry. *Clinical Pediatrics, 30*(4), 50–52.

Roben, N. (1993). Hypertension. In D. L. Carnevali & M. Patrick (Eds.), *Nursing management for the elderly* (3rd ed.). Philadelphia: J.B. Lippincott.

Shinozaki, T., Deane R., & Perkins, F. M. (1988). Infrared tympanic thermometer. Evaluation of a new clinical thermometer. *Critical Care Medicine, 16*(2), 148–150.

Vander, A., Sherman, J., & Luciano, D. (1998). *Human physiology: The mechanisms of body function* (7th ed.). Boston: McGraw-Hill.

Widener, J., Yang, C., Costello, P. & Allen, K. (1999, March). Modifications to standard guidelines and changes in blood pressure readings: Use of an automatic blood pressure device. *AAOHN Journal, 47*(3), 107–113.

Winslow, E. (1997). Tympanic thermometers' accuracy is questionable. *American Journal of Nursing, 97*(5), 71.

Woods, S. L., Sivarajan Froelicher, E. S., & Motzer, S. U. (2000). *Cardiac nursing* (4th ed.). Philadelphia: Lippincott Williams & Wilkins.

BIBLIOGRAPHY

Bayne, G. (1997). Vital signs: Are we monitoring the right parameters? *Nursing Management, 28*(5), 74–76.

McConnell, E. (1998). Automated vital signs monitoring devices. *Nursing Management, 29*(2), 49–51.

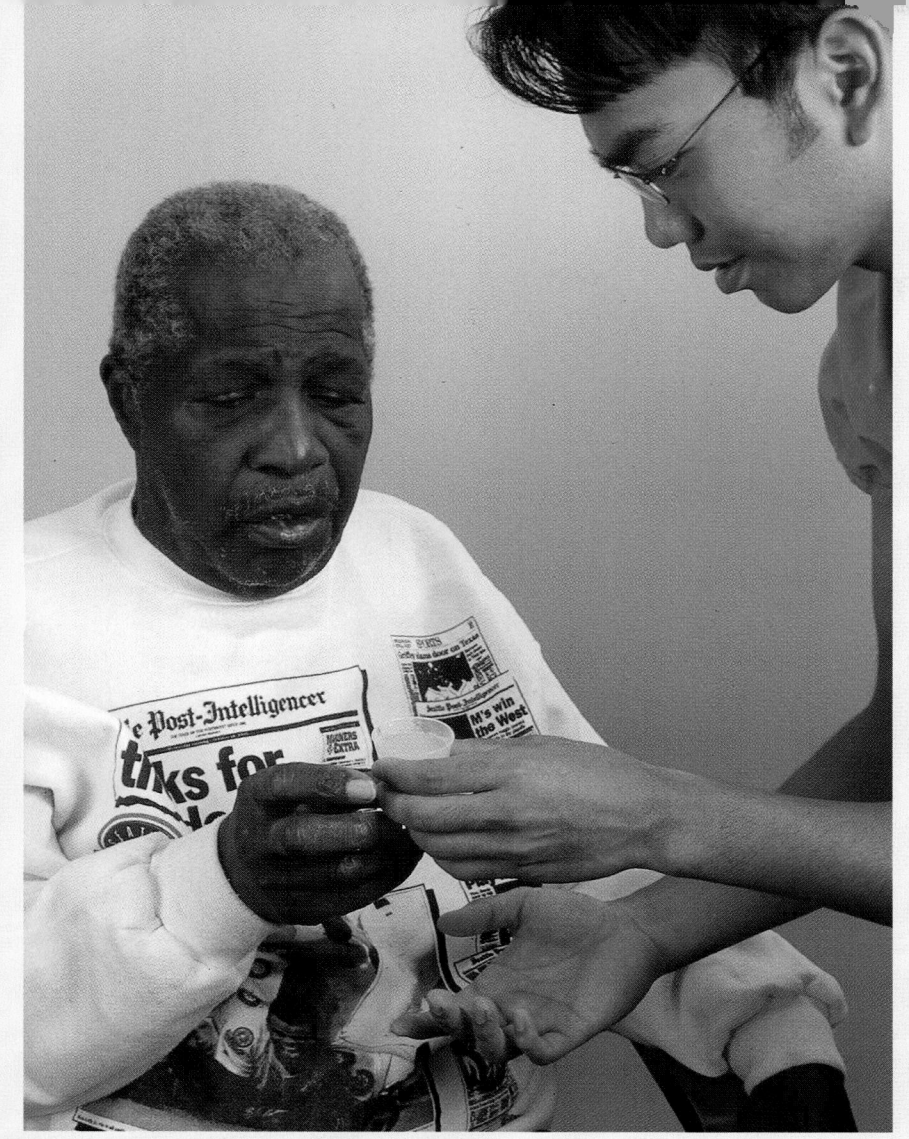

Unit 6

Selected Clinical
Nursing Therapeutics

Chapter

26 Asepsis and Infection Control

Key Terms

antiseptic
asepsis
autoclaving
bactericidal
bacteriostatic
carrier
disinfectant
infectious disease

isolation
medical asepsis
nosocomial infection
pathogens
sepsis
standard precautions
sterilization
surgical asepsis

Learning Objectives

Upon completion of this chapter, the student will be able to do the following:

1. Identify the six components of the chain of infection.
2. Explain examples of ways that infection may occur.
3. Describe factors that increase the risk of infection in various settings.
4. Discuss the role of healthcare personnel and health agencies in infection control.
5. Identify ways that caregivers can increase their protection against infectious exposure.
6. Explain ways that caregivers can decrease the exposure of clients to infection.
7. Differentiate between medical and surgical asepsis.
8. Demonstrate good handwashing technique, incorporating it as an integral part of practice.
9. Describe appropriate situations for using cleaning, disinfection, and sterilization.
10. Discuss the two-tier system of isolation.
11. Identify age-related considerations in preventing the transmission of infectious diseases.

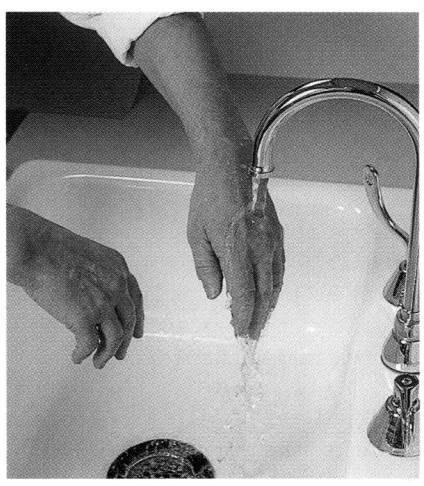

Critical Thinking Challenge

Your client is HIV positive and hospitalized with pneumonia. As you enter the room and start washing your hands, the client asks, "Why do so many of the staff wear gloves when they just come into the room to talk with me?"

Once you have completed this chapter and have incorporated asepsis and infection control into your knowledge base, review the above scenario and reflect on the following areas of Critical Thinking:

1. What Standard Precautions should healthcare workers use when entering a room to talk with a client who is infected with HIV?
2. Identify reasons why staff members may want to avoid this client and any unnecessary touching.
3. Reflect on possible ways to respond to this client. You want to acknowledge the client's concern, yet not act unethically.
4. Decide how you will talk with other members of the healthcare team about the client's observation and concerns. Explore possible ways to approach the subject with other staff members.

Regardless of where they practice, preventing the transmission of microorganisms is a concern of all nurses. One way that nurses accomplish this goal is by asepsis. **Asepsis** means to make free from disease-producing organisms. In homes, schools, clinics, industry, hospitals, and extended-care facilities, nurses strive to teach about, prevent, and treat infections. Promoting healthy lifestyles and preventive health practices is an important focus.

A large number of microorganisms live and multiply on every surface. They are in the air, grow on the skin, and flourish in the digestive tract. Certain microorganisms are necessary for normal body function. Some microorganisms help produce food and maintain the planet's ecology. Most of the time, humans and microorganisms live in harmony. When this balance is upset, however, microorganisms are capable of causing infection.

Infectious disease is the most common reason why people contact healthcare providers and accounts for more clinic and physician office visits than any other cause in the United States. Preventable infectious diseases are common worldwide, resulting in great suffering and the loss of many lives. The economic costs of preventing and treating infection are great. Recent years have shown an alarming increase in resistant organisms, such as tuberculosis and *Staphylococcus aureus,* that antibiotics can no longer easily eradicate. Recent outbreaks of *Escherichia coli,* the ebola virus, and the hantavirus underscore the need for precise infection control practices.

Nursing practice focuses on providing a safe and therapeutic environment to protect clients, family members, and healthcare providers from acquiring infections. The chapters on skin integrity and wound healing (see Chapter 38) and infection (see Chapter 39) provide additional information on specific infectious diseases and diagnostic and treatment procedures.

ROLE OF MICROORGANISMS IN INFECTION

Microorganisms that are capable of harming people are called **pathogens** or pathogenic. When pathogens enter and multiply within body tissues, they disrupt normal physiologic processes and produce an infection. The organisms or their toxins disrupt normal cell function or kill the cells entirely. **Sepsis,** a term that means poisoning of tissues, is often used to describe the presence of infection. Transport of an infection or the products of infection throughout the body by the blood is known as *septicemia.*

In common usage "infected" and "septic" are often used interchangeably. In most instances when a client is said to be infected, it means that he or she has a disease caused by microorganisms. When the client is referred to as septic, it means that he or she is displaying the manifestations of microbial destruction of tissues, such as high fever or hypotension.

Infectious disease refers to the pathology or pathologic events that result from the invasion and multiplication of microorganisms in a host. Toxins and enzymes produced by the microorganisms cause tissue injury. This injury produces manifestations of infection: fever; rashes; malaise; nausea and vomiting; diarrhea; purulent discharge from wounds; a hot, red, tender area around wounds or puncture sites; aches and pains; or total body collapse.

Healthcare practitioners devote a major portion of their time, energy, and talent to developing and maintaining practices to control the spread of microorganisms. These practices, known as aseptic techniques, are used in the broader context of infection control. Aseptic techniques, which start and end with handwashing, include the processes of cleaning, disinfection, and sterilization. The use of barriers to prevent the spread of microorganisms, such as gloves, masks, hair coverings, and gowns, as well as client isolation, is part of aseptic practice.

Agents Causing Infection

Bacteria
Bacteria are single-celled, independently living microorganisms, some of which are capable of causing disease in humans. Bacteria may be transmitted through air, food, water, soil, vectors, or sexual activity. They differ in size and shape, growth and replication requirements, and the method by which they inflict harm to the host. Some are capable of producing metabolic toxins, which they secrete into the host (exotoxin producers). Others can produce poisons that are contained in their cell walls and released after the death of the microorganism (e.g., gram-negative endotoxin producers). In addition, all bacteria are capable of diminishing organ function by invading tissues and initiating inflammation.

Viruses
Viruses are living microorganisms composed of particles of nucleic acid and protein that are often membrane bound. They reproduce inside living cells and cause various diseases. Some infections are acute and are controlled by the host's defense mechanisms; others spread throughout the body and cause severe tissue damage or result in chronic illness.

Fungi
Fungi are single-celled organisms that include molds and yeasts. *Candida albicans,* present as part of the normal human flora on mucous membranes and skin and in the gastrointestinal tract and vagina, can cause yeast infections of the mouth, skin, vagina, and intestinal tract in immunocompromised adults. Fungal infections of the hair, skin, and nails also frequently occur in humans. Fungi also infest and destroy plant life and cause fermentation in food and milk.

Parasites
Parasites are multicellular organisms that live on other organisms without contributing anything to their hosts. Examples of parasites include protozoa, helminth, and arthropod species. Sexual contact, insects, and domestic animals frequently carry parasites to humans.

Protozoa are free-living microorganisms that commonly thrive in water. Humans often contract diseases related to protozoa through unsanitary conditions surrounding food preparation or handling. Malaria and sleeping sickness are examples of diseases caused by protozoa. Helminths are worms that infect the gastrointestinal tract or other body tissues of humans. Examples of helminths include tapeworms, hookworms, and trichinae (or porkworm). Arthropods, including mites, fleas, and ticks, are often responsible for skin and systemic diseases.

Drug-Resistant Microbial Strains

Microbes, just like humans, adapt to an ever-changing environment to compete for survival. In the 1940s, strains of staphylococcus emerged that were immune to the antimicrobial activity of penicillin. Scientists developed new penicillins to treat these drug-resistant strains effectively. In the last few decades, increasing numbers of microbial organisms have developed drug-resistant strains. Specific resistant microbial strains causing a significant challenge to healthcare providers include methicillin-resistant *S. aureus* (MRSA), *Streptococcus pneumoniae*, *Klebsiella pneumoniae*, *Pseudomonas aeruginosa*, *Mycobacterium tuberculosis*, *Neisseria gonorrhoeae*, and *Enterococcus* species (Gold & Moellering, 1996; Tenover & Hughes, 1996; Edmund et al., 1999; Jacobs, 2000; Murthy, 2001). Factors that have contributed to the evolution of resistant microbial strains include the following:

- Overprescription of antibiotics
- Use of inappropriate antibiotics for the infecting organism
- Incomplete use of antibiotic prescriptions as symptoms subside
- Harboring and spreading of resistant organisms by carriers who remain symptom free, usually unaware that they have been infected
- Increased use of antibiotics in farming, thus contaminating milk and meat.

SAFETY ALERT

Drug-resistant microorganisms pose considerable health risks to the general population and specifically to healthcare workers. The infections they cause are increasingly difficult to treat and, in some cases, cannot be effectively destroyed by any known antibiotic. Using effective infection control practices is critical in these instances.

Chain of Infection

The life cycle of pathogens frequently is described as an uninterrupted chain of events. For organisms to spread disease, they must grow, reproduce, and move from one source to another. Nursing interventions are directed at stopping the transmission from the source to the client and at controlling other links in the chain, thereby controlling infection. The "chain of infection" includes the infectious agent, the source, the portal of exit, the mode of transmission, the portal of entry, and a susceptible host (Fig. 26-1).

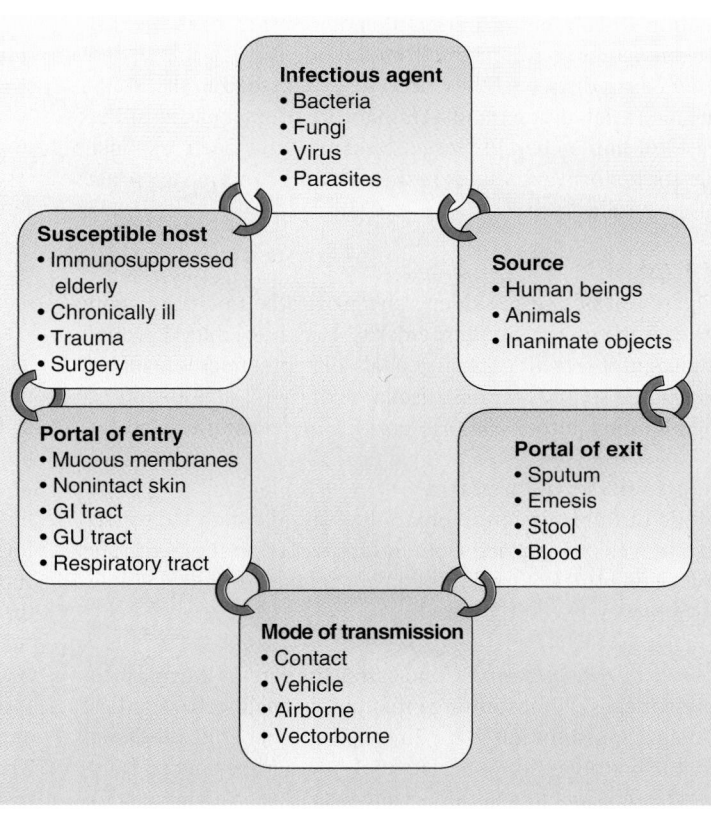

FIGURE 26-1   The chain of infection.

Infectious Agent

The first link in the chain of infection is the microbial agent, which may be a bacterium, virus, fungus, or parasite. The ability of the infectious agent to cause disease depends on its pathogenicity, virulence, invasiveness, and specificity. *Pathogenicity* is the organism's ability to harm and to cause disease. *Virulence* relates to the vigor with which the organism can grow and multiply. *Invasiveness* describes the organism's ability to enter tissues. *Specificity* refers to the organism's attraction to a specific host, which may include humans. The more pathogenic, virulent, and invasive the organism, the more likely that it can overcome normal body defenses, causing an infection. These four characteristics are determined by the structure or chemical composition of the microorganism, which includes the organism's ability to attach to skin and mucous membranes, the production of enzymes that counteract the immune system's response to invasion, and the production of toxins.

Source

The sources of organisms, also called reservoirs, are elements in the environment. Inanimate objects, human beings, and animals are sources. Inanimate objects include medications, air, food, water, or any other material on which organisms can find nourishment or lie dormant and survive. Human sources include other clients, healthcare personnel, family members, visitors, and clients themselves. Clients may become infected from people who have active disease, people in the incubation portion of their own disease, or people who harbor pathogens but have no symptoms of disease (known as **carriers**). A person's own bacterial flora may cause contamination when it is transferred to another organ or tissue. Endogenous microorganisms from the client's gastrointestinal tract cause disease if they become established in the lungs, urinary tract, or a wound. Animals are often sources of disease for human beings. Insects and rats have been responsible for historic epidemics in the past and continue to spread disease today.

Portal of Exit

The portal of exit provides a means for the microorganism to leave the source. Sputum, emesis, stool, urine, blood, wound drainage, or secretions from genitals all permit microorganisms to exit the source. Animal discharge or blood organisms carried by mosquitoes can also provide a means of escape.

Mode of Transmission

Mode of transmission refers to the way in which the organism moves or is carried from the source's portal of exit. The five main routes of transmission are contact, droplet, vehicle, airborne, and vectorborne.

Contact Transmission. Contact transmission is the most frequent means of transmitting infections in healthcare facilities. Contact transmission is by direct or indirect contact. Direct contact involves body surface–to–body surface contact causing the physical transfer of organisms between an infected or colonized person and a susceptible host. Healthcare personnel can transfer organisms to clients during care such as bathing, dressing changes, and inserting invasive devices. Direct transfer also may occur between two clients, with one acting as the source and the other as the host. Indirect contact occurs when a susceptible host is exposed to a contaminated object such as a dressing, needle, or surgical instrument.

Droplet Transmission. Droplet transmission may be considered a type of contact transmission. It occurs when mucous membranes of the nose, mouth, or conjunctiva are exposed to secretions of an infected person who is coughing, sneezing, or talking. It may be considered contact transmission because droplets do not remain suspended in the air for very long and seldom travel more than 3 feet.

Vehicle Transmission. Vehicle transmission involves the transfer of microorganisms by way of vehicles, or contaminated items that transmit pathogens. Food can carry *Salmonella,* water can carry *Legionella,* drugs can carry bacteria from contaminated infusion supplies, and blood can carry hepatitis and human immunodeficiency virus (HIV).

Airborne Transmission. Airborne transmission occurs when fine particles are suspended in the air for a long time or when dust particles contain pathogens. Air currents widely disperse organisms, which can be inhaled by or deposited on the skin of a susceptible host.

Vectorborne Transmission. Vectors can be biologic or mechanical. Biologic vectors are living animals, such as rats or insects, that carry pathogens. Transmission by biologic vectors is of great concern in tropical areas, where mosquitoes transmit diseases such as malaria. Mechanical vectors are inanimate objects that are contaminated with infected body fluids. Examples of mechanical vectors include contaminated needles and syringes shared by intravenous (IV) drug users. Both hepatitis B and HIV are commonly spread in this manner.

Portal of Entry

The portal of entry permits the organism to gain entrance into the host. Pathogens can enter susceptible hosts through body orifices such as the mouth, nose, ears, eyes, vagina, rectum, or urethra. Breaks in the skin or mucous membranes from wounds or abrasions increase opportunities for organisms to enter hosts. The practice in modern medicine of placing tubes for long-term IV or gastric feedings and drainage of body cavities further increases the number of potential routes of entry into the body, thus increasing the risk of infection.

Susceptible Host

A host is a person whose own body defense mechanisms, when exposed, are unable to withstand the invasion of pathogens. The body has numerous defense mechanisms that naturally resist entry and multiplication of pathogens. These factors are discussed in detail in Chapter 39. When infectious disease occurs in a human, the agent of infection has overcome the body's ability to resist infection. A primary focus of nursing practice is identifying clients whose defenses may be compromised and working to enhance their defenses.

Nosocomial Infections

Nosocomial infection refers to "hospital-acquired" infection but may be expanded to include infections acquired in other healthcare delivery settings. At times, the client is exposed to the infection while in the healthcare agency (i.e., hospital, clinic, long-term care center) but the disease does not always become apparent at that time. Each healthcare setting is unique, with its own set of risks for infection. Knowledge of the environment permits nurses to focus efforts on preventing the spread of infection.

Hospital-acquired infections, which number approximately 2 million per year in the United States and cost $4.5 billion annually, are the eleventh leading cause of death in the United States (Crow, 1998; Weinstein, 1998; Gaynes, 2001; Jarvis, 2001). The urinary tract is the most common site for nosocomial infections (34% to 40%). Additional sites are surgical wounds (17% to 24%), the respiratory tract (13%), the bloodstream (15%), and other sites including skin and subcutaneous tissues (21%) (Gaynes, 1998; Matrone et al., 1998; Weinstein, 1998; Burke & Zavasky, 1999; Wong, 1999).

Risk Factors in the Development of Nosocomial Infections

The longer a client is in a healthcare facility, the greater is his or her risk of infection. Exposure to the facility's environment changes the client's own normal body flora. Risk factors that contribute to the development of nosocomial infections can be grouped into three categories: environment, therapeutic regimen, and resistance of the client. They interact in varying patterns of importance, but all must be considered when making attempts to decrease the client's risk.

Environment. Hospitals, outpatient clinics, extended care facilities, the home, and schools are reservoirs of organisms that pose threats to the increasing number of clients who have decreased resistance. The sources of these organisms include the air, other clients, families and visitors, contaminated equipment, food, and personnel. Pneumonia and influenza can spread rapidly among clients and other people in all types of facilities. Equipment that is not thoroughly cleaned, disinfected, or sterilized can spread many pathogens.

Therapeutic Regimen. Multiple factors involved in therapies used to cure clients can also contribute to the risk of infection. Drugs such as steroids, immunosuppressive agents, and cancer therapy, as well as prolonged use of antibiotics, predispose clients to infection. Equipment such as IV catheters, indwelling urinary catheters, and feeding tubes that invade body orifices provide routes for bacterial invasion. Inadequate dressing techniques for wounds can provide media for bacterial growth. Identifying treatments that pose risk and discontinuing their use as soon as possible decrease the chances of nosocomial infection.

Client Resistance. Changes in the physical or psychological status of a client can affect his or her resistance to infection. Any break in the integrity of the skin or mucous membranes increases the chance of infection. Stress, fatigue, poor nutrition, and chronic illness can also decrease the client's ability to ward off infection. Adequate hygiene is important to decrease microorganisms on the skin that could contribute to infection risk.

Infection Risks in Various Healthcare Settings

Acute Care Settings. According to the National Nosocomial Infections Surveillance (NNIS) system of the Centers for Disease Control and Prevention (CDC), the rate of nosocomial infections in hospitals has remained stable over the past 25 years (Weinstein, 1998). There have been declines in some types of infections, but they have been replaced with increases in infections in compromised clients. As people live longer, more extensive surgeries are performed, and more technology is used, rates are expected to rise in the future. This increase in nosocomial infection rates will not only increase healthcare costs but will also place clients at risk for acquiring difficult-to-treat, drug-resistant pathogens.

Extended Care Facilities. Nursing homes, psychiatric care facilities, drug and alcohol treatment centers, and group homes for the mentally or physically impaired are associated with high risks for infection. The most frequent infections that occur in long-term care facilities are urinary tract infections, pneumonia, and skin and soft tissue infections (Makris et al., 2000). Frequently such institutions are understaffed, and available personnel may lack extensive training in infection control measures. Residents, sometimes debilitated from chronic medical or psychiatric conditions, may be incapable of maintaining their own personal hygiene. Communicable diseases are common in these facilities, with the underlying medical problems of clients often placing them at risk for infections. Additionally, many older clients do not mount a febrile response

---

APPLY YOUR KNOWLEDGE

You are making a home visit to a single mother with three children younger than 5 years of age. When you arrive, the mother tells you that the oldest child has had a fever for 2 days, is lethargic, and has little appetite. After assessing the child, you suspect that he has influenza. Based on your knowledge that influenza is an airborne communicable disease, what health teaching regarding infection transmission is appropriate for the mother and family at this time?
Check your answer in Appendix A.

to infection, and increasing agitation or confusion in response to infection may be dismissed as "normal" signs of aging. Also, the immunization status of older adults and other facility residents may not be kept up to date.

Ambulatory Care Settings.   Clients come to ambulatory care settings for wellness visits, diagnoses, and treatment of health problems. Procedures used by personnel frequently involve invasive techniques that increase the risk of infection. Waiting rooms in such facilities may contain people with active infections, increasing the risk for infection. This is especially true for pediatric clinics, where children who are ill often come in contact with well children. Children frequently play with office toys or interact with one another, thus increasing the risk for infection.

Home Care.   Clients being discharged to home care can be seriously ill, requiring sophisticated invasive treatments to be performed in the home setting. Treatments such as indwelling urinary catheters, IV infusions for medications or nutrition, and care of extensive open wounds and drainage collection systems are being seen more frequently in the home setting, providing numerous opportunities for infection. Because people in the home are assuming the primary responsibility for these treatments, they need teaching about how to perform prescribed procedures using aseptic practices to reduce the client's risk. People also must learn how to care for family members with communicable illnesses and to prevent spread.

Schools.   Classrooms, athletic departments, and school health clinics pose risks of infection to students and their teachers. The incidence of communicable illness is high among children who are grouped together for study and play. Schools often employ nurses to teach health classes and to develop and monitor infection control practices and outbreaks of communicable diseases. Their responsibility also includes evaluating children who may be infectious to help ensure their proper treatment.

Workplace.   Employees are exposed to, and can expose their coworkers to, infections. Working conditions and materials that workers use may carry infectious risks. Farmers and other people who work with animals have a high risk of contracting diseases carried by animals. Sinks, bathrooms, lunchrooms, and food utensils may be sources of infection in the workplace. Many industries employ nurses to screen employees for communicable diseases, to collaborate with building maintenance personnel to maintain hygienic conditions, and to supervise waste disposal.

INFECTION CONTROL

Prevention and control of infections are important concerns for all types of healthcare agencies. Acute care hospitals have organized infection control programs. The infection control practitioner is usually a nurse with advanced training in infection

control practices and methods for tracking the source and spread of infections (epidemiologic studies). Each department in the hospital must have written policies and procedures for the control of infection. Caregivers and support personnel (e.g., housekeepers, transport personnel) must have periodic educational updates on infection control, usually mandated annually. Various state and federal regulatory agencies require other healthcare facilities to have infection control policies.

Several studies have demonstrated cost savings to healthcare facilities that practice good infection control (Jarvis, 1996; Kotilainen & Keroack, 1997; Haley, 1998). Approximately one third of the 2.1 million nosocomial infections annually can be prevented with effective infection control programs (Matrone, 1998).

Regulatory Agencies

Several local, state, regional, provincial, and national agencies are involved in the control of institutional safety designed to protect clients, staff, and the community from infectious disease. Physician's offices, school nurses, health clinics, extended care facilities, and various acute care facilities must report episodes of infection to these agencies. Agency statistics on the incidence of the disease in the area provide practitioners with information on control and treatment.

Both the CDC and the Joint Committee on Accreditation of Healthcare Organizations (JCAHO) publish guidelines for storage, cleaning and disinfection, and use of equipment and supplies. JCAHO sets requirements to which healthcare agencies must adhere to obtain accreditation. The CDC does basic research on infectious disease and conducts large multicenter studies on data gathered by local centers. The Occupational Safety and Health Administration (OSHA) of the U.S. Department of Labor develops standards and regulations to protect the safety and health of workers (see Chapter 30).

Healthcare agencies and practitioners are responsible for reporting diseases to appropriate agencies as required by law. Guidelines as to what is a reportable disease vary according to location and circumstance. Good communication and rapport among clinical and regulatory agencies are necessary to optimize infection control and to prevent severe outbreaks of infectious disease.

Employee Health

Healthcare agencies maintain personnel health service programs as part of their infection control programs. Infection control nurses are often involved in employee education programs. The objectives of such programs include stressing good health practices in diet, exercise, rest, and personal hygiene; monitoring and investigating potentially harmful infectious exposures and outbreaks of infections among personnel; providing care to personnel for work-related illnesses or exposures; identifying the infection risks related to employment; and instituting appropriate measures for preventing exposure and transmission of infectious disease.

Monitoring and Counseling of Personnel

Almost all institutions require a personal health and safety education lecture as part of the orientation process and on an annual or semiannual basis. Some institutions require laboratory screening for high-risk diseases and offer their employees routine immunization programs. Mechanisms for prompt diagnosis and management of job-related illnesses and provision for prophylaxis of preventable diseases are important to ensure the health of all employees.

Access to health counseling about infections is especially important for women of childbearing age. Pregnant nurses may not be allowed to care for clients who have diseases that pose risks to unborn babies. Among the diseases that pose particular risks to fetuses if contracted by pregnant women are rubella, hepatitis B, herpes simplex virus, varicella-zoster virus, cytomegalovirus, and HIV (Strodtbeck, 1995).

SAFETY ALERT
Inform any personnel who are or who might become pregnant about potential risks to the fetus due to work assignments and about preventive measures that reduce those risks.

Transmissible Diseases

Because hospital personnel are at risk for contracting and transmitting vaccine-preventable diseases, maintenance of current immunization status is a good health practice. Employees who work in high-risk areas, such as pediatric, dialysis, or transplantation units, usually are required to prove that their immunization status is current as a condition of employment. Chapter 39 contains a list of available vaccines and their effectiveness.

Significant Exposure

Institutional policies and employee restrictions are designed to prevent exposure to and contraction of infectious disease. Any "significant" exposure is investigated to protect employees, clients, and the institution. An exposure's significance is determined by the type and duration of exposure, with consideration of the mode of transmission, whether the host was susceptible, and whether precautions were taken. Exposures to hepatitis, rubella, meningococcal meningitis, tuberculosis, varicella (chickenpox), and HIV are commonly investigated by the infection control nurse. Most exposures require timely reporting by staff members to expedite prophylaxis (if any is available) and to qualify for labor and industry insurance coverage should an illness result. If an employee contracts an infectious disease, it must be reported to the local health department.

Needlesticks. One of the most frequently occurring and potentially serious exposures for healthcare personnel is from needlestick injuries, which may transmit organisms that cause bloodborne diseases, such as hepatitis or acquired immunodeficiency syndrome (AIDS). Accidental needlesticks account for almost one third of all healthcare accidents and billions of dollars in liability and treatment costs. Approximately 800,000 needlestick injuries occur annually to U.S. healthcare workers (Pugliese, 1997, 2000; Rogers, 1997; Reed, 2000).

A significant number of all needlestick injuries (30% to 40%) result from recapping needles after their contact with blood from a client (e.g., after an injection, drawing blood, or starting an IV line (Rogers, 1997; Roudot-Thoraval et al., 1999). In the past, used needles were recapped, bent, or broken. The CDC strongly advises all institutions to educate their employees as to the dangers of these practices (Fig. 26-2). Puncture-proof, plastic units for safe needle disposal (uncapped) immediately after their use are provided in all client care areas (Fig. 26-3). Needle-housing systems and new needleless systems have been developed to decrease the incidence of needlesticks (Fig. 26-4). Several studies have documented a decreased rate of needlestick injuries when needleless systems are used (Cardo & Bell, 1997; Beekman et al., 2001).

Gloves. Gloves cannot protect all personnel in every situation, but increased use of gloves during contact with all mucous membranes, nonintact skin, and moist body substances, in combination with good handwashing practices, makes a difference in cross-contamination between clients and staff. Gloves must be discarded and reapplied between clients to avoid spreading microorganisms from one client to another.

Work Restriction

Ill healthcare employees should not be in contact with clients if their illnesses pose threats to clients or other personnel. Agencies should have well-defined policies directed at restricting or limiting work for personnel with potentially transmissible diseases. Table 26-1 lists the conditions requiring relief from direct client contact or partial work restriction.

SAFETY ALERT
Strongly urge all personnel with diseases characterized by profuse coughing, sneezing, or frequent diarrhea to stay home from work and to care for themselves.

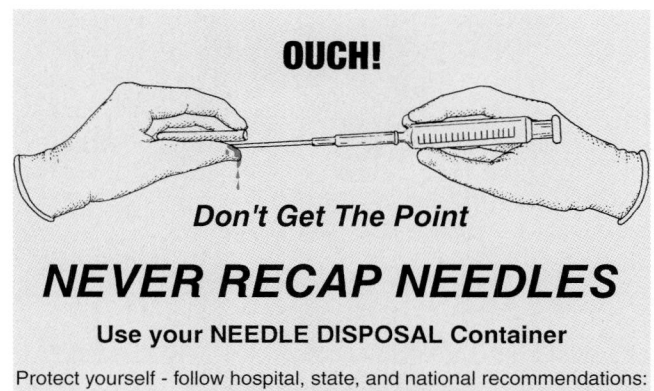

FIGURE 26-2   Sample needlestick hazard poster.

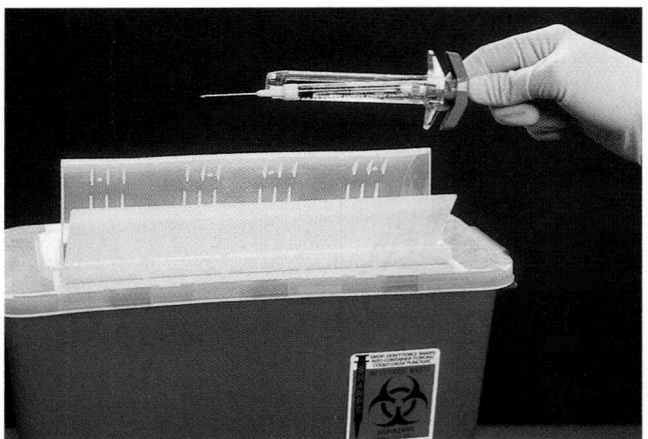

FIGURE 26-3   Disposal container for contaminated sharps.

Healthcare Workers with AIDS. Personnel considered to have any of the clinical features associated with the AIDS spectrum should be counseled about the risks they pose to clients and to themselves in the work environment. Healthcare workers who perform invasive procedures in which a

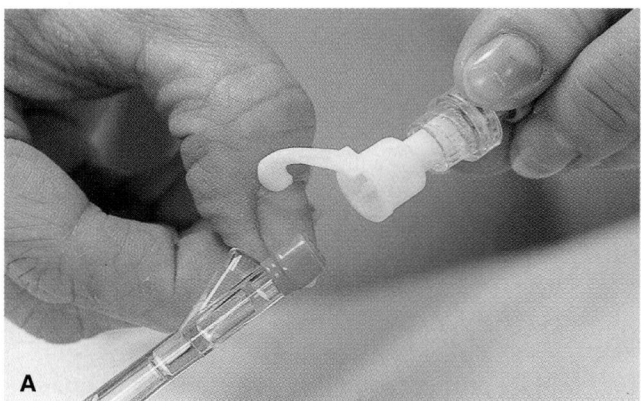

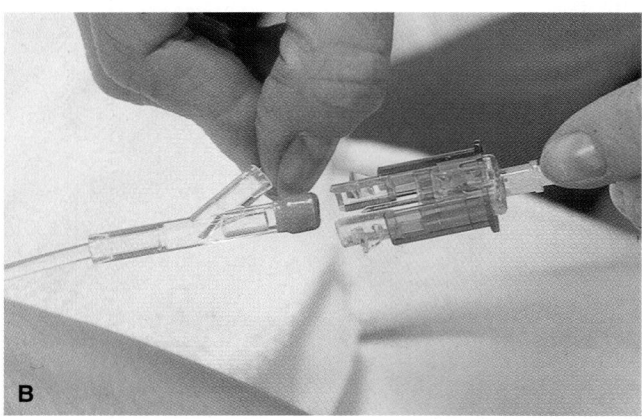

FIGURE 26-4   New systems have been developed to prevent needlestick injuries. **(A)** Needleless system—no needles are used, so stick injuries are avoided. **(B)** Needle housing system keeps the needle within a sheath to limit needlesticks.

needlestick or scalpel injury would expose their blood to that of the client's pose the greatest risk. *All personnel with AIDS should wear gloves for direct contact with mucous membranes or nonintact skin of all clients. Any healthcare worker with AIDS and exudative lesions or weeping dermatitis should refrain from all direct care and handling of client care equipment until the lesions clear* (CDC, 1987, 1988). All healthcare workers with AIDS need to be meticulous in adhering to infection control practices.

HIV impairs the immune system, making people with AIDS more likely to acquire infectious diseases or to experience more serious complications. These staff members should be counseled about potential risks to themselves as well.

Waste Disposal

Several regulatory agencies are involved in identifying and directing acceptable practices for collecting, transporting, and disposing of wastes. Local health agencies and the JCAHO require hospitals to develop programs for disposal of wastes categorized as infectious, injurious, or hazardous to employees, clients, visitors, the general public, and the environment. Display 26-1 lists common materials within each category of institutional waste for which proper waste disposal protocol must be followed. Most waste that hospitals produce is not infectious, injurious, or hazardous. Safe waste includes paper, plastic, metal, and glass products used for a multitude of purposes within the healthcare agency.

A great deal of controversy exists about hospital waste products, much of it caused by the public's fear of HIV infection. The CDC has maintained that hospital waste in general is no more infectious than residential waste. Current CDC recommendations are for incineration or autoclaving of infectious waste before disposal in a sanitary landfill (CDC, 1996). Liquid body fluids (blood, urine, aspirated body fluids) can be flushed down a drain connected to a sewer system. Healthcare agencies use separate waste containers, clearly marked "Biohazard," for infectious waste, such as blood-contaminated items (Fig. 26-5). Because the cost of contaminated waste disposal is great, it is important not to dispose of all waste in such containers.

Another public health concern is the use of disposable diapers for infants and geriatric clients. Although most commercial packages advise rinsing the diaper in the toilet before disposal into garbage containers, it is known that there is little institutional or residential compliance with this advice. The result is millions of tons of carefully wrapped urine or feces lying in sanitary landfills in nonbiodegradable plastic.

ASEPTIC PRACTICES

The dramatic reduction in the incidence of infectious disease that occurred during the late 1800s and early 1900s resulted largely from the understanding that microorganisms cause disease and that they can be controlled through aseptic practices. Established control methods include use of physical agents, such as disinfectants, on agents outside the body; use

TABLE 26-1

Infectious Conditions Requiring Work Restriction	
Infectious Condition	**Direct Client Care Restrictions and Duration**
Conjunctivitis	Until discharge ceases
Diarrhea (with other acute symptoms)	Until symptoms resolve and *Salmonella* infection is ruled out
Hepatitis A	Until 7 days after the onset of jaundice
Hepatitis B (acute)	Partial client care restriction with gloves worn for procedures involving tissue trauma and mucous membrane or nonintact skin contact
Hepatitis B (chronic)	Until antigenemia resolves
Group A streptococcal infection	Until 24 hours after the start of treatment
Herpes simplex (hands)	Until lesions resolve
Herpes zoster (acute)	Exclusion from care of clients at high risk for infection with use of appropriate barriers
Herpes zoster (postexposure)	From days 10 to 21 after exposure or until all lesions dry and crust
Measles (active)	Until 7 days after rash appears
Measles (postexposure)	From days 5 to 21 after exposure
Mumps (active)	Until 9 days after onset of parotitis
Mumps (postexposure)	From days 12 to 26 after exposure
Rubella (active)	Until 5 days after rash appears
Rubella (postexposure)	From days 7 to 21 after exposure
Scabies	Until treated
Staphylococcus aureus skin lesions	Until lesions resolve
Upper respiratory tract infections	Until acute symptoms resolve with exclusion from care of clients at high risk for infection
Varicella (acute)	Until all lesions dry and crust
Varicella (postexposure)	From days 10 to 21 after exposure

ETHICAL/LEGAL ISSUE
Needlesticks

On a clinical rotation as a nursing student, you accidentally stick yourself with a lancet after you perform a capillary fingerstick to obtain a blood glucose level for your client. Your client is 86 years old and has been healthy most of his life but now has been hospitalized with cardiovascular problems and diabetes.

Reflection
- Explore your concerns after the needlestick injury. What risks are there (if any) for you and for the client?
- When you disclose the incident to your clinical instructor, she explains that you and the client must have blood drawn so that testing can be done to make certain you have not been exposed to bloodborne pathogens. You are worried about money and realize these tests will cost more than $100. Do you have the right to refuse testing? Weigh the consequences of having the testing versus not having the testing.
- If testing is done, what measures need to be taken to protect your confidentiality and that of the client?
- Think about measures you or the agency could take to prevent this type of incident from happening in the future.

DISPLAY 26-1

⑤ CATEGORIES OF INSTITUTIONAL WASTE

Infectious Waste
Blood and blood products
Pathology laboratory specimens
Laboratory cultures
Body parts from surgery
Contaminated equipment (e.g., dialysis materials, suction receptacles)
Food
Unrinsed infant and adult diapers

Injurious Waste
Needles
Scalpel blades
Lancets
Broken glass
Pipettes
Aerosol cans

Hazardous Waste
Radioactive materials
Chemotherapy solutions and their containers
Caustic chemicals

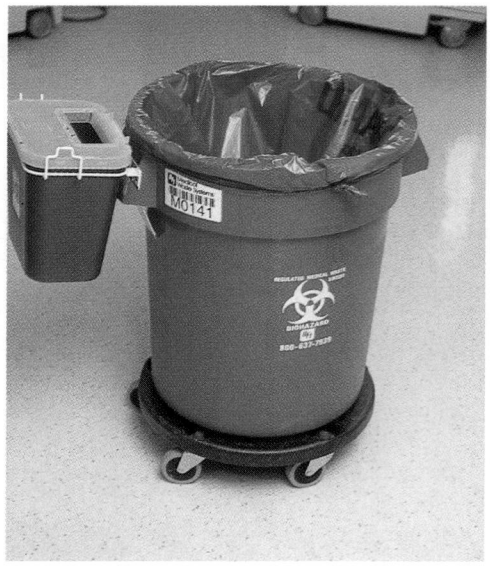

FIGURE 26-5   Waste container used for infectious waste in a dialysis unit.

of chemical agents, such as antiseptics, on inanimate objects and on the body surface; and use of chemotherapeutic agents, such as antibiotics, to combat microorganisms on body surfaces and inside the body.

The two major categories of aseptic practice are medical asepsis and surgical asepsis. **Medical asepsis** refers to measures taken to control and to reduce the number of pathogens present. It is also known as "clean technique." Measures used to prevent the spread of organisms from place to place include handwashing, gloving, gowning, and disinfecting to help contain microbial growth. **Surgical asepsis** refers to "sterile technique." To be sterile, an object must be free of all microorganisms. Sterile technique is used to prevent the introduction or spread of pathogens from the environment into the client. Sterile technique is employed when a body cavity is entered with an object that may damage the mucous membranes, when surgical procedures are performed, and when the client's immune system is already compromised. Procedures requiring sterile technique include insertion of IV catheters, injections, urinary catheterization, irrigation of drainage tubes that enter sterile parts of the body, and all operative procedures.

For clients whose immune systems are compromised, certain procedures that normally would require clean technique should be performed using sterile technique. Premature newborns, burn clients, transplant recipients, and clients receiving chemotherapy or radiation are examples of groups for whom sterile technique for otherwise clean technique procedures may be necessary.

Handwashing

Even with the emphasis on use of gloves for contact with client secretions, nothing is more effective in preventing the spread of infection than handwashing. It is also the least expensive method for decreasing the risk of infecting oneself or others.

Contact transmission, from the hands of healthcare personnel or the clients themselves, is the most common form of contamination because microorganisms are transient flora until the hands are washed. Both soap and water and alcohol-based handrubs are effective preparations for removing transient microorganisms (Larson et al., 2000). Experts agree and studies have demonstrated that handwashing can reduce nosocomial infections, but compliance typically ranges between 10% and 60% (Larson & Kretzer, 1995; Voss & Widmer, 1997; Pittet, 1999). Particularly important are the techniques of washing the entire hand and using paper towels (Larson, 1995; Boyce, 1996; Sneddon et al., 1997; Voss & Widmer, 1997; Ward, 2000).

🔳 SAFETY ALERT
Proper handwashing is the single most effective method to prevent nosocomial infections (Patterson, 1996).

Equipment necessary for handwashing (soap, running water, and paper towels) is inexpensive and should be readily available to all healthcare providers. High-risk areas, such as nurseries; critical care, transplantation, and burn units; and operative suites, may also require the use of antiseptic cleansing agents, nail files or sticks, and antiseptic-impregnated scrub brushes.

Wash hands before and after every client care contact. The use of gloves during client care does not eliminate the need for handwashing. Wash your hands in the following situations:

- At the beginning and end of your shift
- Before contact with a client
- Between contacts with different clients
- Before and after contact with wounds, dressings, specimens, or bedclothes
- Before performing any invasive procedure
- Before administering medications
- After contact with any client secretion or excretion
- Before and after using the bathroom
- After sneezing, coughing, or blowing your nose
- After removing gloves
- Before eating

Medical and surgical asepsis vary in the technique for proper handwashing. Handwashing done to ensure medical asepsis is described in Procedure 26-1. Handwashing for surgical asepsis usually is longer and more methodical. Special antimicrobial agents also are used. These variations are usually defined by institutional protocols. During a surgical scrub of the hands, the hands are held higher than the elbows to avoid contamination from water running back from the forearms to the hands. Studies have demonstrated that effectiveness of handwashing is determined by adequate friction, thoroughness of surfaces cleansed, and minimum duration of use, rather than the particular cleansing agent employed (Kerr, 1998).

Most long-term flora on the hands reside in the nailbed and under the fingernails. Pay special attention to these areas, and

(text continues on page 491)

PROCEDURE 26-1

HANDWASHING

Purpose
1. Reduce the numbers of resident and transient bacteria on the hands.
2. Prevent transfer of microorganisms from the environment to the client and from the client to healthcare personnel.

Assessment
- Inspect hands for breaks or cuts in skin or cuticles.
- Identify appropriate times for handwashing before and after client contact.
- Identify need to repeat handwashing if hands become contaminated during a procedure.

Equipment
Warm, running water
Soap (Most agencies supply liquid soaps, containing a germicidal agent, in dispensers at each sink.)
Paper towels

Procedure
1. Remove all rings except a plain wedding band. Push watch 4 to 5 inches above wrist.
   Rationale: Microorganisms lodge in the irregular surfaces of jewelry.
2. Turn on the water and adjust temperature to warm. Do not splash water or lean against the wet sink.
   Note: Faucets may be controlled by your hands or may be operated by knee levers or foot pedals.
   Rationale: Warm water removes fewer protective oils from the skin than does hot water and reduces chapping of hands from frequent handwashing. Microorganisms need moisture to thrive. Avoid water splashing and sink contact with clothing to prevent contamination.

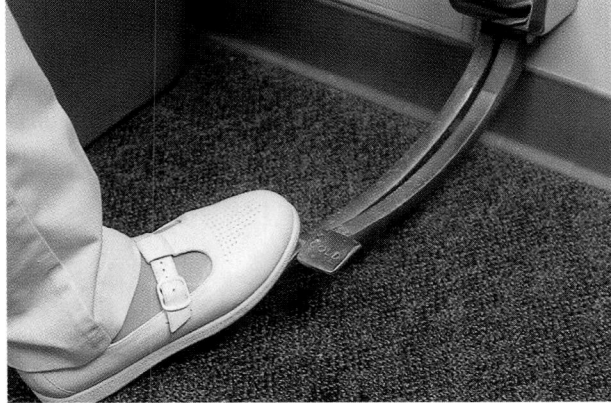

Step 2 Foot pedals may be available to turn on water.

3. Hold hands lower than elbows and thoroughly wet hands and lower arms under running water.
   Rationale: Hands are more contaminated than lower arms; water should flow from least to most contaminated areas.

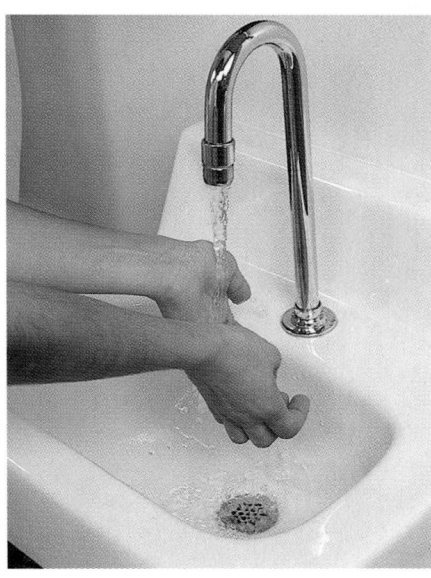

Step 3 Wet hands, holding wrists below elbow.

4. Apply soap and rub palms, wrists, and back of hands firmly with circular movements. Interlace fingers and thumbs, moving hands back and forth. Continue using plenty of lather and friction for 15 to 30 seconds on each hand. Timing of scrub may vary depending on purpose of wash and amount of contamination.
   Rationale: Friction mechanically loosens and removes dirt and microorganisms on all hand surfaces.
5. Clean under fingernails using fingernails of other hand and additional soap. Use orangewood stick if available.
   Rationale: Microorganisms are frequently harbored under nails.
6. Rinse hands and wrists thoroughly with hands held lower than forearms.
   Rationale: Rinsing washes away microorganisms and dirt and prevents recontamination of clean skin surfaces.

PROCEDURE 26-1 (Continued)

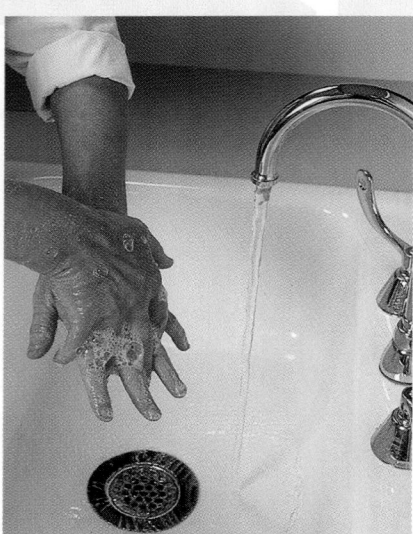

Step 4 Lather soap using friction.

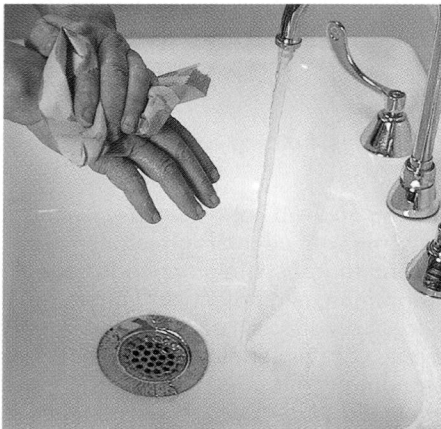

Step 7 Dry hands with paper towel.

7. Dry hands and arms thoroughly with paper towel, wiping from fingertips toward forearm. Discard in proper receptacle.
   Rationale: Drying hands prevents chapping and cracking of skin. Dry from cleanest area (fingertips) toward least clean area to reduce chances of contamination.

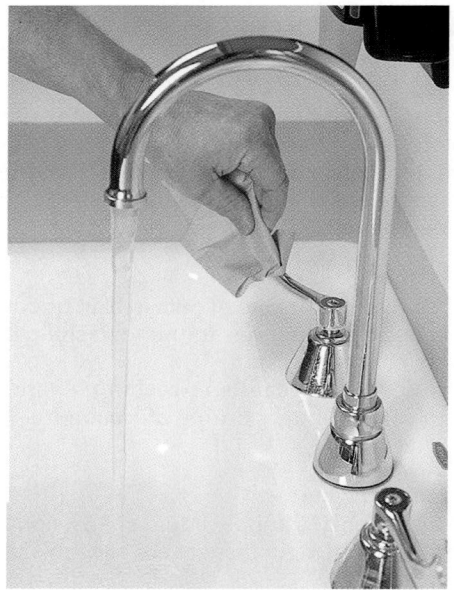

Step 8 Turn off faucet with clean paper towel.

8. Turn off water using clean, dry paper towel on faucets.
   Rationale: Paper towel prevents transfer of microorganisms from faucet to hands.

Home Care Modifications
- Bring bactericidal soap in a plastic container and paper towels with you to the client's home.
- If running water is unavailable, use disposable washcloths or alcohol as an alternative to handwashing. Both of these agents are drying to the hands if used often. Remember to still wash with soap and water as often and as soon as possible.

Collaboration and Delegation
- All healthcare personnel are responsible for following appropriate handwashing technique during care delivery. Monitoring and reminding one another are important to ensure 100% compliance.

use soft sticks or fingernails from the opposite hand to clean them. Keep fingernails short, and avoid nail polish, because cracked or chipped nail polish can harbor bacteria that ordinary handwashing cannot reach. Artificial fingernails present similar reservoirs for infectious agents. Ideally, remove all rings before handwashing and place them in pockets or pin them to the uniform during client care to minimize the potential places for harboring bacteria. If you wear a thin wedding band, slide it up on the finger to cleanse the area under the ring properly.

If the hands become dry or cracked or develop dermatitis, a person may be less apt to wash them as often as necessary. This problem is a frequent complication for people with sensitive skin. Switching to another soap or antiseptic solution, thoroughly drying after every washing, and using skin lotion may help.

SAFETY ALERT
Always wear gloves during client care when your skin is abraded.

All healthcare personnel, clients, and their family members should learn proper handwashing technique. Provide clients with materials to wash their hands before and after toileting. Instruct all visitors to wash their hands before contact with clients and before leaving a client's room. If infection is to be controlled, the paramount importance of adequate hand-washing cannot be stressed too often, no matter how unsophisticated it may seem.

Cleaning, Disinfection, and Sterilization

The removal of potentially pathogenic microorganisms is accomplished by disinfection and sterilization. Cleaning precedes disinfection and sterilization.

Cleaning

Cleaning refers to the physical removal of visible dirt and debris by washing, dusting, or mopping surfaces that are contaminated. Soap, manufactured from fats and chemicals, is used for mechanical cleaning. A lather forms that emulsifies fats and lifts off dirt and other materials and can be rinsed away. Because intact skin is an effective barrier to most microorganisms, items that come in contact with intact skin need not be sterile. Items such as blood pressure cuffs, linens, bedside tables, and room furniture can be cleaned and reused.

Disinfection

Disinfection refers to chemical or physical processes used to reduce the numbers of potential pathogens on an object's surface. These processes do not necessarily remove all potential for infection, because spores, capable of growing at a later time, may remain. A chemical used on lifeless objects is called

---

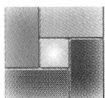

Nursing Research and Critical Thinking

What Interventions Have the Greatest Effects on Increasing the Frequency of Handwashing Among Elementary School Children?

A group of nurses wanted to assess the effectiveness of several interventions on increasing the frequency of handwashing among elementary school children. They designed a study to test four handwashing interventions in five schools: a peer educational program; an introduction of hand wipes with an instructional poster in bathrooms; a combination of the educational program and hand wipes; and a comparison school that had no intervention. Participants in the study were first graders and fourth graders from jurisdictions within a mid-Atlantic metropolitan area. Phase I of the study included a baseline assessment of bathroom cleanliness and adequacy of supplies for handwashing in each school. Phase II included observation and recording of the frequency proportion of handwashing before lunch or after bathroom use during a 2-month period. The researchers compared the preintervention and postintervention handwashing frequencies for each intervention group (wipes; .50 vs .66, $P < .03$; education only, .64 vs .72, $P < .02$; education and wipes, .45 vs .67, $P < .03$;

control group, .42 vs .46; $P < .26$). The researchers concluded from this study that education combined with accessible, convenient hand hygiene materials may result in a sustainable increase in the frequency of handwashing among elementary school children.

Critical Thinking Considerations. Community-based research is complex, presenting both administrative and feasibility challenges. Although uniform enthusiasm for the project existed among school officials and teachers, the researchers say that it took months to negotiate through various school systems. Implications of this study are as follows:

- Education alone was not effective in increasing the frequency of handwashing over time.
- Education combined with accessible, convenient hand hygiene products may result in a sustainable increase in the frequency of handwashing among elementary school children.

From Early, E., Battle, K., Cantwell, E., English, J., Lavin, J. E., & Larson, E. (1998). Effect of several interventions on the frequency of handwashing among elementary public school children. *American Journal of Infection Control, 26*(3), 263–269.

a **disinfectant.** A chemical used on living objects is called an **antiseptic.** Solutions that are disinfectants at higher concentrations may be diluted to be used as antiseptics on living objects. A chemical is **bactericidal** if it kills microorganisms; an agent that prevents bacterial multiplication but does not kill all forms of the organism is called **bacteriostatic.** To be useful, the method chosen must kill or retard growth of the pathogens without damaging the material or person being treated.

Any item that may come in contact with mucous membranes or with skin that is not intact must be free of all microorganisms, with the exception of spores. Respiratory therapy and anesthesia equipment, thermometers, and gastrointestinal endoscopes are examples of items that are disinfected. Table 26-2 lists common disinfectants and antiseptics along with their typical uses. The CDC is an excellent resource for information on the use of these chemicals in relation to objects and humans and the level of disinfection they produce.

Sterilization

Sterilization refers to the complete destruction of all microorganisms, including spores, leaving no viable forms of organisms. Sterilization processes are caustic because they require extremes of heat, potent chemicals, or gas that cannot be used on body tissues. Any process used to sterilize equipment must be effective in killing organisms but not destructive to the equipment.

Most items are purchased as sterile or are sterilized by autoclaving. If the items might be destroyed by the heat used during autoclaving, ethylene oxide gas or chemical solutions may be used. The two most popular methods are steam sterilization and gas sterilization with ethylene oxide. Other sterilization methods include dry heat and ionizing radiation.

Steam Sterilization. Supersaturated steam under pressure, known as **autoclaving,** is the most widely used and dependable method of sterilization. It is nontoxic, inexpensive, sporicidal, and able to penetrate fabrics rapidly. Chemical indicators, which change color when the object being sterilized has been exposed to steam penetration for a specific period, are placed outside and inside the object's package. This practice enables the healthcare worker to know when sterilization of an object has been effective (Fig. 26-6). Contamination can occur at a later time, so packaging should be checked for integrity. Because the object is considered sterile only for a specified period, always check the expiration date.

Gas Sterilization. Ethylene oxide is used to sterilize medical products that cannot be steam sterilized. This colorless gas can penetrate plastic, rubber, cotton, and other substances. Articles must be left to release the gas through aeration before they are used. Liquids may not be sterilized by this process because ethylene oxide is absorbed and not released. This type of sterilization is expensive and requires 2 to 5 hours to be accomplished. In addition, proper safety precautions must be used to prevent exposure of workers to the gas.

Use of Barriers

Techniques that prevent the transfer of pathogens from one person to another are referred to as "barriers." Their aim is to contain pathogens by establishing aseptic barriers around the client and personnel. The most commonly used barriers

SAFETY ALERT

Remember that any item entering sterile tissues or the vascular system, such as surgical instruments, cardiac and urinary catheters, implants, IV fluids, and needles, must be sterile.

TABLE 26-2

Common Disinfectants and Antiseptics		
Agent	**Kills**	**Uses**
Disinfectants		
Chlorine	Most microbes	Countertops and floors
Formaldehyde (formalin)	Bacteria, spores, virus, fungi	Hemodialysis units
Glutaraldehyde	Bacteria	Endoscopes, anesthesia and respiratory equipment
Antiseptics		
Povidone–iodine	Bacteria	Skin decontamination, wound packing, and irrigation
Sodium hypochlorite (Dakin's)	Bacteria, yeasts	Wound irrigation and packing
Chlorhexidine gluconate (Hibiclens)	Gram-positive organisms	Skin scrubs and irrigation
Acetic acid	*Pseudomonas*	Cleaning, packing, irrigating wounds
Hydrogen peroxide (3%)	Decomposes necrotic tissue	Wound irrigation, cleansing of pus and necrotic tissue
Alcohol	Bacteria	Skin prep before injections
Hexachlorophene	Bacteria	Handwashing, skin prep; must be washed off to avoid neurotoxicity

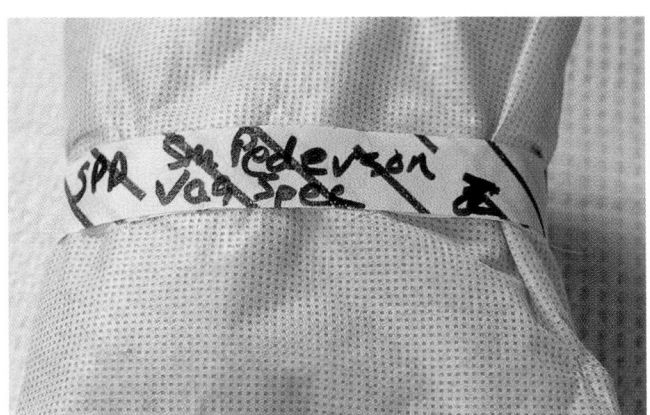

FIGURE 26-6 Color indicator strips change color, indicating that sterilization has occurred.

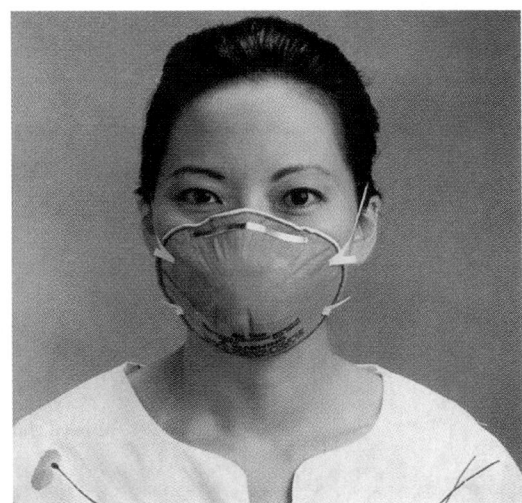

FIGURE 26-7 Particulate respirator fits tightly to the face and filters out organisms as small as 1 μm.

are masks, gowns, gloves, private rooms, waterproof disposal bags for linen and trash, labeling and bagging of contaminated equipment and specimens, and control of airflow into sterile areas and out of contaminated areas. With the advent of AIDS, goggles or face shields have been added to the list, as well as check valves on masks used in mouth-to-mouth resuscitation. Staff awareness about the need to prevent cross-contamination of people, equipment, and supplies is most important.

Some facilities that treat severely immunocompromised clients use laminar flow units that totally isolate clients from the environment. Plastic curtains are assembled in a box around a client's bed and connected to a system that filters the air entering the enclosed space. Ports with sleeves for covering the caregivers' arms are built into the sides of the unit. Some institutions have specially designed laminar flow rooms.

Masks

Masks prevent transmission of infectious agents through the air. They protect the wearer from inhaling both large-particle droplets, which are transmitted by close contact and usually travel only a short distance (up to 3 feet), and small-particle droplets, which remain suspended in air and may travel further. Masks lose their effectiveness if they are wet or are worn for long periods. They also are ineffective when they are not changed after caring for each client. Goggles and face shields also may be worn in high-risk situations where splashing is likely.

Disposable particulate respirators are indicated whenever a caregiver is working with a client who has, or is suspected of having, contagious airborne diseases such as tuberculosis (Fig. 26-7). Respirators look like masks but fit the face more tightly and are able to filter out particles or organisms as small as 1 μm (Decker & Schaffner, 1996; Willeke & Quian, 1998; McCullough & Bousseau, 1999). Individual mask fitting is recommended, because a tight seal must be maintained. Nurses working in communities with high-risk populations need to carry respirators and use them whenever indicated.

Gowns

Gowns should be worn when the caregiver's clothing is likely to be soiled by infected material. Use gowns only once and discard them. Also change your gown when it becomes moist.

Caps and Shoe Coverings

Caps are used to cover the hair, and special covers are available for shoes. New products are being developed for use in high-risk areas (e.g., labor and delivery, emergency room) to shield body parts from accidental exposure to contaminated body secretions.

Gloves

Gloves protect personnel from acquiring infective organisms on their hands. They also reduce the likelihood that personnel will transmit their own or other clients' microbial flora from their hands to clients. Clean, nonsterile gloves should be worn when direct contact with moist body substances from any client is anticipated. Hands are washed and dried before and after gloving. Gloves should be changed and discarded between clients or when they become torn or grossly soiled. Gloves should not be washed and reused.

> **SAFETY ALERT**
> **Never touch with bare hands anything that is wet coming from a body surface.**

Latex and vinyl gloves are two categories of gloves that are widely used clinically. Latex gloves are made of natural rubber and are more flexible and durable. Although they are more expensive, latex gloves are preferred when lengthy exposure is anticipated or fine motor skill is required (Korniewicz & Garzon, 1994; Johnson, 1997). The incidence of latex allergy is increasing among healthcare workers. Healthcare facilities must be sure that neither personnel nor clients are allergic to latex when latex gloves and products are used. If a latex allergy is suspected, special latex-free gloves and other equipment are available. For healthcare providers who are not allergic to latex gloves, washing of hands after gloves are removed may decrease the development of an allergy over time.

Vinyl gloves, made of polyvinyl chloride, a synthetic rubber, fit loosely and offer less protection than latex gloves but are usually adequate for routine client care activities such as emptying bedpans, handling specimens, or providing hygiene. Use of latex gloves for routine care activities is unnecessary, adds to the cost of care, and increases the risk of latex allergy. Double-gloving is indicated during activities when gloves may tear or puncture, such as during surgical procedures (Korniewicz & Garzon, 1994; Marin-Bertolin et al., 1997; Caillot et al., 1999).

Private Rooms

Separation of clients into private rooms decreases the chance of transmission of infection by all routes. If this is impossible, a client with an infection may be placed in the same room as another client who is infected with the same microorganism, as long as they are not infected with other potentially transmissible microorganisms and the likelihood of reinfection with the same microorganism is minimal (Garner, 1996). Special negative-airflow rooms are indicated for patients infected with tuberculosis or other organisms transmitted by the airborne route. High-risk groups include children younger than 5 years of age, clients with altered mental status, and clients with large, draining wounds or blood loss that cannot be contained in dressings.

Transport of clients with infections who need a private room should be avoided whenever possible. If transport to another department is necessary, the client's gown and dressings should be changed before leaving the room and the client should wear appropriate barriers, such as a mask or gown. If the infection is transmitted by the airborne route, the client should wear a mask and the transporters should be immune to the disease. Be sure to notify the department to which the client is being transported so that staff members are aware of the client's status and can take appropriate precautions.

Equipment and Refuse Handling

Special handling of articles and linen soiled by any body fluid is indicated. These articles should be placed in impervious bags before they are removed from the client's bedside. Bagging in watertight containers is indicated to prevent exposure of personnel and contamination of the environment. The outside of the bag should not be contaminated when placing articles inside it. Each hospital and community agency has procedures for labeling and decontaminating exposed articles. Items that are visibly soiled with body substances should be rinsed and placed in plastic bags or clearly marked containers, often labeled as "Contaminated," in dirty utility rooms before returning them to the central processing areas. If the outside of the bag becomes contaminated, placing that bag in another bag (double-bagging) is required.

Isolation Systems

Isolation refers to techniques used to prevent or to limit the spread of infection. Some form of isolation has been used for centuries, whether to protect a high-risk person from exposure to pathogens or to prevent the transmission of pathogens from an infected person to others.

The first two manuals published by the CDC recommended only category-specific isolation. Increased episodes of nosocomial infections (especially among immunocompromised clients) and the AIDS epidemic in the 1980s fostered the development of two new systems—Universal Precautions and body-substance isolation. Universal Precautions relate to blood and certain body fluids to protect healthcare workers from clients possibly carrying HIV, hepatitis B virus, or other bloodborne pathogens. Body-substance isolation involves the use of barriers to provide protection from all moist body secretions. In 1995, the CDC introduced guidelines for a new two-tiered system of isolation precautions that includes Standard Precautions and Transmission-Based Precautions:

1. Standard Precautions for all clients to protect against blood and body fluid transmission of potential infective organisms
2. Transmission-Based Precautions to protect against the spread of highly transmissible or epidemiologically significant pathogens in clients with documented or suspected infection

Isolation systems are costly in terms of equipment, supplies, and the time that they require from caregivers. Even more expensive are breaks in isolation technique that result in infection. All healthcare personnel and staff, physicians, nurses, technicians, students, and housekeepers are responsible for complying with isolation precautions. All personnel are responsible for tactfully calling observed infractions to the attention of those who do not comply. Compliance is best obtained by using a consistent, simple system, educating staff, and instilling a sense of personal responsibility in all caregivers.

Standard Precautions

Standard Precautions synthesizes the major features of Universal Precautions (decreasing risk of transmission from bloodborne pathogens) and body-substance isolation (decreasing risk of transmission from moist body substances). This system protects against the transmission of both undiagnosed and identified infections. Use of Standard Precautions protects healthcare providers as well as clients accessing healthcare services (Display 26-2).

Transmission-Based Precautions

When highly transmissible or significant pathogens have been identified, additional isolation may be required to prevent the spread of infection. Depending on the organism identified and its mode of transmission, Airborne Precautions, Droplet Precautions, or Contact Precautions may be instituted. Combined protocols may be used if the organism has more than one mode of transmission (Table 26-3).

DISPLAY 26-2

⬚ STANDARD PRECAUTIONS

A. Wear clean gloves when touching
1. Blood, body fluids, secretions and excretions, and items containing these body substances
2. Mucous membranes
3. Nonintact skin
B. Perform handwashing immediately
1. When there is direct contact with blood, body fluids, secretions and excretions, or contaminated items
2. After removing gloves
3. Between patient contacts
C. Wear a mask, eye protection, and face shield during procedures and patient care activities that are likely to generate splashes or sprays of blood, body fluids, secretions, and excretions.
D. Wear a cover gown during procedures and patient care activities that are likely to generate splashes or sprays of blood, body fluids, secretions or excretions, or cause soiling of clothing.
E. Remove soiled protective items promptly when the potential for contact with reservoirs of pathogens is no longer present.
F. Clean and reprocess all equipment before reuse by another patient.

G. Discard all single-use items promptly in appropriate containers that prevent contact with blood, body fluids, secretions and excretions, contamination of clothing, and transfer of microorganisms to other patients and the environment.
H. Handle, transport, and process linen soiled with blood, body fluids, and secretions and excretions in such a way as to prevent skin and mucous membrane exposures, contamination of clothing, or transfer to other patients and the environment.
I. Prevent injuries with used needles, scalpels, and other sharp devices by
1. Never removing, recapping, bending, or breaking used needles
2. Never pointing the needle toward a body part
3. Using a one-handed "scoop" method, special syringes with a retractable protective guard or shield for enclosing a needle, or blunt-point needles.
4. Depositing disposable and reusable syringes and needles in puncture-resistant containers
J. Use a private room or consult with an infection control professional for the care of patients who contaminate the environment or who cannot or do not assist with appropriate hygiene or environmental cleanliness measures.

Adapted from Foley, M. (1998). *Lippincott's need to know nursing reference facts.* Philadelphia: Lippincott-Raven, p. 24.

Airborne Precautions. Airborne Precautions are used to protect against microorganisms transmitted by small-particle droplets that can remain suspended and become widely dispersed by air currents. The client should be cared for in a private, negative-airflow room. Caregivers are to wear masks, and the client should wear a mask when transported out of the room.

Droplet Precautions. Droplet Precautions are used for microorganisms transmitted by larger-particle droplets, which disperse into air currents. For Droplet Precautions, the client should be in a private room or with a person who is infected with the same microorganism. A negative-airflow room is not required. Personnel are to use masks when working within 3 feet of the client. The client should wear a mask when outside the room.

Contact Precautions. Contact Precautions are used with organisms that can be transmitted by hand- or skin-to-skin contact, such as during client care activities or when touching the client's environmental surfaces or care items (Garner, 1996). When clients are known to be infected with significant organisms (e.g., drug-resistant pathogens), extra care is required to prevent transmission, and Contact Precautions are instituted.

The client is cared for in a private room or has a roommate who is infected with the same organism. Personnel use gloves when entering the room and change the gloves when exposed to potentially infected material during care delivery. They remove gloves before leaving the client's room. Gowns and other protective barriers are to be used when contamination is likely, either from the client, the environmental surfaces, or the client's room.

Protective Isolation

Protective isolation may still be used in high-risk situations to prevent infection for people whose body defenses are known to be compromised. Clients who are neutropenic (neutrophils less than 500/mm^3) as a result of chemotherapy, radiation therapy, or immunosuppressive medications are prime candidates. Clients with extensive burns or dermatitis are also at high risk. Such clients are placed in private rooms. Meticulous handwashing is strictly practiced by everyone, including the client and his or her family. Visitors are restricted. No fresh fruits or vegetables are allowed, only canned and cooked foods. All of these measures help to ensure that the client's environment stays as free from pathogens as possible, thereby decreasing the chance of infection.

TABLE 26-3

	Transmission-Based Precautions	
	Precautions	Indications
Airborne	Private, negative-airflow room with adequate filtration; mask; mask worn by client during transport out of room	Transmission via airborne route (small-particle droplets); tuberculosis, measles, varicella
Droplet	Private room or cohabitation with client infected with same organism; mask required when working within 3 feet of client; mask worn by client during transport	Transmission of large droplets through sneezing, coughing, or talking. *Haemophilus influenzae,* multidrug-resistant strains, *Neisseria meningitidis,* diphtheria, rubella, *Mycoplasma pneumoniae*
Contact	Private room or cohabitation with client infected with same organism; gloves at all times (don before entering room and remove before leaving) with change after exposure to organism; handwashing immediately after removal of gloves; gown and protective barriers when direct contact with organism occurs; daily cleaning of bedside equipment and client care items; exclusive use of items such as stethoscope and sphygmomanometer for infected client with terminal disinfection when precautions are no longer necessary	Serious infections easily transmitted through direct contact. Any multidrug-resistant strains, *Clostridium difficile, Shigella,* impetigo, and others

Psychological Effects of Isolation

Psychological effects of being separated from healthcare personnel, family, and friends may occur when isolation precautions are used. Clients spend more time alone. The bodies, hands, and faces of caregivers are covered. Clients may mistakenly feel dirty or untouchable, especially if they have diseases that are considered socially unacceptable. Lack of social interaction can be psychologically injurious, especially to children and their parents. Direct care at preventing the spread of microorganisms while maintaining the client's social support by spending time before, during, or after performing procedures to listen to the client's concerns and answer questions.

Surgical Asepsis

The purpose of sterile technique is to prevent the introduction of microorganisms from the environment into the client. Surgical asepsis is used in the following circumstances:

- Surgical procedures
- All procedures that invade the bloodstream
- Procedures that cause a break in skin or mucous membranes (e.g., intramuscular injections)
- Complex dressing changes and wound care
- Procedures involving insertion of catheters or devices into sterile body cavities (e.g., bladder)
- Care for high-risk groups (e.g., transplant recipients, burn clients, immunosuppressed clients)

When all organisms and their spores have been destroyed, the item is deemed sterile. These items are clearly labeled as sterile on their packaging. The packaging must not be torn, punctured, wet, or outdated. During any sterile procedure, care must be taken to keep all sterilized equipment sterile.

Principles of Surgical Asepsis

Surgical asepsis starts with thorough planning and preparation of the environment, supplies, and personnel. Although surgical asepsis is carried out in many settings, the operating room is the area where surgical asepsis is used most extensively. Staff members in the operating room require special training in maintaining aseptic technique for various operative procedures. Operative suites are specially constructed rooms that provide for no-touch handwashing at sinks controlled by foot pedals, have special airflow patterns, and control traffic into and out of areas.

Good personal hygiene is basic behavior for all personnel. Staff members who are ill with respiratory infections or who have conditions that cause diarrhea, vomiting, or skin lesions should not participate in sterile procedures. Street attire is not worn in the operating room or in other hospital areas where sterility is important. Shoes can be covered with shoe covers, and beards and hair must be covered by caps and masks. Jewelry should not be worn on the hands. General principles of surgical asepsis are discussed in Table 26-4.

THERAPEUTIC DIALOGUE
Asepsis

Scene for Thought

Arnie McKellan is 43 years old and has been admitted to the respiratory unit for treatment of AIDS and a serious drug-resistant infection. The nurse is meeting him for the first time and is wearing a mask, gown, and gloves.

Less Effective

Client: Well, well, another astronaut entering the forbidden planet. And who are you, spaceperson?! *(Looks annoyed and depressed but sounds cheerful.)*

Nurse: Well, I'm Sally Ride, the first woman astronaut! How's it going with you today? *(Very cheerful, answers with the same tone of voice.)*

Client: Couldn't be better with all the spacepeople coming in here. I get lots of company and nobody's done anything awful to me yet. How can I complain? *(Looks strained, and his eye contact begins to slip.)*

Nurse: Well, I'm not here to change that part yet. I'm really Sheila Evans, your nurse for the evening shift. I need to take a history and do a nursing assessment. It won't take long. I can see you're tired. *(Sits down in the chair next to the bed, opens his chart, and begins to write.)*

Client: Yes, I really am. I'd appreciate it if you'd make it quick. *(Continues to look strained.)*

Nurse: Sure, no problem. *(Proceeds to ask some assessment questions. Client makes jokes, answers questions shortly, usually with sarcasm.)* You know, I can't tell if you're serious or joking sometimes! Makes it hard to fill out this assessment.

Client: Well, I'll try my best to be serious all the time from now on! Are you done yet? *(Sounds irritated.)*

Nurse: Yes, I am, for now. I'll let you rest now and I'll be back with your dinner tray. We can talk some more then. *(Leaves thinking, "Just what I need. An angry client!")*

Client: *(Turns to the wall and sighs.)*

More Effective

Client: Well, well, another astronaut entering the forbidden planet. And who are you, spaceperson?! *(Looks annoyed and depressed but sounds cheerful.)*

Nurse: I'm Susan O'Shea, Mr. McKellan, your nurse for the evening shift. You sound cheerful today. Are you? *(Stands next to the bed.)*

Client: Of course! Wouldn't you be, getting to spend all this time alone and spacepeople coming to see you every 5 minutes? *(Says this with great sarcasm.)*

Nurse: No, I'd be lonely and annoyed. *(Says this quietly and seriously.)*

Client: *(Looks away and stays quiet for awhile. So does Susan.)* I don't want to feel depressed about this admission, Susan. I know it's going to be one of many. So I guess I've been a little loud and sarcastic. I can tell you won't let me get away with it. *(Smiles.)*

Nurse: *(Laughs.)* We can get loud together later, but we have other work to do first. Maybe I could start with the reason for the "spacesuits," and then we could go on to a short history and physical. How does that sound? *(Makes an alliance with the client, being sure to laugh rather than smile, which is hidden by the mask.)*

Client: Okay, okay. Especially the part about the masks and everything. I'm not used to it. Makes me feel terminal already!

Nurse: Sounds like we have a lot to talk about. Let's get to it. *(Explains about the reason for the isolation, what's involved, how long it will go on, and so forth. Mr. McKellan listens carefully, asks questions, makes a few jokes, but appears more relaxed.)*

Critical Thinking Challenges

- List behaviors that indicate Mr. McKellan is angry, afraid, apprehensive, and annoyed.
- Compare and contrast how Sheila and Susan responded to these behaviors.
- Identify each nurse's concerns.
- Appraise your emotional reaction when you're confronted by an irritated, sarcastic person, and describe what you do.
- Examine the aspects of communication that are lost with a mask.

Skin Preparation

Skin preparation reduces microorganisms present on the skin. The skin cannot be sterilized, because chemicals used to sterilize objects would kill dermal cells. Skin is disinfected by chemicals in a procedure called *degermation.*

Bacteria on the skin include both transient and resident flora. The transient microorganisms are held in place by sweat, oil, and debris. They can be removed easily with soap and water and by the friction of scrubbing. Resident flora adhere to epithelial cells and extend into hair follicles and glands in the skin. Resident flora vary according to location on the body.

Antiseptic agents are used in skin preparation and surgical scrubs to reduce the number of transient microorganisms. They do not penetrate into the dermis, nor are they able to remove all resident flora. The mechanical action of scrubbing and rinsing with water helps remove organisms from deeper layers of the skin, but a portion of these bacteria remains. When surgical gloves are worn, especially for extended periods, resident flora grow and replicate from deeper skin layers.

 SAFETY ALERT
Remember that if your gloves become punctured or torn during a sterile procedure, change them immediately to reduce the chance of contamination. Any puncture or tear of gloves during sterile procedures allows organisms on the hands to contact an open wound.

TABLE 26-4

Principles of Surgical Asepsis	
Technique/Principle	**Rationale**
Moisture causes contamination. • Handle liquids carefully near sterile fields to prevent splashing. • Place wet objects on sterile, water-impermeable surfaces, such as sterile basins.	Microorganisms travel more easily through moist environments. When a sterile surface becomes moist, microorganisms may be transmitted from an unsterile surface by capillary action.
Never assume that an object is sterile. • Check to see that it is labeled as sterile. • Always check the integrity of the packaging. • Always check the expiration date on the package. • If there is any doubt about the sterility of an object, it should be considered unsterile.	Commercially prepared products are labeled as sterile on their packaging. Special indicators are used to show that objects have completed their sterilization process, such as tapes on the outside of packages or chemically impregnated paper inside containers. Packages that are torn, punctured, or moist cannot be considered sterile. All packaging materials should have clearly visible dates that indicate when sterility cannot be guaranteed. Items that have passed that date cannot be used.
Always face the sterile field.	The area defined as sterile for the purposes of the procedure is the "field." Objects that are out of the line of vision may be inadvertently contaminated and their sterility is never guaranteed.
Sterile articles may touch only sterile articles or surfaces if they are to maintain their sterility.	Anything considered unsterile may transfer microorganisms to the sterile object it touches. An object used on an unsterile surface, such as swabs used in cleaning the skin, must be used once and then discarded because skin cannot be sterilized. Keep unsterile objects away from the field.
Sterile equipment or areas must be kept above the waist and on top of the sterile field. • Drapes hanging over the edge of the table are not considered sterile.	Waist level is the limit of good visual field. By defining only the top of the field as sterile, maximum visibility of all sterile objects used in the procedures is ensured.
Prevent unnecessary traffic and air currents around the sterile area. • Close doors. • Unfold drapes or wrappers slowly. • Do not sneeze, cough, or talk excessively over the sterile field. • Do not reach across sterile fields.	Microorganisms cannot be completely excluded from the air even with the best filtration and airflow designs. Movement creates air currents that circulate organisms in the air. Masks do not contain all organisms expelled from the oral or nasal cavities and become moistened more quickly from talking. Move around a sterile field or turn the field slowly by reaching under the drapes if an object is not convenient to a sterile person.
Open, unused sterile articles are no longer sterile after the procedure.	Once the protective wrappings have been removed, the article is being contaminated by the air. Even if it is untouched and resting on a sterile surface, it must be discarded or resterilized before it is used. Liquids opened during the procedure that remain in their original container are also considered to be contaminated.

TABLE 26-4 (Continued)

Principles of Surgical Asepsis	
Technique/Principle	**Rationale**
A person who is considered sterile who becomes contaminated must reestablish sterility.	If a "scrubbed" person punctures the gloves or is contaminated accidentally by touching an unsterile object, he or she must change the contaminated article. If a scrubbed person leaves the area of the sterile field, he or she must go through the procedure of rescrubbing, gowning, and gloving.
Surgical technique is a team effort. • A collective and individual "sterile conscience" is the best method of enhancing sterile technique.	Staff members must rely on one another to maintain sterile technique. Persons who are considered sterile must have access to sterile supplies delivered to them by circulators in the operating room or prepared by themselves at the bedside. Team members must be open to critiques by other members about their technique and respond to their suggestions that objects of their clothing have been contaminated or that they have contaminated an object. Periodic review of procedures and infection control surveillance reports enhance everyone's sterile technique

The following are the objectives of surgical scrubs and client skin preparation:

• Remove dirt, oil, and microorganisms from the skin.
• Reduce bacterial counts to a minimum.
• Avoid abrading the skin.
• Leave a layer of antimicrobial material on the skin that inhibits the growth of microbes for an extended period.

Typically, a client's skin preparation consists of several steps. The first is a bath or shower or washing with soap and water before the planned procedure. Removal of hair with depilatory creams, clipping with sterile scissors, or shaving may be necessary. If shaving is ordered, it should not be performed more than 2 hours before the surgical procedure, because tiny nicks in the skin may predispose the client to infection. In some instances (e.g., same-day surgery), the client may be asked to shave at home before the procedure. After the skin is cleansed and hair has been removed, the skin is scrubbed with an antimicrobial agent. For surgical procedures, this may take place in the operating room.

Surgical Handwashing

Surgical hand scrubs differ from general handwashing that the nurse performs during most client encounters in both technique and length. A disposable scrub brush or sponge is usually impregnated with antimicrobial scrub solutions. The solution of choice in most institutions is an iodophor solution. Sterile nail cleaners made of plastic or metal should also be available. Antiseptic soap containers that dispense solution by knee or foot pressure must be located above or next to a splashproof sink.

Before starting the scrub, remove all nail polish. Keep fingernails short and without sharp edges that can puncture surgical gloves. Make sure your hands are free of lesions, cuts, or abrasions, because traumatized skin can harbor bacteria. Always hold hands higher than the level of the elbows and away from the body to allow water to run off at the elbows. Water running down the arms to the hands can cause contamination. Thoroughly dry your hands when finished. This procedure for surgical hand scrubbing is outlined in Procedure 26-2.

Sterile Gloves

Sterile gloves are mandatory for all procedures that require surgical technique. Gloves are worn to prevent contamination of wounds, equipment, supplies, and the sites of invasive procedures. Sterile gloves are donned after the hands have been thoroughly cleaned. For procedures performed at the bedside, it is common to use the open method of gloving, which is outlined in Procedure 26-3.

In the operative suite or during invasive procedures, the practitioner may use either a closed or an open method for donning gloves. The closed method is preferred when sterile gowns are used for the procedure. In this method, the sterile gown is donned, and the hands are slid into the sleeves until the cuff seam is reached. Then, using the dominant hand, pick up a cuffed glove for the other hand. Draw the glove over the nondominant hand, and pull the sleeve onto the wrist. Glove the dominant hand in the same manner using the sterile glove on the other hand. For Donning a Sterile Gown and Closed Gloving, refer to Procedure 26-4.

Sterile Field

A sterile field is an area free of microorganisms on which sterile items can be placed. This provides a work surface to facilitate maintaining sterility during a sterile procedure. Drapes or sterile wrappers can be used to create a sterile field. Sterile items are transferred to the surface by peeling back packaging and dropping the item onto the field without

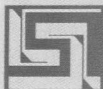

PROCEDURE 26-2

SURGICAL HAND SCRUB

Purpose
1. Remove as many microorganisms from the hands as possible before a sterile procedure.
2. Decrease the risk of infection for high-risk groups (e.g., newborns, transplant recipients).

Assessment
- Assess agency policy regarding surgical hand scrub.
- Assess hands for cuts, abrasions, or traumatized skin that can harbor microorganisms.
- Assess length and conditions of nails and cuticles. Long nails, artificial nails, and nail polish should be avoided.

Equipment
Deep sink with knee or foot controls for soap and water.
Agency-approved antimicrobial soap.
Surgical scrub brush
Plastic nail stick or sterile nail cleaner
Sterile towel for drying

Procedure
1. Remove rings. Apply surgical attire (scrubs, shoe cover, cap or hood, face mask and protective eye wear)
   Rationale: Rings can harbor microorganisms. Applying attire after handwashing would contaminate hands.
2. Wash and rinse hands for the initial wash.
   Rationale: To remove gross contamination and transient microorganisms.
3. Open disposable brush impregnated with antimicrobial soap and adjust water temperature to warm using water control lever.
   Rationale: Antimicrobial soap is more effective at reducing microorganisms. Use of warm water decreases drying of the hands. This is especially important in areas where surgical hand scrubs are performed frequently.
4. Wet hands and arms. Keep elbows bent so that hands remain higher than elbows. Water will flow down hands and off elbows.
   Rationale: Movement of water and dirt will flow from hands to less clean areas, thus not contaminating hands during the scrub.
5. Use nail stick or cleaner to clean under nails of both hands.
   Rationale: The nails can harbor significant bacteria and need to be cleaned thoroughly.
6. Wet scrub brush or apply antibacterial soap if not already impregnated in the brush.

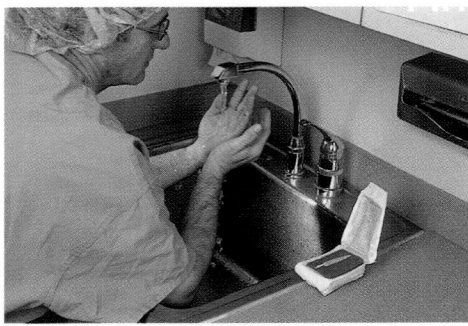

Step 4 When wetting arms and hands, elbows are bent and hands remain higher than the elbows.

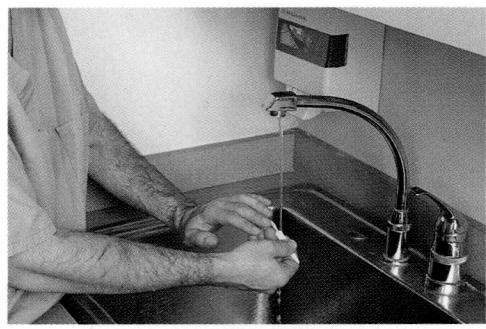

Step 5 Use the nail stick to clean under the nails.

   Rationale: Antibacterial soap assists in removing transient and resident microorganisms.
7. *Anatomic Timed Scrub.* Starting with the fingertips, scrub each anatomic area (nails, fingers each side and web space, palmar surface, dorsal surface, and forearm) for the designated amount of time according to agency policy (total usually around 5 minutes). Scrub vigorously using vertical strokes. Repeat with other hand.

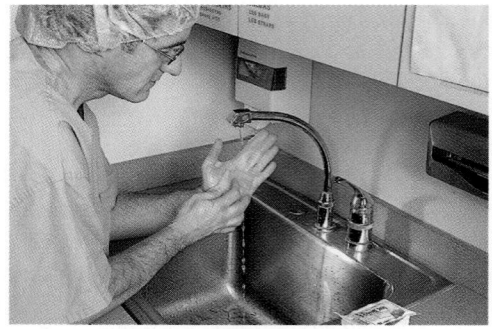

Step 7 Use the scrub brush with vertical strokes.

PROCEDURE 26-2 (Continued)

Rationale: Ensures that all surfaces will be systematically scrubbed to remove transient and resident microorganisms.

8. *Counted Brush Stroke Method.* Starting with the fingertips, scrub each anatomic area (nails, fingers each side and web space, palmar surface, dorsal surface, and forearm) for the designated number of strokes according to agency policy. Scrub vigorously using vertical strokes.
   Rationale: Ensures that all surfaces will be systematically scrubbed to remove transient and resident microorganisms.

9. Do not touch faucet, clothing, or other objects. Avoid splashing. Rinse hands thoroughly under warm running water keeping hands elevated to allow water to drain off at the flexed elbow.
   Rationale: Prevents contamination of the hands from dirtier areas. Touching nonsterile objects would mean the surgical scrub would need to be repeated.

10. Keep hands held upward to allow water to drip from the elbow. Dry with sterile towel.
    Rationale: prevents contamination before gloving.

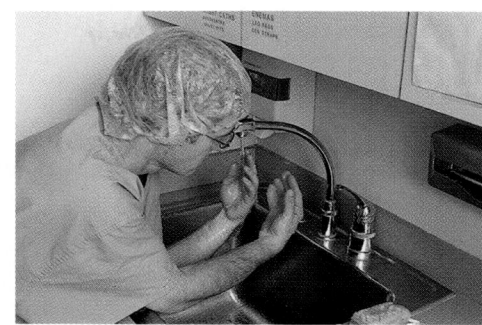

Step 9 Hold hands upward while rinsing.

Collaboration and Delegation:
- Nonprofessional support personnel will keep designated areas stocked with supplies necessary for the surgical scrub.
- Guidelines for the surgical scrub should be posted in appropriate areas, and staff should inform each other of any breaks in technique.

---

contact with anything nonsterile. See Procedure 26-5 for Preparing and Maintaining a Sterile Field.

SAFETY ALERT
Always place sterile objects on a dry surface and avoid splashing liquids when pouring. Moisture causes contamination. Refer to Chapter 38, Procedure 38-1 (Changing a Dressing) for specific guidelines.

LIFESPAN CONSIDERATIONS

Newborn and Infant

Prevention of infection in newborns begins by protecting the fetus from infection exposure during pregnancy. Maternal infections can be transmitted to the fetus during pregnancy, resulting in minor or major congenital anomalies or fetal death, depending on the time of exposure and the organism involved. In general, the earlier in pregnancy the mother is infected, the more severely the fetus is affected. A very mild or asymptomatic infection in the mother can have serious consequences

for the fetus. Very early in pregnancy, when exposure is most dangerous, the mother may be unaware that she is pregnant. Adequate prenatal care is important in decreasing maternal infection.

SAFETY ALERT
All women of childbearing age should have up-to-date immunizations. Urge those trying to get pregnant to avoid exposure to infectious disease whenever possible.

The most frequent mode of transmission of organisms is from direct contact with the skin and hands of caregivers and, to a lesser extent, through contaminated infant formula. Handwashing is the single most important means for preventing nosocomial infection in the newborn (Siegel, 1998). Teaching all caregivers the importance of scrupulous handwashing and general good hygiene has been shown to decrease infection in this age group (Churchill & Pickering, 1997; Siegel, 1998; Hall, 2000). Immunizations begin during infancy and continue

(text continues on page 505)

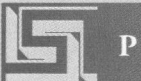

PROCEDURE 26-3

APPLYING AND REMOVING STERILE GLOVES

Purpose
1. Prevent transfer of microorganisms from hands to sterile objects or open wounds.

Assessment
- Identify appropriate time to wear sterile gloves.
- Inspect glove package to determine whether it is dry and intact.
- Assess that nails are filed short and all jewelry is removed from hands.
- Examine ungloved hands for presence of open cuts or lesions, which may harbor microorganisms and prevent the nurse from participating in a sterile procedure.

Equipment
Packaged sterile gloves in correct size
Flat working surface

Procedure
Applying Gloves
1. Wash hands.
   Rationale: Clean hands reduce the number of microorganisms that could be transferred if gloves accidentally puncture or tear.
2. Remove outside wrapper by peeling apart sides.
   Rationale: This protects inner package from inadvertently opening and contaminating the gloves.

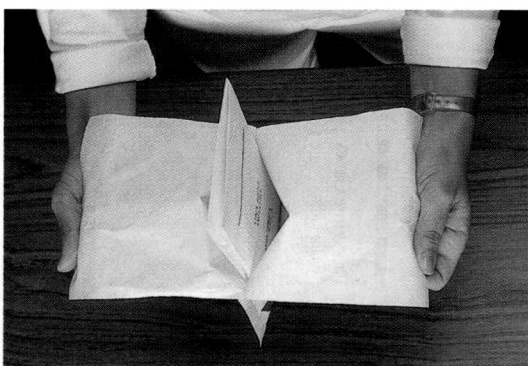

Step 2 Peel down to remove outside wrapper.

3. Lay inner package on clean, flat surface about waist level. Open wrapper from the outside, keeping gloves on inside surface.
   Rationale: Objects below waist level are considered contaminated. Inner surface of wrapper is considered sterile.

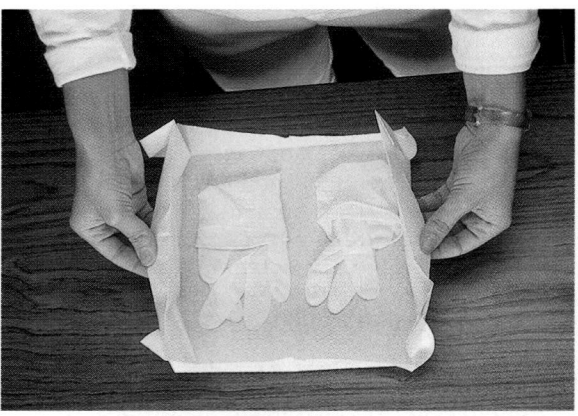

Step 3 Open inner wrapper, providing sterile field for glove application.

4. Grasp inside edge of the glove with thumb and first two fingers of your dominant hand. Holding hands above waist, insert your nondominant hand into glove. Adjust fingers inside glove after both gloves are on.
   Rationale: Inner edge of cuff unfolds against skin of hand and is not sterile once applied. Contamination occurs if ungloved hand contacts gloved hand.

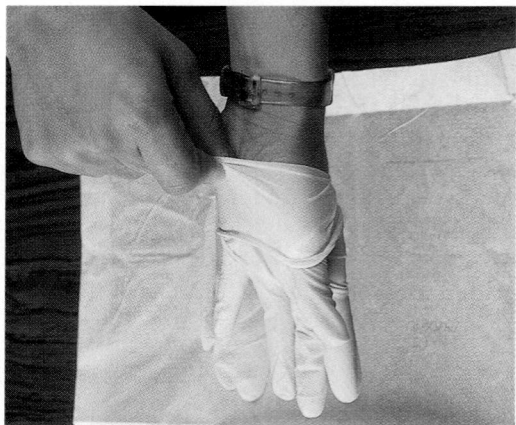

Step 4 Grasp first glove by inside edge of cuff and slide on.

PROCEDURE 26-3 (Continued)

5. Slip gloved hand underneath second gloved cuff still in package and pull over dominant hand.
   Rationale: Sterile cuff protects fingers of gloved hand from being contaminated.

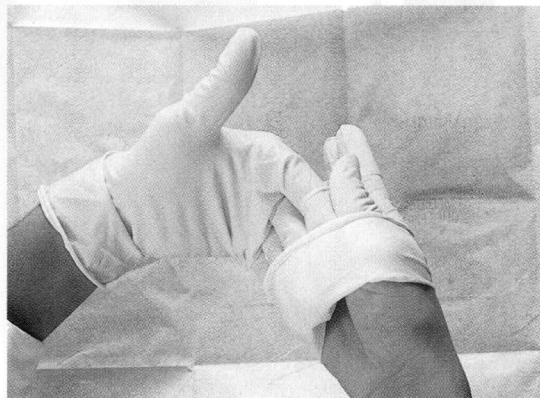

Step 5 Slip gloved fingers underneath cuff of other glove and pull over hand.

6. Keeping hands above waist, adjust glove fit, touching only sterile areas.
   Rationale: These actions prevent potential contamination while ensuring a smooth fit over fingers.

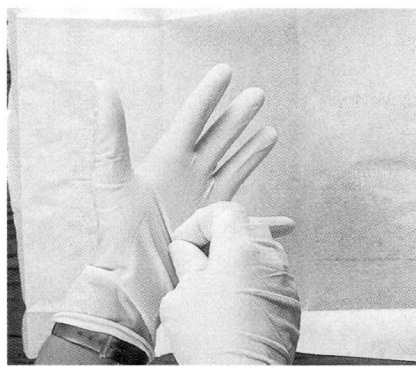

Step 6 Adjust gloves as necessary, taking care to keep both gloves sterile.

Removing Gloves

7. With dominant hand, grasp outer surface of non-dominant glove just below thumb. Peel off without touching exposed wrist.
   Rationale: After use, outer surface of gloves is contaminated and could transfer microorganisms to the nurse's wrist.

8. Place ungloved hand under thumb side of second cuff and peel off toward the fingers, holding first glove inside second glove. Discard into appropriate receptacle.
   Rationale: Folding contaminated glove surfaces toward the inside minimizes the chance of transfer of microorganisms.

9. Wash hands.

Home Care Modifications

- For many procedures in the home, clean gloves are used rather than sterile gloves.

Collaboration and Delegation

- Encourage coworkers to notify one another of any observed breaks in sterility, either when gloves are applied or when breaks in technique cause glove contamination.

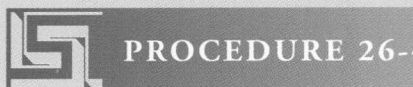

PROCEDURE 26-4

DONNING A STERILE GOWN AND CLOSED GLOVING

Purpose
1. To apply attire necessary to safely carry out sterile procedures

Assessments
- Assess availability of sterile supplies.
- Assess availability of personnel (e.g., circulating nurse) if help is needed.
- Assess location of all sterile fields to avoid contamination.

Equipment
Sterile gown
Sterile gloves
Mayo stand or flat surface area above waist level

Procedure
1. Locate all surgical attire (scrubs, shoe covers, cap or hood, face mask and protective eye wear) and perform the surgical hand scrub as described in Procedure 26-2.
   Rationale: The gown and gloves should be donned last, because it is most important for them to be sterile.

Donning a Sterile Gown
2. Grasp folded sterile gown at the neckline and step away from the sterile field. Allow gown to gently unfold, being careful that it does not touch the floor. The inside of the gown is toward the wearer.
   Rationale: Maintains sterility of the gown and positions it for donning.
3. Holding the arms at shoulder level, grasp the sterile gown just below the neckband near the shoulders and slide arms in the sleeves until the fingers are at the end of the cuffs but not through the cuffs.
   Rationale: The fingers remain in the cuffs to protect the sterility of the gown and prepare for closed gloving.
4. Have someone tie the back of the gown, taking care that only the ties are touched and not the sides or front of the gown.
   Rationale: Maintains sterility of the gown. Gowns are considered sterile in the front from the shoulder to the table level, and sleeves are considered sterile from 2 inches above the elbow to the wrist.

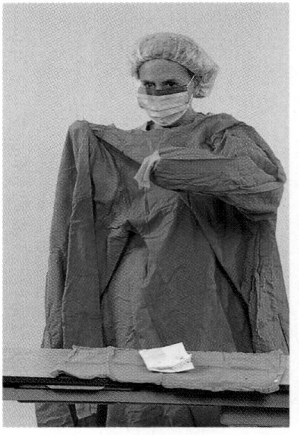

Step 3 Arms are at the end of, but not through, the cuffs.

Closed Gloving
5. With fingers still within the cuff of the gown, open the inner sterile glove package and pick up the first glove by the cuff, using your nondominant hand.
   Rationale: Maintains sterility of the glove.
6. Position the glove over the cuff of the gown so the fingers are in alignment, and stretch the entire glove over the stockinet cuff, being careful not to touch the edge of the stockinet cuff. Fingers remain within the cuff of the gown.
   Rationale: Maintains sterility of the glove.

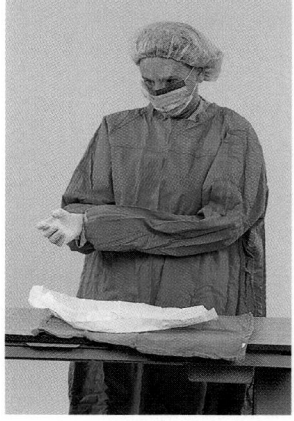

Step 6 The glove is stretched over the cuff of the gown.

7. Work the fingers into the glove and pull the glove up over wrist with the nondominant hand that still remains within the cuff of the gown.
   Rationale: Maintains sterility of the glove.
8. Use the sterile gloved hand to pick up the second glove, placing it over the stockinet cuff of the dominant hand and repeating the glove application process.
   Rationale: Maintains sterility of the glove.

PROCEDURE 26-4 (Continued)

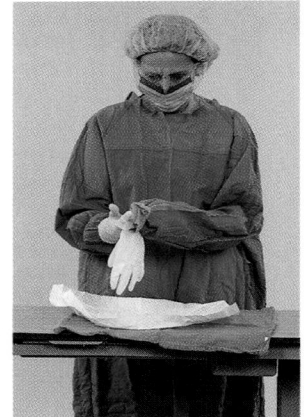

Step 8 Use the sterile glove to pick up the second glove and place it over the stockinet cuff of the other hand.

9. Adjust gloves for comfort and fit, taking care to keep gloved hands above waist level at all times. **Rationale: If gloved hands fall below waist level, they are no longer sterile.**

Collaboration and Delegation
- Operating room personnel, especially circulating nurses, often assist with gowning and gloving.
- It is role of the circulating nurse to notify all personnel of any breaks in sterile technique.

---

on through childhood. Provide parents and other caregivers with immunization schedules and teach them the importance of vaccination in preventing many contagious diseases.

Toddler and Preschooler

Young children frequently become infected, because normal behavior at this age fosters transmission of microorganisms. These children usually are not yet toilet trained and have poor personal hygiene. Playing on the floor, continually putting objects in the mouth, and even playing with bodily secretions all contribute to exposure to potential pathogens. For both toddlers and preschoolers, increased exposure to groups of children in day care or preschool is another factor affecting the spread of infection. Upper respiratory tract and subsequent ear infections are common among these age groups.

Teaching about hygiene practices that limit infectious exposure is important for toddlers and preschoolers. Proper handwashing after use of the bathroom and before meals is an important habit for young children to develop. If children of this age are exhibiting signs of infection, advise parents and other caregivers to avoid exposing them to other children, so that infection transmission can be minimized.

School-Age Child and Adolescent

During the school years, the incidence of many infections decreases because of children's more mature immune systems and completion of routine childhood immunizations. Direct contact and airborne transmission of infections are more common in the winter months because children crowd into schoolrooms and engage in indoor recreational activities. Often, skin eruptions such as impetigo and lice infestations occur because these children may share personal hygiene aids, clothing, and sports equipment.

Adolescence brings new elements of exposure. Injuries become more frequent and may predispose to infection. The incidence of sexually transmitted diseases (STDs) and of mononucleosis starts to rise when adolescents begin sexual activity. Respiratory infections and viral diseases are common because many group activities keep adolescents in close quarters.

School nurses play a significant role in detecting and preventing the spread of infections among older children and adolescents. Health teaching is also important in preventing injury and STDs among these groups.

Adult and Older Adult

By adulthood, most people have acquired immunity to many communicable diseases. However, infection as a complication of injury and STDs continue to be threats. As adults increase their independence and travel, especially to foreign countries, they may be exposed to new infectious organisms.

As adults age, the incidence of infection as a complication of chronic disease increases. The effects of long-standing cardiovascular disease, diabetes, drug and alcohol abuse, and *(text continues on page 508)*

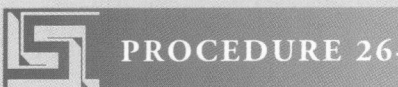

PROCEDURE 26-5

PREPARING AND MAINTAINING A STERILE FIELD

Purpose
1. To create an environment to prevent the transfer of microorganisms during sterile procedures.
2. To create an environment that helps ensure the sterility of supplies and equipment during a sterile procedure.

Assessment
- Assess what sterile supplies are necessary for the procedure
- Select an area at or above waist height that is free from clutter
- Assess the area on which the sterile field will be established for potential sources of contamination (e.g., moisture, soiling) and clean if necessary
- Assess for the sterility of all supplies by noting the package integrity, the color strip indicator (Fig. 26-6), or the expiration date on the package.
- Assess the order in which supplies will be used during the procedure so that supplies used first can be added to the field last

Equipment
Flat work surface
Sterile drape
Sterile supplies as needed (sterile gauze, sterile basin, solutions, scissors, forceps)
Packaged sterile gloves

Procedure
1. Wash your hands.
   Rationale: Reduces the number of transient bacteria on the hands, helping to prevent microbial contamination.
2. Inspect all sterile packages for package integrity, contamination, or moisture.
   Rationale: Moisture, breaks in package integrity, and visible contamination indicate that the contents are no longer sterile and must be discarded.
3. During the entire procedure, never turn your back on the sterile field or lower your hands below the level of the field.
   Rationale: Sterility of the field can not be certain.

Opening a Sterile Drape
4. Remove the sterile drape from the outer wrapper and place the inner drape in the center of the work surface, at or above waist level, with the outer flap facing away from you.
   Rationale: Maintains sterility of the package and allows for opening the drape in a manner that will not contaminate the sterile field.
5. Touching the outside of the flap only, reach around (rather than over) the sterile field to open the flap away from you.
   Rationale: Maintains sterility of the field.

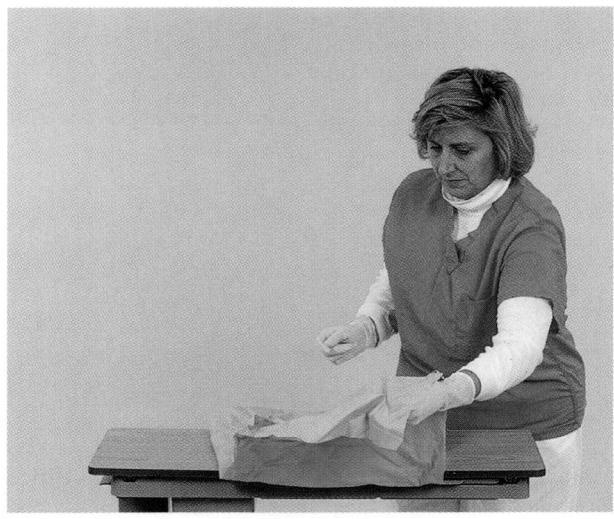

Step 5 Reach around the sterile field to open the flap away from you.

6. Open the side flaps in the same manner, using the right hand for the right flap and the left hand for the left flap.
   Rationale: This maintains sterility by avoiding crossing over the field.
7. Lastly, open the innermost flap that faces you, being careful that it does not touch your clothing or any object.
   Rationale: Maintains sterility of the field.

Adding Sterile Supplies to the Field
8. Prepackaged sterile supplies are opened by peeling back the partially sealed edge with both hands or lifting up the unsealed edge, taking care not to touch the supplies with your hands.
   Rationale: Maintains the sterility of the supplies.
9. Hold supplies 10 to 12 inches above the field and allow them to fall to the middle of the sterile field.
   Rationale: Holding supplies too close to the field may cause hand contact that would contaminate the entire field. Holding supplies too

PROCEDURE 26-5 (Continued)

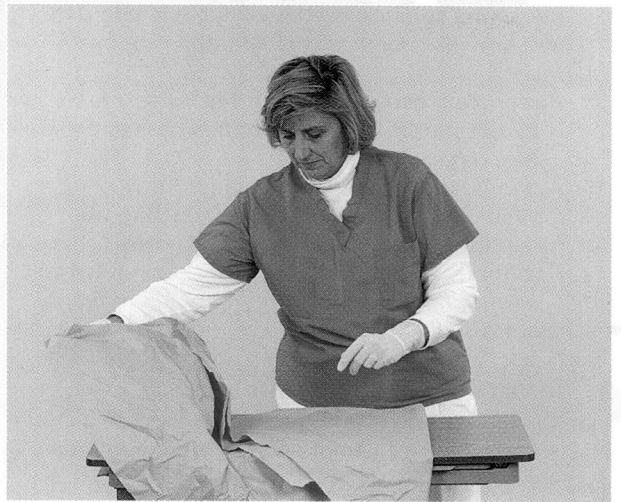

Step 6 Use the right hand to open the right flap and the left hand to open the left flap.

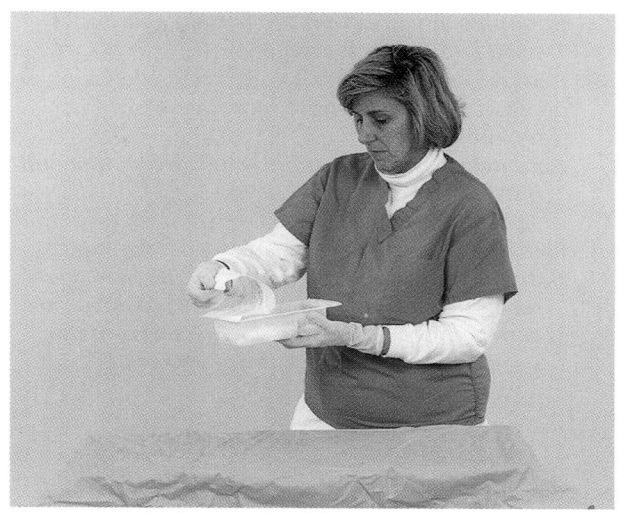

Step 8 Open the unsealed edge, taking care not to touch the supplies with your hands.

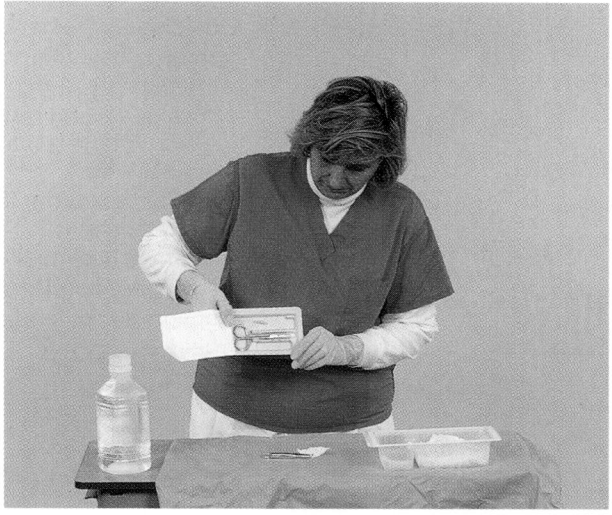

Step 9 Hold supplies 10 to 12 inches above the field and allow them to fall to the middle.

high may cause them to land on the edge of the field, also resulting in contamination. The edges of the field are not considered sterile.
Wrapped sterile supplies are added by grasping the sterile object with one hand and unwrapping the flaps with the other hand.
Rationale: Maintains sterility of the object.

10. Grasp the corners of the wrapper with the free hand and hold them against the wrist of the other hand while you carefully drop the object onto the sterile field.
Rationale: Maintains sterility of the object and the field.

Adding Solutions to a Sterile Field

11. Read the solution label and expiration date. Note any signs of contamination.

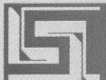

PROCEDURE 26-5 (Continued)

Rationale: Ensures that the correct solution is used and that it is sterile.

12. Remove cap and place it with the inside facing up on a flat surface. Do not touch inside of cap or rim of bottle.
    Rationale: Maintains sterility of the solution and bottle.

13. Hold bottle 6 inches above container on the sterile field and pour slowly to avoid spills.
    Rationale: Spilling fluid on the sterile field could result in contamination because a wet surface allows microorganisms to wick up from the support surface, which is not sterile.

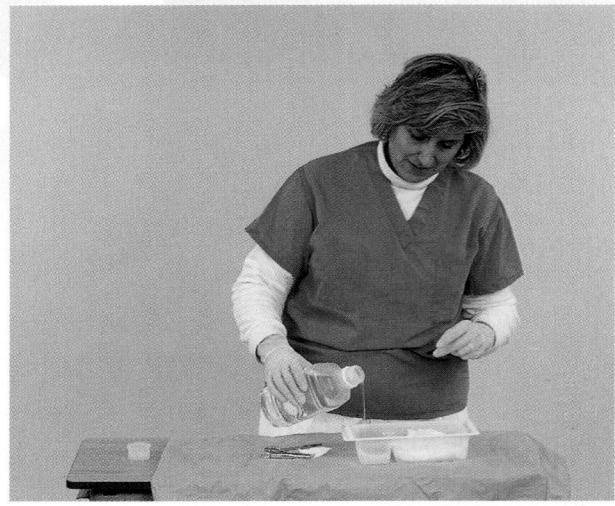

Step 13 Hold the bottle 6 inches above the container and pour slowly.

14. Recap the solution bottle and label it with date and time of opening if the solution is to be reused.
    Rationale: Keeps solution in the bottle sterile and avoids use of solution that has passed expiration date.

15. Add any additional supplies and don sterile gloves (Procedure 26-2) before starting the procedure.
    Rationale: Donning sterile gloves just prior to beginning the procedure helps to ensure sterility.

Home Care Modifications

- Select a clean area in the home to set up a sterile field. Avoid areas that pets frequent and areas that are visibly dirty. Alcohol can be used to clean surface areas.
- Self-contained, prepackaged, disposable sterile kits are convenient for use in the home.
- Use waterproof, plastic bags to dispose of contaminated waste.

Collaboration and Delegation

- Nonprofessional staff with appropriate training often set up sterile fields, especially in areas such as the operating room or delivery room.
- All coworkers must be responsible for informing each other when they observe contamination of the sterile field so that sterility can be reestablished.
- At times it is more convenient to have one person gloved and sterile with another person opening and handing sterile supplies as they are needed.

cancer can predispose adults to infection. Elective surgical procedures can also pose infection risks. In working with adult populations, stress preventive health practices to reduce the risk of chronic disease states and thereby decrease potential infection risk. Monitoring to ensure current immunizations for the adult is also important, because adults frequently forget to update immunizations as necessary.

Older adults are predisposed to serious infections because of decreased nutritional status, waning immunologic responses, decreased activity level, poor circulation, frequent breaks in skin integrity, urinary retention, and impaired mechanical clearance mechanisms. Old diseases such as tuberculosis and herpes zoster can be reactivated, and there is an increased incidence of staphylococcal and streptococcal infections among the elderly (Smith & Rusnak, 1996; Arias, 2000). Severely disabled older adults are at particular risk because they are often unable to perform their own personal hygiene. Immobility and incontinence also greatly increase infection risk.

Hospitalized older adults incur nosocomial infections at two to five times the rate of younger clients. Higher rates of pneumonia, urinary tract infections, bacteremia, and surgical wound infections occur during their hospitalizations, and they usually require treatment with vigorous courses of antibiotics. If clients are placed in extended care facilities on continuing antibiotic regimens, they risk the possibility of developing antibiotic-resistant infections. When these clients, who are potential reservoirs for transmission to others in their nursing home, are readmitted to acute care hospitals, they become reservoirs for the new facility. Thus, they may require several acute care admissions and pass on more virulent organisms with each round trip (Cahill & Rosenberg, 1996; Strausbaugh & Joseph, 1996, 2000; Nicolle, 2000; Strausbaugh, 2001).

KEY CONCEPTS

- Agents that cause infection are everywhere in the environment—on body surfaces, in food, and in products used in normal activities of daily living. Intact skin and mucous membranes are major barriers against organisms and transmission of infection.
- The chain of infection from person to person, from object to person, and from reservoirs in the environment can be broken with infection control practices.
- The incidence of infections associated with healthcare delivery (nosocomial infections) can be decreased with good infection control practices.
- Regulatory agencies at local, state, regional, and national levels are involved in the control of infection and institutional waste to protect clients, staff, and the community.
- Employee health programs to monitor and to counsel personnel are important components of institutional and community infection control programs.
- Institutional waste disposal methods are important factors in infection control programs.
- Effective infection control measures have a favorable cost–benefit ratio.
- Contact transmission of infectious organisms on the hands of caregivers is the most frequent mode of transmission of infection in healthcare facilities.
- Handwashing is the single most important infection control practice. All caregivers, clients, and family members should learn handwashing techniques.
- Aseptic practices are those techniques used to keep people or objects free from microorganisms. Cleaning, disinfection, and sterilization can be accomplished by various methods and agents.
- Isolation precautions involve the use of barriers, which are important in preventing the spread of infection. Gloves should be worn whenever there could be contact with the client's body secretions.
- Sterile technique is used to prevent the introduction of microorganisms from the environment into the client.
- An item is sterile when all organisms and spores on the object are destroyed.
- Infectious exposures and the risk of contracting infectious disease change during a person's lifespan.

REFERENCES

Arias, K. M. (2000). *Quick reference to outbreak investigation and control in health care facilities.* Gaithersburg, MD: Aspen.

Beekman, S. E., et al. (2001). Hospital bloodborne pathogens programs: Program characteristics and blood and body fluid exposure rates. *Infection Control and Hospital Epidemiology, 22*(2), 73–82.

Boyce, J. M. (1996). Treatment and control of colonization in the prevention of nosocomial infections. *Infection Control and Hospital Epidemiology, 17*(4), 256–261.

Burke, J. P., & Zavasky, D. (1999). Nosocomial urinary tract infections. In C. G. Mayhall (Ed.), *Hospital epidemiology and infection control* (2nd ed.). Philadelphia: Lippincott Williams & Wilkins, 173–185.

Cahill, C. K., & Rosenberg, J. (1996). Guidelines for prevention and control of antibiotic resistant microorganisms. *Journal of Gerontological Nursing, 25*(2), 40–47.

Caillot, J. L. et al. (1999). Electronic evaluation of the value of double gloving. *British Journal of Surgery, 86*, 1387–1390.

Cardo, D. M., & Bell, D. M. (1997). Bloodborne pathogen transmission in health care workers. *Infectious Disease Clinics of North America, 11*(2), 331–334.

Centers for Disease Control and Prevention, Hospital Infections Program. (1996). National Nosocomial Infections Surveillance (NNIS) report, data summary from October 1986–April 1996, issued May 1996. *American Journal of Infection Control, 24*, 380–388.

Centers for Disease Control and Prevention. (1996). Guidelines for Isolation Precautions in Hospitals. *MMWR Morbidity and Mortality Weekly Report, 45*, 36.

Centers for Disease Control and Prevention (1988). Perspectives in disease prevention of health promotion update: Universal precautions for prevention of transmission of human immunodeficiency virus, hepatitis B virus, and other bloodborne pathogens. *MMWR Morbidity and Mortality Weekly Report, 37*(24), 377–388.

Centers for Disease Control and Prevention (1987). Recommendations for prevention of HIV transmission in health-care settings. *MMWR Morbidity and Mortality Weekly Report, 36*, (SU02).

Churchill, R. B., & Pickering, L. K. (1997). Infection control challenges in child care centers. *Infectious Disease Clinics of North America, 11*(2), 347–361.

Crow, S. (1998). Asepsis: Back to basics. *Urologic Nursing, 18*(1), 42–46.

Decker, M. D., & Schaffner, W. (1996). TB control in the hospital: Compliance with OSHA requirements. In C. G. Mayhall (Ed.), *Hospital epidemiology and infection control.* Baltimore, MD: Williams & Wilkins.

Edmond, M. B., et al. (1999). Nosocomial bloodstream infections in United States hospitals: A three-year analysis. *Clinical Infectious Diseases, 29*, 239–244.

Garner, J. S. (1996). Hospital Infection Control Practices Advisory Committee: Guidelines for isolation precautions in hospitals. *Infection Control and Hospital Epidemiology, 17*, 53–80.

Gaynes, R. P. (1998). Surveillance of nosocomial infections. In John V. Bennett and Phillip S. Brachman (Eds.), *Hospital Infections* (4th ed.). Philadelphia: Lippincott-Raven, 65–84.

Gaynes, R. P. (2001). Feedback surveillance data to prevent hospital-acquired infections. *Emerging Infectious Diseases, 7*(2), 295–298.

Gold, H. S., & Moellering, R. C. (1996). Antimicrobial-drug resistance. *New England Journal of Medicine, 335*(19), 1445–1453.

Haley, R. W. (1998). Cost-benefit analysis of infection control programs. In John V. Bennett and Phillip S. Brachman (Eds.), *Hospital Infections* (4th ed.). Philadelphia: Lippincott-Raven, 249–267.

Hall, C. B. (2000). Nosocomial respiratory syncytial virus infections: The "cold war" has not ended. *Clinical Infectious Diseases, 31*(2), 590–596.

Jacobs, R. F. (2000). Judicious use of antibiotics for common pediatric respiratory infections. *Pediatric Infectious Disease Journal, 19*(9), 938–943.

Jarvis, W. R. (1996). Selected aspects of the socioeconomic impact of nosocomial infections: Morbidity, mortality, cost, and prevention. *Infection Control and Hospital Epidemiology, 17*(8), 552–557.

Jarvis, W. R. (2001). Infection control and changing health-care systems. *Emerging Infectious Diseases, 7*(2), 170–173.

Johnson, F. (1997). Disposable gloves: Research findings on use in practice. *Nursing Standard, 11*(16), 39–40.

Kerr, J. (1998). Handwashing. *Nursing Standard, 12*(51), 35–39.

Korniewicz, D., & Garzon, L. (1994). Combating infection: How to choose and use gloves. *Nursing '94, 24*(9), 18.

Kotilainen, H. R., & Keroack, M. A. (1997). Cost analysis and clinical impact of weekly ventilator circuit changes in patients in intensive care unit. *American Journal of Infection Control, 25*(2), 117–120.

Larson, E. L. & Kretzer, E. K. (1995). Compliance with hand-washing and hospital environmental control. *Journal of Hospital of Infection, 30,* 88–106.

Larson, E. L., and the Association for Professionals in Infection Control and Epidemiology 1992–1993 and 1994 APIC Guidelines Committee. (1995). APIC guideline for handwashing and hand asepsis in health care settings. *American Journal of Infection Control, 23,* 251–269.

Larson, E. L., et al. (2000). Assessment of alternative hand hygiene regimens to improve skin health among neonatal intensive care unit nurses. *Heart and Lung, 29*(2), 136–142.

Makris, A. T., et al. (2000). Effect of a comprehensive infection control program on the incidence of infections in long-term care facilities. *American Journal of Infection Control, 28*(1), 3–7.

Marin-Bertolin, S., et al. (1997). Does double gloving protect surgical staff from skin contamination during plastic surgery? *Plastic Reconstructive Surgery, 99,* 956–960.

Matrone, W. J., et al. (1998). Incidence and nature of endemic and epidemic nosocomial infections. In John V. Bennett and Phillip S. Brachman (Eds.), *Hospital Infections* (4th ed.). Philadelphia: Lippincott-Raven, 461–476.

McCullough, N. V., & Bousseau, L. M. (1999). Selecting respirators for control of worker exposure to infectious aerosols. *Infection Control and Hospital Epidemiology, 20*(2), 136–144.

Murthy, R. (2001). Implementation of strategies to control antimicrobial resistance. *Chest, 119*(2), 4055–4115.

Nicolle, L. E. (2000). Infection control in long-term care facilities. *Clinical Infectious Diseases, 31,* 752–756.

Patterson, J. E. (1996). Isolation of patients with communicable diseases. In C. G. Mayhall (Ed.), *Hospital epidemiology and infection control.* Baltimore, MD: Williams & Wilkins.

Pittet, D. (1999). Compliance with handwashing in a teaching hospital. *Annals of Internal Medicine, 130*(2), 126–129.

Pugliese, G. (1997). Reducing risks of infection during vascular access. *Journal of Intravenous Nursing, 20*(65), 511–523.

Pugliese, G. (2000). Congress approves needlestick safety bill. *Infection Control and Hospital Epidemiology, 21*(12), 805–807.

Reed, S. (2000). A victory for nurses. *American Journal of Nursing,* (12), 22.

Rogers, B. (1997). State of the science of health hazards in nursing and health care: An overview. *American Journal of Infection Control, 25*(3), 248–261.

Roudot-Thoraval, F., et al. (1999). Costs and benefits of measures to prevent needlestick injuries in a university hospital. *Infection Control and Hospital Epidemiology, 20*(9), 614–617.

Siegel, J. D. (1998). The newborn nursery. In John V. Bennett and Phillip S. Brachman (Eds.), *Hospital Infections* (4th ed.). Philadelphia: Lippincott-Raven.

Smith, P. W., & Rusnak, P. G. (1996). Infection prevention and control in the long-term-care facility. *American Journal of Infection Control, 25*(6), 488–512.

Sneddon, J., et al. (1997). Control of infection: A survey of general medical practices. *Journal of Public Health Medicine, 19*(3), 313–319.

Strausbaugh, L. J. (2001). Emerging health care-associated infections in the geriatric populations. *Emerging Infectious Diseases, 7*(2), 268–271.

Strausbaugh, L. J., & Joseph, C. L. (1996). Epidemiology and prevention of infections in residents of long term care facilities. In C. G. Mayhall (Ed.), *Hospital epidemiology and infection control.* Baltimore, MD: Williams & Wilkins.

Strausbaugh, L. J., and Joseph, C. L. (2000). The burden of infection in long-term care. *Infection Control and Hospital Epidemiology, 21*(10), 674–679.

Strodtbeck, F. (1995). Viral infections of the newborn. *Journal of Obstetrical, Gynecological, and Neonatal Nursing, 24*(7), 659–667.

Tenover, F. C., & Hughes, J. M. (1996). The challenges of emerging infectious diseases. *Journal of the American Medical Association, 275*(4), 300–304.

Voss, A., & Widmer, A. F. (1997). No time for handwashing!? Handwashing versus alcohol rub. Can we afford 100% compliance? *Infection Control and Hospital Epidemiology, 18*(3), 205–208.

Ward, D. (2000). Handwashing facilities in the clinical area: a literature review. *British Journal of Nursing, 9*(2), 82–86.

Weinstein, R. A. (1998). Nosocomial infection update. *Emerging Infectious Diseases, 4*(3), 1–7.

Willeke, K., & Quian, Y. (1998). Tuberculosis control through respirator wear: Performance of National Institute for Occupational Safety and Health- regulated respirators. *American Journal of Infection Control, 26*(2), 139–142.

Wong, E. S. (1999). Surgical site infections. In C. G. Mayhall (Ed.), *Hospital Epidemiology and Infection Control* (2nd ed.). Philadelphia: Lippincott Williams & Wilkins, 189–210.

BIBLIOGRAPHY

Anonymous. (1997). Respiratory protection. *Code of Federal Regulations,* Title 29, Part 1910.134, 413–417. Washington, DC: Office of the Federal Register, National Archives and Records Administration.

Anonymous. (2001). Standard principles for preventing hospital acquired infections. *Journal of Hospital Infection, 47* [Suppl], S21–S37.

Bentley, D. W., et al. (2000). Practice guidelines for evaluation of fever and infection in long-term care facilities. *Clinical Infectious Disease, 31,* 640–653.

Briggs, M., et al. (1996). Infection control: The principles of aseptic technique in wound care. *Professional Nurse, 11*(12), 805–808.

Centers for Disease Control and Prevention. (1994). CDC guidelines for preventing the transmission of TB in health care facilities, 1994. *Federal Register 1994, 59*(208), 54242–54303.

Centers for Disease Control and Prevention. (1994). Guidelines for prevention of nosocomial pneumonia: Part I. Issues on prevention of nosocomial pneumonia; Part II. Recommendations for prevention of nosocomial pneumonia. *American Journal of Infection Control, 22,* 247–292.

Centers for Disease Control and Prevention. (1996). Guidelines for prevention of intravascular device-related infections: Part I. Intravascular device-related infections: an overview. Part II. Recommendations for the prevention of nosocomial intravascular device-related infections. *American Journal of Infection Control, 24,* 262–292.

Centers for Disease Control and Prevention. (1998). Draft guidelines for the prevention of surgical site infection. *Federal Register, 63*(116), 33168–33192.

Centers for Disease Control and Prevention. (1998). Guideline for infection control in health care personnel. *Infection Control and Hospital Epidemiology, 19,* 407–463.

Cotran, R. S., Kumar, V., & Collins, T. (1999). *Pathologic basis of disease.* Philadelphia: W. B. Saunders.

Garcia, B. S., Barnard, B., & Kennedy, V. (2000). The fifth evolutionary era in infection control: International epidemiology. *American Journal of Infection Control, 28*(1), 30–41.

Garner, J. S. (1996). Guideline for isolation precautions in hospitals. The Hospital Infection Control Practices Advisory Committee. *Infection Control and Hospital Epidemiology, 17,* 53–80.

Glover, T. L. (2000). How drug-resistant microorganisms affect nursing. *Orthopedic Nursing, 19*(2), 19–25.

Hattula, J. L., & Stevens, P. E. (1997). A descriptive study of the handwashing environment in a long-term care facility. *Clinical Nursing Research, 6*(4), 363–374.

Ihrig, M., et al. (1997). Evaluation of the acceptability of a needleless vascular-access system by nurses. *American Journal of Infection Control, 25*(6), 434–438.

Jarvis, W. R. (1996). Nosocomial infections in pediatric patients. *Advances in Pediatric Infectious Diseases, 12,* 243–295.

Jones, S. G., & Fraise, A. P. (1997). Coping with nosocomial infections: A nonantibiotic approach. *British Journal of Hospital Medicine, 58*(5), 217–224.

Larson, E. L., and the Association for Professional in Infection Control and Epidemiology. (1995). APIC guideline for handwashing and asepsis in health care settings. *American Journal of Infection Control, 23,* 251–269.

Mayhall, C. G. (Ed.). (1999). *Hospital epidemiology and infection control* (2nd ed.). New York: Williams & Wilkins.

Miller, J. M., et al. (1996). Reduction in nosocomial intravenous device-related bacteremias after institution of an intravenous therapy team. *Journal of Intravenous Nursing, 19*(2), 103–106.

Moore, D. A., & Edwards, K. (1997). Using a portable bladder scan to reduce the incidence of nosocomial urinary tract infections. *MEDSURG Nursing, 6*(1), 39–43.

Occupational Safety and Health Administration. (2001). Occupational exposure to bloodborne pathogens: Needlestick and other sharp injuries, 2001. *Federal Register, 66*(12), 5317–5325.

Sharbaugh, R. J. (1999). The risk of occupational exposure and infection with infectious disease. *Nursing Clinics of North America, 34*(2), 493–507.

Shlaes, D. M., et al. (1997). Society for Healthcare Epidemiology of America and Infectious Diseases Society of America Joint Committee on the Prevention of Antimicrobial Resistance. Guidelines for the prevention of antimicrobial resistance in hospitals. *Infection Control and Hospital Epidemiology, 18*(4), 275–291.

Steed, C. J. (1999). Common infections acquired in the hospital. *Nursing Clinics of North America, 34*(2), 443–461.

Stotts, N. A., et al. (1997). Sterile versus clean technique in postoperative wound care of patients with open surgical wounds: A pilot study. *Journal of Wound, Ostomy, and Continence Nursing, 24*(1), 10–18.

Tortora, G. J., Funke, B. R., & Case, C. L. (1998). *Microbiology: An introduction* (6th ed.). Menlo Park, CA: Addison Wesley Longman.

Wenzel, R. P. (1995). The Lowbury Lecture: The economics of nosocomial infections. *Journal of Hospital Infections, 31*(2), 79–87.

Wenzel, R. P. (1997). *Prevention and control of nosocomial infections* (3rd ed.). Baltimore: Williams & Wilkins.

Wenzel, R. P. (2000). Managing antibiotic resistance. *New England Journal of Medicine, 343*(26), 1961–1963.

West, K. H., & Cohen, M. L. (1997). Standard precautions: A new approach to reducing infection transmission in the hospital setting. *Journal of Intravenous Nursing, 20*(6S), S7.

Wise, L. C., et al. (1997). Nursing wound care survey: Sterile and nonsterile glove choice. *Journal of Wound, Ostomy, and Continence Nursing, 24*(3), 144–150.

Woeltje, K. F. (1998). Preventing nosocomial infections in the intensive care unit: Lessons learned from outcomes research. *New Horizon, 6*(1), 84–90.

27 Medication Administration

Key Terms

absorption
antagonism
buccal
controlled substance
distribution
drug
excretion
intradermal
intramuscular
intravenous
medication

metabolism
parenteral
pharmacodynamics
pharmacokinetics
prescription
subcutaneous
sublingual
synergism
therapeutic effect
transdermal

Learning Objectives

Upon completion of this chapter, the student will be able to do the following:

1. Describe essential components of a medication order.
2. Discuss pharmacokinetic principles of drug action.
3. List the five rights of proper medication administration.
4. Calculate proper drug dosage using different systems of drug measurement.
5. Discuss important assessment data to obtain from the client during the initial interview and before medication administration.
6. Develop an individualized teaching plan to improve client knowledge of medications.
7. Describe recommended guidelines and procedures for medication administration by each route.

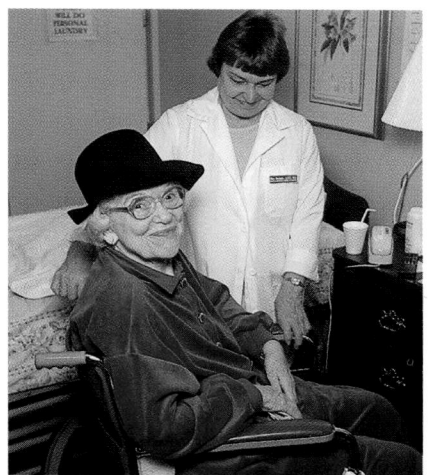

Critical Thinking Challenge

You are making a nursing visit to an older woman in her retirement facility. She was recently discharged from the hospital after treatment for a gastric ulcer that resulted from pain medications she was taking for arthritis. During your initial conversation, as you inquire about her health, you notice that the client appears distracted and seems to have difficulty following questions and giving answers. When you ask about her current medications, her responses indicate that she is unsure about what they are for and how to take them. When you ask her to show you her medications, she produces a large brown paper bag with about ten bottles: two bottles of a diuretic labeled "Take two tablets twice a day," three bottles of potassium chloride labeled "Take five tablets a day in divided doses," one bottle of a histamine blocker labeled "Take one capsule daily," one bottle of analgesic containing oxycodone to take "prn arthritis pain," one bottle of extra-strength acetaminophen, one bottle of stool softener capsules to take "as needed," and one bottle of another analgesic containing codeine to take "every 4 hours prn." As you inquire again about which medications she takes and when, you learn that she has age-related macular degeneration and is legally blind.

Once you have completed this chapter and have incorporated medication administration into your knowledge base, review the above scenario and reflect on the following areas of Critical Thinking:

1. Describe the direction that your assessment might take in this situation.
2. From the information the woman shared with you, identify possible factors that may make it difficult for the client to adhere to her medication regimen, possibly threatening her health.
3. Propose a course of timely and appropriate nursing actions.
4. What other individuals or healthcare professionals might you want to collaborate with concerning this situation?

The nurse's role in administering medications has become increasingly complex and diversified. Administering the correct medication and dosage by the specified route, using proper technique, and taking appropriate precautions were once all that was expected of nurses. Today, these important functions constitute only part of safe medication administration. The level of knowledge and skill now demanded of nurses is much broader. In addition to delivering pills and giving injections, observing and interpreting the client's response to therapy are crucial to recognize possible medication incompatibilities and interactions. Knowledge about the actions and side effects of medications and about the moral, ethical, and legal aspects of drug therapy also is important. Familiarity with sources of medication information, knowing when and how to use them, recognizing unsafe or unclear medication orders, and knowing what to do when such an order is encountered are key components involved with safe medication administration.

Nurses play a major role in promoting and maintaining client health by encouraging clients who need medications to be proactive consumers. By doing so, nurses help clients develop an active understanding of medications, clarify confusing information, insist on being consulted in every aspect of medication prescribing, and responsibly share decision making with other healthcare providers.

In many ways, the success of health promotion depends on clients' seeing themselves as healthcare participants with responsibility for choices about treatment and medications—whether alternative, prescribed, or over-the-counter (OTC) medications. Health promotion and health maintenance are the domain of knowledgeable and responsible consumers encouraged by healthcare professionals, especially nurses.

DRUGS AND MEDICATIONS

A **drug** is any substance that alters physiologic function, with the potential for affecting health. A **medication** is a drug administered for its therapeutic effects. Therefore, all medications are drugs, but not all drugs are medications. To administer medications effectively and safely, nurses must possess a broad range of general and specific knowledge.

Medications or drugs may be known by several names. A medication's *chemical name* describes the constituents that make up its molecular structure. It describes in chemist's terms the placement of atoms or atomic groupings. For example, the chemical name of the anti-inflammatory agent ibuprofen is 2-(4 isobutylphenyl) propionic acid.

The *official* drug name is assigned by the United States Adopted Names Council. Usually, this name is the *generic name,* or nonproprietary name. Each drug has only one generic name, which is simpler than the chemical name from which it is often derived. Examples of medications known by their generic names include morphine sulfate, acetaminophen, and ibuprofen.

The brand name or *trade name* is a registered name assigned by the manufacturer. Brand names are proper nouns with the first letter capitalized and marked with a circled R.

Some medications are manufactured by several companies and so may be known by several different brand names. An example is ampicillin sodium (generic name). This drug is marketed under such trade names as Omnipen-N, Polycillin-N, SK Ampicillin-N, and Totacillin-N.

Medication Standards

Because medications vary, the government establishes and controls standards guiding medication quality. The official list of medications in the United States is contained in two texts, the *United States Pharmacopeia* (USP) and the *National Formulary* (NF). The corresponding Canadian publication is the British Pharmacopoeia. The USP and NF describe medication products according to their source, physical and chemical properties, tests for purity and identity, method of storage, category, and normal dosages. Because medications vary according to their properties of purity, potency, bioavailability, efficacy, and safety and toxicity, medication standards must provide an appropriate range of quality for these properties.

Types and Forms of Drugs

Medications may be classified in many ways (e.g., according to their chemical composition, clinical actions, or therapeutic effect on body systems). Understanding general drug classifications aids in learning about the actions, side effects, and precautions needed for unfamiliar drugs. Table 27-1 lists classes of medications that may be used to promote the client's health.

Medications are prepared in various forms. Table 27-2 lists different drug preparations. Because of the wide range of available medication forms and dosages, nurses must pay close attention to medication orders and administer the specified form requested.

Sources of Information about Medications

A fundamental rule of safe drug administration is, "Never administer an unfamiliar medication." Before giving any drug, first understand the condition of the client for whom the medication is ordered. This knowledge, combined with knowledge of the ordered medication, explains why (and whether) the medication is appropriate for that client. Be familiar with dosage ranges of the medication being given, the expected therapeutic effects, and possible adverse actions or interactions with other medications. Also be prepared to teach the client the medication's purpose and to answer questions about the medication's use.

Making a habit of consulting standard drug reference materials is a way to stay up to date on medications, dosage, purpose, administration, and side effects. The latest developments in medication therapy are published in current journals, such as *American Journal of Nursing* and *Nursing,* as

TABLE 27-1

Classes of Medications to Promote Normal Function		
Health Pattern	**Drug Classes**	**Actions**
Activity and exercise	Antihypertensives	Decrease blood pressure
	Antiarrhythmics	Regulate heart rhythm
	Inotropes	Strengthen cardiac contraction
	Antianginals	Increase coronary blood flow
	Anticoagulants	Decrease clot formation
	Bronchodilators	Open airways
Nutrition and metabolism	Antibiotics	Decrease or prevent infection
	Antiemetics	Decrease nausea
	Antacids	Decrease gastric acidity
	Insulin	Decrease blood glucose levels
	Corticosteroids	Decrease inflammation
	Thyroid	Regulate metabolic rate
	Vitamins and minerals	Supplement inadequate dietary intake
Elimination	Laxatives	Promote stool evacuation
	Antidiarrheals	Decrease diarrhea
	Diuretics	Increase urine production and elimination
Sleep and rest	Sedatives, hypnotics	Induce sleep
Cognition and perception	Analgesics	Decrease pain
	Antipsychotics	Decrease psychotic symptoms (e.g., hallucinations)
Coping and stress tolerance	Antianxiety agents	Decrease anxiety
	Antidepressants	Decrease depression
Sexuality and reproduction	Ovarian hormones	Provide hormone replacement
		Provide birth control

well as monthly newsletters, such as *Nurses' Drug Alert* and *Medical Letter*.

The American Hospital Formulary Service publishes individual monographs on single generic and groups of medications. These monographs organize drug information by pharmacologic properties and index the medications by common brand names, generic name, and therapeutic class. Most hospitals prepare their own formulary, compiling information on all medications available within the individual facility. In addition, drug manufacturers' package inserts provide detailed data on the product contained in a packaged unit. Healthcare agencies frequently have drug information systems on computer for easy access.

The information source that nurses most frequently use is a drug handbook or reference guide. A nursing drug handbook not only provides information about specific medications but also emphasizes the nursing implications for medication administration. Many drug handbooks, which are usually updated annually, are sold with a computer disk or CD-ROM so that information on a specific medication can be downloaded and printed. Most healthcare facilities have several copies of these reference books available. A drug reference book may be kept on the medication cart, in the medication room, or at the nurses' station. Most nursing students are required to purchase a nursing drug handbook and are expected to bring it to clinical classes.

Systems of Medication Distribution

Various systems are used for storage and administration of medications. These systems include stock supply, unit-dose supply, automated medication-dispensing system, self-administered supply, and bar code medication administration (BCMA). Each distribution system varies among institutions depending on their procedures and policies, and a given institution may use a combination of two or more of these systems.

Healthcare facilities have designated areas for medication preparation. Some facilities have a central room with locked cupboards containing supplies; others use mobile medication carts with locked drawers or locked wall cabinets near the clients' rooms. Other facilities have satellite pharmacy units that are located on a particular floor and serve several client-care areas. In accordance with narcotic control laws, controlled substance medications are kept in locked drawers in all client-care areas.

Stock Supply System

A stock supply system in a client-care area provides large quantities of frequently prescribed medications for that particular unit; these are stored in locked cupboards in a storage room. Individual doses are dispensed and administered by nurses, who measure individual doses from the large stock bottles or packaged containers. Examples of stock supply

TABLE 27-2

Drug Preparations	
Type of Preparation	**Description**
Oral Preparations	
Capsule	Gelatinous container to hold powder or liquid medicine
Elixir	Liquid preparation of medication with alcohol base
Emulsion	Suspension within an oil base
Enteric coated	Coating that causes drug absorption in intestines rather than the stomach; prevents stomach irritation
Lozenge (troche)	Tablet held in the mouth to be dissolved
Powder	Finely ground drug; frequently mixed with liquid before administration
Spansule	Timed-release drug capsule, which dissolves more slowly to provide an effect over a long period
Suspension	Medication in liquid, which must be shaken before administration because it separates
Syrup	Medicine dissolved in sugar and water
Tablet	Compressed hard disk of powdered medication; may be scored for easy breaking; may be sugar coated or have film coating for cohesion
Tincture	Potent solution with alcohol base made from plants; dosage usually small
Topical Preparations	
Cream	Nongreasy, semisolid preparation for topical application
Gel or jelly	Translucent or clear semisolid substance that liquefies when applied to the skin
Liniment	Oily liquid used on the skin
Lotion	Emollient liquid, clear solution or suspension, which is applied to the skin
Ointment	Drug combined with oil base for external application
Paste	Thick ointment used for local application to the skin
Suppository	Medicine contained within a gelatinous base (shaped for easy insertion into the body), which dissolves at body temperature, slowly releasing the drug
Transdermal patch	Medicine in a patch, which, when applied to the skin, permits gradual, controlled absorption

medications include acetaminophen, multiple vitamins, and saline solutions. The stock supply system is the least common medication distribution system. When used, it is usually in combination with another system.

Unit-Dose System

A unit-dose system involves the pharmacy or manufacturer in prepackaging and prelabeling an individual client dose. The individual unit dose is a prescribed amount of medication dispensed at a specified time.

This type of system is widely used in large healthcare facilities such as hospitals. Pharmacists and nurses both participate in preparation and administration of medications and evaluation of their effects. The pharmacy dispenses medications that are individually packaged and labeled with the medication name and dose. The pharmacist can provide information to the nurse about potential medication interactions or contraindications. The nurse administers the medications.

In many extended care facilities, a client-specific unit-dose system is used. The pharmacy packages and labels a medication in the specified dose for a specific person in a "bingo card" (Fig. 27-1). Each "bubble" on the bingo card contains one dose; the card as a whole may contain as many as 60 doses. This method is more economic in healthcare settings where the average length of stay for clients is longer than 2 weeks and there is no pharmacy on site.

Automated Medication-Dispensing System

The automated medication-dispensing system is common in healthcare facilities (Fig. 27-2). It is a technologically enhanced combination of the stock supply and unit-dose systems. The system consists of a machine containing a combination of

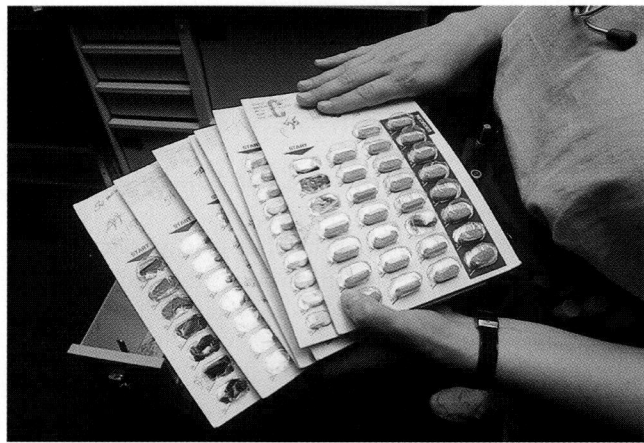

FIGURE 27-1   In long-term care settings, where medication prescriptions remain the same over weeks or months, "bingo" cards are a cost-effective method of dispensing medications. Each bubble contains one dose for the client.

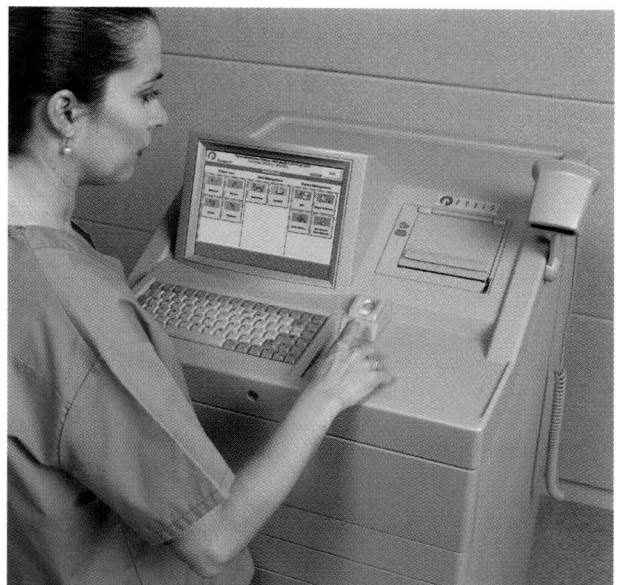

FIGURE 27-2 An automated medication system.

medications frequently used on a unit (to enable immediate administration of newly ordered medications), "as needed" (prn) medications, controlled drugs, and emergency medications. The machine operates similarly to an automated bank machine. Nurses access the system by using a password, then select a function from choices offered by the computerized menus to obtain the desired medication for a client. The medication is delivered in a unit-dose package. The automated medication-dispensing system keeps an account of all medications used for billing and controlled substance record keeping.

Self-Administered Medication System

The self-administered medication system supplies each client with his or her prescribed doses and quantities for a given period. Each medication is supplied in a separate container and is used for one client only. Medications can be stored at the client's bedside, allowing the client to administer his or her own medication doses. This system can be used along with the stock or unit-dose systems. For example, a client may have sublingual nitroglycerin supplied by the self-administered medication system and other medications supplied by the unit-dose system. This combination allows the client to use nitroglycerin immediately if chest pain occurs. Moreover, this method of administration allows the client a greater opportunity to be involved in his or her own care. It also decreases the time the nurse spends administering medications and increases the nurse's ability to evaluate how well the client can manage his or her medication regimen.

Bar Code Medication Administration

This system uses a lightweight handheld laser scanner, a laptop computer attached to a medication cart, and bar codes (Styrcula, 2000). Clients wear bar-coded identification bracelets. The nurse must enter a password to access the computer system. When the nurse passes the scanner over the patient's identification bracelet, the patient's medication record dis-

plays on the computer screen. The nurse then selects medications from the client's drawer on the medication cart and scans the bar code on each unit-dose packaged medication. At this time this system confirms patient identity, medication, dose, and route. It also tracks actual time of administration and the identity of the nurse administering the medication. This system also can display assessment results such as vital signs and laboratory findings (Waldo, 1999). A legible, real-time medication administration record is created and available for review by nurse, pharmacist, and physician. BCMA was conceptualized by Sue Kinnick, B.S.N., M.S., nursing informatics specialist at Eastern Kansas Veterans Administration Health Care System, in the early 1990s (Arquiza, 2001). It is now in use at all of the Veterans Administration system hospitals, as well as various other institutions throughout the United States.

Nonprescription and Prescription Medications

Nonprescription Medications

Many medications can be obtained without a written order from a healthcare provider. They are sold OTC because they are generally regarded as safe enough for use without medical or nursing supervision. Common examples of OTC medications include cold remedies and mild analgesics, such as aspirin and acetaminophen. The U.S. Food and Drug Administration (FDA) maintains control over the safety, effectiveness, and advertising of nonprescription medications.

Nonprescription medications are considered safe when used as directed. The dangers of these readily available medications lie in their misuse, which can cause dangerous side effects. Some people persist in self-medicating with nonprescription drugs and delay seeking professional help, possibly enabling a minor problem to develop into a major one because of early mistreatment. There also is danger of serious drug interactions.

Prescription Medications

A **prescription** is a legal order for the preparation and administration of a medication.

SAFETY ALERT
Always determine which (if any) nonprescription medications the client has been taking and ensure that he or she takes no medications without the healthcare provider's knowledge.

For some clients, certain medications require medical supervision, often because of a narrow margin of safety between a therapeutic and a toxic dose. Physicians and dentists are legally responsible for prescribing medications. In some states, nurse practitioners and physician's assistants may prescribe medications.

Herbs and Other Botanicals

In the United States, use of herbal and other botanical medications fell out of favor in the early 20th century because of the lack of quality standardization and scientific data regarding efficacy and adverse effects. But, in the 1970s interest in herbal preparations re-emerged. The term "natural" was equated with "safe" and therefore implied better medicine (Decker & Myers, 2001). Even though the use of medicinal herbs and other botanicals or plant products is currently widespread, until recently botanical medications have not consistently been included in a client's history. The nurse needs to assess for the use of these products. Some of the most common botanicals are St. John's wort (*Hypericum perfoliatrum*), used for mild depression; *Echinacea* (coneflower), used as a mild antibiotic; and *Gingko biloba* (maidenhair tree), used to increase blood circulation and to improve cognitive function.

People may think that these products are safe because they are advertised as "all natural," but judging their safety and efficacy can be difficult. Unlike other medications, herbs and botanicals lack quality standards and regulation; their ingredients or quantities may or may not be as stated on the label. Dosages are less exact because the potency of a botanical can vary, depending on how it was prepared and the particular plant source used. Herbal preparations are classified by the FDA as "dietary supplements." In 1999, The FDA required all labels on herbal preparations to state which part of the plant (e.g., root, leaf, stem) was used for the active ingredient, to suggest the relative potency of each preparation (Borins, 1999). Some botanicals can cause toxic effects and drug–drug interactions. For example, gingko biloba can cause bleeding when taken with medications such as aspirin or Coumadin. Table 27-3 lists uses and possible side effects of selected herbal preparations.

Controlled, randomized studies have been done on some botanical preparations; other scientific investigations are beginning to provide clinically relevant information (Decker & Myers, 2001). The nurse needs to think about botanical products as drugs. Any time a person puts a substance into the body, it can cause unknown or unexpected effects. Therefore, the nurse needs to assess the client for use of botanical tablets, teas, extracts, and tinctures and to consult herbal formularies as needed for specific information.

Medication Order

Components

The prescriber of a medication conveys an order by specifying the client's name, the medication's name, amount and frequency of the dose, and route of administration. Included with this directive are the date and time the prescription was written and the signature of the prescribing healthcare provider. The client's first and last name must be written with the medication order to avoid confusion between two clients with the same last name. The client's identification or medical number can be written with the order as further identification.

Abbreviations are commonly used in the medication order. Certain standard abbreviations indicate the amount and frequency of a medication dosage. These abbreviations are legal and may be used in the client's chart. The more commonly used abbreviations are listed in Table 27-4.

Medication Name. The name of the medication can be written using the generic or trade name. The name should be written clearly, because many medications are similar in spelling but different in drug action.

🥛 **SAFETY ALERT**
Always clarify with the prescriber any medication order that is unclear or seems inappropriate.

Medication Dosage. The medication dosage can be written using the metric, apothecary, or household measurement systems. The strength and frequency of the dose also are indicated (e.g., digoxin 0.25 mg once a day). If a medication is dispensed in only one dose, the prescriber may indicate the number of tablets or pills to take (e.g., multiple vitamin one daily).

Route of Administration. The route of administration is commonly abbreviated as a part of the written order. Many medications can be given by several routes, such as orally (PO), intravenously (IV), or intramuscularly (IM).

🥛 **SAFETY ALERT**
If an order specifies a certain route of administration and the client's condition changes, making the ordered route inappropriate or possibly unsafe, notify the prescriber so that he or she can change the route of administration.

Signature. Because the written order is a legal request, the prescriber's signature must follow the written order. An unsigned order is invalid and should not be carried out until the prescriber signs the order.

Types of Orders

Routine or Standing Order. The routine medication order is one that should be carried out for a specified number of days (e.g., antibiotic) or until another order cancels it (e.g., diabetic medication). In some healthcare agencies, the standing orders must be reviewed and rewritten within a specified time frame or they are canceled automatically.

PRN Orders. A prn order (from the Latin, *pro re nata*) does not indicate a specific time for administration of a medication. Rather, it states guidelines so that the medication can be administered as needed. Pain medications, nausea medications, and laxatives are often ordered on a prn basis. Good judgment is essential to determine when a medication is needed and when it is safe to administer the medication.

Standing Protocols. Standing protocols are written for medications to be administered in specific situations with criteria for administration outlined clearly for clients on a specific unit

TABLE 27-3

Commonly Used Herbs and their Side Effects/or Drug Interactions		
Herb	**Use**	**Side-Effect or Drug Interaction**
Aloe latex	Constipation; heals bowel inflammation	Binds with other drugs, decreasing absorption; hypokalemia; toxicity for some cardiac medications
Dong Quai	Relieves hot flashes	Increased bleeding, especially when used in combination with other anticoagulants
Echinacea	Improves immune function and wound healing; fights flu and colds	Possible liver inflammation and damage when used with anabolic steroids or methotrexate
Ephedra (Ma-Huang)	Improves respiratory function in asthma or bronchitis; diet aid and appetite suppressant	Could severely increase pulse or blood pressure when taken with antidepressants or antihypertensive agents, possibly causing death
Feverfew	Prevents migraines, treats allergies, and manages arthritis and rheumatic disease	Increased bleeding, especially when used in combination with anticoagulants
Garlic	Lowers cholesterol, triglycerides, and blood pressure	Increased bleeding, especially when used in combination with anticoagulants
Ginger	Decreases nausea, vomiting, and vertigo	Increased bleeding, especially when used in combination with anticoagulants
Ginkgo biloba	Improves memory and mental alertness; increased circulation and oxygenation	Increased bleeding, especially when used in combination with anticoagulants
Ginseng	Increases physical stamina and mental concentration	May increase heart rate and blood pressure; may cause bleeding in some women after menopause; decreases effectiveness of anticoagulant medications
Goldenseal	Decreases inflammation and acts as a laxative	May increase blood pressure or cause swelling
Kava-kava	Muscle relaxant, decreases nervousness and anxiety	Prolongs the effects of some anesthetic agents; increases side effects of some anti-seizure medications; may increase suicide risk for depressed clients; enhances effects of alcohol
Licorice	Treats stomach ulcers	May cause hypertension, swelling, and electrolyte imbalances
Saw palmetto	Treats urinary inflammation and enlarged prostate	Interacts with other hormone therapies
St. John's wort	Treats mild to moderate depression, anxiety, and sleep disorders	May prolong effects of anesthetic agents
Valerian	Mild sedative or sleep aid; muscle relaxant	May prolong effects of anesthetic agents or increase the side effects of antiseizure medications

or service. For example, a standing protocol might be written in a cardiac unit to administer a certain antiarrhythmic agent if the client develops a specific arrhythmia or on a general unit to administer Tylenol if a client complains of a headache.

One-Time Order. The one-time or single order is written for a medication that will be given only once. An order for a preoperative medication, to help calm the client before surgery, is an example of a one-time order.

Stat Order. A stat order (from the Latin *statim*, "immediately") is a single order for a medication that must be given immediately. An example of this order is "furosemide 20 mg IV stat" for fluid volume excess.

Telephone, Verbal, and Fax Orders. At times, the nurse and prescriber may discuss a client's condition over the phone and decide to change the client's medication regimen. Because the prescriber is not available to write and sign the order, the

TABLE 27-4

Common Abbreviations Used in Medication Orders

Abbreviation	Meaning	Abbreviation	Meaning
a or a.	before	mg	milligram
a.c.	before meals	no	number
ad lib	as desired	noct.	night
alt. h.	alternate hours	OD	right eye
AM	in the morning; before noon	os	mouth
A.D.	right ear	OS	left eye
A.S.	left ear	OU	both eyes
A.U.	each ear	oz	ounce
aq.	water	p or p.	after; per
bid	twice a day	p.c.	after meals
c̄	with	per os, PO	by mouth
cap., caps.	capsule	PM	afternoon; evening
cc	cubic centimeter	prn	as needed, according to necessity
d	day	q	each, every
D/C, dc	discontinue	qh	every hour
dil.	dilute	qid	four times a day
dist.	distilled	q1h	every 1 hour
DS	double strength	q2h	every 2 hours
EC	enteric coated	q3h	every 3 hours
elix.	elixir	q4h	every 4 hours
et	and	q6h	every 6 hours
ext.	external, extract	q8h	every 8 hours
fl, fld	fluid	q12h	every 12 hours
g	gram	qod	every other day
gr	grain	qs	as much as needed, quantity sufficient
gtt	drop	qt	quart
H	hypodermic	R. or PR	rectally, per rectum
h, hr	hour	Rx	take, prescription
h.s.	at bedtime	s̄	without
IM	intramuscular	sc	subcutaneously
inj.	injection	sol. or soln.	solution
IV	intravenous	SQ	subcutaneous
IVP	IV push	stat.	immediately, at once
IVPB	IV piggy back	tab.	tablet
kg	kilogram	tbsp, T	tablespoon
L	liter	tid	three times a day
lb	pound	tinct, tr	tincture
liq.	liquid	tsp, t	teaspoon
mcg, μg	microgram	ung.	ointment
mEq	milliequivalent		

nurse may write the order on a physician order sheet. This type of order is usually designated on the sheet as a telephone order (e.g., "T.O. by Dr. Phillips," "Susan Brown, ARNP") and signed by the nurse.

 SAFETY ALERT

To ensure accuracy when taking telephone orders, always repeat the order to the prescriber after writing it down. The prescriber must cosign the order within a specified time, usually 48 hours.

Sometimes nurses and prescribers communicate about a client's condition by fax (facsimile) machine. In writing, the nurse may briefly describe a change in the client's condition and request a new medication order or change in a current medication order. The nurse sends this request to the prescriber's office by fax machine. The prescriber sends a return fax, indicating any necessary changes. The nurse then writes the order in the client's chart. Because the fax machine uses telephone lines, the fax order is considered a telephone order, and the prescriber must cosign it at a later time.

LEGAL ASPECTS OF MEDICATION ADMINISTRATION

Food and Drug Administration

The FDA, a division of the U.S. Department of Health and Human Services, regulates the manufacture, sale, and effectiveness of medications. It also requires drug testing in laboratory animals and in humans (through controlled, three-phase clinical trials) before a drug is approved for use. The FDA also is charged with keeping ineffective or unsafe drugs off the market and recalling inadequately tested or dangerous drugs. Additional functions include identifying which medications can be obtained with or without a prescription, setting and en-

forcing standards of purity and potency, overseeing all drugs, and controlling drug advertising to the medical profession.

Controlled Substances

As a result of rising drug abuse and increasing public concern in the late 1960s, the U.S. Congress enacted the Comprehensive Drug Abuse Prevention and Control Act of 1970, which includes the Controlled Substances Act. **Controlled substances** are drugs that are considered to have either limited medical use or high potential for abuse or addiction. The Controlled Substances Act categorizes controlled substances in five groups (I, II, III, IV, and V) based on their potential for abuse and their medical usefulness. Table 27-5 describes

TABLE 27-5

Schedules of Controlled Substances Categorized by the Controlled Substances Act			
Schedule	**Characteristics**	**Dispensing Restrictions**	**Examples**[a]
I	High abuse potential No accepted medical use—for research, analysis, or instruction only	Approved protocol necessary	Heroin, marijuana, tetrahydrocanabinols, LSD, mescaline, peyote, methaqualone
II	May lead to severe physical or psychological dependence High abuse potential Accepted medical uses	Written Rx necessary—only emergency dispensing permitted without written Rx Only required amount may be prescribed No Rx refills allowed Container must have warning label	Opium, morphine, hydromorphone, meperidine, codeine, oxycodone, methadone, secobarbital, pentobarbital, dextrol, amphetamine, methylphenidate, cocaine
III	Less abuse potential than drugs in Schedules I and II Accepted medical uses May lead to moderate or low physical dependence or high psychological dependence	34-day supply limit Written or oral Rx required Rx expires in 6 months No more than five Rx refills allowed within a 6-month period Container must have warning label[b]	Preparations containing limited quantities of opioids or combined with one or more active ingredients that are non-controlled substances Also pargone, nandrolone, stanozolol, testosterone
IV	Low abuse potential compared with drugs in Schedule III Accepted medical uses May lead to limited physical or psychological dependence	Written or oral Rx required Rx expires in 6 months No more than five Rx refills allowed Container must have warning label	Barbital, phenobarbital, chloral hydrate, meprobamate, fenfluramine, chlordiazepoxide, diazepam, oxazepam, chlorazepate, flurazepam, lorazepam, propoxyphene, pentazocine, mazindol, aprazolam
V	Low abuse potential compared with drugs in Schedule IV Accepted medical uses May lead to limited physical or psychological dependence	May require written Rx or be sold with Rx (check state law)	Medications, generally for relief of coughs or diarrhea, containing limited quantities of certain opioid controlled substances

[a] The examples cited constitute a partial listing. Individual hospital counsel should be consulted for a complete list for a particular state.
[b] Caution: Federal law prohibits the transfer of this drug to any person other than the client for whom it was prescribed.
From DEA pharmacist's manual—An informational outline of the Controlled Substances Act of 1970. U.S. Dept. of Justice. Washington, DC, Red Book, 1996.

the five schedules. Under this law, possession of a controlled substance without a valid prescription is illegal, and the number of times a prescription can be filled is limited. The primary reasons for the Controlled Substances Act were to prevent drug abuse and dependence, provide treatment and rehabilitation for people who are dependent on drugs, and strengthen drug abuse laws.

In hospitals and other healthcare settings, controlled substances are kept in a locked drawer or box as an additional safety measure. Controlled substances may be ordered only by physicians or other healthcare providers registered with the Department of Justice, Bureau of Narcotics and Dangerous Drugs. A record must be kept for each controlled substance administered. Individual pharmacies provide various types of controlled substance sheets. Information generally required includes the name of the client receiving the controlled substance, the date and hour the medication was given, the amount of the controlled medication used, the name of the healthcare provider prescribing the controlled substance, and the name of the nurse administering the controlled substance.

A count of controlled medications is performed at specified times (e.g., at each change of shift). The types and amounts of controlled medications issued by the pharmacy for that particular unit are counted, and any medications administered during the previous shift must be on the control sheet. Before administering a controlled medication, the count in the drawer must be verified and the control sheet must be signed to indicate that the medication has been removed. If all or part of a dose is discarded, a second nurse should witness the discarding and should countersign the control sheet. At the end of the shift, one nurse should record the amount of each controlled medication on the control sheet while another nurse counts the medications aloud. Any discrepancies must be identified and corrected before the nurse leaves the unit; if the discrepancy cannot be resolved, it must be reported to the nurse manager, nursing supervisor, or pharmacy. The use of automated medication-dispensing systems eliminates the need to count and sign out controlled substances, because the system maintains a computerized record each time a medication is removed from the system.

Nurse Practice Acts

Nursing legislation controls the administration of medications by nurses. Nurse practice acts, established to describe legitimate nursing functions, vary from state to state. Be informed about how your state's nurse practice act defines the boundaries of your functions. Also, recognize your own individual limits of knowledge and skill.

Under current nurse practice laws, nurses are responsible for their own actions regardless of the prescriber's written order. If an order is ambiguous or inappropriate, the nurse must clarify the medication order with the prescribing healthcare provider. If dissatisfied with the prescriber's response and still believing that the order is incorrect or unsafe, the nurse must notify a supervisor.

SAFETY ALERT
Know that you have the right and responsibility to decline to administer a medication if you believe it jeopardizes client safety.

Nurses also are expected to practice in a safe and prudent manner. Each nurse is responsible for being knowledgeable about the medication's actions, indications, contraindications, and any adverse effects. Knowledge of appropriate dosages and dosage schedules, routes and methods of administration, and actions to take if the client has an adverse reaction is also important.

Dispensing medications (i.e., preparing a medication that someone else will deliver) is not a legal practice for registered nurses in most states. Whereas physicians and other healthcare providers prescribe and pharmacists dispense therapeutic agents, it is the nurse's legal domain to administer medications in a safe and timely manner.

SAFETY ALERT
Do not give any medication prepared by another nurse unless the unit-dose label identifies the drug and the seals are intact.

Institutional Medication Policies

Nurses work in various settings, including schools, hospitals, nursing homes, home healthcare agencies, and private industries. Each institution develops and oversees its own medication administration policies, and these rules can vary widely.

Some institutions allow only registered nurses to administer medications. Others allow graduate nurses, licensed practical (or vocational) nurses, or nursing students working in the agency to administer medications. Institutions may place restrictions on the types of medications nurses can give or on the degree of supervision or experience they require. Every institution is governed by its own policies and procedures. Be aware of the practice within your institution.

Client's Rights

The client has the right to expect safe and appropriate drug administration by the nurse (see Display 6-2 in Chapter 6—A Patient's Bill of Rights). To accomplish this, the nurse must observe "five rights": the right drug, in the right dose, at the right time, by the right route, to the right client.

In addition to these five rights, the client has the right to refuse to take medications. Under these circumstances, the nurse has the duty to explain to the client as fully and clearly as possible the importance of taking the medication. If a client refuses to comply with prescribed medication therapy, attempt to clarify the client's concern about the medication and notify the prescriber, including information about the client's concerns.

ETHICAL/LEGAL ISSUE
Client's Refusal of Medications

You are a nursing student assigned to care for George Saunders, a 47-year-old homeless man, who was admitted last evening for pneumonia. He has a history of alcohol abuse and mental illness. When you approach his room with his scheduled antibiotic and antipsychotic medications, he starts yelling, telling you to "get that poison away from me." You talk with staff members about his reaction, asking them what to do. One staff person tells you to mix the medications in the client's food when he is not looking. Another tells you to chart that the client refused the medications.

Reflection
- Explore whether Mr. Saunders has the right to refuse his medication.
- Evaluate possible factors that might have affected Mr. Saunders' ability to make an informed decision regarding whether to take his medication.
- Determine whether you have the right to trick him into taking his medications. Discuss why or why not and any possible ramifications in doing so.
- Outline possible positive and negative consequences of allowing Mr. Saunders to refuse medication.
- Would you respond any differently if Mr. Saunders were a middle-class business executive?

ETHICAL/LEGAL ISSUE
Possible Substance Abuse by a Healthcare Worker

You are a charge nurse working the evening shift on a busy surgical unit. For the third time in 3 weeks, the narcotic count is incorrect at the end of shift. You suspect that one of your coworkers may be diverting narcotics based on the following information: she has always been working when the count has been short, she calls in sick frequently, she has mood swings, and she tends to blame others rather than accept responsibility for her errors. You have no objective evidence that she is diverting narcotics, just a suspicion.

Reflection
- Outline responsibilities you have to clients on the unit, the nurse you suspect, the administration, and yourself.
- Identify possible negative and positive consequences of notifying your nurse manager if your assumptions are right. If they are wrong.
- Imagine how you might effectively interact with the nurse involved. Anticipate her possible reaction.

assists the nurse in evaluating therapeutic and adverse effects of medications.

Pharmacokinetics

Pharmacokinetics involves the absorption, distribution, metabolism, and excretion of a medication. Each medication has its own characteristic rate and manner by which it is absorbed by body tissues, delivered to reactive cells, transformed to harmless substances, and removed from the body.

Absorption is the process by which a medication enters the bloodstream. The route of administration affects how quickly and how completely a medication is absorbed. Intravenous administration offers the quickest rate of absorption, followed in descending order by intramuscular, subcutaneous, and oral routes.

Distribution is the process by which the medication is delivered to the target cells and tissues. Effectiveness of the circulatory system, amount of medication bound to protein, and tissue specificity of the drug affect distribution.

Metabolism is the process of chemically changing the drug in the body. Metabolism takes place mainly in the liver. Alterations in liver function, including decreased function that occurs with aging or disease, affect the rate at which drugs are metabolized.

Excretion is the process of removing the drug or its metabolites from the body. The kidneys excrete most drug metabolites. Some excretion also occurs in the lungs and the intestines. Decreased kidney function adversely affects drug excretion.

Substance Abuse

The illegal use of drugs by any health professional jeopardizes client welfare and professional credibility. Stringent rules and procedures help to prevent diversion of client medications to healthcare personnel. Each nurse has the ethical and legal obligation to maintain accurate medication records and to report any discrepancies. The law further requires nurses to report any known diversion of controlled substances by colleagues.

SAFETY ALERT
The chemically impaired nurse cannot be trusted to exercise optimal clinical judgment. Such individuals must be identified so that they can obtain treatment and to protect client safety.

PRINCIPLES OF DRUG ACTION

An understanding of the ways by which drugs exert their effects is an important component of medication administration. **Pharmacokinetics** is the process by which a drug moves through the body and is eventually eliminated. **Pharmacodynamics** refers to the physiologic and biochemical effects of a drug on the body. Understanding these processes

Pharmacodynamics

Drug activity is the result of chemical interactions between a medication and the body's cells to produce a biologic response. Most drugs interact with a cellular component to initiate a series of biochemical and physical changes, resulting in the drug's effectiveness. These biochemical and physiologic effects can be local or systemic. For example, local effects are seen when moisturizing lotion is applied to chapped skin. Systemic effects can affect one or more body systems. For example, when analgesics (pain medications) are administered, effects on sedation (nervous system), respiratory rate and depth (lungs), and constipation (gastrointestinal tract) are seen.

Medication effects are monitored by changes in the client's clinical condition. Generally, improvement in physical or psychological symptoms or laboratory test results occurs when medications are effective. In addition to clinical observations, laboratory measurements of the concentration of medication in the blood can be obtained.

Therapeutic Effects

A medication's desired and intentional effects are called its **therapeutic effects.** These effects vary with the nature of the medication, the length of time the client has been receiving it, and the client's physical condition. Interactions with other medications also can affect a drug's therapeutic action. The onset of action of medications varies widely depending on the medication, the route of administration, and the half-life of the drug.

Adverse Effects

An adverse effect is any effect other than the therapeutic effect. Adverse effects can result from excessive therapeutic effects (e.g., severe hypotension when an antihypertensive agent is administered). Some adverse effects are minor (e.g., constipation) and can be treated easily. Others may pose serious health risks for the client (e.g., respiratory depression). Adverse effects increase in clients who are very ill and receiving many medications (Cleveland, Aschenbrenner, Venable, & Yensen, 1999).

The FDA has developed the MedWatch program to encourage voluntary reporting of any serious adverse drug effects. Any healthcare professional can report, without proof of direct causation, any unexpected response to drug therapy or medical devices. The FDA correlates data collected to update drug information that it gives to the public. An example of the MedWatch form is included in Figure 27-3.

Side Effects. Minor adverse effects are called side effects. Many side effects are essentially harmless and can be ignored. Some, however, are undesirable and potentially harmful. Especially when a new medication is started or added or when a dose is increased, nurses must be alert for adverse drug reactions or side effects in clients.

Hypersensitivity Reactions. Hypersensitivity reactions occur when a client is unusually sensitive to a medication's therapeutic effects or secondary effects. An estimated therapeutic dosage of medication may be too large for the client and may result in a degree of action that is greater than desired. For example, a middle-aged man of normal body weight usually requires 5 to 10 mg of morphine to relieve pain. An underweight elderly client, however, may respond to the same dosage with longer duration and excessive somnolence. Usually, if the medication dose or the dosing interval is decreased, the medication may be administered safely.

Tolerance. Tolerance to a medication occurs when a client develops a decreased response to it, requiring an increased dosage to achieve the therapeutic effects. Some agents that produce tolerance include nicotine, ethyl alcohol, opiates, and barbiturates.

Allergic Reactions. Allergic reactions result from an immunologic response to a medication to which the client has been sensitized. A foreign substance or antigen has been introduced into the body, and the body responds by producing antibodies. Clients respond to certain medications as they would to this foreign substance and develop symptoms of an allergic reaction. These symptoms range from mild to severe.

Mild allergic reactions, commonly manifested by hives (urticaria), pruritus, or rhinitis, can occur within minutes to 2 weeks after medication administration. Skin reactions, including hives, rashes, and lesions, usually improve soon after the medication is discontinued, especially with concomitant use of antihistamines. Severe allergic reactions producing symptoms such as wheezing, dyspnea, angioedema of the tongue and oropharynx, hypotension, and tachycardia occur immediately after the medication is given. A severe allergic reaction, called an *anaphylactic reaction,* requires immediate medical intervention because it can be fatal. Treatment includes discontinuing the medication and administering epinephrine, IV fluids, steroids, and antihistamines.

Toxicity. Medication toxicity results from overdosage or buildup of medication in the blood due to impaired metabolism and excretion. Careful attention must be given specifically to the dosage and to toxicity monitoring, such as assessing laboratory values of liver and kidney function. Some medications can produce toxic effects almost immediately, whereas some do not produce toxic effects for days or weeks.

Toxicity can affect and permanently damage organ function. Common drug toxicities include nephrotoxicity (kidney), neurotoxicity (brain), hepatotoxicity (liver), immunotoxicity (immune system), ototoxicity (hearing), and cardiotoxicity (heart). Knowledge about potential drug toxicity permits focused nursing assessments for early detection, thus preventing permanent damage.

Interactions

Medication interaction occurs when a medication's effects are altered by the concurrent presence of other medications or food. This interaction may result in potentiation or **synergism,** which increases a drug's effects. Interaction also can result in **antagonism,** by which drug effects decrease. Sometimes,

MedWatch

THE FDA MEDICAL PRODUCTS REPORTING PROGRAM

For **VOLUNTARY** reporting
by health professionals of adverse
events and product problems

Page ___ of ___

Form Approved OMB No. 0910-0291 Expires:12/31/94
See OMB statement on reverse

FDA Use Only **[DAVIS]**

Triage unit
sequence #

PLEASE TYPE OR USE BLACK INK

A. Patient information

1. Patient identifier
2. Age at time of event: ___ or Date of birth: ___

In confidence

3. Sex ☐ female ☐ male
4. Weight ___ lbs or ___ kgs

B. Adverse event or product problem

1. ☐ Adverse event and/or ☐ Product problem (e.g., defects/malfunctions)

2. Outcomes attributed to adverse event (check all that apply)
☐ death ___ (mo day yr)
☐ life-threatening
☐ hospitalization – initial or prolonged
☐ disability
☐ congenital anomaly
☐ required intervention to prevent permanent impairment/damage
☐ other: ___

3. Date of event (mo day yr)
4. Date of this report (mo day yr)
5. Describe event or problem
6. Relevant tests/laboratory data, including dates
7. Other relevant history, including preexisting medical conditions (e.g. allergies, race, pregnancy, smoking and alcohol use, hepatic/renal dysfunction, etc.)

C. Suspect medication(s)

1. Name (give labeled strength & mfr/labeler, if known)
#1
#2

2. Dose, frequency & route used
#1
#2

3. Therapy dates (if unknown, give duration) from/to (or best estimate)
#1
#2

4. Diagnosis for use (indication)
#1
#2

5. Event abated after use stopped or dose reduced
#1 ☐ yes ☐ no ☐ doesn't apply
#2 ☐ yes ☐ no ☐ doesn't apply

6. Lot # (if known) #1 #2
7. Exp. date (if known) #1 #2

8. Event reappeared after reintroduction
#1 ☐ yes ☐ no ☐ doesn't apply
#2 ☐ yes ☐ no ☐ doesn't apply

9. NDC # (for product problems only)

10. Concomitant medical products and therapy dates (exclude treatment of event)

D. Suspect medical device

1. Brand name
2. Type of device
3. Manufacturer name & address
4. Operator of device ☐ health professional ☐ lay user/patient ☐ other:
5. Expiration date (mo day yr)

6. model # ___ catalog # ___ serial # ___ lot # ___ other #

7. If implanted, give date (mo day yr)
8. If explanted, give date (mo day yr)

9. Device available for evaluation? (Do not send to FDA) ☐ yes ☐ no ☐ returned to manufacturer on ___ (mo day yr)

10. Concomitant medical products and therapy dates (exclude treatment of event)

E. Reporter (see confidentiality section on back)

1. Name, address & phone #
2. Health professional? ☐ yes ☐ no
3. Occupation
4. Also reported to ☐ manufacturer ☐ user facility ☐ distributor
5. If you do NOT want your identity disclosed to the manufacturer, place an " X " in this box. ☐

Mail to: MedWatch 5600 Fishers Lane Rockville, MD 20852-9787 or FAX to: 1-800-FDA-0178

FDA Form 3500 (6/93) Submission of a report does not constitute an admission that medical personnel or the product caused or contributed to the event.

FIGURE 27-3 MedWatch form for healthcare professionals to report serious adverse effects.

foods influence a drug. An example of a food–drug interaction is the deactivation of the antibiotic tetracycline by dairy products. In some cases, a drug will precipitate from solutions if mixed with other medications. This is known as a *drug incompatibility.*

Almost all drugs interact adversely with at least one other drug. Therefore, it is not always possible to avoid prescribing drugs that interact adversely.

SAFETY ALERT

Always be aware of the possibility of drug incompatibilities and interactions to protect clients from harmful effects. Refer to incompatibility charts, and check with the pharmacist for valuable information.

MEDICATION ASSESSMENT

To administer medications safely to any client, information must be collected during the initial assessment. In addition to these baseline data, a medication-specific assessment should be part of the ongoing nursing assessment to determine medication effectiveness and promptly identify adverse effects. Assessment also is necessary in planning appropriate client teaching to promote compliance with therapy.

Information Collected During Initial Assessment

Medication History

During the initial interview, determine the names, dosages, schedules, and client's understanding of the purposes of any medications he or she takes routinely. If necessary, obtain additional information from family members, who may provide information that the client does not volunteer. An example is, "Mom doesn't take her water pill in the evening because she doesn't like to go to the bathroom at night."

While hospitalized, the client usually is required to send all medications home or store them in a secure location until discharge. Some agencies permit clients to keep their own medications at the bedside once the pharmacy has checked and labeled them and the admitting physician has given an order. Alert the physician or other prescribing provider to all medications the client has been taking so that necessary medications can be ordered. This is especially important if the client is taking antidiabetic agents, anticonvulsant medications, or cardiovascular medications.

Also, discuss the client's use of any OTC medications. A question such as, "What medications do you buy without a prescription?" may help elicit this information. A client may overlook common medications, such as aspirin, acetaminophen, herbal remedies, supplements, or laxatives, when asked to list medications. In particular, clients may not consider eyedrops, nasal sprays, skin lotions, food supplements, and herbal remedies to be medications.

If clients are taking multiple medications or cannot remember the names of all the medications they are taking, or if their medication profile differs from their clinical status, ask the client or family to collect all medications for evaluation.

Access to the client's medications allows the nurse to make a complete list of prescribed medications and to identify actual or potential medication problems. Note whether prescriptions have expired, whether all medications are stored separately in correctly marked containers, whether the prescriptions are actually this client's or another person's, and whether the number of pills in a bottle seems correct (considering the prescription's date and directions).

Allergies and Intolerances

During the initial interview, ask the client about allergies to any medications. If the client indicates any medication allergies, ask follow-up questions about the allergic symptoms noted with each drug. This information allows differentiation between a medication that caused a true allergic response and a medication that caused unpleasant side effects. Nausea and vomiting, although unpleasant, are symptoms of possible side effects to a medication, not an allergic reaction. In some situations, medications that caused unpleasant side effects (e.g., nausea, diarrhea) may be used.

Clients in the hospital or in long-term care facilities should have all allergies listed on their identification bands and on all medication administration records.

SAFETY ALERT

To avoid potentially fatal anaphylaxis, write all stated client allergies on the client's record, on the cover of the client's record, and in any other locations mandated by agency policy.

Medical History

Before administering any medication to a client, be aware of the client's medical diagnosis and general medical history. Any renal, hepatic, cardiac, respiratory, endocrine, or neurologic dysfunction is important to ascertain before administering any medication. This information can be used to identify clients who are at greater risk for drug toxicity or who may require extra care in drug administration.

Drug or alcohol abuse also is important to determine before medication administration. The client who has frequently used opiates or alcohol may require higher doses of sedatives or opiates to obtain the desired effect. Administering aspirin to an alcohol-dependent client may predispose the client to gastric irritation and bleeding. Normal dosages of acetaminophen in such clients occasionally can cause severe hepatic or renal dysfunction.

Pregnancy and Lactation Status

Drugs known to cause birth defects are called *teratogenic.* Women should avoid any known teratogenic drug and any drug that has not been thoroughly evaluated during pregnancy. Rarely (e.g., in a pregnant client with difficult-to-control epilepsy), use of a potentially harmful drug during pregnancy is indicated. The prescriber should discuss the risks and benefits of such treatment with the client before prescribing the drug. This discussion should be documented in the medical record. Late in pregnancy, women should avoid hepatotoxic medications because of increased risk of liver damage to the woman.

A medication may be excreted through breast milk and ingested by a nursing baby. Many medications are excreted in low dosages that do not affect breast-feeding babies, but some (e.g., opiates, antibiotics, anticoagulants, anticonvulsants, histamine antagonists, tranquilizers) can be excreted in amounts great enough to affect babies. If a woman must receive a medication that is excreted in large concentrations in breast milk, bottle feeding is recommended.

Assessment Before Medication Administration

Medication Record

Before giving a client any medication, check the client's medication administration record (MAR). The client may have several medications ordered to treat the same problem. Checking the client's MAR allows the nurse to see which medication has been used most recently and whether it is time for the medication to be administered. Knowing a client's current medications also allows the nurse to avoid giving a medication that may interfere with or add to the effects of another medication the client has received.

Diet and Fluid Orders

A client may have fluids and food withheld in preparation for surgery or for a diagnostic test. When a client is ordered to have nothing by mouth (NPO), remind the client that usually in this situation most oral medications are not given. When the client is receiving important medications that should not be discontinued abruptly (e.g., blood pressure medication, digoxin, anticonvulsants), contact the physician or other provider concerning alternative orders for medication administration. In some situations, prescribers order that oral medications be administered with a small sip of water even though a client is NPO. When a diabetic client is NPO, contact the prescriber concerning specific orders for insulin or oral hypoglycemic medications.

Laboratory Values

Laboratory tests may be used to monitor serum drug levels, medication effects, and medication side effects. Dosages of certain drugs (e.g., digoxin, gentamicin, phenytoin) are evaluated by monitoring serum drug levels to determine proper dosage for the client. Assess these serum drug levels and notify the prescriber about values outside the therapeutic range. Doing so permits the prescriber to change the medication dosage to ensure therapeutic effects without causing undesirable toxicity.

Laboratory tests also may be used to monitor a medication's direct effects. Serum levels can be used to determine proper dosing of medications such as iron, potassium, and thyroid preparations. Anticoagulants also are monitored for therapeutic effects by drawing venous blood to assess coagulation status.

Common or serious side effects of medications may be monitored with the use of laboratory tests. Many diuretics are potassium-wasting; hence, serum potassium levels are measured to detect hypokalemia. Many types of chemotherapy cause leukopenia (decreased numbers of white blood cells) or thrombocytopenia (decreased numbers of platelets). Therefore, blood counts are monitored before and after chemotherapy. If medications are known to cause kidney dysfunction, kidney function tests (e.g., serum creatinine, blood urea nitrogen) are done at regular intervals. If medications can potentially cause liver damage, liver function tests (e.g., alanine aminotransferase [ALT], aspartate aminotransferase [AST]) may be ordered and evaluated.

Physical Assessment

Before giving a medication, quickly assess the client's physical ability to take the medication. The ability to swallow and normal gastrointestinal motility are important considerations for oral medications. Adequate muscle mass and venous access are important for parenteral medications. If the medication is likely to affect vital signs or the function of a body system, appropriate assessments are made before medication administration.

Ability to Swallow. Before administering an oral medication, be sure the client has an adequate swallowing reflex. If suspicion exists that a client cannot swallow, give the client a few sips of water. If the client coughs or chokes on the water, do not give the medication and inform the client's prescribing provider.

Gastrointestinal Motility. If a client's gastrointestinal function is abnormal (e.g., recent surgery, nausea, or vomiting), perform a quick abdominal assessment. If the client's abdomen is distended and firm and bowel sounds are hyperactive or absent, gastrointestinal dysfunction is present. Contact the client's prescriber to check whether oral medications can be given by another route.

Adequate Muscle Mass. Premature babies and debilitated clients may have limited amounts of lean muscle mass. If an irritating medication is given into subcutaneous tissue or into a very small muscle, pain, inadequate absorption of medication, or tissue damage could occur. Contact the client's prescriber to determine whether another route of administration could be used.

Adequate Venous Access. Before giving an IV medication, be sure the IV catheter is located in an adequate vein and is patent. Check the catheter insertion site for temperature, redness, swelling, and pain.

Vital Signs. Medications may affect blood pressure, heart rate, and respiratory rate. Before giving a medication that can affect vital signs, measure and record the value. Measure blood pressure before administering antihypertensive medications or coronary vasodilators (e.g., nitroglycerin, isosorbide dinitrate). If the client's systolic blood pressure is low (usually less than 90 or 100 mm Hg systolic), withhold the medication and notify the prescriber. Counting apical heart rate for 1 minute is necessary before giving digoxin, a medication that slows the heart rate. If the heart rate is slow (usually less than 60 beats/minute), withhold the medication and contact the prescriber. Count the respiratory rate before giving a medication, such as an opiate, that may depress the respiratory rate.

Body System Assessment. To assess the effect of a medication, the appropriate body system must be assessed before it is given. For example, bronchodilators may be inhaled by a client with chronic obstructive lung disease to treat bronchospasm. Before

beginning the treatment, assess the client's respiratory system. This quick assessment includes counting the respiratory rate, asking the client to rate his or her ease of breathing, noting the use of accessory respiratory muscles, and auscultating the client's breath sounds. After the treatment, this assessment is repeated. Judge the effect of the treatment by noting any changes in assessment findings and the length of time the change lasts.

Assessment of Knowledge and Compliance

Client knowledge about a prescribed medication varies with the person and depends on many factors. Some clients desire and receive detailed information about the medications they are taking, whereas other clients want and receive min-

OUTCOME-BASED TEACHING PLAN

Laura Calley, 12 years old, was diagnosed with type I diabetes mellitus. You will provide diabetic teaching for her. Her parents are with her. It is clear that the entire family is upset over Laura's newly diagnosed diabetes.

OUTCOME: Before discharge, Laura and her parents will be able to demonstrate the ability to accurately assess Laura's blood glucose level.
Strategies
- Assess Laura's and her parents' readiness to learn by their interest and comfort while watching you perform blood glucose monitoring.
- As you test Laura's blood glucose, verbally explain the procedure.
- At first, encourage Laura to participate by holding equipment and cleansing her own finger.
- Give Laura and her parents written information detailing blood glucose monitoring.
- Verbally cue Laura and/or the parents through blood glucose monitoring.
- Observe a return demonstration by Laura and by her parents.
- Allow Laura to express fears and feelings regarding how frequent glucose monitoring might affect her life.

OUTCOME: After a teaching session, Laura and her parents can verbalize type, dosage, and time of administration for prescribed insulin and list signs and symptoms of hyperglycemia and hypoglycemia.
Strategies
- Provide Laura and her parents with the insulin order in writing.
- Explain the difference between rapid-acting and intermediate-acting insulin, providing in writing approximate times for onset, peak, and duration for each type.
- Relate signs of hyperglycemia to Laura's symptoms before diagnosis.

- Compare and contrast the signs of hyperglycemia and hypoglycemia, providing a written list.
- Based on the type of insulin Laura is taking, explain when she may experience hypoglycemia.
- Have Laura and her parents verbalize signs of hypoglycemia and hyperglycemia.

OUTCOME: Before discharge, Laura and her parents will demonstrate the ability to accurately draw up and administer insulin.
Strategies
- Provide Laura and her parents with written information, including illustrations, for drawing up insulin, selecting appropriate site, and performing the injection.
- Periodically review written material with Laura and her parents, allowing time for questions.
- To help Laura overcome any fear of self-injection, avoid long explanations and teaching before giving injection.
- Provide Laura with the dose drawn up and supportively guide her insulin injection.
  – Point to appropriate site.
  – Explain the angle to insert the needle.
  – Stretch or pinch to firm skin.
  – Dart needle through skin and inject insulin dose.
- With successive doses, allow Laura to choose appropriate site, assisting as necessary until Laura is confident with site selection.
- After fear of injecting has passed, verbally cue and observe Laura while she draws up the correct insulin dose, including:
  – Gently rotate insulin to mix suspension.
  – Inject an equal amount of air into vial.
  – Accurately withdraw the ordered amount of insulin.
- Observe a return demonstration of insulin injection into the correct site by Laura and by her parents without cuing and prompting.

imal information. Determine what the client already knows and what he or she needs to know to take the medication safely. Then ask questions to elicit this information. Clearly document inadequate knowledge or gaps in important areas so that an individualized teaching plan can be formulated.

Assessing cognitive ability is important for individualizing the teaching plan and determining whether the client can independently manage self-medication. Cognitive impairment, confusion, and psychiatric disorders may increase the potential for difficulty with the medication regimen. Learning disabilities may necessitate creative teaching to ensure understanding and compliance with therapy. Include family members or the caregiver in the teaching sessions.

Compliance with a medication routine means that the client takes the medication exactly as prescribed. Lack of compliance can occur in many ways, for example when the client

- Does not take any of the prescribed drug
- Does not take the proper number of doses of the drug
- Takes extra doses of the drug
- Does not follow the dosage schedule as prescribed
- Discontinues the medication prematurely
- Excessively uses a prn order
- Takes medications that were ordered previously for another condition

Compliance with a medication routine is more likely to occur when the client understands and agrees with the ratio-nale for using the medication, the routine for taking the medication, and the desired effect of the medication. Clients are more likely to follow simple medication routines that suit their lifestyles.

A client's attitude about medical care and about specific medications can influence his or her compliance with drug therapy. Begin by asking general questions, such as, "Do you believe that these medications will help you get better?" Be alert to comments that indicate a client's lack of confidence in prescribed drug treatment.

Lifestyle and financial considerations also affect compliance with drug therapy. The client with a regular income, health insurance, and a stable home is more likely to obtain medications and to organize routines to remember to take them. When a client does not have a home, income, or health insurance, buying, storing, and remembering to take medications regularly can be difficult.

SAFE MEDICATION ADMINISTRATION

To administer medications safely, the following actions are necessary:

- Accurately interpret the prescriber's order.
- Accurately calculate the amount of drug to give for the prescribed dose.

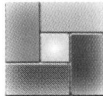 Nursing Research and Critical Thinking
Do Teaching Methods Affect Students' Performance of Medication Administration?

These nursing educators wanted to know the effects of teaching method on the ability of nursing students to learn medication administration. They designed this posttest-only study to ascertain whether a difference existed in baccalaureate nursing students' ability to accurately administer medications when taught using a faculty-assisted method (control group, $n = 50$) versus a self-directed method (experimental group, $n = 48$). The control group received faculty instruction on the skill performance during the laboratory practice. The experimental group viewed a faculty-generated videotape on medication administration before laboratory practice. The participants ($n = 98$) were randomly assigned to the faculty-assisted group or the self-directed group. Student performance in medication administration was measured 1 week after laboratory practice using a 17-item instrument developed by the faculty. Each student was randomly assigned a simulated client's chart that included orders for medication. Some situations involved drug calculations to provide the correct dosage. Within each set of orders, each student was required to administer at least three medications involving different routes (i.e., injection, oral, topical). The data were analyzed using an analysis of variance (ANOVA) and a two-tailed t-test for independent samples at the .05 probability level. No significant difference was found between the faculty-assisted learning group and the self-directed learning group ($t = .48$, df = 96, $P < .05$). Test mean for the faculty-assisted group was 16.81 (SD = 0.57). Test mean for the self-directed group was 16.76 (SD = 0.52).

Critical Thinking Considerations. Random assignment of students to the two groups and teaching both groups the same content helped to control threats to internal validity. Faculty involved in the evaluation of students' performance were unaware to which group the student had been assigned. Implications of this study are as follows:

- The researchers concluded that students could effectively perform the skill of medication administration when taught by either method.
- These findings indicate that other skills could also be taught using a videotape and independent practice approach.

From Powell, S. S., Canterbury, M. A., & McCoy, D. (1998). Medication administration: Does the teaching method really matter? *Journal of Nursing Education, 37*(6), 281–283.

- Develop a systematic and safe procedure, using the "five rights" for drug administration.
- Document medication administration according to agency policy.

Interpretation of the Order

The nurse is responsible for safe interpretation of the medication order. If the order is illegible, the intended medication request can easily be misinterpreted. If the written order is not completely clear or contains unusual abbreviations, always consult the prescriber for clarification. Clarification also may be necessary if important information, such as the route or frequency of administration, is omitted.

Evaluate whether the amount and route ordered are likely to be safe for the client. Know, or look up, the dosage range, route of administration, contraindications, and side effects before giving any medication. If you question the safe use of any prescribed medication, you have the legal responsibility to consult with the prescriber rather than administer a medication that could potentially cause harm.

Computerized automated order entry systems are becoming more common, especially in large healthcare institutions. Errors related to illegibility of medications are virtually eliminated. In addition, these computerized information systems alert prescribers, pharmacists, and nurses to potential errors related to drug–drug interactions, inappropriate dosing, or critical patient allergies (Teich et al., 2000).

Calculating Adult Medication Dosages

Medication orders are usually written in metric units of measure and supplied the same way. Occasionally, liquid medications or commonly used oral medications may be ordered in apothecary or household units of measure. If a medication is ordered in one unit of measure and supplied by the pharmacy in another unit of measure, calculate the amount of medication needed in the measurement system ordered. Expertise in medication calculation and administration is essential for safe medication administration. Regular self-testing of medication calculation skills is recommended.

🥛 SAFETY ALERT

If the calculated dosage of a medication seems unusual (e.g., consists of more than two tablets, less than one half tablet, more than one unit-dose of a liquid medication) or if you have any doubts about the accuracy of your calculation, ask another nurse or a pharmacist to check the dosage calculation.

If the medication is ordered and supplied in the same measurement system, use the following formula to calculate the amount of medication needed:

$$\frac{\text{Dose on hand}}{\text{Quantity on hand}} = \frac{\text{Dose desired}}{X}$$

where X is the quantity desired.

Example: 400 mg of an antibiotic is ordered and you have 200-mg tablets on hand.

$$\frac{200 \text{ mg}}{1 \text{ tablet}} = \frac{400 \text{ mg}}{X}$$
$$200X = 400$$
$$X = 2 \text{ tablets}$$

Example: You have 0.25 mg of digoxin ordered IV. The vial the pharmacy sent says 0.125 mg = 1 cc.

$$\frac{0.125 \text{ mg}}{1 \text{ cc}} = \frac{0.25 \text{ mg}}{X}$$
$$0.125 X = 0.25$$
$$X = 2 \text{ cc}$$

Conversions within the metric system can be calculated using this formula or by remembering that the metric system is based on units of ten. Equivalents are computed by multiplying or dividing—moving the decimal point to the right or left, respectively. Only three basic units in the metric system are used to calculate medication dosages: gram (g), milligram (mg), and microgram (μg). The equivalents among these three units are 1 g = 1000 mg = 1,000,000 μg.

To change grams to milligrams, multiply the grams by 1000 (because there are 1000 mg in 1 g), or move the decimal point three places to the left. An example of this conversion in an equation is 800 mg = 0.8 g.

Calculating Children's Medication Dosages

Children's dosages are most often calculated using the child's weight or body surface area. Most drugs are ordered specifically for a child and are not computed from an adult dose. Take into account the many differences in sizes of children and the individual metabolic rate, which influences the therapeutic dose. Observing the child's response to the medication may determine whether the dosage needs to be adjusted for the benefit of the individual child.

Administering Medications According to the "Five Rights"

After validating the order and calculating the proper drug dose, accurate administration of a medication can be ensured by following the "five rights" of medication administration. These rights are summarized in Display 27-1.

🥛 SAFETY ALERT

Each time you administer a medication, be sure that you give the right client the right medication, in the right dose, by the right route, at the right time.

The Right Client
The first "right" of administering medications, the right client, means that the medication is given to the client for whom it is intended (Fig. 27-4).

DISPLAY 27-1

🖵 "FIVE RIGHTS" OF MEDICATION ADMINISTRATION

- Identify the *right client.*
- Select the *right medication.*
- Give the *right dose.*
- Give the medication at the *right time.*
- Give the medication by the *right route.*

Incorrect identification of clients can occur when a nurse is busy, when clients with similar names are located in the same areas of an agency, and when client identification procedures are not followed. To avoid errors, identify the client by name and check the name band against the client's MAR before giving medications. Follow the institution's "name alert" policy whenever clients with similar names are located in the same unit. Name alert procedures involve a special way of identifying clients with similar names and a way of alerting other departments of the clients' name similarity.

The Right Medication

The second "right" of administering medications, the right medication, means that the medication given is the medication that was ordered and that is appropriate for the client. Medication errors involving this right may occur when

- The pharmacy incorrectly dispenses a medication that looks similar to the ordered medication.
- A pharmacist or nurse incorrectly dispenses or administers a medication that has a similar name to the medication ordered.

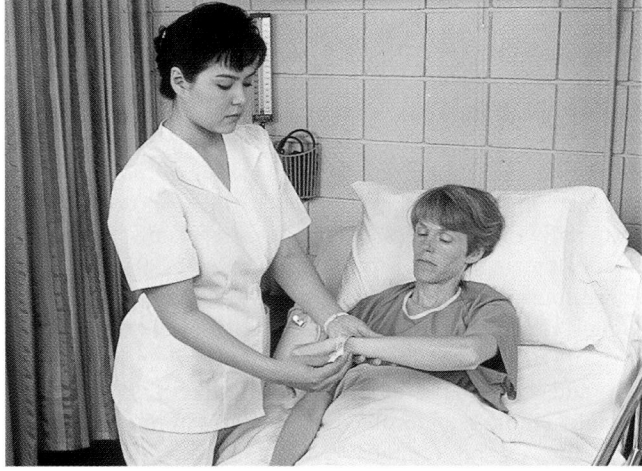

FIGURE 27-4 No matter what the administration route, always check that the right client receives the right medication. Check the medication record, the unit dosage, and the client's identification bracelet. If the client is conscious, also ask the client to state his or her name. (Photograph © B. Proud.)

- The prescribing provider orders a medication that is not appropriate for the client.
- The nurse administers a medication that he or she has not prepared.
- The nurse incorrectly identifies a medication.

Reduce the risk of giving the wrong medication by using a BCMA system, administering only medications that have been prepared and labeled by the nurse or pharmacist, checking the medication label against the medication order, knowing the medication's generic and trade names and the reason it is being given to the client, and listening for client clues. Be alert for clues such as, "This doesn't look like the same pill I took before." After hearing such clues, recheck the medication order immediately.

The Right Dosage

The third "right" of administering medications, the right dosage, means that the medication is given in the dose ordered and that the dose ordered is appropriate for the client. Incorrect dosages may be given if the prescriber orders a dose that is inappropriate for a client; if the pharmacist dispenses or if the nurse administers an incorrect amount of medication; or if a pharmacist, nurse, or support staff transcribes an order incorrectly onto the client's medication record.

These errors may be avoided if the nurse and pharmacist are aware of the usual dosage ranges of medications, the nurse double-checks with the prescriber whenever questions concerning the accuracy of a dosage arise, and the nurse and pharmacist correctly calculate the amount of medication required. In addition, errors may be eliminated if a computerized order entry system is used.

Double-check medication dosages whenever you encounter the following situations, which are suggestive of an incorrect medication dosage:

- A client suggests that the dose he or she is used to taking is different from the dose the nurse is administering.
- Multiple tablets are needed to supply a single medication dose.
- Large or abrupt changes in medication dosages are ordered.
- The amount of medication supplied by the pharmacist does not match the amount needed for the ordered doses.

The Right Route

The fourth "right" of administering medications, the right route, means that the medication is given by the ordered route and that the ordered route is safe and appropriate for the client. The prescriber's medication orders should always specify the route of administration. If a route is not specified or seems inappropriate, check with the prescriber to clarify which route to use.

To ensure that a medication is given by the proper route, know the medication's usual route or routes of administration and the safety of administering the medication by the ordered route. Double-check the route of administration before administering a medication.

The Right Time

The fifth "right" of administering medications, the right time, means that the medication is given with the correct frequency and at the time ordered according to agency policy. Routine medication administration schedules vary among institutions. For example, one agency may specify 9 AM, 1 PM, 5 PM, and 9 PM as times for medications ordered four times a day. Another agency may specify these times as 8 AM, 12 PM, 4 PM, and 8 PM. Policies defining the meaning of "on time" also vary. Many institutions consider a medication to be given "on time" if it is administered within 30 minutes to 1 hour before or after the scheduled dose time.

Many factors influence the schedules a facility uses to administer medications:

- A medication may be more effective if it is given on an "around-the-clock" schedule.
- A medication that interacts with food may need to be given before meals.
- A medication that causes gastric irritation may need to be given with meals.

Be aware of the scheduling requirements of the medication being given and the routine scheduling times the agency uses.

🥛 SAFETY ALERT

Before giving any medication, always check the client's medication administration record (MAR) to note when the medication was last administered and if a change has occurred in medication orders.

Documentation of Medication Administration

An agency's medication policies define the time and type of medication documentation (charting) that is required. Medication documentation includes the time, route, dosage, site of administration (for intradermal, subcutaneous, or intramuscular injections), and the nurse's initials and signature (Fig. 27-5). Specific documentation also is required if a nurse does not give a medication. Many agencies require nurses to circle the normal time of administration when they have withheld a medication. Nurses must indicate why they did not give the medication. At times, this can simply be a matter of indicating NPO next to the designated time for administration. At other times, the reason is more complex, and an explanation needs to be written in other appropriate places on the MAR or client record.

Some medications (e.g., insulin, heparin) may have separate flowsheets on the MAR. Frequently, this flowsheet contains laboratory data or other pertinent information. Such a flowsheet permits nurses and other healthcare providers to visualize patterns of management over time. When numerous injections are administered, a chart documenting the location of each injection is provided to ensure adequate site rotation. Whenever injections are administered, the site used should be documented.

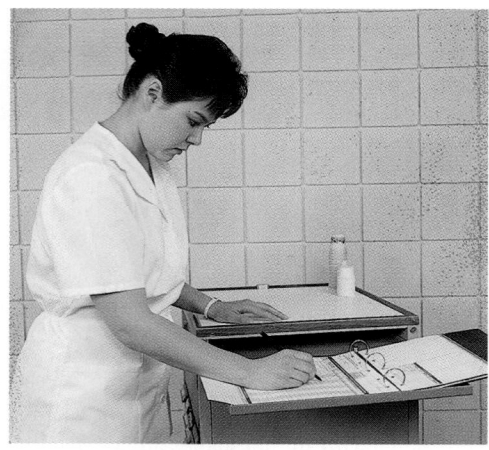

FIGURE 27-5   Documentation of medication administration is an important nursing requirement. (Photograph © B. Proud.)

Nurses also are responsible for documenting the therapeutic effects and side effects of any medication administered. For example, if an opiate is administered for pain, document the amount of pain relief the client obtains, usually on the MAR. If a client develops a rash after the administration of an antibiotic, describe the onset and type of rash in detail in the client's record.

🥛 SAFETY ALERT

To avoid potential medication errors, always document immediately after giving a medication.

Medication Errors

The Institute of Medicine (IOM) is a private, nonprofit institution that provides health policy advice under a congressional charter granted to the National Academy of Sciences. The IOM defines an error as "the failure of a planned action to be completed as intended or the use of a wrong plan to achieve an aim" (IOM, 1999, p. 28) Medication errors are one of the most common types of medical errors. These errors can have untoward outcomes for clients. The prevention of serious injuries to clients resulting from medical errors must be a high priority for health care professionals and institutions. The majority of medical errors do not result from individual recklessness but from basic flaws in the way the healthcare system is organized (IOM, 1999). The IOM, as well as accrediting agencies (JCAHO) and professional organizations, are emphasizing as a top priority efforts within institutions to design systems geared to preventing, detecting, and minimizing hazards and the likelihood of error. Simplified but standardized processes within institutions, as well as use of computerized systems such as automated physician order entry and BCMA, will become more widespread. Quality improvement efforts to analyze root causes of errors and recommend changes in systems to prevent similar errors in the future will be emphasized. Computers and automation will never take the place of critical thinking, clinical judgment, and personal responsibility. However, to improve systems, errors must be recognized, acknowledged, and reported, so that analysis of the cause of the error can be determined and plans for improvement can be implemented.

Examples of medication errors include when a medication is not administered as ordered; when the medication is administered according to the order, but the order is unsafe or inappropriate for the client; or when the documentation in a client's chart does not reflect that a medication was administered as ordered. The most common medication errors are related to documentation errors: the medication was given but not charted. Other common medication errors include administering IV medication at the wrong rate, administering medication in the wrong dose, giving medication at the wrong time, administering the wrong medication, and charting medication that was not given. Errors of medication substitution may occur with increased use of generic medications. Nurses must be sure that the name of the medication supplied is the same as, not just similar to, the name of the medication ordered. Less common errors include giving a medication by the wrong route, or to a client with a known allergy to that medication, or to the wrong client. When a medication error occurs, document it by charting the medication as it was given in the client's MAR and filling out a quality improvement or unusual incident form. Inform your supervisor, the prescriber, and the patient as appropriate.

Medication Administration in the Home

Types of Medications
Oral medications, such as antibiotics and pain relievers, have always been prescribed for clients to take at home, and this practice continues to be common. Long-term antibiotic or antineoplastic medications are also being administered in the home with a variety of portable IV drug infusion devices. Sometimes, home health nurses administer these medications at regular intervals. More often, however, family caregivers must learn to give the medications.

In such situations, client education becomes a major nursing focus for maintaining accuracy and minimizing potential risks. Of equal concern is having help quickly available in case of emergency. In some areas, pharmacies may contract with clients to administer and manage medication administration within the home.

When supervising or administering medications in the home, nurses must be sure that this nursing intervention is within the scope of the state's nurse practice act. Furthermore, if controlled substances are administered in the home, nurses must carefully comply with the law regarding appropriate drug storage, documentation, and disposal. Doing so protects against suggestions of improper diversion of the controlled substances and accounts accurately for controlled substances administered in the home.

Organizing Medication Regimens in the Home
An important aspect of accurate home medication administration is ensuring a schedule, or regimen, that is easy to remember and suits the client's lifestyle. Arranging administration of medications by linking it with normal events in the client's life (e.g., meals, bedtime) promotes compliance and accuracy. Be sure to assess the hours when these events occur so that medication administration is staggered appropriately.

For some clients, especially older ones, remembering to take medications and knowing which ones to take can present worrisome problems, as illustrated in this chapter's Critical Thinking Challenge. When weak vision and poor memory are both factors, a sectioned medication-dispensing device may be helpful. Such a device may be as simple as an egg carton, divided dish, or envelopes or as elaborate as a commercially available medication pill pack with compartments for a one-day supply or a weekly supply. These devices may require someone to set up the medications in the appropriate compartments, usually once a week for the entire week. The client then follows instructions to take medications from the appropriate compartment at the appropriate time. Use of such a device may not prevent all errors, but medication administration with the device may be considerably safer.

Oral Medications

Medications that are given by mouth are designed to be swallowed (*oral* route), held under the tongue until they dissolve (*sublingual* route), or held in the side of the mouth until they dissolve (*buccal* route). Refer to Procedure 27-1, Administering Oral Medications. Oral medications can also be administered into feeding tubes paced into the stomach or jejunum.

Giving medications by mouth is usually the simplest and easiest way. It minimizes client discomfort and is associated with the fewest side effects of any route. Oral medications tend to be less expensive and more widely available than medications given by other routes.

If the client cannot swallow water or fluids or is nauseated or vomiting, oral medications are usually discontinued or given by another route. If a client is NPO before a test or surgery, the prescriber may continue selected oral medications, given with sips of water. If the client is NPO after major surgery, oral medications are usually withheld or administered by another route until intestinal function resumes. If the client is being treated with gastric suction, oral medications usually are withheld or given by another route. Occasionally, a prescriber may order a specific medication to be administered through a nasogastric tube, ordering that the gastric suction be discontinued for a specified time (usually 30 minutes) after medication administration.

Routes of Oral Medications
Oral Administration. With oral medications, position the client standing or sitting, or elevate the head of the bed. Have the client drink liquid to ensure that the medication moves

(text continues on page 537)

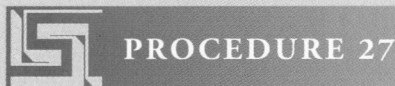

PROCEDURE 27-1

ADMINISTERING ORAL MEDICATIONS

Purpose
1. Provide a safe, effective, economical route for administering medications.
2. Provide a sustained drug action with minimal discomfort.

Assessment
- Review medication orders for accuracy and completeness, including client's name, drug name, dosage, route, and time.
- Consult a nursing drug handbook, drug package inserts, or other standard references about unfamiliar drugs.
- Assess the client's allergy history.
- Assess the client's ability to take oral medications:
  - Level of consciousness, cooperativeness
  - Active swallow reflex
  - Complaints of nausea and vomiting
  - Recent gastrointestinal surgery or bowel obstruction
  - Nasogastric tube connected to suction
  - Current diet order
- Identify and perform individual preadministration assessments of pulse, blood pressure, and other factors as indicated by the medication being administered.
- Ensure that the correct medication and dosage are available at the time scheduled.

Equipment
Medication administration record (MAR)
Medication cart
Disposable medication cups
Water, juice, or milk
Mortar and pestle or other drug-crushing device (when necessary)

Procedure
1. Wash hands.
   Rationale: Reduces transfer of microorganisms from hands to medication.
2. Arrange MAR next to medication cart or cabinet, medication trays, and cups.
   Rationale: Organizes work space to save time and reduce the chance of error.
3. Prepare medications for only one client at a time.
   Rationale: Prevents errors during preparation.
4. Remove ordered medications from cart or shelf. Compare label on medication with the MAR and check the five rights of medication administra-

tion. Scan bar code if using bar code medication administration (BCMA). If a discrepancy exists, recheck the client's chart and medication orders.
Rationale: Check the five rights of medication administration twice. The first check occurs when removing the medication from the storage area.

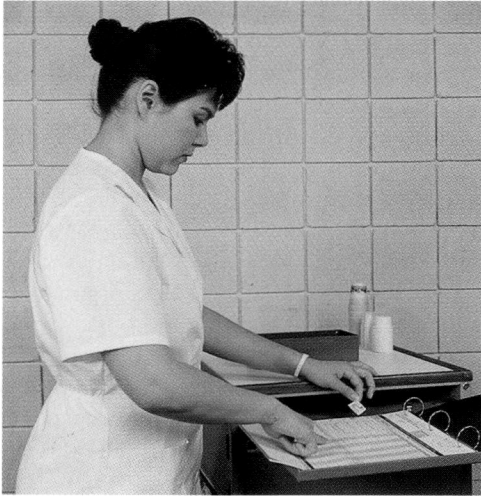

Step 4 Compare medication, container label, and medication record. (Photo © B. Proud.)

5. Calculate correct drug dosage if necessary.
   Rationale: Prevents dosage errors.
6. Prepare selected medications.
   a. Unit dosage: Place packaged medications directly into medicine cup or lay them on tray without unwrapping.
   b. Medications from a multidose bottle: Pour tablets or capsules into the container lid, and transfer them into medicine cup. Return any extra tablets to the bottle.
   c. Medications from a bingo card: Snap the bubble containing the correct medication directly over the medication cup. Do not touch the medication.
   Rationale: Maintains cleanliness of drugs.
   d. Swallowing difficulty: If client has trouble swallowing tablets, grind with mortar and pestle or other drug-crushing device until smooth. Mix powder in small amount of pudding or applesauce. *Do not* crush enteric-coated tablets or extended-release tablets.

PROCEDURE 27-1 (Continued)

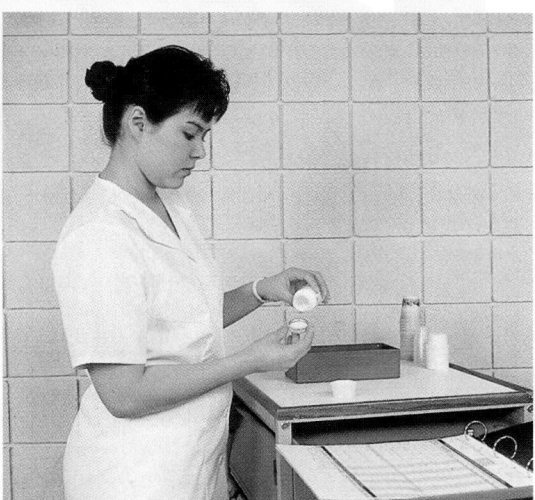

Step 6B Pour medication into medicine cup. (Photo © B. Proud.)

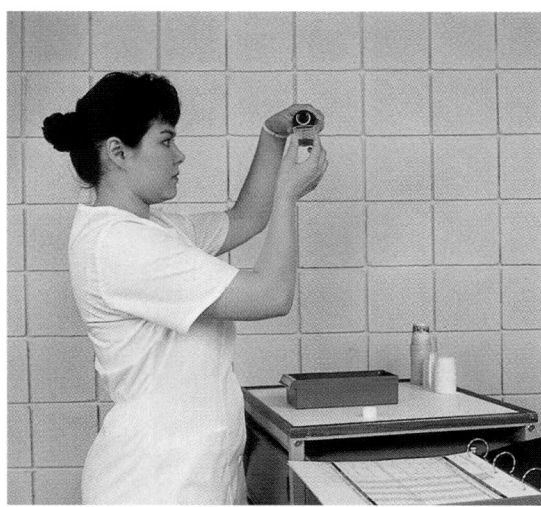

Step 6E Hold liquid medication at eye level to read dosage level at base of meniscus. (Photo © B. Proud.)

Rationale: Crushed enteric-coated tablets irritate gastric mucosa, and crushed extended-release tablets alter drug absorption and duration of drug effects.

e. Liquid medications: Remove cap and place on countertop with the inside up. Hold bottle so label is against palm of hand. Fill until bottom of meniscus (the surface of the fluid that appears curved) is at desired dosage. Discard excess poured liquid from cup into sink; do not pour it back into the bottle.
Rationale: Prevents soiling of label when pouring medication and contamination of the medication in the bottle.

7. Take medication directly to client's room. Do not leave medication unattended.
Rationale: Prevents potential medication errors.

8. Compare name on MAR with name on client's identification band. If the client is not wearing an identification band, ask the client to state his or her name. Scan patient's identification bracelet if using BCMA.
Rationale: Careful checking ensures administration of drugs to proper client.

9. Complete any preadministration assessment (e.g., blood pressure, pulse) required for the specific medication to be given.
Rationale: Medications that have a direct action, such as decreasing pulse rate or blood pressure, require assessment to determine if the medication can be given safely at that time.

10. Compare medication to MAR, and recheck the five rights of medication administration. If using unit-dose medication, unwrap the medication and place it in the cup before checking the five rights of the next medication.
Rationale: The second check of the five rights occurs before administration to the client.

11. Explain the medication's purpose to the client.
Rationale: Protects the client's rights and encourages client's participation in care and compliance.

12. Assist client to sitting position if necessary. Give the medication cup and glass of water to the client.
Rationale: The sitting position assists swallowing and prevents aspiration.

13. If client is unable to hold the medication cup, place pill cup to the client's lips and introduce the medication into his or her mouth. If a tablet or capsule falls on the floor, discard and repeat preparation.
Rationale: Medication that has fallen on the floor is contaminated.

14. Stay with client until he or she swallows all medications. Look inside client's mouth if the client is cognitively impaired or has difficulty swallowing.
Rationale: The nurse is responsible for ensuring that the client receives the ordered medications.

15. Dispose of soiled supplies, and wash hands.

16. Record time at which medication was administered and any preadministration assessment data collected.
Rationale: Maintains legal record and prevents potential medication errors.

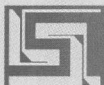

PROCEDURE 27-1 (Continued)

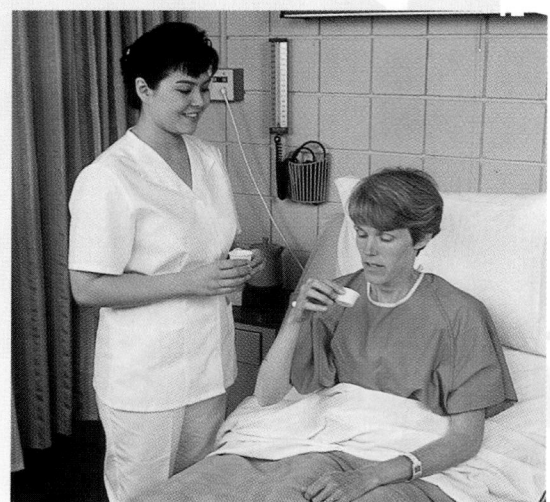

Step 14 Stay with client while medications are swallowed. (Photo © B. Proud.)

Lifespan Considerations
Infant and Child

- Tablets and capsules are not recommended forms of oral medication in children younger than 5 years of age. Young children may not swallow them safely. Use liquid preparations available for most oral medications and measure the preparation appropriately. Some come with calibrated droppers for measuring small amounts of medication for infants. Do not interchange droppers among medications. Different companies use different sized droppers, and medications may be inaccurately measured.
- Always let children know that you are giving them medicine, not candy.
- If appropriate, offer children a choice about what fluid to take with the medication.
  Rationale: Offering choices allows children to participate in care and promotes self-esteem.

Older Adult

- Be aware that normal physiologic changes that occur with aging, such as decreased salivation resulting in a dry mouth and delayed esophageal clearance, may impair swallowing. Such problems may influence a client's ability to take oral medications. Use a liquid form of medication as necessary.

- Additional changes with aging, such as decreased stomach peristalsis, gastric acidity, and colon motility, may affect the client's ability to take oral medications.

Home Care Modifications

- Assess client or caregiver's knowledge of medication therapy.
- Assess client's sensory function (sight, hearing, touch) to determine whether he or she needs special teaching or administration strategies. Be sure client wears eyeglasses or hearing aid during teaching sessions.
- Assess client's ability to read. Client may be unable to read prepared booklets or medication labels.
- Instruct client or caregiver in purpose of medications, dosage schedule, common side effects, whom to call with problems, and what to do about missed doses.
- Give guidelines for drug safety as appropriate: discarding outdated drugs, keeping drugs out of children's reach, refrigerating medications.
- Devise learning aids if needed. Examples include calendars for each week that contain separate ziplock bags with medications to take at specific times, egg cartons with color-coded sections for medications to take at specific times, and commercially available divided containers to provide 1 week of medication at a time.
- Document client teaching, including the use of learning aids.

Collaboration and Delegation

- Clarify with prescriber any unclear orders.
- Notify prescriber of any changes in a client's status that necessitate a change in medication orders.
- Do not ask unlicensed assistive personnel to administer medications to clients. Instruct them in how to observe for and report therapeutic effects and side effects when caring for clients. Also, urge them to notify the nurse caring for the client about any client complaints or changes.

into the stomach and does not lodge in the esophagus. Even clients with normal swallowing reflexes may have problems swallowing and moving tablets or capsules down the esophagus. Drug-induced esophagitis, an inflammation of the esophagus, may occur if a tablet or capsule lodges in the esophagus and begins to dissolve there. Whenever possible, encourage the client to drink about 100 mL of fluid after swallowing a capsule or tablet. If the client senses that a medication is stuck in the throat, offer a small portion of a soft food, such as a piece of bread or banana, to help move the medication.

Antifungal liquid medications, such as nystatin, that work through contact with the mucous membranes in the mouth are given by the "swish and swallow" technique. The client puts the liquid in his or her mouth, moves the liquid back and forth in the mouth several times, and then swallows it.

Several techniques may be used to administer medications to a client who can swallow soft foods but not whole capsules or tablets. A capsule can be opened and the contents added to a small amount of the client's food, such as pudding or applesauce. Some medications have an unpleasant taste when crushed and should be mixed with a soft food to minimize the unpleasantness. Most tablets can be crushed and added to soft foods.

SAFETY ALERT

Never crush enteric-coated or sustained-release tablets. Crushing enteric-coated tablets allows the irritating medication to come in contact with the oral or gastric mucosa, resulting in mucositis or gastric irritation. Crushing a sustained-release medication allows all the medication to be absorbed at the same time, resulting in a higher than expected initial level of the medication and a shorter than expected duration of action.

Facilities provide calibrated medicine cups, droppers, and syringes for accurate measurement of prescribed doses of liquid medications. When measuring liquids in a cup, hold the measuring container at eye level with one hand and use the other hand to pour the medication to the indicated level. An elliptical curve, called the *meniscus,* is produced because the solution clings to the side of the measuring container. The lower part of the meniscus should rest on the calibration line of the dose being measured (see Step 6E in Procedure 27-1).

Administration Through Tubes. Oral medications may be administered through nasogastric or gastric tubes or through nasointestinal or jejunal tubes. When giving oral medications through gastric or intestinal tubes, take care to decrease the risks of client aspiration and clogging of the feeding tube. The risk of *aspiration* (movement of matter into the lungs rather than into the stomach) decreases if the client is properly positioned, for example in a semi-Fowler's or Fowler's position, whenever he or she is receiving food or medications. Additionally, the head of the client's bed should remain elevated for at least 30 minutes after medication administration.

Most liquid medications can be given through feeding tubes. Tablets may be given through a feeding tube if they can be crushed into fine particles and dissolved in water. (Remember that enteric-coated, sustained-release, sublingual, and buccal medications may not be crushed.) A feeding tube can become clogged, however, if medications solidify in it. Before and after administering a medication, flush the feeding tube with a minimum of 30 to 45 mL of warm water. If it becomes difficult to instill fluid into the tube, irrigate the tube with 30 to 50 mL of carbonated beverage. This fluid may help to dissolve food or medication particles within the tube, possibly restoring tube patency. Do not give hydrophyllic gels such as Metamucil through feeding tubes, because these agents tend to attract water and solidify within the feeding tube.

Sublingual Administration. The **sublingual** tablet is placed under the tongue and allowed to dissolve. If the client's mucous membranes are dry, use 1 mL of normal saline solution or water to wet the membranes underneath the tongue so that absorption can occur. Clients should not swallow sublingual tablets. A capsule will not absorb sublingually. When a medication in a capsule is ordered sublingually, the fluid must be aspirated from the capsule and placed under the tongue. Some clients are able to bite into the capsule to free the liquid for absorption under the tongue.

Buccal Administration. The **buccal** route involves placing medications underneath the upper lip or in the side of the mouth. Buccal medications should not be chewed, swallowed, or placed under the tongue. A variety of medications for buccal administration are available, including sustained-release nitroglycerin, opiates, antiemetics, tranquilizers, and sedatives.

Topical Medications

Topical medications are placed on the skin surface or mucous membranes. They may also be placed in body cavities.

Lotions, Creams, and Ointments

Lotions, creams, and ointments may be used to treat a skin or wound infection or skin disease, or to decrease symptoms of skin disorders. Lotions such as hand and body moisturizers prevent complications associated with excessively dry skin. Sunscreens form a protective covering against ultraviolet light. Lotions are rubbed into the skin until no longer visible.

Creams, such as the antifungal agent miconazole, the corticosteroid hydrocortisone, or the antibiotic silver sulfadiazine, may be applied to skin surfaces with a sterile swab, a sterile tongue depressor, or gloved fingers. Clean and dry the skin surface before applying most creams. Silver sulfadiazine is often applied to cleaned, open wounds such as burns or full-thickness pressure ulcers.

Ointments, such as zinc oxide, are applied to protect skin against chafing or maceration associated with bowel and bladder incontinence. Clean the skin and pat it dry before applying ointments.

Transdermal Medications

Medications designed to be absorbed through the skin for systemic effects are called **transdermal** medications. Usually they are prepared as patches. The medication patches are made with special membranes that allow medication to be absorbed slowly. These patches allow controlled amounts of medication to be supplied over a 24- to 72-hour period.

Nitroglycerin, scopolamine, estradiol, nicotine, and fentanyl are examples of commonly used transdermal patches (Fig. 27-6). Although the manufacturer's guidelines for application of specific transdermal patches vary, these are general guidelines:

1. Remove a previously placed patch and any remaining traces of medication.
2. Fold the patch in half and avoid touching the inner surface containing the medication.
3. Apply the new patch to a clean, dry, hairless, intact area of skin.
4. Rotate sites.
5. Apply the patch immediately after removing the protective liner.
6. Wash your hands before and after applying the patch.
7. Dispose of transdermal patches carefully.
8. Note the date, time, and your initials on the patch.

Transdermal patches containing opiate medication should be flushed down a toilet or dropped into a sharps container. Some agencies require two nurses to witness and document disposal of opiate patches. Because heat increases the absorption rate of most transdermal medications, fever greater than 102°F or the use of heating pads, sun lamps, or other sources of direct heat are usually contraindications for continued use of the transdermal patch (Gever, 1998).

Nitroglycerin also comes in an ointment form that is applied to nitroglycerin paper. The paper is marked with half-inch increments, and the ointment is applied to the measuring paper using a continuous motion. The paper is folded in half to spread the ointment evenly on the paper. The paper is applied to a skin surface and, if necessary, secured to the skin with paper tape.

Ophthalmic Medications

Ophthalmic solutions and ointments may be used to treat eye irritation, infections, or glaucoma. The lower eyelid is gently retracted, and the solution or ointment is placed in the conjunctival sac (Display 27-2). Take care to avoid touching the client's eye or eyelid with the tip of the ointment tube or dropper. Instruct the client not to rub the eye after the medication is applied.

Otic Medications

Solutions may be dropped into the ear to treat external ear infections or to soften and remove ear wax. Always use solutions at room temperature, because using hot or cold solutions in the ear can cause vertigo, nausea, and pain (Display 27-3).

Nasal Medications

Solutions are usually sprayed into the nose to treat nasal congestion. OTC nasal sprays may contain decongestant and adrenergic medications (which stimulate the sympathetic nervous system). Frequent use can cause systemic effects, such as increased heart rate and increased blood pressure. Rebound nasal congestion, or nasal congestion that is as bad as or worse than the original symptoms, commonly occurs if a client uses decongestant nasal sprays too frequently or for several days. Corticosteroid nasal sprays are commonly used to treat nasal congestion associated with seasonal or perennial allergies. When consistently used, these nasal sprays are effective as local anti-inflammatory agents to relieve nasal congestion without systemic effects. The nasal route is increasingly used to deliver medications to prevent osteoporosis (calcitonin). When used on a daily basis, alternate nares to avoid irritation.

When administering a nasal spray, have the client sit up and lean his or her head back. While holding the medication bottle in one hand, place the top of the bottle just inside the

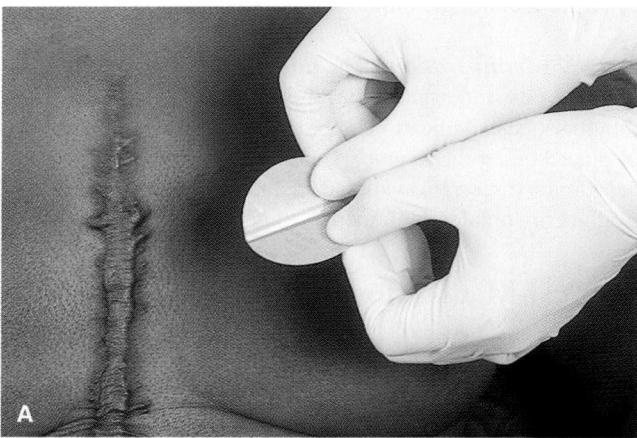

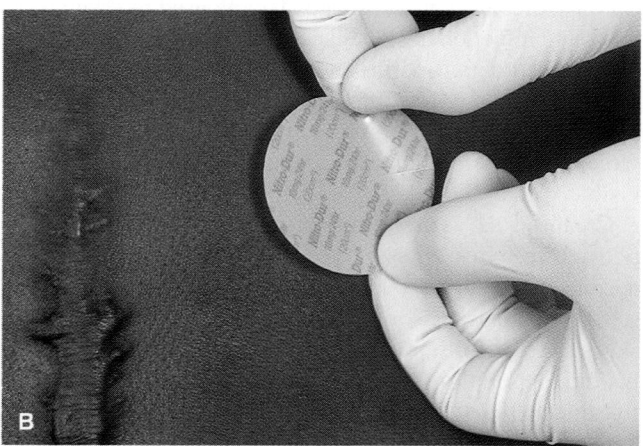

FIGURE 27-6   Transdermal medications absorb through the skin. **(A)** First, bend to break seal. **(B)** Remove protective covering and apply to skin.

INSTILLATION OF EYE MEDICATIONS

- Assist client to sit in an upright position with the head hyperextended.
- Provide client with tissues to blot any medication or tears that spill from the eye during the instillation.
- Ask client to look toward ceiling.
- Place finger or thumb on lower bony orbit and gently pull the lower lid down (as shown).

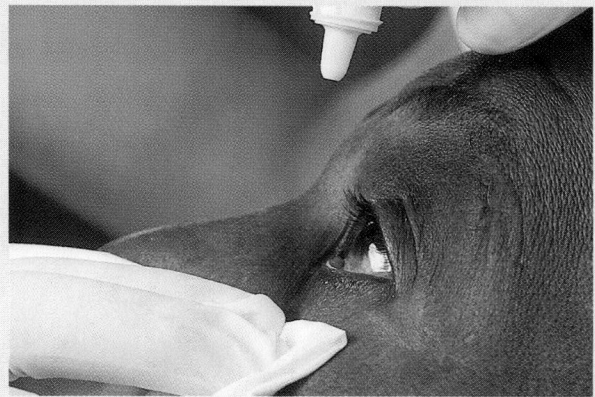

- With other hand resting on the client's forehead, instill the required number of drops or the ointment on the lower conjunctival sac.
- Avoid touching the eyelids, lashes, or the eyeball with either hand or with the applicator.
- Avoid dropping a solution onto the cornea directly because it causes discomfort.
- Release the lower lid, and allow the client to close the eye.
- If the client blinks and the medication is not instilled, repeat the above steps.

INSTILLATION OF EARDROPS

- Have client sit or lie with head turned to unaffected side.
- Warm solution to body temperature to prevent discomfort during instillation.
- Prepare appropriate amount of medication in dropper.
- Straighten the auditory canal by gently pulling the pinna (cartilaginous portion of outer ear) up and back in older children and adults (as shown) and down and back for infants and children younger than 3 years.

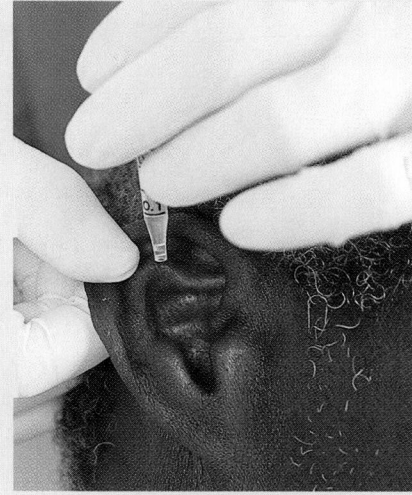

- Instill eardrops on side of the auditory canal to allow the drops to flow in and to continue to adjust to body temperature.
- Release the pinna, and gently massage tragus of the ear.
- If permitted, place a cotton ball or wick in the outer ear to keep medication in the canal.
- If drops are required in the opposite ear, wait a few minutes, and repeat the procedure in that ear.

nostril, aiming the spray applicator top toward the midline of the nose. While the client inhales, squeeze the bottle.

Rectal Medications

Medication in suppository form (a small, cylindrically shaped, waxy base) may be placed in the rectum to treat systemic complaints or as a laxative to encourage bowel movements. Antiemetic suppositories may be used to treat nausea when other routes are not appropriate. The technique for inserting suppositories is shown in Fig. 27-7.

Liquid medications may be instilled into the rectum using an enema to encourage bowel movements or to treat clients with elevated potassium levels. Enema fluids are usually given in volumes of about 100 mL and are usually meant to be retained by the client for 5 to 10 minutes. An enema of resin-containing fluid may be used to remove potassium from the bowel of a client with an elevated potassium level. The pro-

cedure for administering small-volume enemas is discussed in Chapter 41.

Vaginal Medications

Medications given vaginally come in various forms: foams, jellies, liquids (douches), creams, tablets, or suppositories. These medications may be used for contraception, to help kill bacteria in the vaginal area before gynecologic surgery, to treat vaginal itching or infection, or to induce labor. Prostaglandin vaginal suppositories cause uterine contractions and induce labor in women after fetal demise (when death of the fetus occurs early in pregnancy). The technique for instilling vaginal suppositories and creams is shown in Fig. 27-8.

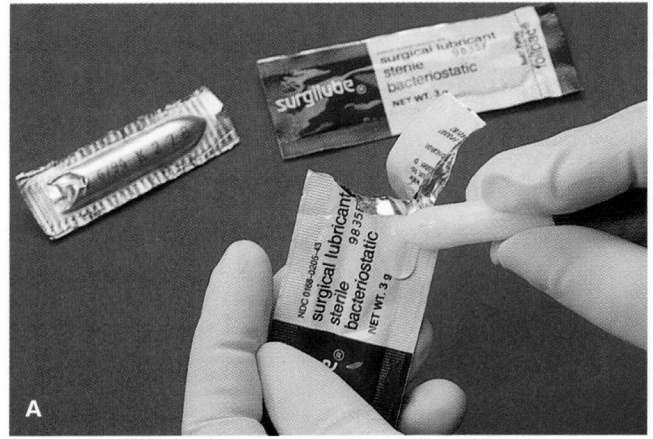

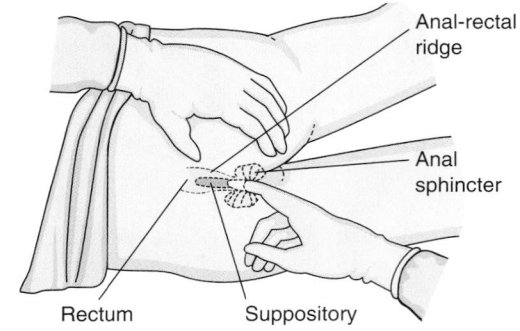

FIGURE 27-7   Insertion of rectal suppositories. **(A)** Prepackaged suppositories. **(B)** Insert the suppository past the internal anal sphincter against the rectal wall.

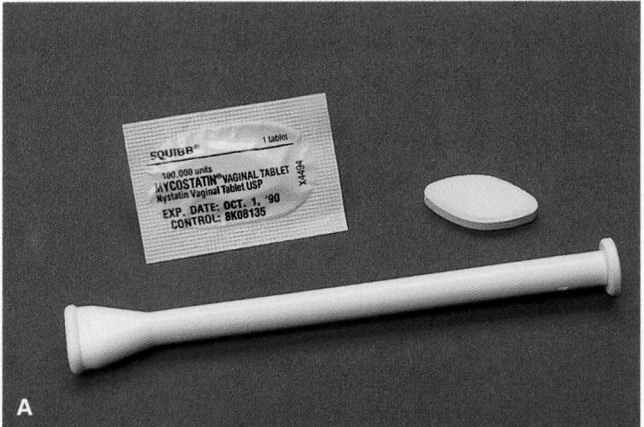

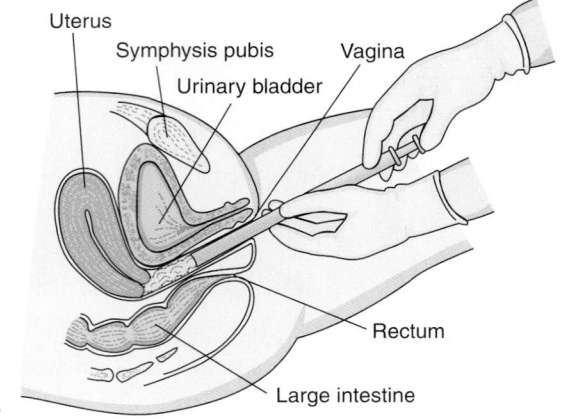

FIGURE 27-8   Insertion of vaginal medication. **(A)** Vaginal suppository and applicator. **(B)** Insertion of vaginal cream using applicator.

Inhaled Medications

Inhaled medications may be used to induce anesthesia during surgery and to treat respiratory disorders. Anesthesiologists or nurse anesthetists administer anesthetic medications through a machine. Nurses may administer other types of inhaled medications through a mechanical ventilator, a handheld nebulizer, or a metered-dose inhaler (MDI). Liquid medications are added to a receptacle in the ventilator or nebulizer and changed into a gas form when air or oxygen flows over them.

An MDI is a small, handheld device that a client presses before inhaling. Each time he or she presses the cartridge, the MDI releases a set dose (metered dose) of medication. Clients can use MDIs with or without a spacer device. Spacers trap the dose of medication and are especially useful for people (e.g., children, older adults) who cannot inhale slowly or cannot press the canister while inhaling. Inhaled medications have rapid effects on the lungs and are rapidly absorbed by the systemic circulation.

Bronchodilator medications, used to open lung airways and to promote easier breathing, are frequently administered through MDIs or nebulizers. Assess the client's respiratory status (reported ease of breathing, breath sounds, respiratory rate, and use of accessory respiratory muscles) before and after administering an inhalable medication (Procedure 27-2).

Parenteral Medications

The **parenteral** route refers to medications that are given by injection or infusion. Parenteral medications may be injected into intradermal (ID), subcutaneous (SC), intramuscular (IM), or intralesional tissue; into intravenous (IV) or intra-arterial circulation; or into intraspinal or intra-articular spaces. The ID, SC, IM, and IV routes are discussed in this chapter.

Medications given by a parenteral route usually are absorbed more completely and begin acting more quickly than medications given by oral or topical routes. Parenteral medications are injected through the skin; bypassing the skin barrier makes infection more likely if aseptic technique is not used when preparing and administering parenteral medications. Complications may occur if parenteral medications are not given into the intended tissue site or space. Tissue damage may occur if the pH, osmotic pressure, or solubility of the medication is not appropriate to the tissue where the medication is given. Specialized equipment required for parenteral administration usually makes medications given by these routes more expensive than medications given by other routes.

(text continues on page 543)

PROCEDURE 27-2

ADMINISTERING MEDICATION BY METERED-DOSE INHALER

Purpose
1. Deliver a premeasured dose of medication to the bronchial airways and lungs.

Assessment
- Review client's medical history, medication history, and allergy status.
- Review medication order for type of medication, dosage, route.
- Assess client's respiratory status including ease of breathing, respiratory rate, accessory muscle use, and breath sounds.

Equipment
Medication administration record (MAR)
Medication canister
Inhaler mouthpiece
Spacer device (optional)

Procedure
1. Check medication order (see Procedure 27-1, Steps 1 to 5).
2. Assemble medication canister, inhalation mouthpiece, and spacer device if needed. Attach the medication canister to the inhaler mouthpiece by inserting the metal stem into the long end of the mouthpiece. Shake the canister several times.
   Rationale: Shaking the canister mixes the medication and ensures uniform dosage delivery.

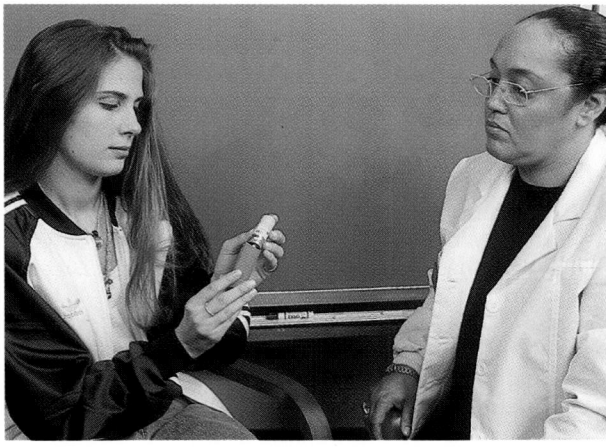

Step 2 The client attaches the medication canister to the inhaler mouthpiece by inserting the metal stem into the long end of the mouthpiece.

3. Assist the client to sitting or standing position. Perform the second medication check of five rights.
   Rationale: Sitting or standing enhances full chest expansion allowing deeper inhalation of the medication. The second check occurs before administration of the medication to the client. Checking the five rights minimizes potential medication errors.
   (The next three steps, although described separately, need to occur smoothly, one right after the other.)
4. Ask client to breathe out through his or her mouth.
   Rationale: Empty lungs enhance subsequent deeper inhalation.
5. Position the mouthpiece 1 to 2 inches from the client's open mouth. Instruct the client to breathe in slowly through the mouth. As the client starts inhaling, press the canister down to release one dose of the medication.
   Rationale: Releasing the medication 1 to 2 inches away from the mouth allows medication to form a mist and to be delivered more accurately by inhalation to the bronchial airways rather than being trapped in the oropharynx and then swallowed.

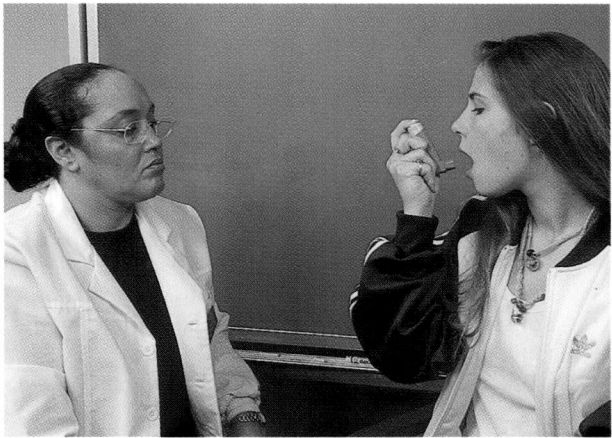

Step 5 As the client starts inhaling, she presses the canister down to release one dose of the medication.

6. Instruct the client to hold his or her breath for 10 seconds (if possible).
   Rationale: Enhances complete absorption of the medication.
7. Wait at least 1 minute before administration of a second dose or inhalation of a different medication by metered-dose inhaler (MDI). Administer bronchodilators by MDI before other inhaled medications.

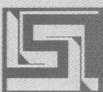

PROCEDURE 27-2 (Continued)

Rationale: Waiting allows medication from the first dose to be distributed and absorbed. Administering the bronchodilator first opens the airway and enhances greater absorption of subsequent inhaled medications.

8. Wash hands and clean mouthpiece. If steroid medication was administered, have client rinse mouth.
   Rationale: Washing hands and equipment minimizes spread of infection and maximizes inhaler efficiency. Oral fungal infections can occur if inhaled steroid medication remains in the oral cavity.

9. Reassess ease of breathing, respiratory rate, accessory muscle use, and breath sounds.
   Rationale: Follow-up assessment provides data to evaluate the effectiveness of inhaled medications.

10. Document medication administration and client status before and after administration.
    Rationale: Documentation helps maintain accurate client records, including effectiveness of the medications, and prevents medication errors.

Modification for Using a Spacer With an MDI

11. Attach the spacer to the inhalation mouthpiece. Instruct the client to exhale and then place the mouthpiece in the mouth, closing his or her lips around the mouthpiece. Depress the medication canister and have the client inhale. If the client cannot take and hold a deep breath, advise the client to take two or three short breaths to get all the medication from the spacer.
    Rationale: A spacer device attached to the inhaler mouthpiece traps the dose of medication and helps ensure adequate inhalation of medication for clients who have difficulty inhaling slowly and deeply or who cannot coordinate pressing on the canister while simultaneously inhaling the medication.

Lifespan Considerations
Infant and Toddler
- Use a spacer or nebulizer with a face mask to deliver medications by inhalation for an infant or toddler.
- Teach caregivers about symptoms that require prn bronchodilator treatment.

Child and Adolescent
- Remember that school-age children often require treatment during school hours or in emergencies. Inform the school nurse of the need for the MDI, and check school policies regarding use of medications at school.

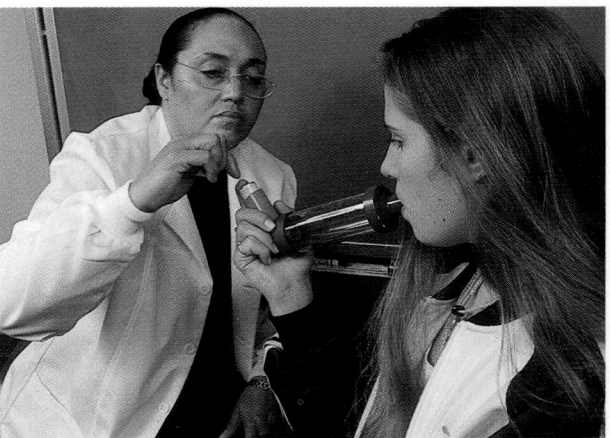

Step 11 The client places the mouthpiece in her mouth and closes her lips around it. Depress the medication canister and have the client inhale.

- Know that, at times, children can be embarrassed to use MDIs in the school setting. Provide encouragement, support, and health teaching regarding respiratory function.

Adult and Older Adult
- Use spacers for older adults, as necessary, especially if a client has difficulty with manual dexterity or deep breathing.

Home Care Considerations
- Stress the importance of which MDI to use in an emergency (β_2-agonist) and when to seek medical treatment.
- Caution against overuse of the MDI.
- Review infection control measures, including daily rinsing of the inhaler in warm, running water and biweekly washing of the mouthpiece with soap and water.
- To avoid running out of medication, teach the client to assess whether medication remains in canister by placing the canister in a container of water. When full, canisters are heavy and they sink to the bottom. If the canister floats, it is almost empty and must be replaced.

Collaboration and Delegation
- Respiratory therapists may provide initial instruction on how to use an MDI. Consult them as needed when problems occur with clients using MDIs.
- Report worsening respiratory symptoms to the physician or pulmonary specialist as soon as possible.

Equipment

Syringes and Needles. Syringes, usually made of plastic, consist of a barrel, a plunger, and a syringe tip (Fig. 27-9). The plunger fits snugly within the syringe barrel. Moving the plunger out of the barrel allows fluid or air to move into the syringe, and pushing the plunger into the barrel allows fluid or air to move out of the syringe. A needle is attached to the syringe tip (the narrow end of the syringe). Syringes may be packaged with or without attached needles. Needle gauge (diameter size) varies from 14 to 29. Needles with the smallest gauges are labeled with the largest number. For example, an 18-gauge needle has a larger diameter than does a 25-gauge needle. Needle length varies from 0.4 to 3 inches (Fig. 27-10).

The three common types of syringes are tuberculin, insulin, and standard syringes. Tuberculin syringes are 1-mL syringes that are calibrated with 0.1-mL markings and supplied with a small-gauge (26- to 28-gauge), short (0.5- to 0.625-inch) needle. Tuberculin syringes are used to administer tuberculin or sensitivity (allergy) tests.

Insulin syringes, calibrated in units of insulin (100 U per 1 mL), are used to administer insulin. Insulin syringes are made in 0.5-, or 1-mL sizes, with very small-gauge needles (26- to 30-gauge) attached.

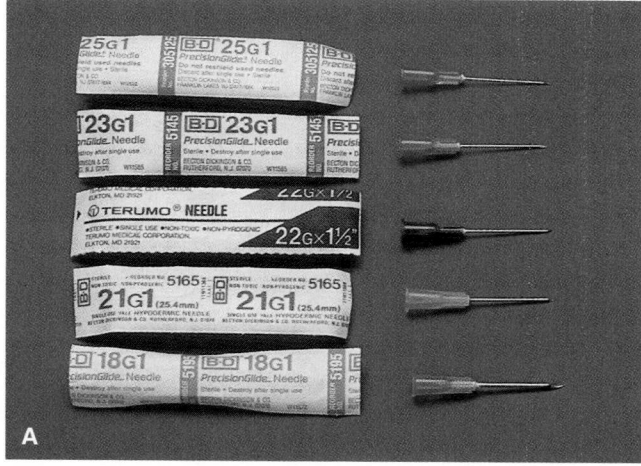

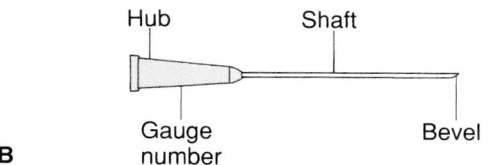

FIGURE 27-10 Needles. **(A)** Needles of different gauges and lengths. **(B)** Parts of a needle.

Standard syringes are supplied in 3-, 5-, or 10-mL sizes. Standard syringes may be supplied without needles or with 18-, 21-, 22-, 23-, or 25-gauge needles that are 0.5 to 3 inches long. IM injections are usually administered to adults via a 3-mL syringe with a long (1- to 2-inch), medium-sized (21-, 22- or 23-gauge) needle. Larger-gauge needles are used to administer viscous medications or to mix IV medications.

Prefilled syringes, prepared by a medication manufacturer or pharmacy, may be used to supply medications. Systems of prefilled syringes that require a specially designed outer injector device are in widespread use. Medications, such as opiate analgesics and heparin, are supplied in a glass syringe with an attached needle. The needle and syringe fit into a metal or plastic injector device with attached plunger (Fig. 27-11). Air and any extra medication are expelled from the syringe, and the medication is injected. Because the needle is fused to the medication syringe, needle gauge and length cannot be changed. The nurse must use the needle supplied, or transfer the medication into a standard syringe if a different needle size is required.

Filter Needles. Some agencies require the use of a filter needle to trap any rubber or glass fragments that may be drawn up with the medication in a vial or ampule. The nurse must replace the filter needle with a regular needle before injecting the medication into the client.

Needleless Systems. To avoid needlestick injuries and to increase safety for healthcare workers, needleless systems have been developed for administration of IV medications. IV tubing is designed with "Y" connectors or injection ports where medication or other tubing can be added without the use of

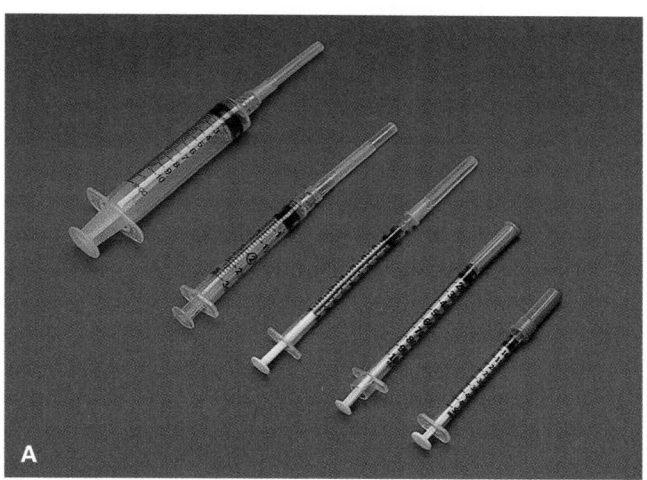

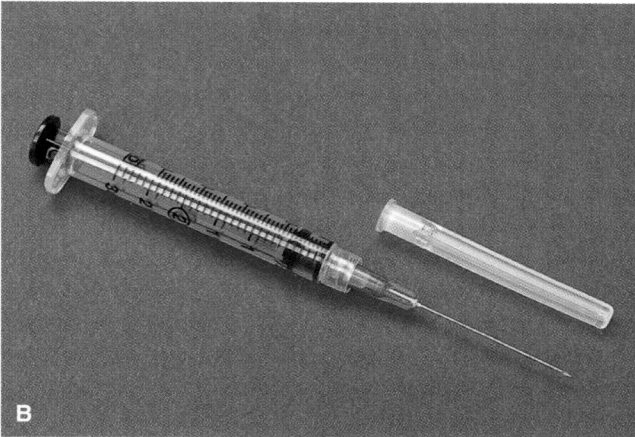

FIGURE 27-9 **(A)** Syringes (*top to bottom*): 10 mL, 3 mL, tuberculin, insulin, and low-dose insulin. **(B)** Syringe and needle.

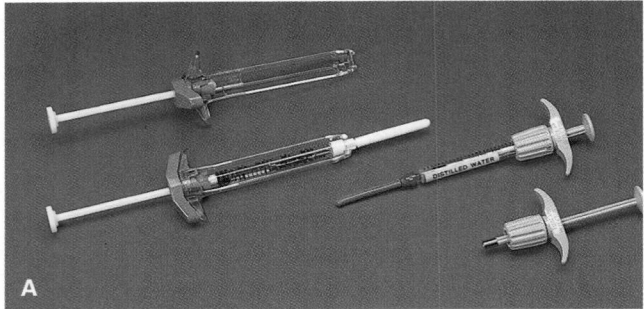

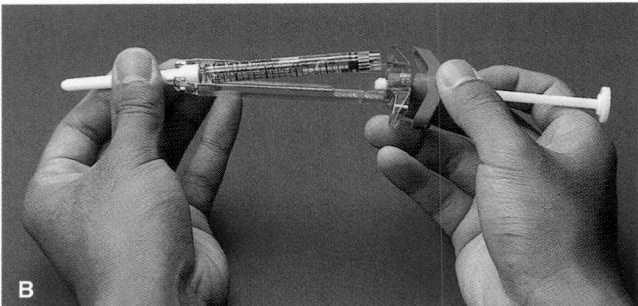

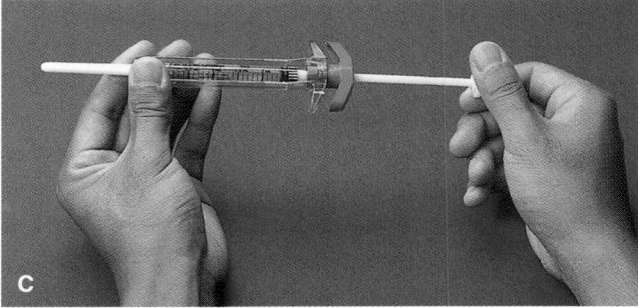

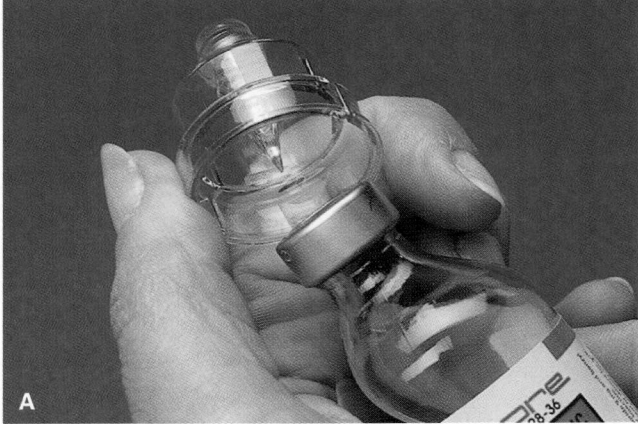

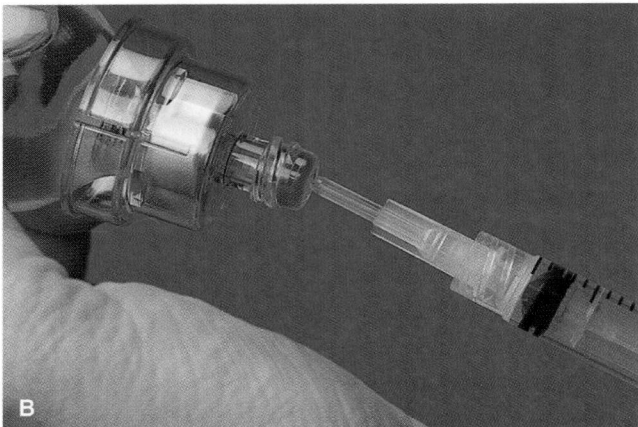

FIGURE 27-12 **(A)** Needleless system adaptor for vial. **(B)** Use syringe (without needle) to withdraw medication.

FIGURE 27-11   Prefilled syringes. **(A)** Prefilled medication cartridges and injector devices. **(B)** Cartridge inserted into injector device. **(C)** Cartridge, after being screwed in place.

needles. Vials can also be fitted with adaptors that permit access through a valve system without a needle (see Chapter 28).

Vials. Vials are plastic or glass containers that hold one or more doses of medication. The vial is opened by removing a plastic cap that covers a rubber diaphragm at the top of the container. A needle is used to pierce the center of the diaphragm, and the correct amount of medication is withdrawn into a syringe. An adaptor, which allows access to the vial without use of a needle, can be used when drawing up IV medications in a needleless system (Fig. 27-12).

Medications that are not stable for long periods may be supplied in a vial in powdered form. A diluent (sterile liquid specified by the drug manufacturer—usually sterile water or saline) is mixed with the powder to reconstitute it.

Ampules. Ampules are thin-walled glass containers that hold a single dose of a liquid medication. An ampule is shaped like a bowling pin; it has a wide base, narrow neck, and pointed top.

Medication Preparation Techniques

Drawing Up Medications. Drawing up medications is the process of moving medications from an ampule or vial into a syringe (Procedures 27-3 and 27-4). When withdrawing medication in this manner, first open the ampule or vial and then remove the needle cap from the syringe. Place the needle directly into the open ampule or vial, and pull the syringe plunger back until all medication enters the syringe. Air is usually drawn into the syringe along with the liquid medication. To dispel the air, hold the syringe, after removing it from the ampule or vial, with the needle pointed upward. If any medication has adhered to the top of the syringe in the air bubble, tap the barrel of the syringe until the liquid moves down the barrel to the rest of the medication. Expel the air and any volume of unneeded medication slowly.

Reconstituting Medications. Medications are reconstituted by adding the proper amount and type of diluent to a powdered medication. Vials of powdered medications may be packaged along with vials of the proper type and volume of diluent. The manufacturer's directions printed on the medication box or vial should indicate the amount and type of diluent to add. To reconstitute the medication, remove the

PROCEDURE 27-3

WITHDRAWING MEDICATION FROM A VIAL

Purpose
1. Withdraw a precise amount of medication from a vial while maintaining asepsis.

Assessment
- Review the prescriber's order, and assess the intended medication administration route (e.g., subcutaneous, intramuscular, intravenous) before selecting the needle and syringe.
- Inspect the ordered medication for clarity, crystals, and expiration date.

Equipment
Medication administration record (MAR)
Vial with medication
Alcohol wipes or antiseptic swabs for cleaning vial
Sterile syringe and needle
Solvent (sterile water or normal saline solution) for reconstituting medication if it is in powder form (optional)
Needle with filter if needed to prevent drawing solid matter into the needle and syringe (optional)

Procedure
1. Check medication order and compare the name of the ordered medication with the label on the medication vial. See Procedure 27-1, and complete Steps 1 through 5.
2. Assemble needle and syringe.
3. Pick up vial. If medication has been reconstituted or is in suspension, place the vial between your palms, rotating or rolling the vial back and forth. Do not shake the vial.
   Rationale: The rolling motion mixes and disperses the medication. Shaking can cause bubbles that interfere with accurate measurement.
4. Remove metal cap from vial, cleanse top of vial with alcohol wipe, remove guard from needle.
   Rationale: Maintain asepsis.
5. Pull back on barrel of syringe to draw in a volume of air equal to the volume of the ordered medication dose. Holding the vial between the thumb and fingers of the nondominant hand, insert needle through the rubber stopper into the air space—not the solution—in the vial and inject air.
   Rationale: Injection of air into the air space in the vial prevents creation of negative pressure within the vial, allowing easy withdrawal of medication. Injection of air into the solution

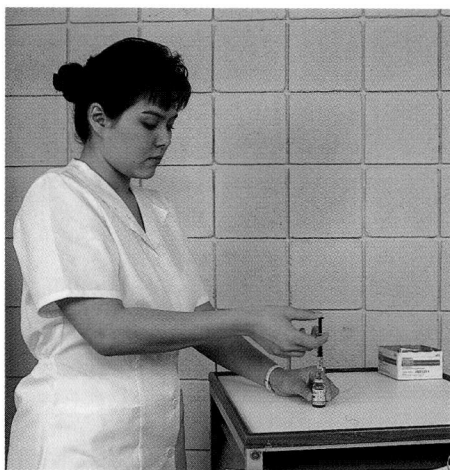

Step 5 Add air to the vial. (Photo © B. Proud.)

creates bubbles and may interfere with withdrawing an accurate dose of medication.
6. Invert the vial and withdraw the ordered dose of medication by pulling back on the plunger. Make sure that the needle is in the solution to be withdrawn.
   Rationale: Inversion of the vial brings the needle in contact with the solution so that medication can be withdrawn.

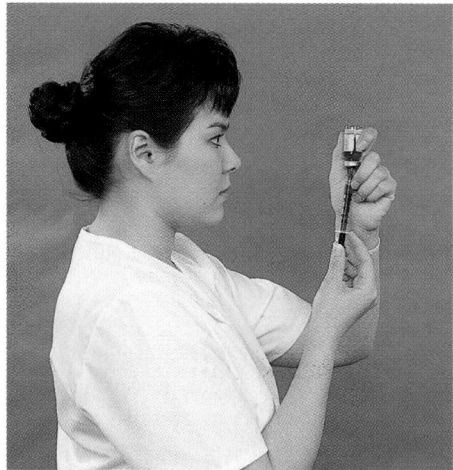

Step 6 Withdraw medication from the vial. (Photo © B. Proud.)

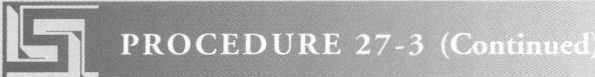

PROCEDURE 27-3 (Continued)

7. Expel air bubbles and adjust dose if necessary.
   Rationale: Air bubbles inadvertently drawn into the medication solution take up space that needs to be occupied by medication in order to deliver the accurate dose.

8. Remove needle from vial and cover the needle with guard. Wash hands.
   Rationale: Maintains asepsis and reduces the risk of needlesticks.

caps from both the medication and diluent vials and clean the tops of both vials with an alcohol wipe. Draw up the diluent into the syringe and inject it into the medication vial. Hold the medication vial and mix the medication and diluent until the medication has dissolved. Draw the reconstituted medication into a syringe (as described in Procedure 27-3), and remove air and unneeded medication from the syringe. Administer the medication as directed.

Mixing Medications. Mixing medications in the same syringe may allow a client to receive fewer injections at a lower cost. Medications may be mixed only if they are compatible. Pharmaceutical companies study the compatibility of medications (the ability to mix medications without affecting their constituents or actions). Package inserts and medication references usually present compatibility information. Medications are mixed in a syringe by first drawing up one medication into the syringe and expelling any air and unneeded medication. The ordered volume of the second medication is then slowly added to the syringe containing the first medication. If the medication is added rapidly, too much of the second medication may be drawn up. If this occurs, the syringe and medications must be discarded. Refer to Procedure 27-5 for more information.

Equipment Disposal. Discarding equipment carefully decreases the risk of inadvertent needlestick injuries and exposure to a client's blood. After administering an injection, place the syringe and needle in a needle disposal box or sharps container (see Chapter 26).

SAFETY ALERT
Avoid recapping a needle (placing the protective cap back onto the needle) after injection because of the increased risk of injury.

Intradermal Injections

Intradermal injections are given into the dermis, the layer of tissue located beneath the skin surface. ID injections are commonly used for allergy testing and tuberculin skin testing (TST). They are administered into the inner forearm area, the upper arm, and across the scapula (Procedure 27-6).

The TST, also referred to as the purified protein derivative (PPD) test or the Mantoux test, is the most commonly administered ID injection. The TST is the standard screening method for identifying persons infected with *Mycobacterium tuberculosis.* The inner forearm is the site for TST. The TST is usually administered with a 1-mL syringe and a short, ½-inch, small-gauge (26- to 28-gauge) needle. Cleansing the skin of the inner forearm is unnecessary unless it is visibly contaminated. If the skin is cleansed with an alcohol wipe, allow the site to dry. While holding the syringe with the bevel of the needle up, almost parallel to the skin, insert the needle until the entire bevel lies under the skin. Slowly inject a small volume of medication (usually 0.10 mL). A wheal (or bleb) will rise under the epidermis.

Do not apply pressure or massage the injection site; the dermal tissue will quickly absorb the medication. Because the medication is administered into dermal tissue and the injection site is not touched after the injection, use of gloves is considered optional. Document the location of the injection and time of the test. Forty-eight to 72 hours after the injection is given, the test area is inspected and palpated for evidence of induration (i.e., palpable swelling). When reading a TST, palpate the site and measure the induration. Measure the diameter of the indurated area in millimeters across the width of the forearm. Do not measure erythema (redness). Interpretation of the TST results (positive or negative) is based on the millimeters of induration and the risk category of the person being tested. An induration of more than 5 mm is classified as positive in high-risk people (e.g., people who have had recent close contact with persons with

PROCEDURE 27-4

WITHDRAWING MEDICATION FROM AN AMPULE

Purpose
1. Withdraw the full dose of medication from an ampule safely while maintaining asepsis.

Assessment
• Same as in Procedure 27-3.

Equipment
Medication administration record (MAR)
Ampule with medication
Sterile syringe and needle (or a filter needle if indicated by agency policy)
Sterile gauze pad or alcohol wipe

Procedure
1. Check medication order and make sure the solution in the ampule matches the ordered solution. See Procedure 27-1, and complete Steps 1 through 5.
2. Assemble needle and syringe. A filter needle may be used.
3. Pick up ampule and flick its upper stem several times with a fingernail.
   Rationale: The sharp, flicking motion releases medication trapped in the ampule's upper chamber.

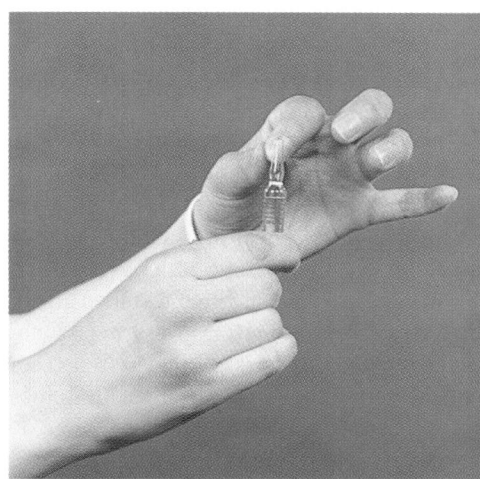

Step 3 Flick upper stem to release medication. (Photo © B. Proud.)

4. Wrap a sterile gauze pad or alcohol wipe around the ampule's neck before breaking the neck with an outward snapping motion.
   Rationale: The sterile gauze barrier protects the fingers from broken glass, possibly trapping

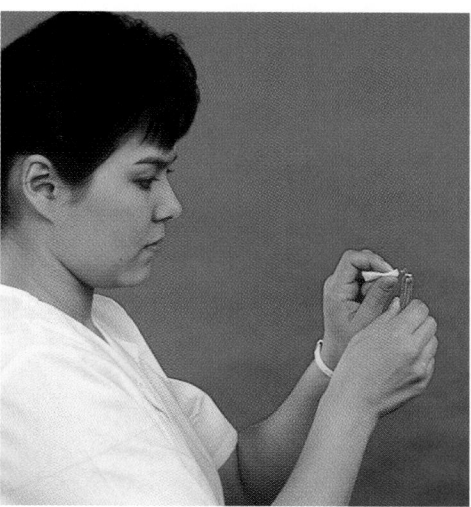

Step 4 Break neck of ampule. (Photo © B. Proud.)

   sharp fragments and preventing accidental injury to the hand.
5. Discard the broken neck appropriately, and prepare to withdraw medication from the ampule using one of the following methods.
   a. Place the ampule upright on a flat surface, insert the needle in the solution, and withdraw the correct amount of medication by pulling up on the plunger. Do not touch the needle to the glass rim.
   Rationale: Contact between needle and ampule contaminates the needle.

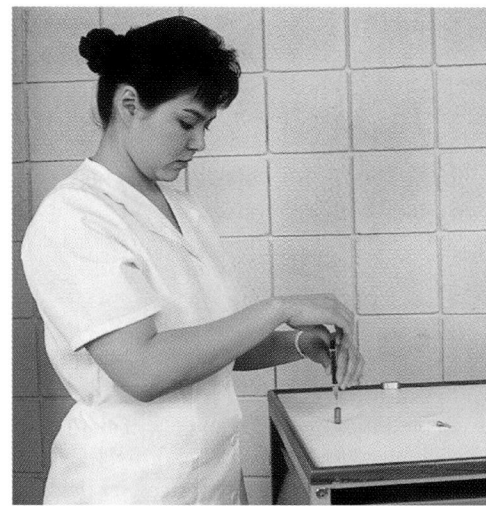

Step 5A Withdraw medication from upright ampule. (Photo © B. Proud.)

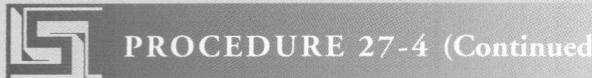

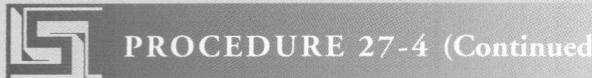

PROCEDURE 27-4 (Continued)

b. Invert the ampule or tilt it sideways. Insert the needle into the solution; pull back on the plunger, and withdraw the proper dose of medication.
   Rationale: Keeping the needle in the solution keeps air out of the dose of medication.

6. Remove the needle from the solution. Hold the needle upright, inspect the syringe, and dispel any air that may have been drawn into the syringe. Make sure that the syringe contains the right amount of medication. Expel any extra into a container.
   Rationale: Doing so ensures accurate measurement of dose.

7. Cover the needle with guard and change needle if a filter needle was used. Discard ampule in sharps container.
   Rationale: Proper disposal protects healthcare personnel from injury. A filter needle is used to trap glass particles and should not be used for injection.

8. Wash hands.
   Rationale: Maintains asepsis and minimizes risk for infection transmission.

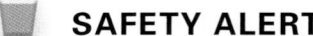

active tuberculosis [TB], people infected with human immunodeficiency virus [HIV]). An induration of more than 10 mm is necessary to classify a positive reaction in people with moderate risk (e.g., injection drug users, immunocompromised people, healthcare workers employed in high-risk settings). An induration of more than 15 mm is required to be considered a positive reaction in people in low-risk groups (Bloch, 1995/1998).

Subcutaneous Injections

Subcutaneous injections are given into the SC tissue, the layer of fat located below the dermis and above the muscle tissue (Fig. 27-13). When a medication is injected into SC tissue, absorption is usually slow, sustained, and complete. Small amounts (0.5 to 1 mL) of medication may be injected SC using a syringe with a short (½- to ⅝-inch), small-gauge (26- to 30-gauge) needle. SC injections may be given in the upper arm, upper back, abdomen, upper buttocks, or thigh (Fig. 27-14).

Speed of absorption varies with the site selected. Medications injected into the abdomen are absorbed most rapidly, those injected into the arms are absorbed intermediately, and those injected into the thigh and upper buttocks are absorbed most slowly. Avoid sites of abnormal SC tissue, such as areas lying underneath burns, birthmarks, inflamed tissue, or scars, because of unpredictable medication absorption. Absorption also may be slow or incomplete if SC medication is administered to a client with generalized edema or severe peripheral vascular disease, or to a client in cardiogenic shock. Medications may be absorbed faster than expected if SC injections are administered to clients with little SC tissue, such as premature babies or cachectic adults.

SAFETY ALERT
If a client has little or abnormal subcutaneous tissue or abnormal blood flow to subcutaneous tissue, check with the prescriber to see whether you can use an alternative route of administration.

Heparin and insulin are the most common SC medications. Nonirritating, water-soluble medications, such as opiates, also may be administered by SC injection. See Procedure 27-7 for guidelines for administering SC injections.

Insulin Administration. Insulin is administered SC, using an insulin syringe (1-mL syringe with 26- to 30-gauge nondetachable needle), to regulate a client's blood glucose levels. The syringe is calibrated in units. Most syringes today contain 100 U/mL (referred to as U-100 syringes). When administering insulin, the number of units rather than the number of milliliters is prescribed and measured in the syringe. Low-dose insulin syringes (0.5 mL, 50 U) permit better visualization when small insulin doses (e.g., less than 10 U) are given.

Insulin pens are also available for the administration of insulin. For patients who wish to self-administer insulin but are either visually impaired or lack the manual dexterity required for a regular syringe (e.g., someone with arthritis), pens are advantageous. Twisting the barrel of the pen sets the dose; an audible click assists with dose identification (Godfrey, 1998). Nurses educate clients in the proper use of insulin pens.

Insulin is available in rapid-, short-, intermediate-, and long-acting formulations. Vials of lispro (rapid) and regular (short) insulin should be clear on visual examination. Vials of NPH (intermediate), Lente (intermediate), and Ultralente

PROCEDURE 27-5

DRAWING UP TWO MEDICATIONS IN A SYRINGE

Purpose
1. Minimize the number of injections a client receives.
2. Prevent contaminating one vial of medication with medication from the other vial.

Assessment
- Review medication order.
- Review drug literature to ensure compatibility of the two medications.

Equipment
Medication administration record (MAR)
Two vials of ordered medication
Sterile 1- to 3-mL syringe with appropriate gauge and length needle
Antiseptic swabs

Procedure
1. Compare medications to the MAR. See Procedure 27-1, and complete Steps 1 through 5.
2. Cleanse tops of both vials with antiseptic.
   Rationale: Maintains asepsis and prevents possible introduction of organisms into vials.
3. With syringe, aspirate a volume of air equal to the medication dose from first medication (Vial A).
4. Inject air into Vial A, being careful that the needle does not touch solution.
   Rationale: Air in vial creates positive pressure to facilitate solution withdrawal. The same needle will be used to withdraw medication from second vial, so it must not have medication from Vial A on it.

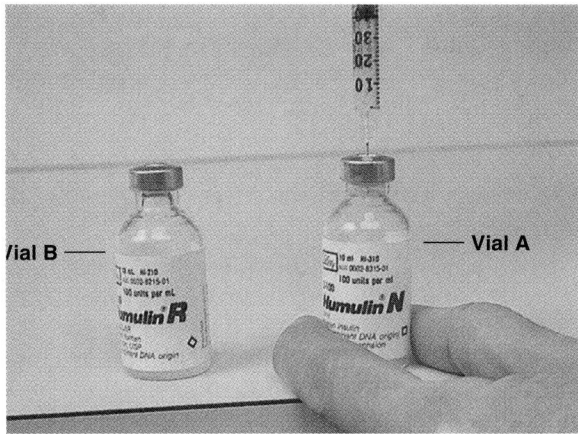

Step 4 Inject air into vial A.

5. Remove syringe from Vial A. Aspirate volume of air equal to the medication dose from second medication (Vial B). Inject air into Vial B.
   Rationale: Same as for Step 4.

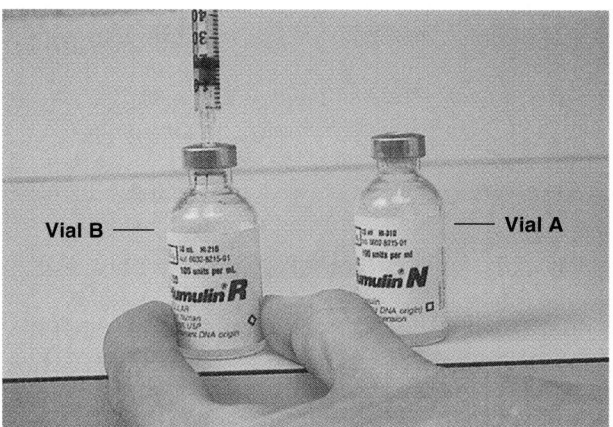

Step 5 Inject air into vial B.

6. Invert Vial B, and withdraw the required volume of medication into syringe. Expel all air bubbles, and withdraw needle from Vial B.
   Rationale: Expelling air permits accurate dosage measurement.

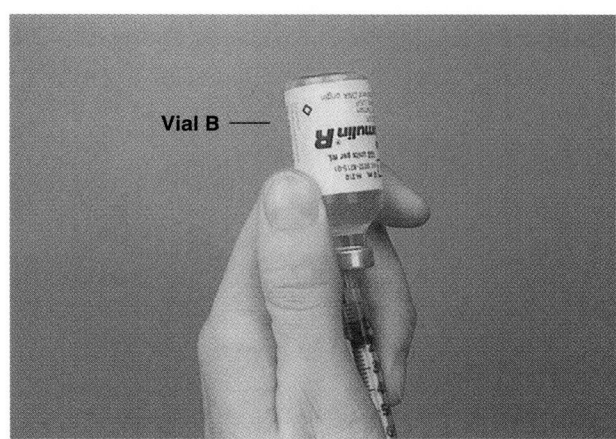

Step 6 Withdraw medication from vial B.

7. Determine what the total combined volume of the two medications would measure on the syringe scale.
   Rationale: Prevents accidental withdrawal of excess medication from Vial A.

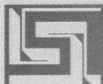

PROCEDURE 27-5 (Continued)

8. Insert needle into Vial A, invert vial, and carefully withdraw required volume of medication (as in Step 6).
9. Withdraw needle from Vial A and replace needle guard.
   Rationale: Prevents injury to healthcare workers.
10. Check medication and dosage before returning or discarding vials.
    Rationale: Rechecking dosage reduces the risk for medication errors.

Modification for Insulin
Equipment
U-100 insulin syringe
Vials of prescribed U-100 insulin

Procedure
1. Wash hands.
2. When preparing insulin in suspension, gently rotate vials between palms of hands to mix the suspension.
   Rationale: Medication separates from suspension during storage. Mixing ensures accurate concen-

trations of medications throughout. Shaking vigorously can cause changes in potency of insulin.
3. Follow Steps 2 through 8 above.
4. Establish a routine order for drawing up insulin.
   Rationale: Use of a standard sequence while mixing insulins prevents errors (Fleming, 1999).

Home Care Considerations
- If clients are having difficulty drawing up medications from two vials, assist with drawing up a week's supply; this is common with insulin.
- Teach caregivers how to draw up insulin and prefill syringes for the client. Insulin pens are devices by which diabetics can program the syringe by clicking on the desired number of units to be delivered.
- Suggest the use of adaptive aids such as syringe holders, magnifiers, or insulin pens to assist the client.
- Mark the vials of medication as Vial #1 and Vial #2 to help the client remember which vial to draw up first.

(long) insulin are in suspension and should be uniformly cloudy on visual examination. Changes such as clumping, frosting, precipitation, or change in clarity or color may signify a loss in potency (American Diabetes Association, 2001). If, after inspection of a vial of insulin, you are uncertain about its potency, obtain a new vial. Gently roll a vial of intermediate- or long-acting insulin in the palms of your hands to uniformly resuspend the insulin solution before drawing the medication into a syringe. Do not vigorously shake the vial. Excess agitation of the vial can lead to loss of potency (American Diabetes Association, 2001).

Insulin may be administered subcutaneously in the upper arm, anterior or lateral aspects of the thigh, buttocks, or abdomen (avoiding a 2-in radius around the umbilicus). If SC injections of insulin are given repeatedly into the same site, unpredictable insulin absorption and lipodystrophy (dimpling in the skin caused by atrophy of SC tissue) may occur. Rotate the site for each injection systematically about 1 inch from the previous injection site. Rotation within one area is preferred to rotation to a new body area with each injection, in order to minimize daily variability in absorption associated

with different sites. Plan and document site rotation well to prevent repeated use of the same site. Additionally, injection of cold insulin has been linked to lipodystrophy formation. Insulin need not be refrigerated for short-term use. A 10-mL vial of insulin will maintain its potency for 1 month without refrigeration, if the vial is kept cool and away from heat and sunlight (Fleming, 1999). Observe clients injecting insulin, because technique problems can affect dose administration and absorption.

Heparin Administration. SC heparin is used to help prevent deep vein thrombosis and subsequent pulmonary embolism. Because SC injections of heparin frequently cause hematoma formation, precautions are necessary. Recommendations for administering heparin are included in the modifications for heparin administration in Procedure 27-7.

Intramuscular Injections

Intramuscular injections are given into the muscle layer beneath the dermis and SC tissue (Fig. 27-15). Medications administered by IM injection usually are absorbed intermediately,

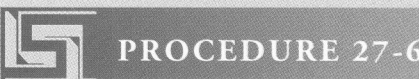

PROCEDURE 27-6

ADMINISTERING INTRADERMAL INJECTIONS

Purpose
1. Administer medication into the dermal tissue to screen for an allergic (antigen–antibody) dermal reaction.

Assessment
- Review medication order for type of medication, dosage, and route.
- Assess client for anxiety related to fear of injections.
- Inspect site for lesions, rash, ecchymosis.
- Review client history for possible allergies.

Equipment
Medication administration record (MAR)
Antiseptic swab
Vial of medication
Sterile syringe and needle (1-mL syringe with 26- to 28-gauge 0.5-inch needle)
Gloves (optional because blood exposure is rare when injection is intradermal)

Procedure
1. Check medication order. See Procedure 27-1, Steps 1 through 5.
2. Assemble needle and syringe.
3. Remove needle guard and withdraw medication from vial (see Procedure 27-3).
4. Identify client by name or identification bracelet. Scan bracelet if using bar code medication administration. Explain procedure to client. Repeat check of five rights.
   Rationale: Repeated checking prevents errors before medication is administered to client.
5. Select injection site that is relatively hairless and free from tenderness, swelling, scarring, and inflammation.
   Rationale: Injection into skin areas with abnormal characteristics could impair drug absorption or interfere with subsequent interpretation of skin reaction.
6. Remove needle guard. Hold syringe in dominant hand. Gently pull skin distal to intended injection site taut with nondominant hand.
   Rationale: Pulling skin taut helps to stabilize injection site and more reliably ensures administration into dermal tissue.
7. Holding syringe from above, at 10- to 15-degree angle (almost parallel to skin), gently insert needle, bevel up, until dermis barely covers bevel.

Rationale: Accurate delivery of medication into dermal tissue is very important. An angle > 15 degrees will inadvertently deliver medication into subcutaneous tissue. Visualization of wheal will occur with needle bevel up and barely covered by dermis.

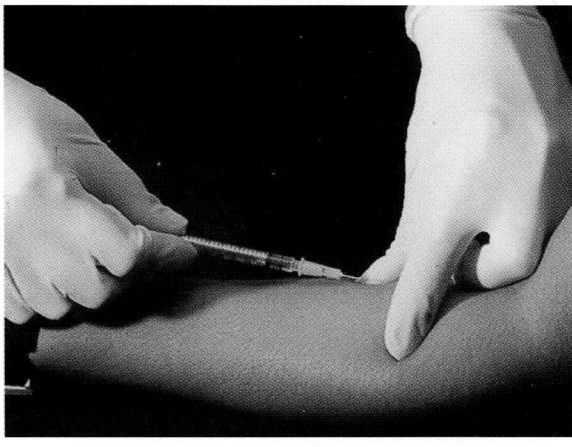

Step 7 Gently insert the needle, with the bevel up, until the dermis barely covers the bevel.

8. Stabilize needle, then inject medication slowly over 3 to 5 seconds.
   Rationale: Slow medication injection prevents discomfort from injection and ensures that medication is being delivered correctly as wheal gradually forms at injection site.
9. Withdraw needle. Do not wipe or massage site.
   Rationale: Wiping or massaging may inadvertently remove or promote absorption into subcutaneous tissue.
10. Do not recap needle. Dispose of syringe and needle in sharps container.
    Rationale: Proper disposal protects nurse and other healthcare workers from accidental needle injury.
11. Record time and site of injection according to agency protocol.
    Rationale: Maintains legal record and communicates to health care team.
12. Instruct client when to return for reading of response—15 to 60 minutes after injection for allergy testing, and usually 48 to 72 hours after injection for tuberculin skin testing.
    Rationale: Appropriate timing of site assessment is necessary to accurately interpret antibody response.

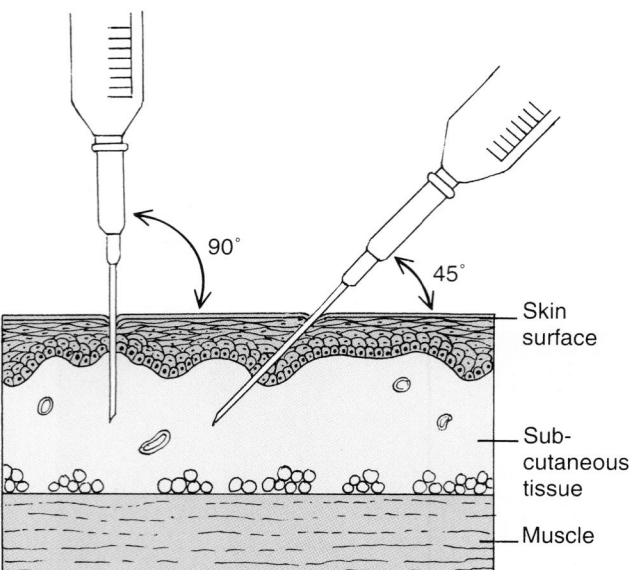

FIGURE 27-13 Subcutaneous injection deposits medication in subcutaneous tissue at a 45- or 90-degree angle.

slower than IV administration but more rapidly than SC injections. A larger volume of medication per injection and a wider variety of medications may be administered into IM sites than into SC sites. Refer to Table 27-6 for appropriate sites and volumes of medication to inject for clients of different ages. Medications in solution or suspension (including

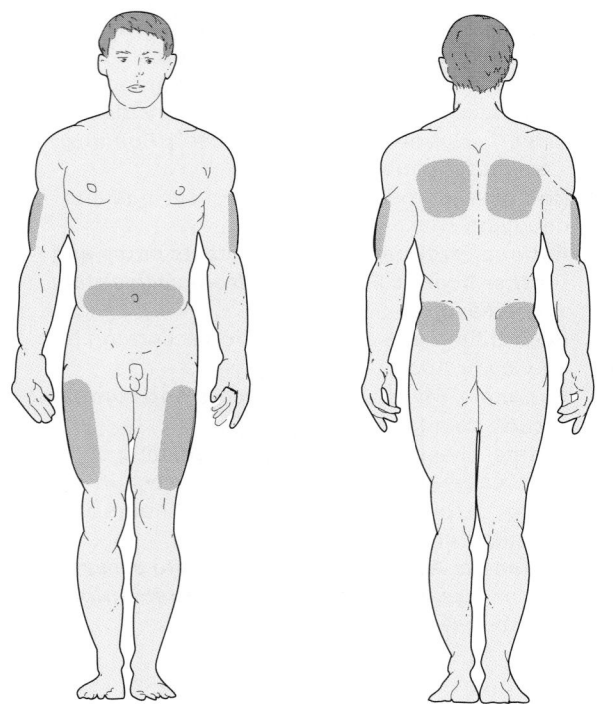

FIGURE 27-14 Sites used for subcutaneous injections.

antibiotics, antiemetics, opiates, and vaccines) may be injected into IM sites. IM injections are administered with a 3-mL syringe and a 19- to 25-gauge, 1- to 3-inch needle. The larger-gauge needles are used when the medication solution is very thick. Longer needles are used for larger adults. A 23-gauge, 1.25-inch needle is commonly used for IM injections for average-sized adult clients. Procedure 27-8 discusses administration of IM injections.

IM injections may be administered into sites in the upper arm (deltoid muscle), hip (ventrogluteal), thigh (vastus lateralis or rectus femoris), or buttocks (dorsogluteal). Age of the client, medication to be injected, amount of medication, and client's general condition influence site choice. Injections should not be given into abnormal muscle tissue, such as tissue underneath burns, scars, or inflamed areas (Table 27-7).

Deltoid Site. The deltoid site has a small amount of muscle mass with little overlying subcutaneous fat. Medication injected into this site is absorbed rapidly. Because the muscle is small and lies close to the radial nerve and the brachial artery, the deltoid site is used infrequently.

🥛 SAFETY ALERT
If you must use the deltoid site, locate the site carefully, using anatomic landmarks to decrease the risk of injury to the radial nerve and brachial artery.

The deltoid site is located by drawing an imaginary line one to three fingerbreadths (2.5 to 5 cm) below the lower edge of the acromion process of the scapula. The injection is given into the thickest area of muscle that lies over the midaxillary line (Fig. 27-16). To give the injection, slightly angle the needle toward the acromion process or insert it at a 90-degree angle.

Rectus Femoris and Vastus Lateralis Sites. Injection sites in the thigh, the vastus lateralis and rectus femoris sites, offer rapid rates of medication absorption. Because these muscles contain no large blood vessels or nerves, they are safe to use for IM injections for most clients.

The rectus femoris is the site of choice for infants and children, but it also may be used for adults. The rectus femoris is located one third of the distance from the knee to the greater trochanter of the femur, in the center of the anterior thigh (Fig. 27-17A). An injection is administered into this site by lifting the muscle away from the bone and inserting the needle at a right angle to the muscle. Use short needles (not exceeding 1 inch) to administer injections into the rectus femoris site in children.

In adults, the vastus lateralis site is the area between one handbreadth above the knee and one handbreadth below the greater trochanter on the medial outer portion of the thigh (Fig. 27-17B). An injection is administered into this site by lifting the muscle away from the bone and inserting the needle at a right angle to the muscle.

The vastus lateralis site is used for IM injections for infants, children, and adults. In infants and children, the vastus lateralis

(text continues on page 555)

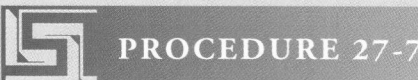

PROCEDURE 27-7

ADMINISTERING SUBCUTANEOUS INJECTIONS

Purpose
1. Ensure more rapid absorption and action of a drug than can be achieved orally.
2. Administer drugs to clients who are unable to take oral medications (e.g., unconscious, nausea/vomiting, NPO status).
3. Administer medications that are not active by the oral route or are inactivated by digestive enzymes (e.g., heparin, insulin).

Assessment
• Review client's medical history, medication history, and allergy status.
• Assess for contraindication to receiving subcutaneous injections, such as circulatory shock or localized body areas of reduced tissue perfusion that would interfere with drug absorption.
• Assess for anxiety related to fear of injections.
• Review chart for documentation of previous injection sites. Note rotation schedule when administering insulin or heparin.
• Inspect administration site for lesions, rash, ecchymoses, lipid dystrophy, and other abnormalities.
• Refer to drug literature to determine appropriateness of medication and dosage, common side effects, and nursing implications.

Equipment
Medication administration record (MAR)
Antiseptic swabs
Vial or ampule of ordered medication
Sterile gauze or cover for opening an ampule
Sterile syringe and needle (1- to 3-mL syringe with 25- to 29-gauge, ½- to ⅝-inch needle)
Gloves

Procedure
1. Check medication order. See Procedure 27-1, Steps 1 through 5.
2. Assemble needle and syringe.
3. Remove needle guard and withdraw medication from container (see Procedures 27-3 and 27-4).
4. Identify client by name or identification bracelet. Scan bracelet if using bar code medication administration. Explain procedure to client. Recheck five rights.
   Rationale: Checking five rights before medication is administered to client prevents errors.

5. Don gloves.
   Rationale: Gloving maintains Standard Precautions in case blood leaks from injection site.
6. Select an injection site that is free from tenderness, swelling, scarring, and inflammation.
   Rationale: Injection into skin areas with abnormal characteristics could impair drug absorption or increase chance of abscess or infection.
7. Cleanse site with antiseptic swab, using a circular motion from center toward outside. Allow area to dry thoroughly.
   Rationale: Cleanse site from cleanest toward more contaminated areas, pulling any contamination away from the intended injection site.

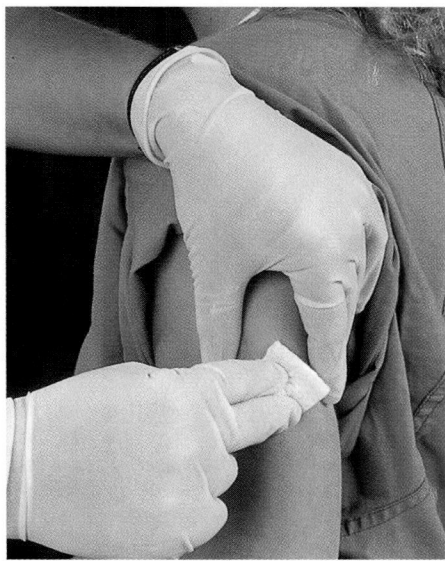

Step 7 Cleanse site with a circular motion. (Photo © B. Proud.)

8. Remove needle guard. Hold syringe in dominant hand. Place nondominant hand on either side of injection site. Spread or bunch skin to stabilize site and identify subcutaneous tissue.
   Rationale: The amount of subcutaneous tissue varies among sites and individuals. Nursing judgment is necessary to decide if spreading or bunching the skin will more accurately deliver the medication into subcutaneous tissue.
9. Hold syringe between thumb and forefinger of dominant hand. Inject needle quickly at a 45- to 90-degree angle depending on the amount of subcutaneous tissue. Release bunched skin.

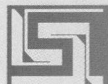

PROCEDURE 27-7 (Continued)

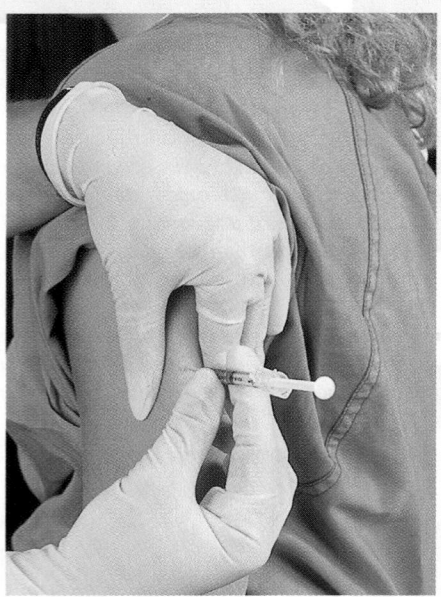

Step 9 Inject at a 45- to 90-degree angle. (Photo © B. Proud.)

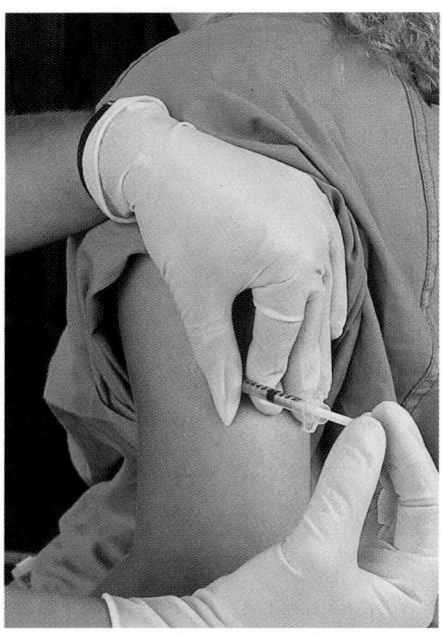

Step 10 Aspirate for blood return. (Photo © B. Proud.)

Rationale: Quick insertion minimizes discomfort. Use of the appropriate angle more accurately delivers medication into subcutaneous tissue.

10. Aspirate by slowly pulling back on plunger. If blood appears in syringe, withdraw needle, discard syringe, and prepare a new injection.
    Rationale: Aspiration of blood indicates needle is in a vein and medication would be delivered intravenously instead of subcutaneously.
    Do not aspirate when administering heparin or insulin.
11. If no blood appears, inject medication with slow, even pressure.
    Rationale: Slow, even pressure promotes client comfort and prevents tissue damage.
12. Remove needle quickly while pressing antiseptic swab over site.
    Rationale: Client discomfort is minimized by supporting tissues while withdrawing needle.
13. Gently massage site with antiseptic swab.
    Rationale: Massage stimulates circulation to the injection site and may facilitate drug absorption. (**Note:** See modifications for administering heparin.)
14. Assist client to a position of comfort.
15. Do not recap needle. Dispose of syringe and needle in sharps container.
    Rationale: Protects healthcare workers from accidental needle injury.

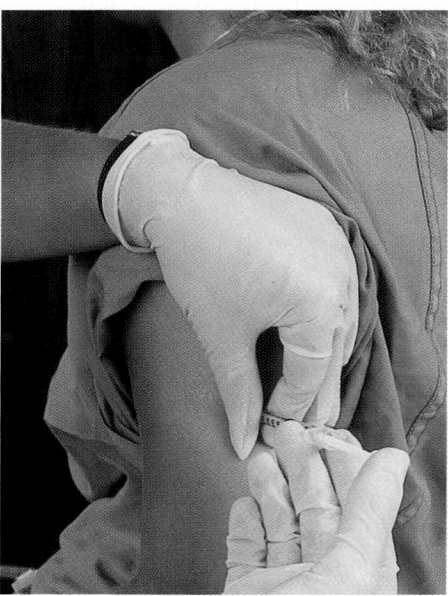

Step 11 Inject medication slowly. (Photo © B. Proud.)

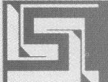

PROCEDURE 27-7 (Continued)

16. Wash hands.
    Rationale: Maintain asepsis and minimizes the risk for infection transmission.
17. Record according to agency protocol.
    Rationale: Documentation maintains accurate client records and prevents possible medication errors.

Modifications for Insulin Administration

- Know that routine aspiration is not necessary.
- Systematically rotate injection sites to prevent lipodystrophy and variable insulin absorption.
- Instruct clients who self-administer insulin about not needing to cleanse the site with alcohol before injection or to wear gloves.

Modifications for Heparin Administration

- The abdomen (avoiding the area 1 to 2 in on either side of the umbilicus) is the most frequently used site because the lack of major muscle groups or muscle activity in the abdomen is thought to reduce the chance of hematoma formation.
- Roll or gently bunch the tissue between thumb and forefinger to ensure that heparin is administered into subcutaneous tissue. Do not tightly pinch the skin.
- Because heparin is an anticoagulant, do not aspirate for a blood return or massage the site after injection.
- After injection, slowly and smoothly withdraw the needle to prevent leakage into subcutaneous tissue.

Lifespan Considerations
Infant and Child

- Securely restrain infants and children up to about 5 years of age for injections. Quick movement by the child once the needle is injected could cause trauma and loss of medication.

- Enlist the help of an assistant to restrain the child. Tell the child, "I will help you to hold still," to convey that you are asking for cooperation.
- Do not perform painful procedures in the child's bed, which is a "safe zone." And remember that parents also are regarded as "safe protectors" and should not help restrain the child during a painful procedure. Let the parent comfort the child after the injection.
- Offer praise, bandages, and "good kid" stickers as effective rewards for children for a job well done.

Obese Adult

- Know that obese clients have a layer of fatty tissue above the subcutaneous layer.
- Select an appropriate needle length to deliver medication to the subcutaneous skin layer.
- Bunch the skin at the site and inject the needle below the tissue fold to facilitate delivery of medication to the subcutaneous layer.

Home Care Modifications

- If a visually impaired client must self-administer injections, teach family members how to pre-load several syringes to help increase the client's independence.
- Assist a client who requires multiple or daily injections to develop a pattern of site rotation to minimize trauma and scarring of body tissues. Provide the client with a sheet to record each site.
- Know that the client may be taught not to cleanse the skin with alcohol when giving self-injections. However, always stress the need for proper handwashing.

---

site is located in the middle third of the area between the greater trochanter and the knee on the medial outer aspect of the thigh (Fig. 27-18). Use short needles (not exceeding 1 inch) to administer injections into the vastus lateralis site in children.

Ventrogluteal Site. The ventrogluteal site on the lateral hip is free of major blood vessels, nerves, and fat. It is consid-

ered the safest and least painful site for delivering IM injections. To locate the ventrogluteal site, place the heel of the opposite hand (for right hip, use left hand; for left hip, use right hand) over the greater trochanter, with the index and middle fingers angled toward the anterior superior iliac spine and toward the iliac crest, respectively. Give the injection in the center of the triangular area thus formed, with

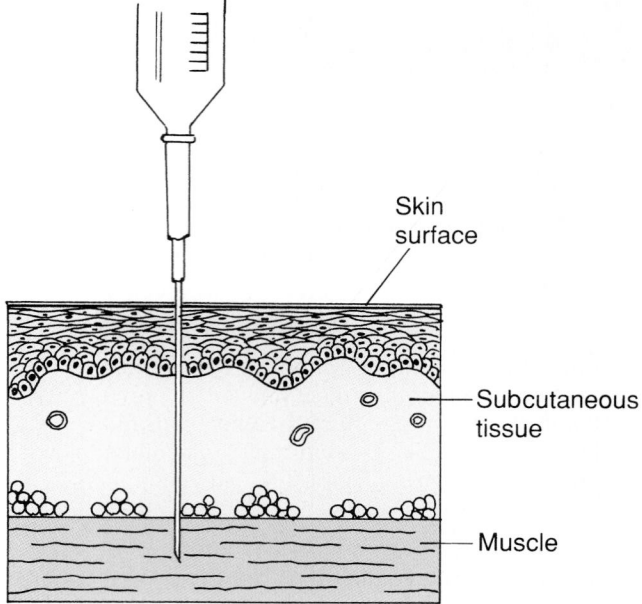

FIGURE 27-15   The intramuscular injection deposits medication into the muscle at a 90-degree angle.

the needle directed at a 90-degree angle to the skin or angled slightly toward the iliac crest (Fig. 27-19).

The Dorsogluteal Site. The dorsogluteal site of the buttocks has been used commonly for IM injections. Because of its proximity to the sciatic nerve and superior gluteal artery and the possibility of administering the injection subcutaneously into the thick layer of fat over the dorsal gluteal muscle, the routine use of this site for IM injections is not recommended.

🔲 SAFETY ALERT

Limit use of the dorsogluteal site to medications that can be safely given into subcutaneous fat. Give irritating medications and medications that must be more rapidly and consistently absorbed, such as hepatitis B vaccine, into the vastus lateralis or ventrogluteal sites.

Properly identifying the site by palpating bony landmarks helps to ensure safe use of this site. To locate the dorsogluteal site, use the index fingers to find the greater trochanter and the posterior superior iliac spine. Draw an imaginary straight line between these landmarks, and give the injection with the needle at a 90-degree angle lateral and superior to the midpoint of this line (Fig. 27-20). Pain and bleeding that may occur when injections are administered into the dorsogluteal site are less likely if clients are in the prone position with the toes pointing inward.

🔲 SAFETY ALERT

Do not use the dorsogluteal site in infants and toddlers. Muscles in this site are not well developed until children begin to walk. Older and debilitated clients who have lost muscle mass elsewhere usually have enough muscle in the dorsogluteal site to allow safe intramuscular injections.

Most medications that are appropriate for IM injection can be given using the technique described in Procedure 27-9. Medications that irritate SC tissue (e.g., hydroxyzine) or that discolor SC tissue (e.g., iron) should be given by the Z-track method (Fig. 27-21), which also is described in Proce-

dure 27-8. Although the Z-track technique is generally used with medications that are irritating to the tissues, it can be used routinely for all IM injections. Z-track technique allows medication to be administered into the muscle tissue with no tracking of medication in the SC tissues as the needle is removed. To ensure that medication does not leak back into the SC tissues, an air lock of 0.2 mL is added to the syringe. If these techniques are not followed or if site selection is not accurate, complications can occur (see Table 27-6).

Intravenous Administration

Intravenous medications are given by way of catheters inserted into veins. The IV route is advantageous for the following reasons:

- The onset of medication action is rapid.
- Predictable, therapeutic blood levels of medications can be obtained.
- The route can be used when gastrointestinal dysfunction or compromised peripheral circulation makes medication absorption unpredictable by oral, SC, or IM routes.
- Medications that cannot be given by other routes may be delivered IV.
- Larger doses of medications can be administered by this route than by SC or IM injection.

The disadvantages of the IV route include the high cost of treatment, complexity of administering IV medications outside healthcare settings, difficulty of maintaining patent peripheral IV catheters, and increased risk of complications. Complications related to IV administration of medications are given in Table 27-8.

IV medications must be prepared and packaged in a sterile manner to prevent an infection within the vein (phlebitis) or

TABLE 27-6

Intramuscular Sites: Safe Volumes to Administer (mL)					
	Infants <18 Mo	Toddlers <3 Yr	Preschoolers <6 Yr	School Age <13 Yr	Adolescents and Adults
Deltoid	N.R.	0.5	0.5	0.5–1	1.0
Rectus femorus	0.5	1	1.5	1.5	2.0
Vastus lateralis	0.5	1.0	1.5	2.0	5.0
Ventogluteal	0.5	1.0	1.5	2.0	2.5–3
Dorsogluteal	N.R.	N.R.	1.5	2.0	2.5–3

N.R., Not recommended.

Note: Individual assessment of muscle mass is necessary before giving injection. For small or wasted muscles, the volumes listed may be inappropriate.

a generalized infection (sepsis). Medications prepared in an oil base and insoluble substances cannot be administered by the IV route. Medications prepared in oil suspension (e.g., penicillin G benzathine) contain large particles suspended in a solution; if they were given by the IV route, the large medication particles might act as emboli and lodge in small veins. Examples of medications commonly given by the IV route include antibiotics, opiate analgesics, antiarrhythmics, and antiulcer medications.

IV catheters are placed in the peripheral or the central circulation. IV medications are administered through various access devices that have been placed in a vein after venipuncture. Intermittent infusion devices or lock devices, sometimes referred to as "heparin locks," "hep locks," or "saline locks," are used for short-term intermittent therapy. The intermittent infusion device is a small, dead-end connector attached to the proximal end of an IV catheter. About 1 to 3 mL of solution is instilled ("flushed") through the catheter every 8 hours or after any medication is infused through the lock. This maintains catheter patency. The fluid used to flush lock devices is usually a normal (isotonic) saline solution. Central venous access devices (Hickman or Groshong catheters) are selected for more long-term, continuous, or intermittent therapy. Venous access devices are discussed more completely in Chapter 28.

IV medications may be given by IV push (bolus), intermittent infusion, or continuous infusion. IV pain medication may be self-delivered with equipment known as a patient-controlled analgesia (PCA) device (see Chapter 43).

Intravenous Push Technique. The IV push technique is used to administer medications that can be given rapidly (over 1 to 5 minutes) for desired therapeutic effects. Most medications supplied by IV push can be administered following the steps in Procedure 27-9.

If a medication ordered to be given by IV push is not prepackaged in a syringe, draw up the medication into a syringe. If the total volume of medication is less than 1 mL, use a 1-mL syringe to allow more accurate measurement of medication volume.

IV push medications also may be given into a continuously infusing IV set or into a capped IV port. The infusion rate may be ordered by the physician or other prescriber; more commonly, the exact infusion rate is not specified, so check a medication reference manual for the infusion time recommended by the pharmaceutical company. Once the recommended total infusion time is known, calculate the infusion rate by dividing the total volume of medication that is ordered by the recommended total time of infusion.

SAFETY ALERT

To avoid speed shock and possible cardiac arrest, give most IV push medications over 3 to 5 minutes (Konick-McMahan, 1996).

Intermittent Infusion Technique. The intermittent infusion technique is most common for infusing IV medications. It is used to administer medications that need to be infused for an intermediate length of time (usually, 20 to 60 minutes). Medications administered by intermittent infusion are supplied either in bags that contain 50 to 250 mL of IV fluid (0.9 normal saline or 5% dextrose in water) or in 20- to 60-mL syringes to be used with an infusion pump. The pharmacist or nurse who prepares the medication labels the bag or syringe with the client's name, medication name, type of IV fluid or diluent, and suggested infusion rate (Procedure 27-10).

When administering IV medication, be sure the medication supplied is the medication ordered; that the medication, as ordered, is safe for the individual client; that the IV catheter is patent (i.e., the catheter is still in the vein, the catheter is not clogged, and the catheter site is not reddened or swollen); and that the medication is infused at the proper rate and time.

Continuous Infusion Technique. The continuous infusion technique is used to infuse medications that must be given continuously to achieve the desired effect (e.g., heparin) and medications that are toxic if given over short periods (e.g., cisplatin, potassium). Medications ordered by continuous infusion are supplied in IV bags containing 250 to 1000 mL of IV fluid.

Most agency protocols require the use of an IV pump or controller for administration of continuous IV medications.

(text continues on page 560)

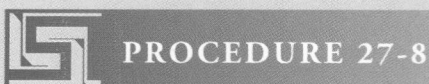

PROCEDURE 27-8

ADMINISTERING INTRAMUSCULAR INJECTIONS

Purpose
1. Administer medication deeply into muscle tissue, without injury to the client.
2. Administer a medication that requires absorption and onset of action quicker than the oral route and that may be irritating to the subcutaneous tissues.

Assessment
- Review client's medical history, medication history, and allergy status.
- Assess for contraindications to receiving intramuscular injections, such as circulatory shock, reduced blood flow, or muscle atrophy.
- Assess for anxiety related to fear of injection.
- Review chart for documentation of previous injection sites, if client is receiving multiple injections.
- Refer to drug literature to determine appropriateness of medication and dosage, common side effects, and nursing implications.
- Assess adipose tissue and muscle mass of client to determine needle size.

Equipment
Medication administration record (MAR)
Antiseptic swabs
Vial, ampule, or prefilled cartridge syringe of medication
Syringe or tubex: 2 to 3 mL for adult
Sterile needle (1.5- to 3-in, 21- to 23-gauge for adult)

Procedure
1. Check medication order. See Procedure 27-1, Steps 1 through 5. Assemble needle and syringe.
2. Prepare needle, syringe, and medication by following the appropriate steps in Procedures 27-3 or 27-4. If medication is known to be irritating to subcutaneous tissues, replace needle after withdrawing medication.
   Rationale: Prevents medication that adheres to outside of needle from irritating and burning subcutaneous tissues as needle passes into muscle.
3. Identify client by name or identification bracelet. Scan bracelet if using bar code medication administration. Explain procedure to client. Recheck five rights.
   Rationale: Proper identification and rechecking prevent errors before administration of the medication to the client.

4. Don gloves. Assist client to a comfortable position, and expose only the area to be injected.
   Rationale: Maintains Standard Precautions should blood leak from injection site. Exposing as little area as possible promotes comfort and privacy.
5. Select appropriate injection site by inspecting muscle size and integrity. Consider volume of medication to be injected.
   Rationale: Larger muscles can absorb larger volumes of medication.
6. Use anatomic landmarks to locate the exact injection site, as shown in the accompanying photos (see also Figs. 27-16 through 27-20).
   Rationale: Injection into proper site prevents trauma to bones, nerves, or blood vessels.

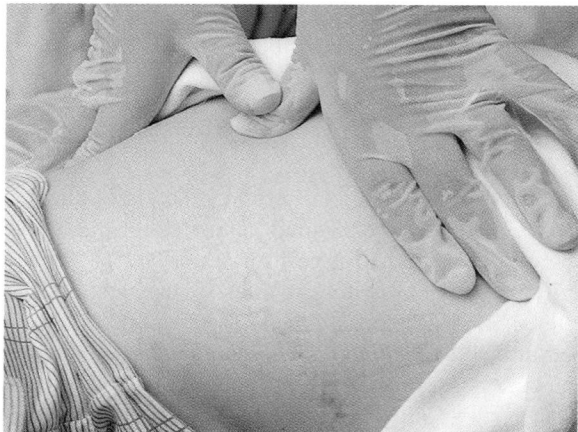

Step 6 Identify anatomic landmarks for dorsogluteal site.

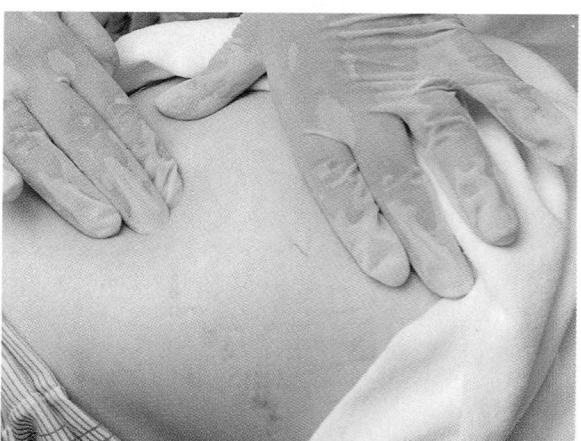

Step 6 Locate the exact injection site.

PROCEDURE 27-8 (Continued)

7. Cleanse the site with antiseptic swab, wiping from center of site and rotating outward.
   Rationale: Cleanse site from cleanest to most contaminated areas, pulling any contamination away from the intended injection site.
8. Remove needle guard. Hold syringe between thumb and forefinger of dominant hand (like a dart). Spread skin at the site with nondominant hand.
   Rationale: Facilitates needle insertion by firming skin surface and flattens tissue so needle penetrates into muscle. (Note: If client has very small muscle mass, bunch muscle before insertion.)
9. Insert needle quickly at a 90-degree angle to the client's skin surface.
   Rationale: Insertion at a 90-degree angle enables needle to reach deep muscle layers (see Fig. 27-15). Rapid needle insertion minimizes client discomfort.

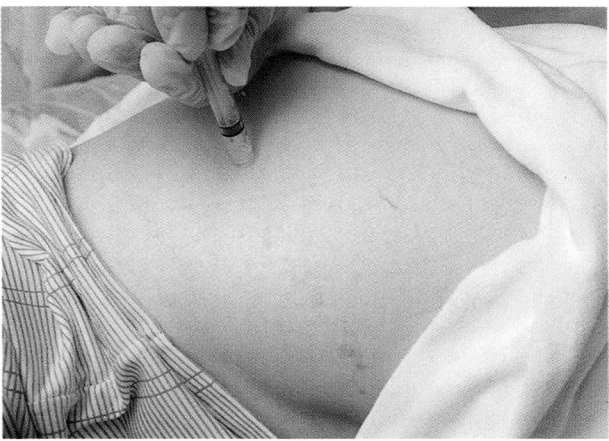

Step 10A Aspirate slowly for blood return.

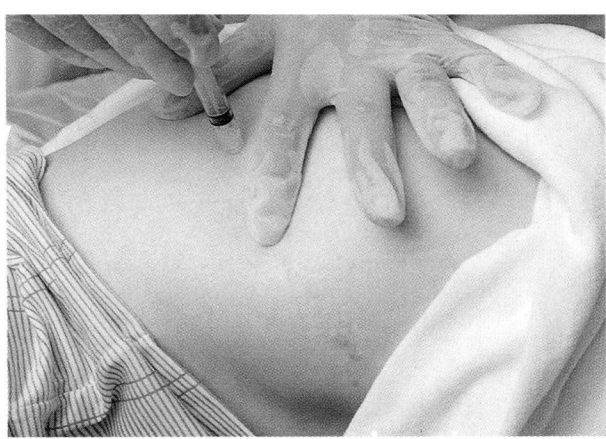

Step 9 Quickly insert needle at a 90-degree angle.

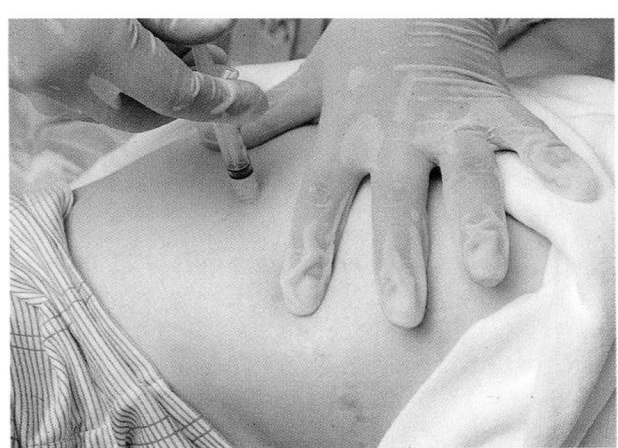

Step 10B Slowly inject medication.

10. Stabilize syringe barrel by grasping with nondominant hand.
    a. Aspirate slowly by pulling back on plunger with dominant hand.
    b. If no blood appears, inject medication slowly.
    c. If blood appears in syringe, remove needle, dispose of syringe, and prepare new medication.
       Rationale: Aspiration of blood indicates needle is placed intravascularly and must not be given.
11. Withdraw needle while pressing antiseptic swab above site.
    Rationale: Minimizes discomfort by supporting tissues during needle withdrawal.

12. Gently massage site.
    Rationale: Massage stimulates local circulation and enhances drug absorption.
13. Do not recap needle. Dispose of equipment in sharps container.
    Rationale: Proper disposal protects nurse and healthcare workers from accidental needle injury.
14. Wash hands.
    Rationale: Maintains asepsis and minimizes the risk for infection transmission.
15. Record medication and client response according to agency protocol.
    Rationale: Proper documentation provides information about the client's status, maintains accurate client records, and reduces the risk for medication errors.

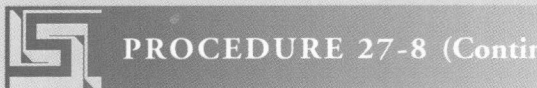

PROCEDURE 27-8 (Continued)

Variations for Air Lock Injection Technique

The air lock technique, which clears excess medication from the needle after injection, is thought to prevent medication from leaking into the subcutaneous tissues and skin surface as the needle is withdrawn, thereby preventing irritation and staining of tissues. Air lock technique is recommended in combination with Z-track technique but may also be used for non–Z-track IM injections. If an airlock variation is selected:

1. Withdraw desired volume of medication into syringe.
2. Draw in an additional 0.2 mL of air.
   Rationale: Adding 0.2 mL of air ensures an air lock.
3. Check medication dose in syringe; expel excess amount of medication from syringe.
   Rationale: Checking the medication dose ensures accurate measurement and prevents errors.
4. Redraw in 0.2 mL of air, and recheck dose accuracy.
5. Insert the needle, entering at a 90-degree angle to the client's skin surface and the floor. Position the client so the proper anatomic landmarks can be located for the chosen site and still allow the needle to enter the client at a 90-degree angle to the floor. For example, when using either the ventrogluteal or deltoid sites, the client must be lying on the side.
   Rationale: This ensures that the air bubble follows the solution during the injection and maintains the "air lock" to protect the subcutaneous tissues.

Variations for Z-Track Injection

Manufacturer's guidelines for certain medications advise "for deep IM use only" or "given deeply into the body of a relatively large muscle." Z-track method is then the recommended technique:

1. When preparing the injection site, pull the skin and subcutaneous tissues about 1 to 1.5 inches to one side of the selected site (see Fig. 27-21).
   Rationale: Creates a zig-zag track through the tissues, which prevents back-leaking of medication when needle is withdrawn.
2. Insert the syringe at a 90-degree angle.
3. Aspirate and administer medication while continuing traction on skin.
4. Leave needle inserted an additional 10 seconds.
   Rationale: Allows medication to disperse and muscle to begin absorption.
5. Simultaneously remove needle and release traction on skin.
   Rationale: Zig-zag pathway seals medication into the muscle tissue.

Lifespan Considerations
Infant and Child
- See Procedure 27-7.
- Use a 1- to 2-mL syringe, 0.5- to 1-inch, 25- to 27-gauge needle for a child.
- Know that the rectus femoris site is preferred in infants and children.

Home Care Considerations
- Teaching injection technique to caregivers requires time to decrease anxiety and master psychomotor skills.
- Use a plastic jug for safe collection of used needles.

These machines can be programmed to deliver a set volume of IV fluid over a specific time frame, usually a certain number of milliliters per hour. Controlled delivery is important to prevent inadvertent overdose of IV medication. The machines also have audible alarms that temporarily stop the infusion while simultaneously alerting the nurse to check the system. Possible problems that set off the alarm include air in the tubing, occlusion (kinked tubing, possible clot formation at the catheter tip, bent catheter), infusion complete, and bag empty.

Patient-Controlled Analgesia. PCA devices permit clients to administer opiates intravenously as needed for pain control. A PCA device is programmed electronically to deliver a set amount of medication (usually a controlled substance) through a prefilled syringe connected to IV tubing. Specific dosages and time intervals can be programmed into the machine to prevent overdosage; medication is delivered when the client pushes a control button. Refer to Chapter 43 for more information on PCA.

TABLE 27-7

Complications Associated with Intramuscular Medication Administration

Complication (Signs/Symptoms)	Causes	Nursing Measures
Pain with injection (client reports discomfort)	Muscle tensing during injection Medication irritating to IM tissue Inadvertent tracking of medication or alcohol through SC tissue	Encourage client to relax muscles during injection and point toes inward. Use Z-track technique when administering medications that are irritating to SC tissue. Change needle after drawing up medication. Use an air lock when giving irritating medications. Let alcohol skin prep dry before giving injection.
Damage to SC or IM tissue, including sterile abscesses (collection of undissolved medication), SC tissue discoloration, hematomas, and muscle contractions (tissue nodules or indurations [indentations], bruising, brown discoloration, or pain in IM injection site; muscle contracture [in infants] characterized by difficulty crawling 4 weeks to 1 year after receiving IM injections)	Multiple injections given into same area Injection given into abnormal tissue Injection of drug that is not water soluble (e.g., dilantin, Valium) IM administration of heparin IM route used for client with a low platelet count SC deposition of iron supplements (e.g., Imferon)	Give an injection at least 1 inch away from recently administered injections or from scars, burns, or areas of abnormal SC or IM tissue. Rotate injection sites (give injections at least 1 inch away from recent injection). Record sites used for all injections. As soon as possible, change from IM route to another route. Be sure that medication is recommended for IM administration. Check with physician before administering IM injection to a client whose platelet count is under 30,000/mL. Do not administer IM injections into atrophied muscle. Decrease risk of knee contractures for infants with passive range-of-motion exercises and applying warm soaks and massage to the thighs. Give iron supplements (e.g., Imferon) using the Z-track technique.
Nerve injury (shooting pain down limb, temporary or permanent paralysis)	Nerve struck during injection Medication injected close to nerve	Use careful visual inspection and palpation to locate injection site. Avoid use of deltoid and dorsogluteal sites whenever possible.
Bone injury (pain or bone damage)	Bone struck during IM injection	Use a short needle (1.25 in) when giving injections into the deltoid or ventrogluteal sites. Use visual inspection and palpation to locate injection sites.
Speed shock or rapid absorption of medication (unexpectedly rapid onset of action of medication; may lead to increased heart rate and respiratory rate, decreased level of consciousness, and cardiovascular collapse)	Medication administered directly into a vein or artery	After inserting needle into muscle, aspirate (pull back on plunger of syringe) to check for blood. If blood appears in syringe barrel, remove syringe and needle and discard. Draw up another dose of medication and administer in a new site.
Infection of muscle or bone (muscle or bone pain in injection site, skin redness or warmth, localized swelling)	Organism introduced into tissue or bone during injection	Follow strict aseptic technique when administering IM injections.

IM, intramuscular; SC, subcutaneous.

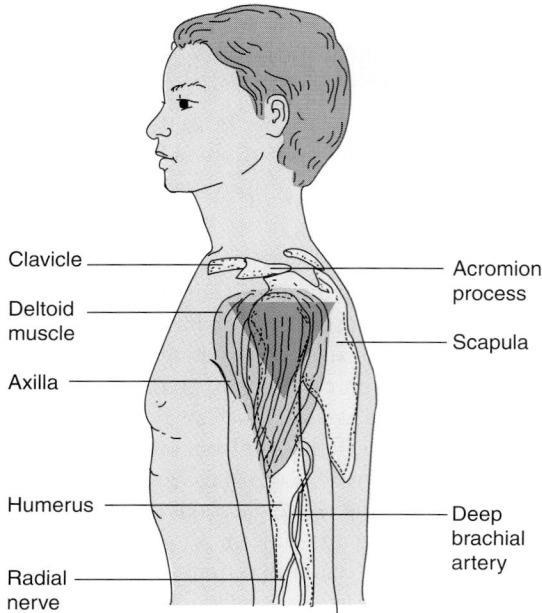

FIGURE 27-16   Deltoid muscle injection site. The site is located by imagining a line extending 1 to 2 fingerbreadths (or 2.5–5 cm) from the acromion process. A triangle is formed that indicates the injection site.

Healthcare Planning and Home or Community-Based Care

Community-based nursing care describes a philosophy of care reflective of how nursing care is provided, not where. The National League for Nursing (NLN) has defined the essential components of community care as advocating for self-

care; prevention; consideration of family, culture, and community; and continuity of care through collaboration (NLN, 1993). Likelihood of compliance with medication routines can be difficult to predict. Many researchers estimate that as many as one fourth to one half of clients may stop taking their medications early. Assessment and risk identification for possible factors influencing a client's ability to adhere to the medication regimen and client teaching are key to successful community-based care.

Clients are most likely to follow medication routines that are specific to individuals and integrated into their daily routines. To tailor medication routines and teaching plans to a client, assess the client's physical and psychosocial status, financial situation, daily routine before the illness, learning style, and manner of coping with previous therapeutic regimens. This information usually can be gathered informally by talking with the client and family.

The client's physical condition may influence his or her ability to take medications as prescribed. The physical senses of sight and hearing may deteriorate with disease or advancing age, evoking the question, "Does the client see and hear well enough to follow the daily medication routine?" A diabetic client with retinopathy and blurred vision may be unable to draw insulin accurately into a syringe. The ability to perform fine motor movements also may change with illness or advancing age. Most people can learn the coordinated motor movements needed to administer injections. Expect to spend more time teaching this technique to older clients.

The client's psychosocial condition influences the ability to take medications correctly. People without supportive friends or family members may be less likely to follow medical regimens. Awareness of this situation can allow the nurse to help the client problem-solve or get support or counseling, and the medication routine can be simplified to fit the client's situation.

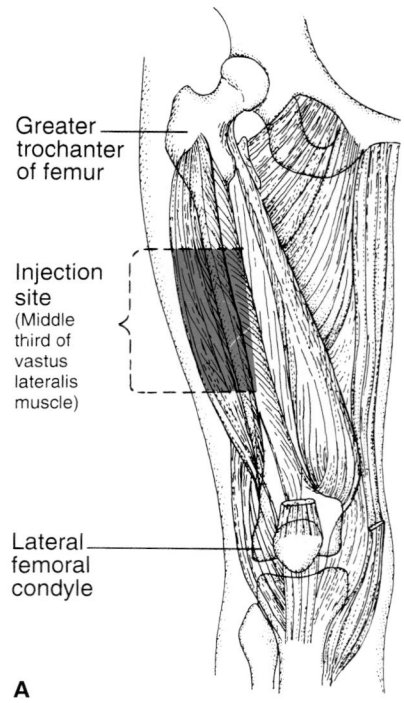

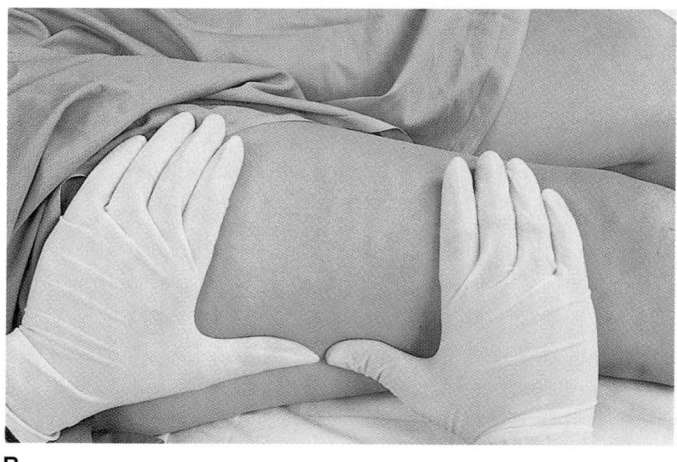

B

FIGURE 27-17   (**A**) Location of rectus femorus and vastus lateralis sites for injection. (**B**) The thigh is divided into thirds; the middle third is the injection site.

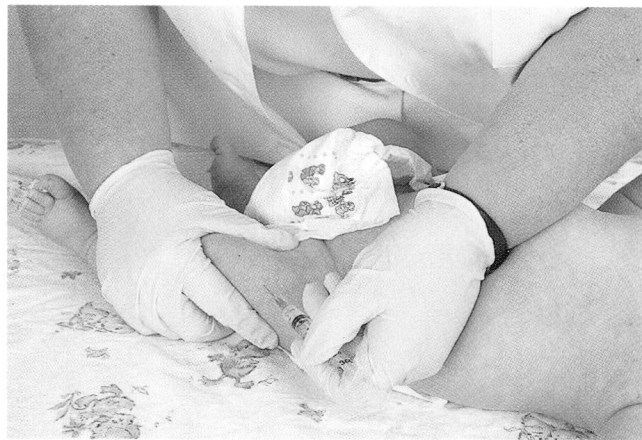

FIGURE 27-18 Administration of an injection to an infant in the vastus lateralis site. Note the right angle of short needle.

The client's finances may limit his or her ability to obtain medications or to take them as prescribed. Use of the least expensive, simplest medication routine possible is preferred for clients with limited resources. Make sure clients understand the possible consequences of discontinuing medications. Contact resources for financial support when need is evident.

The complexity of a medication routine also may make a client's compliance difficult. Medication regimens that involve multiple dosing intervals of multiple medications or through-the-night dosing can be difficult to remember. Given a client's abilities and limitations, consider whether he or she can self-administer medications safely. Simplifying routines and eliminating unnecessary or ritualistic steps can make self-medication at home easier. For example, diabetics who must self-administer insulin can eliminate the use of alcohol wipes when giving injections and can reuse syringes (Fleming, 1999). If more than one insulin injection per day is necessary, teach the client to rotate sites by using a certain body area at the same time each day (e.g., using the abdomen for morning insulin and the thigh for evening insulin). If concerns about the client's ability to take medications safely arise, consult the client's primary care provider to see whether the medication routine can be changed or help can be authorized for the client at home. After discussing the planned home medication routine with the client, ask about his or her plan for taking medications. If the client does not have such a plan, useful techniques include prefilled medication boxes or syringes, calendars with the medications written on them, and storage of medications in places that prompt the client to remember them.

Guide priorities for teaching by determining what the client needs to know to take medications safely. Present the information in everyday, nontechnical language, both verbally and in writing. Provide brief but practical information about the following topics:

- Name of the medication
- Reason for taking the medication
- How and when to take the medication
- How long to take the medication

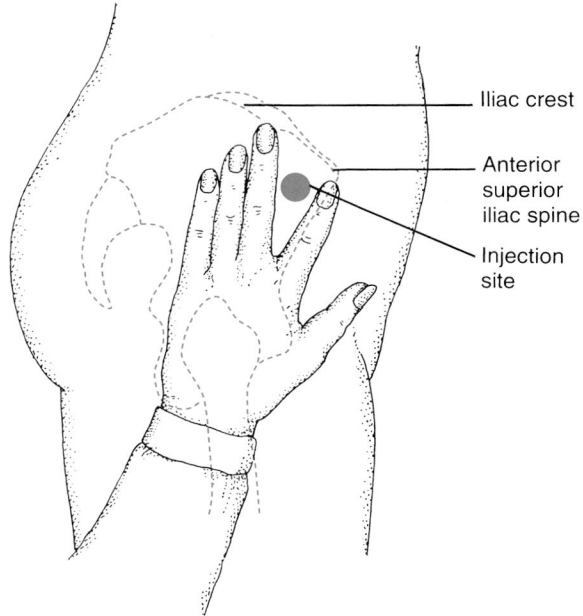

FIGURE 27-19 Ventrogluteal site injection. The heel of the hand is placed over the greater trochanter, and the middle finger reaches toward the iliac crest while the index finger is angled toward the anterior superior iliac spine. The injection is given in the center of the resulting triangle.

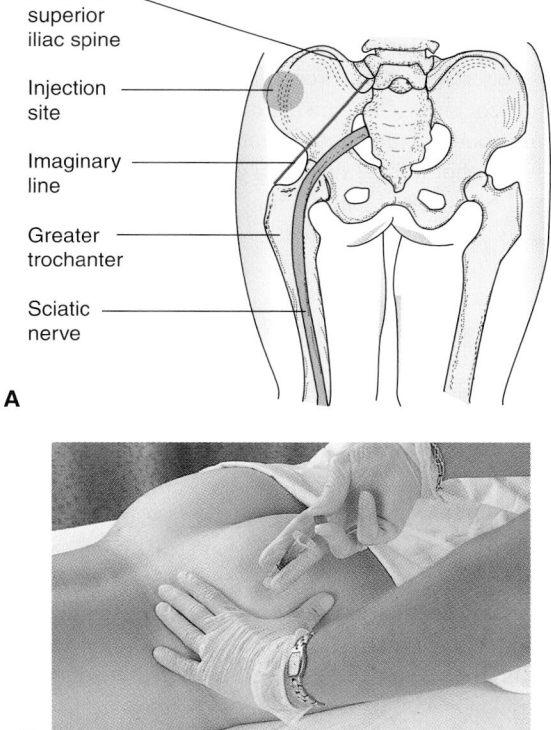

FIGURE 27-20 **(A)** Dorsogluteal site for intramuscular injection. The injection is given lateral and superior to the midpoint of an imaginary line drawn between the greater trochanter and the posterior superior iliac spine. **(B)** Locating the dorsogluteal site for injection. (Photograph © B. Proud.)

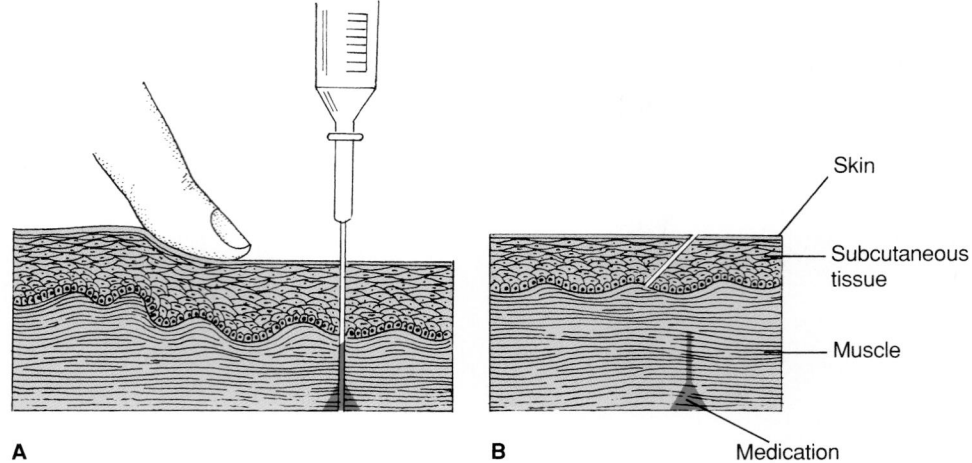

A   **B**

FIGURE 27-21 Z-track method. **(A)** Pull skin and subcutaneous tissue 1 to 1.5 inches to one side of the injection site while injecting medication. **(B)** Release traction to allow skin to fall back, sealing medication in site.

- Foods, drinks, and prescription or OTC medications that may affect the medication's action
- Any activities that may be affected when taking this medication
- Usual adverse effects of the medication and their treatment

If a medication is being given to improve a bothersome symptom (e.g., an MDI to treat shortness of breath), provide specific warnings about using more than the ordered dosage. Without this warning, a client who thinks "if a little is good, more is better" may take excessive amounts.

Begin teaching about medications as soon as possible. Teaching about administration techniques that require learning new psychomotor skills, such as those used for injecting insulin, should start at least 24 hours before discharge from a hospital or extended-care facility. The client is unlikely to learn a complex psychomotor skill without frequent demonstrations and practice. Learning complex psychomotor skills typically requires several clinic or home visits for reinforcement and refinement.

Document any client teaching. Indicate topics discussed, to whom the teaching was given (client only, or client and family members), use of any audiovisual aids or written materials given, any learning barriers (e.g., poor command of English, visual or hearing impairment), and what was done to address them. Matching medication routines and teaching materials to individual clients; ensuring frequent, ongoing follow-up; encouraging involvement of family or friends in assisting the person with medication compliance; and discussing compliance issues with the client may help improve clients' adherence to and compliance with their medication routines.

Evaluation

Assessing the client's response to medications is an important nursing function. Evaluation should include therapeutic effects, unexpected adverse effects, the client's adherence to and compliance with the medication regimen, and the client's knowledge level concerning prescribed medications.

Ask the client if the prescribed medication seems to be working. Subjective feelings of improvement are important indicators of therapeutic effect for many medications. Use physical assessment data (e.g., vital signs, lung auscultation) to identify physical improvements. Laboratory test values provide additional objective data and are useful in evaluating many medications. Be knowledgeable about the adverse effects of any drug administered. Document signs of toxicity or unpleasant side effects and report them to the healthcare provider.

Assessment of the client's understanding and compliance with drug therapy is another important part of evaluation. Having the client describe the dose, frequency, action, and side effects of each medication is one way to evaluate knowledge level. Clients administering injections for the first time should demonstrate the skill safely and correctly. Clients should be able to explain how they plan to purchase, store, and take their medications after discharge.

LIFESPAN CONSIDERATIONS

Newborn and Infant

Special considerations are important when giving oral, SC, IM, and IV medications to newborns and infants. Liquid oral medications are preferred for newborns and infants. If such medications are unavailable, crush the solid medication and dissolve it in water. Using a syringe to draw up and give oral medications also may be helpful. Babies should receive oral medications on an empty stomach unless otherwise noted. Infant formulas may alter medication absorption, and infants are less likely to spit up medications they receive before feedings.

Administer parenteral medications to newborns and infants with special care. The SC route is rarely used for administering medications to babies, who have little or no subcutaneous tissue. See Table 27-5 for information on appropriate

TABLE 27-8

Complications Associated with Intravenous (IV) Medication Administration		
Complication (Signs/Symptoms)	**Causes**	**Nursing Measures**
Speed shock (headache, tightness in chest, shock, cardiac arrest)	Medication administered more rapidly than intended	Know time period recommended for medication administration. If administering by IV bolus technique, time infusion with a watch with a second hand. If administering by continuous drip or intermittent drip methods, regulate drip rate accurately. Check rate of infusion of medication at least several times per hour. Infuse any medications with serious or toxic side effects using an infusion control device. Infuse all medications that are titrated at a consistent rate using an infusion control device.
Infection (redness, warmth, or pain at catheter insertion site; fever, increased leukocyte count, organisms present on blood culture samples, chills, shaking, increase in body temperature)	Break in aseptic technique when preparing or administering IV medications. Contamination of IV catheter site when IV dressing is changed. IV equipment changed infrequently. Contaminated IV solution	Tape catheter securely to skin. Check catheter insertion site at least once per shift and before and after infusion of medications. Change IV tubing every 48 to 72 hr.
Extravasation during which medication leaks out of the vein lumen (pain, swelling at distal end of catheter, slowed rate of infusion, increase in size of one extremity [with IV] over the other extremity, severe tissue sloughing)	Catheter migrated out of vein during client movement	Avoid placing IV catheter close to client's wrist or elbow whenever possible. Tape catheter securely to skin.
Thrombophlebitis (redness and warmth along cannulated vein; burning pain; slow flow rate; when palpated, vein feels hard, cordlike)	Trauma to vein during catheter insertion or from catheter movement. Irritation of vein resulting from medication administered	Inspect IV site at least once per shift. Whenever possible, avoid infusing irritating medications into the small veins of the hands and forearms. Whenever possible, avoid placing catheters near the wrist or elbow. If placement in these areas is necessary, decrease catheter movement by securing arm to an arm board. Check catheter insertion site at least once per shift and before and after infusion of IV medications.

IM injection sites and amounts of medication that are safe to inject for various IM sites.

When giving IV medications to newborns and infants, follow these guidelines:

- Calculate the dose accurately and make sure the dose is appropriate for the infant or young child.
- Monitor infusions with the use of electronic controllers.

- Use IV sites in the hand, scalp, forearm, foot, or central circulation.
- Monitor the catheter insertion site carefully and frequently.

Teaching about medication administration is geared toward caregivers. In addition to routine medications, teaching (text continues on page 570)

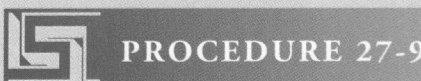

PROCEDURE 27-9

ADMINISTERING MEDICATIONS BY INTRAVENOUS PUSH

Purpose
1. Achieve high blood levels of a medication in a short period.
2. Achieve immediate and maximal effects of a medication.

Assessment
- Check medication orders for type of medication, dosage, route, and time scheduled for administration.
- Assess for compatibilities of medications and solutions to be administered.
- Identify all pertinent allergies.
- Assess intravenous (IV) site for patency and signs of erythema, pain, tenderness, or edema.
- Collect all information to administer medication safely, including action, purpose, side effects, normal dosage, time of peak onset, and nursing implications.
- Obtain pertinent physical assessments (e.g., pulse rate, blood pressure) and laboratory data (e.g., potassium level)

Equipment
Medication administration record (MAR)
Antiseptic swab
Medication vial or ampule
Watch with second hand or digital display
Syringe; two 5- to 10-mL syringes (if medication is not compatible with IV solution)
Syringe of appropriate size for medication volume
Sterile needle (if nurse is preparing medication from vial or ampule)
Gloves

Procedure
1. Check medication order. See Procedure 27-1, Steps 1 through 5.
2. If medication has not been prepared and labeled by pharmacy, the nurse prepares the medication. Draw up ordered medication from vial or ampule. Read package insert for proper amount and solution for dilution. Remove needle and dispose of it properly.
   Rationale: Needleless equipment is used for IV procedures to prevent accidental needlesticks and decrease risk of infection.
3. Identify the client by looking at nameband or asking name, and recheck five rights. Scan client's

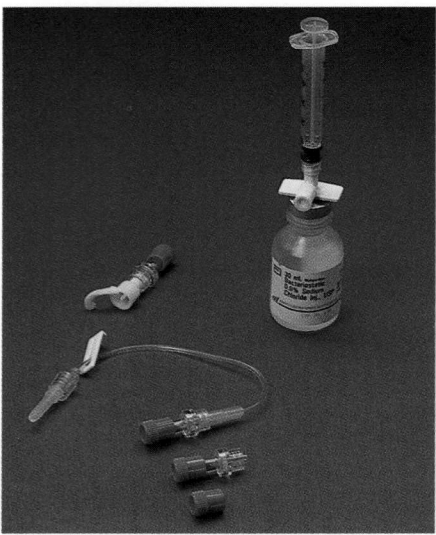

Step 2 Prepare ordered medication.

identification bracelet if using bar code medication administration.
   Rationale: Rechecking before administering the medication to the client prevents errors.
4. Explain procedure to the client.
   Rationale: Explanations allay client anxiety.
5. Don gloves.
   Rationale: Barriers such as gloves are necessary to comply with Standard Precautions.

Administering Medication Into an Existing Intravenous Line
1. Select injection port or "Y" site in IV tubing closest to the IV insertion site.
   Rationale: Minimizes dilution of the medication and increases transit of medication into client's vascular system. Close proximity to the insertion site also makes it easier to assess catheter placement by blood return.
2. Attach syringe to injection port.
3. Occlude the IV tubing above the injection port by pinching the tubing.
   Rationale: Prevents backflow of medication into primary IV tubing.
4. Inject the medication slowly into the IV port at the prescribed rate. Use a watch to time administration rate.
   Rationale: Timing ensures safe infusion of drug. Too rapid injection of some IV medications can be fatal.
5. If IV medication and IV solution in tubing are incompatible, flush line with normal saline solution while occluding catheter above port. Administer

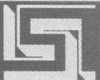

PROCEDURE 27-9 (Continued)

medication at prescribed rate; reflush with 10 mL of sterile normal saline solution, and release occlusion.
Rationale: Flushing before and after with normal saline keeps incompatible solutions from mixing.

Administering the Drug Into an Intermittent Infusion Device or Lock Device

1. Don gloves.
   Rationale: Maintains asepsis.
2. Attach syringe with 1 mL normal saline solution into injection port and flush. Remove syringe.
   Rationale: Flushing confirms patency of catheter, assesses for signs of infiltration or phlebitis at IV site.
3. Attach syringe with medication into injection port. Inject medication slowly at the prescribed rate. Use watch to time safe administration rate. Remove syringe.
   Rationale: Careful timing ensures safe medication infusion. Too rapid injection of some IV medications can be fatal.
4. Attach syringe with 1 to 3 mL of normal saline into injection port and flush the port with saline.
   Rationale: Maintains patency of the IV site.

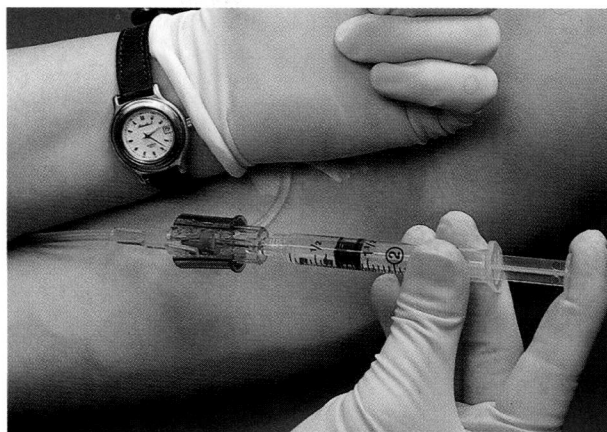

Step 3 Use a watch to time the slow injection of medication at the prescribed rate.

5. Dispose of used syringes properly and wash hands.
   Rationale: Maintains asepsis.
6. Document medication administration.
   Rationale: Accurate documentation is mandatory to prevent medication errors.
7. Evaluate the client's response to medication therapy.
   Rationale: Careful and timely assessment is necessary because medications given by IV bolus can have a rapid action.

Lifespan Considerations
Infant and Child
- Anticipate that medication dosages for infants and children are greatly reduced and based on their body weight.
- Cross-check computations of weight-based medications with another nurse to verify accuracy and decrease errors in administration.

Older Adult
- Medication doses for older adults may be decreased related to diminished renal and liver capacities to excrete and metabolize drugs.

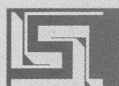

PROCEDURE 27-10

ADMINISTERING INTRAVENOUS MEDICATIONS USING INTERMITTENT INFUSION TECHNIQUE

Purpose
1. Maintain therapeutic levels of medication in client's blood.
2. Dilute irritating intravenous (IV) solutions.
3. Prevent complications associated with bolus administration by delivering medications over a longer period.
4. Prevent combining incompatible medications.

Assessment
- Review medication order and appropriate rate of infusion.
- Assess patency of existing IV line.
- Inspect insertion site for infiltration or phlebitis.
- Determine client's drug allergy status.
- Check for possible drug incompatibilities.

Procedure When Using Syringe Pump and Heparin Lock
Equipment
Medication administration record (MAR)
Medication prepared and labeled in a 20- to 60-mL syringe
IV syringe pump
Microbore extension tubing
Two sterile syringes with 1 to 3 mL normal saline solution each
Intravenous lock adaptor or cap

Procedure
1. Check medication order. See Procedure 27-1, Steps 1 through 5.
2. Prepare the medication syringe and IV tubing. Examine the syringe for any air bubbles and expel any that are present. Attach the syringe to the extension tubing, and gently push the syringe plunger to prime the tubing. Cover adaptor.
   *Rationale: Primed IV tubing prevents air bubble from entering client's vein. Guard on needle or cover on adaptor maintains the sterility of the system before connection to the primary intravenous line. (**Note:** Many types of needleless systems are available. Be sure to follow the manufacturer's instructions for use.)*

3. Secure the medication syringe into the pump with the flange of the syringe in the clamp's groove.
   Rationale: The syringe must fit snugly in the pump according to manufacturer's guidelines to function properly.
4. Confirm the client's identity by looking at the identification bracelet or asking his or her name. Scan the patient's bracelet if using bar code medication administration. Recheck the five rights and explain the procedure to the client.
   Rationale: Rechecking the five rights prevents potential errors.

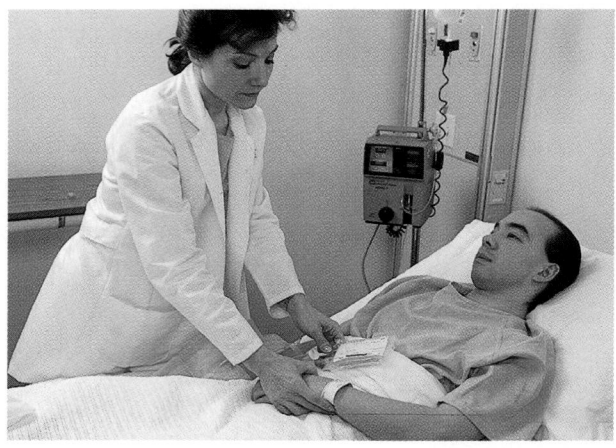

Step 4 Confirm client's identity verbally and by checking identification bracelet.

5. Don gloves.
   Rationale: Prevents spread of microorganisms and adheres to Standard Precautions.
6. Attach syringe with normal saline into the lock device. Flush lock with normal saline.
   Rationale: Confirms patency of IV catheter, assesses for signs of infiltration or phlebitis at IV site.
7. Attach tubing to lock device. Secure IV tubing to IV site with tape.
   Rationale: Prevents inadvertent dislodgement of the IV catheter.
8. Program the pump for the appropriate infusion speed and press the start key. The medication syringe label often indicates the suggested infusion speed, typically 30 to 60 minutes. If uncertain, consult a drug reference handbook or pharmacist.
   Rationale: Careful timing ensures safe medication infusion. Too rapid injection of some IV medication causes serious side effects.

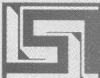

PROCEDURE 27-10 (Continued)

9. Document medication administration.
   Rationale: Proper documentation reduces the risk for medication errors.
10. Assess the client and infusion device 5 to 10 minutes after infusion has begun.
    Rationale: Assessment provides information about any adverse reactions to the medication and proper functioning of the infusion pump.
11. When the completion alarm sounds, return to client's room and press the pump's stop key.
12. Don gloves. Remove tubing from lock device. Attach syringe with 1 to 3 mL normal saline or heparin flush solution and flush lock.
    Rationale: Flushing the lock immediately after the IV infusion is complete ensures infusion of the entire dose of medication and ensures catheter patency.
13. Replace lock with new sterile cap.
    Rationale: Using a new cap maintains sterile system.
14. Dispose of syringes in proper container. Wash hands.

Variation Using IV Bag and Gravity IV Tubing
Equipment
Medication administration record (MAR)
Medication prepared and labeled in 50- to 250-mL IV bag
IV infusion tubing
Two sterile syringes with 1 to 3 mL normal saline solution each
Intravenous lock adaptor or cap

Procedure
1. Check medication order. See Procedure 27-1, Steps 1 through 5.
2. Connect IV tubing to medication bag. (See Procedure 28-2 in Chapter 28, Changing Intravenous Solution and Tubing.)
   Rationale: Primed IV tubing prevents air bubble from entering client's vein.
3. Follow Steps 4 through 7 above.
4. Set IV drip rate to infuse medication over prescribed time. Monitor periodically.
5. Document medication administration.
6. When medication has infused, turn off flow clamp.
7. Follow Steps 12 through 14 above.

Variation When Administering Intermittent IV Medication into Primary IV Line
Equipment
Medication administration record (MAR)
Medication prepared and labeled in a syringe or IV bag

IV syringe pump and microbore extension tubing *or* gravity IV tubing
20-mL syringe of sterile normal saline flush solution (*Optional*—used only if medication is incompatible with primary infusing IV solution to flush IV line of incompatible primary solution both before and after medication is infused)

Procedure
1. Check medication order. See Procedure 27-1, Steps 1 through 5.
2. Prepare medication, tubing, and pump, if used, according to procedures described earlier.
3. Confirm client's identity and check five rights again.
   Rationale: Decreases potential medication errors.
4. Hang syringe pump or medication bag at or above level of primary IV solution. Insert secondary line into the adaptor port. *Note: Some infusion sets include backcheck valves that stop primary IV solution flow while medication infuses, then automatically open when medication infusion stops. When using these devices, the primary bag is hung lower, as illustrated here.*

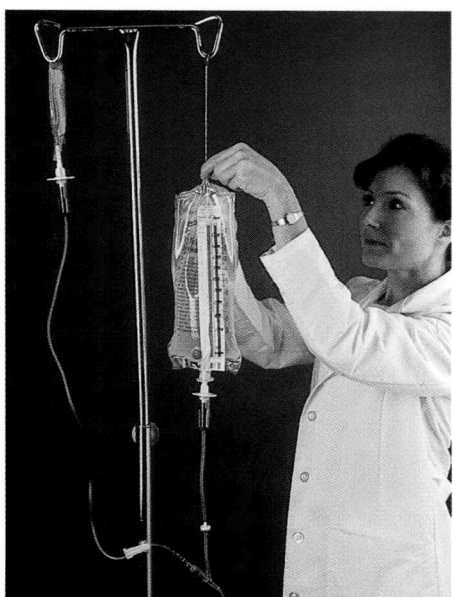

Step 4 Hang primary bag lower during IV piggyback administration when backcheck valve system is used.

5. Check compatibility of medications to be administered with the IV solution being infused and any other infusing medications. If medication is not compatible with primary IV solution, clamp

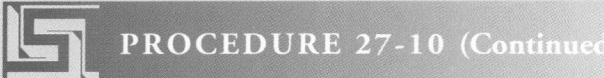

PROCEDURE 27-10 (Continued)

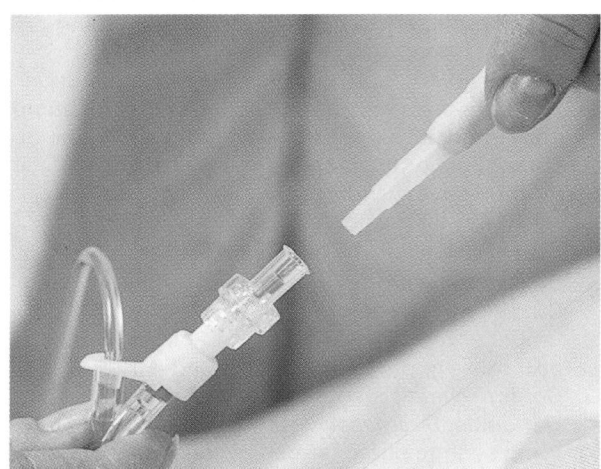

Step 4 Insert secondary tubing into adaptor.

primary IV tubing above injection port, attach syringe with 20-mL of normal saline flush solution, and flush IV line.
Rationale: Flushing prevents reactions and precipitation of incompatible solutions.

6. Connect secondary (piggyback) line to injection port or "Y" site on IV tubing closest to IV insertion site.

7. Start syringe pump or set drip rate.
8. When medication has infused, stop syringe pump or turn off flow clamp. Flush IV line with saline as needed. Regulate primary infusion as necessary.
Rationale: Medication infusion may alter flow rate of primary solution. Flushing after the infusion may be necessary to prevent medication and primary IV solution incompatibility.
9. Discard medication syringe or bag and tubing (or reserve for next medication infusion) according to agency guidelines.
10. Wash hands.
Rationale: Handwashing maintains asepsis.
11. Document medication administration and add IV volume to IV intake.
Rationale: Proper documentation maintains accurate client records and reduces the risk for medication errors.

Lifespan Considerations
Infant and Child
- Know that infants receive much smaller volumes of fluid than adults.
- Infuse intravenous medications through a volume-control IV unit to avoid potentially serious fluid overload.

also encompasses the methods of measuring the dosage (e.g., syringe, dropper), the dosage schedule in relation to feedings, and what to do if the child spits up the medication. If an infant spits up a volume of medication that looks like the total dose within 5 to 10 minutes after receiving it, the medication is usually repeated.

Toddler and Preschooler

Physical changes during the toddler and preschool years also have implications for medication administration. Oral medications are still given in liquid form, or, if necessary, tablets are crushed and mixed with food. Children younger than 3 years of age have straighter, stiffer external auditory canals than older children and adults do. Therefore, when administering eardrops to this age group, pull the pinna of the ear down and back before dropping the medication into the ear canal.

Many young children fear injections, so give them as promptly as possible to avoid escalating anxiety and fear. Often, children must be carefully immobilized, usually by another person, to ensure safety during the procedure. EMLA cream, a cream containing a mixture of local anesthetics, can be applied to the skin 1 hour before painful procedures such as IV insertions. The area of application is covered with clear plastic. EMLA cream is helpful only when painful procedures can be anticipated.

Children in these age groups are beginning to explore their world and learn about themselves and their environment. Accidental medication poisoning is a particular risk. Urge parents to store all medications in a protected area out of children's reach and make sure that medications are packaged in containers with childproof caps. Make sure that children are aware that medications are not candy. Also, instruct caregivers to have the telephone number of a Poison Control Center readily

THERAPEUTIC DIALOGUE
Medication Administration

Scene for Thought
As the nurse brings Mr. Abramson, age 58, his cardiac pills, he turns his attention from the television on the wall to her.

Less Effective

Client: Kirsten, I don't want those pills. I told the doctor I don't need them. They give me headaches, and I don't want them.
Nurse: *(Stops in surprise just inside the room. Sits in chair next to client.)* You sure seem upset about this. Tell me what happened.
Client: I just get headaches from them, that's all. And she said I'd have to take them for the rest of my life! I can't live with headaches for the rest of my life. *(Looks angry and powerless.)*
Nurse: I can tell this bothers you a lot. Do you have a headache now?
Client: No, but after I take that little white pill, I always do.
Nurse: Which pill is it? I don't seem to have one to give you right now. *(Shows him the three capsules in the cup, two blue and one white with a yellow stripe.)*
Client: *(Looks in confusion.)* It isn't there. Maybe she changed it already.
Nurse: I think that's what happened. There was a medication order change this morning after she made rounds, and the pharmacy just sent these new blue capsules for you. Do you feel better about it now? *(Pours fresh water into a glass so he can take the medication.)*
Client: Sure, sure. At least I won't have those headaches. *(Looks somewhat relieved, but still skeptical.)*
Nurse: Yes. I'm glad we got that straightened out! Call me if you need me. *(Goes out to finish giving meds.)*

More Effective

Client: Christine, I don't want those pills. I told the doctor I don't need them. They give me headaches, and I don't want them.
Nurse: *(Stops in surprise just inside the room. Sits in chair next to client.)* You seem upset about this. Tell me what happened.
Client: I just get headaches from them, that's all. And she said I'd have to take them for the rest of my life! I can't live with headaches for the rest of my life. *(Looks angry and powerless.)*
Nurse: I can tell this bothers you a lot. Did you mention the reason you don't want this medication to your physician?
Client: Yes. She said she'd change it. *(Sounds irritated.)*
Nurse: Let me check for you. *(Checks the med order physician wrote that morning. The medication has been changed.)* Well, she did change it, Mr. Abramson. This is the new medication she ordered. *(Shows him the capsule.)*
Client: *(Takes it reluctantly.)* How do I know this won't affect me the same way?
Nurse: I would like to come back and give you some information about it after I've given out the other medications on the unit. Would that help?
Client: Yes, indeed. *(Looks relieved but still a little skeptical.)*
Nurse: And maybe we can talk about your concerns that you'll have to take it for the rest of your life. That sounds like a separate issue but still important. Have I read that right?
Client: I think so, Christine. I'll think about that while you're gone. *(Gives a small smile, almost sheepish.)*

Critical Thinking Challenge
- In both dialogues, the client received the correct medication. Detect what the client didn't receive in the first dialogue.
- Explain what concerned Christine about Mr. Abramson's remark about having to take the medication for the rest of his life.

---

available and syrup of ipecac on hand in case accidental ingestion of medications occurs.

Explain procedures in simple terms, appropriate to a child's experiences and level of understanding. Reassure children that the medication is not a punishment. Whenever possible, allow children to make choices about therapy (e.g., which arm to use for the IV, which fluid to drink with the oral medication).

Effective teaching materials for toddlers and preschoolers include texts fashioned like coloring books and dolls or puppets. Dolls and puppets can be used to demonstrate a procedure, and, if necessary, children can return the demonstration on the doll.

School-Age Child and Adolescent

As children mature and develop, nurses can direct more teaching and responsibility for medication administration toward them. Most school-age children can swallow tablets and cap-

sules. To increase compliance, the dosage schedule should avoid school hours whenever possible. When medication administration is necessary during school hours, most schools require that medications be deposited with the school nurse in the original prescription container.

Many school-age children still fear injections and worry about crying or losing control when injections are administered. Although these children understand the importance of remaining still during injections, sudden movement may occur as the needle pierces the skin. Support of the extremity and judicious positioning help ensure safety during the injection. By the time children have reached school age, all injection sites may be used, because all muscles have adequately developed.

Teaching during the adolescent years should emphasize the importance of not taking any prescription medication that has not been ordered specifically for the person. Nurses need to explore possible use of illegal drugs or alcohol with adolescents.

Adult and Older Adult

As adults age, the need for more medications to treat chronic health problems may become a reality. Compliance with complex medication schedules can be difficult, especially for those older people who have cognitive deficits. Most adults can swallow tablets, but neurologic problems may interfere with swallowing.

Physical conditions (e.g., cachexia, obesity) may influence which IM sites are chosen for adults. Cachectic adults may retain muscle mass in the ventrogluteal site longer than in other IM sites. The least desirable IM site for obese adults is the dorsogluteal site, where a thick fat layer often causes the medication to be deposited in the SC tissue.

Visual deficits may make reading drug information and prescription labels difficult. Decreased fine motor skill and tactile sensation may increase the difficulty of administering eyedrops or injections such as insulin.

Older people are at increased risk for drug toxicity because of altered renal excretion and hepatic metabolism of drugs. Decreased circulation can affect absorption of ingested drugs. Watch older adults very carefully for drug toxicity, especially if renal or hepatic disease is present.

Drug misuse can occur when adults save medications for future use. Older people may share their prescription drugs with friends who complain of similar symptoms. Older clients on a fixed income may find that the expense of many medications stresses an already limited budget. Although these problems can occur among all age groups, they are more common among older adults because of their increasing dependence on medications to improve health and functioning.

KEY CONCEPTS

- Medication administration is a significant nursing responsibility that requires solid understanding of pharmacologic principles, assessment skills, and ability to individualize client teaching.
- A drug is a substance that alters physiologic function. A medication is a drug that is administered for its therapeutic effects.
- Medications can be identified by three different names: chemical name, generic name, and brand name.
- Drug references are available to provide healthcare professionals with specific information on each medication. Nurses are responsible to use drug reference resources for knowledge about each drug they administer.
- Medication distribution systems include the stock supply system, unit-dose system, automated medication-dispensing system, self-administered medication, and BCMA.
- A medication order must include the client's name, the date of the order, the medication's name, the dose, the frequency, the route of administration, and the prescriber's signature.
- Types of medication orders include standing orders, prn orders, one-time orders, stat orders, and telephone and verbal orders. It is the nurse's responsibility to interpret accurately and carry out safely the prescriber's orders.
- Federal legislation controls the way medications are manufactured, marketed, and controlled. The nurse must practice within the state's nurse practice act and the agency's policies and procedures concerning medication administration.
- To ensure client safety, the nurse must follow the "five rights" (the right drug, in the right dose, at the right time, by the right route, to the right client) whenever a medication is administered.
- Drug activity is the result of chemical interactions between a medication and the cells of the body, which produce a biologic or physiologic response. This response can be altered by drug absorption, distribution, metabolism, or excretion.
- Therapeutic effects are the desired effects obtained from medication administration. Adverse effects are any effects other than therapeutic effects and may include side effects, toxicity, tolerance, hypersensitivity reaction, and allergic reaction. Interactions with other drugs or food also can occur.
- Nursing assessments are done to obtain baseline information concerning a client's medications, before any administration of medications, and to individualize client teaching concerning medications.
- Many forms of medications, such as tablets, capsules, syrups, and elixirs, are appropriate for oral administration. Oral medications may be swallowed, administered through gastric or intestinal tubes, or given by the sublingual or buccal route.
- Topical medications include those that are applied to the skin or inserted in a body cavity. Solutions, creams, lotions, ointments, and transdermal patches are applied to the skin. Topical medications can be administered into the eye, ear, nose, rectum, or vagina.
- Parenteral medications are given by injection or infusion into ID tissue, SC tissue, IM tissue, or the venous or arterial circulation.
- Sites commonly used for IM injections include the deltoid, ventrogluteal, vastus lateralis, rectus femoris, and dorsogluteal muscles. Anatomic landmarks must be used to identify each site properly.
- IV medications enter the venous circulation by IV push, intermittent infusion, or continuous drip. The client may self-deliver IV medications by using a PCA device.
- Changes occurring during the lifespan are important to consider when administering medications and may necessitate adjustments in the techniques for administration.

REFERENCES

American Diabetes Association. (2001). Insulin administration. *Diabetes Care, 24*[Suppl 1], S94–S97.

Arquiza, E. E. (2001, February 5). Bar codes aren't just for supermarkets. *Nursing Spectrum: Career Fitness Online.* Available at: www.nursingspectrum.com/MagazineArticles. Accessed 1/14/02.

Bloch, A. B. (September 8, 1995; updated November 17, 1998). Screening for tuberculosis and tuberculosis infection in high risk populations: Recommendations of the Advisory Council for the Elimination of Tuberculosis. *MMWR Morbidity and Mortality Weekly Report, 44*(RR-11), 18–34.

Borins, M. (1999). What to tell your patients about herbs. *Hospital Medicine, 8,* 27–32, 53–54.

Cleveland, L., Aschenbrenner, D., Venable, S., & Yensen, J. (1999). *Nursing management in drug therapy.* Philadelphia: Lippincott Williams & Wilkins.

Decker, G. M., & Myers, J. (2001). Commonly used herbs: Implications for clinical practice. *Clinical Journal of Oncology Nursing, 5*(2), 13.

Fleming, D. R. (1999). Challenging traditional insulin injection practices. *American Journal of Nursing, 99*(2), 72–74.

Gever, M. P. (1998). Transdermal patches: What's in a brand name? *Nursing, 27*(5), 58–59.

Godfrey, K. (1998). Diabetes: Syringes and pens. *Community Nurse, 4*(8), 25–26.

Institute of Medicine, Committee on Quality of Health Care in America. (1999). *To err is human: Building a safer health system.* Washington, DC: National Academy Press.

Koncik-McMahan, J. (1996). Full speed ahead—with caution: Pushing intravenous medications. *Nursing, 26*(6), 26–32.

National League for Nursing. (1993). *A vision for nursing education.* New York, NY: NLN Press.

Styrcula, L. (2000, December 11). VA barcoding system reduces medication errors. *Nursing Spectrum: Career Fitness Online.* Available at: www.nursingspectrum.com/MagazineArticles. Accessed 1/14/02.

Teich, J. M., Merchia, P. R., Schmiz, J. L., et al. (2000). Effects of computerized physician order entry on prescribing practices. *Archives of Internal Medicine, 160,* 2741–2747.

Waldo, B. H. (1999). Preventing adverse drug reactions through automation. *Nursing Economics, 17*(5), 276–279.

BIBLIOGRAPHY

Abrams, A. (2001). *Clinical drug therapy: Rationale for nursing practice* (6th ed.). Philadelphia: Lippincott Williams & Wilkins.

Arquiza, E. E. (2001, February 5). Bar codes aren't just for supermarkets. *Nursing Spectrum: Career Fitness Online.* Available at: www.nursingspectrum.com. Accessed 1/14/02.

Ashby, D. A. (1997). Medication calculation skills of the medical-surgical nurse. *Medical-Surgical Nursing, 6*(2), 90–94.

Brumley, C. (2000). Herbs and the perioperative patient. *AORN Journal, 72*(5), 783, 785–6, 788–794.

Covington, T. P., & Trattler, M. R. (1997). Bull's-eye! Finding the right target for I.M. injections. *Nursing, 26*(1), 62–63.

Curtin, L., & Simpson, R. L. (2001). Making the leap to avoid medication errors. *Health Management Technology, 22*(1), 28.

Edwards, J. (1997). Guarding against adverse drug events. *American Journal of Nursing, 97*(5), 26–31.

Eggland, E. T. (1997). Documenting discharge teaching. *Nursing, 26*(3), 26.

Fiesta, J. (1998). Legal aspects of medication administration. *Nursing Management, 29*(1), 22–23.

Hadaway, L. C. (2001). How to safeguard delivery of high-alert I.V. drugs. *Nursing, 31*(2), 36–41.

Johnson, C., & Horton, S. (2001). Owning up to error: Put an end to the blame game. *Nursing 2001, 31*(6), 54–55.

Lehne, R. (2001). *Pharmacology for nursing care* (4th ed.). Philadelphia: Lippincott Williams & Wilkins.

McConnell, E. A. (1998). Admixing drugs in a syringe. *Nursing, 27*(5), 20.

McConnell, E. A. (1998). How to choose and use needle-stick prevention devices. *Nursing, 27*(5), 32hn6–32hn8.

Miller, D., & Miller H. (2000). To crush or not to crush? *Nursing, 30*(2), 50–52.

Power, L. (1999). Boning up on IV push. *The Canadian Nurse, 95*(10), 36–39.

Styrcula, L. (2000, December 11). VA bar coding system reduces medication errors. *Nursing Spectrum: Career Fitness Online.* Available at: www.nursingspectrum.com. Accessed 1/14/02.

Waddell, D. L., Hummel, M. E., & Summers, A. D. (2001). Three herbs you should get to know. *American Journal of Nursing, 101*(4), 48–54.

Ward-Collins, D. (1998). "Noncompliant": Isn't there a better way to say it? *American Journal of Nursing, 98*(5), 27–32.

28 Intravenous Therapy

Key Terms

air embolism
central venous catheter
colloid
crystalloid
cycling
electronic infusion device
  (EID)
hemolysis
hemolytic transfusion
  reaction
hypertonic
hypotonic
infiltration

intravenous therapy
isotonic
needleless systems adapters
osmolarity
parenteral nutrition
peripherally inserted central
  catheter (PICC)
phlebitis
positional IV
thrombophlebitis
total parenteral nutrition
transfusion
venipuncture

Learning Objectives

Upon completion of this chapter, the student will be able to do the following:
1. Explain the purpose of intravenous infusion therapy.
2. Identify the two major types of solutions administered intravenously.
3. List equipment necessary to administer peripheral and central intravenous therapy.
4. State guidelines for site selection in venipuncture.
5. Outline the nurse's role in initiating, monitoring, maintaining, and discontinuing intravenous therapy.
6. Describe potential complications of intravenous therapy, total parenteral nutrition, and blood transfusions.
7. Identify principles of client and family education associated with intravenous therapy.

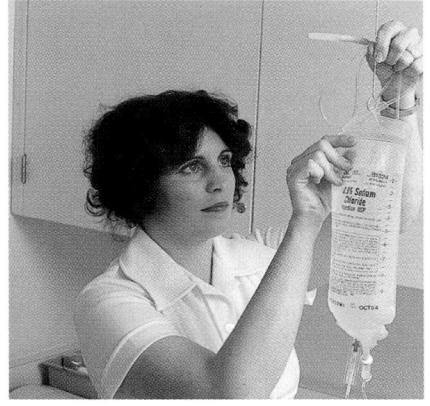

Critical Thinking Challenge

You are assigned to care for an older man who is receiving intravenous (IV) therapy. The solution is isotonic saline (0.9% saline) and is being administered through a microdrip system. While counting the drops per minute, you notice that it is dripping slower than ordered and that opening the flow clamp does not increase the rate. You must decide what to do.

Once you have completed this chapter and have incorporated IV therapy into your knowledge base, review the above scenario and reflect on the following areas of Critical Thinking:

1. Describe further assessment data you will collect.
2. List the factors to check in the infusion system, giving rationales.
3. Identify other information you would want to know about this client's IV therapy.
4. Outline possible problems that may exist in this situation.
5. Given your answers to the above, indicate how you will proceed.

Clients in a variety of healthcare settings receive intravenous therapies. **Intravenous (IV) therapy** is the infusion of a fluid into a vein to prevent or to treat fluid or electrolyte imbalance or to deliver medications, nutrition, or blood products. The therapeutic goal may be maintenance, replacement, treatment, diagnosis, monitoring, palliation, or a combination. Intravenous therapy may be prescribed for many reasons including provision of the following:

- Maintenance or replacement fluids for daily body fluid requirements
- Electrolytes to maintain normal electrolyte balance
- Glucose and nutrients for client use as an energy source
- An access route to administer medications intravenously
- Venous access to administer blood products
- Venous access for emergencies.

IV therapy may be administered in outpatient settings, acute and long-term care facilities, and in client's homes.

Venipuncture is the technique that permits insertion of a needle or catheter into a vein. Because skin is broken, venipuncture must be a sterile procedure. In most facilities, nurses are responsible for starting IV therapy. In some agencies, a special IV team is responsible for all IV starts; in some cases, this team also oversees general IV maintenance. Usually the IV team is composed of nurses with specialized training and extensive experience with venipuncture. In facilities that do not employ IV teams, nurses usually are certified in venipuncture technique by the institution.

The most common method of accessing the venous system is through percutaneous insertion of a needle or flexible catheter into a peripheral vein (vein in the extremities). The peripheral veins usually provide the quickest and easiest approach to establishing IV access for administration of solutions and medications. This process differs from central venous therapy, which involves placement of a flexible catheter into one of the client's large veins, with the tip of the catheter placed in either the superior vena cava or the right atrium. Central venous therapy may be required when infusing hypertonic solutions or when the client's peripheral venous access is inadequate for the duration or type of IV therapy required.

INTRAVENOUS THERAPY

Types of Intravenous Solutions

IV solutions are classified as **crystalloid** (fluids that are clear) or **colloid** (fluids that contain proteins or starch molecules). Crystalloids can be further classified as isotonic, hypotonic, or hypertonic according to how closely the solution's osmolarity matches that of plasma, which is between 275 and 295 mOsm/L. **Osmolarity** refers to the number of particles or amount of substance that is in a liter of solutions. Therefore, osmolarity is measured in milliosmoles per liter (mOsm/L). Specific client fluid and electrolyte needs will determine which solution is prescribed.

Crystalloid Solutions

Due to the permeability of cellular membranes, water will move across membranes based on the osmolarity within the body's three fluid compartments. Figure 28-1 presents an artist's conception of the relationship of osmotic pressure to isotonic, hypotonic, and hypertonic solutions.

Isotonic Fluids. **Isotonic** fluids have an osmolarity of 250–375 mOsm/L, which is the same osmotic pressure as that found within the cell. Isotonic fluids are used to expand the intravascular compartment and thus increase circulating volume. Because these solutions do not alter serum osmolarity, interstitial and intracellular compartments remain unchanged (Josephson, 1999). An isotonic solution would be helpful for hypotension caused by hypovolemia. Examples of an isotonic solution include normal saline (0.9% NaCl) and lactated Ringer's.

Hypotonic Fluids. **Hypotonic** fluids have an osmolarity below 250 mOsm/L, or a lower osmotic pressure than the cell. When a hypotonic solution is infused, it lowers serum osmolarity, causing body fluids to shift out of the blood vessels and into the cells and interstitial space. For this reason, hypotonic fluids are administered when a client needs cellular hydration. One-half normal saline (0.45 NaCl) is an example of a hypotonic solution. Five percent dextrose in water, although an isotonic solution before administration, quickly becomes a hypotonic solution once in the body, because the dextrose is quickly metabolized, leaving only the water.

Hypertonic Fluids. **Hypertonic** fluids have an osmolarity of 375 mOsm/L or higher and a greater osmotic pressure than the cell. When a hypertonic solution is infused, it raises serum osmolarity, pulling fluid from the cells and the interstitial tissues into the vascular space. Examples of hypertonic solutions include 3% saline (NaCl) and 5% saline (NaCl). These solutions should be administered slowly to prevent circulatory overload and are rarely used clinically (Kuhn, 1999). Table 28-1 presents nursing considerations relative to the osmolarity of intravenous solutions.

Colloid Solutions

Infusion of a colloid solution increases intravascular osmotic pressure (pressure of plasma protein). Colloid solutions remain within the intravascular space, and the pressure gradient pulls fluids into the vascular space.

Blood Products. Whole blood or specific components of blood may be infused directly into a person's circulatory system. Blood components include packed red cells, white blood cells, platelets, plasma, albumin (as a volume expander), and cryoprecipitate (a clotting factor). Nursing responsibilities associated with transfusion therapy are discussed in greater detail later in this chapter.

Parenteral Nutrition. **Parenteral nutrition** refers to nutritional elements supplied through an IV route, usually a central vein. **Total parenteral nutrition** (TPN) is a hypertonic solution containing 20% to 50% dextrose, proteins, vitamins,

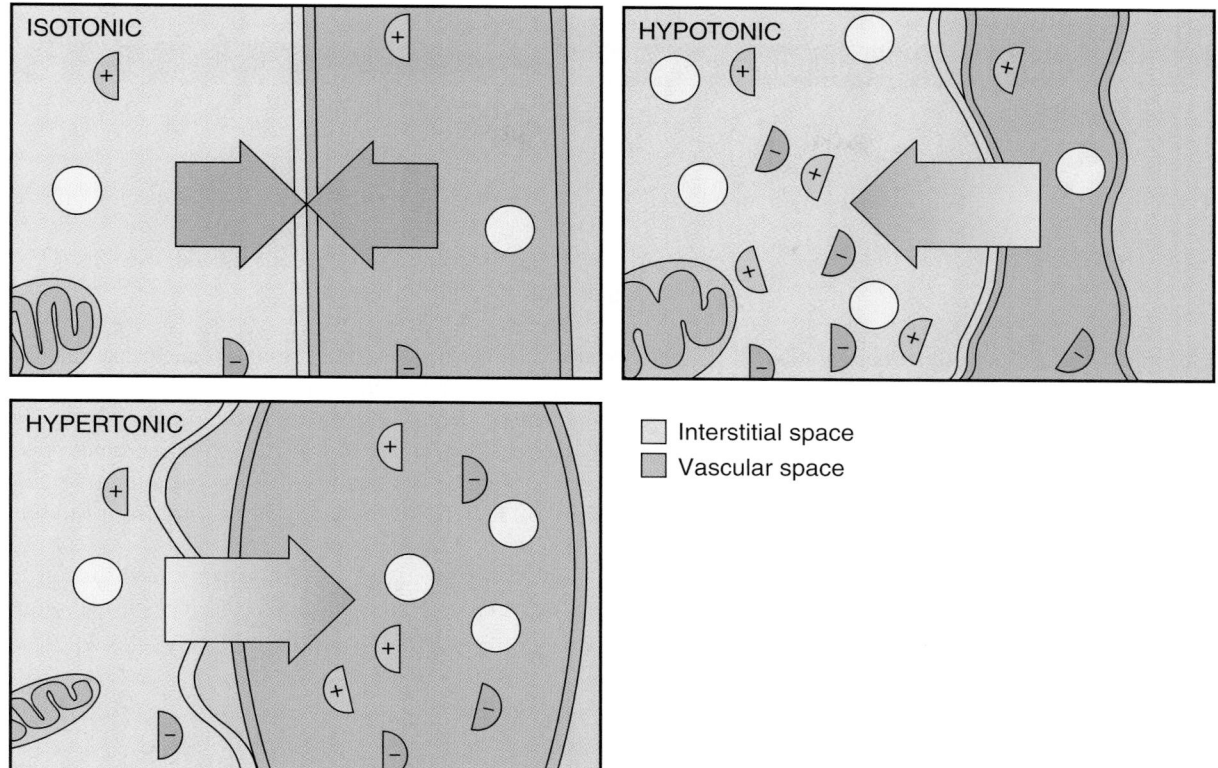

FIGURE 28-1   Isotonic, hypotonic, and hypertonic solutions. In isotonic fluids, cells maintain normal size because of fluid balance. In hypotonic solutions, the body fluids shift out of the blood vessels and into cells and the interstitial space. In hypertonic solutions, the fluid is pulled from the cells and the interstitial tissues into the vascular space.

and minerals that is administered into the venous system. TPN is indicated when there is interference with nutrient absorption from the gastrointestinal tract or when complete bowel rest is necessary for healing. Parenteral nutrition is discussed later in this chapter.

Equipment for Intravenous Infusion

A variety of equipment is available to meet the IV therapeutic needs of diverse clients. Brands may vary slightly among different manufacturers. However, most IV setups contain the following:

- An access device that gains entry to a vein
- A plastic or glass container with the IV solution
- An administration set that connects the IV bag with the access device
- Needleless system accessories for administration sets
- Electronic infusion devices

Sterility of IV equipment must be maintained during use to prevent potentially life-threatening infection.

Venous Access Devices
Peripheral Insertion Devices. Winged infusion needles and over-the-needle IV catheters are among access devices most commonly used for peripheral IV therapy. Winged infusion

needles are short, beveled needles with plastic flaps or wings. They may be used for short-term therapy or when therapy is given to a child or infant. Winged infusion needles also are referred to as small vein needles. Over-the-needle catheters are plastic catheters that are placed over metal stylets or introducer needles (Fig. 28-2). The metal stylet is used to pierce the skin and enter the vein, then the plastic catheter is threaded into the vein, and the metal stylet is removed.

Both the winged infusion needle and the over-the-needle catheter come in a variety of sizes. The lumen size is measured in gauges; odd numbers designate winged infusion needles (19, 21, 23), whereas even numbers designate catheter sizes. The most common adult catheter sizes are 22, 20, and 18. As the numbers increase, the lumen size decreases; thus a 22-gauge needle is smaller in diameter than an 18-gauge needle. A variety of catheter lengths are also available. Usually the shortest length possible is used. Most catheters are 1 or $1\frac{1}{4}$ inches long. The small vein needles are approximately $\frac{3}{4}$ inch long and range in diameter from 16- to 27-gauge bore.

Intermittent Infusion Devices. Intermittent infusion devices are available as winged needle sets or as over-the-needle catheters; each has an attached latex cap adaptor (Fig. 28-3). These are used when the client is to receive solutions or medications intermittently. The devices are irrigated with a small

TABLE 28-1

Nursing Considerations in Administering IV Solutions		
Solution Type and Examples	**Indications**	**Nursing Considerations**
Isotonic Normal saline Lactated Ringer's	Intravascular dehydration	Monitor closely for signs of fluid overload, especially if client has a history of cardiovascular disease. Avoid use of lactated Ringer's in clients with liver disease or those in metabolic alkalosis.
Hypotonic 0.45% Saline	Cellular dehydration	Monitor regularly because these solutions can cause a sudden shift of fluid into the cells. This can lead to intravascular fluid depletion and cardiovascular collapse. Don't give to clients at risk for increased intracranial pressure (ICP)—(head trauma, neurosurgery, cerebrovascular accident). Increased ICP can result from shift of fluid into brain cells. Don't give to clients at risk for abnormal fluid shifts into the interstitial compartment (third spacing) or abdominal cavity (burn victims, trauma, liver failure, severe protein malnutrition). Rarely used clinically
Hypertonic 3% NaCl	Intravascular dehydration with interstitial and intracellular fluid overload	Closely monitor client for fluid overload because these solutions expand the intravascular compartment. Avoid use in clients with renal or cardiac impairment. Avoid use in clients with intracellular dehydration such as diabetic ketoacidosis. Hypertonic solutions draw fluid from intracellular to the intravascular compartments.

quantity (1–3 mL) of sterile saline to prevent blood clot formation. Previously, intermittent infusion devices were irrigated with heparinized normal saline; thus they can be referred to as heparin locks. Nursing research demonstrated that flushing with positive pressure, not the dilute heparin solution, kept the device patent. With an adaptor, any type of peripheral venipuncture device can be converted to an intermittent infusion device. Intermittent infusion devices maintain venous access without requiring the client to receive continuous infusion, thus minimizing danger of fluid overload.

Central Venous Access Devices. Access to central veins is often necessary for infusion of concentrated medications and TPN, when peripheral vein access is not available or when long-term venous therapy is anticipated. When central access is necessary, a wide assortment of products may be used to facilitate cannulation of the central vein. Physicians usually insert central venous catheters. However, nurses with advance training may insert some types. Central venous access devices are associated with a high risk of complications such as pneumothorax and air embolism because the tip lies in the superior vena cava or right atrium. The risk of catheter-related infection is high in clients with central venous devices. This is thought to be related to a fibrin sheath developing

along the catheter's inner lumen (Schmid, 2000). Recent advances in the development of catheters impregnated with bacteriocidal chemicals show reduced risk of catheter related infections (Mermel, 2001).

Multilumen Central Catheters. The most frequently used **central venous catheter** includes either the basic single-lumen catheter or the multilumen catheter, which are either double or triple lumen and made of nonthrombogenic Silastic materials. Some catheters are coated with antimicrobial agents to decrease the risk of infection. Because the catheter tip is placed in the superior vena cava or at the entrance of the right atrium, central venous catheters also allow the nurse to monitor central venous pressure in specialized client populations. The multilumen catheter's obvious advantage is that multiple drugs can be administered simultaneously without the risk of incompatibility of solutions. Due to the risk of complications, the multilumen non-tunneled catheters are only used in the hospitalized client population. If a client's condition necessitates long-term IV therapy, numerous additional options are available.

Tunneled Central Venous Catheters. When IV therapy is needed for a long time, a more permanent type of catheter can be used. Hickman, Groshong, and Broviac are common brand names of these catheters. The catheters, which may be single-

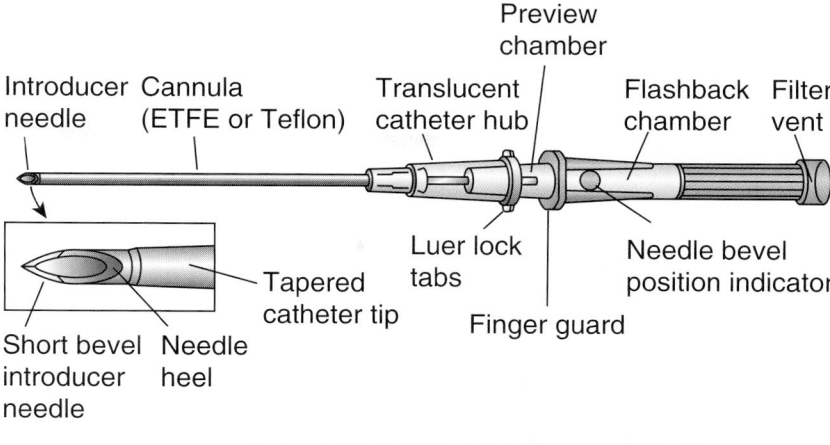

Introducer needle
Cannula (ETFE or Teflon)
Translucent catheter hub
Preview chamber
Flashback chamber
Filter vent
Tapered catheter tip
Short bevel introducer needle
Needle heel
Luer lock tabs
Finger guard
Needle bevel position indicator

A

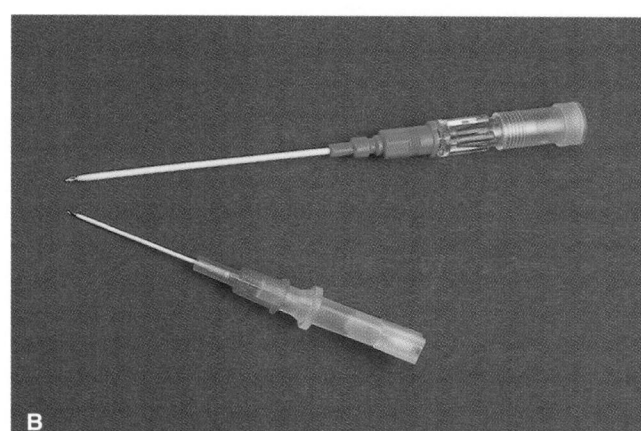

B

FIGURE 28-2 (A) Parts of the over-the-needle catheter. (B) Over-the-needle catheter.

or multilumen, are approximately 90 cm in length and contain a Dacron cuff (Fig. 28-4).

The catheter is implanted by surgical procedure through an incision made in the deltopectoral groove and by isolating the subclavian vein. A subcutaneous pathway or tunnel is gently formed with a long forceps to a point between the nipple and the sternum. Thus the term *tunneled catheter*. The Dacron cuff is positioned between the skin incision and the vein. The catheter is threaded into the lower part of the vena cava at the entrance to the right atrium. Dressings placed at both incision sites require simple cleaning, application of an antimicrobial agent, and a sterile occlusive dressing. The catheter is taped to the person's chest to lessen tension and tugging. Eventually, fibrous tissue grows around the Dacron cuff, which stabilizes the catheter in place, decreases infection rates, and permits use as a long-term venous access route (Fig. 28-5).

Tunneled catheters may be used for months, even years, for continuous or intermittent therapy. Intermittent therapy

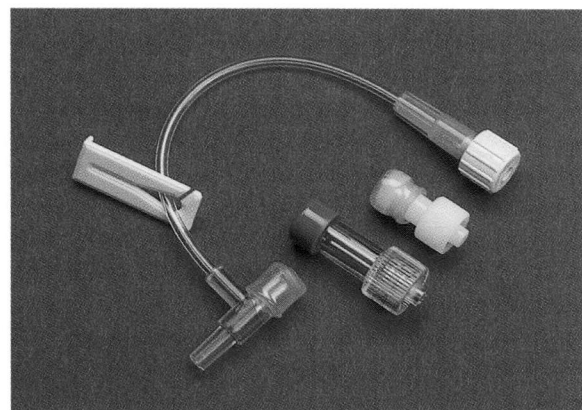

FIGURE 28-3 Adapters used to convert indwelling IV catheters or infusion sets to intermittent infusion devices.

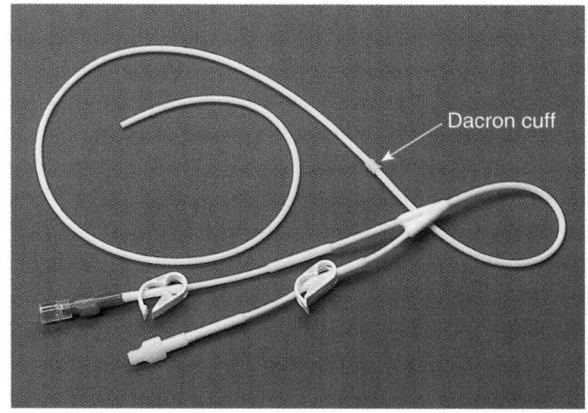

Dacron cuff

FIGURE 28-4 Double lumen Hickman catheter showing the two ports and clamps.

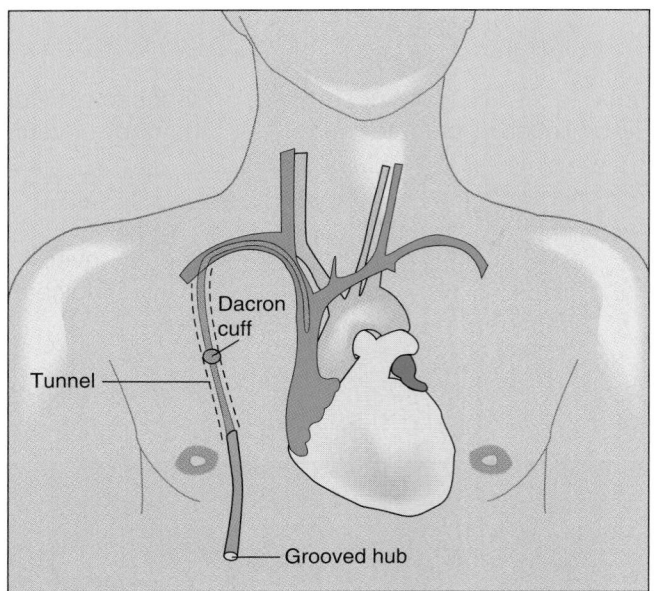

FIGURE 28-5   Insertion technique of indwelling tunneled catheter. A tunnel is formed from the vein to an area between the sternum and the nipple. The catheter tip is placed in the superior vena cava.

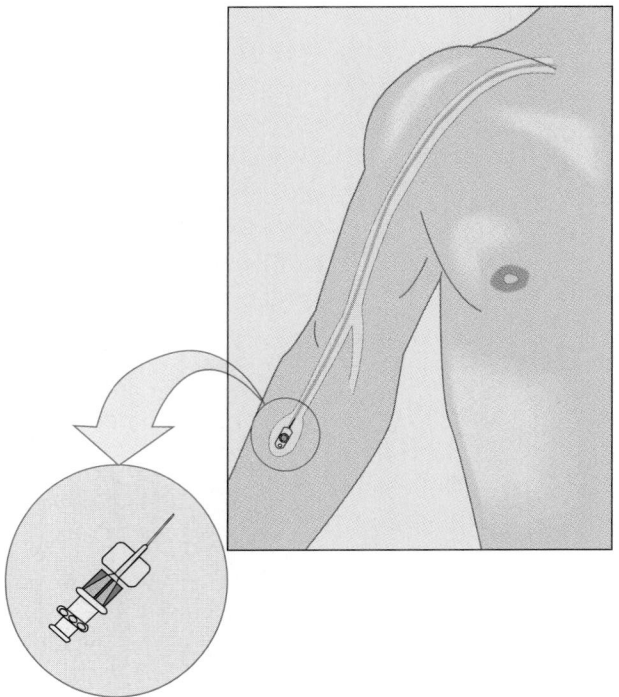

FIGURE 28-6   PICC access device.

requires the catheter to be fitted with an intermittent infusion device to allow access as needed and to keep the system otherwise closed and intact. Catheter patency is maintained with periodic heparin flushing. Because of its unique design, the Groshong catheter requires irrigation with normal saline rather than heparin.

Peripherally Inserted Central Catheters. **Peripherally inserted central catheters** (PICCs) are long-line catheters made of soft silicone or Silastic material; they are placed peripherally but deliver medications and solutions centrally (Fig. 28-6). The basilic vein is usually used, but the median cubital and cephalic veins in the antecubital area can be used also. PICC lines are threaded so the catheter tip may terminate in either the axillary or subclavian vein or the superior vena cava. A nurse specially trained in PICC insertion will insert the catheter and usually will anchor the line with sutures. A radiograph confirms correct placement of the catheter tip.

PICC lines are used for clients who require intermediate to long-term venous access. Because PICC lines can be left in place for several months, they are very useful for home as well as acute care. PICC lines have a small diameter, which makes them ideal for use in the very young and the elderly. The catheter flexibility does not restrict arm movement or normal activity; these lines also carry fewer risks of pneumothorax, air embolism, and sepsis than are associated with other central lines. Clients and their caregivers require instructions on the care and maintenance of the PICC as well as information about potential complications and appropriate interventions should complications occur.

Implanted Vascular Access Devices. Totally implantable access devices have been developed to allow long-term access without having a catheter protrude from the skin (Fig. 28-7). The system includes the subcutaneous injection port and a Silastic catheter, which is usually inserted into the superior vena cava. The device has a self-sealing septum or port, which allows repeated use without the risk of air entering the system.

With the client under local anesthetic, the system is surgically implanted and sutured into a subcutaneous pocket (see Fig. 28-7A). When venous access is desired, the location of the injection port must be palpated. The system is then accessed with a noncoring needle such as a Huber point needle (see Fig. 28-7B). As with other central venous systems, patency is maintained by periodic flushing with a diluted heparin solution.

Solution Containers

Containers for IV fluid include glass bottles and plastic bags, as shown in Figure 28-8. Plastic bags have become the industry standard unless a particular infusate is unstable in plastic. Plastic bags collapse as they empty and therefore require no vent to equalize pressure. However, the plastic bag's semirigid nature makes it difficult for healthcare personnel to accurately measure the amount of remaining fluid. Another disadvantage of plastic bags is that certain drugs (e.g., insulin) bind with the plastic; this makes IV administration of these drugs in plastic bags difficult.

Bottles and bags come in a variety of sizes. Usually 1,000 mL containers are used for routine hydration purposes. Smaller bags (e.g., 250–500 mL) may be used for children or when fluid is infusing at a very slow rate. Smaller quantity containers (50, 100, or 250 mL) also are used to dilute and dispense medications.

OUTCOME-BASED TEACHING PLAN

Mr. Tambuli is being discharged home after treatment for a serious bone infection. He requires IV antibiotic therapy for 4 more weeks. Mr. Tambuli has a peripherally inserted central catheter (PICC) line in place. He and his wife will be caring for the PICC line and administering the antibiotics through it at home.

OUTCOME: Before discharge, Mr. Tambuli and his wife can demonstrate safe care and flushing of the PICC line.
Strategies
- Assess Mr. and Mrs. Tambuli's readiness to learn, cognitive ability, and psychomotor dexterity.
- Provide the Tambulis with a pamphlet about PICC line care, using the illustrations to explain where the catheter is placed and why it is important to use strict asepsis and prevent any air from entering the system.
- Ask them to read the pamphlet together then review it with them.
- Arrange for a time with the Tambulis for demonstration on how to flush the catheter using aseptic technique.
- Verbally list the steps as they are completed. Provide them with a written list of steps to review. Allow them time to practice with additional equipment.
- Have both Mr. and Mrs. Tambuli demonstrate the flushing procedure repeatedly until they voice comfort and confidence with the procedure.
- Positively reinforce behaviors; answer questions and provide feedback as necessary.

OUTCOME: Before discharge, Mr. Tambuli and his wife will demonstrate safe administration of antibiotics through the PICC catheter.
Strategies
- Review their knowledge of the PICC catheter.
- Discuss the antibiotic ordered, how it is to be prepared, and frequency of IV administration.

- Develop a schedule for administration based on their usual daily routine.
- When administering Mr. Tambuli's IV antibiotic, verbally list the steps as you complete them.
- Provide a written list of information about the medication and the procedure of administering it IV through a PICC line. Allow them time to practice with equipment.
- Ask Mr. and Mrs. Tambuli to describe the procedure with administration of next dose.
- Have both Mr. and Mrs. Tambuli demonstrate administration of the IV antibiotic until they can voice comfort and confidence with the procedure.
- Give positive feedback and repeat instructions as necessary.

OUTCOME: Mr. and Mrs. Tambuli can verbalize when to call for help and how to contact the IV home management company should the need arise.
Strategies
- Provide Mr. and Mrs. Tambuli with the number of the IV home management agency that will be working with them after discharge and with the name of the nurse who will manage their care. (*Note:* Often this nurse does the IV teaching while the client is still in the hospital.)
- Review the signs and symptoms of possible complications that may occur.
- Provide written guidelines for complications that require notification of this nurse (inability to flush the line, redness or pain at the site, signs of infection).
- Provide the Tambulis with some hypothetical problems that might occur and ask them to discuss what they would do.
- Ask if the Tambulis have any questions, and encourage them to call if they have any questions or concerns.

Administration Sets

An IV administration set is tubing that connects the IV bag or bottle to the access device. Parts of the administration set are shown in Figure 28-9. Normally an IV administration set includes the following features:

- A piercing pin or spike to permit the tubing to access the IV container
- A slide clamp to stop fluid flow and a roller clamp to manually regulate the flow rate
- An inline filter to trap any particles and prevent entry into the client's bloodstream
- A drip chamber to allow the nurse to visualize and count the drops of IV fluid as they enter the system

- Injection sites or ports to permit the administration of medications, blood products, or other IV therapies
- A connector at the end of the tubing for connecting the tubing to the needle or cannula. Although the connectors have a variety of designs (slip tip or Luer Lok), the dimensions are standard and fit all needle and cannula hubs.

In addition to these features, individual manufacturers produce tubing that delivers a different number of drops per milliliter of fluid based on the size of the drop (called the drop factor). Two general classifications of tubing are macrodrip and microdrip (or minidrip; Fig. 28-10). Macrodrip tubing delivers 10, 15, or 20 drops/mL, depending on the manufacturer.

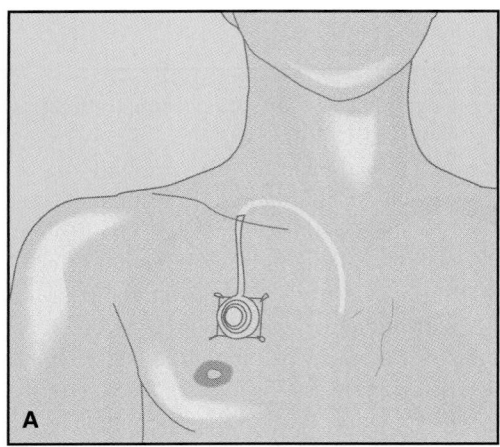
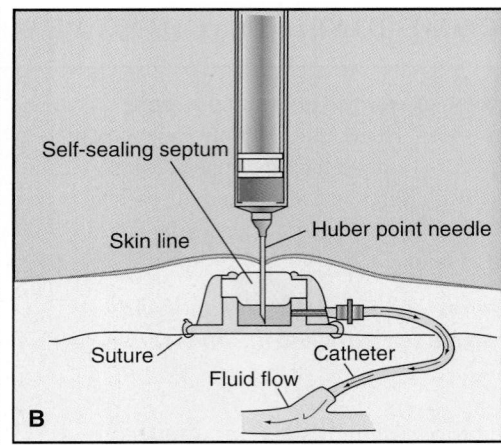

FIGURE 28-7   Implantable access system. (**A**) Placement of the implantable system beneath the skin. (**B**) Access to the system with a noncoring needle.

Macrodrip tubing is generally used for adult clients, especially when large volume replacement may be required (e.g., during surgery). Microdrip tubing delivers 60 drops/mL and is used for infants, children, or when fluids are infused slowly.

Specialized administration sets also are available. Volume-controlled sets, such as Buretrol or Soluset, may be used to provide greater accuracy and safety in controlling fluid volume (Fig. 28-11). For an unvented bottle system, there is tubing available that provides an air vent in the drip chamber to equalize pressure and provide easy fluid flow from the bottle to the client. Also available are a variety of electronic infusion devices (EID; discussed later in the chapter) with tubing and cassettes unique to the particular equipment brand. Additionally, programmable syringe pumps are useful for precise administration of small dose, high potency medications at rates of 0.01–99.9 ml/hr. (Phillips, 2001). These pumps are useful alone or piggybacked to a continuous infusion.

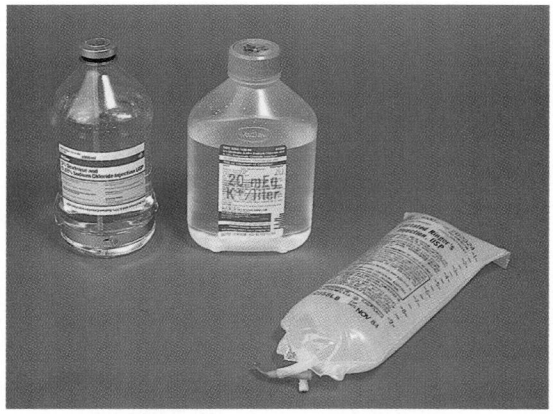

FIGURE 28-8   Examples of solution containers.

Needleless System Accessories

A variety of **needleless access adapters** are available to help protect the healthcare provider from accidental needlesticks during IV procedures (Fig. 28-12). These systems consist of adapters that connect easily to a standard syringe or IV tubing. Some adapters contain an antireflux valve that opens in response to either infusion or aspiration pressures. The antireflux valve is designed to reduce the risk of "backflow of blood" and air embolism. Many manufacturers make these products: Some are set-specific and require the use of a manufacturer's products; others are universal. Any add-on device should be of a Leur Lok–type configuration; add-on devices also require the healthcare staff to use aseptic technique.

Intravenous Flow Rates

Calculating Flow Rate

Calculating flow rate is the first step in ensuring the proper infusion of IV fluids. After the administration set is selected or known, the infusion drip rate can be calculated from the physician's order using the following formula:

$$\text{Drops/min} = \frac{\text{Total volume infused}}{\text{minute}} \times \text{drop factor}$$

The drop factor, which can be found on the administration set packaging, represents the size of the drop that the administration set creates. This factor may change with different manufacturers, because macrodrip tubing can deliver 10, 15, or 20 drops/mL. To calculate the drip rate of an IV that is to infuse 1000 mL in 8 hours using tubing that has a drop factor of 10, the nurse would use the previous formula, obtaining a rate of 21 drops/min.

This is calculated as follows:

$$\text{Drops/min} = \frac{1000 \times 10}{8 \text{ hr} \times 60} = \frac{10,000}{480} = 21 \text{ drops/min}$$

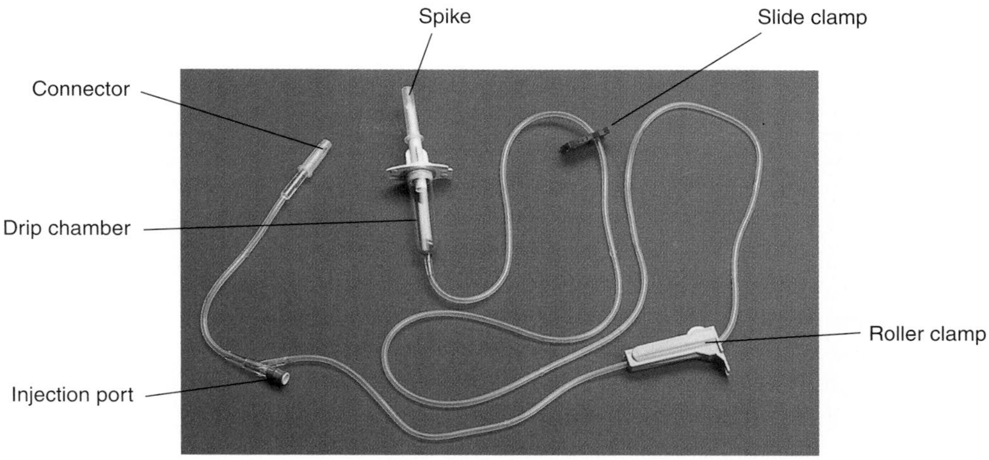

Spike · Slide clamp · Connector · Drip chamber · Roller clamp · Injection port

FIGURE 28-9 Administration set. (Courtesy of Abbott Laboratories, North Chicago, IL.)

Regulating Flow Rate

Manual Regulation of an IV Rate. Once the IV drip rate has been calculated, the infusion can be regulated manually. A roller clamp adjusts the flow rate according to drops per minute counted in the drip chamber. Count the drops as they fall into the drip chamber for 15 seconds, then multiply this number by 4 to determine the rate of flow for 1 full minute. Use the roller clamp to adjust the flow rate until it corresponds with the prescribed rate of flow.

A time strip, which can be made from adhesive tape or purchased commercially, also can help ensure accurate infusion of IV fluids. An example of an IV time tape is illustrated in Figure 28-13. The time strip is placed along the IV bag or bottle next to the calibrated numbers that indicate the volume remaining in the container. The strip is marked in hourly increments, indicating where the fluid level will be at specific times. This device permits the nurse to assess at a glance when the IV is getting behind or ahead of schedule. Monitor IV infusions every hour to ensure proper infusion of fluid.

Factors Affecting Flow Rate

Height of the Solution Container. Height of the IV bag or bottle can affect the rate of infusion. As the height of the container from the infusion site is increased, the gravitational force will be greater, thus the fluid will flow faster. Conversely, as the distance between the bottle and IV site decreases, the fluid will infuse more slowly. This often occurs when the client gets up and walks in the hall, pushing his or her IV pole with the hand into which the IV is flowing. In such a case, the drip rate slows and often stops altogether. Blood may flow back into the tubing. Frequent assessment and readjustment of the regulating clamp will ensure proper infusion rate.

Position of the Extremity. When the extremity is elevated, the fluid will infuse more slowly. Bending the extremity at a

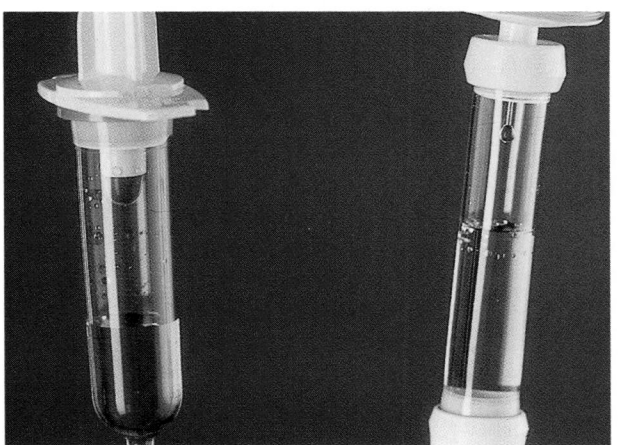

FIGURE 28-10 Drip chambers for macrodrip and microdrip IV tubing.

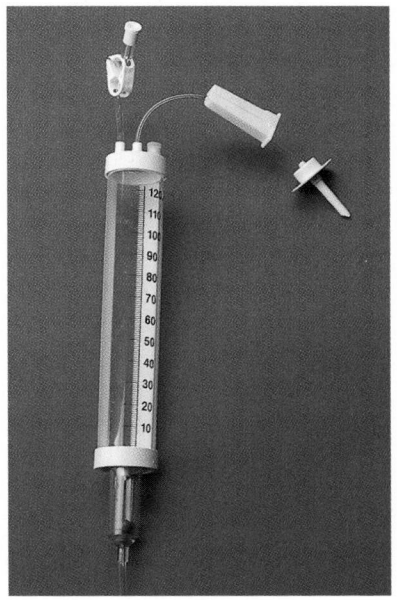

FIGURE 28-11 Volume-controlled set.

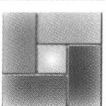

Nursing Research and Critical Thinking
How Often Should IV Administration Sets Be Changed?

Nurses caring for clients with cancer wanted to know how often to change the IV administration sets. In many settings, the IV administration sets of neutropenic clients with cancer are changed daily. But the nurses found that no study had been done of the variables associated with higher rates of infusate colonization within a neutropenic cancer client population. The nurses designed a randomized clinical trial with repeated measures to examine the effects of changing IV administration sets at 48 versus 24 hours on rate of infusion-related septicemia in neutropenic clients with cancer. Fifty subjects for the study were recruited at a large urban cancer center. Twenty-five subjects were included in each of two groups: Group A with IV administration sets changed every 24 hours; Group B with IV administration sets changed every 48 hours. A table of random numbers was used to assign subjects to one of the two treatment groups. The researchers examined 413 administration sets during the study. The study results showed that subjects with colonized IV sets were equally distributed between the two groups. Changing IV administration sets at 48 hours did not result in colo-

nization rates significantly different than the rate of colonization occurring in IV administration sets changed every 24 hours. Within-subject variability or differences in colonization rates among the five measurements used to evaluate risks of infection were not statistically significant.

Critical Thinking Considerations. Although the sample size (N = 50) for this study was small and determining the risk of infusion therapy involves multiple variables, the researchers were able to make several recommendations that are applicable to nursing practice:

- Infusion-related septicemia is not only possible, but probable, given the frequency with which IV therapy is indicated and IV sets manipulated.
- With no obvious benefit from changing IV administration sets every 24 hours, the cost of this practice in terms of client comfort, nursing hours, and physical resources warrants reconsideration.
- Changing administration sets every 48 hours rather than every 24 hours is recommended.

From deMoissac, D., & Jensen, L. (1998). Changing IV administration sets: Is 48 versus 24 hours safe for neutropenic patients with cancer? *Oncology Nursing Forum, 25*(5), 907–913.

point of flexion, such as the wrist or the elbow, or leaning on the arm can slow the rate of infusion. Caution the client not to raise her or his arm over the head and not to sleep on the side where the IV is infusing.

Tubing Obstruction. Constriction or kinking of IV tubing also can contribute to altered flow rates. Tubing can become kinked if inadvertently placed under the client. Tubing also can be obstructed if tape is applied too tightly or if edema develops when the tape interferes with venous blood return in the extremity.

Position of the IV Access. The position of the needle or catheter within the vein can affect the rate of flow. Position changes can cause the needle bevel or catheter to rest against a vein wall. This is known as a **positional IV.**

🔲 SAFETY ALERT
Take extra care to monitor an IV that appears to be positional. When the IV slows down, adjust the rate. Remember, though, that if the client moves again and the bevel becomes free of the vein wall, the infusion rate will increase again. Use an armboard to help immobilize the joint and decrease the chance of needle movement.

IV Patency. Catheter patency is important to ensure proper infusion of fluids. Whenever fluid flow is interrupted for any reason (e.g., bending at a joint, kinking of tubing), a blood clot can form at the end of the catheter, stopping the infusion. If the clot does not completely obstruct the lumen of the catheter, the flow rate may slow and become sluggish.

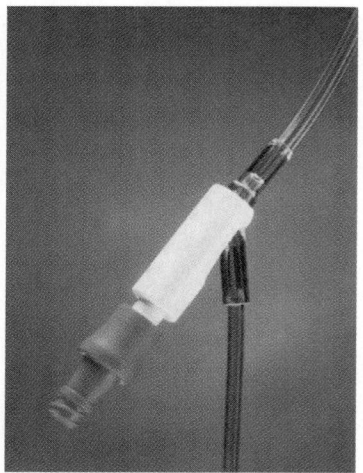

FIGURE 28-12   Needleless system.

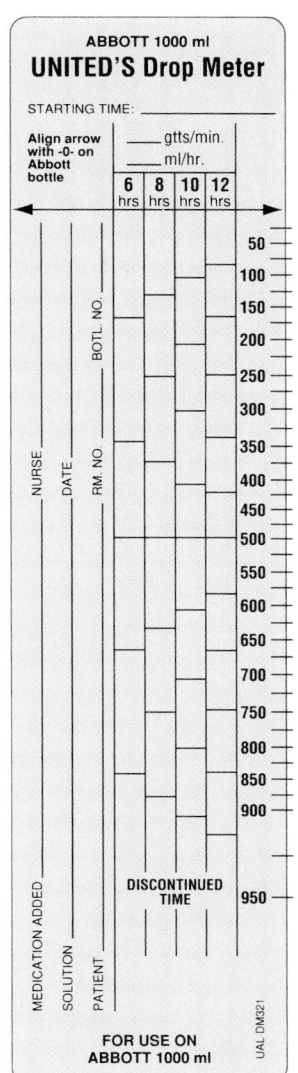

ABBOTT 1000 ml
UNITED'S Drop Meter

STARTING TIME: _____

Align arrow
with -0- on
Abbott
bottle

| | ____ gtts/min. |
| | ____ ml/hr. |

| 6 hrs | 8 hrs | 10 hrs | 12 hrs |

NURSE   DATE   BOTL. NO.   RM. NO.

50
100
150
200
250
300
350
400
450
500
550
600
650
700
750
800
850
900

DISCONTINUED TIME   950

MEDICATION ADDED   SOLUTION   PATIENT

UAL DM321

FOR USE ON
ABBOTT 1000 ml

FIGURE 28-13   Sample time tape.

This is often a problem when IVs are infusing very slowly to keep the vein open (TKO [to keep open] or KVO [keep vein open]). When a KVO rate is ordered, intermittently increase the flow rate to flush the catheter and prevent clot formation. If the flow has stopped completely, gently aspirate the catheter.

SAFETY ALERT
Never irrigate the catheter if you meet pressure when attempting to flush, because irrigation pushes the clot into the circulatory system.

Clogged Air Vents. If the air vent on a solution bottle or volume control chamber becomes clogged or wet, fluid cannot leave the system because air is unable to enter to replace it. Changing the tubing may be necessary to correct this problem.

APPLY YOUR KNOWLEDGE

Your surgical client has an IV order for 3000 cc 5%D/NS every 24 hours.

- Calculate the infusion rate for an IV controller to be programmed using cc/h.
- Calculate the drip rate using a gravity infusion with a drop factor of 20 drops per cc.
- Calculate the drip rate for a gravity infusion with a microdrip (60 drops per cc) tubing using a simplified formula.

Check your answers in Appendix A.

Electronic Regulation of IV Rate. An IV **electronic infusion device** (EID) is useful to regulate the infusion rate accurately, especially if fluid administration must be watched very carefully such as when infusing fluid to an infant or administering certain medications. The Intravenous Nurse's Society (INS) standards state that EIDs should be used when warranted by the client's age, condition, setting, and prescribed therapy (Intravenous Nursing Society [INS], 2000). Various types of EIDs are available commercially. In general, the EID pump uses positive pressure to deliver the prescribed fluid volume, whereas the controller uses gravity to maintain a precise flow rate (Fig. 28-14).

SAFETY ALERT
Because many different types and models of EIDs are used, be knowledgeable about specific operating guidelines for the machine you are using. Always review the instructions for use that are permanently affixed to the particular EID. Never turn off the alarm until the underlying problem has been discovered and resolved.

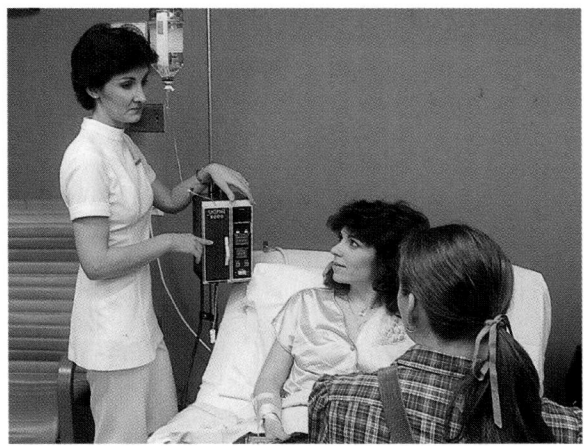

FIGURE 28-14   The nurse teaches the client about the electronic infusion device (EID).

The pump regulates the flow by volume, whereas the controller senses the drops infusing. Most new models of pumps and controllers can be electronically programmed. The healthcare provider enters the amount of fluid (e.g., 1,000 mL) and the rate of infusion in milliliters (or ccs; 1 cc 5 1 mL) per hour. The instrument displays how many milliliters have infused and how much fluid in ccs remains in the IV container at any given time.

Electronic regulating devices also have alarms that indicate when fluid cannot be delivered at the prescribed rate for any reason (e.g., the container is empty; the tubing is kinked; air is in the line; the vein is occluded). Regulating pumps do not replace diligent nursing assessment of the IV system. The nurse is still responsible for identifying the cause of any problems and making corrections to ensure proper fluid infusion. Because there are many EIDs on the market, refer to the manufacturer's guidelines for setting up and troubleshooting each device.

ROLE OF THE NURSE IN INTRAVENOUS THERAPY

Nurses are responsible for initiating, monitoring, maintaining, and discontinuing the IV infusion and for client teaching related to the infusion. Although many clients who receive IV fluids are admitted to healthcare facilities, it is increasingly common for clients to receive IV fluids at home or in special ambulatory or short-stay settings. The physician orders the type and amount of IV fluid and electrolyte replacement. Components of an IV order include the following:

- Type and amount of solution
- Other medications or electrolytes to be added to the solution
- Length of time for infusion to be given or infusion rate

Initiating Intravenous Therapy

IV therapy requires an order from a licensed physician. The nurse is responsible for checking the order to determine its correctness (e.g., the volume of solution to be infused, the rate of flow per hour, any additives to the solution). When the solution has been prepared consistent with the physician's order, the nurse gathers all needed equipment and prepares the client for venipuncture.

Preparing the Client
Teaching the client about why the therapy is ordered and what is expected including any positioning limitations, such as don't bend your right arm or sleep on that side, is a major component of client preparation. Continuous nursing supervision is available during IV therapy in the hospital or nursing home setting, but the client at home requires in-depth instruction and support from a home health nurse.

Before the procedure, the nurse makes sure that the curtains are drawn for privacy. The nurse may also ask visitors to leave the treatment room. Position the client comfortably with the arm on a flat surface.

Selecting the Site
Assessment of the client's history, diagnosis, activity level, vein condition, therapy type, and duration are all important to consider when determining the IV placement site. In the adult, the veins of the hand and forearm are commonly used for IV infusion (Fig. 28-15). When the basilic or cephalic vein is used, the ulna and radius act as natural splints, allowing the client greater freedom of movement. Whenever possible, larger veins are used and the distal portion of the vein is punctured first, leaving the more proximal sites for later venipunctures (INS, 2000). Avoid veins located directly over movable joints because their use increases the possibility that the IV will dislodge and infiltrate or that the client will develop phlebitis. Also avoid veins of the lower extremities whenever possible because they limit mobility and increase the incidence of thrombophlebitis.

Various techniques are helpful to locate and visualize veins before venipuncture. First, determine the type and duration of therapy and visually inspect the client's veins, avoiding any areas that appear bruised or sclerosed. Place a tourniquet on the extremity 4 to 6 inches above the intended venipuncture site to distend the vein with blood. This will make the vein more visible. Additionally, lower the extremity below the level of the heart, ask the client to open and close his or her fist several times, tap lightly over the selected vein, or use warm soaks for 5 minutes before venipuncture to vasodilate the selected vessel. All these techniques may help fill the vein with blood.

Preparing the Site
Adequate site preparation is necessary to avoid infection. Clip any hair around the site as necessary. Avoid shaving because small microscopic nicks or abrasions can provide entry for microorganisms. Prepare the site using a vigorous circular motion with 70% alcohol as a defatting agent; work from the center outward to a diameter of 2 to 3 inches; follow with an application of povidone-iodine (INS, 2000). Allow the solutions to air dry. Although povidone-iodine is a better bactericide, some people are sensitive to this preparation and may have an allergic response. If the client is allergic to iodine, prepare the site with 70% alcohol with friction for at least 30 seconds.

Performing the Venipuncture
Assemble all equipment before attempting venipuncture. Cut tape and have all equipment within reach. Wear gloves as in any invasive procedure. Stretch the skin taut over the intended venipuncture site with the thumb and index finger. With the bevel up, hold the needle to enter the skin at a 45-degree angle. As the skin is pierced, decrease the angle of the needle to 30 degrees. This will permit entry into the vein at an angle and decrease the likelihood of accidentally puncturing a vein. Watch for a blood return that indicates placement in the vein. When using an IV catheter, thread the plastic catheter into the vein, usually after the needle and cannula have been inserted $\frac{1}{2}$ inch. Then remove the stylet while the catheter is fully inserted within the lumen of the vessel. When placement of the needle or catheter in the vein is ensured, attach the tubing and release the tourniquet.

THERAPEUTIC DIALOGUE
Intravenous Therapy

Scene for Thought

The evening nurse enters the room of Delores Davis, a 65-year-old social worker with a wide smile who has an IV in her left arm. She greets the nurse warmly as she assesses the IV site, drip rate, and IV pump function.

Less Effective

Client: Hi there. How are you this evening? *(Big smile.)*

Nurse: Just fine, Ms. Davis. How are you this evening? *(Gently palpates the area around the IV site.)*

Client: Don't touch that, please. *(Winces and pulls back.)*

Nurse: *(Stands still; hand moves to rest on client's hand gently.)* Is the IV bothering you?

Client: Well, yes, it is, actually. *(Her face now looks worried, her eyes searching the nurse's.)*

Nurse: Let me check everything out now. *(Thoroughly examines the site, pump, drip rate, tubing.)* I can untangle this tubing a bit for you, but I don't see anything else wrong. Tell you what, I'll be back later on this evening to check on it again, and, if something is wrong, we'll fix it. Okay? *(Pats her hand reassuringly and smiles as she leaves.)*

Client: Okay, I guess. *(Face has no expression except for two frown lines between her eyes.)*

More Effective

Client: Hi there. How are you this evening? *(Big smile.)*

Nurse: Just fine, Ms. Davis. How are you this evening? *(Gently palpates the area around the IV site.)*

Client: Don't touch that, please. *(Winces and pulls back.)*

Nurse: *(Stands still; moves hand to rest on client's hand gently.)* Is the IV bothering you?

Client: Well, yes, it is, actually. *(Her face now looks worried, her eyes searching the nurse's.)*

Nurse: Tell me a little more.

Client: It started this evening after supper. I'm afraid I pulled on it when I was reaching for my tea. The other nurse put the tray where I couldn't reach it, and I didn't want to bother her, so I just reached for it, and then the skin felt a little sore there. Did I do something wrong? *(Face is still worried.)*

Nurse: Well, let's see what the area is like. *(Talks to Ms. Davis while examining.)* I don't see any redness or swelling where the needle enters your skin, the pump seems to be functioning fine, and the fluid is dripping at just the right rate. I think everything is working properly. One thing I can do is untangle the tubing a little so you'll have more room to move. How's that?

Client: *(Looks more relieved.)* Better. I'm pleased to hear that I didn't do any damage. I've never had one of these before. *(Smiles but not as widely as before.)*

Nurse: Sound like you're still a little worried about it. Anything I can help with?

Client: No, I'm fine. But could you come back and check again later? It would put my mind at ease.

Nurse: I'd be delighted. I was going to suggest that myself. By the way, it isn't a bother to set your tray up more comfortably for you. Please ask next time. We're here to make you feel better, not to make you struggle!

Client: Thank you so much. I appreciate it. *(Big smile).*

Critical Thinking Challenge

- Analyze how the second nurse reassured Ms. Davis.
- Explain how you can tell from behavior that a person is reassured.
- Determine when reassurance becomes patronizing.
- Assess what was missing between the nurse and client in the first dialogue.

SAFETY ALERT

When performing venipuncture, observe standard precautions to limit exposure to bloodborne pathogens, especially hepatitis B and human immunodeficiency virus (HIV). Be sure your hepatitis B vaccinations are current. To avoid needlestick injuries, dispose of needles in appropriate biohazard containers and make no attempt to recap needles.

Securing the Venipuncture Device

Tape the cannula flush with the skin with ½-inch wide tape. Place another strip of tape under the hub, adhesive side up. Secure one end tightly and diagonally over the cannula and repeat with the other end. Repeat this with the other end of the tape crossing the first. This secures the cannula and prevents sideways movement. Then loop the tubing and anchor it with tape. Apply a transparent dressing over the infusion site.

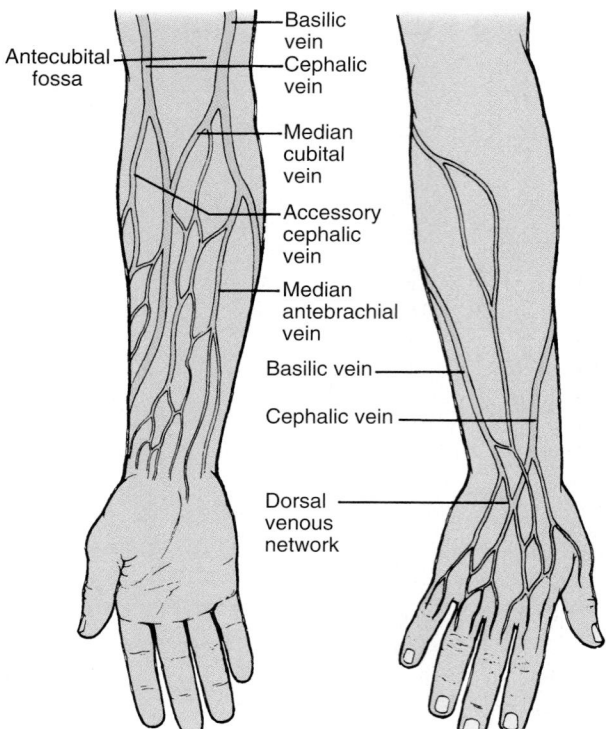

Basilic
vein

Cephalic
vein

Antecubital
fossa

Median
cubital
vein

Accessory
cephalic
vein

Median
antebrachial
vein

Basilic vein

Cephalic vein

Dorsal
venous
network

FIGURE 28-15 Adult IV insertion sites.

Use an armboard to help immobilize the extremity when motion can lead to infiltration or phlebitis. Armboards are useful when clients are uncooperative or disoriented, are children, or when the cannula is inserted in the dorsum of the hand. When using an armboard, be careful to position it properly to ensure adequate hand functioning.

Maintaining Intravenous Infusions

The nurse is responsible for maintaining and monitoring IV infusions to ensure that the fluid infuses at the proper rate and that complications of IV therapy are detected promptly. The steps in monitoring the IV infusion are outlined in Procedure 28-1.

Monitoring and Documentation

The client's condition, type of access device, practice setting, and agency protocols all determine the frequency of monitoring an IV device.

🔲 SAFETY ALERT

In an acute care, clinic, or long-term care facility, evaluate the client's IV at least once each hour. If the client is a child, perform this assessment more frequently.

Document pertinent assessment data including condition of the IV site, infusion rate, vital signs, intake/output data, and the client's response to therapy.

In the home setting, clients and their caregivers are instructed to monitor the IV site for redness, swelling, and patency. If problems are noted, a home healthcare nurse should be notified.

Dressing Changes

Institutional and agency policies specify expectations for site care, in accordance with the Nursing Standards of Practice defined by the INS. The site should be visually inspected and palpated for tenderness daily. If tenderness, fever without obvious source, or symptoms of local or bloodstream infection are present, remove the dressing and inspect the site directly. Gauze dressing should be changed every 48 hours on peripheral sites or whenever the integrity of the dressing is compromised (INS, 2000). Apply the dressing aseptically and securely tape all edges of the dressing. Transparent, semipermeable membrane (TSM) dressings allow continuous inspection of the site, are more comfortable than gauze, and allow the client to shower without saturating the dressing. TSM dressings are, however, more expensive. TSM dressings should be changed every 48 to 72 hours, depending on the standard of practice within the institution (Phillips, 2001). TSM dressings on central catheters should be changed at least every 3 days or sooner if the integrity has been compromised. Whenever performing site care, take extra care not to dislodge the catheter.

Changing Intravenous Bottles and Tubing

The nurse is responsible for changing the IV bag or bottle as needed and changing IV tubing according to institutional or agency policy. The IV bag or bottle is changed when the previous container is empty, when there is a change in IV orders, or when the IV container has been hanging for more than 24 hours.

All IV bag and tubing changes must be done under strict aseptic technique to prevent infection. Most facilities have policies that indicate the frequency and protocol for these procedures. Procedure 28-2 outlines changing IV solution and tubing.

Intermittent Flushing of an Intravenous Lock

An existing IV catheter may be converted to an intermittent infusion device by using a "plug" (Procedure 28-3). Peripheral intermittent lines are usually flushed with saline before and after each medication administration and every 8 hours when medications are not being given. Intermittent injection caps or ports may also be used to plug an unused line of a multilumen central line catheter. Most central line catheters are flushed with a heparinized saline solution. The quantity and type of flush solution instilled depend on the manufacturer's recommendation.

Assessing for Complications

Monitoring the client for possible complications of IV therapy is an important nursing responsibility. The most significant complications of IV therapy include infiltration, phlebitis,

(text continues on page 594)

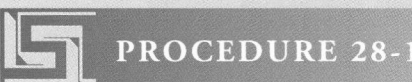

PROCEDURE 28-1

MONITORING AN INTRAVENOUS INFUSION

Purpose
1. Provide a safe, patent route for infusion of IV therapy.
2. Ensure correct infusion of IV fluids.
3. Detect IV complications promptly.

Assessment
- Review client's chart for diagnosis and medical plan for IV therapy.
- Assess client for clinical signs of fluid or electrolyte imbalances.
- Check physician's order for type of IV solution, additives, and infusion rate.
- Calculate hourly infusion rate or drops/min or cc/hr when an EID is used.

Equipment
May need:
3-mL sterile syringe
Heparinized NaCl
Sterile NaCl
Alcohol or Betadine wipe (according to hospital policy)
Clean, disposable gloves
Dressing supplies

Procedure
1. Compare IV fluid currently infusing with the ordered solution.
   Rationale: Comparison ensures prompt recognition and correction of errors.
2. Inspect the rate of flow at least every hour. For gravity-regulated IVs, check actual flow rate for 15 seconds and compare with prescribed flow rate. If the infusion is ahead of schedule, slow it so the infusion will complete at the planned time. If infusion is behind schedule, review hospital policy before increasing flow rate. Many agencies require a physician's order to increase the rate of flow. If electronic infusion device (EID) is used, the hourly infusion rate in milliliters per hour is programmed into the machine. Most EID manufacturers require use of cassette tubing unique to their machines.
   Rationale: IV therapies that are not on schedule can be detrimental to the client. Fluids that are infused too rapidly may cause circulatory overload with resultant pulmonary edema and cardiac failure. Fluids that are behind schedule deliver insufficient fluids and nutrients.

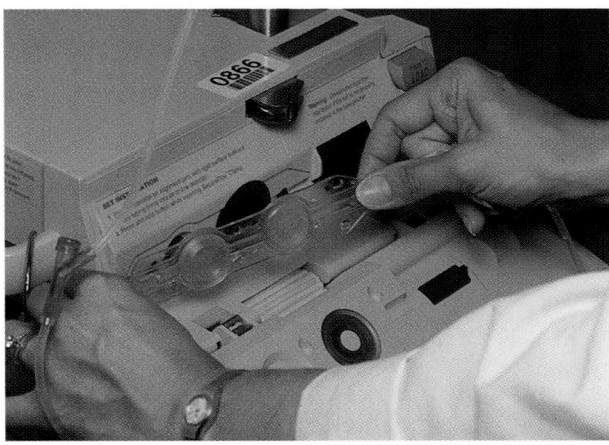

Step 2A Cassette tubing is placed in EID pumping chamber.

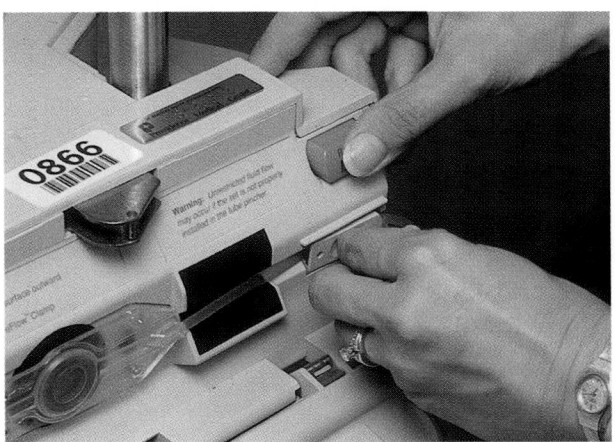

Step 2B Tubing is threaded through the EID.

3. Inspect the system for leakage; if present, locate the source. Tighten all connections within the system. If leak persists, slow IV flow rate to keep vein open and replace tubing with sterile set.
   Rationale: IV therapy is a sterile procedure. A break or leak in the tubing allows microorganisms to enter and contaminate the entire system.
4. Inspect the tubing for kinks or blockages. Loosely coil tubing and place it on the bed.
   Rationale: Blockages in the tubing impede the solution flow, and the client may not receive the necessary fluids and nutrients.
5. Observe the fluid level in the drip chamber. If it is less than half full, squeeze the chamber gently to allow in more fluid.

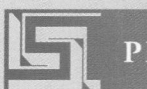

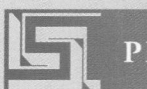

PROCEDURE 28-1 (Continued)

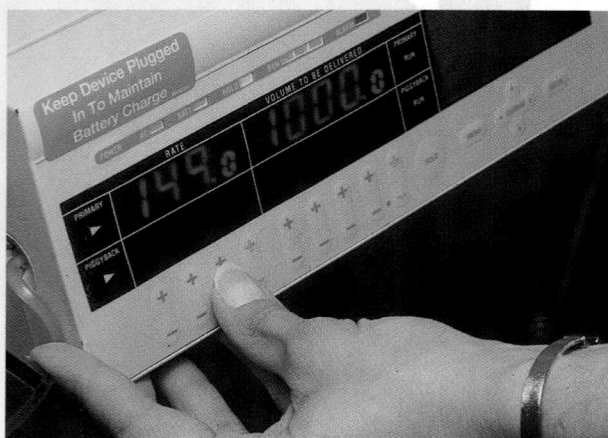

Step 3 IV rate is programmed into EID in mL/hr.

Rationale: If the fluid level in the drip chamber is too low, turbulence from the fluid dripping into the chamber may create air bubbles that may enter the tubing.

6. Inspect the infusion site for infiltration. Infiltration occurs when the needle becomes dislodged from the vein and IV fluid flows into the interstitial tissue. Look for signs of infiltration including decreased flow rate, swelling, pallor, coolness, and discomfort at or above needle insertion site. If signs are present, change the IV site. If a large amount of fluid infiltrated, elevate the arm above the heart on several pillows.
   Rationale: Prompt detection is important to promote client comfort and permit early treatment. Site elevation facilitates venous and lymphatic drainage.

7. Inspect arm above the insertion point for signs of phlebitis including redness, swelling, warmth, and pain along the vein above IV insertion site. If present, discontinue the IV and restart in another area.
   Rationale: This may occur as a result of trauma or chemical irritation secondary to intravenous additives or solution pH.

8. Inspect the insertion site for bleeding.

9. Although monitoring IV therapy is a nursing responsibility, if the client is able to comply, teach him or her to contact the nurse if the following occur:
   a. The flow rate changes suddenly.
   b. The fluid container is almost empty.
   c. Blood is in the tubing.
   d. The site becomes uncomfortable.
      Rationale: Allowing the client to participate in care helps to detect and prevent complica-

tions and enhances the client's feelings of control.

10. Chart any findings indicating complications of IV therapy (e.g., infiltration).
    Rationale: Charting maintains legal record and communicates with all health care team members.

Lifespan Considerations
Infants and Children
- Remember that children change position frequently, and their tubing can easily become kinked or disconnected. Tape all connections and protect the insertion site with a medicine cup and rigid armboard to help prolong the patency of the IV. Offer emotional support. IV therapy can be stressful for the child and the parents.

Additional
- Use airboards and soft wrist restraints or mitt restraints to protect the IV site in any client, regardless of age, who is at risk for purposefully disrupting the IV system.

Home Care Modifications
- Collaborate with the home care agency that will provide home follow-up. Give the client the agency's name and phone number and the name of the nurse who will coordinate care.
- Teach the client or caregiver the following:
- Inspect the insertion site at least four times daily through the transparent dressing.
- Assess for infiltration, phlebitis, or obvious dislodged catheter. If any of these occur, the caregiver should clamp the IV tubing, remove the catheter, and call the nurse.
- Observe flow rate for sluggishness or lack of dripping. Should this occur, the caregiver should open roller clamp and look for kinked tubing. If problem continues, contact healthcare provider.

Collaboration and Delegation
- In acute care agencies, work closely with members of the IV team to ensure safe, efficient IV management.
- If an agency does not have an IV team, consult the anesthesia department for problems with IVs or difficult IV starts.
- Teach unlicensed personnel how to safely provide hygiene care and ambulation for clients receiving IV therapy. Instruct them to notify the nurse if the alarm is ringing or the IV bag needs to be changed.

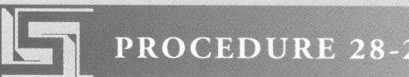

PROCEDURE 28-2

CHANGING INTRAVENOUS SOLUTION AND TUBING

Purpose
1. Deliver IV therapy as ordered.
2. Decrease risk of client infection.

Assessment
- Determine what time next solution container is due. Prepare next solution 1 hour before it is due. Plan to change container when less than 50 mL remains.
- Review physician's orders for current IV fluid orders.
- Check label on currently infusing solution and tubing for the date and time they were hung. (IV solutions are not considered sterile if they are open longer than 24 hours.)
- Determine date and time of last tubing change. It is recommended that IV tubing be changed every 72 hours to ensure sterility of system. Review the policy of your agency.
- Inspect IV system to determine type of tubing required. Many different administration sets are available. Some infusion pumps use specially designed cassette tubing. Review the policy of your agency and manufacturer's recommendations.

Equipment
Sterile container of ordered amount and type of solution
Appropriate sterile tubing administration set
Adhesive tape or premarked strips for labeling and timing solution container and tubing
Tape for securing tubing
Clean, disposable gloves (for tubing change)
Dressing material and antiseptic solution if IV site dressing is to be changed (follow agency procedure)

Procedure
Changing Solution Container
1. Wash hands.
2. Compare solution with physician's order. Adhere to five rights of medication administration.
   Rationale: IV solutions are considered medications. Errors in administration could have serious negative consequences for the client.
3. Remove IV bag from outer wrapper. Look for leaks or impurities in the bag.
   Rationale: Some dampness may occur as plastic on plastic sweats, but distinct leaks would destroy IV bag sterility.
4. Label solution container with client's name, solution type, additives, date, and time hung. If not

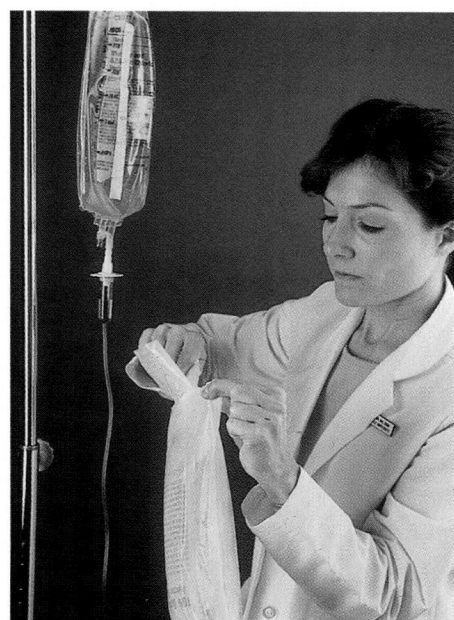

Step 3 Remove IV bag from outer wrapper.

already done, check prelabeled container with physician's order. Line up time strip with volume amount on bag or bottle. Record solution change in the client's record.
   Rationale: Proper labeling helps prevent errors in administration. Time strip will alert the nurse if IV is not on time.
5. Prepare container for spiking:
   a. If solution is in a plastic bag, remove plastic cover from entry nipple. Maintain sterility of nipple end.
   b. If solution is in a bottle, remove metal cap, metal disk, and rubber disk. Maintain sterility of bottle top.
   Rationale: Sterility prevents transmission of microorganisms into container when spike is inserted.
6. Close the clamp on the existing tubing.
   Rationale: Clamping prevents fluid in drip chamber from emptying and air from entering tubing during changing procedure.
7. Take old solution container from pole and invert it.
   Rationale: This position prevents fluid remaining in container from emptying onto floor when tubing is removed.
8. Remove spike from used container, maintaining its sterility. Spike new IV container with firm push/twist motion.

PROCEDURE 28-2 (Continued)

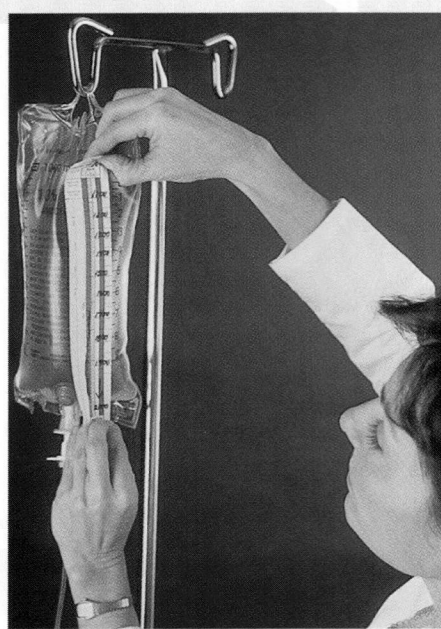

Step 4 Place time label on side of IV container.

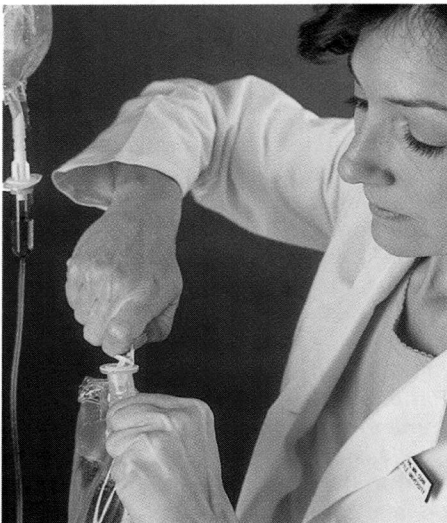

Step 5 Remove plastic cover from entry nipple.

9. Hang new container on IV pole.
   Rationale: This action allows gravity to augment fluid filling drip chamber.
10. Inspect tubing for air bubbles, and assess that drip chamber is one-half full of solution.

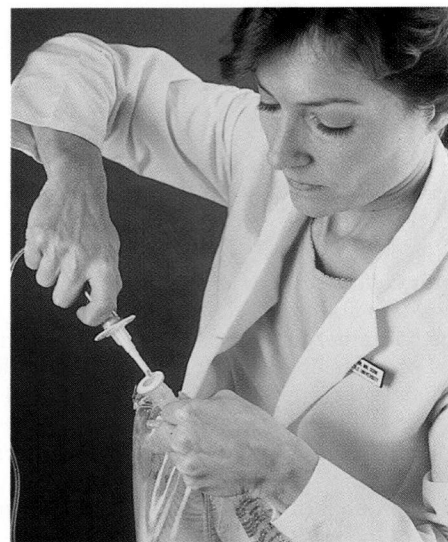

Step 8 Insert spike into IV bag.

Rationale: This action decreases the risk of air embolism.
11. Adjust clamp to regulate flow rate or program EID, according to orders.
   Rationale: IV fluids are delivered as ordered to restore fluid balance.

Changing Solution and Tubing
1. Follow first three steps of Changing Solution Container only.
2. Open new tubing package, keeping protective covers on spike and catheter adapter.
   Rationale: Sterility of new tubing set must be maintained.
3. Adjust roller clamp on new tubing to fully closed position.
   Rationale: Closed clamp prevents air from entering the tubing.
4. Prepare new solution container as directed in Step 5 of Changing Solution Container.
5. Maintaining sterility, remove protective cover from spike and insert spike into new solution container.
6. Hang container and "prime" drip chamber by squeezing gently, allowing to fill one-half full.
   Rationale: This action prevents air bubbles from entering tubing with the solution.
7. Remove protective cap from catheter adapter, and adjust roller clamp to flush tubing with fluid. Replace protective cap.
   Rationale: Air removal from tubing protects client from risk of air embolus. Protective cap maintains sterility of system.

PROCEDURE 28-2 (Continued)

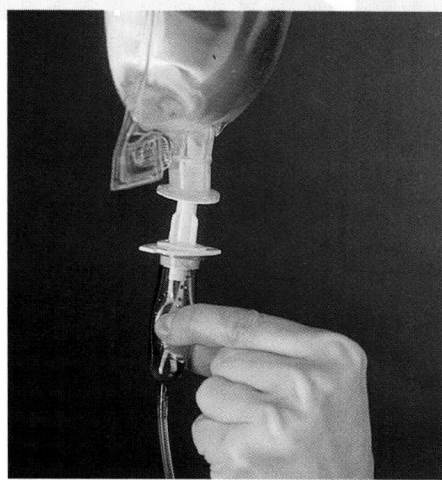

Step 6 Squeeze drip chamber gently to prime.

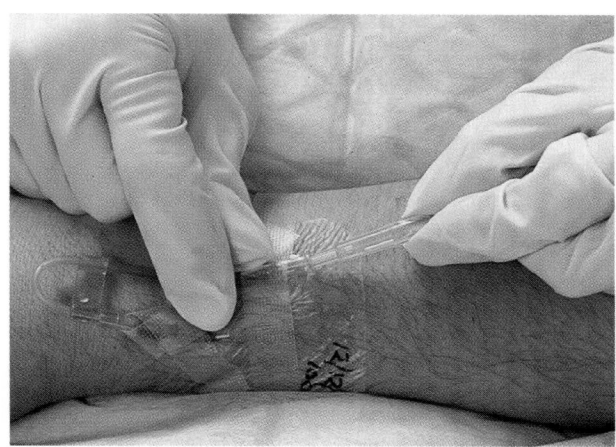

Step 11 Stabilize IV catheter hub while connecting new tubing tightly.

8. Adjust roller clamp on old tubing to close fully.
   Rationale: Fluid leakage should be prevented when tubing is disconnected.
9. Place towel or disposable underpad under extremity. Don clean, disposable gloves.
   Rationale: Towel or underpad protects the client's skin. Nurse is protected from transfer of microorganisms if blood inadvertently gets on hands.
10. Hold catheter hub with fingers of one hand (may use hemostat). With other hand, loosen tubing using gently twisting motion. *Note:* The dressing may have to be removed.
    Rationale: Holding catheter hub firmly maintains needle position in the vein.
11. Grasp new tubing, remove protective catheter cap, and insert tightly into needle hub, while continuing to stabilize catheter hub with other hand.
12. Adjust roller clamp to start solution flowing according to physician's order.
13. Discard gloves.
14. Secure tubing with tape.
    Rationale: Secure tubing prevents accidental dislodging of catheter in the vein.
15. If dressing was removed, apply new dressing to IV site according to agency policy.
16. Label new tubing with date, and time and your initials.
17. Label solution container with client's name, solution type, additives, date and time hung. Time label side of container (if not already done). Record solution and tubing change.

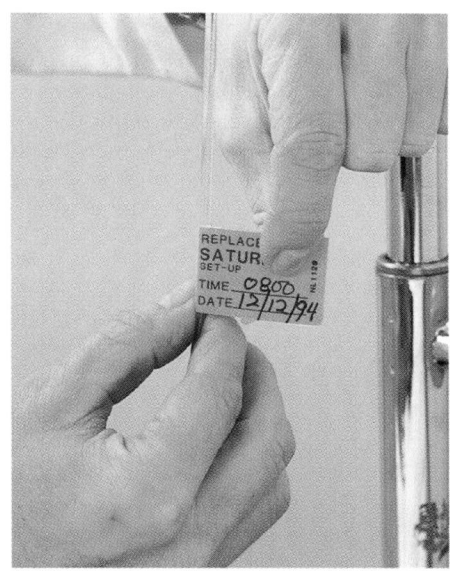

Step 16 Attach date and time label to tubing.

Rationale: Documentation facilitates monitoring by other staff members.

Lifespan Considerations
Infants and Children
- Remember that infants and children are at risk for circulatory overload if IV fluids are accidentally infused too rapidly. Use IV solutions available in 250- and 500-mL containers to guard against such accidents.

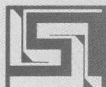

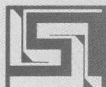

PROCEDURE 28-2 (Continued)

- Always use volume control administration sets to allow only a preset amount of fluid to be infused in children, especially those younger than 2 years.

Home Care Modifications
- Have client/caregiver practice changing IV containers using aseptic technique. Allow time for practice and return demonstration.

- Make sure client and caregiver have the name and number of their home care company should problems arise.

Collaboration and Delegation
- Know that IV teams may be responsible for routine tubing and dressing changes. Check your agency's policies.

---

infection, and fluid overload. Air embolism and pneumothorax are potentially life-threatening complications associated more commonly with central venous therapy. Catheter breakage is another complication occasionally seen with long-term therapy and central venous access devices. For more information, see Table 28-2.

Infiltration
When fluid enters the subcutaneous tissues, it is called **infiltration.** Infiltration can occur if the needle or catheter slips out of the vein or if IV fluid leaks from the vein into subcutaneous tissue. When infiltration occurs, the client may complain of pain and may have swelling around the infusion site, which usually becomes cool to the touch. When infiltration occurs, the IV usually infuses more slowly because of increased pressure within the subcutaneous tissues. Absence of blood return into the tubing when the IV bag is lowered below the infusion level further supports the possibility that infiltration may have occurred. Absence of blood return is not diagnostic, however, because some catheters do not readily permit the backflow of blood and the location of the needle bevel may make backflow difficult.

Phlebitis
Phlebitis refers to inflammation of a vein. If a blood clot accompanies the inflammation, it is referred to as **thrombophlebitis.** Factors that contribute to the development of phlebitis include catheter gauge, size, and material; length of time the catheter is in a vein; type and pH of solution administered; and use of small veins or veins of the lower extremities where blood flow is relatively sluggish. Clinical manifestations of phlebitis include complaints of discomfort and a vein that appears red and feels warm and hard (almost

cordlike) when palpated. The IV will be sluggish, especially if a clot is present. To prevent or decrease development of phlebitis, all peripheral IV catheters should be changed every 72 hours (Phillips, 2001).

SAFETY ALERT
Do not irrigate the IV because irrigation could push the clot into the systemic circulation.

Infection
Infection can occur at the IV infusion site or systemically. The longer an IV is in one site, the greater the chance for infection. Thus IV sites often are routinely changed according to guidelines given in agency policies. Infection can occur with central venous catheters, especially when the client is immunosuppressed. Meticulous handwashing, site preparation, and use of sterile technique during insertion and maintenance are essential to minimize the risk of infection. Multilumen catheters should be used only when necessary as they are associated with increased infection risk (Schmid, 2000). Signs and symptoms of infection can be local or systemic. If infection is suspected, notify the physician.

Fluid Overload
Fluid overload may occur if the client, especially the very young or the very old, receives IV fluid too rapidly. Fluid overload can occur if the nurse tries to "catch up" when the IV infusion gets behind. Preventing fluid overload is crucial by carefully monitoring all IVs and using electronic infusion devices. Assessments such as increased weight, decreased

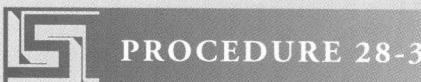

PROCEDURE 28-3

CONVERTING TO AN INTERMITTENT INFUSION DEVICE (IID) AND FLUSHING

Purpose
1. Maintain patency of intermittently used intravenous access.

Assessment
- Check for order for converting IV line to an intermittent infusion port.
- Check medication orders for types of medications, dosage, and time scheduled to be administered by way of the Intermittent Infusion Device (IID).
- Assess for compatibilities of medications with solutions to be flushed through lock.
- Identify all pertinent allergies.
- Assess site for signs of erythema, pain, tenderness, edema.
- Assess label and documentation for date and time of IV device placement.
- Review procedure manual for specific policies regarding flushing locks with saline or heparin.

Equipment
Medication documentation sheets
Gloves
Antiseptic swab
Appropriate intermittent infusion port adapter
Sterile 3-cc syringe with 21- to 25-gauge needle (use high-risk needles if available)
Many facilities are promoting needleless equipment for procedures. If available, will require sterile end protectors.
Vial of heparin flush solution, concentration depends on agency policy: (1 mL = 10 units sodium heparin or 1 mL = 100 units sodium heparin for central lines) or vial of sterile normal saline for peripheral lines. (Saline and heparin flush solutions may be available in prefilled syringes.)

Procedure
Beginning the Procedure
1. Wash hands.
   Rationale: Clean hands help prevent spread of microorganisms.
2. Explain procedure to client.
3. Prepare syringe with heparin flush solution or saline solution according to agency policy and manufacturer's recommendations for the type of device in place (may use between 0.5 and 1 mL

[peripheral], 2.5 and 3 mL [central line] heparin flush, or 1 and 3 mL normal saline). *Note:* If flushing lock after administering a prescribed medication, a saline flush may be required, followed by a heparin flush to completely clear the medication from the catheter to prevent incompatibilities with heparin.
   Rationale: Heparin is incompatible with many medications. Normal saline has been shown to be as effective as heparin in maintaining patency of peripherally inserted intravenous locks. Most central lines require patency to be maintained by intermittent heparin flushes.
4. Obtain appropriate IID.
5. Don clean gloves.
   Rationale: Gloves are worn to prevent transmission of microorganisms.

Converting IV to an Intermittent Infusion Device
6. Clamp tubing of IV infusion with roller clamp.
   Rationale: Clamping prevents backflow and IV fluid from spilling over bed and client when IID is connected.
7. Hold the catheter hub firmly with your nondominant hand (a hemostat may be used if necessary). With dominant hand, quickly twist IV tubing to the left to loosen but not disconnect from IV catheter.
   Rationale: Loosening this connector allows you to get ready for quick conversion to IID.
8. Take IID out of package, keeping tip sterile. Hold in dominant hand between thumb and finger.
   Rationale: Maintaining sterility is essential to prevent the spread of infection.
9. Stabilize IV catheter with nondominant hand as you disconnect IV tubing. Quickly insert IID into IV catheter, twisting to the right to tighten.
   Rationale: Quick transfer helps maintain sterility and prevent blood backflow if IV access is not clamped.
10. Tape IID to stabilize. Redress using transparent dressing if necessary.
    Rationale: Taping prevents accidental dislocation of IV access.

Flushing With Needle Type System
Perform Steps 1 to 5 above.
11. Swab injection port with antiseptic swab and allow to dry.
    Rationale: This prevents introduction of microorganisms during flushing.
12. Insert the needleless syringe into the port and aspirate gently for evidence of blood return.
    Rationale: Clear aspiration determines if IV catheter is correctly positioned in the vein.

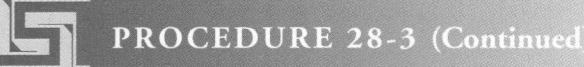

PROCEDURE 28-3 (Continued)

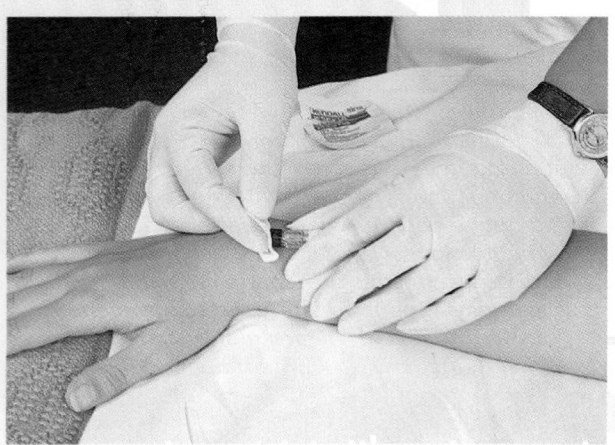

Step 11 Swab the injection port. (© B. Proud.)

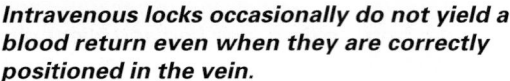

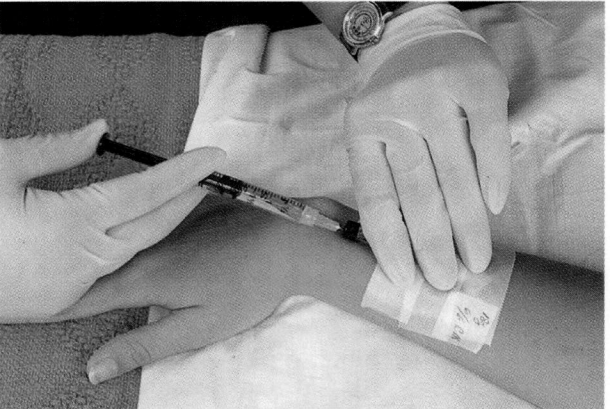

Step 13 Inject the recommended amount of saline or heparin flush. (© B. Proud.)

Intravenous locks occasionally do not yield a blood return even when they are correctly positioned in the vein.

13. Inject the recommended amount of saline or heparin flush ending with 0.5 mL of solution remaining in syringe.

Rationale: Positive pressure is maintained, preventing backflow of blood into the catheter, which carries chance of occlusion. Note: This procedure must be done at least every 8 hours or after each use of the catheter for IV medications to ensure catheter patency. Most agencies recommend changing intravenous locks every 72 hours to ensure patency and to prevent commonly associated complications of IV therapy (e.g., phlebitis).

14. Dispose of uncapped needles and syringes in proper container.

Rationale: Proper disposal prevents accidental needlesticks.

15. Wash hands.

16. Document date, time, route, amount, and type of flush solution. Also document assessment of site.

Rationale: Documentation facilitates monitoring by other staff members.

Lifespan Considerations
Infants and Children
- Check unit policy and physician orders carefully to determine type and required amount of flushing solution to be used.

Home Care Modifications
- Check the type of IV device used. Clients requiring long-term intravenous access usually have devices placed that are especially designed for long-term use (i.e., tunneled catheters such as the Hickman or Groshong and implantable catheters such as the Port-a-Cath). Each of these catheters has unique flushing requirements and procedures. Refer to manufacturer's recommendations or agency protocols for use.

Collaboration and Delegation
- Flushing IVs is usually not delegated to unlicensed personnel because breaks in aseptic technique could result in sepsis.

TABLE 28-2

Complications of IV Therapy

Complication	Signs/Symptoms	Action	Prevention
Infiltration	Swelling, coolness, and discomfort at site Slowed infusion rate Absence of blood return	Discontinue IV and restart in another location. Apply warm soaks to decrease swelling.	Select site that is over long bones that act as splint. Avoid sites over joints. Use armboards to stabilize. Use long-term catheters.
Phlebitis	Pain, warmth, and redness at site Vein may feel hard and cordlike Slowed infusion rate	Discontinue IV and restart in another location. Apply warm soaks to decrease discomfort. Do not irrigate.	Change IV sites every 72 hours. Use large veins and large-gauge needles rather than catheters. Dilute medications well and infuse slowly. Use central line for very irritating solutions.
Infection	*Local:* redness, warmth, and purulent drainage at the IV site *Systemic:* fever, chills, malaise, and elevated WBC	Discontinue IV and restart in another location. Culture catheter tip and draw blood cultures. Treat with appropriate antibiotics.	Maintain strict asepsis when dealing with IVs. Use good handwashing. Change tubing and dressings every 72 hours or according to protocol.
Fluid overload	Elevated B/P, increased pulse and respirations, dyspnea, rales, neck vein distention, weight.	Slow IV to "keep open" rate and notify doctor. Place client in high or semi-Fowler's position. Administer oxygen as needed.	Monitor rates carefully especially for high-risk clients (elderly, infants, CHF or renal disease). Use EID. Don't catch up when IV gets behind for high-risk clients.
Air embolism (central venous catheters, seldom seen with peripheral venous lines)	Pain in chest, shoulder, or back; dyspnea, hypotension; thready pulse; cyanosis; loss of consciousness	Place on left side in Trendelenburg position. Notify physician. Monitor vital signs closely.	Tape all connectors or use leur lock connectors. Use EID for all central venous catheters. Instruct client to use Valsalva maneuver when changing tubing on a central line.

urine output compared to intake, and crackles (rales) upon lung auscultation often indicate fluid overload.

Air Embolism

The entry of air into the client's circulatory system is called an **air embolism.** Air embolism is more common when central venous catheters are used; air entry is due to the change in intrathoracic pressures during respiration. A significant amount of air (usually more than 5 mL) must enter the peripheral venous circulation before it poses a significant health risk for the client. Smaller amounts of air are significant when a central venous catheter is used for IV therapy. The most common causes of air embolism are air in the tubing and loose IV connections. Symptoms of air embolism include complaints of chest, shoulder, or back pain; dyspnea; hy-

potension; cyanosis; thready pulse; and loss of consciousness. At the first sign of air embolism, position the client on her or his left side in the Trendelenburg position to allow the air to rise into the right ventricle and allow blood to pass into the lungs. Refer to Table 28-2 for strategies to prevent air embolism.

Pneumothorax

Pneumothorax may occur during insertion of a central venous catheter. This results when the catheter inadvertently punctures the pleural membrane. Symptoms of pneumothorax include chest or shoulder pain, sudden shortness of breath, tachycardia, and absence of breath sounds on the affected side. After all central venous catheter insertions, the client must undergo a chest radiograph to verify the position of the catheter before infusion of any solutions or medications. The chest radiograph also will detect pneumothorax.

Catheter Breakage or Damage

Catheter breakage or damage may occur at any point along the central venous catheter. This damage can be in the form of tiny pinholes or a complete fracture of the catheter. If the damage is external to the insertion site, the catheter may be repaired. If the repair is unsuccessful, the catheter must be removed.

The most serious risk to the client is if the catheter breaks and the fractured fragment embolizes to the heart or pulmonary artery. All IV devices are made of radiopaque materials so radiographic evaluation will assist in locating the catheter fragments. To avoid catheter damage, remove all sharp objects and scissors and use needleless systems and syringes 5 cc or greater to flush the catheter whenever possible.

Discontinuing an Intravenous Infusion

An infusion is discontinued when all ordered fluids have infused or when complications develop. Before discontinuing an infusion, don disposable gloves because contact with blood can occur. Stop the flow of fluid by moving the roller clamp to the off position. Carefully remove the tape, while supporting the catheter. Place a gauze pad over the venipuncture site while withdrawing the catheter, then apply pressure over the site. Apply a bandage if necessary, but remember that does not take the place of pressure. Ascertain the integrity of the catheter. Document the amount of fluid infused, the time the infusion was discontinued, the condition of the site, complications of therapy that occurred, and any nursing measures taken (such as application of a warm compress).

When removing a central venous catheter (CVC) or a peripherally inserted central catheter (PICC), it's important to take special precautions to prevent complications related to air embolism and catheter breakage. To prevent air embolism, follow the recommended guidelines for catheter removal:

Place the client in Trendelenburg position and remove the catheter while the client performs the Valsalva maneuver during the beginning of the expiratory phase. If you encounter resistance while attempting to remove the catheter, stop the procedure and notify the physician. Immediately after catheter removal, cover the site with an occlusive dressing. An occlusive dressing consists of an ointment-based antibiotic gel, gauze, and an airtight adhesive covering that should remain in place for 24 to 72 hours (Dumont, 2001). Inspect the integrity of the catheter after removal. If a defect is noted, document and report the finding according to agency policy.

Lifespan Considerations

Newborn and Infant

Newborns and infants present the nurse with unique challenges regarding IV therapy. Veins are very tiny and are difficult to locate and cannulate. For the newborn and infant, scalp veins in the temporal region are often used (Fig. 28-16). Seeing venipuncture or IV therapy delivered into the head can be very upsetting for parents so provide them with support and comfort, answer their questions, and allay their fears. Never ask parents to restrain a baby, but allow them to be involved in comforting the child during or after the procedure. Secure the IV site well so that the parents can hold and comfort their infant without fear of dislodging the IV.

> ### 🔲 SAFETY ALERT
> **For very young clients, always use an electronic infusion device for continuous IV infusions to prevent too rapid an infusion of fluid, which could be lethal.**

Toddler and Preschooler

After explaining the IV procedure to both parents, ask them if they would like to stay. The parent's presence is for the child's comfort; their role is not to restrain the child. Be honest in your explanations to the young child and provide information

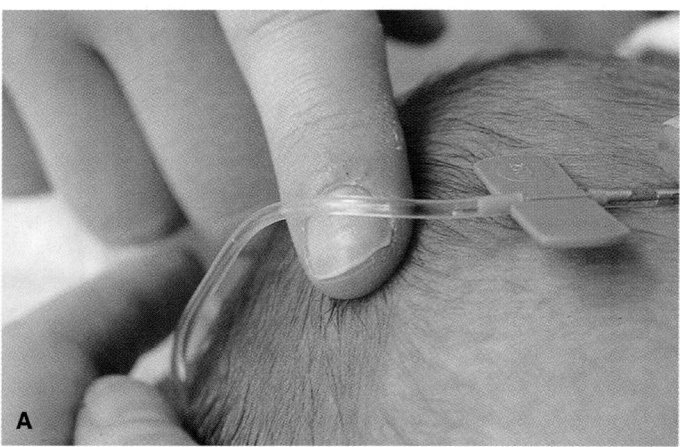
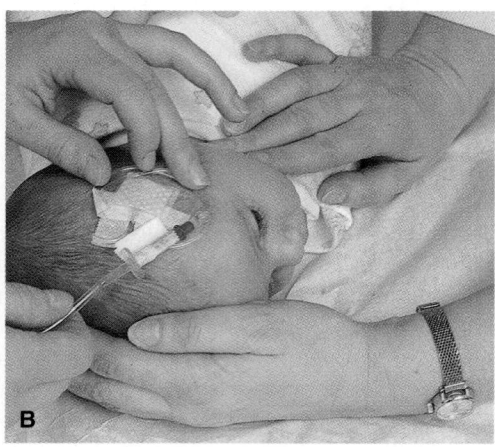

FIGURE 28-16   Site of IV therapy in infants. **(A)** Butterfly scalp vein needles are used in infants. **(B)** The nurse monitors the patency of the infant's scalp vein infusion site.

in terms she or he can understand. Perform the procedure as soon as possible after your explanation to prevent delays during which anxiety can build.

The child's room, whether at home or in the hospital, should be a place where the child can feel safe and comfortable. For this reason, perform painful or unpleasant procedures in a different room.

Selecting appropriate IV sites for children can be a challenge. Avoiding the areas over joints is even more important with children than with the adult because of children's increased activity level. Because infants and young children have very small veins, IV sites may include the metacarpal and cephalic veins in the upper extremities and the dorsalis pedis and great saphenous veins in the lower extremities. Use small-gauge catheters and monitor IV infusions with an electronic infusion device. Smiley faces or stickers can be placed close to the IV site.

School-Age Child or Adolescent

Fear of invasive procedures, such as injections or IVs, is common for the older child who may have had previous experience or heard about it from classmates. Individualize explanations based on the child's developmental level and readiness. Demonstrating the procedure using dolls or coloring books that outline the treatment can be helpful. Giving the child or adolescent some choice, if possible, decreases the sense of loss of control. Body image is very important for the adolescent, and IV treatment, especially with long-term catheters, can be stressful.

Adult and Older Adult

The older adult client receiving IV therapy requires special care because of the normal age-related changes in the skin and vessels. As people age, subcutaneous fat and elasticity decrease, the dermis thins, and the collagen tissue diminishes. For these reasons, the veins become more fragile, appear tortuous, and are likely to roll. These changes require the nurse to alter the insertion technique.

Using a tourniquet may cause blood to leak around the puncture site into surrounding tissue. The older adult client's veins might fill sufficiently for the IV start simply by placing the client's arm in a dependent position without using a tourniquet. To stabilize the large, tortuous veins during IV insertion, apply tension or downward pressure on the vein below the insertion site. Avoid using veins in the feet and lower extremities; impaired circulation at those sites increases the potential for complications. To prevent tearing fragile skin, take special care with the site dressing and tape. Older people, especially those with poor cardiac or renal function, are prone to fluid overload.

PARENTERAL NUTRITION

Parenteral nutrition is a form of nutritional support that supplies protein, carbohydrate, fat, electrolytes, vitamins, minerals, and fluids via the IV route. With the addition of lipid emulsion to the solution, nutrients essential to the repair and maintenance of body tissues are delivered.

Total Parenteral Nutrition (TPN) constitutes a hyperosmolar solution exceeding 10% dextrose and/or 5% protein. TPN must be administered through a central venous catheter. Peripheral parenteral nutrition (PPN) contains the same components as TPN except the final concentrations are dextrose 10% or lower and/or protein 5% or lower. This provides a formula that is less than 900 mOsm/L to prevent thrombosis of the peripheral vein. As PPN contains a lower concentration of dextrose and protein, it provides fewer calories than TPN and is used more commonly for supplemental nutrition.

The indications for parenteral nutrition have greatly expanded since the late 1960s when Dudrick first demonstrated the efficacy of parenteral nutrition in the pediatric populations with short gut and failure to thrive (Dudrick, Wilmore, & Vars, 1968). Currently, parenteral nutrition is indicated when enteral nutrition is contraindicated, such as in bowel obstruction and severe acute pancreatitis, or when enteral nutrition is not meeting the client's nutrition requirements such as with malabsorption, chronic diarrhea or vomiting, or short bowel syndrome. A comprehensive nutritional assessment of all clients is recommended as a means to screen for clients who are either malnourished or are nutritionally at risk (Worthington, Gilbert, & Wagner, 2000). Early identification of clients who are at risk for malnutrition is especially important for clients scheduled for surgery because the relationship between nutritional status and decreased morbidity, mortality, and length of stay in the hospital have been well described in the literature (Konstantinides, 1998). The laboratory evaluation of prealbumin or transferrin as well as assessment of height, weight, and anthropometrics are recommended as indicators of the client's current nutritional status (Smeltzer & Bare, 2000). Nutritional assessment is further discussed in Chapter 37.

Total Parenteral Nutrition (TPN)

All TPN solutions contain essential nutrients including protein, carbohydrates, electrolytes, vitamins, water, and trace elements. The proportion of each ingredient is individualized based on the client's clinical condition. The carbohydrate source is often a 50% dextrose solution. Protein is provided as synthetic crystalline amino acids. The client's caloric need is carefully assessed to provide the number of calories required to maintain an anabolic state. Electrolytes, vitamins, and trace elements are added based on laboratory assays. Additionally, some common medications such as histamine blockers and insulin can be added to the parenteral nutrition solutions. Compatibility data should be carefully evaluated before adding any medications to parenteral nutrition solutions. To supply all necessary nutrients, fat in the form of 10% or 20% lipid emulsion is often given with TPN. These isotonic solutions, which are milky in appearance, are compatible with TPN and can be infused simultaneously. Single-solution containers with admixtures of dextrose, amino acids, and lipid emulsions are also available.

Administration

TPN must be administered through central venous access because it is a highly osmotic solution. Irritation and sclerosing of the vein and sudden fluid shifts are less likely to occur when the hypertonic solutions are infused into large vessels with rapid blood flow and dilution. When TPN is a short-term intervention (less than 4 weeks), the subclavian and jugular veins are commonly used. When TPN is anticipated for an extended period (greater than 4 weeks), a more permanent catheter such as a PICC line, a tunneled catheter, or an implanted vascular access device may be surgically placed, as shown in Figure 28-7.

TPN and PPN must be administered through a tubing with an in-line filter and monitored with an electronic infusion device (INS, 2000). A 0.22-fm filter is sufficient for administering solutions without lipid additives. The lipids then are administered through separate tubing attached below the filter of the main IV administration set to prevent separation of the emulsified fats in solution. If the parenteral solution has lipids added to the container, a 1.2-fm filter tubing should be used.

Usually in the beginning of a client's TPN therapy, the solution is administered at a consistent rate over 24 hours. Use of an electronic control device ensures accurate rate administration. Change the parenteral solution container and tubing every 24 hours to decrease the risk of microbial growth; discard the used container and tubing (INS, 2000). See Procedure 28-4 for more information.

Cyclic Infusions

After the client has stabilized in tolerance of the TPN prescription, the physician may prescribe a cyclic infusion. Orders for cycling vary but usually mean that the client receives a 24-hour volume of TPN over a 10- to 14-hour period. **Cycling,** or the interruption of infusion for a period of time, is routinely used for clients receiving home infusion therapy. It permits increased freedom because nutrition is delivered during the sleeping hours, and the client is able to continue with activities of daily living during "off" hours. When instituting cyclic infusions, increase rates gradually to avoid sudden fluid shifts or hyperglycemia. To protect the client from sudden changes in blood glucose during cyclic infusion, the physician may order a ramping administration schedule. A ramping schedule allows the administration rate to begin slowly over 2 hours, reach and sustain the peak hourly rate over a period of time, then decrease slowly over the last 2 hours of the infusion. Tapering the TPN rate allows the body's endogenous insulin production to increase or decrease as the body's biofeedback system dictates.

Complications of TPN

Clients receiving parenteral nutrition are at risk for a variety of complications. Many potentially serious complications, such as pneumothorax and air embolism, are associated with central line placement and have been previously discussed. Other complications include infection, fluid overload, or metabolic alterations, which are usually due to the parenteral nutrition solution.

Infection. Infection is a potentially serious complication of parenteral nutrition due to the very high glucose concentrations that readily support microbial growth. Prevention of infection at the site and in the solution is accomplished by using strict aseptic technique during catheter manipulations, dressing changes, and tubing and bottle changes. Before hanging a new container, observe the solutions for any changes in color or cloudiness. Institutional protocol determines the frequency and technique to be used for routine care of the site and tubing. Assess the insertion site frequently (Fig. 28-17). Document any signs and symptoms of inflammation at the site. Culture any drainage; if present, the catheter may need to be removed.

🥛 SAFETY ALERT

When using a multilumen central venous catheter, keep one lumen dedicated strictly for administering parenteral nutrition. Never draw blood, administer other medications, or determine central venous pressure measurements through the TPN lumen.

Clients receiving TPN are often immune-compromised as a result of malnutrition; these clients are highly susceptible to infections. The infection's origin may be the catheter-related sepsis. If the client spikes a temperature during TPN therapy, blood cultures are usually drawn to evaluate for sepsis. If the

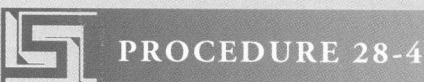

PROCEDURE 28-4

ADMINISTERING TOTAL PARENTERAL NUTRITION

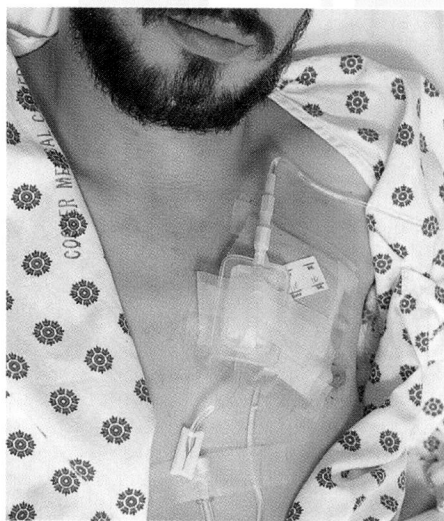

Patient receiving TPN.

Purpose
1. Provide parenteral nutritional support to malnourished clients.
2. Provide parenteral nutritional support to clients requiring bypass of the GI tract for prolonged periods.
3. Provide parenteral nutritional support to clients who have excessive metabolic needs due to trauma, cancer, or hypermetabolic states.

Assessment
- Assess client's nutritional needs.
- Check pattern of weight loss or gain, and intake and output balance.
- Check physician's order for TPN, noting additives and rate of infusion.
- Compare container of TPN with physician's order to ensure that it is correct.
- Assess client's knowledge of TPN and need for client teaching.

Equipment
TPN solution (usually prepared by pharmacy)
Appropriate IV tubing with filter
Infusion control pump
TPN dressing kit as per hospital protocol (usually contains transparent dressing, acetone swabs, Betadine swabs)

Sterile gloves and mask
Blood glucose monitoring equipment

Procedure
Monitoring TPN Therapy
1. Schedule and assist client with chest x-ray after central catheter insertion.
   Rationale: X-ray documents that catheter is in correct position and whether or not pneumothorax occurred during insertion.
2. Confirm correct solution is running at ordered rate. Check solution's expiration date. Use infusion controller to monitor and regulate flow rate.
   Rationale: Careful checking helps prevent medication errors. Note: Solutions with more than 10% dextrose must be infused directly into the subclavian or internal jugular vein to rapidly dilute the solution and prevent thrombophlebitis. Constant flow rate helps prevent hyperglycemia and electrolyte imbalances.
3. Inspect tubing and catheter connection for leaks or kinks. Tape all connections. Change tubing every 24 hours according to agency policy.
   Rationale: Leaks prevent client from receiving prescribed volume of solution and are a potential entry site for bacteria. Kinks in tubing can obstruct flow of solution and result in clotting of catheter. Taping connections prevents accidental disconnection.
4. Inspect insertion site for infiltration, thrombophlebitis, or drainage. If present, notify physician. *Note:* The physician may order removal of the catheter and culture of the catheter tip.
   Rationale: Complications are best detected and treated early.
5. Monitor vital signs, including temperature, every 4 hours.
   Rationale: Unexplained elevated temperature may indicate catheter-related sepsis.
6. Assess for symptoms of air embolism (i.e., decreased level of consciousness, tachycardia, dyspnea, anxiety, "feeling of impending doom," chest pain, cyanosis, hypotension). *Note:* If suspected, lay client on left side with head in Trendelenburg position.
   Rationale: Lying on left side may prevent air from flowing into the pulmonary veins. Lying in Trendelenburg position increases intrathoracic pressure, which decreases the amount of blood pulled into the vena cava during inhalation.
7. Use the TPN line only for administration of TPN and lipids. Do not use the line for any other reason.
   Rationale: Dedicating the IV line minimizes breaks in integrity of line to prevent infection.

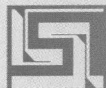

PROCEDURE 28-4 (Continued)

8. Perform test for glucose every 6 hours. Notify physician if abnormal.
   *Rationale: **Hyperglycemia may indicate that client needs insulin to help metabolize glucose or may be an early indication of sepsis.***
9. Monitor laboratory tests of electrolytes, BUN, glucose, as ordered, and report abnormal findings.
   *Rationale: **Constant checking and reporting of various factors are a means of preventing complications or treating them immediately**.*
10. Maintain accurate record of intake and output to monitor fluid balance.
    *Rationale: **Intake and output records are important documentation for observance of early occurrences of complications.***
11. Weigh client daily and record.
    *Rationale: **Consistent record keeping helps the nurse compare and observe for complications**.*
12. Inspect dressing once a shift for drainage and intactness. Change whenever loose or moist and at least every 48 hours.
    *Rationale: **Intact and dry dressings help prevent infection and keep client comfortable.***

Administering Intralipids
1. Check solution against physician's order. Inspect solution for separation of emulsion into layers or for froth. Do not use if present.
   *Rationale: **Solution may become contaminated or spoiled.***
2. Wash your hands.
   *Rationale: **Clean hands help prevent spread of microorganisms**.*
3. Attach fat emulsion tubing to bottle. Prime tubing as for a conventional IV.
   *Rationale: **Tubing has no in-line filter to cause separation of the emulsion.***
4. Identify client.
   *Rationale: **Correct client identification is important for medication administration.***
5. Identify Y-port on hyperalimentation tubing (below in-line filter).
6. Cleanse Y-port with antiseptic swab. Allow to dry. Insert connector into port. Secure with tape.
   Note: Lipids can be infused into a peripheral IV.
7. Adjust flow rate to infuse at 1.0 mL/min for adults and 0.1 mL/min for children. Infuse at this rate for 30 minutes while monitoring the client and vital signs every 10 minutes. *Note:* If any adverse reactions occur, stop infusion and notify physician.

8. If no adverse reactions occur, adjust flow rate:
   a. Adults: 500 mL intralipid over 4 to 6 hours.
   b. Children: up to 1 g/kg over 4 hours.

Lifespan Considerations
Infants and Children
- TPN solutions for children generally start with a 10% dextrose solution, increased to 25% dextrose. Exogenous insulin is usually not needed because a child's pancreas adapts easily to higher glucose levels. TPN solutions also usually contain higher concentrations of calcium, phosphorus, magnesium, and vitamins.
- Children are usually more active than adults and require frequent assessment of the tubing to prevent disconnections or obstruction during ambulation or play.
- Instruct parents about preventing accidental disconnection or obstruction of tubing.
- Soft restraints may be necessary to prevent the child from pulling out the catheter. Provide play therapy, books, and stimulation to distract the child.

Home Care Modifications
- The healthcare team must determine that the client or a guardian is responsible and able to be present during therapy.
- Identify and consult with a home health nurse who can be available 24 hours a day to troubleshoot complications.
- A long-term infusion device, such as a Hickman or Groshung catheter, should be in place before the client's discharge.
- Teach the client or caregiver how to initiate, monitor, and maintain an IV catheter and infusion according to the above protocol.
- Weigh the client daily. Record intake and output. Monitor blood values at least every other week. Have the client keep a log.

Collaboration and Delegation
- Nutritionists and pharmacists may be consulted, may write TPN orders, or may complete teaching before client is discharged for home management.
- IV teams or home IV companies may be involved in teaching and monitoring.

detect and treat imbalances of potassium, sodium, calcium, magnesium, phosphate, and trace minerals promptly.

BLOOD TRANSFUSION

Blood **transfusion** refers to the introduction of whole blood or blood components (packed red cells, plasma, platelets) directly into a client's circulatory system. Transfusions are given primarily to restore circulating blood volume, restore coagulation factor deficiencies, improve oxygen-carrying capacity of the blood, and increase white blood cells to decrease the chance of infection.

Blood Components

Whole Blood

Whole blood contains all blood components and is usually transfused to people who need both red blood cells and volume replacement, e.g., after significant blood loss. A unit of whole blood is approximately 500 mL. If whole blood isn't available, combinations of red blood cells, platelets, and fresh frozen plasma can be given.

Packed Red Blood Cells (RBCs)

Packed RBCs contain a concentration of RBCs with most plasma removed. A unit of packed cells is approximately 250 mL. Packed RBCs provide the same oxygen-carrying capacity as whole blood but without the volume. They are especially useful in the treatment of chronic anemia. Problems of fluid overload and electrolyte imbalances can be avoided because packed cells contain less volume and also less sodium and potassium. To prevent an allergic response, the packed RBCs can be washed to remove most antibodies from the cells.

White Blood Cells (WBCs)

WBCs, also called granulocytes, can be administered to clients with a low or abnormal WBC count. Infusion of white cells is helpful in fighting infection. They are frequently given to cancer clients who have low white cell counts due to chemotherapy or the effects of the cancer.

Platelets

Platelets, transfused more than any other blood component, consist of platelet concentrates and platelet-rich plasma. The major function of platelets is to initiate blood clotting and hemostasis. One common indication for platelet transfusion is thrombocytopenia following chemotherapy.

Fresh Frozen Plasma (FFP)

FFP is administered to provide clotting factors to clients with coagulation deficiencies who are bleeding or about to undergo an invasive procedure. FFP is sometimes used inappropriately as a volume expander or as a nutrient source.

Albumin

Albumin is a plasma protein contained within the plasma. It is used to restore intravascular volume and to maintain cardiac output in clients with hypoproteinemia. Another advantage of

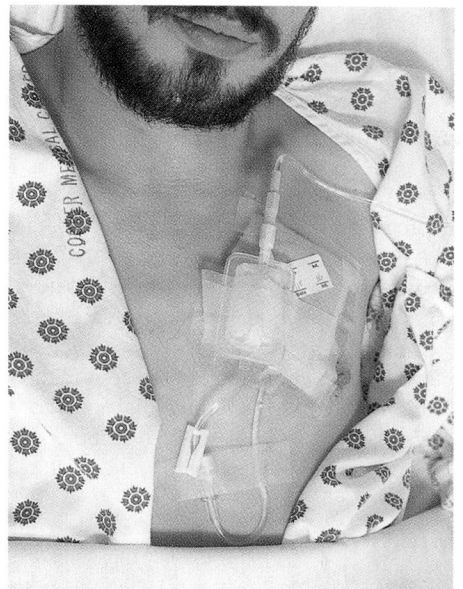

FIGURE 28-17 The nurse assesses the insertion site regularly for signs of inflammation.

fever source cannot be identified, the catheter may be removed and cultured. There is also increasing opinion that use of parenteral nutrition may predispose clients to an increased risk of non-catheter related infection because they are not being fed enterally. This predisposition is thought to be related to changes in intestinal morphology and increased permeability of the intestinal mucosa due to lack of nutrients passing through the gut. The increased permeability allows translocation of endotoxin and bacteria from the gut to cross into the vascular system. To prevent sepsis from this cause, nutritional support administered by way of the enteral route is recommended whenever possible rather than the more complicated and costly parenteral route (Silk & Green, 1998).

Fluid Overload. Fluid overload can occur if the hyperosmolar solution is infused too quickly, drawing fluid into the circulatory system. This risk is increased for clients who have a history of congestive heart failure or renal insufficiency and who cannot tolerate rapid fluid shifts. Always use an EID to regulate TPN infusions and avoid sudden shifts in fluid rate. Monitor fluid balance through serum electrolytes, daily weights, and intake and output measurements.

Metabolic Complications. Metabolic complications also may present a problem for the client receiving TPN. Most commonly, clients experience hyperglycemia if they are unable to tolerate the high glucose content of the TPN solution. When therapy is initiated, the infusion rate is usually tapered up over a period of a day or two. Blood glucose is monitored at least once a day or more frequently if unstable. Insulin is administered as needed. Hypoglycemia may occur when the TPN is discontinued, especially if the infusion rate is not tapered gradually. Electrolyte values are assessed daily to

albumin is that, unlike whole plasma, it carries no risk of hepatitis transmission and may be given without regard to the client's ABO group or Rh factor.

Cryoprecipitate

Cryoprecipitate is a plasma protein rich in fibrinogen and blood clotting factor VIII. Cryoprecipitate is concentrated from many units of blood and administered to control bleeding in clients with fibrinogen deficiencies, such as those with hemophilia or von Willebrand's disease, who are predisposed to bleeding problems because genetically they lack factor VIII. Commercially prepared factor VIII concentrates are also available in a powder purified from human plasma. The concentrate is heat or detergent-solvent treated to reduce the risk of virus transmission. Alternatively, a synthetic protein purified from genetically engineered nonhuman cells is also available for transfusion.

Blood Compatibility

Blood typing refers to testing the client's blood type. Crossmatching is the process of ensuring that the client's blood type is compatible with the donor blood. Prior to administering blood products, the products are tested for infectious diseases and ABO typing (Brown & Whalen, 2000).

🟦 SAFETY ALERT
Remember that, except in life-threatening circumstances, compatibility or cross-match testing is required on all RBC transfusions to ensure that donor blood is compatible with the client's blood.

Compatibility testing is not required before giving platelets, FFP, or cryoprecipitate.

Blood Groups

ABO blood groups can be determined by testing for antigens on the erythrocyte. The population can be divided into four blood groups: types A, B, AB, and O. The erythrocytes of a person in group A have the A antigen; group B, the B antigen; group AB, both A and B antigens; and group O, neither A nor B antigens. In addition to antigens, each blood group also contains naturally occurring antibodies (agglutinins) in the serum. Group A has anti-B antibodies, group B has anti-A antibodies, group AB has no A or B antibodies, and group O has anti-A and anti-B antibodies in the serum. Anti-A antibodies destroy A antigens, and anti-B antibodies destroy B antigens. This results in red cell destruction, known as **hemolysis.** People with type O blood are often referred to as universal donors because type O blood has neither A nor B antigens and it can be given safely to people with other blood types. Likewise, AB blood is often referred to as the universal recipient because the lack of antibodies enables accepting transfusions from other blood types.

Rh Factor.   Before transfusion, it is important to determine Rh factor to prevent blood incompatibility. Five antigens in the Rh system, the most important of which is D, are located on the surface of the erythrocyte. The presence of D antigen determines that a person is Rh positive (85% of Caucasian people), whereas the lack of this antigen designates a person as Rh negative (15% of Caucasian people). Antibodies against Rh factor do not occur naturally; those antibodies form only when Rh-negative blood is exposed to Rh-positive cells. After antibodies form, it is only on subsequent exposure to Rh-positive blood that a reaction (agglutination) occurs, in which there is hemolysis of cells. Rh factor is especially important in obstetrics. If an Rh-negative mother carries an Rh-positive fetus, antibodies can form in the mother's blood. If the mother should become pregnant again with an Rh-positive fetus, Rh agglutinogens can enter the circulation of the fetus and cause a hemolytic reaction. RhoGAM, a commercial name for antibodies directed against Rh factor, is given to the mother after the first miscarriage, abortion, or pregnancy to prevent future problems.

Selection of Blood Donors

Nurses are frequently responsible for screening prospective blood donors and overseeing the blood collection process. The nurse is responsible for ensuring the safety of both the blood donor and the blood recipient. To do this, the nurse interviews the prospective donor to rule out any history of hepatitis or recent hepatitis exposure, recent infectious exposure, syphilis or malaria, recent immunizations, and any recent blood product transfusions. Exposure to HIV or risky behaviors, such as IV drug abuse or homosexual or bisexual activities, is also ascertained. Screening ensures the safety of the blood supply by identifying and preventing high-risk people from donating blood. To protect the blood donor, people are not permitted to donate if they are pregnant, anemic, don't meet weight restrictions, have abnormal blood pressure, or have donated whole blood within the last 56 days.

Blood is tested for antibodies to HIV, hepatitis B, hepatitis C (non-A, non-B), and syphilis. The chance of contracting acquired immunodeficiency virus (AIDS) through blood transfusions has been significantly reduced since the development and implementation of testing all blood for antibodies to HIV. The blood donor is not at risk for acquiring any infectious disease, including AIDS, because all blood procurement is done under strict aseptic conditions.

Transfusion Technique

Before administering any blood product, it is essential to understand correct administration technique and to be aware of complications (Bradbury & Cruickshank, 2000). Steps for administering a blood transfusion are given in Procedure 28-5.

Important considerations when administering blood products include properly identifying the client and the blood, using a 170-micron standard blood filter, using a large enough IV access device (usually 18-gauge or larger) to avoid damage to the infusing blood cells, and using only compatible IV solutions of normal saline to prevent cell hemolysis (INS, 2000). PICC lines are prone to clotting due to the length and small lumen of the catheter. Instead of using an existing PICC

PROCEDURE 28-5

ADMINISTERING A BLOOD TRANSFUSION

Purpose
1. Replace blood volume or blood components lost through trauma, surgery, or a disease process.
2. Prevent complications from transfusing incompatible blood products.

Assessment
- Review physician's order for transfusion.
- Review chart for pertinent, baseline laboratory values (i.e., CBC, platelets).
- Review chart for previous transfusion history, noting if client has ever had a transfusion reaction.
- Inspect client's current IV for patency and intactness. Assess that IV catheter is an 18- or 19-gauge cannula, which will facilitate transfusion flow and prevent hemolysis of red blood cells. Restart if necessary.

Equipment
Packaged blood component from blood bank according to agency protocol
250-mL IV container of sterile 0.9 normal saline
Blood administration set with filter
Blood warmer and pressure bag (optional) may be used if infusing large volumes of blood rapidly
Alcohol swabs and tape

Procedure
1. Explain procedure to client. Have client sign consent form if required by hospital policy.
   Rationale: Keeping client informed increases participation in care.
2. Obtain client's vital signs including temperature.
   Rationale: Baseline pretransfusion vital signs can be compared against vital signs taken during and after transfusion to detect reactions.
3. With another RN at the client's bedside, verify the blood product and the client's identity by comparing the laboratory blood record with:
   a. The client's name and identification number both verbally and against client's wrist band.
   b. The blood unit number on the blood bag label.
   c. The blood group and RH type on the blood bag label.
      Also verify the type of blood component and the expiration date noted on the blood label. Document verification by both RN signatures on transfusion record.
   Rationale: Strict adherence to verification before blood administration greatly reduces the risk of infusing the wrong blood type.

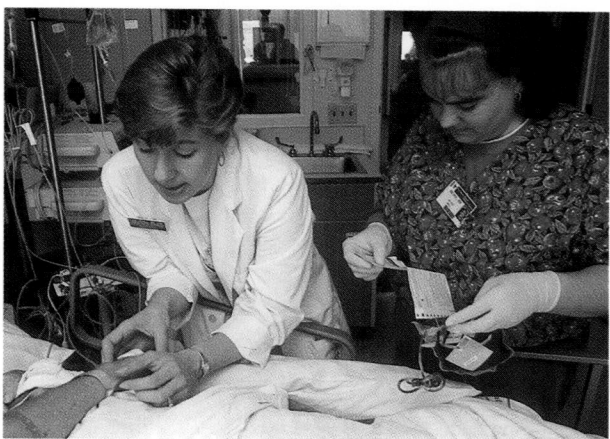

Step 3 Two registered nurses verify client's identity, blood product, and laboratory record.

4. Wash your hands.
   Rationale: Prevents transmission of microorganisms.
5. Open Y-type blood administration set, and clamp both rollers completely.
   Rationale: Clamping prevents spilling and wasting blood.
6. Spike 0.9% NaCl container. Prime drip chamber and tubing with saline.
   Rationale: Normal saline is compatible with blood. Dextrose solutions will cause hemolysis.
7. Spike blood or blood component unit with second spike. Keep roller clamp shut.
8. Remove primary IV tubing from catheter hub, and cover end with sterile protector.
   Rationale: If sterility of IV is ensured, it can be reconnected after transfusion.
9. Attach blood administration tubing to catheter hub, and secure with tape.
10. Flush line with NS. Open clamp to blood product. Open roller clamp below drip chamber and begin transfusion.
    Rationale: Flushing line with NS prevents blood from mixing with IV solutions containing dextrose, which will hemolyze cells and clog tubing.
11. Infuse blood slowly for first 15 minutes (10 drops per minute).
    Rationale: Most blood reactions occur within first 15 to 20 minutes of transfusion.
12. Monitor and document vital signs every 5 minutes during first 15 minutes, assessing for chilling, back pain, headache, nausea or vomiting, tachycardia, hypotension, tachypnea, or skin rash.

PROCEDURE 28-5 (Continued)

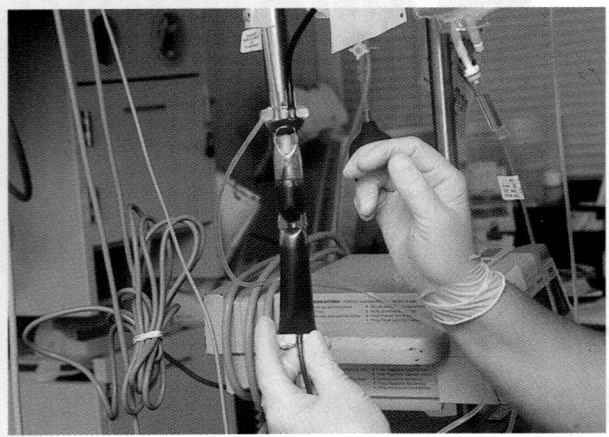

Step 11 Infuse slowly for first 15 minutes.

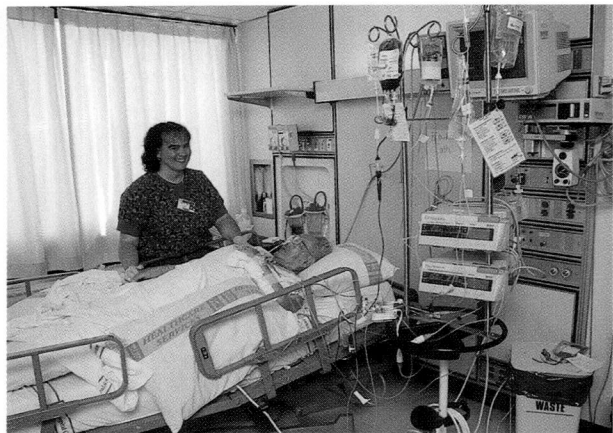

Step 12 Monitor and document vital signs every 5 minutes during first 15 minutes.

Rationale: Altered vital signs or other adverse reactions are early indications of a transfusion reaction. Infusing blood slowly during this period limits the amount of blood the client receives if there is a reaction. Note: If any adverse reactions occur, close clamp to blood, open clamp to 0.9% NaCl, and notify physician immediately. Follow agency policy for laboratory notification and obtaining blood and urine specimens.

13. If no adverse reactions occur after 15 minutes, regulate clamp to increase infusion according to physician's orders. A unit of blood is administered usually over 2 hours. Monitor vital signs hourly until transfusion is complete.

Rationale: Altered vital signs may indicate transfusion reactions or fluid volume overload.

14. When blood transfusion is complete, clamp roller to blood and open roller to 0.9% NaCl. Infuse until tubing is clear.
    Rationale: This action prevents wasting blood product and prevents hemolysis of cells from incompatible IV solutions.

15. Obtain and document post-transfusion vital signs.

16. If second blood component unit is to be transfused, slow 0.9% NaCl to keep vein open until next unit is available. Follow verification procedure and vital sign monitoring for each unit.

17. If transfusion orders are complete, disconnect the blood administration tubing from the catheter hub. Reconnect the primary IV solution and tubing and adjust to desired rate.

18. Wash hands and document procedure.
    Rationale: Facilitates communication with health care team.

Lifespan Considerations
Infants and Children
- Be aware that many blood banks have "pedi-packs" of blood available in 50 and 100 mL for infusing to children.
- Follow agency protocol for administering blood and blood components to children.

Older Adult
- If the client has cardiac failure, carefully assess to prevent fluid overload. Keep in mind that packed red blood cells are frequently infused to limit the volume being infused. The infusion of 0.9% NaCl may be limited to the minimum needed to irrigate the tubing. The infusion time may be increased to decrease the load on the heart.

Home Care Modifications
- Know that blood products are only administered in the home to stable clients. The home care nurse can transport the blood in a special cooler. The caregiver can help verify the client and check the serial number. Home care clients can also receive transfusions in short stay or special procedures units; they leave after the transfusion.

Collaboration and Delegation
- Do not allow unlicensed personnel to verify clients or blood products before transfusion. Allow them to monitor and record client's vital signs during transfusion.

line, insert a temporary peripheral IV for blood transfusion. Also, frequently assess the client for signs of a transfusion reaction, which can range from mild to life threatening (Whitsett & Robichaux, 2001).

Complications of Blood Transfusion

Febrile Reactions. Febrile reactions to blood products can occur because of the recipient's hypersensitivity to the donor's white blood cells. In this reaction, the client develops a fever and chills and complains of headache and malaise. Sometimes antipyretics and meperidine are administered before the transfusion to prevent the shaking and chills. If symptoms occur after the infusion has been started, stop the infusion immediately and keep the IV open with normal saline. Notify the physician and monitor vital signs. Leukocyte-reduced blood components can be ordered for clients with a history of febrile reactions.

Allergic Reactions. Allergic reactions may occur because the client has a sensitivity to the donor blood's plasma protein. Symptoms of an allergic reaction include flushing, urticaria (hives), wheezing, and a rash with itching. Once again, the infusion must be stopped, the IV kept open with normal saline, and the physician notified. An antihistamine may be ordered to decrease the severity of the reaction and make the client more comfortable. If hives are the only manifestation, the physician may elect to continue the infusion at a slower rate. Monitor the client carefully for manifestations of a more severe reaction that could cause respiratory difficulty. Washed red blood cells and premedication with antihistamines can prevent allergic reactions in subsequent transfusions.

Hemolytic Reactions. Acute hemolytic transfusion reactions, the most serious of the acute complications, can be life-threatening. A **hemolytic transfusion reaction** occurs when the donor's blood is incompatible with the recipient's blood. This can occur if the wrong blood is mistakenly administered to a client. Hemolysis, or destruction of red cells, occurs when the antibodies in the recipient's blood quickly react to the donor's blood cells. Symptoms are immediate and include facial flushing, fever, chills, headache, low back pain, tachycardia, dyspnea, hypotension, and blood in the urine. Prompt intervention is essential to decrease mortality in hemolytic reactions.

⬚ SAFETY ALERT
Always monitor vital signs before starting the infusion and during the first 5 minutes when the blood is infusing slowly. If you suspect a hemolytic reaction, stop the transfusion immediately and keep the IV open with normal saline.

The physician will order drugs to treat the hypotension and have the client monitored closely. Blood from the donor and recipient will be tested to assess whether or not a hemolytic reaction has occurred. A urine specimen also is collected to determine if renal involvement is present.

Fluid Volume Overload. Fluid overload can occur when blood products are infused too quickly or in too much volume. Fluid overload is more likely to occur in the very young or the older adult with poor cardiac or renal function. Symptoms include increased venous pressure, distended neck veins, dyspnea, coughing, and abnormal breath sounds. Fluid volume overload can be minimized by infusing packed RBCs rather than whole blood for high-risk clients and carefully monitoring the infusion rate of blood products. If fluid overload is suspected, slow the infusion of blood, position the client in an upright position with feet dependent, and notify the physician.

Septic Reactions. Septic reactions can occur if the blood products have been contaminated with bacteria. The client will likely have a rapid onset of fever and chills and perhaps vomiting, diarrhea, and hypotension. If this occurs, stop the transfusion and notify the physician. To minimize time for bacterial growth within the blood product, the product should be refrigerated until used and then infused within 4 hours. The longer blood products remain at room temperature, the more likely bacteria will grow and multiply.

COMMUNITY-BASED NURSING

Home IV therapy and nutritional support have become a thriving part of the home care industry over the past 2 decades. Long-term antibiotic therapies, once only given in the acute care facility, are frequently administered in the home setting, avoiding long periods of hospitalization. The ability to provide home IV and nutritional support has increased due to the technologic advances with IV catheter materials, placement techniques, and the simplicity and portability of the electronic infusion devices.

Planning for home IV or nutritional support requires a careful assessment of the client, family/caregiver, and the home environment. Clients receive their medications or TPN solutions in the privacy of their residences with the support of an interdisciplinary team including the physician, nurse, dietitian, and pharmacist (American Society of Parenteral and Enteral Nutrition, 1998). Successful home therapy depends on the following: medical stability, emotional stability, patient's lifestyle, intellectual ability, the client or primary caregiver's visual acuity and manual dexterity, and evaluation of the home environment (Phillips, 2001).

Client Teaching

Teaching the client and/or caregiver should ideally begin in the hospital with continued follow-up at home. Training should include aseptic technique, preparation and storage of solutions, operation of the infusion device, self-monitoring, detection of complications, and appropriate troubleshooting techniques. A plan should be in place about handling equipment malfunctions or problems with IV therapy, and telephone numbers for the supplier and nurse should be provided. Developing hypothetical problems and asking the client to think of possible solutions is a good method of evaluating problem-solving abilities and skills. Pharmacists who prepare

Home Health Record

Guidelines For Patient TPN Home Health Record
This form will be available to the Home Health Nurse to help monitor patient's progress.

1. Patient's name.
2. Enter date daily.
3. Enter weight daily (same time).
4. Enter temperature reading twice a day.
5. Enter urine results (if appropriate) per physician's order.
6. Enter blood sugar value (if appropriate) per physician's order.
7. Enter amount of TPN infused.
8. Enter rate/amount of lipids infused.
9. Enter oral intake.
10. Enter urine output.
11. Enter other output.
12. Enter stool frequency/consistency.
13. Note dressing change by a check mark in the box. Indicate appearance of site by use of the key letter:
    C = clean/dry
    R = red
    D = drainage
    P = pain
    S = swelling
    L = loose
14. Enter information as noted in parentheses.
15. Enter any other situations/problems not addressed.
16. Save this record for Home Health Nurse.

Name:						
Date:						
Weight: _____ lbs. _____ kg.						
Temperature: a.m.						
p.m.						
Urine: A						
Sugar and acetone M						
P						
M						
Blood Sugar:						
Intake Rate/amount of TPN infused (cc's/24 hours)						
Lipids						
Albumin						
Antibiotics						
Oral fluid intake/24 hours (Total cc's)						
Output - Urine Other output (cc's) Type						
Stool frequency/ consistency L/F						
Dressing changed/site: C = clean/dry R = red D = drainage P = pain S = swelling L = loose						
General: (include problems, appetite, how you feel, foods eaten, supply problems, etc.)						

FIGURE 28-18   Sample of a home health report to be used in TPN, with guidelines for use. (Courtesy of Midwestern Regional Medical Center, Zion, IL.)

IV medications or TPN solutions for home must use extra caution with aseptic technique, because solutions are often stored for extended periods before they are infused.

Monitoring

The client receiving home IV or nutritional support is monitored by both a home care nurse and the physician. The nurse should be present to start the initial nutritional support at home, set up all equipment, and make sure that all supplies including glucose monitoring equipment are present. This is an opportunity to teach the client to watch for symptoms that she or he needs to report to the physician. The client and/or caregiver must learn to detect and report fever, catheter redness, or any unusual symptoms.

Frequency of monitoring varies widely. Stable long-term clients need infrequent laboratory studies and monthly weights, whereas other clients may require weekly intake and output measurements and more frequent laboratory studies. Outcomes of nutritional support therapy are an important focus of monitoring. Often a client is taught how to keep a record in her or

his own home (Fig. 28-18). The prescribed regimen's nutritional adequacy and achievements in weight gain are included as objective outcome measures.

KEY CONCEPTS

- Homeostasis of body fluids, electrolytes, and nutrition may need to be supported through the use of IV therapy, parenteral nutrition, or transfusions.
- Important nursing interventions include client teaching and initiating, regulating, monitoring, and discontinuing an IV infusion.
- Bottle height, extremity position, catheter position in the vein, and catheter and tubing patency are all factors that can affect the infusion rate.
- Potential complications of IV therapy include infiltration, phlebitis, infection, air embolism, and fluid overload.
- Blood transfusions are administered to restore circulating volume, to improve the blood's oxygen-carrying capacity, to restore coagulation factors, and to increase white blood cell count to decrease the risk of infection.
- To prevent serious adverse reactions from blood administration, careful screening and matching of donor and recipient blood are necessary.

REFERENCES

American Society for Parenteral and Enteral Nutrition (ASPEN). Board of Directors (1999). Standards for home nutrition support. *Nutrition in Clinical Practice, 14*(96), 151–161.

Bradbury, M., & Cruickshank, J. (2000). Blood transfusion: Crucial steps in maintaining safe practice. *British Journal of Nursing, 9*(3), 134–138.

Brown, M., & Whalen, P. (2000). Red blood cell transfusion in critically ill patients. *Critical Care Nurse, Supp.*(12), 1–14.

Dudrick, S. J., Wilmore, D. S., Vars, H. M., et al. (1968). Long-term parenteral nutrition with growth development and nitrogen balance. *Surgery, 64,* 134–142.

Dumont, C. (2001). Procedures nurses use to remove central venous catheters and complications they observe: A pilot study. *American Journal of Critical Care, 10*(3), 151–155.

Intravenous Nursing Society (INS). (2000). Intravenous nursing standards of practice. *Journal of Intravenous Nursing, 21,* S35–42.

Josephson, D. (1999). *Intravenous infection therapy for nurses: Principles and practice.* Albany, NY: Delmar.

Konstantinides, F. (1998, February). Nutritional assessment of hospitalized patients, a long overlooked area of lab testing. *Clinical Laboratory News* (On-line). Available at: *www.aacc.org.*

Kuhn, M. (1999). *Pharmacotherapeutics: A nursing process approach* (4th Ed). Philadelphia: F. A. Davis.

Mermel, L. (2001). New technologies to prevent intravascular catheter-related bloodstream infections. *Emerging Infectious Diseases, 7*(2). U.S. Department of Health and Human Services Centers for Disease Control.

Phillips, L. (2001). *Manual of IV Therapeutics* (3rd Ed). Philadelphia: F. A. Davis.

Schmid, M. (2000, June). Risks and complications of peripherally and centrally inserted intravenous catheters. *Critical Care Nursing Clinics of North America, 12*(2), 165–174.

Silk, D. B., & Green, C. J. (1998). Perioperative nutrition: Parenteral versus enteral. *Current Opinion in Clinical Nutrition and Metabolic Care, 1*(1), 21–25.

Smeltzer, S., & Bare, B. (2000). Health assessment. *Brunner & Suddarth's textbook of medical-surgical nursing.* Philadelphia: Lippincott.

Whitsett, C., & Robichaux, M. (2001, May). Assessment of blood administration procedures: problems identified by direct observation and administrative incident reporting. *Transfusion, 41*(5), 575–576.

Worthington, P., Gilbert, K. A., & Wagner, B. A. (2000). Parenteral nutrition for the acutely ill. *AACN Clinical Issues, 11*(4), 559–579.

BIBLIOGRAPHY

American Society for Parenteral and Enteral Nutrition (ASPEN). (1998). *Clinical pathways and algorithms for delivery of parenteral and enteral nutrition support in adults.* Silver Spring, MD: Aspen.

Blackburn-Capel, J. (1998). *Nutritional assessment: Determining metabolic needs of the TPN patient.* Intravenous Nurses Society Annual Conference. Houston, Texas.

Breier S. (2000, January–February). Ethics and total parenteral nutrition: issues for intravenous nurse professionals. *Journal of Intravenous Nursing, 23*(1), 52–57.

Corrigan, A., Pelletier, G., & Alexander, M. (Eds.). (2000). *Intravenous Nurses Society: Core Curriculum for Intravenous Nursing.* Philadelphia: Lippincott.

Gilio A., Stape A., Pereira, C., et al. (2000, May). Risk factors for nosocomial infections in a critically ill pediatric population: A 25-month prospective cohort study. *Infection Control Hospital Epidemiology, 21*(5), 340–342.

Goode, C. J., Titler, M., & Rakel, B. (1991). A meta-analysis of effects of heparin flush and saline flush: quality and cost implications. *Nursing Research, 40*(6), 324–330.

Hadaway, L. (1999). Choosing the right vascular access device, part 1. *Nursing 99, 99*(2), 18.

Hadaway, L. (1999). Choosing the right vascular access device, part 2. *Nursing 99, 99*(7), 28.

Hamilton, H. (2000). Selecting the correct intravenous device: Nursing assessment. *British Journal of Nursing, 9*(15), 968–978.

Himberger, J., & Himberger, L. (2001). Accuracy of drawing blood through infusing intravenous lines. *Heart and Lung, 30*(1), 66–73.

Hoffmann, K., Weber, D., Samsa, G., et al. (1992). Transparent polyurethane film as an intravenous catheter dressing: A meta-analysis of the infection risks. *Journal of the American Medical Association, 267,* 2072–2076.

Intravenous Nursing Society. (2000). *Revised standards of practice.* Philadelphia: Lippincott Williams & Wilkins.

Jacob, E. (1999). Making the transition from hospital to home: Caring for the newly diagnosed child with cancer. *Home Care Provider, 4*(2), 67–73.

Oyama, A. (2000). *Journal of Intravenous Nursing, 23*(3), 170–175.

Raad, I., Hanna, H., Awad A., et al. (2001). Optimal frequency of changing intravenous administration sets: Is it safe to prolong use beyond 72 hours? *Infection Control Hospital Epidemiology, 22*(3), 136–139.

Rossetto, C., & McMahon, J. (2000, July). Current and future trends in transfusion therapy. *Journal of Pediatric Oncology Nursing, 17*(3), 160–173.

Internet Resources

www.aspen.org.

Internetworking Strategies Ltd. Available at: *www.ins1.org*

29 Perioperative Nursing

🖺 Key Terms

anesthesiologist
certified registered nurse
  anesthetist
circulating nurse
conscious sedation
general anesthetic
intraoperative phase
local anesthetic
malignant hyperthermia

paralytic ileus
postanesthesia care unit
postoperative phase
preoperative care unit
preoperative phase
regional anesthetic
scrub person
skin staple
suture

🖺 Learning Objectives

Upon completion of this chapter, the student will be able to do the following:
1. Describe the three phases of perioperative client management.
2. Discuss the impact of surgery on health and function.
3. Identify lifespan considerations for the client undergoing a surgical procedure.
4. Describe appropriate perioperative client teaching.
5. Discuss emotional support, safety, and asepsis during the intraoperative phase.
6. Identify appropriate nursing assessments in the recovery facility and during the postoperative period.
7. List common postoperative complications and appropriate nursing care to promote normal function.
8. Develop an appropriate discharge plan for the surgical client.

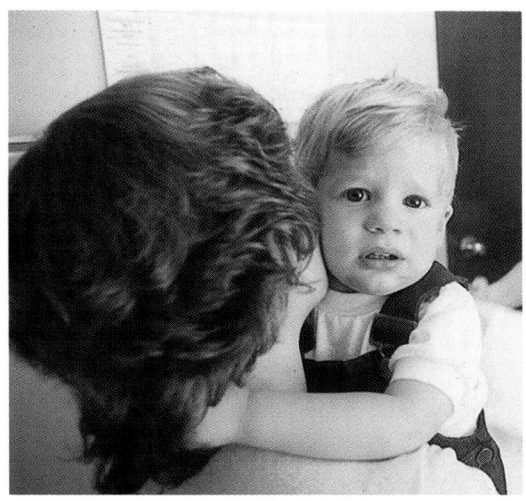

🖺 Critical Thinking Challenge

You are a nurse working in the preadmission surgical unit where preoperative assessment and teaching are performed. A young mother brings in her 2-year-old son, who is scheduled for a myringotomy (tubes inserted in the eardrums). You talk with the mother about the surgery and then proceed to collect the following information:

- *A 12-month history of repeated ear infections, averaging usually between one and two per month*
- *No known drug allergies*
- *Currently on no medications*
- *Vital signs: temperature 37.9°C, pulse 108, respirations 22*
- *Tenacious, dark tan nasal drainage for last 48 hours*
- *Lungs clear on auscultation*
- *Remainder of physical assessment within normal limits*

You observe that the mother–child interaction appears good, noting that the mother comforts the child when he begins to cry and actively interacts with him.

Once you have completed this chapter and have incorporated perioperative nursing into your knowledge base, review the above scenario and reflect on the following areas of Critical Thinking:

1. Reflect on age-related considerations for a 2-year-old child having surgery. How will you individualize care for this toddler and his family?
2. Reviewing the data collected, prioritize the most significant data, explaining why you think they are most significant.
3. Plan what teaching is important at this time, and role play how you will individualize the teaching for this family.
4. Demonstrate how you will document or report this information to other team members by preparing a written or oral report to be shared, focusing on the most significant assessment data.

In modern culture, surgery has become a common method of treating disease and promoting health. In the last few decades, the complexities of surgery have increased greatly, and entire organ systems can be transplanted to replace nonfunctioning body parts. All surgical procedures can potentially affect a person's functional abilities. The impact can be great and permanent or brief and temporary.

The goal of perioperative nursing practice is to assist clients and their families and significant others to achieve a level of wellness equal to or greater than that which they had before the procedure (Association of periOperating Room Nurses [AORN], 2001). Perioperative nurses provide specialized care to surgical clients, promoting their return to optimal function. As appropriate, nurses include family members and significant others in this specialized care.

SURGICAL INTERVENTION
Phases of Perioperative Nursing

Perioperative nursing includes three distinct phases: preoperative, intraoperative, and postoperative. The **preoperative phase** includes all activities that prepare the client for surgery. It begins when the decision for surgery is made and ends when the client is transferred to the operating room bed. The **intraoperative phase** includes all those activities that occur from the time the client is transferred to the operating room until he or she is transferred to the recovery facility. The **postoperative phase** involves the period after the client is discharged from the recovery facility and ends with the resolution of all surgical consequences. This phase may be short (less than 1 day) or lengthy (several months or longer), depending on the nature and extent of the surgical procedure and the client's ability to recover from it. Immediate postoperative care usually is given in a designated area of the hospital or ambulatory care facility. This area is referred to as the **postanesthesia care unit (PACU).**

In each phase, the nurse plays an integral role, using the nursing process to individualize care and meet the surgical client's specific needs. Collaborative care paths may be used in the perioperative surgical unit. A sample care path used for the client with abdominal surgery is included here.

Classification of Surgery

Surgery may be performed for many specific reasons: to investigate a problem or set of symptoms, alleviate pain, prolong life, improve mobility, provide vascular access for medications or nutrition, improve function, or improve appearance. Table 29-1 provides general classifications of surgery according to purpose and urgency.

Surgical Facilities
Clinics and Physicians' Offices

Surgery performed in a clinic or in a physician's office is usually limited to minor procedures, such as diagnostic, oral, or gynecologic procedures or removal of skin lesions. Usually

TABLE 29-1

Types of Surgery Based on Purpose and Urgency		
Classification	**Purpose**	**Examples**
Purpose		
Diagnostic	Confirmation of suspected diagnosis	Biopsy, culture, endoscopy, fluid tap
Explorative	Confirms the type and extent of a disease process	Laparotomy, joint exploration
Reconstructive	Repairs physical deformities or improves appearance	Rhinoplasty, mammoplasty, skin grafting
Curative	Diseased or damaged body organ or structure is removed or repaired and the client is cured	Appendectomy, hysterectomy, fixation of fractures
Transplant	Diseased or damaged body organs and structures replaced with donated or artificial organs	Heart, kidney, cornea, bone, liver, lung, pancreas, or skin transplants
Palliative	Alleviates pain or other disease symptoms, slows progression of diseases but does not cure	Tumor debulking, nerve blocks, placement of feeding tubes
Urgency		
Emergent	Preserves function of body parts or life of client	Repair of major vessel to stop severe bleeding
Urgent	Requires prompt attention within 24–48 hours	Repair of fracture, incision and drainage of wound infection
Required	Indicated for health problem but immediacy not necessary to preserve function or life	Gallbladder removal, excision of cancerous growth
Elective	Satisfies client's desire but not needed to preserve life or function	Cosmetic surgery

these procedures require either no anesthesia, local anesthesia, or regional blocks. Surgery done here is least expensive, because complex equipment is not used and inpatient recovery is not needed. As technology advances and procedures become less invasive, the number of surgeries performed in clinics and physicians' offices continues to grow.

Ambulatory Surgical Centers

Ambulatory surgical centers, also known as one-day surgical units or surgicenters, have proliferated in an attempt to keep down rising surgical costs. These facilities may be affiliated with and located in or near hospitals. Clients typically are admitted on the day of surgery and discharged that same day.

Because ambulatory surgical centers can save time and money, many hospitals are increasing the number of surgeries performed here. This trend is likely to continue in the next decade until the majority of all surgery is performed on an ambulatory basis. The anesthetic and surgical risks and the client's ability to safely care for himself or herself after discharge from the short-stay facility are important determinants. Increasingly, surgeries once performed only in the hospital, such as cholecystectomies (gallbladder removal), appendectomies, and hernia repairs, are being performed with the use of a laparoscope (a tubular optical and surgical instrument) in ambulatory surgical centers. Clients who have procedures using this minimally invasive technology are usually able to avoid the complications often associated with more extensive "open" procedures and are able to return to previous activity levels much sooner. However, ambulatory surgery provides a special challenge to perioperative and postanesthesia nurses, who must provide optimal client care and teaching within limited time frames.

Hospitals

Hospitals are comprehensive facilities for all types of surgery and postsurgical recovery. They have the necessary equipment and personnel available for surgeries requiring intensive monitoring, complex technology, and prolonged recovery periods. Hospitals provide a wide range of services and have extensive emergency backup systems, should they be necessary. Hospital surgeries are generally more expensive than surgeries at either ambulatory surgery centers or clinics. Emphasis on cost containment may prevent admission to a hospital for minor surgical procedures because insurance companies may be unwilling to reimburse for the cost of inpatient hospital care.

Impact of Surgery on Health and Function

Health Perception and Health Maintenance

The decision to have surgery is made jointly by the client and healthcare provider to promote health or improve function. This individual decision is based on a person's perception of health and what actions are appropriate to manage current problems.

Surgery involves many aspects of safety, both psychological and physical. Psychological safety is a feeling of comfort, security, and well-being, which are feelings of trust and confidence in the client's healthcare that providers and caregivers can enhance. Nurses can do much to promote these feelings. Providing emotional support and promoting an understanding of procedures greatly facilitate this process. When possible, nurses should include family members and significant others in the explanation of surgical procedures. Physical safety considerations include safety with anesthesia, medications, chemicals, electricity, procedures, special equipment (e.g., lasers, radiation units), surgical positioning, and client transport.

Activity and Exercise

Depending on the nature of the surgery, the impact on exercise and activity levels can be significant. Such alterations in activity levels may be either temporary or permanent. The woman who is to have a breast biopsy in an ambulatory surgery center will probably need to curtail her regular activities for only a few hours, whereas the client who is to have surgery on a fractured leg will need to alter activity for several weeks to months, depending on the extent of rehabilitation needed to return to a previous level of functioning. Both clients will experience relatively temporary changes in their activity levels.

Permanent changes in a client's activity level may also occur as a result of surgery. A person who has a leg amputated secondary to trauma or peripheral vascular disease will need to make permanent changes in activity patterns. Regardless of the specific nature of the changes that surgery brings, all clients will benefit from well-planned and well-implemented nursing interventions directed at returning them to their highest possible level of activity.

During the immediate postoperative period, respiratory and cardiovascular complications may result from inactivity and immobility. Deep breathing and incentive spirometry are beneficial in maximizing air exchange and in preventing atelectasis (alveoli collapse) and pneumonia. Leg exercises, antiembolic hose, and sequential compression devices help maintain peripheral circulation, promote venous return to the heart, and prevent deep vein thrombosis and subsequent pulmonary emboli.

Nutrition and Metabolism

Nutrition. An optimal nutritional state is essential for safe and successful surgery. It promotes wound healing, increases resistance to infection, promotes physical and psychological well-being, and maintains an adequate energy level and optimal fluid and electrolyte balance. After surgery, a diet with sufficient amounts of protein and vitamins A and C helps rebuild tissues and promotes wound healing. Adequate amounts of carbohydrates and fat are also important to avoid depleting protein stores. Metabolic disorders, such as diabetes mellitus, need to be assessed preoperatively and managed well to avoid intraoperative and postoperative complications.

Postoperatively, nutrition may be affected. For example, nausea and vomiting can occur postoperatively from the effects of anesthetic agents, pain medications, or manipulation of intestinal organs. In addition, oral fluid and food

(text continues on page 618)

COLLABORATIVE CARE PLAN Critical Pathway

Total Abdominal Hysterectomy (TAH)

Client Name: _____

Case Type: _____ Admit Date: _____ Expected LOS: 4–5 days

DRG: _____ Date Path Actual LOS: _____ Physician: _____

ICD-9: _____ Initiated: _____ Discharge Date: _____ Case Manager: _____

Outcome Criteria

Client Problems	Pre-Op Office/Pre Hosp	D	E	N	Surg Day 1 Surgery/PACU/Floor	D	E	N	PO Day 2–5 Floor	D	E	N
Anxiety related to impending surgery, lack of knowledge of preoperative care activities, expectation of pain, and altered reproductive/sexual function	Verbalizes fears and concerns related to surgery Identifies previous coping mechanisms and support system				Verbalizes concerns related to hysterectomy, expectations for recovery, effects on sexual function				Acknowledges acceptance of surgery, changes in anatomy and function Participates in self-care Identifies concerns re body image, sexual function, menopause, hormone therapy			
Knowledge deficit related to lack of information about surgical procedure, sensations, preoperative and postcare activities, effect on sexual function	Verbalizes understanding of surgical experience, precare and postcare activities Demonstrates postcare exercises: turn, cough, deep breathe (TCDB), incentive spirometry (IS), leg exercises States effects of surgery on sexual function				Performs postcare exercises (TCDB, IS, splinting) leg exercises				Verbalizes activity restrictions (avoid heavy lifting, straining, prolonged sitting or standing, tub baths, douches) States signs and symptoms to report to doctor (fever, chills, abnormal vaginal wound dressing, bright red bleeding) States wound care and perineal hygiene techniques Identifies dietary needs			

Pain related to surgical trauma to tissues and nerves	Verbalizes how to use pain rating scale of 0–10 Verbalizes knowledge when to notify nurse with request for pain medication	Rates pain <4 on scale of 0–10 15–30 min after IV or IM administration of pain medication	Rates pain <2 on scale of 0–10 30 min after oral pain medication Ambulates in hall without excessive pain (<2 pain rating)
Risk for altered tissue perfusion related to trauma to tissues, blood loss, venous stasis, lithotomy position	Verbalizes rationale for post-care leg exercises	Stable vital signs Peripheral pulses palpable: bilateral capillary refill <3 sec Skin pink/warm Incision intact Small amount of vaginal bleeding Adequate urine output >30 mL/hr	Hemoglobin (Hb) >10, hematocrit (Hct) >30 Incision dry and intact without bleeding Scant vaginal bleeding after packing No leg pain, edema, redness; pedal pulses palpable
Body image disturbance related to loss of body part and sexual function	Verbalizes understanding of changes in sexual anatomy/function and effect of hysterectomy Verbalizes fears and concerns related to surgical procedure and effect on body image	Verbalizes feelings about hysterectomy Asks appropriate questions	Acknowledges acceptance of self related to inability to bear children, effect on sexuality and surgical menopause Participates in self-care
Interventions			
Consult/Referral	Gynecologist/history and physical examination (H&P)/consult		Follow up with gynecologist for estrogen therapy, Pap smears
Diagnostic Test	Schedule laboratory tests, complete blood count, electrolytes, coagulation profile, chemistry profile, chest radiography, electrocardiogram (ECG), type and cross-match units Pap smear/pregnancy test Ultrasound/computed tomography scan	Validate laboratory/radiology reports for chart	Hb & Hct as indicated

COLLABORATIVE CARE PLAN   Critical Pathway (Continued)

Client Problems	Pre-Op				Surg Day 1				PO Day 2–5			
	Office/Pre Hosp	D	E	N	Surgery/PACU/Floor	D	E	N	Floor	D	E	N
Assessment	Vital signs Allergies H&P/past experience with surgery/hospital				Vital signs q 1–2 h I&O q 1° Foley catheter ECG rhythm Peripheral pulses O₂ saturation Assess incision/vaginal bleeding				Vital signs q8h Intake and output q8h—urinalysis for blood urine. Discontinue Foley—catheterize PRN—Assess voiding after discontinuing Foley; peripheral pulses, Homans' sign, pain in calf, redness, edema, chest pain Assess bowel sounds, abdominal distention, nausea, vomiting			
Treatments	OR permit Surgical scrub Hibiclens shower Foley catheter				O₂ 2–4 L by nasal cannula Head of bed ↑30° TCDB. IS q1h IV fluids/blood products Antiembolism hose—remove q shift				Discontinue O₂ if O₂ sat >92% Wound care/perineal hygiene after packing removed TCDB/IS/leg exercises, discontinue IV—if sufficient oral intake—Saline lock Antiembolism hose—remove q shift Shower if incision intact			
Activity	Upright posture ad lib				TCDB, q1h Head of bed ↑ 30–45° Dangle—chair in PM Leg exercises (calf pumps) Antiembolism stockings/sequential compression device				Ambulate QID independently—encourage frequent position changes Leg/foot exercises, antiembolism stockings			

Diet	Diet as tolerated NPO after midnight before OR	Clear liquid as tolerated IV fluids Assess bowel sounds	Diet as tolerated Discontinue IV fluids Assess bowel sounds before advancing diet
Meds	Hypnotic half strength Antianxiety agent as needed	Administer IV/IM pain meds as needed	Administer PO pain meds as needed (Tylenol, Percocet) (No ASA) Bowel care of choice
Teaching	Precare/postcare teaching, related to surgical procedure, TCDB, sensation, pain rating	Teach sustained maximal inspiration (SMI), splinting while coughing, activity and diet progression	Discharge teaching re wound care, vaginal bleeding, perioperative care, complications, signs of infection, activity progression, pain management Discuss misconceptions re sexuality, menopause, estrogen
Discharge/Transfer Planning	Assess discharge needs, home situation, support system, needs for assistance after discharge	Discuss home care needs/concerns of patient with family/significant others Provide patient/family support	Discuss estrogen, menopause, sexuality Discuss follow up care and when to report complication to MD Follow up appt with MD

Write "V" for variance in box if expected outcome not met or staff intervention not performed as stated. Patient variances need to be explained in progress notes.

D = Day
E = Evening
N = Night

Initials/Signatures: _____

may be withheld until intestinal motility resumes. Once active bowel sounds are present, the diet is usually advanced as tolerated.

Infection. The skin is the primary defense against infection. Before surgery, detection and treatment of any infection are necessary to promote healing and lessen the chance that the infection will spread or become systemic. During surgical procedures, the risk of infection increases because the skin barrier is broken and trauma occurs. Meticulous intraoperative aseptic practices are necessary to prevent infection.

Preoperative skin scrubs can decrease endogenous flora (microorganisms that normally live on the skin), which might otherwise increase the infection risk. Antibiotic prophylaxis is especially important with intestinal surgery or joint replacement, but it can be used for many other types of surgery or for clients who are considered to be at high risk. Usually a cephalosporin antibiotic is administered just before the surgical procedure so that the level of medication circulating in the client's blood will be high during surgery (Fortunato, 2000).

During the postoperative period, key nursing responsibilities focus on monitoring the wound for infection and instituting measures to prevent other infectious complications, such as respiratory or urinary tract infections.

Thermoregulation. Normally, body temperature is maintained without difficulty. During surgery, a number of factors, including decreased ambient temperature in the operating room, vasodilation secondary to the use of certain anesthetic agents, blood loss, intravenous (IV) fluid administration, exposure of body surface area, cool skin preparation solutions, and decreased consciousness, can lead to hypothermia. In addition, the client's age can affect thermoregulation. The risk for hypothermia increases in the very young and the very old. Interventions such as providing warm blankets, using electric warming devices, warming skin preparations and IV solutions, and minimizing body surface exposure help to alleviate body heat loss.

Another potential surgical problem of body temperature regulation is **malignant hyperthermia,** a hypermetabolic disorder of skeletal muscle that can be induced by some anesthetic agents, including certain inhalants and muscle relaxants (Stoelting & Miller, 2000). Because malignant hyperthermia has been identified as an inherited disease, clients who have a positive family history are particularly susceptible. This complication is manifested by masseter (jaw) muscle rigidity and ventricular dysrhythmias, which are associated with tachypnea (rapid respirations), cyanosis, skin mottling, and unstable blood pressure. These symptoms are followed by an increase in body temperature (possibly 1°C every 5 minutes if untreated), although fever may be a late sign of malignant hyperthermia. Consequently, in addition to identifying susceptible people, nurses must monitor muscle rigidity and body temperature closely during surgery for all clients and have emergency medications and equipment immediately available.

Elimination

Surgery can affect both bladder and bowel elimination. Before surgery, the client usually receives no food or fluid orally (known as NPO status) to decrease the risk of aspiration during the surgical procedure. NPO status decreases urine production and bowel function.

Urinary Function. Output of 30 to 60 mL/hour usually indicates adequate intravascular volume and blood pressure (Fortunato, 2000). The client may have an indwelling urinary catheter placed in the bladder before surgery. If a urinary catheter is not in place, the client should void immediately before going to the operating room to help prevent bladder distention during or after the procedure. Emptying the bladder also helps to make the abdominal organs more accessible during abdominal surgery and prevents accidental injury to the bladder.

During surgery, urine output is monitored closely for all clients with indwelling catheters. Clients who are undergoing shorter procedures (less than 2 to 4 hours) may not have a urinary catheter. For clients with urinary catheters and those without, blood pressure and fluid and electrolyte balance are carefully monitored intraoperatively, because these measurements provide information that helps evaluate the adequacy of renal function and circulation.

Postoperatively, urine output is closely monitored. In this stage, inadequate output may indicate hypovolemia, hemorrhage, electrolyte imbalance, inadequate circulation, hypoxia, or impending shock. Clients without a urinary catheter in place should void within 8 hours after the surgical procedure. Clients without a urinary catheter can have difficulty voiding postoperatively due to decreased level of consciousness, pain, medications, or edema in the pelvic area.

Bowel Function. A client who is NPO preoperatively has less active bowel function. In addition, bowel preparation may include use of "enemas until clear" or laxatives to clean the bowel of fecal material, further affecting bowel function. The preoperative bowel preparation is especially important for clients undergoing gastrointestinal surgery, because it helps prevent the possible intraoperative spillage of bowel contents, which could lead to peritonitis.

Postoperatively, the bowel may take several days or longer to resume normal activity and function. A combination of factors causes this delay, including decreased intestinal peristalsis, decreased food and fluid intake, decreased dietary bulk, pain medications, decreased physical activity, stress, lack of a normal routine, and decreased privacy. Frequently, stool softeners are prescribed after surgery once bowel sounds are present, especially if the client is receiving large doses of opioid analgesics. Sometimes, laxatives and enemas are necessary.

A potential complication after surgery is **paralytic ileus,** a condition in which there is significantly decreased bowel functioning. In some cases, intestinal peristalsis may temporarily cease altogether. The bowel becomes distended and partially paralyzed. Bowel sounds are usually absent. This condition, possibly a result of bowel manipulation during surgery, is commonly associated with gastrointestinal surgery. Metabolic disturbances, which can occur in the postoperative client, also contribute to paralytic ileus (DeWit, 1998). Paralytic ileus is very painful for the client and usually responds to treatment with a nasogastric tube, bowel rest, and IV therapy.

Sleep and Rest

The surgical client may experience disrupted sleep owing to preoperative preparation activities, changes in schedule, stress or anxiety related to the impending procedure, medication therapy, physical or emotional pain, separation from family and others, money worries and job uncertainties, and changes in normal diet and activity level. Nursing interventions that can help promote rest include providing a calm environment, relieving anxiety through client teaching and emotional support, making referrals to other professionals as appropriate (mental health professionals, financial counselors, chaplains), and administering medications and treatments as appropriate. Sedatives or antianxiety agents may be administered the evening before surgery and during the postoperative period.

After surgery, adequate sleep and rest are important for wound healing and emotional well-being. The client who can rest sufficiently and maintain adequate amounts of rapid eye movement or dream sleep (REM sleep) can better handle the stress associated with surgery and recovery. Planning for adequate periods of rest and sleep and maintaining a quiet, restful environment are essential.

Cognition and Perception

Pain. Pain has both physical and psychological components. Pain may occur before surgery secondary to a disease process or to a traumatic injury and also after surgery secondary to the surgical incision or procedure. Nursing interventions vital in helping clients cope with pain include administering medications, positioning, relaxation techniques, psychological support, distraction techniques, and appropriate referrals to other health professionals. Maintaining a restful and comfortable environment is also helpful.

Analgesics often are administered by the IV route, either IV push or via patient-controlled analgesia (PCA), or by epidural administration. These forms of administration are more successful in controlling pain than intramuscular or subcutaneous injections are. Many hospitals now have a pain service or clinic that may be consulted.

Confusion. The surgical client may experience confusion secondary to medication therapy, unfamiliar surroundings and people, sensory overload, electrolyte imbalances, pain, anxiety, or sleep deprivation. Nursing interventions to assist confused clients include orienting and reorienting clients to unfamiliar surroundings and people, maintaining a safe and comfortable environment, promoting increased visual and auditory input (pictures of family and friends, calendars, radio, television) during waking hours, promoting a quiet and restful environment during the hours set aside for sleep and rest, and monitoring medication therapy.

Self-Concept

For many people, self-concept is closely related to physical appearance, which surgical procedures may alter. The impact of surgery on self-concept depends on the client's perception of his or her value or image rather than a specific objective measure. The alteration may be minor, such as a small scar, or it may be major, such as a limb amputation or breast removal. Surgical alterations may also involve removal of certain organs (e.g., uterus, portions of the colon), which may result in significant emotional and psychological changes. Such alterations may extensively affect a person's self-concept, which may necessitate intensive, long-term rehabilitation, both physical and emotional.

In addition to providing the client with the necessary technical care, teaching, extensive rehabilitation, and emotional support, nursing interventions may also include referral to agencies and support groups that can benefit the client after surgery and discharge from the acute care facility. Such groups include the American Cancer Society and its numerous affiliates, the American Heart Association, and the American Red Cross. These organizations sponsor support groups that can assist the client and family to cope with changes in self-concept.

Roles and Relationships

Surgery and the separation that it may entail can affect personal, family, and business relationships. Changes may be temporary or permanent. Usually procedures from which one recovers quickly allow a person to resume previous roles and relationships without any long-range changes or conflicts. Chronic illnesses and major procedures, however, may lead to long-lasting changes that require much adaptation. Surgery may directly affect energy level, so that fulfilling the role of provider, sexual partner, or parent may be more difficult. Moreover, a prolonged recovery period may create problems in a person's work relationships, which can have an impact on financial security.

Appropriate nursing interventions depend on the specific role or relationship and the values or beliefs that are creating conflict. Providing the client and family members with emotional support and appropriate client teaching can positively affect role relationships. Referring the client to another healthcare team professional, such as a social worker, mental health counselor, or a chaplain, may be necessary.

Coping and Stress Tolerance

Surgery, even a minor procedure, entails significant stress. Coping behaviors and stress tolerance are closely related to how a person defines stress and how that person has managed stress in the past. Nursing interventions should include attempts to identify stress management strategies that were effective for the client in the past, because these strategies may be effective again during the perioperative period. Keep in mind that stress tolerance and coping behaviors are individual matters. What is effective for one person may not be effective for another.

Other interventions to assist a person in coping and managing stress include identifying and promoting effective stress

THERAPEUTIC DIALOGUE
Postoperative Pain

Scene for Thought

Alicia Martin, a 52-year-old woman, returned from the operating room last evening. A right leg fracture was repaired and her spleen was removed after a skiing injury yesterday. She has been awake and sitting up in a chair for the last few hours.

Less Effective

Nurse: Hello, Ms. Martin, I'm Robert Henderson, your nurse for the day shift. How are you? *(Good eye contact to indicate that the question is a real one.)*

Client: Hello, Robert. Call me Alicia. I'm okay, I guess. *(Looks tired, leaning against the back of the chair.)*

Nurse: You look tired. Do you want to get back into bed?

Client: Yes, please. Amazing how just sitting can tire you out. *(Gets back into bed slowly, with help.)*

Nurse: *(Gets Alicia settled and comfortably positioned.)* How does that feel? *(She smiles and nods okay.)* Good. I was wondering if I could talk with you to see if you have any particular questions about the operation or your injuries.

Client: I don't have any questions. I just want to go home. *(Looks like she's going to cry.)*

Nurse: I can understand that. No one likes to be in the hospital, especially in the middle of a vacation. *(Puts hand on client's arm in sympathy.)* But I thought you might have some questions that I could help you with. You had quite a difficult accident, and I know it must be hard on you.

Client: *(Starts to cry.)* That's true, it is hard on me. And all I want to do is rest right now, I'm not feeling very well at all.

Nurse: Can I get you anything before I go?

Client: No, I'll be okay if I just rest a little. *(Closes her eyes.)*

Nurse: Okay, I'll check back with you in a little while.

More Effective

Nurse: Hello, Ms. Martin, I'm Richard Hines, your nurse for the day shift. How are you? *(Good eye contact to indicate that the question is a real one.)*

Client: Hello, Richard. Call me Alicia. I'm okay, I guess. *(Looks tired, leaning against the back of the chair.)*

Nurse: You look tired. Do you want to get back into bed?

Client: Yes, please. Amazing how just sitting can tire you out. *(Gets back into bed slowly, with help.)*

Nurse: *(Gets Alicia settled and comfortably positioned.)* How does that feel? *(She smiles and nods okay.)* Good. I was wondering if I could talk with you for a while to see if you have any particular questions about the operation or your injuries.

Client: I don't have any questions. I just want to go home. *(Looks like she's going to cry.)*

Nurse: *(Pulls up a chair.)* Tell me a little more about that. *(Leans forward.)*

Client: I don't live here; I was just visiting with my husband and children, and I had the accident. And I hurt, a lot. *(Crying while splinting the incision.)* I'm not used to being sick.

Nurse: How about if I get you some pain medication first; then we can talk about the rest after you're a bit more comfortable?

Client: That's a good idea. It's hard for me to think clearly with the pain. *(Wipes her eyes.)*

Nurse: I'll be right back. *(Returns with pain medication, which he administers. Alicia reports relief after a few minutes, and they begin to discuss her questions, worries, and fears.)*

Client: Thank you, Richard. I think I'll be able to rest now.

Nurse: I'll check back with you in an hour or so to see how you are.

Critical Thinking Challenge

• Both nurses showed caring and sensitivity, but determine what the second nurse did that the first nurse did not do.

• Detect what information the second nurse gathered that the first nurse did not.

• Using Ms. Martin's behavior, analyze the ways pain affects a person psychologically.

---

management strategies and coping behaviors, providing emotional support and instruction for the client and family, and making referrals to other health professionals as necessary.

Sexuality

Surgery may temporarily or permanently affect sexuality and reproduction. Separation, prolonged convalescence, and actual surgical alterations all may significantly affect a person's sexuality and sexual identity. The impact may be physical, psychological, or both. Physical changes that may affect a person's sexuality can result from surgeries that alter appearance, limit mobility, alter reproductive capacity, and limit physiologic functioning.

Display 29-1 lists surgeries that may affect a person's physical appearance, mobility, and functioning, either temporarily or permanently. Although any of the surgeries listed may affect a person's psychological and physical functioning, some in particular affect sexual functioning. In addition, some procedures, such as certain types of prostatectomies, orchiectomies (removal of the testes), and certain urinary diversion procedures, may lead to impotence. Surgically corrective procedures may be available to restore sexual functioning.

DISPLAY 29-1

SURGICAL PROCEDURES AFFECTING APPEARANCE, MOBILITY, AND FUNCTIONING

Physical Appearance
Radical neck surgery
Mastectomy
Amputations
Facial surgeries
Oral surgery

Mobility
Bone fusions
Dislocations
Spinal surgeries
Amputations
Joint replacement

Functioning
Vaginectomy
Hysterectomy
Prostatectomy
Ostomies (colostomy, ileostomy)
Oral surgeries

Clients need to be fully informed of options regarding surgery or alternative treatments. Nursing interventions focus on performing a thorough assessment of the potential sexual or psychological impact and providing client teaching, technical skills, emotional support, and referrals as appropriate. The client also needs to understand clearly the depth and scope of any limitations that the surgical procedure imposes. Some clients may feel uncomfortable discussing sexual matters with healthcare professionals. When working with clients, create as open and comfortable an environment as possible and initiate discussion when appropriate.

Values and Beliefs

The client's value–belief system is significant because it guides personal choices and life decisions. A person's cultural background, philosophy, and religious orientation typically affect choices made with regard to surgery and treatment options. An example is the decision involving blood transfusions. Some religions prohibit their members from receiving blood products. This factor is significant for a person who has experienced major trauma, blood loss, or surgery.

Choices a person is required to make should be made only when the person is fully informed of the alternatives and the expected consequences of any decisions. After the client arrives at a decision, expert care, knowledgeable instruction, and emotional support are important nursing interventions. A chaplain or other religious or cultural leader may be useful at this time. Even if healthcare professionals oppose or do not understand the client's decision, they must maintain a non-judgmental and supportive approach.

Lifespan Considerations

Newborn and Infant

For newborns and infants, separation from their primary caregivers during a surgical experience is traumatic. Their ability to understand what is happening is limited, and they may perceive the experience as strange, frightening, and lonely. Promote a calm, comfortable environment by holding babies, keeping background noises to a minimum, and providing a stuffed animal, toy, or other diversion as appropriate. Provide careful explanations to the parents and other caregivers, and include them in their child's care as much as possible. Doing so helps to foster a sense of control over the situation.

An infant's ability to tolerate blood loss and alterations in temperature is significantly less than an adult's (Fortunato, 2000). Therefore, make every attempt to minimize both blood loss and heat loss from the body throughout the perioperative experience. In addition, infant skin is sensitive and easily traumatized. Items such as skin preparation solutions, tape, and dressings can impair skin integrity. Use items that are gentle to the skin and use extra care when applying and removing dressings. In addition, because of the infant's physical size, instruments, equipment, and medications need to be appropriate to size and physiologic status.

SAFETY ALERT
Always ensure that the medication dosages are calculated correctly for the child's size and weight.

Toddler and Preschooler

Many of the same factors that apply to infants also apply to toddlers and preschoolers. At these ages, separation anxiety may be more pronounced because children are more aware of their surroundings. Although these children have an expanded capacity to understand what is going on, they may still perceive the situation as frightening and lonely. Provide careful explanations to children and their families, and elicit their cooperation as needed. Having all instruments and equipment ready in the operating room before a child arrives helps shorten the waiting time before induction of anesthesia. It also helps to maintain a calm, quiet environment. In some situations, allowing the parents to hold the child while medications are being administered is helpful. For example, a suppository may be prescribed to promote relaxation and anesthesia before the child is taken into the operating room. This causes sufficient relaxation so that the child does not perceive other procedures as quite so frightening. Removing the child's clothing, applying the grounding pad, and applying monitoring devices after the child is anesthetized also are helpful. As with the infant, use of appropriately sized instruments and equipment, correct medication dosages, and measures to minimize blood loss and ensure temperature control are essential in promoting a safe and efficient surgical experience.

Planning for a safe recovery phase is another important consideration for both infants and toddlers. A crib with side rails provides a safe environment. If necessary, soft restraints may be used to prevent pulling on an IV line or dressing. As with all clients, monitor the airway and vital signs carefully and keep children warm postoperatively. In many situations, allowing the parents in the recovery room as children regain awareness of their surroundings helps to keep the children calm. This also may help ensure children's cooperation with necessary procedures and promote parental perception of inclusion in care (Ireland, 2000).

School-Age Child and Adolescent

School-age children and adolescents may have an increased understanding of surgery and many of the activities that a surgical procedure will entail. These children usually benefit from a more detailed preoperative teaching program. Many hospitals include a tour of the operating room for school-age children and adolescents and their parents during the preoperative teaching period. A child who has seen the operating room, the operating room bed, the anesthesia machine, and the mask used to administer an anesthetic is usually less frightened than a child who has not had this experience. In addition, because older children are better able to understand the surgery, they are likely to cope better with separation from parents.

Allow children of these age groups to participate in the administration of anesthesia by holding the mask or counting as the anesthetic is administered. Simple choices (e.g., selecting the arm for the IV line) may help give children a sense of control.

Adolescents requiring surgery have special needs. Teenagers usually are concerned with body image and possible disfigurement. They are often self-conscious and embarrassed when private body areas are exposed. Adolescents vary markedly in their ability to cope with the stress of the surgical experience. In striving for identity and independence, they may attempt to hide their feelings. In addition to providing extensive teaching to both adolescents and their families, demonstrate support and acceptance of such feelings and behaviors.

Adult and Older Adult

Although surgical intervention is becoming more common for older adults, the risks of surgery and anesthesia are increased for older people with chronic illness (Bailes, 2000). In addition, certain adults may require special considerations when having surgery because of alterations in vision, hearing, or mobility or the presence of chronic disease.

If an adult client is visually impaired, leave the client's glasses on until just before an anesthetic is administered. Doing so maintains visual orientation and helps to decrease fear and increase confidence. If a client is having a regional or local anesthetic, operating room personnel may allow the client to wear glasses or contact lenses during the procedure. Glasses should be placed with the client's belongings, if they will be needed in the immediate postoperative period, or cared for according to the agency's policy. Note any visual impairment on the chart so that operating room personnel are aware of this significant deficit.

Older clients may also have hearing impairments. The operating room staff can speak clearly and directly to such a client or allow the client to wear a hearing aid until the anesthetic is delivered. Being able to hear members of the healthcare team fosters teaching and helps alleviate fear, keeping the client oriented to the environment. After removal, care for the hearing aid according to the agency's policy.

Document the disposition of glasses or hearing aids in the operative record brought to the operating room. If the client's glasses are kept in the operating room so that the client can use them in the recovery unit, take special care to avoid losing or misplacing them, because the agency may be held liable for their replacement.

Clients with altered mobility, such as those with limited joint mobility, obesity, extreme thinness or fragility, or back problems, may require individualized planning for positioning during the surgical experience. Specific positions necessary for surgical procedures (such as the lithotomy, prone, and lateral positions) may need modification or require special padding, positioning devices, or restraints to assist in maintaining required positions.

Alterations imposed by chronic illness, a common consideration in older adults, require specific planning and special monitoring during surgery. Respiratory and cardiovascular problems may affect a person's ability to tolerate certain anatomic positions (e.g., head-down positions may impede breathing for a person with respiratory problems). Kidney or liver dysfunction can affect excretion and metabolism of anesthetic agents. Therefore, the elderly person with severe chronic organ dysfunction is at greater surgical risk. As a result, only essential surgical procedures usually are permitted.

PREOPERATIVE NURSING

Nursing Assessment

History and Physical Examination

Preoperative assessment provides valuable information directly affecting the client's safety and well-being throughout the perioperative experience. Some of the most significant assessment information in the client's medical record includes the hematology report, allergy history, chronic disease history, current cardiovascular and respiratory status, history of past surgeries and anesthesias, height and weight, and the results of diagnostic studies. Table 29-2 lists rationales for obtaining these data before surgery. Current medication use, especially use of medications that can affect coagulation status (e.g., warfarin, nonsteroidal anti-inflammatory drugs, aspirin), is important and should be reported to the surgeon. In addition, any herbal preparations or nutritional supplements that the client is taking should be reported. Some of these may interact with other medications or anesthetic agents and need to be discontinued for as long as several weeks before surgery. Refer to

TABLE 29-2

Preoperative Assessment Data and Rationale	
Data	**Rationale**
Interview and Physical Assessment	
Proposed surgery	Individualize client teaching and preoperative preparation
History of previous surgery	Recognize and avoid problems previously encountered
History of allergies	Avoid client exposure to allergens eliciting allergic response
Chronic disease history	Provide competent care and necessary medications; alert to possible complications
Smoking history	Identify increased risk for postoperative respiratory complications
Current respiratory and cardiac status	Assess safety of anesthetic and medication administration; minimize risk for postoperative complications
Current height and weight	Determine body surface area for drug dosage calculations
Vital signs	Detect abnormalities; provide baseline data
Mobility restriction	Plan for surgical positioning needs and safe transport
Laboratory and Diagnostic Tests	
Blood studies (CBC, electrolytes, coagulation studies)	Evaluate for actual or potential problems with anemia, infection, fluid and electrolyte imbalances, cardiac dysrhythmias, or bleeding disorders
Urinalysis	Evaluate renal function and absence of urinary tract infection
Electrocardiogram (ECG)	Evaluate cardiac function and absence of dysrhythmias
Chest radiograph	Evaluate respiratory status
Blood type and cross-match	Identify blood type; match with potential donor should transfusion be needed

Table 27-3 in Chapter 27 for a list of common herbs and potential interactions. The collection of physical data is an integral part of the preoperative assessment for many healthcare providers. The physician completes an in-depth client medical history and physical examination. The anesthesia provider completes a preanesthetic assessment form (Fig. 29-1). Data collected on this form are particularly important in selecting and preparing safe administration of anesthetic agents.

The nurse also completes an in-depth interview and physical assessment of the client during the preoperative period. This may be completed days or weeks before surgery during a preoperative visit, by telephone, or in the preoperative care unit just before surgery. With the increasing number of ambulatory surgeries resulting in decreased access to the client, completion of the preoperative assessment may be a challenge. However, the information obtained is critical; it provides data needed to identify potential and actual nursing diagnoses and to individualize the perioperative nursing plan of care.

Allergies
Assess client allergies to medications, food, and latex before the surgical procedure, and clearly mark them on the client record and on the client identification band. Allergies to latex, tape, and iodine-based solutions (e.g., radiopaque dyes, skin prep solutions) are especially important to note, because exposure to these substances is common during surgery.

A recent increase in the number of clients (and staff) sensitized to natural rubber latex products is of concern throughout surgery. The sensitivity may be manifested by a mild-type IV allergic reaction (local inflammation, redness, and pruritus),

or it may cause a full-blown type I anaphylactic response. Clients at risk include those with many allergies, those who have had multiple surgeries, those with neural tube defects (e.g., spina bifida, myelomeningocele), healthcare workers, and people with a stated intolerance to objects containing natural rubber latex (e.g., latex balloons, condoms, gloves, underwear). A Latex Risk Tool may be used to screen surgical clients (Figure 29-2). Once a client is known to be at risk, members of the operating room team should be notified and a latex-safe environment provided for the client (AORN, 2001).

Learning and Discharge Needs
The preoperative assessment also helps to identify learning and discharge needs of the client and the family. Client teaching begins during the preoperative period and continues throughout all perioperative phases of care. In the preoperative phase, assess the client's and family's readiness to learn and their knowledge base so that teaching can be individualized. If the client will be discharged on the day of surgery, be sure to identify someone who can take the client home and assist during the postoperative recovery period.

Nursing Diagnoses and Outcome Identification

With the use of the preoperative nursing assessment, actual and potential problems can be identified for the surgical client. Knowledge deficit, anxiety, pain, and sleep pattern disturbance are common. These problems, stated as nursing diagnoses, are listed in Table 29-3, along with appropriate outcomes.

| DATE | TIME | Inpatient Limited Stay | HT | WT (Kg) | BP | HR | RR | T | SaO₂ | O.R. DATE |
| | | Out Patient   AM | | | | | | | | |

DIAGNOSIS | PROPOSED OPERATION | SURGEON

COMMUNICATION: Patient prefers to be called:_____
Language: ☐ English ☐ Other_____
Interpreter ordered DOS, ☐ Pre ☐ Intra ☐ Post-op

PRE-OP TEACHING: Review with Patient
☐ OP/ ☐ AM, Brochure ☐ Housing Opt. ☐ NPO instructions ☐ Ride
☐ Pain management ☐ Pre-op shower ☐ Other_____
☐ **ADVANCE DIRECTIVES / DNAR** _____
☐ AM Meds _____
RN Print & Sign: _____

PRE-OP PHONE CALL (remind patient) Local Phone No. _____
☐ NPO ☐ Arrival Time ☐ AM Meds ☐ Ride/Escort ☐ Other_____
RN Signature _____ Date _____

LIMITATIONS: Impairment(s): ☐ Prosthesis_____
☐ Speech ☐ Dev. delayed ☐ Implant / Pacemaker_____
☐ Hearing ☐ Mobility ☐ Vision
Functional Status: ☐ Independent ☐ Needs assist_____
Devices: _____

DISCHARGE PLANNING   Name
Support system(s): ☐ Family/SO _____
☐ None identified ☐ Care giver_____
Pre-op day before surgery, patient will be at: _____
(home, motel, friend)   (phone #)
Post-op: Escort: _____ Phone: _____ ☐ None identified
Transportation: ☐ Escort ☐ Cabulance/paratransit ☐ None identified
If no escort, patient change to LS? ☐ No ☐ Yes   (date)

MEDICATIONS | **ALLERGIES** | **HABITS** | **PHYSICAL EXAM**
| Meds: Y N____ | ETOH: Y N____ | Chest:____
| Latex: Y N____ | | Cardiovascular:____
| Food: Y N____ | Drug Use: Y N____ |
| Tape: Y N____ | | Neuromuscular:____
Anticipate Pain Management Problem: N Y | Prep Soln/Contrast: Y N____ | Smoking: Y N____ |

RESP
| | No Yes Comments: |
Asthma/Bronchitis ☐ ☐
COPD/Dyspnea ☐ ☐
Productive Cough ☐ ☐
Recent URI ☐ ☐
Sleep Apnea ☐ ☐

CARDIO
Valve Dis/MVP ☐ ☐
Exercise Tolerance ☐ ☐
Abnormal EKG ☐ ☐
CHF/Orthopnea ☐ ☐
Angina/MI ☐ ☐
Hypertension ☐ ☐

GAST
Bowel Obstruction ☐ ☐
Hepatitis/Jaundice ☐ ☐
Cirrhosis ☐ ☐
Hiatal Hernia/Reflux ☐ ☐

REN/ENDO
Diabetes ☐ ☐
Renal Failure ☐ ☐
Thyroid Disease ☐ ☐
Pregnancy/EDLMP ☐ ☐

NEURO
Arthritis ☐ ☐
Muscle Weakness ☐ ☐
CVA/Stroke/TIA ☐ ☐
Paresthesia ☐ ☐
Headaches/ICP ☐ ☐
Syncope/Seizures ☐ ☐

HEM/ONC
Anemia ☐ ☐
Bleeding ☐ ☐
Cancer ☐ ☐

PREVIOUS ANESTHETICS
☐ General ☐ Regional ☐ Sedation
Difficulties: Family Anesthesia History:

AIRWAY EXAM
Mallampati I II III IV
Thyromental <6 cm   >6 cm
Mouth Opening _____ cm
Prominent Incisors Y N
AO Extention 0 1/2 Full
Neck Mobility- Ext 0 < 2.5 cm > 2.5 cm
Flex 0 < 5 cm > 5 cm
Prior Difficult Intubation Y N Unknown
Anticipate Difficult Intubation Y N

DENTITION: Good   Poor
R 6 7 8 9 10 11 L
27 26 25 24 23 22
Chipped_____ Missing_____
Loose_____ Bridge_____
Capped_____ Denture_____
Patient Informed of Dental Risk Y N

EVALUATOR SUMMARY   CRITICAL ISSUES FOR THE ANESTHESIA TEAM

EVALUATOR PRINT & SIGN | ASA STATUS

PRE-OP TESTING: | ☐ Pregnancy Test | DISCUSSED: | **ANESTHESIA PLAN**
Hct/K⁺ _____ | CXR _____ | ☐ Ride ☐ NPO ☐ AM Meds |
EKG _____ | Other Labs _____ | ☐ Contact Lenses/Dentures ☐ Other |

PT.NO.

NAME

DOB

UNIVERSITY OF WASHINGTON MEDICAL CENTERS
HARBORVIEW MEDICAL CENTER - UW MEDICAL CENTER
SEATTLE, WASHINGTON
PRE-SURGICAL PATIENT ASSESSMENT

* U 0 0 0 4 *

UH 0004 REV SEP 96

WHITE - MEDICAL RECORD
CANARY - DEPT. COPY
PINK - RESIDENT COPY

FIGURE 29-1   Example of a preanesthetic assessment form. The preadmission nurse completes the boxes above the first heavy black line. The anesthesia provider completes the remainder of the form. The circulating nurse uses this information in planning care during the intraoperative phase.

Nursing Interventions

Client Teaching

Preoperative teaching helps clients understand what will occur during each phase of the surgical experience and how they can participate in their own recovery. Preoperative teaching includes a general orientation and explanation of the sur-

gical experience, discussion of preoperative activities to prepare the client for surgery, and description of postoperative care to promote optimal function and recovery. Whenever possible, include family members in the preoperative teaching sessions.

Preoperative teaching can occur after the client has been admitted to the surgical unit. However, the client who is hav-

LATEX RISK ASSESSMENT TOOL
MULTIDISCIPLINARY CLIENT EDUCATION RECORD

Who must learn prior to discharge? (circle & code) Client ____ Spouse ____ Mother ____ Father ____ Other ____

Previous knowledge/experience _____

CHALLENGES (document interventions in narrative)			WHO	LEVEL OF PARTICIPATION
*1. Language (list)____	5. Fatigue	12. Cognitive Impairment	C = Client	A = Active
*2. Hearing Impaired	6. Stress	13. Withdrawn	S = Spouse	PC = Poor Concentration
*3. Visually Impaired	7. Pain	14. Chemical Dependency	M = Mother	D = Declined
*4. Literacy	8. Refusal of Teaching	15. Other ____	F = Father	UA = Unavailable
	9. Anxiety	16. None	O = Other, define	
	10. Fear			
	11. Physical Limitations			

*For #1-4 only, circle if applicable & document interventions

TEACHING CONTENT/ DISCHARGE LEARNING GOALS	INITIAL TEACHING				INSTRUCTIONAL STRATEGIES				TEACHING REINFORCEMENTS								GOALS MET	
	Challenges	Date/Initials	WHO	Participation	Audio Visuals	EZ-TV	Demo/Verbal	Written Information	Challenges	Date/Initials	WHO	Participation	Challenges	Date/Initials	WHO	Participation	Date	Initials
Describe the need to prevent exposure to latex.																		
Identifies common items that contain latex.																		
States responsibilities for reporting latex allergy risk status with each encounter.																		
States responsibilities for reporting latex risk status in the community setting.																		
Latex content in products used during each encounter.																		
Symptoms of allergic reaction.																		
Seek medical care for signs & symptoms of reaction.																		
The connection between other allergies and latex allergy.																		

Signature	Initial	Signature	Initial

FIGURE 29-2 Example of a Latex Allergy Risk Assessment tool.

TABLE 29-3

Selected Preoperative Nursing Diagnoses and Client Outcomes	
Nursing Diagnosis	**Client Outcome**
Deficient Knowledge regarding perioperative procedures related to verbalization of lack of knowledge	Client will verbalize understanding of perioperative care.
Anxiety related to insufficient knowledge, separation from family, fear of death or disfigurement	Client will report decreased anxiety level regarding surgery.
Acute Pain related to disease process or injury	Client will experience adequate control of pain.
Disturbed Sleep Pattern related to preoperative activities and anxiety	Client will demonstrate signs of sufficient rest before surgery.

ing ambulatory surgery may be instructed before admission. Usually, when the client is admitted the morning of surgery, little time is available for client teaching. Moreover, the client may be anxious and unable to process the information given. Some surgical centers preadmit clients a few days or a week before the scheduled surgery. At this time, the nurse can begin preoperative teaching while obtaining a nursing assessment and compiling necessary laboratory test results. Audiovisual materials may be available for the client to view. Frequently, the client is sent home with written material explaining what will happen before, during, and after surgery and what the client can do to participate in his or her own surgical recovery. When the client is admitted for surgery, any new questions can be answered and a review (reinforcement) of previous teaching can occur.

Because of the fears of hepatitis B and human immunodeficiency virus infection associated with blood transfusion, donation of autologous blood (one's own blood) for surgery is becoming a common practice. If the client wishes, provide the necessary information about blood donation if the client is seen a number of weeks before surgery.

General Information. A general orientation to the surgical experience should include the following:

- The expected time at which the procedure will begin
- How long the procedure will take
- When the client will probably return to his or her room (or to the waiting area for same-day surgery)
- Where the family and friends of the client can wait during the surgery
- How the client will be transported to the operating room
- What type of medications and anesthesia will be administered
- Other factors specific to the surgical procedure

If the client will be transferred to an intensive care unit after surgery, some facilities offer a tour of the unit for the client and family.

Preoperative Protocols. Review all preoperative activities and their importance for a successful surgical outcome. Address any specific procedures that must be performed preoperatively, such as bowel preparation, skin preparation, and the insertion of urinary or IV catheters or nasogastric tubes. Discuss possible dietary or fluid restrictions, including NPO status.

Postoperative Protocols. Preoperative teaching also provides the client with information concerning what conditions will be like after surgery. Frequently, clients have specific questions such as, "How much pain will I have?" or "What will my scar look like?" Begin by asking clients what questions or concerns they have about their upcoming surgery and deal with these issues before proceeding with the information that should be presented to each surgical client.

Before surgery, explain what tubes (IV lines, catheters, nasogastric tubes) will be in place during the postoperative period, the size and location of the incision, which medications will be ordered to control pain and nausea, and activities that the client will participate in, such as turning, deep breathing, using incentive spirometry, coughing, getting out of bed, performing leg exercises, or using a PCA device, to promote recovery and prevent complications.

Because these therapeutic procedures are used for a wide variety of clients, specific guidelines are included in appropriate clinical chapters in this text and in Table 29-4.

Informed Consent

The informed consent obtained before any surgical procedure is an important legal document. The surgeon is legally responsible for obtaining the client's informed consent. He or she fully explains the proposed surgical procedure by providing the client with all the information needed to make the decision, discussed in language the client can understand, and obtains the client's signature on the consent form. If the client does not speak or understand the physician's language, an interpreter should be used.

The information usually discussed includes a description of the proposed surgery, the possible risks and benefits of the procedure, the reason why the surgery is indicated, the probability of success, the consequences of nonsurgical treatment or no treatment, and any other information that will help the client reach an informed decision. The client has the right to ask any questions and to withdraw consent at any point before the surgery begins. Figure 29-3 gives an example of a consent form.

OUTCOME-BASED TEACHING PLAN

Susan Stone is a 15-year-old girl who is pre-admitted for a tonsillectomy that will take place in 2 weeks. She has never had surgery before and voices some apprehension. You have 15 minutes to complete preoperative teaching for Susan and her parents.

OUTCOME: At the end of the teaching session, Susan can describe preoperative protocols (informed consent, NPO status, and when to arrive at the surgical center) necessary before her surgery.
Strategies
- Question Susan about what she knows or understands about her upcoming surgery.
- Ask Susan whether she has any questions about her upcoming surgery to address her concerns before any teaching.
- Provide Susan with a preoperative booklet outlining general preoperative and postoperative routines for a tonsillectomy.
- Focus and discuss the preoperative procedures that will be ordered before Susan's surgery. Highlight the information in the booklet for her to review.
- Answer any questions.
- Ask her to verbalize important preoperative procedures.

OUTCOME: Before surgery, Susan can verbalize discharge care important during the postoperative recovery period (pain management, diet, when to notify her physician)

Strategies
- Review postoperative care in the booklet, including what will happen after surgery; why vital signs are monitored; medications that will be ordered for pain and nausea; what to expect when she wakes up in the recovery facility; expectation of some pain, throat soreness, and drainage.
- Reinforce actions that could irritate surgical site and delay healing.
- Have Susan and her parents verbalize plan for after-discharge care including pain management, and food and fluids to be included in the diet for the first week after surgery.
- Ask Susan to state actions to avoid that could irritate surgical site and delay healing (citrus juices, gargling with mouthwash, coughing and clearing of throat).

OUTCOME: Before discharge, Susan and her parents can verbalize appropriate follow-up care and indications that require physician notification during postoperative period.
Strategies
- Review symptoms (bright red bleeding, signs of infection such as temperature above 38°C (100.5°F); provide them with a written list of danger signs to report.
- Give Susan and her parents telephone numbers to call in case of questions or concerns.
- Provide Susan and her parents with written information regarding follow-up appointment with surgeon.

In addition to the proposed procedure, the consent form also lists the name of the surgeon and assisting surgeons and the surgical site (e.g., left or right eye, knee, kidney, ear). The surgeon, the client, and a witness must sign and date the consent form. If the client is a minor or is not mentally or physically competent to give consent, the consent should be obtained from the client's parents, spouse, legal guardian, or next of kin. Do not administer any medications that might alter judgment or perception before the client signs the consent form, because many drugs commonly administered as preoperative medications, such as narcotics or barbiturates, can alter cognitive abilities and invalidate informed consent.

The nurse may be involved in obtaining consent, usually by witnessing the client's signature on the consent document. Be knowledgeable about the healthcare agency's policy regarding informed consent and ensure that the policy is strictly followed. If the client seems unsure or indicates lack of understanding, notify the surgeon so that more information can be provided. The nurse is responsible for making sure that the consent form contains all correct, necessary information; is properly signed and witnessed; and is part of the client's medical record before the surgical procedure begins.

Client Preparation
Nurses are responsible for preparing clients physically and emotionally to ensure optimal condition for surgery. Specific client preparation is prescribed by the physician or indicated by healthcare facility policy, but usually it includes placing the client on NPO status, starting an IV line, inserting a nasogastric tube, preparing the intestinal tract and skin, and administering preoperative medications.

NPO Status. For any client receiving general anesthesia, foods and fluids are restricted and the client is held NPO before surgery. However, it is becoming more common to allow clear liquids until as late as 2 hours before the time of surgery (Stoelting & Miller, 2000). The institutional policy and the type of procedure planned dictate these guidelines. To help ensure safe anesthetic administration and prevent vomiting and aspiration, the client should not have a full stomach. If the surgical client is receiving necessary medications (such as antihypertensive, anticonvulsant, or antiarrhythmic agents) that should not be suddenly discontinued, clarify with the physician how and whether these medications should be administered. Some medications may be taken with a sip of water in certain

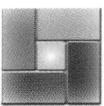

Nursing Research and Critical Thinking

What Model of Education for Preoperative Teaching Results in the Best Outcomes for Orthopedic Surgery Clients?

Orthopedic clinical nurses recognized a growing need for preoperative education for clients undergoing elective orthopedic procedures. However, most clients were admitted to the hospital the morning of surgery or were treated as outpatients for their procedures. A small number of clients were referred to a Learning Center for preoperative teaching before their hospital admission. Because the opportunity for contact with the clients before their surgeries was so limited, the nurses wanted the clients to receive the most effective preoperative teaching possible. These nurses designed an experimental (empowerment teaching method) group versus a comparison (traditional teaching method) group for a posttest research study to examine whether clients who received the empowerment model of education for preoperative orthopedic teaching had improved outcomes. Each client scheduled for a preoperative clinic visit was randomly assigned to receive teaching in the clinic (control group) or in the Learning Center (experimental group). Thirty-nine clients in the experimental group and 35 in the comparison group had complete preoperative data and were included in the analysis. The investigators developed an instrument to measure empowerment in the education process. Results of the study were that clients in the experimental group had higher self-efficacy scores than clients in the comparison group ($t = 4.27$, $P < .001$), and the experimental group reported feeling better able to perform preoperative and postoperative care ($t = 2.16$, $P < .05$).

Critical Thinking Considerations. The fact that the sample was limited to Caucasian adults undergoing orthopedic procedures was a major limitation of this study. It would be informative to further test the model with more diverse populations. The nurse researchers pointed out several issues of relevance to perioperative nursing practice, including the following:

- An empowerment approach to client and family education results in more favorable outcomes than the traditional medical model approach to preoperative teaching.
- Enhanced continuity of care across settings was an unexpected benefit of the new preoperative education program.

From Pellino, T., Tluczek, A., Collins, M., Trimborn, S., Norwick, H., Engelke, Z. K., & Broad, J. (1998). Increasing self-efficacy through empowerment: Preoperative education for orthopaedic patients. *Orthopaedic Nursing, 17*(4), 48–51, 54–59.

---

situations; others may need to be administered parenterally. If the client is diabetic, insulin orders should also be clarified. Dosages may be reduced, or the insulin may be given intravenously immediately before or during the surgery.

Intravenous Access. IV access in any surgical client is important for providing fluid and electrolyte replacement, administering IV medications, providing a route for emergency medication, and administering blood products. Vascular access may be obtained through a peripheral line or a central line. In certain situations, both are indicated. In other situations (e.g., surgery requiring only local anesthesia), an intermittent access device (heparin lock) may be adequate. The IV line may be started in the preoperative period to ensure adequate hydration status. For those clients who are well hydrated, IV insertion may be delayed until the client is in the operating room. For

TABLE 29-4

Preoperative Client Teaching of Postoperative Protocols		
Procedure	**Rationale**	**Related Chapter**
Turning, getting out of bed	Improve postoperative mobility to minimize impact of immobility	Chapter 33: Mobility and Body Mechanics
Deep breathing, coughing, use of incentive spirometer	Improved postoperative gas exchange and prevent respiratory complications	Chapter 34: Oxygenation: Respiratory Function
Leg exercises	Improve venous return and prevent deep venous thrombosis postoperatively	Chapter 35: Oxygenation: Cardiovascular Function
Using patient-controlled analgesia	Provide optimal pain control postoperatively	Chapter 43: Pain Perception and Management

> I HEREBY AUTHORIZE DR. _____, AND SUCH ASSISTANTS AS MAY
> BE DESIGNATED, TO PERFORM:
>
> _____
> (NAME OF TREATMENT / PROCEDURE)
> AND ANY OTHER RELATED PROCEDURES OR FORMS OF TREATMENT THAT THEY DEEM NECESSARY FOR THE WELFARE OF
>
> _____
> (NAME OF PATIENT)
> I CONSENT TO THE ADMINISTRATION OF ANESTHESIA AND/OR SUCH DRUGS AS MAY BE NECESSARY. I UNDERSTAND
> THAT ALL ANESTHETICS INVOLVE RISKS OF COMPLICATION, SERIOUS INJURY, OR RARELY DEATH FROM BOTH KNOWN
> AND UNKNOWN CAUSES.
>
> I CONSENT TO THE ADMINISTRATION OF BLOOD AND/OR BLOOD PRODUCTS IF DEEMED MEDICALLY NECESSARY. I
> UNDERSTAND THAT ALL BLOOD AND BLOOD PRODUCTS INVOLVE RISKS OF ALLERGIC REACTION, FEVER, HIVES,
> AND IN RARE CIRCUMSTANCES INFECTIOUS DISEASES SUCH AS HEPATITIS AND HIV/AIDS. I UNDERSTAND THAT
> PRECAUTIONS ARE TAKEN BY THE BLOOD BANK IN SCREENING DONORS AND IN MATCHING BLOOD FOR TRANSFUSION
> TO MINIMIZE THOSE RISKS.
>
> **OR, I REFUSE CONSENT FOR BLOOD AND BLOOD PRODUCTS (DOCUMENT ON CONSENT FORM UH 0399)** | PATIENT INITIALS |
>
> I CONSENT TO THE EXAMINATION, USE AND DISTRIBUTION FOR EDUCATIONAL, SCIENTIFIC AND RESEARCH PURPOSES
> BY THE UNIVERSITY OF WASHINGTON MEDICAL STAFF OF ALL BIOLOGICAL MATERIALS SUCH AS BODY FLUIDS, TISSUES
> AND ORGANS REMOVED DURING THE COURSE OF THE ABOVE TREATMENT/PROCEDURE WITH PRIVILEGE OF ULTIMATE
> USE AND DISPOSAL RESTING WITH SAID MEDICAL STAFF. I HEREBY ACKNOWLEDGE THAT ALL SUCH BIOLOGICAL
> MATERIALS MAY BE USED FOR THE DEVELOPMENT OF ONE OR MORE RESEARCH, DIAGNOSTIC, OR THERAPEUTIC
> PRODUCTS. I AUTHORIZE SUCH POTENTIAL USE AND DISTRIBUTION AT THE DISCRETION OF UNIVERSITY OF
> WASHINGTON MEDICAL STAFF.
>
> I UNDERSTAND THAT EACH PERSON REACTS DIFFERENTLY TO TREATMENTS/PROCEDURES, THEREFORE, THE
> EXPECTED RESULTS OF SAID TREATMENT CANNOT BE GUARANTEED. THE PHYSICIANS, SURGEONS, OR DENTISTS OF
> THE UNIVERSITY OF WASHINGTON HAVE DISCUSSED TO MY SATISFACTION THE FOLLOWING:
>
>   A.   THE NATURE AND CHARACTER OF THE PROPOSED TREATMENT/PROCEDURE.
>
>   B.   THE ANTICIPATED RESULTS OF THE PROPOSED TREATMENT/PROCEDURE.
>
>   C.   THE RECOGNIZED ALTERNATIVE FORMS OF TREATMENT/PROCEDURE.
>
>   D.   THE RECOGNIZED SERIOUS POSSIBLE RISKS AND COMPLICATIONS OF THE TREATMENT/
>   PROCEDURE AND OF THE RECOGNIZED ALTERNATIVE FORMS OF TREATMENT/
>   PROCEDURE, INCLUDING NON-TREATMENT.
>
>   E.   THE ANTICIPATED DATE AND TIME OF THE PROPOSED TREATMENT/PROCEDURE.
>
> ADDITIONAL COMMENTS: _____
>
> _____
> | | PATIENT INITIAL |
>
> MY PHYSICIAN HAS OFFERED TO ANSWER ALL INQUIRIES CONCERNING THE PROPOSED TREATMENT/PROCEDURE. I
> UNDERSTAND THAT I AM FREE TO DECLINE CONSENT TO THE PROPOSED TREATMENT/PROCEDURE AT ANY TIME.
>
> | HEALTH CARE PROVIDER OBTAINING CONSENT (**PRINT NAME & INITIAL**) | SIGNATURE OF PERSON GIVING CONSENT |
>
> | DATE SIGNED | TIME | ☐ A.M. ☐ P.M. | RELATIONSHIP TO PATIENT (IF APPLICABLE) |
>
> ☐ PLEASE CHECK IF THIS IS A TELEPHONE MONITORED CONSENT.
>   THIS CONSENT WILL BE PERMANENTLY FILED IN THE PATIENT'S MEDICAL RECORD.
>
> PT.NO.   **UNIVERSITY OF WASHINGTON MEDICAL CENTERS**
>   HARBORVIEW MEDICAL CENTER - UW MEDICAL CENTER
>   SEATTLE, WASHINGTON
>   **SPECIAL CONSENT TO TREATMENT**(DIAGNOSTIC & SURGICAL
> NAME   PROCEDURES, ANESTHESIA, MEDICAL TREATMENT & OTHER PROCEDURES)
>
> D.O.B.   * U 0 1 7 3 *
>
> UH 0173 REV FEB 95

FIGURE 29–3 Example of a consent form, which must be signed before surgery.

any surgical client, a large-gauge (e.g., 18-gauge) IV device should be used in case a blood transfusion is necessary during the surgical or postoperative period.

Nasogastric Decompression. For selected surgical clients, a nasogastric tube may be inserted to decompress the stomach and allow removal of its contents. Nasogastric decompres-sion may be necessary for clients who have not been NPO before surgery, such as those undergoing emergency surgery. Nasogastric decompression is also indicated when surgery is performed on the stomach or the intestines.

Bowel Preparation. Enemas, suppositories, laxatives, and oral antibiotics (e.g., neomycin) may be given preoperatively to help clear the colon and reduce the level of endogenous bacteria. This decreases the possibility of intraoperative bowel content spillage, which could lead to peritonitis and other complications. Bowel preparation is most important when surgery is performed on the intestines, but it can be indicated for general abdominal surgery.

Skin Preparation. Preoperative skin preparation removes soil and transient microorganisms from the skin, decreasing the number of resident microbes and the chance of infection. Depending on the type of surgery, the healthcare policy, and the surgeon's preference, the client may need shaving, clipping of body hair, scrubbing of the surgical area, or showering with antimicrobial soap. Usually, the skin preparation focuses on the area that will be involved in the surgery itself and surrounding wide margins. A surgical "prep," or shaving of the hair in the affected area, was a common preoperative procedure a decade ago. Today, most surgeons no longer recommend shaving hair on or near the surgical site, because tiny breaks in skin integrity can increase the risk of postoperative infection. Much literature supports leaving hair at the operative site. However, the necessity for hair removal depends on the amount of hair, the location of the incision, and the type of procedure to be performed. When hair removal is necessary, skillful personnel should perform it as close as possible to the time of surgery and in a manner that preserves skin integrity. Hair clippers and chemical depilatory agents

are less likely to disrupt skin integrity and are the preferred methods of hair removal when absence of hair at the operative site is desired (AORN, 2001).

Preoperative Medications. Medications, such as those to promote relaxation, decrease nasal and salivary secretions, assist delivery of the anesthetic, relieve pain, and promote sedation, are given just before surgery. The trend in recent years has been to give fewer preoperative medications, except for antibiotics. However, it is important to administer any prescribed preoperative medication on time so that maximum effect can be coordinated with the time of surgery.

Whenever medications that can impede cognition are administered, keep the client in bed with the side rails up.

Preoperative Checklist

Many hospitals use a preoperative assessment checklist on the day of surgery to summarize the client's preoperative preparation. These checklists provide such preoperative baseline measurements as level of consciousness, vital signs, and skin integrity and ensure that all information is in the client's record before transport to the operating room. Figure 29-4 is an example of a preoperative assessment checklist. Completing the preoperative checklist is a quick way to show that all client preparation activities have been accomplished and safety measures have been taken. The nurse usually checks off each item as it is completed and then signs the form in the appropriate place.

ETHICAL/LEGAL ISSUE
Informed Consent

Mr. Willis, a 46-year-old man, is brought to your trauma center after a severe accident. He needs surgery to evaluate abdominal trauma and repair multiple fractures. His vital signs have been unstable, and shock is suspected. His wife is notified and enters the emergency room very distraught. The physician is trying to explain the surgery that needs to be performed and get her consent. Mrs. Willis agrees to the surgery, but explains that they are Jehovah's Witnesses and she will not agree to any blood transfusions.

Reflection
- Discuss factors that are significant for Mrs. Willis at this time in making a decision on her husband's behalf.
- Explore how making a decision for next of kin is different and more complex than making a decision for yourself.
- Role play how Mrs. Willis can receive the information she needs to make an informed decision about her husband's surgery, yet support her in the decision-making process.
- Try to verbalize your own feelings when dealing with clients who have cultural or religious beliefs that differ significantly from your own.

🔲 SAFETY ALERT
Make sure that all activities requiring the client to be out of bed (such as showering and voiding before surgery) are accomplished before administering any medications that can alter the level of consciousness. After such medications are given, instruct the client to stay in bed and keep the side rails up to prevent falling and possible injury.

After all preparation for surgery is completed, the preoperative checklist is filled out, and documentation is completed according to protocol, the client is ready for transport to the preoperative care unit.

In the **preoperative care unit,** where the client remains until entering the operating room, final presurgical assessments are completed. The preoperative care unit nurse and the operating room nurse check the following: the client's name band, site and type of surgery, location of valuables, allergies, appropriate dress of the client, surgical consent obtained, NPO status, appropriate records and paperwork, laboratory and diagnostic study results entered on the chart, blood availability, preoperative medication administration, and any additional physician's orders. At this time, IV access and, if necessary, an arterial line may be established. The arterial line provides continual monitoring of blood pressure during the procedure and allows ready access for laboratory studies such as arterial blood gases, hematocrit, and electrolytes. Also during this time in the preoperative care unit, the anes-

PATIENT CHECKLIST / INITIATING NURSE

NPO SINCE	BP	PULSE	RESPIRATION	TEMPERATURE	IV/LOCK	☐ EXISTING ☐ SEE PARENTERAL FLUID SHEET	☐ INITIATED - SEE BELOW
					GAUGE:	SITE: LENGTH: SOLUTION:	AMOUNT:

DENTURES/PARTIALS/BRIDGE WORK ☐ NONE ☐ REMOVED ☐ IN PLACE
HEARING AID/SPEAKING DEVICE ☐ NONE ☐ REMOVED ☐ IN PLACE
EYEGLASSES OR CONTACTS ☐ NONE ☐ REMOVED ☐ IN PLACE
JEWELRY/HAIRPINS ☐ NONE ☐ REMOVED ☐ IN PLACE
MAKE-UP/NAIL POLISH ☐ NONE ☐ REMOVED ☐ IN PLACE
OTHER PROSTHESIS ☐ NONE ☐ REMOVED ☐ IN PLACE
☐ GOWN ONLY
☐ DISPOSITION OF BELONGINGS _____

COMMENTS

☐ I.D. AND ALLERGY BANDS ON PATIENT
☐ ADDRESSOGRAPH
☐ CONSENTS SIGNED AND DATED
☐ LAB / EKG
☐ HISTORY AND PHYSICAL
☐ PHYSICIANS ORDERS
☐ INPATIENT FLOW SHEETS
☐ PROGRESS REPORT
☐ OLD CHART SENT
☐ VOIDED AT ☐ FOLEY

PRE-OP MEDICATIONS	TIME	DOSAGE	INITIALS

ADDITIONAL NURSING NOTES
AUTOLOGOUS BLOOD DONATED: ☐ YES ☐ NO
AUTOLOGOUS ARMBAND IN PLACE: ☐ YES ☐ NO

MEDICATIONS SENT TO OR ☐ YES ☐ NO ☐ NONE ORDERED
FAMILY/SIGNIFICANT OTHER
NAME: RELATION: TELEPHONE NUMBER:
☐ PRESENT
☐ NOBODY AVAILABLE LOCATION: ☐ WILL CALL US ☐ WE NEED TO CALL TRAVEL TIME:
UNIT RN SIGNATURE DATE

PREOP CARE UNIT

TIME IN PREOP HOLDING AREA VITALS ☐ NOT INDICATED BP PULSE O_2 SAT
INDWELLING LINES/TUBES: ☐ NONE ☐ DRAINS ☐ TRACH ☐ O_2 ☐ CHEST TUBE ☐ OTHER:
AWARENESS LEVEL ☐ ALERT ☐ DROWSY ☐ SEDATED ☐ UNRESPONSIVE ☐ ORIENTED ☐ CONFUSED ☐ OTHER:
ANXIETY LEVEL ☐ RELAXED ☐ COOPERATIVE ☐ NERVOUS ☐ TALKATIVE ☐ CRYING ☐ AGITATED ☐ WITHDRAWN ☐ OTHER:
COMMUNICATION LIMITATIONS ☐ NONE ☐ APHASIC ☐ UNCONSCIOUS ☐ HEARING IMPAIRED ☐ BLIND ☐ FOREIGN LANGUAGE ☐ INTERPRETER PRESENT ☐ OTHER:
ADDITIONAL NURSING NOTES
UNIT RN SIGNATURE DATE

OR ASSESSMENT

☐ I.D. AND ALLERGY BANDS ON PATIENT ☐ CONSENTS SIGNED AND DATED ☐ LAB / EKG ☐ CONFIRM CHECKLIST ☐ CONFIRM PLANNED PROCEDURE ☐ CONFIRM SITE
SKIN ☐ WARM/DRY ☐ COLD ☐ RASH ☐ MOTTLED ☐ BRUISED ☐ REDDENED ☐ OTHER:
MOBILITY LIMITATIONS ☐ NONE ☐ CAST ☐ TRACTION ☐ PARALYZED ☐ AMPUTEE ☐ OBESITY ☐ OTHER:
ADDITIONAL NURSING NOTES
AUTOLOGOUS BLOOD DONATED: ☐ YES ☐ NO
AUTOLOGOUS ARMBAND IN PLACE: ☐ YES ☐ NO
AUTOLOGOUS BLOOD HERE: ☐ YES ☐ NO CIRCULATOR SIGNATURE DATE

PT.NO.

UNIVERSITY OF WASHINGTON MEDICAL CENTERS
HARBORVIEW MEDICAL CENTER - UW MEDICAL CENTER
SEATTLE, WASHINGTON
PREOPERATIVE SURGICAL DATA / ASSESSMENT

NAME

U 0 8 3 3

D.O.B.

UH 0833 REV FEB 94

FIGURE 29-4 Example of a preoperative assessment checklist. The nurse sending the client to surgery completes the Patient Checklist section. The nurse in the holding area completes the Preop Care section, providing evidence of continued assessment while the client is awaiting transportation to the surgical suite. The circulating nurse completes the OR Assessment section as preparation for the intraoperative phase.

thesia provider may administer the regional block (spinal or epidural), if appropriate. In the operating room, the scrub person and the circulating nurse are preparing the instruments, supplies, and the operating suite (OR) environment for the individualized needs of the client.

In the preoperative care unit, provide a warm, caring environment and offer appropriate emotional support. In some facilities, a limited number of family members may stay in the preoperative care unit with the client until the client's transfer to the operating room.

Evaluation

While performing interventions in the preoperative phase, continually evaluate the client's response and document it in the client's chart. This information is essential for formulating an individualized plan of care in succeeding phases of the surgical experience. Selected outcome criteria are provided here for each of the general preoperative client goals.

Goal

The client will verbalize understanding of perioperative care.

Possible Outcome Criteria

- During preoperative preparation, the client asks questions about the impending surgical procedure.
- During preoperative preparation, the client describes what will happen during the surgical experience.
- After receiving instruction, client demonstrates effective turning, coughing, deep breathing, and leg exercises and states why they are important in postoperative recovery.

Goal

The client will report a decreased anxiety level regarding surgery.

Possible Outcome Criteria

- During preoperative teaching, the client discusses fears and concerns regarding the surgical procedure.
- After client teaching, the client verbalizes decreased anxiety.
- The client identifies a support system and strategies to use to reduce stress and anxiety imposed by the surgical experience.

Goal

The client will experience adequate control of pain.

Possible Outcome Criteria

- The client reports an acceptable pain level during the preoperative period.
- The client completes presurgical activities without limitation caused by pain.

Goal

The client will demonstrate signs of sufficient rest before surgery.

Possible Outcome Criteria

- The client verbalizes feeling adequately rested on the morning of surgery.
- The client sleeps restfully the night before surgery, as observed by the nurse during the night.

INTRAOPERATIVE NURSING

Nursing Assessment

Assessment continues in the intraoperative period. In addition to planning for the client's intraoperative needs, assessment allows initial planning for the recovery phase. The operating room nurse is responsible for communicating specific assessment data to the recovery facility, so that recovery personnel can anticipate the client's individualized needs.

When the client arrives in the operating room, the operating room nurse reviews the client's record and notes any new physician orders. A brief assessment is conducted to determine the client's physical and emotional status, communication ability, emotional needs, and ability to cope with the planned surgery. Any questions the client may have are identified and answered. Tubes such as IV lines and a urinary catheter are checked for patency.

During surgery, assessment is continuous, because of the client's dynamic condition and the potential for serious complications. Monitor all clients appropriately based on the procedure and the client's condition. Essential assessment parameters include vital signs (blood pressure, heart rate, respiratory rate, temperature), oxygen saturation, electrocardiogram (ECG), and estimated blood loss. Other parameters that may be monitored, depending on the procedure and the client's condition, include arterial and central line pressures, laboratory values (hematocrit, blood glucose level, sodium and potassium levels, arterial blood gases, blood pH, and clotting factors), and urinary output. Continuous monitoring is necessary to detect and treat any abnormalities immediately. These values and any interventions are recorded in the client's medical record.

Nursing Diagnoses and Outcome Identification

Although nursing diagnoses and outcomes vary depending on the client, some common areas are Risk for Injury, Risk for Imbalanced Body Temperature, Risk for Infection, Risk for Latex Allergy Response, and Risk for Perioperative Positioning Injury. Table 29-5 lists possible nursing diagnoses and client outcomes for the intraoperative period.

Nursing Interventions

Nursing interventions during the intraoperative period focus on providing emotional support, ensuring a safe environment and preventing injury, providing anesthesia or monitoring the client during anesthetic administration, maintaining asepsis, and promoting wound healing. Both the scrub person and the circulating nurse carry out these interventions.

Role of the Scrub Person and Circulating Nurse

The **scrub person** wears a sterile gown, mask, headgear, gloves, disposable shoe covers, and eye protection and provides the surgeon with required instruments, sponges, drains,

TABLE 29-5

Selected Intraoperative Nursing Diagnoses and Client Outcomes	
Nursing Diagnosis	**Client Outcomes**
Risk for Perioperative Positioning Injury related to length of surgery and obesity	Client will remain free of positioning-related injury.
Risk for Injury related to equipment, electrical, or physical hazards during surgery	Client will maintain injury-free status during the surgical procedure.
Risk for Infection related to breaches in asepsis or individual risk factors	Client will maintain an infection-free wound site post-operatively.
Risk for Latex Allergy Response	Client will not experience an allergic response from exposure to latex.
Risk for Imbalanced Body Temperature	Client's temperature will remain within 2°F of baseline.

and other equipment, anticipating what will be needed throughout surgery (Fig. 29-5). Anticipation helps to minimize the time the client is anesthetized and the wound is open, decreasing potential complications. Other scrub person responsibilities include preparing the sterile tables before surgery. A thorough understanding of the principles of asepsis, anatomy, tissue care, and the surgical objectives is necessary. The scrub person also must have the knowledge and skills to anticipate needs of other members of the surgical team and the ability to make decisions and perform interventions in an emergency situation (Kane, 2000).

The **circulating nurse** manages client care in the operating room environment and protects the client's safety and health needs (Kane, 2000).

Protection involves controlling the environment for cleanliness, temperature, humidity, and lighting. The circulating nurse ensures that the client's rights are protected and coordinates client care in the operating room. Coordinating activities

of related personnel (e.g., laboratory, x-ray) and monitoring aseptic practices are also the circulating nurse's responsibilities (Kane, 2000). The circulating nurse and the scrub person are responsible for accounting for all sponges and instruments at the close of surgery.

Emotional Support

Providing emotional support for the client in the operating room can be vital to the success of the procedure. Although some clients may be awake only a short time (half an hour or less) before induction of anesthesia, others are awake during the entire procedure. Attempt to elicit the client's cooperation, and make the client as comfortable as possible. Doing so helps the client to tolerate the procedure in a calmer, more relaxed manner, which should result in a better outcome. Providing appropriate information and explanations for each phase of the procedure helps prevent unexpected, stressful surprises and promotes a more relaxed, cooperative environment.

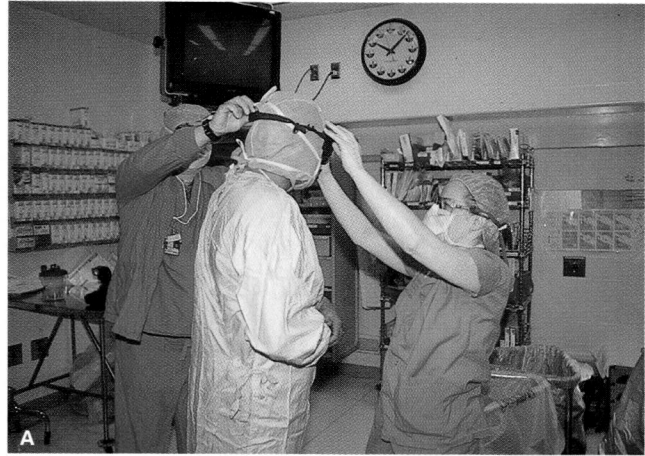

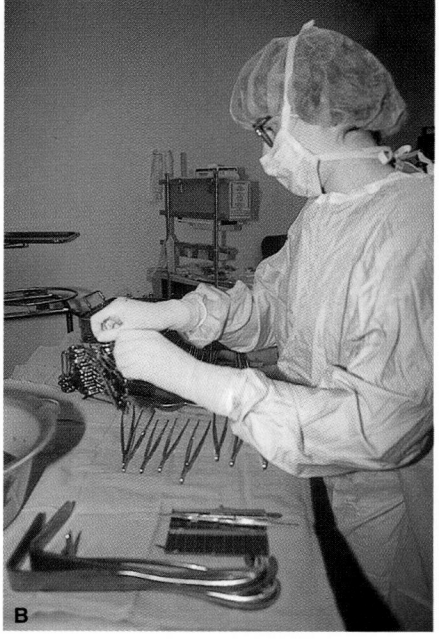

FIGURE 29-5   Safety is maintained for both the client and the operating room personnel. **(A)** U.S. Occupational Safety and Health Administration (OSHA) requirements mandate protective eyewear in addition to masks to protect personnel from splash exposure to blood. **(B)** The scrub person prepares needed surgical instruments.

Providing emotional support for the client's family is equally important. Answer the family's questions, provide them with information on the progress of the procedure, and give more detailed information if indicated and if time permits. Also, let the family know when the procedure is completed, how long the client will be in the recovery facility, and where the client will go after discharge from the recovery facility. For ambulatory clients who are to be discharged home after their surgical procedure, the intraoperative nurse may also be involved in planning for discharge and in discharge teaching.

Client and Staff Safety

Although safety is important in all phases of the surgical experience, equipment safety, electrical safety, chemical safety, radiation safety, client transport and positioning, and continuous asepsis are particularly important in the intraoperative phase.

Equipment Safety. The operating room nurse routinely checks and maintains equipment used during surgical procedures. Safety policies for client care equipment should include the following principles and activities:

- Written procedures for the use of equipment
- Special classes and education for those people required to operate and care for equipment
- Routine, periodic maintenance programs for equipment to meet or exceed the manufacturers' recommendations
- Inspection and testing of equipment (such as connectors, grounding pads, and settings as required) before each use
- Easily accessed, current, written instructional materials for all people required to use the equipment
- Rapidly available professional assistance if equipment problems arise
- Written documentation for the use, settings, and care of special equipment

Electrical Safety. One of the most significant potential hazards to the client in the operating room is electricity. To avoid sparking, all client jewelry is removed or taped before transfer to the operating room. Electrical equipment is used in many surgical procedures. Common devices that rely on electricity include lasers, x-ray machines, electrosurgical units (electrocautery), video equipment, physiologic monitors, microscopes, heart bypass machines, cell savers, blood warmers, heating–cooling blankets, ultrasonic devices, cryosurgery units, and surgical spotlights.

🔲 **SAFETY ALERT**

The most common potential threats to client safety related to electrical devices are electric shock and burns. Appropriate operating room personnel should know how to use the equipment safely, check the equipment for proper functioning, and report and handle problems, especially emergency problems such as fire or explosion. In addition, personnel using electrical equipment should be familiar with the safe use of backup systems should a power failure occur.

Chemical Safety. Chemical safety is another important area of client and staff safety in the operating room. Common hazardous chemicals found in the operating room include ethylene oxide, used for sterilizing purposes (an eye irritant, also potentially explosive and flammable); alcohol, used as a disinfectant (flammable); methyl methacrylate, used as a bone cement (an eye and respiratory tract irritant, also potentially flammable and explosive); housekeeping products used for cleaning and disinfecting (potential eye, skin, and respiratory tract irritants); and various gases (e.g., halothane, nitrous oxide, nitrogen, carbon dioxide), used as anesthetics or fuels for gas-powered equipment (potentially combustible and asphyxiating); (Fortunato, 2000). Personnel working with these chemicals must understand their potential hazards, how to read and follow warning labels, how to use the chemicals safely, how to dispose of them safely, and what to do should an accident occur.

Because of the increase in the number of people who are sensitive to natural rubber latex proteins, perioperative nurses should constantly assess clients for potential risk factors.

🔲 **SAFETY ALERT**

Perioperative nurses should continually assess the operating room environment for products that may contain latex so that they can be removed when a potentially sensitive client is undergoing surgery.

Radiation Safety. Radiation hazards in the operating room may come from the portable x-ray machine, fluoroscopic equipment, diagnostic radiologic devices, radiation implants, and other instruments and compounds used in radiation therapy. Radiation is potentially hazardous because it changes or modifies cells and can lead to genetic defects, thyroid disorders, and cancer.

🔲 **SAFETY ALERT**

All personnel who work with radiation sources must strictly adhere to the policies and procedures set forth by the healthcare facility's radiation safety officer. Such practices include wearing monitoring badges, lead aprons, and other shielding devices. Always maintain a safe distance away from the radioactive source, because the amount of radiation exposure decreases inversely with the square of the distance from the source.

Positioning. Proper positioning of the client is another important safety consideration in the operating room. The ideal position can be defined as the position that provides the best possible exposure for the surgeon, for airway management and monitoring for the anesthetist, and for the client's physiologic safety. The responsibility for positioning is shared by the anesthesia provider, the surgeon, and the circulating nurse.

Proper positioning helps prevent skin, nerve, and muscle damage, which can be temporary or lead to permanent dysfunction. Circulation is altered during surgery because anesthetic agents disrupt normal vasodilation and constriction, reducing perfusion to elevated or dependent limbs and to bony prominences (Fortunato, 2000).

SAFETY ALERT
Use appropriate padding for all body prominences and joints to avoid excessive pressure on the skin and to ensure optimal functioning of the respiratory, nervous, and circulatory systems.

Some common surgical positions are the supine, Trendelenburg, reverse Trendelenburg, lithotomy, sitting, prone, and lateral or side-lying positions. Chapter 33 provides illustrations of selected surgical positions. Clients in each of these positions require special padding or support devices to ensure physiologic safety.

Anesthesia Monitoring

Monitoring the client's status during and after the administration of anesthesia is an important responsibility for the nurse in the operating room and in the recovery facility. Knowledge concerning specific anesthetic agents is essential to focus assessment parameters.

Anesthesia may be classified as general, regional, or local. A **general anesthetic** effectively produces analgesia, relaxes muscles, and results in a sleeplike state. A **regional anesthetic** produces decreased sensation and pain in selected body parts by way of nerve blocks, intrathecal blocks, or epidural blocks. A **local anesthetic** depresses superficial peripheral nerves and blocks conduction of pain impulses from their site of origin.

The administration of general or regional anesthesia may be performed by an **anesthesiologist** or a **certified registered nurse anesthetist (CRNA).** Both of these professionals have specialized education and skills in the administration of anesthetic agents and in monitoring clients during surgical and other procedures. An anesthesiologist is a physician who has specialized education in the administration of anesthesia. Similarly, a CRNA is a registered nurse who has specialized education and certification in the administration of anesthesia. Both professionals are also skilled in managing pain and in placing vascular access lines. The surgeon usually administers local anesthesia at the surgical site.

General Anesthesia. General anesthesia may be administered either intravenously or by inhalation. Inhalation agents (gases) are delivered from the anesthesia machine and tubing by a face mask, endotracheal tube, laryngeal mask airway, or endonasal tube. Some commonly used inhalation agents include nitrous oxide, oxygen, halothane, enflurane, and isoflurane. IV agents can also be delivered through an established vascular access. These agents include barbiturates (thiopental), narcotics (morphine, meperidine, fentanyl), tranquilizers (diazepam, propofol), and phencyclidines (ketamine).

Muscle relaxants are also commonly administered during surgical procedures and are especially beneficial during wound closure. When an abdominal incision is to be closed with sutures, relaxed abdominal muscles allow the wound edges to be approximated (brought together) more easily than when muscles are tense.

Close monitoring of the client is necessary during induction of, maintenance of, and emergence from general anesthesia. Table 29-6 describes the four stages of anesthesia, beginning with induction of anesthesia or analgesia and ending with the toxic stage. The type of anesthesia administered may vary the transition. Clients who are receiving general anesthesia normally go through the first three stages, which are observed by the anesthetist. However, the nurse may assist by taking vital signs, applying cricoid pressure to occlude the esophagus and prevent regurgitation and aspiration of stomach contents, and assisting the anesthetist as needed to maintain the client's airway during intubation and extubation. As the client emerges from anesthesia, the sequence of stages is reversed.

Regional Anesthesia. Regional anesthesia can be a useful alternative to general anesthesia. Instead of placing the entire body in a sleeplike condition, regional anesthesia affects only selected body parts. This type of anesthesia can be used for surgeries of the lower extremities (feet, ankle, knees, hips) and other localized sites, such as the hands and arms. Regional anesthetics are advantageous because they minimize the pulmonary and gastrointestinal complications (pulmonary congestion, atelectasis, nausea and vomiting) that sometimes occur with general anesthetics. A client receiving a regional anesthetic usually recovers more quickly from the anesthetic than a client receiving a general anesthetic. Remember that the client having a regional anesthesia may be awake during the surgery. Therefore, keep any conversation appropriate to the situation. Regional anesthesia may also be used for postoperative pain control. Table 29-7 provides examples of regional anesthesia.

Local Anesthesia. Local anesthesia is actually a type of regional anesthesia. It is differentiated here by the people responsible for administering the agent and monitoring the client. Instead of the anesthetist, the surgeon is usually responsible for administering local anesthetics, and a perioperative nurse is responsible for monitoring the physiologic and psychological status of the client.

Methods used to provide local anesthesia include topical or direct application of an anesthetic agent to the skin or mucosal surfaces and injection of a local anesthetic agent into the areas surrounding the operative site. This type of anesthesia can be used for localized operations, such as breast biopsies, central line insertions, and surgery of the fingers, hands, nose, eyes, or ears. Clients who are candidates for local anesthetics usually are calm, able to cooperate with the surgical procedure, and have no major systemic medical problems. Local anesthesia has the advantages of regional anesthesia, enhanced by decreased cost to the client because some healthcare facilities do not charge for local anesthesia services.

The choice of local anesthesia for a client has many implications for the perioperative nurse. In the absence of an anesthetist, the nurse is totally responsible for monitoring the

TABLE 29-6

Client Responses in the Stages of Anesthesia					
Stage	Reflexes	Heart Rate	Respiration	Blood Pressure	Eyes
I. Analgesia amnesia	Present	Normal	Slow rate Increased depth	Normal	Some dilation Reacts to light
II. Dreams and excitement (frequently bypassed with intravenous induction agents)	Active	Increased	Irregular breathing Breath holding	Increased	Pupils widely dilated and divergent
III. Surgical Involves four planes: plane 2 and plane 3 best for surgery	In progression of loss: Lid reflex Pharyngeal (swallowing) Laryngeal (can tolerate oral airway, suctioning, and then intubation) Gag and corneal reflexes lost	Decreased	Progressively depressed until apneic	Normal to decreased	Early plane: constricted pupils, then slightly dilated and centrally fixed
IV. Toxic Extreme depression	No reflexes	Weak and thready	Completely flaccid	Decreased	Widely dilated pupils

client (Hoffer, 1999). Monitoring includes blood pressure, level of consciousness, respiratory rate, oxygen saturation, skin condition, cardiac rate and rhythm, and maintaining a patent IV access line.

Conscious Sedation. **Conscious sedation** involves the use of IV sedation administered during a surgical or diagnostic procedure to alter the client's conscious state, thereby allaying fear and anxiety (AORN, 2001). Combinations of IV opioids

and sedatives are employed to decrease consciousness but to a degree where the client still can respond to verbal commands and maintain a patent airway (Foster, 2000). Commonly used drugs include morphine, meperidine (Demerol), fentanyl, diazepam (Valium), and midazolam (Versed). Frequently, the nurse is responsible for administering these agents and monitoring the client. Assess each client receiving IV conscious sedation physiologically and psychologically, monitoring for reaction to the drugs. A working knowledge of resuscitation and

TABLE 29-7

Regional Anesthesia		
Type	Definition and Uses	Examples of Use
Topical	The direct application of an anesthetic agent to skin or mucosal surfaces (mouth, throat, nose, cornea)	Often used before injections (nerve blocks, epidurals) or endotracheal tube placement
Nerve or nerve bundle block (local)	The injection of a local anesthetic agent into a nerve bundle or the nerve supply of the operative site	Breast biopsy, lymph node biopsy, ear procedure, cataract extraction, or cornea transplantation
Epidural or peridural	The injection of a local anesthetic agent into the potential space outside the dura	Lower extremity surgery (foot, ankle, knee), lower abdominal procedures, or for postoperative pain relief
Spinal	The injection of a local anesthetic agent into the subarachnoid space	Useful for surgeries below the xyphoid process, or abdominal surgery

monitoring equipment and the ability to interpret the data obtained are crucial (AORN, 2001).

Asepsis

Maintaining asepsis to avoid contamination of the surgical site by microorganisms is the responsibility of all other members of the surgical team. AORN, the professional organization for perioperative nurses, has established guidelines for maintaining asepsis and for sterilization of equipment, instruments, and supplies (AORN, 2001). Display 29-2 highlights these guidelines.

Additional policies and procedures have been established in the operating room to ensure asepsis. Every operating room nurse should be familiar with policies concerning the surgical hand scrub, cleaning and preparation of the client's skin before surgery, special considerations for cleaning the operating room environment and disposing of waste products, procedures for sterilizing instruments and supplies, and methods for draping the surgical client and establishing the sterile field (Fig. 29-6).

DISPLAY 29-2

⑤ MAINTAINING ASEPSIS DURING SURGICAL PROCEDURES

- Keep all items within a sterile field. Resterilize items of questionable sterility. Inspect all sterile packages for damage to package integrity. Protect packages from moisture, tearing, sharp objects, or other threats to the integrity of the wrapping material. In addition, unwrap and dispense according to acceptable sterile procedure.
- Ensure that gowns and gloves used by the scrubbed personnel are sterile and donned correctly. Caution scrubbed personnel to always maintain the sterility of their gowns at the level of the sterile field and their gloves, arms, and hands between the level of the sterile field (table) and the scrubbed person's shoulder level.
- Consider tables and ring stands draped with sterile drapes sterile only at the table level.
- Use drapes impervious to moisture. Consider items dropping over the sides of the table to be unsterile.
- Ensure that scrubbed personnel remain close to the sterile field. Have unscrubbed personnel stay at least 1 foot away from the sterile field. Allow scrubbed personnel to move around a sterile field in such a way as to maintain the sterility of the sterile field.
- Do not allow unscrubbed personnel to move between two sterile fields.

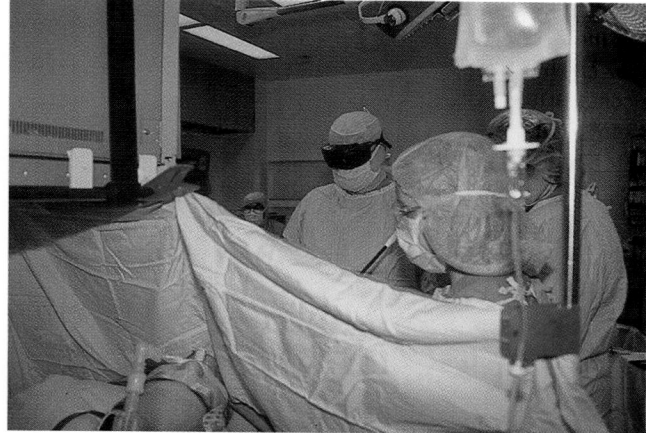

FIGURE 29-6 Proper draping exposes only the surgical site, which decreases infection risk.

Wound Closure

Nurses often assist surgeons in accomplishing wound closure, and they may be directed to remove wound closure devices during the postoperative period. The type of material used for wound closure affects wound healing. In some situations, sutures or staples (or both) are used. For example, a client may have absorbable sutures closing the viscera and staples approximating the wound edges.

Sutures. A **suture** is the material used to sew an incision together. Sutures can be absorbable (e.g., catgut, chromic) or nonabsorbable (e.g., synthetic nylon or polypropylene, silk). Absorbable sutures used in skin closure absorb into the skin so that removal is not necessary. Nonabsorbable sutures used for closing the skin must be removed after the incision has healed. When used internally, nonabsorbable sutures remain in place.

The type of suture used depends on the size and location of the wound being closed, how strong the suture material needs to be for the type of wound being repaired, the desired cosmetic result, and the surgeon's preference. In general, the less suture material used and the smaller the suture size, the better the wound closure. Sutures represent a foreign body that can potentially lead to infections, such as stitch abscesses.

Staples. The use of skin staples is also an effective wound-closure method. **Skin staples** (see Fig. 38-12 in Chapter 38) are made of stainless steel, look like paper staples flat against the skin, and are inserted close to the incision with a staple gun. Skin staples are minimally reactive to the body as a foreign substance and therefore minimize the risk of infection. Use of staples reduces tissue handling and accomplishes wound closure faster than suturing does. Skin staples usually are removed with a staple remover within the first week after surgery, after the incision has healed.

Transport to the Recovery Facility

After the intraoperative phase of the surgical procedure has been completed, the circulating nurse, the anesthetist, and the surgeon safely transport the client to the recovery facility, taking care to maintain the client's airway during this critical time. Each completes written documentation and provides the recovery facility with reports of the surgical experience. The nurses in the recovery facility have been notified of the client's impending arrival and have prepared for the client accordingly.

Evaluation

During the intraoperative period, the results are evaluated and revised as needed. Selected outcome criteria are provided here.

Goal

The client will maintain injury-free status during the surgical procedure.

Possible Outcome Criteria

- The client exhibits no skin injury due to electrical devices or chemicals used during surgery.
- The client evidences no injury from defective or improper use of surgical equipment.

Goal

The client will remain free of signs of positioning-related injury.

Possible Outcome Criteria

- The client maintains full range of motion and adequate sensation postoperatively.
- The client exhibits no signs of nerve or muscle damage from inadequate or improper padding or positioning during surgery.

Goal

The client will experience an infection-free wound site postoperatively.

Possible Outcome Criteria

- The client's wound site is clean and dry without signs of inflammation or purulent drainage within 24 hours after surgery.
- The client's wound site appears well approximated and shows signs of normal wound healing 24 hours after surgery.

POSTOPERATIVE NURSING

Nursing Assessment

Systematic assessment is essential during the postoperative period to detect quickly any complications and to individualize nursing care that promotes optimal recovery from the surgery.

Assessment in the Recovery Facility

The nurse in the recovery facility usually obtains a verbal report from the operating room staff and reads the written documentation of the surgery and the physician's postoperative

orders. To plan care effectively, the following information is needed: type and extent of the surgical procedure performed, type of anesthesia used, dosages and times at which medications were given, amount of blood lost, whether the client is still intubated, and any surgical or anesthetic complications that may have occurred. Knowing whether the client will be an inpatient or will return home after recovery from anesthesia is also important. During the immediate postoperative period, assessments are made frequently (Fig. 29-7). Table 29-8 shows these assessments.

> ### 🛡 SAFETY ALERT
> **Assessment of cardiovascular function is necessary to detect bleeding promptly. Monitor vital signs every 15 minutes, or more frequently if the client's condition warrants.**

Assess respirations during the immediate postoperative period to detect promptly any signs of hypoxia or airway obstruction. Evaluate respiratory rate and depth and pulse oximetry values, which denote arterial oxygen levels, and compare with baseline data. Hypoxia may be first detected as apprehension, anxiety, or restlessness. Loud, irregular respirations may indicate obstruction of the airway, possibly from emesis, accumulated secretions, or client positioning that allows the tongue to fall to the back of the throat.

Assess the electrocardiogram for cardiac rhythm and rate. Evaluate both the blood pressure and the pulse for trends rather than absolute values. Decreasing blood pressure and an increased pulse rate in the postoperative client are significant because they may signify hemorrhage or shock. Certain anesthetic agents and muscle relaxants can also cause hypotension. Also inspect the client's skin for color (e.g., pale, cyanotic), temperature, and diaphoresis (perspiration). Pale, cyanotic, cool, or clammy skin can indicate impaired tissue perfusion, possibly from shock.

Inspect the dressing for drainage. When present, circle the area of drainage on the dressing with a marking pen and note the time. This provides a baseline from which to track the

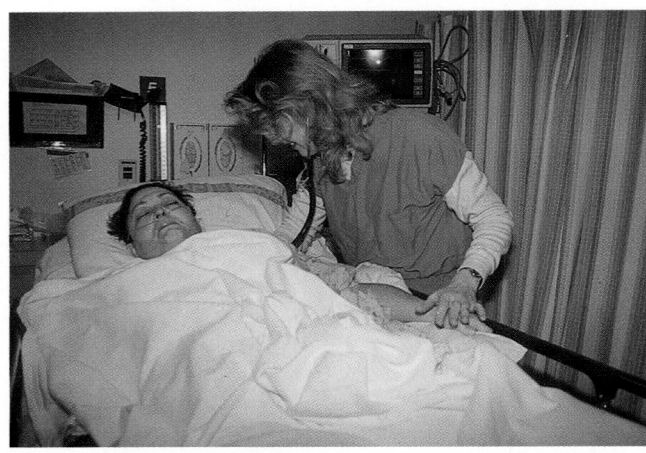

FIGURE 29-7   Close monitoring is needed in the recovery facility.

TABLE 29-8

Assessments in the Immediate Postoperative Period (Recovery Facility)	
Focus Area	**Assessments**
Respiratory	Check airway patency and monitor respiratory rate and depth
	Auscultate breath sounds
	Inspect skin color
	Observe chest expansion
Cardiac	Monitor blood pressure and heart rate and rhythm at least every 15 min
Neurologic	Check pupillary response
	Monitor muscle strength to determine muscle relaxant reversal, if used
Dressings	Monitor for drainage
	Observe for hemorrhage or hematoma formation
Pain management	Assess for both subjective and objective manifestations of pain
	Administer analgesics as appropriate
Renal function	Monitor amounts of urinary output for clients with indwelling catheter (at least 30 mL per hr)
	For clients without a urinary catheter, palpate and percuss for bladder distention or scan with portable bladder ultrasound.

amount of bleeding. When evaluating incisional bleeding, check for drainage under the client, where bleeding may not be readily apparent. Catheters, drains, and chest tubes are also assessed for the amount and type of drainage present. Laboratory values (e.g., hematocrit) may also be requested during this period to help evaluate circulatory status.

APPLY YOUR KNOWLEDGE

Mr. Johnson is admitted to the postanesthesia care unit immediately after surgery for a bowel resection. He is unresponsive to verbal commands but is breathing on his own. Preoperative vital signs are 134/86, 76, 16. Postoperative vital signs for the last 30 minutes are 128/78, 74, 14 and 142/82, 88, 18. What, if any, conclusions can you draw from these assessment data? What additional assessment data would be important for you to collect?
Check your answers in Appendix A.

Perform neurologic assessments to evaluate recovery from the anesthetic agent. Return of reflexes, indicated by swallowing and gagging, occurs when the effects of a general anesthetic are ending. Level of consciousness also changes as the anesthetic agent wears off. Initially, the client is unconscious and does not respond to verbal or tactile stimuli. As the anesthetic agent begins to wear off, the client will respond to loud noises or to his or her name. Finally, the client becomes oriented to person and place. During this period, the client may still appear sleepy and will fall into a sleep when not stimulated.

After regional anesthesia, assess the client for the return of sensory and motor ability. Sensation can be plotted on a dermatome chart (see Chapter 24).

SAFETY ALERT
Autonomic blockade may persist after regional anesthesia, causing severe postural hypotension when the client assumes an upright position (Spitzer, 1996).

Also, assess the client's fluid balance, urine output, and pain level during the immediate postoperative period. When administering pain medication, it is important to document whether pain was relieved and what further measures, if any, were needed. Ensure that all tubes and drains are patent and that all equipment works properly.

Assessment during the Postoperative Period
During the remainder of the postoperative recovery period, systematically assess the client's functional health patterns. Table 29-9 lists possible postoperative complications and appropriate nursing assessments for each area.

Each assessment is individualized based on the client, the surgery that was performed, and the length of time since the surgery occurred. During the first few days after a major surgery, assessments may focus on pain, tissue perfusion, and respiratory function; later in the postoperative course, the client's ability to perform self-care and to manage at home after discharge may be more important. For an ambulatory surgical client, self-care capability is a priority in the immediate postoperative period.

Nursing Diagnoses and Outcome Identification

The overall goal for any postoperative client is to prevent or minimize complications and return the client to optimal functioning. Although the specific nursing diagnoses vary from client to client, Table 29-10 lists some of the more common diagnoses.

Nursing Interventions in the Recovery Facility

The primary responsibilities of the nurse in the recovery facility are assessment and continual monitoring of the client's condition until the effects of anesthesia subside and the client's

TABLE 29-9

Postoperative Assessment of Functional Health

Function	Potential Complication	Assessments
Health perception–health maintenance	Injury secondary to equipment or body positioning or inadequate recovery from anesthesia	Skin, CMS (color, movement, sensation), patent airway, safe environment (side rails up)
Activity–exercise	Hemorrhage/shock	Vital signs, skin color, bleeding from wound, hematocrit, urine output
	Atelectasis	Respiratory rate and depth, breath sounds, color, arterial blood gases, pulse oximetry, temperature
	Deep vein thrombosis	Circulation, calf pain or swelling
	Pulmonary emboli	Respiratory rate and depth, other vital signs, breath sounds
Nutrition–metabolism	Wound infection	Temperature and other vital signs, wound observation for redness, warmth, swelling, and purulent drainage
	Poor wound healing Dehiscence Evisceration	Wound appearance
	Fluid volume deficit	Postural blood pressure and pulse, intake and output, weight, skin turgor
	Nausea/vomiting	Bowel sounds, abdominal distention
	Malignant hyperthermia	Temperature and other vital signs
	Hypothermia	Temperature
Elimination	Urinary retention	Urine output (especially first 8 hours after surgery), bladder distention or discomfort
	Paralytic ileus	Absent bowel sounds, abdominal distention
	Constipation	Lack of stool, abdominal distention, hypoactive bowel sounds
Sleep–rest	Sleep deficit	Sleep duration and quality
Cognition–perception	Pain	Pain level and pain relief after medication, nonverbal indicators
	Confusion	Orientation to person, place, time; level of consciousness
Self-concept	Altered self-concept	Reaction to wound, drains, tubes, and so forth
Roles–relationships	Altered role relationship	Perception of alteration in roles or relationships
Coping	Ineffective coping	Anxiety, stress, and lack of coping
Sexuality	Altered sexual function	Impact on sexuality and sexual function
Values–beliefs	Spiritual distress	Surgery or recovery period effects on spiritual beliefs or values

physiologic status stabilizes. A safe client environment is essential to prevent injury. Family members usually are not permitted in the PACU, but some researchers have challenged this policy, especially for young children. In their experience, the client's anxiety decreased when family members were permitted to visit in the PACU (Leack, 2000).

The PACU nurse maintains a patent airway for the client through positioning, suctioning, and care of the endotracheal tube, if one is still in place. Fluid replacement and blood administration may be necessary to maintain adequate circulating volume. Pain medications are frequently administered to control postoperative discomfort. As the client regains consciousness, encouraging deep breathing and moving improves ventilation and circulation.

For the client to be discharged from the recovery facility to the postsurgical nursing unit, certain conditions must be met. These conditions usually include stable vital signs, patent airway, control of bleeding and wound drainage, normal thermal

state, absence or control of any anesthetic or surgical complications, full or almost full recovery from the anesthetic, adequate respiratory function, orientation to the environment, adequate fluid balance and urinary output, and ability to request assistance if needed (Stoelting & Miller, 2000).

After the client meets the recovery facility's discharge criteria, transfer to the postsurgical nursing unit may occur. The postanesthesia nurse gives a report to the nurse responsible for the surgical client. This report includes the following information: type of surgery performed and the client's tolerance of the procedure, type of anesthesia used, vital signs, IV lines, blood loss, blood and fluid replacement, dressings, tubes and drains, urinary and drainage output, medications administered, level of pain and method of pain control, and any complications that occurred. If family members or friends are waiting in the surgery waiting area, they should be informed that the client is being transferred to another unit.

TABLE 29-10

Postoperative Nursing Diagnoses and Possible Client Outcomes

Nursing Diagnosis	Client Outcomes
Risk for Aspiration related to anesthesia, decreased level of consciousness	Client will maintain a patent airway and remains free from aspiration.
Impaired Gas Exchange related to anesthesia, decreased mobility, pain, pain medications	Client will demonstrate adequate oxygenation of body tissues.
Ineffective Tissue Perfusion related to loss of blood, postoperative edema, anesthetic agents, immobility	Client will maintain adequate circulation of blood to all body tissues.
Deficient Fluid Volume related to loss of fluids during surgery, decreased oral intake, and abnormal postoperative drainage	Client will maintain adequate fluid volume.
Risk for Infection related to surgical wounds, invasive lines, decreased nutritional status	Client will remain free of any postoperative infection.
Urinary Retention related to anesthesia, immobility, and edema	Client will void within 8 hours of surgery and without difficulty thereafter.
Constipation related to anesthesia, pain medication, decreased mobility	Client will resume normal bowel function when normal diet resumes.
Acute Pain related to surgical trauma, inflammation, edema, and invasive procedures	Client will report that postoperative pain is well controlled.
Impaired Physical Mobility related to pain, fatigue, and tubes, catheters, and drains	Client will maintain optimal state of mobility, progressively increasing activity daily.
Anxiety related to pain and separation from family, job, and normal activities	Client will demonstrate adequate coping during the postoperative period.
Deficient Knowledge related to lack of instruction in postoperative activities to prevent complications and promote return to normal function	Client will verbalize and participate in postoperative activities to prevent complications.
Impaired Home Maintenance related to decreased mobility and decreased energy	Client will manage normal daily activities at home with necessary assistance from family and friends.
Delayed Surgical Recovery related to length of surgery, age, chronic health problems	Client will not develop postoperative complications that will delay return to normal activities.
Nausea related to pain medication, anesthetic agents, decreased gut motility	Client will not experience nausea or vomiting during postoperative period.

Discharge from the Ambulatory Surgical Center

Most ambulatory surgical centers have two recovery areas for surgical clients: (a) a traditional recovery area where clients are kept recumbent on stretchers and monitored closely until significant effects of anesthesia have subsided, and (b) an area with recliner chairs where clients are encouraged to ambulate, drink fluids, and eat some solids until they meet all the criteria for discharge.

Recovery from anesthesia is usually much quicker when shorter-acting IV anesthetic agents, such as propofol (Diprivan), are administered. Before discharge from an ambulatory surgical unit (Marley & Moline, 2000), the client should:

- Void (after a spinal or epidural anesthetic or after pelvic surgery)
- Be able to ambulate
- Be alert and oriented
- Have minimal nausea and vomiting
- Require no pain medication within the last hour
- Exhibit no excess bleeding or drainage

Discharge teaching for the client also must be completed, and a responsible person must be available to accompany the client home (Fig. 29-8).

Nursing Interventions on the Surgical Unit

Nursing interventions after the client arrives on the surgical unit build on client teaching during the preoperative period. A brief overview of nursing interventions is provided here; in-depth information is provided in selected clinical chapters throughout this text.

Respiratory Maintenance

Aggressive treatment, especially in the immediate postoperative period, is needed to minimize the risk of atelectasis and prevent possible respiratory complications. Deep breathing

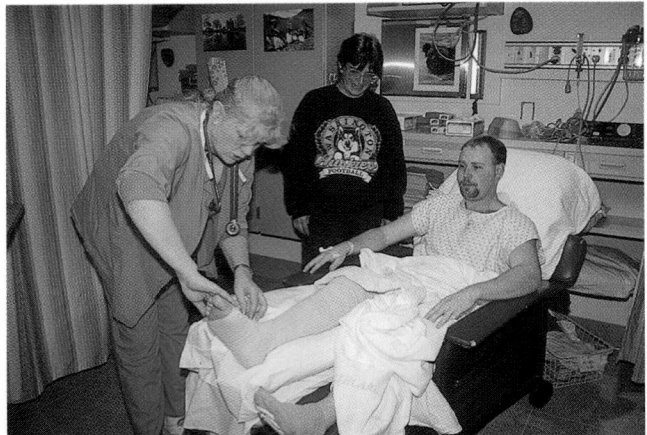

FIGURE 29-8   The client is assessed in ambulatory day surgery to determine whether criteria for discharge have been met. Client and family teaching is an important part of care before discharge in the ambulatory surgery facility.

and coughing, turning and positioning, early and aggressive ambulation, and the use of incentive spirometry are all helpful in preventing postoperative respiratory complications. Refer to Chapter 34 for detailed descriptions of these interventions.

Circulatory Maintenance
Venous stasis resulting from immobility increases the incidence of blood clot formation in the lower extremities. If blood clots lodge in the pulmonary artery (a pulmonary embolus), gas exchange can be severely curtailed and death may occur. Leg exercises, frequent turning and positioning, the use of sequential compression devices and antiembolic stockings, adequate hydration, and early ambulation all decrease the risk of deep vein thrombosis.

Hydration and Nutrition
IV fluids are provided during the postoperative period to ensure adequate hydration until the client can take fluids orally. Fluid volume deficit may occur because of excessive loss of fluids and inadequate fluid replacement. Monitor postural blood pressure on all postoperative clients to detect fluid volume deficits. How long IV fluids will be required depends on the surgery and the client. Before IV fluids are discontinued, normal bowel sounds should be present, indicating that normal intestinal peristalsis has resumed after the surgery. Peristalsis may resume more slowly if surgery was performed on the gastrointestinal tract.

Progressive dietary intake is ordered postoperatively depending on the client's recovery. Frequently, the physician orders "diet as tolerated" (DAT), and the nurse orders the appropriate diet based on client assessment. After peristalsis resumes, a clear liquid diet is ordered, progressively followed by full liquids, a soft diet, and a regular diet. As the diet is advanced, continually assess the client for nausea, vomiting, abnormal bowel sounds, and abdominal distention. Abnormal findings may necessitate a change in diet orders.

Elimination
During the postoperative period, the client is expected to void within 8 hours after surgery. If the postoperative client may be unable to void because of edema, trauma, medications, or the inability to ambulate to the bathroom, an order for intermittent catheterization may be necessary to relieve urinary retention. An indwelling catheter may be indicated for clients undergoing urologic or gynecologic surgery. Urine output should be at least 30 mL/hour during the postoperative period. Urine volumes less than this amount should be reported to the surgeon. When low urine output occurs, challenging the client with increased IV fluid or administering diuretics may be necessary to ensure adequate urine output.

Surgery may also affect bowel elimination. Normal bowel movements are not expected until normal intestinal motility resumes and the client has begun eating. Rectal tubes and return-flow enemas may be ordered to help relieve intestinal gas and promote the passage of flatus. Postoperative constipation may occur because of decreased activity, side effects of medications (especially pain medications), fluid volume deficit, or fear of painful evacuation. When the client has started eating, stool softeners are commonly ordered. Encourage activity, adequate fluid intake, and a diet that promotes normal bowel evacuation. If a bowel movement has not occurred within 3 days after resuming normal dietary intake, laxatives, suppositories, and enemas may be necessary.

Wound Care
Wound assessment, aseptic care of the wound, and monitoring of wound drainage systems are all important nursing interventions. Inspect dressings regularly and note the amount and type of wound drainage. Some surgeons prefer to change the first postoperative dressing, but if the nurse makes the first change, remove it carefully to avoid inadvertent removal of drains. Increasingly, surgeons leave wounds undressed and open to the air to heal. Report symptoms of wound infection (redness, warmth, or purulent drainage) to the physician. Finally, removal of sutures and staples is often the responsibility of nursing personnel.

Mobility and Self-Care
During the early postoperative period, the client may require assistance with mobility and self-care. Encourage the client to increase mobility and independence in self-care progressively to prepare the way for discharge. Early ambulation is indicated for most surgical clients to minimize potential complications. The client usually sits in a chair or may even ambulate for a brief period on the evening of surgery. Administering pain medication before activity and providing instructions on how best to get out of bed will increase client comfort. Encourage the client to ambulate progressively longer distances each postoperative day.

SAFETY ALERT
Always provide standby assistance if the client is weak or unsteady when ambulating. If the client complains of dizziness or feels diaphoretic when ambulating, he or she should return to bed.

Adequate hygiene after surgery is important to ensure client comfort. If the client has many tubes and has had major surgery, a bed bath may be given on the first postoperative day. Wash off any solutions used to prepare the skin before surgery (e.g., povidone-iodine). Remove compression devices and antiembolic stockings at bath time and inspect the skin. Always encourage the client to perform as much self-care as possible. Usually, the surgical client may shower if surgical dressings and IV sites are covered with a protective, waterproof barrier. Care should be taken when the client is showering, however, because the warm water can promote vasodilation and hypotension.

Comfort and Rest

Pain management is an important nursing intervention during the postoperative period. Nonpharmacologic interventions such as positioning, back massage, distraction, and emotional support help the postoperative client feel more comfortable. Pain medications are administered as needed to control postoperative discomfort. Teaching the client to recognize and report pain is an important part of pain management. If the dose, frequency, or type of medication ordered by the physician for pain control is ineffective, notify the physician. Many facilities have a pain service whose staff members routinely see postoperative clients and assist physicians in determining appropriate pain management regimens.

Rest is important to promote healing. Hypnotics and barbiturates may be ordered to help ensure rest. Providing a quiet, comfortable environment encourages sleep and rest. Whenever possible, nursing activities, especially during the night, should be grouped together to allow for uninterrupted periods of rest.

Community-Based Nursing

During the last decade, in-hospital recovery from surgical procedures has been significantly shortened, and an increasing number of surgeries are performed on an ambulatory basis. Much surgical recovery occurs in the client's home, with family or friends assisting in postsurgical care. Discharge needs vary depending on the surgical procedure and the individual client. Whereas many clients are discharged and recuperate in the home, others may need to be transferred to an extended-care facility. Some clients who have sufficiently recovered from their surgical procedure to be discharged home may need the assistance of home care nurses.

Many hospitals and surgical centers have developed special discharge procedures and forms for use when preparing the client for discharge. Discharge concerns for the surgical client include pain management, wound care and dressing changes, monitoring for infection, dietary needs, bowel and bladder function, activity restriction, recommended sexual activity, and ability to perform self-care activities. The client or a responsible caregiver learns to manage any special equipment that is required at home and to perform necessary procedures (e.g., dressing changes) independently. The client needs to know where to buy needed supplies and how to obtain specialized equipment. A limited number of supplies may be given to the client to ensure continuing care until the client can obtain these necessary items.

Include the client's family or caregiver in the client teaching session, as appropriate, and give written guidelines. Such guidelines usually include limitations on activity and diet, treatments, and medications necessary during postoperative recovery, as well as symptoms necessitating notification of the healthcare provider. Use verbal and written instructions for any prescribed medications, and allow time to answer any questions. Provide the client, family, or caregiver with instructions concerning a follow-up appointment with the surgeon, along with a phone number.

Explore with the client what assistance he or she will have after discharge and how he or she plans to manage once home. Asking questions such as, "How do you envision your first few days at home?" may help to identify how the client will cope after discharge. When the identified plan does not seem realistic, help the client explore alternative approaches or encourage the recruitment of family, friends, or community resources for help.

Evaluation

During postoperative evaluation, determine whether goals have been met. Goals and outcome criteria relate to preventing postoperative complications and returning the client to optimal functioning. Table 29-10 lists the more common postoperative nursing diagnoses and outcomes. Outcome criteria for four goals are presented here.

Goal

The client will experience normal bowel function when normal diet orders are resumed.

Possible Outcome Criteria

- The client verbalizes decrease in abdominal (gas) pain.
- The client reports passage of usual bowel movement 24 hours after regular diet resumes.

Goal

The client will state that postoperative pain is well controlled.

Possible Outcome Criteria

- During postoperative period, the client reports that pain does not interfere with turning, positioning, ambulating, or self-care activities.
- The client verbalizes good pain control on oral medications by the time of discharge from acute care facility.

Goal

The client will maintain optimal mobility, progressively increasing activity daily.

Possible Outcome Criteria

- The client sits up in a chair, with the nurse's help, on the evening after surgery.

- The client walks to the bathroom, with the nurse's help, by 24 hours after surgery.
- The client walks 24 feet in the hallway on the day after surgery.

Goal

The client will manage postoperative treatments and normal daily activities in the home with assistance from family and friends.

Possible Outcome Criteria

- The client can state discharge instructions before discharge from the hospital.
- The client or responsible caregiver can demonstrate dressing change and wound drain management before discharge.
- The client can satisfactorily complete activities of daily living with necessary assistance from a responsible caregiver during the first week after discharge.

KEY CONCEPTS

- Perioperative nursing provides individualized care for the surgical client during the preoperative, intraoperative, and postoperative phases of the surgical experience.
- Surgery may be performed in a variety of clinical facilities, including a physician's office, a clinic, an ambulatory surgical center, or a hospital.
- Surgical procedures can affect all areas of function.
- Lifespan considerations are important when individualizing care for the surgical client.
- Preoperative teaching is important to minimize postoperative complications, increase client compliance, and decrease client anxiety.
- Informed consent must be obtained before any surgical procedure is performed.
- Preoperative preparation of the client includes ensuring NPO status, starting IV access, initiating bowel preparation and skin preparation, administering preoperative medications, and, at times, inserting a nasogastric tube.
- Nursing personnel in the operating room provide emotional support, ensure a safe client environment, and maintain asepsis.
- Anesthesia may be administered by an anesthesiologist or by a certified registered nurse anesthetist.
- General anesthesia produces a sleeplike state, whereas regional anesthesia decreases pain and sensation in certain areas.
- Sutures or staples may be used to approximate wound edges and promote healing.
- Continual nursing assessment is important in the recovery facility to detect complications promptly and monitor recovery from anesthesia.
- Nursing care during the postoperative period focuses on preventing surgical complications and promoting optimal return of normal function.
- Potential complications during the postoperative period include hemorrhage, shock, atelectasis, deep vein thrombosis, pulmonary emboli, wound infection, fluid volume deficit, nausea, vomiting, malignant hyperthermia, hypothermia,

urinary retention, paralytic ileus, sleep deficit, pain, confusion, altered self-concept, altered role relationships, ineffective coping, and altered sexual function.
- To prepare for discharge, instructions regarding activity restrictions, incisional care, and symptoms to be reported to a physician should be addressed.

REFERENCES

American Society of Anesthesiologists. (1999). *What you should know about herbal use and anesthesia* [Brochure]. Park Ridge, IL: Author.

Association of periOperating Room Nurses, Inc. (2001). *AORN standards and recommended practices for perioperative nursing.* Denver: Author.

Bailes, B. K. (2000). Perioperative care of the elderly surgical patient. *AORN Journal, 72,* 186–207.

DeFazio-Quinn, D. M. (1997). Ambulatory surgery: An evolution. *Nursing Clinics of North America, 3s,* 357–386.

DeWit, S. C. (1998). *Fundamentals of medical-surgical nursing* (4th ed.). Philadelphia: W. B. Saunders.

Fortunato, N. (2000). *Berry & Kohn's operating techniques* (9th ed.). St. Louis: C. V. Mosby.

Foster, F. (2000). Conscious sedation . . . coming to a unit near you. *Nursing Management, 31,* 45, 48–52.

Hoffer, J. L. (1999). Anesthesia. In M. Meeker & J. Rothrock (Eds.), *Alexander's care of the client in surgery* (11th ed.). St. Louis: C. V. Mosby.

Ireland, D. (2000). Pediatric patients and their families. In N. Burden, D. M. DeFazio-Quinn, D. O'Brien, & B. S. Dawes (Eds.), *Ambulatory surgical nursing* (2nd ed., pp. 613–642). Philadelphia: W. B. Saunders.

Kane, H. L. (2000). In S. Smeltzer & B. G. Bare (Eds.), *Brunner & Suddarths's textbook of medical–surgical nursing* (7th ed., pp. 329–346). Philadelphia: Lippincott-Raven.

Leack, K. M. (2000). In B. V. Wise, C. McKenna, G. Garvin, & B. J. Harmon (Eds.), *Nursing care of the general pediatric surgical patient* (pp. 16–23). Gaithersburg, MD: Aspen.

Marley, R. A., & Moline, B. M. (2000). Patient discharge issues. In N. Burden, D. M. DeFazio-Quinn, D. O'Brien, & B. S. Dawes (Eds.), *Ambulatory surgical nursing* (2nd ed., pp. 504–526). Philadelphia: W. B. Saunders.

Stoelting, R. K., & Miller, R. D. (2000). *Basics of anesthesia* (4th ed.). New York: Churchill Livingstone.

BIBLIOGRAPHY

Adkins, R. B., Jr., & Scott, H. W., Jr. (Eds.). (1998). *Surgical care of the elderly* (2nd ed.). Philadelphia: Lippincott-Raven.

Cuschieri, A., Steele, R. J. C., & Moossa, A. R. (Eds.). (2000). Essential surgical practice, vol. 1 (4th ed.). Oxford, England: Butterworth-Heinemann.

Fortunato, N. (2000). *Berry & Kohn's operating techniques* (9th ed.). St. Louis: C. V. Mosby.

Meeker, M., & Rothrock, J. (1999). *Alexander's care of the client in surgery* (11th ed.). St. Louis: C. V. Mosby.

North American Nursing Diagnosis Association (NANDA). (2001). *NANDA nursing diagnoses: Definitions and classification 2001–2002.* Philadelphia: Author.

Pandit, U. A., & Pandit, S. K. (1997). Fasting before and after ambulatory surgery. *Journal of PeriAnesthesia Nursing 12,* 181–187.

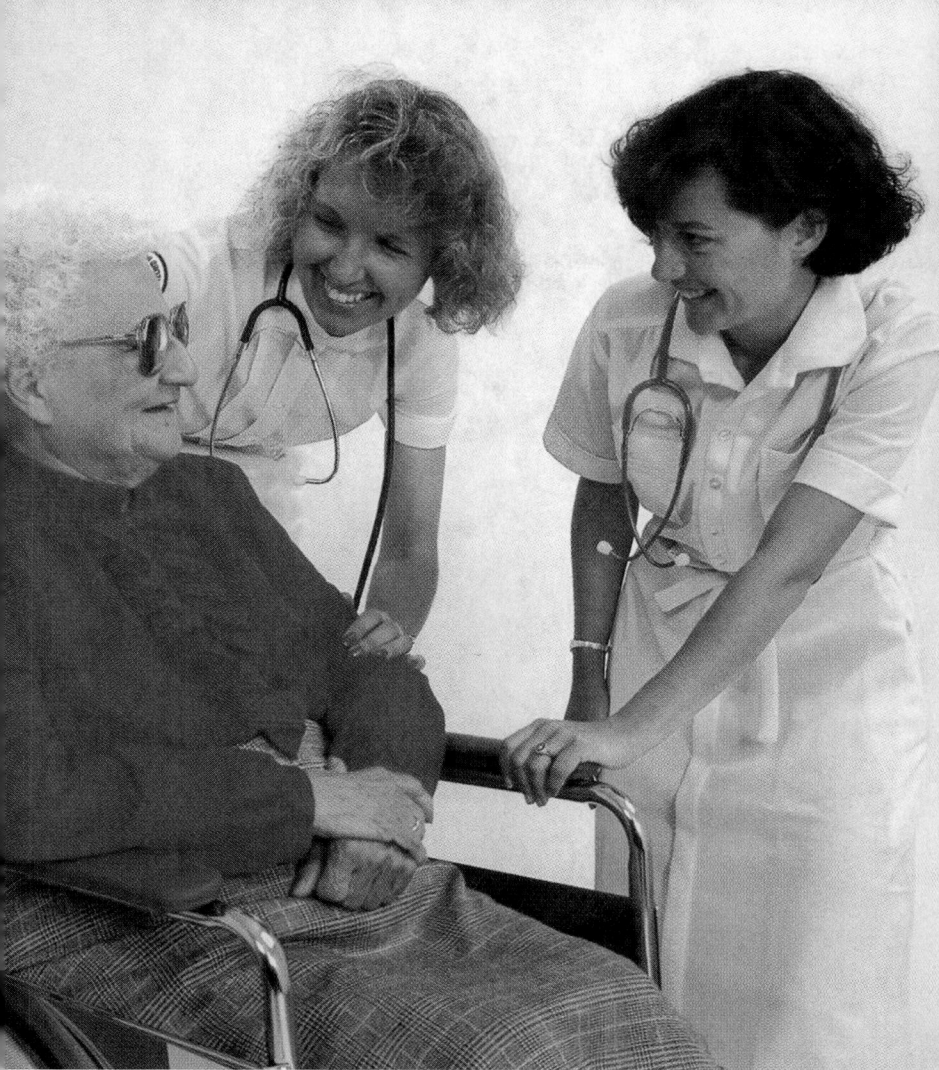

Human Function and Clinical Nursing Therapeutics

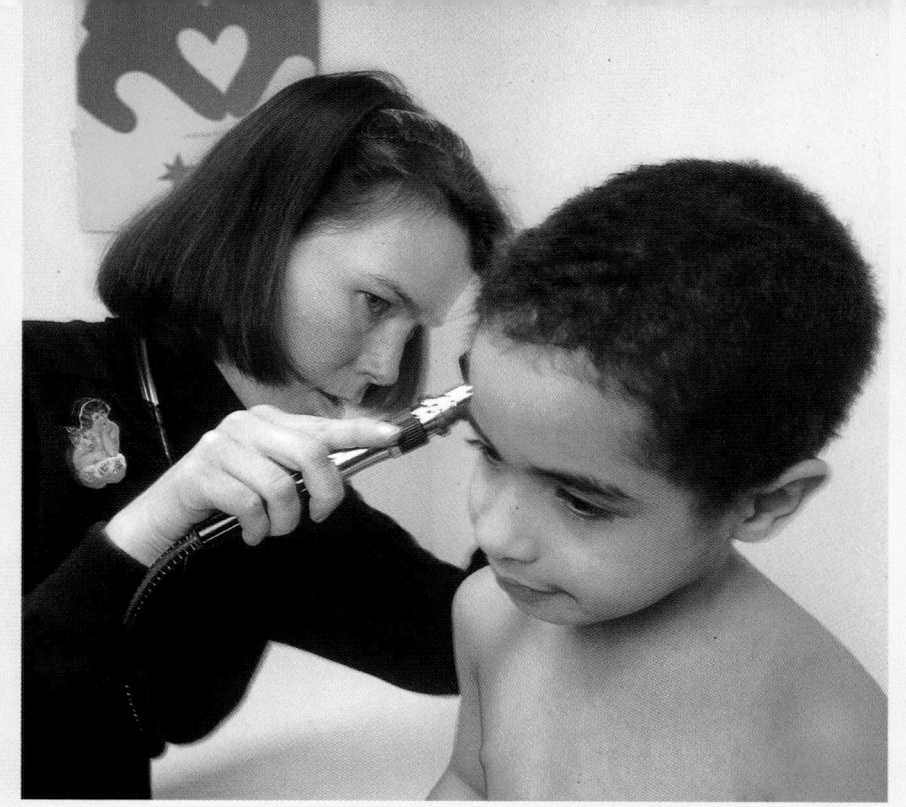

Health Perception and Health Management

30 Safety

⌐ Key Terms

asphyxiation
burns
electrical shock
falls
ground

nosocomial infections
poisoning
pollution
restraints
suffocation

⌐ Learning Objectives

Upon completion of this chapter, the student will be able to do the following:

1. Recognize the importance of safety in the home and healthcare environments.
2. Relate special safety considerations to specific developmental stages.
3. Identify factors that affect safety and describe common manifestations of altered safety.
4. Identify individual safety patterns through assessment.
5. Using assessment, identify people at risk for safety dysfunction.
6. Characterize the appropriate nursing diagnoses for altered safety.
7. Discuss teaching topics and nursing interventions to promote safe homes and healthcare environments.
8. Identify nursing interventions for altered safety.

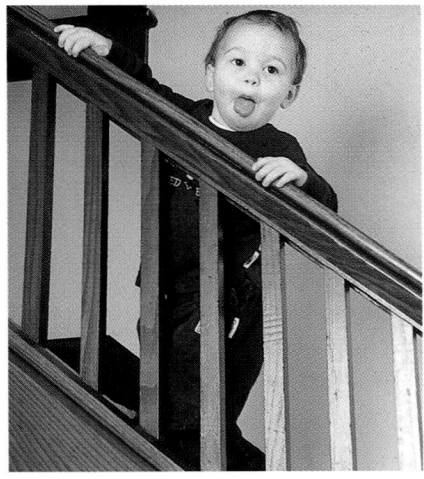

⌐ Critical Thinking Challenge

You are a nurse in a pediatric primary care clinic conducting a well-child assessment for an active toddler and his young mother. As you discuss the home environment, the mother tells you that they live in a two-story house with bedrooms on the second floor and the other rooms on the main floor. The mother tells you that the toddler climbs up and down the stairs and on chairs, gets up on counters and table tops, and is very curious about boxes and bottles of all types. The mother seems tired and somewhat irritated as she tries to hold the toddler still on her lap. He is fussing and struggling to get down.

Once you have completed this chapter and have added safety to your knowledge base, review the above scenario and reflect on the following areas of Critical Thinking.

1. List and analyze your immediate impressions of this family. Describe how you think the mother feels at this time.
2. Propose how you will proceed with your assessment of the mother, toddler, and home environment.
3. Summarize additional information you need to provide further anticipatory guidance to this family.
4. Plan methods for improving the toddler's safety.
5. Reflect on how you can follow up with the mother and her coping strategies.

Unintentional injuries were the fifth leading cause of death in the United States in 2000, exceeded only by heart disease, cancer, stroke, and chronic obstructive lung disease (National Safety Council [NSC], 2001). In that same year, unintentional injuries were the leading cause of death among people age 1 to 38 years. The leading causes of unintentional injuries in 2000 were motor vehicle incidents; falls; poisonings by solids or liquids; drownings; fires, burns, and fire-associated injuries; suffocation by ingested object; and firearms (NSC, 2001). For minority populations, unintentional injuries took an even greater toll. For instance, among Native Americans, unintentional injuries were the second leading cause of death for men and the third leading cause of death for women in 1999 (U.S. Department of Health and Human Services, 2001).

Unintentional injury incidents may result in permanent disability, pain, emotional distress, and financial hardship. Approximately 25% of those who suffer a nonfatal injury seek medical attention or endure at least 1 day of activity restriction from the injury (NSC, 2001).

Safety is important on every level of human interaction. Teaching and applying the concepts of safety are part of a seamless approach to injury prevention, regardless of setting. Safety is an individual, community, national, and worldwide concern.

A truly danger-free environment is rare. Consequently, safety promotion involves awareness and implementation. Traditionally, nursing's realm of safety care involved only the hospital environment. Today, however, nursing care is broad and specific. Not only is maintaining a safe healthcare environment one of the nurse's most important roles, but so is teaching the client and family about safety precautions at home, in the workplace, and in the community. The healthcare environment no longer refers solely to an inpatient hospital facility. It includes hospice and home care, assisted living settings, senior centers, and school health clinics, to name a few. Nurses work in many different environments, some of which are hazardous. They must minimize their own potential for injury. Safety habits for both clients and nurses will ensure an optimal therapeutic environment and promote health.

NORMAL SAFETY

The science of injury control has emerged in recent years to address the components of safety hazards that contribute to nonfatal and fatal injuries. The term *accident* is no longer used in discussing injury prevention, because "accident" implies an event that occurred as a random act of God or bad luck, was unforeseeable, and therefore was unpreventable. Unlike accidents, injuries have recognizable patterns of occurrence with corresponding controls. The principles of injury control include education about safety hazards and prevention strategies; engineering and environmental controls (active or passive safety features that may prevent injury from product or equipment use); and enforcement of regulations to mandate changes among manufacturers, retailers, employers, workers, and product users.

Active safety features are devices that rely on a person's behavior to derive their benefits. Passive or automatic safety features are devices that are engineered into a location, machine, or piece of equipment and do not require specific human behaviors to become activated. Air bags in automobiles, guard rails, and electrical fuses and circuit breakers are examples of passive safety features. Passive safety measures work better than active ones do: That is, where possible, engineering works better than education (Glass, Segui-Gomez, Graham, 2000; McLoughlin & Fennell, 2000).

Safety and security are basic human needs, second in priority only to physiologic needs in Maslow's hierarchy (Maslow, 1970; see Chapter 4). Safety not only prevents harm and injury but also allows people to feel secure in their actions. Safety reduces stress, promoting general health. Safety allows people to meet other basic human needs, such as love, belonging, and self-esteem, and to accomplish personal goals. A positive outlook on life, in turn, results in better mental health and more effective functioning.

Characteristics of Safety

Pervasiveness
Safety is pervasive, affecting everything. Subconsciously, people are concerned with safety in all their activities, including eating, breathing, sleeping, working, and playing. Consciously, people assume or neglect responsibility for their own safety.

Perception
A person's perception of danger influences his or her incorporation of safety into daily activities. Safety measures are effective only insofar as a person accurately understands and perceives hazards. Humans do not innately understand safety factors, but they learn them from others throughout life. Maturity brings a recognition of possible dangers and a realization of the importance of practicing safety. Parents, teachers, healthcare workers, and laws contribute by increasing the level of knowledge and awareness of safety concerns and the principles of injury control.

Management
Once a person recognizes dangers in the environment, he or she takes measures to prevent those dangers and thus practices safety. Prevention is a major characteristic of safety. Self-care is involved in safety practices, but safety for others should be provided as well.

Lifespan Considerations

Safety concerns are individualized to fit developmental stages. The diverse physiologic and psychological capabilities and encounters with various safety hazards across the lifespan put different age groups at risk for different injuries. Interventions must be geared toward specific age-related concerns.

Newborn and Infant

Because they lack life experience and musculoskeletal and neurologic maturity, newborns and infants are susceptible to burns, falls, choking, and other traumatic injuries. Their thermoregulation capability is immature, and their ability to satisfy basic needs depends on inarticulate cries and nonverbal communication. With limited ability to respond to environmental challenges and no clear method of communication, newborns and infants depend on their caregivers to create safe environments for normal, injury-free growth and development. Providing such safety is a major task of parenting.

Babies explore by pulling things and placing almost everything in their mouths. Cords, tablecloths, plastic bags, bottles, and cans are tempting and dangerous objects for exploration that caregivers must strive to keep out of reach. A safe environment for newborns and infants also includes a comfortable temperature range; nonrestrictive, nonflammable, adequate clothing; warm bath water; clean air; safe toys; guard rails at staircases and steps; protection with locked, padded rungs or rails for cribs or changing tables; covered electrical outlets; and appropriate car seats for automobile travel (Fig. 30-1).

Toddler and Preschooler

Falls, bumps, and bruises are common during these ages of curiosity and exuberance. Increasing mobility, lack of life experience, and still immature musculoskeletal and neurologic systems are potentially hazardous for toddlers and preschoolers. Caregivers must anticipate the wide-ranging interests of their young explorers. Once upright, toddlers can reach up to new sources of interesting items. Curiosity still reigns; pets and other animals become new, moveable objects of exploration. Life

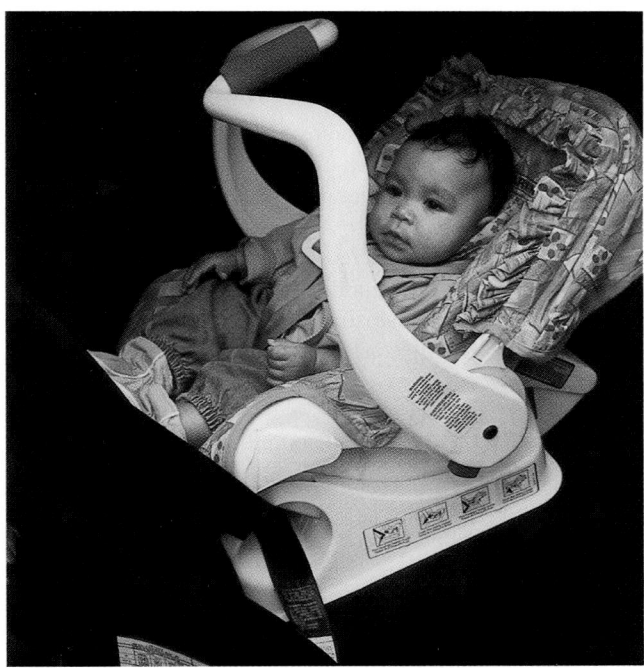

FIGURE 30-1 Car seats are an important safety measure for caregivers of children to practice. The seat must be appropriate for the child's age and size.

experiences begin to accumulate, however, and learning safe and dangerous behaviors begins. Setting a safe example is an important first step for caregivers of toddlers and preschoolers.

Improving eye–hand coordination and increasing strength and speed characterize these developmental stages. Toddlers and preschoolers delight in opening and closing doors, turning knobs, climbing furniture, and engaging in all sorts of active play. Although these young children usually are able to communicate their basic needs in words or actions, caregivers must still ensure a comfortable environmental temperature; adequate, nonflammable, nonrestrictive clothing; and warm bath water. Bathtubs should have nonskid mats or decals to prevent slipping when standing up.

Toddler toys must be sturdy, without sharp or rough edges, and free of small, removable, or breakable parts that could be swallowed or could damage an eye. Toddlers and preschoolers usually enjoy tricycles, push cycles, rocking horses, and other active toys that use large muscle groups. Children should use such toys under adult supervision until they understand safety limits. Toddlers need guard rails at staircases and steps.

As the transition to preschool occurs, children begin to learn safety rules and gain better motor control. Preschoolers usually can avoid bumps and learn to climb safely up and down stairs. Preschoolers also benefit from learning about safety zones, which are safe places to stand or sit when a potentially dangerous activity is underway. For instance, a kitchen should have a safety zone where children may watch activity but are out of reach of the stove, oven, and knives.

Outside the home, toddlers and preschoolers need supervision. With caregiver guidance, they will learn about playing out of the way of automobile traffic and avoiding strange animals. Car seats are necessary for travel in motor vehicles.

Preschoolers learn the rules of safe social interaction by trial and error. Striking out and aggression that may occur usually result from the natural exuberance of this stage rather than any malicious intent. Caregivers, however, can help their preschoolers by teaching cooperation and sharing. This also is the age at which caregivers should encourage caution toward strangers. Some law enforcement agencies recommend identification bracelets, fingerprinting, and frequent photographs.

Fire safety is a family concern when children reach this age. Learning about matches, electrical cords, stoves, and ovens is important for curious preschoolers who might be tempted to experiment. The whole family should regularly practice crawling on the floor, using escape routes, and having a meeting place outside the home in case of fire. Local fire departments often have useful information about planning alternative escape routes and other safety procedures.

School Age Child and Adolescent

Physiologic maturity is almost complete for school-age children. Motor control of large muscles and rapidly developing fine motor control enable them to accomplish complex tasks. Learning occurs at an astounding rate. Life experiences accumulate, and children use them to make judgments about the appropriateness of behaviors. Their expanding world demands flexible responses and presents opportunities for independent action.

School-age children can make their needs known verbally. Their usually quick reflexes help to protect them from burns, falls, and other unintentional traumatic injuries. New activities require new skills, and children of this age group may learn to ski, ride horseback, swim, bicycle, sail, or participate in team sports. Safety precautions are important. Children should wear helmets when cycling, riding, or playing contact sports and life jackets when sailing or boating. All children should learn to swim or at least float and tread water. The buddy system is an important outdoor and water safety strategy. The buddy system is a prearranged agreement between two or more people to provide mutual companionship and to monitor each other's whereabouts and well-being during certain high-risk activities. The buddy system is also used in many occupational settings.

Safe examples from adult caregivers continue to influence school-age children. A home environment in which alcohol is used in moderation; guns, if any, are kept locked away; and discussion rather than force is used to resolve conflicts demonstrates safety habits that children will need in later years. On a family farm where children participate in many work activities (including use of dangerous equipment), adults must also teach their children safety skills and demonstrate safe work habits.

Growth and development spurt during adolescence. Physical maturity of the musculoskeletal system is nearing completion, and the nervous and cardiovascular systems are fully mature. Adolescents have a physiologic need for more sleep during this time of accelerated growth and development (Wolfson & Carskadon, 1998). Sleep deprivation as a result of trying to balance many activities can compromise safety. While life experience is accumulating rapidly, so are new responsibilities. Autonomy develops in response to social and societal pressures. Driving a car, coping with drugs, beginning to explore sexually, babysitting, working after school, and developing expertise are activities that require judgment and independent action. As they explore opportunities, adolescents may know that certain behaviors are unsafe, but social pressure may persuade them to act against their better judgment. Experimentation is also a common trait of adolescents in order to explore their limits and capabilities. Supportive families who allow discussion and expression of conflict provide safe home environments. Increasingly, schools are developing programs on violence prevention to teach teens constructive methods for solving problems and disputes.

Adult and Older Adult

With physical maturity complete, adults move at will in a world full of potential dangers. Unintentional injuries at home, in the workplace, and during sports are common. Safety habits may become rusty, and overconfidence or ignorance can place adults in danger's path.

Between 1986 and 1996, motor vehicle deaths decreased by 110%; however, motor vehicles continue to be the major cause of unintentional injury deaths for all age groups up to 80 years (NSC, 2001). Use of safety belts with shoulder harnesses is mandatory in most states, as is the use of helmets when riding motorcycles. Many cars are equipped with air bags for increased safety.

Boaters, hikers, skiers, hunters, and mountain climbers are lost every year when they travel alone. For such outdoor enthusiasts, the buddy system continues to be the best safety measure. Every sport has experts who can share safety information with beginners, often through clubs or associations.

Advancing age entails some loss in physical function and usually in acuity of sensory–perceptual function. Older adults may have impaired eyesight and hearing and decreased proprioception and sensitivity to touch. The ability to thermoregulate may be impaired; older adults are at higher risk than younger adults for hypothermia and heatstroke (Ramsey & Kernvitz, 1998). Reflex responses slow, and the musculoskeletal system may lose flexibility and strength. Various conditions, such as arthritis, osteoporosis, or congestive heart failure, may limit the ability to endure sustained physical activity. Medications taken to control conditions such as high blood pressure or Parkinson's disease may result in orthostatic hypotension and the potential for falling. Some older adults experience cognitive impairment, with severity ranging from mild memory loss to dementia that prevents safe independent living. The principles of a safe environment for older adults follow the same general guidelines as for all ages: comfortable temperature range; adequate clothing; bath water of the right temperature (the setting on the hot water heater may need to be turned down); adequate ventilation; lighting that allows for safe navigation throughout the house at all times of day; nonskid surfaces on stairs, in the kitchen, and in the bathroom (throw rugs should be removed); and stable supports for climbing (firm stair rails, grab bars if needed).

FACTORS AFFECTING SAFETY

Physiologic Factors

The complex physiologic systems of the human body normally work together to allow a person to avoid or minimize injury. For example, reflexes withdraw the hand from the flame before conscious thought can do so. A loud noise causes a startle reaction and an immediate increase in level of alertness. The sensation of pain provides important feedback that an activity or situation is dangerous. Impairments to various systems can affect the body's overall capacity to help maintain safety.

Musculoskeletal System

Musculoskeletal integrity is essential for normal posture and movement. Disruption inhibits mobility and the ability to respond to hazards, and it increases the risk of unintentional injuries. Musculoskeletal alteration that impairs safety can result from fractures, osteoporosis, muscular dystrophy, arthritis, or strains and sprains.

Neurologic System

Peripheral nerves sense hazards in the environment. The spinal cord relays impulses that allow the reflex arc to function. The brain coordinates activities, processes information, and initiates responses. Complex cognitive and perceptual functions, such as judgment, orientation, and socially appropriate behaviors, depend on the accumulation and accurate interpretation of information. The abilities to think clearly, to recall past problems and solutions, to imagine feasible solutions to current problems, and to solve problems are cognitive functions needed to promote safety. The perception of danger based on past experience and accumulated knowledge also is essential for promoting safety. Neurologic impairment, which may alter these abilities and thus impair safety, can result from head injury, medications, alcohol and drugs, stroke, spinal cord injury, degenerative diseases (e.g., Parkinson's disease and Alzheimer's disease), or brain tumors.

Cardiovascular and Respiratory Systems

Functioning cardiovascular and respiratory systems provide oxygen and nutrients to the rest of the body as needed for quick response. Cardiovascular dysfunction that may impair safety can result from hypertension, congestive heart failure, congenital cardiac anomalies, or peripheral vascular disease. Respiratory illnesses that contribute to shortness of breath, wheezing, and fatigue cause a diminished tolerance for activity, limit mobility, and, in turn, impair safety.

Activity and Exercise

Activity and exercise condition the body to react quickly in an emergency. Deficient activity and exercise may impair the ability to protect oneself from outside hazards.

Fatigue

Fatigue can cause poor perception of danger, faulty judgment, and inadequate problem solving. Careless driving, irresponsible taking of medication, and inadvertent overexposure to sunlight are possible results. Fatigue arises from poor sleep habits, lifestyle patterns, work schedules, stress, or a variety of medical or other unknown conditions.

Coping and Stress Tolerance

Factors such as anxiety and depression alter one's ability to perceive hazards, express concerns, and follow safety precautions. For example, a person may be anxious about a surgical procedure and may not process information about postoperative procedures and home care. The result could be injury or complications after surgery. Coping mechanisms a person uses in times of stress have a direct relationship to safety. Personality factors may play a part in responsiveness. Impulsiveness, distrust, or shyness may affect safety promotion. Psychological factors may be inborn or learned, or they may result from mental illness.

Environmental Factors

Home

A safe home environment features adequate ventilation, a reliable heating system, nonskid bathtub surfaces, well-maintained electrical appliances and electrical cords, sturdy stepstools and

ladders, and careful labeling, handling, and storing of all potentially toxic substances. Guns are safely locked out of children's reach. Foods and medications are discarded on their expiration date. Fire escape routes are practiced. Smoke alarms function and are strategically located. Outdoor areas have effective lighting, maintained fences, and proper security for potential hazards (e.g., swimming pools). Family members use personal protective equipment, such as earplugs and eyewear, when operating power equipment (e.g., saws, lawn mowers).

Hazards in the home include poorly lighted stairways, throw rugs, slippery floors, cluttered areas, and unstable ladders, all of which can cause falls. The risk of falls is compounded when an aged person or a person with impaired mobility encounters these hazards. Other home hazards include poorly secured medications, household cleansers and other hazardous chemicals; guns left within children's reach; careless smoking; and lack of supervision of children. People are often unaware of the hazards in their homes until an injury occurs. Display 30-1 presents a summary of possible home hazards.

Workplace

Health and safety hazards and risk of injury are inherent in many jobs. Examples of exposures for some occupations include noise, hazardous dusts (e.g., asbestos, lead, coal) and chemicals, working at heights, dangerous machines, biologically infectious agents, and violence. Ergonomic hazards, such as heavy lifting and repetitive motion, also contribute to many disabling injuries. Other dangers result when employers or workers do not follow safety precautions, such as wearing protective gear and following safe work practices.

The Occupational Safety and Health Administration (OSHA) requires employers to provide their workers with a safe and healthy work environment (Occupational Safety and Health Act, 1970). An employer must identify hazardous conditions and exposures present in the workplace, inform workers of their presence, and educate them about the preventive strategies necessary to avoid injury. OSHA also investigates worker complaints about health and safety issues (Occupational Safety and Health Act, 1970).

Community

The community in which one lives, works, shops, and plays may present safety concerns. Noise (e.g., from trains or planes), air pollution, crime, poor lighting, presence of hazardous waste sites or landfills, busy intersections, dilapidated houses, cliffs, and unprotected creeks are hazards. The community should be free from most of these hazards to lend a feeling of safety and security.

The level of sanitation affects a community's safety. Sanitation includes a clean water supply, an adequate sewage system, absence of insects and rodents, and refrigeration of food supplies. Lack of sanitation may result in increased spread of disease and infection. Sanitation may be lacking in impoverished or poorly developed areas.

DISPLAY 30-1

POSSIBLE HOME HAZARDS

- Poor lighting inside or outside
- Uneven walking areas
- Steps with broken concrete
- Steps without hand rails
- Loose mats on steps
- Cluttered steps or clutter near head of stairs
- Slippery tub or shower
- Extension cords across open spaces where people may trip
- Throw rugs on slippery floors
- Folding chairs and cribs that are not properly balanced or secured in place
- Insecure stools or stepladders
- Standing on chairs rather than stools or stepladders
- Items placed precariously on closet shelves
- Bookcases or heavy pieces of furniture that might topple
- Defective smoke detectors
- Oily or dirty rags near heat source
- Stacks of old newspapers or boxes in basement or garage
- Flammable liquids in illegal containers
- Items placed too close to the heat source of the kitchen stove
- Loose-fitting clothes worn while cooking
- Water temperatures that are too hot

- Defective wiring
- Overloaded outlets or frayed cords
- Smoking in bed or alone at night in living room
- Electrical appliances in the bathroom, where they may fall in the bathtub or sink
- Obstructed doorways or pathways in case of fire
- Many medications, or unlabeled medications, in medicine cabinet
- Unlocked cupboards or cabinets with potential poisons
- Improper use of pesticides or other chemicals
- Presence of cracked or peeling lead-based paint
- Poisonous plants where children can reach them
- Unsafe sexual practices
- Pets that may harm children, older adults, or visitors
- Cigarette smoking in a closed area in the presence of nonsmokers
- Plastic bags where children may find them
- Cribs near windows or near Venetian blind cords
- Unsupervised children in the bathtub
- Poor hygiene, especially in the bathroom and kitchen
- Improper food preparation
- Rodents or insect infestation
- Guns improperly stored and locked

Healthcare Setting

The healthcare environment contains many potential hazards. Falls, fires, and poisonings occur because of problems with equipment, procedural errors, and impairment of clients. Examples of equipment problems include a wheelchair with nonlocking wheels that causes a fall when the client attempts to sit down and a malfunctioning heating pad unit that causes a fire. The frequent use of oxygen in client care areas increases the risk of fire; therefore, smoking is prohibited wherever oxygen is in use. Many healthcare sites have adopted totally smoke-free environments to promote safety and health. Procedural errors, such as failure to check client identification bands before administering medications or forgetting to monitor intravenous (IV) infusion rates, may harm clients as well. Clients may suffer falls or burns because they are impaired by medication that causes central nervous system depression; sensory dysfunction, such as blindness or hearing loss; decreased mobility due to musculoskeletal or neurologic illness; language or other communication barriers; or confusion due to mental or physical illness.

Healthcare facilities have developed procedures and policies for client care and equipment operation to minimize hazards. Facilities should review these measures periodically to promote the safety of clients and staff. Nursing assessment of factors that put clients at risk for injuries should help identify safety concerns and the precautions necessary to minimize risks.

Healthcare workers must also be aware of the risks to their own safety in any healthcare environment. Common risks include exposure to bloodborne pathogens from needlestick injuries, back injuries as a result of heavy lifting, and potential adverse reproductive outcomes as a result of overexposure to antineoplastic medications. Threats of violence and assaults from clients and visitors have also emerged in recent years as a serious hazard for healthcare workers (Anderson & Stamper, 2001; Runyan, 2001; Worthington & Franklin, 2001). More assaults occur in healthcare and social service industries than in any other; and such violence continues to increase (U.S. Department of Labor, 1996). All hazardous exposures or conditions require some type of intervention to protect workers. Training regarding strategies for prevention is essential. Use of safer needle devices can prevent needlesticks. Proper lifting devices can prevent back injuries. Chemical exposures often require the use of some type of personal protective equipment and special handling procedures. Controls to prevent violence in the healthcare setting may include use of alarms, increased security measures, improved lighting, and increased staffing.

Temperature

The temperature of outdoor and indoor environments affects safety. Extremes in temperature and other climate conditions (e.g., wind, humidity, snow, rain, ice) present hazards. Inappropriate dress or protection against these conditions increases safety risks. Indoor thermoregulation problems may result from inadequate finances or lack of help maintaining a heating or cooling system in the home.

Pollution

Pollution is the presence of harmful or unnatural substances in the air, water, or land. Such toxic substances, which are frequently byproducts of manufacturing, increase risks of cancer. Air pollution increases the risk for and severity of respiratory problems, such as asthma and chronic bronchitis. Poor air quality due to pollution often increases allergic symptoms. Polluted water may lead to the spread of disease and infection, either from the direct effects of drinking contaminated water or from contamination of the food supply. Noise pollution from airplanes, trains, heavy automobile traffic, loud music, or public stadiums may harm people by increasing stress and blood pressure levels and by contributing to hearing loss.

Radon, a gas resulting from natural radioactive decay processes, has been linked to lung cancer and may be present in excess in many homes (Environmental Protection Agency [EPA], 1993). The website for the EPA has many resources available for consumers and professionals alike (EPA, 1998). Increasing government and public awareness of environmental health issues has led to many cleanup programs for known pollutants and health and safety guidelines to prevent further pollution. Safety and health risks from pollutants may be hidden for many years after their emission into the environment.

Electrical Hazards

Electrical hazards can be found in all settings. Overloading outlets, using appliances with frayed cords, and allowing infants or children to play with plugs or near electrical outlets may result in electrical shock or burns. New parents may be unaware of these household risks for their children and require safety education from healthcare professionals.

In the healthcare setting, heavy use or misuse of equipment may lead to flaws that result in excessive leakage of electricity. A nurse who simultaneously touches a damaged or ungrounded electrical appliance and a client with wet skin or a central IV line may create a potentially dangerous electrical circuit. The client whose skin surface is broken by a wound, invasive line, abrasion, or puncture or who has wet skin is more vulnerable to electric current flow. Such clients should be considered electrically sensitive, and nurses must avoid creating a potentially hazardous circuit. The use of faulty or ungrounded electrical equipment also increases the risk of electrical shock.

Radiation

Ionizing radiation consists of high-frequency electromagnetic radiation of short wavelength (e.g., x-rays, gamma rays). Such radiation may occur naturally or in devices such as nuclear reactors. The many adverse health effects related to excess exposure to radiation include birth defects, tissue cell destruction, and cancer. Most human exposure occurs either in occupational settings or as the result of radioactive contamination from a nuclear facility into the surrounding community.

Many healthcare facilities use radiation in diagnosis and treatment. X-ray machines and pharmaceuticals for injection or implantation emit small doses of radiation into the environment. While clients receive the intended dose of radiation, nurses and x-ray technicians are exposed to small doses repeatedly. Procedures for preventing unanticipated exposures are discussed later in this chapter.

Disease

Disease is pervasive. Injury and unsafe behaviors facilitate a pathogen's ability to overwhelm the body's defenses. Unsafe sex is associated with sexually transmitted diseases, including human immunodeficiency virus/acquired immunodeficiency syndrome (HIV/AIDS). Sharing of needles by IV drug abusers is associated with hepatitis B, hepatitis C, and HIV/AIDS. Use of contaminated water and food is associated with typhoid fever, hepatitis A, and parasite infections. Poor hygiene is associated with urinary tract infections, colds, and tuberculosis. Being bitten by an infected tick can result in Lyme disease. Hanta virus, which is contracted through exposure to dried droppings from infected deer mice, sometimes causes death.

Clients are exposed to microorganisms in the healthcare environment. Infection may result, especially if fatigue, stress, poor nutrition, or other conditions impair a client's immunity. Clients are at risk for **nosocomial infections** (infections acquired in the healthcare environment) when the facility does not follow safety precautions. Medical and surgical asepsis are the primary safety precautions for preventing disease in the healthcare environment (see Chapter 26). Nurses and other healthcare workers also are at risk for contracting infections such as hepatitis B, hepatitis C, HIV/AIDS, and tuberculosis.

Viruses, such as herpes, cytomegalovirus, and human T-lymphotropic virus, along with multidrug-resistant bacteria and yeast, cause dangerous infections in susceptible people. Following Standard and Transmission-Based Precautions is vital to prevent the spread of these organisms in healthcare settings. All human blood and other potentially infectious material containing blood or blood components (i.e., semen, vaginal secretions, cerebrospinal fluid, pleural fluid, pericardial fluid, peritoneal fluid, amniotic fluid, synovial fluid) are treated as if they were known to be infected. In that way, all people are treated the same and protected the same, regardless of the presence of infection. This approach considers any body substance—urine, stool, saliva, blood, or sputum—to be contaminated.

All healthcare staff must protect themselves and other clients by wearing disposable gloves when handling any of these substances. If aerosolization is suspected, goggles, respirator, and gown must be worn. Nurses should be especially careful when bathing clients, because any open or fluid-filled lesion is a potential source of pathogens. Each healthcare agency has an infection control manual to help guide nurses in caring for clients safely and protectively. OSHA adopted the Bloodborne Pathogen Standard in 1991 (OSHA, 1991). This standard describes the requirements of employers to prevent employee exposure to blood or other bodily fluids potentially infected with blood.

With the increased use of gloves, there has been an increase in the occurrence of allergies to the natural rubber latex used to manufacture latex gloves. These allergies can range from minor symptoms to major disabilities. Use of either powderless, low-antigen latex gloves or synthetic (vinyl or nitrile) gloves is now being recommended (National Institute of Occupational Health and Safety, 1997).

Disregard for Safety

Individuals or groups who disregard safety may jeopardize the safety of others. Unsafe driving practices can potentially injure others in automobile crashes. Disregard for safety leads to bicycle, skateboard, and other recreation and sports injuries. Disregard may be intentional, or it may be a result of ignorance of risks and safety precautions. Employers may cause harm to workers or the general population when they fail to supply safety gear for operating dangerous machinery, dispose of toxic wastes improperly, or sell products with potential safety flaws.

Some people are at greater risk for safety problems because of lifestyle and behavior patterns. A person's lifestyle may involve risky or impulsive behaviors, such as walking alone at night or high-speed driving. Some people enjoy potentially dangerous sports, such as skydiving or mountain climbing, and may not follow usual safety precautions. Cigarette smoking, use of alcohol and illicit drugs, unsafe sexual practices, and poor diets also impair safety. These practices may result from lack of awareness of risks, addiction, or neglect of health and safety.

ALTERED SAFETY

Manifestations of Altered Safety

Altered safety is manifested in a variety of harmful and preventable injuries and illnesses. Unintentional injuries include motor vehicle incidents; falls; poisonings; drownings and suffocation; fires and burns; firearm injuries; electrical shocks; radiation exposures; infections; illnesses such as respiratory problems, allergies, and effects of hazardous chemicals or pollution; and stress-related illnesses.

Motor Vehicle Incidents
Motor vehicle incidents frequently result from hazardous driving. They may involve one or more drivers or passengers, bicycle riders, skateboarders, and pedestrians.

Motor vehicle incidents are the leading cause of unintentional injury death in the United States, accounting for 43,200 deaths in 1999 (NSC, 2001). Motor vehicle incidents also cause permanent disability, pain, and suffering. Factors that contribute to motor vehicle incidents include speeding, lack

of defensive driving techniques, failure of bicycle riders and skateboarders to use helmets, fatigue, and use of alcohol and other substances that cause impairment while driving. About 41% of deaths related to motor vehicles in 1995 were alcohol related. Alcohol-related fatalities decreased by 1% between 1995 and 1996 and declined by 29% from 1986 to 1996. In 1986, 52% of traffic deaths involved alcohol. Alcohol was involved in 7% of all traffic injury incidents, fatal and nonfatal, in 1999 (NSC, 2001).

Falls
Falls are common inside and outside the healthcare environment, especially among older adults and ill or disoriented people. Falls can cause pain, permanent disability, and even death. Sometimes, falls in older adults result in hip fractures; conversely, spontaneous hip fractures may lead to falls. Falls were the second leading cause of unintentional injury death overall in the United States in 1999 and the leading cause among people aged 79 and older (NSC, 2001). Variables that increase a client's risk for falls include gait and balance disorders, weakness, dizziness, environmental hazards, decreased mobility of the lower extremities, sleeplessness, incontinence, confusion, visual impairment, sedating medications, depression, and substance abuse. A cardiovascular problem that causes syncope or hypotension may also lead to a fall. A common scenario involves the older or impaired client who falls on the way to the bathroom at night. The client may be disoriented and not see obstacles cluttering the path from the bed to the bathroom. Falls at home commonly involve stairways. Poor lighting, obstacles on the stairs, and slippery or poorly repaired steps are common culprits. In the workplace, risk factors for falls include the presence of cluttered or slippery floors and working at heights in construction, such as on a ladder, roof, or scaffold.

Poisoning
Poisoning occurs by ingesting, inhaling, or absorbing potentially hazardous substances (Fig. 30-2). Poisoning by solids and liquids was the third leading cause of unintentional injury death in the United States in 1999 (NSC, 2001). Poisoning compromises the cardiovascular, respiratory, central nervous, hepatic, gastrointestinal, and renal systems through chemical reactions. Young children are at high risk for poisoning, as are adults who have sensory impairment and communication barriers.

In the home, children may ingest household cleansers, lawn and garden chemicals, or medicines that are improperly labeled and stored. Plants and paint products are examples of other potential household poisons. In older homes, lead-based paint that is chipping or peeling is a hazard to young children who are prone to putting things into their mouths. Adolescents and young adults frequently experiment with alcohol and drugs and may overdose inadvertently. Older adults may ingest an overdose of medication because of mental impairment or difficulty reading the label as a result of

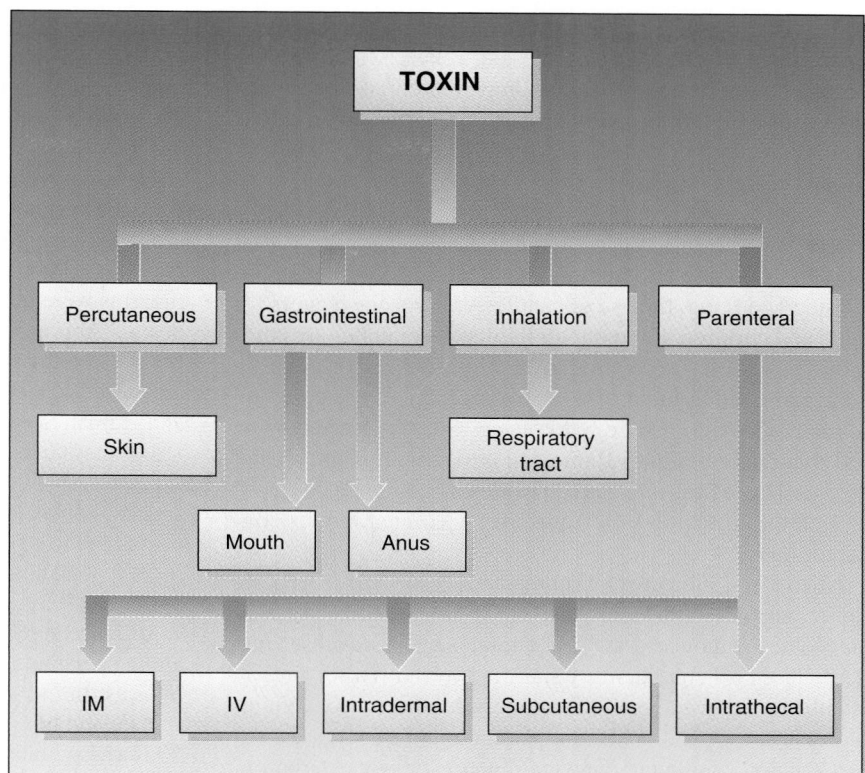

FIGURE 30-2 Routes by which toxins may enter the body.

poor eyesight, illiteracy, or language barrier. Display 30-2 lists common toxins in the home.

Poisoning may occur in the healthcare environment when pharmaceutical products are administered improperly. They may be given to the wrong client, in excessive dosage, or by the wrong route. Cardiac medications, narcotics, cancer chemotherapy agents, and IV medications are all potentially lethal. Shortcuts taken when preparing and administering medications contribute to errors.

Drowning and Suffocation

Suffocation or **asphyxiation** occurs as a result of drowning, smothering, strangling, airway obstruction, or entrapment in a confined space. Drowning was the fourth leading cause of un-intentional injury death in the United States in 1999 (National Safety Council, 2001). It usually occurs in children.

In the home, these injuries include infants suffocating in a pillow or blanket; toddlers suffocating from a plastic bag over the face or strangling by a shoulder harness, clothesline, or cord from a window shade; a child trapped in an abandoned refrigerator; and older adults choking on poorly chewed food. Drownings occur in natural bodies of water, pools, bathtubs, and even large pails or toilets. Lack of supervision, hazardous swimming conditions, careless boating and water sports, and impairment by drugs and alcohol contribute to the risk of drowning.

Suffocation in the healthcare environment frequently occurs because of airway obstruction, either by choking on foreign

DISPLAY 30-2

⑤ COMMON HOME TOXINS

Living Room/Den
Air freshener
Glass cleaner
Rug and upholstery shampoo
Houseplant insecticides
Flea collar, bomb
Furniture polish
Permanent ink markers
Typewriter correction fluid
Carbonless copy paper
Bathroom
Toilet bowl cleaner
Disinfectant
Mildew remover
Medicines
Hairspray
Hair color
Home permanent
Nail polish/remover
Lice/flea shampoo

Kitchen/Laundry
Scouring powder, ammonia
Oven cleaner, drain cleaner
Dishwashing detergent
Moth balls
Bleach
Metal polish
Insect spray, rodent killer
Laundry detergent
Spot remover
Garage/Basement
Latex, oil-base paints
Paint stripper
Wood preservative
Adhesives, glues, epoxys
Herbicides, insecticides
Insect repellents, poisons
Fertilizers
Gasoline, fuels
Other chemicals

objects or aspirating fluid into the small airways of the lungs. Impairment of chewing and the gag reflex, which usually occur in older or neurologically impaired clients, cause airway obstruction. Improperly fitting dentures and overzealous feeding of older or neurologically impaired clients can lead to choking and aspiration.

Fires

Careless smoking practices, faulty electrical equipment, unattended cooking, the use of candles or kerosene heaters for heat, and children playing with lighters or matches are common causes of fire in the home. Grease fires originating from faulty equipment or poor work practices are common in the home and in some workplaces. Stoves in use may be left unattended; a high flame can easily ignite, splattering grease. These fires may spread to curtains, kitchen cabinets, and clothing. Children left unsupervised near stoves contribute to risks.

Clients in healthcare environments are especially at risk for fire-related injuries because they may be incapacitated and unable to flee without assistance. Flammable gases, such as oxygen and anesthetic agents, contribute to the risk of fires in healthcare environments. Commonly used electrical equipment, such as monitors, heating or cooling units, and respiratory therapy equipment, may malfunction or be used improperly, causing sparks that ignite linens easily in the presence of oxygen. Regular servicing of and education about electrical equipment and strict smoking policies may help reduce the risk of fires.

Four classes of fires exist, based on the type of material burning:

- Class A: Paper, wood, cloth
- Class B: Flammable liquids, such as fuel oil, cooking oil or grease, paint or solvents, and gases, such anesthesia gases
- Class C: Electrical fires
- Class D: Combustible metals

Firefighting measures, discussed later in this chapter, vary according to fire classification.

Burns

Burns are a major cause of injury and death in the home for infants and children. In 1999, burns were the third leading cause of unintentional injuries among children from 1 to 14 years of age (NSC, 2001). Children may sustain burns in the home by playing with matches or candles, pulling a teakettle off the stove, being fed formula that is too hot, or playing outdoors without sunscreen protection. Adolescents working in fast food restaurants are at risk for burn injuries from hot grease or food. Burns also occur in the healthcare environment due to scalds and fires. The person with sensory impairment is at risk for scalds from hot water or steam. A person with diabetic peripheral neuropathy may place hands under or step into very hot water and not feel the excessive temperature. Burns also may be sustained from cardioversion during resuscitation efforts.

Firearms

Firearms are involved in a significant number of unintentional injuries and deaths as well as homicide and suicide deaths. There were 35,279 firearm-related deaths in the United States in 1997, making it the second leading cause of injury death after motor vehicles (43,363 fatalities). In 1999, firearms were the seventh leading cause of unintentional fatal injuries among all age groups and totaled 1,500 deaths (NSC, 2001). Among children and young adults aged 5 to 24 years, however, firearms were the fourth leading cause of unintentional injury death. Approximately 40% of U.S. households contain firearms of any type (Cook & Ludwig, 1996), many of which are stored loaded and unlocked (U.S. Department of Health and Human Services, 1998).

Deaths due to firearms increased by 4% over the 10-year period from 1987 to 1997 but increased by 15% between 1996 and 1997 (NSC, 1998). In 1995, 86% of unintentional firearm deaths occurred in boys and men. Firearms were also involved in 69% of all homicides and 59% of all suicide deaths between 1997 and 1999 (NSC, 1998). In 1997, homicide and suicide were, respectively, the second and third leading causes of death among persons age 15 to 24 years, after all other unintentional injuries. In the same year, among those aged 25 to 34 years, suicide and homicide were the leading causes of death (NSC, 2001) after unintentional injuries and AIDS. Firearms also pose a serious occupational hazard among law enforcement officers, taxi drivers, and others in retail sales where money is present. Between 1980 and 1992, 76% of work-related homicides involved the use of firearms (Jenkins, 1996).

In a national survey of high school students, many (24.1%) stated they had been a victim of violent behavior (Resnick et al., 1997). In the same study, household access to guns and a recent suicide attempt or completion by a family member were associated with a higher level of violence for students. Gun control is typically handled as a state and local concern. Estimates are that 20,000 separate firearm laws exist in the United States, more than in any other country in the world. Although debate exists over the effectiveness of gun control laws, several studies have shown a decrease in assaults and deaths involving the use of a firearm. Sloan et al. (1988) found a seven times higher assault rate involving firearms in Seattle, Washington (where gun laws are more liberal) than in Vancouver, British Columbia (where the sale and possession of guns are restricted). Using these data, Dresang (2001) suggested that healthcare providers might want to focus their firearm safety efforts on preventing handgun deaths and suicides. In Washington, D. C., homicide and suicide deaths by firearms declined by approximately 25% after a restrictive gun control law went into effect. Some states have adopted laws that make gun owners responsible for storing firearms out of children's reach. Cummings et al. (1997) found that, among children younger than 15 years of age, unintentional shooting deaths were reduced by 23% in states where such laws were in effect.

Electrical Shock

Electrical equipment and outlets present common hazards in the home and healthcare environments. Lighting and electric power lines in the community create a threat as well.

Electrical shock occurs when a current travels to the ground through the body rather than through electrical wiring or from static electricity that accumulates on the body's surface. A macroshock may cause superficial and deep burns, muscle contractions, and cardiac and respiratory arrest.

In the home, the use of frayed cords or overloaded outlets, use of electrical appliances near the sink or bathtub, and lack of supervision of children near uncovered electrical outlets or electrical appliances present hazards.

In the healthcare environment, electrical shock is a danger because of the abundant electrical equipment in proximity to the client. Water from a spilled pitcher, diaphoretic skin, or a leaking IV line increases electricity conduction. Three-pronged plugs that ground electrical equipment help prevent electrical shocks. A **ground** is an electrical connection with a large conducting body (e.g., the earth) that allows dissipation of the electrical charge.

Radiation Injury

Radiation injury may occur as a result of leakage of ionizing radiation into the community from power plants and industrial sources or excessive exposure to radiation used to diagnose or treat illness in the healthcare environment. Radiation can injure the skin, reproductive organs, bone marrow, gastrointestinal tract, and other parts of the body. Closer proximity and longer exposure to radiation increase the risk of injury.

Nuclear releases and exposures that occur in communities place large groups of people at risk for injury. Psychological stress may be incurred even if physical injury is avoided. Federal agencies, such as the Department of Energy and the Nuclear Regulatory Commission, are primarily responsible for establishing and enforcing guidelines for radiation safety.

In healthcare environments, the potential for radiation injury exists when nurses must care for clients with radioactive implants and when technicians or nurses must restrain clients during radiography. Failure to use lead shielding for staff and clients and or failure to follow radiation safety procedures when caring for clients with implants contributes to the risk of injury.

Infection

Infection may occur when safety precautions against the transmission of microorganisms are altered. Infectious illnesses include gastroenteritis, hepatitis, tuberculosis, sexually transmitted diseases, Lyme disease, and hanta virus infection. Practices in the home that place a person at risk for infection are unsafe sex, lack of immunization, improper food preparation, and poor hygiene. Community problems such as water supply contaminated by sewage or tick infestations near residential areas also may result in infection. Nosocomial infections include urinary tract infections, pneumonia, hepatitis, and gastroenteritis. Debilitated clients, clients on mechanical ventilators, and those with chronic illnesses are at risk for nosocomial infection. Lack of asepsis, unsafe needle devices, poor handwashing practices, and disregard for necessary precautions contribute to exposures for clients and healthcare workers alike.

Respiratory problems may result from unsafe air pollution levels in the community or occupational exposure to chemicals, wood dust, asbestos, or other airborne substances. Passive smoke inhalation from living or working with persons who smoke cigarettes is a recognized potential cause of respiratory disease. Cigarette smoking and asbestos exposure have been linked to lung cancer, and smog and dust worsen respiratory allergy symptoms and cause chronic bronchitis. Coal dust from mining causes fibrosis of the lungs, known as "black lung." OSHA has established guidelines to prevent injury to workers from chemical exposures and other hazardous conditions.

Stress-Related Illnesses

Stress-related illnesses include peptic ulcer disease, anxiety, depression, and psoriasis. Fear of the environment, caused by feeling unsafe and insecure at home, at work, or in the healthcare environment, can lead to stress-related illnesses. Stress-related illnesses can develop due to noise, crime in the community, job demands, or fear of environmental hazards. Unions and community action groups help people work together to overcome these safety concerns and avoid undue stress. Unfamiliar surroundings, invasive procedures, and absence of close family members and friends contribute to client stress in the healthcare environment. Competent, caring nurses can alleviate much of the client's stress.

Impact on Activities of Daily Living

Many people, intentionally or as a result of physiologic dysfunction, behave unsafely. In addition, their environments may not have been engineered to prevent hazardous conditions. The specific source of safety concern affect corresponding activities of daily living (ADLs). A person's inability to complete ADLs indicates the need for nursing intervention. Decreased ability to perform personal hygiene, prepare meals, participate in activities, or engage in usual vocational or social activities may result from altered safety. Loss of income or increased expenses may stem from work absences and the need to purchase equipment or to hire people to assist with care and ADLs.

Fear of falls, fires, job-related injuries, or crime may impair normal functioning. Fear of real or imagined safety hazards may actually contribute to altered safety by increasing a person's stress and anxiety. Emotional tension may impair perception and judgment, placing a person at risk for injury. Altered safety may lead to social isolation—rather than risk harm from potential safety hazards, a person may begin to avoid activities and contact with others. Staying at home, where the client feels safest, isolates the client from needed support systems.

Nutritional deficits may arise from contaminated food and water that are unsafe to consume, fear of disease from polluted or contaminated food or water, or inability to shop for food due to fear of crime or of falls outside the home. Many older adults have difficulty shopping for food and preparing balanced meals, resulting in weight loss and vitamin and iron deficiencies. Family members may help prevent nutritional problems by preparing food and encouraging eating. However,

ETHICAL/LEGAL ISSUE

Ability of Older Adults to Remain Independent Despite Declining Health Status

Georgia McMaster, 83, was admitted to your facility 2 days ago to rule out a fractured hip after a fall. The radiology studies came back negative, and discharge is planned for tomorrow. Her son approaches you with a very worried look on his face, saying, "I know the doctor is going to send my mother home tomorrow, but our family worries about her all the time. She has fallen three times in the last month. Her house is cluttered with all sorts of junk, and she is no longer able to keep up. Her memory is failing, and she often leaves pans on the stove, forgetting to turn off the burner. She's so stubborn, she refuses to even talk about going into a nursing home. Can we force her to go into a nursing home for her own good?"

Reflection
- Explore the concerns and feelings of Mrs. McMaster and her family in this situation.
- Legally, can the family force Mrs. McMaster to move into a nursing home? If so, under what conditions?
- What responsibility do healthcare providers have to ensure that Mrs. McMaster remains safe?

if an affected person was the primary food provider or preparer, the family may encounter problems with affording, obtaining, or preparing food.

Altered safety may result in compromised sleep and rest due to anxiety and fear of potential danger. The person remains overly vigilant to safety hazards in the environment, preventing normal relaxation and proper sleep. Lack of sleep leads to poor job performance and loss of interest in recreation and sex. An entire family's sleep and rest can potentially be disrupted if one person is having such troubles. If a client's primary caregiver does not get enough sleep and rest, taking care of the client during the day becomes increasingly difficult and may predispose the caregiver to potentially altered safety.

Altered safety can impair self-concept. People may believe they are "accident prone" and may perform poorly at their job or sports activities; they may feel unworthy of enjoying usual activities as a result. Problems in self-concept and self-esteem can lead to substance abuse and personality disorders.

A family might fear that a member who has experienced an unintentional injury is not the same person he or she was before the event. For example, if the event that endangered safety was related to employment, the family might fear that the client will be unable to return to work or unable to find work due to the fear and anxiety that the memory or disability engenders. Adequate return-to-work programs are not always available, delaying a person's return to a normal level of work activity. The family's economy and financial support may be disrupted, increasing social isolation.

The family may need to provide extra support and encouragement to the person who has lost self-confidence. If the person is not performing well or fears not performing well at work or in leisure activities, he or she may be reluctant to resume an active lifestyle. If poor self-concept progresses to depression, the family has a more serious problem to handle.

ASSESSMENT

Assessment of a person's ability to function safely involves careful investigation of individual and environmental aspects. Questions about safety reveal the ways clients act at home, at work, and in public. Building trust by being nonjudgmental and supportive will elicit the most accurate information.

Subjective Data

Safety assessment begins with a careful investigation of the client's concerns or perceptions of hazards, including injury history. The person who is at risk for altered safety may report a history of falls, bruises, broken bones, burns, cuts, scratches, and restricted activities. The pattern of past injuries is important; such incidents often relate to periods of emotional stress, fatigue, diminished health, or lack of awareness about hazards associated with various activities. People may share their fears about unsafe conditions or activities and their concerns about the potential for injury. Many people are aware of their risk factors for injury and will share this information if offered nonjudgmental assistance.

Normal Pattern Identification
Current safety practices or plans for management of hazards are part of the assessment.

Consider the following:

- Does the client use appropriate restraints when in a car?
- Can the client read traffic signs and danger warnings?
- Does the pediatric client have a childproofed home?
- Does the client have up-to-date immunizations?
- Does the client understand the health and safety hazards in the workplace?

Keep in mind the special concerns for each age group to direct questions appropriately. Explore recent changes in the environment (home, school, workplace), the support system (divorce, change in caregivers, death of family member), or the developmental stage (transition from infant to toddler). Gather data not only from the client but also from family members, caregivers, referring health professionals, and others. Be sure to have the client's permission to solicit data from other sources, unless he or she is underage or declared incompetent. This approach ensures client confidentiality and promotes trust.

Risk Identification

When assessing current safety concerns, consider the client's reason for seeking healthcare. A recent change in health status related to cognition, perception, sensation, or activity and exercise may have placed the client at risk for injury. Explore these areas fully, and question the client about occupation, home environment, lifestyle, habits, and level of knowledge of safety practices. Some questions to ask include the following:

- What medications does the client take?
- Do side effects, such as drowsiness or dizziness, contribute to injury?
- What medical conditions may place the client at increased risk for injury?

Nurses are responsible for assessing for injuries related to abuse or neglect. This skill requires sensitivity and the ability to evaluate the explanations that clients give. Often, conferring with other health professionals is essential, and a diagnostic workup may be ordered (see Physical Assessment). Injuries that seem disproportionate to the reported cause or occur with unexpected frequency warrant further investigation. No age group is immune to abuse or neglect, and people with higher dependency needs are at higher risk. The highest risk groups include children, older adults, the developmentally disabled, and the debilitated.

Dysfunction Identification

Nurses may determine dysfunctional patterns of safety when the client reports a serious, preventable injury or a recent change in ability to participate safely in ADLs. A dysfunctional pattern also may be evident in the presence of unsafe behaviors that the nurse observes or the client describes. Using specialized knowledge, the healthcare team may determine that the client is at risk for injury, illness, or infection because of unsafe behaviors or physiologic dysfunction. Unless the client shares a concern for preventing such developments, there may be no agreement on the existence of a dysfunctional pattern. In such a case, help the client realize the importance of safety before trying to change safety dysfunction.

As part of the nursing health history, ask about previous injuries and hospitalizations. Find out the cause of these injuries and whether any unsafe behaviors or hazards have been rectified. For example, a client may report a history of burns from a fire. Ask the client what caused the fire. If smoking in bed contributed to the injury, has the client altered careless smoking practices? If not, does the client realize the potential for further problems?

Objective Data

Physical Assessment

Objective data contribute to safety function assessment. Physical assessment techniques can help nurses assess clients for injuries and risk factors for injury. Physical assessment should focus on the neurologic system, cardiovascular and respiratory systems, skin integrity, and mobility.

Assessment of the Neurologic System. Assessment of the neurologic system includes determination of mental status, sensory function, reflexes, and coordination. Assessment of mental status begins with observation of the client's appearance and general behavior. For the purposes of safety promotion, focus attention on the client's ability to detect danger and rapidly avoid hazards. Note any impulsive behavior or behavior that suggests impaired or unsafe judgment. Determine the client's level of alertness; orientation to time, person, and location; attention span; and basic cognitive function by asking simple questions. Determine decision-making capabilities by asking "what if" questions appropriate to the client's age and life experiences.

Examination of sensory function allows the nurse to verify the accuracy and quality of sensory input. Testing should at least include ability to balance, sensitivity to sharp versus dull stimulation, and sensitivity to light touch of the extremities. If sensation is impaired, the client is deprived of important information that may warn of danger or impending injury.

Assessment should include testing of vision, hearing, taste, and smell. Impaired taste or smell may prevent the client from detecting spoiled food or a natural gas leak. Alterations in visual acuity may prevent the client from differentiating pills, detecting uneven terrain or stairs, and reading traffic signs or telephone numbers. Impaired hearing acuity has profound implications when it prevents a person from hearing cars, smoke alarms, or other warning sounds. The gag reflex also should be tested before feeding a client with decreased alertness or muscle strength. A review of important withdrawal reflex arcs will provide clues to the client's ability to respond reflexively to potentially harmful stimuli by pulling away from danger. Reflex arcs to test include biceps, triceps, knees, and ankles. Coordination is important to prevent falls. Observing the client's gait, muscle strength, and repetitive motions can test coordination.

Observe changes in the client's awareness and sensitivity to the environment. The person with delirium may have limited awareness of the environment and poor integration of information. He or she may move inappropriately to discontinue IV medication lines, feeding tubes, or ventilation tubing. Ongoing neurologic assessment of some clients is essential.

Assessment of Cardiovascular and Respiratory Systems. Assess cardiovascular and respiratory integrity as it relates to safety by determining the person's mobility and activity tolerance and the presence of any conditions that impair function. If a client can walk only 50 feet before shortness of breath or chest pain (exertional angina) becomes severe, the ability to accomplish many daily tasks is limited. If this person lives more than 50 feet from the emergency exit of his or her apartment building, escape during a fire may be impossible. Activity tolerance is usually stated as distance or duration of activity (walking, standing) before fatigue or other symptoms interrupt the activity; it is an important assessment in discharge planning for a client's safety outside the hospital environment.

THERAPEUTIC DIALOGUE
Safety Assessment

Scene for Thought

Mrs. Jennie Adobo, 45 years old, has been receiving home healthcare for 6 months. During that time, Martha Davis, a community health nurse, has noticed that Jennie's small house has become increasingly cluttered with newspapers, saved paper bags, plastic bags, clean rags, and so forth. Everything is clean and orderly, but the piles seem to be growing at an alarming rate, especially since Jennie's husband left her and her two adolescent children. Jennie has controlled hypertension and is working on controlling her diabetes through diet.

Less Effective

Nurse: Hi, Jennie, how are you this week? *(Acknowledges client by name.)*

Client: Not too good, Martha. I can't seem to get enough sleep or enough to eat lately. *(Fidgets with string she's winding into a ball.)*

Nurse: Let me just get your blood pressure and do a glucose test on you for a minute. *(Does the procedures concentrating on getting the readings correctly. Jennie watches fearfully.)*

Nurse: Everything seems to be okay with your pressure and blood sugar, especially since you seem to have lost some weight. How much would you say you've lost? *(Puts away the equipment and smiles at Jennie.)*

Client: About 10 pounds, I think. That's good, isn't it? My husband will be so glad when he comes back. He's always saying I should lose some weight. *(Starts to cry and wring her hands.)*

Nurse: Now, don't you worry. Everything will be fine. Your pressure and sugar are down, you look much better than you did with the weight you lost, and I know your kids are helping out with jobs. You'll see. Anything else you'd like to talk about? *(Packs equipment bag.)*

Client: No, I'll be fine. I just need to look on the bright side. *(Smiles with her lips.)*

Nurse: That's the ticket. I'll see you in a couple of weeks. Stay well!

More Effective

Nurse: Hi, Jennie. How are you this week? *(Acknowledges client by name.)*

Client: Not too good, Martha. I can't seem to get enough sleep or enough to eat lately. *(Fidgets with string she's winding into a ball.)*

Nurse: Tell me more about that, Jennie. *(Takes blood pressure, keeping an eye on Jennie's face.)*

Client: It's just so hard for me to go to sleep at night. I hear noises and the sirens go off, and I just can't sleep. *(Sounds annoyed.)*

Nurse: Sounds difficult for you. How long has this been going on? *(Puts away the cuff and sits down facing her.)*

Client: Since he went away. *(Starts to cry.)*

Nurse: That's been 2 months now, hasn't it? *(Jennie nods.)* Anything else you've noticed besides the sleeping problem? *(Quietly watches Jennie.)*

Client: I can't eat. I have no appetite. *(Still fiddling with the string.)*

Nurse: I noticed that you're looking a little thinner. How much weight have you lost?

Client: About 10 pounds. Actually, I needed to lose the weight, but not this way. *(Crying.)*

Nurse: Something else I've noticed, you've collected a lot more bags and stuff since the last time I was here. Can you tell me about that?

Client: I just can't throw them away. We may need them. He's not sending any money. We could sell them and get money to eat! *(Sounds a little panicky.)*

Nurse: You really do seem worried about a lot of things, Jennie. Would it help if we talked about them one at a time? I think we can work together on some resources to help you with the problems you're having.

Client: Okay. *(Wipes her eyes.)* I need some help; I can see that. I'm not used to having all these problems all at once.

Critical Thinking Challenge

- Analyze intrinsic and extrinsic factors that are affecting Jennie's behavior with respect to the accumulation of bags, string, and so forth.
- Detect the safety hazards associated with these items.
- Determine what the second nurse attended to that the first nurse did not.
- Identify with what common human emotion insomnia, anorexia, weeping, and sadness are associated.
- Predict what the first nurse might discover when she returns in 2 weeks.

Assessment of Skin Integrity. A brief physical examination of the integument (see Chapter 16) provides important clues to the client's history of accidents or injuries. Inspect the skin for bruises, cuts, scratches, and scars. Carefully note the location and distribution of the lesions and correlate them with the client's explanation of their origin. A bath is an excellent opportunity for assessing the integument while providing a refreshing comfort measure.

Assessment of Mobility. Inspect and palpate the client's muscles, joints, and bones to assess mobility. Range-of-motion testing of joints, muscle strength testing of the extremities, and observation of ambulation are important for determining risk for altered safety. Any joint showing limited range of motion and any muscle group showing weakness place the client at a disadvantage when trying to avoid hazards. For example, a person with arthritis in the knees may be safely active on level surfaces but unable to use stairs in an emergency. Observation of posture and gait can provide valuable information about the stability of balance and the presence of sway.

Gather information about the client's ADLs from caregivers and family, but supplement this information with direct observation when possible. Observe the client moving from bed to chair or commode (and back) when appropriate; for more mobile people, observe them walking from bedroom to bathroom, front door, kitchen, and telephone locations.

Toileting includes the ability to safely get on and off a toilet or commode. Weakness or pain in the hips may create the need for a raised toilet seat to make access safer. Assess for safe footing and transfers (position changes) in showers or at sinks, and for the need for grab bars or special benches if standing is difficult. Some people can get into the bathtub but are unable to get out without assistance.

Because assessment of the ability to dress safely is difficult when a person is allowed only a hospital-type gown, observe the client dressing in street clothes before discharge. Regardless of healthcare setting, assess the client's ability to put on clothes in the correct sequence, maintain balance, and avoid pinching with zippers or shoelaces.

Diagnostic Tests and Procedures

Diagnostic tests and procedures are used to determine a person's health status by assessing for the presence of medical conditions that may place the person at risk for injury. Neuropsychological testing may be used to determine the type and source of a cognitive abnormality. Blood pressure assessment, electrocardiogram (ECG) testing, and pulmonary function tests may be used to detect cardiopulmonary abnormalities. Specific blood tests can identify the presence of certain conditions, such as a complete blood count (CBC) and kidney function tests to detect an infection or kidney damage. The blood glucose concentration can help assess for diabetes, and cholesterol levels can assess cardiac risk.

NURSING DIAGNOSES

The accepted nursing diagnosis involving alterations in safety is Risk for Injury. Data from the subjective and objective assessments will help determine whether the client is at risk for injury.

Diagnostic Statement: Risk for Injury

Definition. Risk for Injury is a state in which a person is at risk for injury as a result of environmental conditions interacting with his or her adaptive and defensive resources (North American Nursing Diagnosis Association [NANDA], 2001).

Defining Characteristics. The defining characteristics include presence of internal risk factors, such as changes in the biochemical or regulatory functions (e.g., sensory dysfunction, integrative dysfunction, effector dysfunction, tissue hypoxia); presence of malnutrition; an immune–autoimmune status; an abnormal blood profile (leukocytosis/leukopenia; altered clotting factors; thrombocytopenia; sickle cell, thalassemia; decreased hemoglobin). Physical alterations (broken skin, altered mobility) can contribute to the risk for injury by creating conditions conducive to infections or other agents that increase the potential for injury. Developmental age (physiologic, psychosocial) and psychological state (affective, orientation) can increase the risk for injury because of the possibility of errors in judgment or cognition (NANDA, 2001).

The environment can increase the risk for injury through biologic (immunization level of community, microorganisms), chemical (pollutants, poisons, drugs, pharmaceutical agents, alcohol, caffeine, nicotine, preservatives, cosmetics, dyes), nutritional (vitamins, food types), and physical (design, structure, and arrangement of community, building, or equipment) factors. Additionally, the mode of transport of people or caregivers (nosocomial agents; staffing patterns; cognitive, affective, and psychomotor factors) contribute to the risk for injury (NANDA, 2001).

Related Factors. As described in the previous paragraphs, many factors can interact and interrelate, creating increased opportunities or risks for injury. For example, a person who is malnourished, has respiratory problems, and is exposed to large numbers of people with common respiratory infections is at high risk for contracting a respiratory tract infection.

Related Nursing Diagnoses

Other nursing diagnoses may be evident in people who are at risk for injury or have altered safety function. These include Risk for Aspiration, Ineffective Breathing Pattern, Fatigue, Risk for Infection, Risk for Poisoning, Risk for Suffocation, and Risk for Trauma. Safety dysfunction also affects the person's ability to perform ADLs. Nursing diagnoses in these situations may include Impaired Home Maintenance, Imbalanced Nutrition: Less Than Body Requirements, Situational Low Self-Esteem, and Disturbed Sleep Pattern. Psychological reactions may include nursing diagnoses such as Anxiety, Defensive Coping, Fear, and Hopelessness.

OUTCOME IDENTIFICATION AND PLANNING

After the nursing diagnosis and related factors have been formulated, client goals and nursing interventions are identified. Common goals for the client who is at risk for injury include the following:

- The client will identify actual and high-risk environmental hazards.

- The client will demonstrate safety habits appropriate to selected environments (home, healthcare setting, workplace, community).
- The client will experience a decrease in the frequency and severity of injury events.

These goals must be individualized to reflect the unique needs of the person at risk. Once they are individualized, specific nursing interventions support the goals.

Planning for nursing interventions to promote safety is based on assessment data and resulting nursing diagnoses and client goals. Nursing interventions related to safety fall into two broad categories: providing safety education for the home, workplace, and community, and providing a safe environment in the healthcare setting. Nurses promote these safety interventions wherever they practice. Examples of nursing interventions commonly used to promote safety are listed in the accompanying display and discussed in the next section.

IMPLEMENTATION

Health Promotion

Nurses must help clients develop personal safety habits. The Centers for Disease Control and Prevention (CDC) and OSHA provide guidelines for promotion of health and safety. Each accredited healthcare setting must have an ongoing health and safety program.

The client is at risk for injury in the healthcare environment because of its unfamiliarity and the procedures the client undergoes. Nurses are responsible for protecting the client from environmental hazards wherever they provide services. Nurses are also responsible for anticipating and minimizing the adverse consequences of procedures and treatments. Many nursing policies and procedures are intended to protect the client, and a familiarity with these policies assists the nurse in the healthcare environment.

Initial nursing actions to promote safety and security in a healthcare setting are to introduce staff to the client and orient the client to the immediate environment. If the client is staying overnight, orientation includes instruction on the use of call-light system and bed controls, location of personal care supplies in the bedside stand, location of bathroom, operation of lights, and schedule of unit activities. Ensure that the room is uncluttered and free of obstacles between the bed and the bathroom. Use of a night light and bedside rails is standard. Instruct each client about activity limitations and assist with ambulation as needed. Talk to the client and answer questions calmly and confidently to increase the client's security.

Motor Vehicle Safety

Nursing intervention for motor vehicle safety involves client education about potential hazards and safety measures. Use of seat belts has greatly decreased morbidity and mortality on the highways. Seatbelts have been found to reduce the risk of fatal injury in passenger cars by 45% and in light trucks by 60%. As of December 1996, 49 states and the District of Columbia (New Hampshire being the one exception) required the use of seatbelts (NSC, 2001). Car safety seats or restraint devices for young children are required by law in all 50 states. Despite the existence of such laws, hundreds of children die each year because of improper use or lack of restraints (American Academy of Pediatrics, 1996).

Infants and children should be properly restrained in approved car seats when in automobiles. Infants weighing up to 20 lb require rear-facing car seats that are semireclined and provide good support for their heads. Rear-facing car seats should never be placed in front seats of cars with passenger-side airbags. Toddlers and preschoolers (20 to 40 lb) should be secured in forward-facing car seats. Parents and caregivers should use booster seats when children outgrow standard car seats, preferably those that use combination shoulder and lap belts (American Academy of Pediatrics, 1996). Children weighing more than 60 lb need to wear properly applied lap and shoulder harnesses.

Motor vehicle safety also includes maintaining a safe driving speed for road and weather conditions. Educate clients about the effects of alcohol on driving. All people should avoid any substance that impairs alertness and reaction time (e.g., antihistamines) while driving motor vehicles. Teach adolescents about the danger of riding with friends who are impaired by alcohol or drugs.

Fall Prevention

In the home, teach adults, especially older adults, the following measures to prevent falls:

- Remove throw rugs.
- Make sure stairways are well lighted and repaired.
- Remove clutter from stairways and walkways.
- Install handrails wherever needed.
- Avoid use of unstable ladders and stepstools.
- Never attempt to do anything beyond reach or physical ability.
- Clean up damp areas promptly.

In all healthcare environments, ensure the client's safety from falls. The room needs to be free of clutter and well lighted

---

PLANNING: NIC/NOC

Accepted Safety Nursing Interventions Classification (NIC)
Risk Identification
Risk Identification: Childbearing Family
Physical Restraint

Accepted Safety Nursing Outcomes Classification (NOC)
Risk Detection, Risk Control
Safety Behavior: Fall Prevention

Refer to the following for specifics regarding NIC/NOC:
  McCloskey, J., & Bulechek, G. (2000). *Iowa Intervention Project: Nursing Interventions Classification (NIC)*. 2nd ed. St. Louis, MO: C.V. Mosby.
  Johnson, M., & Maas, M. (2000). *Iowa Outcomes Project: Nursing Outcomes Classification (NOC)*. 2nd ed. St. Louis, MO: C.V. Mosby.

during transfers and ambulation. Side rails and grab bars must be firmly anchored (Fig. 30-3A). The floor must be nonskid, either carpeted or free of liquid. Wheelchairs, beds, commode chairs, and shower chairs must have working brakes (Fig. 30-3B). These devices must be free of any sharp edges and have a support surface that is comfortable. Teach clients with orthostatic hypotension to change position slowly to allow for blood pressure stabilization. Use night lights, and respond promptly to call lights. During the daytime, encourage family members to help weak clients to the bathroom, unless doing so would be unsafe. In some cases, two or more professionals are needed to support very weak clients.

Nurses and other healthcare workers are at high risk for back injuries due to frequent lifting and transfer of clients, often in awkward positions. When necessary, complete an assessment of the type of lift or transfer required for each client

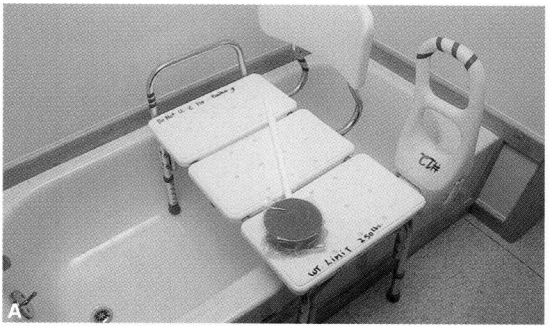

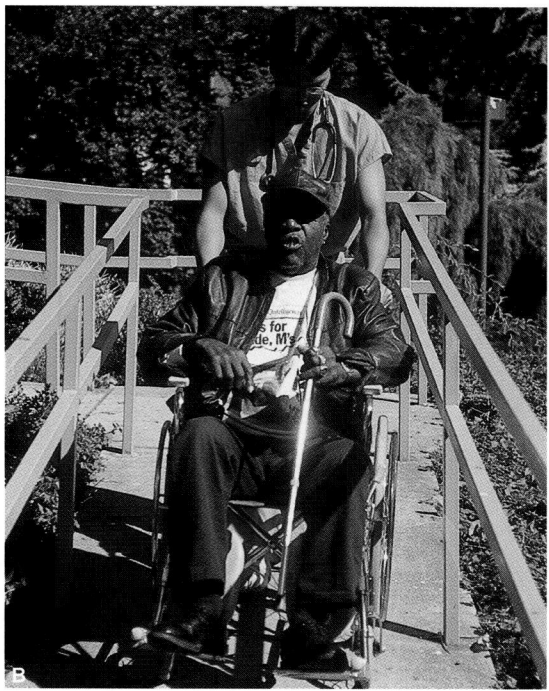

FIGURE 30-3 The healthcare facility must provide safety for the client. **(A)** This shower protects the client with grab bars, safety rails, shower seat, and transfer seat. **(B)** The nurse checks wheelchair brakes for safe use.

on admission. In many instances, a mechanical lifting device is used to assist nursing staff to lift or transfer a client.

Use of Restraints. A **restraint** is a protective device, material, or equipment, attached or adjacent to the body, that restricts freedom of movement or normal access to one's body (Omnibus Budget Reconciliation Act, 1990). Restraints may be physical, mechanical, or chemical. The latter involves medication to relax a client or to make him or her sleep.

Generally, the use of physical restraints is not advocated and is illegal when not used within the guidelines of the Omnibus Budget Reconciliation Act of 1990. These guidelines require that restraints be part of the medical treatment after all less restrictive interventions have been tried first, other appropriate disciplines have been consulted, and supporting documentation for their use has been provided (Health Care Financing Administration, 1989). There is little evidence that restraints prevent injury, particularly from falls, and they have many unintended negative consequences (Frank, Hodgetts, & Puxty, 1996; Sullivan-Marx, Strumpf, Evans, Baumgarten, & Maislin, 1999a, 1999b).

Restraints may be necessary, however, to limit a client's physical activity to prevent movement that would disrupt therapy, such as pulling out an IV line or mechanical ventilator tubing. Use restraints cautiously to prevent agitation, preserve dignity, prevent physical injury from the restraining device, and avoid abuse of a client's right to move freely. Display 30-3 lists guidelines from the U.S. Food and Drug Administration (FDA) for the use of restraints (FDA, 1992). The Joint Commission on Accreditation of Healthcare Organizations (1999) has set standards for use of restraints for nonpsychiatric clients that limit restraint use to clinically appropriate and adequately justified situations. Follow healthcare institution guidelines regarding the use of restraints. Be sure to describe the reason for their application in the client's care record. Nurses may apply restraints in an emergency without a primary healthcare provider's order; however, they should obtain such an order as soon as possible. Use direct supervision and communication to reassure and reorient the client. Use of restraints is not a substitute for vigilant nursing care.

Types of restraints include a jacket or vest restraint, which is worn on the chest and tied to the bed frame or legs of a chair; a belt restraint on stretchers or wheelchairs used in transporting; mitt or hand restraints that prevent confused clients from using their hands; wrist or ankle restraints that immobilize one or more limbs; and mummy restraints that are wrapped around a child's body to prevent movement during a procedure. Figure 30-4 shows some examples of restraints.

A common form of restraint is side rails, which are used on beds, stretchers, and similar equipment. Side rails remind clients not to roll too far to the side, and they provide clients with bars to assist them when turning to the side. When they are used on beds, the bed must be in the lowest position with the wheels locked. Having side rails up does not replace careful and frequent observation, because clients may still attempt to get out of bed by climbing over the side rails or over the foot of the bed. Deaths have occurred as the result of entrapment of

DISPLAY 30-3

🔲 FDA RECOMMENDATIONS TO DECREASE THE INCIDENCE OF DEATHS AND INJURIES WITH THE USE OF RESTRAINTS

- Assess the cause for which the restraint is being considered, develop alternatives to restraint use, and implement these alternatives before applying restraints.
- Allow the use of restraints only under the supervision of a licensed healthcare provider and for a strictly defined period of time.
- Define and communicate a clear institutional policy on the use of restraints (e.g., alternatives to restraint use, appropriate conditions for restraint use, length of wear time). This written policy also should be available for any client/resident or any family member.
- Obtain informed consent from client/resident or guardian before use. Clients have the right to be free from restraints. However, if it is determined that a restraint is necessary, explain the reason for the device to the client/resident and guardian to prevent misinterpretation and to ensure cooperation.
- Display instructions for use in a highly visible location and interpret in foreign languages as necessary.
- Provide in-service training for staff as regularly as possible, which should include a return demonstration of proper application of restraints.
- Before use, read and follow the manufacturer's directions for use.

- Select the type of restraint that is appropriate to the client's condition.
- Use the correct size restraint.
- Note the "front" and "back" of the restraint, and apply correctly.
- Secure restraints designed for use in bed to the bed springs or frame, *never* to the mattress or the bed rails.
- Tie knots with appropriate hitches so they may be released quickly.
- Emphasize good nursing, rehabilitative, and client care practices.
- Observe clients in restraints frequently.
- Remove the restraints at least every 2 hours and more often if necessary. Allow for activities of daily living.
- Carefully apply the device and adjust properly so it maintains body alignment and ensures client comfort.
- Continue assessment even after a restraint is used, and discontinue use as soon as feasible. Restraint use should be considered a temporary solution to a situation.
- Clearly document in the client's record the medical reason for use of the restraint, the type selected, and the length of time for treatment.
- Follow local and state laws regarding the use of protective restraint devices.

From U.S. Food and Drug Administration. (1992). *FDA safety alert: Potential hazards with restraint devices.* Rockville, MD: Department of Health and Human Services.

the face or neck between the mattress and rails or within the rails (Parker & Miles, 1997; Hanger, Ball, & Wood, 1999). The need to go to the bathroom is the most frequent reason for clients' trying to get out of bed, no matter what kind of restraint may be in place. Anticipating the client's need to urinate is the primary safety measure that nurses can use.

Many restraints require tying to an object: the bed, a chair, or a wheelchair. Knots should be tied so that clients cannot release them but healthcare providers can do so quickly in an emergency. Knots and restraints are tied to the movable part of the bed frame and not to the side rails or mattress. Two basic types of knots can be used; they are both hitches. (A square knot is not used for restraints, but it is a useful knot in first aid and bandaging.) Figure 30-5 gives directions for tying these knots, which are described in more detail below.

Half-Hitch or Half-Bow Knot. A half-hitch is safer than a traditional knot. It may be used with wheelchairs or on beds. Wrap the strap twice around the frame. Make a loop by folding the remainder of the strap in half. Slip the middle of this loop under the part wrapped around the frame and tighten. A single knot will be formed, which can be slipped open easily for release. Keep the free end out of the client's reach, especially children.

Clove-Hitch Knot. A clove-hitch may be used with limb restraints. Make a "figure 8" with the free ends extending in

each direction. Pick up the loops and bring them together, then slip them over the padded extremity. Make adjustments so that there is one fingerbreadth of space between the extremity and the restraint. Although it cannot be released as easily as the half-hitch, it can be cut easily in an emergency.

Nonrestraint Safety Devices. Increasingly, nonrestraint safety environments and devices are being developed and used to increase client safety without the use of typical restraints. Such devices include alarm systems and pressure devices. Pressure devices are placed on the bed under the client's back. When the person sits up, he or she triggers an alarm that alerts the staff that the client is attempting to get out of bed. Other alarm devices allow the person free movement in bed but trigger an alarm if he or she is about to transfer from the bed. Special cushions may be placed on chairs; these cushions are comfortable to sit on, but because of the angle of the cushion and the material inside, it is extremely difficult for the client to rise without assistance. Both of these devices permit safety without the use of restraints and involve the nurse or caregiver when the client ambulates, thereby improving the safety of the client.

The decision to use restraints is influenced by the knowledge, attitudes, and beliefs of nursing personnel (Karlsson,

POSEY

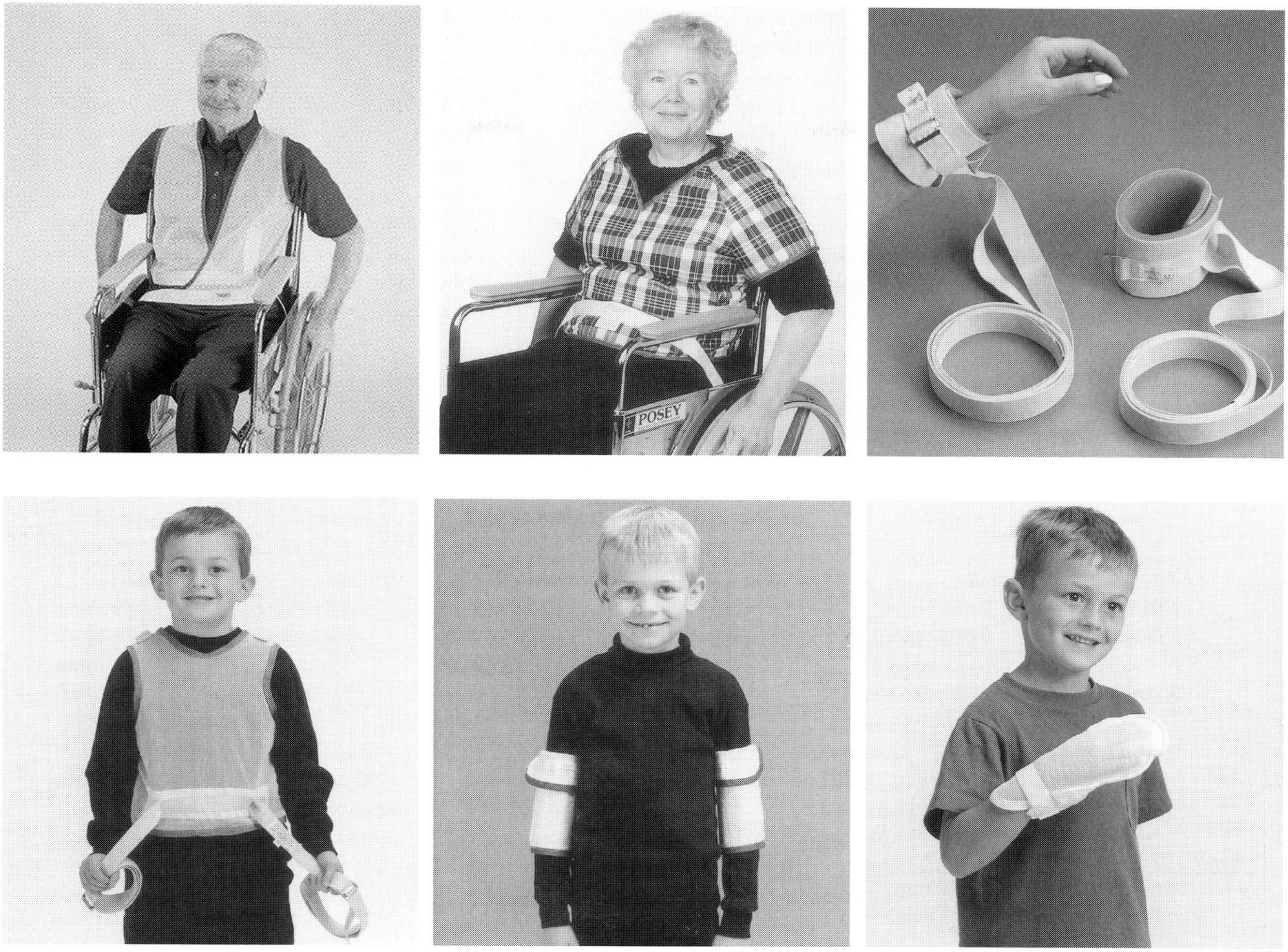

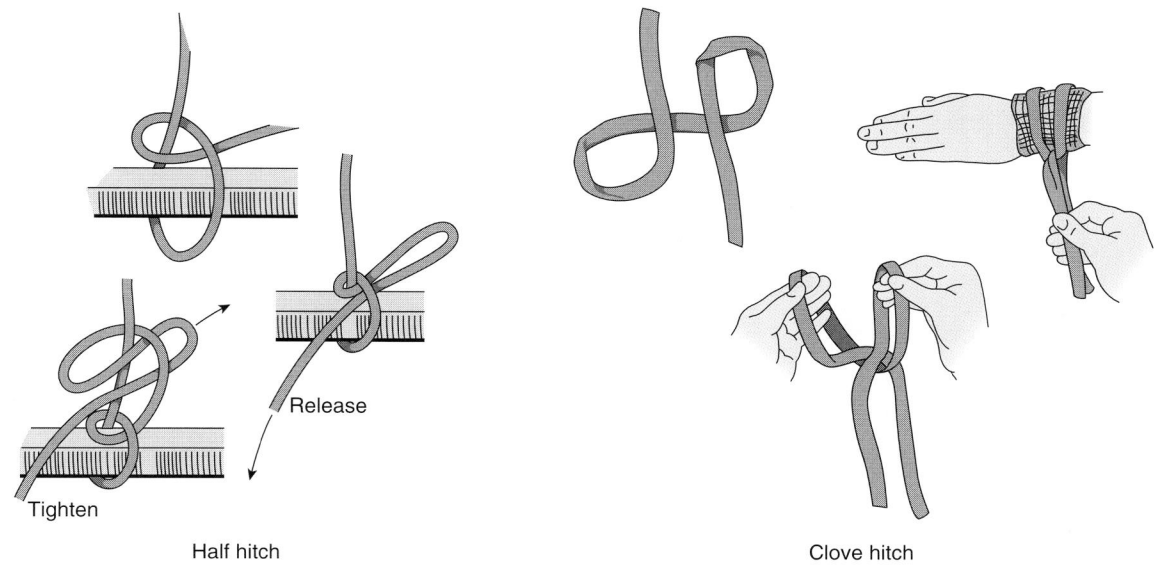

FIGURE 30-4 Safety devices used to prevent clients from injuring themselves or others. (Product photos provided by Posey Company, Arcadia, CA.)

Release
Tighten
Half hitch
Clove hitch

FIGURE 30-5 Two types of hitch knots used with restraints.

Bucht, & Sandman, 1998; Terpstra, Terpstra, & Van Doren, 1998). In particular, level of practice and knowledge of alternatives among nursing personnel, as well as institutional policy regarding the use of restraints, contribute to this decision. Many nursing homes and some hospitals have been successful in implementing restraint-reduction programs; more acute care settings could benefit from these models (Bryant & Fernald, 1997; Dunbar, Neufeld, White, & Libow, 1996; Fletcher, 1996; Jensen et al., 1998). With a comprehensive assessment of the client and careful and imaginative attention to the environment, nurses can reduce environmental risks and improve safety. Anticipating client needs for assistance with transfers and responding to the client's need to go to the bathroom or to change position or location are ways the nurse can help the client prevent falls and reduce the need for restraints (Sullivan-Marx, 1996; Sullivan-Marx et al., 1999a and

1999b). Display 30-4 provides guidelines for using alternatives to restraints.

Prevention of Childhood Falls. Educate parents and other caregivers about children's potential for falling. Prevention includes not leaving infants unattended in the bath, in the bed, or on a table where they may roll or fall off; keeping side rails up on cribs; using guard rails or gates at the top and bottom of stairs when infants crawl; and supervising children in jumpers, swings, and high chairs. Walkers are particularly dangerous for toddlers, and many have been withdrawn from the market.

Poison Prevention

Remind adult caregivers to store all medications, including over-the-counter products, in childproof containers out of children's reach. Caregivers should not treat medications as

DISPLAY 30-4

🔲   **ALTERNATIVES TO RESTRAINTS**

- Use alternatives to restraints (i.e., less restrictive devices) before resorting to restraints.
- Assess and address reasons for agitation or confusion to find another solution to the problem.
- Keep the client's room orderly. Lower the bed and push overbed table and chairs out of the way so the client will not fall if he or she gets up during the night.
- Provide sufficient light so the client can see, especially when the surroundings are strange.
- Place the client in a room near the nurses' station if the client needs frequent observation or supervision. Nurses can take turns checking on the client.
- Use a barrier, such as a chair, to inhibit the client from wandering out of the room or area.

- Provide warm milk, soothing music, or a back massage to help the client relax and sleep.
- Use side rails when the client is in bed. However, if the client tends to climb over the rails, this can be unsafe.
- Provide a rocking chair during the day to help the client use up some energy.
- Use alarm systems that notify the nurse or nurses' station when the client is attempting to get out of bed or out of a chair.
- Use nonslip matting to hold cushions in place on chairs so the client will not slip off the chair.
- Use a pelvic-tilt wedge cushion to maintain proper seating alignment while preventing sliding by gently tilting the resident back in the chair.

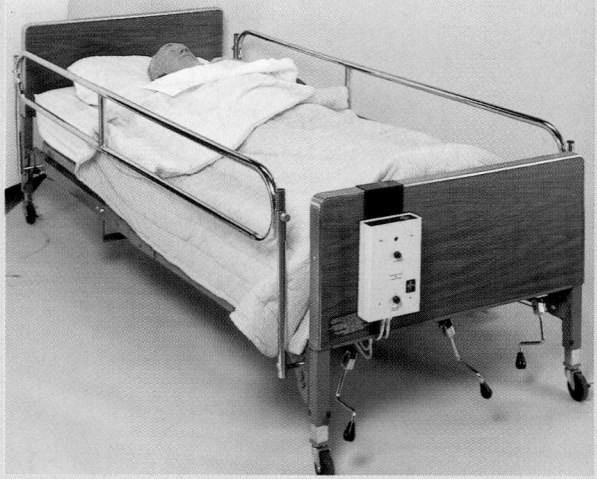 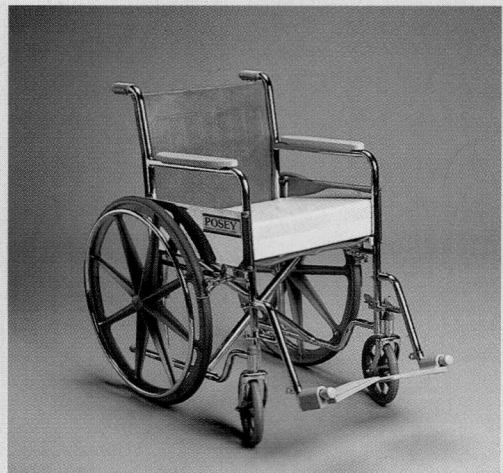

Side rails can be considered a restraint and a nonrestraint. A pelvic tilt (wedge) cushion helps maintain proper seating alignment and prevents sliding by gently tilting the client back. (Product photos provided by Posey Company, Arcadia, CA.)

APPLY YOUR KNOWLEDGE

At change-of-shift report, you are told that Mr. Rau was acutely confused during the night shift and that wrist restraints were applied to prevent him from pulling out his IV. When you make rounds, you find Mr. Rau very agitated, pulling hard against the restraints. His fingers are slightly blue and appear swollen. What is the best way to maintain safety for this client?

Check your answer in Appendix A.

candy. They should store household cleansers and other potentially toxic products in childproofed or locked cupboards or on shelves out of children's reach. Remind them to keep all household chemical products in their original containers with warning labels and emergency information intact.

Caregivers should keep all poisonous house plants out of young children's reach, and should supervise children outdoors. Some poisonous plants include azaleas, buttercups, daffodils, mistletoe berries, philodendrons, poinsettias, potato sprouts, tomato greens, and tulip bulbs. Teach children never to eat berries, mushrooms, seeds, or plants found in the wild.

Teach clients to keep poison control center phone numbers posted near telephones. An integrated system of local centers across the United States and Canada can provide emergency information whenever a substance is ingested, inhaled, or splashed in the eyes or on the skin.

Poison prevention in the healthcare environment can be accomplished primarily through safe medication preparation and administration practices. Nurses are responsible for checking that the healthcare provider's orders for medications are signed and updated appropriately and have been transcribed accurately. Identify the client by checking his or her identification band before administering any medication. Document any significant side effects and report them to the healthcare provider.

Suffocation and Drowning Prevention
Drowning can occur not only in pools but also in bathtubs and other sources of water around the home. Caregivers should never leave young children unattended in bathtubs or kiddie pools. They should not leave pails or basins of water within children's reach. Pools should be fenced in, and children of all ages should be supervised at pools and beaches. Encourage swimming lessons for children of all ages. Children should wear life jackets for boating and fishing and should be warned not to ice skate or play on ice unless ice thickness is proven safe.

Fire Safety
Fire extinguishers are designed to fight specific types of fires and are labeled appropriately. Table 30-1 describes the various classes of fires and the type of fire extinguisher used for each. Review these topics with children and adults as appropriate.

OUTCOME-BASED TEACHING PLAN

When Julie Michaels, the mother of a 1½-year-old toddler named Paula, comes to the clinic for a routine well-child visit, you learn that Paula is becoming increasingly inquisitive. Her mother reports that she has found her getting into the cabinet under the sink and pulling open drawers in the bathroom. She states, "I'm really concerned that she might put something into her mouth before I get to her."

OUTCOME: Julie will verbalize a realistic plan to decrease potential danger of accidental injury from ingestion and to prevent childhood poisoning.
Strategies
- Discuss with Julie common safety measures to prevent Paula's access to potential poisons.
- Review the appropriate handling of medications:
  - Maintain childproof caps on all medications and toxic products.
  - Keep medications and toxic products in their original containers and out of Paula's reach.
  - Measure and give medications in well-lit areas to avoid errors in amount and type of medication.
  - Read labels of medications carefully before administering.
  - Destroy all medications not in use by flushing them down toilet.
- Encourage Julie to think of other potential poisoning situations:
  - Keep cleaning products and garden chemicals out of the reach of children.
  - Use chemical and cleaning products in well-ventilated areas.
  - Do not mix chemicals or common household cleaning products.
  - Remove or keep out of Paula's reach any houseplants or natural materials that may be poisonous.
- Review with Julie a plan of response in the event of accidental poisoning, giving positive feedback regarding her concerns:
  - Keep emergency drugs in the home (e.g., syrup of ipecac).
  - Have the phone number of the poison control center available.

Healthcare agency safety programs emphasize reducing fire hazards by strictly limiting smoking, using nonflammable materials whenever possible, and practicing fire drills and firefighting skills. In the client care area, each nurse should become familiar with emergency phone numbers; the locations of fire alarms, fire extinguishers, and fire hoses; shut-off valves for oxygen and other flammable gases; evacuation equipment; and exits. Posted wall maps should show evacuation routes.

TABLE 30-1

Correct Fire Extinguishers to Use with Specific Classes of Fires		
Class	**Type of Material**	**Type of Fire Extinguishers**
A	Paper, wood, cloth	Water (stored pressure, gas cartridge, soda acid, pump)
		Multipurpose dry chemical (stored pressure, gas cartridge)
		Loaded stream
B	Flammable liquids, such as fuel oil, cooking oil or grease, paint, solvents; gases, such as anesthesia gases	Carbon dioxide
		Regular and multipurpose dry chemical (stored pressure, foam, loaded stream, gas cartridge)
C	Electrical fires	Regular and multipurpose dry chemical (stored pressure, gas cartridge)
		Carbon dioxide
		Liquefied gas
D	Combustible metals	Special dry powder

Burn Prevention

Teach clients with sensory impairment to monitor water temperature at home. They may need to adjust the thermostat on the hot water heater. Adults should keep pot handles turned away from the front of the stove top, where young children might reach. They should never allow young children to play unsupervised in the kitchen or near burning fireplaces, barbecue grills, or containers of gasoline. Remind parents to apply sunscreen to children playing outdoors to prevent sunburn.

Teach adults never to smoke while using lighter fluid to start a charcoal fire or when filling lawnmowers with gasoline. Smoking in bed or late at night in a chair is hazardous. Smoking materials should be properly extinguished.

All people should use sunscreen protection (either barrier creams or clothing) and sunglasses in all outdoor recreation and work activities where exposure to ultraviolet sunlight is a potential hazard. In addition to burns to the skin, extensive exposure to sunlight poses risks for cancer as well as eye damage.

Burns can be prevented in the healthcare environment by testing bath water for temperature when the client has sensory impairment; checking heating pads, heat lamps, and other electrical equipment to be sure they are functioning properly; and assisting clients when handling hot beverages as needed.

Firearm Safety

Prevention of injuries and fatalities from firearms is an important public health responsibility of nurses. Anticipatory guidance about violence in general, and firearms in particular, is a crucial part of any client encounter.

Among physicians and nurse practitioners surveyed, up to 84% believed that healthcare providers should be involved with firearm injury prevention. However, only 20% to 38% reported counseling their clients (Barkin, Duan, Fink, Brook, & Gelberg, 1998; Cassel, Nelson, Smith, Schwab, Barlow, & Gary, 1998). Healthcare professionals must ask clients (children and adults alike) about their experience with violence and the presence of handguns or other firearms in the home. Advise adults to store guns unloaded in a secured (preferably

locked) area with special attention to keeping them out of children's reach. Warn children not to handle guns unless given instruction and supervision by an adult.

In addition to increasing counseling efforts during client care activities, nurses and other healthcare professionals should join community efforts to regulate handguns. Promote product designs that modify guns to make them more childproof (e.g., trigger safety locks, designs that increase the force necessary to discharge a weapon). Such a product-oriented approach has been successful in decreasing other types of childhood injuries. For instance, injuries from poisonings have been reduced with the use of child safety caps on medication bottles, and use of car seats has reduced injuries from motor vehicles (Freed, Vernick, & Hargarten, 1998).

Injury prevention experts recommend a comprehensive approach to reduce firearm injuries. Elements include firearm surveillance and safety regulation, research, enforcement of restrictions limiting access by minors and other unlawful purchasers, local and state prevention programs, and development of public support. More emphasis is also needed on building community coalitions to make youth environments safer (Institute of Medicine, 1999). Nurses can play important roles in all these steps.

Electrical Safety

Nurses must protect themselves and clients from dangerous shocks by keeping their hands dry when manipulating machinery, mopping up spilled fluid, ensuring that all plugs are grounded (three-pronged), and reporting any equipment damage. Electrical equipment should be serviced regularly.

Radiation Safety

Although the risk of radiation injury in most communities is low, nurses should let the community know about the sources and effects of radiation. Greater public awareness and understanding of radioactive waste and nuclear power can lead to stricter regulation of radiation used in industry.

Areas where radioactive substances are used are marked by an international symbol (Fig. 30-6). Radioactive implants or

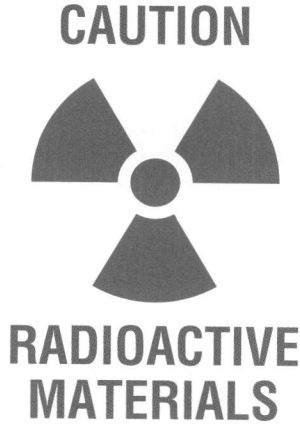

CAUTION
RADIOACTIVE
MATERIALS

FIGURE 30-6 International radiation symbol.

ingestion of radioactive materials may make a client a source of radioactive contamination. Nurses routinely wear radiation detection badges to assist the institution's radiation safety officer in monitoring exposure levels. These badges are collected periodically, and the exposure levels are calculated to ensure that staff are staying within safety limits of exposure. The three cardinal rules of radiation protection are (a) minimize time of exposure to the source, (b) maximize distance from the source, and (c) use appropriate shielding.

Safety precautions for staff include distancing and shielding themselves from the radiation source and measuring accumulated dose. Regular inspection and servicing of equipment and licensing of x-ray and pharmacy technicians help minimize risks to the clients and staff. Proper training on safe work procedures is essential for nursing personnel.

Nursing care for radiation therapy clients must be well organized so that assistance and support are given efficiently without needless exposure of nurses. Lead shields or lead aprons should be available if close contact with the client is required. Gloves should be worn to prevent skin contact with any body substances (urine, stool, saliva, blood). Clients may be encouraged to do as much of their own care as possible. If the client is admitted to a healthcare facility, a private room with private bath is essential to prevent exposure of other clients. Linens should be kept in the room until the radioactive source is removed. Soiled linens, excreta, and other wastes may require special labeling and disposal.

After cessation of therapy, the radiation safety officer will sweep the room with a radiation detector to assess for spills or contamination. After clearance, the room may be cleaned and linens sent to the laundry. If the client is to go home while receiving radiation therapy through an ingested substance (e.g., iodine 131), the hospital radiation safety manual will list directions for protection of the family, caregivers, and home environment.

Infection Control

Immunization against infections (communicable diseases) is important for children, adults, and healthcare workers. Influenza and hepatitis B vaccines are frequently offered to healthcare employees who work in close contact with clients, blood, or other potentially infectious materials. Because no immunization for tuberculosis is available, healthcare workers are usually tested yearly for exposure. If a person has been infected with tuberculosis (as indicated by a positive skin test), treatment is implemented to prevent active illness and spread to others. With the increasing incidence of tuberculosis, this testing is becoming especially important. Use of special respiratory protection and isolation procedures is required when working around persons with suspected or confirmed tuberculosis (OSHA, 1996). The *Guidelines for Preventing the Transmission of Mycobacterium Tuberculosis in Health-Care Facilities* (CDC, 1994) is the basis of these requirements.

Nurses play an important role in advocating timely vaccination of at-risk people. Childhood vaccination programs are mandatory in many states and provide protection against diphtheria, polio, measles, mumps, rubella, pertussis (whooping cough), varicella (chickenpox), hepatitis B, and tetanus. Some vaccinations require booster doses throughout life. The recommendation for a tetanus booster is once every 10 years (Hawker, Begg, & Weinberg, 2001). Remind adults about the need for boosters, and evaluate tetanus status periodically, especially when clients have incurred wounds. Vaccinations for influenza are generally suggested for older adults and for people with underlying chronic disease. The influenza vaccine changes annually to anticipate the most likely virulent strains and may need to be administered annually for those at risk. The pneumococcal vaccine is recommended for people older than 65 years and for those between 2 and 65 years with asplenia, sickle cell disease, chronic illness, or immunosuppression due to illness or therapy (Hawker, Begg, & Weinberg, 2001).

Teach sexually active adolescents and adults safe sex practices to prevent sexually transmitted diseases. Such practices include following abstinence, limiting the number of partners, using condoms and other barrier contraceptives, and using spermicide containing nonoxynol-9 (Cates & Raymond, 1998; Speroff & Darney, 2001). Women should receive regular gynecologic checkups, and men and women should seek medical attention for possible exposure or at the first sign of a sexually transmitted disease.

Infection control is a high priority in the healthcare environment. Most healthcare agencies, particularly hospitals, have full-time staff (usually nurses) devoted to teaching and implementing employee health programs and infection control practices throughout the facility. The principles of asepsis help prevent the spread of microorganisms. Handwashing, glove use, disinfection, sterilization, isolation precautions, and immunization are standard infection control procedures (see Chapter 26). Safer needle devices to prevent needlestick injuries, such as syringes with retractable needles or needleless IV systems, are essential. Use of alternatives to latex gloves prevent the development of latex allergy.

Childhood Safety

Make parents and other adult caregivers aware of the need to childproof the home and to supervise children in any potentially hazardous outside area. Teach caregivers to use only cribs and other equipment approved by the U.S. Consumer Products Safety Commission or other regulatory agency. The use of older equipment that is worn or poorly designed may present a hazard. Toys should be age appropriate.

Teach children bicycle safety. Among clients younger than 14 years old admitted to trauma centers as a result of bicycle-related injuries, more than half sustained head injuries—concussions and skull fractures (Li, Baker, Fowler, & DiScala, 1995). Children should wear helmets to protect against head injury in the event of a fall. Proper signaling and illumination of children and bicycles at night are important measures for injury prevention. Teach adults to check for small children riding low vehicles before driving a car out of a driveway or parking space. Warn children about riding in streets or near driveways.

The care of children in the healthcare environment requires special safety precautions. High staff-to-client ratios, use of cribs and beds with side rails, carpeting on the floor, play areas with age-appropriate toys and furnishings, locked medications and supply rooms, and protected exits contribute to safety.

Occupational Health and Safety

The work environment brings many rewards and frustrations to both nurses and clients alike. People spend a large portion of their time on the job—approximately 40% of their waking hours (Leigh, Markowitz, Fahs, Shin, & Landrigan, 1997).

Workplace hazards take a high toll on employees' lives due to disability and death. Estimates are that approximately 6500 job-related deaths from injury, 13.2 million nonfatal injuries, 63,000 deaths from occupational disease, and 862,200 illnesses occur each year (Leigh et al., 1997). The costs of medical care and lost work time are enormous; however, such estimates do not begin to address the costs associated with pain and suffering or with care provided by family members. Furthermore, researchers believe the actual number of injuries and illnesses to be much higher than these figures suggest, because underreporting of work-related conditions is a significant problem.

The leading causes of work-related deaths in 1995 were motor vehicles in the transportation and public utilities industries; homicides in wholesale and retail trade, government, and service industries; falls to lower level in the construction industry; and being struck by objects in manufacturing and construction industries. More than half of the nonfatal work-related injuries in 1999 were caused either by trauma that resulted from contact with objects or equipment (e.g., lacerations, contusions, fractures) or by overexertion injuries, primarily from heavy lifting (NSC, 2001).

The healthcare industry has many occupational hazards, some of which have already been mentioned. The Bureau of Labor Statistics data in 1996 found an overall injury rate for all private sector industries of 7.4 per 100 full-time employees

---

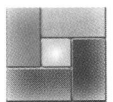

Nursing Research and Critical Thinking
Can a Community-Based Childhood Injury Prevention Program Reduce the Number of Safety Hazards in Peoples' Homes?

Public health nurses conduct home safety assessments as a part of their routine home visits. In this study, the nurses wanted to know if a new community-based childhood injury prevention program would reduce the number of safety hazards they found during their assessments. The nurses worked with the healthcare team of a large urban community-based home visiting program to evaluate the effectiveness of their injury prevention program on the reduction of home hazards. A one group pretest-posttest design was used to evaluate the differences between initial and discharge home safety assessment. Participants for this pilot study consisted of 72 families enrolled in the Healthy Baby Program. Women are referred to this program based on risk assessments conducted during prenatal care visits at neighborhood health center and hospital clinics. Forty-four potential home hazards were assessed before the intervention. On completion of the initial assessments, nurses and neighborhood health advocates provided education and counseling to clients about injury prevention practices, in addition to dispensing specific safety supplies. To evaluate the impact of the initial home

safety assessments, 14 of the original 44 home hazards were reassessed after discharge of the clients from the program. The mean length of time from initial home safety assessment to discharge was 3½ months. Eight home hazards did not show a statistically significant change from initial assessment to discharge. On average, 85% of homes that did not show statistically significant changes were assessed as safe at both initial assessment and discharge, leaving little room for improvement. However, 5 of the 13 discharge situations evaluated displayed a statistically significant improvement from initial assessment.

Critical Thinking Considerations. The study was limited because it was not ethical to withhold the intervention from eligible participants, and, therefore, no control group was included. Implications of the study are as follows:

- This community-based childhood injury prevention program appears to reduce the prevalence of home hazards and, therefore, to increase home safety.
- The program is most effective at reducing home hazards for which safety supplies are provided.

From Bablouzian, L., Freedman, E. S., Wolski, K. E., & Fried, L. E. (1997). Evaluation of a community-based childhood injury prevention program. *Injury Prevention, 3,* 14–16.

(FTEs). Healthcare industry sectors were substantially higher, with a rate of 9.1/100 FTEs. Nursing and personal care facilities had a rate of 16.5/100 FTEs, hospitals 11.00.1/100 FTEs, and residential care 11.0/100 FTEs (NSC, 2001). These figures are higher than rates found in mining and many sectors of construction and agriculture, all industries that have historically been associated with the highest rates of injury. Little information is currently available for home care, although back injury rates have been found to be three times greater among home care nurses compared with nurses in acute care (Myers, Jensen, Nestor, and Rattiner, 1993).

Workers younger than 18 years of age have been found to have higher rates of injury than adult workers (Miller & Kaufman, 1998). Probably, this finding is in large part the result of inexperience and possible immaturity of adolescents working in an adult setting.

Be aware of the contribution of occupational hazards to the incidence of injuries and illnesses that clients experience. Including an occupational history as part of the basic subjective assessment provides information about the source of certain health conditions, as well as the impact that other medical conditions or injuries may have on the client's ability to resume normal work activities. Client education should include basic principles about injury prevention, use of personal protective equipment, and safe work practices when dealing with hazardous exposures.

Nursing Interventions for Altered Safety

Harm to a person or group occurs when safety is not maintained. In the healthcare environment, specific nursing interventions are carried out when preventive measures fail. Nursing interventions for altered safety function include fire evacuation, emergency first aid for poisoning, administration of obstructed airway and cardiopulmonary resuscitation techniques, and filing an incident report.

Disaster Plans

Some areas of the country are prone to tornadoes, earthquakes, floods, and hurricanes. Nurses are responsible for knowing the disaster plans for such emergencies where they work. Understanding and practicing the plan help nurses to remain calm in emergencies. The two basic types of healthcare agency disasters are internal or external. Internal disasters are those in which the facility itself is in danger. Personnel must take actions to protect employees and clients. In an external disaster, many people are brought to a hospital or clinic for care after a large-scale emergency. Personnel must carry out specific plans when the healthcare agency is notified of any emergency.

Fire Evacuation

In the event of a fire in a client care area, nurses are responsible for determining which clients are in immediate danger. Direct ambulatory clients toward exits to wait in a safe area or enlist them to help evacuate bedridden clients. Use stretch-

ers and wheelchairs; if necessary, clients can be carried or dragged on sheets. Do not use elevators in the event of a fire. Activate the fire alarm and notify the healthcare agency's switchboard of the fire's location. The local fire department will be notified automatically. If the fire is small, a fire extinguisher can be used, but do not neglect other interventions, because small fires can quickly escalate out of control. Close windows and doors and turn off oxygen in the area to reduce the fire's oxygen supply. Evacuate clients in surrounding areas, if necessary, and give them wet washcloths to breathe through to reduce smoke inhalation.

Healthcare facilities are required to have fire evacuation plans with exits clearly marked. Additional staff from the facility and firefighters will respond quickly to help nurses evacuate clients. Never attempt to extinguish fires if the safety of yourself or your clients is in jeopardy. When evacuating clients who require mechanical ventilation, an ambubag can be used for manual respiration. Clamp tubes connected to suction before disconnecting them, and transport IV fluids with the client.

Emergency Care in Unintentional Poisoning

In the healthcare environment, ingestion of dangerous substances, overdosage, or incorrect medication administration can be treated as in the home. Notify the client's healthcare provider, but if the substance is potentially toxic, notify the poison control center without delay. The center will require information about the specific poison (the ingredients section on the label may provide this information), quantity ingested, person's age and weight, and apparent symptoms. Nurses may be instructed to induce vomiting with syrup of ipecac if the client is not unconscious or convulsing or if the substance was not a strong corrosive or petroleum product. Display 30-5 gives appropriate doses. Position the client on his or her side or with the head placed between the legs to prevent aspiration. Gather urine, vomitus, or blood samples as instructed.

If poisonous substances have been instilled into the eye or on the skin, immediate irrigation with lukewarm water for

DISPLAY 30-5

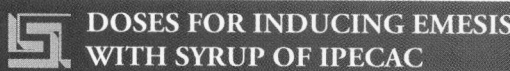

DOSES FOR INDUCING EMESIS WITH SYRUP OF IPECAC

Pediatric
- 6–12 months—administer 10 mL orally.
- Older than 1 year—administer 15 mL orally, followed by one to two glassfuls of whatever fluid the child will tolerate (ipecac is not effective on an empty stomach). Maintain activity level. Results should occur within 30 minutes.

Adult
- Administer 30 mL. The same procedure as above is applied to the adult victim.

10 to 15 minutes may reduce harmful effects. Remove contaminated clothing from the skin. Instruct the person to blink as much as possible during eye irrigation. Depending on the type of chemical exposure, be cautious about potential skin contact with the client or the client's clothing. Special procedures for handling hazardous materials may be necessary to protect staff and other clients in the area.

Cardiopulmonary Resuscitation

If a client chokes, aspirates, or is found cyanotic and apneic, the nurse is responsible for initiating resuscitation efforts (see Chapter 34). Electrical shock also may lead to cardiac arrest requiring cardiopulmonary resuscitation.

Filing an Incident Report

An incident report is filed whenever an injury event occurs in the healthcare environment. It is a confidential document filed with the institution's legal, insurance, or quality assurance department for internal use only. In it, the nurse describes how an injury occurred, what the effects were on the client, and what was done for the client. Incident reports are commonly used for falls, medication errors, and needlestick injuries.

In addition to filing an incident report, the nurse must enter on the client's medical record a description of the incident and its effects on the client. Notify the client's healthcare provider of the incident, and he or she will document the client's condition. The nurse does not make note of the incident report on the medical record because it is used internally. The incident report can be reviewed by the institution's attorneys in the event of a lawsuit, and it may be collected by the risk manager to see whether trends in injuries in the workplace are developing. When an injury to the nurse occurs, a workers' compensation claim usually is filed to cover the medical costs of the injury as well as the costs of any lost work time.

Healthcare Planning and Home/Community-Based Nursing

Nurses promote safety interventions wherever they practice. For example, school nurses function as safety educators for school-age children. They teach children drug-prevention measures and how to tell someone when they do not want to be touched. In many states, school nurses are required to report suspected child abuse. School nurses also may identify children who seem to be at high risk for injury. These children may have a neuromuscular or a sensory-perceptual basis for their injuries and should be evaluated. Screening for problems with vision and hearing is especially important.

The occupational health nurse may be involved in health and safety education and injury prevention at the worksite. Adults often need to learn proper body mechanics and may need to use transfer or lifting devices for lifting heavy loads. For the sedentary worker, principles of body alignment and stretching may help prevent muscle strain from prolonged static posture. Proper lighting may improve productivity and prevent eye strain. Occupational health nurses identify ergonomic hazards (e.g., repetitive strain injuries) and hazardous materials in the workplace and encourage appropriate worker protection (adequate ventilation, respiratory protection, ear plugs, protective clothing and eyewear); they also develop instructional health and safety promotion programs to prevent back injury, on-the-job injuries (e.g., falls, needlestick injuries), and illness.

All nurses may act as community activists and advocates for environmental safety in such areas as promoting clean air and water; cleanup of hazardous waste sites; safe, well-lighted pedestrian walkways; and laws supporting seatbelts, air bags, helmet use, and gun control.

Home Care Management

Home care nurses identify areas in which the client is unsafe when performing essential ADLs. They devise a plan that prepares the client, home caregivers, and the home itself for optimal safety. Display 30-1 lists potential hazards in the home. Other health professionals, such as social workers, occupational therapists, and physical therapists, are involved in the planning process and home care, but the nurse is often considered the most accurate source of information about the client's function in ADLs. If you work as a home care nurse, observe the client engaging in transfers and mobility, toileting, hygiene, eating and feeding, and dressing. Observations made during assessments allow the nurse to anticipate the measures that need to be taken to promote safety in these activities at home (Fig. 30-7).

The nurse working with a newly disabled client in a rehabilitation facility helps the healthcare team anticipate en-

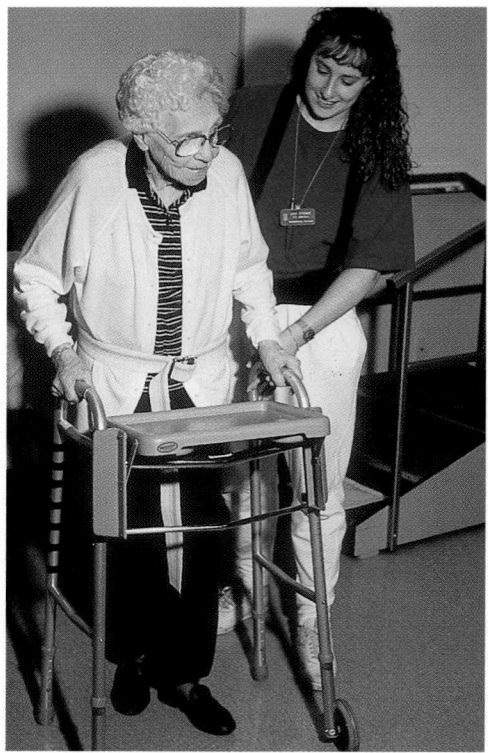

FIGURE 30-7   Use of a walker promotes safety when walking. The nurse may observe the client and her ability to use the walker before she is discharged.

vironmental changes that may be needed after discharge. Often, the client, family, or other caregivers are asked to draw a floor plan of the house, noting especially the width of doorways, configuration of the bathroom and kitchen, stairs approaching the home and within the home, and access to transportation from the home. Special equipment used during the hospitalization may need to be used in the home, and hospital beds, wheelchairs, tub benches, and mechanical lifts may not fit in the home. Early identification of the client's postdischarge equipment needs will help the family and caregivers to modify the home before the client is discharged.

Essential to overall safety is the support system. Actively involved caregivers or supportive friends can provide assistance with assessing the availability of caregivers, their level of desired participation, and their own capacity for safe judgment. Identify who will be providing care and whether they will be available occasionally, part-time, or 24 hours a day. Ask what care the caregivers can provide: assistance with mobility and transfers; with other ADLs (e.g., toileting, hygiene, dressing, eating); with laundry, shopping, and bill paying; or with supervision during inactive times. Determine what training the caregivers need to provide safe care. A home health referral may be needed to allow a home health nurse to visit the client and caregivers in the home and provide training there.

Community Services

Community health nurses may help older adults safety-proof their homes against falls by removing loose rugs and obstacles in hallways and stairwells. Community health nurses often educate members of the community about safety promotion through health fairs and lectures. Some communities offer a service that telephones the single older adult daily and responds to a help signal activated by a medallion worn around the neck. This system or a buddy system of telephone calls can provide a quick response to injury events for the older adult.

EVALUATION

The effectiveness of nursing interventions to promote safety is determined through nursing observation and feedback from clients, caregivers, and healthcare professionals in the community. Long-term goals include the identification of actual and potential environmental hazards, demonstration of safety habits, reduction in frequency and severity of injuries, and development of safe compensatory strategies for physical deficits. To measure the progress toward these goals, question the client and caregivers, using "what if" and "what would you do if" questions. Ask for and evaluate the client's performance of selected safety habits (e.g., transfers in and out of the bathtub). Gather data on the frequency and type of injury incidents. Determine the effectiveness of compensatory strategies: Is the client using the suggested strategies? What are the potential obstacles to their use? Is the client satisfied? Does the strategy make the activity eas-

ier, safer, or faster to accomplish? Any incident, fall, scrape, bruise, or other trauma requires a nurse's analysis to identify the cause and the best means to prevent recurrence. Nurses have a fundamental responsibility to promote continuous client safety, and every interaction with the client is an opportunity to promote and evaluate his or her safety habits.

Goal

The client will identify actual and high-risk environmental hazards.

Possible Outcome Criteria

- In the healthcare setting, the client verbalizes difficulty walking to the bathroom within 24 hours after being admitted as a client or resident.
- At home, the client verbalizes difficulty using stairs to access the bathroom.
- Before discharge, the client expresses fear of falling over obstacles at home or in the healthcare facility.

Goal

The client will demonstrate safety habits when performing ADLs.

Possible Outcome Criteria

- Immediately after instructions by the nurse, the client uses nurse call light system for assistance each time he or she needs to use the bathroom.
- The client uses over-the-bed lights, nonskid slippers, and eyeglasses when transferring to chair at first and subsequent times out of bed.
- The client identifies modifications for home safety (removal of throw rugs, installation of hand rails in hallway, better lighting of hallway and stairway) 24 hours after nurse's instruction about home safety.
- The client demonstrates appropriate use of bedside commode or availability of other appropriate accommodation for toileting while recuperating at home.
- The client demonstrates safety practices in dressing and hygiene.

Goal

The client will experience decreased frequency and severity of injury events.

Possible Outcome Criteria

- The client practices safety precautions, as evidenced by absence of falls or other trauma in the 48 hours before discharge.

NURSING PLAN OF CARE
THE CLIENT AT RISK FOR INJURY

Nursing Diagnosis
Risk for Injury related to sensory and integrative dysfunction manifested by altered mobility and faulty judgment.

Client Goal
Client will demonstrate safety habits when performing ADLs and injury prevention.

Client Outcome Criteria
- Client uses nurse call light system for assistance at each need to use bathroom immediately after instruction by the nurse.
- Client demonstrates safety practices in dressing and hygiene.
- Client uses over-the-bed lights, nonskid slippers each time when transferring to chair or out of bed.
- Client identifies modification for home safety (removal of throw rugs, installation of hand rails in hallway, better lighting of hallway and stairway) 12 hours after nurse's instruction about home safety.

Nursing Interventions	Scientific Rationale
1. Position bed in lowest position.	1. Low position minimizes distance to floor if client falls.
2. Place client call light within reach of hand, and give instructions.	2. A call light allows client to call for help.
3. Explain all safety modifications of the client's room: removal of clutter, providing a clear path to bathroom, use of a night light, installing brakes on bed and chairs, placement of call light.	3. Client and family will feel safer if they are aware of safety promotion strategies.
4. Perform frequent visual checks of client.	4. Client may attempt to get out of bed or chair without calling for assistance.
5. Use safety belt in all transfers if the client is unsteady or has difficulty with balance.	5. A safety belt allows for control/monitoring of client movement without trauma to any body part.
6. Evaluate the client's ability to use toilet; obtain raised toilet seat or grab bars if indicated.	6. Clients with hip muscle weakness may be unable to rise from low toilet seat. Grab bars may assist the weak person to move slowly and safely.
7. Assist client to perform hygiene at sink with large mirror; encourage client to scan the whole visual field.	7. Mirror provides client with visual reinforcement of activity.
8. Discuss floor plan of home with client and support person. Make suggestions for modifications that will lead to a safer environment.	8. Client and support person need to be involved in planning for client's safety in the home.

KEY CONCEPTS

- Safety is a basic human need that is essential in the healthcare environment, home, workplace, and community.
- Individual and environmental factors affect safety.
- Manifestations of altered safety include falls, fires, burns, lacerations, poisoning, suffocation, electrical shock, radiation injury, infection, allergies, respiratory problems, stress-related illness, and motor vehicle incidents.
- Infants, older adults, and those impaired by illness or medications are at greatest risk for falls.
- Falls in the healthcare environment are frequently associated with walking to the bathroom or early ambulation after illness, injury, or surgery.
- Nursing interventions to promote health and safety function involve client education and providing a safe environment in a healthcare setting, in the workplace, at home, and in the community.
- Nurses must educate parents about the developmental capabilities of infants and children and the special safety precautions needed for their care.
- Nurses must be familiar with emergency interventions for disasters, including fire evacuation and filing an incident report.
- Nurses must be knowledgeable about the health and safety hazards they face in healthcare settings in order to prevent their own injury and illness.

REFERENCES

American Academy of Pediatrics. (1996). Selecting and using the most appropriate car safety seats for growing children: Guidelines for counseling parents. *Pediatrics, 97,* 761–763.

Anderson, C., Stamper, M. (2001). Workplace violence. *RN, 64*(2), 71–74.

Barkin, S., Duan, N., Fink, A., Brook, R. H., & Gelberg, L. (1998). The smoking gun: Do clinicians follow guidelines on firearm safety counseling? *Archives of Pediatrics and Adolescent Medicine, 152*(8), 749–756.

Bryant, H., & Fernald, L. (1997). Nursing knowledge and use of restraint alternatives: Acute and chronic care. *Geriatric Nursing, 18*(2), 57–60.

Cassel, C. K., Nelson, E. A., Smith, T. W., Schwab, C. W., Barlow, B., & Gary, N. E. (1998). Internists' and surgeons' attitudes toward guns and firearm injury prevention. *Annals of Internal Medicine, 128*(3), 224–230.

Cates, W., & Raymond, E. (1998). Vaginal spermicides. In R. A. Hatcher, J. Trussell, F. Stewart, W. Cates, G. Stewart, & D. Kowal (Eds.). *Contraceptive technology* (17th rev. ed.; pp. 357–369). New York: Ardent Media.

Centers for Disease Control and Prevention. (1994). Guidelines for preventing the transmission of *Mycobacterium tuberculosis* in health-care facilities. *MMWR Morb Mortal Wkly Rep, 43*(RR-13), 1–132.

Cook, P. J., & Ludwig, J. (1996). *Guns in America.* Washington, DC: Police Foundation.

Cummings, P., Grossman, D. C., Rivara, F. P., & Koepsell, T. D. (1997). State gun safe storage laws and child mortality due to firearms. *Journal of the American Medical Association, 278*(13), 1084–1086.

Dresang, LT. (2001) Gun deaths in rural and urban settings: Recommendations for prevention. *Journal of the American Board of Family Practitioners, 14*(2), 107–115.

Dunbar, J. M., Neufeld, R. R., White, H. C., & Libow, L. S. (1996). Retrain, don't restrain: The educational intervention of the National Nursing Home Restraint Removal Project. *Gerontologist, 36*(4), 539–542.

Environmental Protection Agency. (1993). *A physician's guide. Radon: The health threat with a simple solution.* EPA Document #402-K-93-008. Washington, DC: U.S. Government Printing Office.

Environmental Protection Agency. (1998). Sources of information on indoor air quality. Available at: http://www.epa.gov/iaq/radon. Accessed 1/2/02.

Fletcher, K. (1996). Use of restraints in the elderly. *AACN Clinical Issues, 7*(4), 611–635.

Food and Drug Administration. (1992). *FDA safety alert: Potential hazards with restraint devices.* Rockville, MD: Author.

Frank, C., Hodgetts, G., & Puxty, J. (1996). Safety and efficacy of physical restraints for the elderly: Review of the evidence. *Canadian Family Physician, 42,* 2402–2409.

Freed, L. H., Vernick, J. S., & Hargarten, S. W. (1998). Prevention of firearm-related injuries and deaths among youth: A product-oriented approach. In H. Hennes & A. D. Calhoun (Eds.), *The Pediatric Clinics of North America: Violence among children and adolescents, 45*(2), 427–438.

Glass, R. J., Segui-Gomez, M., & Graham, J. D. (2000). Child passenger safety: Decisions about seating location, airbag exposure, and restraint use. *Risk Analysis, 20*(4), 521–527.

Hanger, H. C., Ball, M. C., & Wood, L. A. (1999). An analysis of falls in the hospital: Can we do without bedrails? *Journal of the American Geriatrics Society, 47*(5), 627–628.

Hawker, J., Begg, N., & Weinberg, J. (2001). *Communicable Disease Control Handbook.* Boston: Blackwell Scientific.

Health Care Financing Administration. (1989). Medicare and Medicaid: Requirements for long term care facilities. *Federal Register, 54*(21), 1.

Institute of Medicine. (1999). *Reducing the burden of injury.* Bonnie, R. J., Fulco, C. E., & Liverman, C. T. (Eds.). Washington, DC: National Academy Press. Available at: http://www.nap.edu. Accessed 1/2/02.

Jensen, B., Hess-Zak, A., Johnston, S. K., Otto, D. C., Tebbe, L., Russell, C. L., & Waller, A. S. (1998). Restraint reduction: A new philosophy for a new millennium. *Journal of Nursing Administration, 28*(7–8), 32–38.

Jenkins, E. L. (1996). Workplace homicide: Industries and occupations at high risk. In R. Harrison (Ed.), *Occupational medicine state of the art reviews: Violence in the workplace, 11*(2), 219–225.

Joint Commission on Accreditation of Healthcare Organizations. (1999). *Revised restraint standards for nonpsychiatric patients.* Oakbrook Terrace, IL: Author.

Karlsson, S., Bucht, G., & Sandman, P. O. (1998). Physical restraints in geriatric care: Knowledge, attitudes and use. *Scandinavian Journal of Caring Sciences, 12*(1), 48–56.

Leigh, J. P., Markowitz, S. B., Fahs, M., Shin, C., & Landrigan, P. J. (1997). Occupational injury and illness in the United States. *Archives of Internal Medicine, 157,* 1557–1568.

Li, G., Baker, S. P., Fowler, C., & DiScala, C. (1995). Factors related to the presence of head injury in bicycle-related pediatric trauma patients. *Journal of Trauma, 38*(6), 871–875.

Maslow, A. H. (1970). *Motivation and personality* (2nd ed.). New York: Harper and Row.

McLoughlin, E, Fennell, J. (2000). The power of survivor advocacy: Making car trunks escapable. *Injury Prevention, 6*(3), 167–170.

Miller, M. E., & Kaufman, J. (1998). Occupational injuries among adolescents in Washington State, 1988–1991. *American Journal of Industrial Medicine, 34*(2), 121–132.

Myers, A., Jensen, R. C., Nestor, D., & Rattiner, J. (1993). Low back injuries among home health aides compared with hospital nursing aides. *Home Health Care Services Quarterly, 14*(2–3), 149–155.

National Institute of Occupational Health and Safety. (1997). *NIOSH alert: Preventing allergic reactions to natural rubber latex in the workplace.* DHHS (NIOSH) publication no. 97-135. Cincinnati: U.S. Department of Health and Human Services, Public Health Services, Centers for Disease Control and Prevention.

National Safety Council. (2001). *Injury facts.* Itasca, IL: Author.

North American Nursing Diagnosis Association. (2001). *Nursing diagnoses: Definitions and classification 2001–2001.* Philadelphia: Author.

Occupational Safety and Health Act. (1970). *General Duty Clause, Public Law 91-596, Section 5(a)(1).*

Occupational Safety and Health Administration (OSHA). (1991). *Occupational exposure to bloodborne pathogens, final rule. 29 CFR Part 1910.1030.* Washington, DC: Office of the Federal Register, U.S. Government Printing Office.

Occupational Safety and Health Administration (OSHA). (1996). *CPL 2.106: Enforcement procedures and scheduling for occupational exposure to tuberculosis.* Washington DC: Author.

Omnibus Budget Reconciliation Act of 1990. (1990). *Act to provide for reconciliation pursuant to section 4 of the concurrent resolution on the budget for fiscal year 1991.* Washington, DC: U.S. Government Printing Office.

Parker, K., & Miles, S. H. (1997). Deaths caused by bed rails. *Journal of American Geriatrics Society, 45*(7), 797–802.

Ramsey, J. J., & Kernvitz, J. W. (1998). Bioenergetics. In J. E. Birren (Ed.), *Encyclopedia of gerontology: Age, aging, and the aged.* San Diego, CA: Academic Press.

Resnick, M. D., Bearman, P. S., Blum, R. W., Bauman, K. E., Harris, K. M., Jones, J., Tabor, J., Beuhring, T., Sieving, R. E., Shew, M., Ireland, M., Bearinger, L. H., & Udry, J. R. (1997). Protecting adolescents from harm: Findings from the National Longitudinal Study on Adolescent Health. *Journal of the American Medical Association, 278*(10), 823–832.

Runyan, C. W. (2001). Moving forward with research on the prevention of violence against workers. *American Journal of Preventive Medicine, 20*(2), 169–172.

Sloan, J. H., Kellerman, A. L., Reay, D. T., Ferris, J. A., Koepsell, T., Rivara, F. P., Rice, C., Gray, L., & LoGerfo, J. (1988). Handgun regulations, crimes, assaults, and homicide: A tale of two cities. *New England Journal of Medicine, 319*(19), 1256–1262.

Speroff, L., & Darney, P. (2001). *A clinical guide for contraception* (3rd ed.). Philadelphia: Lippincott Williams & Wilkins.

Sullivan-Marx, E. M. (1996). Restraint-free care: How does a nurse decide? *Journal of Gerontological Nursing, 22*(9), 7–14.

Sullivan-Marx, E. M., Strumpf, N. E., Evans, L. K., Baumgarten, M., & Maislin, G. (1999a). Initiation of physical restraint in nursing home residents following restraint reduction efforts. *Research in nursing and health, 22*(5), 369–379.

Sullivan-Marx, E. M., Strumpf, N. E., Evans, L. K., Baumgarten, M., & Maislin, G. (1999b). Predictors of continued physical restraint use in nursing home residents following restraint reduction efforts. *Journal of the American Geriatrics Society, 47*(3), 342–348.

Terpstra, T. L., Terpstra, T. L., & Van Doren, E. (1998). Reducing restraints: Where to start. *Journal of Continuing Education in Nursing, 29*(1), 10–16.

U.S. Department of Health and Human Services, Public Health Service. (2000). *Healthy people 2010: Understanding and improving health* (2nd ed.): Available at: http://www.health.gov/healthypeople/Document/tableofcontents.htm#under. Accessed 1/2/02.

U.S. Department of Labor. (1996). *Guidelines for preventing workplace violence for health care and social service workers.* OSHA document #3148. Washington, DC: U.S. Government Printing Office.

Wolfson, A. R., & Carskadon, M. A. (1998). Sleep schedules and daytime functioning in adolescents. *Child Development, 69*(4), 875–887.

Worthington, K., & Franklin, P. (2001). Workplace violence. *American Journal of Nursing, 101*(4), 73.

BIBLIOGRAPHY

Castle, N. G., & Mor, V. (1998). Physical restraints in nursing homes: A review of the literature since the Nursing Home Reform Act of 1987. *Medical Care Research & Review, 55*(2), 139–176.

Kane, R., Ouslander, J., & Abrass, I. (1999). *Essentials of clinical geriatrics* (4th ed.). New York: McGraw-Hill.

Maki, B. E., & Fernie, G. R. (1998). Accidents: Falls. In J. E. Birren (Ed.), *Encyclopedia of gerontology: Age, aging, and the aged.* San Diego, CA: Academic Press.

McGreevy, J. C., & Decina, L. E. (1996). Child safety misuse. *Journal of Emergency Medical Services, 21*(3), 118–119.

Reigle, J. (1997). Limiting use of physical restraints: New guidelines present a challenge. Joint Commission on Accreditation of Healthcare Organizations. *Critical Care Nurse, 17*(4), 80–85.

Spencer, R. T., et al. (1998). *Clinical pharmacology and nursing management* (5th ed.). Philadelphia: Lippincott-Raven.

31 Health Maintenance

Chapter

Key Terms

disease-prevention activities
health-maintenance activities

health-promotion activities
health-protection activities

Learning Objectives

Upon completion of this chapter, the student will be able to do the following:

1. Describe characteristics essential for normal health.
2. Give examples of health-promotion and disease-prevention behaviors.
3. Describe important lifespan development considerations related to health maintenance.
4. Recognize major factors that affect motivation and health maintenance.
5. Describe factors that place an individual's health at risk.
6. Characterize manifestations of altered health maintenance.
7. Obtain subjective data through a nursing history to assess health maintenance.
8. Provide appropriate information about common illnesses that may result from altered health maintenance.
9. List resources for client-teaching information on health maintenance.
10. Value health-promotion concepts and act as a role model for clients.

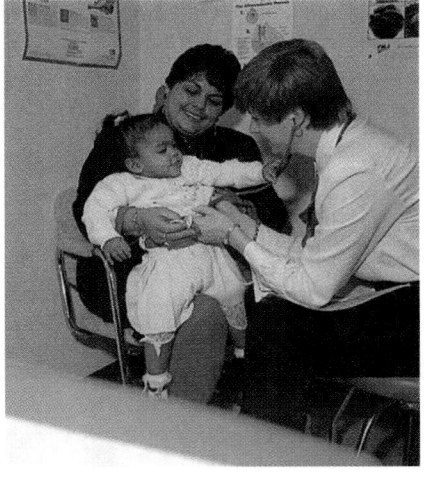

Critical Thinking Challenge

Patricia, a 28-year-old mother, has brought Evita, age 15 months, into the family health clinic for a well-child assessment. On this first encounter, you start a family database because all family members will visit the clinic. You also consider Patricia's parenting skills, possible stressors to successful parenting, and health knowledge.

The family has recently moved to the city; the husband and father, Hector, has his first job after college graduation. In obtaining the family history, you note the following health problems: diabetes mellitus (paternal father and maternal mother and father); hypertension and emphysema (paternal father); and obesity (maternal and paternal mothers). One of Patricia's brothers died at age 16 years in an auto accident; all other siblings (total of eight) of Hector and Patricia are living and well. Hector smokes a pack of cigarettes and two cigars a day. Patricia has recently read material about family risks for diabetes, cancer, and heart disease. She is concerned about her own health (she now weighs 50 lb more than she did 3 years ago) and her family's health.

Once you have completed this chapter and added health maintenance to your knowledge base, return to the above scenario and reflect on the following areas of Critical Thinking:

1. Reflect on the information you know about Patricia and her family, your own values, and your initial impression of the client and her situation.
2. Consider additional data you will need to determine necessary health teaching.
3. Analyze risky behaviors and health-seeking behaviors in your client's situation.
4. Based on your analysis of risky behaviors, recommend health information your client needs.
5. Based on your identification of health information needs, what Internet sites would you recommend to your client?

Florence Nightingale believed the following:

- Health is the ability to use well every power one has.
- Preventable disease should be a crime.
- It is cheaper to promote health than it is to care for illness.
- Goals of nursing should include health maintenance, health teaching, and disease prevention.

More than 150 years later, nurses continue to address these issues and have the potential and social responsibility to assist individuals, families, and communities to maintain and improve their health. Nursing activities of health education and client teaching focus on enhancing the abilities of clients to engage in effective and efficient health behaviors. Nurses engage in promoting health in a variety of settings, including the workplace, schools, homes, camps, rehabilitation units, nursing homes, and hospitals. Although nurses promote healthy behaviors, it is the individual's option to accept or reject those behaviors. For example, the nurse may teach the client Patricia about ways to reduce health risks associated with diabetes, hypertension, and cancer, but she and her family must decide whether they will use all, some, or none of the information.

Health promotion and disease prevention have become increasingly popular concepts in healthcare reform in the United States, Canada, and internationally. At the Fourth International Conference on Health Promotion of the World Health Organization (WHO), social responsibility for the promotion of health was emphasized in the following priorities: to promote health through policies and practices that avoid harming the health of other individuals; to protect the environment and ensure sustainable use of resources; to restrict production and trade in inherently harmful goods and substances such as tobacco and armaments, as well as unhealthy marketing practices; to safeguard both the citizen in the marketplace and the individual in the workplace; and to include equity-focused health impact assessments as an integral part of policy development. Other priorities included increasing health development, developing community partnerships between different sectors of government and society, and securing funding for health promotion activities (WHO, 2001). The increasing emphasis on community partnerships places responsibilities on nurses to work cooperatively with all levels of government, college programs, community and business organizations, and neighborhoods to improve the health of groups of people.

NORMAL HEALTH MAINTENANCE

Health-maintenance activities are the behaviors that a person in stable health uses to maintain or improve that state over time. To understand health maintenance, recall the concepts of health and wellness from Chapter 16. Health and wellness involve assuming responsibility for oneself, making informed choices, feeling a sense of self-worth, and managing healthcare regimens and stress. Health maintenance, then, is the continuity and harmony of those beliefs and behaviors.

As discussed in Chapter 16, individuals have their own definitions of health and wellness, which relate to their personal expectations and values. Healthcare workers may define health and wellness in one way, but clients may define them differently. If a person believes that health means being free of disease, his or her parameters of health are narrow. If a person believes that health is the optimal functioning of biologic, psychosocial, economic, and spiritual factors within the environment, the meaning of health becomes quite broad.

Characteristics of Normal Health Maintenance

To maintain a level of health and to strive for higher levels of well-being, a person may need to alter health habits and the environment. He or she may seek new support sources, both formal (agencies) and informal (friends). Normal health maintenance requires four characteristics:

- Perception of health
- Motivation to change direction, if necessary
- Adherence to management goals
- Available social and economic resources

Perception
A person's ability to maintain a desired level of health depends on that person's perception of his or her current health status, knowledge of how to manage positive health behaviors, and the economic and social resources to implement desired interventions. For example, many older adults mistakenly believe joint pain to be a normal part of aging and therefore do not seek medical attention for it. When asked about their health status, these people may say they are in good health, forgetting about or ignoring the joint pain.

The person who believes that health is a gift from God may believe that little can be done to change health. This perception influences how the person rates personal health and the options available for management. The person's perception and understanding of health determine the accountability and responsibility that he or she assumes for health.

People who believe that exercise programs and low-fat diets are too expensive or not readily available may dismiss options because of the fear of the cost. Additionally, many people are not aware of low-cost or free programs available in their community that can assist with health activities, such as Medicaid and the Children Health Insurance Program, both federal- and state-subsidized insurance programs for the medically indigent. Or pride may prevent a person from accepting social help, which may limit access to health services.

Motivation
When a person is strongly motivated toward realizing an optimal level of wellness or maintaining current health status, he or she actively seeks health information, teaching, and activities that help achieve that goal. A person who is less strongly motivated may not succeed in achieving those goals and behaviors, no matter what the nurse counsels.

Because each person defines health in relation to personal expectations and values, the degree of motivation for change depends on those expectations and values. Motivation is internally generated; although the nurse can support and enhance motivation, the client is the ultimate determinant.

Biologic capabilities influence both the initiation of motivation and the potential for success. For example, even a person who is highly motivated toward a healthy lifestyle with optimal nutrition, regular exercise, and stress management may not succeed in achieving wellness because of the limitations (barriers) posed by his or her genetic inheritance, available resources, or environmental exposures.

Management

Reducing health risks is not always easy. Reducing risks usually entails making a decision to change one's lifestyle and to break old habits (e.g., quitting smoking, losing weight, controlling alcohol intake, exercising regularly). Often, it is far easier to continue risky behaviors, hoping for the best. The initiative to change is sometimes motivated by situational factors (e.g., marriage, pregnancy, a friend's newly diagnosed lifestyle disease), new awareness that a behavior is risky, or the availability of a new resource.

Once a person makes the decision to change, the next step is to set realistic and achievable goals. Momentary overenthusiasm may lead to goals that are unrealistic and difficult to achieve, which can ultimately result in discouragement and failure. For example, a person who is 60 lb overweight decides to lose 80 lb within 6 months; for this person, the goal is unrealistic and unhealthy and needs to be modified.

Adapting and adhering to new health behaviors can be trying and frustrating. During the transition, people may need social support to comply with their goals. They can obtain such support from nurses and other healthcare professionals, friends, family, and support groups such as Alcoholics Anonymous, Weight Watchers, and Parents Anonymous. In some situations, changes may be necessary in the person's social and physical environment. For instance, someone who takes illicit drugs probably has friends who do drugs. The person who wants to stop using drugs may need to seek new friends as well as a new lifestyle and physical environment.

Managing health-maintenance goals is similar to the nursing process: it requires assessing the need for change, determining weaknesses and strengths, setting goals, planning and implementing interventions, and evaluating outcomes. The client may continue selected health behaviors or choose different health behaviors if the first selections are not useful or possible.

Available Economic and Social Resources

Over the last several decades in the United States, the number of people with adequate health insurance coverage has diminished. Businesses are requiring increasing cost sharing for employer-sponsored health insurance, while the cost of deductibles and copayments has increased. This has occurred during a time when medical costs (including prescription drugs) has increased at a rate faster than inflation. The increased cost of health insurance often places individuals with low income out of the insurance market. People of lower socioeconomic status often have fewer economic and social resources for health activities than others do. Poverty is the greatest threat to good health; it is associated with increased incidence of preventable diseases, tooth loss, and premature death. In countries without a national health insurance enrollment, the lack of health insurance limits access to health care services. Often people on limited incomes must decide between paying for housing and food or paying for medications and healthcare.

Poor communities are less likely to have parks, bike trails, and other resources that encourage healthy behaviors. Rural communities also have fewer health care resources than urban areas, causing individuals to travel great distances to access health care services. Many rural areas are also economically depressed, thereby compounding health resource deficits.

Normal Health-Maintenance Patterns

Health-maintenance patterns are a synthesis of all the other functional patterns. Marjorie Gordon (1994) referred to health maintenance as the "umbrella." The other function areas, she said, "can be viewed as specific areas of health management. The goal . . . is to identify health strengths, health beliefs, health risks, and health deficits for which improvements are possible to maximize health status" (pp. 106–107).

The basic components of health maintenance are health promotion and disease prevention. **Health-promotion activities** are approach behaviors that seek to expand the potential for health and are often associated with lifestyle choices; **disease-prevention activities** are avoidance behaviors that seek to prevent specific diseases or conditions (Pender, 1996; Murray & Zentner, 2001). Approach behaviors require a decision to make positive lifestyle changes in an effort to increase the level of wellness. Avoidance behaviors (e.g., immunizations) are used to avoid illness, rather than to promote health per se. The focus of health differs between these two concepts: health promotion implies a positive and multidimensional concept of health involving lifestyle choices, whereas disease prevention implies that health equals the absence of disease (Pender, 1996). The two behaviors often overlap.

Health maintenance also is influenced by **health-protection activities** that occur at a community level. Health-protection activities are environmental or regulatory measures that seek to protect the health of a community or large population. Examples of health-protection activities include air and water quality regulations and food and drug regulations promulgated by federal, state, and local governments. Health-protection activities usually fall within the realm of public health and community or public health nursing.

Health Promotion

Put simply, people use health-promotion activities to feel better. Health-promotion behaviors enhance overall well-being. Examples include increasing dietary fiber and decreasing intake of fats and refined carbohydrates, avoiding tobacco products, developing regular patterns of exercise and sleep, controlling stress, seeking wellness information, establishing and maintaining friendships, and being environmentally concerned. Nola Pender (1996) suggested that defining health promotion as lifestyle modification is narrow and in the tradition of clinical medicine interventions. People who use health-promotion behaviors want to move beyond the absence of disease in their lives toward high-level wellness by evaluating their lifestyle, learning about options, and striving to become all they can be. Health promotion is not about any particular disease or condition: people using health-promotion behaviors do so to pursue their highest level of wellness, not to prevent a specific disease.

Pender (1996) proposed a theory to explain the health-promoting activities of people (Fig. 31-1). Work is being done to expand this theory to include health-promoting activities of families and communities. This model comprises three components: behavior-specific cognitions and affect, individual characteristics, and behavioral outcome. Behavior-specific cognitions include the variables of perceived benefits and barriers to action, perceived self-efficacy (belief that one can perform a skill or behavior), activity-related affect (feelings about the activity), interpersonal influences (family, friends, norms, supports), and situational influences (options, environment). Individual characteristics include prior related behaviors and personal factors (biologic, sociocultural,

and psychological). Behavioral outcomes include competing demands, a commitment to a plan of action, and a health-promoting behavior.

Disease Prevention

People use preventive behaviors to protect themselves from certain diseases or conditions. Disease prevention is targeted at three levels (Table 31-1). Primary disease prevention includes activities and lifestyle factors directed toward high-level wellness, such as adequate nutrition, adequate immunization status, regular exercise, and stress management. Maintaining health is the primary mode for preventing illness.

Secondary prevention includes all health screening clinics, such as well-child assessments and checks for blood pressure abnormalities or for cervical or uterine, breast, testicular, or prostate cancers. The goal is to identify abnormalities within a population. The clinics tend to have one focus, and those with abnormal results are referred elsewhere for follow-up and treatment. Secondary prevention also includes self-examination techniques such as breast and testicular self-examinations and checking one's skin for lesions.

Tertiary prevention is directed toward minimizing individual disability from disease or dysfunction. Its goal is to assist the person to obtain optimal health or to learn to live with limitations. Diabetes education and cardiac rehabilitation are examples of tertiary prevention measures.

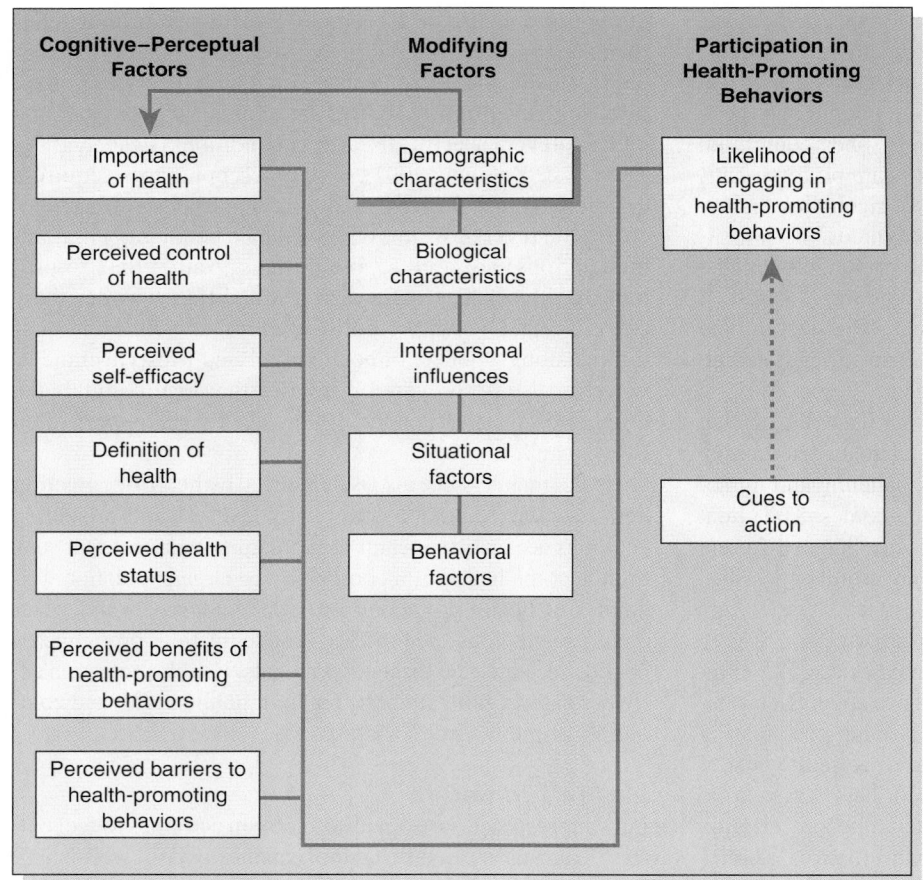

FIGURE 31-1 Characteristics of normal functional health maintenance. (Adapted from Pender, N. [1996]. *Health promotion in nursing practice* [3rd ed.]. Norwalk, CT: Appleton & Lange.)

TABLE 31-1

Three Levels of Disease Prevention		
Level	Description	Examples
Primary prevention	Seeks to prevent a disease or condition at a prepathologic state; to stop something from ever happening	Immunizations, fluoride supplements, car seat restraints, oral contraceptives, education in elementary schools about drug addiction
Secondary prevention	Seeks to identify specific illnesses or conditions at an early stage with prompt intervention to prevent or limit disability; to prevent catastrophic effects that could occur if proper attention and treatment are not provided	Physical assessments, developmental screening, vision screening, breast and testicular self-examinations, pregnancy testing
Tertiary prevention	Occurs after a disease or disability has occurred and the recovery process has begun; intent is to halt the disease or injury process and assist the person in obtaining an optimal health status	Habilitation for handicapped children, support groups such as Reach for Recovery and Alcoholics Anonymous, cardiac rehabilitation, health education for a newly diagnosed diabetic

Combination of Promotion and Prevention

Display 31-1 lists examples of health-promotion and disease-prevention activities for the functional health patterns. It is often difficult to differentiate between the two types of activities because they overlap and work in combination. For instance, daily jogging may be a health-promotion behavior for one person and a disease-prevention behavior for another. A person who begins to jog because of a risk of cardiovascular disease and then continues because she feels better may switch from disease prevention to health promotion. A person may be involved with health promotion and all three levels of disease prevention. For example, a woman with diabetes mellitus may give herself insulin (tertiary prevention), perform a monthly breast self-examination (secondary prevention), brush her teeth daily (primary prevention), and exercise regularly to feel good (health promotion).

Lifespan Considerations

Health-maintenance opportunities begin before conception and continue until death. Characteristics of development at various stages call for specific health-maintenance behaviors.

Newborn and Infant

Health maintenance begins during the prenatal period. Low birth weight and congenital defects—which put babies at risk for additional health problems—have been linked to lack of prenatal care, poor nutrition, and use of alcohol, tobacco, or drugs during pregnancy. Because their immune systems are immature, newborns and infants are at risk for infectious diseases, so immunizations are of primary importance. (The schedule of recommended immunizations is given in Chapter 39.) The nervous system develops rapidly, and bones, muscles, and other organ systems grow during infancy, so proper nutrition and regular developmental and health check-ups are important.

Toddler and Preschooler

Toddlers and preschoolers develop and learn through exploration and imitation. Curiosity and lack of experience predispose them to accidents and injuries. Exposure to other children in day care centers, school, or play groups puts them at risk for infection. Safety practices, proper sleep and nutrition, avoidance of second-hand tobacco smoke, and regular immunization schedules are important for health maintenance. Toddlers and preschoolers begin to learn healthy and unhealthy practices by imitating their parents and other caregivers.

School-Age Child and Adolescent

School-age children begin to form beliefs about health. They are still influenced primarily by their parents and caregivers, but teachers and friends become increasingly important. School-age children may begin to experience problems such as obesity, high cholesterol levels, and poor stress management, which can become symptomatic in adulthood. Physical and intellectual development are rapid. Health-maintenance concerns include proper nutrition, sleep, and exercise; safety; and learning to deal with stress and frustration.

Adolescents must deal with sexual development and confirmation of their identity. Struggles for independence and the physical changes accompanying sexual development make adolescence a time for experimenting with healthy and unhealthy practices. Peer influence is so strong for adolescents that they may adopt unhealthy practices, such as smoking or drinking. Peer pressure also can have positive influences—for example, when the peer group does not use tobacco or alcohol. Overconcern about image and weight can lead to anorexia or steroid abuse. Driving safely, preventing sexually

DISPLAY 31-1

🗐 **NORMAL FUNCTIONAL HEALTH MANAGEMENT**

Health Perception and Health Management
- Has a personal perception of health and all it entails
- Has a strong motivation for an optimal level of wellness
- Sets health goals and seeks help in managing them
- Has sufficient financial resources to maintain health
- Maintains a safe environment at home and work
- Performs activities of daily living

Activity and Exercise
- Maintains good hygiene through self-care
- Uses good body mechanics in activities of daily living
- Maintains optimal motor function
- Uses leisure hours in a healthy manner
- Uses oxygen efficiently

Nutrition and Metabolism
- Has sufficient knowledge of nutrition
- Plans daily menu carefully
- Obtains and digests appropriate amounts of nutrients to promote optimal nutrition
- Protects body against infection
- Maintains homeostatic thermoregulation

Elimination
- Maintains a regular schedule for elimination
- Understands body processes in digestion and elimination
- Practices hygiene after elimination

Sleep and Rest
- Maintains a regular sleep pattern
- Maintains balance of work and rest
- Provides time for relaxation

Cognition and Perception
- Demonstrates optimal cerebral function
- Builds knowledge and skills
- Develops quality sensory perception

Self-Perception and Self-Concept
- Displays activities appropriate for developmental level
- Demonstrates positive self-concept
- Has a stable body image
- Recognizes and cherishes personal identity as unique
- Recognizes uniqueness of other people

Roles and Relationships
- Demonstrates functional verbal and nonverbal communication
- Participates in social interactions
- Builds and maintains meaningful relationships
- Has intrinsic mechanisms or support people to help with coping during grieving

Coping and Stress Tolerance
- Makes decisions reflecting understanding of personal limitations
- Protects self against overwhelming situations and changes
- Manages to keep in touch with personal needs while balancing life's roles with minimal conflict

Sexuality and Reproduction
- Has valid knowledge about sexual functioning and human sexuality
- Accepts sexual functions and sexuality as normal
- Recognizes and accepts personal sexual feelings
- Maintains healthy lifestyle during pregnancy

Values and Beliefs
- Expresses respect for all life and the quality of life
- Maintains realistic goals for self based on value decisions
- Demonstrates a zeal for life
- Provides for spiritual sustenance

transmitted diseases (STDs) including acquired immunodeficiency syndrome (AIDS), preventing pregnancy, avoiding drugs and alcohol, avoiding gang-related violence, and maintaining mental health are primary health-maintenance concerns during adolescence.

Adult and Older Adult

With rapid physical and intellectual growth completed and health beliefs ingrained, adults should enjoy productive and satisfying years. They may now, however, become at risk for lifestyle-related chronic conditions, such as heart disease, hypertension, cancer, and diabetes, depending on health beliefs and practices and genetic factors. The responsibilities of raising a family, holding a job, and being a productive

member of society may lead to addictions or stress-related illnesses. Health-maintenance concerns include exercise, nutrition, self-examinations, prenatal care for women, health screening, stress management, and reduction or cessation of alcohol and smoking.

Primary prevention continues in adulthood. Many adults have an inadequate immunization status because they forget or are unaware of necessary boosters and new immunizations such as influenza and pneumonia. Health maintenance with adults, nevertheless, focuses more on secondary prevention than the other levels, except during pregnancy. Exercise, nutrition, social stimulation, and regular medical checkups are important because of the normal physiologic changes of aging and the increased risk of chronic illness in older adults. Using medications safely and identifying community resources and support groups are also important health-maintenance considerations.

FACTORS AFFECTING HEALTH MAINTENANCE

Many factors influence health maintenance positively or negatively. These factors affect what people believe about health, as well as what healthy and unhealthy practices they perform.

Cognition and Perception

Cognitive and perceptual factors include what health means to a person, how important it is, and how the person perceives control over health, self-efficacy, health status, benefits, and barriers. The more a person values health, the more likely he or she is to participate in health-promoting and health-maintaining behaviors (Pender, 1996; Edelman & Mandel, 1998; Arnold & Boggs, 1999). Peers, family, and society influence values. A person may believe that he or she primarily controls health (internal) or that factors beyond his or her control are responsible for health (external). People with an internal perception of control are more likely to engage in health-seeking behaviors on their own, but people with an external perception of control are more likely to do so with social pressure and encouragement.

A person's belief about self-efficacy or the ability to accomplish a certain behavior affects his or her willingness to try the behavior. As the person's mastery of behaviors increases, he or she may be more likely to engage in additional activities. Success with one activity can motivate the person to try other activities (Bandura, 1977).

People may define health negatively (not being ill) or positively (an optimal state of well-being). That definition influences how the person perceives health and the mechanics of maintaining health (Gorin & Arnold, 1998; Murray & Zentner, 2001). People who see themselves as having a positive health status may be more likely to continue behaviors that promote and maintain that level of health. However, two people with the same health status may have different perceptions of that health status. Those who see the benefits of health behaviors are more likely to begin or continue those behaviors; those who see the effects as negative or neutral are less likely to do so (Gorin & Arnold, 1998).

People with low perceived barriers to health behaviors are more likely to pursue healthy behaviors than are those with high perceived barriers. Barriers can include time, finances, access, location, convenience, attitude, culture, and social support.

Age and Developmental Level

Age can have a significant impact on a person's ability to manage his or her health status. A 17-year-old woman with arthritis or diabetes mellitus may perceive her health status as low and may not engage in proper health-maintenance prac-

tices, whereas an 80-year-old woman may see such conditions as acceptable and may carry out practices to promote optimum health.

Developmental level also affects a person's ability to manage health. Although infants and young children must rely on their caregivers for health maintenance, school-age children can learn proper behaviors and may be able to carry them out independently or with little supervision. Common problems in older adults may also affect health maintenance. For example, loss of teeth may preclude proper nutrition, arthritis may affect the ability to exercise, or dementia may affect self-responsibility. In these cases, increasing age hinders health maintenance because of functional limitations.

Previous Experiences

A person's past experiences with health and the healthcare system affect health maintenance. If a person has had a negative experience with an agency or program, he or she may refuse to participate again, even if no alternatives are available. If a particular health practice (e.g., a low-calorie diet) worked well for the person or for a family member in the past, the person is likely to try again. Also, a person's health maintenance may be affected by a relative's or friend's experience (e.g., a family history of cancer, a close friend who had a heart attack). It may take many different attempts for a person to be successful with lifestyle changes; for example, very few people are successful in their first attempt to eliminate the use of tobacco products.

Lifestyle and Habits

A person's lifestyle and habits strongly affect health maintenance. People with an unhealthy lifestyle and habits are considered to have poor health maintenance. Unhealthy habits include lack of exercise, poor diet (in terms of fiber, cholesterol, fat, mineral, vitamin, and protein content), use of tobacco, use of alcohol (except in moderation), use of illegal drugs or abuse of prescription drugs, multiple sexual partners, lack of sleep, lack of contraception, poor dental hygiene, and disregard for safety. Although most people can have some unhealthy habits without suffering health problems, all unhealthy habits carry some increased risk for illness. Repeated, multiple unhealthy habits usually lead to at least one preventable health problem and contribute to a foreshortened life. A person whose lifestyle conveniently incorporates adequate sleep, exercise, and nutrition and avoidance of unhealthy practices may more easily achieve good health maintenance and fewer illnesses.

Environment

Pollution, nearby highways, lack of safe play areas, inadequate housing, and unsanitary conditions lead to poor health maintenance and set the stage for illness. The work environment may lead to health-maintenance problems if conditions

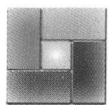

Nursing Research and Critical Thinking
What Role Do Cognitive-Perceptual Factors and Modifying Factors Play in Understanding Participation of Older Adult Women in Health-Promotion Behaviors?

Nurses are concerned with the increased incidence of health problems such as cancer and cardiovascular disease among women. Younger women have been the focus of health-promotion activities, but women older than 64 years of age have not been receiving the same considerations. These nurse researchers reviewed the few studies on health promotion among older adults and realized that they have not explained the continued low rate of participation in health-promotion activities in this age group despite identified potential benefits of these activities. They designed a study to evaluate the roles that potential antecedents and predictors have in older adult women's participation and maintenance of health-promotion behaviors. The investigators made contacts with management staff of community and senior recreation centers, independent living apartments, women's health fairs, and volunteer service programs to obtain a convenience sample of 107 women between the ages of 65 and 95 years (mean age, 76.7 years). They designed a study using Pender's Health Promotion Model to investigate through canonical correlation analysis the role that selected cognitive-perceptual factors (health self-determination, learned helplessness, self-esteem, and perceived health) and modifying factors (age, race, marital status, education, and income) play in the participation of community-living older adult women in the health-promotion behaviors of health responsibility, physical activity, nutrition, spiritual growth, interpersonal relations, and stress management. The results of the data analysis

indicated that age, marital status, race, education, self-esteem, and the two health-related factors of perceived health and health self-determination made statistically significant contributions to the health-promotion behaviors of physical activity, nutrition, spiritual growth, and interpersonal relations. Internal barriers to participation in health-promotion behaviors focused on perceived physical difficulties with all types of activities.

Critical Thinking Considerations. Although society tends to view older women as a homogeneous group, in this study the demographic and cognitive-perceptual factors clustered with four of the six health-promotion domains, suggesting that there are multiple factors influencing participation or nonparticipation in health-promotion behaviors. Implications for nursing are as follows:

- Support of older women's participation in health promotion could be best accomplished by nurses through identification of each woman's goals for health and ongoing assessment of her individual capabilities.
- By first teaching ways to self-manage chronic health problems and physical limitations, internal physical barriers may be decreased and self-motivation toward health-promotion activities increased.
- Modifying a recommended activity according to an individual's capabilities may help these women enhance their self-competence.

Lucas, J. A., Orshan, S. A., & Cook, F. (2000). Determinants of health-promoting behavior among women ages 65 and above living in the community. *Scholarly Inquiry for Nursing Practice: An International Journal, 14*(1), 77–97.

include long working hours, poor ventilation, poor lighting, loud noises, lack of nutritious food, or sedentary or repetitious tasks. Social environments that support domestic and civil violence also negatively affect the health maintenance efforts of people.

Economic Resources

Economics plays a large role in health maintenance and access to healthcare. People who live in poverty may be unable to afford nutritious food and adequate housing. They may not receive routine medical care and screenings and may seek healthcare only when a serious illness develops. Poverty may cause homelessness or may force people to live in overcrowded conditions with poor sanitation and heating. Children may sleep poorly if they share beds with other family members. Nutrition may be inadequate, leading to poor school performance. Unemployment and dropping out of school cause

boredom, and boredom and frustration about such conditions may lead to substance abuse and crime. Homeless children do not receive immunizations, dental care, or the usual safety and security required for health promotion.

Poverty is inversely correlated with health status. People living in poverty have higher rates of mortality (death) and morbidity (illness) than other groups of people regardless of race or ethnicity. Additionally, people in poverty are more likely than others to die from preventable diseases (Stanhope & Lancaster, 2001). Knowledge deficits about health maintenance, lack of motivation to improve practices related to unpleasant past experiences, lack of health insurance, and difficulty obtaining adequate resources are some reasons for these increased rates of morbidity and mortality. Wealthier people have greater financial access to medical care, nutritious food, and preventive programs such as aerobics classes, health-related books and videos, and health lectures.

Culture, Values, and Beliefs

The culture in which a person was raised influences his or her health beliefs and practices, including diet, childbearing and child-rearing customs, self-medication, and alternate therapies. A language barrier may prevent people from entering the healthcare system. Spiritual beliefs and personal or family values also affect health maintenance. Some people place great value on physical health to achieve spiritual health. Others may have religious beliefs that prohibit certain medical practices and treatments (e.g., Christian Scientists prohibit the use of medications). A belief that health depends solely on God's will may hinder health maintenance.

Roles and Relationships

People who are comfortable in their roles and relationships with others often form strong support systems and use available resources to promote health. Having role models and relationships with others who have good health-maintenance practices may benefit one's own health maintenance efforts.

Difficulty with roles and relationships can act as a stressor, which can compromise a person's respect for others and self-esteem. Possible negative outcomes include decreased coping skills, increased isolation, depressive symptoms, violence toward self or others, and negative health behaviors.

ETHICAL/LEGAL ISSUE
Parental Refusal of Immunizations for Child

You are an RN at the public health department, in charge of the child health conferences. In reviewing the records for today's appointments, you notice that MaryBeth Cooper, age 18 months, has not had any immunizations. You make a note to discuss this with her parents, especially because a rubella outbreak has been documented in one of the area schools. Your state has laws mandating immunizations, with few exceptions, for children in day care and school. In talking with Mrs. Cooper, you discover that she is opposed to immunizations for safety and spiritual reasons. She does not belong to any specific religious organization. Mrs. Cooper also tells you that she might be pregnant.

Reflection
• Consider your own views of immunizations and how your spiritual values influence your thinking.
• Identify who is at risk and what those risks are for MaryBeth, her mother, and others if MaryBeth contracts rubella.
• Consider Mrs. Cooper's rights versus the state immunization mandate.
• Identify two approaches to this situation and the ethical pros and cons of both.

Coping and Stress Tolerance

Coping mechanisms people use to handle everyday events may help or harm their health. Stress-reducing techniques such as relaxation breathing or imagery promote health; other coping mechanisms, such as denial and use of alcohol, may lead to health problems.

ALTERED HEALTH MAINTENANCE
Manifestations of Altered Function

Altered health maintenance may result in physical and/or psychological problems. Common manifestations include chronic illnesses, injuries, developmental problems, and psychosocial disruptions. Some manifestations are the result of prolonged exposure to poor health-maintenance practices (e.g., years of smoking that leads to lung cancer). Other conditions, however, may be the result of a one-time exposure (e.g., an adolescent who becomes pregnant after failing to use contraception just one time).

Chronic Illnesses

Many chronic illnesses have been linked to altered health maintenance. Hypertension and cardiovascular disease are associated with diet, stress, lack of exercise, tobacco use, and obesity. The Framingham Study identified risk factors for cardiovascular disease that are the basis for most cardiac prevention and rehabilitation programs (Gorin & Arnold, 1998). Such risk factors as tobacco use, sedentary lifestyle, high-cholesterol diet, obesity, and stress can be modified, but family history cannot. People with multiple risk factors are at a much greater risk for coronary artery disease and myocardial infarction.

Cancer has been linked to a number of practices now considered poor health maintenance behaviors, although its exact cause is yet unknown. A low-fiber diet is associated with colon cancer, tobacco smoking is directly related to lung cancer, chewing tobacco is related to oral cancer, and excessive exposure to ultraviolet light is related to skin cancer. A direct cause-and-effect relationship has not been established in many cancers, but continuing research will ultimately reinforce health-maintenance beliefs. Practices once considered healthy and desirable (e.g., eating large amounts of red meat, sunbathing) have now fallen out of favor because of research findings.

Gastrointestinal illnesses are also related to altered health maintenance. Stress contributes to the development of colitis and can exacerbate irritable bowel syndrome. Ingestion of alcohol or other irritants can cause gastritis. Obesity is considered an illness in itself because the person's general health is poor and his or her risk for other chronic conditions is increased. Obesity may have a genetic component, but it is directly related to diet and exercise patterns.

Musculoskeletal and dermatologic illnesses also result from altered health maintenance. Osteoporosis, which often occurs in postmenopausal women, has been linked to inadequate calcium intake and lack of exercise as the woman ages. Stress and dietary factors aggravate psoriasis, eczema, and other rashes.

Injuries

Many preventable injuries result from single episodes of altered health maintenance. They may result when safety practices are disregarded. Motor vehicle crashes, falls, drownings, and job-related injuries are leading causes of death and disability. Injuries include sprains, strains, fractures, lacerations, burns, and other trauma. (See Chapter 30 for more information on safety issues.)

Unwanted pregnancy and transmission of STDs may result when people disregard safe sex and contraception practices. Adolescents who become pregnant are at higher risk for having babies with low birth weight, congenital defects, and additional health problems. Unwanted pregnancies and STDs can cause psychological distress and may isolate the victim from society.

Developmental Problems

Problems that children experience because of altered health maintenance include tooth decay, infectious diseases, growth retardation, and learning difficulties. Tooth decay results from poor dental hygiene and ingestion of sugary foods and beverages. Infectious diseases such as mumps, measles, rubella, polio, diphtheria, varicella (chickenpox), and meningitis result from lack of immunization. The risk of bronchitis and asthma increases with exposure to second-hand smoke. Growth retardation and improper neurologic and musculoskeletal development may result from inadequate nutrition. Obesity may begin in infancy from an improper diet. Learning and intellectual development may be slowed by poor nutrition, lack of discipline, and lack of sleep.

Psychosocial Problems

Psychosocial problems may result from specific illnesses caused by altered health maintenance or from a more general loss of well-being. Addiction is both a psychological problem and a physical illness. Behavioral changes often occur in the addicted person, including abusive and violent behavior, withdrawal, and mood swings. Other psychosocial manifestations of altered health maintenance include anxiety, depression, and social rejection. Anxiety often accompanies unhealthy lifestyles that include stress, excessive caffeine intake, lack of sleep, alcohol consumption, and tobacco use. Depression may accompany obesity.

Family and friends may reject people who show disregard for their own health. Today, society values people who lead healthy lifestyles. Many smokers feel like outcasts in today's nonsmoking environments.

Impact on Activities of Daily Living

Altered health maintenance may marginally or greatly affect activities of daily living (ADLs). The nurse must be able to identify the effect of altered health maintenance on both the individual and the family. Assessing the family's strengths and limitations can help both the client and the family develop a realistic perspective for coping with the disruptions accompanying the person's altered health maintenance.

Poor sleep habits can affect work or school performance. Poor nutrition reduces the energy a person has to carry out ADLs and affects normal growth and development. Ingestion of alcohol impairs the drinker's cognitive and physical performance. Cigarette smoking can impair oxygenation and lead to frequent respiratory infections or chronic lung impairment, making ADLs more difficult to perform.

Any illness, injury, or other problem not prevented by health-maintenance activities disrupts a person's usual level of functioning. An athlete, for example, tries to maintain optimum health by getting enough sleep, not using tobacco, eating a nutritious diet, and doing physical conditioning. Any disruption in these health-maintenance activities would place him or her at a disadvantage in competition. Similarly, anyone with altered health maintenance does not perform ADLs optimally.

Family functioning in ADLs becomes a significant focus as members alter their normal patterns to meet the person's altered health state. Family relationships change as members adapt usual roles. For example, someone must assume the household functions of cooking, cleaning, child care, and income production when the person who normally performs such activities can no longer do so.

ASSESSMENT

The nurse's assessment of a client's health maintenance tends to be more abstract than other assessments. The objectives of this assessment are to evaluate how well the individual and family can manage health behaviors and to identify deficiencies, risks, potential for improvement, and motivation to change. Information about other functions, such as nutrition, mobility, and values, is used in the health-maintenance assessment. Much of this assessment is done through the health history interview, observations, validation of self-assessment techniques, and a synthesis of all other functional areas.

Subjective Data

Subjective data are obtained in an organized interview. During the interview, note the person's verbal and nonverbal communication and use observation skills to guide the data collection. Subjective data identify normal patterns of health maintenance, risk factors for altered health maintenance, and active health-maintenance dysfunction. Nurses collect data from individuals, family members or significant others, parents and caregivers (if the client is a child), and medical records.

Normal Pattern Identification

People in all settings should be assessed for health maintenance, even if no problems are suspected. Information on normal patterns of health maintenance helps reinforce the client's state of health, and information can also be gained on areas that need further work. For example, the nurse may learn while discussing exercise that the client walks three times a

THERAPEUTIC DIALOGUE
Concerns About Altered Health

Scene for Thought

Abby Sinclair is 25 years old and has come to the community clinic for her annual physical. The nurse practitioner has known Abby since she was 21. The practitioner knows that Abby is bright, has a good job, and is concerned about keeping healthy. Abby is sitting on the examining table when the nurse comes in, and she quickly puts away the magazine she has been reading.

Less Effective

Nurse: Hi, Abby. I'm glad to see you. How's it going for you?

Client: Um, fine, I guess. *(Looks at her hands in her lap.)*

Nurse: You don't sound too sure. What's up? *(Looks through the chart while standing at the foot of the table.)*

Client: I've been having really bad cramps every month and sometimes in between. *(Looks worried.)*

Nurse: I know you worry about your periods and cramps because your mom died of cancer when you were little. How long have these been going on? *(Still reads the chart.)*

Client: For the last 3 months. *(Begins to sound unsure of symptoms.)* I even missed work because the pain was so bad. *(Tries to convince the nurse of how she suffered.)*

Nurse: *(Looks at client.)* I'm going to examine you and then we'll see what we really have here. *(Does further nursing assessment; diagnosis of endometriosis is confirmed by the gynecologist.)*

Client: What a relief! What do I do now? I can't miss any more work from the pain. *(Looks interested in learning more.)*

Nurse: Don't worry too much about it; it's a pretty common problem, Abby. I have some pamphlets and articles you can take home with you. And there's a prescription for the pain and bleeding. We'll want to see you back here next month. Okay? *(Doesn't wait for a reply. Abby takes the reading materials and slowly leaves the clinic.)*

More Effective

Nurse: Hi, Abby. I'm glad to see you. How's it going for you?

Client: Um, fine, I guess. *(Looks at her hands in her lap.)*

Nurse: You don't sound too sure. What's up? *(Sits down next to the table and pays attention, exploring.)*

Client: I've been having really bad cramps every month and sometimes in between my periods, too. *(Looks worried.)*

Nurse: How long has this been going on? *(Asking for data.)*

Client: For the last 3 months. Last month, I couldn't go to work for 2 days, they were so bad. I take ibuprofen, but sometimes it doesn't relieve the pain. *(Begins to cry.)*

Nurse: What worries you about this pain? *(Requesting evaluation.)*

Client: My mother had cramps like these, and they found ovarian cancer. I'm so afraid I have it, too. *(Cries.)*

Nurse: I remember you told me she died when you were 10 or 11.

Client: I remember her being in pain and having the operation and radiation, and then she died anyway.

Nurse: I know you're scared, Abby. But before you decide you have cancer, I'd like to examine you, get some more facts about your periods, and then we'll talk. *(After further nursing assessment and confirmation by the gynecologist, endometriosis is diagnosed.)*

Client: What a relief! But what do I do now? I can't miss any more work from this pain. *(Now looks interested and ready to learn how to cope.)*

Nurse: I have some pamphlets and articles on endometriosis. How about if you read them in the waiting room, and I'll come talk to you in about half an hour to answer any questions you might have. Do you have time today? *(Offers teaching materials and self.)*

Critical Thinking Challenge

- Formulate the NANDA nursing diagnosis pertaining to Abby.
- Detect what the first nurse seems to be implying when she referred to Abby's worry of cancer.
- Relate Abby's response.
- Compare and contrast the nurses' approaches to Abby before and after the medical diagnosis.

---

week for 20 minutes and places high value on cardiovascular health. This information could be used to encourage the client to reduce the amount of fat in the diet.

Questions to ask include the following (Gordon, 1994):

- What is your perception of your health status?
- How do you define health?
- What value do you place on health?
- How could your health be improved?
- What are you doing to maintain your health?

- What prevents you from engaging in a desired health behavior?
- How much control do you have over your own health?
- What is your perceived ability to perform health behaviors?

The person's perception of health and ability to manage health are important. Validate all information obtained in this area, because miscommunication can hurt the client–nurse relationship and can create barriers against healthy behavior.

Risk Identification

Cues from the nursing history can alert the nurse to risk factors, which are traits that increase the client's vulnerability to a certain condition or disease. Risk factors can be classified as genetic background, age, biologic characteristics, personal habits, and environment. They vary in intensity, and multiple risk factors may interact to develop additional risk factors (Pender, 1996). Behaviors such as dieting, exercising, avoiding tobacco, genetic testing, or leaving a particular environment or situation can modify the intensity of the risk factor. Abolishing the behavior may eliminate the risk factor. Risky behavior has been defined as any irresponsible behavior that leads to negative health outcomes. For example, the risky behavior of a sedentary lifestyle has health consequences of obesity, coronary heart disease, hypertension, and osteoporosis.

Risk identification can be done with the help of several assessment tools. A computer program called *Healthier People,* developed by the Centers for Disease Control and Prevention and Emory University (Atlanta, GA), helps the client and nurse identify risk factors; another computer program, *Health Predict: Personal Health Analysis,* is available from Compuhealth Associates (St. Louis, MO). *The Health Hazard Appraisal* (1981; Health Care Service, Inc., San Diego, CA) and *Lifestyle Assessment Questionnaire* (1981; University of Wisconsin at Stevens Point, WI, available at http://www.testwell.org/) are risk appraisals that are sent to the respective company for scoring. A self-test for risk appraisal is *Health Style: A Self-Test* (1981) by the U.S. Department of Health and Human Services, Office of Disease Prevention and Health Promotion.

These risk appraisals are designed to help the client and nurse identify common threats to health and to motivate behavioral change. Some items are difficult for the client to answer; however, errors may result if the person cannot answer or selects an inappropriate answer. These appraisals are not a substitute for, but may be a component of, a nursing health assessment. Many health risk appraisals are now available on-line to individuals with access to the Internet. For example, the following sites contain free self-administered tools: You First Health Risk Assessment (www.youfirst.com), Continuum Health Partners: Assessment: Interactive Health Evaluation (www.wehealny.com), American Heart Association: Health Risk Awareness (www.americanheart.org), and UW Physicians On Line: Health Risk Assessment (www.uwphysicians.org/healthcalc.html). This represents only a small number of the sites that can be found with an Internet search.

Dysfunction Identification

A dysfunction is any behavior that alters health maintenance. In many cases, the client perceives the dysfunction and may or may not want to change, or the client may learn that a behavior is dysfunctional through health education. Many people are unaware of their dysfunctional behavior; for instance, some-

one immunized in 1965 for measles may not know that he or she did not obtain adequate immunity and now requires a second dose. As researchers learn more about risks to health, nurses must transmit that information.

Identifying dysfunction goes beyond identifying risk factors. Assess not only the risk factor but also how that factor has altered the client's health maintenance. For example, when assessing the client's diet, ask the following questions:

- How do you feel on your new diet? or, How would you evaluate your energy level since you have been on this diet?
- Have you had your blood pressure checked since you stopped restricting your salt intake?
- I see that you eat two or three eggs each morning for breakfast. Have you ever had your cholesterol level checked?

By asking such questions and having the client describe the possible effects of risky practices, the nurse identifies actual health-maintenance dysfunctions.

🖳 **SAFETY ALERT**

Advise clients who are dieting for weight loss that the diet must still meet nutritional needs. Make sure meals contain foods from all the basic groups and that clients do not skip meals.

Objective Data

Objective data include results of the physical assessment and diagnostic tests that focus on general health management and prevention. Objective data are used to identify the client's health maintenance through screening techniques.

Physical Assessment

There is no specific physical assessment skill for health maintenance; instead, data obtained from other assessments are used (Fig. 31-2). The screening assessments in the accompanying health assessment display (see next section) can be pooled to assess health maintenance comprehensively.

During the physical assessment, validate the client's self-examination skills (e.g., breast or testicular self-examination) to ensure that he or she is effectively performing each skill. Assess clients who engage in risky behaviors for their ability to spot potential abnormalities; for example users of spit tobacco (chewing and snuff) should be able to perform oral screening, and intravenous drug users should be able to assess for phlebitis.

Many clients have health-assessment equipment at home, such as scales, thermometers, or machines to measure blood pressure or monitor blood glucose levels (Fig. 31-3). Inspecting the equipment for accuracy and assessing the client's ability to use the equipment safely increase the accuracy and reduce the risk of injury or incorrect data. The client should know what to do with the data obtained: does he or she know normal and abnormal readings? If the client obtains abnormal data, when should he or she consult a professional?

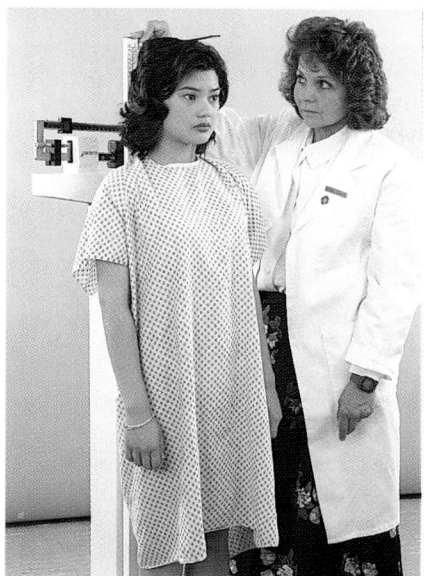

FIGURE 31-2 The adolescent undergoes a growth spurt, which the nurse monitors as a part of health assessment.

Diagnostic Tests

Many diagnostic tests can be used to assess health maintenance, including urine tests for protein and glucose, a complete blood count for hematocrit and hemoglobin, an electrocardiogram, a chest radiograph, a stool test for occult blood, and a mammogram. The U.S. Preventive Services Task Force (1996) has identified specific screening and counseling services for people across the lifespan (Display 31-2). Nurses may initiate some screening tests independently; other tests require a order by a physician or nurse practitioner. Some tests are performed on the nursing unit, some in the office or home, and still others in a laboratory. Some, such as cholesterol screening and mammograms, can be obtained in a community practice. Agency policies vary on physician's orders, written consent, and protocols. Nurses should review all di-

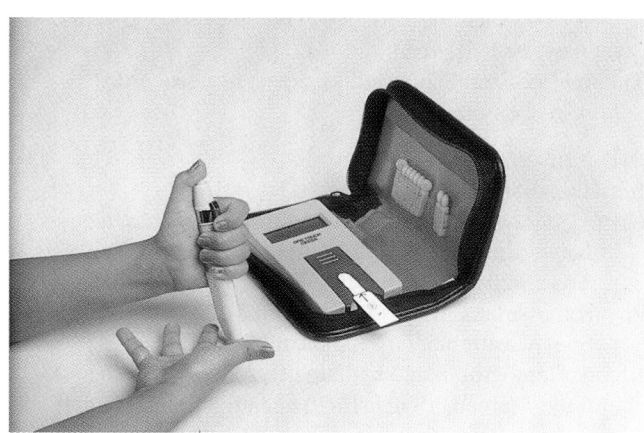

FIGURE 31-3 Equipment for monitoring blood glucose increases the health-maintenance abilities of the person with diabetes.

agnostic test results and incorporate them into the health-maintenance assessment.

Many screening diagnostic tests are available to the public. These include mail-in human immunodeficiency virus (HIV) testing, measurements of cholesterol levels, drug screening tests, and at-home pregnancy tests. The availability of these useful tools has expanded in the last few years. If individuals are going to use these tests, they need to know what to do with both the positive and the negative results. For example, there are just as many implications for a negative result on a HIV or drug screening test as there are for a positive result.

NURSING DIAGNOSES

North American Nursing Diagnosis Association (NANDA) lists three diagnoses involving health maintenance: Ineffective Health Maintenance, Health-Seeking Behaviors, and Therapeutic Regimen Management.

Diagnostic Statement— Ineffective Health Maintenance

Definition. Ineffective health maintenance is the inability to identify, manage, and/or seek out help to maintain health (NANDA, 2001).

Defining Characteristics. Of the defining characteristics or clinical cues that point to this nursing diagnosis, the following should be present:

- Demonstrated lack of knowledge regarding basic health practices
- Demonstrated lack of adaptive behaviors to internal or external changes
- Reported or observed inability to take responsibility for meeting basic health practices in any, or all, functional pattern areas
- Reported or observed lack of equipment, finances, or other resources for health maintenance
- Reported or observed impairment of personal support system
- History of lack of health-seeking behavior
- Expressions of interest in improving health behaviors

Related Factors. Numerous factors contribute to a person's difficulty with health maintenance. They may include lack of or significant alteration in communication skills (written, verbal, and gestural), which may interfere with the ability to receive and process health information. The lack of ability to make deliberate and thoughtful judgments or perceptual or cognitive impairment may interfere with the person's ability to choose and participate in healthy behaviors. Ineffective coping, dysfunctional grieving, ineffective family coping, and disabling spiritual distress also may interfere with the ability to make appropriate health behavior choices or consume the energy necessary to engage in healthy behaviors. The lack of material resources may make

DISPLAY 31-2

SELECTED HEALTH ASSESSMENT ACROSS THE LIFESPAN

Infant, Toddler, and Preschool Child (Birth–5 Years)

Health history and family history: Initially and then update as needed

Vision: Infancy—follows objects, corneal light reflex, turn to light

Toddler—cornea light reflex, cover test

Preschool—Snellen E, screenings as for toddler

Hearing: Infants—startle reflex (birth), tracking sounds (3–6 months), recognizes sounds (6–8 months), location of sound (8–12 months)

Preschool—pure tone audiometry beginning at age 4 years. Inability to cooperate and understand instructions hinders this screening in younger children

Speech: Assess in infancy and early preschool with Denver II and Denver Articulation Screening Examination for children 2.5–6 years

General development: Denver II in ages newborn to 6 years can be done along with physical assessments

Congenital hip dislocation: Newborn through age 23 months

Blood pressure: Before age 1 year, then yearly

Dental: Infancy—Presence of teeth and oral care, screening by dentist at age 2 years and then every 6–12 months

General physical assessment: At ages 1, 2, 4, 6, 12, 18, 24 months, then yearly, including height and weight

Urine: Phenylketonuria before age 4 weeks; glucose and protein at same time as physical assessment; between 2 and 5 years analysis for bacteriuria

Nutrition: Same as for physical assessment

Blood: Sickle cell if indicated at 6 months; hemoglobin or hematocrit at 9 months, and then every 6 months through 24 months; yearly thereafter

Tuberculin: Baseline at 12 months if at risk, secondary to endemic status; repeat before beginning school year

Environment: Ask parents about age-appropriate injury risks in environment

School-Age Child (6–12 Years)

Health history: Update

Vision: Visual acuity every 1–2 years

Hearing: Pure tone audiometry ages 6, 8, and 11 years

Dental: Assessed by dentist every 6–12 months

General physical assessment: Including blood pressure, general development, height, weight, and nutrition every year

Urine: Glucose, protein yearly

Blood: Hematocrit or hemoglobin every 1–3 years as indicated by nutritional status and history

Tuberculin: If in an at-risk environment, every 1–3 years

Environment: Ask parents about age-appropriate injury risks in environment

Adolescent (13–18 Years)

Health history: Update; include tobacco and sexual practices

Vision: Visual acuity every 1–2 years; usually odd year age (i.e., 13, 15, 17)

Hearing: Pure tone audiometry ages 14 and 18 years

General physical assessment: Including blood pressure, general and sexual development, height, weight, nutrition every 1–2 years

Scoliosis: Age 11 and then yearly through age 14 or completion of growth spurts

Self-examination technique: Girls—breast at age 14–15 years. Boys—testicular at age 14–15 years

Urine: Analysis every 3 years

Blood: Hemoglobin or hematocrit every 1–3 years; others as indicated

Dental: By dentist every 6–12 months

Emotional: Be alert for depressive symptoms and need for screening

Young Adult (19–39 Years)

Health history: Update as needed

Vision: Visual acuity every 1–5 years, glaucoma every 3 years beginning at age 35

Hearing: Gross screening yearly

Physical assessment: Including risk appraisal, height, weight, and nutrition every 3–5 years

Blood pressure: Every 2–3 years

Dental: Every 6–12 months

Self-examinations: Women—breast every month with professional evaluation every 1–2 years. Men—testicular monthly

Mammogram: Women, once between 35 and 39 years

Pap smears: Women, every 3 years after two successive normal results

Urine: Complete analysis every 5–10 years

Blood: Cholesterol every 5–10 years; blood glucose every 10 years; hematocrit—women every 3–5 years, men every 5–10 years

Tuberculin: Establish baseline, repeat as needed if in high-risk environment

Pregnant Women

Initial assessment

History: Genetic and obstetric; nutrition; tobacco, alcohol, and drug use. Risk factors for low birth weight, prior sexually transmitted diseases (STDs)

Physical assessment: Height, weight, blood pressure, pelvic measurements, Pap smear

Blood: Hemoglobin and hematocrit, ABO/Rh typing, antibody screen, VDRL/PRP, hepatitis B surface antigens, human immunodeficiency virus (if at risk)

Urine: Analysis for bacteriuria, protein, and glucose

DISPLAY 31-2 (Continued)

SELECTED HEALTH ASSESSMENT ACROSS THE LIFESPAN

Other: Gonorrhea culture and other STDs
Follow-up
History: Update
Physical assessment: Blood pressure, weight, fetal heart sounds
Urine: Analysis for protein and glucose
Other: May be necessary because of risks, including maternal serum alpha-fetoprotein, ultrasound, glucose tolerance, STD screening, hepatitis screening

Middle Adult (40–64 Years)
Health history: Update as needed
Vision: Visual acuity every 5 years, glaucoma every 3 years
Hearing: Every 3–5 years, more frequently if in noisy environment
General physical assessment: Every 2–3 years including height, weight, and nutrition
Blood pressure: Every 2–3 years
Dental: Every 6–12 months
Women only: Breast self-examination monthly, with professional evaluation every 1–2 years, mammogram every 1–2 years, Pap smear every 1–3 years, bone mineral analysis after menopause
Urine: Complete analysis every 5–10 years
Blood: Cholesterol, blood glucose, hematocrit every 5 years, prostate-specific antigen (PSA) for men yearly beginning at age 55 (controversial)

Other: Stool guaiac yearly, sigmoidoscopy for bowel cancer every 5 years beginning at age 50, baseline electrocardiogram (ECG), and medication evaluation
Skin: Yearly for malignant skin disorders

Older Adults (65 and Over)
Health history: Update as needed
Vision: Acuity and glaucoma every 2–3 years
Hearing: Every 3–5 years
Blood pressure: Yearly
General physical assessment: Every 2–3 years including height, weight, and nutrition
Cancer screenings: Stool guaiac yearly, sigmoidoscopy every 5 years, skin for malignant tumors yearly. Women only—cervical/uterine every 1–3 years depending on risk, monthly breast self-examination, mammogram yearly until age 75, unless pathology found. Men only—prostate every 1–2 years, PSA yearly
Urine: Complete analysis every 2 years
Blood: Chemistry, lipid, complete blood count thyroid function, and glucose every 2–3 years
Dental: Every 6–12 months
Other: ECG as indicated or at risk, medication evaluation, especially for polypharmacy and drugs that may cause confusion or increase risk for falls

some healthy behaviors difficult to perform, such as purchasing medication for chronic health problems, purchasing nutritious foods, or obtaining necessary immunizations (NANDA, 2001).

Diagnostic Statement— Health-Seeking Behaviors

Definition. Health-seeking behaviors are a state in which a person in stable health is actively seeking ways to alter personal health habits and/or the environment to move toward a higher level of health. (Stable health status is defined as age-appropriate disease-prevention measures achieved; client reports good or excellent health; and signs and symptoms of disease, if present, are controlled [NANDA, 2001].)

Defining Characteristics. Of the defining characteristics or clinical cues that point to this nursing diagnosis, the following must be present:

- Expressed or observed desire to seek a higher level of wellness

- Expressed or observed desire for increased control of health practice
- Expression of concern about effect of current environmental conditions or health status
- Stated or observed unfamiliarity with wellness community resources
- Demonstrated or observed lack of knowledge in health-promotion behaviors

Minor characteristics also may be present but are not required for this diagnosis.

Related Factors. Several situational variables or changes in roles generally increase a person's desire to seek health information. These include marriage, parenthood, changes in living situation (e.g., children leaving home), and retirement. Health-seeking behaviors can also be increased when the media bring to the person's awareness the need for specific behaviors such as mammograms, testicular self-examinations, and immunizations. In addition, the advertisement of new resources such as exercise equipment in city parks piques interest in health-seeking behavior (NANDA, 2001).

Diagnostic Statement—Therapeutic Regimen Management: Effective and Ineffective—Focus: Individual, Family, and Community

Definition. Effective management by an individual entails effective integration of a program of treatment of an illness and sequelae into daily activities to meet health goals. Ineffective management by an individual, family, or community occurs when the client has difficulty or is at risk for difficulty incorporating a treatment program for an illness into daily living to meet health goals (Carpenito, 2001).

Defining Characteristics
Effective
- Appropriate choices to meet goals
- Symptoms within expectations
- Verbalized desire to manage treatment and reduce risk factors for complications

Ineffective
- Desire to manage treatment of illness
- Verbalized difficulty with regulation/management of one or more treatment regimens for illness
- Lack of attention to illness
- Acceleration of symptoms
- Morbidity/mortality rate above expected (community)

Related Factors. Many factors affect the ability to manage a therapeutic regimen. The more complex the regimen, the less the chance of success. For example, the chances of a client's compliance with a medication regimen are greater if he or she is taking one dose per day instead of two or more doses per day. The cost of some medications is beyond the reach of individuals, especially those on fixed incomes and those without prescription medication insurance coverage. Side effects of medication, such as depression, weight gain, and nausea, result in stopping of medication. Additional barriers include motivation, cognitive defects (memory loss), family conflicts, previous experiences (both bad and good), lack of transportation, unavailability of services (i.e., immunization program) in the community, and lack of awareness of importance or seriousness of the situation.

Related Nursing Diagnoses

Nursing diagnoses closely related to health maintenance include Risk for Infection, Risk for Injury (trauma, poisoning, suffocation), Deficient Knowledge, and Noncompliance. Although Deficient Knowledge is an accepted nursing diagnosis, it more often is considered to be a related or contributing factor. Noncompliance is a situation in which the client has expressed a desire to comply but does not do so because of barriers. Noncompliance is not used when the person makes an informed decision not to comply with suggestions (Carpenito, 2001). This nursing diagnosis must be used carefully to ensure that the client is not labeled "noncompliant" before complete data collection is done.

OUTCOME IDENTIFICATION AND PLANNING

After the nursing diagnoses and related factors have been identified, client goals and nursing interventions are planned. Common goals in health maintenance include the following:

- The client will identify areas for improvement in health maintenance.
- The client will adopt appropriate health-seeking behaviors.
- The client will maintain or improve current health status.

Planning will evolve around the client's motivation to be healthy. Did the client actively seek help, or was altered health discovered during an assessment or examination? The client's cooperation is needed in planning and setting goals, because it is the client who will manage appropriate care. Most nursing interventions for health maintenance are educational. Examples of nursing interventions commonly used in health promotion are listed in the accompanying NIC/NOC display and are discussed in the next section of this chapter.

IMPLEMENTATION

The nurse uses educational interventions to help the client explore alternatives in health practices. Such education can take place in acute care or long-term care settings, the home, school, workplace, or ambulatory clinics. Use the teaching–learning process to educate the client about self-care (Fig. 31-4). Share knowledge with the client and lead the client through the learning process. Assess the client's knowledge deficit and, together with the client, set priorities, goals, and outcome criteria. Allow the individual or family to set the pace and create a supportive learning environment. Both nurse and client evaluate the process by observing progress toward goals.

Health Promotion

Nursing interventions to promote proper health maintenance include the following:

- Educating clients about common illnesses and how to prevent illness
- Teaching self-examination techniques
- Encouraging routine physical examinations, health screenings, and immunizations

Educating about Common Illnesses
Teaching clients about common illnesses can help improve health maintenance and prevent illness. Nurses should know how to teach clients about common conditions such as hypertension, heart disease, cancer, osteoporosis, STDs, lung disease, and childhood infectious diseases. When working with people of different ethnicities, the nurse needs to be aware of which health problems pose the greatest risks for those people. Client education involves teaching clients about risk factors for and warning signs of common illnesses, as well as

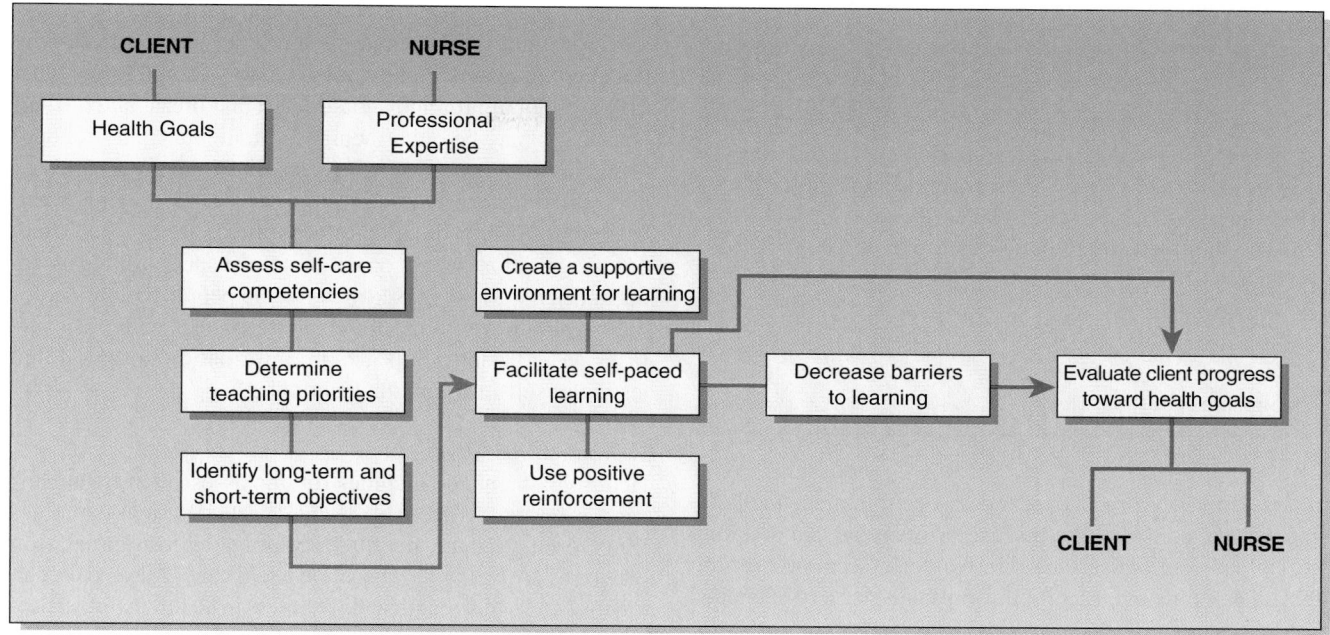

FIGURE 31-4 The self-care education process. (Adapted from Pender, N. [1996]. *Health promotion in nursing practice* [3rd ed.]. Norwalk, CT: Appleton & Lange, p. 106.)

ways to prevent those conditions. Information should be appropriate for the client's age and likelihood of contracting an illness. For example, teach adults and older adults about hypertension and heart disease; warn adolescents and sexually active adults who are not monogamous about STDs (includ-

ing HIV infection); advise parents about childhood infectious diseases. Clients can also be referred to agencies such as the American Cancer Society for information.

Hypertension and Heart Disease. Hypertension and heart disease share many risk factors. Clients should learn that they cannot alter hereditary predisposition but can change other risk factors that may aid in preventing such illness. Eliminating risky behaviors such as using tobacco products, eating a high-fat and high-cholesterol diet, having a high sodium intake, being overweight, and failing to exercise may prevent subsequent illness. Give information on healthy diet and exercise. Clients with one or two risk factors should learn the symptoms of myocardial infarction, as listed in Display 31-3. Advise them to seek medical attention immediately if symptoms occur, because identification of early signs and prompt medical intervention reduce mortality. Teaching cardiopulmonary resuscitation to family members and close friends can be life-saving.

SAFETY ALERT

Advise clients who are beginning exercise programs to start slowly and proceed cautiously, never overexerting themselves. Pregnant women and those with a history of cardiac problems, diabetes, or hypertension should consult their physicians before beginning an exercise program.

Cancer. Because cancer comes in many forms and can invade virtually any body tissue, there are many risk factors and warning signs (Display 31-4). Cancer education and screening programs have traditionally been age and gender

---

PLANNING: Examples of NIC/NOC Interventions

Accepted Health Maintenance Nursing Interventions Classification (NIC)
Health Education
Health Screening
Risk Identification
Self-Modification Assistance
Self-Responsibility Facilitation
Smoking Cessation Assistance

Accepted Health Maintenance Nursing Outcomes Classification (NOC)
Adherence Behavior
Health Beliefs: Perceived Ability to Perform
Health Beliefs: Perceived Control
Health Beliefs: Perceived Resources
Health Beliefs: Perceived Threat
Health Orientation
Health-Promoting Behavior
Health-Seeking Behavior
Knowledge: Substance Use Control
Risk Control: Tobacco Use

Refer to the following for specifics regarding NIC/NOC:
  McCloskey, J., & Bulechek, G. (2000). *Iowa Intervention
  Project: Nursing Interventions Classification (NIC)* (2nd ed.).
  St. Louis, MO: C.V. Mosby.
Johnson, M., & Maas, M. (2000). *Iowa Outcomes Project:
  Nursing Outcomes Classification (NOC)* (2nd ed.).
  St. Louis, MO: C.V. Mosby.

DISPLAY 31-3

SYMPTOMS OF MYOCARDIAL INFARCTION

Cardinal symptom is persistent chest pain. Clients may describe it as heaviness, squeezing, or crushing. Pain may radiate to the left side of the jaw or neck or left shoulder/arm. Other symptoms:

- Anxiety
- Dizziness
- Sweating
- Nausea
- Shortness of breath

related. However, breast cancer does occur in men, and lung cancer, long considered a disease of men, has become the leading cause of cancer death in women (Gorin & Arnold, 1998). Therefore, nurses must inform a wide variety of clients about the risks and warning signs of cancer; education should begin in childhood and carry on into old age. Risks include diet, sun exposure, tobacco use, exposure to asbestos, pollution, and genetics. Teach clients practices that are believed to prevent cancer, such as eating a high-fiber diet, using sunscreen, and avoiding chemical products associated with cancer.

Osteoporosis. Teach clients, especially women, that practices to prevent osteoporosis begin in childhood with adequate calcium intake. People must maintain calcium intake throughout adulthood. Older women should learn the importance of weight-bearing exercise and estrogen replacement (for postmenopausal women) to decrease bone decalcification.

Self-Examination Techniques

Self-examinations of the breasts, testicles, and skin are important health-maintenance practices that clients should start by age 18 years in women and age 15 in men. Clients can

DISPLAY 31-4

SEVEN WARNING SIGNS OF CANCER

- **C**hanges in bowel or bladder habits
- **A** sore that does not heal
- **U**nusual bleeding or discharge
- **T**hickening or lump in breast, testicle, or elsewhere
- **I**ndigestion or difficulty swallowing
- **O**bvious change in wart or mole
- **N**agging cough or hoarseness

learn the techniques earlier if they desire. Education includes a demonstration by the nurse and a return demonstration by the client to ensure competency. Clients should know what they are looking for and should learn that breast and testicular masses may be either benign or malignant. They should bring any mass, no matter how small, to the physician's or nurse practitioner's attention to aid in early diagnosis and treatment. Skin lesions that do not heal, are multicolored, or change color, shape, or texture are suspect. Skin cancers occur often in sun-exposed areas and in people with fair complexions, but everyone should carefully inspect all skin surfaces. (See Chapter 50 for more information on breast and testicular self-examination techniques.)

Routine Healthcare

Health maintenance includes routine assessment by healthcare providers. Well-baby visits, yearly physical examinations, prenatal care, health screenings, and immunization programs are examples of routine healthcare. These visits can identify areas of strength and weakness in health maintenance, and education can be provided to improve health-maintenance practices, if necessary (Fig. 31-5). The content of the physical examination may vary according to the client's age, family history, and previous health status. Encourage clients to comply with routine healthcare visits and to seek care sooner if problems arise.

Health screenings include blood pressure measurement, cholesterol screening, blood sugar testing, vision and hearing assessment, obesity screening, and stool testing for blood. There are additional screenings for pregnant women. Screenings are often aimed at high-risk populations, but all clients should be encouraged to participate. Screenings take place in hospitals, physicians' offices, clinics, schools, workplaces, community agencies, and even shopping malls. Provide information about screenings and the implications of their results.

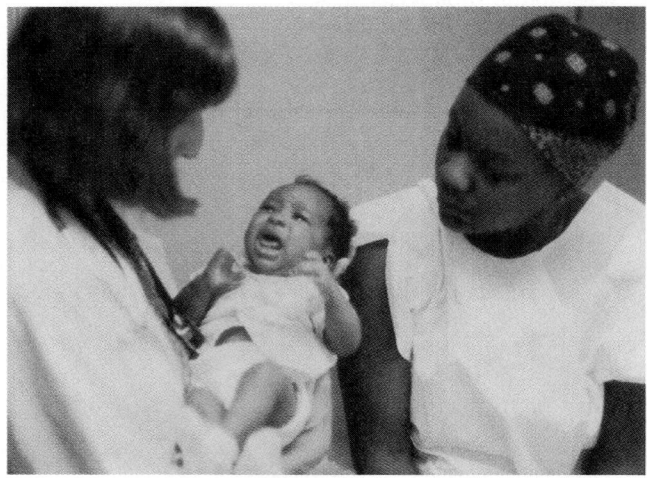

FIGURE 31-5 Assisting the new mother in understanding her newborn's development helps prevent altered function.

Immunization programs are health-maintenance concerns for children and adults. All new parents should be familiar with the immunization schedules for their children; adults often do not realize that they themselves need periodic immunizations for protection from specific infectious diseases throughout their life span. Review immunization histories, particularly for tetanus, rubella, and measles, and advise clients appropriately (see Chapter 39).

Nursing Interventions for Altered Function

Nursing interventions for altered function also tend to be educational in nature and may include information about smoking cessation, diet modification, exercise programs, stress management, and alcohol and drug rehabilitation. The nurse may lead a program on smoking cessation or diet modification, for example, or may simply provide background information and referrals to such programs.

The primary nursing goal is to help the client assume responsibility for self-care in these areas and to connect the individual to needed resources. To help a client assume responsibility, the nurse not only imparts knowledge but may need to change the client's attitudes and instill motivation. Teaching the client the potential outcomes of altered health-maintenance practices may increase his or her motivation to change. The nurse provides emotional support to clients making changes in their health maintenance.

Interventions also address related and contributing factors as a way to correct the disruption in health-maintenance practices. Barriers to health protection and promotion (e.g., misinformation, lack of transportation, lack of health insurance) guide the type of interventions used. A client with financial problems can use a public clinic and the Department of Social (Human) Services. Giving the client information about public or volunteer transportation may solve transportation problems. Clients who cannot afford a commercial exercise or diet program may borrow books and videotapes from a public library or attend free community lectures.

Healthcare Planning and Home- or Community-Based Nursing

The Nursing Plan of Care should reflect the client's educational needs. Goals are set and prioritized so that essential information is taught first and then reinforced. Nurses can enlist the help of other members of the healthcare team, such as a dietitian to help with meal planning or a clinical nurse specialist to provide information on smoking cessation. Family members and significant others should be included in the teaching so that they can offer support. Reference materials (e.g., printed menus for a low-cholesterol diet) should be provided.

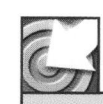

OUTCOME-BASED TEACHING PLAN

Patricia, whom you met in the Critical Thinking Challenge, returns to the clinic a few months later for Evita's routine well-child visit. You learn that Patricia is becoming increasingly concerned about health promotion for herself and her husband. With family histories of diabetes, high blood pressure, emphysema, and obesity, Patricia realizes that she and Hector need to make some lifestyle changes if they want to be healthy parents. Patricia is 50 lb overweight and says that Hector smokes a pack of cigarettes a day. She wants guidance on how to approach changes in their lives.

OUTCOME: Review with Patricia the causes of the many problems in her family's history, and ask her what is reasonable to work on as lifestyle changes, such as food intake and activity level.
Strategies
- Discuss with Patricia how to become aware of her daily food intake.
- Instruct Patricia on how to keep and to review the content of a daily food diary:
  — Keep track of all food that she eats during the day.
  — Note the time of day that she eats.
  — Examine and record her feelings, activities, or emotions connected with eating or the desire to eat.
  — Encourage her to take the diary with her to her next healthcare provider appointment so she can discuss appropriate next steps.
- Encourage Patricia to think of ways in which to increase her activity:
  — Go for walks with the children.
  — Participate with her children in active play.
  — Trade childcare with Hector, another relative, or family friend so that she has some time to herself for vigorous exercise.

If the client needs extensive care or continuing help, additional interventions are indicated. For instance, the client may be referred to a community education series for new parents, to a cardiac rehabilitation program after a heart attack, or to a home health agency for in-home nursing assistance. Home health nurses can help clients monitor their health status and manage diet and exercise. Often, clients can take responsibility for health maintenance with additional support and contact with the healthcare provider or referral agency on an ambulatory basis. A home health nurse or public health nurse may assist the client who is learning new skills or who needs reinforcement or continuation of learning.

EVALUATION

Nursing interventions related to health maintenance are successful if the nurse and client agree that the client has made progress toward the identified outcomes. Progress is easily measured by outcome criteria established in the planning phase. The following are general goals and outcome criteria for clients with altered health maintenance, although these topics are always individualized.

Goal

The client will identify areas for improvement in health maintenance.

Possible Outcome Criteria

The client identifies at least three problems in health maintenance (e.g., overweight, sedentary lifestyle, cholesterol level above normal) by this afternoon.

Goal

The client will adopt appropriate health-seeking behaviors.

Possible Outcome Criteria

- The client asks for information about weight loss programs at the next meeting.

- At the next meeting, the client reports scheduling walks for 30 minutes four times a week.
- At the next meeting, the client uses the stairs instead of the elevator and parks his or her car in the lot rather than using valet parking.
- The client and the client's spouse or partner read a complete book on low-cholesterol diets within the next week.
- The client says he or she will eliminate high-cholesterol foods from the diet beginning immediately.

If no progress toward the goal occurs, the nurse and client need to reassess the goal. The following are possible conclusions:

- The goal was too difficult to attain, and appropriate adjustments should be made.
- The client did not want the goal but agreed to it out of courtesy or because of intimidation or fear.
- Barriers exist, and interventions are needed to reduce them.
- The goal was established without the client's knowledge.
- The goal was established on the basis of insufficient information; additional information is needed to establish a desired goal.

After conclusions are reached, the client and nurse can mutually decide whether to readjust previous goals, establish new goals, or terminate goals related to health maintenance.

KEY CONCEPTS

- Health-maintenance activities are those behaviors that the person in a stable state of health uses to maintain or improve that state of health over time.
- A person's ability to maintain health depends on his or her perception of health, motivation to change, and adherence to management goals.
- Health promotion and disease prevention are components of health maintenance. Health promotion is characterized by approach behaviors, disease prevention by avoidance behaviors.
- Environmental factors, poverty, and unhealthy lifestyle and habits create a potential for altered health maintenance.
- The manifestations of altered health maintenance are chronic illnesses, injuries, developmental problems, and psychosocial problems.
- Three categories of altered health maintenance are approved by NANDA as nursing diagnoses: Ineffective Health Maintenance, Health-Seeking Behaviors, and Therapeutic Regimen Management: Effective and Ineffective.
- The nurse can diagnose and treat health-maintenance alterations; most nursing interventions involve teaching the client appropriate health behaviors and knowledge to manage self-care.
- Nursing interventions to promote health and function include education about risk factors for, and warning signs of, common illnesses.
- Routine healthcare, including prenatal care, well-baby visits, immunizations, yearly physical examinations, and health screenings can be nursing interventions to promote health and function.

NURSING PLAN OF CARE
THE CLIENT WITH HEALTH-SEEKING BEHAVIOR

Nursing Diagnosis

Health-seeking behaviors as evidenced by lack of knowledge of testicular self-examination and a desire to learn.

Client Goal

Client will learn testicular self-examination techniques.

Client Outcome Criteria

* Client lists risks of and needs for regular self-examinations immediately after nurse's explanations.
* Client demonstrates effective self-assessment skills on return demonstration immediately after instruction.
* Client demonstrates normal from abnormal findings in discussion with nurse immediately after teaching session.
* Client performs monthly assessments as reported back to nurse at regular examinations.

Nursing Interventions	Scientific Rationale
1. Develop a teaching plan.	1. Individualized teaching plans meet unique learning needs as related to the diagnosis.
a. Testicular cancer rates, risks, and survivor rates when treated early	
b. Skill	
c. Normal and abnormal findings	
2. Provide written material for information.	2. This allows client to refer back to material and not rely on memory alone.
3. Demonstrate skill initially and on return.	3. Demonstration aids in learning of new skills, whereas return demonstration aids in validating proficiency of skill acquisition.
4. Assess performance with routine assessments.	4. Assessments reinforce need for health-promoting behavior.

REFERENCES

Arnold, E., & Boggs, K. (1999). *Interpersonal relationships: Professional communication skills for nurses.* Philadelphia: Saunders.

Bandura, A. (1977). Self-efficacy: Toward a unifying theory of behavioral change. *Psychological Review, 84*(2), 191–215.

Carpenito, L. (2001). *Nursing diagnosis: Application to clinical practice* (9th ed.). Philadelphia: Lippincott.

Edelman, C., & Mandle, C. (1998). *Health promotion throughout the lifespan.* St. Louis, MO: C.V. Mosby.

Gordon, M. (1994). *Nursing diagnosis: Process and application* (3rd ed.). St. Louis, MO: Mosby.

Gorin, S., & Arnold, J. (1998). *Health promotion handbook.* St. Louis, MO: C.V. Mosby.

Murray, R., & Zentner, J. (2001). *Nursing assessment and health promotion through the lifespan* (6th ed.). Englewood Cliffs, NJ: Prentice-Hall.

North American Nursing Diagnosis Association. (2001). *Nursing diagnoses: Definitions and classification 2001–2002.* Philadelphia: Author.

Pender, N. (1996). *Health promotion in nursing practice* (3rd ed.). Norwalk, CT: Appleton & Lange.

Stanhope, M., & Lancaster, J. (2001). *Community health nursing: Process and practice for promoting health* (5th ed.). St. Louis, MO: C.V. Mosby.

U.S. Preventive Services Task Force. (1996). *Guide to clinical preventive services* (2nd ed.). Baltimore, MD: Williams & Wilkins.

World Health Organization. Jakarta Declaration on Health Promotion. Available at: http://www.who.int/dsa/cat95/zjak.htm. Accessed November 16, 2001.

BIBLIOGRAPHY

Cody, W. (1997). Theoretical concerns. Persistence in health patterns: The mystery of being human. *Nursing Science Quarterly, 10*(4), 152–153.

Eisenberg, D. (1997). Advising patients who seek alternative medical therapies. *Annals of Internal Medicine, 127,* 61–69.

Fitch, M., Greenberg, M., Fevstein, L., Muir, M., Plante, S., & King, E. (1997). Health promotion and early detection of cancer in older adults: Needs assessment for program development. *Cancer Nursing, 20*(6), 381–388.

Foxall, M., Barron, C., & Houfek, J. (1998). Ethnic differences in breast self-examination practice and health beliefs. *Journal of Advanced Nursing, 27*(2), 419–428.

Goeppinger, J., & Lorig, K. (1997). Interventions to reduce the impact of chronic disease: Community-based arthritis patient education. *Annual Review of Nursing Research, 15,* 101–122.

Health Insurance Association of America. (1996). *Source book of health insurance data.* Washington, DC: Author.

Nelson, K. (1997). Health service applications: The needs of children and the role of school nurses. *Journal of School Health, 67*(5), 187–188.

Stolte, K. (1996). *Wellness: Nursing diagnosis for health promotion.* Philadelphia: Lippincott-Raven.

U.S. Department of Health and Human Services, Office of Disease Prevention and Health Promotion. (2000). *Healthy People 2010.* (Stock No. 017-001-00547-9). Washington, DC: U.S. Government Printing Office.

Woolf, S., Jonas, S., & Lawrence, R. (Eds.). *Health promotion and prevention in clinical practice.* Baltimore, MD: Williams & Wilkins.

Relevant Web Sites:

This is just a short list; many more sites can be found using any search engine on the Internet.

American Journal of Health Promotion. Available at: http://www.healthpromotionjournal.com. Accessed November 16, 2001.

Australian Health Promotion site. Available at: http://www.achp.health.usyd.edu.au/achp. Accessed March 4, 2002.

Center for Disease Control and Prevention. Available at: http://www.cdc.gov. Accessed November 16, 2001.

Center for Disease Control and Prevention: Mortality and Morbidity Weekly Report (MMWR). Available at: http://www.cdc.gov/mmwr. Accessed November 16, 2001.

Chronic Disease Prevention. Available at: http://www.cdc.gov/nccdphp. Accessed November 16, 2001.

Communicable Disease Prevention and Control. Available at: http://www.cdpc.com/. Accessed November 16, 2001.

Department of Noncommunicable Disease Prevention and Health Promotion. Available at: http://www.who.int/hpr.

Disease Prevention and Control Guidelines (Canada). Available at: http://www.hc-sc.gc.ca. Accessed March 4, 2002.

Disease Prevention News. Available at: http://www.tdh.state.tx.us/phpep/dpn/dpnhome.htm. Accessed November 16, 2001.

England's Health Promotion home page. Available at: http://www.hpe.org.uk/. Accessed November 16, 2001.

Health Promotion Clearinghouse. Available at: http://www.heart-health.ns.ca. Accessed March 4, 2002.

Health Promotion International. Available at http://heapro.oup.journals.org

Healthy People 2010. Available at: http://www.health.gov/healthypeople. Accessed November 16, 2001.

Hope Health: A Health Promotion Guide. Available at: http://www.hithope.com/corp/main.php3?dir=content&file=hpromo.txt. Accessed November 16, 2001.

National Center for Chronic Disease Prevention and Health Promotion (US). Available at: http://www.cdc.gov/nccdphp/. Accessed November 16, 2001.

Nola Pender: Most frequently asked questions about the Health Promotion Model. Available at: http://www.nursing.umich.edu/faculty/pender_questions.html. Accessed November 16, 2001.

Office of Disease Prevention and Health Promotion (US). Available at: http://www.odphp.osophs.ddhs.gov. Accessed November 16, 2001.

Ottawa Charter for Health Promotion (First International Conference). Available at: http://www.who.dk/policy/ottawa.htm. Accessed November 16, 2001.

US Army Center for Health Promotion. Available at: http://www.apgea.army.mil/.

University of Arizona's Health Source Center: Health Promotion Tips. Available at: http://www.ahsc.arizona.edu/opa/health. Accessed November 16, 2001.

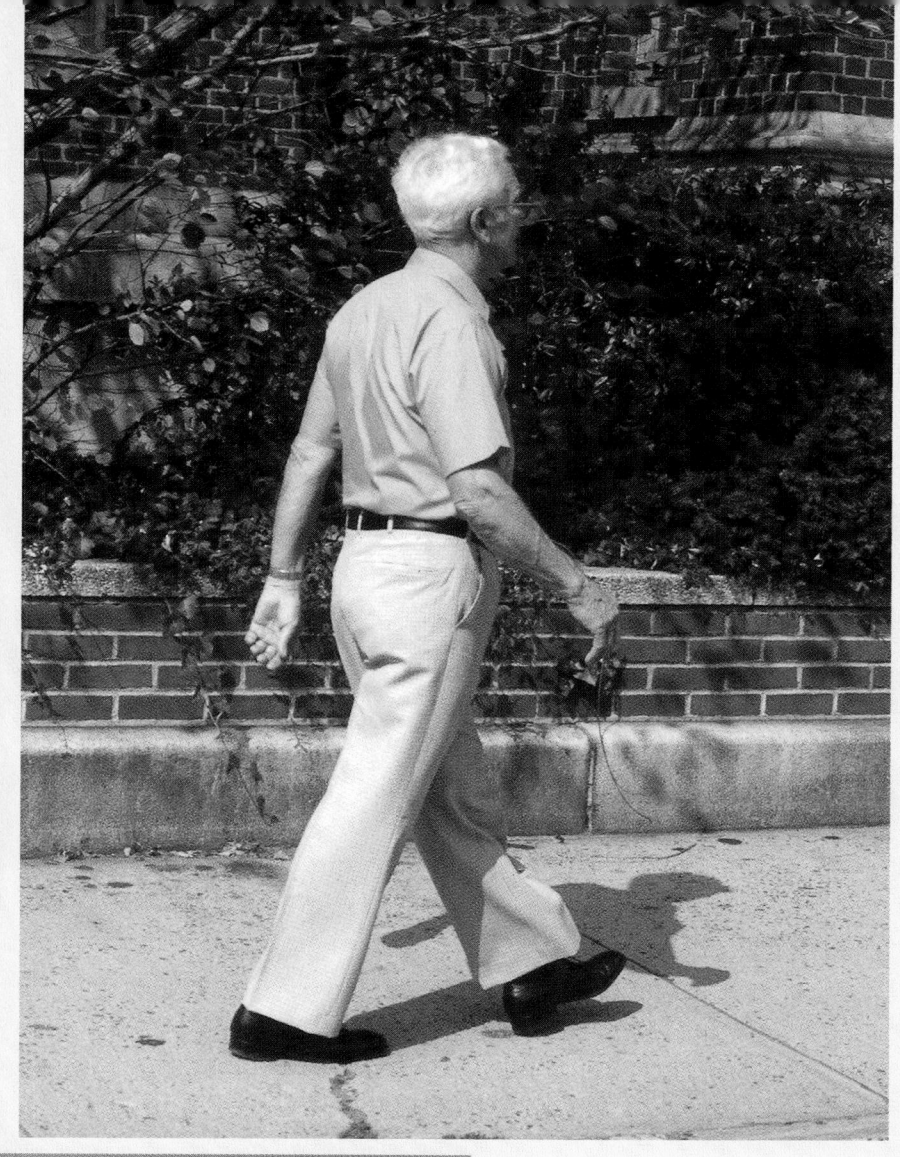

Activity and Exercise

32 Self-Care and Hygiene

⌧ Key Terms

alopecia	hygiene
caries	pediculosis
cerumen	plaque
commode	proprioception
condom catheter	self-care
dysphagia	tartar
gingiva	urinal

⌧ Learning Objectives

Upon completion of this chapter, the student will be able to do the following:
1. Discuss the importance of self-care and hygiene in health and illness.
2. Identify factors that may affect self-care.
3. Discuss important subjective and objective areas of assessment when identifying self-care deficits and individualizing a plan for self-care.
4. Demonstrate basic self-care skills such as bathing, perineal care, foot care, back massage, toileting, and bedmaking.
5. Demonstrate proper care of eyes, ears, and teeth including aids such as dentures, glasses, contact lenses, and hearing aids.
6. List beneficial client teaching for each of the four areas of self-care.

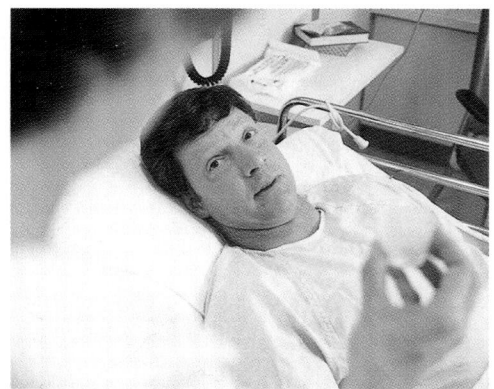

⌧ Critical Thinking Challenge

You are caring for a 37-year-old bachelor, who is recovering from urologic surgery. He lived with his mother until her death a few years ago. He works independently as an accountant. This is your client's first surgery and, although the pathology reports are not back, there is some concern that your client may have bladder cancer. After your morning assessment, you tell your client you will help him wash. He states he does not want to wash and just wants to be left alone. Your assessment reveals dirt under his fingernails, which are untrimmed and jagged; body odor and bad breath, which is easily detected; and dirty tissues all over his bed.

Once you have completed this chapter and have incorporated self-care and hygiene into your knowledge base, review the above scenario and reflect on the following areas of Critical Thinking:

1. Identify factors that might make your client reluctant to participate in morning care.
2. Discuss reasons why you as a nurse believe he should participate in morning care.
3. Reflect on your feelings when you encounter a client who is dirty and smells bad.
4. Identify two or three conclusions you might draw before obtaining more information from the client.
5. Predict positive and negative potential consequences of directly approaching this client and "forcing" him to wash.

Self-care refers to a person's ability to perform primary care functions in the four areas of bathing, feeding, toileting, and dressing without the help of others; hygiene is the observance of health rules relating to these self-care activities. Because these activities are so basic, many people take them for granted. The ability to independently perform appropriate self-care and hygiene practices greatly enhances a person's health status and emotional well-being.

Nurses can play a crucial role in helping clients learn or relearn self-care techniques. Because nurses focus on clients' responses to health and illness rather than on disease itself, helping clients gain or regain independence in self-care is one of the most important goals of nursing. When illness or injury interferes with the ability to perform self-care, nurses assist or perform tasks that clients cannot manage or offer support to family members or other caregivers. The main focus, however, is to help clients achieve as much independence in self-care as possible.

NORMAL SELF-CARE
Characteristics of Normal Self-Care

Normal self-care is the ability to bathe and perform normal grooming functions and to dress, feed, and toilet oneself.

Bathing and Hygiene

The skin is the first line of defense against microorganisms entering the body. Thus, keeping skin intact and healthy is important in preventing infection. Increased perspiration interacts with bacteria on the skin to cause body odor, which can be offensive and promote bacterial growth. Regular bathing removes excess oil, perspiration, and bacteria from the skin surface.

Bathing also increases circulation (from the friction of a washcloth) and helps maintain muscle tone and joint mobility (from the movement of limbs during the bath). In addition, bathing provides relaxation and comfort and gives most people a sense of well-being. A warm or hot bath increases circulation by dilating blood vessels near the skin surface, allowing more blood to flow to the skin.

Bathing promotes assessment of the client's physical condition by noting injured areas, bruises, rashes, or any other unusual signs. Bathing also can promote conversation and interaction between the client and the nurse, facilitating a trusting, satisfying relationship.

Feet and Nail Care. Healthy feet are crucial in helping people stand and walk. Most people wash their feet along with the rest of the body when showering or bathing. Nails are trimmed as needed. There are many tiny bones, ligaments, and muscles in the foot, and comfortable, properly fitting shoes are essential to healthy feet. Shoes should accommodate the size and shape of the foot and should be large enough so that toenails do not rub on the shoes, causing skin breakdown or ingrown nails. Many people ignore their feet until problems occur. The feet are vulnerable to injury because of their susceptibility to skin breakdown. Seemingly minor problems, such as ingrown nails, ill-fitting shoes, swollen feet, corns, or abrasions, can jeopardize mobility.

The client's general condition and health habits affect the nails. Improper diet or fever may cause brittle, broken nails. Water and strong soaps or solutions dry nails. Torn cuticles around the edges of the nail can be a source of infection. Dirt under the nails can spread infection.

Well-maintained nails are pleasing to see and give protection. Daily care involves cleaning beneath the nails and pushing back the cuticles. Fingernails should be filed rather than cut. Convalescing clients may be able to care for their own nails.

Hair Care. Shampooing removes dirt and oil from the hair and scalp. It also increases scalp circulation. For most people, having their hair shampooed is relaxing. Clean hair makes clients feel good about their appearance and enhances feelings of self-worth. Daily hair brushing and combing help maintain healthy hair by distributing oil across the hair shafts and massaging the scalp. Neatly groomed hair also promotes a good self-image.

Oral Care. Proper care of teeth and gums helps prevent gum deterioration and tooth loss. Cavities in the enamel (**caries**) are caused by deposits of **plaque,** a substance that forms and hardens on the teeth and is composed primarily of bacteria and saliva. Bacterial enzymes from the plaque combine with carbohydrates from food and organic acids to ferment and break down enamel. Caries form more often when food and plaque remain on the teeth for long periods. When plaque remains on the teeth, it hardens into **tartar,** which cannot be removed by simple brushing; a professional must scrape it off with dental instruments.

Fluoride in small amounts strengthens teeth during their formation and helps prevent caries. Fluoride is added to most water-treatment systems at the appropriate concentration—1.0 part per million. Adult caregivers may want to ask the dentist how to give children appropriate supplements of fluoride until the age of 14 if their water system is not fluoridated.

Healthy gums are important because they provide support for the teeth. The gums are made up of the oral mucosa (**gingiva**), which covers the bone supporting the tooth; the alveolar bone, which forms sockets around the teeth; and the periodontal ligament, which joins the teeth to the bone. Inflammation in these tissues, called gingivitis or periodontitis, can be caused by local irritation from bacteria, plaque, tartar, food impaction, or mechanical, chemical, or thermal extremes.

Proper oral **hygiene** includes daily brushing, flossing, and rinsing of teeth and care of dentures or other appliances. Regular dental checkups ensure the health of the teeth and gums.

Eye, Ear, and Nose Care. Under normal conditions, the eyes require little care because the lacrimal fluid bathes them continually, and the lids and lashes prevent foreign material from entering the eye. Special care may be needed for clients who wear glasses, contact lenses, or prostheses; those who have other visual problems; or those who use eye medications.

Ears need little attention, although the external ear should be cleaned while bathing. Clients wearing hearing aids may need special care. Some people may have excess accumulation of earwax (**cerumen**), which often requires careful removal. A sharp object, such as a hairpin or toothpick, should never be used to extract wax because this can damage the tympanic membrane. Cotton-tipped applicators should not be used on the inner ear because they can force wax further into the ear canal.

Nostrils can be cleaned by gentle blowing with both nostrils open. Closing one nostril while blowing can force foreign material into the eustachian tube or cause other damage to the inner canal.

Feeding

The ability to feed oneself may be the most important self-care skill in terms of independence. Independence or even partial independence in making food choices and being able to feed oneself can be immensely gratifying and can enhance self-concept for people of all ages. Feeding requires the following activities:

- Desire to make food choices and eat
- Energy and muscular coordination to move food from the plate to the mouth
- Ability to chew and swallow

Toileting

Normal toileting includes feeling the urge to void and defecate, moving to the toilet or bedpan, rearranging clothing, voiding or defecating, and effectively cleaning the perineal and rectal areas. Although these activities are usually done independently, assistance may be required during periods following injury, acute illness, or chronic debilitating conditions.

Dressing and Grooming

Dressing oneself includes being able to get clothes from the closet or drawers, put them on, manage fasteners (such as zippers and buttons), and put on socks and shoes. Normal grooming patterns include the daily brushing and combing of hair. Depending on cultural or personal preferences, some women wear makeup and many shave underarms and legs as an important part of grooming. For men, shaving can be extremely important to their physical appearance and self-image. Personal preference and the amount of beard growth may dictate how often shaving is needed. Men with beards or mustaches may need to trim them periodically and remove spilled food particles from them.

Normal Self-Care Patterns

Self-care and hygiene techniques vary depending on cultural or personal preferences. In general, patterns include independence in eating and toileting; daily bathing or cleansing of the skin and perineal areas; daily brushing, flossing, and rinsing of teeth; special care for dentures or other oral appliances; brushing or combing hair; and other grooming preferences. Men may shave or trim facial hair; women may put on makeup. Some people prefer to bathe in the morning, others bathe before going to bed.

The hair, feet, and nails are other areas that require attention and care. The hair should be shampooed as frequently as needed to keep it clean, depending on its texture and oiliness. People with dry hair may need to moisturize it with conditioners or other commercial products. Shoes should be comfortable and fit properly. Toenails should be trimmed so they do not rub against the shoes. Fingernails should be cleaned and trimmed periodically. Most people dress and groom themselves in the morning, soon after arising. Clothes may need to be changed during the day depending on activities and weather.

Lifespan Considerations

Newborn and Infant

Newborns participate in self-care only by crying and letting others know when they need to be fed or diapered. Parents or other caregivers supply feeding, bathing, dressing, and grooming. Newborns are born with sucking, rooting, and swallowing reflexes that allow them to ingest milk and liquids. They communicate hunger by crying and indicate satiety by falling asleep. By 3 to 4 months, infants begin to develop eye–hand coordination; by 5 to 6 months, many children can grasp and eat pieces of food. As gross motor function develops around 7 to 9 months, children can hold a spoon or drink from a cup with help. At 9 to 12 months, children usually can pick up finger food and feed themselves, hold and drink from a bottle, drink from a cup with some spilling, and spoon-feed themselves with quite a bit of spilling.

Infants are totally dependent on caregivers for toileting. Urination may occur as frequently as 20 times a day. Stools also are frequent and can be soft or liquid. Keeping the skin as dry and clean as possible helps preserve its integrity.

Changing an infant's diaper is relatively easy in early infancy and becomes more difficult as the child becomes more active. During a diaper change, adults should never leave an infant unattended where the child could roll or fall.

Toddler and Preschooler

Self-care abilities increase considerably during this stage, particularly in feeding and toileting. As gross motor development increases, toddlers and preschoolers gain more mastery of their environment. Toddlers' eating patterns are erratic, but most can drink from a cup and use a spoon without spilling (Pillitteri, 1999). Small portions of easy-to-handle food are appropriate.

Many children achieve daytime bowel and bladder control between 2 and 3 years. Staying dry through the night is usually achieved by 4 years, but some children still wet the bed at night until 5 years after which time further nursing intervention may be necessary (World Council of Enterostomal Therapists, 2001).

Preschoolers can manage most aspects of bathing and grooming with some support, but children younger than 4 years need support with wiping after toileting, handwashing, and dressing and undressing.

During illness or stress, most children regress in their toileting and feeding habits. Children who are toilet trained may revert to wetting their pants or the bed at night. Older children who can feed themselves may want to be fed or drink from a bottle again.

Regression is a common coping mechanism, especially for toddlers and preschoolers. During a stressful period, a child may revert from the most recently learned behavior to an earlier behavior that is more comfortable and satisfying. This "time-out" behavior permits the child to withdraw, conserve energy, and regain control. Regression is a normal reaction, and caregivers should understand and permit it.

Child and Adolescent

Although independent in self-care, some school-age children and adolescents may require reminders to bathe, brush their teeth, and change clothes appropriately. They still need direction and encouragement to eat healthy foods and use appropriate table skills. As children approach adolescence, self-care activities become more important as the body begins to mature and physiologic changes start to occur.

Hormonal changes stimulate the growth of axillary (underarm) and pubic hair during adolescence. Boys develop facial hair and may begin shaving. Sebaceous glands become more active and often produce excess oil on the skin. Many adolescents suffer minor skin problems and some experience acne, which can be psychologically devastating to the adolescent's self-image. Sweat glands become fully developed and functional, and adolescents may need to begin using a deodorant or antiperspirant. Daily bathing and shampooing become important to counteract body odor.

Along with these physiologic changes, adolescents undergo extreme psychological and emotional changes. Adolescence is a time of burgeoning independence and self-discovery, as teens begin to develop their own identities. Girls and boys become interested in looking attractive to the opposite sex. Peer behavior heavily influences dressing and grooming practices, because adolescents want others to accept them. Magazine advertisements and media celebrities also influence adolescents, who may copy such hairstyles, make-up, and fashions.

Adult and Older Adult

Young and middle-aged adults usually independently perform self-care. By this stage, people have established self-care techniques that enhance their appearance and health. Busy lifestyles that include working and raising families may leave little time for self-care and health maintenance.

Special problems in self-care arise in older adults. Skin becomes drier, less elastic, and less resilient because glands reduce oil production. The skin may develop brown discolorations, called liver spots, on the hands and feet. Hair becomes thinner and grows more slowly, and hair loss is common. Men and women experience changes in hair color. Teeth may gradually deteriorate from periodontal disease or caries, and many older people wear dentures. The oral mucosa tends to become drier as saliva production lessens; some older people experience receding gums.

The feet of older adults require special attention, because foot problems relate to reduced peripheral blood flow. Poor circulation makes the feet more vulnerable to infection and skin breakdown, particularly after trauma. Some older adults are not mobile enough to care for their feet and may be unable to inspect them easily.

Older adults may need to care for appliances such as hearing aids, glasses, dentures, contact lenses, or artificial eyes. Reduced circulation and decreased muscular flexibility may impair agility and increase the time older adults need to perform tasks. Older people generally are at greater risk for injury because of decreased perception and altered sensation. This age group has the greatest number of people with physically disabling chronic diseases that impact self-care abilities.

FACTORS AFFECTING SELF-CARE

Many people take self-care activities for granted because self-care seems simple and is accomplished routinely throughout life. However, many factors influence how and if a person performs these tasks of daily living.

Self-care requires adequate neuromuscular functioning, muscle strength, mobility, fine motor control, adequate energy, and intact sensory capabilities. Cognitive functioning, psychological factors (motivation, mental status), and sociocultural factors (values, cultural grooming practices) also influence performance of self-care activities.

Culture, Values, and Beliefs

Individuals largely learn self-care routines and practices from the family and community. They form habits around the frequency of bathing, brushing teeth, and changing clothes or eating patterns based on the patterns of family members, friends, and peers within the community. Such preferences may vary widely among individuals and across cultures. For instance, many people in the United States do not feel clean unless they bathe daily and use a deodorant, but people from other countries consider bathing once a week to be normal and do not feel the need to mask natural body odors. Some people are extremely sensitive regarding privacy during bathing; others are used to communal baths. Selected cultures and religions prohibit personal hygiene being provided by members of the opposite gender, especially males providing such care for females. There is a vast difference in family customs and personal preferences in relation to self-care practices.

Environment

Lack of access to facilities or proper resources for self-care (e.g., poverty or poor living conditions) may affect a person's ability to provide for adequate self-care. Homeless people, migrant workers, and the rural poor may not have access to adequate bathroom facilities or running water to bathe properly and wash their clothes. They may not have adequate money to purchase nutritional foods, enough food to ensure a proper diet, or access to adequate cooking facilities to prepare a nutritious meal.

People in wheelchairs may have problems finding wheelchair-accessible facilities. Bathrooms must be designed so wheelchairs can move in and out of stalls. Sinks must be at the right height for a wheelchair-bound person. Home alterations may be necessary to allow the person to perform self-care. Legislation within the last decade has ensured free access to public facilities for disabled persons with mobility restrictions.

Motivation

Motivation can be a powerful factor in achieving independence in self-care. Even though a person is physically capable of self-care, he or she must be motivated to perform self-care and must believe that self-care is important. People with a positive self-image and those who perceive themselves as worthy of attention and care have a greater motivation to attend to self-care.

The nurse or caregiver must value and support the client in becoming as independent in self-care as possible. Efforts must be made to avoid doing something "for" the person that he or she can really do independently. The caregiver may do this to save time and effort, but performing a task independently to the fullest extent possible enables a person to gain independence and self-confidence and bolsters self-concept.

Emotional Disturbance and Depression

Emotional factors can result in self-care deficits. The inability to perceive reality because of psychosis or schizophrenia may cause inattentiveness to the need for personal care. Being highly distractible with short attention spans, these people are unable to concentrate on such basic needs as eating, grooming, and toileting. Severe dysfunction may be reflected by wearing inappropriate or no clothes in public or refusing to eat due to a fear of being poisoned.

Depressed people may lack the energy or interest to care for themselves and may be poorly groomed, poorly nourished, or constipated. In addition, poor grooming may exacerbate feelings of depression. Depression may greatly complicate self-care problems in older people.

Cognitive Abilities

People with normal cognitive and perceptive abilities are usually motivated to perform self-care. Those with limited or altered cognitive abilities may be unaware of the need for self-care, may not know appropriate methods of achieving it, or may be unable to assess what they can safely perform independently.

Careful assessment of clients with a decreased level of consciousness or confusion due to injury or illness is necessary to determine how much assistance they will need. Although these clients may be physically capable of feeding, dressing, bathing, and toileting, they may not be alert enough to know when they should perform these activities and how to do them safely. Clients with minor deficits need to be reminded to provide self-care, but those with severe disabilities (such as severe head trauma or injuries) are often totally dependent on others and mechanical aids for self-care. Clients with cognitive deficits need careful and individual assessment to determine what self-care skills they can accomplish or learn to accomplish with assistance.

Energy

Energy must be available at the cellular level for muscle movement. Adequate nutrition and the ability to break down food for absorption and use by the cells are important in providing energy for self-care. This process also requires adequate oxygen, so respiration plays a significant role. The circulatory system delivers nutrients, oxygen, and other substances to the cells to produce adenosine triphosphate, a nucleotide used to store energy and remove waste products produced by cellular metabolism. Adequate energy stores also prevent fatigue during self-care.

Acute or chronic illness or injury can jeopardize independence in self-care by decreasing energy levels. Compromised respiratory or cardiac function reduces the body's ability to provide sufficient oxygen to the cells, limiting the ability to participate in self-care without fatigue. Decreased energy and weakness can also result from disrupted diet, infection, disturbed gastrointestinal function, fluid and electrolyte imbalance, or a response to a medication.

Acute Illness and Surgery

People who have undergone surgery or who have been acutely ill often need assistance with self-care. The amount of help needed varies depending on the illness or surgery, the client's general health, and any sociocultural expectations. Analgesics, fluid and electrolyte imbalance, and hypoxemia can lead to drowsiness and confusion. Nausea and vomiting add to the general malaise and produce a lack of motivation to perform self-care. Postoperatively, a temporary decrease in cellular oxygenation resulting from anesthesia, hypovolemia, lowered hematocrit level, and atelectasis can lead to weakness. Weakness combined with pain also impedes self-care. Casts, splints, intravenous lines, incisions, urinary catheters, nasogastric tubes, surgical drains, and anxiety constitute encumbrances to mobility and interfere with the ability to perform activities of self-care.

Pain

Clients may experience so much pain that they are unable to care for themselves because their ability or willingness to move may be significantly curtailed. Most analgesics given for pain also cause drowsiness and lightheadedness, placing the client at risk for falls. Therefore, clients taking such medications should be closely monitored to avoid falls during self-care activities. Bathing may offer some pain relief. Clients often find bathing or being bathed a relaxing experience and a distraction from the pain.

Neuromuscular Function

Self-care activities, such as swallowing, getting to the toilet, and dressing, require a well-functioning neuromuscular system. To accomplish these tasks, the central nervous system sends messages to the peripheral nervous system and the muscle fibers to coordinate the necessary fine and gross motor activities. Normal muscle strength and normal contraction and relaxation of muscles also are necessary.

Fine motor control allows the person to have command of small, precise movements (usually of the hands). Fine motor control requires coordination of muscle groups to facilitate activities such as cutting food, opening a milk carton, buttoning a shirt, applying makeup, and wiping after toileting. Gross motor activity involves the coordinated movement of large muscle groups (e.g., climbing in and out of the bathtub, walking or driving to the grocery store, carrying groceries home, getting on and off the toilet). Normal alignment, awareness of the body's spatial position (**proprioception**), and balance are needed to coordinate these large motor movements.

Permanent neuromuscular impairment from conditions such as stroke, spinal cord injury, and some nervous system disorders (parkinsonism, cerebral palsy, myasthenia gravis, and muscular dystrophy) are serious threats to independent self-care. Many of these conditions produce muscle weakness, muscle atrophy, lack of coordination, spasticity, partial or total paralysis, and joint contractures that make walking, talking, eating, and using the extremities difficult or impossible. However, many people with these conditions progress to a high level of independence in self-care with the aid of appliances or other creative adaptations.

Sensorimotor Deficits

People who suffer sensorimotor deficits because of surgery, injury, or infection may need assistance in self-care. Those who have lost some sight may need help with eating or getting to the bathroom. If the visual impairment is prolonged or permanent, the client may learn to compensate by making adjustments to the environment. For example, placing food and utensils on a tray in a consistent manner makes it easier for a visually impaired person to eat independently. Furniture can be arranged so the person does not bump into objects or fall on the way to the bathroom.

Hearing-impaired people may have difficulty carrying out self-care activities because they cannot hear instructions or verbal cues. Devising alternate methods of cuing and communicating proper instructions can help them to perform self-care independently.

ALTERED SELF-CARE

Nurses often encounter people with deficits in self-care in the community and acute care settings. Problems with self-care range from short-term and simple to long-term and complex.

Manifestations of Altered Self-Care

Poor Hygiene and Grooming
Often the senses provide clues to poor hygiene and grooming and problems with self-care. On visual inspection, the skin may be soiled, dry, or flaky or may have rashes and excoriated areas. Hair may be oily, unwashed, and uncombed. Nails may be dirty and broken. Clothes may be soiled, torn, or inappropriate. Inspection of the mouth may reveal sores, caries, inflamed gums, plaque build-up, and stained teeth. Mouth odor (halitosis) is common. There may be an offensive body odor. The smell of urine or feces on soiled clothing may indicate difficulty in toileting.

Inability to Demonstrate Self-Care Activities
Inability to demonstrate gross and fine motor coordination needed for self-care activities indicates impaired ability to perform these functions independently. The ability to get to the bathroom, bathe, dress, and eat is evidence of gross motor skills. The ability to fasten garments, apply makeup, open food containers, and cut food demonstrates fine motor skills. The client should be able to perform self-care activities without cuing and without excessive fatigue.

Verbalization of Reluctance to Perform Self-Care
Listening to what the client says provides important clues to self-care. If the client expresses reluctance or fear to perform self-care activities, a deficit usually is present. Some clients may be reluctant due to depression, altered cognition, or dependent personality. Some may be too fatigued, while others may be in too much pain or have fear of performing the activity successfully. Lack of interest in self-care may be evident because the client's value system does not attach significance to conventional grooming activities.

Impact on Activities of Daily Living

By definition, a self-care deficit causes an alteration in ability to perform activities of daily living. In a culture that values independence, the inability to perform personal care tasks for oneself has significant psychological and physical implications. Often the person has to depend on family or friends for physical help and psychological support. If needed assistance is not available within the client's support system, people may be hired to assist with basic daily needs. Finding qualified help is difficult and expensive, often beyond the budgets of many.

Often a female child or spouse is thrust into the role of caretaker. Willingness to perform these functions can vary depending on many factors including relationship with the client, comfort with such physical tasks, other obligations such as work or children, and the degree and length of time assistance is required. If self-care deficits are short-term (e.g., recovery from orthopedic surgery), family members can often arrange their schedules to provide care. If self-care deficits are extensive and long-term, caregiver demands

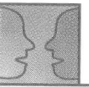

THERAPEUTIC DIALOGUE
Self-Care

Scene for Thought

Rick Newfield, 32 years old, was admitted to the rehabilitation unit 2 days ago after being stabilized in the acute unit with a spinal cord injury. He had been in a motorcycle accident, and today is the first day the nurse is meeting him.

Less Effective

Nurse: Hi, Rick. I'm Sarah James, your nurse for the day shift. How's it going today?

Client: Just great! How do you think, Sarah? I'm a paraplegic, or didn't you know this?! *(Sarcastic tone of voice, swearing, angry face, glaring eye contact.)*

Nurse: I knew. It sounds like you just found out. *(Calm tone and body language.)*

Client: Yeah, they told me yesterday that all the testing they did showed that paralysis is permanent. I won't be able to walk, go to the bathroom by myself, have sex with my wife, run with my little boy, none of that. *(Turns his head to the wall.)*

Nurse: *(Sits in chair next to the bed.)* Pretty devastated by it all right now, aren't you?

Client: Wouldn't you be? God, what a waste. *(Lies back in the bed.)*

Nurse: Sure, I'd be devastated, but I wouldn't be so hopeless. There's lots of stuff we can do to help. *(Still sits quietly.)*

Client: Sure, sure, I know. The doc told me all about the physical therapy and that stuff. Big deal. I'll still be crippled! *(Angry face and voice.)*

Nurse: We don't use that word around here. It means you can't do anything, and there'll be lots you can do. Just hang tight for a bit, and you'll begin to see a big change in yourself. *(Smiles encouragingly.)*

Client: Yeah, yeah. *(Turns face to the wall again.)*

Nurse: *(Notes his body language.)* I can see you'd rather be alone right now. I'll be back in a bit to check on the incision from the operation and to see if you need anything.

Client: *(Cries quietly with his face to the wall.)*

More Effective

Nurse: Hello, Rick. I'm Susan Jacobs, your nurse for the day shift. How's it going today?

Client: Just great! How do you think, Susan? I'm a paraplegic, or didn't you know this?! *(Sarcastic tone of voice, swearing, angry face, glaring eye contact.)*

Nurse: I knew. It sounds like you just found out. *(Calm tone and body language.)*

Client: Yeah, they told me yesterday that all the testing they did showed that paralysis is permanent. I won't be able to walk, go to the bathroom by myself, have sex with my wife, run with my little boy, none of that. *(Turns his head to the wall.)*

Nurse: *(Sits in chair next to the bed.)* Pretty devastated by it all right now, aren't you?

Client: Wouldn't you be? God, what a waste. *(Lies back in the bed.)*

Nurse: *(Sits quietly and says nothing.)*

Client: Well, what are you in here for? I'm not in pain; I don't need help with anything.

Nurse: You're saying you want to be left alone? *(Continues to sit quietly.)*

Client: *(Looks up in surprise.)* What do you mean?

Nurse: It seems to me that you're pretty discouraged and angry right now and are having trouble seeing anything but the worst, and so you want to be left alone. Is that right?

Client: *(Begins to cry quietly and tries to hide it.)* No. I want someone to tell me I'm going to be fine.

Nurse: You will be fine, but you'll be different.

Client: Don't con me, whoever you are. I don't want to hear any of this.

Nurse: I wouldn't con you. You have lots of work to do on yourself, and some of it won't be easy. We'll be around to help and so will the other guys in the PG.

Client: What's that?

Nurse: It's a group called the Paraplegia Group. They help each other through the rehab you all have to go through, like the bowel and bladder training, upper body strength exercises, wheelchair races, skin inspection rounds, how to have great sex, and so forth.

Client: Sounds like fun. *(Said sarcastically but with a spark of interest.)*

Nurse: Jimmy Saguro will be by this afternoon to talk to you about it. Meanwhile, tell me about how your body really feels. You and I have to work together too, you know. *(Smiles.)*

Client: *(Smiles back.)*

Critical Thinking Challenge

- Name obstacles that are in the way of Rick's self-care abilities.
- Detect what Susan did that helped him change his perspective that he wouldn't be able to do anything.
- Detect what Sarah did that did not change his perspective.
- Critique timing and how each nurse used or ignored it.

on the family are great. If deficits are long-term, the client may need to move to the designated caregiver's residence. Although at times this can be a positive experience for the entire family, it also can create much strain and difficulty for every family member including the client. Inability to perform self-care is a leading cause of nursing home placement.

ASSESSMENT
Subjective Data

By asking questions, the nurse can learn what the client considers normal self-care activity and determine which areas are problematic. These questions are designed to elicit the client's feelings about the problem, what he or she sees as the solution, and his or her level of motivation to alter self-care ability. If family members are present, they may give their perceptions of the client's self-care abilities.

Normal Pattern Identification

Interviewing the client permits the nurse to collect information about normal self-care patterns. Examples of questions to elicit this information are the following:

- How do you manage bathing or hygiene (dressing, eating, toileting)? Are you satisfied with your ability to bathe (dress, eat, and toilet)?
- Describe any factors that interfere with bathing (dressing, eating, and toileting)?
- What are your expectations about performing self-care?
- Do you foresee any problems with your ability to care for yourself?
- How independent do you want to be with self-care?
- How would you feel if you were unable to perform self-care independently?

Such information helps to determine how the client normally manages self-care and what his or her feelings and values are about self-care. Use such information to individualize client care. Schedule bathing in the morning or evening, according to client preference. Oral care can be provided before or after breakfast with cold or warm water. Clients who sleep late may want to delay self-care activities, but others prefer to wash and apply makeup early in the morning before seeing anyone.

Normal self-care patterns can be categorized according to the assistance required by the client; Table 32-1 summarizes the levels and gives examples. Level 0 reflects complete independence; level 4 reflects complete dependence on others.

Risk Identification

As the nurse gathers self-care information from the client, she or he identifies factors that could put the client at risk for self-care deficits. Observe and interview the client for possible factors affecting self-care, being especially alert for the following risk factors:

- Pain
- Immobility or limited use of an extremity
- Neuromuscular impairment
- Mental confusion or decreased mental alertness
- Decreased visual acuity or other sensory deficits
- Inability to control bowel or bladder function
- Decreased energy levels or fatigue
- Socioeconomic factors

The client's responses should be corroborated by a physical examination. For example, if the client says he or she does not have problems with bathing and shampooing but the nurse observes skin breakdown, body odors, and dirty fingernails, this would indicate that the person is likely to be at risk for self-care deficits.

Dysfunction Identification

The nurse should be familiar with the signs indicating inability to perform self-care. The nurse can use an Index of Activities of Daily Living (Table 32-2), developed by Katz

TABLE 32-1

Levels of Self-Care		
Level	**Description**	**Example**
Level 0	Client is independent in self-care activities.	Healthy college student lives alone in an apartment.
Level 1	Client uses equipment or devices to perform self-care activities independently.	An elderly man uses a cane for extra support during walking.
Level 2	Client requires assistance or supervision from another to complete self-care activities.	Postoperative client needs help in bathing first day after surgery.
Level 3	Client requires assistance or supervision from another and uses devices or equipment.	Client ambulates using a walker and needs contact supervision.
Level 4	Client is completely dependent on another to perform self-care activities.	Comatose client requires complete care from nursing staff.

TABLE 32-2

Index of Independence in Activities of Daily Living*		
ADL	**Independent**	**Dependent**
Bathing (sponge, shower, or tub)	Client needs assistance only in bathing a single part (such as back or disabled extremity) or bathes self completely.	Client needs assistance in bathing more than one part of body; needs assistance in getting in or out of tub or does not bathe self.
Dressing	Client gets clothes from closets and drawers; puts on clothes, outer garments, braces; manages fasteners (act of tying shoes is excluded).	Client does not dress self or remains partly undressed.
Toileting	Client gets to toilet, gets on and off toilet, arranges clothes, cleans organs of excretion (may manage own bedpan at night or may not be using mechanical supports).	Client uses bedpan or commode or needs assistance getting to and using toilet.
Transferring	Client moves in and out of bed and chair independently (may be using mechanical supports).	Client needs assistance in moving in or out of bed or chair; does not perform one or more transfers.
Continence	Client has self-control over urination and defecation.	Client has partial or total incontinence in urination or defecation; partial or total control by enemas, catheters, or regulated use of urinals or bedpans.
Feeding	Client gets food from plate into mouth; precutting of meat and preparation of food (such as buttering bread) are excluded from evaluation).	Client needs assistance in feeding; does not eat at all or uses parenteral feeding.

* Independence means without supervision, direction, or active personal assistance, based on actual status and not on ability. A client who refuses to perform is considered as not performing even though he or she is deemed able.

(1963; 1983), to aid in this assessment and determine the level of functional independence in self-care practices of feeding, continence, transferring, going to the toilet, dressing, and bathing. This standardized assessment guide allows the nurse to compare self-care deficits with normal patterns. Katz believed that loss of self-care is a natural part of aging and proceeds in an orderly fashion with more complex activities being lost first. He also argued that people regain functional self-care abilities in patterns similar to the development of these skills in children. For example, they achieve feeding and continence skills first, then transfer and toileting abilities, and finally dressing and bathing abilities.

Objective Data

Validate information obtained during the client interview by objectively observing the client engaged in self-care functions. Look for the following:

- Evidence of inability to manage self-care (i.e., poor grooming, body odor, lice, skin lesions, poor nutrition)
- Ability to process sensory input by hearing, sight, smell, and touch
- Evidence of disabilities such as weakness, cognitive deficits, immobility or spasticity, or mental lethargy
- Manual dexterity

- Use of sensory or mechanical aids (i.e., glasses or contact lenses, dentures, hearing aid, cane or walker, condom catheter, raised toilet seat, or special eating utensils)

When activity intolerance or fatigue is suspected, evaluate the client's cardiopulmonary response before, during, and after each self-care activity by assessing pulse rate, respiratory rate, and quality of breathing and by observing for changes in skin color. At the same time, note any alterations in the client's normal physical status.

To formulate realistic goals and interventions, the nurse must assess the resources available to the client. This can mean internal resources (psychological, intellectual, and emotional factors) and external resources (living arrangements, finances). Display 32-1 lists external and internal resources to evaluate and their influence on self-care.

NURSING DIAGNOSES

Self-care deficit nursing diagnoses accepted by the North American Nursing Diagnosis Association (NANDA) are Bathing/Hygiene, Dressing/Grooming, Feeding, and Toileting Self-Care Deficits. The diagnosis Self-Care Deficit is broad and can be used for problems involving a variety of body systems.

DISPLAY 32-1

🖵 EVALUATING EXTERNAL AND INTERNAL RESOURCES AND INFLUENCES

External Resources

Housing

Location, design, access by elevators/stairs, special equipment, kitchen and bathroom facilities, access to telephone, how many people share facilities

- Mobility around home
- Ability to shop for and prepare food
- Access to bathroom for self-care

Water

- Availability of water for bathing and drinking
- Hot water for bathing

Neighborhood

Proximity of shops, hospitals/clinics, available transportation

- Ability to obtain groceries
- Access to healthcare and assistance
- Public transportation

Financial Resources

- Ability to purchase food and self-care products
- Ability to afford healthcare

Support Network and Community Resources

- Family and friends
- Support groups and volunteers such as Meals on Wheels
- Home healthcare

Government and Social Services

- Help with shopping, getting to doctor's appointments, self-care, and meal preparation
- Financial or material assistance for supplies and special equipment

Internal Resources

Inner Strength

Ability to handle physical, mental, and emotional work

Endurance

Stamina or "staying power" to cope with physical, mental, or emotional difficulties

Sensory Input

Ability to attend to and process environmental stimuli to provide a safe environment when attending to self-care needs

Cognitive Abilities

Amount and use of knowledge regarding self-care

Desire

Will or motivation to participate in self-care

Courage

Willingness to take risks and bear hardship to achieve self-care independence

Skills

Abilities regarding psychomotor functions, dexterity, or communication and interpersonal relationships

Communication

Ability to make others understand and make needs known

Diagnostic Statement: Bathing/Hygiene Self-Care Deficit

Definition. Bathing/Hygiene Self-Care Deficit is the inability to perform or complete bathing or hygiene activities for oneself (NANDA, 2001).

Defining Characteristics. Defining characteristics are inability to wash body or body part, obtain water, regulate temperature or flow of water, get in or out of bathroom, dry body, or obtain bath supplies (NANDA, 2001).

Related Factors. Related factors include intolerance to activity, decreased strength and endurance, pain, discomfort, perceptual/cognitive impairment, neuromuscular impairment, depression, severe anxiety, decreased or lack of motivation, weakness and tiredness, and environmental barriers (NANDA, 1999).

Diagnostic Statement: Feeding Self-Care Deficit

Definition. Feeding Self-Care Deficit is the inability to perform or complete feeding activities for oneself (NANDA, 2001).

Defining Characteristics. Defining characteristics include inability to cut, swallow, prepare, manipulate, or chew food; or the inability to bring food from receptacle to mouth, open containers, get food onto a utensil, pick up a cup or glass, ingest food safely or in a sufficient manner, or ingest food in a socially acceptable manner (NANDA, 2001).

Related Factors. Related factors include weakness, tiredness, pain, discomfort, perceptual/cognitive impairment, musculoskeletal or neuromuscular impairment, depression, environmental barriers, decreased motivation, and severe anxiety (NANDA, 2001).

Diagnostic Statement: Toileting Self-Care Deficit

Definition. Toileting Self-Care Deficit is the inability to perform or complete toileting activities for oneself (NANDA, 2001).

Defining Characteristics. Defining characteristics include inability to get to the toilet or commode, inability to sit on or rise from a toilet or commode, inability to manipulate clothing for toileting, inability to carry out proper toilet hygiene, or inability to flush toilet or empty commode (NANDA, 2001).

Related Factors. Related factors include impaired transfer ability, impaired mobility, intolerance to activity, decreased strength and endurance, pain, discomfort, perceptual/cognitive impairment, neuromuscular impairment, depression, and severe anxiety (NANDA, 2001).

Diagnostic Statement: Dressing/Grooming Self-Care Deficit

Definition. Dressing/Grooming Self-Care Deficit is the impaired ability to perform or complete dressing or grooming activities for self (NANDA, 2001).

Defining Characteristics. Defining characteristics include impaired ability to put on or take off necessary items of clothing, fasten clothing, choose clothing, put on socks or shoes, use assistive devices, or maintain appearance at a satisfactory level (NANDA, 2001).

Related Factors. Related factors include decreased or lack of motivation, weakness or tiredness, pain, discomfort, perceptual/cognitive impairment, neuromuscular or musculoskeletal impairment, or environmental barriers (NANDA, 2001).

Related Nursing Diagnoses

Other nursing diagnoses frequently exist along with Self-Care Deficit and may include Impaired Skin Integrity (related to inability to provide hygiene and clean oneself after toileting); Imbalanced Nutrition: Less than Body Requirements, and Deficient Fluid Volume (related to inability to feed oneself); Impaired Oral Mucous Membrane (related to inability to manage mouth care and feed oneself); Ineffective Coping (related to depression about limitation in self-care abilities); Anxiety (related to inability to reach the toilet reliably or perform other self-care activities); Powerlessness (related to difficulty in maintaining usual schedule); and Caregiver Role Strain and Interrupted Family Processes (related to stress).

OUTCOME IDENTIFICATION AND PLANNING

The following may be included when formulating goals for clients with the four self-care deficits:

- Client will actively participate in hygiene measures.
- Client will safely increase level of independence in eating.
- Client will actively participate in dressing.
- Client will manage toileting as independently as possible.

Examples of nursing interventions to help in planning are listed in the accompanying display and discussed in the following section.

In practice, outcomes are highly personalized and specific. Because of their personal nature, outcomes reflect the client's wishes and the stage of illness. For example, a chronically ill person who looks at death as a release may have a different response to working toward independence than a person with a favorable prognosis for complete recovery.

IMPLEMENTATION
Health Promotion

Frequently the nurse is able to stress the relationship of good hygiene, optimal health, and infection prevention. In preschools, nurses can teach young children the importance of

---

PLANNING: NIC/NOC Suggested Interventions

Accepted Self-Care and Hygiene Nursing Interventions Classification (NIC)
Self-Care Assistance
Self-Care Assistance: Bathing/Hygiene
Self-Care Assistance: Dressing/Grooming
Self-Care Assistance: Feeding
Self-Care Assistance: Toileting

Accepted Self-Care and Hygiene Nursing Outcomes Classification (NOC)
Self-Care: Activities of Daily Living (ADL)
Self-Care Bathing
Self-Care Dressing
Self-Care Feeding
Self-Care Grooming
Self-Care Hygiene
Self-Care Toileting

Refer to the following for specifics regarding NIC/NOC: McCloskey, J., & Bulechek, G. (2000). *Iowa intervention project: Nursing interventions classification* (NIC) (2nd ed.). St. Louis, MO: Mosby.
Johnson, M., & Maas, M. (2000). *Iowa outcomes project: Nursing outcomes classification* (NOC) (2nd ed.). St. Louis, MO: Mosby.

proper hygiene after toileting or older children how to detect and prevent the transmission of lice. In prenatal classes, nurses can teach the new mother how to bathe a newborn and prevent scalp problems; and in a community health center, the nurse can teach proper foot care to an aging population. Teaching about dental health and regular dental visits also is important.

Nurses can support community and governmental programs to promote self-care for high-risk groups. For example, promoting increased support for shelters and relief agencies so the homeless and mentally ill will have access to showers and bathroom facilities is one way a nurse might support self-care on a community level. Some communities with a large homeless population are encouraging the placement of portable toilets, so toileting can be private and sanitary. Free clinics need to be available and accessible to provide foot care for diabetic clients and dental care for low-income families.

Nursing Interventions for Altered Self-Care

Emphasize to all clients the importance of increasing their independence in self-care. Client teaching is a cooperative venture that requires the nurse's knowledge, patience, and effort and the client's motivation to learn and offer information regarding personal preference. Some people have an innate desire to be independent and, therefore, have a willingness to learn. Others are more inclined to be dependent and, thus, may be less willing to relearn how to care for themselves.

People with self-care deficits often must learn new skills or methods of overcoming or coping with difficulties. Rehabilitation involves many health team members working together to promote optimal functioning. Table 32-3 lists health team professionals who commonly work with clients to improve self-care abilities.

Work collaboratively with these healthcare professionals when teaching and reinforcing skills and nurturing the client's desire for self-care independence. Careful assessment of client values and interests often reveals motivating factors that might encourage a client to achieve independence.

Careful communication is necessary when providing assistance or teaching self-care. Explain techniques as simply as possible, avoiding technical or medical terms. Learning or relearning self-care skills takes time and effort. Be patient, supportive, and reassuring. Do not criticize the client when he or she is unsuccessful. When the client is successful, regardless of how small or insignificant the task may seem, give reinforcement and encouragement. Do not provide care for clients that they can perform for themselves; receiving unnecessary help fosters dependence and a helpless role. Focus on patiently teaching toward independent self-care.

A study by Buck (2001) demonstrates that when the healthcare worker promotes a positive self-image and cooperation in treating clients faced with long-term rehabilitation, those clients have greatly improved ability for self-care. Ultimately, the client has control over participation in self-care. Positive interventions to encourage self-care include coaxing, rewarding, and educating. Providing assistance with self-care activities gives the nurse an opportunity to develop a trusting, satisfying relationship with the client. Many of these activities, such as bathing, shampooing, or combing hair, are relaxing and soothing to the client. Pleasant conversation during these activities can enhance feelings of comfort and self-worth. These activities give hospitalized or long-term care clients a chance to interact with people.

Scheduled Care

Clients with self-care deficits may require the nurse's assistance in performing hygiene. For the client's comfort and the nurse's planning, specific types of hygienic care are given at regular intervals. Routine times for providing hygiene care in an inpatient setting include early morning, morn-

TABLE 32-3

Collaboration to Promote Self-Care	
Health Professional	**Role**
Registered nurse	Assesses abilities and deficits in self-care; coordinates and supports rehabilitation through individualized plan of care and client teaching
Rehabilitation physician	Directs rehabilitation and medical management of client enrolled in a rehabilitation program
Physical therapist	Assesses mobility, strengthens muscle groups, and works to improve motor function
Occupational therapist	Assesses ability to perform ADLs; helps clients relearn basic care skills and energy conservation methods
Social worker	Coordinates placement for clients unable to remain in the home; identifies community resources to help client stay in the home despite deficits
Speech therapist	Evaluates swallowing and retrains safe eating for clients with deficits
Home health nurse	Provides follow-up and coordination for self-care deficits in the home by accessing community resources, teaching, and providing support and direct care

OUTCOME-BASED TEACHING PLAN

Mr. George is experiencing weakness on his right side (he is right-handed) and is having difficulty understanding complex verbal commands as a result of a cerebrovascular accident (CVA). He is on the rehabilitation unit and would like to be able to independently dress himself using aids before discharge.

OUTCOME: By the end of the second teaching session, client can verbalize three energy-saving techniques to use while dressing.
Strategies
- Ask Mr. George to describe his usual dressing routine.
- Evaluate this routine for areas that increase energy expenditure.
- Describe methods that Mr. George can use to reduce energy expenditure.
- Explain the connection between energy expenditure, Mr. George's condition, and success or failure with self-care.
- Develop a written list for Mr. George, identifying measures appropriate for him to use; incorporate use of pictures depicting those measures as necessary.
  - Stress sitting position while dressing.
  - Allow enough time for dressing.

- Schedule dressing for times when Mr. George is well rested.
- Use loose-fitting clothes with Velcro fasteners.
- Instruct Mr. George to refer to the list and review it periodically, especially before he dresses each day.
- Provide for assistive devices, such as a long-handled reacher to slip on shoes, as necessary.
- Instruct Mr. George in how to use assistive devices.

OUTCOME: By third week of rehabilitation, Mr. George demonstrates ability to put on shoes and loose-fitting clothes with Velcro fasteners without complaints of fatigue or dyspnea.
Strategies
- Tell Mr. George to sit on a chair next to the bed.
- Lay out clothes in the order that Mr. George will put them on.
- Place assistive devices, if used, within easy reach.
- Give simple, concise verbal cues. Provide positive reinforcement as Mr. George completes each step.
- Encourage use of assistive devices as appropriate.
- Assess Mr. George's fatigue level and dyspnea during dressing.
- Provide positive feedback and encouragement even for the smallest accomplishments.

---

ing, afternoon, or evening. Display 32-2 includes common hygiene measures provided. Hygienic procedures should be individualized according to personal and cultural preferences. Because hospital stays are decreasing in length, client acuity is increasing and staffing ratios are decreasing. These changes challenge the ability to provide complete hygiene care to all clients. Due to staffing and cost constraints, hygiene measures frequently are delegated to nursing assistants. Specific guidelines for delegating are provided in the procedures. Delegating hygiene for a confused or aggressive client is complex and should be done judiciously, especially if this intervention is to be therapeutic as well as cleansing. Aggression by cognitively impaired clients was shown to decrease when bathing was individualized and client-centered (Whall, Black, Groh, Yankou, Kupferschmid, & Foster, 1997).

Bathing and Skin Care
The usual time of day for bathing varies greatly. Some people prefer to bathe in the morning; others find that an evening bath is relaxing and promotes a good night's sleep. It is not always possible to satisfy personal preferences, but clients appreciate the opportunity to wash their face and hands in the morning before breakfast and before going to sleep at night. The frequency of bathing should be determined by the client's needs, rather than by adhering to a rigid bathing schedule that meets the staff's convenience. Frequent bathing for the older client can dry skin and contribute to breakdown. The comatose client or

the client who has excessive body excretions or wound drainage requires bathing every day (sometimes more frequently) to avoid skin irritation, breakdown, and infection.

Some clients are anxious or embarrassed about needing assistance with bathing, grooming, dressing, and toileting. Be sensitive to the client's preferences and respect the client's sense of privacy and modesty. To ensure privacy, curtains should be pulled around beds and doors closed when bathing or dressing clients. Some clients are sensitive to having these activities performed by someone of the opposite sex.

The environment in the long-term care facility should promote self-care independence. Have supplies or equipment available, such as a walker if the client needs support in getting to the bathroom. When bathrooms in these facilities are designed in a homelike manner, bathing is a more pleasant experience; this helps ensure the resident's cooperation and dignity (Baker, Smith & Stead, 1999).

Types of Baths. There are two types of baths: cleansing baths and therapeutic baths. Cleansing baths are needed to keep the skin free of secretions, microorganisms, perspiration, and debris. All body parts should be cleansed but areas requiring particular attention to prevent skin breakdown, odors, or discomfort are the face, hands, axillae, and perineum. Therapeutic baths soothe skin irritation or promote healing (Table 32-4).

DISPLAY 32-2

 SCHEDULING HYGIENE CARE

Early Morning Care
Comfort Measures and Preparation for the Day
- Bedpan, urinal, or assistance to bathroom
- Preparation for diagnostic tests or early surgery
- Washing hands and face
- Oral care
- Preparation for breakfast

Morning Care (AM Care)
Morning Hygiene and Grooming
- Bedpan, urinal, or assistance to bathroom
- Bath, shower, or bathing
- Back massage
- Hair care and shaving
- Oral care
- Care for feet and nails
- Dressing
- Bed linen change
- Straightening bedside unit
- Positioning (bed or chair)

Afternoon Care
After Tests, After Lunch, and Before Visitors
- Bedpan, urinal, or assistance to bathroom
- Washing hands and face
- Oral care
- Bed linens and repositioning if needed

Hour-of-Sleep (HS) Care
Comfort Measures and Bedtime
- Bedpan, urinal, or assistance to bathroom
- Washing hands and face
- Oral care
- Back massage
- Bed linens (change soiled linens, fluff pillow, pull out wrinkles)
- Bedclothes
- Straightening unit (place needed night objects within reach)

Methods of Bathing. There are several methods of bathing depending on the client's condition and abilities:

- Tub bath
- Stand-up shower
- Sit-down shower with shower chair
- Bed bath (partial or complete)
- Towel or bag bath
- Partial bath at a nearby sink or washbasin

When assessing the type of bath to use, take into account the client's abilities then adopt the method that allows the most independence in self-care. Consider the client's energy level and need to conserve energy for other activities, surgical dressings or body parts that may need to be kept dry, the client's preference, and the need to encourage independent self-care.

Some methods are easier for the client to perform independently or with limited assistance. If the nurse provides the needed equipment, some clients can bathe themselves although they may need assistance to reach the back and feet. Tub baths or showers are more effective for cleaning and ensuring that the skin is thoroughly rinsed but they require more mobility and agility. Procedure 32-1 gives steps in assisting with a bath or shower.

SAFETY ALERT
Clients who suffer dizziness, weakness, or mental confusion should not be allowed to take stand-up showers. Obese clients may find it difficult to maneuver into a bathtub and might risk falling. For these clients, a shower may be more appropriate.

Towel baths, sometimes referred to as bag baths, are given with a quick-drying solution (Septi-Soft) that evaporates from the body so rinsing is not necessary. Towels or multiple washcloths are placed in a plastic bag with the warmed solution and wrung out before being placed on the client. The damp towels are used to cleanse and massage body areas. A towel bath is advantageous because it decreases bathing time, decreases client's energy expenditure, and decreases skin drying because of the oil in the solution. Clients report feeling clean and refreshed from this type of bath. Skewes (1994) also reports a decreased spread of gram-negative organisms when the bag bath or towel bath is used. Gram-negative organisms can proliferate when wet washbasins are stored between bed baths. The use of multiple washcloths ensures that organisms are less likely to be transferred from a contaminated area to a clean area, because a new cloth can be used for each area of the body.

SAFETY ALERT
To ensure asepsis, always wash from clean areas to dirty areas when possible.

Washing extremities from distal to proximal stimulates circulation and venous blood return. Preventing excess skin dryness is important for the skin's health and integrity. Dry skin is increased by inadequate fluid intake, too frequent bathing with soaps or detergents, and use of defatting solutions such as alcohol on the skin. Use practices that reduce skin dryness, and teach the client to do the same.

Some clients are weak or comatose and cannot bathe themselves. Their weakness may necessitate the nurse bathing the client in bed. Procedure 32-2 outlines steps for this. Often, bathing a client is delegated to unlicensed personnel.

Perineal Care
If the client cannot perform adequate perineal and genital care, the nurse must do so. Cleaning the perineum and genitals is usually a part of the bath but may need to be done more

TABLE 32-4

Types of Therapeutic Baths		
Type	**Purpose**	**Nursing Considerations**
Sitz bath	To cleanse, soothe, and reduce inflammation of perineal or vaginal area after childbirth, vaginal or rectal surgery, or from local irritation of hemorrhoids and fissures	Water temperature depends on the client's condition and personal preference but is usually 105°–113°F.
Hot-water bath	To relieve muscle spasms and soreness by total immersion	Water temperature should be 113°–114.8°F but may be individualized to client condition and preference. Be alert for vasodilation with resultant orthostatic blood pressure drop and for scalding of skin.
Warm-water bath	To cleanse, promote relaxation, and relieve tension	Adjust water temperature to client's preference.
Cool-water bath	To relieve muscle tension or decrease body temperature in febrile clients	Water should be tepid (98.6°F), not cold. Avoid chilling; shivering may increase body temperature.
Soaks	To soften and loosen secretions during dressing changes or to reduce pain and swelling or itching of inflamed or irritated skin	Medications or topical agents may be added to the water. Apply hot, warm, or cold water to an isolated body part.

frequently if the person is incontinent of urine or feces or has drainage from the perineal area. Also teach perineal and genital care while bathing the client.

Perineal care for women involves cleansing the upper inner thighs, the labia majora, and the folds between the labia majora and minora.

SAFETY ALERT
Always wipe from front to back to avoid contaminating the vagina or urethra with microorganisms from the anus (Fig. 32-1A).

For men, perineal care involves washing the upper inner thighs, the penis, and the scrotum; in uncircumcised men, the foreskin must be retracted and the glans penis washed (Fig. 32-1B). For both sexes, the buttocks are cleaned after the genitals, from a side-lying position.

Perineal tissue is more sensitive than other skin so avoid temperature extremes. Pouring water over the perineum while the client sits on the toilet or a bedpan is a comfortable way of rinsing for the client who is between baths or cannot use a tub or shower. Certain people are at greater risk for infection and irritation of these areas including clients with indwelling catheters; those with perineal, rectal, or lower urinary tract surgery; incontinent clients; and women after childbirth. Perineal care is routinely performed frequently by or for these clients.

Many clients can do their own perineal care with minimal assistance. When giving perineal care to a client of the opposite sex, be direct and professional to help allay embarrassment. Always wear gloves during perineal care and

while handling items that may contain exudate from the perineal area.

Back Massage
Back massage is given to clients to enhance the blood supply to the skin and muscles, to promote comfort, and to promote relaxation. The degree of pressure used varies and should be determined by observing the client's response or verbal cues. Research has demonstrated that the therapeutic effects of massage include a shortened labor with decreased pain and anxiety (Field et al., 1997); decreased systolic and diastolic blood pressure (Cady-Jones, 1997); and decreased pain and increased length of sleep (Richards, 1998). The psychophysiologic benefits of back massage may be shown through a decreased stress response in hospitalized clients (Gauthier, 1999). To prevent pressure ulcers, back massage is no longer indicated for high-risk clients (Agency for Health Care Policy and Research, 1992; Buss, Halfens, & Abu-Saad, 1997) because excessive pressure over bony prominences can damaging the underlying tissue. A lubricant (cream or lotion) permits the hands to glide over the skin. Some young people with oily skin find that alcohol is a cooling and refreshing lubricant but alcohol is drying to the skin and can cause cracking and skin breakdown in dehydrated clients and older adults.

If possible, have the client assume a prone position for a backrub. If this is contraindicated or inconvenient, use a side-lying position. With immobile clients, it may be effective to perform a partial backrub after turning him or her from one side to the other to enhance circulation to the lateral aspect of the hips. Procedure 32-3 summarizes the back massage.

(text continues on page 723)

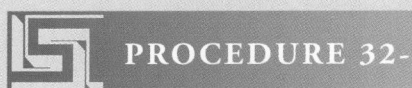

PROCEDURE 32-1

ASSISTING WITH THE BATH OR SHOWER

Purpose
1. Cleanse the skin, control body odors, and promote self-esteem.
2. Stimulate circulation.
3. Provide an opportunity to assess skin and physical mobility.
4. Provide range-of-motion exercises for joints.
5. Promote relaxation and comfort.

Assessment
- Assess client's ability to perform self-care and amount of assistance he or she needs. Evaluate activity tolerance, cognitive function, musculoskeletal function, and level of discomfort to determine type of bath. Note: Encourage the client to be as independent as possible but not to become excessively fatigued. Pain should not be intensified.
- Assess the client's preferences for bathing (i.e., frequency, time of day, type of skin-care products).
- Review chart to determine other procedures or therapies the client is receiving to coordinate scheduling and prevent fatigue.
- Identify clients with special considerations for bathing:
- Older clients: Susceptible to dry skin
- Immobilized clients: Pressure areas on dependent and bony parts; need for range-of-motion exercises to joints
- Clients with altered sensation: Risk for burns from hot water
- Obese or diaphoretic clients: Excessive perspiration or moisture on skin surfaces that rub against each other and provide medium for excoriation and bacterial growth
- Review history for precautions regarding movement or positioning.
- Assess client's knowledge and practice of hygiene to determine learning needs.

Equipment
1–2 bath towel(s)
Bathmat
One washcloth
Soap, soap dish, or liquid (nonsoap) cleanser
Personal skin-care products (deodorant, powder, lotions, cologne)
Clean gown or pajamas
Laundry bag

Procedure
1. Make sure the tub or shower is clean.
2. Prepare bathroom by placing towel or disposable bathmat on floor by tub or shower.
   Rationale: Maintain cleanliness and safety for the client.
3. Accompany or transport client to the bathroom. Some clients may need to use a shower chair for transportation.
   Rationale: Showering or bathing will be tiring. Transportation in a chair will conserve energy.
4. Place "occupied" sign on door.
   Rationale: Client needs privacy while bathing. Doors are not usually locked, so nurse can come in to assist client as necessary.
5. Keep client covered with a bath blanket until water is ready.
   Rationale: Keep the client warm to prevent chills.

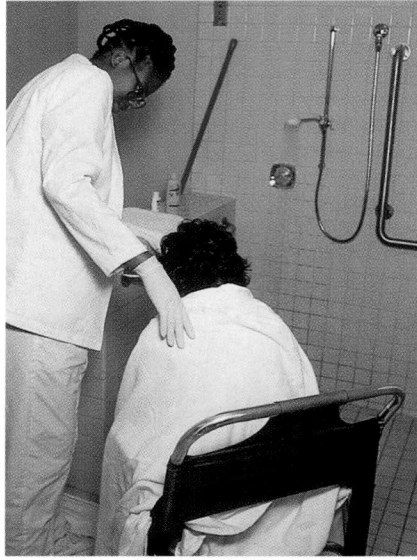

Step 5 Wrap client in bath blanket.

6. Fill bathtub halfway with warm water (105°F, 40.6°C). Test water or have client test water. If the client is taking a shower, turn on shower and adjust water temperature.
   Rationale: Testing temperature before entering water prevents burns.
7. Help client into shower or tub, providing necessary assistance.
   Rationale: Falls can occur in the shower or tub; provide safety for the client.

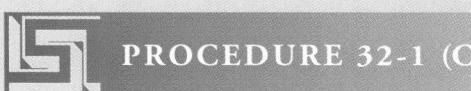

PROCEDURE 32-1 (Continued)

8. Instruct the client in use of safety bars and call bell signal. Client may prefer to sit in shower chair to prevent fatigue.
   Rationale: Provide for the client's safety and comfort.
9. If the client is unable to shower independently, stay with the client at all times. (Two nurses may be necessary for some clients.) Use handheld shower to wash client.
   Rationale: Hand-held shower allows nurse to stay dry.
10. If client is showering or bathing independently, check on client within 15 minutes. Wash any areas he or she could not reach.
    Rationale: Prolonged exposure to warm water may cause vasodilation and pooling of blood, which can result in lightheadedness or dizziness.
11. Help client out of tub or shower. Assist with drying. Note: If client is unsteady, drain water before helping client out of tub.
    Rationale: Draining water and assisting the client with getting out of tub helps to prevent falls.
12. Assist client with dressing and grooming.
13. Help client to room. Return to bathroom then clean tub or shower according to agency policy. Discard soiled linen. Place "unoccupied" sign on door.
    Rationale: Maintain cleanliness and good infection control practices.

Lifespan Considerations
Newborn and Infant
- To prevent infection, do not submerge an infant in water until the umbilical cord has fallen off (around 7–10 days of age).

Child
- To prevent drowning, do not leave children younger than 8 years unattended in a bath.
- Although children often enjoy washing themselves, be sure to supervise so they wash thoroughly.

Adolescent
- Sebaceous glands become active during puberty. Special cleansing agents may be necessary to treat facial acne. Antiperspirants and more frequent baths will help control body odors.

Older Adult
- Older adults are susceptible to dry skin due to reduced sebaceous gland activity, epidermal thinning, and decreased fluid intake. Use lotions, bath oil, and less soap to reduce the drying effects of aging. Bathing may occur weekly to decrease drying of the skin.
- Check water temperature carefully. Older adults may have decreased sensation and are at risk for burns from hot water.

Home Care Modifications
- Instruct clients at risk for falling to apply lotions and oils after the bath and not put them in bath water. Oils can make the bathtub or shower surfaces more slippery.
- Encourage installation of safety devices, such as tub bars, nonskid tub surfaces, and bathroom carpeting, to reduce the chance of falls and promote independence.

Collaboration and Delegation
- Because unlicensed personnel often assist with showers or bathing, be sure to provide assistants with the following information regarding the client:
- Any physical limitations or special safety precautions needed
- Amount of help the client will require
- The presence of any drains, casts, IVs along with any precautions or limitations they will impose during the shower/bath
- Any assessments to report to you (e.g., skin condition under breasts)
- Collaborate with occupational therapy if an occupational therapist is seeing the client. Often, occupational therapists want to assess and work with a client's ability to perform hygiene, so coordination is important.

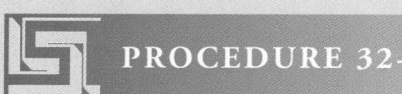

PROCEDURE 32-2

BATHING A CLIENT IN BED

Purpose
Same as Procedure 32-1.

Assessment
Same as Procedure 32-1.

Equipment
Two bath towels
Two washcloths
Bath blanket
Washbasin with warm water (110°–115°F; 43.3°–46.1°C). Test by measuring with bath thermometer or by placing several drops on your inner forearm.
Soap, soap dish, or liquid (nonsoap) cleanser
Personal skin-care products (deodorant, powder, lotions, cologne)
Clean gown or pajamas
Bedpan or urinal
Laundry bag
Disposable clean gloves for perineal care

Procedure
1. Close curtains around bed or shut room door.
   Rationale: Privacy is important to maintain the client's dignity.
2. Help client use bedpan, urinal, or commode if needed.
   Rationale: Client will be more comfortable and relaxed after elimination.
3. Close window and doors to decrease drafts.
   Rationale: Provide client comfort and minimize chilling.
4. Wash your hands.
   Rationale: Handwashing reduces transmission of microorganisms.
5. Raise bed to high position. Lock up side rail on opposite side of bed from your work.
   Rationale: Prevent back strain while preventing client from falling out of bed.
6. Remove top sheet and bedspread, then place bath blanket on client. Help client move closer to you, and remove client's gown. If client has an IV line, remove gown from arm, lower IV container, and slide it through gown with tubing. Rehang IV container, and check flow rate.
   Rationale: Bath blanket provides for client comfort, warmth, and privacy. Bringing client closer to you prevents undue muscle strain.
   Note: If top linen is to be reused, place it on back of chair; otherwise place it in laundry bag.

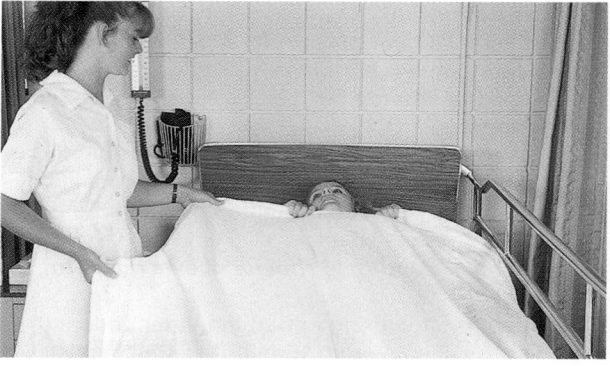

Step 6 Place bath blanket on client.

7. Lay towel across client's chest.
8. Wet washcloth and fold around your finger to make a mitt.
   a. Fold washcloth in thirds.

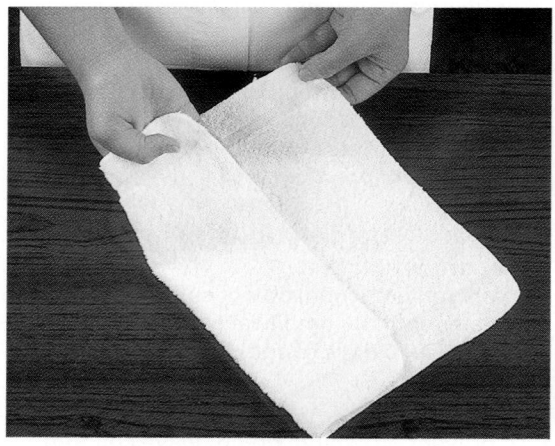

Step 8a Fold washcloth into thirds.

   b. Straighten washcloth to take out wrinkles.
   c. Fold washcloth over to fit hand.
   d. Tuck loose ends under edge of washcloth on palm.
      Rationale: Mitt retains heat and water better than a loosely held washcloth and prevents water from dripping on client.
9. Cleanse eyes with water only, wiping from inner to outer canthus. Use separate corner of mitt for each eye.
   Rationale: Washing eye from inner to outer canthus prevents secretions from entering and irritating nasolacrimal ducts. Using separate

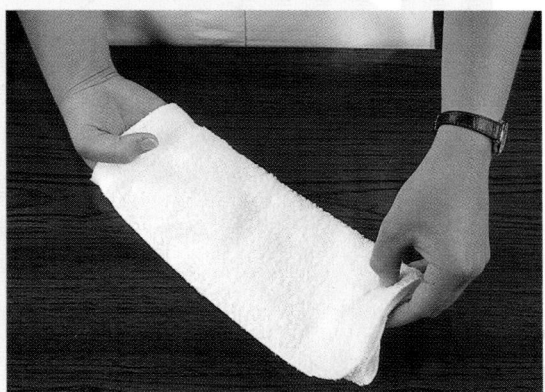

Step 8c Fold washcloth over to fit hand.

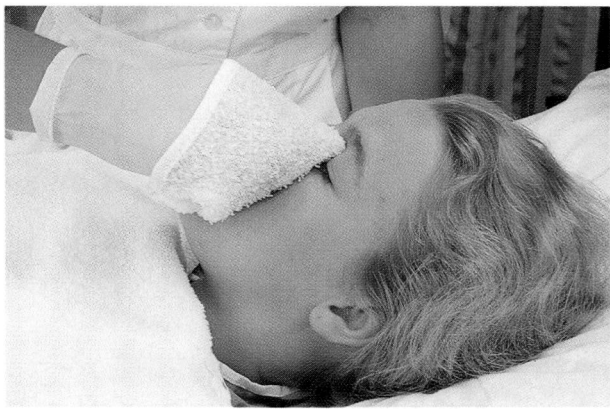

Step 9 Wipe each eye with separate corners of cloth.

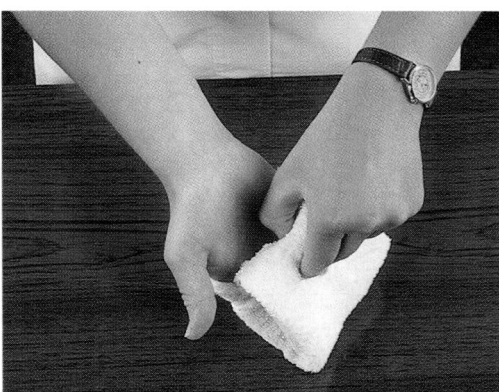

Step 8d Tuck end in to make mitt.

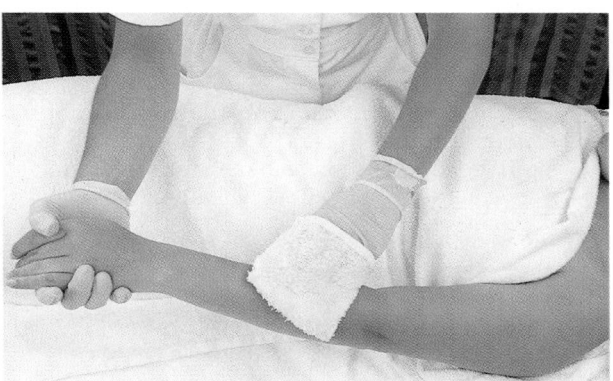

Step 11 Wash arm, stroking from fingers toward axilla.

corners for each eye prevents transfer of micro-organisms from one eye to the other.

10. Determine if client would like soap used on face. Wash face, neck, and ears. Avoid letting soap bar sit in washbasin or water will become too soapy for rinse. Liquid nondetergent cleansing agents are available in many institutions to mix directly into bath water. These products are nondrying and need not be rinsed from the skin.
    Rationale: Soap can be drying especially to the face.
11. Fold bath blanket off arm away from you. Place towel lengthwise under arm. Wash, rinse, and dry the arm using long, firm strokes from the fingers toward the axilla. Wash axilla.
    Rationale: Stroking from distal to proximal stimulates circulation and facilitates venous blood return.
12. (Optional) Place bath towel on bed and put washbasin on it. Immerse client's hand and allow to

soak for several minutes. Wash, rinse, and dry hand well. Repeat on other side. Apply lotion.
Rationale: Soaking softens cuticles and loosens dirt under nails.
13. Repeat for hand and arm nearest you.
14. Apply deodorant or powder according to client's preferences. Avoid excessive use of powder or inhalation of powder.
    Rationale: Hygiene products control excess body moisture and odor. Excessive powder can cause caking, which leads to skin irritation; inhalation can cause respiratory difficulty.
15. Assess bath water temperature and change water if necessary. Side rails should be up.
    Rationale: Precaution prevents accidental falls when nurse leaves the client to change water.
16. Place bath towel over chest. Fold bath blanket down to below umbilicus.

PROCEDURE 32-2 (Continued)

Rationale: Keep the client warm while preventing unnecessary exposure of body parts.

17. Lift bath towel off chest, and bathe chest and abdomen with mitted hand using long, firm strokes. Give special attention to skin under the breasts and any other skin folds if client is overweight. Rinse and dry well. Apply a light dusting of bath powder under the breasts or between skin folds.
Rationale: Toweling and powdering absorb excess moisture and prevent skin maceration and irritation.

18. Help client don a clean gown.
Rationale: Gown prevents exposure of upper body area.

19. Expose leg away from you by folding over bath blanket. Be careful to keep perineum covered.
Rationale: Preventing unnecessary exposure of body parts maintains the client's dignity.

20. Lift leg, and place bath towel lengthwise under leg. Wash, rinse, and dry leg using long, firm strokes from ankle to thigh.
Rationale: Washing from distal to proximal stimulates circulation and facilitates venous blood return.

21. Wash feet or place in basin of water as for hands. Rinse and dry well. Pay special attention to space between toes.

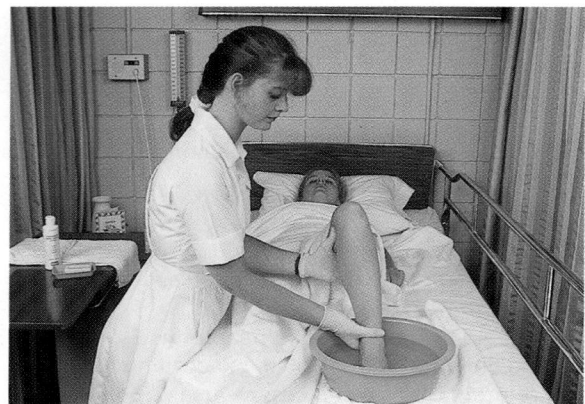

Step 21 Place foot in basin of water to soak.

22. Repeat for other leg and foot.
23. Assess bath water for warmth. Change water if necessary.
24. Assist client to side-lying position. Apply gloves. Place bath towel along side of back and buttocks to protect linen. Wash, rinse, and dry back and buttocks. Give a backrub with lotion.
Rationale: Backrub stimulates circulation and promotes comfort.

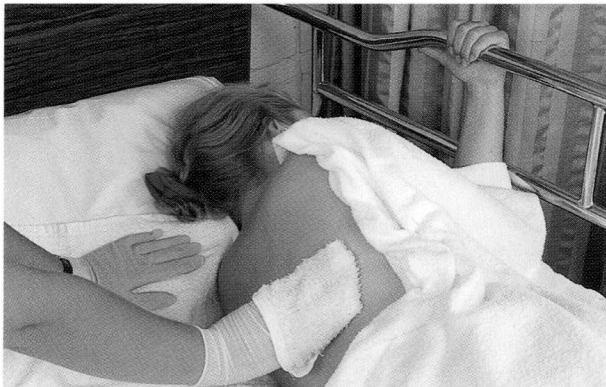

Step 24 Assist to side-lying position to wash back and buttocks.

25. Assist client to supine position. Assess if client can wash genitals and perineal area independently. If client needs care, drape with blanket so that only genitals are exposed. Don disposable, clean gloves. Using fresh water and a new cloth, wash, rinse, and dry genitalia and perineum (see text for instructions).

26. Complete care according to client's preference. Apply powder, lotion, cologne. Assist with hair and mouth care. Make bed with clean linen.
Rationale: Involving client nurtures self-esteem and self-care efforts.

27. Clean equipment and return to appropriate storage area. Wash your hands.
Rationale: Maintain cleanliness.

28. Chart significant observations.
Rationale: Charting communicates information to health team members.

Home Care Modifications
- Arrange for a hospital bed to help prevent caregiver back strain and assist with turning and moving the client in bed.

Collaboration and Delegation
- Same as indications for Procedure 32-1.

Mrs. Ramirez, an 87-year-old client, was admitted last evening after a fall in her home. Due to mobility problems and cognitive changes, she has neglected basic hygiene care in recent weeks. Mrs. Ramirez is confused. She has a sore right hip, but all x-rays have been negative for fractures. Develop a plan for providing hygiene care this morning including strategies for encouraging her participation.

Check your answer in Appendix A.

Care of Feet and Nails

Assess the appearance of the feet and nails to identify existing problems or clients at risk for foot or nail problems. Table 32-5 lists common foot problems, and their causes and treatment.

The skin's color and temperature give clues to the quality of perfusion (blood flow). Cold feet with a dusky skin color may signal poor circulation. People with diabetes mellitus, older people, and clients with poor circulation are at special risk for foot difficulties so good foot care and education about self-care are essential. Combining teaching with care is a good way to motivate a person with foot problems.

ETHICAL/LEGAL ISSUE
Delegation of Care to Unlicensed Personnel

You are the RN at a long-term care facility, supervising care for over 30 residents. You have one LPN and three nursing assistants working with you. When you are passing medications, you enter a room where a nursing assistant and the LPN are bathing a comatose client. They are discussing their boyfriends and their social plans for the upcoming weekend. The client is completely uncovered and appears cold. At no time do you observe them talking with the client. They appear rough in the way they move and position him.

Reflection

- Reflect on your own feelings as you encounter this situation, trying to identify those elements that make you feel uncomfortable.
- Identify underlying assumptions you have concerning what you think is ethically appropriate behavior.
- Refer to the Patient's Bill of Rights in Chapter 6. Do you believe this situation illustrates a breach of this contract?
- Think about three different ways to respond to this situation. Identify a possible approach that might bring about long-term changes in behavior that would improve the quality of care.

To protect the feet of people with peripheral vascular disease from trauma during foot care, avoid cutting nails too short and cutting into calluses. Some hospital policies forbid nurses from cutting the toenails of diabetic clients or people with peripheral vascular disease because healing is slow and the risk of infection after accidental injury is high. These clients often have thick, distorted toenails that are difficult to cut safely, but the nails can be safely filed.

SAFETY ALERT
Soaking the feet of diabetic clients is no longer encouraged because excessive moisture can contribute to skin breakdown (VanRijswijk, 1998).

Procedure 32-4 outlines nursing care of feet and nails.

Client education concerning foot care should include the following:

- Inspect feet daily. You may need a mirror to visualize all areas.
- Never use razors, sharp instruments, or caustic solutions on your feet. File nails straight across rather than cutting.
- Avoid habits that will decrease circulation to your feet (smoking, garters, crossing legs).
- Notify your healthcare provider if you notice abnormal sores or drainage, pain, changes in temperature, color, or sensation of the foot.
- Select sturdy, well-fitting footwear with a nonskid sole. Shop for shoes in the afternoon or evening when feet are often larger due to swelling. Break shoes in gradually, carefully observing for signs of irritation or skin breakdown.
- Do not walk barefoot.

Hair Care

Brushing and Combing. Clients who can brush and comb their hair should be given the equipment and encouraged to do so independently, but clients who cannot comb their own hair need assistance. Brushing hair massages the scalp, stimulates circulation, and facilitates oil distribution along the hair shaft more effectively than combing. Clients with long hair who must spend an extended time in bed need a hairstyle that minimizes matting; combing the hair daily, braiding it, or tying it back helps (Fig. 32-2). If tangles occur, hair is divided into small sections, brushed, then combed. Tightly curled hair usually requires a wide-toothed comb or a pick and a firm-bristled brush. Combing with the fingers can loosen tangles. A lubricating conditioner or petroleum jelly may be used to soften hair and avoid breakage.

Shampooing. Shampooing cleans the hair and scalp and helps get rid of excess oil. It promotes circulation to the scalp and provides a relaxing, soothing experience for the client. Use this opportunity to inspect the hair for dandruff or lice. Shampooing can be done while the client sits in the shower chair, leans back over the sink, leans forward over a pan of

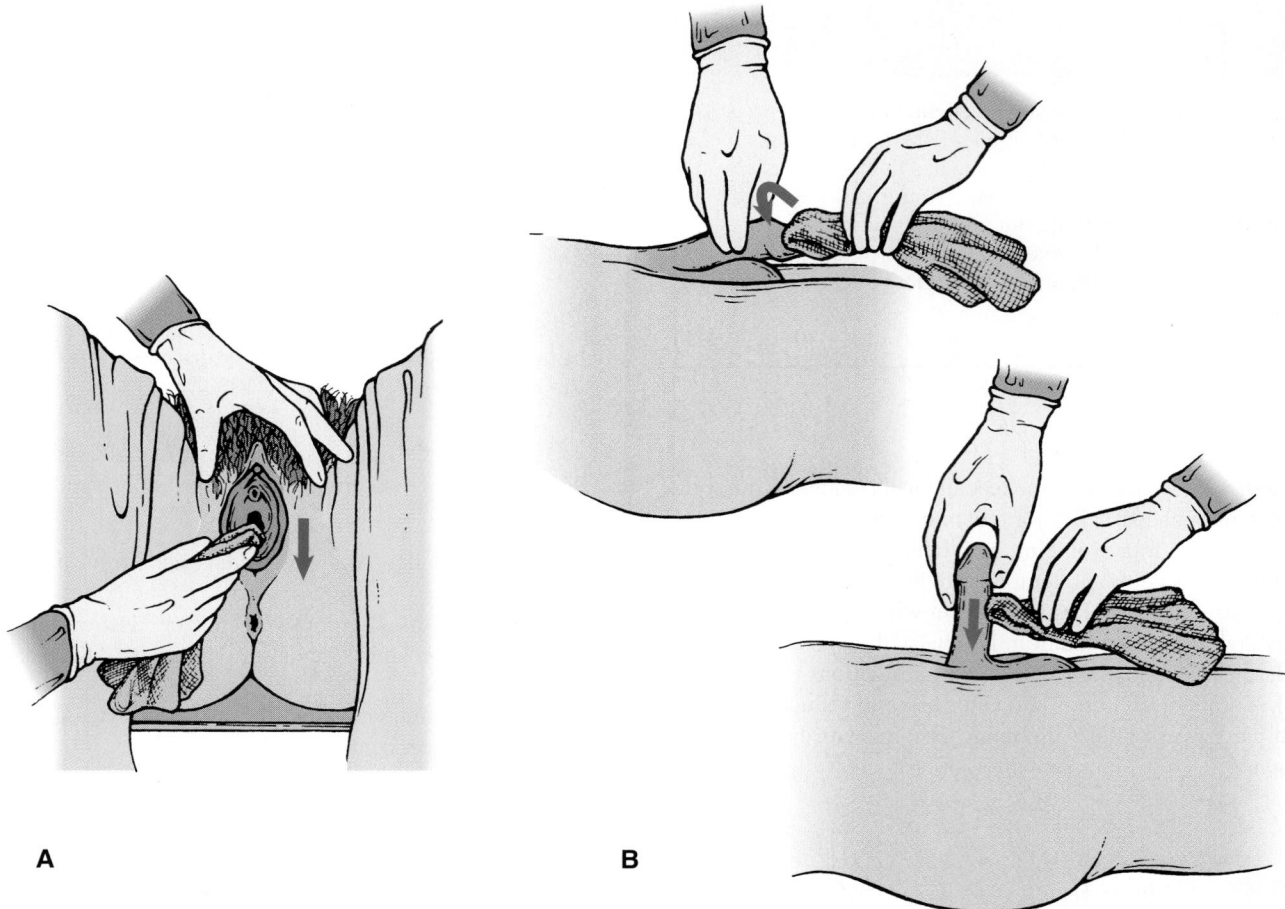

FIGURE 32-1   Perineal care. **(A)** Female: Spread the labia to expose the urethral meatus and the vaginal orifice. Cleanse the area from the pubic area toward the anus in one stroke. Repeat several times, always using a clean area of the washcloth. **(B)** Male: Cleanse the tip of the penis from the urethral meatus downward in a circular motion. Cleanse the penile shaft from the tip downward toward the scrotum.

water on the bedside table, lies on a stretcher over a sink (if unable to sit), or is in bed with a tray to drain the water. Protect the client from fatigue and chilling during shampooing. Procedure 32-5 summarizes steps in shampooing the hair of a bedridden client. Dry shampoo is a powder that can be combed or brushed through the hair to remove excess oils and dirt. Cleansing quality is less effective than traditional methods of shampooing, so this treatment is used only when wetting the hair is contraindicated or not feasible.

Lice. Infestation with lice is called **pediculosis.** Lice found on the hair of the head, eyebrows, eyelashes, and beard is known as pediculosis capitis; hair on the body is pediculosis corporis; and hair in the perineal area is pediculosis pubis.

Head lice and pubic lice attach their eggs, called nits, to hairs with a tenacious substance that makes them hard to remove. Nits, which may be visible with a light and magnifying glass, resemble shiny ovals. To the naked eye, they appear similar to dandruff. Lice live on the skin, and their bites cause itching. Inflamed bites can be seen along the hair-

line. Body lice suck blood from the skin and tend to live in the clothing, making them hard to detect. Clues to the presence of body lice are scratching and hemorrhagic lesions on the skin.

The usual treatment for pediculosis is gamma benzene hexachloride (Kwell), which comes in lotion, cream, and shampoo form. Lice can be treated by showering with Kwell. Recently there have been some reports of resistance and difficulty successfully treating infestations (Hensel, 2000). Because of the area's heavy hair growth, pubic lice are often difficult to remove; the shampoo may be applied and left on for 12 to 24 hours. Linens and clothing used by the client must be washed in hot water. Blankets, furniture, and carpets can be sprayed with insecticide. People with whom the client has had sexual or intimate contact also should be treated.

Dandruff. Dandruff is a chronic, diffuse scaling of the epidermis of the scalp. It is characterized by itching and flaking of whitish scales that are annoying and embarrassing. Frequent brushing and daily shampooing with a keratolytic sham-

PROCEDURE 32-3

MASSAGING THE BACK

Purpose
1. Stimulate circulation to the skin.
2. Relieve muscle tension.
3. Promote comfort and relaxation.

Assessment
- Assess client for muscle fatigue or stiffness, complaints of back discomfort or tension.
- Identify clients with impaired physical mobility who may benefit from back massage.
- Assess skin for localized areas of redness on the back, shoulders, or hips.
- Assess client's desire for back massage.
- Identify conditions that may contraindicate backrub (rib and vertebral fractures, burns, or open wounds).
- Determine any limitations to positioning.

Equipment
Bath blanket
Bath towel (to absorb excess moisture)
Lotion, powder, or alcohol. Lotion is used to lubricate skin and prevents friction during massage. Powder reduces friction and prevents "sticky" feeling on diaphoretic clients. Powder and lotion are not used together. Alcohol cools the skin but can be drying.

Procedure
1. Help client to side-lying or prone position.
2. Expose back, shoulders, upper arms, and sacral area. Cover remainder of body with bath blanket.
   Rationale: Covering areas not being massaged prevents unnecessary exposure and chilling while maintaining dignity.
3. Wash hands in warm water. Warm lotion by holding container under running warm water.
   Rationale: Warm hands and lotion prevent startle response and muscle tension from cold lotion and hands. *Note:* Alcohol is applied cold, but warn the client before application.
4. Pour small amount of lotion into palms.
   Rationale: Lubricating palms decreases friction on skin during massage.
5. Begin massage in sacral area with circular motion. Move hands upward to shoulders, massaging over scapulae in smooth, firm strokes. Without removing hands from skin, continue in smooth strokes to upper arms and down sides of back to iliac crest. Continue for 3 to 5 minutes.
   Rationale: Continuous, firm pressure promotes relaxation and stimulates circulation.

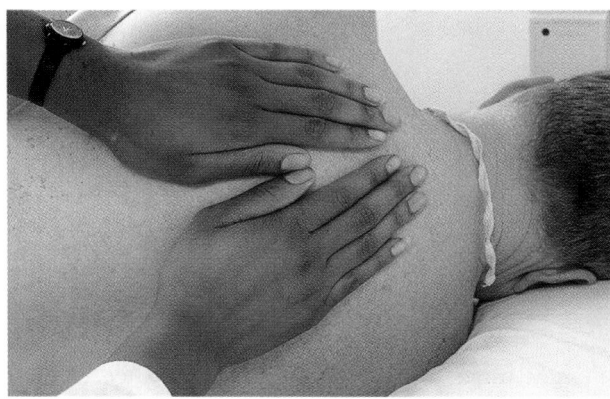

Step 5 Move hands upward with firm, circular motion.

6. While massaging, assess for broken skin areas and whitish or reddened areas that do not disappear. Avoid pressure over areas of breakdown or redness.
   Rationale: Pressure from massage can traumatize and damage tissues.
7. If additional stimulation is desired, nurse can use petrissage (kneading) over the shoulders and gluteal area and tapotement (tapping) up and down the spine.
8. End massage with long, continuous, stroking movements.
   Rationale: Stroking is the most relaxing of the massage movements.
9. Pat excess lubricant dry with towel. Retie client's gown, and assist to comfortable position.
   Rationale: Massage promotes client comfort.
10. Wash your hands.

Collaboration and Delegation
- Encourage unlicensed personnel to provide back massage especially at bedtime. In some facilities, volunteers are trained to provide back massage for receptive clients. Communicate any positioning restrictions and assessments that they should report.

TABLE 32-5

Common Foot Problems			
Type	Description	Possible Causes	Treatment
Calluses	Flattened thickening of epidermis, often on bottom or side of foot over a bony prominence	Tight shoes or inadequate padding in shoes	Soften by soaking in warm water and abrade with pumice stone.
Corns	Cone-shaped lesion (thickening of epidermis) usually on fourth or fifth toe over toe joint	Pressure from tight shoes	Client should purchase and wear softer, better-fitting shoes or foam protective pads. Apply keratolytic agents with salicylic acid to keratinous skin.
Plantar warts	Round or irregular, flattened by pressure, surrounded by cornified epithelium; often painful	Virus, but may be worsened by inadequate circulation or pressure from tight shoes	Remove by curettage, freezing with solid carbon dioxide, or application of salicylic acid.
Bunions (hallax valgus)	Inflammation and thickening of bursa of the great toe joint; enlargement of joint and displacement of toe	Heredity, degenerative bone and joint disease, and tight shoes or high heels	Surgical intervention may be needed, or client can achieve symptomatic relief by wearing shoes that are wide at the front.
Ringworm, tinea pedis (athlete's foot)	Redness, scaling, and cracking of skin especially between toes	Fungus, worsened by moist, unventilated environment	Apply antifungal powder or ointment. Change socks daily; wear 100% cotton socks to absorb moisture.
Ingrown nails	Inflammation, swelling, and tissue pain at edge of nail	Improper nail trimming, poorly fitting shoes	Prevent by trimming nails straight across and wearing well-fitted shoes. Pain and inflammation are treated with anti-inflammatory agents. Surgical removal of nail may be required.
Foot odor	Excessive foul odor of feet	Possibly from fungal foot infections; exacerbated by hot, moist environment	Decrease excess moisture; use deodorant foot powders, 100% cotton socks, well-ventilated shoes.

poo may control the problem, but persistent, severe cases may require medical attention.

Hair Loss. Hair continually grows and renews itself. To promote healthy hair, chemical treatments and excessive heat (drying on the high setting, electric rollers) should be avoided. Cream rinses can be helpful in keeping hair untangled.

Male-pattern baldness occurs in middle or older age but can appear much earlier in some men. Premature loss of hair can be stressful, impacting self-image and sexual identity. Treatment includes hair pieces, hair transplants, or drugs that stimulate hair growth.

Acute hair loss can occur due to stress, high fever, certain medications, general anesthesia, or childbirth. Most commonly, hair loss (**alopecia**) is caused by cancer treatment. Warn clients that hair loss may be gradual or sudden and may continue a

few weeks after treatment is started. After treatment completion, hair usually regenerates although it may grow back a different color or texture. Support the client during this time and help with selecting a hat, wig, or decorative scarf to wear and/or refer the client to a community agency, such as the American Cancer Society, for support.

Shaving

Shaving may make men feel good about their physical appearance. Most men without beards shave every day; receiving help with shaving can boost the client's morale. To avoid cuts, soften the beard with warm towels before shaving. Use soap lather or shaving cream, pull the skin taut, and shave in the direction in which the hair grows to decrease irritation (Fig. 32-3). Men with decreased energy and impaired fine

(text continues on page 729)

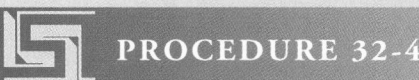

PROCEDURE 32-4

PERFORMING FOOT AND NAIL CARE

Purpose
1. Maintain skin integrity around nails.
2. Provide for client's comfort and sense of well-being.
3. Maintain foot function.
4. Encourage self-care.

Assessment
- Note client's gait for limping or unusual position. Unnatural gait can be caused by painful feet or bone and muscle disorders.
- Assess footwear worn by client. Socks should be worn to absorb excess perspiration and avoid fungal infections.
- Identify clients at risk for foot or nail problems:
- Diabetes is associated with changes in microcirculation to peripheral tissues. The diabetic client is at high risk for infection from breaks in skin integrity and may have decreased sensation to pain as a result of neuropathy.
- Older adult clients' ability to perform foot and nail care may be impeded by poor vision, obesity, or musculoskeletal conditions that limit their ability to bend and maintain balance.
- Cerebrovascular accident may alter the client's gait due to foot drop, muscle weakness, or paralysis.
- Conditions associated with foot and ankle edema (renal failure, congestive heart failure) interfere with blood flow to surrounding tissues and impede proper shoe fit.
- Determine client's ability to perform self-care.
- Inspect nails and skin of fingers, toes, and feet. Assess areas between toes for dryness and cracking.
- Assess client's knowledge of foot and nail care practices.
- Review agency policy for trimming nails. Many agencies require a physician's order to perform nail trimming on high-risk clients.

Equipment
Waterproof pad
Washcloth, towels
Washbasin, warm water, soap
Lotion
Disposable gloves
Nail clippers, file
Orange stick

Procedure
1. Wash your hands.
2. Identify client and help to chair if possible. Elevate head of bed for bedridden client.
3. Fill washbasin with warm water (100°–104°F; 37.7°–40°C). Place waterproof pad under basin. Soak client's hands or feet in basin. Diabetic clients should *not* soak feet.
   Rationale: Warm water softens nails, increases local circulation, and reduces inflammation. Prolonged soaking increases risk of infection and tissue maceration for diabetic clients.
4. Place call bell within reach. Allow hands or feet to soak for 10 to 20 minutes.
   Rationale: Softening allows easier removal of dead epithelial cells and reduces possibility of nails cracking during trimming.

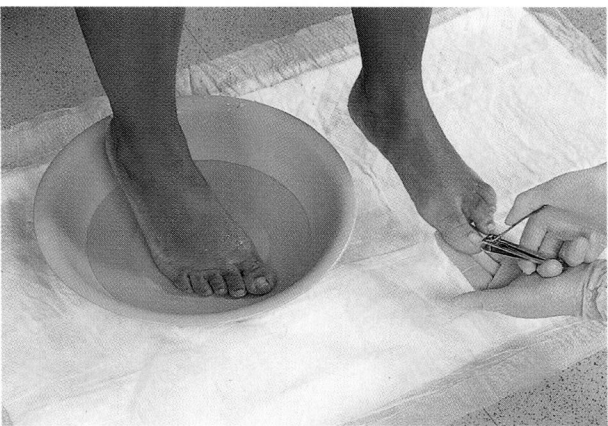

Step 5 Continue to soak other extremity while working on softened nails.

5. Dry the hand or foot that has been soaking. Rewarm water, and allow other extremity to soak while you work on the softened nails.
   Rationale: Soaking the second hand or foot while the nurse works on the first is efficient use of time.
6. Gently clean under nails with orange stick. If nails are thickened and yellow, client may have fungal infection. Wear disposable gloves.
   Rationale: Gloves prevent transmission of infection.
7. Beginning with large toe or thumb, clip nail straight across. Shape nail with file. File rather than cut nails of clients with diabetes or circulatory problems.
   Rationale: Trimming straight across prevents nail splitting and tissue injury around nail.

PROCEDURE 32-4 (Continued)

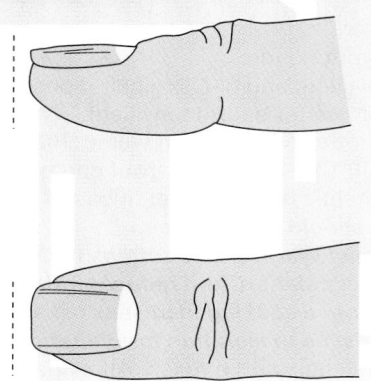

Step 7 Cut nails straight across.

8. Push back cuticle gently with orange stick.
   Rationale: Cuticle care reduces inflamed cuticle and hangnail formation.
9. Repeat procedure with other nails.
10. Rinse foot or hand in warm water.
11. Dry thoroughly with towel especially between digits.
    Rationale: Removing excess moisture inhibits bacterial growth.
12. Apply lotion to hands or feet.
13. Help client to comfortable position.
14. Remove and dispose of equipment.
15. Wash your hands.

Lifespan Considerations

Infant

- Teach parents to care for their infant's nails to prevent the infant from scratching. Instruct parents to cut nails straight across using blunt scissors. It is easiest to trim the nails when the baby is asleep.

Child

- Observe for nail biting, which is often a concern in school-age children. It may be a learned behavior or a symptom of nervous tension. Bad-tasting over-the-counter preparations are available to paint on the nails to discourage nail biting. Other measures may include positive reinforcement and rewards for "good" days with no nail biting.

Older Adult

- Inspect the older adult's nails closely. Older clients often have thickened, horny nails due to poor peripheral perfusion. Mobility problems may make nail care difficult for the elderly.

Collaboration and Delegation

- Refer high-risk clients or those with severely hypertrophied nails to a podiatrist or foot clinic for care. In some institutions, be aware that the diabetic clinician can provide foot care for high-risk clients.

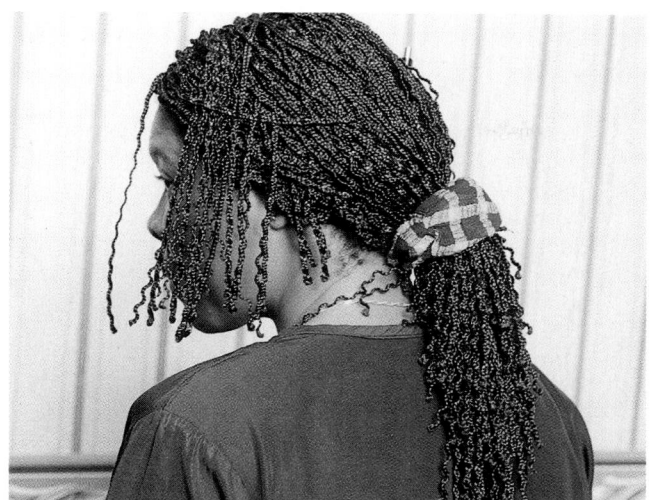

FIGURE 32-2 Braiding is stylish and helps decrease tangling and matting in clients with long hair.

motor skills find it easier to use electric shavers, which some agencies provide. Urge clients at risk for excessive bleeding (i.e., those with bleeding disorders or who are taking anticoagulants) to use an electric razor rather than a safety razor to avoid cuts. Men with beards or mustaches may need help trimming them and keeping them clean and free from food particles. Facial hair can be washed during a bath or shower. Mustaches or beards are shaved off only at the client's request.

Shaving underarm and leg hair is an important part of grooming for many women. This is done using the same shaving technique as for men.

Oral Care

Brushing the teeth and cleansing and rinsing the mouth are comfort measures. Rinsing is soothing to the client with a dry mouth. An unclean mouth can harbor bacteria that can multiply and cause other problems. Procedure 32-6 gives guidelines for providing oral care.

The nurse or caregiver may need to assist or perform brushing and flossing for clients who are unable to do so. Encourage regular brushing and flossing, which contribute to the prevention of caries and periodontal disease and help prevent tooth loss. Providing oral care also permits assessment of the oral cavity.

Brushing and Flossing. Encourage clients who can brush and floss independently to do so. If the client cannot get out of bed to use the sink, provide the necessary equipment including a basin for spitting.

For the client who has difficulty grasping the small handle of an ordinary toothbrush, an electric toothbrush is useful because its larger handle is easier to grasp and requires less manipulation. The handle of a regular toothbrush can be built up with tape, a bicycle handlebar grip, or a split rubber ball. Ultrasonic toothbrush systems, which require less manual dexterity, have been demonstrated effective for the older adult (Jahn, 2001).

Flossing finishes the task of removing plaque and debris from between teeth. Unwaxed dental floss is used to avoid traumatizing the gums. The floss should be long enough so the client can move easily from a frayed floss section to a new intact section of the floss.

Other oral hygiene measures include cleansing and moisturizing the oral mucosa by rinsing with water, saline, dilute mouthwash, or an anesthetic mouthwash. Caustic agents such as hydrogen peroxide and sodium bicarbonate once commonly used for oral care are no longer recommended because nursing research demonstrates mucosal alterations and increased potential for fungal infections (Stiefel, Damron, Sowers, & Velez, 2000). Clients at risk for altered oral mucous membranes include clients who are NPO or dehydrated; undergoing chemotherapy or radiation therapy for cancer treatment; experiencing trauma or surgery to the oral cavity; malnourished or immunosuppressed; or unable to perform oral care. High-risk clients should avoid alcohol-based products, such as commercial mouthwashes or lemon glycerin swabs, because these products are drying to tissues. Clients with drainage or lesions in the oral cavity and those who cannot take fluids by mouth may need rinsing and cleansing as often as every 2 hours. Such clients may have dry lips; a water-based lubricant or petroleum jelly can be applied.

Oral Care in the Unconscious Client. Feeding tubes, nasogastric tubes, and constant breathing through the mouth can dry mucous membranes. External surfaces of the teeth are brushed in the usual way. To protect fingers, place a padded tongue blade between the upper and lower teeth toward the back on one side. Then, using a toothbrush, sponge-tipped applicator, or gauze on a tongue blade, clean the interior of the teeth and the chewing surfaces. To prevent aspiration, use only small amounts of liquid. An oral suction device can be used to remove the fluid safely. See "Variation for the Unconscious Client" in Procedure 32-6.

🛢 SAFETY ALERT

Because of the risk of fluid aspiration into the lungs, the unconscious client should be turned on the side during mouth care so fluids can drain easily.

Denture Care. Determine if the client wears dentures. If so, encouraging the client to wear them improves eating, talking, and appearance and may boost the client's self-image.

Dentures collect the same debris, plaque, and tartar as natural teeth. If the client cannot care for the dentures, the nurse or caregiver needs to do so, using a brushing technique similar to that for natural teeth. Whenever possible, have the client remove his or her own dentures. If the client is unable, grasp dentures with a gauze pad to prevent slippage. Bottom dentures usually remove easily; upper dentures may need to be gently rocked forward or from side to side to break the vacuum seal created with the upper palate. A soft toothbrush is recommended because hard-bristled brushes can produce grooves in dentures. Soap and water is effective although a

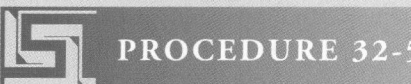

PROCEDURE 32-5

SHAMPOOING HAIR OF A BEDRIDDEN CLIENT

Purpose
1. Cleanse hair and scalp.
2. Promote comfort and self-esteem.
3. Apply medication to scalp and hair.

Assessment
- Assess condition of hair and scalp.
- Determine agency policy about shampooing hair of some clients (e.g., head trauma). Some agencies require a physician's order.
- Assess client's activity level and identify positioning restrictions.
- Assess client's preference for hair-care products. Determine if medicated shampoo has been ordered and is available.

Equipment
Comb and brush
Hair dryer (optional)
Two bath towels, one washcloth
Shampoo (cream rinse is optional)
Water pitcher
Plastic shampoo basin
Washbasin or bucket
Bath blanket
Waterproof pads
Cotton balls (optional)
Hydrogen peroxide (optional, to cleanse matted blood from hair)

Procedure
1. Place waterproof pads under client's head and shoulders, and remove pillow.
   Rationale: Bed linen can be kept clean and dry.
2. Raise bed to highest position.
   Rationale: This position reduces strain on nurse's back.
3. Remove any pins from hair. Comb and brush hair thoroughly.
   Rationale: Removing tangles and distributing scalp oils through hair result in thorough cleansing.
4. Adjust bed to flat position. Place shampooing basin under head. Place bath towel around shoulders and folded washcloth where neck rests on basin.
   Rationale: Shoulder padding protects client from becoming wet. Washcloth protects neck from strain and discomfort.

5. Fold bed linens down to waist. Cover upper body with bath blanket.
   Rationale: Client should be kept warm and linen protected from water.
6. Place waste basket with plastic bag under spout of shampoo basin on a chair or table at the bedside.
   Rationale: Water should flow from face and head into a receptacle.
7. Using water pitcher, wet hair thoroughly with warm water (approximately 110°F or 43.3°C). Check temperature by placing small amount of water on your wrist.
   Rationale: Wetting the hair in this manner protects the face and scalp from becoming wet or burned.

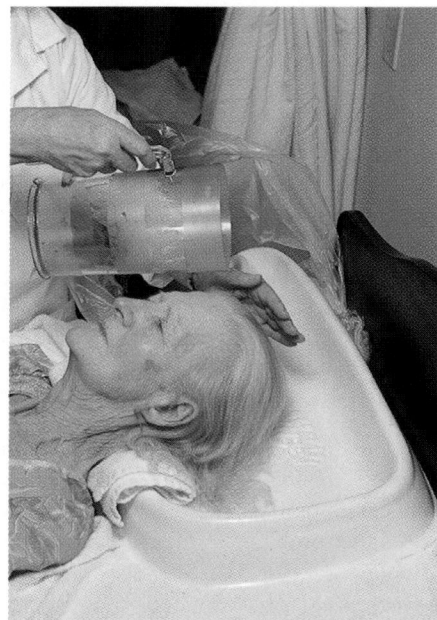

Step 7 Run warm water over hair.

8. Apply small amount of shampoo. Before shampooing, hydrogen peroxide may be used to dissolve matted blood in hair. Peroxide normally feels bubbly and warm. Reassure client that it will not bleach hair.
9. Massage scalp with fingertips while making shampoo lather. Start at hairline and work toward neck.
   Rationale: Massage stimulates circulation to the scalp; systematic lathering ensures thorough cleansing.
10. Rinse hair with warm water. Reapply shampoo and repeat massage.

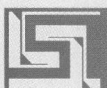

PROCEDURE 32-5 (Continued)

11. Rinse hair thoroughly with warm water. Clean hair "squeaks" when rubbed between fingers.
    Rationale: Soap residue in hair may dry and irritate hair and scalp.
12. Apply small amount of conditioner per client request. Rinse well.
    Rationale: Conditioner decreases tangles and makes combing easier.
13. Squeeze excess moisture from hair. Wrap bath towel around hair. Rub to dry hair and scalp. Use second towel if necessary.
14. Remove equipment and wet towels from bed. Place dry towel around client's shoulders.
    Rationale: These activities prevent client from getting a chill.
15. Dry hair with hair dryer. Comb and style.
16. Help client to comfortable position.
17. Dispose of soiled equipment and linen.

Lifespan Considerations
Infant
- Perform shampooing usually during the daily bath to prevent seborrhea (cradle cap), a gray, scaly scalp condition.
- Warm the room and use warmed towels to prevent chilling infant during bath.
- Use baby shampoo to decrease eye irritation.

Child
- Assess hair carefully for nits (lice eggs). Pediculosis infestations are common in school-age children.

Adolescent
- Many adolescents shampoo their hair daily. Offering to shampoo their hair may improve their self-esteem and help them feel better than many other nursing interventions do.

Older Adult
- Use warm towels to thoroughly dry hair after a shampoo to prevent chilling. Many older adults have decreased subcutaneous tissue and chill quickly.
- Older adults may have decreased sensation to heat. Use a hair dryer cautiously on a low-heat setting to prevent burning the scalp.

Home Care Modifications
- Ask the family if a relative or friend might provide hair-care services. Inform the family about helpful equipment, such as a shampoo tray, to purchase.
- Assist the family with adapting things in the home (e.g., a dish drainer mat or rolled plastic trash bags) for use as a shampoo tray.

Collaboration and Delegation
- Know that many long-term care facilities and community-based centers of care contract with a beautician to provide hair services for clients. Encourage and make arrangements for such services.

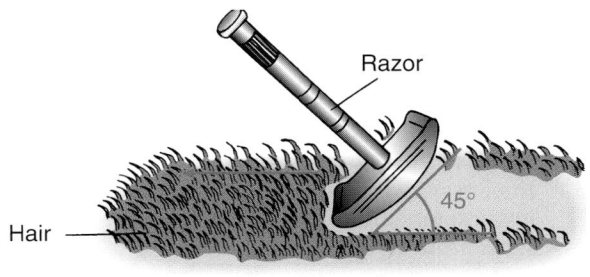

FIGURE 32-3 Shave in the direction of hair growth.

mild commercial cleaning agent can be used. To protect dentures from breakage, keep them in a denture cup while carrying them to the sink, and store them in water in a covered container if not worn continuously (Fig. 32-4).

The client should rinse the mouth before reinserting the dentures. Gums and tongue should be cleaned with a soft brush when the dentures are out. Massaging the gums with a brush or thumb and forefinger helps to stimulate circulation and toughen the oral mucosa. Dentures should be removed at night to expose tissues to air.

(text continues on page 734)

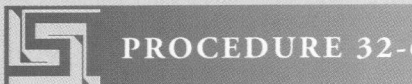

PROCEDURE 32-6

PROVIDING ORAL CARE

Purpose
1. Cleanse tooth surfaces to prevent odor and caries.
2. Maintain hydrated, intact oral mucosa.
3. Promote self-esteem and comfort.

Assessment
- Inspect lips, buccal membrane, gums, palate, and tongue for lesions or inflammation.
- Assess for presence of caries or halitosis (bad breath).
- Identify clients at risk for oral hygiene complications:
- Dehydration, NPO status, nasogastric tubes dry the oral mucosa.
- Oral airways accumulate secretions and irritate the mucosa.
- Chemotherapy often results in stomatitis and ulcerations.
- Anticoagulant therapy or clotting disorders predispose the client to gum bleeding.
- Oral surgery or trauma may contraindicate tooth brushing; special rinses may be ordered.
- Determine client's ability to assist with procedure.
- Assess client's risk for aspiration.

Equipment
Toothbrush (sponge-ended swabs may be used for clients at risk for bleeding)
Toothpaste
Cup with water, straw
Emesis basin
Washcloth, towel
Mouthwash (optional)
Dental floss
Disposable gloves (if the nurse provides oral care)

Procedure
1. Wash your hands.
2. Close bedside curtains or room door, identify client, and explain procedure.
   Rationale: Provide privacy.
3. Help client to a sitting position. If client cannot sit, help to a side-lying position.
   Rationale: High or semi-Fowler's or side-lying position helps prevent choking and aspiration.
4. Place towel under client's chin.
   Rationale: Protect bed linens and gown from soiling.
5. Moisten toothbrush with water. Apply small amount of toothpaste. *Note:* If client is anticoagulated or has a clotting disorder, use a very soft toothbrush or a sponge-ended swab to prevent gum bleeding.
6. Hand toothbrush to client or don disposable gloves and brush client's teeth as follows:
   a. Hold toothbrush at a 45-degree angle to the gum line.

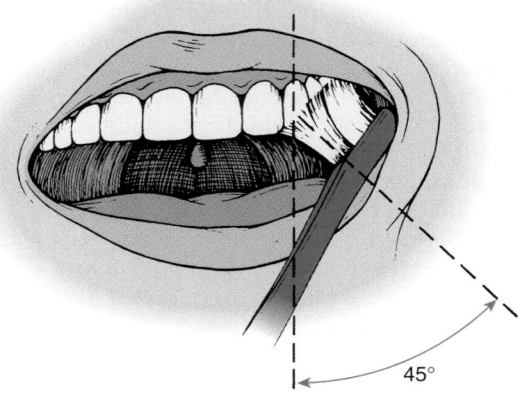

Step 6a Brush teeth at a 45-degree angle to the gum line.

   b. Using short, vibrating motions, brush from the gum line to the crown of each tooth. Repeat until outside and inside of teeth and gums are cleaned.
   Rationale: Angling the toothbrush allows brush to reach all tooth surfaces and to penetrate and cleanse under the gum line, where plaque and tartar accumulate.
   c. Cleanse biting surfaces by brushing with a back-and-forth stroke.
   d. Brush the tongue lightly. Avoid stimulating the gag reflex.
   Rationale: Bacteria accumulate and grow on the tongue surface.
7. Have client rinse mouth thoroughly with water and spit into emesis basin.
8. Remove emesis basin, set aside, and dry client's mouth with washcloth.
9. Floss client's teeth.
   Rationale: Flossing removes particulate matter trapped between the teeth and below the gum line.
   a. Cut 10-inch piece of dental floss. Wind ends of floss around middle finger of each hand.
   b. Using index fingers to stretch the floss, move the floss up and down around and between lower teeth. Start at the back lower teeth and work around to the other side.

PROCEDURE 32-6 (Continued)

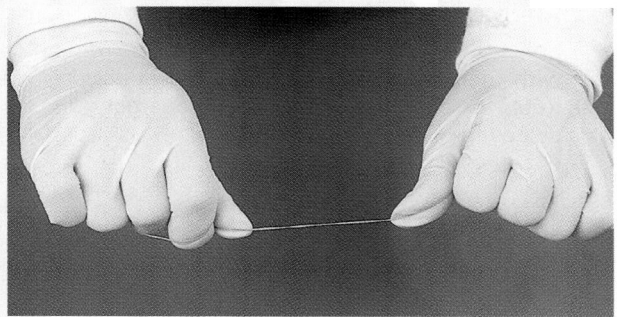

Step 9a Grasp dental floss tightly.

   c. Using thumb and index fingers to stretch the floss, repeat procedure on upper teeth.
   d. Have client rinse mouth thoroughly and spit into emesis basin.
10. Remove basin; dry client's mouth.
11. Remove and dispose of supplies. Help client to comfortable position.
12. Wash your hands.

Variation for the Unconscious Client

1. Gather equipment.
2. Place client in a side-lying position. **Rationale: Side-lying position prevents aspiration.**
3. Place towel or waterproof pad under client's chin.
4. Place emesis basin against client's mouth or have suction catheter positioned to remove secretions from mouth.
5. Use padded tongue blade to open teeth gently. Leave in place between the back molars. Never put your fingers in an unconscious client's mouth. **Rationale: Unconscious clients often respond to oral stimulation by biting down.**

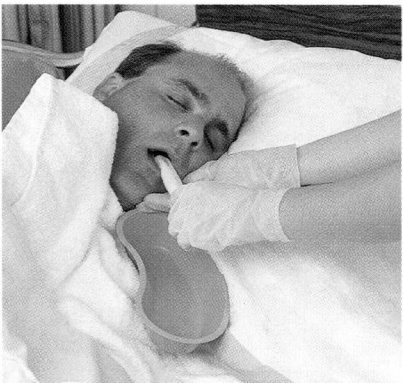

Step 5 Using a padded tongue blade, gently open the client's mouth.

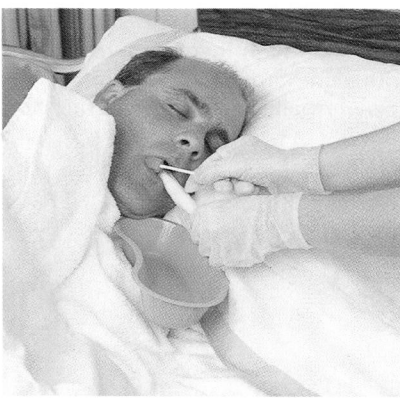

Step 6 Using a soft sponge-ended swab, cleanse teeth and mouth.

6. Brush teeth and gums as directed previously, using toothbrush or soft sponge-ended swab.
7. Swab or suction to remove pooled secretions. A small bulb syringe or syringe without needle may be used to rinse oral cavity.
8. Apply thin layer of petroleum jelly to lips to prevent drying or cracking. *Note:* Lemon glycerin swabs can be drying to the oral mucosa if used for extended periods.

Lifespan Considerations

Infant
- Use a dry gauze or washcloth to remove accumulated secretions from an infant's gums.
- Use a small, soft-bristled brush after first teeth have erupted.

Child
- Remember that children younger than 3 or 4 years may not understand what "rinse" or "spit" means. Do not offer them water to rinse with if they are NPO because they will swallow the rinse.
- Pay special attention to children or teens wearing braces to ensure removal of food particles from the wires.

Older Adult
- Because many older adults wear full or partial dentures, be sure dentures are removed and cleaned regularly. Special denture cleansers are available. Brush the gums or any remaining teeth well.

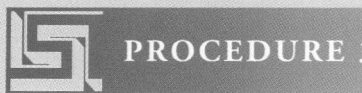

Home Care Modifications
- When teaching family members who are working with a comatose family member, be sure they can verbalize and demonstrate how to avoid aspiration.

Collaboration and Delegation
- Enlist the aid of occupational therapists to work with clients to relearn oral care procedures.
- Refer the client to a dentist if you detect gum disease or caries.

Eye Care

Some clients need help with eye care, particularly those who have had eye surgery, injury, infection, or who are unconscious and have lost the blink reflex. Assessments include noting if the eyelids are edematous, crusted with secretions, or inflamed with sties and if the lacrimal ducts are inflamed or tearing excessively. Examine the sclera for discoloration and the conjunctiva for inflammation and degree of redness.

Clients with eye inflammation, draining, or crusting need help cleaning these secretions from the eyes. Eyes should be cleaned with a washcloth or cotton ball soaked with saline or sterile water.

SAFETY ALERT

Clean from the inside of the eye toward the outside. If infection is not suspected, use a different part of the washcloth for each eye; if infection is present, use a different cloth for each eye. This reduces the potential for spreading infection from one eye to the other.

Eyeglasses and Contact Lenses. Determine if a visual aid is used; locate the aid and encourage its use. Safeguarding these aids contributes to the client's independence and safety.

Glasses should be cleaned daily, but clients do not often ask for this kind of help. Glass lenses can be washed under warm water, but plastic ones should be washed with a special cleaning solution. Both can be dried with facial tissue or a lens cloth. Store glasses in a secure place where the client can reach them. When clients are too ill to manage these activities or have other physical limitations to self-care, the nurse must take responsibility for glasses. Include the glasses' location in the nurses' notes or the Kardex. This allows the nurse on the next shift or in the next unit to which the client is transferred to locate them.

Contact lenses are a common alternative to glasses. These concave plastic disks cover the pupil and float on the tear layer. Contact lenses may be hard, soft, or gas-permeable hard or soft. Hard lenses are made of rigid plastic that does not absorb air or liquid. Because they restrict oxygen supply to the

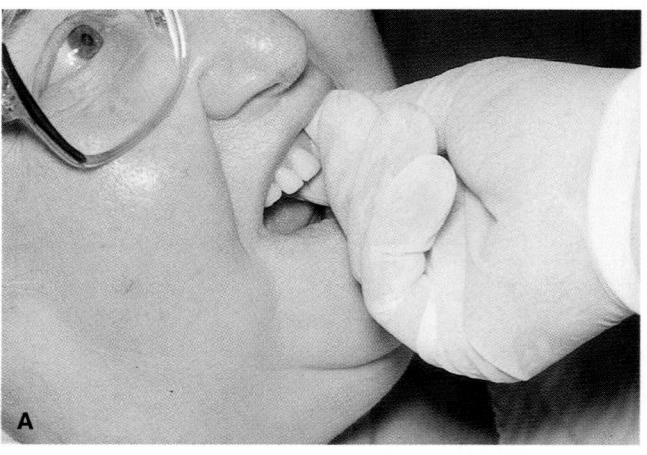
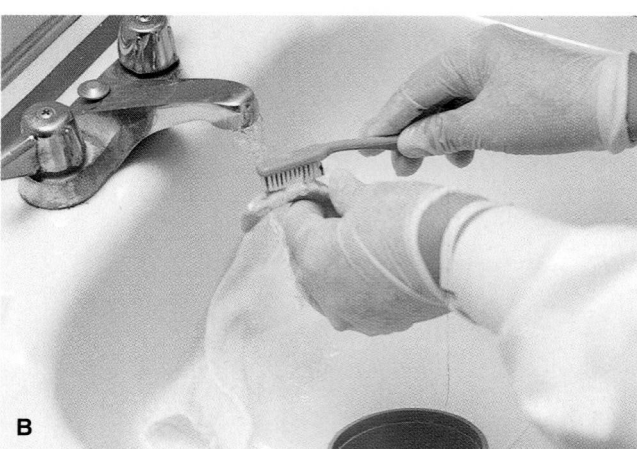

FIGURE 32-4   Denture care. **(A)** Remove dentures from mouth by gently rocking to break seal. **(B)** Place a towel in the sink and hold dentures firmly to prevent breakage. Brush as you would do with natural teeth.

cornea, their use is limited to 14 hours per day. Some kinds of soft lenses are worn during the day and removed at night, but others can be worn for as long as 14 to 30 days. Disposable contact lenses, a recent innovation, require less care.

Red conjunctiva, excess tearing, and burning pain are symptoms of lens overwear. Secretions and foreign matter (dust, pollen) accumulate under the lenses as they are worn. These substances are irritating to the eye and result in distorted vision and increased risk of infection. Because all contact lenses decrease the flow of oxygen to the cornea to some extent, corneal damage can occur if they are left in place for too long.

Contact lenses must be cleaned and disinfected after removal, using the appropriate method for the type of lens. If the client cannot do so, the nurse must remove and care for the lenses. Refer to Procedure 44-1 for Care of Contact Lenses. To care for soft lenses, a cleaning solution is used to loosen and remove film and debris. After cleaning, rinsing with a rinsing and disinfecting solution is necessary to remove loosened deposits. Then the lenses are covered with rinsing solution for storage. Before insertion, each lens is rinsed again with the rinsing solution to ensure removal of particulate matter. Recommended care may include a weekly heat or chemical lens cleaning to remove accumulated protein, lipids, and mucin. The client should bring contact lens supplies from home.

SAFETY ALERT
Do not use sterile saline commonly found in healthcare agencies. It may contain additives and may be inappropriate for use in contact lens care.

Artificial Eyes. Artificial eyes are made of glass or plastic. Some are permanent, others require daily removal for cleaning. Most clients prefer to provide eye care for themselves; the nurse may need to assist by removing the artificial eye if there is evidence of inflammation, if the client is scheduled for surgery, or if the client is dependent due to injury or immobility.

To remove an artificial eye, pull down on the lower eyelid and exert slight pressure below the eyelid to overcome the suction holding the eye in place. To ease removal, a small bulb syringe may be used to create a suction great enough to counteract the suction holding the eye in the socket. Clean the eye with saline and store it in saline or water in a covered, labeled container. Clean the edges of the eye socket with saline or tap water and inspect for redness, swelling, or drainage. Because of the proximity of the eye to the sinuses and underlying brain tissue, infection in this area is of great concern. To reinsert the eye, pull down on the lower lid and slip the eye into the socket, lifting the upper lid to permit the eye to slide in.

Eye Care in the Unconscious Client. Comatose clients are at risk for corneal ulceration, which can cause blindness. When the blink reflex is lost, eyes may remain open and become dry. To prevent these complications, eyes should be kept moist and protected from the air. Liquid tear solution (methylcellulose) or saline can be instilled to prevent drying, or the eyes can be closed and covered with a protective eye patch.

Ear Care
Healthy ears require little care. Check the external ear for inflamed tissue, drainage, and discomfort. Clean the auricles with a washcloth-covered finger. Excessive cerumen can be removed with the twisted end of a clean washcloth while pulling down the auricle. If this method fails, irrigation may be necessary.

SAFETY ALERT
Emphasize the danger of using bobby pins, cotton-tipped applicators, toothpicks, or other sharp objects to remove cerumen. Bobby pins or toothpicks can rupture the tympanic membrane or traumatize the ear canal; cotton-tipped applicators can push wax into the ear canal, which can cause blockage.

Care of Hearing Aids. A hearing aid is a sound-amplifying device powered by batteries. The aid contains a microphone that picks up sound waves, changes them into electric signals, and transmits them. It also includes an amplifier for magnifying sound, a receiver that transforms the electric signals back to sound energy, and an ear mold that channels the sound to the tympanic membrane. There are several kinds of hearing aids, as Display 32-3 describes.

Hearing aids are expensive and significant to their owners. These devices must be handled and stored safely. Note the type of device, how well it functions, how the client cares for it, and what problems the client has with it. Care includes careful handling to prevent damage, appropriate use, cleaning of the ear mold, and replacement of dead batteries. To check the batteries, remove the hearing aid from client and turn volume slowly to high. A harsh whistling noise is apparent if batteries are in working order. No sound at all indicates that the batteries should be replaced.

When placing the hearing aid in the ear, turn off the device to protect the ear from any sudden loud sound. When the hearing aid is snugly in the ear canal, the volume can be adjusted as needed to promote hearing. See Procedure 44-2.

Although the hearing aid amplifies the sound of voices, it also amplifies background sounds. Clients may continue to have difficulty hearing especially in a noisy setting. To foster optimal hearing, face the client, speak slowly and clearly, and rephrase what is said if the client does not understand. Some hearing-impaired people can lip-read; careful enunciation improves their ability to understand. The telephone company can provide phone amplification for the hearing impaired.

Feeding
A self-care deficit involving feeding may occur in clients who are weak, fatigued, paralyzed, or have neuromuscular impairments. Assess the client's feeding ability and the level of support he or she needs for eating; plan assistance and institute a teaching program if appropriate.

Often clients are spoon fed in institutional settings even though they are capable of self-feeding if given adequate time. Verbal prompts and physical guiding can assist the cognitively impaired client to maintain independent eating,

DISPLAY 32-3

⑤ TYPES OF HEARING AIDS

- **Behind-the-ear aid:** the most common type; fits over the ear. An ear mold fits into the ear, and the case containing the microphone, amplifier, receiver volume control, batteries, and T/M switch fits behind the ear.
- **In-the-ear aid:** the most compact; has all of the elements located in the ear mold.
- **Eyeglass aid:** involves a hearing aid in one or both temples of a pair of eyeglasses. It functions similarly to the behind-the-ear aid, but the components are located in the temples of the glasses.
- **Body-type hearing aid:** used for the most severe hearing losses. The case looks like a pocket-sized transistor radio and can be clipped into a pocket, undergarment, or harness. The case contains the microphone and amplifier and is connected to a receiver that snaps into an ear mold.

Behind-the-ear   **In-the-ear**

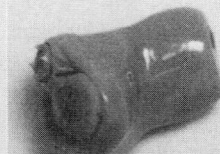
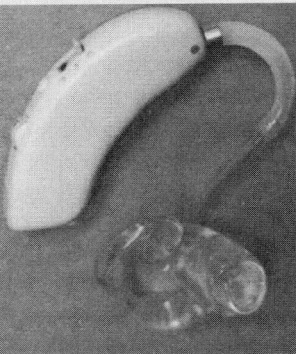

DISPLAY 32-4

⑤ MEETING THE CLIENT'S FEEDING NEEDS

- Check chart, Kardex, or diet list to determine if the client has limitations on eating (e.g., fasting for laboratory tests or procedures).
- Check each tray for the client's name and the type of diet. Verify the client's name by checking the wristband.
- If pain is a factor limiting food intake or self-feeding ability, time analgesia to permit pain relief at mealtime.
- If fatigue is a problem, schedule a rest period before eating to enhance appetite and increase independence.
- Help the client urinate or defecate before meals.
- Enhance the setting. Turn on the lights if needed. Provide good ventilation. Remove room odors and disturbing sights such as soiled dressings.
- Prepare the client for mealtime by finding dentures and eyeglasses, brushing teeth, rinsing mouth, and washing hands.
- Help the client to a comfortable position for eating, usually sitting in high Fowler's position in bed or a chair.
- Clear the overbed table of extraneous items.
- Determine how much help the client needs (i.e., uncovering containers, removing food from plastic bags, buttering bread, cutting meat).
- Plan ahead so that you help clients who need assistance while their food is still hot. Food that has cooled can be microwaved.

which is preferred over spoon feeding. Quiet, soothing music is thought to be therapeutic during mealtime and in other areas of patient care such as decreasing pain, anxiety, and stress from hospitalization (White, 2001).

Because being fed represents a loss of control, allow the client some way to participate if possible. This is true for people of all ages. Giving the client a choice—for instance, the order in which food is eaten—may relieve some helpless feelings. Using bibs and mixing food together decrease the client's dignity (Galvan, 2001). Because the process of helping with eating is time consuming, the client may feel like a burden. The person feeding the client must avoid reinforcing this belief and should always give the client ample time to chew and swallow.

Interventions to meet feeding needs vary; Display 32-4 lists examples. Raise the head of the bed if the client cannot sit on the side of the bed. A high sitting position is necessary to reduce the danger of choking and aspirating food. Research has demonstrated that when the caregiver who is feeding the client sits (rather than stands) consumption of food and fluids increases (Galvan, 2001). See Procedure 37-1 for details on helping a client to eat.

Blind clients can be oriented to the location of food on a plate by referring to the numbers on a clock. The client may use clockwise references to develop a mental map of the tray by doing a survey with his or her fingertips; then she or he can locate food by gently probing with a fork. Knowing what the foods are helps a blind person plan how best to eat them. For example, knowing that peas and mashed potatoes are on the plate enables a blind person to eat the peas more easily by pushing them against the mashed potatoes.

Many eating aids are available (Fig. 32-5). Plates with guards or lips help the client get food onto a utensil. Utensil handles can be padded to make them easier to grasp. Cups with spouts help with drinking. Straws may help clients drink without dribbling.

For infant feeding, the atmosphere should be relaxed and free of interruptions. Parents or other relatives should feed children if possible. For feeding solid food, position the infant to face the feeder at eye level. Finger foods allow the older infant to participate in feeding before fine motor skills are developed sufficiently to enable self-feeding with utensils.

When the meal is finished, assess the food and fluid intake and record it if indicated. If a calorie count is ordered, record

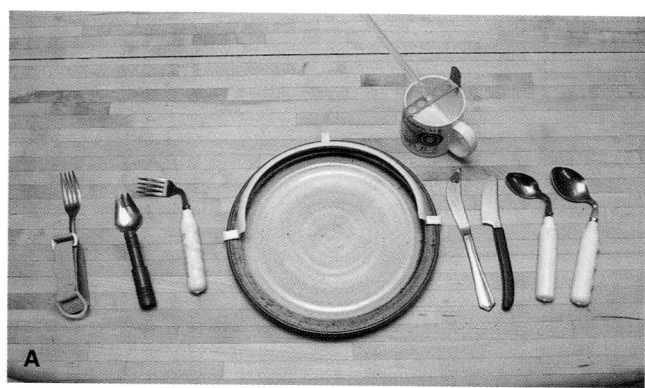

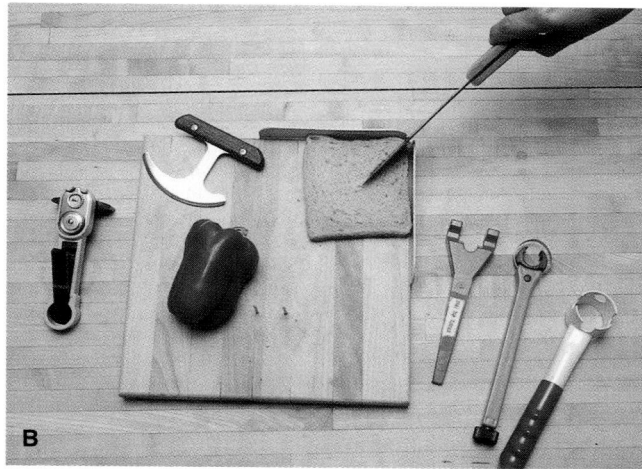

FIGURE 32-5 **(A)** Assistive feeding devices. Such devices are made to be easy for clients to grasp and to get food on the utensils. **(B)** Assistive food preparation devices. Many devices are available to aid in opening containers and cutting and preparing food.

the precise amount of food eaten. Record any pertinent reaction to the meal. Make necessary adjustments in the diet and the plan of care.

Swallowing Impairment. Adequate swallowing is essential for safe eating. Difficulty swallowing (**dysphagia**) may occur as a result of disease or trauma to cranial nerves. Such damage commonly occurs after a cerebrovascular accident (stroke) or head injury. Diseases such as myasthenia gravis and muscular dystrophy, which cause muscle weakness, also may result in dysphagia. After a stroke or surgical removal of part of the larynx, the client may need to relearn how to initiate swallowing. Consulting a speech therapist or an occupational therapist is important in planning a safe rehabilitation program.

To avoid food aspiration, carefully assess the client's ability to swallow before feeding. Elicit the gag reflex by stroking the inside of the throat with a tongue depressor. This will cause the pharynx to rise and constrict while the tongue retracts.

🥛 **SAFETY ALERT**
When there is any doubt as to the client's ability to swallow, do not try to feed him or her until obtaining an expert opinion.

If a client needs supervision during feeding, this should be indicated on the plan of care. If supervision is delegated to auxiliary personal or family members, the nurse must assess that they understand proper feeding technique and emergency care in case of choking.

Keep verbal cues short and simple while feeding. Multiple verbal cues or conversation during feeding may distract and confuse the client who is cognitively impaired. Use directions like "chew" and "swallow" rather than complete sentences.

Food consistency is important for clients who have difficulty swallowing. Liquids may have to be thickened; dry food, such as crackers and toast, and sticky food, such as peanut butter, should be avoided. The dysphagic client should not use straws. Remaining in an upright position after a meal will prevent gastric reflux and possible aspiration. Check the oral cavity to detect food pocketing that might have occurred and could led to aspiration.

Toileting

Clients often require assistance with toileting (i.e., walking to the bathroom or being placed on a bedpan). Needing help with these intimate functions may provoke discomfort for some clients; a kind approach helps allay embarrassment. Helping clients to be as independent as possible with toileting is an important nursing intervention.

The following measures can help clients manage self-care of elimination. Teach these methods and help clients determine which ones work best.

Exercise can affect micturition by strengthening abdominal and perineal muscles, which enhances voiding and helps to prevent urinary incontinence. For example, Kegel exercises strengthen the perineum muscles. These exercises involve contracting the perineal muscles as if trying to stop micturition or by actually practicing stopping the urine stream while voiding.

Privacy and an opportunity to relax enhance most people's ability to urinate and defecate. Worrying about being able to void or have a bowel movement, especially after surgery or giving birth, may produce tension, so do not pressure clients to eliminate on schedule. If the client is having difficulty urinating, the following may help:

- Turn on the bathroom water.
- Have the client visualize his or her bathroom at home.
- Warm the bedpan.
- Have the client assume a comfortable position (standing for men).
- Provide analgesia for pain.
- Pour warm water over the perineum.
- Always provide call light within easy reach.

(For measures to assist with bowel elimination, see Chapter 41.)

Toilet. Ambulatory clients can walk to and from the bathroom to use the toilet for voiding and defecation with nursing assistance as necessary. For some clients who have difficulty sitting down on and arising from a conventional-height toilet, a raised or elevated toilet seat can be attached, so that the client has a decreased distance to lower and raise himself or herself (Fig. 32-6). A raised toilet seat may be required after some types of hip surgery. Based on previous assessment, provide necessary comfort measures for the client using the bathroom, and give the opportunity after voiding for the client to wash the hands.

Bedside Commode. A bedside **commode** is a portable chair with a toilet seat and a waste receptacle beneath that can be emptied. In this way, a client who cannot walk to the bathroom but can transfer out of bed to a chair can manage toileting. A commode chair can often be wheeled into the bathroom and placed over the toilet after the waste receptacle has been removed (Fig. 32-7). Some commodes are made with their own receptacles; others have a place for attaching a conventional bedpan. Many commodes have a flat seat that covers the toilet seat so it can also be used as a chair. Commodes can be rented for use at home if access to the bathroom (e.g., upstairs) or ambulation is difficult during recovery from acute illness or during chronic illness. Before assisting the client to the commode, assess whether or not the client can safely transfer independently and, if not, determine the support he or she needs. If the client is at risk for falling, the nurse or a caregiver should remain with the client or stand just beyond to give privacy. Provide comfort measures as needed. Give support by providing water, a washcloth, and a towel for self-cleaning or by performing the cleaning as necessary.

Urinal. A male client who is on strict bed rest or confined to bed due to weakness or disability may use a **urinal,** a metal or plastic receptacle into which the penis can be

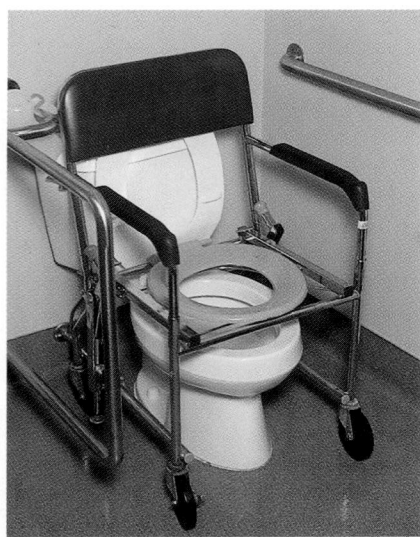

FIGURE 32-7   The commode chair can slide over the toilet when the waste receptacle is removed, allowing clients with mobility problems greater access to the privacy of a bathroom.

placed to facilitate urinating without spilling. The urinal needs to be emptied frequently into a toilet to prevent spilling and odors. Assisting the client to stand at the bedside when using the urinal is physiologically advantageous; sometimes, however, standing is contraindicated and the client must be positioned in bed in as close to an upright position as feasible. In most instances, the client is able to place and hold the urinal himself. If he is unable to do so, hold the urinal in place while the client urinates or place the urinal and leave the client alone for a few moments. When the client has completed voiding, the client may place the urinal on an overbed table. This should be avoided whenever possible because the client's tray is placed on the same overbed table and the nurse uses the table for sterile procedures. Be sure to empty the urinal in a timely manner; this eliminates the possibility of anyone bumping or knocking the urinal and spilling its contents and also avoids the embarrassment of having the client's urine clearly visible at the bedside. Men who are incontinent may be more comfortable if the urinal is left in place. If this is done, the urinal should be plastic and the scrotum should be padded for protection. Provide comfort measures as needed and a means of handwashing after voiding.

Bedpans. There are two types of bedpans: a regular bedpan has a high rim, and a fracture pan has a lower rim for clients who cannot raise their buttocks or in whom such movement is contraindicated (Fig. 32-8).

Many clients need help to get on a bedpan. Sitting is the most effective position for passing urine or stool. Some clients can use a bedpan alone if it is left on the bed or covered on a nearby chair; encourage such independence. A trapeze on the bed frame also facilitates moving on and off a bedpan. Procedure 32-7 outlines bedpan use.

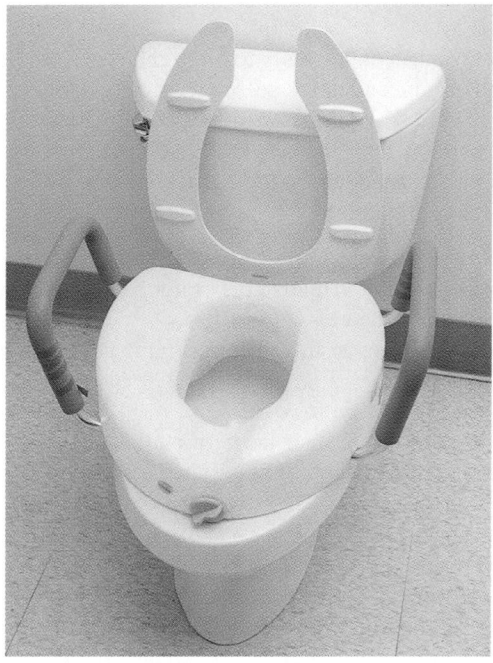

FIGURE 32-6   A raised toilet seat allows a client who has had hip surgery to safely use the toilet at home.

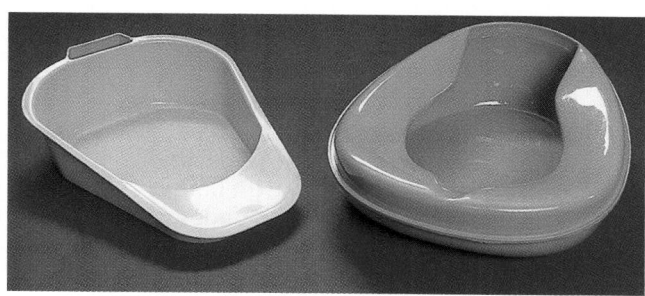

FIGURE 32-8 Two types of bedpans. *(Left)* The fracture bedpan. *(Right)* Regular bedpan.

Condom Catheter. A **condom catheter** is a heavy rubber sheath that fits over the penis and is connected to a collection tube and bag. A small bag that can be strapped to the leg may promote self-care for the ambulatory man. Procedure 40-2 outlines and illustrates application.

Dressing

Dressing and undressing consume a great deal of time and energy, which is why chronically and acutely ill people often become fatigued and discouraged. The following interventions are designed to help clients relearn dressing skills:

- Schedule dressing or undressing in conjunction with bathing.
- Encourage the client to use his or her eyeglasses or hearing aid.
- Provide analgesia if needed.
- Organize carefully and allow ample time.
- Lay clothes out in the order in which they will be needed, and place them within easy reach.
- Choose clothes that are loose and easy to get on and off, that have wide sleeves and pant legs, and front fasteners. Use Velcro closures when possible. Shoes should have elastic laces or Velcro closures.
- Encourage the client to help select clothes. Suggest street clothes rather than night clothes when appropriate.
- Assess the client's ability to maintain balance.
- Ensure privacy (within the limits of safety).
- If the client has cognitive deficits, develop a routine to lessen confusion, keep instructions clear and simple, and avoid distractions. Research demonstrates that clients respond positively to a combination of simple words and non-verbal communication leading to increased trust, confidence, and cooperation in the nurse-client relationship (Sundin, Jansson, & Norberg, 2000).
- Teach the use of aids for dressing (e.g., long-handled shoehorn, zipper pull, long-handled reacher, buttonhook). Help the client adapt to available equipment to meet specific needs.

Care of Unit Environment

The equipment and supplies that clients use while in the healthcare facility are kept in what is called the client's unit.

Overbed tables, which provide a surface for eating and a work space for nurses, have wheels so they can be maneuvered to fit over the bed or over a chair. Some overbed tables have a mirror and storage space for toilet articles.

Small stands are placed at the side of the bed to provide storage space for personal belongings, a basin for bath water, a small curved basin (emesis basin), supplies for oral care, soap, bedpan, urinal, and toilet paper. A towel bar may be attached to the stand. Closet storage for belongings also is usually provided. A chair, either lightly padded and straight or upholstered, is often provided for the client or visitors.

In many agencies, oxygen and suction outlets are installed on the wall above the bed, and often a sphygmomanometer with a blood pressure cuff is mounted on the wall. The unit lighting usually includes diffuse, less intense lighting for general use; a brighter light for client reading; and an intense light for use during procedures and when visualization is needed for diagnostic purposes.

A call light with which the client can summon the nurse is attached to the bed. Often, the call light is part of the sound receiver for the television set and the television channel selector. A television and telephone are commonly available free or for a small fee. Televisions are usually mounted on the wall to facilitate viewing from a Fowler's or flat position. Explain all this equipment to the client and family at admission.

Beds. Hospital beds can be moved to a variety of positions, providing comfort for the client, therapy for some conditions, and proper body mechanics for the nurse. Adjustments in height usually can be made. The high setting permits nurses to perform their tasks without back strain; the low setting permits clients to get in and out of bed easily and safely. Be familiar with prescribed bed positions (Display 32-5) and how to achieve them. Because bed controls are usually accessible to clients, teaching them how to use the bed enhances independence. Other adjustments that can be made in the beds include the following:

- Elevating the head of the bed to permit eating and other activities
- Simultaneously elevating the head and foot of the bed to prevent sliding toward the foot
- Elevating the foot of the bed when the legs need to be placed above the level of the heart to reduce swelling

Several kinds of beds are available for clients who cannot turn themselves and are at risk for skin breakdown; these are discussed in Chapter 38.

Mattresses, usually constructed of inner springs to provide good support, are covered with a water- and soil-resistant material to permit cleaning. Foam-rubber mattresses with an eggcrate configuration can be placed on top of the inner spring mattress for clients who must stay in bed for a long time or who find the mattress uncomfortable. Eggcrate mattresses are often not needed with the new types of mattresses that distribute pressure more evenly. Bedboards can be placed under the mattress for added firmness. People with back problems may require additional support.

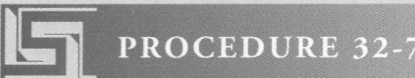

PROCEDURE 32-7

USING A BEDPAN

Purpose
1. Provide a means for elimination for clients who are confined to bed or unable to get to the bathroom or bedside commode independently or safely.

Assessment
- Assess the client's normal elimination habits and when he or she last voided or defecated.
- Assess level of mobility, positioning restrictions, and degree of assistance required.
- Review orders to determine if urine or fecal specimens are needed.
- Identify medications the client is receiving that would alter the color, consistency, or amount of urine or feces obtained.

Equipment
Clean bedpan or fracture pan (see Fig. 32-8 for two types of bedpans)
Toilet tissue
Washcloth, towel, soap
Air freshener (optional)
Specimen container (if needed)
Cover for bedpan (if toilet for discarding is not in client's room)
Disposable gloves

Procedure

Placing the Bedpan
1. Wash your hands. Don clean gloves.
   Rationale: Maintain good infection control practices.
2. Close curtain around bed or shut door.
   Rationale: Provide privacy and reduce embarrassment.
3. Run warm water over rim of pan; dry with towel.
   Rationale: Warming the pan facilitates client relaxation and encourages elimination.
4. Position and lock side rail up on opposite side of bed from which you will work.
   Rationale: Prevent the client from rolling out of bed when turning on and off bedpan.
5. Raise bed to height appropriate for nurse.
   Rationale: Prevent muscle strain and promote proper body mechanics.
6. For client who can raise buttocks and assist with procedure:
   a. Fold top linen down on your side to expose the client's hips.

Rationale: Minimally expose the client to decrease embarrassment and preserve dignity.
   b. Have client flex knees and lift buttocks. Assist client by placing your hand under sacrum, elbow on mattress, and lifting as a lever.
   Rationale: Lower legs and feet support the client's body weight. Proper body mechanics prevent muscle strain.
   c. Slide rounded, smooth rim of regular bedpan under client. If using a fracture pan, slide narrow, flat end under buttocks.
   Rationale: Proper placement prevents spillage and shearing trauma of skin in sacral area.
7. For client unable to assist by raising buttocks:
   a. Lower head of bed to flat position.
   b. Fold top bed linens down to expose client minimally.
   c. Help client to roll to side-lying position.
   d. Place bedpan against buttocks and tucked down against mattress. Hold firmly in place and roll client onto back as bedpan positions under buttocks.
   Rationale: Correct placement prevents spillage.

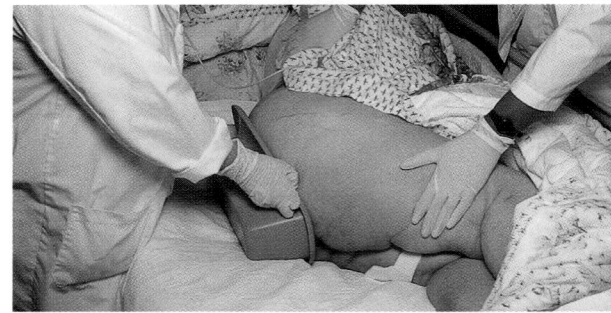

Step 7d Placing bedpan from side-lying position.

8. Cover client with linen. Place call bell and toilet paper within reach.
   Rationale: Privacy, warmth, independence, and self-dignity are important for the client.
9. Raise head of bed 45 to 80 degrees unless contraindicated.
   Rationale: Sitting position reduces discomfort and strain on lower back and facilitates elimination.
10. Lower bed to lowest position. Place side rails up if indicated.
    Rationale: These measures help to ensure client safety.
11. Wash your hands. Allow client to be alone.

PROCEDURE 32-7 (Continued)

Removing the Bedpan

12. Answer call bell promptly.
 Rationale: Sitting for long periods on a bedpan is uncomfortable and can cause pressure on skin.
13. Place soap, wet washcloth, and towel at bedside.
14. Raise bed to appropriate working height for nurse.
 Rationale: Prevent muscle strain and promote proper body mechanics.
15. Fold back top linens to expose client minimally.
16. Put on disposable clean gloves.
 Rationale: Gloves help prevent contamination of hands with body substances.
17. Assess if client can wipe perineal area. If not, wipe area with several layers of toilet tissue. If specimen is to be measured or collected, dispose of soiled toilet tissue in separate receptacle, not bedpan. For female clients, wipe from urethra toward anus.
 Rationale: Prevent tracking of rectal micro-organisms into the urinary meatus. Use as an informal teaching session to reinforce good hygiene practices.
18. For client who can raise buttocks and assist with procedure:
 a. Lower head of bed.
 b. Have client flex knees and lift buttocks. Assist client by placing one hand under sacrum and supporting bedpan with other hand to prevent spillage. Remove bedpan and place on bed-side chair.
 c. Offer soap, warm water, washcloth, and towel for client to wash hands or perineal area.
 Rationale: Washing prevents transfer of micro-organisms, promotes good hygiene practices, and prevents skin breakdown.
19. For client unable to assist by raising buttocks:
 a. Lower head of bed to flat position.
 b. Fold top linen down to expose client minimally.
 c. Help client to roll off bedpan and onto side. Use one hand to stabilize bedpan during turning to prevent spillage.

 d. Wipe anal area with tissue. Wash perineum with soap and warm water. Pat dry.
 Rationale: Prevent skin breakdown and excoriation.
20. Assist client to comfortable position.
21. Cover bedpan, and remove from bedside. Obtain specimen if required. Empty and clean bedpan, and return it to bedside.
 Rationale: A clean pan minimizes spread of offensive odor.
22. Remove and discard gloves. Wash your hands.
 Rationale: Washing reduces spread of micro-organisms.
23. Spray air freshener if necessary to control odor, unless contraindicated (client with respiratory conditions, allergies).
 Rationale: Odor is embarrassing to client and visitors. Minimizing embarrassment preserves self-dignity.

Lifespan Considerations
Child
• If possible, use a potty chair at the bedside for a toddler. A toilet-trained child may be reluctant to use a bedpan because he or she has learned not to toilet in bed.

Older Adult
• Keep in mind that older adults may find using a regular bedpan difficult because of body movement limitations and arthritis. A fracture pan is less difficult and less painful to use.

Collaboration and Delegation
• Because nurses frequently delegate placing and removing a bedpan to unlicensed personnel, be sure to review client mobility restrictions and the need to measure or collect urine or feces.

Side rails, a standard part of beds and stretchers, help to prevent accidents caused by clients falling out of bed or getting out of bed by themselves when they are not able to do so safely. They also provide a support for clients to hold while moving in bed and getting up. When all side rails are up they can be considered a restraint, so it is important to be informed of and follow agency guidelines.

Footboards are boards of wood or plastic placed to form a right angle at the foot of the bed. They remove the weight of bedclothes from feet and legs and support the feet to prevent

DISPLAY 32-5

⬒ BED POSITIONS

Flat position: Mattress is completely flat.

Fowler's position: The lower part of the bed is raised to the following positions:

- *Low Fowler's position:* Head of bed is elevated to semisitting position of 15 to 45 degrees. This position also is called semi-Fowler's position.
- *High Fowler's position:* Head and trunk are elevated to 80 to 90 degrees. This position also is called simply the Fowler's position.

Trendelenburg position: The entire bed is tilted with the head downward. This position is not often used because it causes blood pressure to rise and causes hypotension on return to the supine position.

Reverse Trendelenburg position: Entire bed is tilted with feet downward. Prevents gastric reflux.

---

foot drop. Bed cradles also can remove the pressure of bedclothes from the feet and legs. For clients with injured or swollen legs, feet, or toes, removing the pressure of bedclothes may relieve pain and improve circulation.

Poles used for hanging IV containers are located near the bedside in most units. A pole can be free-standing or inserted into a hole in the bed frame. Or the IV containers can be hung from hooks suspended from the ceiling.

Bedmaking. A clean, dry, smooth bed enhances the client's feeling of well-being. Linens are changed on the basis of client need and cost, rather than a fixed routine. Linens that are soiled, wet, or stained need to be changed. When deciding whether or not to change linens, however, consider the client's other needs and the other clients' demands. For instance, if the client is tired and weak, it may be better to pad slightly damp or soiled areas immediately, then wait until the client has rested to change the linens. Sometimes, straightening and tightening the sheets are adequate. Procedures 32-8 and 32-9 give guidelines regarding making unoccupied and occupied beds.

To conserve time and energy, pick up all the necessary linens from the linen supply before beginning. Make one side of the bed as completely as possible before moving to the other side. Lowering the head of the bed and raising the bed to a comfortable working height help prevent back strain.

🠦 SAFETY ALERT

Asepsis is an important consideration in bedmaking. Drainage onto used linens may contain microorganisms that can be transmitted through the air when the linens are shaken or through contact with the nurse's hands or clothing. Handle linens carefully without shaking them. Wear gloves during bedmaking if linen soiling is likely. Avoid touching your clothing and wash your hands after handling soiled linens.

Put soiled linens immediately into a linen bag. Do not put soiled linens on the floor. If a linen bag is not available, slip a pillowcase over the back of a standard chair to provide a handy receptacle for dirty linens.

Healthcare Planning and Home/ Community-Based Nursing

Many people who are unable to provide for their own hygiene, feeding, grooming, and toileting independently live in the community. Family and community support are often needed to ensure adequate functioning. Rehabilitation promotes optimal return of function and ability to cope with limitations while supporting a range of independence.

Before the client is discharged from the acute care facility, promote as much independence in self-care activities as possible. An occupational therapist often helps the client develop self-care skills. Support this learning on a daily basis. Help the client anticipate self-care problems at home and plan how to manage them.

Bathing

The home environment may need to be altered to enhance self-care. For most clients, getting in and out of the tub poses the greatest problem. In the bathtub or shower, hand grips and nonskid mats can protect against falls. Tub seats can be installed so clients need not lower themselves down into the tub. Hand-held shower appliances also can assist with bathing.

🠦 SAFETY ALERT

The hot water tank thermostat should be set below 48°C (120°F) to avoid burns during bathing.

For the client who cannot shower or use the bathtub, place a chair in the bathroom so he or she can sit and wash by the sink. This aid may help to conserve energy. Relatives may be available to visit on a weekly basis to supervise or assist with bathing, but often clients are embarrassed to ask relatives or friends to assist with this private, personal activity. If family support is inadequate, home health aides can visit on a routine basis to provide hygiene care.

Grooming and Dressing

Assess and promote independent grooming and dressing before discharge. Many clients do not dress in the hospital and are surprised at how draining this activity can be. Before discharge, encourage clients to practice dressing using energy-conserving measures. The client should sit as much as possible while dressing and should wear clothes that are easy to put on and remove. Because they have no buttons or zippers, sweat suits are often ideal for clients who have difficulty with fine motor skills. Slip-on shoes with nonskid soles are easy to put on and they help prevent falls. Assess the need for assistive devices to help promote independence with dressing. Discuss with the client the psychological benefits of getting dressed,

(text continues on page 746)

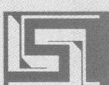

PROCEDURE 32-8

MAKING AN UNOCCUPIED BED

Purpose
1. Provide clean linen and remove sources of skin irritation.
2. Promote comfort.

Assessment
- Assess client's activity level and ability to get out of bed.
- Determine nursing interventions needed in assisting client out of bed:
- Vital sign check for orthostatic hypotension
- Analgesia
- Position precautions (i.e., elevation of body parts)
- Assess client's potential for excessive perspiration, drainage, or incontinence in determining special linen requirements.

Equipment
Bottom sheet
Top sheet
Draw sheet
Blanket
Bedspread (changed only if soiled)
Mattress pad (changed only if soiled)
Pillowcases
Waterproof pads or bath blanket (optional for incontinent or diaphoretic clients)
Linen bag
Bedside table or chair

Procedure
1. Wash your hands. Assemble equipment on bedside table or chair. Do not place on another client's bed.
   Rationale: Prevention of contamination with microorganisms helps maintain a safe environment.
2. Help client to chair at bedside.
3. Raise bed to comfortable working position.
   Rationale: Promote good body mechanics and reduce muscle strain to back.
4. Loosen linen on one side of bed. Move to other side of bed and loosen all linen.
5. Remove bedspread and blanket, and fold each separately if they are to be reused. Place over back of chair.
   Rationale: To reduce cost, most agencies change blanket and bedspread only when soiled.
6. Remove pillowcases by grasping seamed end with one hand and pulling out pillow with the other. Place pillows on chair. Discard pillowcases in linen bag.
7. Remove each piece of linen separately by rolling into a ball and discarding into linen bag. Be careful to prevent soiled linen from touching your uniform.
   Rationale: Disposing of linen separately minimizes the chance of nurse's uniform being contaminated by soiled linen. Rolling linen into compact unit prevents microorganisms from shaking off during transfer to linen bag.
8. Slide mattress to head of bed if it has slipped to the foot. Wipe mattress with antiseptic solution if grossly soiled. Dry thoroughly.
   Rationale: Prevents transfer of microorganisms.
9. Working from side of bed where linen is stored, spread mattress pad over mattress and smooth out wrinkles.
   Rationale: Wrinkles in linen irritate the skin, can cause pressure areas, and are uncomfortable.
10. Unfold bottom sheet lengthwise on bed with vertical center crease along center of bed. Unfold top layer toward opposite side of mattress. Pull remaining top of the sheet over head of mattress, leaving bottom edge of sheet even with mattress edge. Smooth bottom sheet with hand.
    Rationale: If not using a contour sheet, tuck the bottom sheet in only at the top of the bed so you can change linen without undoing the top sheet.

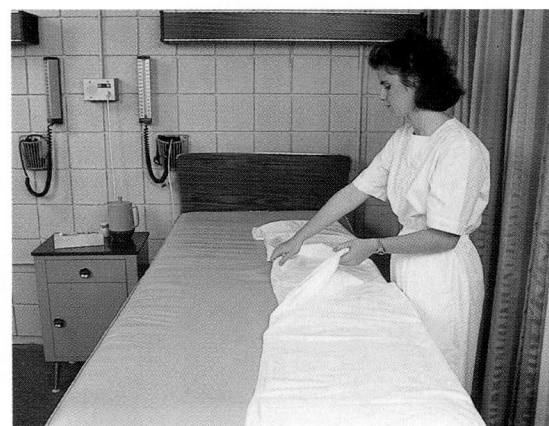

Step 10 Center bottom sheet on bed.

11. Standing near head of bed, tuck the excess sheet under the mattress on your side at the end of the bed.

PROCEDURE 32-8 (Continued)

12. Miter the corner on your side:
    a. Grasp side edge of sheet about 18 in down from mattress top.
    b. Lay sheet on top of mattress to form a triangular, flat fold.
    c. Tuck sheet hanging loose below mattress under the mattress without pulling on the triangular fold.
    d. Pick up top of triangular fold, and place it over side of the mattress.
    e. Tuck this loose portion of sheet under the mattress.
        Rationale: Mitered corners do not loosen easily when client moves in bed. Note: If using a contour sheet, fit elastic edges under corner of mattress.

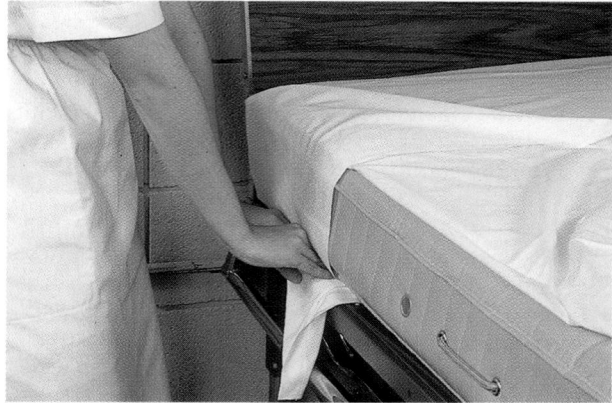

Step 12c Tuck hanging part under mattress.

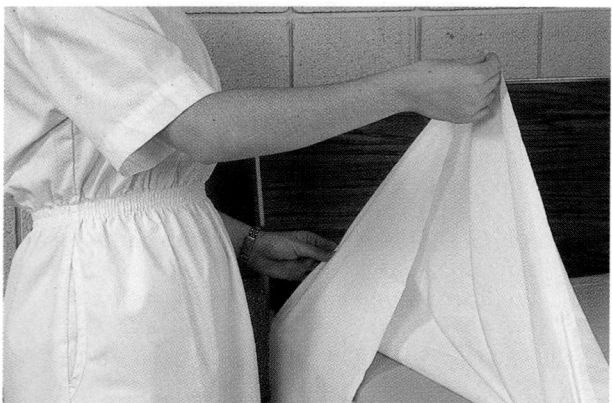

Step 12a Pick up selvage edge of sheet.

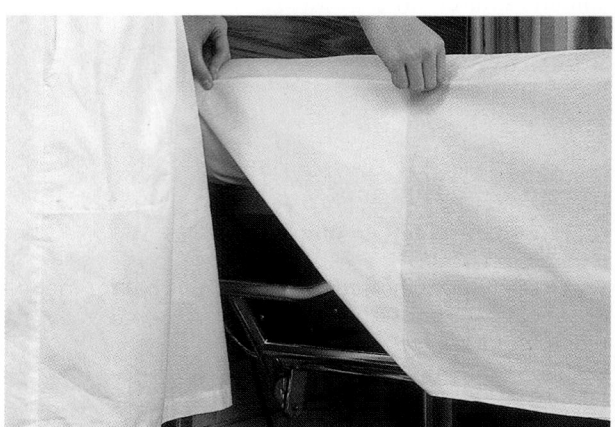

Step 12d Drop triangle over side of bed and tuck in.

13. Tuck remaining sheet on that side under the mattress.
14. Lay draw sheet (folded in half) on the bed with the center fold at center of bed. Place top edge of draw sheet about 12 to 15 inches from head of bed. Tuck excess draw sheet under mattress.
    Rationale: Draw sheet secures bottom sheet in place to decrease wrinkling.
15. Move to opposite side of bed.
    Rationale: Completing work on one side of bed at a time saves time and decreases energy expenditure.
16. Spread bottom sheet over mattress edge and miter top corner.
17. Tuck excess bottom sheet tightly under mattress, pulling gently to smooth out wrinkles.

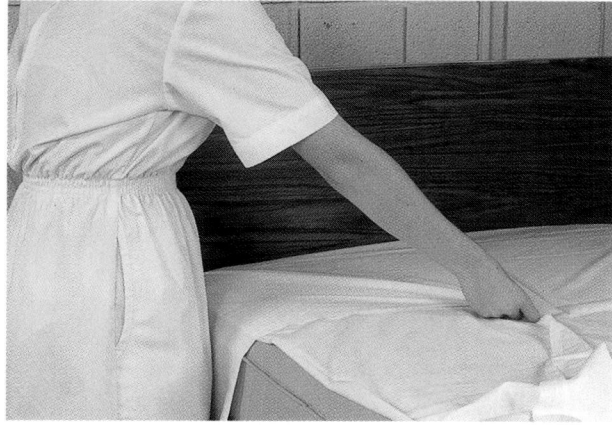

Step 12b Lay triangle back on bed.

PROCEDURE 32-8 (Continued)

Rationale: A taut sheet eliminates wrinkles that irritate and cause pressure on the skin.

18. Grasp draw sheet, pulling gently. Beginning at middle, tuck draw sheet under mattress firmly. Finish tucking top and bottom.
    Rationale: Tucking middle of draw sheet first prevents wrinkling and poor fit.

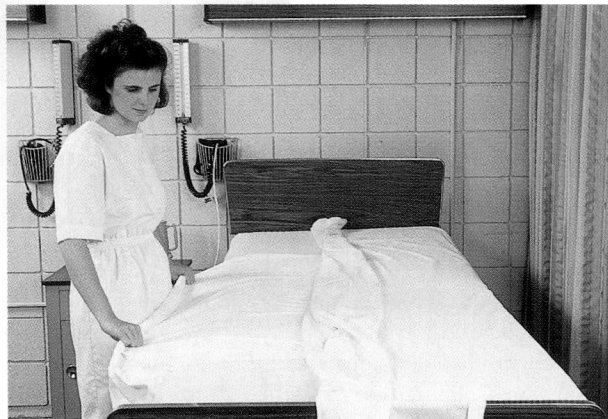

Step 18 Tuck draw sheet firmly under mattress.

19. Return to side of bed where linen is placed.
20. Place top sheet on bed with vertical center fold at center of bed. Unfold sheet with seams facing out and top edge even with top of mattress. Smooth sheet, with excess falling over bottom edge of mattress.
    Rationale: Placing seam side up prevents edges from rubbing and irritating client's skin.

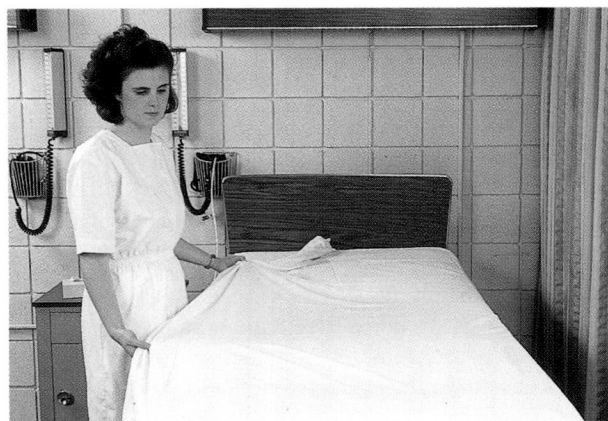

Step 20 Center top sheet on bed.

21. Spread blanket and bedspread evenly over bed. Miter the bottom corner, using all three layers of linen (sheet, blanket, bedspread). Leave sides untucked.
22. Move to opposite side of bed and miter bottom corner using all three layers of linen.
    Rationale: Mitering all three layers together saves time and energy. Mitered corners secure top covers but allow easy access in and out of bed by leaving sides free.
23. Standing at bottom of bed, grasp top covers about 10 inches from bottom of mattress. Loosen linen slightly by pulling on top covers or forming a pleat.
    Rationale: Additional room for client's feet gives comfort and prevents pressure on toes.
24. Put on clean pillowcases:
    a. Grasp center of pillowcase with one hand on seamed end.
    b. Gather case, turning it inside out over the hand holding it.
    c. With same hand, grasp middle of one end of pillow.
    d. Pull case over pillow with free hand.
    e. Adjust case so corners fit over pillow.
    Rationale: This method prevents shaking of pillowcase and linen and distributing micro-organisms in room.

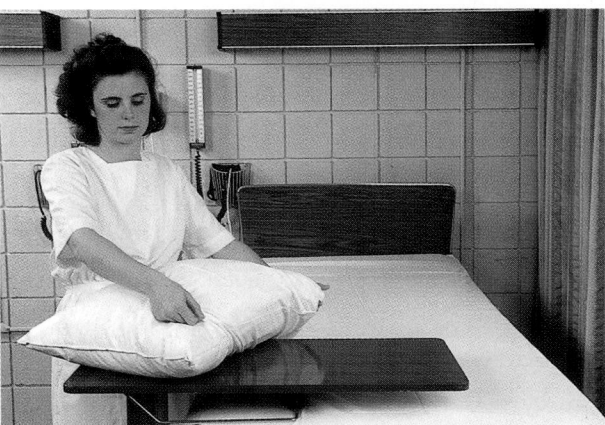

Step 24 Replace pillowcase.

25. Place pillows in center at head of bed.
26. Fold top linen back to one side or fanfold at bottom of bed.
27. Secure call bell within client's reach, and lower bed.

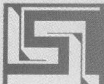

PROCEDURE 32-8 (Continued)

Rationale: A call bell within reach helps provide safety for the client.

28. Arrange the bedside table, night stand, and personal items within easy reach.
29. Discard soiled linen according to agency policy.
30. Wash your hands.

Collaboration and Delegation
- Because nurses frequently delegate bedmaking to unlicensed personnel, prioritize and communicate when beds need to be made. Doing so permits coordination of care and efficient management of discharges and admissions.

and work out a plan so he or she can avoid wearing nightclothes during the day.

Hair care provides a morale boost to homebound clients. Hair should be washed before discharge for clients who might have difficulty with this task. Relatives can take the client to a local hairdresser for shampoos and hair care, and some beauticians make house calls. Frequently a family member or friend can be encouraged to provide such a service. Applying makeup is important to some women, and lack of coordination or energy can make this activity difficult.

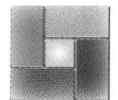

Nursing Research and Critical Thinking
Can Nurses Provide Discharge Teaching in a Way That Improves Their Clients' Ability to Follow the Instructions?

Nurses who care for clients in the hospital emergency department (ED) know the importance of the ability of clients to follow through with the recommendations of the healthcare staff. Adherence rates to discharge treatment plans, however, are generally low at 28%. Nurses developed a program of instructions based within a geragogy framework that provided clients with individualized computer-generated instruction. The information was presented at a fifth-grade reading level and printed with a size 14 font. To test the new instruction program, the nurses designed a study to compare the effectiveness of the new program with that of the preprinted discharge instructions usually given to clients. The study was conducted as a two-group, experimental, posttest-only trial of the new instruction program. The control group and experimental groups contained 30 subjects each. The study took place in three rural midwestern hospitals. All the subjects were Caucasian, could speak and read English, ranged between 60 and 98 years of age, were deemed stable by the triage nurse, and discharged home from the ED with at least one prescribed or recommended medication. Once all the subject inclusion criteria had been met, the subjects were tested with the Short Portable Mental Status Questionnaire

(SPMSQ) to evaluate that their cognitive status was intact. Other instruments used in the study were the Knowledge of Medication Subtest (KMS), the Medication Complexity Index (MCI), and the Rapid Estimate of Adult Literacy in Medicine (REALM). Clients receiving the new education program had significantly greater knowledge than the control group ($t = 2.19$, $df = 58$, $P = .016$) 48 to 72 hours after discharge from the ED.

Critical Thinking Considerations. In this study, the treatment was delivered and controlled by one investigator. A study in which investigators were blinded to the treatment and control groups would add to the reliability of the findings. Implications of the study applicable to nursing practice are as follows:

- Written medication instructions that are large print, on a fifth-grade reading level, and organized in the elderly schema for remembering medications appear to be successful in the teaching and learning of medication information.
- The findings from this study may also have implications for older clients being discharged from other settings.

From Hayes, K. S. (1998). Randomized trial of geragogy-based medication instruction in the emergency department. *Nursing Research, 47*(4), 211–218.

PROCEDURE 32-9

MAKING AN OCCUPIED BED

Purpose
1. Provide clean linen for client who is unable to get out of bed.
2. Promote comfort.

Assessment
Same as Procedure 32-8.

Equipment
Same as Procedure 32-8.

Procedure
1. Wash your hands.
2. Assemble equipment on bedside table or chair. Do not place on another client's bed.
   Rationale: Placing linen on clean surface prevents contamination with microorganisms.
3. Close room door or bedside curtains.
   Rationale: Maintain the client's privacy.
4. Lock up side rails on side of bed opposite from where you stack the clean linen.
   Rationale: Side rails prevent the client from rolling out of bed and give the client a bar to grasp to assist with turning.
5. Raise bed to comfortable working position. Lower side rail on your side of bed.
   Rationale: Use good body mechanics to reduce muscle strain on back.
6. Loosen all top linen from foot of bed. Remove bedspread and blanket separately. Without shaking, fold each piece and place over back of chair if they are to be reused. If they are soiled, hold them away from your uniform, and place in linen bag.
   Rationale: Folding linen enables nurse to discard or handle without contaminating uniform. Shaking linen spreads microorganisms through the air.
7. Leave top sheet on client or cover client with a bath blanket; remove and discard top sheet.
   Rationale: Provide warmth and prevent unnecessary body exposure during linen change.
8. Loosen the bottom sheet on your side. Lower head of bed to flat position. *Note:* If client cannot tolerate flat position, lower head of bed as far as client can tolerate.
   Rationale: Changing linen is easier when bed is flat.
9. Help client to roll onto side facing away from you. Client may grasp side rail to assist. Additional personnel may be needed to assist with client positioning. Adjust pillow under head.

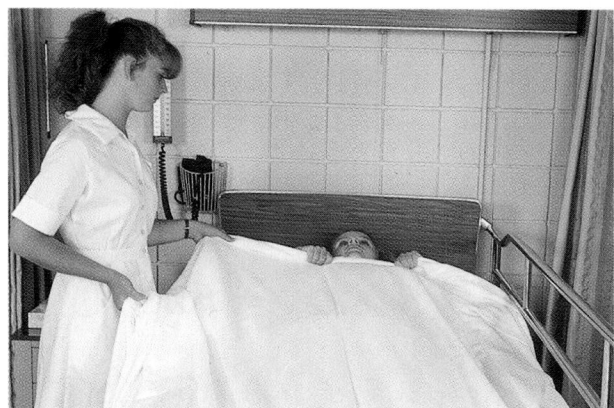

Step 7 Cover with bath blanket or leave top sheet in place.

Rationale: Side-lying position provides space for placing clean linen on mattress.

10. Tightly fanfold soiled draw sheet and tuck under buttocks, back, and shoulders. Repeat with soiled bottom sheet and tuck under client. Do not fanfold mattress pad unless it is soiled.
    Rationale: Fanfolds under client should be as tight and smooth as possible to provide space for clean linen and enable client to eventually roll back over folds.

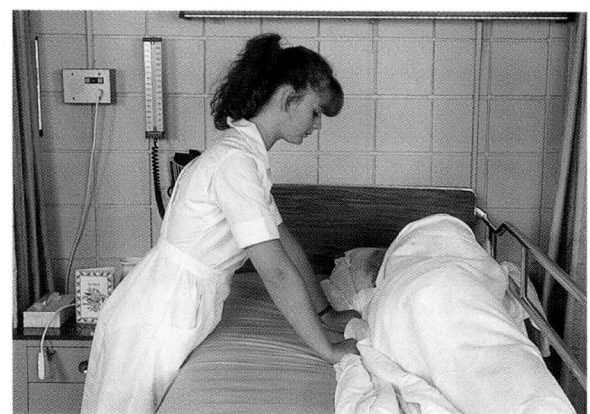

Step 10 Fanfold soiled linens and tuck under client.

11. Place clean bottom sheet on bed. Unfold lengthwise so bottom edge is even with end of mattress and vertical center crease is at center of bed.
    Rationale: Ensure sheet will fit properly on mattress.

PROCEDURE 32-9 (Continued)

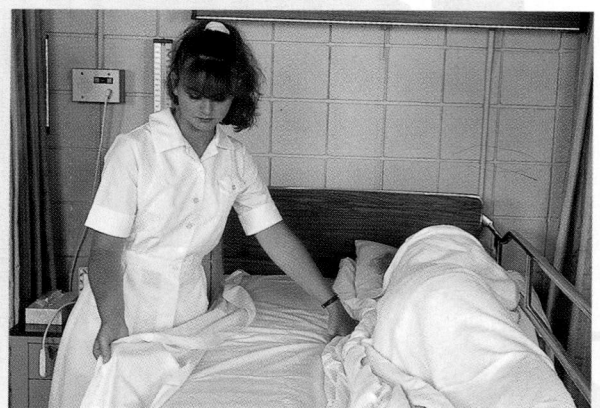

Step 11 Unfold and center clean linen.

12. Bring sheet's bottom edge over mattress sides and fanfold top of sheet toward center of mattress and place next to client.
13. Tuck top edge of sheet under mattress. Miter top corner on your side (as in Procedure 32-8). Tuck remaining portion of sheet under mattress. *Note:* If using a contour sheet, fit elastic edges under corner of mattress.
14. Place draw sheet on bed with center fold at center of bed. Position sheet so it will extend from the client's back to below the buttocks. Fanfold the top edge and place next to client. Tuck excess under mattress.
    Rationale: Draw sheet is used to reposition client and absorb excess perspiration.
15. Lock up side rails on your side and move to other side of bed.
    Rationale: Side rails maintain client's safety.
16. Lower side rail. Help client to roll over folds of linen onto his or her other side. You may need additional help if client is unable to move easily.
    Rationale: When second half of bed is exposed, soiled linen can be removed and clean linen replaced.
17. Move pillow under client's head.
18. Remove soiled linen by folding into a square or bundle with soiled side turned in. Place in linen bag.
    Rationale: These actions reduce transmission of microorganisms and prevent client embarrassment at seeing soiled sheets.
19. Grasp edge of fanfolded bottom sheet and pull from under the client.
20. Tuck top of sheet under top of mattress. Miter top corner.

21. Facing bed, pull bottom sheet tight and tuck excess linen under mattress from top to bottom.
    Rationale: Tucking linen under mattress maintains a sheet's tight fit and eliminates wrinkles.

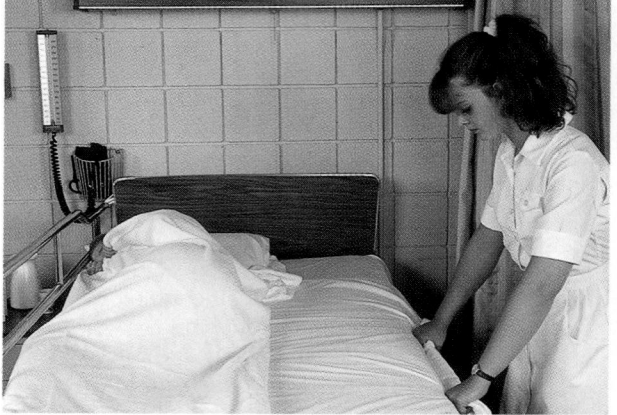

Step 21 Smoothly tuck sheets under mattress.

22. Unfold draw sheet by grasping at center. Tuck excess tightly under mattress. Tuck the middle first, then the top, and finally the bottom.
    Rationale: Tucking the center first prevents the draw sheet from pulling sideways and causing a poor fit and wrinkles.
23. Help client to center of bed.
24. Raise side rail if necessary and move to side of bed where remainder of linen is stored.
25. Place top sheet over client with center crease lengthwise at center of bed with seam side up. Unfold sheet from head to toe.
26. Have client grasp top edge of clean top sheet. Remove bath blanket or soiled top linen by pulling from beneath clean top sheet.
27. Discard in linen bag.
    Rationale: Limiting exposure of body parts gives client dignity.
28. Complete top covers as described in Procedure 32-8.

Collaboration and Delegation
See Procedure 32-8.
• In addition, communicate positioning restrictions and the amount of assistance that may be required to ensure the client's safety. If family members/caregivers are learning this skill for the first time, allow them to practice before discharging the client to home.

Food Preparation and Eating

Buying and preparing food can be exhausting, so provide instructions for easy, nutritious meals. Frozen foods have improved dramatically in recent years and can be nutritious. Relatives can package single-serving meals to be reheated. Stress safety (i.e., burn prevention). Meals on Wheels is a community service that provides hot, well-balanced meals for the homebound person for a nominal fee. Few supermarkets deliver groceries, but friends, relatives, and neighborhood young people can shop for the homebound person.

Eating can consume energy. Encourage rest before and after meals. Clients with fine motor impairment can use special utensils.

Toileting

Self-care deficit in toileting is an important consideration; so assess home bathroom facilities before the client is discharged. If the bathroom is on a different floor from the bedroom, the client may need a bedside commode or a urinal. For the client who is wheelchair-bound, the bathroom doorway must be wide enough for the wheelchair and the bathroom must be large enough to permit the client to transfer from the wheelchair to the toilet. Some clients find it difficult to lower themselves onto the toilet and get up again. A high-rise toilet seat can be helpful and is indicated for most clients after hip surgery. Hand grips next to the toilet also are helpful. Clients must be able to wipe themselves and wash their hands after toileting. Prepackaged towelettes can be an easy way to wash hands.

Incontinence can be managed with a Foley catheter or disposable diapers. If a catheter is used, a client can wear a leg bag under clothes to promote self-image and can use a larger collection bag at night. A condom catheter also can be used with the same urine collection system. Disposable incontinent briefs for adults are now widely available although more costly than infant diapers. A more streamlined adult incontinence pad (Depends) also is available.

Coordination of Care

Clients with self-care deficits and inadequate support may be unable to manage safely at home and may require transfer to an extended care facility or nursing home. When a client is transferred to another healthcare agency, communicate his or her level of self-care function to that staff. Transfer forms usually have a place to indicate the client's abilities in bathing, feeding, grooming, and toileting. Be specific so the client can maintain optimum independence.

A designated caregiver may have to provide much assistance for a client with severe self-care deficit to remain in the community. The nurse's role expands to include teaching and support for the caregiver. Providing 24-hour care for a client with severe self-care deficits can be emotionally and physically draining. Providing respite care (e.g., adult day care) or support groups for the caregiver is important to prevent burnout and improve quality of life for all involved.

EVALUATION

Evaluation of self-care deficit is based on the outcome criteria developed from the client goals. Collect objective and subjective data from the client to support successful attainment of client outcomes. Ideally, the client should exhibit increased independence in bathing, grooming, feeding, and toileting. The client should be able to state any limitations and should feel comfortable accepting necessary assistance. The client should demonstrate a positive self-image and satisfaction with accomplishments in self-care despite any limitations. The client should be able to use adaptive devices to facilitate self-care, and self-care should occur without injury.

Examples of outcome criteria are listed below. Although some criteria may be important for more than one goal, they should be specific for each client.

Goal

Client will safely increase level of independence in eating.

Possible Outcome Criteria

- Before discharge, client verbalizes a plan for managing food preparation at home.
- During next home visit, client demonstrates using a cup with a built-up handle held with both hands to drink thick liquids.

Goal

Client will participate in dressing himself or herself.

Possible Outcome Criteria

- By the third week of rehabilitation, client demonstrates the ability to put on a loose-fitting dress with Velcro fasteners.
- By the fourth week of rehabilitation, client uses a long-handled reacher to put on slip-on shoes.
- Before discharge from the rehabilitation unit, client expresses a positive approach to solving problems inherent in relearning to dress self.
- Before discharge, client demonstrates dressing using energy conservation techniques.

Goal

Client will manage toileting as independently as possible.

Possible Outcome Criteria

- Within 48 hours, client is able to recognize and communicate the need to go to the toilet.
- Within 5 days, client transfers from bed to wheelchair to toilet or from bed to commode with standby assistance.
- Before discharge, client states plan for managing toileting at home.

NURSING PLAN OF CARE
THE CLIENT WITH SELF-CARE DEFICIT

Nursing Diagnosis
Bathing/Hygiene Self-Care Deficit related to right-sided weakness manifested by impaired ability to wash most body parts.

Client Goal
Client will willingly participate in hygiene measures.

Client Outcome Criteria
- During care, client states need for assistance to perform hygiene activities that he or she cannot perform alone.
- After teaching session, client demonstrates bathing face, trunk, and upper extremities, with verbal cuing.
- Before discharge, client verbalizes a realistic plan for bathing at home.

Nursing Intervention	Scientific Rationale
1. Assist client to identify self-care deficits in hygiene.	1. Maximum self-participation can occur with improved self-esteem.
2. Encourage client to communicate needs and concerns to nursing staff and significant others.	2. Communication reduces the presence of energy-consuming stressors such as isolation and worry.
3. Permit and encourage client to accept some dependency and verbalize feelings.	3. A degree of dependence is a necessary part of recovery and rehabilitation for most people.
4. Ensure safety through monitoring and assistance during bathing and hygiene activities.	4. Safety measures reduce the possibility of increased injury due to falls.
5. Schedule hygiene self-care 1 hour after breakfast when client feels rested.	5. Hygiene self-care is a tiring procedure; fatigue can produce confusion.
6. Lay out objects for hygiene care in the order to be used and place them within client's reach and sight. Don't hurry client.	6. Nurse gives support and conserves his or her energy. Placement enables easy access with decreased energy expenditure.
7. Provide for the greatest amount of privacy possible.	7. Privacy enhances feeling of dignity and self-worth.
8. Assist client to use unaffected hand to wash self, comb hair, and brush teeth within the limits of ability.	8. Activities enhance independence while providing help and support as needed. Some programs encourage use of affected side to strengthen and regain function.
9. Evaluate frequently for indications of fatigue by checking pulse and respiratory rate.	9. Ability to sustain concentrated effort may be limited until endurance is developed.
10. Coordinate self-care rehabilitation with occupational and physical therapy and any other involved health professionals.	10. Necessary techniques and assistive devices are used in the most beneficial manner. Represent client in negotiations and making arrangements for care.

- By first home visit, client demonstrates toileting in own bathroom without experiencing fatigue or activity intolerance.

Key Concepts

- Self-care and hygiene are important factors in promoting health.
- During stress or illness, children and adults often regress to a lower developmental level that requires more assistance with self-care.
- Factors affecting self-care include culture, values and beliefs, environment, motivation, emotional status, cognitive abilities, energy, acute illness or surgery, pain, and motor deficits.
- Although the primary reason for bathing is to enhance cleanliness, warm water and friction enhance circulation, and movement during bathing provides an opportunity for range of motion. The experience also can be relaxing.
- Care of the eyes, ears, and teeth is important in maintaining optimal health. Care must be taken to avoid damage or loss of glasses, contact lenses, hearing aids, or dentures because they are significant to the client's functioning and expensive to replace.
- Identification of inability to self-feed is important to promote nutrition and prevent possible aspiration.

- Providing a clean environment and a smooth, wrinkle-free bed helps promote comfort.

REFERENCES

Agency for Health Care Policy and Research (AHCPR). (1992). *Pressure ulcers in adults: Prediction and prevention* (Publication No. 92-0047, 92-0050). Rockville, MD: Public Health Service, U.S. Department of Health and Human Services.

Baker F., Smith, L., & Stead, L. (1999, January 20–26). Practical procedures for nurses: Giving a blanket bath, part I. *Nursing Times, 75*(3), insert.

Baker F., Smith, L., & Stead, L. (1999, January 27–Feb 4). Practical procedures for nurses: Giving a blanket bath, part II. *Nursing Times, 75*(4), insert.

Buck, S. (2001, February). Long term rehabilitation all by myself: Innovative thinking and cooperation can lead to seating and mobility solutions for even the most difficult cases. *Rehab Management: The Interdisciplinary Journal of Rehabilitation, 14*(1), 36, 38, 40.

Buss, I., Halfens, R., & Abu-Saad, H. (1997). The effectiveness of massage in preventing pressure sores: A literature review. *Rehabilitation Nursing, 22*(5), 229–234.

Cady-Jones, G. (1997). Massage therapy as a workplace intervention for the reduction of stress. *Perceptual and Motor Skills, 84*(1), 157–158.

Field, T, Hernandez-Reif, M., Taylor, S., Quintino, O., & Burman, I. (1997). Labor pain is reduced by massage therapy. *Journal of Psychosomatic Obstetrics & Gynaecology, 18,* 286–291.

Galvan, T. (2001, January). Dysphagia: Going down and staying down. *American Journal of Nursing, 101*(1), 37–42.

Gauthier, D. M. (1999, June 17). The healing potential of back massage. *Online Journal of Knowledge Synthesis for Nursing, 6*(5).

Hensel, P. (2000, July–August). The challenge of choosing a pediculicide. *Public Health Nursing, 17*(4), 300–304.

Jahn, C. A. (2001, Spring). Automated oral hygiene self-care devices: Making evidence based choices to increase client outcomes. *Journal of Dental Hygiene, 75*(2), 171–189.

Katz, S. (1983). Assessing self-maintenance: Activities of daily living, mobility and instrumental activities of daily living. *Journal of the American Geriatric Society, 31*(12), 721–725.

North America Nursing Diagnosis Association. (2001). *NANDA nursing diagnoses: Definitions & classification 2001–2002.* Philadelphia: Author.

Pillitteri, S. (1999). *Child health nursing: Care of the child and family.* Philadelphia: Lippincott.

Richards, K. (1998). Effect of a back massage and relaxation intervention on sleep in critically ill patients. *American Journal of Critical Care, 7*(2), 288–298.

Stiefell, K., Damron, S., Sowers, N., & Velez, L. (2000). Improving oral hygiene for the seriously ill patient: Implementing researched-based practice. *Medical-Surgical Nursing Journal, 9*(1), 40–43.

Sundin, K., Jansson, L., & Norberg, A. (2000, July). Communication with people with stroke and aphasia: Understanding through sensation without words. *Journal of Clinical Nursing, 9*(4), 481–488.

Whall, A. L., Black, M. E., Groh, C. J., Yankou, D. J., Kupferschmid, B. J., & Foster, N. L. (1997, September–October). Effect of natural environments upon agitation and aggression in late state dementia patients. *American Journal of Alzheimer's Disease, 12*(5), 216–220.

White, J. M. (2001, March). Music as an intervention: A notable endeavor to improve patient outcomes. *Nursing Clinics of North America, 36*(1), 83–92.

White, J. M. (2001, January–March). Nocturnal enuresis and appropriate management for children. *World Council of Enterostomal Therapists Journal, 21*(1), 14–18.

BIBLIOGRAPHY

Hektor, L. M., & Touhy, T. A. (1997, May). The history of the bath: From art to task? Reflections for the future. *Journal of Gerontological Nursing, 23*(5), 7–15, 53–59.

Lavelle, A. (2000, September). Head lice: The truth, the myths, the update. *School Nurse News, 17*(4), 35–36.

McHale, J., Phipps, M., Horvath, K., & Schmelz, J. (1998). Expert nursing knowledge in the care of patients at risk of impaired swallowing. *Image: Journal of Nursing Scholarship, 30*(2), 137–141.

Ramponi, D. (2001). Eye on contact lens removal. *Nursing 2001, 31*(8), 56–57.

Satterly, L., Grizzle, M., & Fortener, L. (2000). Individuals' perspectives regarding hospital based self-care instruction and its effect on ability to perform self-care at home. *Physical and Occupational Therapy in Geriatrics, 17*(3), 23–26.

Steele, J. (1997). Strategies to improve the quality of oral care for frail and dependent older people. *Quality Health Care, 6*(3), 165–169.

33 Mobility and Body Mechanics

Key Terms

activity intolerance
aerobic exercise
anaerobic exercise
arthroscopy
atrophy
body mechanics
contracture
dangling

deep vein thrombosis
flaccidity
foot drop
gait
isometric exercise
isotonic exercise
range of motion
spasticity

Learning Objectives

Upon completion of this chapter, the student will be able to do the following:
1. Explain normal functions of the musculoskeletal system and characteristics of normal movement.
2. Identify factors, including lifespan considerations that can affect or alter mobility.
3. Describe the impact of immobility on physiologic and psychological functioning.
4. Discuss appropriate subjective and objective data to collect to assess mobility status.
5. Demonstrate nursing interventions such as positioning, ambulating, providing range of motion, and using assistive devices.
6. Plan strategies to avoid musculoskeletal injury to the nurse and client during client care.
7. Develop appropriate community-based nursing interventions for preventing and managing mobility problems.

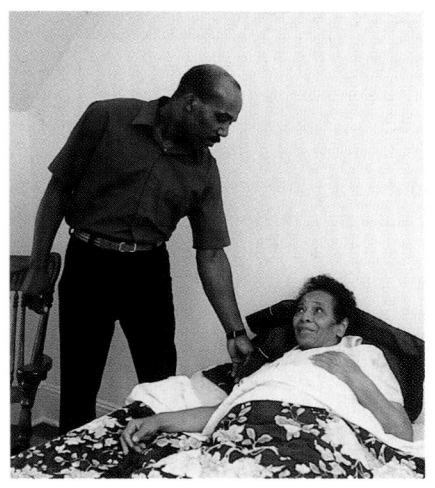

Critical Thinking Challenge

You are a home health nurse visiting a new client, a retired woman recently discharged from the hospital after knee replacement surgery. Her son meets you at the door, looking tired and anxious. He explains that his mother is reluctant to do anything for herself because it still hurts to move. She has been sleeping on the sofa bed in the living room and spends much of the day there. She uses a bedpan rather than walking to a nearby bathroom. Helping her to a recliner has been very difficult for the son, who fears his mother may fall even while using the walker. The son adds that his mother becomes very upset and yells when he encourages her to do more for herself.

Mobility and body mechanics are important factors in preventing injury for your clients, your coworkers, and you. Mobility allows people to remain independent and to participate actively in normal activities that add pleasure to life. After you have completed this chapter, return to the above scenario and reflect on the following areas of Critical Thinking:

1. Considering the mobility and safety concerns apparent in this scenario, prioritize your assessment.
2. Identify possible causes underlying this client's reluctance to move. How might this information affect your plan?
3. From the information provided, consider possible nursing diagnoses. Prioritize them, and give rationales for your choices.
4. Propose ways in which collaboration with other healthcare professionals would be beneficial.
5. As you work with this family, discuss ways to ensure their safety.

Mobility, or the ability to move freely within the environment, is fundamental to normal daily functioning. In a highly mobile society, problems affecting mobility are especially significant. Independence is usually defined by a person's ability to perform activities of daily living (ADLs), job-related activities, and role-related activities (e.g., as a parent or spouse). Limitations in a person's ability to move normally and spontaneously can affect all these areas.

Changes in mobility also create more subtle psychological effects especially in communication. Facial expressions and gestures are significant in nonverbal communication, and talking with someone at eye level promotes equality between those talking. The person who must look up at someone from a chair or bed may feel that he or she is at a psychological disadvantage. Movement also is significant in dispersing negative feelings and tension. Many people find that jogging and other forms of exercise help to relieve stress and anxiety. Being able to leave uncomfortable or dangerous situations gives most people a feeling of control. Conversely, people confined to bed usually see themselves as sick and may feel less able to participate in the recovery process. Disabilities that affect mobility, such as amputation or a musculoskeletal defect, may impair self-image.

Most people associate mobility with health. Like many aspects of health, mobility can be viewed along a continuum from full mobility to immobility. Full mobility occurs when the person has no physical or psychological factors that limit mobility. Immobility occurs when the person cannot move his or her entire body or a specific body part.

Clients move along this continuum as their abilities change:

- Therapeutic treatments, such as traction to repair a fracture, may cause temporary changes in mobility.
- Some conditions lead to progressive disability; examples are muscular dystrophy and severe crippling rheumatoid arthritis.
- Permanent changes in mobility occur when physiologic dysfunction that interferes with normal body movement cannot be reversed (e.g., spinal cord injuries that result in paralysis or cerebrovascular accidents [strokes] that cause weakness or paralysis on one side of the body).

Rehabilitation is the key to restoring a person with certain disabilities to optimal health. Nurses can play a significant role in this process.

NORMAL MOBILITY

The musculoskeletal system is the supporting framework for the body. The bones and muscles are involved in movement and are responsible for the body's form and shape. Central and peripheral nerves coordinate movement's complex activity. Maintaining posture and balance against the force of gravity requires smooth coordination of muscles, joints, and nerves and a stable center of gravity.

Structures of the Musculoskeletal System

Bones

Bones are a framework on which muscles, tendons, and ligaments are attached. They facilitate movement, protect vital organs (brain, heart, lungs, liver), store and regulate calcium and phosphate, and form blood cells.

The structure of bones provides for minimum weight and maximum structural strength. Bone tissue is either woven or lamellar. Woven bone is characterized by rapid growth, as occurs in infancy, and is generally found where ligaments and tendons insert into the bones of adults. Lamellar bone is mature with highly organized mineralized plates.

The 206 bones in the body also can be classified by shape: long (arms, legs), short (tarsals, carpals), flat (cranium), and irregular (vertebral). Basic components of the long bones are the diaphysis (shaft) and the epiphyses (ends). Most bone is covered by periosteum, which contains nerves and blood vessels. The outer portion of long bones is composed of dense, compact bone with a marrow cavity in the center where the blood-forming cells are located.

Muscles

Skeletal muscles are connected to bones at or across joints. Muscles are composed of striated, long muscle fibers usually in parallel alignment. The fibers' formation allows muscle to contract (shorten) or extend (lengthen) as required by movement. Contraction occurs when the overlapping striated fibers slide toward each other, thereby shortening and increasing the muscle's strength.

Muscle contraction requires a complex mechanical, chemical, and electrical interaction. The contraction is initiated when an action potential (electrical charge) moves along a nerve and across the neuromuscular junction to the muscle. Neurotransmitters, which are chemical substances such as acetylcholine, permit neurologic impulses to be transmitted to muscle. The transmitting activity occurs when calcium is released into the sarcoplasmic reticulum (site of storage and release for calcium in the muscle), which initiates a complex series of biochemical events that result in muscle contraction. Energy for the work of contraction comes from the metabolism of food, especially fats and carbohydrates.

Muscles are covered by a layer of connective tissue that joins with tendon fibers at the end of the muscle fiber where muscle joins bone. Muscle fibers are innervated by motor neurons originating from the anterior horn of the spinal cord. All muscle fibers connected to a single motor nerve are called a motor unit.

During a lifetime, the body has only the number of muscle cells with which it was born; however, the work of the muscle determines the size of the muscle cells. When forceful activity is demanded of the muscle, the muscle hypertrophies (the muscle's diameter increases) increasing the muscle's strength. **Atrophy,** the opposite of hypertrophy, causes the muscle to decrease in strength and size because of disuse.

Disuse may be related to lack of exercise, aging, enforced rest, or use of immobilizing devices.

Joints

Joints are the areas where bones meet. The types of joints are fibrous, which do not move (cranial); cartilaginous, which allow minimal movement (costochondral); and synovial, which are movable (joints of the extremities). Synovial joints are lined with synovial tissue, which has a rich blood supply and produces synovial fluid. Synovial fluid lubricates joints, allowing smooth articulation and easy motion. Terms used to describe joint motion are provided in Display 33-1.

Ligaments and tendons connect and support joints. Ligaments stabilize the bones in the joints and are more elastic than tendons. Tendons are specialized tissues. They connect muscle to bone and are surrounded by synovial-like tissues.

Normal Physiologic Function

Carrying out coordinated movement is a complex process. Even with a framework of bones held together by ligaments and covered with soft tissue and skin, normal function cannot occur without coordinated muscle activity and neurologic integration.

Alignment and Posture

Maintaining upright posture requires proper alignment of the bones, muscles, and joints and a stable center of gravity. Alignment is achieved when the joints and muscles are not experiencing extremes in extension or flexion or unusual stress when the person is lying down, sitting, or standing.

Upright posture and movement require a balanced center of gravity: the weight of the body is centered and the downward forces of gravity are balanced. The usual line of gravity starts at the top of the head and bisects the shoulders, trunk, weight-bearing joints, and base of support; it runs slightly anterior to the sacrum. In older people, the lumbar spine tends to flatten and the upper spine and head tend to tilt forward causing the head to fall forward from the usual line of gravity (Fig. 33-1).

Balance

Maintaining balance is a complex function of counteracting gravity and reflexes to maintain posture. The reticular formation, a neural network through the brainstem, integrates neural input that is important for maintaining balance. If a person begins to fall to one side, the extensor muscles on that side stiffen whereas the extensor muscles on the opposite side relax to prevent the fall.

Equilibrium is provided mainly by the vestibular apparatus of the ear. The vestibular apparatus consists of the cochlear duct, the three semicircular canals, and two large chambers known as the utricle and the saccule. The utricle, saccule, and semicircular canals contain tiny hair cells connected to sensory nerve fibers that pass into the vestibular nerve. When the head moves, these hair cells are bent, pulled, or compressed, transmitting signals to the sensory nerves over the appropriate nerve tracts to the area that controls equilibrium and balance.

Coordinated Movement

The cerebellum, cerebral cortex, and basal ganglia are responsible for the control of motor functions. The cerebellum coordinates the motor activities of movement, the cerebral cortex initiates voluntary motor activity, and the basal ganglia maintain posture. These systems make up the pyramidal and extrapyramidal tracts. The pyramidal tract (the direct corticospinal pathway) initiates transmission of impulses to the spinal cord for voluntary movements. The extrapyramidal tract (the indirect corticospinal pathway) dampens and inhibits impulses to promote smooth and coordinated movement.

The cerebellum has a special role in controlling movement: it controls muscles used to maintain steady posture and coordinated, detailed movements. The cerebellum coordinates rapid, automatic adjustments that maintain balance and

DISPLAY 33-1

🔄 TERMS DESCRIBING JOINT MOTION

Adduction	Moving a joint or extremity toward the midline of the body
Abduction	Moving a joint or extremity away from the midline of the body
Rotation, internal	Turning a joint or extremity on its axis toward the body's midline
Rotation, external	Turning a joint or extremity on its axis away from the body's midline
Flexion	Decreasing the angle between two bones
Extension	Straightening a joint
Hyperextension	Moving a joint past normal extension
Supination	Turning the body or a body part to face upward
Pronation	Turning the body or a body part to face downward
Circumduction	Moving a body part in widening circles
Inversion	Turning the feet inward so toes point toward the midline
Eversion	Turning the feet outward so toes point away from the midline
Opposition	Touching the thumb to each finger

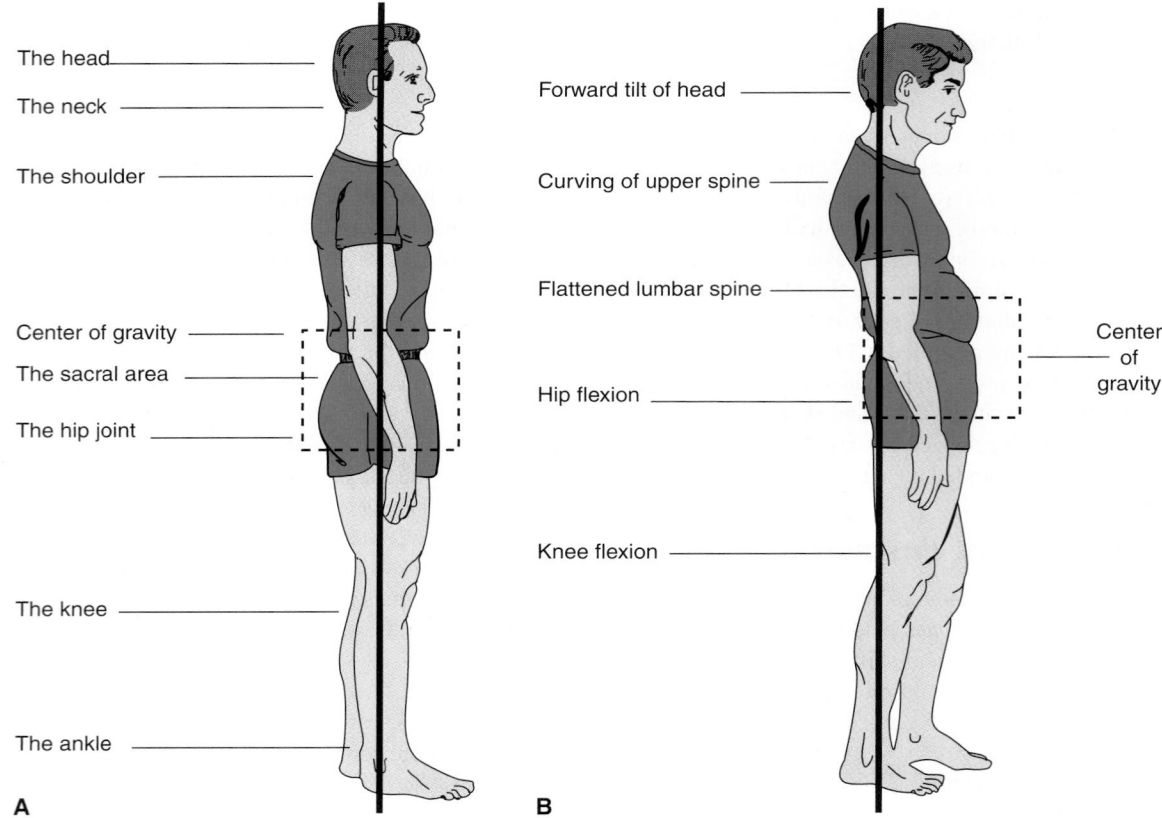

The head

The neck

The shoulder

Center of gravity

The sacral area

The hip joint

The knee

The ankle

A

Forward tilt of head

Curving of upper spine

Flattened lumbar spine

Hip flexion

Center of gravity

Knee flexion

B

FIGURE 33-1   Vertical gravity line and posture. **(A)** Vertical gravity line and center of gravity. **(B)** Postural changes with age.

equilibrium. It refines learned movement patterns. The cerebellum compares the motor commands with proprioceptive information (position sense) and performs any adjustments needed (Martini, Ober, Garrison, Welch, & Hutchings, 2000). The result is smooth, coordinated movement and developed, fine-motor function, rather than uncoordinated, arrhythmic movement.

Body Mechanics

Body mechanics can be defined as using alignment, posture, and balance in a coordinated effort to perform activities such as lifting, bending, and moving. Proper use of body mechanics promotes safe musculoskeletal function and maintains balance without placing undue strain on muscles (Metules, 2001). When nurses use their bodies to perform therapies, assist clients with movement, or move equipment, they benefit from effective use of body mechanics to prevent injury to themselves or others. Proper use of body mechanics is explained in Procedure 33-1.

Components of Body Mechanics.   Using body mechanics effectively means using gravity advantageously in body alignment, posture, balance, and movement. Maintaining a balanced center of gravity, which tends to be in the area of the pelvis slightly anterior to the sacrum, is essential to this process.

Maintaining balance involves keeping the spine in vertical alignment, the feet positioned for a broad base of support, and the body weight close to the center of gravity. When a person lifts or carries a load, that weight becomes part of the body weight; therefore that additional weight must be balanced over the center of gravity (Fig. 33-2).

The greater the support base, the more stability the person has for changing body position while maintaining alignment, posture, and balance. The weight-bearing joints and skeletal muscles of the legs provide a stable base of support that a person can widen by placing the feet farther apart and flexing the hip and knee joints. These adjustments lower the center of gravity, making a person more stable and allowing flexibility to avoid muscle strain.

Opposing voluntary muscle groups and neuromuscular reflexes coordinate movement. The flexor and extensor muscle groups provide opposing tensions for movement. When the flexors contract to move a joint, the extensors relax; when the flexors relax, the extensors contract. The legs' flexors are among the largest and strongest muscles in the body and are used for leverage in good body mechanics. The neuromuscular reflexes maintain posture by enabling opposing muscle groups to coordinate movement.

Principles of Body Mechanics.   Nurses and clients may fall or incur back injuries as clients are moved from one position

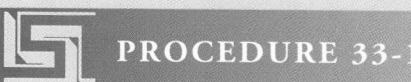

PROCEDURE 33-1

USING BODY MECHANICS TO MOVE CLIENTS

Purpose
1. Prevent injury to the nurse's musculoskeletal system.
2. Prevent injury to the client during transfer.

Assessment
- Evaluate weight of client to be lifted. Arrange for assistance if necessary.
- Assess position and height of client to be lifted.
- Assess client's balance and ability to bear weight.
- Assess client's knowledge about body alignment and how to maintain it with position changes.

Procedure
1. Plan movement before doing it.
   a. Always lock wheels on bed, stretcher, or wheelchair.
      Rationale: Unexpected movements may move bed, stretcher, or wheelchair and result in injury to yourself or client.

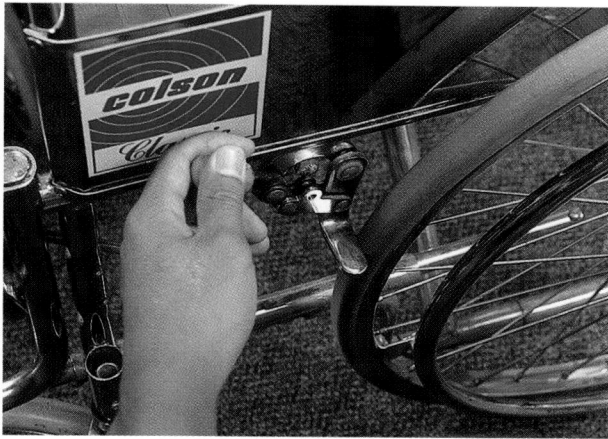

Step 1a Lock wheels on wheelchair.

   b. Allow client to assist during move.
      Rationale: Client participation helps overcome forces resisting the move, encourages client's sense of independence, and provides exercise for client.
   c. Use mechanical aids (e.g., lifters, slide boards, body mobilizers) or additional personnel to move heavy clients.

Rationale: Having assistance decreases stress of movement for client and nurse thus reducing risk of injury.
   d. When possible, slide, push, or pull client rather than lifting and carrying.
      Rationale: Your body weight adds power to muscle work. Rocking your own body weight can balance the client's weight when assisting to a standing position.
   e. Tighten abdominal and gluteal muscles before lifting or moving client.
      Rationale: Tightening supports the abdomen and stabilizes the pelvis to provide a firm base of support.
   f. Use smooth, rhythmic, coordinated motions.
      Rationale: Smooth motions use less energy and lead to less muscle strain than jerky motions.
   g. If another person is assisting, plan your movements before beginning.
      Rationale: Planning prevents uncoordinated movements that may result in muscle strain or injury.
2. Begin all movements with body aligned and balanced.
   a. Face client to be moved, and plan to pivot your entire body without twisting your back.
      Rationale: Proper positioning avoids back strain and injury.
   b. Place both feet flat on floor; bend knees slightly with one foot slightly in front of the other or one step apart.
      Rationale: Balanced positioning increases base of support and stability.
   c. Bend knees to lower center of gravity toward client to be moved.
      Rationale: This maintains body balance, reduces risk of falling, and allows larger muscle groups to work together.
3. When possible, elevate adjustable beds to waist level and lower side rails.
   Rationale: Adjusting the bed and side rails prevents stretching and muscle strain.
4. Carry objects close to body, and stand as close as possible to work area.
   Rationale: This maintains the workload near the center of gravity to prevent muscle strain and fatigue caused by hyperextension.

Home Care Modifications
- Teach caregivers the above guidelines for body movements. Redemonstration of learning provides a good opportunity to evaluate technique.

PROCEDURE 33-1 (Continued)

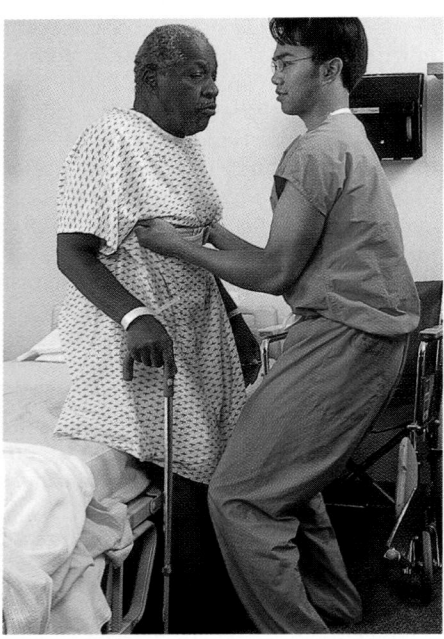

Step 2b and c With feet flat and slightly apart, lower center of gravity.

Collaboration and Delegation

• Injuries, especially to the back, are common for unlicensed healthcare workers who do much lifting. Continually reinforce body mechanics while expressing concern for the health and well-being of coworkers.

• Identify high-risk clients (e.g., clients who suffered previous back injury, obese clients, older adults) who may need more intensive follow-up. Physical therapy can provide classes on proper body mechanics.

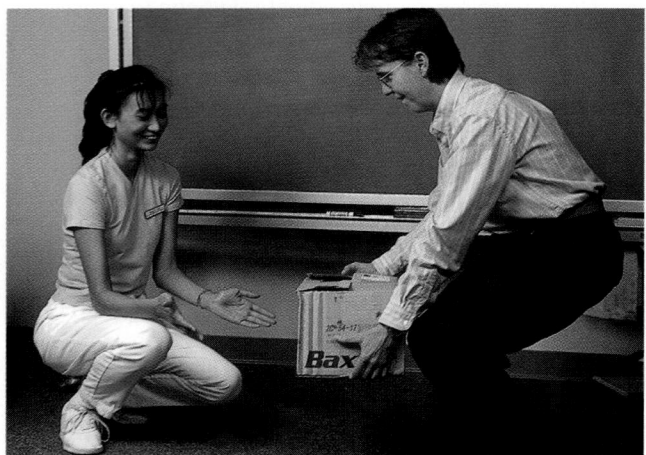

FIGURE 33-2   The nurse instructs a client on proper lifting technique to prevent back strain and injury.

or location to another. The more limited the client's mobility, the more the nurse must rely on good body mechanics. Using assistive devices (e.g., friction reducers) to enhance an ergonomic approach to the necessary lifting in nursing can decrease occupational injuries (Owen, 2000). Display 33-2 lists the principles of body mechanics. Some general rules for body mechanics are presented below.

Rule one is to assess the situation carefully before acting. Planning is crucial. Necessary equipment should be out of the way of the nurse and client, usually near the head or foot of the bed. Ventilator tubing, catheters, intravenous (IV) tubing, and wires for cardiac and ventilatory monitoring must be handled by an assistant or positioned to prevent accidental disconnection during a turn or transfer. Using a counting method helps to coordinate the actions of everyone involved in the movement. Counting "one, two, three" with the position change on "three" helps focus everyone's attention and invites the client's active participation.

DISPLAY 33-2

🔄 PRINCIPLES OF BODY MECHANICS

Scientific Principles Underlying Body Mechanics
- Less energy is used if all body parts are balanced appropriately.
- The greater the base of support, the more stable the body.
- Pelvic tilt (contraction of the abdominal and gluteal muscles to stabilize the pelvis) before activity helps protect the lower back from strain and injury.
- Facing the direction of work reduces the chance of injury.
- Less energy is needed to keep an object moving (momentum) than to initiate movement (inertia).
- Moving an object on a level surface requires less effort.
- Reducing friction between the object moved and the surface on which it is moved requires less energy.
- Holding an object close to the body requires less energy than holding it farther away.
- Muscle strain can be avoided by using the strong leg muscles when lifting, pushing, and pulling.
- Smooth, continuous movements are easier and safer than sudden, sharp, or uncontrolled movements.

- Using rhythmic movements at a normal speed requires less energy.

Applied Principles of Body Mechanics
- Adjust the height of the work area when possible.
- Assume a starting position that will permit freedom of movement in range, direction, and position.
- Keep body balanced over the base of support with knees relaxed and trunk erect (in relation to the pelvis).
- Bend hips and knees to alter position of body, widening the base of support as needed, for effective leverage and use of energy.
- Face the direction of motion, using the muscles of the lower extremities and shifting body weight for lifting, pushing, and pulling actions.
- Hold objects close to the body when lifting.
- Use rhythmic, smooth, and coordinated motions at a reasonable speed.
- Use elbows, hips, and knees as levers when lifting.
- Use mechanical devices when appropriate.
- Holding the breath during a physical activity is an indication of muscle strain and inefficient use of body mechanics.

🬚 SAFETY ALERT

When in doubt, seek assistance before beginning to move a client. Examine the surroundings for potential obstacles to the desired movement (e.g., equipment, cords, tubing, or other items that could trip the nurse or hamper the client's free movement).

The second rule is to use the legs' large muscle groups whenever possible to provide the force for the movement. The back stays straight, the arms maintain a strong grip with elbows slightly flexed, and the hips and knees are bent. Pushing, pulling, or lifting is then accomplished by orienting the torso in the desired direction of movement and straightening the legs. Back injuries that result from moving clients can usually be traced to asymmetric muscle use. Avoid twisting or moving diagonally.

The third rule is to perform work at the appropriate height for body position. When helping a client to move in bed, raise the bed height to a level close to the nurse's center of gravity, which is usually between the hips and waist. Usually, lowering the side rails allows the nurse to move the client as close as possible and avoid awkward positioning involved in reaching over side rails to perform tasks. When moving the client from a bed to a stretcher, the two surfaces should be at the same height so the client does not need to be lifted.

The fourth rule is to use mechanical lifts or assistance whenever needed to ease a move. Mechanical lifts are recommended when the client cannot assist or cooperate or when the nurse is uncertain about the safety of the transfer. Stand-up lifts, used when clients can bear some weight, have decreased injury to staff and clients in long-term care settings. Overhead trapezes may provide handholds for clients who wish to assist. In many situations, a lift sheet (also called a turn or draw sheet) is helpful. This sturdy sheet is positioned under the client in bed so it extends from the shoulders to just below the hips. Depending on the client's weight, two or more nurses (equally placed on each side of the bed) can use the lift sheet to move the client anywhere on the mattress and then to position the client onto either side. The key to successful use of the lift sheet is coordinated movement by the lifters.

Exercise

Exercise that actively requires alignment, posture, balance, and coordinated movement offers many physiologic and psychological benefits. Exercise must be regular and integrated into the person's lifestyle for maximum benefits. A person's family, culture, job, and health may influence his or her participation in and appreciation for exercise. In recent years, exercise has become more popular as people have taken responsibility for decreasing risk factors and leading healthier lives.

Types of Exercise. Exercise may be classified by the source of energy (aerobic or anaerobic) and by the type of muscle tension (isotonic or isometric) required:

- **Aerobic exercise** requires oxygen to use the energy provided by the metabolic activities of the skeletal muscles. Vigorous, continuous muscle movement (as in walking, running, cycling, cross-country skiing, aerobic dancing, and playing tennis) is aerobic exercise when the person's heart rate is high enough to promote cardiovascular conditioning.
- **Anaerobic exercise** occurs when the muscle cannot extract enough oxygen from the blood and anaerobic pathways provide additional energy for a short time. This type of exercise is useful in athletic endurance training. All endurance exercise can become anaerobic when oxygen sources are depleted.
- **Isotonic exercise** is a dynamic form of exercise with constant muscle tension, muscle contraction, and active movement. Most activities (e.g., walking, running, performing ADLs) are isotonic.
- **Isometric exercise** is static exercise in which the muscle undergoes tension and contraction but no change in length and no joint movement. Examples of isometric exercise are quadriceps setting to strengthen the quadriceps muscle, maintaining strength in immobilized muscles (casts, traction), and endurance training.

Benefits of Exercise. Exercise strengthens muscles, increases endurance, and promotes joint mobility. Cardiovascular health improves as lung capacity increases, resting pulse rate and blood pressure decrease, and the risk of atherosclerosis decreases. Exercise helps to prevent constipation, enhance appetite, and improve sleep quality. Exercise contributes to a feeling of well-being because activity increases circulating endorphins and promotes tension and stress release. Weight loss and improved physical appearance frequently motivate people to continue exercising regularly. The person who does not exercise regularly is at risk for health problems, just as the immobile client is at risk for problems related to disuse.

Characteristics of Normal Movement

Full Range of Motion
Range of motion (ROM) is the ability to move all joints through the full extent of intended function. Each joint must be kept actively moving for the joints to maintain mobility, the muscles to maintain strength, and the cardiovascular system to function adequately.

Active ROM means that the person can initiate and perform exercises in which each joint moves through its complete ROM. The healthy person may complete active ROM as a part of everyday activities and exercise.

Joints move through various planes and ROMs depending on the type of joint. Table 33-1 shows the types of joints and their designated ROMs.

Normal Gait
Walking is the most common form of locomotion. Although most people take the ability to walk for granted, the normal walking **gait,** which is the style and character of a person's walk, is a coordinated process requiring equilibrium and balanced posture. Normal human ambulation requires a complex interactive control between multiple limb and body segments that work congruently to provide the most shock-absorbing and energy-efficient forward movement possible (Ayyappa, 2001).

The normal walking gait has two phases:

- The stance phase is composed of three events: heel strike, midstance, and push-off.
- The swing phase completes the walking gait with another three events: acceleration, swing through, and deceleration.

Walking is initiated by stepping with a slight forward tilt. The weight of the body is rolled off the ball and toes of one foot and shifted to the heel of the opposite foot and extended leg. In the process, the center of gravity moves from one side to the other and forward at the same time. The body weight is balanced on a narrow base, shifted from one side to the other, and supported alternately on one foot and then the other.

Lifespan Considerations

Newborn and Infant
Movements of newborns are random and reflexive. Survival reflexes include rooting (turning toward the breast when the baby's cheek is stroked) and sucking. Subcortical reflexes (Moro, startle, tonic neck, Babinski) subside as higher brain function matures and exerts an inhibitory influence. Protective reflexes (gag, blink, and withdrawal) persist into adulthood.

The stepping response can be evoked in newborns by holding them on a solid surface and leaning them slightly forward. The shift in the center of gravity and change in equilibrium initiate the stepping reflex. With maturity, infants learn to control and use the same reflex when learning to walk.

Neuromuscular assessment of newborns is important to detect deformities or abnormalities that respond well to early treatment. Some deformities result from the position the baby had in utero and will correct spontaneously as the child grows. Because hip dislocation/subluxation can occur any time during the first year of life, assessing all infants for hip abnormalities during well-baby examinations is crucial.

Control over movement progresses during the infant's first year as the neurologic system matures. Development proceeds from proximal to distal parts and in a head-to-toe fashion; babies progress from being able to control their heads, to rolling over, to crawling, to pulling themselves up to a standing position, to standing, and, finally, to walking.

TABLE 33-1

Normal Movement of Body Joints

Location in Body	Type of Joint	Normal Movement
Neck, cervical spine	Pivotal Supine Cervical	Flexion, extension, lateral flexion, rotation

Supine

Cervical

Lateral flexion   Rotation   Flexion extension hyperextension

| **Shoulder** | Ball and socket | Flexion, extension, hyperextension, abduction, adduction, internal rotation, external rotation, circumduction |

Shoulder

Abduction

Adduction

Rotation: outward inward

Flexion extension hyperextension

| **Elbow** | Hinge joints | |

Elbow

Supination   Pronation

Flexion   Extension

| **Forearm** | Pivotal | Supination, pronation |
| **Wrist** | Condyloid | Flexion, extension, hyperextension, adduction, abduction |

Wrist

Ulnar flexion (adduction)   Radial flexion (abduction)

Flexion   Extension   Hyperextension

| **Fingers** | Condyloidal hinge | Flexion, extension, hyperextension, abduction, adduction |

Fingers

Adduction Abduction   Flexion   Extension

(continues)

TABLE 33-1 (Continued)

Normal Movement of Body Joints		
Location in Body	**Type of Joint**	**Normal Movement**
Thumb	Saddle	Flexion, extension, abduction, adduction, apposition
Hip	Ball and socket	Flexion, extension, hyperextension, abduction, adduction, internal rotation, external rotation, circumduction
Knee	Hinge joint	Flexion, extension
Ankle	Hinge joint	Dorsal flexion, plantar flexion
Foot	Gliding	Inversion, eversion
Toes	Condyloid	Flexion, extension, abduction, adduction

Each successive task requires increasingly coordinated movement. Refinement of gross motor skills precedes fine motor skills. The ages at which babies accomplish specific tasks vary, but the development always occurs in an orderly progression. Motor activity during the first year characterizes many changes that occur in infants. For this reason, parents and other caregivers frequently rely on motor development as a yardstick to evaluate their infants' progress. Many parents need reassurance that their children master certain physical traits within the usual age range. Physical milestones provide the order but not the exact time for mastering new physical traits.

Toddler and Preschooler

Refinement of gross and fine motor skills and nearly boundless energy mark the developmental stages of the toddler and preschooler. Most children usually master walking soon after the first birthday. Walking begins with a wide stance and unsteady gait, hence the term *toddler*. In the second and third years of life, common developmental tasks mastered include coordinated walking, running, jumping, climbing stairs, throwing a ball, self-feeding, and scribbling with crayons. Fine motor skills generally develop more rapidly in girls than in boys. Young children use their physical abilities to explore their environment and to develop cognitively.

Preschoolers continue to increase gross and fine motor skills rapidly. Gross motor activities mastered before school typically include riding a tricycle, walking backward, dancing, skipping, running, jumping, and climbing well. Fine motor skills include using crayons to draw or make letters, catching a ball, stringing beads, brushing teeth, doing puzzles, fastening or using zippers, and washing hands.

Child and Adolescent

Physical growth slows between 6 and 12 years. Refinement of gross and fine motor skills continues, however, and is often enhanced by group activities (e.g., sports, dancing, and swimming lessons). Exercise patterns for later life are often determined at this time. Families should encourage regular physical exercise while avoiding excessive pressure on children to excel. Unrealistic expectations can be emotionally and physically damaging for youngsters whose muscles are not fully developed.

Adolescence is a period of rapid physical and sexual development. Because of varied growth in different body parts, teenagers typically appear gangly and awkward. Consequently, resulting uneven motor function affects body image, which can be especially distressing for adolescents. Most schools require some physical education as a graduation requirement, and many students engage in competitive sports or other school-sponsored physical activities such as dancing.

Adult and Older Adult

Between ages 20 and 40 years, relatively few physical changes occur that affect mobility, although late-term pregnancy can limit vigorous physical activity. Young adults may experience altered mobility when trauma (e.g., sprains or fractures) limits normal function. Adults with jobs that require repetitive movement (e.g., typists, assembly line workers, supermarket checkers, computer operators) may develop carpal tunnel syndrome, a nerve compression that causes pain and decreases hand mobility. As adults approach middle age (40 to 60 years), muscle tone and bone density and mass decrease. Joints lose elasticity and flexibility. Bone mass decreases, especially in women with osteoporosis, resulting in an increased incidence of fractures. Additionally, altered coordination affects normal gait, and a slowing reaction time delays the overall body response to stressors.

Aging brings postural changes and chronic joint disorders. Flattening of the lumbar spine and changes in the intervertebral disks and vertebral bodies may cause the head and upper spine to tilt forward, shifting the center of gravity. Joint degeneration and bone demineralization also affect balance and gait. As a result, older adults usually have less extension and swing through and more side-to-side sway; weight is transferred from the ball of one foot to the ball of the other foot, leading to a wide-based, short-stepped, shuffling gait.

Many older people have more difficulty overcoming inertia and using gravity efficiently. One contributing factor is the shift in the center of gravity. To compensate for the shift, the knees flex slightly for support. The resulting posture is a forward-leaning crouch with a widened base. Chronic health problems or injuries from falls also affect the mobility of older adults. Fear of falling causes some older adults to restrict activity voluntarily. If this results in increased caution, it can be a positive response; taken to the extreme though, severely restricting activity results in muscle atrophy or deconditioning.

FACTORS AFFECTING MOBILITY
Lifestyle and Habits

Regular exercise and optimal nutrition are essential to maintain mobility and musculoskeletal functioning. If a person has a balanced approach to activity, nutrition, and exercise, he or she should maintain mobility. The maxim "use it or lose it" is particularly true regarding the musculoskeletal system: the person must use it regularly to maintain function. Regular, ongoing exercise is required for optimal conditioning. About 30 minutes of strenuous aerobic exercise three times weekly promotes conditioning. Without this ongoing conditioning, 6 hours of vigorous exercise once a month for a sedentary person may overtax an unconditioned body.

Intact Musculoskeletal System

Anything that interrupts muscle strength, bone resiliency and strength, and full ROM of the joints may impair the musculoskeletal system's ability to facilitate mobility. Fluid and electrolyte levels, exercise, conditioning, nutrition, and condition of tendons, ligaments, or soft tissue influence muscle strength. Exercise increases muscle tone, mass, and strength and enhances the condition of other musculoskeletal tissues and body organs.

The function of the bones and joints depends on the bone's mineral content, which gives them adequate resilience, and on the flexibility of joints and their tendons and ligaments. Adequate dietary calcium, phosphorus, and vitamin B are essential to maintain bone resilience and an intact skeletal system. Joints must be able to move through their entire ROM so the body can move freely and maintain mobility.

Trauma usually results in accidental injury to joints, tendons, ligaments, muscles, or bones. The damage may be minor, affecting mobility for only a short time (e.g., a strain caused by overexerting a muscle or a sprain caused by twisting a joint), or it may be more extensive by involving a dislocated joint, torn tendons, broken bones, or joint replacements.

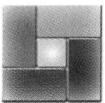

Nursing Research and Critical Thinking
Does the Competition Between Cognitive and Postural Tasks Contribute to Instability and Falls in Some Older Adults?

Research has shown that many aspects of postural control decline with age, and that postural deficits are a contributing factor to an increased likelihood for falls. These researchers designed a dual-task investigative study to test the effects of two different types of cognitive tasks on stability in young versus older adults with and without a history of falls. Twenty young adults (mean age 31), 20 older adults (mean age 78) with a self-reported history of falls, and 20 older adults (mean age 74) without a history of falls were recruited for the study by means of a newspaper advertisement. Two secondary cognitive tasks (sentence completion and visual perception matching) were used to produce changes in attention during quiet stance on a flat surface. Postural stability was quantified using forceplate measures of center of pressure (COP). Speed and accuracy of verbal response on the cognitive tasks were also quantified. No differences were found between the young adults and the older adults without a fall history on the firm surface, no task condition. When task complexity increased, either through the introduction of a secondary cognitive task or a more challenging postural condition, significant differences in postural stability between these two groups became apparent. In contrast to the young adults and the older adults without a fall history, postural stability in older adults with a history of falls was significantly affected by both cognitive tasks.

Critical Thinking Considerations. The use of volunteers limits the generalizability of the study. The information, however, is relevant to the nursing care of older adults with a history of falls. The study's implications are as follows:

- When postural stability is impaired, even relatively simple cognitive tasks can further impact balance.
- Other factors could possibly account for the differences in the two groups of older adults. An example is differences in health and mental status.

From Shumway-Cook, A., Woollacott, M., Kerns, K. A., & Baldwin, M. (1997). The effects of two types of cognitive tasks on postural stability in older adults with and without a history of falls. *Journal of Gerontology, Series A: Biological Sciences, 52A*(4), 232–240.

Immobilizing devices are usually used to keep healing body parts in normal alignment.

Demineralization of the bone, as in osteoporosis, increases the risk of fractures. Rheumatoid arthritis, degenerative joint disease (osteoarthritis), and gout also limit mobility because movement causes pain. Bone tumors may cause pain as well and may require amputation of an affected limb.

Nervous System Control

Normal mobility requires the smooth control of movement provided by the nervous system. Motor ability depends on the integrity of the multisynaptic pathways of the afferent and efferent nerves and the central integration provided by the cerebral cortex. Nerve conduction, in turn, requires adequate circulation and appropriate fluid and electrolyte balance. Balance and stability are the products of equilibrium, which can be affected by some medications, fatigue, or situations that temporarily impair vision and visual input to the vestibular system in the semicircular canals.

Any disorder that impairs the nervous system's ability to control muscular movement and coordination hinders functional mobility. Usually these disorders (e.g., muscular dystrophy, Parkinson's disease, and multiple sclerosis) are progressive; they slowly erode and eventually destroy the ability to move normally until the person is confined to bed or a wheelchair.

Impairments of the brain or spinal cord can also affect movement. When the spinal cord is severed or severely damaged, paralysis occurs below the level of injury. The term *paraplegia* describes decreased motor and sensory function to the legs. *Quadriplegia* describes paralysis of the arms and the legs.

Infectious processes (e.g., meningitis), tumors, or cerebrovascular accidents (strokes) can disrupt central nervous system control over movement. Treatment can limit or reverse some damage to the central nervous system, but, at times, dysfunction is permanent and severe.

Circulation and Oxygenation

The skeletal muscles need adequate amounts of oxygen to function optimally. The lungs must provide oxygen while removing carbon dioxide, the byproduct of aerobic metabolism in the muscles. The heart must adequately pump blood to the muscles and supply other body organs with enough blood to meet the increased demands imposed by exercise. The vasculature must redirect proportionally larger amounts of blood to the muscles, often shunting blood flow away from the gut, during periods of extreme exercise.

Many chronic disorders limit the supply of oxygen and nutrients needed for muscle contraction and movement. Chronic cardiovascular conditions, such as congestive heart failure or peripheral vascular disease, limit effective blood flow especially during periods of increased need such as aerobic exercise. Lung disorders decrease the amount of oxygen delivered to all body tissues including skeletal muscles. Anemia decreases the amount of hemoglobin available for oxygen binding.

Energy

Cancer or other conditions that strain nutritional stores deplete energy necessary for movement. Energy for muscle function is derived from using oxygen and the breakdown products of food to produce muscle contraction. There are two primary types of metabolism: aerobic and anaerobic. In aerobic metabolism, the oxidative processes that produce energy occur in the mitochondria of cells; water and carbon dioxide are the byproducts. Aerobic metabolism is the most efficient form of energy production for long-term activity.

In anaerobic metabolism, a process known as glycolysis converts stored glycogen to energy. This process provides energy when the oxygen supply is inadequate or delayed; lactic acid is the byproduct. The depletion of stored glycogen in the presence of lactic acid produces fatigue in a short time so this type of metabolism is useful only for short bursts of energy.

Congenital Problems

Some conditions, such as spina bifida or cerebral palsy, are present at birth and cannot be cured. Treatment goals are maximal functional mobility and minimal complications.

Affective Disorders

Severe affective disorders can hinder mobility. Depression and catatonic states result in limited mobility not because of physical impairments but because the person lacks the desire to move. Fear, especially of pain on movement, may cause some people to restrict their movements as well.

Therapeutic Modalities

Sometimes limited movement is the treatment for a medical problem. Restrictive devices, such as casts, braces, and splints, can immobilize certain areas of the body to promote healing. Bed rest is another treatment whereby mobility is restricted for therapeutic benefits. A client may be placed on bed rest for the following reasons:

- To promote healing and tissue repair by decreasing metabolic needs
- To relieve edema (swelling)
- To reduce the body's oxygen requirements
- To decrease pain
- To support a weak, exhausted, or febrile client
- To avoid dislodging a deep vein thrombosis.

The definition of bed rest may vary: Some healthcare providers permit clients on bed rest to use bedside commodes; others insist on strict confinement to bed.

ALTERED MOBILITY
Manifestations of Altered Mobility

The client with altered mobility may have various symptoms including decreased muscle strength and tone, lack of coordination, altered gait, falls, decreased joint flexibility, pain on movement, and decreased ability to tolerate activity.

Decreased Muscle Strength and Tone

Frequent muscle contraction, which occurs during movement, maintains muscle strength. When movement is limited or abnormal, maximal tension is not applied to muscle groups, which decreases the muscles' ability to contract. Disuse may be accompanied by muscle atrophy, which is a decrease in muscle size.

Decreased strength is apparent when the client cannot grasp the nurse's hand strongly or can push only weakly with the legs. Weakness may be so severe that the client's leg muscles cannot support his or her body weight. At other times, decreased strength is less obvious. For example, a client may be able to extend his or her arms in front of the body, but, after a few minutes, the arms begin to drift down as the muscles become too fatigued to provide adequate support.

Muscle tone, or the normal resistance to stretch, also decreases with inactivity. Decreased muscle tone is called hypotonicity or **flaccidity.** Decreased tone can cause the muscles to stretch (if they are held in a lengthened position) or contract (if they are held in a shortened position). Neurologic impairment that results in increased muscle tone, often called **spasticity,** also can affect normal movement. Nursing care can be pivotal in caring for the client with spasticity (Porter, 2001).

Lack of Coordination

Lack of coordination occurs when neurologic control and movement regulation are impaired. Usually this is the case when trauma or disease affects the cerebellum. Alcohol and certain drugs, such as barbiturates, also may interfere with normal coordinated movement. Uncoordinated movements appear jerky and uneven and affect the person's ability to move purposefully and efficiently. Many terms are used to describe alterations in coordinated, purposeful movement:

- *Ataxia* is a general term used to describe defective muscle coordination.
- A *tremor* is a rhythmic, repetitive movement that can occur at rest or when movement is initiated. A tremor usually interferes with fine motor control, but in Parkinson's disease it also can interfere with coordinated ambulation.
- *Chorea* is spontaneous, brief, involuntary muscle twitching of the limbs or facial muscles; severe chorea hinders mobility.
- *Athetosis* is movement characterized by slow, irregular, twisting motions.
- *Dystonia* is similar to athetosis but usually involves larger areas of the body.

Altered Gait

Abnormal gait can affect the rhythm, steadiness, and speed of walking:

- An *ataxic gait* is characterized by staggering and unsteadiness.
- The gait is called *spastic* when walking appears stiff and toes appear to catch and drag.
- A *waddling gait* is walking with feet wide apart in a duck-like fashion.
- A *hemiplegic gait* occurs when one leg is paralyzed or neurologically damaged, so the leg is dragged or swung around to propel it forward.
- A *festinating gait,* typified by walking on the toes as if being pushed, is common in Parkinson's disease.

Falls

Clients with mobility limitations are likely to fall from gait changes, weakness, postural hypotension, or diminished coordination. Falls can result in musculoskeletal trauma, such as fractures, which can further decrease mobility. Sensory and cognitive changes in older adults, combined with medication usage, further increase the risk of falls for this age group. Fear of repeated falls may cause some clients to limit their mobility.

Decreased Joint Flexibility

Decreased joint flexibility typically occurs with altered mobility because decreased movement causes joints to stiffen. Normal ROM decreases because fibrosis and fixation affect the joint structures. Muscles atrophy when they do not regu-

ETHICAL/LEGAL ISSUE
Following Orders

You are an RN working at a nursing home. When you arrive for duty, the nursing supervisor asks to see you. She tells you that Mrs. Johnson fell yesterday afternoon and was found shortly after you left. She would like you to fill out the Quality Assurance Form (QAF) that outlines the incident. You start to explain that you feel uncomfortable doing this, but the supervisor stops you and states, "I believe I have made myself clear."

Reflection
- Discuss ways that a healthcare agency may use a QAF.
- If you were in this situation, identify some of your concerns.
- Explore positive and negative consequences of filling out the QAF.
- Explore positive and negative consequences of not filling out the QAF.
- Did the manner in which the supervisor made the request influence your response to the situation?

larly shorten and lengthen during normal muscle contraction. Initially decreased flexibility and altered ROM occur in affected joints, but if the joints remain immobilized, contractures can occur. A **contracture** is the progressive shortening of a muscle and loss of joint mobility resulting from fibrotic changes in tissues surrounding the joint.

Pain on Movement

Impaired mobility is often caused by or accompanied by pain on movement. Pain can result from physical injury, as in sprains, strains, or torn ligaments, or it may result from degenerative and inflammatory processes. Osteoarthritis (degeneration of the articular surface of weight-bearing joints) and rheumatoid arthritis (an inflammatory disorder that affects joints) are two common disorders that limit mobility secondary to discomfort/pain on movement.

Incisional pain decreases most clients' willingness to ambulate during the postoperative period. Pain caused by inadequate blood flow to the extremities (intermittent claudication) also can severely decrease mobility. Cancer, low back pain, and other disorders associated with chronic pain also limit movement.

Activity Intolerance

Decreased ability to tolerate activity often accompanies impaired mobility. **Activity intolerance** is when a person has inadequate physiologic or psychological energy to endure or to complete an activity. A balance must occur between the activity and the client's energy. Symptoms associated with activity intolerance are dyspnea, tachycardia, discomfort, weakness, and fatigue.

Commonly, disorders that affect oxygenation, such as respiratory or cardiac problems, decrease a client's ability to tolerate increases in activity. Some activity intolerance, however, can be noted in anyone who has been inactive. For example, a 46-year-old man who has been inactive since college will experience activity intolerance if he tries to run 2 miles. Even short periods of immobility can impair activity tolerance.

Impact of Immobility on Function

Immobility affects most areas of function (Table 33-2). Recognizing the possible consequences of immobility allows the nurse to intervene to limit or prevent problems.

Activity and Exercise

Muscle Atrophy and Weakness. Reduction in muscle cell size (atrophy) results from the alterations in metabolism that occur during immobility; the body breaks down muscle mass to obtain energy (catabolic metabolism). The resulting changes in strength and mass are substantial and last even after immobility is reversed. Immobility affects the leg muscles more than other muscles. This is thought to be due to the effects of gravity in maintaining muscle tone. The evidence of atrophy can be seen dramatically when a cast is removed and the limbs are compared.

TABLE 33-2

Comparison of the Effects of Exercise and Immobility on Function		
Functional Area	**Effects of Exercise**	**Effects of Immobility/Inactivity**
Health perception/ health maintenance	Promotes optimal health and well-being	Increases risk of various health problems (e.g., cardiovascular, diabetes)
Activity/exercise	Strengthens muscles and increases muscle tone	Causes muscle weakness and atrophy, activity intolerance, contractures
	Increases endurance	Decreases range of motion
	Promotes joint mobility	Increases cardiac workload
	Increases cardiac efficiency	Causes orthostatic hypotension
	Decreases resting pulse rate and blood pressure	Increases risk of thrombus formation
	Improves circulation	Decreases lung expansion
	Increases respiratory rate	Promotes retained secretions
	Increases depth of respirations	Impairs gas exchange
	Improves gas exchange	
Nutritional/metabolic	Increases metabolic rate, appetite, energy	Decreases metabolic rate
	Improves skin tone and turgor	Causes anorexia, negative nitrogen balance, disuse osteoporosis, impaired immunity, skin breakdown, and pressure sore development
Elimination	Increases intestinal tone and motility	Decreases intestinal tone and motility
	Increases blood flow to kidneys, promoting optimal excretion of waste products	Causes constipation, urinary stasis
		Increases risk of urinary tract infection, renal calculi
		Decreases bladder tone
Sleep/rest	Improves sleep quality	Decreases sleep quality
Cognitive/perceptual	Increases vitality and well-being	Causes sensory deprivation, confusion, hallucinations, pain, and discomfort
Self-perception/ self-concept	Improves appearance, body image, self-concept	Impairs appearance, body image, self-concept
Roles and relationships	Fosters relationships if exercise done in groups	Interferes with roles requiring mobility (e.g., going to work, caring for child)
Coping/stress	Reduces stress	Increases stress
		Produces anxiety, anger, depression, powerlessness
Sexuality	Increases energy available for sexual expression	Can hinder normal sexual expression
		Immobilizing devices may interfere

Endurance (the ability to tolerate activity) decreases as the muscle atrophies. In many cases, a vicious cycle ensues. Decreased endurance can discourage the client from engaging in activity, which contributes to further atrophy.

Contractures and Joint Pain. In the active, mobile person, movement promotes the formation of new connective tissue deposited around joints and muscles. This tissue is loose and pliable and remains so as long as normal body movement occurs. During immobility, stretching of muscles and movement of joints cease; this results in the deposition of denser, less pliable fibrotic tissue, and renders joints fixed and unable to move normally.

A contracture (progressive shortening of a muscle and loss of joint mobility) results from fibrotic changes that occur

when normal mobility is not maintained. Impaired blood flow to the muscle or joint hastens the formation of contractures. Without appropriate intervention, increasing damage occurs, and a contracture can become irreversible. An irreversible contracture further decreases the person's mobility because it makes moving the involved muscle difficult or impossible. Contractures also cause disfigurement, which can increase social isolation. Research is inconclusive as to the value of positioning as an effective nursing intervention for the care of contractures (Atwood, 1999; Fox, Richardson, McInnes, Tait, & Bedard, 2000). Some research suggests that the use of splints is effective in treating contractures (Seebeck, 2000).

Flexion contractures are most common in immobilized clients. Clients may assume positions of flexion naturally because these positions require less muscle stress and tension to maintain. Also, flexor muscles (those that allow joints to bend) are usually stronger than their extensor counterparts. Common flexor contractures occur at the joints of the elbow, hip, knee, shoulder, wrist, and ankle. **Foot drop** is a contracture in which the foot is fixed in plantar flexion. A footboard is used to maintain dorsiflexion and tendon flexibility. A nurse should position the patient's feet so they rest firmly against the footboard (Ludwig, 1995).

Immobility can decrease joint stability as a result of decreased tension exerted by ligaments and muscles secondary to loss of muscle tone. Decreased joint stability is thought to cause the aches and pains that immobilized clients often experience. It also may account for the difficulty ambulating and general stiffness that follow inactivity and bed rest.

Increased Cardiac Workload.

Cardiac workload is increased in the immobilized client because the heart must work harder when the body is supine than when it is erect. Pooling of blood in the legs usually does not occur in the supine position. With less gravitational pull, blood can be redistributed from the legs to the trunk. This subsequent increase in venous blood returning to the heart means the heart must work harder to circulate the increased volume. The heart rate also increases in the immobilized client to accommodate the greater amount of blood that must be pumped.

Orthostatic Hypotension.

Orthostatic hypotension is the decreased ability to maintain systemic blood pressure when changing from a supine to an upright position (see Chapter 25). It is commonly seen after a period of immobility. Position changes do not normally cause systemic blood pressure to drop substantially because arteriolar vasoconstriction prevents large amounts of blood from pooling in the extremities when the person assumes an upright posture. Baroreceptors are stimulated when blood flow decreases in the aortic arch and carotid arteries (when, for instance, the person stands up). This, in turn, triggers increased sympathetic activity, which causes vasoconstriction.

Immobility decreases the effectiveness of this neurovascular reflex. During inactivity, the body's regulatory adjustments are not used and become inactive. Sympathetic stimulation may still occur in response to standing upright, but peripheral vessels do not respond to this stimulation. Therefore, vasoconstriction does not occur, and a drop in blood pressure results.

Another factor that may contribute to orthostatic hypotension is the ineffectiveness of the muscle pump in promoting venous return. This is especially true of muscles atrophied by immobility. As the calf muscles weaken, they are less effective in compressing the leg veins and less able to promote venous return. Blood pooling in the legs increases, which intensifies postural hypotension.

Thrombus Formation and Embolism.

A thrombus is a blood clot, which is composed of platelets, fibrin, and cellular elements, that attaches to the wall of an artery or vein. A thrombus most commonly originates in the large veins of the legs because of the leg's relatively low velocity of blood flow. This condition is called **deep vein thrombosis** (DVT). Embolus is when the clot breaks away from the vessel wall and enters circulating blood. The clot lodges in the circulatory system as the blood vessel diameter decreases. This most commonly occurs when the thrombus enters the pulmonary vasculature, where it interferes with blood flow to the lung (a pulmonary embolus). Large pulmonary emboli can cause immediate death, but small emboli may produce no clinical symptoms.

Immobility promotes venous stasis, which contributes to the development of DVT. When leg muscles are inactive, venous return to the heart decreases; with time the gravitational effect of the supine position results in the redistribution of body fluids with a net decrease in venous return. The vein's numerous bifurcations and valves are thought to promote further stasis. Poor positioning can cause external pressure on blood vessels, which also contributes to inadequate blood flow and promotes development of thrombi.

Hypercoagulability does not directly result from immobility, but sometimes immobilized clients become dehydrated, which can increase blood viscosity. Dehydration may partly result from the client's inability to obtain fluids without assistance. Use of heparin prophylactically has been shown to decrease incidence of DVTs in the immobile patient (Cook, Attia, Weaver, McDonald, Meade, & Crowther, 2000).

Decreased Lung Expansion.

The immobilized client experiences greater-than-normal resistance to breathing, resulting in underinflation of the lungs and increased work of breathing.

The healthy person keeps the lungs well inflated with practically no effort. In an upright position, the diaphragm can move up and down freely. An efficient mechanism known as the mucociliary escalator keeps airways cleared of mucous secretions. Periodic sighing and coughing help to keep even the smallest air sacs (alveoli) open and available for gas exchange. Finally, ordinary activity produces enough carbon dioxide to stimulate a smooth, effective breathing pattern.

The immobile client, however, breathes less deeply and with greater effort. The supine client must overcome two resistances that do not ordinarily work against breathing. First, the diaphragm is prohibited from free movement by the abdominal organs, which shift against the diaphragm when the client lies down. To achieve full lung expansion, the client's diaphragm must push the organs out of the way with each breath. Second, the pressure of the bed against the chest wall limits the client's chest movement. Together, these factors result in diminished depth of breathing. Because the immobilized client's activity level is less than normal, less carbon dioxide is produced. This results in a lower level of stimulation for breathing, causing further reduction of tidal volume.

Decreased depth of breathing can result in the collapse of alveoli, which, in turn, hinders the exchange of oxygen and carbon dioxide. This condition of alveolar collapse is known as atelectasis. In addition to limiting the lungs' ability to exchange gases, atelectasis predisposes the client to pneumonia. The client's ability to cough deeply is often limited; thus mucus may become trapped in the lung, which provides a rich medium for microbial growth.

Nutrition and Metabolism

Decreased Metabolic Rate. The basal metabolic rate decreases during immobility. Severely restricted activity affects the production amount and pattern of thyroid hormone, adrenocorticotropic hormone, aldosterone, and insulin. It also alters drug metabolism. Weight loss is thought to result from loss of muscle mass and diuresis.

Negative Nitrogen Balance. In an active person, a balance exists between protein breakdown and protein synthesis. However, immobility raises the rate of protein breakdown probably because of muscle atrophy. One way to monitor this process is to measure nitrogen, which is excreted in urine as a waste product of protein breakdown. Elevated urine nitrogen levels occur in most immobilized clients. A negative nitrogen balance results when nitrogen excretion exceeds dietary intake. In such cases, the body lacks adequate nitrogen for protein synthesis, which results in nutritional depletion; this, in turn, interferes with wound healing and restoring muscle mass when mobility resumes. More insulin is required during immobility to maintain normal blood glucose levels. Insulin resistance also occurs, which contributes to negative nitrogen balance (Porth, 1998).

Immobilized clients often have concomitant factors that further deplete nitrogen such as trauma, burns, surgery, coma, cancer, fever, or infection. Clients with chronic illness or poor nutritional balance before immobilization are at increased risk for negative nitrogen balance.

Anorexia. Anorexia (loss of appetite) is common in immobilized clients. Decreased metabolic rate is accompanied by decreased caloric need. Moreover, if the client is confined to a healthcare facility, the institutional food, eating in a supine position, environmental factors, and psychological state can inhibit the appetite.

Disuse Osteoporosis. In disuse osteoporosis, bone demineralization occurs secondary to immobility. The bone matrix is always in a dynamic state of formation and destruction. Osteoblastic cells are responsible for the proliferation of bone matrix. In contrast, osteoclastic cells destroy bone matrix by absorbing and removing osseous tissue from the bone. Immobility results in an imbalance between osteoblastic and osteoclastic activity because normal stress and strain imposed on bone through movement are an important part of osteoblastic processes. In the immobilized client, osteoblasts continue to lay down bony matrix but osteoclasts break down bone faster than osteoblasts can build it. The result is a loss of bony matrix. Disuse osteoporosis results in bones that are more porous, brittle, and susceptible to fractures.

Impaired Immunity. The immune system is weakened during immobility. Catabolism of immunoglobulin G doubles, significantly decreasing the normal concentration of circulating antibodies. Leukocytes are less able to engulf and destroy microorganisms. Lymphatic transport may be decreased as well when skeletal muscles are inactive.

Pressure Ulcers. Pressure ulcers form when pressure exerted over an area of skin or subcutaneous tissue exceeds the pressure required for adequate blood flow to the area. Cells die because they do not receive oxygen and nutrients and because waste products accumulate. Pressure is usually concentrated on bony prominences but can occur anywhere pressure is great. In the supine position, pressure is greatest over the back of the skull and at the elbows, sacrum, ischial tuberosities, and heels. In the sitting position, the greatest pressure is at the ischial tuberosities and the sacrum.

Reactive hyperemia is a compensatory mechanism that responds to inadequate blood flow. When pressure is removed, blood floods the area in an attempt to prevent tissue necrosis. Reactive hyperemia is only effective if it occurs before cellular damage occurs. The critical time varies from one person to another. Usually the normal person can sense pressure buildup and can change position to reduce discomfort. The client with impaired mobility, such as a person with neurologic impairment, may be incapable of movement or unable to sense the need to change positions.

Healing of pressure sores is difficult and slow especially in the immobilized client. Pressure sores can prolong immobility and increase the cost and length of confinement. See Chapter 38 for more information.

Elimination

Urinary Stasis. The immobilized client may not heed the urge to void. Clients in institutional settings may not want to bother the nurse by asking for a bedpan. Some clients try to void when they feel the need but have difficulty relaxing the perineal muscles when in the supine position. Delaying micturition causes urine to collect in the bladder. Chronic delay can lead to overstretching the detrusor muscle in the bladder wall, permanent changes in bladder tone, and long-term consequences for normal voiding patterns.

Urinary retention poses significant problems for the immobilized client. One problem, urinary stasis, contributes to urinary tract infections and renal calculi. Bladder distention, another problem, leads to overflow incontinence, which is embarrassing for the client and can contribute to skin breakdown.

Urinary Tract Infection. Stagnant urine makes a good medium for bacterial growth. Bladder distention can cause small tears in the delicate bladder mucosa, which contribute to the incidence of urinary tract infection. When the client experiences distention, catheterization may be necessary to empty the bladder. With any type of catheterization comes the risk of introducing pathogens and infection into the body.

Renal Calculi. Urinary stasis and an increased serum calcium level promote the formation of renal calculi (kidney stones). As serum calcium levels rise (the result of calcium loss from the bones), the kidney excretes more calcium. This raises urinary calcium levels. Because calcium can precipitate from solution to form crystals and because stagnant urine encourages the aggregation of crystals, renal calculi pose a significant problem. Dehydration, common in the immobilized client, also increases the incidence of calculi formation. Additionally, some urinary infections make the urine more alkaline, which also promotes calculi development.

Constipation. Even in a healthy person, dietary changes, activity variations, and emotional stress affect normal bowel patterns. The immobilized client faces additional changes. Abdominal and perineal muscles can be weakened by muscle atrophy, making it more difficult for the client to bear down and exert pressure to evacuate stool. As stool descends against the rectum, the person feels the stimulus to defecate. In an upright posture, stool descends more quickly into the rectal area, eliciting a strong stimulus. In the supine position, rectal filling is slow, which weakens the stimulus for defecation.

The defecation reflex also can be affected if the person postpones defecation after recognizing the stimulus to defecate. This happens frequently in the immobilized client, who may feel embarrassed or may need assistance to use a bedpan. When a person delays defecation, the intestine absorbs more water from the feces, making stool passage even more difficult. Dehydration, common in the immobile client, also can contribute to constipation. The result may be fecal impaction (hard stool in the rectum that cannot be removed naturally by defecation). Often, liquid stool seeps around the obstruction formed by the impaction.

Sleep and Rest
Immobility can interfere with normal sleep patterns. Normal activity, especially physical work, and aerobic exercise produce a sense of fatigue that helps the person fall asleep and obtain restful sleep. The immobilized client may doze frequently during the day, which disrupts normal nighttime sleep patterns. The immobilized client may need to be awakened frequently to be turned, monitored, or given treatments and medications. Such wakings, especially when numerous, impair the quality of sleep. In addition, the immobilized client may sleep in an unfamiliar, noisy environment and may have stressful health concerns that further reduce the amount and quality of sleep.

Cognition and Perception
Because immobility decreases the freedom to interact normally with the environment, the client receives less sensory information. Preoccupation with somatic complaints, difficulty with time perception, difficulty with understanding and following directions, crying, and other emotional outbursts can occur. Confusion is common but reversible if normal sensory input returns. In severe cases, sensory deprivation can occur, causing the client to experience visual and auditory hallucinations.

Pain may result from physiologic changes that occur with immobility. Joint stiffness, pneumonia, pressure ulcers, thrombosis, and emboli can contribute to discomfort. The perception of pain also may intensify because focusing on discomfort is more common when diversions are limited.

Self-Perception and Self-Concept
Changes in self-perception and self-concept commonly accompany functional motor impairment or immobility. Immobility contributes to a feeling of powerlessness especially when the client must depend on others. Motor impairment can alter body image especially if the impairment results from loss of a body part. Self-concept is altered when the client must depend on devices such as crutches, wheelchairs, or walkers. Problems with coordination can cause embarrassment (e.g., the client may worry about appearing awkward or even intoxicated). Altered body image can negatively impact self-esteem and can lead to a feeling of lowered self-worth.

Roles and Relationships
Immobility affects role function for many people. For children and adolescents, it disrupts school and social activities (Fig. 33-3). For adults, immobility may interfere with the ability to work, resulting in temporary or permanent unemployment with corresponding financial stress. Immobility also disrupts various parental or spousal activities. Child care may be impossible when a parent is hospitalized or immobilized at home.

Coping and Stress Tolerance
Loss of mobility is not something the client chooses or desires. With trauma, the loss occurs suddenly. In some cases, the loss is permanent and requires the client to adapt to different functional abilities. Despite supportive social inter-

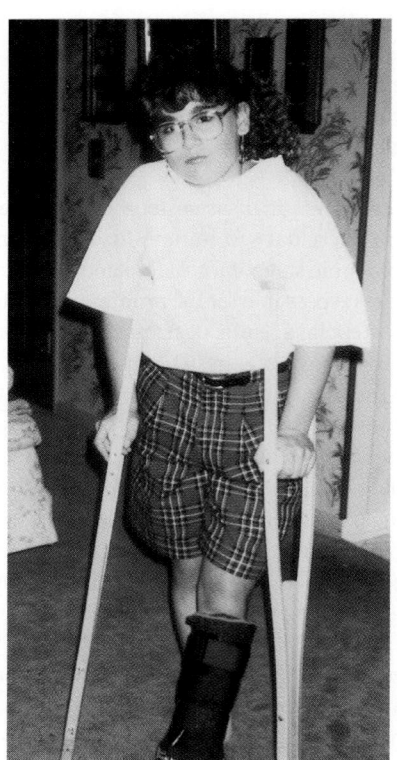

FIGURE 33-3 A broken leg can seem very significant to an adolescent when school and social activities are disrupted.

actions with family and friends, immobilized clients may spend many hours alone and can be bored or lonely. Depression, anger, and anxiety are common.

Clients who experience stress due to immobility exhibit various behaviors. Some withdraw, limiting social contact even further. Some complain and become demanding. The client who constantly requests assistance may be responding negatively to the stress of immobility.

Sexuality

Mobility limitations may affect sexual feelings and activities. Lack of privacy, depression, fatigue, and physical limitations can contribute to decreased sexual function. Immobility may impede grooming activities that are often important in maintaining sexual identity. For some clients with long-term motor impairments such as paraplegia, sexual function may be permanently altered, so the client needs to learn new methods of sexual expression.

Impact on Activities of Daily Living

Impaired mobility can severely restrict the client's ability to perform normal daily activities either temporarily or permanently. Coordination and muscle strength are necessary for eating, dressing, and grooming. Usually the nurse can show the client ways to function successfully and independently despite physical limitations. Setting short-term, achievable goals and developing a long-range plan in collaboration with the healthcare team (e.g., physician, physical therapist, occupational therapist, psychologist, social worker) usually achieve the best results. For example, ambulatory physical therapy sessions may help the client with mobility problems regain function and independence (Fig. 33-4).

Because hygiene and self-care activities are a personal matter, most clients may find it stressful to depend on family members or nursing personnel for this care. Clients who can perform some care independently may report doing so to be

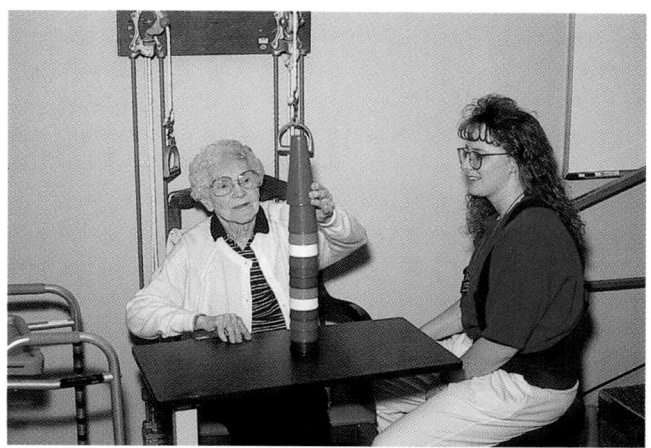

FIGURE 33-4 Outpatient physical therapy sessions can help an older person remain independent as mobility improves after a cerebral vascular accident (stroke).

physically taxing. Sometimes fatigue and lack of endurance limit performance of self-care tasks.

Impaired mobility affects other daily activities as well. Performing housework, driving a car, buying groceries, and paying bills may be difficult; social activities may be curtailed; and participation in athletic or exercise programs may be impossible.

Whether temporary or permanent, mobility problems affect the family members. A spouse who breaks a leg skiing may need to be in a long leg cast for several weeks. This may interfere with job-related tasks and the ability to perform tasks at home. Inability to drive a car or board a bus limits independence, so the more mobile spouse (or other family members) will assume additional responsibilities. Many mobility problems are chronic and progressive, especially in older adults. In such cases, family members in caretaker roles may feel excessively burdened. Full-time, 24-hour care of a bedridden client in the home is an exhausting experience even for a few days. With chronic impairment, such care is required for months or years. Adequate support of the primary caregiver, either from other family members, friends, or community agencies, is significant in enabling the immobilized client to remain in the home. Clients without an adequate support system or those who need special care (e.g., quadriplegic clients) may need to employ a caregiver or consider seeking care in an intermediate or long-term care facility.

ASSESSMENT

Assessment data help identify the client's normal mobility, risk factors for potential alterations in mobility, actual mobility impairments, and management techniques or devices the client uses.

Subjective Data

Normal Pattern Identification

First, determine the client's normal activity pattern. Have the client describe his or her ability to move normally and perform ADLs. A rating scale may be useful for documenting the client's independence, partial independence, and complete dependence in various activities involving mobility such as ambulation, toileting, dressing, bathing, and household chores. Ask the client to describe any recent change in mobility or activity level. Determine the client's normal patterns of exercise and leisure. If the client actively engages in aerobic exercise, determine the frequency and appropriateness of the activity.

Discuss the client's lifestyle. Some people enjoy sedentary activities and work at sedentary jobs. Others work at jobs that require vigorous physical exertion and take part in sports and physical activities. People who grew up in a family that valued quiet activities commonly carry the pattern of inactivity into adulthood. Assess the client's satisfaction with his or her current activity level, and note any desire on the client's part to change the activity pattern.

(text continues on page 776)

COLLABORATIVE CARE PLAN

Critical Pathway (Home Health)

Total Hip Replacement

Client Name: _____

Case Type: Ttl Hip Rplcmnt   (THR)

Expected LOS: 2 wks po–2 mo

DRG: _____   Date Path
Initiated: _____

Actual LOS: _____

ICD-9: _____

Discharge Date: _____

Physician: _____

Case Manager: _____

Home Health—Outcome Criteria

Client Problems	Post Hospital 2 wk	D	E	N	Post Hospital 6 wk	D	E	N	Post Hospital 3 mo	D	E	N
Deficient Knowledge related to postop activity & exercise regimen & hip precaution	Client/family will verbalize understanding of exercise pgm, activity progression, hip precautions, safety, medication, diet, and wound care				Client/family will state S & S of complications of hip dislocation (sig. ↑ pain, & loss of sensation) Demonstrates safe transfers, ambulation, & chair activity				Client/family verbalizes understanding of po complications (deep vein thrombosis [DVT], hip dislocation) & when to notify health provider			
Pain related to surgical trauma, edema, muscle spasms	Rates pain <2 on scale of 0–10 after po pain med. Performs exercises & ambulation s̄ excessive hip pain (<5)				No pain or pain controlled c̄ po pain med. No significant increase in pain with exercises or ambulation				No pain at rest or with activity No significant increase in pain with exercises or ambulation			
Altered Mobility related to pain, weakness, & activity restriction	Performs isotonic/isometric exercises & ADL c̄ caregiver assistance Adheres to position limits of <80-degree hip flexion, no internal rotation or adduction Weight-bearing ambulation as ordered c̄ assistive devices (walker, crutches) Sits in reclining chair c̄ feet apart; does not cross legs.				Ambulates independently c̄/s̄ assistive devices Performs isotonic & isometric exercises independently Performs ADLs independently Returns to work & ambulates in community (no longer homebound)				Transfers & ambulates safely at home Attains PT outcomes hip flexion >110 degrees c̄ full extension–PT Dcd if outcomes achieved. Performs ADLs/household/ work tasks s̄ limitations			

High risk for injury related to falls, hip dislocation, bleeding due to anticoagulants	No injury or falls will occur / No hip dislocation (no extreme pain) / No bleeding, urine & stools neg for blood / Follows hip & safety precaution	Demonstrates safety in transfers/ambulation →	→
Critical Path			
Consult/Referral	Home PT visit 2×/wk output PT/OT (adaptive aids) / Evaluate need for home health aide / Home health RN phone call 1–2 wk PO	Home Health visit by RN/case manager for assessment/evaluation of progress / Continue outpt PT services 2–3×/wk / Office visit to orthopedic surgeon	Follow-up office visit to orthopedic surgeon 3, 6, 12 mo. / Follow-up X-rays 2 yr & 5 yr / Return to family MD / Evaluate need for PT services
Diagnostic Tests	Pro Time 2×/wk for 4–6 wk	Pro Time 1×/wk until Coumadin DC'd or 6 wks	Possible X-rays hip & pelvis
Assessment	Safety of home & mobility; hip precautions assessed by PT in home. / Neurovascular assessment (6P's); degree of flexion & mobility, status of wound, S&S of complications / Assess need for assistive devices.	Home health RN to assess NV (6P's) status in affected extremity (polar [cold] pallor, pain, pulselessness, paresthesia, paralysis) / Condition of wound, assess ROM of hip/leg, functional mobility.	Assess NV status of affected extremity, S&S of complication (hip dislocation, DVT) / Condition of wound (S&S of infection) & functional mobility
Treatment	Home PT for 2 wk / Implement prescribed exercise pgm all affected joints (isometric—or quad, gluteal sets) & isotonic (or calf pumping). / TED hose when OOB for dependent edema / Remove staples/steristrips	Outpt PT 2×/wk for 6 wk–3 mo. / Continue advancing exercises & ambulation / Home health visit by RN to evaluate compliance c̄ exercise pgm, hip precautions, functional mobility, incision, & complications. / TED hose for dependent edema—remove at night / Assess wound	Home health RN evaluate exercise/activity progression & need for further PT if functional outcome not met, or need for further physician follow-up

COLLABORATIVE CARE PLAN
Critical Pathway (Home Health) (Continued)

Client Problems	Post Hospital 2 wk	D	E	N	Post Hospital 6 wk	D	E	N	Post Hospital 3 mo	D	E	N
Activity	No abduction pillow—Use regular pillow between knees when in bed.				Continue pillow between knees when in bed				→			
	Full wt bearing on standard THR. If cementless THR, partial wt bearing & no resistive exercise c̄ assistive device (walker)				Advance activity & ambulation c̄ or s̄ assistive device (walker if needed)				Independent ambulation c̄ or s̄ assist devices (if needed for safety)			
	Sit with high chair, feet together, knees apart Reinforce exercises/ strengthening & ROM				Evaluate & advance exercises for strengthening & ROM				Continue strengthening & ROM exercises			
Diet	Diet as tol				→				→			
	Adeq. fluids & fiber to prevent constipation				→				→			
	Low calorie—avoid obesity				→				→			
Meds	Instruct client to take po analgesics before exercise & ambulation				PO pain meds PRN & before exercises & ambulation.				PO pain meds PRN			
	Assess understanding of meds & side effects											
	Instruct in bowel mgt (LOC, stool softener), anticoagulants (Coumadin)				Stool softener as needed DC anticoagulant at 6 wk				→			

Teaching	Teach position limits <80-degree hip flexion	Reinforce hip & safety precaution	→
	No internal rotation or adduction for 6 wk po	Bleeding precaution with Coumadin	Instruct client in need for antibiotics before dental work, invasive procedures, or surgery
	No crossing legs for 3 mo. Reinforce exercises	Reinforce home exercise pgm—gradually increase strengthening & ROM & progress with ambulation	→
	Reinforce safety precautions (handles, grab bars, raised toilet seat, high chair, no throw rugs)		
Discharge/ Transfer Planning	Reinforce need for keeping appts c̄ PT/OT.	Evaluate whether PT outcomes met & need to continue to 3 mo.	DC from PT if functional outcomes met
	Instruct in resources for assistive/adaptive devices	Continue exercises & activity progression	Return to family MD for further follow-up care.
	Provide information on community resources (Meals on Wheels, home health aide)	Reinforce need for continued safety precautions	

* Variance reporting: Write initials of nurse/health provider in box if outcome met or intervention performed. Write "V" for variance if outcome not met or intervention not performed. Explain client variance in progress notes.

Initials/Signatures: Shift: D = Day

       E = Evening

       N = Night

_____

_____

_____

Risk Identification

Interviewing the client also can help the nurse identify risk factors that can contribute to impaired mobility. For example, inadequate aerobic activity may increase the risks for chronic disease and deconditioning. Determine if the client feels weak or fatigued after routine exercise and activity. Ask the client to describe any distressing symptoms (such as difficulty breathing, pain, or increased heart rate) with activity; document the degree of exercise and the degree of stress. Ask the client how long the symptoms have occurred and how long they persist after the activity ends.

Evaluate the client's risk for falls. Factors that increase this risk include decreased mobility, muscle weakness or atrophy, altered cognition, postural hypotension, and a cluttered environment. Ascertain alcohol or drug use that might impair mobility and contribute to falls. Hypotensive agents and pain medications lower blood pressure and can contribute to falls; anticonvulsants can cause ataxia; antidepressants can contribute to postural hypotension; and corticosteroids can result in muscle weakness and wasting (Hieber, 1998).

Document current or chronic health problems that may limit mobility or decrease activity tolerance. Common and notable medical conditions are respiratory disease, cardiac disease, anemia, peripheral vascular disease, arthritis, cerebrovascular accidents, multiple sclerosis, Parkinson's disease, brain tumors, head injuries, fractures, spinal cord injuries, and amputations. Evaluate the impact of medical conditions on mobility.

Dysfunction Identification

Document any inability of the client to move normally and easily. Encourage the client to explain any problems with mobility or activity tolerance and any adaptations he or she uses to promote optimal functioning at home. If the client reports any limitation in mobility, determine the extent of the problem, when it first occurred, and if the client knows the cause.

Ask the client if the mobility problem has been improving or worsening and how it affects his or her functional abilities in other areas. Document what the client can do independently so that independence within his or her capabilities can be encouraged.

Ask the client if he or she uses devices to assist with ambulation (e.g., prostheses, canes, walkers, crutches). If surgery is planned and if assistive devices will be used afterward, the client may be asked to demonstrate skills previously learned.

Perform a comprehensive functional health assessment to determine the impact of decreased mobility on all functional health areas. Note any complications resulting from limited mobility (e.g., pressure ulcers or renal calculi). To guide the assessment, review Table 33-2, which describes the effects of immobility on functional health patterns.

Discuss how impaired mobility has affected the client's roles and relationships, self-concept, self-esteem, and body image. Identify family and community support services and evaluate past and present coping strategies.

Objective Data

Physical Assessment

Physical examination findings contribute information about alignment; balance; coordination; gait; joint structure and function; muscle mass, tone, and strength; and activity tolerance. For the most part, the nurse uses the technique of inspection to visualize these qualities. When mobility appears normal, more extensive assessment techniques are usually unnecessary; if mobility is impaired, a more detailed assessment may be indicated.

Alignment. The client should maintain proper alignment while sitting and standing. When alignment is normal, an imaginary line can be drawn through the earlobe, shoulder, hip, femoral trochanter, knee, and front of the ankle. Note the symmetry of organs and bones. Normal spinal alignment is characterized by concave curvature of the cervical spine, convex curvature of the thoracic spine, and concave curvature of the lumbar spine. Extreme curvature of the spine may be abnormal. Scoliosis, a lateral deviation of the thoracic spine, can be detected by watching the client bend at the waist from a standing position. Lordosis, an abnormal concavity of the lumbar spine, and kyphosis, an exaggerated curvature of the thoracic spine, are less common spinal deviations.

Balance. Assess balance by asking the client to sit or stand with eyes closed. Observe his or her ability to maintain a normal erect posture through postural adjustments. Swaying to one side indicates an inability to maintain balance through normal physiologic mechanisms.

Coordination. Watching the client perform normal activities, including ambulation, allows the nurse to evaluate the coordination of movement. Look for fluid, well-controlled movement. The client should be able to initiate the desired movement quickly without hesitation. Assess fine motor skills by asking the client to perform a simple skill such as unbuttoning a shirt or signing papers.

Gait. To evaluate a client's gait, watch the client walk. Normal gait should be rhythmic and even; the stride should be symmetric with full extension. The head should remain erect and the knees and feet should point forward. Arms should swing alternately with leg movements. The full body weight should be easily supported. For more information about gait, observe the client's shoes to detect patterns of wear.

Joint Structure and Function. Observation and palpation can detect redness, swelling, or warmth around the joint. Listen for a crunching or grating sound (crepitus), which can occur when bones rub against one another during movement because of inadequate protection or insufficient joint lubrication. Observe the client's facial expression and nonverbal signs of discomfort during movement. If observation discloses stiffness or guarding during certain body movements, evaluate joint mobility by moving the involved joint through its full ROM (see Table 33-1). When doing this, note the

THERAPEUTIC DIALOGUE
Mobility

Scene for Thought

Jeannette Frost is a 73-year-old woman who has suffered shoulder problems during the last year and who had a surgical repair of her right shoulder 6 months ago. She comes to the clinic for assessment of her ROM and pain in the affected shoulder. She drove herself to the clinic.

Less Effective

Nurse: Hello, Mrs. Frost. I'm Nancy Robertson, the nurse practitioner you'll be seeing today. How are you? *(Looks at the chart.)*
Client: Fine. *(She sits quietly and doesn't smile.)*
Nurse: *(Sits down at the desk and pays attention.)* What can I help you with today?
Client: I want to see how much more I can do with my arm. I can only raise it this high. *(Demonstrates, using her left arm to help the right. Looks serious.)*
Nurse: You're concerned about that arm. *(Uses good eye contact.)*
Client: Yes. I live alone.
Nurse: I see that your husband is listed as your emergency contact, but he has a different address. *(Looks through the chart and then at the client questioningly.)*
Client: Yes. I live by myself. *(Looks embarrassed and annoyed.)*
Nurse: *(Realizes this is not a safe subject.)* Well, I can understand you're concerned about doing your housework and cooking and so forth. Let me examine your shoulder and see how much more you might be able to do with your arm. *(Assesses range of motion and discusses swimming and physical therapy that Mrs. Frost is already doing and how they're helping to maintain her current functioning.)* It seems that this is as good as this shoulder's going to get, Mrs. Frost. But it sounds as though you're doing everything you can to keep it in good shape, so I wouldn't worry if I were you. If it gets any worse, feel free to call me, and we'll go over it again. Okay?
Client: *(Gets dressed.)* Fine. *(No eye contact.)*
Nurse: 'Bye now.

More Effective

Nurse: Hello, Mrs. Frost. I'm Natalie Richmond, the nurse practitioner you'll be seeing today. How are you? *(Looks at the chart.)*
Client: Fine. *(She sits quietly and doesn't smile.)*
Nurse: *(Sits down at the desk and pays attention.)* What can I help you with today?
Client: I want to see how much more I can do with my arm. I can only raise it this high. *(Demonstrates, using her left arm to help the right. Looks serious.)*
Nurse: You're concerned about that arm. *(Uses good eye contact.)*
Client: Yes. I live alone.
Nurse: You live alone, and you're worried you won't be able to manage with your arm the way it is? Am I getting that right? *(Maintains good eye contact.)*
Client: No, I can manage the way it is. I don't want it to get worse. *(Looks more serious.)*
Nurse: I can see how concerned you are. I'd like to examine your shoulder and ask you a few questions, then we can talk about the answers to your questions. Does that sound OK?
Client: Yes, that will be fine. *(After the assessment, Natalie discusses swimming and physical therapy that Mrs. Frost is doing and how they're helping to maintain the ROM in her shoulder.)*
Nurse: It seems that the exercises you're doing are keeping your shoulder in the shape it is now. If you stop the exercises, you risk losing motion, and it will be harder for you to do your cooking, housework, and entertaining. Otherwise, you're doing a good job. *(Pause.)* Is there something you want to say?
Client: No, I think you answered everything I had on my mind. *(Pause.)* Could I come back and see you again so you can check to see that the shoulder is still OK?
Nurse: Certainly. You can call me, too. Here's my card.
Client: Thank you very much. *(Smiles.)*

Critical Thinking Challenge
- Compare and contrast Nancy's and Natalie's actions and assessment styles.
- Analyze how Nancy talked to Mrs. Frost.
- Recognize the emotions Mrs. Frost exhibited, and infer emotions from her nonverbal behavior.
- Determine how you might feel working with a client who is reserved and does not show emotions readily.
- Formulate some helpful skills that could be used when working with Mrs. Frost.

amount of resistance encountered and whether or not the client complains of discomfort. Compare the right and left sides for symmetry (Hieber, 1998).

Muscle Mass, Tone, and Strength. Normal muscle mass, tone, and strength can vary greatly among individuals. Athletes may have bulging, well-defined muscles and great strength and endurance. Older adults may have weak, small muscles with little tone. Increased strength and tone are usually found on the person's dominant side.

Assess muscle strength by evaluating the client's ability to perform activities of self-care such as feeding, dressing, toileting, and grooming. Estimate strength and coordination by observing the ease with which the client performs these tasks. Evaluate the strength of specific muscle groups by asking the client to grip your hand or to use certain muscle groups to push against resistance.

Muscle size in the arms and legs is determined by observation and by comparing measurements. A decrease in circumference in the affected limb usually reflects muscle atrophy from immobility. Atrophy indicates a loss of muscle tone, which decreases endurance.

Postural Blood Pressure. To help determine if a client can safely ambulate, measure postural blood pressure (see Chapter 25 for instructions). A significant drop in blood pressure when the client changes from a supine to a sitting position suggests a risk for falls. Complaints of dizziness, lightheadedness, diaphoresis, and tachycardia may accompany orthostatic hypotension and are indications that fainting may occur if ambulation continues.

Risk for Falls. Determine whether or not independent ambulation is safe. Some healthcare facilities list risk factors contributing to falls and ask the nurse to calculate a score to determine clients at greatest risk (for more information, see Chapter 30). Risk factors include the following:

- Advanced age (especially older than 70 years)
- Visual impairment
- History of falls
- History of dizziness, postural hypotension, or syncope
- Cognitive impairments such as confusion
- Use of drugs or alcohol that can impair balance, coordination, or cognitive abilities
- Incontinence
- Muscle atrophy or weakness

Activity Tolerance. In assessing activity tolerance, observe the client before, during, and after activity to detect abnormal responses. The most common parameters measured are the pulse rate and the respiratory rate. Normally, both increase during activity. Resting vital signs should be within a normal range before activity starts. If activity begins when the client is experiencing hypotension, tachycardia, or tachypnea (rapid, irregular breathing), he or she has little energy in reserve to meet the body's increased need for oxygen during exercise.

When activity resumes after bed rest or the level of prescribed activity increases, observe the client carefully for signs of distress such as dyspnea, diaphoresis, or dizziness. In high-risk clients, such as those with cardiac or respiratory conditions, the nurse may be directed to monitor pulse, respiratory rate, or oxygen saturation during activity and to discontinue the activity if values are outside the prescribed range. After activity, pulse and respiratory rates should return to preactivity baseline values within 3 minutes.

Diagnostic Tests and Procedures
Common diagnostic tests used to evaluate musculoskeletal function are radiographic studies and direct visualization of joints. Laboratory values, such as hemoglobin and hematocrit, may be helpful when assessing activity tolerance.

Radiographic Studies. X-rays are useful in differentiating traumatic injuries such as sprains, dislocations, and fractures. X-rays also help assess the demineralization of bone that occurs in osteoporosis. Radiographic studies using injected, radiopaque dye can help evaluate problems with the spine or joints.

Defects are revealed by an abnormal pattern of dye distribution in the body part. Arthrograms permit visualization of joints and are often used to diagnose tears in ligaments or cartilage. Myelograms rely on radiopaque dye to highlight the spinal column to detect ruptured vertebral disks or other structural defects.

Arthroscopy. **Arthroscopy** is the examination of a joint with a fiberoptic instrument to diagnose abnormalities. Minor corrective surgery also can be performed to remove torn cartilage or repair torn ligaments.

Hematologic Studies. Hemoglobin and hematocrit values can be used to evaluate the client's reserve for activity. Clients with low hemoglobin values have difficulty transporting adequate oxygen to body tissues. Activity expectations may need to be modified for clients with hemoglobin values of less than 10 g/dL. Low hematocrit values often reflect blood loss or inadequate volume replacement. When clients have low hematocrit values, they are likely to experience postural hypotension and activity intolerance.

NURSING DIAGNOSES

North American Nursing Diagnosis Association (NANDA, 2001) diagnoses that relate to mobility are Impaired Physical Mobility, Impaired Walking, Impaired Wheelchair Mobility, Impaired Transfer Ability, Impaired Bed Mobility, Activity Intolerance, and Risk for Disuse Syndrome.

Diagnostic Statement: Impaired Physical Mobility

Definition. Impaired physical mobility is a state in which the person experiences a limitation in independent, purposeful physical movement of the body or one or more extremities (NANDA, 2001).

Defining Characteristics. Defining characteristics include postural instability during performance of routine ADLs, limited ability to perform gross or fine motor skills, uncoordinated or jerky movements, limited ROM, difficulty turning, decreased reaction time, movement-induced shortness of breath, gait changes, substitutions for movement, slowed movement, and movement-induced tremor (NANDA, 2001).

Related Factors. Related factors include medications, prescribed movement restrictions, pain or discomfort, intolerance to activity or decreased strength and endurance, pain or discomfort, perceptual/cognitive impairment, neuromuscular impairment, musculoskeletal impairment, depression or severe anxiety, lack of knowledge regarding value of physical activity, body mass index above 75th age-appropriate percentile, reluctance to initiate movement, sedentary lifestyle, selective or generalized malnutrition, loss of integrity of bone structures, developmental delay, joint stiffness or contractures, limited cardiovascular endurance, altered cellular metabolism, lack of physical or social environmental support, and cultural beliefs regarding age appropriate activity (NANDA, 2001).

Diagnostic Statement: Impaired Walking

Definition. Impaired walking is a state in which the person experiences limited independent movement within the environment on foot (NANDA, 2001).

Defining Characteristics. Defining characteristics include impaired ability to climb stairs, to walk required distances, to walk on an incline or decline, to walk on uneven surfaces, and/or to navigate curbs (NANDA, 2001).

Related Factors. NANDA has not yet developed related factors for this diagnosis.

Diagnostic Statement: Impaired Wheelchair Mobility

Definition. Impaired wheelchair mobility is a state in which the person experiences limitation in independent operation of a wheelchair within the environment (NANDA, 2001).

Defining Characteristics. Defining characteristics include the impaired ability to operate a manual or power wheelchair on an even or uneven surface, on an incline or decline, and/or on curbs (NANDA, 2001).

Related Factors. NANDA has not yet developed related factors for this diagnosis.

Diagnostic Statement: Impaired Transfer Ability

Definition. Impaired transfer ability is a state in which the person experiences limitation of independent movement between two nearby surfaces (NANDA, 2001).

Defining Characteristics. Defining characteristics include the impaired ability to transfer in any of the following situations: from bed to chair or chair to bed; on or off a toilet/commode; in and out of tub/shower; between uneven levels; from chair to car or car to chair; from chair to floor or floor to chair; from standing to floor or floor to standing (NANDA, 2001).

Related Factors. NANDA has not yet developed related factors for this diagnosis.

Diagnostic Statement: Impaired Bed Mobility

Definition. Impaired bed mobility is a state in which the person experiences limitation of independent movement from one bed position to another (NANDA, 2001).

Defining Characteristics. Defining characteristics include impaired ability in any of the following situations: to turn side to side, to move from supine to sitting or sitting to supine, to reposition oneself in bed, to move from supine to prone or prone to supine, to move from supine to long sitting or long sitting to supine (NANDA, 2001).

Related Factors. NANDA has not yet developed related factors for this diagnosis.

Diagnostic Statement: Activity Intolerance

Definition. Activity intolerance is a state in which a person has insufficient physiologic or psychological energy to endure or complete required or desired daily activities (NANDA, 2001).

Defining Characteristics. Defining characteristics include verbal report of fatigue or weakness, abnormal heart rate or blood pressure response to activity, exertional discomfort or dyspnea, electrocardiographic changes reflecting arrhythmias or ischemia (NANDA, 2001).

Related Factors. Related factors include bed rest or immobility, generalized weakness, sedentary lifestyle, and imbalance between oxygen supply and demand (NANDA, 2001).

Diagnostic Statement: Risk for Disuse Syndrome

Definition. Risk for disuse syndrome is a state in which a person is at risk for deterioration of body systems as the result of prescribed or unavoidable musculoskeletal inactivity (NANDA, 2001).

Risk Factors. Risk factors include paralysis, mechanical immobilization, prescribed immobilization, severe pain, altered level of consciousness (NANDA, 2001). Complications from immobility can include pressure ulcers, constipation, stasis of pulmonary secretions, thrombosis, urinary tract infection or retention, decreased strength and endurance, orthostatic hypotension, decreased range of joint motion, disorientation, body image disturbance, and powerlessness (NANDA, 2001).

Related Nursing Diagnoses

Lack of normal movement affects all areas of function. The client with a nursing diagnosis of Impaired Physical Activity or Activity Intolerance is usually at risk for many other problems. Self-Care Deficits in Bathing/Hygiene, Feeding, Dressing/Grooming, Toileting are common because these tasks require normal movement and coordination. The disruption of various body systems can result in Impaired Skin Integrity, Risk for Infection, Urinary Retention, Constipation, Imbalanced Nutrition: Less Than Body Requirements, Impaired Gas Exchange, or Ineffective Airway Clearance. Risk for Injury is greater because the risk for falls increases with impaired mobility. Disturbed Sensory Perception can occur, and Pain may increase. Sexual Dysfunction may be an appropriate diagnosis if spontaneous, normal movement is limited and results in a negative change in sexual expression.

Because mobility directly relates to a person's sense of independence, decreased mobility affects personal feelings. Disturbed Body Image, Situational or Chronic Low Self-Esteem, Anxiety, and Powerlessness can occur when normal movement is impaired. Ineffective Role Performance results because some responsibilities as a spouse, parent, or employee may require normal movement. Social Isolation and Impaired Verbal Communication can occur when the client withdraws from social interaction. Ineffective Coping often results from the stress imposed by altered mobility or the need to adjust to permanent disability.

OUTCOME IDENTIFICATION AND PLANNING

After nursing diagnoses and related factors have been identified, the nurse, client, and family plan interventions and

PLANNING: Examples of NIC/NOC Interventions

Accepted Mobility and Body Mechanics Nursing Interventions Classification (NIC)
Activity Therapy
Body Mechanics Promotion
Energy Management
Exercise Promotion
Exercise Therapy: Ambulation
Exercise Therapy: Balance
Exercise Therapy: Joint Mobility
Exercise Therapy: Muscle Control
Fall Prevention
Positioning
Positioning: Wheelchair
Traction/Immobilization Care
Tracking: Prescribed Activity/Exercise

Accepted Mobility and Body Mechanics Nursing Outcomes Classification (NOC)
Ambulation: Walking
Ambulation: Wheelchair
Balance
Body Positioning: Self-Initiated
Endurance
Immobility Consequences: Physiological
Immobility Consequences: Psycho-Cognitive
Joint Movement: Active
Joint Movement: Passive
Knowledge: Prescribed Activity
Mobility Level
Muscle Function
Self Care: Activities of Daily Living
Sensory Function: Proprioception
Transfer Performance

Refer to the following for specifics regarding NIC/NOC:
  McCloskey, J., & Bulechek, G. (2000). *Iowa intervention project: Nursing interventions classification* (NIC) (3rd ed.). St. Louis, MO: Mosby.
  Johnson, M., & Maas, M. (2000). *Iowa outcomes project: Nursing outcomes classification* (NOC) (2nd ed.). St. Louis, MO: Mosby.

expected outcomes. The accompanying display summarizes some interventions that are used in problems with mobility.
General goals for clients with impaired mobility might include the following:

- Client will increase endurance and tolerance for physical activity.
- Client will participate actively in prescribed therapies to promote optimal healing and restoration of mobility.
- Client will participate in measures to prevent potential complications of immobility.
- Client will maintain optimal function despite mobility restrictions.

IMPLEMENTATION
Health Promotion
Physical Fitness Promotion

In the United States, machines have reduced the need for physical labor, which has led many people into sedentary lifestyles. This activity decrease has been implicated in the rising incidence of many diseases. Recently, however, the benefits of physical fitness have become more appreciated, spurring many people to walk, jog, and participate in exercise programs. Health clubs are available in most communities, and some employers are incorporating gymnasiums into the workplace for after-hour use. Nonetheless, a relatively small percentage of the population is physically fit. Exercise rates among older adults remain especially low. Research suggests that an older person's perception of how integrated exercise is in daily activities impacts adherence to regular exercise (Conn, 1998). Research is quite conclusive that regular exercise improves the quality of life for older adults (Ellingson & Conn, 2000).

Nurses are frequently in a position to promote physical fitness. By stressing the importance of exercise for physical and emotional health, they help prevent mobility problems. Physical fitness teaching opportunities occur in many areas of nursing. For example, school nurses can help young people develop good exercise habits. Physical education should be part of the curriculum in all grades, and school nurses should work with physical education teachers and coaches to promote well-balanced programs. Nurses in clinical practice can teach clients about the value of exercise when they make routine visits to private physicians and clinics. Nurses are often part of the team for weight reduction programs. Nurses can be role models by remaining physically fit.

Exercise Programs. People must perform exercise programs regularly for them to be effective. For example, aerobic exercise is most beneficial when performed three to five times a week for at least 30 minutes of accelerated heart rate. People may drop out of an exercise program because of pain and soreness if they begin too aggressively.

SAFETY ALERT
Clients should increase exercise tolerance gradually to avoid excessive stress on muscles and joints. Pain during exercise is a signal to stop.

Exercise programs are part of many clients' rehabilitation processes. Extended-care facilities often plan group exercise activities. Strength training has been effectively used, with older adults in some settings, to increase ROM, strength, and balance (Gleberzon & Annis, 2000). Research suggests that high intensity, individualized strength training using machines with older adults produces dramatic strength gains (Connelly, 2000). A specific exercise program is recommended after a heart attack or cardiac surgery. After a stroke, exercise is useful to strengthen affected muscles (Dobkin, 1999). Many diabetic clients follow an exercise program to obtain better control over blood glucose levels. The client who has undergone orthopedic surgery is encouraged to exercise certain muscles and joints. In many healthcare facilities, the physical therapy staff is usually responsible for supervising exercise programs, but nurses can encourage and reinforce the prescribed therapies.

Osteoporosis Prevention
Osteoporosis is characterized by decreased bone mass and increased susceptibility to fractures. After age 30, bone mass gradually declines for everyone, but this process greatly accelerates for women after menopause due to a decline in estrogen production. Primary risk factors for osteoporosis include the following:

- Postmenopausal status
- Caucasian or Asian race
- Premature or surgical menopause
- Family history of osteoporosis
- History of fragility fractures
- Alcohol abuse or cigarette smoking
- Prolonged immobility or inactivity

(Theiler, Stahelin, Kranzlin, Tyndall, & Bischoff, 1999)

To counter osteoporosis, prevention must begin early to promote adequate mineralization of the bone. New techniques can measure bone density in high-risk individuals. Lifestyle changes recommended for the prevention or management of osteoporosis include smoking cessation, no or limited alcohol and caffeine consumption, diet rich in calcium and vitamin D, and regular weight-bearing exercise. High sodium intake and low protein intake have also been associated with loss of bone mass. Postmenopausal estrogen replacement is a useful treatment to reduce the incidence and progression of osteoporosis. Increasing research is being done on osteoporosis in men (Kenny & Taxel, 2000). Other pharmacologic modalities include calcium supplementation (1,000 to 1,500 mg/day), vitamin D, calcitonin and bisphosphonates to inhibit bone reabsorption, and new selective estrogen receptor modulators (SERM) that cause estrogen-like effects (Huether & McCance, 2000).

Injury Prevention
Injuries commonly cause impaired mobility, but many injuries can be prevented (see Chapter 30). The nurse can play a significant role in unintentional injury prevention:

- Promote automobile safety and instruct clients to wear seat belts and use proper restraint devices for young children.
- Counsel clients about drug and alcohol use.
- Help clients provide a safe environment for themselves and their families.
- Provide instruction about injury prevention in the workplace.

Decreasing fall rates and decreasing the severity of injury for older adults are important interventions. By identifying older adults at greatest risk, the nurse can increase and individualize surveillance. One effective preventive device is a hip protector consisting of a polymer cup surrounded by polymer foam that is fitted into an undergarment worn on the hip; this protects against injury should a fall occur. Hip fractures have been reduced by 50% in some nursing home residents using the hip protector (Lappe, 1998).

Nursing Interventions for Altered Mobility

Positioning
Therapeutic positioning is used to prevent complications when mobility is limited. The client may be placed in specific positions to facilitate diagnostic tests or surgical intervention (Fig. 33-5). Common positioning postures include prone (face down), supine (lying on back), high Fowler's (head of the bed elevated 80 to 90 degrees), semi-Fowler's (head of the bed elevated 30 to 45 degrees), dorsal recumbent (supine with legs flexed in an elevated position), knee–chest position, Trendelenburg's (supine with head lower than feet), lateral or side-lying position, and Sims' (semiprone between a prone and side-lying position). Positions most commonly used for the immobile client include supine, Fowler's, semi-Fowler's, prone, side-lying, and Sims'.

Regardless of the specific position, general principles of body mechanics should be used in any position change. Maintain proper body alignment and support all body parts. Avoid pressure, especially over body prominences, by adequately padding these areas. Positioning aids, such as pillows, splints, footboards, foam rubber, and sheepskin protectors, are helpful (Table 33-3). Turning and positioning clients requires various organizational skills. Examples of those skills are the following:

- Think through the task before beginning.
- Ensure that all needed equipment is within easy reach.
- Explain to the client exactly what will happen before beginning the position change.

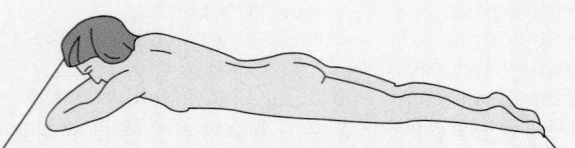

Prone: The client lies face down. Arms may cushion the head or may be flexed. An alternative position for an immobilized client, the prone position is contraindicated after abdominal surgery and in clients with respiratory or spinal problems.

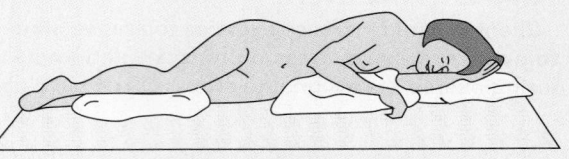

Side-lying: The client lies on the side with weight on hip and shoulder. Pillows support and stabilize uppermost leg, arm, head, and back. A choice position for clients with pressure on bony prominences of the back and sacral pressure sores, side-lying is not used after hip replacement and other orthopedic surgery.

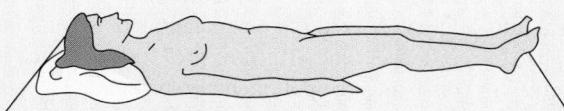

Supine: The client lies flat on back. Pillows may be used under the head, knees, and calves to raise heels off the mattress. An alternative position for a client on bedrest, the prone position is used after spine surgery and some spinal anesthesia. It is not used for clients with dyspnea or at risk for aspiration.

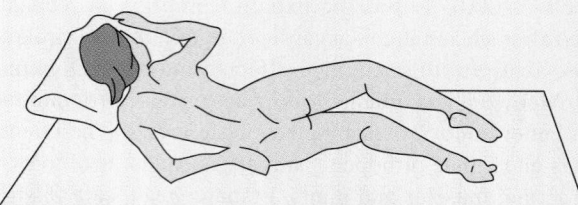

Sims': In this semiprone position the client lies on the side with weight distributed toward the anterior ileum, humerus, and clavicle. Pillows support the flexed arms and legs. The position is contraindicated by many spine or orthopedic conditions.

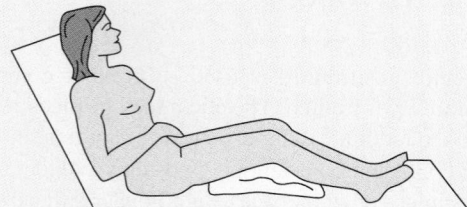

Fowler's: This sitting position raises the client's head 80°–90°. Pillows can be used under the head and arms and a footboard may also be used. The position improves cardiac output, promotes ventilation, and eases eating, talking, and watching TV. It is not used after spine or brain surgery.

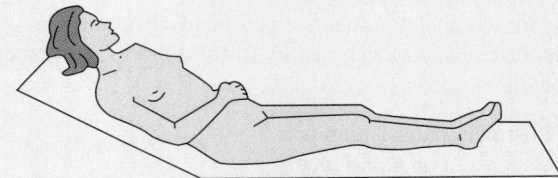

Semi–Fowler's: In this semisitting position the client's head is elevated 30°–45°. This position has the same advantages and contraindications as Fowler's position.

FIGURE 33-5   Common client positions. Among selected body positions, the prone, supine, Fowler's, semi-Fowler's, side-lying, and Sims' positions are commonly used for clients in healthcare facilities, whereas the dorsal recumbent, lithotomy, knee–chest, Trendelenburg's, and Reverse Trendelenburg's positions are often used during certain tests and surgical procedures.

- Enlist the client's assistance whenever possible, giving instructions and encouragement as necessary.
- When the position change has been completed, ask if the client is comfortable. Reposition as necessary.
- Tell the client how long he or she will remain in the position. Provide a call device within easy reach. Document position changes and the client's tolerance of specific positions in the chart.

 SAFETY ALERT

Decide if you need help from other staff members. If so, ensure that they are in the room before beginning the position change. If there is any possibility that you need help, always request it.

Proper positioning, outlined in Procedure 33-2, is important in preventing complications. A client with partial mobil-

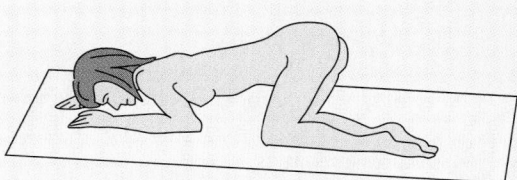

Dorsal recumbent: The client lies supine with legs flexed and rotated outward. This position is used extensively for vaginal examination but not for abdominal assessment because it promotes contraction of abdominal muscles.

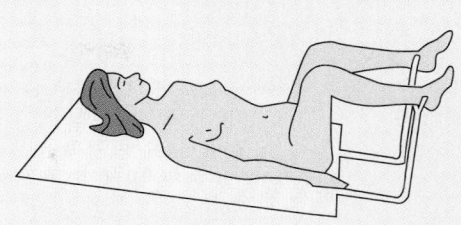

Lithotomy: The client lies supine with hips flexed and calves and heels parallel to the floor. This uncomfortable and embarrassing position requires draping the client for privacy. It is used for vaginal and rectal examination and may pose great difficulty for clients with immobilizing arthritis or a joint deformity.

Knee–chest: The client lies prone with buttocks elevated and knees drawn to the chest to accommodate a rectal procedure or examination. A client with arthritis or other joint deformity may be unable to lie in this position.

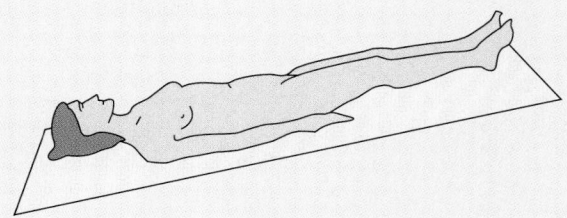

Trendelenburg's: The client lies supine with head 30°–40° lower than feet. The position may be used for postural drainage and to promote venous return. Hypotension may be an after effect of this position.

FIGURE 33-5 (*Continued*)

ity can usually learn positioning techniques to use with or without the nurse's assistance, but immobile clients rely on the nursing staff or caregiver to reposition them. Helping promote functional mobility is an important independent responsibility of the nurse, who works within mobility restrictions ordered by the healthcare provider or physical therapist. Unless contraindicated, clients should be moved to a chair twice a day (Display 33-3).

Turning Schedules. According to most reports in the nursing literature, immobile clients should be turned and repositioned every 2 hours, but little research shows that this schedule is therapeutic for all clients. More frequent turning may be needed. Significant factors include the amount of adipose tissue, skeletal structure, underlying pathophysiology, comfort level, skin condition, and mobility level. Assessing for skin condition and signs of pressure is important in determining the turning schedule. Decreased capillary refill and blanched or reddened areas indicate the need for more frequent turning.

Turning schedules should be incorporated in the plan of care and posted at the bedside if the client is receiving care in

the home, a long-term care facility, or a hospital. This helps ensure consistency of care between different shifts and different caregivers. In extended-care facilities where many clients require frequent position changes, a specific rotation pattern may be developed to ensure that various positions are used in an orderly fashion.

Logrolling. Logrolling (as described in Procedure 33-2) is a technique used for turning clients who have had surgery or an injury involving the back or spine. Instruct the client to keep his or her body as stiff as possible and to avoid any sudden moves during the procedure. A draw sheet can be helpful in logrolling clients smoothly, especially if they are obese. When turning a client, place pillows between the legs. Leave the pillows in place if the client remains in the side-lying position.

🮐 SAFETY ALERT
To prevent further trauma and injury, move the body as a unit so the spinal column does not bend or twist.

TABLE 33-3

Positioning Aids		
Aid	**Purpose**	**Nursing Considerations**
Pillow (feather, foam, or fiber-filled); various sizes	Elevates body part Supports client on side Prevents pressure on skin Increases comfort by decreasing stress and strain on body parts	Use pillows small enough to maintain proper body alignment. Assess for allergies to feathers before using.
Bed cradle	Keeps pressure of linen off feet	Position properly over feet.
Footboard	Maintains dorsiflexion of the feet, preventing foot drop. If board has antirotation blocks, it also can prevent hip rotation	Pad board with bath blanket. Position client's heels over mattress or use heel protectors.
Trochanter roll	Prevents external rotation of legs when in a supine position.	Trochanter roll should be placed from client's iliac crest to mid-thigh. Can be made by rolling bath blanket.
Hand roll	Keeps hand in functional position; prevents finger contractures	Roll should be large enough to prevent finger flexion and keep thumb in opposition. Rolled washcloth may be used if manufactured hand roll is unavailable.
Hand-wrist splint	Keeps arm and hand in normal functioning position (slight adduction of thumb and dorsiflexion of wrist)	Individually made for each client: Pad inside of splint. Remove every 4 hours to check for pressure areas.
Heel or elbow protectors (sheepskin or foam)	Reduces mattress pressure on heels or elbows; helps remove elbow friction when client moves in bed	Launder as necessary. Remove every 4 hours to check for pressure areas.
Abduction pillow	Maintains hip abduction after hip surgery to prevent hip dislocation	Pad pillow straps. Remove every 4 hours to assess for pressure points. Check pedal pulse to detect interference with circulation.
Trapeze bar	Helps client raise trunk from bed Allows client to help in transfers and position changes Allows client to strengthen upper arms through exercise	Teach client how to use the bar. Avoid hitting your head when you are assisting client with care.
Side rail	Helps weak client turn independently Protects client from falling out of bed	Keep in raised position to aid client mobility and ensure client safety.
Turn sheet	Helps reposition client; can be secured to side rail to support client in side-laying position	Position from midthorax to below hips. Roll sheet close to client to obtain better support when moving client. Can be made from bath blankets if manufactured models are unavailable.

Managing Clients With Hip Surgery. Turn clients who have had hip replacement surgery on the non-operative side only (Leininger, 1998), and take special care to prevent adduction of the affected hip and leg. Hip dislocation can result from movement of the leg toward or past the midline of the body (adduction). To avoid this, use abductor pillows. If unavailable, place regular pillows between the client's legs, and an additional staff member should support the affected leg so it will not fall, even momentarily, during the move. Avoid hip flexion of greater than 90 degrees and keep the operative leg in a neutral position with the toes pointing up (Leininger, 1998).

Joint Mobility Maintenance

Types of ROM. A client who can perform ROM unassisted is said to have active ROM. A client who needs the nurse's assistance to perform ROM is said to have passive ROM. Assistive ROM indicates that the client can participate in ROM exercises with assistance. For example, after a stroke the client may have weakness on one side of the body. With direction, the client may use the strong muscles on the unaffected side to exercise the weaker muscles on the affected side.

(text continues on page 788)

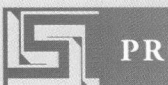

PROCEDURE 33-2

POSITIONING A CLIENT IN BED

Purpose
1. Maintain proper body alignment.
2. Maintain skin integrity and prevent deformities of the musculoskeletal system.
3. Provide comfort.
4. Maintain optimal position for ventilation and lung expansion.

Assessment
- Assess client's body alignment and comfort level in current position.
- Review chart for conditions that influence ability to move or to be positioned (e.g., fractures, paralysis, spinal injury).
- Assess for tubes, IV lines, incisions, or equipment that may alter the positioning procedure.
- Assess client's level of consciousness and ability to understand and follow directions.
- Assess client's ability to assist with positioning.
- Assess client's weight and your strength. Determine if additional assistance is needed.

Equipment
Pillows
Draw sheet or turning sheet
Side rails

Procedure

Moving a Client Up in Bed (One Nurse)

1. Identify client and any positioning restrictions. Explain procedure and rationale to client.
   Rationale: Explanation reduces anxiety and increases cooperation.
2. Lower head of bed to flat position and raise level of bed to comfortable working height.
   Rationale: This decreases gravitational pull of upper body and promotes good body mechanics by decreasing back strain.
3. Remove all pillows from under client. Leave one at head of bed.
   Rationale: Pillows prevent accidental head injury against top of bed frame.
4. Instruct client to bend legs and put feet flat on bed.
   Rationale: Client will be able to assist by pushing legs against bed.
5. Place your feet in broad stance with one foot in front of the other. Flex your knees and thighs.
   Rationale: Lowering center of gravity ensures using the legs' large muscle groups.

6. Place one arm under client's shoulders and one arm under thighs. Keep head up and back straight.
   Rationale: The heaviest parts of client's body are supported. Avoiding twisting the back prevents injury.
7. Rock back and forth on front and back legs to count of three. On third count, have client push with feet as you lift and pull the client up in bed.
   Rationale: Rocking motion develops momentum, which promotes smooth lifting with minimal exertion by the nurse.
8. Elevate head of bed and place pillows under head. Raise side rails and lower bed to lowest level.
   Rationale: These actions provide for client comfort and safety.

Moving Helpless Client Up in Bed (Two Nurses)

1. Identify client and note any mobility restrictions. Explain procedure and rationale to client.
   Rationale: Rechecking information provides for safety. Explanation reduces anxiety.
2. Lower head of bed to flat position and raise level of bed to comfortable working height.
   Rationale: Positioning equipment minimizes required effort and back strain.
3. Remove all pillows from under client. Leave one at head of bed.
   Rationale: Pillow prevents accidental head injury against top of bed frame.
4. One nurse stands on each side of bed with legs positioned for wide base of support and one foot slightly in front of the other.
   Rationale: Proper positioning lowers center of gravity and reduces risk of injury.
5. Each nurse rolls up and grasps edges of turn sheet close to client's shoulders and buttocks.
   Rationale: Turn sheet distributes client's weight and prevents shearing injury to skin by reducing friction during move.
6. Flex knees and hips. Tighten abdominal and gluteal muscles and keep back straight.
   Rationale: Using the legs' large muscle groups and tightening muscles during transfer prevent back injury.
7. Rock back and forth on front and back legs to count of three. On third count, both nurses shift weight to front leg as they simultaneously lift client toward head of bed.
   Rationale: Rocking motion develops momentum, which provides a smooth lift of client with minimal exertion by nurses.

PROCEDURE 33-2 (Continued)

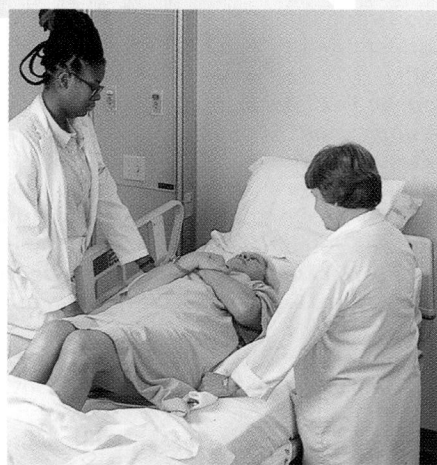

Step 5 Moving a helpless client up in bed: Grasp turn sheet near client's shoulders and buttocks.

8. Elevate head of bed and place pillows under client's head. Adjust other positioning pillows as necessary. Put up side rails and lower bed to lowest level.
   Rationale: Positioning equipment provides for client comfort and safety.

Positioning Client in Side-Lying Position

1. Identify client and note any mobility restrictions. Lower head of bed as flat as client can tolerate.
   Rationale: Client turns easier from flat position.
2. Elevate and lock side rail on side client will face when turned.
   Rationale: Locking opposing side rail prevents accidental injury from the client falling out of bed during turn.
3. Using draw sheet, move client to the edge of the bed, opposite the side on which he or she will be turned.
   Rationale: Provides room so when the client is turned he or she will be positioned in the center of the bed.
4. Place arm that client will turn toward away from his or her body. Fold other arm across chest.
   Rationale: Positioning arms facilitates turning by preventing client from rolling onto bottom arm.
5. Flex client's knee that will not be next to mattress after turn. Have client reach toward side rail with opposite arm.
   Rationale: Encourage client to assist with position change.
6. Assume a broad stance with knees slightly flexed.

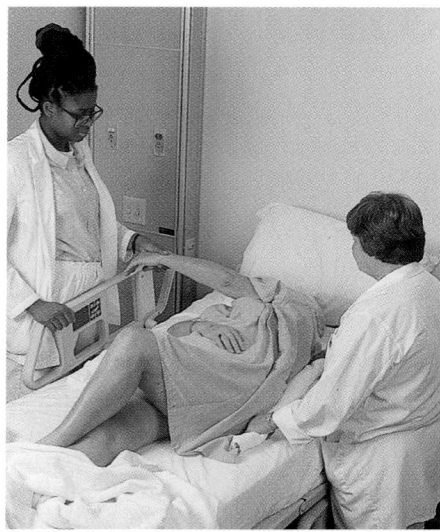

Step 5 Positioning client in side-lying position: Have client reach toward side rail with opposite arm.

   Rationale: This stance increases balance, lowers center of gravity, and encourages use of large muscle groups during movement.
7. Using draw sheet, gently pull client over on side.
   Rationale: You can evenly support heaviest part of client during turn.
8. Align client properly then place pillows behind back and under head.
   Rationale: Support the client in a side-lying position to maintain proper alignment.

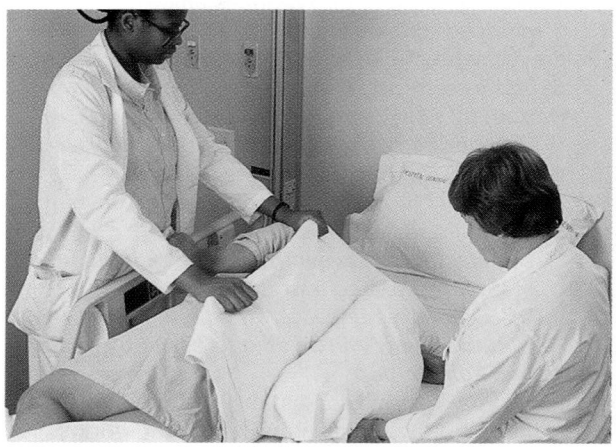

Steps 7 and 8 Using draw sheet, pull client onto side and place pillow behind back.

PROCEDURE 33-2 (Continued)

9. Pull shoulder blade forward and out from under client. Support client's upper arm with pillow.
   Rationale: Joints are protected from weight and strain. Ventilation also may improve because chest can expand more fully.
10. Place pillow lengthwise between client's legs from thighs to foot.
    Rationale: This keeps leg aligned and prevents pressure on bony prominences.

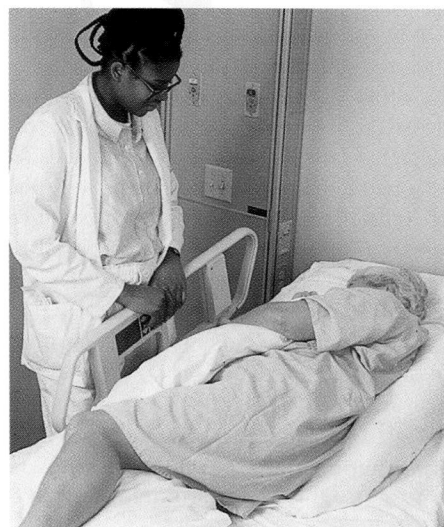

Steps 9 and 10 Support arm and legs with pillows.

Logrolling

1. Obtain assistance.
   Rationale: Two or three nurses are usually required.
2. All nurses stand on same side of bed with feet apart, one foot slightly ahead of the other. Flex knees and hips.
   Rationale: This stance increases balance and stability and ensures use of large muscle groups when turning client.

3. Use one pillow to support client's head during and after turn.
   Rationale: Pillow maintains alignment of cervical spine.
4. Place pillows between client's legs.
   Rationale: Pillows support the uppermost leg and prevent adduction during turn.
5. Instruct client to fold arms over chest and keep body stiff.
   Rationale: Spine is kept in alignment during turn.
6. Reach across client and support head, thorax, trunk, and legs. On count of three, roll client in one coordinated movement to lateral position.
   Rationale: Alignment of whole body is maintained during turn.
7. Support client in alignment with pillows as described in "Side-lying position." Clients with suspected or known cervical spinal injuries should wear cervical collars.
   Rationale: Support prevents injury to the spinal cord whenever client is turned or moved in bed.

Home Care Modifications
- Teach caregivers principles of body alignment.
- Demonstrate how to turn and position a person in bed. Have caregiver perform a return demonstration of positioning techniques.
- Beds can be placed on blocks to prevent back strain for caregivers.

Collaboration and Delegation
- Frequently, positioning clients is delegated to unlicensed assistive personnel. Provide clear guidelines regarding limitations and amount of assistance required.
- Consult with a physical therapist to develop a collaborative plan for any client with complex positioning problems due to injury or spasticity.

DISPLAY 33-3

🔄 GUIDELINES FOR MOVING CLIENTS

- Assess the client's abilities and limitations.
- Medicate client to provide optimal pain relief.
- Organize environment, and request needed help to ensure safety.
- Explain what you are going to do and how you expect the client to help.
- Permit client to do as much as his or her capabilities allow.
- Consider safety precautions (e.g., lock wheels, use transfer belt).
- Follow the principles of body mechanics.
- Keep movements smooth and rhythmic.
- Prevent trauma (e.g., friction against skin, pulling joints, grabbing muscles).
- Check client for proper body alignment and comfort, and provide client with call bell before leaving.

General Principles of ROM Exercises. ROM exercises should be initiated as soon as possible because changes in affected joints can occur after only 3 days of impaired mobility. Allow the client to participate as fully as he or she can. Perform ROM exercises in a systematic order at a designated time each day (usually during morning care). For high-risk clients, ROM exercises may be indicated more often. In some facilities, physical therapists help immobile clients perform ROM exercises at the bedside.

🔲 SAFETY ALERT
ROM exercises should be done smoothly and gently. Stop movement if the client complains of pain or if there is resistance.

Support the joint distal to the one being exercised. A healthcare provider's order and specific instructions should be obtained to perform ROM for clients with acute arthritis, fractures, torn ligaments, joint dislocation, or acute myocardial infarction. Procedure 33-3 details ROM technique.

Automatic ROM Equipment. Mechanical devices, such as continuous passive range-of-motion machines, have been developed to provide continuous ROM to a specific joint. Such devices are most commonly used after orthopedic surgery, usually of the knee, when such exercise promotes joint mobility and permits rapid rehabilitation. The equipment extends the joint to a prescribed angle for a prescribed period, continuously cycling according to parameters set by the healthcare provider.

Ambulation

Early ambulation significantly reduces complications of immobility. Walking exercises almost all body muscles and promotes joint flexibility. Most surgical clients are permitted and encour-

aged to get out of bed and walk on their first postoperative day. Early ambulation significantly reduces the formation of venous clots and atelectasis, thereby decreasing respiratory and circulatory complications after surgery. Even a short period of immobility decreases a client's exercise tolerance, so assistance is usually required when the client resumes walking. Musculoskeletal or neurologic alterations typically require temporary or permanent assistance with ambulation (Procedure 33-4).

Dangling the Legs. **Dangling** is a preliminary step to ambulation, especially for clients who may be unable to ambulate initially. The activity involves sitting on the side of the bed with the legs dependent. Often dangling is recommended on the evening after surgery or when weight bearing is not permitted. When it precedes the client's first ambulatory steps, dangling helps to prevent postural hypotension.

When assisting the client to dangle his or her legs, raise the head of the bed slowly as high as the client can tolerate. This not only decreases the distance the client needs to move but also uses the bed to help the client into a sitting position. To further assist the client to an upright position, have the client move as close to the edge of the bed as possible. Face the client and establish a broad base of support, flexing your hips, knees, and ankles. While supporting the client under the knees and around the shoulders, move her or him to a sitting position in one smooth movement.

🔲 SAFETY ALERT
When supporting the client during dangling, tighten your gluteal and abdominal muscles to avoid back strain or injury.

Some clients can independently reach a sitting position. The easiest way to accomplish this is to have the client roll onto his or her side, grasp the mattress with the lower arm, and use the other hand to push up while swinging the legs over the side of the mattress (Fig. 33-6). After achieving this position, the client can maintain it by placing the hands palm down on the mattress for balance.

Assisting the Client With Ambulation. Assisting the client to ambulate safely begins by thoroughly assessing his or her muscle strength and coordination. Assist the client to a sitting position on the side of the bed. If the client complains of dizziness, is diaphoretic, or has orthostatic hypotension (confirmed by blood pressure measurement), postpone ambulation. If dangling is well tolerated, proceed with ambulation.

🔲 SAFETY ALERT
Have the client wear shoes or slippers with non-skid soles, and clear the path of obstacles that might cause the client to trip. Many hallways have railings the client can grip. A weak or unstable client may prefer to push a chair or wheelchair to provide extra support and balance. Encourage the client to look straight ahead to promote balance and prevent dizziness.

(text continues on page 793)

PROCEDURE 33-3

PROVIDING RANGE-OF-MOTION EXERCISES

Purpose
1. Maintain joint mobility.
2. Improve or maintain muscle strength.
3. Prevent muscle atrophy and contractures.

Assessment
- Review medical history to determine specific limitations to joint mobility.
- Assess client's level of consciousness and physical ability to assist or independently perform range-of-motion (ROM) exercises.
- Assess for redness, tenderness, pain, swelling, or deformities around joints.

Equipment
No special equipment is required except a bed.

Procedure
1. Identify client and client's movement limitations. Explain procedure and purpose to client.
   Rationale: Explanation reduces anxiety and encourages cooperation.
2. Position client on back with head of bed as flat as possible. Elevate bed to comfortable working height.
   Rationale: Adjusting bed promotes proper body mechanics to prevent muscle strain for nurse.
3. Stand on side of bed where joints are to be exercised. Uncover only the limb to be exercised.
   Rationale: This provides warmth and privacy.
4. Refer to Table 33-1 for illustrations of normal movement for each joint. Perform exercises slowly and gently, providing support by holding areas proximal and distal to the joint.
   Rationale: This prevents discomfort and muscle spasms from jerky movements.
5. Repeat each exercise five times. Discontinue or decrease ROM if client complains of discomfort or muscle spasm.
   Rationale: Pain may indicate ROM is causing damage.
6. Neck:
   a. Move chin to chest.
   b. Bend head toward back.
   c. Tilt head toward each shoulder.
   d. Rotate head in circular motion.
   e. Return head to erect position.

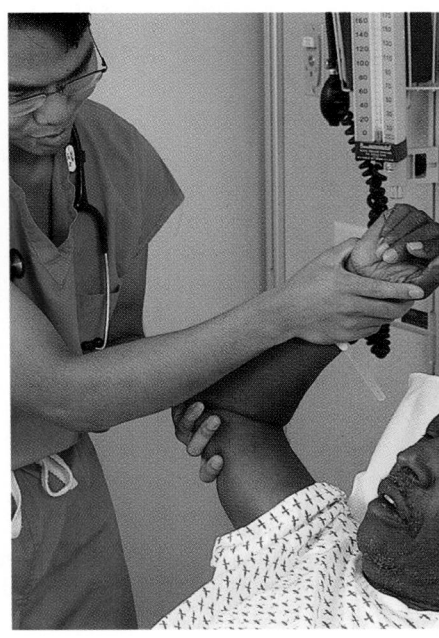

Step 7a Raise client's arm from side to above head.

7. Shoulder:
   a. Raise client's arm from side to above head.
   b. Abduct and rotate shoulder by raising arm above head with palm up.
   c. Adduct shoulder by moving arm across body as far as possible.
   d. Rotate shoulder internally and externally by flexing elbow and moving forearm so the palm touches mattress; then reverse the motion so that back of client's hand touches mattress.
   e. Move shoulder in a full circle.
8. Elbow:
   a. Bend elbow so that forearm moves toward shoulder.
   b. Hyperextend elbow as far as possible.
9. Wrist and hand:
   a. Move hand toward inner aspect of forearm.
   b. Bend dorsal surface of hand backward.
   c. Abduct wrist by bending toward thumb.
   d. Adduct wrist by bending toward fifth finger.
   e. Make a fist; extend the fingers.
   f. Spread fingers apart, then together.
   g. Move thumb across hand to base of fifth finger.

PROCEDURE 33-3 (Continued)

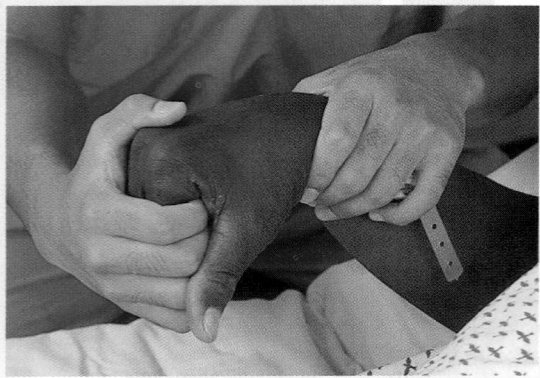

Step 9e Flex fingers by making a fist.

10. Hip and knee:
    a. Lift leg and bend knee toward chest.
    b. Abduct and adduct leg, moving leg laterally away from body and returning to medial position.
    c. Internally and externally rotate hip by turning leg inward, then outward.
    d. Take special care to support joints of larger limbs.

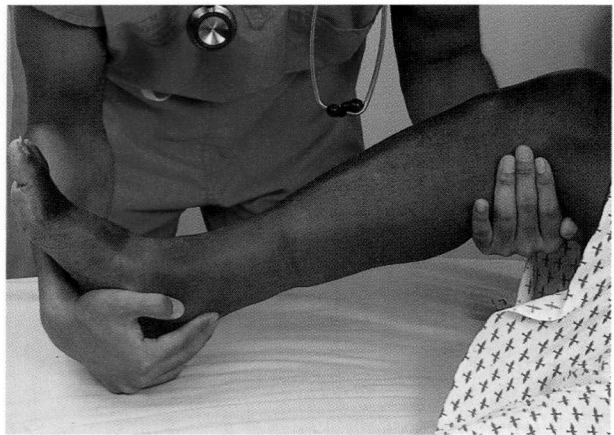

Step 10a Lift leg and bend knee.

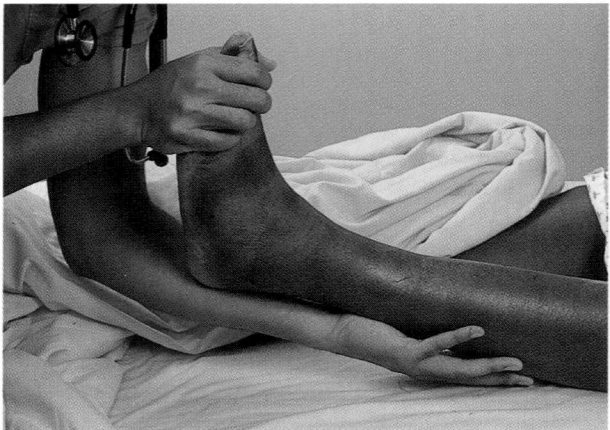

Step 11a Dorsiflex foot.

11. Ankle and foot:
    a. Dorsiflex foot by moving it so toes point upward.
    b. Plantarflex by moving foot so toes point downward.
    c. Curl toes down, then extend.
    d. Spread toes apart, then bring together.
    e. Invert by turning sole of foot medially.
    f. Evert by turning sole of foot laterally.
12. Move to other side of bed and repeat exercises.
13. Reposition client comfortably.
14. Document ROM.

Home Care Modifications
• Demonstrate to caregivers how to perform ROM and use return demonstration to evaluate technique.

Collaboration and Delegation
• Encourage unlicensed assistive personnel to provide ROM during hygiene care. Inform them of any client limitation and stress that they stop activity whenever a client experiences pain.
• A physical therapist may be consulted to develop an individualized plan for a client with contractures or spasticity.

PROCEDURE 33-4

ASSISTING WITH AMBULATION

Purpose
1. Promote safe ambulation free of falls or injury.
2. Increase muscle strength and joint mobility.
3. Prevent complications of immobility.
4. Promote self-esteem and independence.

Assessment
- Review chart for conditions that impair ambulation (arthritis, fractures, paralysis) and for healthcare provider's orders for ambulation or ambulating aids (walkers, canes, crutches).
- Assess comfort level. Medicate as ordered with analgesics. Plan ambulation for time when analgesics have peak action.
- Assess range of motion and muscle strength. Determine if extra assistance is required.
- Obtain baseline vital signs. Obtain postural vital signs if client has been on prolonged bedrest or is at risk for orthostatic hypotension for other reasons.

Equipment
Ambulation aid (crutches, cane, walker) if required
Transfer belt (optional), clothing, or robe
Well-fitting shoes or slippers with nonskid soles

Procedure
1. Identify client. Explain procedure and purpose of ambulation to client. Decide together how far and where to walk.
   Rationale: Explanation reduces anxiety and facilitates cooperation. Planning helps to ensure safety.
2. Place bed in lowest position.
   Rationale: Allow client to get out of bed safely.
3. Assist client to sitting position on side of bed. Assess for dizziness. Obtain orthostatic vital signs if complaints are present. Allow client to remain in this position until he or she feels secure.
   Rationale: This minimizes orthostatic hypotension upon standing, which could result in falls or injury.
4. Help client with clothing and footwear.
   Rationale: Being comfortably dressed maintains dignity and safety during ambulation.

One Nurse
1. Wrap transfer belt around client's waist (optional according to previous assessment).
   Rationale: Transfer belt provides a firm hold for the nurse and prevents injury to the client.

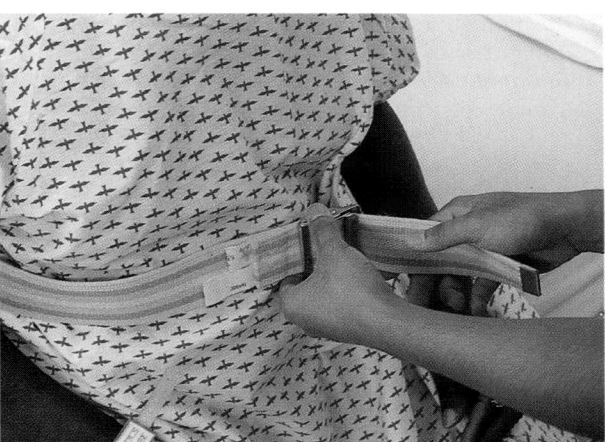

Step 1 Place transfer belt snugly around waist.

2. Assist client to standing position and assess client's balance. Return client to bed or transfer to chair if he or she is very weak or unsteady. Be sure client does not grasp your neck for support but places his or her hands around your shoulders or at your waist.

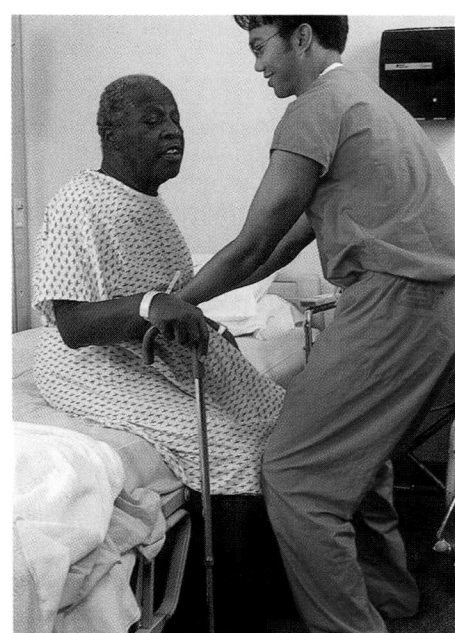

Step 2 Assist client to standing position, using a wide base of support and with knees flexed.

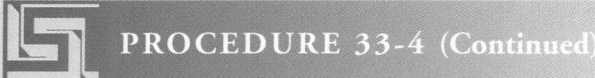

PROCEDURE 33-4 (Continued)

3. Position yourself behind client while supporting him or her by waist or transfer belt.
   Rationale: Client can stand erect and does not lean to one side for support from nurse.

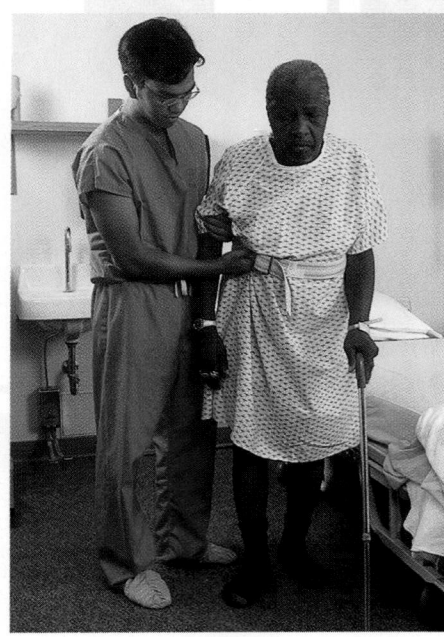

Step 3 The nurse should walk behind and to the side of the client.

4. Take several steps forward with client. Assess strength and balance. Encourage client to use good posture and to look ahead, not down at feet.
   Rationale: Starting carefully and slowly promotes good balance.
5. Ambulate for planned distance or time. If client becomes weak or dizzy, return client to bed or assist to chair.
   Rationale: Monitoring the walking encourages exercise tolerance while maintaining client safety.
6. If the client begins to fall, place your feet wide apart with one foot in front. Support the client by pulling his or her weight backward against your body. Lower gently to floor, protecting head.
   Rationale: Nurse's foot position widens and stabilizes the base of support and enables nurse to support client's weight with large muscle groups. This protects nurse from back strain.

Two Nurses
1. Assist client to sitting position as described.
2. Assist client to standing position with one nurse on each side.
3. One nurse grasps the transfer belt to support the client. The other nurse may carry and manage equipment.
   Rationale: Support is provided during ambulation and equipment is managed to prevent falls.
4. Walk with client using slow, even steps. Assess strength and balance. Encourage client to look forward rather than down at floor.
   Rationale: This promotes client's stability.

Using a Walker
1. Assist client to standing position. Have client keep one hand on the arm of the chair or bed while she or he assumes an upright posture.
   Rationale: Using bed or chair for support maintains balance and stability to promote safety.
2. Have client grasp walker handles. Client moves walker ahead 6 to 8 inches placing all four feet of walker on floor. Client moves forward to walker.
   Rationale: Using walker handles stabilizes walker and promotes safety.
3. Nurse should walk closely behind and slightly to side of client.
   Rationale: If client begins to fall, nurse can support him or her and prevent injury (see Fig. 33-7).
4. Repeat above sequence until walk is complete.

Home Care Modifications
- To provide safety and prevent falls at home, throw rugs and small pieces of furniture should be removed so client will not trip on them.
- Client should always wear shoes with nonskid soles.
- The bathroom is a common place for falls and injury. Placing a large rug with a skid-resistant backing on the floor can prevent falls from slipping on wet floors.

Collaboration and Delegation
- Physical therapists often teach and supervise ambulation for high-risk clients (e.g., those who have had orthopedic surgery, amputation, CVA). Collaborative, individualized ambulations plans can be developed.

APPLY YOUR KNOWLEDGE

Mrs. Jones, an 82-year-old retired librarian, had major abdominal surgery yesterday and has not been out of bed. Her vital signs are stable, but her blood pressure is lower than her baseline. She has a hydration IV and a PCA (patient-controlled analgesia). Her pain is well controlled with morphine sulphate via the PCA. She has complained of some nausea postoperatively and received an antiemetic. She has a Foley catheter in place and has only had 200 cc of urine during the last 8 hours. Before getting Mrs. Jones out of bed, review factors that may contribute to unsteadiness and difficulty ambulating. How can you promote safety during Mrs. Jones' first time out of bed ambulating?

Check your answer in Appendix A.

All equipment (IV tubing, indwelling catheter, drains) must be secured to a pole. Do not carry equipment while assisting the client. Keep your hands free to provide support in case the client falls.

Watch IV lines carefully to promptly detect any problems. Nasogastric suction can usually be discontinued while the client is ambulating then reconnected on return to the room.

Transfer Belts. Transfer belts (sometimes called safety belts or ambulation belts) should be used if the client is weak or has problems with coordination. The transfer belt is a canvas belt applied around the waist and tightened over clothing (see the example in Procedure 33-4).

SAFETY ALERT

Grip the transfer belt as the client walks so you can provide aid if the client begins to fall. If the client becomes dizzy or starts to fall, slowly and gently lower the client to the floor and call for help. If the client is at high risk for falls, two nurses may be required to assist with ambulation.

Mechanical Aids. Mechanical devices can help the client with certain limitations to ambulate safely. During ambulation, walkers, canes, quad canes, and crutches help bear a portion of the client's weight, promote stability, and maintain balance. The physical therapist is usually responsible for instructing the client initially with use of these devices; however, the client often requires additional instruction or supervision from the nurse.

Canes are useful for clients who can bear weight but need support for balance or who have decreased strength in one leg. Canes are made of wood or metal and should be about waist high. A variety of canes is available ranging from a simple straight-leg cane to a three- or four-pronged cane (often called a quad cane).

The cane acts as an additional "leg" by providing the client with three points of support during ambulation. The client holds the cane in the hand opposite the weak or injured leg, then moves the affected or weak foot forward with the cane as the weight of the body remains on the stronger extremity. When climbing stairs, the strongest leg advances up the stair first, followed by the cane and the weaker leg. This process is reversed when descending stairs: The cane and the weaker leg are followed by the stronger leg. Instruct the client to look straight ahead rather than at the feet while walking.

Walkers are lightweight, tubular metal structures that provide more support than canes. Four rubber-tipped legs give walkers a wide base of support. The client grips the walker, picks it up, and moves it forward (Fig. 33-7). The client may use a two-point or three-point gait when ambulating with the walker. Be sure to clear hallways of obstructions before the client uses the walker. Some walkers have wheels and a seat so clients who tire can sit and rest or propel themselves by pushing with their feet.

Crutches allow the client to walk without weight bearing on the legs. Crutches may be indicated when the client has a sprain, fracture, or nonwalking cast. Underarm crutches usually serve these short-term purposes. The client must use the arms, not the shoulders, to support the body weight. Using the shoulders can cause skin breakdown at the axilla and nerve damage to the brachial plexus. Underarm crutches must be fitted correctly. About 2 inches should remain between the axilla and the top of the crutch when the crutch is placed 2 inches in front of and 6 inches to the side of the foot.

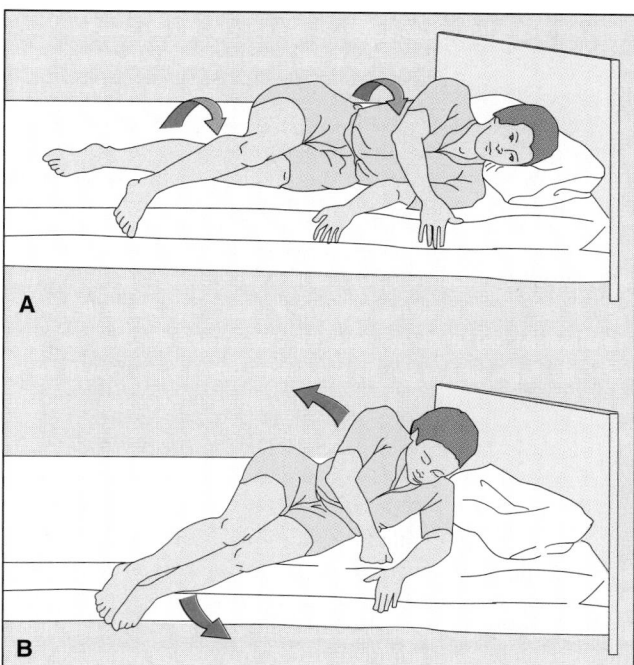

FIGURE 33-6 Many clients can reach a sitting position independently when taught the proper method. **(A)** The client rolls over onto his or her side. **(B)** The client grasps the mattress with the lower arm and uses the other hand to push up while swinging the legs over the side of the bed.

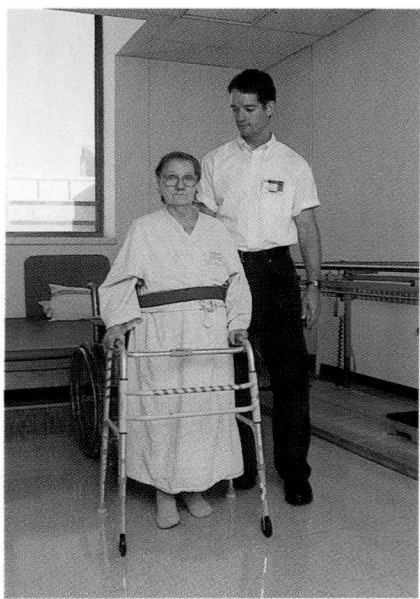

FIGURE 33-7   When assisting a client using a walker, stand behind and to the side. Use a transfer belt if the client is not steady or is at risk for falling.

Crutches also may be used for additional support that weak or paralyzed legs cannot provide for walking. For long-term use, Lofstrand crutches, which have metal bands encircling the forearms, are used. The client on crutches may use several gaits (Procedure 33-5):

- When the client can bear partial weight on both feet, the four-point gait may be used. The right crutch is placed forward, followed by the left foot, then the left crutch is moved forward, followed by the right foot.
- When the client can bear weight on only one foot, the three-point gait is used. Both crutches and the weaker leg move forward first, followed by the stronger leg.
- The two-point gait requires at least partial weight bearing on each foot, as each crutch moves at the same time as the opposing leg.
- The swing-through gait is often used by paraplegics, who move both crutches forward then swing the body beyond the crutches to propel themselves forward.

To function independently, the client on crutches must learn how to rise from a sitting position then climb and descend stairs. This instruction is usually done by a physical therapist. The client also should be taught to inspect the rubber tips of crutches for wear.

🥛 SAFETY ALERT
Prompt replacement of worn tips on crutches can prevent falls.

Muscle Strengthening to Facilitate Ambulation. Certain muscle groups may need strengthening before some clients can walk. Clients on bed rest should learn to contract their quadriceps and gluteal and abdominal muscles regularly because these muscles are important for ambulation. Clients who will use crutches or walkers need to strengthen their arm muscles as well because increased arm strength will be necessary to support their body weight. *Setting* is a term used to refer to isometric strengthening of muscles. The client concentrates on one muscle at a time, contracting it for 10 seconds and then permitting it to relax completely. This is repeated a prescribed number of times.

Transfers

Assisted transfers are necessary when the client is unconscious, extremely weak, or has decreased muscle strength or paralysis in the legs. Transfers usually involve moving the client from one flat surface to another, for example, from the bed to the stretcher or vice versa (Procedure 33-6). Another transfer involves moving the client from the bed to a sitting position either in a chair or wheelchair (Procedure 33-7).

🥛 SAFETY ALERT
Safety is important during transfers. Doing an assessment to identify client abilities and limitations permits the nurse to individualize the transfer technique and plan for extra help as needed. Body mechanics will help to prevent injury to the client and nurse.

Equipment (transfer belts, transfer boards or sleds, roller boards, hydraulic lifts) can make transfers easier and safer. Table 33-4 describes common transfer aids.

Two- or Three-Person Lifts. Lifts or carries by staff are seldom used in hospitals because they are usually uncomfortable for the client and pose safety risks for the nurse. However, such carries can be used in emergencies or when the client being transferred is light. When lifting a client, place the client's arms over his or her chest and have colleagues available to lift each body area. When moving the client to another flat surface, one nurse grasps the client under the head and shoulders, one under the hips, and a third under the thighs and legs. If the client is being lifted to a chair, one nurse holds the client under the arms around the chest, and the second supports the hips and legs. Synchronize the lift by counting to three. Using body mechanics is essential to prevent injury to the lifters.

🥛 SAFETY ALERT
The under-axilla lift techniques, where care providers pull the client by grasping the arms and under the axilla, should never be employed. This technique should never be used because it exerts pressure on the brachial plexus that can affect the nerve function to the neck, shoulder, arm and hands. It can also subluxate the shoulder. Also this technique is the cause of poor body mechanics for the nurse and has been associated with L5-S1 back injuries (Owens, 2000).

(text continues on page 801)

HELPING CLIENTS WITH CRUTCHWALKING

Purpose

1. Increase client's level of activity after musculo-skeletal injury.
2. Assist client to walk safely with crutches using the least amount of energy.

Assessment

- Review medical history to determine reason for crutches and instructions for weight bearing.
- Determine if client has experience with crutchwalking.
- Assess client's ability to balance himself or herself.
- Observe for unilateral or unusual weakness.
- Assess muscle strength, especially in legs and arms.
- Determine appropriate size crutch. There should be 2 inches between axilla and top of crutch.

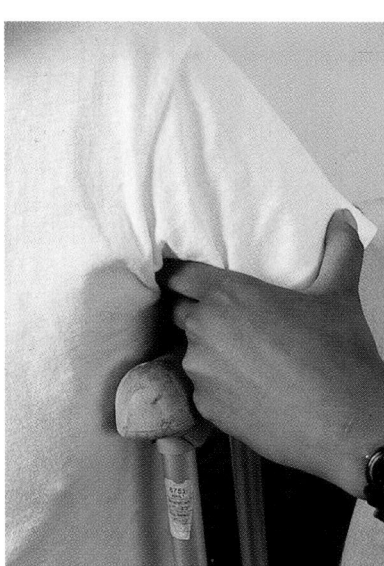

Assessment: Measuring crutches for proper fit.

Equipment

Crutches with suction tips, hand grips, and axillary pads
Shoes with nonskid soles

Procedure

Four-Point Gait

1. Client stands erect, face forward in tripod position. Client places crutch tips 6 inches in front of feet and 6 inches to side of each foot.

Rationale: This is the position used to start crutchwalking. It provides a wide base of support so stability and balance are increased.

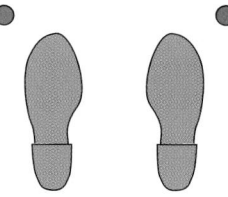

Step 1 To assume beginning tripod position, place crutch tips 6 inches ahead and to the side of each foot.

2. Client moves right crutch forward 6 inches.

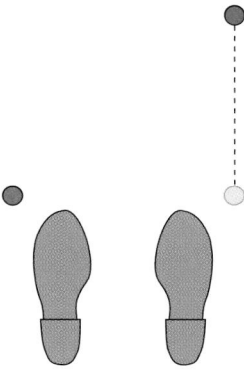

Step 2 Move right crutch forward.

3. Client moves left foot forward to level of right crutch.

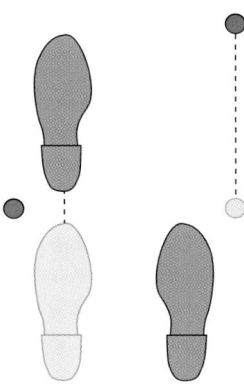

Step 3 Move left foot forward.

4. Client moves left crutch forward 4 to 6 inches.

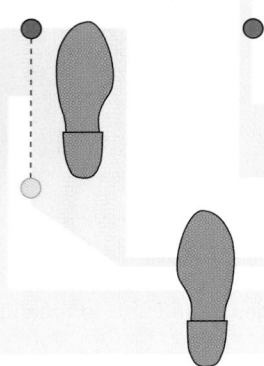

Step 4 Move left crutch forward.

5. Client moves right foot forward to level of left crutch.

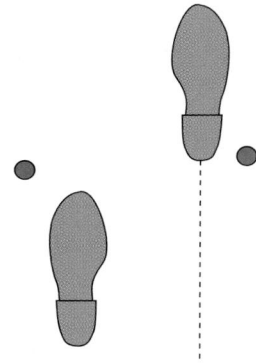

Step 5 Move right foot forward.

6. Repeat sequence.
   Rationale: This gait is the safest and most stable because three points are always on the ground. The crutch and foot positions mimic arm and foot positions during regular walking. The client must be able to bear weight partially on the affected side to perform this gait.

Three-Point Gait

1. Beginning in the tripod position, client moves both crutches and affected leg forward.

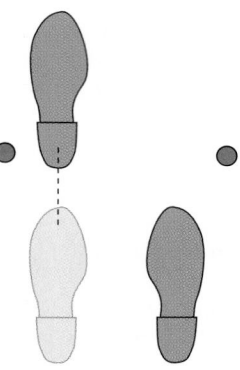

Step 1 Move both crutches and the affected leg.

2. Client moves stronger leg forward.

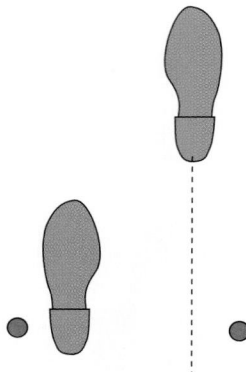

Step 2 Move stronger leg forward.

3. Repeat sequence.
   Rationale: Client must bear his or her entire weight on the stronger leg to perform this gait.

PROCEDURE 33-5 (Continued)

Two-Point Gait

1. Beginning in the tripod position, client moves left crutch and right foot forward.

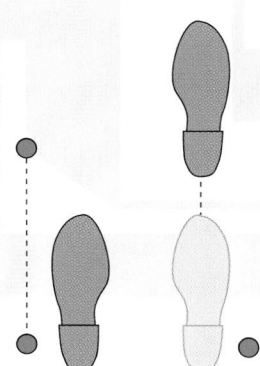

Step 1 Move left crutch and right leg forward.

2. Client moves right crutch and left foot forward.

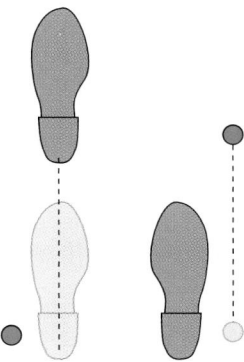

Step 2 Move right crutch and left leg forward.

3. Repeat sequence.
    Rationale: Crutch and foot movement is similar to arm and leg movement in normal walking. This gait requires partial weight bearing on both feet and is faster than the four-point gait.

Swing-To Gait

1. Client forms tripod position and moves both crutches forward.
2. Client lifts legs and swings to crutches, supporting body weight on crutches.
    Rationale: This alternative is used by clients with non–weight-bearing precautions or paralysis of legs and hips or those wearing weight-supporting braces on their legs.

Swing-Through Gait

1. Client forms tripod position and moves both crutches forward.
2. Client lifts legs and swings through and ahead of crutches, supporting weight on crutches.
    Rationale: Although similar to swing-to gait, this requires much more strength and coordination.

Climbing Stairs

1. Use one crutch and the railing. Beginning in tripod position facing stairs, client transfers body weight to crutches and holds onto the railing.
2. Client places unaffected leg on stair.
3. Client transfers body weight to unaffected leg.
4. Client moves crutches and affected leg to stair.
5. Repeat sequence to top of stairs.
    Rationale: The crutches always support the affected leg.

Lifespan Considerations
- Older clients may not have the strength or balance necessary to feel comfortable or safe using crutches. A walker may be preferable.

Home Care Modifications
- The client using crutches must anticipate problems. If he or she carries books to school or a briefcase to work, a backpack may be a solution until crutches are no longer needed.
- Throw rugs, small pieces of furniture, and toys should be removed from the traffic pattern to provide for safety and ease of walking with crutches.

Collaboration and Delegation
- Physical therapist and orthopedic nurses teach clients the proper use of crutches. After initial instruction, reinforcement and follow-up are required. A home health nurse may evaluate the home setting for safety.

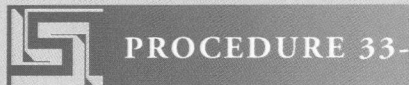

PROCEDURE 33-6

TRANSFERRING A CLIENT TO A STRETCHER

Purpose
Transfer a client without injuring nurse or client

Assessment
- Review medical history for conditions that influence or contraindicate ability to move (i.e., fractures, paralysis, spinal injury, generalized muscle weakness, cardiac or respiratory disease that limits exertion).
- Assess client's range of motion and muscle strength.
- Assess cognitive function or ability to understand and follow directions.
- Assess comfort level. Medicate as ordered with analgesics.
- Assess client's weight and your strength. Determine if assistance is needed.

Equipment
Stretcher
Transfer board

Procedure
1. Identify client. Explain procedure and purpose.
   Rationale: Explanation reduces anxiety and increases cooperation.
2. Place stretcher parallel to bed. Raise bed to same level as stretcher. Lower side rails. Lock wheels.
   Rationale: Positioning equipment makes transfer easier and decreases risk of injury.
3. One or two nurses stand on side of bed without stretcher. Two nurses stand on side of bed with stretcher.
   Rationale: Team coordination provides for client safety during transfer.
4. Loosen draw sheet on both sides of bed.
   Rationale: Draw sheet assists in transferring client.
5. Nurse on side without stretcher helps client to move toward them onto his or her side. They may use draw sheet to pull client closer.
   Rationale: Getting client closer to stretcher enables a smooth transfer.
6. Nurse on stretcher side of bed slides transfer board under draw sheet and under client's buttocks and back.
   Rationale: Transfer board helps slide client from bed to stretcher.
7. Slide client onto transfer board into supine position. Place client's arms across his or her chest.
   Rationale: This prevents injury to arms during transfer.
8. Wrap end of draw sheet over curved end of transfer sled and slide client onto stretcher on count of three.

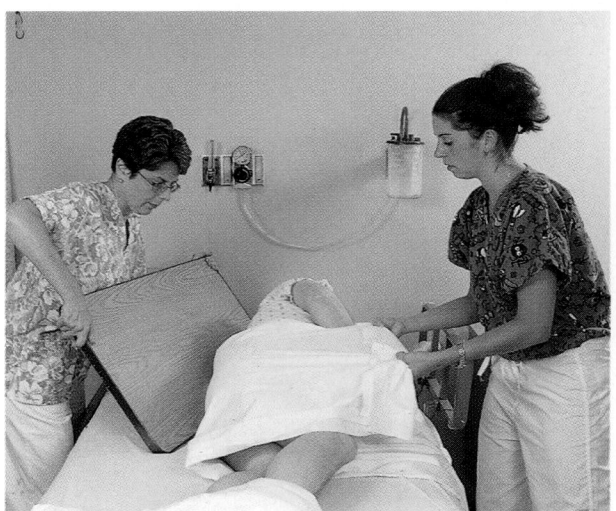

Step 6 Use of a draw sheet and transfer board helps in correctly positioning a client for movement. (©B. Proud.)

   Rationale: This provides smooth motion for transfer.
9. Roll client slightly up onto side, and pull transfer sled out from under him or her.
10. Lock up side rails on bed side of stretcher and move stretcher away from bed.
    Rationale: This provides for client's safety.
11. Place sheet over client and lock safety belts across client's chest and waist. Adjust head of stretcher according to client limitations.
    Rationale: Comfort, warmth, and safety are provided.

Lifespan Considerations
Infant and Child
- Infants can be safely held and moved by one person.
- Children may be moved by one or two people.

Adult
- Depending on level of musculoskeletal function, adults may be able to slide onto a stretcher with minimal assistance.

Collaboration and Delegation
- Acute care facilities and surgical centers often have transport aides that transfer clients via stretcher from one department to another. The nurse communicates any activity restrictions or special precautions (e.g., need for oxygen during transport).

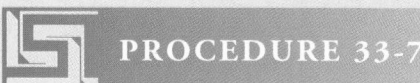

PROCEDURE 33-7

TRANSFERRING A CLIENT TO A WHEELCHAIR

Purpose
1. Prevent complications of immobility.
2. Increase independence and promote self-esteem.
3. Increase mobility status using a wheelchair.

Assessment
- Assess musculoskeletal function: joint mobility; paresis or paralysis of extremities; fractures, amputations.
- Assess cognitive function: ability to understand and follow directions; short-term memory and recognition of physical limitations to movement.
- Assess comfort level. Medicate as ordered with analgesics, and plan transfer when pain is relieved.
- Assess baseline vital signs. Assess for history of orthostatic hypotension.
- Review physician's orders for activity level.

Equipment
Wheelchair
Robe or appropriate clothing
Slippers or shoes with nonskid soles
Transfer belt

Procedure
1. Identify client and explain procedure.
   Rationale: Explanation reduces anxiety and gains client's cooperation.
2. Position wheelchair at 45-degree angle or parallel to bed. Remove footrest and lock brakes.
   Rationale: This facilitates a smooth, safe transfer.
3. Lock bed brakes; lower bed to lowest level, and raise head of bed as far as client can tolerate.
   Rationale: Amount of energy needed to move to a sitting position is decreased.
4. Assist client to side-lying position, facing the side of bed he or she will sit on. Lower side rail and stand near client's hips with foot near head of bed in front of and apart from other foot.
   Rationale: Nurse's center of gravity is placed near client's greatest weight to safely assist client to a sitting position.
5. Apply transfer belt. Grip belt to assist with transfer.
   Rationale: Transfer belt ensures the client's safety during transfer.
6. Swing client's legs over side of bed. At the same time, pivot on your back leg to lift client's trunk and shoulders. Keep back straight, avoid twisting.
   Rationale: Gravity lowers client's legs over bed while nurse transfers weight in the direction of motion and protects back from injury.

7. Stand in front of client, and assess for balance and dizziness.
   Rationale: Assessment prevents falls or injuries from orthostatic hypotension.
8. Help client to don robe and nonskid footwear.
   Rationale: Nonskid soles reduce risk of falling.
9. Spread your feet apart and flex your hips and knees.
   Rationale: Position lowers center of gravity and broadens base of support to provide stability and smooth movement using the legs' large muscle groups.
10. Have client slide buttocks to edge of bed until feet touch floor.
    Rationale: Position provides balance and support.
11. Rock back and forth until client stands on the count of three.
    Rationale: Rocking motion prevents muscle strain by giving client's weight momentum and requiring less of the nurse's energy to lift.
12. Brace your front knee against client's weak knee as client stands.
    Rationale: Position prevents weak knee from buckling and client from falling.
13. Pivot on back foot until client feels wheelchair against back of legs; keep your knee against the client's knee.
    Rationale: Ensure proper position before sitting.

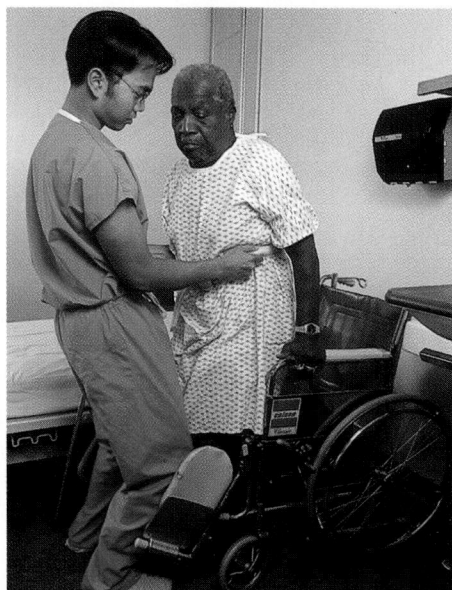

Step 13 Pivot client into wheelchair; have client grasp armrests.

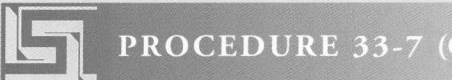

PROCEDURE 33-7 (Continued)

14. Instruct client to place hands on chair armrests for support. Flex your knees and hips while assisting client into chair.
    Rationale: Good body mechanics prevent back injury by supporting weight with large muscle groups.
15. Adjust foot pedal and leg supports.
    Rationale: Adjustments provide comfort and prevent injury to leg and foot.
16. Assess client's alignment in chair. Provide call light.
    Rationale: This promotes comfort and provides for safety.

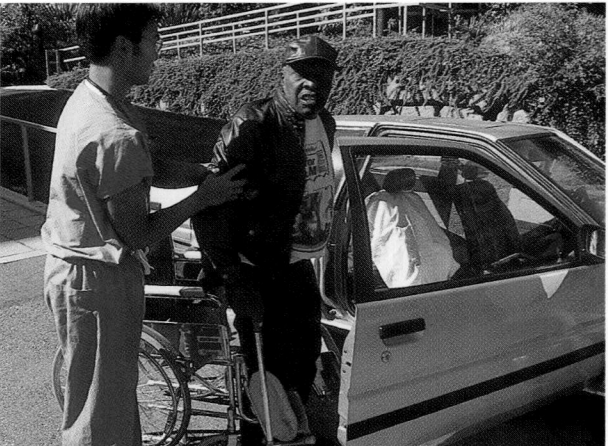

Help client master transfer from chair to car.

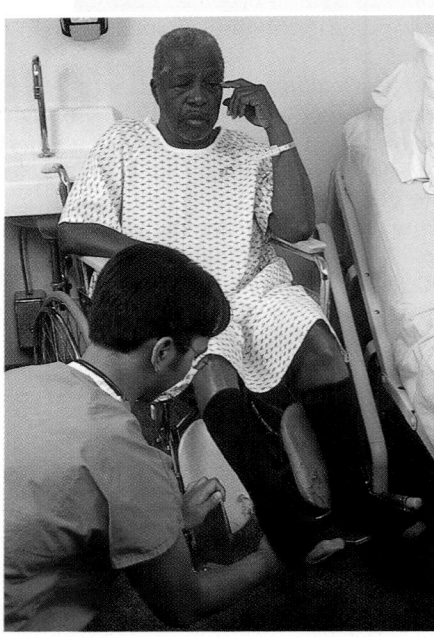

Step 16 Assess client's alignment and comfort.

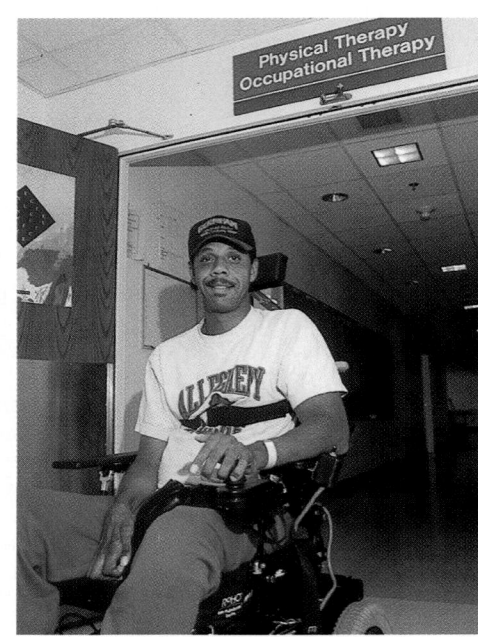

This client uses a motorized wheelchair.

Home Care Considerations
• Before client is discharged, client/caregiver should demonstrate safe transfer technique. Client should master transferring from a wheelchair to a car or van (see photograph). Motorized wheelchairs, designed for clients who have permanent injuries, permit a greater degree of mobility (see photograph).

Collaboration and Delegation
• Physical therapy may provide assessment and teaching for clients recently experiencing problems that significantly decrease mobility; increased assistance is required for safe transfers.
• Unlicensed assistive personnel should be required to get assistance when necessary to safely transfer a client.

TABLE 33-4

Transfer Equipment		
Device	**Purpose**	**Nursing Considerations**
Transfer board (also called transfer sled)	Smooth, flat surface placed under a supine client to ease the transfer to another flat surface	Use only when transfer surfaces are at the same height. Avoid pinching client's skin when positioning board.
Roller board	Also assists with transfers from one flat surface to another; consists of metal frame covered with longitudinal rollers encased in a fabric covering	Board is placed in the gap between the bed and the stretcher. Draw sheet is used to slide client across.
Transfer belt	Used for support during transfers or ambulation, especially for clients who are weak or dizzy, or have poor balance	Fasten belt snugly over clothing. Use whenever ambulation may be unsteady.
Hydraulic lift	Used to transfer immobile clients from bed to chair or bathtub. Lift has a canvas sling that fits under client and hooks into metal frame. Client can then be elevated and transferred using the hydraulic mechanism.	Reassure clients that they will not fall.

Hydraulic Lifts. A hydraulic lift is a mechanical device that permits a client to be transferred from the bed to a chair (Procedure 33-8). It is used when transferring a client may pose a safety risk to the client or the nurse. The lift has a canvas or fabric sling that fits under the client and hooks into a metal frame. Before using any hydraulic device, read the manufacturer's guidelines for proper operation. The client may become frightened when lifted away from the bed, so provide verbal support.

Stand-Up Assist Lifts. Stand-up lifts are helpful in assisting clients who can bear weight to assume a standing position. The sling in this lift is placed behind the back and under the arms (without causing pressure in the axillary area), the knees and legs are positioned against a padded support, and the fabric loops are attached to the lift frame (Figure 33-8). The lift then gently assists the client to assume an upright position or transfers the client to another location. The client is often unaware of the degree of support the lift provides and thus feels more independent than when moved by a hydraulic lift. The consistent use of stand-up lifts for all high-risk clients can decrease the incidence of back injury to the healthcare provider.

Healthcare Planning and Home/Community-Based Nursing

Most people with mobility problems manage independently in the community and at home. Acute injuries, such as fractures or sprains, are often treated with immobilizing braces until they heal. Most orthopedic surgery is now performed in same-day surgery centers, allowing the client to be discharged a few hours after the surgery. With adequate support, even chronic neuromuscular problems, e.g., from cerebrovascular accident, Parkinson's disease, or multiple sclerosis, can be managed at home.

Client teaching aims at helping the client learn to use special equipment and to live with motor limitations. The client and family should learn about transfer techniques, ambulation techniques, and special equipment. The physical therapist may provide much of this instruction with reinforcement from the nursing staff. Written instructions help reinforce initial learning and are useful for reference at home.

In some situations, the nurse may assess the client's home especially for safety. Ask about the physical layout of the house including the number of stairs, the location of bedrooms and bathrooms in relation to living areas, and the ability to accommodate special equipment in the house (e.g., if a wheelchair can fit through doorways). If disabilities are permanent, reconstruction may be necessary (e.g., ramps built to permit easy wheelchair access).

Stress the importance of safety to the client returning home with impaired motor function. Clutter and area rugs should be removed to prevent falls. Plans should be developed for emergencies. Smoke detectors should be installed, and the person's bedroom should be on the ground floor. The local fire department can provide a special alert sign to place in the handicapped person's bedroom window. Arrangements may be made for someone to telephone or check on the person daily; this is especially important for older adults living alone who are at high risk for falls.

Arrangements for special equipment and home services may be necessary. Sometimes equipment can be rented, or customized equipment may be made. Written referrals to home health agencies for nursing care, physical therapy, or other support services may be made as well. Telephoning such personnel to relay preliminary information promotes communication before discharge.

Modifications may be necessary for continued care in the home setting. When possible, the home situation should be simulated in the hospital before discharge. For example, if a hospital bed will not be available at home, practice transferring

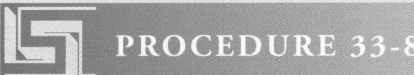

PROCEDURE 33-8

PROCEDURE FOR TRANSFERRING A CLIENT FROM BED TO A CHAIR USING A HYDRAULIC LIFT

Purpose
To safely transfer a client from a bed to a chair when safe transfer is not possible without using a hydraulic lift.

Assessment
- Assess knowledge of hydraulic lift being used.
- Assess musculoskeletal function: joint mobility; paresis or paralysis of extremities; fractures, amputations.
- Assess cognitive function or ability to understand and follow directions
- Assess comfort level. Medicate as ordered with analgesics before transfer
- Assess client's weight and your strength. Determine if assistance is needed.

Equipment
Hydraulic lift

Procedure
1. Identify client and any mobility restrictions. Explain procedure and purpose to client.
   Rationale: Explanation reduces anxiety and increases cooperation.
2. Place the fabric sling evenly under the client.
   Rationale: Even distribution of client's weight in the fabric sling provides for client comfort and safety.

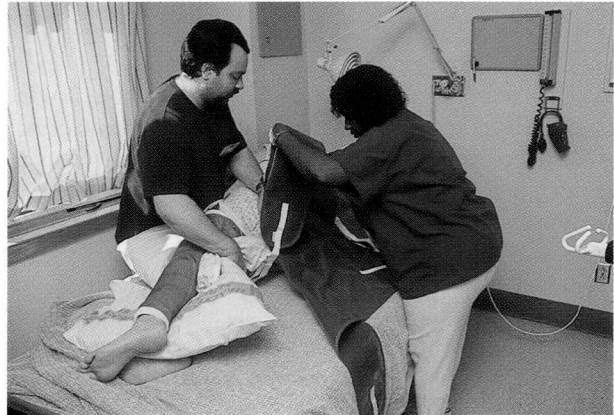

Step 2 Place the fabric sling under the client.

3. Position the hydraulic lift so the frame can be centered over the client. Attach the fabric sling to the frame. Note manufacturer's instructions for the specifics of how the sling should be attached to the frame.
   Rationale: Improper attachment of the sling to the frame can result in unequal distribution of body weight and possible injury.

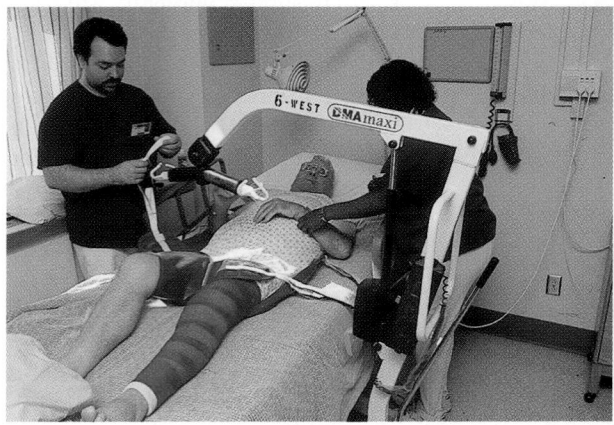

Step 3 Attach the fabric sling to the frame.

4. Have a nurse on each side of the hydraulic lift. Warn the client that he or she will be lifted from the bed. Support head of heavy casts as needed. Engage the hydraulic system to raise the client from the bed.
   Rationale: Supporting the client physically and verbally provides for client safety and helps reduce fear that often accompanies being lifted from the bed and suspended in mid-air.
5. Carefully wheel the client in hydraulic lift away from the bed, supporting limbs as needed. Position client over chair and gently lower to chair using the hydraulic mechanism.
   Rationale: Provides for client safety during transfer.
6. The sling remains in place under the client and is reattached to the frame when the client is moved back to bed.
   Rationale: Prevents unnecessary removal and replacing of sling under the client, which is difficult when client is sitting in the chair.

PROCEDURE 33-8 (Continued)

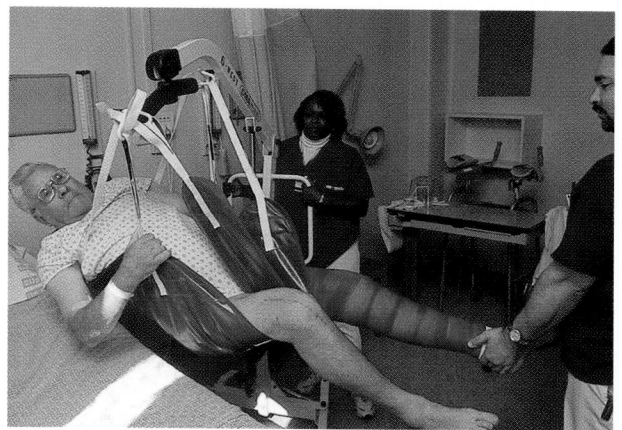

Step 5 Engage hydraulic system to raise the client from the bed and move the client to the chair.

Lifespan Considerations
Older Adult
- Being moved using a hydraulic lift is especially frightening for the older adult who is confused. Physical contact and verbal reassurance is helpful.

Collaboration and Delegation
- Often unlicensed personnel use hydraulic lifts to move clients especially in long term care facilities. All personnel need to complete instruction and be able to provide return demonstration prior to use with clients. Communicate clearly any mobility restrictions or special care in client transfer using the hydraulic lift.

the client in a high-bed position using a transfer sled or board. The client should discuss how he or she will manage such activities as bathing and cooking. The client who is place-bound due to mobility restriction can use a special reacher (Fig. 33-9) to achieve greater independence.

Often much family support is necessary for the client to manage at home. Family members should feel knowledgeable and comfortable in assuming this responsibility. They also should schedule time for respite from such responsibilities; time off will allow them to recover their strength and enthusiasm. Give relatives a telephone number of support groups to contact if problems arise. A physical therapist may provide education to caregivers to prevent back and neck injuries, improve general strength and balance, and facilitate the safety and

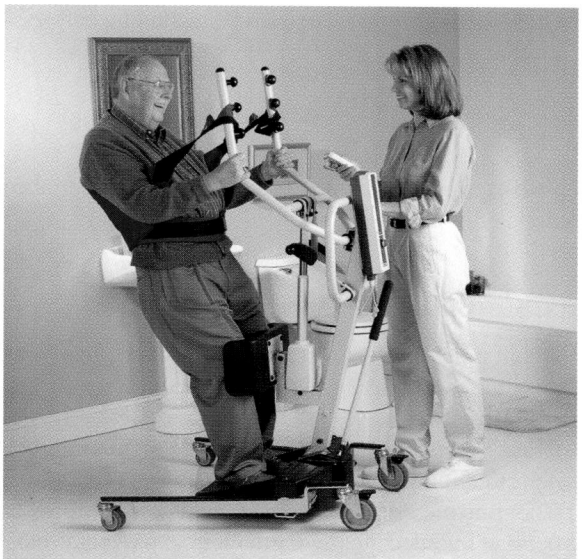

FIGURE 33-8 A Stand-Up Assist lift supports the client to an upright position when he or she can bear weight.

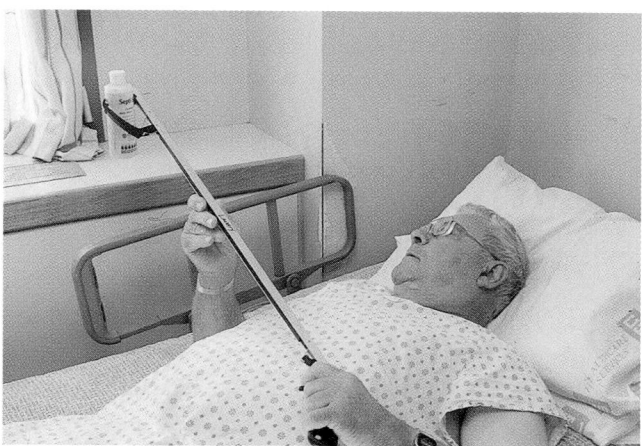

FIGURE 33-9 A reacher is a handy device for the client with mobility restriction.

mobility of care recipients (Cornman-Levy, Gitlin, Corcoran, & Schinfeld, 2001).

Great strides have been made in the United States to accommodate people with disabilities. Public buildings have wheelchair access, and special facilities can be found in some public restrooms. Some buses and vans are equipped to handle wheelchairs. Barrier-free, equal accessibility to public buildings is a right guaranteed to all people under the 1990 Americans with Disabilities Act.

 OUTCOME-BASED TEACHING PLAN

You are responsible for discharge teaching for Mr. Block, a 69-year-old retired plumber, who had a total hip replacement 2 days ago. He is a an independent man who lives with his wife in a two-story home.

OUTCOME: Mr. and Mrs. Block can verbalize precautions to avoid dislocation of new hip prosthesis.
Strategies

- Assess the Blocks' readiness to learn and their preferred learning styles.
- Collaborate with the physical therapist to understand the individualized mobility plan that has been developed and how Mr. Block has been doing.
- Review written sheet outlining hip dislocation precautions with Mr. and Mrs. Block (keep legs abducted or apart, never cross affected leg to midline, never flex hip more than 90 degrees, keep affected leg in neutral position).
- Demonstrate, on a model of the hip, how crossing legs or flexing at the hip joint causes dislocation.
- Have Mr. and Mrs. Block reverbalize precautions, providing praise when accurately done.

OUTCOME: Mr. Block will demonstrate hip dislocation precautions and verbalize how he will do this after discharge.
Strategies

- When Mr. Block gets out of bed, verbally cue him regarding proper movement of the affected hip.
- Provide a raised toilet seat and demonstrate how to use it.
- Have the Blocks describe their home and plans after discharge. Stress the following measures:
  – Take showers rather than baths.
  – Avoid using any low, soft chairs or sofas; reclining chairs are good.
  – Don't bend over to tie shoes or wash feet.
  – Never cross legs.
- Discuss plans for safe transport in the car to the home. (Place the seat in the farthest back position, lead with the unaffected leg when getting into the car, avoid bucket seats, incline the seat back to avoid a 90-degree angle.)

EVALUATION

Measuring outcome criteria helps determine whether or not the client has achieved mobility goals. Outcome criteria must be individualized for each client, but the outcome criteria listed here may be appropriate.

Goal

Client will exhibit increased endurance and tolerance for physical activity.

Possible Outcome Criteria

- Within 24 hours, client states the importance of gradually increasing activity or exercise.
- Client increases amount of exercise or degree of activity daily according to preset parameters.
- Client discontinues exercise or activity if experiencing adverse symptoms (e.g., dyspnea, tachycardia, pain, vertigo).

Goal

Client will actively participate in prescribed therapies to promote optimal healing and restored mobility.

Possible Outcome Criteria

- Client assists with turning by using trapeze and pushing with legs as instructed during repositioning.
- Client increases ambulation for a longer period each day.
- Client demonstrates use of crutches or walker before discharge.
- Client demonstrates safe transfer technique before discharge.

Goal

Client will participate in measures to prevent potential complications of immobility.

Possible Outcome Criteria

- Client practices leg exercises every hour to prevent possible thrombus formation during activity restriction.
- Client practices deep breathing and coughing every hour to minimize pooling of secretions.
- Client increases fluid intake to eight glasses of water per day for adequate hydration and to prevent urinary tract infections and renal calculi.
- Client performs ROM exercises daily as instructed to maintain joint flexibility.

NURSING PLAN OF CARE
THE CLIENT WITH IMPAIRED PHYSICAL MOBILITY

Nursing Diagnosis
Impaired Physical Mobility related to right-leg above-the-knee amputation, as manifested by inability to move the body purposefully and independently.

Client Goal
The client will learn how to move safely after above-the-knee amputation.

Client Outcome Criteria
• Client maintains balance and support by standing on left leg (with help of crutches or walker) 1 week after surgery.
• Client demonstrates safe transfer technique (in and out of bed, commode, wheelchair) by 1 week after surgery.

Nursing Interventions	Scientific Rationale
1. Keep stump flat and unrotated; do not place pillows under stump.	1. Keeping stump flat prevents contracture.
2. Encourage active ROM exercises every 8 hours.	2. ROM exercises improves joint flexibility.
3. Provide a program of frequent position changes that includes having client lie prone for ½-hour intervals every 8 hours.	3. Frequent position changes enhance mobility and prevent contractures.
4. Avoid long periods of sitting in bed or in a chair.	4. Sitting up flexes the stump and can cause contractures.
5. Take postural blood pressure measurements before client rises.	5. This will detect orthostatic hypotension and prevent falls.
6. Encourage client's active participation in physical therapy.	6. Encouraging physical therapy sessions should motivate client.
a. Discuss value of increasing muscle strength in the remaining leg.	
b. Note time when physical therapy is scheduled and ensure that client has eaten and is medicated (if needed) by that time.	
7. Remind client to use abdominal and gluteal muscles to avoid leaning to right side of body when standing.	7. Reminding client which muscles to use while standing promotes better balance.
8. Encourage client to wear a shoe that provides good support and has a nonskid sole.	8. Proper footwear prevents falls and promotes ambulation.
9. Instruct client to perform good foot care daily.	9. Injury to remaining foot will greatly reduce mobility and independence.
10. Show client how to use trapeze for exercise and in preparation for transfer.	10. Increase client compliance with self-transfers. Using trapeze for exercise should strengthen upper extremity muscles.
a. Attach trapeze above bed.	
b. Demonstrate use of trapeze to maneuver in bed and to transfer from bed to sitting position.	
c. Encourage strength in the upper extremities by having client pull on trapeze to lift body off bed, then lowering himself or herself slowly.	
11. When client is in wheelchair, encourage him or her to lift body by pushing down on the arms of the wheelchair.	11. Muscle strength is increased in upper extremities, preventing prolonged pressure and development of pressure sores.

(continued)

NURSING PLAN OF CARE
THE CLIENT WITH IMPAIRED PHYSICAL MOBILITY (*Continued*)

12. Develop a program of isometric exercises, and have client perform 10 repetitions three times a day. For example:
    a. Lie on back, squeeze cushion between legs.
    b. Lie on back, spread legs apart against belt buckled around thighs.
    c. Lie on stomach, lift stump toward ceiling.
    d. Lie on back, raise stump, then lower stump and hip, pushing down toward bed.
13. Teach transfer from bed to chair using stand–pivot technique.
    a. Use transfer belt.
    b. Client should wear shoe with nonskid sole.
    c. Verbally guide client through procedure.

    d. Praise successful efforts.

12. Isometric exercise should maintain muscle tone in right stump and left leg; spelling out exercises reinforces client's understanding of them.

13. A client with good strength in remaining leg should be able to transfer safely to chair using this technique.
    a. Enables you to grip client better during transfer.
    b. Decreases chance of slipping during transfer.
    c. Provides cuing for movement necessary during transfer.
    d. Psychological support and praise increase client motivation and reinforce client's effort.

KEY CONCEPTS

- The normal functions of the musculoskeletal system are proper body alignment, posture, balance, and coordinated movement.
- Proper body mechanics use alignment, balance, and coordinated movement to perform activities such as lifting, bending, and moving safely and efficiently.
- ROM is the ability to move a joint through the full extent of its normal movement. Active ROM is when a client can independently move the joint; passive ROM is when another person must do this for the client.
- Normal walking gait consists of the stance phase and the swing phase. Walking requires coordinated effort, balance, and equilibrium.
- Normal mobility requires an intact musculoskeletal system, nervous system control, adequate circulation and oxygenation, adequate energy, appropriate lifestyle values, and a suitable emotional state.
- Symptoms of altered mobility are decreased muscle strength or tone, lack of coordination, altered gait, decreased joint flexibility, pain on movement, and decreased activity tolerance.
- Immobility affects all areas of function and can contribute to many serious complications.
- Nursing assessment includes subjective data collection to determine normal mobility, risk factors for altered mobility, and any current impairments to mobility. Objective data provide information about body alignment, balance, coordination, gait, joint flexibility, muscle tone and strength, and blood pressure affected by positional changes.
- NANDA nursing diagnoses in the area of mobility are Impaired Physical Mobility, Impaired Walking, Impaired Wheelchair Mobility, Impaired Wheelchair Transfer Ability, Impaired Bed Mobility, Activity Intolerance, and Risk for Disuse Syndrome.
- Nursing interventions to assist the client with mobility problems include turning and positioning, providing ROM exercises, transferring, assisting with ambulation, and teaching how to use ambulation aids.
- Client goals concerning mobility should focus on promoting optimal mobility, increasing endurance and tolerance to exercise, preventing complications from immobility, and adapting to mobility restrictions.

REFERENCES

Atwood, R. M. (1999). Managing contractures in a long-term care setting. *OT Practice, 4*(4), 20–25.

Ayyappa, E. (2001). Normal human ambulation. *Orthopaedic Physical Therapy Clinics of North America, 10*(1), 1–15.

Conn, V. S. (1998). Older women's beliefs about physical activity. *Physical Health Nursing, 15*(5), 370–378.

Connelly, D. M. (2000). Resisted exercise training of institutionalized older adults for improved strength and function mobility: A review. *Topics in Geriatric Rehabilitation, 15*(3), 6–28.

Cook, D., Attia, J., Weaver, B., McDonald, E., Meade, M., & Crowther, M. (2000). Venous thromboembolic disease: An observational study in medical-surgical intensive care unit patients. *Journal of Critical Care, 15*(4), 127–132.

Cornman-Levy, D., Gitlin, L. N., Corcoran, M. A., & Schinfled, S. (2001). Caregiver's aches and pains: The role of physical therapy in helping families provide daily care. *Alzheimer's Care Quarterly,* (1), 47–55.

Dobkin, B. H. (1999). Disabling stroke: Managing common symptoms. *Family Practice Recertification, 21*(12), 31–34, 39–40, 45.

Ellingson, T., & Conn, V. S. (2000). Exercise and quality of life in elderly individuals. *Journal of Gerontological Nursing, 26*(3), 17–25.

Fox, P., Richardson, J., McInnes, B., Tait, D., & Bedard, M. (2000). Effectiveness of bed positioning program for treating older adults with knee contractures who are institutionalized. *Physical Therapy, 80*(4), 363–372.

Gleberzon, B. J., & Annis, R. S. (2000). The necessity of strength training for the older patient. *Journal of Canadian Chiropractic Association, 44*(2), 98–102.

Hieber, K. (1998). Mobility health assessment. *Orthopaedic Nursing, 17*(4), 30–35.

Huether, S. E., & McCance, K. L. (2000). *Understanding pathophysiology.* St. Louis: Mosby.

Kenny, A., & Taxel, P. (2000). Osteoporosis in older men. *Clinical Cornerstone, 2*(6), 45–51, 56–60.

Lappe, J. (1998). Prevention of hip fractures: A nursing imperative. *Orthopaedic Nursing, 19*(3), 15–24.

Leninger, S. (1998). Caring for a patient with a total hip replacement. *Nursing '98, 28*(4), 72–74.

Ludwig, L. M. (1995). Preventing footdrop when your patient's on the mend. *Nursing, 25*(8), 32C–32D, 32F, 32J.

Martini, F. H., Ober, W. C., Garrison, C. W., Welch, K., & Hutchings, R. T. (2001). *Fundamentals of anatomy & physiology.* Upper Saddle River: Prentice-Hall.

Metules, T. J. (2001). Occupational hazards. Watch your back! *RN, 64*(6), 65–66, 82.

North American Nursing Diagnosis Association. (2001). *Nursing diagnoses: Definitions and classification 2000–2001.* Philadelphia: Author.

Owen, B. (2000). Teaching students safer methods of patient transfers. *Nurse Educator, 25*(6), 288–293.

Porter, B. (2001). Nursing management of spasticity. *Primary Health Care, 11*(1), 25–28.

Porth, C. (1998). *Pathophysiology: Concepts of altered health states* (5th ed.). Philadelphia: Lippincott Williams & Wilkins.

Seebeck, A. (2000). Management of knee flexion contracture in elderly nursing home residents using the Contrac-Tree static positioning splint: A case report. *Issues on Aging, 23*(2), 19–22.

Theiler, R., Stahelin, H. B., Kranzlin, M., Tyndall, A., & Bischoff, H. A. (1999). High bone turnover in the elderly. *Archives of Physical Medicine & Rehabilitation, 80*(5), 485–489.

BIBLIOGRAPHY

Alexander, N. B., Galecki, A. T., Nyquist, L. V., Lofmeyer, M. R., Grunawalt, J. C., Grenier, M. L., & Medell, J. L. (2000). Chair and bed rise performance in ADL-impaired congregate housing residents. *Journal of the American Geriatric Society, 48*(5), 526–533.

Barnes, S., Gregson, J., Leathley, M., Smith, T., Sharma, A., & Watkins, C. (2000). Development and inter-rater reliability of an assessment tool for measuring muscle tone in people with hemiplegia after a stroke. *Physiotherapy, 85*(8), 405–409.

Bauman, W. A., Adkins, R. H., Spungen, A. M., Herbert, R., Schecter, C., Smith, D., Kemp, B. J., Gambino, R., Maloney, P., & Waters, R. L. (1999). Is immobilization associated with an abnormal lipoprotein profile? Observations from a diverse cohort. *Spinal Cord, 37*(7), 485–493.

Capezuti, E., Talerico, K. A., Cochran, I., Becker, H., Strumpf, N., & Evans, L. (1999). Individualized interventions to prevent bed-related falls and reduce siderail use. *Journal of Gerontological Nursing, 25*(11), 26–34, 52–53.

Jett, A. M., Lachman, M., Giorgetti, M. M., Assmann, S. F., Harris, B. A., Levenson, C., Wernick, M., & Krebs, D. (1999). Exercise—It's never too late: The Strong-for-Life program. *American Journal of Public Health, 89*(1), 66–72.

Kessenich, C. R., Guyatt, G. H., Patton, C. L., Griffith, L. E., Hamilin, A., & Rosen, C. J. (2000). Support group intervention for women with osteoporosis. *Rehabilitation Nursing, 25*(3), 88–92.

Leff, E. W., Hagenback, G. L., & Marn, K. K. (2000). Preventing home health nursing assistant back and shoulder injuries. *Joint Commission Journal on Quality Improvement, 26*(10), 587–600.

Lieber, S. J., Rudy, T. E., & Boston, J. R. (2000). Effects of body mechanics training on performance of repetitive lifting. *American Journal of Occupational Therapy, 54*(2), 166–175.

Neumann, D. A. (1999). Joint deformity and dysfunction: a basic review of underlying mechanisms. *Arthritis Care & Research, 12*(2), 139–151.

Resnick, B. (1999). Reliability and validity testing of the Self-Efficacy for Functional Activities Scale. *Journal of Nursing Measurement, 7*(1), 5–20.

Smith, A. (1999). Exercise in the management of mental health. *Sportex Medicine,* (3), 18–21.

Teixeira-Salmela, L. F., Olney, S. J., Nadeau, S., & Brouwer, B. (1999). Muscle strengthening and physical conditioning to reduce impairment and disability in chronic stroke survivors. *Archives of Physical Medicine & Rehabilitation, 80*(10), 1211–1218.

White, C. (1999). Pressure sore prevention: The latest in beds and mattresses. *Nursing Times, 95*(23), 54, 56.

34 Oxygenation
Respiratory Function

⑤ Key Terms

alveoli
apnea
atelectasis
bronchioles
bronchospasm
diffusion
dyspnea
hyperventilation

hypoventilation
hypoxemia
hypoxia
oxygen saturation
pulse oximetry
respiration
tracheostomy
ventilation

⑤ Learning Objectives

Upon completion of this chapter, the student will be able to do the following:

1. Identify factors that can interfere with effective oxygenation of body tissues.
2. Describe common manifestations of altered respiratory function.
3. Discuss lifespan-related changes and problems in respiratory function.
4. Describe important elements in the respiratory assessment.
5. List three appropriate nursing diagnoses and outcomes for the client with altered respiratory function.
6. Describe nursing measures to ensure a patent airway.
7. Discuss safe administration of oxygen using different modes of delivery.
8. Describe the impact of respiratory dysfunction on activities of daily living.
9. Identify home care considerations for the respiratory client.

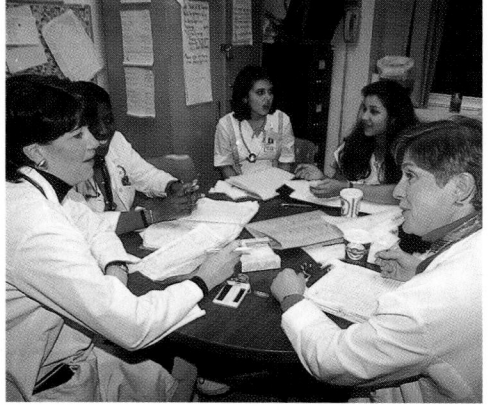

⑤ Critical Thinking Challenge

You are a nurse working in an intermediate care facility. In the past, your facility has served primarily geriatric clients. Recently the facility has begun to care for stable, ventilator-dependent clients. Although staff respiratory therapists regularly monitor the ventilator-dependent clients, the clients' arrival has caused considerable anxiety among the nurses. You have volunteered to serve on a committee to address their concerns.

After you have completed this chapter, return to the above scenario and reflect on the following areas of Critical Thinking:

1. Identify the nurses' concerns about the clients and about themselves that may contribute to their feelings of anxiety.
2. Compare and contrast special needs of these ventilator-dependent clients with those of the average geriatric client.
3. Describe how nursing personnel may collaborate with respiratory care personnel to optimize care for these clients.
4. Identify and plan strategies that may make the nursing staff feel more comfortable caring for the new clients.

The respiratory system replenishes the body's oxygen supply and eliminates waste from the blood in the form of carbon dioxide. During assessment of respiratory function, nurses gather information from clients, listen to breath sounds with stethoscopes, interpret laboratory tests, and make important observations to determine the effectiveness of clients' breathing. Assessment also allows nurses to identify risk factors that could cause respiratory impairment.

Nurses are responsible for promoting normal respiratory function regardless of the practice area. School nurses conduct classes about the hazards of smoking. Perioperative nurses instruct clients in deep-breathing techniques. Community nurses screen for and teach about tuberculosis prevention.

Nurses also help to improve breathing in clients with altered respiratory function. From positioning the debilitated client to managing sophisticated life-supporting ventilator systems, nurses play a vital role in assisting the client with respiratory disease.

NORMAL RESPIRATORY FUNCTION

Structure of the Respiratory System

Breathing delivers air to the lungs, where gas exchange occurs. Before reaching the lungs, air passes through a series of structures and tubes collectively called the airways (Fig. 34-1). The major organs of the upper respiratory tract are the mouth, nose, and pharynx. They are connected by the nasopharynx, which funnels incoming air through the mouth and nose into the lower portions of the pharynx.

The major organs of the lower respiratory tract are the trachea, lobar bronchi, segmental bronchi, and the lungs. The bronchi continue to branch in treelike fashion into **bronchioles,** which connect the larger conducting airways with the lung parenchyma. This gas-exchanging portion of the lung is made up of millions of tiny air sacs called **alveoli.** These thin-walled epithelial structures are in contact with a lush capillary network. Oxygen reaching the alveoli crosses the epithelium into the blood for transport to the heart then to body tissues.

The tracheobronchial tree and the lungs occupy the thoracic cavity. Lung inflation and deflation depend on complex, coordinated neuromuscular activity. The lungs move only passively: they stretch and recoil in response to muscular movement. The diaphragm (which separates the chest from the abdominal cavity) and the intercostal muscles (which lie between the ribs) are the primary muscles of breathing. These muscles respond to impulses from the central nervous system, which uses information obtained from specialized nerve centers in the aorta and carotid arteries.

Function of the Respiratory System

Ventilation

Breathing, or **ventilation,** is the physical process of moving air into and out of the lungs so gas exchange can take place. The mechanical process of ventilation is the result of volume and pressure changes in the chest cavity.

During inspiration, the diaphragm and external intercostal muscles contract. Their contraction enlarges the thorax volume and decreases intrathoracic pressure. The expanding chest wall pulls the lungs outward. As the lungs expand, pressure drops within the airways. As airway pressure falls below atmospheric pressure, air rushes into the lungs.

During exhalation, the process reverses. The diaphragm and intercostal muscles relax, causing the thorax to return to its smaller resting size. Pressure in the chest increases, allowing air to flow out of the lungs.

Ordinarily, little effort is required to draw air through the conducting airways. Cartilage holds open the larger airways sized for air to flow freely. The smallest conducting tubes of the lower airway, the bronchioles, are made primarily of smooth muscle. Smooth muscle tone helps them remain open and usually provides little resistance to breathing. Because there are millions of bronchioles, they have a collectively large diameter; thus, pulling air through these tiny tubes is easy. Inspired air finally reaches the alveoli in the lung parenchyma, which provide an amazingly large surface area for gas exchange.

Gas Diffusion

Oxygen and carbon dioxide move between the alveoli and the blood by **diffusion,** the process in which molecules move from an area of greater concentration or pressure to an area of lower concentration or pressure.

Breathing continually replenishes the lungs' oxygen supply, so the partial pressure of oxygen (PO_2) in the alveoli is relatively high. Simultaneously, breathing removes carbon dioxide from the lungs, so the partial pressure of carbon dioxide (PCO_2) in the alveoli is low. Blood returning to the lungs via the pulmonary circulation is the blood that the body's tissues have used, so it is low in oxygen and rich in carbon dioxide. Oxygen diffuses from the alveoli into the blood because PO_2 is higher in the alveoli than in the capillary blood. For similar reasons, carbon dioxide diffuses from the blood into the alveolar space. Figure 34-2 illustrates the exchange of gases across the alveolar-capillary membrane.

The blood passing through the pulmonary capillaries enters the systemic circulation as freshly oxygenated arterial blood. When oxygenated blood reaches the tissues, the exchange process occurs again but in the opposite direction.

Gas Transport

As oxygen crosses the alveolar-capillary membrane into the blood, the blood transports it to the tissues in two forms. Small amounts of oxygen are physically dissolved in plasma, but most oxygen that the blood carries to the tissues is attached to hemoglobin molecules on red blood cells. Hemoglobin has the unique ability to carry oxygen in its molecular form rather than as an ion. This difference is significant because tissues require molecular oxygen for metabolism.

The blood carries carbon dioxide in several forms. Blood transports carbon dioxide in a dissolved state, but carbon dioxide also can combine with some amino acids to form carbamino compounds. The most important transport mechanism for carbon dioxide is in its dissociated form. When

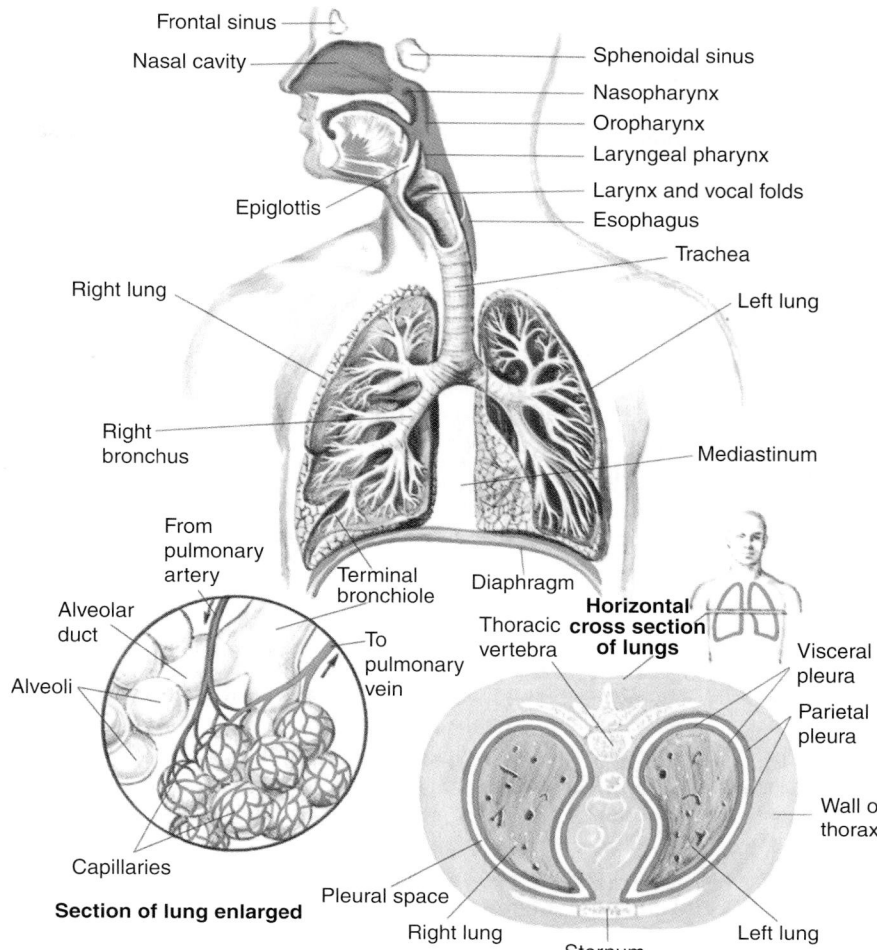

FIGURE 34-1   Respiratory system.

chemically combined with water, carbon dioxide dissociates into bicarbonate ions. These ions form the primary component of the bicarbonate buffer system, which plays a major role in maintaining the body's acid–base balance.

Control of Ventilation

The process of ventilation is regulated through neural pathways. Specialized neurons in the brain stem, known collectively as the respiratory centers, generate regular impulses. These impulses are transmitted to the respiratory muscles, causing them to contract and relax rhythmically.

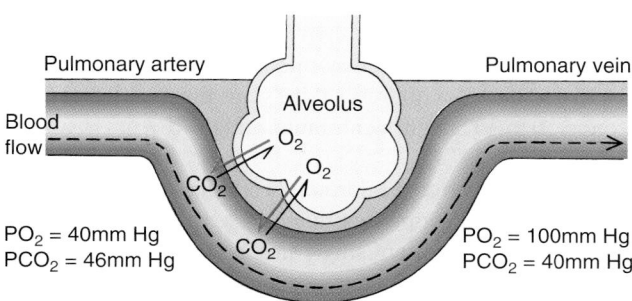

FIGURE 34-2   Gas exchange in the pulmonary capillary.

Peripheral and central chemoreceptors in the aortic arch and carotid arteries (peripheral receptors) and the medulla (central receptors) are sensitive to circulating blood levels of carbon dioxide and hydrogen ions. Decreases in the partial pressure of oxygen in arterial blood (PaO_2) also stimulate the peripheral receptors.

Carbon dioxide plays the primary role in determining the frequency and depth of ventilation. If carbon dioxide levels in the blood increase, the chemoreceptors are stimulated causing more deep and rapid breathing. The opposite is also true: Breathing decreases when carbon dioxide levels decrease. Normal breathing is usually regular and smooth because carbon dioxide levels remain fairly constant. The chemoreceptors also increase ventilation if arterial blood pH or PaO_2 falls substantially. In general, though, the degree of response to these conditions is less than when alterations occur in the partial pressure of carbon dioxide in arterial blood ($PaCO_2$) (Vander, Sherman, & Luciano, 2001).

Defenses of the Respiratory System

A major function of the upper respiratory tract is to warm and humidify inspired air. This moisture and warmth are necessary to maintain the fluid character of the mucus in the lower respiratory tract. The upper respiratory tract also cleans air.

The nose is a highly effective filter for foreign particles. It traps dust and irritants in hairs lining the nostrils or in the mucous layer of the nasal passages. The upper respiratory tract protects the lower respiratory tract from infection and from injury due to aspiration. The epiglottis acts as a trapdoor by preventing large particles of food or foreign matter from being accidentally aspirated. Below the epiglottis, the vocal cords, false cords, and aryepiglottic folds act as secondary protections against aspiration.

The lower respiratory tract's conducting tubes further filter and clean incoming air. An epithelial layer containing millions of ciliated cells and mucus-producing glands lines these conduction tubes (airways). The mucous membrane produces a "mucous blanket" that efficiently traps bacteria and microscopic foreign particles. The ciliated cells provide motion to the mucous blanket, allowing it to carry trapped matter upward and out of the respiratory tract. This "mucociliary elevator" protects the airways by constantly sweeping potentially harmful material out of the lungs. At the alveolar level, specialized scavenger cells called macrophages help decrease the risk of infection by eating bacteria and any minute particles that may have bypassed the mucous blanket.

The sneeze and cough reflexes also protect the lungs and airways. Irritants trapped in the nose stimulate sneezing; that reaction helps to expel trapped material from the nasal passages, thereby decreasing irritation and helping to prevent infection.

The lungs' most important defense is a strong and effective cough (Shapiro, Harrison, Kacmarek, & Cane, 1995). Coughing clears the lower airways much like sneezing helps to cleanse the nose. A forceful expulsion of air from the lungs can remove large amounts of germ-laden mucus. This action is vital for keeping the lungs free of infection. Coughing also helps to prevent mucous plugs from forming and to remove plugs already formed. In this way, airways remain open so all areas are available for gas exchange.

Normal Breathing Pattern

Although it varies depending on a person's age, normal breathing generally is smooth, even, and regular. It occurs at a rate of 12 to 20 breaths per minute in the older child and adult (Table 34-1). The rate does not vary significantly from one minute to the next unless the person's activity level changes.

TABLE 34-1

Respiratory Rates Through the Lifespan	
Age Group	Breathing Rate (breaths/minute)
Newborn and infant	30–60
1–5 years	20–30
6–10 years	18–26
10–adult	12–20
Older adult (60 years and older)	16–25

Exhaling normally takes twice as long as inhaling. Usually a person who is awake breathes slightly faster than one who is asleep.

Normally, each breath is about the same size. Despite an occasional sigh or yawn, the chest of a person who is breathing quietly will be seen to rise and fall the same amount from breath to breath. People who use their diaphragms effectively to breathe make their abdomens rise and fall. The average adult moves about a half a liter of air per breath.

Normal breathing is nearly effortless. Little muscular work is required to move air through the lungs. That is why quiet breathing is almost unnoticeable and ordinarily has no associated sounds. The rate and depth of ventilation increase during exercise to provide more oxygen to the tissues and to remove excess carbon dioxide. An athlete normally breathes more slowly and deeply while at rest than someone who is less fit.

Lifespan Considerations

Like the heart, the lungs perform a lifetime of continual work; however, the structure and function of the respiratory system undergo normal changes across the lifespan.

Newborn and Infant

In the uterus, the fetus' lungs grow rapidly as alveoli continue to develop throughout pregnancy. Until the 24th or 25th week of pregnancy, the fetus' lungs do not have enough properly functioning alveoli to make breathing effective (Avery, Fletcher, & MacDonald, 1999). It takes another 10 weeks or more for fully functional lungs to develop in the fetus. Surfactant, which decreases surface tension and permits alveolar expansion, is not produced in sufficient quantities until late in gestation. For this reason, babies born prematurely may require ventilatory support. Surfactant replacement therapy used in premature newborns has been shown to decrease the severity of respiratory distress syndrome (Lockridge, 1999).

Newborns breathe rapidly (30 to 60 breaths per minute), and, in general, larger newborns breathe more slowly than smaller ones (Avery, Fletcher, & MacDonald, 1999). The newborn's breathing pattern is characterized by occasional pauses of several seconds between breaths. This periodic breathing is normal during the first 3 months of life but frequent or prolonged periods of **apnea** (cessation of breathing of 20 seconds or longer) are abnormal.

Toddler and Preschooler

As children leave infancy, their breathing pattern evens out considerably. The respiratory rate of young children continues to decline. By children's third year, the rate decreases to around 20 to 30 breaths per minute, and the rhythm is smooth and regular.

During this period, children place things in their mouths, and caregivers must protect them against aspirating foreign objects that can obstruct small air passages. Providing safe toys and avoiding hard candy or small, hard pieces of food are important ways to ensure normal respiratory function for children in this age group.

Child and Adolescent

In growing school-age children, the breathing rate steadily slows to the adult rate of around 12 to 20 breaths per minute. During this period, good respiratory health is the general rule.

During adolescence, 3000 young men and women begin smoking every day and most will become addicted before age 20 (Hanson, 1999). One reason for this finding is that adolescents don't believe they will become addicted to tobacco when they start to smoke. The adolescents' sense of invulnerability leads them to believe that they are not at risk for lung cancer or heart disease because these diseases are commonly associated with older adults. The use of smokeless tobacco has dramatically increased over the last decade especially among 16- to 19-year-old males. One of the nurse's most valuable (and most difficult) functions is to educate adolescents about the health risks of smoking.

Adult and Older Adult

Structural and functional changes occur in the respiratory system in the later decades of life. The thoracic wall becomes more rigid, and the lungs become less able to stretch. There is no significant decrease in total lung capacity, but ventilation of non–gas-exchange areas of the lungs increases. The lungs' protective functions are impaired: There is decreased ciliary activity, and the cough is less propulsive and effective in airway clearance. Finally, gas exchange is affected: Normal PaO_2 decreases by 10% to 15% (Kidd & Wagner, 2001). These respiratory changes contribute to the activity intolerance and increased incidence of respiratory infections in older adults.

FACTORS AFFECTING RESPIRATORY FUNCTION

Respiration is highly complex and depends on many factors. Specific physiologic conditions, level of general health, lifestyle, and environment affect the process.

Body Position

An upright posture (standing or sitting erectly) allows for the greatest ease of lung expansion. The diaphragm can move up and down most readily when the abdominal organs are not pressing against it. Breathing requires more effort when lying down because the abdominal contents push against the diaphragm (Grap, Cantley, Munro, & Corley, 1999). This is especially evident in people with compromised respiratory function. During the last weeks of pregnancy, breathing may become increasingly difficult in a supine position because the fetus displaces the diaphragm upward.

Environment

The percentage of oxygen humans breathe, referred to as the forced inspired oxygen concentration (FIO_2), remains stable at around 21% when breathing "room air" (no supplemental oxygen). The atmosphere contains about 21% oxygen. Although the oxygen concentration does not change appreciably, its partial pressure decreases steadily as altitude increases. Lower oxygen pressure at higher elevations means that less oxygen is available to the lungs for gas diffusion. Thus, even healthy people are likely to experience shortness of breath and activity intolerance at higher elevations.

People's reactions to weather conditions are highly personalized. Some tolerate heat and humidity well; others may complain of difficulty breathing under these conditions. People who move to different climates may experience slight changes in breathing patterns until they acclimate to their new surroundings. People with chronic respiratory diseases often find breathing more difficult when the weather is hot and humid because humidity contributes to air viscosity. Some asthmatics breathe more easily in warm, dry climates; others find a damp climate more soothing.

Air Pollution

Industrialized urban areas may have elevated levels of air pollutants. Substances such as hydrocarbons and oxidants emitted by cars and factories interfere with oxygenation by directly damaging the lungs. Carbon monoxide inhibits oxygen attachment onto hemoglobin. Because they are respiratory irritants, pollutants cause increased mucus production and may contribute to bronchitis and asthma. Workers in industrial plants or in certain occupations may be exposed to strong concentrations of specific pollutants and harmful dust. These workers may be prone to development of breathing problems. The role of second-hand smoke (smoke from someone else's cigarette) continues to attract the attention of researchers for its negative impact on respiratory health.

Pollens and Allergens

Specific substances that cause allergic responses can affect respiration, sometimes severely. The body attempts to rid itself of substances perceived as harmful by releasing chemical mediators that cause an inflammatory response. Substances that trigger an inflammatory response are called allergens. Almost any substance can be an allergen; pollens, dust, and foods are common allergy triggers. The allergic response precipitates a series of events that lead to tissue damage.

Hay fever is the result of allergies confined to the nose and upper airways. Symptoms include dripping nose, itchy eyes, and swollen mucous membranes; they are annoying and uncomfortable but not life-threatening. When allergic responses take place in the lungs, breathing difficulties are far more severe. Small airways become edematous, mucus production increases, and inflammatory chemical mediators cause **bronchospasm.** These are the hallmarks of common allergic asthma. Severe and uncontrolled allergic asthma can be fatal.

Lifestyle and Habits

Smoking

Smoking is the most important lifestyle choice affecting respiration. Smokers are far more likely than nonsmokers to acquire emphysema, chronic bronchitis, lung cancer, oral cancer, and cardiovascular diseases. By producing more mucus and by slowing the mucociliary escalator, smoking inhibits mucus removal and can cause airway blockage, promoting bacterial colonization and infection. Regardless of whether or not a clinically identifiable lung disease is present, smokers usually breathe more rapidly than nonsmokers do.

Drugs and Alcohol

Barbiturates, narcotics, and some sedatives (legal or illegal) can depress the central nervous system with a resulting decrease in respiration. Alcohol in large doses can achieve the same effect. The intoxicated person is in danger of vomiting and aspirating stomach contents into the lungs. Alcohol depresses the reflexes that protect the airways, so if vomiting occurs, stomach contents can easily slip into the trachea and choke the victim. If the victim is revived, aspiration is likely to cause pneumonia.

Nutrition

Without proper diet, the body cannot effectively produce plasma proteins and hemoglobin. In addition, sufficient caloric and protein intake is required for respiratory muscle strength (Williams, 1999). People with diminished muscle strength work harder at breathing with even slight activity. For airways to remain patent, adequate fluid intake is necessary to keep secretions thin and easy to expectorate.

Adequate nutrition is also essential for maintaining a competent immune system. Alcohol abusers and malnourished people (e.g., from poverty or eating disorders) are at greater risk than well-nourished people for contracting pneumonia and other respiratory infections.

In the obese person, chest movement is restricted especially in the supine position; this restriction causes shallow respirations and increased respiratory rate. The extra work required to carry extra body weight increases oxygen demands.

Increased Work of Breathing

All bodily functions that require muscle movement involve a certain amount of work. For the healthy person, the work of breathing is minimal. Breathing becomes noticeable only during strenuous exercise because normal lung tissue is stretchy and the airways are open to allow air to flow through them.

In altered respiratory function, the amount of work required for breathing becomes significant because oxygen needs increase for respiratory muscles. Although these muscles ordinarily use less than 5% of the oxygen available in the blood, under extreme conditions (when the work of breathing is very high) muscles may use up to 50% of all oxygen available to body tissues (Shapiro et al., 1995). Because blood oxygen supply is limited, increased work of breathing can deprive other tissues of needed oxygen. The client who experiences increased work of breathing is at risk for oxygen deprivation and exhaustion. The two general causes of increased work of breathing are restricted lung movement and airway obstruction.

Restricted Lung Movement

Certain conditions and diseases may cause the lungs to stiffen or may restrict expansion of the chest. Stiffer lungs (or lungs not allowed to expand fully) tend to collapse and their alveoli also collapse. This condition is called **atelectasis.** The amount of space available for gas exchange in the lungs decreases. Some diseases cause lung tissue to swell and thicken. Oxygen has greater difficulty passing through thickened alveolar walls. Because stiff lungs require more work to expand, the respiratory muscles must consume a disproportionate amount of oxygen. In any of these situations, less oxygen is available to the blood for the tissues.

Actual stiffening of the lung tissues can result from acute or chronic lung injuries. Smoke inhalation, pulmonary fibrosis, respiratory distress syndrome (of the adult or infant), and infections such as pneumonia are examples of disorders that make lung tissues swell and stiffen. These types of problems are classified as restrictive lung disorders.

Not all restrictive problems are caused by lung injuries or lung diseases. A client can have perfectly healthy lungs but other factors may prevent the lungs from expanding completely. While the reasons for restriction may vary, the same problems with oxygenation can result. Pain from a surgical incision is a common example of this. For the client with a high abdominal incision, the discomfort of breathing deeply often forces shallow breathing; this is why atelectasis is common in postsurgical clients. Other factors that can restrict breathing include severe obesity, chest or abdominal binders, abdominal distention by gas or fluid, medications or anesthesia, rib injuries, musculoskeletal chest deformities, and severe weakness or neuromuscular disorders.

Airway Obstruction

Any process that reduces the diameter of the conducting airways causes increased airway resistance. Breathing then requires more effort because air must move through a narrower passageway.

Airways become obstructed in several ways. Airway lumen become plugged by foreign material, mucus, or abnormal growths. Children who aspirate small objects experience airway obstruction. The client who has chronic bronchitis, cystic fibrosis, or asthma may experience airway obstruction from excessive mucus production. Clients with lung cancer may experience difficulty breathing as tumors obstruct large bronchi.

Inflammation caused by chemical or physical irritants also can increase airway resistance. Inflammation makes airways swollen and edematous. As the walls of the airways thicken, lumen size decreases. Asthma, bronchitis, and bronchiolitis are examples of conditions in which small airways become inflamed and narrowed. Croup and epiglottitis, most common in young children, obstruct upper airways by swelling the throat tissues.

Finally, altered bronchial smooth muscle tone also causes airway obstruction. Normal smooth muscle tone maintains the patency of the smallest airways, the bronchioles. Allergy or injury may cause the smooth muscle to become hyperreactive to stimuli. This greatly increases smooth muscle tone, which narrows airway lumens and makes breathing difficult. Airway hyperreactivity, or bronchospasm, is a common problem for clients with asthma. By contrast, clients with emphysema experience breathing problems because of abnormally low bronchial smooth muscle tone. Years of damage to the bronchiole walls make them floppy and unable to remain open during exhalation. Air becomes trapped in the alveoli, leaving little space for newly inspired air and making full inspiration difficult (Copstead & Banasik, 2000).

ALTERED RESPIRATORY FUNCTION

Manifestations of Altered Respiratory Function

Cough

A cough is usually a reflexive response to irritation in the airways. Smoke is certainly an irritant, and coughing is the natural response to smoke. Coughs can be triggered by many chemical and physical substances or by physical conditions such as hot, dry air. There is no such thing as a "normal" cough. Any cough, regardless of how obvious its origin, is most often an indication that the lungs or airways are being subjected to some form of irritation. A cough's primary function is to help clear offending substances from the airways. A cough also serves as a warning signal: it should alert the person that possibly harmful stimuli are assaulting the airways, and that he or she should take measures to prevent further irritation. A cough that accompanies a disease may come from mediators released from inflamed tissues. These mediators, such as histamine, irritate the airways and can trigger a cough.

Not all coughs originate from lung problems. The client with borderline heart failure, for example, often has a chronic cough. Some people may cough for no apparent reason as a nervous habit.

Because coughs are so prevalent, their value as a diagnostic sign is limited. Many people live with a cough, expressing concern only when it changes in severity or frequency. By contrast, some people may have a serious lung disease but a minimal cough.

Sputum Production

As with a cough, sputum production may be a natural consequence of irritation, but it is never really normal. Respiratory mucus, or sputum, is another protective feature of the airways. However, mucus is normally produced in such small amounts that a cough from a healthy person is dry and nonproductive. Raising mucus with a deep cough indicates that the lungs are attempting to clear away irritants. Although the lungs may seem to be the obvious source of expectorated sputum, sometimes coughed-up secretions originate in the nose or throat. It is necessary to determine if the client raises the secretions with a genuine deep cough or if he or she snorts and clears them from the nasal passage. When a cough is productive, it is important to establish the source of the sputum and to assess its color, volume, consistency, and any other noteworthy characteristics.

Especially frightening can be the coughing up of blood, or hemoptysis. Blood-filled secretions that originate in the lungs may indicate a serious condition such as lung cancer or tuberculosis. Often, however, bloody secretions originate in the nose. Drainage from the nose or mouth can drip backward into the throat, staining the mucus of the lower airways. These sources of bleeding should be ruled out before the lungs are assumed to be hemorrhaging.

Shortness of Breath

A person who is unable to breathe sufficiently to meet the body's oxygen and metabolic demands experiences the discomfort of breathlessness. This subjective feeling of labored breathing and breathlessness is known as **dyspnea.** Display 34-1 outlines the various levels of dyspnea.

The most common cause of dyspnea is the increased work of breathing that occurs with lung disease. Along with increased work of breathing, other causes of dyspnea may need to be assessed. Reduced lung capacity, alterations in oxygen and carbon dioxide levels, or stimulation of receptors on the intercostals or diaphragm can contribute to dyspnea (Frownfelter & Ryan, 2000). People with chronic congestive heart failure often experience shortness of breath because of excess fluid in the lungs and low blood oxygen levels. People who become dyspneic during anxiety attacks often have no heart or lung disease.

Shortness of breath is a subjective symptom of lung problems. Some clients with severe lung disease appear to breathe with great difficulty, yet at such times they may report that their breathing is fine. Others may complain of severe dyspnea even when objective data (such as blood gas values or pulmonary function tests) indicate no apparent problem.

Chest Pain

Chest pain can be associated with a wide variety of conditions, some of which are respiratory disorders. Diseases characterized by inflammation or infection often cause pain. Inflammatory mediators such as histamine may directly stimulate nerve endings, some of which may be exposed and made

DISPLAY 34-1

⌐⌐ LEVELS OF DYSPNEA

Level I:	Client can walk 1 mile at own pace before experiencing shortness of breath.
Level II:	Client becomes short of breath after walking 100 yards on level ground or climbing a flight of stairs.
Level III:	Client becomes short of breath while talking or performing ADLs.
Level IV:	Client is short of breath during periods of no activity.
Orthopnea:	Client is short of breath lying down.

hypersensitive by the disease process. This occurs in the airways of the client with bronchitis who complains of a burning sensation with each cough. Acute bronchitis can make the simple act of breathing painful because the flow of cooler air across sensitized nerves can cause them to react violently. Mediators may also be responsible for edema formation, which can further contribute to pain as swollen tissues exert pressure on nerves. Clients with pneumonia often experience pain with deep breathing because each breath increases pressure on pain receptors that are already compressed and irritated by swollen, inflamed lung tissue.

Abnormal Breath Sounds

The breath sounds heard through a stethoscope can change as a result of lung changes. Crackles, wheezes, and pleural friction rub are examples of abnormal breath sounds. These are described in Table 34-2 and in the assessment section of this chapter.

Accessory Muscle Use

Healthy people use the muscles of the neck and upper chest to help them breathe deeply during vigorous exercise. The client with breathing problems may consistently use accessory muscles to ease dyspnea and improve breathing. Accessory muscle use is often evident by a forward-leaning posture. The nurse can readily observe the client raising the shoulders with each breath and straining the neck muscles to maximize chest expansion. Often, clients with chronic breathing problems use accessory muscles habitually, even at rest.

Cyanosis

Cyanosis is a bluish skin discoloration caused by a decreased amount of oxygen in the blood. Hemoglobin, the major carrier of oxygen in the blood, is bright red when saturated with oxygen. When not carrying oxygen, it becomes deep blue. This bluish state should be distinguished from peripheral cyanosis, e.g., blue fingertips on a cold day. Such problems are relatively benign and indicate only local vasoconstriction.

🖳 SAFETY ALERT

Central cyanosis, seen in the mucous membranes of the eyes and mouth, must never be ignored because it indicates the presence of serious oxygenation problems. (Griffey, Brown, & Nadel, 2000)

Clubbing

Clubbing is an unusual phenomenon seen in many clients with lung, heart, liver, or gastrointestinal disease. For reasons that are unclear, the tips of the fingers and toes become rounded and enlarged (see Chapter 24, Fig. 24-11). It is thought that long-term tissue **hypoxia** causes the release of a substance that causes dilation of the vessels of the fingertips (Copstead & Banasik, 2000). Clubbing occurs in lung cancer, cystic fibrosis, and in lung diseases such as lung abscess and chronic obstructive pulmonary disease.

Impact on Activities of Daily Living

Debilitation caused by lung disease can range from mild to severe. The client's ability to perform common day-to-day activities may be impaired because of breathlessness or oxygen dependence. Some clients become dyspneic with simple tasks such as shaving, cooking, or talking.

Meals can pose a problem for the respiratory client. Unless help is available, preparing meals can be exhausting work. Eating is an energy-expending activity. Many people with advanced lung disease cannot eat three large meals daily without feeling severely dyspneic. Many clients will prefer to avoid dyspnea by avoiding eating but this leads to a vicious cycle: The client who has insufficient energy to eat will continue to lose weight and have even less energy to expend eating. Some respiratory clients solve this dilemma by eating several smaller but nutritionally balanced meals; this approach helps to conserve oxygen and prevents the excessive buildup of pressure against the diaphragm caused by larger meals. This regimen provides needed nutrition without causing the breathlessness brought on by a full stomach.

Dressing is also tiring for some respiratory clients. Whenever dressing is physically possible, encourage the client to dress daily. Dressing is important for self-esteem and helps keep clients from thinking of themselves as invalids. Garments should be loose-fitting and easy to slip into. Dressing should be done slowly while sitting down.

Getting into and out of a bathtub can exhaust the breathless client, so showering may be preferred. The client with a laryngectomy or permanent tracheostomy tube can shower but should take care to avoid flooding the stoma with water. A washcloth held over the tube prevents this. A shower also imparts humidity to the mucous lining of the airways.

Elimination concerns of the respiratory client are important to consider. Constipation can cause abdominal distention, thereby limiting diaphragm movement. Extra straining also can tire the client and cause shortness of breath. Prescribed stool softeners and good hydration can help to prevent constipation.

Mobility within the home can be a problem for the client with extreme dyspnea. Use of prescribed oxygen during periods of daily in-home activity is helpful in building up tolerance to exertion. Use of stairs can be especially difficult and may necessitate moving sleeping areas to the main floor of the house. The client may need to rest frequently during periods of activity.

Mobility outside the home can also present special problems for the client with poor respiratory function. If public transportation is available, it may be several blocks from the client's home. Thus the client may have to rely on taxis or a private car. If the client uses oxygen and wants to fly, advance arrangements must be made with the airline. The client who is a marginal candidate for oxygen therapy may find a greater need for it on an airplane or at a high elevation.

Respiratory clients often are less communicative than other clients. This may be because of depression and feelings of isolation. However, some are less talkative because the act

TABLE 34-2 Adventitious Breath Sounds

Abnormal Sound	Characteristics	Location	Source	Conditions
Discontinuous Sounds				
Crackles (fine) Also called fine rales	High-pitched, short, popping sounds heard during inspiration and not cleared with coughing; sounds are discontinuous and can be simulated by rolling a strand of hair between your fingers near your ear.	Alveoli	Inhaled air suddenly opens the small deflated air passages that are coated and sticky with exudate	Crackles occurring late in inspiration are associated with restrictive diseases such as pneumonia and congestive heart failure. Crackles occurring early in inspiration are associated with obstructive disorders such as bronchitis, asthma, or emphysema.
Crackles (coarse) Also called coarse rales	Low-pitched, bubbling, moist sounds that may persist from early inspiration to early expiration	Peripheral airways	Inhaled air comes into contact with secretions in the large bronchi and trachea	Can indicate such conditions as pneumonia, pulmonary edema, and pulmonary fibrosis.
Continuous Sounds				
Wheeze (sonorous) Also called rhonchi or gurgles	Low-pitched snoring or moaning sounds heard primarily during expiration but may be heard throughout the respiratory cycle. These wheezes may clear with coughing.	Large airways	Same as sibilant wheeze. The pitch of the wheeze cannot be correlated to the size of the passageway that generates it.	Sonorous wheezes are often heard in cases of bronchitis or single-bronchus obstructions.
Wheeze (sibilant)	High-pitched, musical sounds heard primarily during expiration but may also be heard on inspiration.	Large or small airways	Air passing through constricted passages caused by swelling, secretions, or tumor	Sibilant wheezes are often heard in cases of acute asthma or chronic emphysema.
Pleural friction rub	Low-pitched, dry grating sound. Sound is much like crackles, only more superficial, and occurs during both inspiration and expiration.	Pleural surfaces	Sound is the result of rubbing of two inflamed pleural surfaces	Pleuritis

Adapted from Weber, J., & Kelly, J. (1998). *Health assessment in nursing.* Philadelphia: Lippincott-Raven.

of speaking can cause shortness of breath. It is difficult to inhale while speaking, so the dyspneic client typically speaks in short, terse sentences to conserve energy.

Respiratory dysfunction can impact the entire family, especially if the dysfunction is severe or chronic. Listening to or staying with a loved one in respiratory distress can cause much anxiety. Family members should know emergency cardiopulmonary resuscitation (CPR) to deal with a respiratory arrest until emergency medical help arrive.

The caregiver's burden depends on the degree of respiratory dysfunction. End-stage respiratory disease or chronic conditions can involve 24-hour care of the ventilator- or oxygen-dependent family member. Premature infants or children with cystic fibrosis often require continual ventilatory support for many years. In such situations, the parent also may grieve over the loss of the opportunity to parent a "normal" child.

ASSESSMENT

Although it is essential to obtain the client's history and perform a physical examination, the nurse may find that the client who is severely short of breath may be unable to respond fully to a battery of questions. The hypoxic client may respond with confused answers; forcing the dyspneic client to speak can worsen shortness of breath. Be sensitive to the client's ability to answer questions; if necessary, defer some questions until a more opportune time.

Subjective Data

Normal Pattern Identification
Unlike eating, sleeping, or elimination patterns, normal breathing is usually nondescript. Unless a person has experienced previous breathing problems, he or she is likely to have taken no notice of the normal breathing pattern. Few people can provide specific information about how often or how deeply they breathe. The nurse may generally assume that the client with no previous history of lung disorders breathes normally.

The normal breathing pattern of the person with chronic respiratory problems may differ greatly from that of the healthy person. For example, the client with chronic asthma ordinarily may breathe with a slight wheeze. Similarly the client with chronic obstructive pulmonary disease (COPD) may grow to accept shortness of breath after walking two city blocks as normal. The client begins to consider that something is wrong only if exercise tolerance decreases below this standard.

These examples show that the nurse must take care in eliciting information about normal breathing patterns. Clients who indicate that their breathing is ordinarily fine or unremarkable may have adjusted to a baseline breathing pattern that is abnormal for most people.

Risk Identification
Causes of the client's breathing problem may be rooted in long-term habits, occupational exposure, or past illnesses. Information about smoking habits is most important for providing insight into the client's condition. The duration and

extent of cigarette smoking is sometimes expressed in terms of "pack-years": 1 pack-year is equal to smoking one pack of cigarettes a day for a year. A person who has smoked two packs a day for 40 years would thus be said to have an 80 pack-year smoking history. Chronic bronchitis, emphysema, and lung cancer are directly related to smoking and are more likely to occur in clients with a long history of heavy smoking.

Other lifestyle factors can also affect lung health. The client who has lived in poverty and is malnourished, for example, is more at risk for infections such as tuberculosis. Tuberculosis and other respiratory infections also are more common in alcohol abusers. People with substance abuse are likely to have problems fighting infection because of self-neglect and the lowered effectiveness of their immune systems.

Work history often provides relevant information. Many occupations involve exposure to fumes or dust such as silicon and asbestos, which are toxic to lung tissue. Agricultural workers are exposed to organic dusts such as molds that can cause infections and asthma-like symptoms.

Family and personal history are also essential to a thorough evaluation. Cystic fibrosis is genetically transmitted, as is α_1-antitrypsin deficiency, which causes emphysema that develops in early adulthood. The client with asthma often recalls a childhood with allergies and eczema. A history of dental problems may explain a client's bronchiectasis or lung abscess.

Investigate a sleep history by including information about excessive daytime sleepiness, morning headache or sore throat, personality changes, or loud snoring or frequent periods of apnea during sleep reported by the spouse. These symptoms commonly occur in sleep apnea, which is common in obese, middle-aged adults. Sleep apnea causes a significant decrease in oxygenation due to multiple apneic periods during sleep.

Dysfunction Identification
When gathering information about the onset and duration of a recent breathing problem, determine if the problem is continuous or intermittent. If the problem seems to be continuous, perhaps some new exposure, such as new carpeting or a new pet, has triggered an allergic reaction. The client may have contracted an infection that has progressed or has remained subacute. If the problem is intermittent, ask if the client can identify the circumstances that bring on the difficulty. Perhaps the client's breathing worsens at certain times of the day or when the client engages in certain activities. Assess cough, dyspnea, sputum production, and discomfort or pain.

Establish if a cough is ordinarily present, for example, and, if so, at what times of the day it usually occurs. The client may deny being usually short of breath unless you can specify degrees of dyspnea to which he or she can relate. Ask how far the client can walk before needing to rest ("A mile; a city block; a flight of stairs; 20 feet?"). Ask the client how much sputum he or she usually coughs up ("A teaspoon; a tablespoon; a half cup?") and about its color. Family members and people close to the client may be helpful in providing supportive information.

A variety of emotions accompanies breathing problems. Acute episodes of dyspnea bring anxiety and fear. Panic often accompanies severe dyspnea. Clients with chronic respiratory problems may experience self-consciousness and embarrassment. Because breathlessness may interfere with communication ability, the chronic respiratory client may feel isolated and appear aloof. This can contribute to frustration, irritability, and eventual depression caused by continued illness and loss of independence.

Objective Data

Physical Assessment

The primary techniques used in physical assessment are inspection, palpation, percussion, and auscultation. Sputum is visually examined.

Inspection. An essential observation is the rate and pattern of respiration. Excessively slow breathing can cause **hypoxemia** (low oxygen levels in the blood) and hypercapnia (abnormally high carbon dioxide in the blood). Conversely, breathing too fast causes excessive elimination of carbon dioxide, which causes dizziness and possibly respiratory alkalosis. Rapid breathing by the severely debilitated client may lead to exhaustion.

Normal respirations should be smooth and regular. Except in the newborn, uneven or irregular breathing can indicate airway obstruction or signal neurologic or muscle problems. Assessment of breathing rate and pattern is described in Chapter 25.

Observe the client's breathing effort by noting obvious use of shoulder or neck muscles. The client with COPD often sits in a forward-leaning position, which uses the accessory muscles to help enlarge the chest cavity for more air. This indicates shortness of breath and may be seen as well in clients without COPD who are having other respiratory or cardiac problems. Note other obvious signs of dyspnea such as gasping, audible wheezing, or panting respirations. In the infant, flaring of the nostrils and retractions of the ribs during inspiration are notable signs of air hunger and extraordinary work of breathing.

In addition to describing the breathing pattern, observe the client's color. Cyanosis around the lips and under the tongue indicates serious hypoxemia.

Finally, inspect the chest to detect obvious chest deformities, wounds, or masses. The chest's overall shape is important but less obvious. In COPD, the client's chest becomes hyperinflated over time because of an inability to exhale fully. This increases the anterior–posterior chest diameter, resulting in a barrel-shaped appearance.

Palpation. The hands are used to assess abnormalities such as swelling or tenderness. Palpation is also used to determine the extent and pattern of thoracic expansion and to note the position of the trachea. Palpation may detect abnormal chest wall vibrations transmitted through inflamed or fluid-filled lung tissues. Fremitus (the vibration of air movement through the chest wall) is best felt by placing the balls of the palms of your hand on the client's back as he or she says "99." The intrascapular space is the best area to feel tactile fremitus because it dimin-

ishes as you move out in the lung fields (O'Hanlon-Nichols, 1998). Increased tactile fremitus can be present in consolidation in the lung, whereas decreased fremitus may occur with pleural effusion, pulmonary edema, emphysema, or bronchial obstruction.

Percussion. Percussion is used to detect fluid-filled or consolidated portions of the lung. A keen ear and experience with pulmonary assessment are needed to interpret correctly the various alterations in pitch, intensity, duration, and quality of percussion notes.

Auscultation. Listening to breath sounds with a stethoscope provides vital information for evaluating the client's respiratory status. Chapter 24 describes normal breath sounds classified as bronchial, bronchovesicular, and vesicular.

The most important reason for listening to the chest is to determine if air is moving through all areas of the lung. When auscultating with a sensitive stethoscope, you should be able to hear air moving in all lung fields. Breath sounds should be equally loud on both sides of the chest.

Absent or distant-sounding breath sounds in any area of the lung can indicate airway obstruction or can mean that fluid or air has accumulated in the pleural space. A "quiet chest" in an asthmatic who is experiencing severe shortness of breath is a grave sign of poor ventilation and impending respiratory failure (Reinke & Hoffman, 2000).

The quality of breath sounds can also be assessed by auscultation. Normal breathing should make soft, rustling sounds like a breeze blowing gently through leaves on trees. Only inspiratory sounds should be noticeable; expiration should be quiet.

Nurses must also become familiar with abnormal breath sounds (see Table 34-2). They have been described in a variety of terms through the years. Official nomenclature (as developed by the American Thoracic Society) is presented here, but be aware that alternative terminology is commonly used.

Crackles (also called rales) are discontinuous sounds heard on inspiration; they indicate the presence of fluid in the lungs. These sounds are often heard in clients with obstructive diseases or pneumonia. Crackles range from soft, fine sounds to coarse, rattling sounds. When they are coarse and loud and occur with severe dyspnea, crackles may be a telling sign of pulmonary fibrosis, congestive heart failure, and pulmonary edema.

A coarse crackle is a low-pitched, rumbling sound that indicates sputum in the airways. These sounds, often called gurgles or rhonchi, are common in clients with chronic bronchitis or cystic fibrosis or in any disorder that produces an excess of mucous secretions. Often rhonchi clear with a strong cough. If the client has a weak cough and cannot clear the secretions, coarse wheezes can indicate the need for airway suctioning.

Wheezes are continuous sounds created by air passing through narrowed airways. They are differentiated by pitch and sound quality. High-pitched, musical sounds are caused by air traveling through bronchospastic or edematous airways. Expiratory wheezes are common in the client with asthma and COPD. Coughing does not usually make this type of wheeze disappear. In many cases, bronchodilators and corticosteroids are required to open the client's airways and ease breathing. Inspiratory wheezes can be heard when the upper airways are swollen and edematous. The most severe type of inspiratory wheeze is called stridor, heard most commonly in children with croup or epiglottitis. If upper airway obstruction becomes too severe, an artificial airway (such as an endotracheal tube or a tracheostomy) must be used to ensure an open passage for breathing.

A pleural friction rub produces a dry rubbing or grating sound caused by inflammation of pleural surfaces rubbing against the chest wall. A pleural friction rub can be heard best on inspiration but also is present during expiration; the rub does not disappear with a cough. This abnormal breath sound is loudest over the lung's lower lateral anterior surface. Unlike a pericardial friction rub, a pleural friction rub disappears when breathing stops.

Sputum Assessment. Any sputum that the client coughs up should be inspected. Normal respiratory secretions are clear or white. Normal sputum has no odor and medium consistency. Thick and sticky sputum is usually difficult to expectorate and may indicate that the client is poorly hydrated. Sputum produced by clients with asthma is stringy, like thickened egg white. Life-threatening pulmonary edema produces frothy, pinkish secretions.

Sputum that is yellow or greenish or has a putrid or musty odor usually indicates infection. When you suspect infection, collect a sputum sample in a sterile container and send the sample to the laboratory for examination.

Blood-streaked mucus indicates airway inflammation; although alarming, it usually is not serious. It commonly occurs during harsh coughing episodes in clients with bronchitis. Frankly red, bloody mucus (hemoptysis) is a sign of continual bleeding somewhere in the airways that requires thorough investigation.

Diagnostic Tests and Procedures

The most commonly used tests for assessing respiratory status are chest x-ray, pulmonary function tests, sputum culture, and arterial blood gas analysis. Pulse oximetry now permits noninvasive measurement of oxygen saturation to monitor and direct clinical management. More specialized tests include lung scans and pulmonary angiography, bronchoscopy, skin testing for allergies in asthma, and skin tests for tuberculosis.

Chest X-ray. The chest x-ray is widely used to identify pathologic changes in the lung and chest that may explain the client's breathing problems. From a chest x-ray, the radiologist can detect abnormal fluid or air in the pleural space or the presence of a collapsed lung (pneumothorax). The x-ray can also show if portions of the lungs are consolidated (as in pneumonia) or underinflated (as in atelectasis). Sometimes routine x-rays initially detect tumors. The chest x-ray is also used to determine the position of catheters and tubes and to monitor a client's response to therapy.

Lung scans and angiography are specialized radiographic techniques used to study blood flow and ventilation in the lung.

Pulmonary Function Tests. Specialized breathing tests measure lung size and airway patency. Spirometry produces graphic representations of lung volumes and flows. These graphs are essential in determining the severity of a client's restrictive or obstructive lung disease. Common measurements include tidal volume, vital capacity, and forced expiratory volume in 1 second (FEV-1). More highly specialized pulmonary function tests can provide additional information on lung characteristics.

Sputum Culture. The client who has a productive cough, is febrile, and shows other signs of infection should have a sputum sample evaluated by the laboratory. A Gram's stain can be performed quickly to determine the presence of an infection and classify it as gram positive or gram negative. Sputum is cultured to identify the specific agent causing the infection. A sensitivity test done at the same time will indicate the best antibiotic to use against the causative agent, but treatment for 2 to 3 days is needed for results.

Arterial Blood Gas Monitoring. Arterial blood levels of oxygen, carbon dioxide, and pH are the most reliable indicators of gas exchange. PaO_2 is one of the best indicators of how much oxygen is available to tissues. When the PaO_2 is lower than normal, tissues may experience hypoxia. This development is dangerous to all tissues and organs but can be especially damaging to the heart and the brain, where hypoxia can result in a myocardial infarction or a cerebrovascular accident. Although PaO_2 normally declines with age, an abnormally low PaO_2 always indicates gas exchange problems (Kidd & Wagner, 2001). PaO_2 decreases in direct proportion to the severity of lung impairment (Display 34-2).

In addition to oxygenation, arterial blood sampling also indicates how effectively the lungs are removing carbon dioxide. The lungs' regulation of this metabolic waste product is essential for the blood's normal acid-base balance. The carbon dioxide level affects many functions including the drive to breathe,

DISPLAY 34-2

🔢 **LEVELS OF HYPOXEMIA**

Mild:	PaO_2 of 60–80 mm Hg
Moderate:	PaO_2 of 40–60 mm Hg
Severe:	PaO_2 of less than 40 mm Hg

Note: PaO_2 naturally declines with age. For every year over 60, subtract 1 mm Hg from the normal range. For example, a man of 70 would be expected to have a PaO_2 of 70–90 mm Hg.

Also, the newborn is normally hypoxemic during the first 12–24 hours of life. A PaO_2 of 80–100 mm Hg is achieved after this time.

affinity of hemoglobin for oxygen, and cardiac function. The $PaCO_2$ stays nearly constant in the person with healthy lungs. A $PaCO_2$ lower than 35 mm Hg indicates **hyperventilation,** or breathing in excess of metabolic needs. Healthy people are able to hyperventilate voluntarily. Hyperventilation is common during an asthma attack and occurs in some clients with head injuries. It may also occur involuntarily during extreme anxiety.

A $PaCO_2$ above 45 mm Hg indicates **hypoventilation,** in which breathing rate and depth are insufficient to clear carbon dioxide adequately from the blood. Severe airway obstruction causes hypoventilation, which is a serious problem for clients with advanced COPD. Respiratory failure is another cause of hypoventilation in clients whose respiratory drive has been diminished by narcotics, barbiturates, or trauma.

Arterial blood sampling also indicates the blood's acidity or alkalinity. The pH is a measure of the blood's acid-base balance. Biochemical processes essential to all cellular life require a close balance of acids and bases. Normally, arterial blood pH ranges from 7.35 to 7.45. Arterial pH below 7.35 is described as acidosis, whereas pH above 7.45 indicates alkalosis (Table 34-3). Chapter 36 presents a more detailed discussion of acid-base balance.

Pulse Oximetry. **Pulse oximetry** offers a noninvasive means for approximating oxygenation, whereas arterial blood sampling provides precise information about blood gases. The pulse oximeter uses infrared light to determine the percentage of hemoglobin that combines with oxygen. A sensor attached to the client's finger or earlobe allows assessment of heart rate and oxygen saturation either intermittently or continuously. Oximetry is a convenient and painless alternative to needlesticks, is simple to use, and provides immediate data. These advantages make oximetry an invaluable tool for determining the client's need for oxygen therapy and assessing the therapy's effectiveness.

The oximeter registers arterial **oxygen saturation** (SaO_2). An SaO_2 greater than 95% is considered normal, whereas values lower than 93% usually indicate the need for oxygen therapy and further assessment.

Several factors affect the accuracy and proper interpretation of oximetry. The client must have adequate peripheral blood flow for the oximeter to detect a pulse. Conditions such as room lighting, client motion, cigarette smoking, or dark polish on the client's fingernails can affect sensor accuracy. Carbon monoxide poisoning results in false high readings; edema at the sensor site produces false low readings (Ehrhardt & Daleiden, 1994). Most importantly, interpretation of SaO_2 depends on the

operator's understanding of hemoglobin and its unique properties. Because of the manner in which hemoglobin combines with oxygen, relatively slight changes in SaO_2 may actually reflect large changes in blood oxygenation. Experience and clinical judgment help the skilled practitioner relate oximetry readings to client condition. Refer to Procedure 34-1 for guidance using pulse oximetry.

Bronchoscopy. Bronchoscopy allows the physician to visualize the airways directly. A flexible fiberoptic tube connected to a viewing screen is inserted through the client's nose. A hand-held control directs the scope into the trachea and bronchi. The bronchoscope can be used to collect sterile sputum specimens or tissue samples for laboratory examination or to withdraw large sputum plugs or aspirated objects obstructing the airways.

Nursing interventions for a bronchoscopy include ensuring informed consent, preprocedure teaching, and maintaining NPO status until the gag reflex returns after the procedure. Postprocedure assessments include frequent assessment for dyspnea, hemoptysis, or cardiac arrhythmias.

Skin Tests. Skin tests can be performed to identify a client's allergies to specific substances. By determining possible sources of airway hypersensitivity in asthmatic clients, allergists can help these people avoid the offending substances. These tests also help the allergist devise serums for desensitizing the client. Another type of skin test is used to establish whether or not a client has been exposed to tuberculosis. The purified protein derivative (PPD) test is a vital screening tool that helps identify people who may have been exposed to tuberculosis.

NURSING DIAGNOSES

Respiratory nursing diagnoses include Ineffective Breathing Pattern, Ineffective Airway Clearance, and Impaired Gas Exchange. In 1992, the North American Nursing Diagnosis Association (NANDA) added Inability to Sustain Spontaneous Ventilation and Dysfunctional Ventilatory Weaning Response, but because these are nursing diagnoses encountered in critical care units, they will not be developed in depth here.

Diagnostic Statement: Ineffective Breathing Pattern

Definition. Ineffective Breathing Pattern is the state in which a person's inspiration and/or expiration pattern does not provide adequate ventilation (NANDA, 2001).

Defining Characteristics. Defining characteristics include decreased inspiratory/expiratory pressure, decreased minute ventilation, dyspnea, shortness of breath, tachypnea, fremitus, abnormal arterial blood gas values, cyanosis, cough, nasal flaring, respiratory depth changes, assumption of three-point position, pursed-lip breathing or prolonged expiratory phase,

(text continues on page 824)

TABLE 34-3

Normal Arterial Blood Gas Values	
PaO_2	80–100 mm Hg
$PaCO_2$	35–45 mm Hg
pH	7.35–7.45
HCO_3^-	22–26 mEq/L
Base excess	±2

PROCEDURE 34-1

MONITORING WITH PULSE OXIMETRY

Purpose
1. Monitor arterial oxygen saturation (SaO_2) non-invasively.
2. Detect clinical hypoxemia promptly.
3. Assess client's tolerance to tapering of oxygen therapy or activity.

Assessment
- Identify clients at risk for hypoxemia (i.e., respiratory and cardiac disease) who would benefit from pulse oximetry.
- Identify indications for continuous or intermittent oximetry monitoring.
- Assess client's baseline respiratory status including vital signs, skin and nailbed color, breath sounds, shortness of breath, alterations in breathing patterns, current oxygen supplementation, presence of dysrhythmias, and tissue perfusion of extremities.
- Review laboratory hemoglobin values to identify anemic clients whose oxygen content in the blood may be low although their SaO_2 is within normal levels.
- To choose appropriate sensor, observe client's height, weight, and size, and note any allergies to adhesive.

Equipment
Pulse oximeter
Nail polish remover, if needed

Procedure
1. Select appropriate type of sensor. A wide variety of sensors are available in sizes for neonates, infants, children, and adults. In addition, there are clip-on, adhesive, and disposable sensors. To select the appropriate sensor, consider the client's weight, activity level, if infection control is a concern, tape allergies, and anticipated duration of monitoring.
   Rationale: Proper sensor will increase accuracy of reading.
2. Explain purpose of procedure to client and family.
   Rationale: Understanding the procedure increases compliance and prevents anxiety.
3. Instruct client to breathe normally.
   Rationale: Consistent breathing prevents large fluctuations in minute ventilation and inaccurate reflections of SaO_2 levels.

4. Select appropriate site to place sensor. Avoid using lower extremities that may have compromised circulation, or extremities receiving infusions or other invasive monitoring. If client has poor tissue perfusion due to peripheral vascular disease or is receiving vasoconstrictor medications, a nasal sensor or forehead sensor may be considered.
   Rationale: Decreased circulation can falsely alter the SaO_2 measurements from the pulse oximeter.
5. Remove nail polish or acrylic nail from digit to be used.
   Rationale: Polish and artificial nails can interfere with accurate measurements.
6. Attach sensor probe and connect it to the pulse oximeter. Make sure the photosensors are accurately aligned.
   Rationale: Proper alignment is essential for accurate SaO_2 measurement.

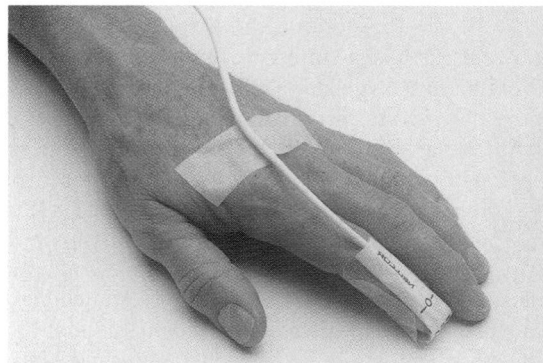

Step 6 Attach sensor probe.

7. Watch for pulse sensing bar on face of oximeter to fluctuate with each pulsation and reflect pulse strength. Double-check machine pulsations with client's radial or apical pulse.
   Rationale: A weak signal or missed pulsations will not produce an accurate measurement.
8. If continuous pulse oximetry is desired, set the alarm limits on the monitor to reflect the high and low oxygen saturation **and** pulse rates. Ensure that the alarms are audible before leaving the client. Inspect the sensor site every 4 hours for tissue irritation or pressure from the sensor.
   Rationale: Ensure client safety by prompt detection of low critical oxygen saturation values or tissue irritation.
9. Read saturation on monitor and document as appropriate with all relevant information on client's chart. Report SaO_2 less than 93% to physician.

PROCEDURE 34-1 (Continued)

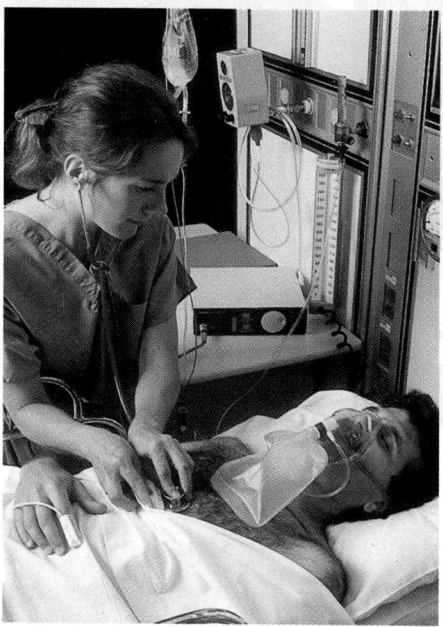

Step 7 Compare apical pulse with pulsations detected by oximeter.

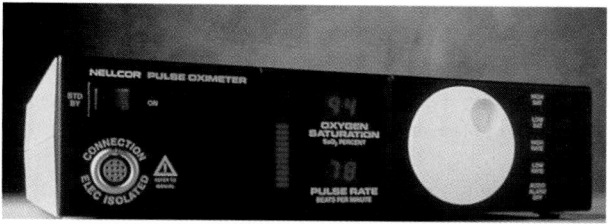

Step 9 Read oxygen saturation from monitor.

Rationale: Documentation provides healthcare team with baseline information and response to therapy. SaO₂ of less than 93% usually indicates need for increased supplemental oxygen.

Lifespan Considerations
Infant and Child
- Use a sensor that is appropriate for the client's weight and size.
- Young children may express fear of being burned or hurt by the light on the sensor. Show the sensor to the child or place it on Mom or Dad's finger before placing it on the child.

Older Adult
- Clients who have peripheral vascular disease or who smoke cigarettes or use nicotine gum may have reduced tissue perfusion. This can make monitoring difficult and interfere with the accuracy of the readings.

Home Care Modifications
- Because they are portable, pulse oximeters may be used in home care to monitor oxygen therapy. When intermittent monitoring is needed, the home nurse may assess pulse oximetry on each visit.

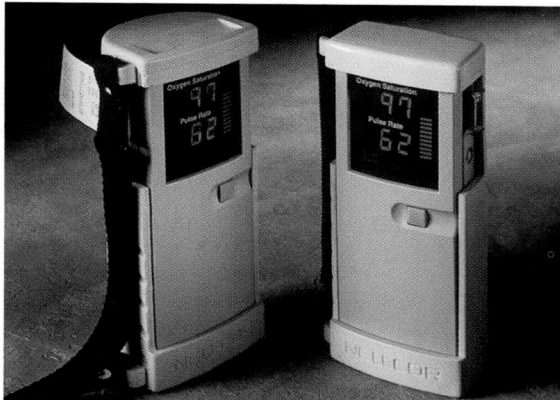

Portable oximeters are convenient for monitoring oxygen saturation in the home.

Collaboration and Delegation
- In some acute care agencies, respiratory therapy is responsible for monitoring pulse oximetry outside of intensive care units. Consult a respiratory therapist to develop a plan for the client with O₂ saturations below 93%. Frequently, respiratory therapists will titrate oxygen levels as needed.
- When delegating O₂ saturation monitoring to unlicensed nursing personnel, tell them to promptly report any values less than 93%. Validate any unusual values they obtain.

increased anteroposterior diameter, use of accessory muscles, altered chest excursion, and decreased vital capacity (NANDA, 2001).

Related Factors. Many factors, such as hyperventilation, hypoventilation, obesity, spinal cord injury, neuromuscular dysfunction, pain, musculoskeletal impairment, perceptual or cognitive impairment, anxiety, decreased energy/fatigue, respiratory muscle fatigue, and neurological immaturity, can contribute to Ineffective Breathing Pattern (NANDA, 2001).

Diagnostic Statement: Ineffective Airway Clearance

Definition. Ineffective Airway Clearance is the state in which a person is unable to clear secretions or obstructions from the respiratory tract to maintain a clear airway (NANDA, 2001).

Defining Characteristics. Defining characteristics are adventitious breath sounds (rales [crackles], rhonchi [wheezes]); diminished breath sounds, changes in rate or rhythm of respiration; ineffective or absent cough; sputum production; cyanosis; and dyspnea; difficulty vocalizing, restlessness, wide-eyed (NANDA, 2001).

Related Factors. Related factors for Ineffective Airway Clearance include smoke, airway spasm, retained secretions, foreign body in the airway, excessive mucus or secretions in the bronchi, neuromuscular dysfunction, COPD, asthma, infection, obstruction, allergic airways (NANDA, 2001).

Diagnostic Statement: Impaired Gas Exchange

Definition. Impaired Gas Exchange is the state in which a person experiences an excess or deficit in oxygenation and/or carbon dioxide elimination at an alveolar-capillary level (NANDA, 2001).

Defining Characteristics. Defining characteristics include confusion, somnolence, restlessness, irritability, hypercapnia/hypercarbia, dyspnea, abnormal rate rhythm, depth of breathing, and/or hypoxia/hypoxemia, abnormal skin color, cyanosis in the neonate, nasal flaring, abnormal arterial pH, visual disturbance or headache upon awakening (NANDA, 1999).

Related Factor. Imbalance of ventilation and perfusion and alveolar-capillary membrane changes contributes to impaired gas exchange (NANDA, 2001).

Related Nursing Diagnoses

Other nursing diagnoses for people with respiratory dysfunction include Risk for Infection, Imbalanced Nutrition: Less than Body Requirements, Chronic or Acute Pain, and Disturbed Sleep Pattern. Breathing difficulties and respiratory dis-

ease also affect the client's ability to carry out ADLs; possible related nursing diagnoses include Risk for Activity Intolerance and Self-Care Deficit. Anxiety, Chronic Low Self-Esteem, and Ineffective Coping or Ineffective Family Coping are examples of possible psychosocial nursing diagnoses. Deficient Knowledge regarding treatment plan and Impaired Adjustment are also potential nursing diagnoses for many clients with respiratory dysfunction.

OUTCOME IDENTIFICATION AND PLANNING

After nursing diagnoses and related factors have been established, the nurse and client identify outcomes. The following general areas should be included in the formulation of client goals and outcomes:

- Client will demonstrate knowledge regarding prevention of respiratory dysfunction.
- Client's tissues will have adequate oxygenation.
- Client will mobilize pulmonary secretions.
- Client will effectively cope with changes in self-concept and lifestyle.

Client outcomes differ substantially depending on the prognosis. For the client with an acute respiratory problem, the goal is recovery without any residual respiratory complications. Goals for the chronic respiratory client focus on the client's ability to live within the limitations the disease imposes and to accept changes in lifestyle and self-concept. For the terminal respiratory client, goals are to maintain adequate comfort and to accept impending death.

Aim interventions at restoring, maintaining, and promoting respiratory health. Examples of nursing interventions often used in respiratory dysfunction are listed in the display and discussed in the following section.

IMPLEMENTATION
Health Promotion

Health promotion to prevent respiratory dysfunction has become an increasingly important nursing role. The nurse and other healthcare professionals can work with organizations such as the American Lung Association to provide programs to reduce smoking and pollution and to improve working conditions contributing to lung disease. More commonly, the nurse works with people in a variety of settings (ambulatory clinics, schools, industry, public health) to teach and promote pulmonary health.

Preventing Respiratory Infections

Health teaching can limit both exposure to and occurrence of acute respiratory infections such as influenza and pneumonia. Promote optimal immune function by encouraging good nutrition. Remind the client to avoid exposure to known infected people or large crowds during peak flu season. Good hygiene practices, especially handwashing, covering the mouth and nose when sneezing or coughing, and proper

THERAPEUTIC DIALOGUE
Respiratory Care

Scene for Thought
Marvin Ottaway is a 60-year-old man in the hospital for stabilization of his pneumonia. He's sitting up in bed with the O_2 nasal prongs lying on his chest, somewhat short of breath but smiles when he sees the nurse at the door.

Less Effective

Client: Hello, Nancy, it's good to see you again today! I haven't seen you for a week! *(Smiles broadly, breathes rapidly.)*

Nurse: Hello, Mr. Ottaway. *(Speaks slowly and clearly.)* My name is Betsy, actually, and this is the second time I've met you. Who is Nancy?

Client: *(Looks confused and somewhat alarmed.)* But . . . you're Nancy, my sister-in-law!

Nurse: *(Gently replaces the O_2 prongs.)* I'm Betsy, your nurse, Mr. Ottaway. You really need to keep this oxygen on. If you don't have enough oxygen you're going to get confused. That's why you think I'm Nancy. *(Smiles and speaks in a gentle tone.)*

Client: But you are! I know my own kin! Why are you telling me you're not?! *(Becomes agitated and frightened.)*

Nurse: Quiet down, now. The oxygen will start to work soon, then you'll recognize me. *(Still speaks quietly, putting hand on his arm.)*

Client: No, I want Nancy! What have you done with her?! *(Becomes more agitated. Finally calms down after nurse administers oxygen and a mild sedative.)*

More Effective

Client: Hello, Nancy, it's good to see you again today! I haven't seen you for a week! *(Smiles broadly, breathes rapidly.)*

Nurse: Hello, Mr. Ottaway. *(Speaks slowly and clearly.)* My name is Barbara, actually, and this is the second time I've met you. Who is Nancy?

Client: *(Looks confused and somewhat alarmed.)* But . . . you're Nancy, my sister-in-law!

Nurse: *(Stands quietly by the bed with hand on his arm. Gently replaces the O_2 prongs.)* I'm Barbara, your nurse, Mr. Ottaway. Tell me a little about Nancy.

Client: *(Still breathes somewhat quickly but begins to warm to the subject.)* Oh, she's lovely; been married to my brother for 30 years, and always treats me like one of the family. You know, Sunday dinner, Christmas at their place with all the kids. I miss her. She hasn't been to see me lately. *(Looks worried.)*

Nurse: You really like her, don't you? *(Still stands next to the bed.)*

Client: *(Looks at Barbara with sudden recognition.)* Oh, now, I remember you. I'm sorry. Sometimes my mind isn't clear. I can't remember things like I used to. *(Looks embarrassed.)*

Nurse: No need to apologize. Sometimes lack of oxygen from pneumonia can play tricks with your memory. It's important to keep the oxygen in place so you can get the benefit.

Client: Okay, I'll try to remember.

Nurse: Would it be okay if I reminded you?

Client: Sure! That'd be great! *(Smiles broadly.)*

Critical Thinking Challenge
- Explain the relationship between oxygen deprivation, confusion, and anxiety.
- Compare and contrast how the two nurses presented reality.
- Identify dialogue that caused Mr. Ottaway's anxiety level to increase or decrease.

---

used tissue disposal, prevents the spread of communicable respiratory infections.

High-risk people (older adults; people with diagnosed respiratory disorders such as asthma or COPD; people with immune system dysfunction such as clients with AIDS, clients undergoing cancer chemotherapy, transplant recipients, healthcare workers) should receive annual influenza vaccinations. Influenza vaccines are formulated annually based on anticipated new strains; revaccination every fall before flu season is required to produce effective immunity. Pneumococcal vaccination is also recommended for high-risk people. Revaccination is only required for adults over 65 or people who are immuno-compromised (Centers for Disease Control and Prevention [CDC], 2001).

Encouraging Smoking Cessation
Smoking cessation is a positive step toward health regardless of the length of time a person has been a smoker. State-of-change theory provides a basis for understanding the process underlying changing an addictive habit. The five stages outlined in the process are:

1. Precontemplation (not thinking about quitting)
2. Contemplation (thinking about quitting in the next 6 months)
3. Preparation (thinking about quitting in the next 30 days)
4. Action (in the process of quitting)
5. Maintenance (abstaining from tobacco use for 6 months or more)

PLANNING: NIC/NOC Suggested Interventions

Accepted Respiratory Nursing Interventions Classification (NIC)
Acid–Base Management: Respiratory Acidosis
Acid–Base Management: Respiratory Alkalosis
Airway Insertion and Stabilization
Airway Management
Airway Suctioning
Allergy Management
Artificial Airway Management
Code Management
Endotracheal Extubation
Mechanical Ventilation
Mechanical Ventilation Weaning
Oxygen Therapy
Smoking Cessation Assistance
Ventilation Assistance

Accepted Respiratory Nursing Outcomes Classification (NOC)
Energy Conservation
Knowledge: Energy Conservation
Respiratory Status: Gas Exchange
Respiratory Status: Ventilation
Risk Control: Tobacco Use
Tissue Perfusion: Pulmonary

Refer to the following for specifics regarding NIC/NOC:
McCloskey, J., & Bulechek, G. (2000). *Iowa Intervention Project: Nursing Interventions Classification (NIC)* 3rd ed. St. Louis, MO: C. V. Mosby.
Johnson, M., & Maas, M. (2000). *Iowa Outcomes Project: Nursing Outcomes Classification (NOC)* 2nd ed. St. Louis, MO: C. V. Mosby.

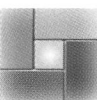

Clinical Research
AHCPR Guidelines for Helping Smokers Quit

1. Ask client about smoking, and advise smoker to quit.
2. Assist the client with a plan for quitting.
   * Set a date, ideally within 2 weeks.
   * Encourage the client to inform family, friends, and coworkers of the plan.
3. Help smoker quit.
   * Remove cigarettes from home, car, and workplace.
   * Review previous attempts (what helped? what didn't?).
   * Anticipate challenges.
   * Recommend total abstinence.
   * Remind the client to avoid alcohol.
   * Recommend nicotine replacement therapy (patch for 8 weeks or gum for up to 3 months).
4. Offer intensive smoking cessation program to increase success rate.
5. Follow up.
   * Visit within 2 weeks of quit date.
   * Congratulate success.
   * If lapse occurs, ask for recommitment.
   * Use lapse as a learning experience.
6. Prevent relapse.
   * Provide positive reinforcement for success.
   * Discuss potential problems (e.g., weight gain; prolonged nicotine withdrawal—unpleasant symptoms; negative mood/depression; lack of support for cessation).
   * Assist the client to develop potential solutions.

From Agency for Health Care Policy and Research. (1996). *Helping smokers quit: A guide of primary care clinicians. Clinical Practice Guideline, Number 18.* AHCPR Publication No. 96-0693. Rockville, MD: Author.

Relapse is common during smoking cessation attempts (Lindell & Reinke, 1999). Provide positive encouragement and explain that it often takes more than one attempt to successfully stop smoking. Ultimately it is up to the smoker to be responsible for choosing and carrying out personal change.

The Agency for Health Care Policy and Research (AHCPR) has developed guidelines (Agency for Health Care Policy and Research [AHCPR], 1996) for primary care providers to use for helping smokers quit. These guidelines reflect a thorough review of evidence from the CDC and clinical studies spanning the years from 1978 to 1994. The guidelines are summarized in the Clinical Research Display.

Reducing Allergens

Reducing exposure to allergens that can trigger bronchoconstriction and inflammation is an important preventive measure. The mortality rate from asthma has increased dramatically in the last 2 decades and is the sixth leading cause of hospital admissions in the United States (Miracle & Winston, 2000). Over 200 occupational asthma triggers have been identified; the most common triggers are chemical vapors found in workplaces such as paper and textile mills, chemical plants, printing plants, and hair salons (Copstead & Banasik, 2000). Most businesses and workplaces ban smoking, which has significantly reduced exposure to second-hand smoke. Aspirin sensitivity, cold air, or exercise can induce an attack. Seasonal pollens from trees, grasses, and flowering plants frequently exacerbate asthma symptoms in the spring or late summer. Indoor allergens include dust mites, pet dander, cockroach eggs and droppings, and molds. Nurses can be instrumental in working with the client and family to identify individual asthma triggers and motivate the family to restructure the environment to limit allergen exposure. See some specific guidelines for allergen reduction in the Outcome Based Teaching Display. Allergens can be identified through skin testing, and a program of allergen desensitization (allergy shots) can be instituted.

OUTCOME-BASED TEACHING PLAN

You are a clinic nurse for an allergist. Gina, 8 years old, and her mom are coming in for a follow-up visit. Gina was hospitalized 2 weeks ago for an acute asthma attack. In the hospital, a definitive diagnosis of asthma was made and teaching began on asthma management. You are now responsible for continuing this teaching.

OUTCOME: Gina/mother will verbalize preventive measures to decrease exposure to allergens by the next clinic visit.
Strategies
- Assess the client's and family's knowledge base regarding possible triggers of Gina's asthma attacks.
- Review methods to decrease animal dander (e.g., remove furred or feathered animals from the home or at least prohibit from bedroom; use HEPA filter air cleaners).
- Review methods to decrease dust mite allergens (e.g., encase pillows and mattress in an allergen-proof cover; wash bedding and stuffed animals weekly; remove carpets; vacuum daily using HEPA filter).
- Review methods to decrease environmental pollutants (e.g., no smoking in the home; avoid woodburning fires; avoid exposure to very cold air, perfumes, chemicals, and automobile exhaust).
- Offer to set up home evaluation for allergens.
- Discuss with the family those preventive measures that fit best with their lifestyle and willingness to try.

OUTCOME: Gina/mother will recognize a worsening of respiratory status and verbalize when they need to consult healthcare professionals by the end of teaching session.
Strategies
- Allow Gina and her mother to express concerns or anxiety they have concerning managing an asthma attack.
- Review peak flow monitoring, asking Gina to demonstrate and verbalize personal "green," "yellow," and "red" zones.
- Review peak flow monitoring log to assess Gina's status, providing positive feedback to her and her parents.
- Review symptoms of respiratory distress that warrant medical attention (peak flow in red zone, dyspnea that is not relieved with MDI use of fast-acting bronchodilator, symptoms of respiratory tract infection).
- Demonstrate how to administer epinephrine via an epi pen should acute symptoms fail to resolve, then call 911.
- Remind the family to alert appropriate people (e.g., teacher, school nurse, babysitter) of asthma and what to do during an attack.

Providing Adequate Hydration

Inadequate moisture in the airways makes respiratory mucus thick and difficult to cough up. Sticky, tenacious sputum that coats the respiratory tract increases work of breathing for any client and makes breathing especially difficult for those with chronic lung disease. Mucus that is hard to expectorate promotes infection because the bacteria it traps have time to multiply. Dried, sticky mucus also causes excessive coughing, which worsens pain in postoperative or trauma clients. Finally, mucous plugs in the airways can lead to atelectasis and decreased oxygenation.

The nurse can help maintain the mobility of mucus by encouraging fluids in all clients who are at risk for dried secretions. Fluid intake should ideally be 6 to 8 glasses of fluid, preferably water, every day. Caffeinated beverages (coffee, tea, cola) and alcohol can have a diuretic effect, thus dehydrating the client. In some clients, milk products tend to thicken secretions so these clients should avoid dairy products. Clients whose oral intake is restricted may require additional aerosol therapy to ensure secretion mobility.

Positioning and Ambulation

Changing positions and movement in general help to shift respiratory mucus into portions of the airways where it may generate a cough, making expectoration easier. Positioning and movement prevent mucus from pooling, which, in turn, decreases the risk of bacterial colonization and infection. Mucus tends to pool in the airways of people with limited mobility. Bedridden clients, clients experiencing pain, and clients with limited exercise tolerance (because of heart or lung disease) often retain secretions.

Encourage changing positions frequently. Whenever possible, position the client with unilateral lung problems with the good lung down to promote optimal matching of ventilation and perfusion (Scanlan, Wilkins, & Stoller, 1999). Moving the client from one side to another or assisting with ambulation when possible aids the lung's natural clearance mechanisms.

Ambulation is difficult for some respiratory clients because of dyspnea with exertion. Whenever possible, help promote exercise tolerance by encouraging progressive ambulation. Additional benefits of increased exercise tolerance include decreased oxygen consumption and extra strength for effective coughing. Some clients may need portable oxygen during periods of ambulation.

APPLY YOUR KNOWLEDGE

You are caring for Mr. Jacob one day postoperatively following abdominal surgery. On your morning assessment, you obtain the following vital signs data: B/P 142/80, pulse 84, respirations 14 and shallow, temperature 38.2°C. Pain is well controlled on PCA morphine, breath sounds are diminished at the bases with a few crackles, O_2 at 94%. Based on this information, how will you individualize your plan of care for Mr. Jacob?
Check your answer in Appendix A.

Deep Breathing

Shallow breathing or an ineffective cough can lead to mucous plugging, atelectasis, hypoxemia, and pneumonia. Taking deep breaths helps to expand alveoli and promote an effective cough, which decreases the risk of atelectasis.

Deep breathing is essential for the prevention of pulmonary complications in the at-risk client. Pain, lung disease, muscle weakness, or neurologic impairment can hinder a client's ability to breathe deeply. A major nursing task is to coach and encourage the client in deep-breathing techniques. Procedure 34-2 explains this technique.

Deep breathing is useful for all clients, especially postoperatively. There are no contraindications to deep breathing: Anyone can do it at any time. Deep breathing may cause discomfort for the client with an abdominal incision or broken ribs, but it is only beneficial. Deep breathing decreases the risk of postoperative complications by opening collapsed alveoli (Brenner, 1999). A deep breath also strengthens the cough and aids in moving mucus in the airways. Instruct the client to deep breathe by inhaling slowly through the nose then holding the breath for 2 or 3 seconds at the peak of inspiration to allow the air to distribute throughout the airways. Then the client can exhale passively through the mouth.

Assisting With Incentive Spirometry

The incentive spirometer motivates the client to breathe deeply by offering the incentive of measuring progress. Models of incentive spirometers vary greatly, but all provide the client with some observable indicator of how deep a breath he or she has taken. Some models use a bellows-like device that deflates as the client inspires; others use ping-pong balls that float. Regardless of the device, the client is visually motivated to take increasingly deeper breaths. The client and nurse set realistic goals for each breathing session, and the client works independently toward achieving each goal. Incentive spirometry motivates the client to take responsibility for the progress of deep-breathing therapy. A reasonable therapy schedule is 8 to 10 breaths hourly during waking hours (Lezon, 1999). To avoid hyperventilation, encourage the client to perform the exercises slowly. Procedure 34-3 explains the details of this technique.

Monitoring Peak Flow

A peak flow meter is a hand-held device that measures the highest flow during maximal expiration; the meter indicates how rapidly the client can breathe out air. Changes in peak flow measurements reflect changes in airway diameter; they occur before symptoms of respiratory distress such as dyspnea, wheezing, or increased coughing. Peak flow measurement can be used to individualize therapy and prevent the onset of an acute asthma attack.

Instruct clients to perform and record peak flow measurement twice a day, once in the morning and once in the evening. Clients should take measurements before using any bronchodilators. Initially the client will determine his or her "personal best" (the highest peak flow measure he or she obtains over a 2-week period during which the asthma was well-

controlled). Once this "personal best" value is obtained, the following zones can be determined:

- Green zone—80% to 100% of personal best (Asthma is well-controlled; proceed on routine treatment plan.)
- Yellow zone—50% to 80% of personal best (Asthma is not well-controlled and treatment plan may need to be increased.)
- Red zone—below 50% of personal best (Take a fast-acting beta$_2$ agonist and contact a healthcare provider immediately.)

Refer to Procedure 33-4 for detailed instruction outlining how to use a peak flow meter.

Nursing Interventions for Altered Respiratory Function

When atelectasis, excess secretions, or bronchoconstriction occur, nurses can use many therapies to support the client and improve oxygen status. Some of these techniques, such as coughing, are simple. Others, such as ventilators and tracheostomy care, are more complex and reserved for people with severe respiratory dysfunction.

Coughing

Retained secretions increase the work of breathing and may contribute to atelectasis and hypoxemia. No single measure controls respiratory secretions more effectively than a strong cough that pushes secretions upward. To cough effectively, the client must be able to take a deep breath and generate rapid airflow (see Procedure 34-2).

For many clients, producing a strong cough is difficult or impossible. The client experiencing postoperative or trauma-related pain may be unable or unwilling to take the deep breath needed to cough. Clients with COPD are often unable to exhale quickly enough to generate an effective cough. Some clients are simply too weak to cough, and others do not understand how to produce an effective cough. Finally, a client with a tracheostomy or endotracheal tube cannot cough with optimal efficiency because the glottis cannot close.

Deep Cough. Encourage the postoperative client who does not have lung disease to cough deeply. Deep coughing will help to mobilize secretions and to open collapsed alveoli. The client should inspire as deeply as possible then hold the breath a second or so while closing the glottis. He or she should then release the air while suddenly opening the glottis.

The deep cough can cause pain around the incisional area in clients who have had abdominal or thoracic surgery. To help control the pain, the client can support the incisional area with a pillow by using it as a splint to immobilize the wound. In clients with severe incisional discomfort, scheduling coughing sessions after pain medications have been administered may be helpful.

Stacked Cough. Some clients find coughing painful despite premedication. For them, a stacked cough may cause less pain and be almost as effective. Stacked coughing is the release of

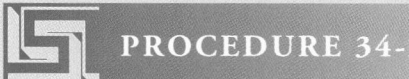

PROCEDURE 34-2

TEACHING COUGHING AND DEEP-BREATHING EXERCISES

Purpose
1. Facilitate respiratory functioning by increasing lung expansion and preventing alveolar collapse.
2. Encourage expectoration of mucus and secretions that accumulate in the airways after general anesthesia and immobility.

Assessment
- Assess client's risk factors for development of respiratory complications (e.g., general anesthesia, history of pulmonary disease or smoking, chest wall trauma, cold or respiratory infection within past week).
- Assess quality, rate, and depth of respiration.
- Auscultate breath sounds.
- Inspect placement of incision and evaluate whether or not it interferes with chest expansion.
- Evaluate client's physical ability to cooperate and perform pulmonary exercises:
   Level of consciousness
   Language or communication barriers
   Ability to assume Fowler's position
   Expression of pain (medicate as ordered)

Equipment
Pillows for positioning and to splint incision

Procedure

Deep Breathing
1. Assist client to Fowler's or sitting position.
   Rationale: Upright position allows increased diaphragmatic excursion secondary to downward shift of internal organs from gravity.
2. Have client place hands palm down, with middle fingers touching, along lower border of rib cage.
   Rationale: This position allows client to feel movement of diaphragm, indicating a deep breath.
3. Ask client to inhale slowly through the nose, feeling middle fingers separate. Hold breath for 2 or 3 seconds.
   Rationale: Inhaling through the nose allows air to be filtered, warmed, and humidified. Holding breath allows lungs to expand fully.
4. Have client exhale slowly through mouth. Repeat three to five times.
   Rationale: Slow expulsion of air frequently initiates the coughing reflex, which facilitates

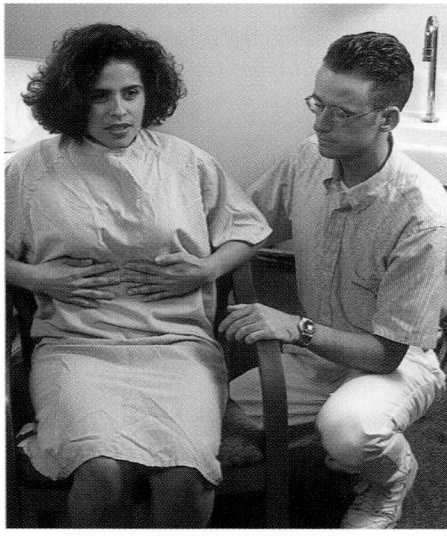

Step 2 Deep breathing: Client places hands along the lower rib cage to feel diaphragm movement.

expectoration of mucus and prevents hyperventilation.

Controlled Coughing
1. If adventitious breath sounds or sputum is present, have client take a deep breath, hold for 3 seconds, and cough deeply two or three times. Stand to the client's side to ensure the cough is not directed at you. Client must cough deeply, not just clear the throat.
   Rationale: Several consecutive coughs are more effective than one single cough at moving mucus up and out of the respiratory tract.
2. If the client has an abdominal or chest incision that will cause pain during coughing, instruct the client to hold a pillow firmly over the incision (splinting) when coughing.
   Rationale: Coughing uses abdominal and accessory respiratory muscles, which may have been cut during surgery. Splinting supports the incision and surrounding tissues and reduces pain during coughing.
3. Instruct, reinforce, and supervise deep-breathing and coughing exercises every 2 to 3 hours postoperatively.
   Rationale: Performing these exercises every 2 to 3 hours will facilitate pulmonary ventilation and promote airway clearance without overtiring the client.

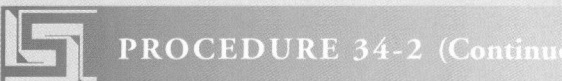

PROCEDURE 34-2 (Continued)

4. Document procedure.
   Rationale: Maintains legal record and communicates with healthcare team.

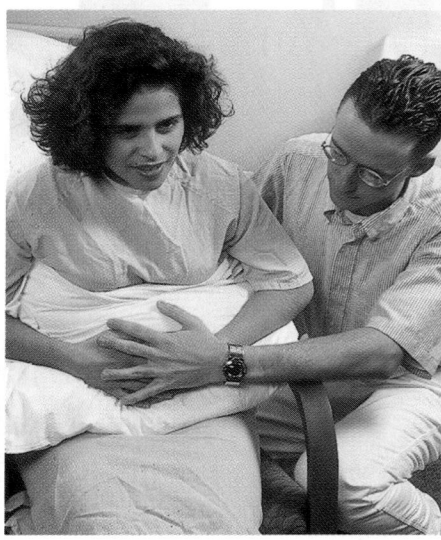

Step 2 Controlled coughing: Splinting with a pillow during coughing promotes comfort.

Lifespan Considerations
Infants and Children
- Infants cannot cooperate with coughing and deep-breathing exercises, but crying is thought to hyperinflate the lungs.
- Young children learn through games and imitation. A preoperative game of "Simon Says" is one way to teach them lung exercises: "Simon says touch your nose," "Simon says stick out your tongue," "Simon says take a deep breath," "Simon says cough."

Collaboration and Delegation
- Unlicensed nursing personnel can remind and assist clients to deep breathe and cough. Identify clearly to such personnel those clients who need aggressive coughing and deep breathing to promote optimal pulmonary status.

---

several short blasts of air instead of one deep cough. This type of cough prevents excessive stretching of the incisional area and also minimizes the airway collapse that may accompany deep coughing.

Low-Flow (Huff) Cough. A third type of cough is called low-flow or "huff" coughing. The low-flow cough is most effective for clients with COPD whose airways tend to collapse with rapid exhalation. Slowing the airflow actually is more helpful in expelling secretions. Instruct the client to inhale deeply. Instead of closing the glottis and generating high pressure, the client says "huff" three or four times while exhaling.

Quad Cough. Clients with neuromuscular disease and quadriplegic clients often need direct assistance to generate an effective cough. The client takes a deep breath, or the nurse provides a deep breath with a manual resuscitation bag. The client then holds the deep breath for a moment. With your hands placed just below the client's rib cage, assist the client by quickly pushing in and upward, much like performing the Heimlich maneuver. The resultant rush of air acts as a cough by helping to dislodge mucus from the airways.

Pursed-Lip Breathing. Pursed-lip breathing helps clients with obstructive lung diseases such as COPD or asthma by causing a back pressure in the airways, which eases exhalation.

To perform pursed-lip breathing, the client takes a deep breath and holds it for a moment, then exhales slowly through lips held almost closed. By pushing the air against the small orifice made by the pursed lips, pressure builds backward through the airways. This back pressure prevents airway collapse by pushing the airways open throughout exhalation. Thus, more air escapes during exhalation and helps prevent air trapping.

PROCEDURE 34-3

PROMOTING BREATHING WITH THE INCENTIVE SPIROMETER

Purpose
1. Improve pulmonary ventilation and oxygenation.
2. Loosen respiratory secretions.
3. Prevent or treat atelectasis by expanding collapsed alveoli.

Assessment
- Identify clients at risk for atelectasis.
- Complete respiratory assessment (i.e., history of smoking, breath sounds, respiratory rate and rhythm, sputum production).

Equipment
Incentive spirometer (flow-oriented or volume-oriented; type of incentive spirometer is usually determined by equipment available through respiratory therapy)

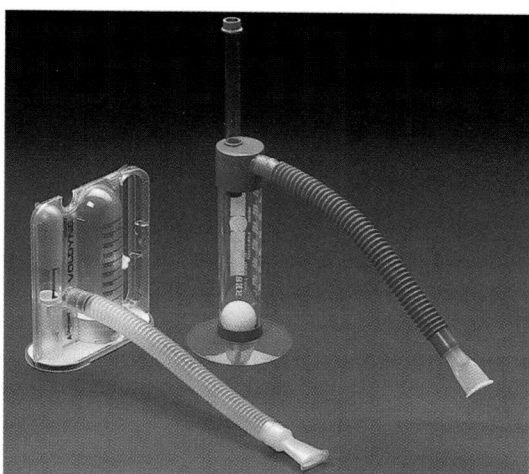

Mouthpiece (if not already connected to spirometer)
Nose clip (optional)

Procedure
1. Verify the physician order and identify the client.
   Rationale: Prevents potential errors.
2. Wash your hands.
   Rationale: Handwashing reduces transfer of microorganisms.
3. Assist client to high Fowler's or sitting position.
   Rationale: These positions facilitate optimal lung expansion.
4. Determine the volume to set incentive spirometry goal based on calculated lung volumes. You may use chart or have respiratory therapy calculated. Set volume indicator.
   Rationale: People of different sizes have different lung capacities. Individualize preset goal to promote optimal lung inflation and provide realistic motivation.
5. Instruct client in procedure:
   a. Seal lips tightly around mouthpiece.
      Rationale: A sealed mouthpiece prevents leakage of air around mouthpiece.
   b. Inhale slowly and deeply through mouth. Hold breath for 2 or 3 seconds.
      Rationale: Holding the breath maintains maximal inflation of alveoli.

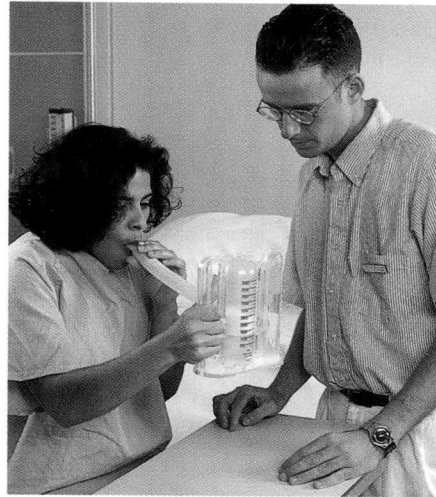

Step 5b Client inhales slowly and deeply through the mouth, holding breath for 2 to 3 seconds.

   c. Have client observe his or her progress by watching the balls elevate or lights go on, depending on type of equipment used.
      Rationale: Observing progress provides visual feedback to the client regarding depth of inspiration, which motivates client to breathe deeply.
   d. Exhale slowly around mouthpiece and breathe normally for several breaths.
      Rationale: Prevents hyperventilation.
6. Repeat procedure 5 to 10 times every 1 to 2 hours, per physician's orders.
   Rationale: Frequent use will prevent alveoli collapse.

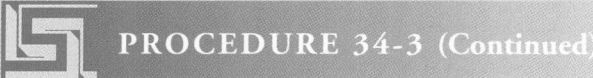

PROCEDURE 34-3 (Continued)

Lifespan Considerations
- Clients who are too young to follow directions, are cognitively impaired or malnourished, or lack necessary motor skills are likely to be unsuccessful at using incentive spirometry.

Collaboration and Delegation
- Respiratory therapy often provides the initial instruction on how to use the incentive spirometer, calculating a realistic lung volume. For preoperative clients, try to coordinate teaching before surgery.

Chest Physiotherapy

This treatment commonly is prescribed to help clear excessive bronchial secretions from airways. It is based on the premise that mucus can be shaken from the walls of the airways and helped to drain from the lungs. Chest physiotherapy is a mainstay of treatment for many clients with cystic fibrosis, COPD, and pneumonia.

The primary techniques of this method of secretion mobilization are percussion, vibration, and postural drainage. Any of these physiotherapy techniques can be used alone, but they are most effective when used together. The client's ability to tolerate these procedures may limit the vigor with which they are applied, so positioning and clapping techniques may need to be modified. Often the respiratory therapist or physical therapist provides chest physiotherapy in the acute care setting.

Percussion. Percussion produces a mechanical wave of energy that is transmitted through the chest wall to the mucus-coated bronchial tubes. Strike the chest rhythmically with cupped hands over the area where secretions are located. Take care to avoid striking over the spine or kidneys, on female breasts, or on incisions or broken ribs. Pneumatic or electrical chest percussors are effective substitutes for manual percussion.

Vibration. Vibration works in much the same manner as percussion. In this technique, use your hands like a gentle jack-hammer: Place them on the client's chest and rapidly and vigorously vibrate them while the client exhales. This technique may help dislodge secretions and stimulate a cough.

Postural Drainage. Postural drainage uses gravity to assist in the movement of secretions. The client is placed in various positions to facilitate mucus flow from different segments of the lung (Fig. 34-3). Placing a mucus-filled segment of the lung higher than the rest of the lung allows the mucus in that segment to flow more readily downward toward larger airways. In this way, coughing or suctioning more easily removes the mucus.

Not all postural drainage positions are well tolerated by all clients. The Trendelenburg (head-down) position can increase shortness of breath in the client with COPD because the abdominal organs limit diaphragm movement. Lying head-down can increase intracranial pressure and should be used cautiously for clients with head injuries. It can also be very stressful for clients with cardiac problems. The nurse or therapist who administers postural drainage may need to modify the treatment for clients who cannot tolerate the prescribed positions.

Aerosol Therapy

An aerosol is a suspension of microscopic liquid droplets in air or oxygen. Aerosol therapy may be given for any of the following reasons:

- To add moisture to oxygen delivery systems
- To hydrate thick sputum and prevent mucous plugging
- To administer various drugs to the airways

A large-volume nebulizer or an ultrasonic nebulizer will deliver a moist fog continuously to the airways. While absorbing the water, the mucous blanket loosens, which facilitates its removal. The watery mist also soothes inflamed airways. Heating the water in the nebulizer increases the amount of moisture delivered.

Check the reservoir frequently to ensure that it is filled with sterile water. Parts must be screwed together tightly to ensure full delivery of the prescribed level of oxygen. The large-bore tubing must be drained often to prevent buildup of condensation. Monitor the mist temperature to prevent possible injury. Finally, because aerosols loosen dried secretions, help the client remove them by coughing or suctioning.

Aerosol Medications. A variety of drugs are administered by aerosol. Bronchodilators reverse bronchospasm most quickly when administered directly to the lungs. Although commonly

PROCEDURE 34-4

MONITORING PEAK FLOW

Purpose
1. Measure peak expiratory flow rate (PEFR), which is the point of highest flow during maximal exhalation.
2. Better control asthma by quickly detecting subtle changes in airway diameter so preventive interventions can be instituted.
3. Provide objective data to assess respiratory function.

Assessment/Preparation
- Identify clients who would benefit from or have been prescribed peak flow monitoring (e.g., asthmatics).
- Assess client's baseline oxygenation status including vital signs, skin and nailbed color, breath sounds, shortness of breath, alterations in breathing pattern, cognitive changes.
- Note any subjective verbalizations regarding respiratory status (e.g., tightness in the chest, more difficult to breathe).
- Note new or recent exposure to factors that could alter airway diameter (e.g., smoke, chemicals, animal dander, pollens, and molds).
- Note any use of medications that could alter airway diameter (e.g., sympathomimetics, anticholinergics, corticosteroids).

Equipment
Peak flowmeter
Charts to calculate green, yellow, and red zones based on personal best data
Daily log to record peak flow values obtained

Procedure
1. Verify the physician order and identify the client.
   Rationale: Prevents potential errors.
2. Explain the purpose of peak flow monitoring to the client and family.
   Rationale: Understanding the procedure increases compliance and decreases anxiety. Measurements taken before using bronchodilators will provide more accurate data regarding baseline airway diameter.
3. Place indicator at the base of the numbered scale. Have client stand up.
   Rationale: Having indicator in the correct position will ensure accurate measurement of peak expiratory flow. Standing position allows full expansion of lungs.
4. Tell the client to take a deep breath. Place the meter in his or her mouth. The client should close the lips around the mouthpiece. Remind the client not to put the tongue in the hole.
   Rationale: Close fit around the mouthpiece and unobstructed mouthpiece are necessary for proper measurement of exhaled air.
5. Tell the client to exhale as fast and as hard as he or she can, keeping a tight fit around the mouthpiece.
   Rationale: Motivation and proper technique will obtain highest peak flow.

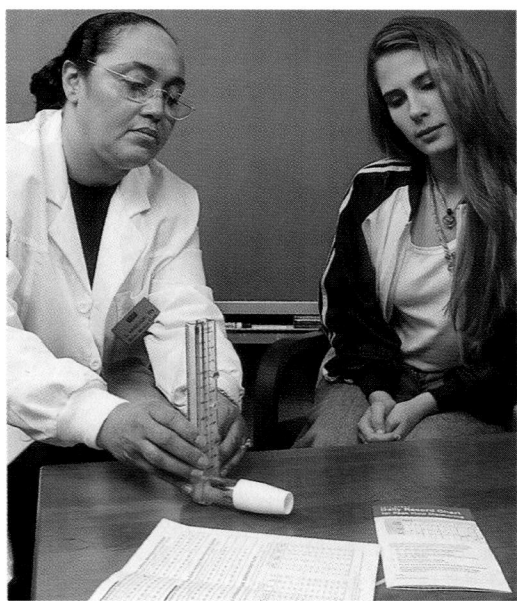

Gather peak flowmeter; chart indicating green, yellow, and red zones; and daily log before teaching.

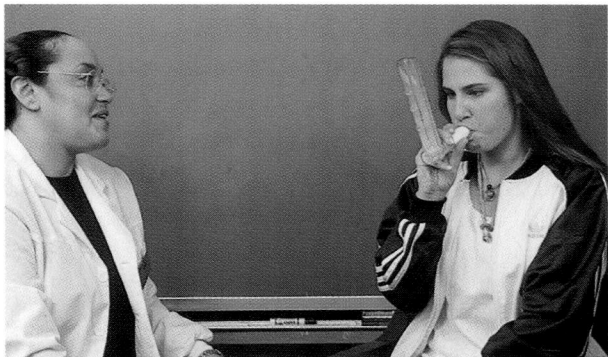

Step 5 Verbally encourage client to exhale as fast and as hard as he or she can.

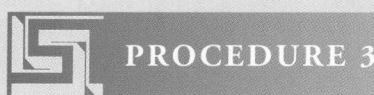

PROCEDURE 34-4 (Continued)

6. Repeat steps 2 through 4 twice more, and record the highest peak flow obtained in the three attempts. *Rationale: Peak flow varies from one attempt to another. The highest number represents the client's best effort.*

7. To determine "personal best" when beginning peak flow monitoring, obtain peak flow measurements in the morning and again in the evening over a 2-week period of good asthma control (feel good without any asthma symptoms). The client should take measurements before using bronchodilators. *Rationale: "Personal best" represents the client's best effort during a period of good control, which will provide a baseline from which to predict green, yellow, and red zones.*

8. Healthcare provider will calculate zones based on percentage of personal best (green 80%–100%; yellow 50%–80%; red below 50%) and give instructions for what to do when in each zone. *Rationale: Zones determine how well asthma is controlled and provide guidelines for client to adjust treatment or contact healthcare provider.*

9. Encourage client to comply with twice-a-day (morning and evening) peak flow monitoring before bronchodilator therapy and follow healthcare provider's instructions for peak flows in each zone. Follow steps 2 through 5.

Rationale: Consistent use of peak flow monitoring allows the client to detect subtle changes in airway diameter and institute appropriate therapy to avoid acute asthma exacerbations.

Lifespan Considerations
Child and Adolescent
- Peak flow monitoring is appropriate for children who are able to follow directions and use effective technique. Baseline values need to be recalculated every 6 months during growth spurts. Children may need reminders from family members and help keeping a daily log. Adolescents need to assume more responsibility and control over their asthma management.

Home Care Modifications
- Most peak flow monitoring is done in the home setting. Initial teaching is usually done in the clinic or physician's office. Follow-up is important. Home care nurses use peak flow logs to assess asthma control.

Collaboration and Delegation
- Respiratory therapists may be responsible for initial teaching and calculation of zones.

used and highly effective, these agents are powerful medications that may have serious side effects. Closely monitor all clients receiving bronchodilators for signs of increased heart rate, nervous agitation, and restlessness. Inhaled corticosteroids are used to fight lung inflammation. For clients with asthma and chronic lung disease, aerosol steroids offer a safe alternative to oral steroids with long-term negative systemic effects. Other types of medications delivered by aerosol include cromolyn (Intal) and nedocromil (Tilade), which are used to prevent asthma attacks. Antibiotics also may be delivered by aerosol to clients with cystic fibrosis to counter stubborn lung infections. Table 34-4 lists common respiratory medications.

Metered-Dose Inhalers. Gas-powered, cartridge-type nebulizers called metered-dose inhalers (MDIs) provide the client with a premeasured dose of aerosolized medication. Squeezing the gas cartridge discharges a single puff of medication

that the client inhales deeply into the lungs. Usually, two puffs provide a single dose. MDIs are ordinarily self-administered by the client, but nurses are usually responsible for providing instruction in their use. These devices are portable, compact, and highly convenient to use. For many people, the MDI is simple to operate but others find it difficult to activate the inhaler and inhale simultaneously. A chamber (or "spacer") that attaches to the MDI helps to minimize this problem and improves the MDI's efficiency. Figure 34-4 shows an MDI and an MDI with a spacer, and Chapter 27, Procedure 27-2, illustrates step-by-step guidelines for using an MDI to deliver medication.

Because MDIs are used to deliver practically any type of respiratory medication, clients may use several MDIs in their medication regimen. A complete understanding of each medication's actions and dosing schedule is essential for optimal management of respiratory symptoms.

POSTURAL DRAINAGE POSITIONS

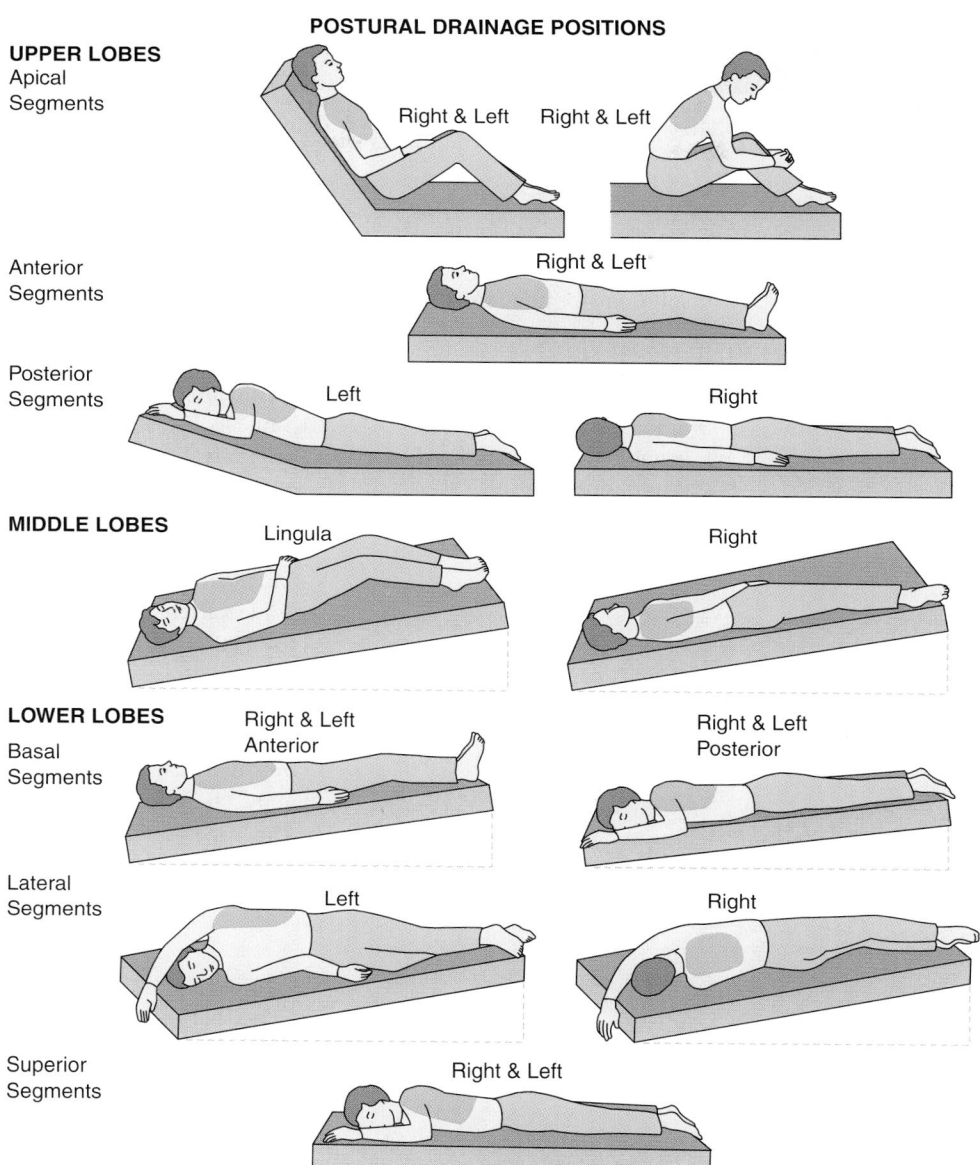

UPPER LOBES
Apical Segments
Right & Left   Right & Left

Anterior Segments
Right & Left

Posterior Segments
Left   Right

MIDDLE LOBES
Lingula   Right

LOWER LOBES
Basal Segments
Right & Left Anterior   Right & Left Posterior

Lateral Segments
Left   Right

Superior Segments
Right & Left

FIGURE 34-3   Various postural drainage positions are used to mobilize secretions from specific lobes and segments of the lung.

Hand-Held Nebulizers. Small-volume nebulizers (Fig. 34-5) offer an alternative to clients who are unable to operate MDIs. Instead of providing a full dose of medication in one or two breaths, the hand-held nebulizer delivers a steady stream of aerosolized medicine that the client breathes over the course of several minutes. Use of nebulizers eliminates the problem of trying to coordinate inspiration with cartridge activation. These devices are operated by means of a compressor, or by oxygen at 4 to 5 L/min.

The client inhales deeply and holds each breath for a moment, which allows for more effective aerosol deposition into distant portions of the airways. The client continues breathing slowly in this manner until the nebulizer is empty.

Oxygen Therapy

Some clients need oxygen therapy to maintain adequate arterial blood oxygen levels. Lung disease, cardiovascular problems, blood disorders such as anemia, and high metabolic demands of healing tissues can limit the body's oxygen supply.

TABLE 34-4

Common Medications for Clients With Respiratory Conditions		
Agent	**How Provided**	**Clinical Notes**
Bronchodilators Isoetharine (Bronkosol) Metaproterenol (Alupent) Terbutaline (Brethine, Bricanyl) Albuterol (Ventolin, Proventil) Ipratropium (Atrovent)	MDI; unit-dose packs; solution for administration via hand-held nebulizer or IPPB; some solutions for injection	1. Used to treat wheezing from asthma, COPD 2. May cause nervousness and tremors 3. May cause tachycardia; note heart rate before and after treatment 4. Aerosol chamber (or "spacer") improves medication dispersal
Theophylline (Theo-Dur, Slo-bid), aminophylline, many others	Oral via tabs and liquids; injectable intravenous solution is aminophylline	1. Same as 1–3 above 2. Side effects include nausea, headache, agitation 3. Toxic effects may include cardiac dysrhythmias and seizures 4. Monitor blood levels; keep at 10–20 µg/dL 5. Wide variety of available preparations; use extra caution in administration
Anti-inflammatory Agents Beclomethasone (Beclovent, Vanceril) Flunisolide (AeroBid) Triamcinolone (Azmacort)	MDI	1. These agents are locally acting steroids; they decrease inflammation in asthma and COPD 2. These agents are not effective in acute dyspnea attacks 3. Client should rinse mouth after use
Leukotriene Inhibitors Zafirlukast (Accolate) Zileuton (Zyflo)	Oral	1. Inhibits leukotriene formation, which selectively decreases inflammatory response 2. Used to prevent asthma attacks 3. Contraindications: hepatic impairment, pregnancy
Antiasthmatic Agent Cromolyn sodium (Intal) Nedocromil (Tilade)	MDI; solution for administration via hand-held nebulizer; powdered for administration via Spinhaler	1. Maintenance drug used to decrease frequency and intensity of asthma attacks 2. NOT to be used during acute asthma attack 3. May require several weeks for noticeable effects 4. Few side effects (cough, dry mouth)

MDI, metered dose inhaler; IPPB, intermittent positive pressure breathing; COPD, chronic obstructive pulmonary disease.

Oxygen therapy is used primarily to reverse hypoxemia. It can help to accomplish three fundamental goals:

- Improved tissue oxygenation
- Decreased work of breathing in dyspneic clients
- Decreased work of the heart in clients with cardiac disease

General Principles of Oxygen Administration. For many clients with lung disease, oxygen therapy helps eliminate dyspnea and improves comfort. For the critically ill client, meticulous oxygen therapy can be life-saving.

Oxygen is prescribed either in terms of flow or concentration, depending on the client's needs and the delivery device's capabilities. Oxygen flow is expressed in liters per

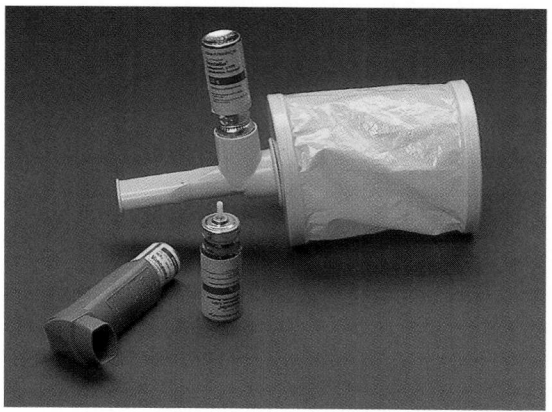

FIGURE 34-4 Metered-dose inhaler (MDI) and MDI with spacer.

minute. Concentration is expressed as a percentage, or as a fraction of inspired oxygen. A general rule for safe oxygen therapy is to use the lowest oxygen concentration or flow possible to achieve an acceptable blood oxygen level.

When administering oxygen, assess the client's response regularly to determine the need for continuation or adjustment of therapy. The client's color, alertness, heart rate, and breathing effort are general indicators of the effectiveness of oxygen therapy. Arterial blood gas monitoring and pulse oximetry provide more specific information concerning client response to oxygen therapy. For most clients, the aim of oxygen therapy should be to maintain the PaO_2 above 60 mm Hg, or the SaO_2 above 93%. It is rarely necessary to exceed a PaO_2 of 90 mm Hg, or an SaO_2 greater than 97%. Most often, clients use oxygen continuously for as short a time as possible until they can maintain satisfactory blood oxygenation without it. Most clients require relatively low concentrations of oxygen to correct hypoxemia. See Procedure 34-5 for a general guide to administering oxygen.

Selection of Oxygen Systems. A variety of equipment is available to provide oxygen in a wide range of flows and concentrations (Fig. 34-6). Nurses should be familiar with the proper operation and capabilities of various oxygen devices.

The client's oxygenation status determines which oxygen delivery device is most appropriate. Although comfort is also

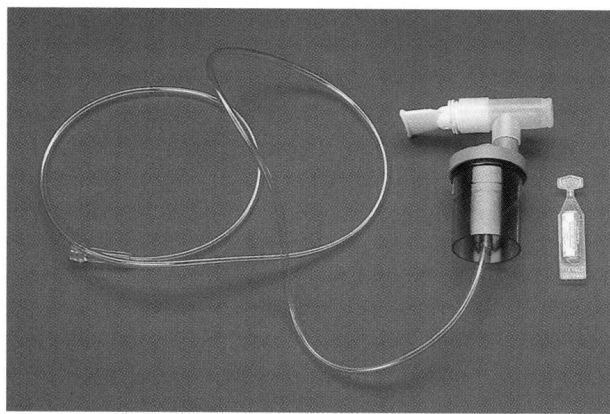

FIGURE 34-5 Hand-held nebulizer.

a factor, the best oxygen device for each client is the one capable of providing his or her oxygen needs. If a client needs only a small amount of additional oxygen to maintain adequate oxygenation, he or she can use a cannula or low-concentration Venturi-type mask. If the client requires a moderate amount of oxygen, a simple mask is suitable. When a client needs a high concentration of oxygen, a reservoir-type mask or more sophisticated system is required. Table 34-5 compares and contrasts a variety of commonly used oxygen delivery systems.

Transtracheal catheters, implanted surgically, are becoming more common. These catheters (12 Fr or smaller) are inserted through the client's neck into the trachea. They are attached to a portable oxygen system. With this oxygen delivery device, less oxygen is wasted because the catheter enters the lung directly. The client is managed well on less oxygen.

Safety Considerations. Because oxygen is a drug, a prescription is required for its use. Although oxygen is generally safe when used properly, certain precautions must be observed. As with all drugs, potential exists for causing harm with misuse.

When a client begins oxygen therapy, inform him or her of the importance of wearing the oxygen device.

SAFETY ALERT
A "no smoking" sign must be posted in the client's room. Strictly enforce this warning. Although oxygen is not flammable, it greatly accelerates combustion and could cause a fire from a small spark.

Check the oxygen flow often to ensure that the prescribed amount is being delivered. If the client is using a humidifier or nebulizer (to minimize the drying effect of oxygen on the airways), ensure that the reservoir is filled with water and is attached properly. A leak in the delivery system can prevent the client from receiving the full amount of oxygen, so all connections must be tight.

Oxygen therapy has the potential for causing serious health consequences in some clients. Relatively low oxygen concentrations can damage the newborn's retina and result in blindness. For this reason, meticulously monitor all newborns receiving oxygen therapy.

High oxygen concentrations are toxic to lung tissue. Severely ill clients who require intense oxygen therapy for extended periods may suffer resultant lung damage. Although this concern is not serious for the average client who uses a nasal cannula, oxygen toxicity poses a danger for the client who needs intensive respiratory care. Oxygen can cause hypoventilation in some clients with advanced COPD.

SAFETY ALERT
Some clients with COPD breathe as a response to hypoxemia. If they receive too much oxygen, their PaO_2 rises excessively and their drive to breathe decreases. This causes hypoventilation, which can lead to respiratory arrest. For this reason, clients with COPD must be maintained only with low concentrations of oxygen.

(text continues on page 840)

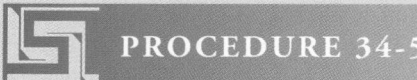

PROCEDURE 34-5

ADMINISTERING OXYGEN BY NASAL CANNULA OR MASK

Purpose
1. Deliver low to moderate levels of oxygen to relieve hypoxia.

Assessment/Preparation
* Assess respiratory status (i.e., breath sounds, respiratory rate and depth, presence of sputum, arterial blood gases if available).
* Assess past medical history, noting chronic obstructive pulmonary disease (COPD). For clients with COPD, hypoxemia is often the stimulus to breathe because they chronically have high blood levels of carbon dioxide. If additional oxygen is needed, a low-flow system is essential to maintain slight hypoxemia so breathing is stimulated.
* Assess for clinical signs and symptoms of hypoxia: anxiety, decreased level of consciousness, inability to concentrate, fatigue, dizziness, cardiac dysrhythmias, pallor or cyanosis, dyspnea.

Equipment
Appropriate oxygen delivery system:
* Nasal cannula and tubing (O_2 concentrations: 22%–44%)
* Simple oxygen mask (O_2 concentrations: 40%–60%)
* Venturi mask—delivers O_2 concentrations accurate within 1% (24%–50%). Frequently used with clients with COPD.
* Partial rebreather mask—low-flow system (O_2 concentrations: 50%–70%). Reservoir bag allows client to rebreathe a portion of exhaled air. (Bag must not totally deflate during inspiration, or O_2 flow rate should be increased.)
* Nonrebreather mask—delivers the highest O_2 concentrations possible without mechanical ventilation (80%–90%). One-way valve prevents room air or exhaled air from being inspired.

Oxygen source
Flowmeter
"No smoking" sign
Humidifier and distilled water (for high-flow O_2 therapy)

Procedure
1. Review chart for physician's order for oxygen to ensure that it includes method of delivery, flow rate, duration of therapy; identify client.
    Rationale: Prevents potential errors.

2. Wash your hands.
    Rationale: Handwashing reduces transmission of microorganisms.
3. Explain procedure to client. Explain that oxygen will ease dyspnea or discomfort, and inform client concerning safety precautions associated with oxygen use. If the client is using the cannula, encourage him or her to breathe through the nose.
    Rationale: Teaching helps ensure compliance with therapy.
4. Assist client to semi- or high Fowler's position, if tolerated.
    Rationale: These positions facilitate optimal lung expansion.
5. Insert flowmeter into wall outlet. Attach oxygen tubing to nozzle on flowmeter. If using a high O_2 flow, attach humidifier.
    Rationale: Oxygen in high concentrations can be drying to the mucosa.

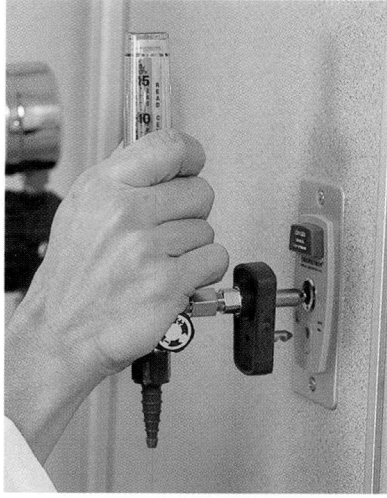

Step 5 Insert flowmeter into wall outlet.

6. Turn on the oxygen at the prescribed rate. Check that oxygen is flowing through tubing.
    Rationale: Oxygen must be administered as prescribed.
7. Cannula.
    a. Place cannula prongs into nares.
    b. Wrap tubing over and behind ears.
    c. Adjust plastic slide under chin until cannula fits snugly.
    Note: The cannula permits some freedom of movement and does not interfere with the client's ability to eat or talk.

PROCEDURE 34-5 (Continued)

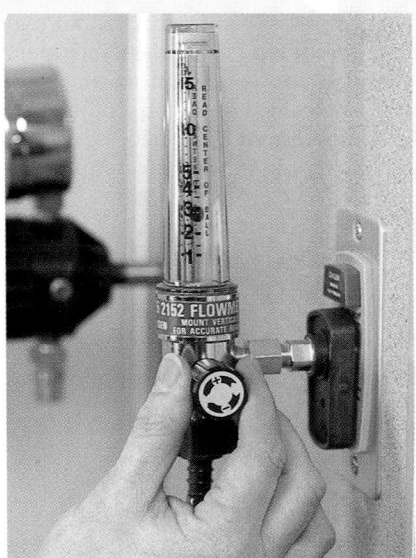

Step 6 Turn on oxygen at prescribed rate.

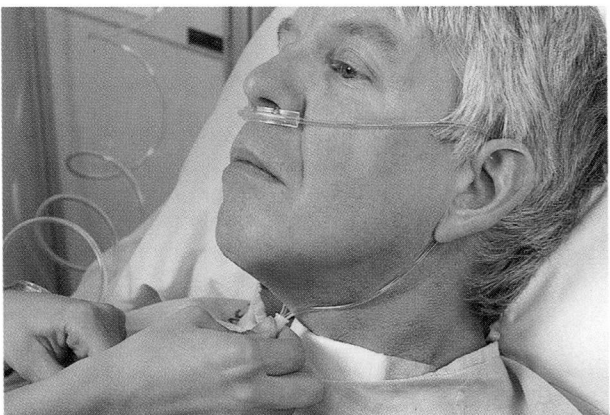

Step 7c Adjust plastic slide under chin until cannula fits snugly.

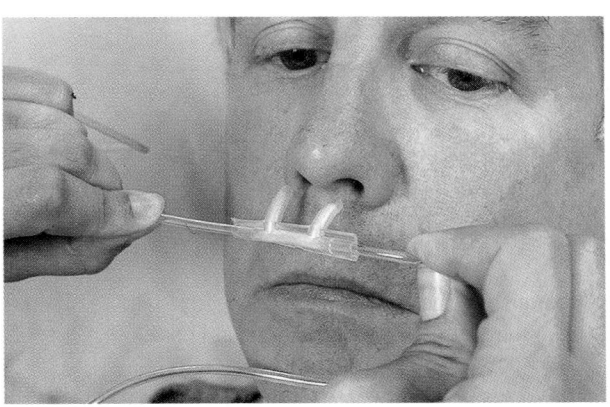

Step 7a Place cannula prongs into nares.

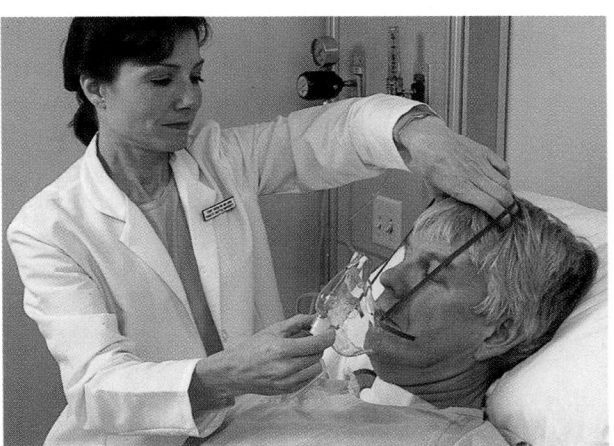

Step 8a Apply oxygen mask over mouth and nose.

8. Mask.
   a. Place mask on face, applying from the nose and over the chin.
   b. Adjust the metal rim over the nose and contour the mask to the face.
      Rationale: When the mask fits the face properly, little oxygen escapes.
   c. Adjust elastic band around head so mask fits snugly.
      Rationale: Client is more likely to comply with therapy if equipment fits comfortably.
9. Assess for proper functioning of equipment and observe client's initial response to therapy.

Rationale: Assessment of vital signs, oxygen saturation, color, breathing pattern, and orientation helps the nurse evaluate effectiveness of therapy and detect clinical evidence of hypoxia.

10. Monitor continuous therapy by assessing for pressure areas on the skin and nares every 2 hours and rechecking flow rate every 4 to 8 hours.
    Rationale: Permit early detection of skin breakdown or inadequate flow rate.
11. Document procedure and observations.
    Rationale: Maintains legal record and communicates with healthcare team members.

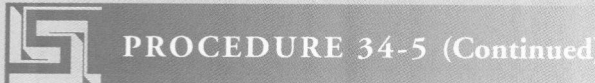

PROCEDURE 34-5 (Continued)

Lifespan Considerations
Infant and Child
- Isolettes (incubators) and tents may be used for administering oxygen and humidity to infants and newborns. It is difficult to maintain high concentrations of oxygen in an isolette or tent, but it is nonintrusive and nonirritating.
- Plan nursing care so tent or isolette is entered as little as possible to prevent oxygen levels from dropping.
- Children frightened by the oxygen tent may feel more secure with their favorite toy or blanket.

Home Care Modifications
- In-home oxygen supply is delivered by cylinders, liquid oxygen, or oxygen concentrators. Portable oxygen systems are available to increase independence and social activities.
- Equipment vendor and home care nurse should instruct client on how to use home oxygen equipment and how often the equipment must be filled.

- The client should be informed about using an oxygen vendor whose services include:
    Trained personnel to instruct the client in use and maintenance of the equipment
    24-hour emergency service
    Monthly follow-up visits for equipment maintenance and client instruction
    Vendor insurance billing
- Needing oxygen at home can be stressful for the client. Clients should be encouraged to share their fears and concerns. A local support group of clients using home oxygen may help them to discuss their feelings.
- For insurance to cover home oxygen, clients must have oxygen saturation below 88% to 90%.

Collaboration and Delegation
- Respiratory therapists often titrate oxygen concentrations per protocols and oxygen saturations.

Although hypoventilation is relatively uncommon, it is difficult to predict which clients may be affected, so all clients with COPD must be considered at risk. A client with COPD who requires higher concentrations of oxygen to achieve minimally acceptable blood gases should be observed carefully.

Chest Tubes

A chest tube is a drainage device the surgeon places in the pleural space to drain fluid, air, or blood. Although the tube is placed and removed by a physician, the nurse is responsible for assisting with tube insertion and continually monitoring and assessing the status of a client with a chest tube.

Normally, the pressure within the thoracic cavity is negative compared to atmospheric pressure. This negative pressure moves air into a person's lungs on inhalation. Any interruption in this negative pressure gradient may necessitate the need for a chest tube. The fluid build-up from a disease process may inhibit the lung's ability to expand normally; the fluid must be drained from the pleural space. An injury may result in blood in the pleural space (a hemothorax). Surgery involving the chest wall almost always results in the collapse of a lung (a pneumothorax); a chest tube is used to re-expand the collapsed lung and remove fluid. When a lung collapses spontaneously (a spontaneous pneumothorax), a chest tube is used to remove air from the pleural space and re-expand the lung.

Components of a Chest Drainage System. The surgeon inserts the chest tube into the intrapleural space. It is sutured in place and covered with an occlusive sterile dressing. The chest tube is connected to the collection/water seal system by a rubber tube that can be up to two feet long. Suction can be ordered if additional pressure is required to re-expand the lung. The water seal prevents air from entering the pleural space as the client inspires. It is important to keep the extra tubing looped at the level of the patient; otherwise fluid can accumulate in dependent loops.

The chest drainage systems currently used in the hospital are single-unit, disposable systems composed of a collection chamber, a water seal chamber, and a suction chamber (Figure 34-7).

The collection chamber collects any fluid that drains from the chest tube. The chamber is composed of a series of graduated columns that fill sequentially. Because of this filling sequence, it is important to keep the chest collection system upright at all times. If the system is overturned, the drainage spills into all the collection columns. The nurse marks the amount of drainage accrued in the collection chamber during each shift.

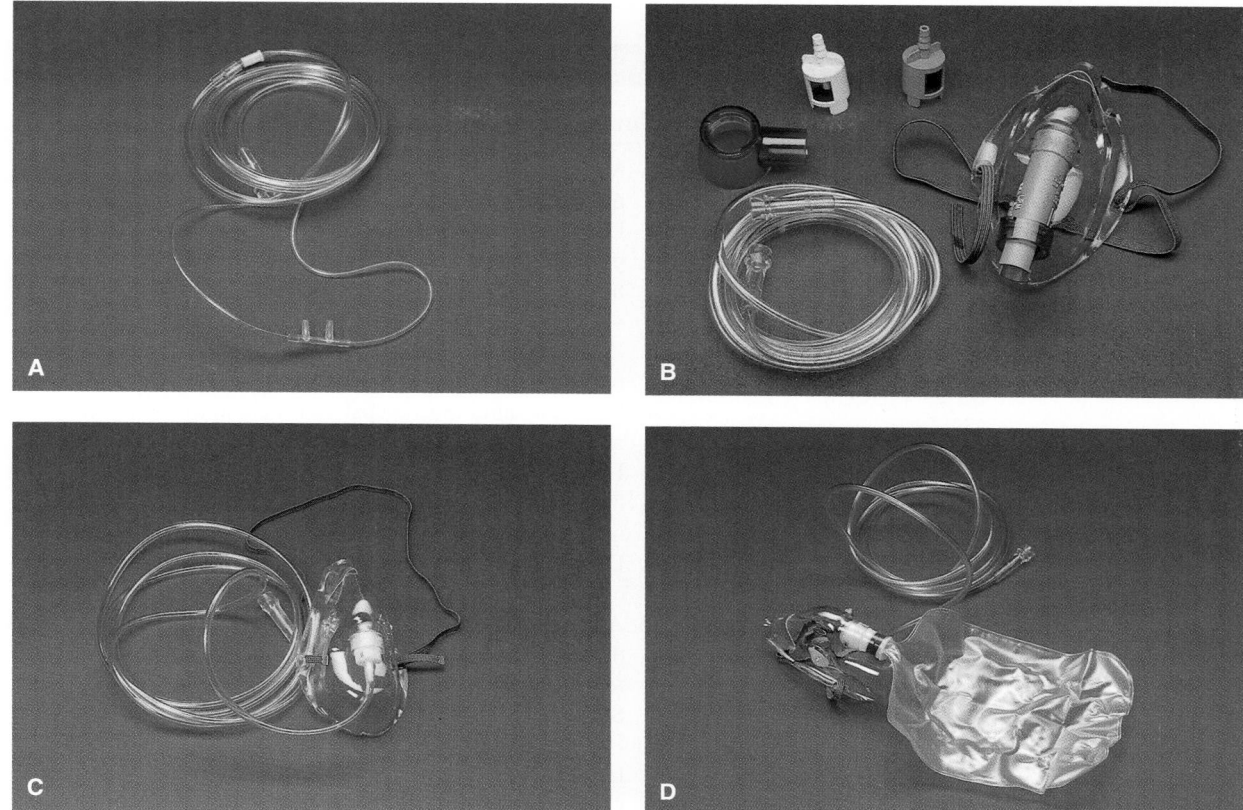

FIGURE 34-6   Common oxygen delivery devices. **(A)** Cannula. **(B)** Venturi mask. **(C)** Simple oxygen mask. **(D)** Reservoir mask.

The water seal chamber allows drainage and air to drain into the collection chamber without air entering the chest tube. The water seal chamber is filled with sterile water up to the mark identified by the manufacturer. Mild fluctuation in the water seal chamber is normal as the patient breathes. Bubbles in the water seal chamber when a client coughs may indicate an intermittent air leak. Continuous bubbling in the water seal chamber indicates an ongoing air leak and should be reported to the physician.

The suction chamber also is partially filled with sterile water and connected to suction. The physician orders the amount of suction to be used (usually 20 cm suction), and the suction chamber is adjusted so that there is gentle bubbling of the sterile water up to the line corresponding to the amount of suction ordered. The inclusion of suction in a chest drainage system establishes negative pressure to more readily reinflate a collapsed lung or encourage fluid removal from the pleural space. As a pneumothorax begins to re-inflate or if there is only minimal amount of fluid to be drained, sometimes a chest tube will be ordered to be disconnected from suction. Refer to Procedure 34-6 for details on monitoring a client with a chest tube.

Assisted Ventilation

Positive Pressure Breathing. Intermittent positive pressure breathing (IPPB) or bilevel positive airway pressure (BiPAP) therapy uses a mechanical ventilator to assist inspiration. The client's inspiratory effort triggers the ventilator, which pushes air into the lungs. The positive pressure helps to prevent and treat atelectasis by helping to open underinflated alveoli. Continuous positive airway pressure (CPAP) uses oxygen under constant pressure to accomplish this objective. CPAP is often used at night to decrease periodic hypoxemia associated with sleep apnea.

To optimize the benefits, experienced personnel should administer positive pressure therapy. The nurse or respiratory care practitioner (RCP) must assess each client's breathing needs and individualize treatment accordingly. When performing such care, adjust the ventilator to provide the best breathing pattern for each client. Allow for rest periods at appropriate times and assess the client continuously for adverse effects.

Positive pressure breathing usually is not ordered unless other, more simple hyperinflation therapies, such as deep breathing and incentive spirometry, have been ineffective. The equipment is expensive and specially trained personnel need to provide and monitor therapy. Complications can be serious and include hyperventilation, spread of infection, air swallowing with resultant gastric distention, danger of causing or worsening a pneumothorax, and the possibility of increasing air trapping in clients with obstructive diseases.

Manual Resuscitation Bag and Mask. When the client is unable to sustain adequate ventilation, use a manual resuscitation

TABLE 34-5

Oxygen Therapy Equipment		
Device	**Oxygen Capability**	**Nursing Considerations**
Cannula (nasal prongs)	22%–44% when operated at 1–6 L/min	1. Most commonly used oxygen device because of convenience and client comfort 2. Delivered oxygen concentration can vary with client breathing pattern. "Rule of Four" used to estimate concentration: for each L/min of O_2, concentration increases by 4% (e.g., 1 L/min provides 22%, 2 L/min provides 26%) 3. Limit maximum O_2 flow to 6 L/min to minimize drying of nasal mucosa; use humidifier prn 4. Nasal passages must be patent for client to receive O_2: mouth breathing does not appreciably diminish delivered O_2 5. Delivered O_2 concentration can vary depending on client's breathing pattern. Relatively consistent O_2 delivery with quiet, steady breathing
Transtracheal catheter	0.5–2 L/min	1. Device is surgically implanted in trachea of O_2-dependent client as alternative to cannula 2. Advantages: efficient use of O_2 (no waste because all O_2 is delivered directly to lungs); practically invisible so client feels less self-conscious 3. Suitable only for clients who can care for device
Venturi mask	24%–50% when operated at 3–8 L/min as specified by manufacturer	1. Provides precise and consistent O_2 concentration 2. Essential to adjust mask according to specifications to ensure accurate O_2 delivery 3. Noisy; like all masks, may cause claustrophobia
Simple mask	40%–60% when operated at 6–10 L/min	1. Most common midrange O_2 delivery device 2. Minimum of 5 L/min O_2 required to prevent client from rebreathing exhaled carbon dioxide 3. As with cannula, actual delivered O_2 concentration varies with breathing pattern 4. Not suitable for client with COPD because of potential for excessive oxygenation
Reservoir mask	Up to 90%+ when operated at 10–15 L/min	1. Used for critically ill client 2. Use sufficient flow to keep O_2 reservoir inflated
Large volume pneumatic nebulizer	21%–100% when operated at 12–15 L/min	1. Used to deliver O_2 with continuous aerosol therapy; required by many clients with artificial airways (e.g., tracheostomies) 2. Temperature must be monitored and tubing must be drained frequently
Incubator	22%–40%+	1. Enclosure used for environmental control for newborn infants 2. Extremely imprecise O_2 delivery; accuracy varies each time unit is opened
Oxyhood	22%–90%+ when operated at 7–12 L/min	1. Precise O_2 delivery for newborns and small infants 2. Minimum O_2 flow of 7 L/min flushes infant's exhaled carbon dioxide 3. Oxygen must be prewarmed and humidified to prevent infant heat loss 4. Frequent analysis needed to prevent excessive oxygenation
Oxygen tent	21%–30%+	1. Primarily used by small child unable to wear mask or cannula 2. Mainly used as "mist tent" to deliver high humidity to children with croup 3. Extremely inefficient O_2 delivery system; O_2 delivery fluctuates because leaks are common

COPD, chronic obstructive pulmonary disease.

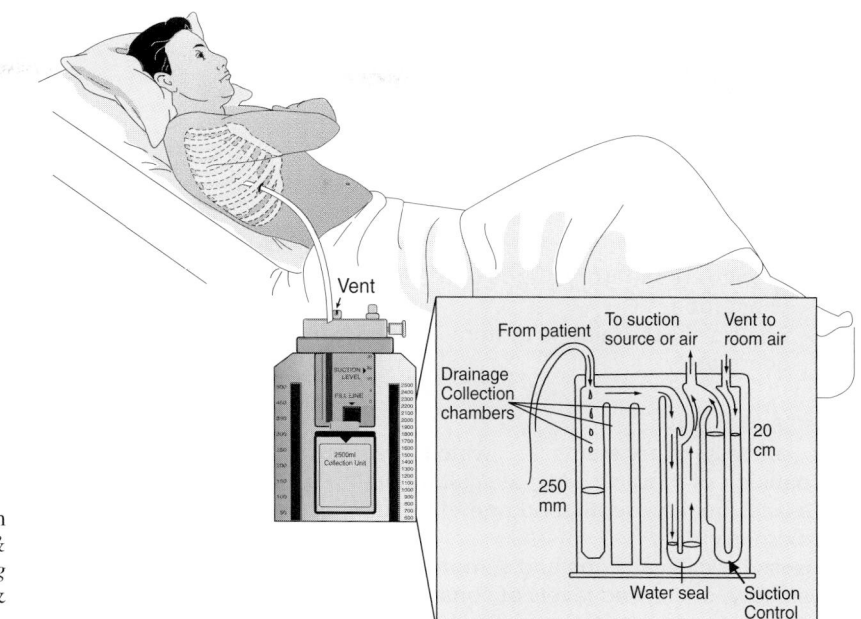

FIGURE 34-7 Chest drainage system. (From Smeltzer, S. C. & Bare, B. G. (2000). *Brunner & Suddarth's textbook of medical–surgical nursing* [9th ed.]. Philadelphia: Lippincott Williams & Wilkins.)

bag and mask until recovery occurs or an airway can be inserted and mechanical ventilation begun or death is pronounced. A manual resuscitation bag is basic emergency equipment. This bag can also be used to hyperinflate lungs just before suctioning and can be adapted to attach to a tracheostomy or endotracheal tube if the face mask is removed. (A resuscitation bag is pictured in Procedure 34-8, Step 7.)

To deliver effective ventilation, tilt the client's chin back and pull the jaw forward to open the airway. Hold the mask tightly over the client's mouth and nose, maintaining a good seal with one hand as you use the other hand to compress the bag and deliver air into the lungs. The bag is self-inflating and a one-way valve allows exhaled air to escape. A normal rate of inflations for an adult is 16 to 20 breaths per minute. The tidal volume delivered, as well as the amount of oxygen, can vary depending on the rate and technique used to compress the bag (Glass, Grap, Corley, & Wallace, 1993).

Ventilators

Ventilators are mechanical devices used to provide artificial breathing for clients who cannot breathe effectively. Until recently, these machines were used only in the intensive care unit. Now ventilator clients increasingly are cared for on general medical-surgical and rehabilitation units. Intermediate care facilities that deal exclusively with ventilator-dependent clients are becoming common, and the use of ventilators in the home is growing steadily.

Positive-pressure ventilators deliver oxygen under pressure to clients who cannot breathe effectively. These machines range from simple pressure-limited devices to microprocessor-driven, volume-limited ventilators. Their uses range from full ventilatory support to simply assisting the client who is too weak to maintain effective ventilation for long periods.

Ventilators require frequent monitoring by specially trained personnel. The person who is caring for a ventilator client must become familiar with the ventilator's alarm system. The ventilator's alarms indicate changes in the client's condition or possible machine malfunction. Alarms should never be turned off.

More information on negative-pressure ventilators follows in the Community-Based Nursing section of this chapter. For additional information on intensive ventilator care, consult texts on respiratory therapy or critical care nursing.

Artificial Airways

An artificial airway is a device inserted through the mouth, nose, or throat to provide direct access to the lungs. Oropharyngeal airways, nasopharyngeal airways ("nasal trumpets"), endotracheal tubes, and tracheostomy tubes are examples of artificial airways.

Oral or Nasal Pharyngeal Airways. These airways are used to bypass upper airway obstructions or to facilitate secretion removal (Fig. 34-8). Oropharyngeal airways (see Fig. 34-8A) are simple to insert but are poorly tolerated by all but the comatose client. The noncomatose client is likely to gag on an oropharyngeal airway, so a nasal trumpet (see Fig. 34-8B) is preferable. These airways should be well-lubricated with water-soluble gel before they are inserted.

Endotracheal Tubes. An endotracheal tube is a plastic tube inserted through the nose or mouth into the trachea (Fig. 34-9). These airways are used to ventilate a client during surgery or when mechanical ventilation is necessary. They are also used to protect the airway in a comatose person.

Tracheostomy. The **tracheostomy** is an artificial airway consisting of a plastic tube surgically implanted just below the larynx into the trachea; the tube bypasses the mouth and upper airway. The surgical procedure that establishes the

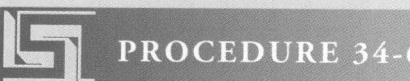

PROCEDURE 34-6

MONITORING A CLIENT WITH A CHEST DRAINAGE SYSTEM

Purpose
1. Monitor respiratory status of a patient with a chest tube.
2. Ensure chest drainage system is functioning adequately.

Assessment
Assess respiratory status (i.e., watch symmetrical expansion of thoracic cage; auscultate breath sounds; assess quality, depth, and rate of breaths, pulse oximetry).

Assess for clinical signs and symptoms of hypoxia: anxiety, decreased levels of consciousness, inability to concentrate, fatigue, dizziness, cardiac dysrhythmias, pallor or cyanosis, dyspnea. Notify physician immediately of any significant changes in patient's respiratory status.

Equipment
Occlusive sterile dressing (if needed).

Procedure
1. Confirm physician's order including amount of suction.
   Rationale: Prevents potential errors.
2. Assist patient to semi- or high Fowler's position.
   Rationale: These positions assist with optimal lung expansion.
3. Assess insertion site of chest tube. Note and document amount and color of drainage on dressing around insertion site. Feel insertion site for krepitis—air leaking into the subcutaneous tissue. Document any krepitis found. Reinforce insertion dressing as needed.
   Rationale: Excessive drainage around the insertion site can indicate bleeding. The insertion site dressing may need to be changed by the surgeon who inserted the chest tube. Development of krepitis can indicate a small air leak into the subcutaneous tissue. Krepitis may indicate a need for the surgeon to adjust the chest tube placement.
4. Assess status of chest tubing. Be sure tubing remains at the level of the patient and no dependent loops are present. Assess that there are no visible clots in the tubing. You may gently "milk" (compress tubing with fingers) the clots to encourage movement into the drainage system, but you never want to strip chest tubing.

Rationale: Dependent loops of tubing may collect fluid and prevent drainage of fluid from the chest cavity. Stripping chest tubing can create dangerous intrathoracic negative pressure, injuring the patient.

5. Assess the drainage collection chamber. Be sure to keep chest drainage system upright. Assess for amount, color, and character of drainage. Mark the collection chamber to accurately reflect the amount of drainage accumulated during your shift.
   Rationale: Keeping the drainage system upright will ensure proper sequential filling of the collection chambers. Marking the collection chamber at the end of each shift will allow evaluation of output to detect excessive bleeding or healing.

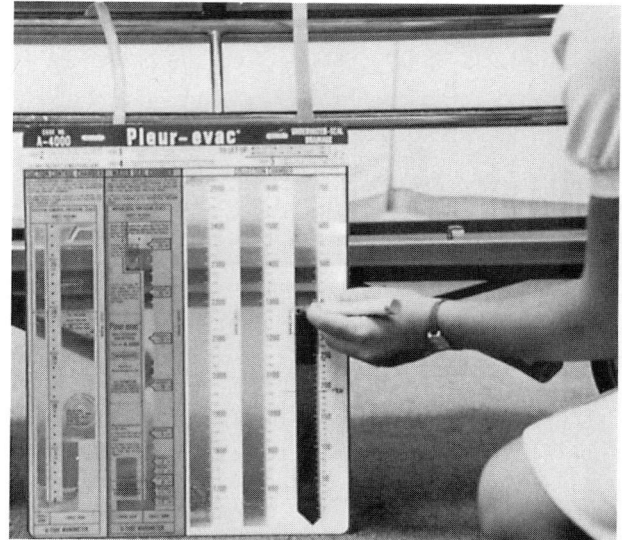

Step 5 Marking the chamber.

6. Assess suction chamber. Make sure the water level in the suction chamber is at the prescribed amount of suction and that it is connected to the wall suction that is turned on to continuous suction. Usually the suction is set at 10 to 20 mmHg.
   Rationale: The amount of suction is determined by the water level in the suction chamber rather than the suction setting on the wall unit. Gentle bubbling is normal in the suction chamber.
7. Assess the system for any airleaks. Check all external connections (i.e., the chest tube's connection to the drainage system, the suction tubing's connection to the drainage system). Examine the water seal chamber as the patient breathes normally and as he or she coughs.

PROCEDURE 34-6 (Continued)

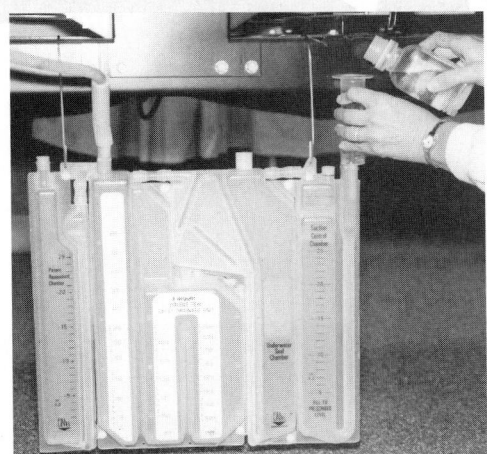

Step 6 Adding water to the suction chamber.

Rationale: A chest drainage system needs to be a continuously closed system to maintain the negative pressure necessary for normal respiratory function. Any air leak interrupts this closed system. Bubbling in the water seal chamber may indicate an intermittent or continuous air-leak. Bubbling when a patient coughs indicates an intermittent air leak. Ongoing bubbling in the water seal chamber indicates a continuous air leak. Air leaks need to be reported to the physician.

8. Encourage the patient to cough, deep breathe, and use an incentive spirometer frequently. Provide analgesics as necessary.

Rationale: Coughing and deep breathing will increase intrapleural pressure, facilitating fluid drainage from the pleural space and enhancing lung expansion. Analgesics will assist with pain control as the patient coughs, deep breathes, and uses an incentive spirometer.

9. If the chest tube becomes expelled, do not leave the patient. Cover the opening where the chest tube had been inserted with the sterile 4″ × 4″ gauze, and keep direct pressure on the site. Send a colleague to call the physician immediately.

Rationale: Leaving the chest tube insertion site open will create an open pneumothorax and can result in respiratory distress. A physician will need to replace the chest tube as soon as possible.

10. Document chest tube drainage, chest tube patency, presence of an air leak, amount of suction, pain level, dressing status, and respiratory status.

Rationale: Documenting maintains legal record and communicates with health team members.

Collaboration and Delegation

- Notify the physician immediately if the chest tube dislodges, a sudden air leak occurs, significant unexpected drainage occurs, or if the client is experiencing dyspnea. Caution all personnel to maintain upright position of the chest tube drainage system and to keep it stable, often hooked to the bed. Take care that system does not get under the bed where it could be accidentally cracked if the bed position were lowered.

---

artificial airway is called a tracheotomy; the resultant airway is a tracheostomy. This procedure is most often done as a temporary measure. Unlike a permanent laryngectomy in which the entire larynx is removed, a tracheotomy leaves the structure of the airway intact.

Indications. A client may require this procedure to bypass a severe or recurrent upper airway obstruction. The client who regularly aspirates food or stomach contents may need a tracheostomy to protect the airway. A few clients may need this type of airway to help with secretion control because a tracheostomy provides ready access for suctioning. Finally, the client who requires long-term mechanical ventilation may be

tracheotomized to provide the safest and most stable artificial airway available. Many tracheotomized clients on the general nursing unit are former clients of the intensive care unit or have had head and neck surgery.

Equipment. Tracheostomy tubes come in a variety of types (Fig. 34-10). All tubes contain an outer cannula that fits into the trachea and a flange that rests against the neck and allows the tube to be fastened in place. An obturator is a guide that is inserted into the tracheostomy tube to ease insertion then removed. Some tracheostomy tubes contain an inner cannula that locks into place and can be removed for cleaning. Cuffed tracheostomy tubes contain an inflatable cuff (or balloon) that

ETHICAL/LEGAL ISSUE
Withdrawal of Ventilator Support

You are working in an intensive care unit, caring for an 18-year-old girl who was in a very serious automobile accident 2 nights ago. Prognosis is very poor because two EEGs demonstrated no brain wave activity. She is being supported by a mechanical ventilator. The doctor tells you he plans to talk with her distraught parents about removing the ventilator and possibly donating the daughter's organs for transplantation.

Reflection
- Try to identify factors that healthcare providers need to consider when requesting organs for transplantation.
- Visualize how you would feel if present with the physician and family at this time. Identify ways that you could be supportive.
- Do the parents have the right to refuse a request for organ transplantation? If so, how would you support them in this decision?
- How might consenting to organ transplantation assist this family in the grieving process?

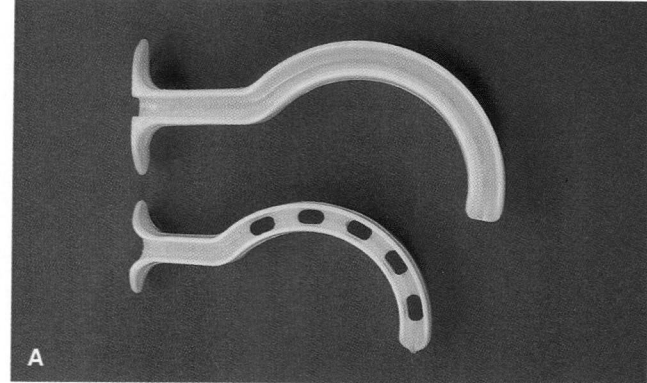
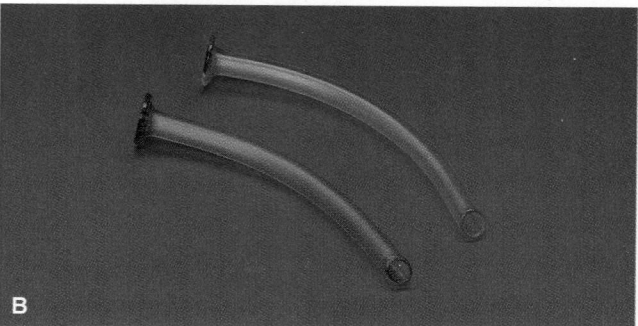

FIGURE 34-8   Artificial airways. **(A)** Oral airways. **(B)** Nasal trumpets.

is inflated to stabilize the tube in the trachea. Advantages of a cuffed tracheostomy tube include decreased risk of aspiration, prevention of air leakage, and access to mechanical ventilation. Low-pressure cuffs also decrease the incidence of tracheal mucosal damage. Fenestrated tracheostomy tubes are tubes with holes in the outer cannula. When the client is being ventilated, the inner cannula remains in place. When weaning is attempted, the inner cannula can be removed and the cuff deflated; this allows the client to breathe around the tube and through the fenestration. Another advantage of the fenestrated tube is that speaking is possible when the tracheostomy is plugged because the hole permits exhaled air to flow over the vocal cords.

SAFETY ALERT
The tube must never be plugged if the cuff is inflated because this could cause suffocation and possible death. (Tamburri, 2000)

Risks. Risks of a tracheostomy are numerous. Immediately after surgery, bleeding of the incision is common. Change dressings frequently during this period. Assess the extent of blood loss and be prepared to call the surgeon if bleeding is excessive.

Fastidious care of the stoma is necessary to keep it free of infection. Because the tracheostomy bypasses the defenses of the upper airway, the client is at risk for pneumonia. Thus, during the postoperative hospitalization period, use sterile technique when cleaning the tracheostomy site and when suctioning the client.

Clients who are tracheotomized often have marginal breathing ability. The client with this condition must be protected most diligently against the tube plugging. Dried secretions can completely occlude the tube, creating a respiratory emergency. For this reason, tracheostomy clients must be well-hydrated and the air they breathe must be completely humidified by a nebulizer or high-output humidifier.

A tracheostomy also poses communication problems. Because the vocal cords are above the level of the tracheostomy tube, the client cannot speak. A tablet and pencil can eliminate a great deal of frustration and confusion. Specialized tra-

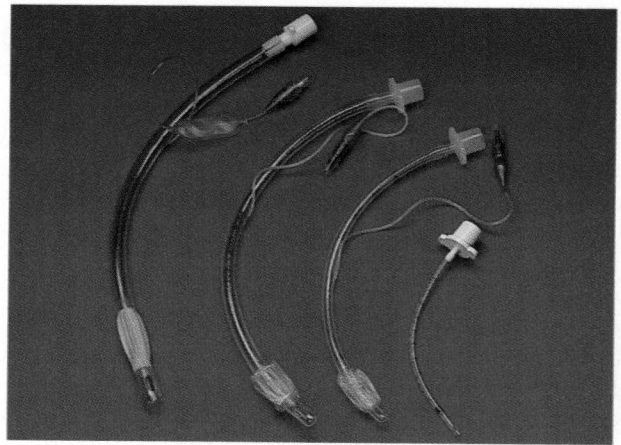

FIGURE 34-9   Endotracheal tubes.

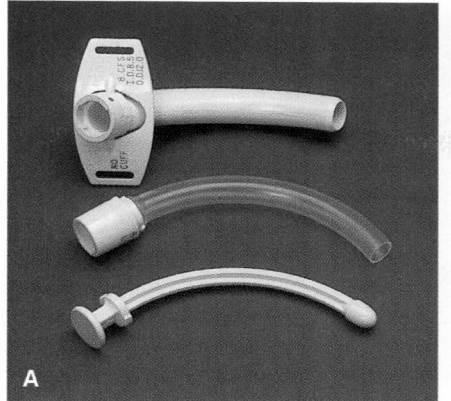
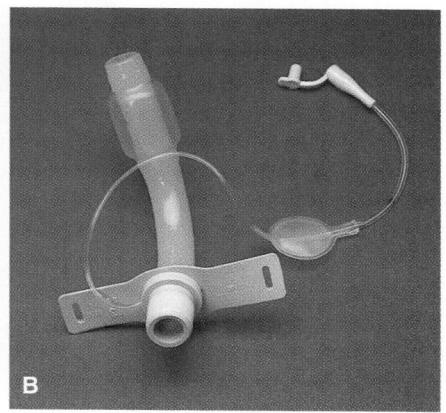

FIGURE 34-10 Tracheostomy tubes. **(A)** Uncuffed tube with inner cannula and obturator. **(B)** Cuffed tracheostomy tube.

cheostomy tubes, such as the Olympic Trach-Talk (Olympic Medical, Seattle, WA), can be attached to a standard tracheostomy tube, making speech possible. Tracheostomy buttons are used temporarily to plug the tracheostomy so the client's ability to breathe through the natural airway can be assessed. When these buttons are in place, the client can once again speak.

Such devices are appropriate for use only by the client with strong spontaneous respirations. Scrupulously follow the directions for each of these specialized devices. Improperly applied, they are unlikely to work and may cause complete airway blockage.

Body image is a potential problem for these clients. The tracheotomized client may feel embarrassed or inadequate because of the stoma. The client may perceive the stoma as ugly and disfiguring and may be embarrassed by its messy, bubbling secretions. Feelings of failure and depression may result from the inability to perform such a basic life function as breathing without assistance. The client is also likely to feel fear and anxiety about the inability to speak. Refer to Chapter 46 for therapeutic interventions for altered body image.

Tracheostomy Care. Tracheostomy care is necessary to decrease infection risk and to ensure that crusted secretions do not plug the tube. Remove dried mucus from the inner cannula of the tube and from around the incision site. Change stoma dressings regularly. Commercially made tracheostomy dressings are available or gauze may be folded to size. Do not cut dressings with scissors because threads from the gauze can cause an inflammatory reaction at the stoma. If the client has large amounts of secretions, change tracheostomy dressings as often as necessary. If the tracheostomy produces few secretions, the dressing may need changing only once or twice a day. Well-established, dry tracheostomies may require no dressing. Procedure 34-7 gives detailed instructions on tracheostomy care.

🔲 SAFETY ALERT
Take great care while changing the security ties that hold the tracheostomy tube in place because the client can easily cough out an unsecured tube. To minimize the danger of accidental extubation, tracheostomy care often is best performed by pairs of nurses.

Suctioning
Atelectasis and pneumonia may develop in clients who cannot cough effectively to expectorate mucus. Excessive mucus can even cause asphyxiation from choking. To prevent this, you may have to suction the airways.

Suctioning is appropriate only when secretions are present in the upper airways as indicated by coarse crackles, diminished breath sounds, increased inspiratory pressure, increased respiratory rate, or decreased oxygen saturation (Tamburri, 2000).

To suction the airways, insert a catheter through the nose, mouth, or tracheal tube. Attach the catheter to a portable or wall unit suction device, which provides the suction pressure for secretion removal. Effective suctioning can clear the oral cavity and nasopharyngeal areas of secretions. Secretions deep in the trachea are more difficult to remove, but the suctioning procedure is similar regardless of where the secretions are found. Procedure 34-8 gives complete instructions on secretion removal by suctioning.

Some clients produce excessive amounts of oral secretions. These clients can use a "tonsil-tip" (Yankauer) suction tube (Fig. 34-11) to evacuate excess saliva and thick mucus from the back of the throat. This suction catheter is also attached to wall or portable suction.

Potential Hazards of Suctioning. Clients with deep bronchial secretions may require deep endobronchial suctioning. Properly performed, suctioning can greatly improve airflow in the lungs, which promotes oxygenation. However the procedure carries several risks. Because oxygen as well as mucus is withdrawn from the airways, suctioning can cause temporary hypoxia.

🔲 SAFETY ALERT
Many studies over the last decade have demonstrated the significance of hyperinflation and hyperoxygenation before each suctioning attempt to minimize hypoxemia and atelectasis. (Marion, 2001)

Apply suction intermittently to help minimize catheter damage to the trachea's delicate mucosal lining. Limit suctioning passes to three for each suctioning procedure with 10 seconds

(text continues on page 851)

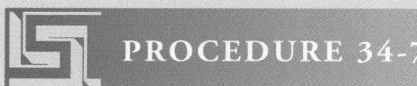

PROCEDURE 34-7

PROVIDING TRACHEOSTOMY CARE

Purpose
1. Maintain airway patency by removing mucus and encrusted secretions.
2. Promote cleanliness and prevent infection and skin breakdown at stoma site.

Assessment
- Assess for excess peristomal secretions, excess intratracheal secretions, or soiled tracheostomy dressing and ties.
- Assess respiratory status: breath sounds, respiratory rate, skin color, labored breathing, flared nares or sternal retractions, arterial blood gases.
- Identify factors that influence tracheostomy care:
  Inadequate nutritional status predisposes client to infection, poor healing, and weak cough reflex.
  Respiratory infection: pulmonary secretions increase in amount. Note color, amount, and odor.
  Fluid status: inadequate hydration increases tenaciousness of secretions. Client may have difficulty coughing up thick secretions.
  Humidity: tracheostomy collars deliver humidified air to prevent dry, cracked membranes and thickened secretions.
- Identify type of tracheostomy tube used and if inner cannula is present. Identify if tracheostomy tube is cuffed and if the cuff is inflated.
- Assess client's ability to understand and perform independent tracheostomy care.

Equipment
Sterile tracheostomy care kit containing:
  Two basins
  Small brush or pipe cleaners
  4″ × 4″ gauze
  Commercially available tracheostomy dressing
  Twill tape or tracheostomy ties
Hydrogen peroxide
Normal saline
Sterile gloves
Scissors
Tracheostomy suction supplies

Procedure
1. Verify the physician order and identify the client.
   Rationale: Prevents potential errors.
2. Wash your hands and don gloves.
   Rationale: Handwashing and gloves reduce transmission of microorganisms.

3. Explain procedure to client. Place the client in semi- to high Fowler's position.
   Rationale: Teaching decreases client anxiety and increases compliance.
4. Suction tracheostomy tube. Before discarding gloves, remove soiled tracheostomy dressing and discard with catheter inside glove. *Note:* Follow Procedure 34-8, Suctioning Secretions From Airways, but insert catheter through tracheostomy tube and advance about 10 to 12 cm in an adult.
   Rationale: Removing secretions maintains a patent airway while doing tracheostomy cleaning.
5. Replace oxygen or humidification source and encourage client to deep-breathe as you prepare sterile supplies.
   Rationale: Maintain good oxygenation status.
6. Open sterile tracheostomy kit. Don sterile gloves. Pour normal saline into one basin, hydrogen peroxide into the second. Open several sterile cotton-tipped applicators and one sterile precut tracheostomy dressing and place on sterile field. If kit does not contain tracheostomy ties, cut two 15-inch pieces of twill tape and set aside.
   Rationale: Preparing equipment allows for smooth, organized performance of tracheostomy care.

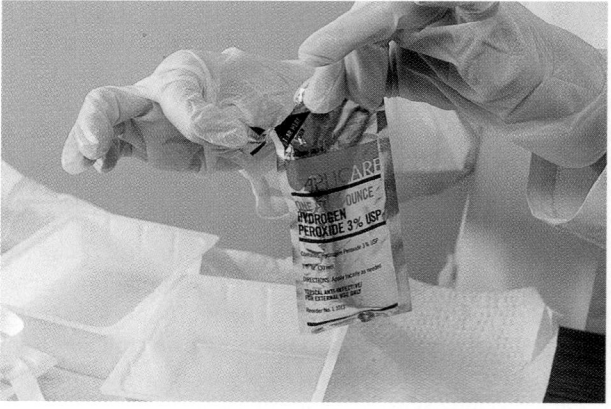

Step 6 Pour sterile hydrogen peroxide into basin.

7. Remove oxygen or humidity source. *Note:* For tracheostomy tube with inner cannula, complete Steps 7 to 25. For tracheostomy tube without inner cannula or plugged with a button, complete Steps 13 to 25.
8. Unlock inner cannula by turning counterclockwise. Remove inner cannula.
9. Place inner cannula in basin with hydrogen peroxide.

PROCEDURE 34-7 (Continued)

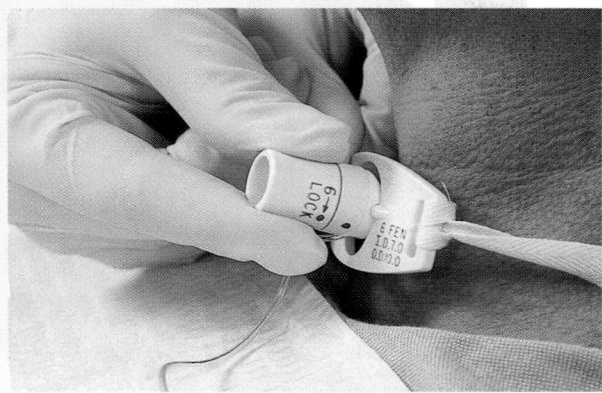

Step 8 Unlock inner cannula by turning counter-clockwise.

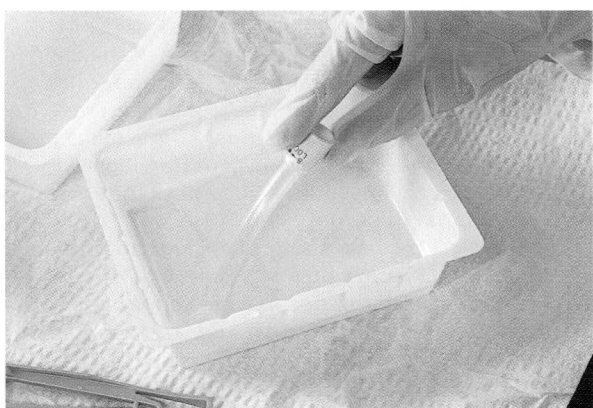

Step 9 Place inner cannula into basin with hydrogen peroxide.

Rationale: Hydrogen peroxide loosens and removes secretions from inner cannula.

10. Replace oxygen source over or near outer cannula.
    Rationale: Maintain a constant supply of oxygen to prevent respiratory or cardiac distress.
    Note: Not all clients require a constant oxygen supply during tracheostomy care.
11. Clean lumen and sides of inner cannula using pipe cleaners or sterile brush.
    Rationale: Mechanical force and friction are needed to remove thick or dried secretions.
12. Rinse inner cannula thoroughly by agitating in normal saline for several seconds.
    Rationale: Rinsing and agitation remove secretions and water from cannula and provide lubrication for each insertion.

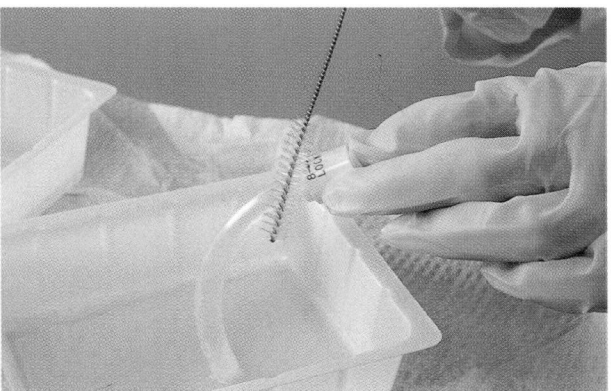

Step 11 Clean inner cannula with brush.

13. Remove oxygen source and replace inner cannula into outer cannula. "Lock" by turning clockwise until the two blue dots align. Replace oxygen or humidity source.
    Rationale: Oxygen is reestablished to a secured inner cannula.

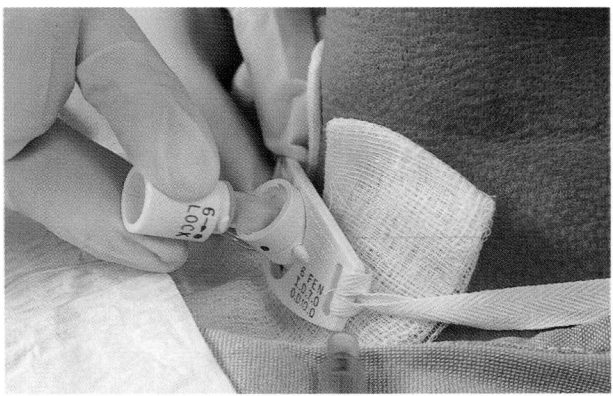

Step 13 Replace inner cannula, then lock into place.

14. Clean stoma under faceplate with circular motion using hydrogen peroxide-soaked cotton applicators. Clean dried secretions from all exposed outer cannula surfaces.
    Rationale: Dried secretions are a good medium for bacterial growth.
15. Remove foaming secretions using normal saline-soaked, cotton-tipped applicators.
    Rationale: Hydrogen peroxide can be irritating to the skin.
16. Pat moist surfaces dry with 4" × 4" gauze.
    Rationale: Moist surfaces support growth of microorganisms and skin excoriation.

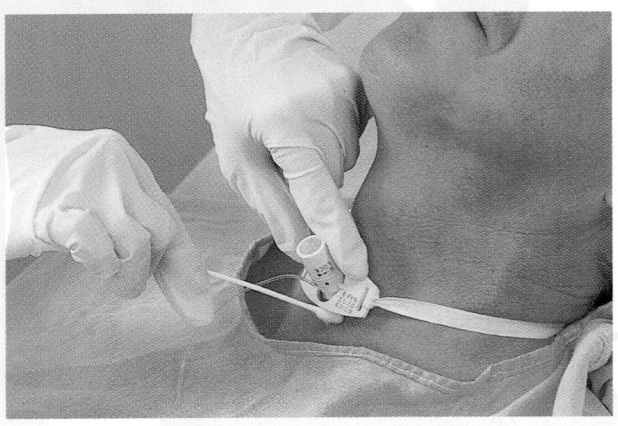

Step 14 Clean secretions from tracheostomy site with cotton applicator.

17. Place dry, sterile, precut tracheostomy dressing around tracheostomy stoma and under faceplate. Do not use cut 4″ × 4″ gauze.
    Rationale: Frayed cotton fibers could be aspirated into the trachea.

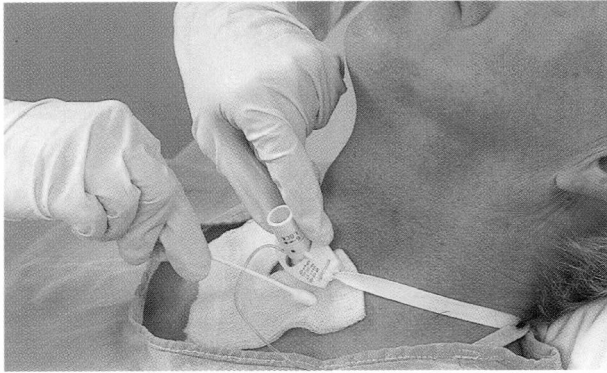

Step 17 Replace new precut tracheostomy dressing.

18. If tracheostomy ties are to be changed, have an assistant don a sterile glove and hold the tracheostomy tube in place.
    Rationale: This action prevents accidental displacement of the tracheostomy tube if the client moves or coughs when the ties are not secure.
19. Cut a ½-inch slit approximately 1 inch from one end of both clean tracheostomy ties. This is easily done by folding back on itself 1 inch of the tie and cutting a small slit in the middle.
20. Remove and discard soiled tracheostomy ties.
21. Thread end of tie through cut slit in tie. Pull tight.

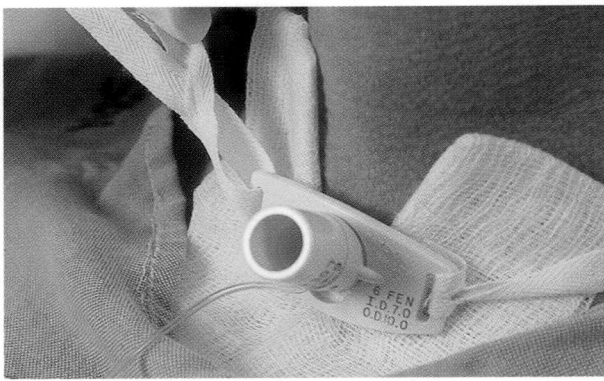

Step 21 Thread end of tie through cut slit in tie. Pull tight.

Rationale: The tie is secured to the faceplate without using knots.
22. Repeat Step 19 with the second tie.
23. Bring both ties together at one side of the client's neck. Assess that ties are only tight enough to allow one finger between tie and neck. Use two square knots to secure the ties. Trim excess tie length. *Note:* Assess tautness of tracheostomy ties frequently in clients whose neck may swell from trauma or surgery.
    Rationale: Ties must be taut enough to prevent accidental dislodging of tracheostomy tube but loose enough not to cause choking or pressure on the jugular veins. Ties at side of neck are more comfortable for the client.
24. Remove gloves and discard disposable equipment. Label with date and time, and store reusable supplies.
    Rationale: Opened normal saline is considered sterile for 24 hours.
25. Assist client to comfortable position and offer oral hygiene.
    Rationale: Promotes client comfort.
26. Wash your hands. Document procedure and observations.
    Rationale: Maintains infection control and communicates with other healthcare team members.

Lifespan Considerations
Infant and Child
- Additional assistants may be necessary during tracheostomy care to prevent active children from dislodging or expelling their tracheostomy tubes.
- Encourage parents to participate with the procedure in an effort to comfort the child and promote client teaching.

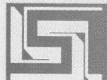

PROCEDURE 34-7 (Continued)

Home Care Modifications

- Teach the client or caregiver the following:
    Handwashing is the most important step before touching the tracheostomy.
    The function of each part of the tracheostomy tube.
    To remove, change, and replace the inner cannula.
    To clean the inner cannula two or three times a day.
    To clean the tracheostomy stoma.
    To suction tracheal secretions.
    To assess for symptoms of infection (i.e., increased temperature, increased amount of secretions, change in color or odor of secretions).
    To use a mirror for better visualization.
- A vaporizer may be used in the home to replace moisture into the air.
- The client may wear a scarf or 4″ × 4″ over the tracheostomy if the air is dusty.
- Home care may be a clean rather than sterile procedure:
    Plain, single-use paper cups may be used for soaking the inner cannula.
    Tap water may be used to rinse secretions from the inner cannula.
    Gloves need not be worn, but thorough handwashing is imperative.
- A list of needed supplies and equipment and the names of medical supply houses is useful.
- Names and telephone numbers of healthcare professionals who are available for emergencies or advice 24 hours a day should be readily available.

Collaboration and Delegation

- Respiratory therapists are responsible for tracheostomy care in some agencies. Communicate with therapists if secretions are excessive or crusted so that they provide tracheostomy care promptly to prevent airway occlusion.

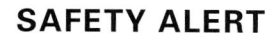

---

as the recommended time limit for each suction attempt (Elkin, Perry, & Potter, 2000). Usually the suction regulator is set between 80 and 120 mm Hg for larger children and adults and between 60 to 80 mm Hg for infants.

SAFETY ALERT
Saline lavage, a practice commonly used to loosen thick secretions, can cause a significant (although temporary) drop in oxygenation, so use this procedure only with caution in selected clients. It is recommended that saline lavage only be done by a respiratory therapist or nurse trained in suctioning procedures. (Sievers & Adams, 2000)

In addition to causing hypoxia, suctioning can cause cardiac dysrhythmias, hypotension, and atelectasis. Because suctioning can stimulate a gag reflex, vomiting (with the potential for aspiration) is possible. Suctioning can greatly relieve the dyspnea that accompanies excessive secretions, but the process is frightening and unpleasant for nearly all clients. Be prepared to offer a great deal of reassurance.

Emergency Airway Measures
Airway obstruction is a medical emergency requiring immediate attention. Because airway obstruction hinders breathing, the airway must be cleared to prevent suffocation and cardiorespiratory arrest.

SAFETY ALERT
The most common cause of airway obstruction is the tongue, which can fall back into the airway and interfere with ventilation and gas exchange. Positioning the client on either side can relieve the obstruction. If such a position is undesirable or impractical, an oral or nasal airway may be needed.

The neurologically impaired client, such as the comatose client or a person with a cerebral vascular accident, is most at risk for airway obstruction. Because the airway is only partially occluded, the person is able to breathe with effort. The partial obstruction is identified by loud snoring sounds as the client inspires.

(text continues on page 855)

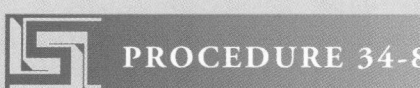

PROCEDURE 34-8

SUCTIONING SECRETIONS FROM AIRWAYS

Purpose
1. Remove excess mucous secretions to maintain patent airway.
2. Collect sputum or secretions for diagnostic testing.

Assessment/Preparation
- Assess respiratory system:
  Note rate, depth, rhythm of respirations.
  Note noisy, wet, or gurgling respirations.
  Auscultate breath sounds.
- Assess client's ability to cough. Note amount and character of sputum.
- Assess vital signs. Compare to baseline vital signs. Note an elevation in temperature.
- Assess level of consciousness and ability to protect airway (i.e., presence of cough reflex). Note any drainage from mouth.

Equipment
Portable or wall suction apparatus with tubing and reservoir
Sterile suction kit containing:
  Appropriate-sized catheter: infants, 5 to 8 Fr; children, 8 to 10 Fr; adults, 12 to 18 Fr
  Pair of gloves
  Container for saline to flush and lubricate catheter
Sterile saline (may be provided in kit)
Water-resistant disposal bag
Facial tissues
Towel (optional)

Procedure
1. Verify the physician order and identify the client.
   Rationale: Prevents potential errors.
2. Wash your hands.
   Rationale: Handwashing prevents transmission of microorganisms.
3. Explain procedure and purpose to client.
   Rationale: Explanations reduce anxiety and encourage cooperation with procedure.
4. a. Position the conscious client with an intact gag reflex in a semi-Fowler's position.
      Rationale: The semi-Fowler's position helps prevent aspiration of secretions.
   b. Position the unconscious client in a side-lying position facing you.
      Rationale: A side-lying position facilitates drainage of secretions by gravity and prevents aspiration.

5. Turn on suction device and adjust pressure: infants and children, 50 to 75 mmHg; adults, 100 to 120 mmHg.
   Rationale: Excessive negative pressure traumatizes mucosa and can induce hypoxia.
6. Open and prepare sterile suction catheter kit.
   a. Unfold sterile cup, touching only the outside. Place on bedside table.
   b. Pour sterile saline into cup.

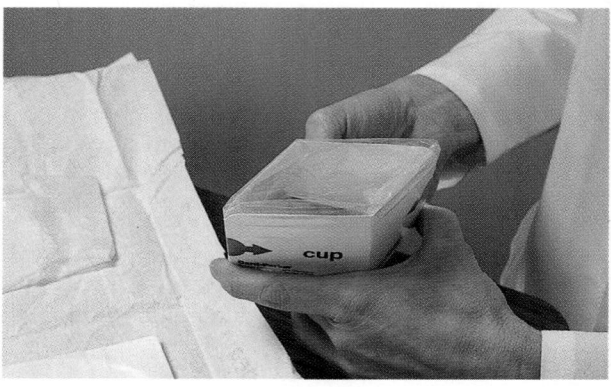

Step 6a Open and prepare sterile suction catheter kit.

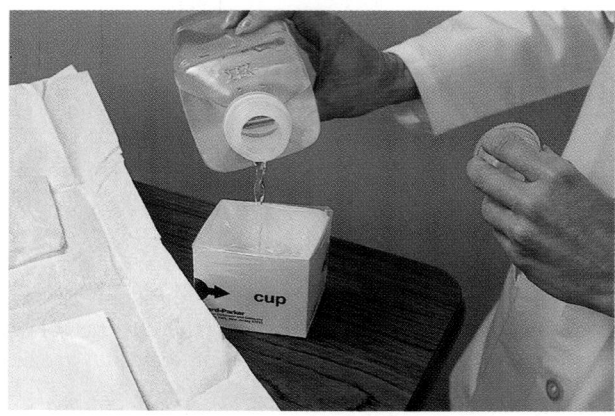

Step 6b Pour sterile saline into cup.

7. Preoxygenate client with 100% oxygen. Hyperinflate with manual resuscitation bag.
   Rationale: Preoxygenation helps prevent hypoxia; hyperinflation decreases atelectasis caused by suctioning.
8. Don sterile gloves. If kit provides only one glove, place on dominant hand.
   Rationale: Dominant hand will remain sterile.
   You may use a clean disposable glove on the nondominant hand to protect yourself from exposure to mucous membranes and sputum.

PROCEDURE 34-8 (Continued)

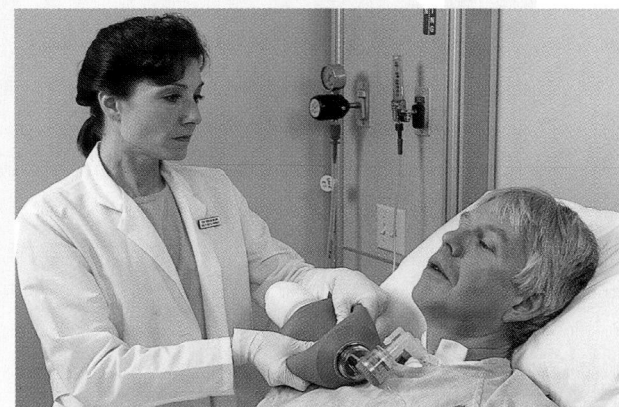

Step 7 Preoxygenate and hyperinflate before suctioning.

9. Pick up catheter with dominant hand. Pick up connecting tubing with nondominant hand. Attach catheter to tubing without contaminating sterile hand.

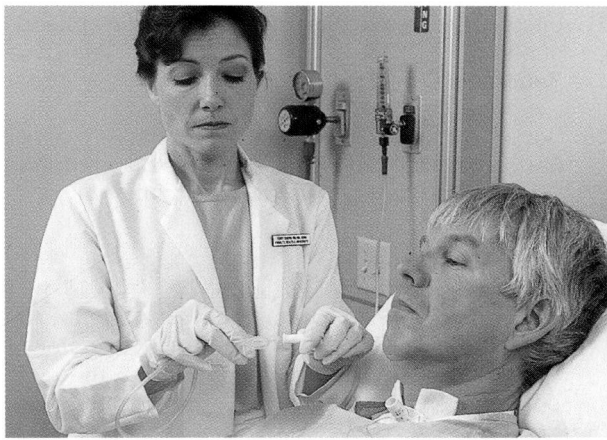

Step 9 Attach catheter to suction tubing.

10. Place catheter end into cup of saline. Test functioning of equipment by applying thumb from nondominant hand over open port to create suction. Return catheter to sterile field.
    Rationale: Lubrication makes catheter insertion easier and ensures proper functioning of suction equipment.
11. Insert catheter into trachea through nostril, nasal trumpet, or artificial airway during inspiration.
    Rationale: Inspiration opens epiglottis and facilitates catheter movement into trachea.
12. Advance catheter until you feel resistance. Retract catheter 1 cm before applying suction.

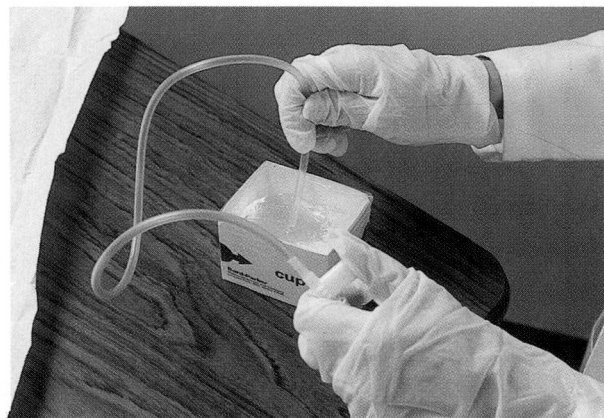

Step 10 Flush saline through catheter.

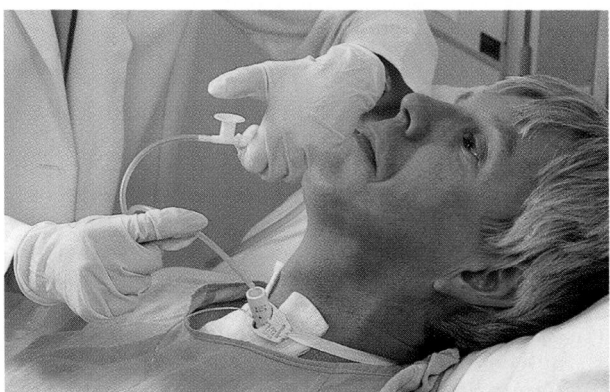

Step 11 Insert catheter into trachea without applying suction.

Note: Client usually will cough when catheter enters trachea.
Rationale: Retracting catheter slightly prevents mucosal damage.
13. Apply suction by placing thumb of nondominant hand over open port. Rotate the catheter with your dominant hand as you withdraw the catheter. This should take 5 to 10 seconds.
    Rationale: Rotation of catheter prevents trauma to mucous membrane from prolonged suctioning of one area. Limiting the suction time to 10 seconds or less prevents hypoxia.
14. Hyperoxygenate and hyperinflate using manual resuscitation bag for a full minute between subsequent suction passes. Encourage deep breathing.
    Rationale: Prolonged suctioning can induce hypoxia.

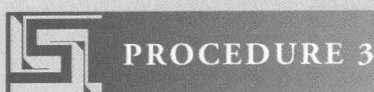

PROCEDURE 34-8 (Continued)

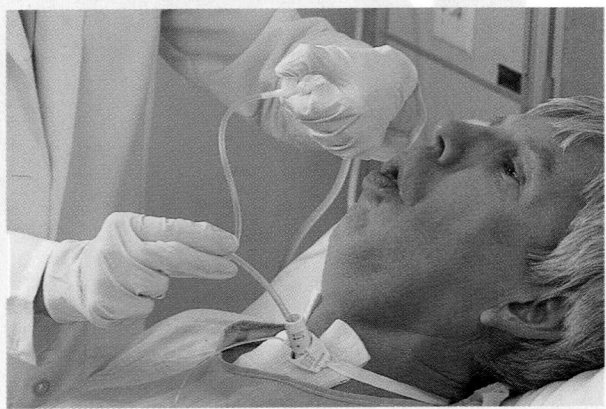

Step 13 Apply suction, as you withdraw the catheter.

15. Rinse catheter thoroughly with saline.
    Rationale: Rinsing clears secretions from catheter.
16. Repeat Steps 10 to 14 until airway is clear.
17. Without applying suction, insert the catheter gently along one side of the mouth. Advance to the oropharynx.
    Rationale: Suction the oropharynx after trachea because the mouth is less clean than the trachea. Directing the catheter along the side of the mouth prevents stimulation of the gag reflex.
18. Apply suction for 5 to 10 seconds as you rotate and withdraw catheter.
    Rationale: Rotation of the catheter prevents trauma to the mucous membrane. Be sure to remove secretions that pool beneath the tongue and in the vestibule of the mouth.
19. Allow 1 to 2 minutes between passes for the client to ventilate. Encourage deep breathing. Replace oxygen if applicable.
20. Repeat Steps 16 and 17 as necessary to clear oropharynx.
21. Rinse catheter and tubing by suctioning saline through.
22. Remove gloves by holding catheter with dominant hand and pulling glove off inside-out. Catheter will remain coiled inside the glove. Pull other glove off inside-out. Dispose of in trash receptacle.
    Rationale: Contain client secretions inside gloves to reduce transmission of microorganisms.
23. Turn off suction device.
24. Assist client to comfortable position. Offer assistance with oral and nasal hygiene. Replace oxygen device if used.

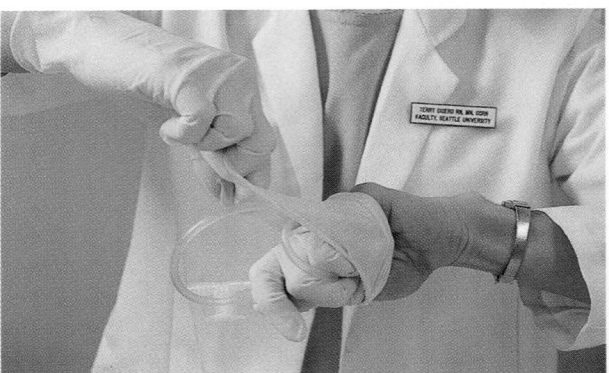

Step 22 Remove glove, pulling it over the catheter in other hand.

Rationale: Accumulated respiratory secretions irritate the mucous membranes and are unpleasant for the client.
25. Dispose of disposable supplies.
26. Wash your hands.
27. Ensure that sterile suction kit is available at head of bed.
    Rationale: Provides immediate access to suction equipment when needed.
28. Document procedure and observations.
    Rationale: Maintains legal record and communicates with other healthcare team members.

Lifespan Considerations
Infant and Child
- Infants and young children have airways that are easily occluded by a small amount of secretions. The nasal airway is smaller in diameter, the epiglottis is higher, and the tongue is proportionately larger.
- A bulb syringe is often used to aspirate secretions from an infant's nasal and oral cavities. This procedure is clean rather than sterile because the trachea is not entered.

Home Care Modifications
- Clients may need to learn to suction their secretions if they have difficulty coughing them effectively. Maintaining adequate hydration thins secretions and facilitates their removal.
- The type and number of microorganisms available to contaminate the respiratory system are different at home than in the acute care setting. Teach the client or caregiver to use plain paper cups for suctioning, not a sterile basin. Keep the cups in a sealable package. The client or care-

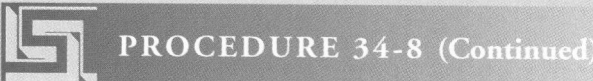

PROCEDURE 34-8 (Continued)

giver should remove a clean cup from the bottom of the package for each suctioning effort and reseal the package between uses.
• Suction catheters can be clean, not sterile. They should be washed in soapy water, rinsed well, and soaked in a vinegar-and-water solution.
• To decrease expenses, saline solution can be made by boiling water and adding salt.

Collaboration and Delegation
• Respiratory therapists frequently suction clients in the acute care setting. Nurses need to maintain skill in suctioning so that suctioning can occur quickly to maintain a patent airway if a respiratory therapist is unavailable.

The choking victim who has aspirated foreign matter such as food into the airway is in grave danger. Quickly assess the situation and be ready to initiate steps to open the airway. On discovering the choking victim, quickly determine the relative extent of airway obstruction. If the choking victim is coughing loudly and gasping for breath, the airway is only partially obstructed. In this case, allow the victim to cough with no assistance. The cough will be more effective than any other intervention. Do not slap the victim's back; it may lodge the obstructing material even more deeply in the airway.

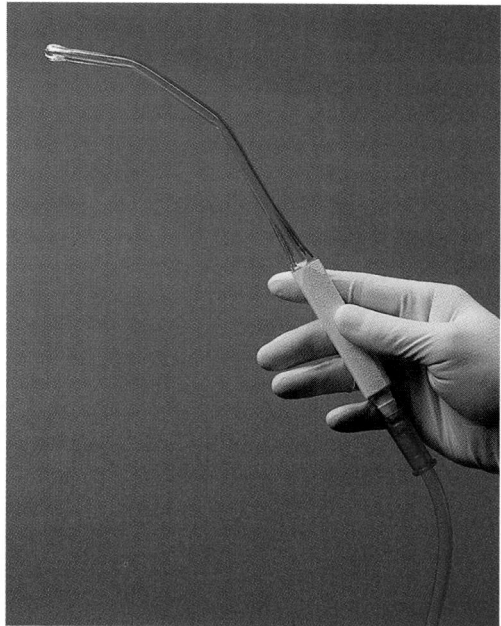

FIGURE 34-11 Tonsil-tip (Yankauer) suction catheter to clear oral cavity of excess secretions.

If you hear high-pitched inspiratory stridor, the airway is near-totally obstructed. At best, the victim can produce only a very weak cough. If the victim cannot cough at all and makes no sounds, the airway is totally obstructed. In either case, treatment is the same as follows.

 SAFETY ALERT
The nurse who discovers the choking victim should stay with the victim while calling for help. The person arriving first to help will be ready to alert the cardiopulmonary resuscitation team, if necessary, and to offer other support. The nurse must then take immediate action to clear the obstruction by using the Heimlich maneuver.

Heimlich Maneuver. The American Heart Association (AHA) recommends the Heimlich maneuver for the treatment of foreign body obstruction in adults and children (American Heart Association [AHA], 2001). In this procedure, abdominal thrusts are used to generate high pressures that can dislodge an aspirated obstruction. After establishing that the choking person cannot cough or speak, you must act quickly. Stand behind the person and wrap your arms around her or his waist. With one fist against the abdomen and the other grasping the opposite wrist, squeeze rapidly and tightly with an upward thrusting motion. Repeat this movement until you have successfully dislodged the obstruction or until the person loses consciousness. Procedure 34-9 outlines managing an obstructed airway.

If unconsciousness occurs, lay the victim in a supine position. Sweep the victim's mouth with the fingers in an attempt to pull out any obstruction. If no obstruction is evident, try to ventilate the victim with a manual resuscitator or with mouth-to-mouth breathing. Follow with abdominal thrusts and repeat the sequence until it is successful.

(text continues on page 858)

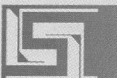

PROCEDURE 34-9

MANAGING AN OBSTRUCTED AIRWAY (HEIMLICH MANEUVER)

Purpose
1. Remove a foreign body from obstructing the airway to prevent anoxia and cardiopulmonary arrest.

Assessment/Preparation
- Identify disorders that put clients at greater risk for airway obstruction:
    Cerebral vascular accident with hemiparesis
    Neuromuscular disorders
    Seizure disorders
    Tumors of neck or esophagus
    Decreased level of consciousness
    Heavy narcotic or sedative use
    Alcohol intoxication
    Diminished or absent cough and gag reflex
- Assess client for signs and symptoms of airway obstruction.
    Symptoms not needing immediate intervention:
    Ability to speak
    Ability to breathe in and out
    Ability to cough
    Stable vital signs
    Note: Stay with the client and allow him or her to cough to clear airway.
    Symptoms needing immediate intervention:
    Universal distress signal for complete airway obstruction
    Irregular, slow, shallow breathing
    Apnea
    High-pitched sounds or no sounds while inhaling
    Inability to cough forcibly or at all
    Inability to speak
    Cyanosis
    Abnormal pulse (irregular, rapid, or slow)
- Determine which variation of the Heimlich maneuver (chest thrusts, finger sweep) to use.

Equipment
No equipment is mandatory; suction equipment and emergency cart are useful if in hospital setting.

Procedure
Conscious Child or Adult (Heimlich Maneuver)

1. The client will be standing or sitting.
2. Stand behind the client.
3. Wrap your arms around client's waist.
4. Make a fist with one hand. Place thumb side of fist against client's abdomen, above the navel but below the xiphoid process.

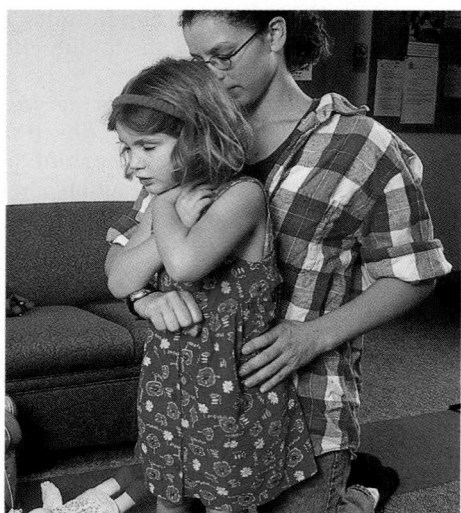

Step 4 Place thumb side of fist against client's abdomen below xiphoid process.

> *Rationale: Proper positioning is important to avoid injury and to successfully clear the airway.*

5. Grasp fist with other hand.
6. Press fist into abdomen with a quick upward thrust.
> *Rationale: A quick upward thrust increases intrathoracic pressure and creates an artificial cough, which forces air and foreign objects out of the airway.*

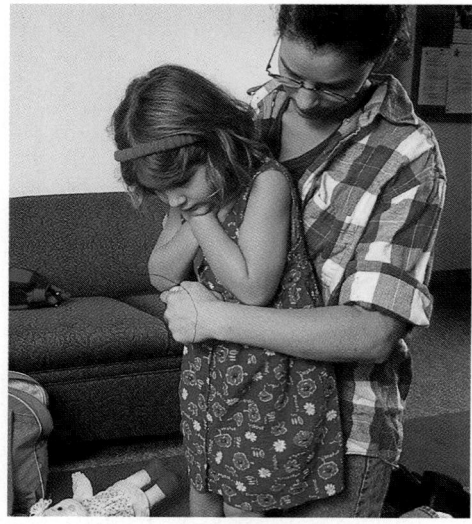

Step 6 Press fist into abdomen with quick upward thrust.

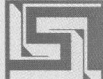

PROCEDURE 34-9 (Continued)

7. Repeat distinct separate thrusts until the client expels the foreign body or becomes unconscious.

Unconscious Client (Heimlich Maneuver, Abdominal Thrust)

1. Client will be lying on the ground.
2. Turn client on back and call for help. Activate emergency response system.
   Rationale: Prompt access to trained emergency professionals can be life-saving.
3. Finger sweep.
   a. Use tongue-jaw lift to open mouth.
      Rationale: Tongue-jaw lift draws tongue away from back of throat to relieve obstruction or visualize foreign body.
   b. Insert index finger inside cheek and sweep to base of tongue. Use a hooking motion if possible to dislodge and remove the foreign body. *Note:* Avoid finger sweeps in infants and children because you can easily push the foreign body further into the airway. Remove only if clearly visible and easy to reach.
   c. If there is no effective breathing, attempt to provide 2 rescue breaths. If unsuccessful, reposition and try to ventilate again.
      Rationale: Ventilation, if possible, would reduce hypoxia.
4. Straddle client's thighs or kneel to the side of thighs.
5. Place heel of one hand on epigastric area, midline above the navel but below the xiphoid process.
6. Place second hand on top of first hand.
   Rationale: Proper positioning is important to avoid injury and successfully clear the airway.
7. Press heel of hand into abdomen with a quick upward thrust. *Note:* Be careful to thrust in the midline to prevent injury to the liver or spleen.
   Rationale: A quick upward thrust increases intrathoracic pressure and creates an artificial cough to force air and foreign body out of airway.
8. Repeat abdominal thrusts 5 times.
9. If airway is still obstructed, attempt to ventilate using mouth-to-mouth respiration and head tilt/chin lift.
10. Repeat Steps 5 through 8 until successful.

Children Younger Than 1 Year of Age (Back Blows and Chest Thrusts)

1. Straddle infant over your arm with head lower than trunk.
2. Support head by holding jaw firmly in your hand.
3. Rest your forearm on your thigh and deliver five back blows with the heel of your hand between the infant's scapula.

4. Place free hand on infant's back and support neck while turning to supine position.
5. Place two fingers over sternum in same location as for external chest compression (one finger-width below nipple line).
6. Administer five chest thrusts.
7. Repeat Steps 1 through 6 until airway is not obstructed.

Children Older Than 1 Year of Age

1. Perform Heimlich maneuver with child standing, sitting, or lying as for adult, but more gently.
2. You may need to kneel behind child or have child stand on a table.
3. Prevent foreign body airway obstruction in infants and children by teaching parents or caregivers to:
   a. Restrict children from walking, running, or playing with food or foreign objects in their mouths.
   b. Keep small objects (e.g., marbles, beads, beans, thumb tacks) away from children younger than 3 years of age.
   c. Avoid feeding popcorn and peanuts to children younger than 3 years of age, and cut other foods into small pieces.
4. Instruct parents and caregivers in the management of foreign body airway obstruction.

Pregnant Women or Very Obese Adults (Chest Thrusts)

1. Stand behind client.
2. Bring your arms under client's armpits and around chest.
3. Make a fist and place thumb side against middle of sternum.
4. Grasp fist with other hand and deliver a quick backward thrust.
5. Repeat thrusts until airway is cleared.
6. Chest thrusts may be performed with client supine and hands positioned with heel over lower half of sternum (as for cardiac compression). Administer separate downward thrusts until airway is clear.

Collaboration and Delegation

- All healthcare personnel should be trained and proficient in the Heimlich maneuver, especially those who are working with high-risk groups (e.g., feeding CVA or neurologically impaired clients). Yearly updates and validation for proficiency should be mandatory.

Dyspnea Management

Causes of Dyspnea. Exertion causes most dyspnea. The range of activity required to precipitate dyspnea varies widely among individuals. Some clients with lung disease live relatively unrestricted lifestyles and experience dyspnea infrequently. For others, dyspnea is almost constant and can be brought on by the simplest ADLs.

Anxiety and emotional distress are also common causes of dyspnea. Regardless of its initial source, anxiety that causes dyspnea is, in turn, worsened by dyspnea; this creates a vicious cycle.

Finally, dyspnea not caused by exertion or anxiety may result from organic problems. Infection, pulmonary embolism, bronchospasm, or changes in the client's underlying condition may trigger difficulty breathing.

Assisting the Dyspneic Client. Effective treatment of dyspnea addresses both its physical and psychological components. Common interventions used to manage dyspnea include anxiety control, activity modification, and comfort measures that modify the client's breathing pattern.

Regardless of its specific cause, dyspnea can be extremely frightening, both for the client who is experiencing it and for the nurse who must treat it. To help the client, remain calm while offering reassurance. Speak calmly and slowly, offering one simple direction at a time to minimize the client's anxiety. Listening empathically and helping the client relax are sometimes all that he or she needs to relieve dyspnea. When uncontrolled anxiety is the primary cause of a client's dyspnea, the physician may prescribe mild antianxiety medication.

Comfort measures include the use of positioning. Usually the client is most comfortable sitting upright, which allows the diaphragm to move freely. If oxygen is ordered, see that it is operating as prescribed. Also focus the client's efforts on slowing the breathing rate. The client should breathe through the nose if possible, using the diaphragm for inspiration. Assist by gently pushing down on the client's shoulders; this discourages the inefficient use of accessory muscles. Usually, with gentle encouragement and reassurance, the client's breathing rate will gradually decrease and the dyspnea will pass. Whenever dyspnea occurs, try to establish its immediate cause and its severity. Comfort measures are always appropriate, as is oxygen when a standing order is available. Most institutions have policies allowing nurses to begin oxygen therapy for the dyspneic client while they are seeking a physician's order. When oxygen and comfort measures do not decrease dyspnea within a short period or when dyspnea appears suddenly and without warning, notify the physician.

Hyperventilation Management

The client who hyperventilates exhibits rapid breathing and symptoms such as dizziness and tingling sensations; arterial blood gases indicate a $PaCO_2$ below 35 mm Hg. The client may experience subjective feelings of dyspnea. Direct nursing efforts at decreasing client anxiety and getting the client to breathe at a slower rate.

If simple encouragement cannot accomplish this, the client may use a paper bag as a rebreathing device. The client breathes in and out of the bag for several breaths. In the process of rebreathing the exhaled carbon dioxide from the bag, the client's $PaCO_2$ can gradually slow the rate of breathing until it returns to normal. The dizziness and tingling sensations should disappear. As with dyspnea, a complete assessment of hyperventilation is needed and referral to the physician may be required.

Healthcare Planning and Home Care/Community-Based Nursing

Most respiratory clients are managed in the community except for those experiencing periods of acute respiratory dysfunction or who have exacerbation of a chronic respiratory condition. Home respiratory therapy can include peak flow monitoring, hand-held aerosol treatments, chest physiotherapy, oxygen, or ventilator care. How much and what kind of home therapy the client receives depends on many factors including the client's age, ability to learn procedures, family support, degree of impairment, and motivation. The nurse is often the one to assess these characteristics for the purpose of making recommendations to the physician. Often the nurse is also responsible for making home care arrangements and for much of the teaching involved.

Infection Control

Clients are likely to use pieces of equipment normally considered disposable after 2 or 3 days in the hospital, such as cannulas or small-volume nebulizers, for much longer periods in the home. Hospital procedures performed under sterile conditions, such as tracheostomy care and suctioning, may be done using clean technique at home. Although cost considerations and limited facilities make sterilization difficult, infection control at home can be practically as effective as it is in the hospital.

Ensure that the client clearly understands the importance of infection control, because potentially lethal pneumonia may result from respiratory infection. Stress the important of handwashing. Teach the client effective cleaning of all equipment.

The client must learn the signs of impending respiratory infection. Increased sputum production, change of sputum color to yellow or green, fever, and increasing difficulty in raising sputum often signal the onset of infection. If the client has a standing order for antibiotics, it is appropriate to begin taking the medication when these signs appear. If there is no relief within a day or two, the client should contact the physician. The client should complete the full prescription of antibiotics to avoid fostering the development of drug-resistant organisms. He or she should immediately report appreciable amounts of blood in the sputum, a severe increase in shortness of breath, or any other severe symptoms to the physician.

Medications

Home use of respiratory medications can be simplified by prepackaged unit-dose medications, but these are more expensive than stock bottles of medications. If the client can learn to measure dosages, stock bottles may be more cost-effective.

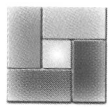

Nursing Research and Critical Thinking
Is The Numeric Rating Scale a Valid Measure of Dyspnea?

Standards for respiratory nursing recommend assessment of dyspnea in clients with chronic pulmonary disease, but implementation of this recommendation in clinical practice has been largely ignored. Some nurse researchers believed that one reason the intensity of dyspnea is not routinely monitored in clinical practice is the lack of a standardized measure for dyspnea. The nurses developed a study to establish the validity of the numeric rating scale (NRS) as a measure of present dyspnea (dyspnea at rest). The study was done in two phases. Phase 1 established the concurrent validity of the NRS as a measure of present dyspnea in clients visiting a pulmonary clinic by comparing scores between the NRS and the Visual Analog Dyspnea Scale (VADS), which has been validated as a measure of shortness of breath. In phase 2, the NRS was used to measure present dyspnea in clients in a home care setting before and after ambulation. Clients were asked to rate their shortness of breath by circling a number from 0 to 10, with 0 being no shortness of breath and 10 being shortness of breath as bad as can be. In phase 2 of the study, usual dyspnea was assessed by using the American Thoracic Society (ATS) Breathlessness Scale from the Pulmonary Functional Status Scale (PFSS) and standard pulmonary function tests. Phase 1 included 68 sub-

jects, and phase 2 included 120 subjects. All subjects had been hospitalized for chronic obstructive pulmonary disease and were participating in a home care study. Results of phase 1 found concurrent validity of the NRS as a measure of present dyspnea; the scores of the NRS and the VADS were not significantly different ($t = 0.74$, $P > .05$). Phase 2 comparison of NRS scores for dyspnea before and after ambulation showed a significant difference between resting scores and post-ambulation scores ($t = 20.5$, $P < .01$).

Critical Thinking Considerations. The researchers point out that the distinction between present dyspnea and usual dyspnea is important. Recalled perception of dyspnea tends to focus on the total dyspnea experience, not that occurring at the present moment. Implications relevant to nursing practice are as follows:

- The NRS scale is easy for clients to use and is recommended as a clinical measure of dyspnea in an outpatient or home care setting.
- Verbal administration of the scale would probably be most useful in a critical care setting, but verbal administration of the NRS as well as its use in critical care requires further study.

From Gift, A. G., & Narsavage, G. (1998). Validity of the numeric rating scale as a measure of dyspnea. *American Journal of Critical Care, 7*(3), 200–204.

Teach the client to recognize side effects of medications and to understand why they are dangerous. Stress the dangers of taking medications more frequently than ordered. If the medications provide no relief, the client should call the physician.

Home Oxygen Systems
The respiratory equipment that clients use at home also differs from hospital equipment. At home, the client can receive oxygen from high-pressure cylinders, liquid gas systems, or electrically powered concentrators. Compressed oxygen from high-pressure tanks is best for the client who only occasionally requires supplemental oxygen. Liquid oxygen systems allow the client to leave home. Portable "walkers" can be filled from a stationary unit at home. The walkers are small enough to be carried or wheeled in a small cart, yet they hold up to several hours' worth of oxygen (Fig. 34-12). A concentrator is a device that chemically separates oxygen from room air. It is an excellent choice for the client who requires continuous oxygen in low concentrations.

Home ventilators are also quite different from those found in intensive care units. Choices range from wrap-around pulmonary-aid belts, which assist clients whose breathing is weak, to negative-pressure chest shells and positive-pressure portable ventilators that provide full ventilatory support.

The companies that rent these items or supply the oxygen should be well-established and reliable. They should be able to provide service 24 hours every day. The client should have the telephone numbers of the suppliers and must be able to get service whenever necessary. Reputable suppliers often hire respiratory therapists to visit the client routinely at home and to assess respiratory status and equipment function. The nurse or discharge planner coordinates these services.

Energy Conservation
Respiratory dysfunction can seriously affect a client's ADLs, but with slight modifications most clients can perform them. Energy conservation and the motivation to be independent are keys to success.

Make suggestions for modifying ADLs based on thoroughly assessing the extent to which respiratory dysfunction has affected each activity. For example, consider the following:

- If meal preparation is a problem, a referral to a Meals on Wheels program may be appropriate.
- If mobility is impaired, sponge baths may be a practical alternative to tub bathing.
- An elevated toilet seat may help decrease the work needed to rise from the toilet.

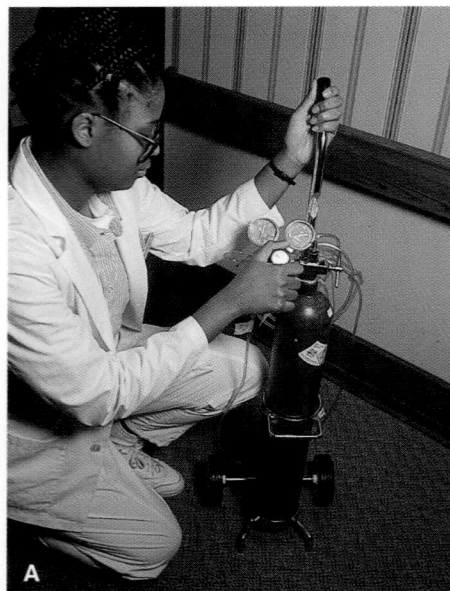 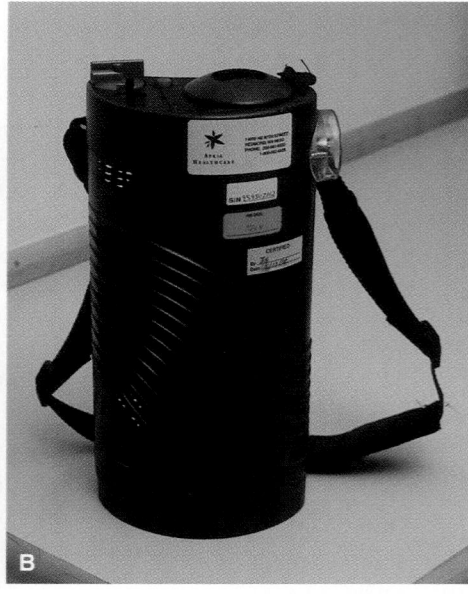

FIGURE 34-12 Portable oxygen. **(A)** E cylinder used as back-up emergency oxygen supply or for short period of ambulation. **(B)** Portable oxygen walker—fill with liquid oxygen for longer period of ambulation.

It is neither practical nor desirable for the client to avoid activity, but modifications may be necessary to prevent activity from causing dyspnea. The client may require assistance either in performing activities or in approaching them more efficiently. The nurse should assess the client's level of ADL functioning and assist him/her to develop positive means for living with dyspnea and fatigue (Small & Lamb, 1999). Help the client establish an activity schedule that allows for more time than the healthy person would require. Energy-saving measures such as sitting while performing basic tasks help to eliminate one source of breathlessness. Clients should space activities between rest periods to prevent overexertion. Activity should be limited to one hour after meals.

Clients must take care not to exceed their physical abilities. Encourage them to work gradually toward increasing exercise tolerance. Helping the client to set realistic goals is of utmost importance. Conversely, goals should provide enough challenge to allow the client to feel the endeavor is worthwhile. Recognize the value of small accomplishments. Offer praise and encouragement because progress at building endurance is often slow.

Fostering Self-Esteem

Like most people, the person with lung disease wants to be independent, contribute to society, feel self-reliant, and not burden others. The ability to get around independently and to do meaningful work can help foster these feelings. These activities are also essential to avoid the debilitating effects of depression.

The diagnosis of pulmonary disease does not mean the person is automatically unable to work. If the client derives satisfaction from a job, he or she should continue to work for as long as possible. Frequent illness can make it difficult for the severely dyspneic client to hold a demanding job. Although it is not always feasible for the client's employer to offer schedule flexibility, the client should explore this option.

Respiratory disease can severely inhibit both sexual desire and sexual performance. Chronic fatigue, shortness of breath, and embarrassment caused by excessive mucus or dyspnea are often reasons the client with respiratory problems loses sexual function. The client should use prescribed bronchodilators before beginning sexual relations, because they will help the client avoid dyspnea throughout sexual activity. Inform the client that passive positions save energy. Finally, stress the importance of open communication between the client and his or her partner, and help the client recognize that adjustments will be necessary.

Offer suggestions for activities outside the home. Social outlets can help the client to cope with the day-to-day frustrations of lung disease. The American Lung Association sponsors classes and support groups for people with respiratory disease. Nurses, physicians, or therapists often are guest speakers at such gatherings. Rehabilitation programs offer more structured activities. Their purpose is to increase the client's ability to function with lung disease. Such programs may provide breathing retraining, exercise, and diet and occupational counseling.

EVALUATION

Work with the client to develop goals and individualized outcome criteria depending on the client's current breathing status.

Goal

Client will demonstrate knowledge regarding prevention of respiratory dysfunction.

Possible Outcome Criteria

- After the teaching session, client demonstrates deep-breathing or coughing techniques.
- After the teaching session, client discusses the physiologic effects of smoking.

NURSING PLAN OF CARE

THE CLIENT WITH INEFFECTIVE AIRWAY CLEARANCE

Nursing Diagnosis
Ineffective Airway Clearance related to tracheobronchial infection as manifested by weak cough, adventitious breath sounds, and copious green sputum production.

Client Goal
Client will mobilize pulmonary secretions.

Client Outcome Criteria
- After teaching session, client demonstrates proper coughing techniques.
- Client drinks at least six glasses of water per day while in hospital.
- Client demonstrates correct self-suctioning technique before discharge.

Nursing Interventions

1. Provide and teach the client the importance of adequate hydration.
   Encourage fluids (2,000–3,000 mL per 24 hours).
   Monitor intake and output.
   Avoid milk and milk products.
   Ultrasonic nebulizer treatment.
2. Position and encourage client to cough to promote mobilization of secretions.
   Deep breathing every 2 hours.
   Huff coughing.
   Have client assume sitting position if possible.
3. Administer analgesic before cough session if pain limits coughing effectiveness.
4. Provide or teach client tracheal suctioning if he or she is unable to remove secretions with effective coughing.
   Hyperoxygenate with 100% O_2 before and after suctioning procedure.
   Suction for no longer than 10 seconds per suctioning attempt.
   Provide opportunities for client to practice and demonstrate suctioning technique if self-suctioning is necessary.
5. Provide or teach postural chest physiotherapy as ordered. Have client or family members demonstrate when comfortable with skill mastery.

Scientific Rationale

1. Adequate hydration thins secretions, which prevents mucus from plugging airways.
   Evaluate hydration status of client.
   Milk products tend to thicken secretions.
   Moisten and aid mobility of respiratory secretions.
2. Open alveoli and prevent further atelectasis.
   Prevent airway collapse.
   Permit deep inspiration and forceful abdominal contractions necessary for coughing.
3. If client fears pain, he or she hesitates to breathe deeply and cough effectively.
4. A weak, nonproductive cough causes secretions to be retained in airways and interfere with gas exchange.
   Hypoxemia, which can occur during the suctioning procedure, is prevented.
   Longer periods of suction can contribute to tissue trauma and hypoxemia.
   Suctioning is a complex motor skill that requires practice for skill acquisition and comfort.

5. Secretions drain from major airways using the force of gravity.

- Client joins and regularly attends meetings of a stop-smoking program for 6 months.

Goal

Client will demonstrate knowledge regarding optimal management of respiratory dysfunction.

Possible Outcome Criteria

- After the teaching session, client lists signs of respiratory infection and knows when to call the physician.
- After the teaching session about any medication administered for respiratory problems, client describes the name, action, and side effects of the drug;

dose to be taken, and any special considerations for administration.

- Before discharge, client demonstrates the safe use of home oxygen equipment.
- After teaching session, client demonstrates pursed-lip breathing.

Goal

Client will mobilize pulmonary secretions.

Possible Outcome Criteria

- After the teaching session, client demonstrates proper coughing technique.
- Client drinks at least six glasses of water a day, as indicated in daily log.
- Caregiver or parent demonstrates proper techniques of chest physiotherapy including percussion, vibration, and postural drainage, by the next home visit.
- Client demonstrates correct self-suctioning technique before discharge.

Goal

Client will effectively cope with changes in self-concept and lifestyle.

Possible Outcome Criteria

- Within 6 months of diagnosis, client verbalizes how the respiratory condition has caused changes in lifestyle.
- Within a week of diagnosis, client identifies support people to provide emotional strength.
- By end of teaching session, client lists community agencies and services that he or she plans to use.
- Before discharge, client demonstrates oxygen-conserving measures such as sitting while dressing and planning rest periods.
- Before discharge, client verbalizes sexual positions requiring less oxygen expenditure.

KEY CONCEPTS

- The primary functions of breathing are the delivery of oxygen to the blood, the removal of carbon dioxide from the blood, and the maintenance of acid–base balance.
- Although almost always effortless, the work required for breathing increases tremendously when the airways are obstructed by inflammation, bronchospasm, or excessive mucous secretions.
- Deep breathing and coughing are the two most important measures for preventing pulmonary complications such as atelectasis and pneumonia.
- Adequate hydration is essential to keep respiratory secretions moist and easily expectorated from the respiratory tract.
- Clients with COPD must not receive too much oxygen because it can cause hypoventilation. They normally require only 2 to 3 L/min through a nasal cannula or 28% through a Venturi mask.

- Smoking is the single most important factor affecting pulmonary health.
- Common manifestations of respiratory dysfunction are cough, dyspnea, chest pain, and sputum production.
- Health promotion for respiratory health includes smoking cessation, peak flow monitoring, allergen reduction, and appropriate vaccination.
- Major nursing interventions for the respiratory client are measures to promote airway patency, improve air distribution in the lungs, and promote oxygenation.
- Airway maintenance interventions include hydration, aerosol therapy, positioning, coughing, chest physiotherapy, suctioning, and management of artificial airways.
- Hyperinflation techniques, such as deep breathing, incentive spirometry, and intermittent positive pressure breathing or BiPAP, help prevent atelectasis and promote a strong cough.
- Oxygen therapy raises the amount of oxygen in the lungs, thereby making more oxygen available to the blood and tissues.
- Dyspnea, excessive mucous secretions, dried secretions, hyperventilation, and hypoventilation are common nursing problems of the respiratory client.
- Home care must be individualized for the respiratory client. Ability to perform activities of daily living and manage home procedures must be considered carefully before discharge.

REFERENCES

Agency for Health Care Policy and Research (AHCPR). (1996). *Smoking cessation: A guide for primary care clinicians.* (Clinical Practice Guideline, Number 18. AHCPR Publication No. 96-0693). Rockville, MD: Author.

American Heart Association. (2001). *BLS for healthcare providers.* Dallas, TX: Author.

Avery, G., Fletcher, M., & MacDonald M. (1999). *Neonatology: Pathophysiology and management of the newborn.* Philadelphia: Lippincott.

Brenner, Z. (1999, Oct.). Preventing post-operative complications. *Nursing, 29*(1), 34–40.

Centers for Disease Control and Prevention. (2001). *Influenza vaccine.* U.S. Department of Health and Human Services. [On-line]. Available at: www.cdc.gov/ncidod/diseases/flu/fluvac.htm.

Copstead, L. & Banasik, J. (2000). *Pathophysiology: Biological and behavioral perspectives* (2nd ed.). Philadelphia: WB Saunders Co.

Ehrhardt, B., & Daleiden, J. (1994). Pulse oximeters: Follow these tips to ensure accurate readings. *Nursing '94, 24*(8), 32V–32X.

Elkin, M., Perry, A., & Potter, P. (2000). *Nursing interventions and clinical skills.* St. Louis: Mosby.

Frownfelter, D., & Ryan, J. (2000). Dyspnea: Measurement and evaluation. *Cardiopulmonary Physical Therapy Journal, 11*(1), 7–15.

Glass, C., Grap, M., Corley, M., & Wallace, D. (1993). Nurses' ability to achieve hyperinflation and hyperoxygenation with a manual resuscitation bag during endotracheal suctioning. *Heart and Lung, 22,* 158–165.

Grap, M., Cantley, M., Munro, C., & Corley, M. (1999, January). Use of backrest elevation in critical care: A pilot study. *American Journal of Critical Care, 8*(1), 475–480.

Griffey, R., Brown, D., & Nadel, E. (2000, April). Cyanosis. *Journal of Emergency Medicine, 18*(3), 369–371.

Hanson, M. (1999, November). Which straw will break the camel's back. *American Journal of Nursing, 99*(11), 63–69.

Kidd, P., & Wagner, K. (2001). *High acuity nursing.* Upper Saddle River, NJ: Prentice Hall.

Lezon, T. (1999, January). Teaching Incentive Spirometry. *Nursing, 29*(1), 60–61.

Lindell, K. & Reinke, L. (1999, July-August). Nursing strategies for smoking cessation. *Heart and Lung, 28*(4), 295–302.

Lokeridge, T. (1999, July-August). Following the learning curve: The evolution of kinder, gentler neonatal respiratory technology. *Journal of Obstetric, Gynecologic, and Neonatal Nursing, 28*(4), 443–455.

Marion, B. (2001) A turn for the better: Prone positioning of patients with ARDS. *American Journal of Nursing, 101*(5), 26–34.

Miracle, V. & Winston, M. (2000). Take the wind out of asthma. *Nursing, 30*(8), 34–41.

North American Nursing Diagnosis Association. (2001). *NANDA nursing diagnoses: Definitions & classification 2001–2002.* Philadelphia: Author.

O'Hanlon-Nichols, T. (1998). Basic assessment series: the adult pulmonary system. *American Journal of Nursing, 98*(2), 39–45.

Reinke, L. & Hoffman, L. (2000, May–June). Asthma education: Creating a partnership. *Heart and Lung, 29*(3), 225–236.

Scanlan, C., Wilkins, R., & Stoller, J. (Eds.) (1999). *Egan's fundamentals of respiratory care* (7th ed.). St. Louis: Mosby.

Shapiro, B., Harrison, R., Kacmarek, R., & Cane, R. (1995). *Clinical application of blood gases* (5th ed.). St. Louis: Mosby-Year Book.

Sievers, A. & Adams, J. (2000, Spring). Instillation of normal saline during endotracheal suctioning: effects on mixed venous oxygen saturation. *ORL-Head and Neck Nursing, 18*(2), 22.

Small, S. & Lamb, M. (1999, August). Fatigue in chronic illness: The experience of individuals with chronic obstructive pulmonary disease and with asthma. *Journal of Advanced Nursing, 30*(2), 469–478.

Tamburri, L. (2000, March–April). Care of the patient with a tracheostomy. *Orthopaedic Nursing, 19*(2), 49–60.

Vander, A., Sherman, J., & Luciano, D. (2001). Human physiology: The mechanisms of body function (8th ed.). Boston: McGraw-Hill.

Williams, S. R. (1999). *Essentials of nutrition and diet therapy* (7th ed.). St. Louis: Mosby.

BIBLIOGRAPHY

Bulechek, G. M. & McCloskey, J. C. (1999). *Nursing interventions: Effective nursing treatments* (3rd ed.). Philadelphia: W.B. Saunders Co.

Carroll, P. (2001). How to intervene before asthma turns deadly. *RN, 64*(5), 53–58.

Connolly, M. (2001). Chest x-rays: Completing the picture. *RN, 64*(6), 56–62.

Drummond Hayes, D. (2001). Stemming the tide of pleural effusion. *Nursing 2001, 30*(5), 49–52.

Lazzara, D. (2001). Respiratory distress: Loosening the grip. *Nursing 2001, 31*(6), 58–63.

Ruppert, R. (1999). The last smoke. *American Journal of Nursing, 99*(11), pp. 26–32.

Sheppard, M. & Davis, K. (2000). Practical procedures for nurses using oxygen therapy. *Nursing Times, 96*(26), 43–44.

Siquirea, L., Diab, M., Bodian, C., & Rolnitzky, L. (2000). Adolescents and becoming smokers: The roles of stress and coping mechanisms. *Journal of Adolescent Health, 27*(6), 399–408.

Woo, K. (2000, December). Physical activity as a mediator between dyspnea and fatigue. *Canadian Journal of Nursing Research, 32*(3), 85–98.

35 Oxygenation
Cardiovascular Function

Key Terms

angina
automaticity
contractility
diastole
dysrhythmia
myocardial infarction
intermittent claudication
ischemia

myocardium
perfusion
shock
stroke
systole
thrombus
transient ischemic attack

Learning Objectives

Upon completion of this chapter, the student will be able to do the following:

1. Discuss factors that contribute to normal cardiac output and tissue perfusion.
2. Discuss cardiovascular changes that occur across the lifespan.
3. Describe the causes of altered cardiovascular function.
4. Describe how altered cardiovascular function can affect normal activities.
5. Perform a basic nursing assessment of cardiovascular function.
6. Identify common procedures and diagnostic tests used in the evaluation of the cardiovascular client.
7. State relevant nursing diagnoses for the client with cardiovascular dysfunction.
8. Discuss nursing measures directed at promoting and restoring cardiovascular function.

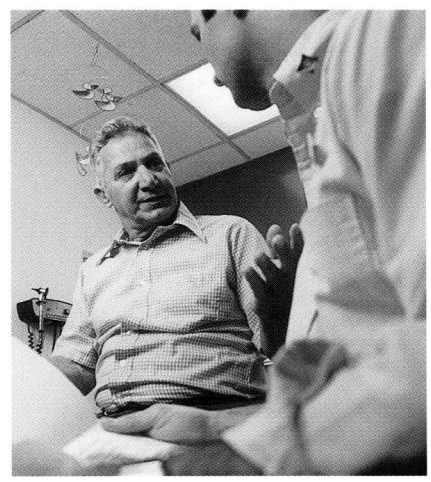

Critical Thinking Challenge

A 59-year-old client comes in for his yearly physical. His family history is positive for cardiac disease, and his father died at 60 years of age from a massive myocardial infarction (MI). The client has been under stress lately at work (a very important trial) and at home (his 24-year-old daughter has returned home with two young children after a recent divorce). He used to play golf twice a week but recently has not had time to exercise. Physical examination reveals BP of 178/94 (last BP a year ago 184/96), pulse 94, and respirations 14. When you tell your client his vital signs, he states, "Now don't you start yelling at me about my blood pressure. I'm as healthy as they come, and I am not about to go on any crazy vegetarian diet." He travels frequently and eats often at fast food restaurants. He has gained 25 lb in the last 6 months, and his BMI is now between 28 and 29. He is a nonsmoker and drinks 1 to 2 beers a week.

Once you have completed this chapter, review the above scenario and reflect on the following areas of Critical Thinking:

1. Evaluate the risk factors that negatively affect this client's cardiovascular health. How can the client change these risk factors?
2. Describe some health promotion measures that can be implemented to improve this client's health.
3. Discuss the impact of his lifestyle on his cardiovascular health.
4. Plan two possible approaches to encourage the client's compliance with necessary lifestyle changes.
5. Reflect on how you as a nurse would feel if a client were reluctant to make positive lifestyle changes.

The primary function of the cardiovascular system is to transport oxygen and nutrients to the body tissues and to deliver the waste products to appropriate organs for their excretion. The heart acts as a pump to deliver blood through the blood vessels. The proper function of every organ and tissue depends on the efficiency and effectiveness of the cardiovascular system. This chapter focuses on the importance of the cardiovascular system in the maintenance of health.

NORMAL CARDIOVASCULAR FUNCTION

Structure of the Cardiovascular System

The heart and blood vessels are part of the cardiovascular system. The system is a closed circuit with two major divisions: the pulmonary circulation and the systemic circulation. It is really a double pump, with the right side going to the lungs, and the left side going to the body. The pulmonary circulation carries blood through the lungs, where carbon dioxide is released and oxygen is absorbed. The systemic circulation then transports oxygenated blood and nutrients to all body tissues (Fig. 35-1).

Heart

The heart is a hollow, muscular pump that is a little larger than a fist. It is an amazing organ, pumping about 5 quarts of blood a minute (American Heart Association [AHA], 2001a). In general, women have a smaller body size than do men and therefore have smaller hearts (Wingate, 1997). The heart's job is to circulate blood throughout the body. The heart is responsible for providing all tissues with a constant blood supply.

Heart Layers. The heart consists of three layers. The innermost layer of the heart, the endocardium, is made of tissue that lines the heart. The thick muscular middle layer is called the **myocardium.** It produces the muscular contraction of the heart. The outer layer of the heart, or epicardium, is a thin-walled sac that surrounds the heart and attaches it to the diaphragm and sternal wall of the thorax (Fig. 35-1).

Heart Structure. The heart has two main walls that divide the heart into four chambers. A strong muscular wall, or septum, divides the heart into left and right halves. These halves are further divided crosswise into upper chambers (atria) and lower chambers (ventricles).

The muscle on the left side of the heart is much thicker than the muscle on the right because the left side of the heart must generate higher pressures to pump blood to all body tissues. The right side of the heart serves the lower-resistance pulmonary system.

Conduction System. The heart is unique because of its property of automaticity. **Automaticity** means that the heart is capable of generating its own electrical impulse, which is then conducted through specialized conduction fibers. Impulses that

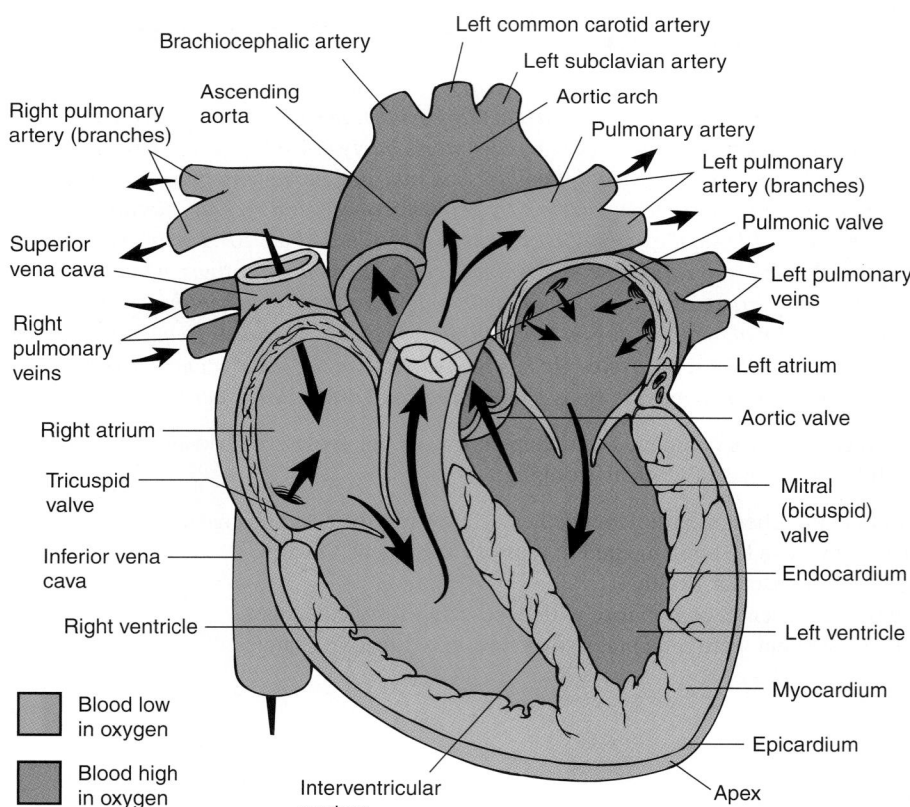

FIGURE 35-1   Heart chamber, valves, and circulation.

Brachiocephalic artery
Left common carotid artery
Left subclavian artery
Ascending aorta
Aortic arch
Pulmonary artery
Right pulmonary artery (branches)
Left pulmonary artery (branches)
Pulmonic valve
Superior vena cava
Left pulmonary veins
Right pulmonary veins
Left atrium
Right atrium
Aortic valve
Tricuspid valve
Mitral (bicuspid) valve
Inferior vena cava
Endocardium
Right ventricle
Left ventricle
Myocardium
Epicardium
Blood low in oxygen
Blood high in oxygen
Interventricular septum
Apex

stimulate contraction normally originate in specialized cells (sinoatrial [SA] node) near the top of the right atrium. Through the atria, the impulse is channeled into the atrioventricular (AV) junction, and then to the bundle of His, and into its right and left branches. It finally enters the many Purkinje fibers that extend throughout the ventricular muscle (Fig. 35-2).

Valves. The heart has four valves. They allow blood to flow in one direction, maximizing efficiency and preventing the backflow of blood. Two valves separate the atria from the ventricles. The tricuspid valve separates the right atrium from the right ventricle; the mitral valve separates the left atrium from the left ventricle (Fig. 35-1).

The other two valves separate the ventricles from the large blood vessels they fill. The pulmonic valve separates the right ventricle from the pulmonary system, and the aortic valve separates the left ventricle from the aorta. These valves are called semilunar valves, because of the half-moon shape of their leaflets.

Coronary Circulation. The coronary circulation provides the heart muscle with oxygenated blood. The right and left coronary arteries with their multiple branches deliver fresh blood to all layers of the heart. One artery serves the right side of the heart; the other serves the left. Because the left side of the heart is more muscular, it has a greater blood supply.

Function of the Cardiovascular System

The heart's effectiveness as a pump depends on several factors. Among the most important factors are its ability to generate and conduct electrical impulses, its ability to fill and empty properly, and the strength with which it can contract.

Heart

The normal heartbeat is a rhythmic cycle of contraction and relaxation. The cardiac cycle begins with the generation of a small electrical impulse in the SA node. This impulse spreads throughout the heart, which then causes the muscle contraction

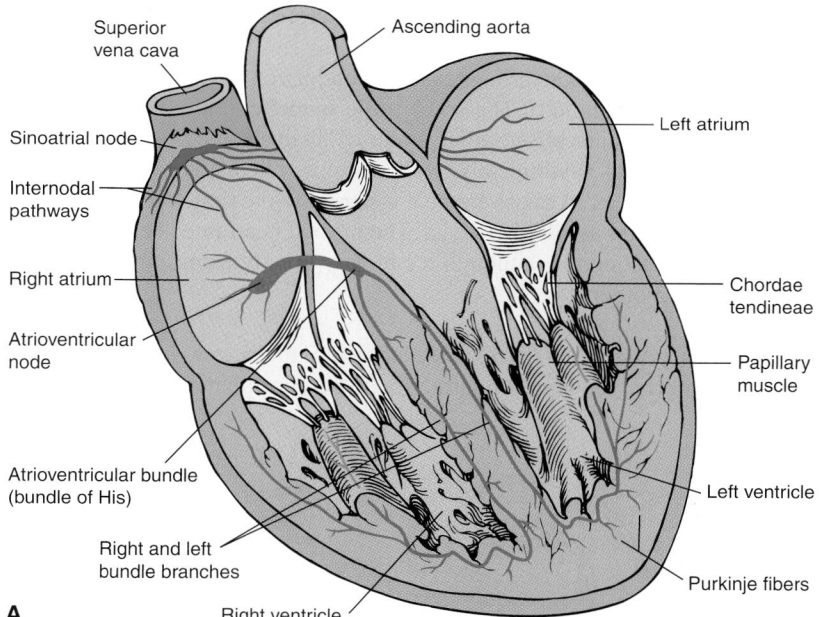

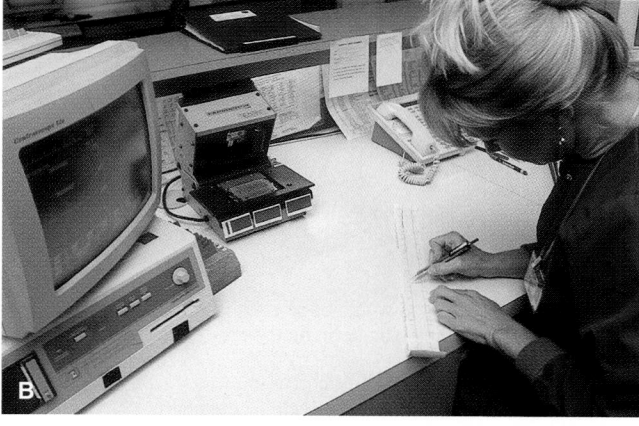

FIGURE 35-2 **(A)** The electrical conduction system of the heart. **(B)** Nurse evaluating electrocardiographic tracing in the coronary care unit to promptly detect dysrhythmias.

and pumping motion. With each contraction, during the period called **systole,** the ventricles eject blood. The period between contractions, called **diastole,** is twice as long as systole. This extra time allows the heart muscle to relax, and its chambers to fill with blood. The blood is thrust through the arteries into the capillaries, where the exchange of O_2 and CO_2 occurs before the blood travels back to the heart in the veins (Fig. 35-3).

Impulse Conduction. In the SA node, small but significant changes in the concentrations of potassium, sodium, and calcium generate a small electrical impulse. This impulse (depolarization) travels through special conduction tissue and normally causes the muscles to contract. After the impulse has passed over the cells, their ionic concentrations return to previous levels (repolarization), and the muscle relaxes. Because the SA node establishes impulses that determine the rate at which the heart beats, it is often called the pacemaker of the heart.

When the impulse reaches the lower portion of the atria, it is delayed briefly at the AV junction before it continues into the ventricles. This delay is important because it allows time for the atria to contract fully. In this way, the atria can add 20% more blood volume to the ventricles before the ventricles contract.

As the impulse spreads through special conduction tissue in the ventricles (bundle of His and bundle branches), the ventricular myocardial cells normally contract. In the healthy adult, the heart beats rhythmically, with an equal time interval between each beat. Also, every beat is normally the same strength or intensity as all other beats. The normal heart rate is 60 to 100 beats/minute, although it can vary greatly from one person to another.

Blood Flow through the Heart. The electrical impulse generates an orderly, sequential contraction. The coordinated contraction of all muscle fibers is essential for maximum cardiac pumping power.

Between heartbeats, the heart is at rest. During this time, the atria fill passively, receiving blood from the venae cavae (on the right side of the heart) and the pulmonary veins (on the left). When the atrial muscle cells contract, pressure builds within the atrial chambers. The pressure forces the AV valves to open, and the blood is pushed into the ventricle below each atrium.

After a brief pause at the AV junction, the ventricular muscle cells begin to contract. The rising pressure within the ventricles forces the AV valves to close and the valves to the pulmonary artery and the aorta to open. The blood from the right ventricle is ejected into the pulmonary artery for gas exchange, and the blood from the left ventricle enters the aorta for transport to body tissues.

Proper valve function is another essential element for effective pumping. The unidirectional action of the valves allows the heart chambers to pump forcefully. This is necessary to ensure that blood is ejected with sufficient pressure to reach the furthest tissues of the body.

Cardiac Output. Cardiac output (CO) refers to the amount of blood pumped by the heart each minute. In the normal resting adult, CO is approximately 5 to 6 L/minute (AHA, 2001a). The healthy person is able to increase CO to several times this amount in response to changing metabolic demands, such as with exercise.

CO is a function of two factors, heart rate (HR) and stroke volume (SV): $CO = HR \times SV$. Heart rate is simply the number of times the heart beats each minute. Stroke volume refers to the amount of blood the heart ejects with each beat. An increase or decrease in either of these factors may change CO.

Heart rate is primarily determined by the heart's pacemaker, the SA node. This tissue receives information constantly from

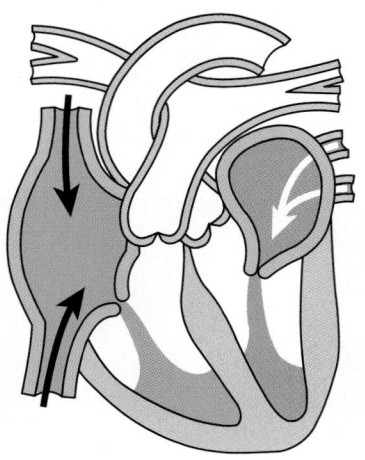

Diastole
Atria fill with blood which begins to flow into ventricles as soon as their walls relax.

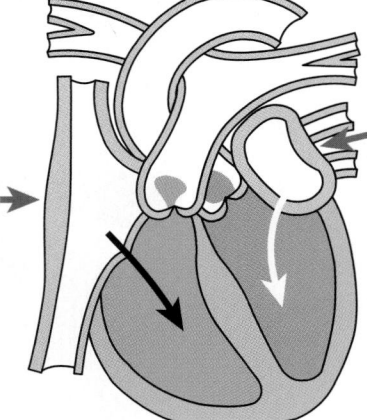

Atrial Systole
Contraction of atria pumps blood into the ventricles.

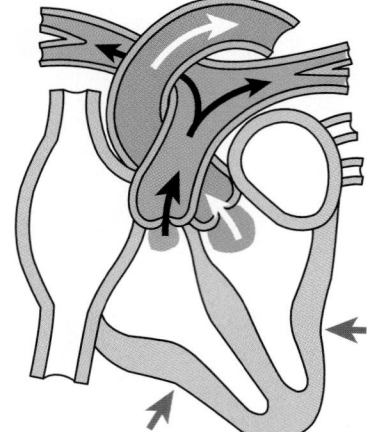

Ventricular Systole
Contraction of ventricles pumps blood into aorta and pulmonary arteries.

FIGURE 35-3   Pumping cycle of the heart.

the autonomic nervous system. The parasympathetic branch slows heart rate; the sympathetic branch increases it. Increased metabolic activity (e.g., vigorous exercise) produces cardiac-stimulating metabolites; it also stimulates the sympathetic nervous system. Therefore, CO increases under these conditions to meet the extra demands of the tissues.

Stroke volume depends on three factors. First, the amount of blood that enters the heart determines how much the heart can pump out. Healthy heart muscle is usually able to stretch to accommodate the volume of blood returning to it. Second, stroke volume depends on the natural strength of the heart muscle, or its **contractility.** Like any muscle, the healthy, well-exercised heart is stronger and more efficient than the weak and flabby heart, so it is able to eject a larger volume of blood with each beat. Finally, stroke volume depends on the resistance to blood flow in the circulatory system. The main resistance is in the diameter of the arterial system, which is measured by blood pressure (BP). If the BP (resistance) is high, the stroke volume will decrease (Copsead & Banasik, 2000).

Blood Vessels

The heart empties its contents into an interconnected network of arteries, arterioles, capillaries, venules, and veins. Collectively, the members of this network are called the blood vessels. These vessels range from more than 1 inch in diameter to microscopic size. In general, because of women's smaller body size, their blood vessels are also smaller than men's (Wingate, 1997). Arteries and arterioles carry blood away from the heart to the tissues; venules and veins carry blood from the tissues back to the heart. The capillaries, which are the smallest vessels, link them together (Fig. 35-4). Arteries, capillaries, and

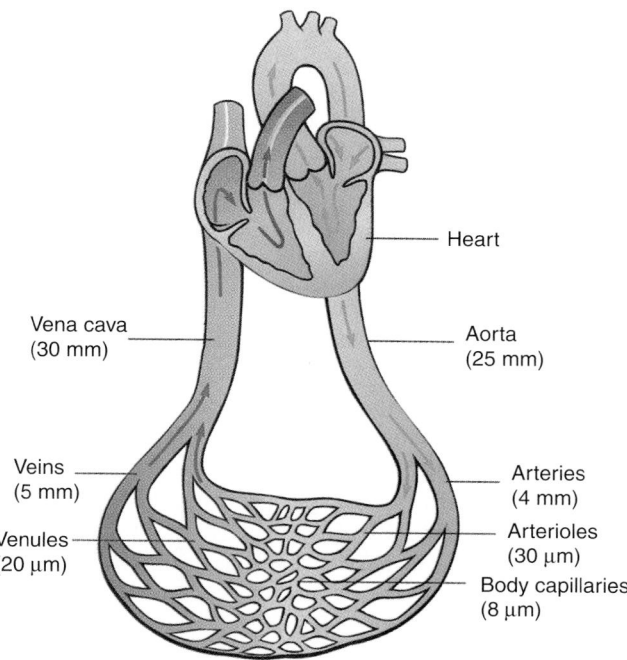

FIGURE 35-4   Systemic circulation with blood traveling from the heart through the aorta, arteries, arterioles, capillaries, venules, and veins. Blood returns to the heart in the vena cava.

veins are dynamic structures that are essential for adequate distribution and perfusion of blood to body tissues.

Distribution of Blood Flow. As the heart ejects blood, the thick, muscular walls of the arteries stretch slightly, then rebound. This is important to ensure that the blood has enough force to reach the tissues. The pressure generated in the arterial system is called blood pressure (BP). Like heart rate, BP varies with age. Normal BP ranges from 100 (systolic)/60 (diastolic) mm Hg (in the healthy young adult) to 135/85 mm Hg in the healthy elderly adult. The average man has a higher BP than the average woman. In women, BP may increase slightly after menopause, probably as a result of hormonal changes. In the healthy person, the supine position usually causes a drop in systolic BP with a slight rise in diastolic BP.

Arteries. Arteries are relatively thick-walled, muscular vessels. This characteristic provides them with strength and elasticity, which allows them to withstand the high pressure of blood that the heart constantly forces into them. The smallest arteries, called arterioles, connect to the capillaries and regulate blood flow into them. The arterioles contain smooth muscle cells, so they can expand (vasodilate) and contract (vasoconstrict). The arterioles are the primary regulators of blood flow, and they play a key role in the moment-to-moment regulation of BP. These tiny vessels are able to increase or decrease their diameter to meet local tissue needs. For example, a jogger's active leg muscles require more oxygen and nutrients than do the digestive tract organs. Metabolites from the working leg muscles, rapid depletion of the local muscle oxygen supply, and the autonomic nervous system cause the arterioles serving the leg muscles to dilate. By opening wider, the vessels allow more blood to flow into the legs to meet the tissue needs. At the same time, arterioles within the digestive tract may actually constrict, limiting the amount of blood entering it. Thus, the body is able to direct blood flow to where it is needed most.

Capillaries. These near-microscopic vessels run through all the body's tissues. Their thin endothelial walls are permeable, which allows for the exchange of nutrients and waste products between the blood and tissues. By the time blood enters the capillaries, its pressure and velocity have decreased greatly. The slower flow rate of blood through the single-layered epithelium of capillaries is necessary to allow sufficient time for tissues to extract oxygen and nutrients. The slow flow also allows the tissues adequate time to deposit their wastes into the blood for removal.

Veins. After blood passes through capillaries, it drains into the venules and veins. Veins are less muscular than arteries and therefore expand more easily. At their junction with capillaries, venules are small. They empty into successively larger veins, finally ending in the superior and inferior venae cavae. Together, these vessels return deoxygenated blood from the systemic circulation to the heart's right atrium.

Blood flows slowly in the venules and veins; the initial force of the heartbeat is greatly diminished by this time. In addition, venous blood must overcome gravity in the upright person. Because of their distensibility, veins can stretch to accommodate relatively large blood volumes. Backward flow of the venous blood would be a problem were it not for one-way valves in the veins. Skeletal muscles, particularly those of the legs, squeeze the veins, pushing blood forward and opening the valves. As the muscles relax, the valves of the veins snap shut, preventing backflow (Copsead & Banasik, 2000).

Tissue Perfusion.   To maintain life, all living body cells must receive a constant supply of oxygen and nutrients. The flow of blood through the body tissues is called tissue **perfusion.**

Individual cells and tissues receive oxygen, glucose, and various ions through the walls of capillaries. At the arterial end of the capillary, the forward force of the blood helps to push fluid and soluble particles out of the vessel. This fluid surrounds the cells, and nutrients are exchanged for wastes. Oxygen and other molecules enter the cells primarily by diffusion, moving from an area of higher concentration (the fluid) to an area of lower concentration (the cell). Metabolites such as carbon dioxide diffuse from the cell into the fluid, also in response to a concentration difference.

At the venous end of the capillary, tissue hydrostatic pressure forces some fluid back into the vessel. Large protein molecules in the plasma pull the remaining fluid into the capillary. This spongelike action of the plasma proteins is called oncotic pressure. Skin temperature is one indicator of cardiovascular tissue perfusion. The person with normal circulatory status is warm, but cooler further from the heart, especially in the feet.

The vital organs require continuous perfusion for their optimal function. The kidneys must receive a steady flow of blood to effectively filter and cleanse it. An adequate BP (mean, at least 60 mm Hg) is needed to keep the renal arteries patent and to ensure continuous blood flow and urine production.

The brain relies on a sophisticated network of neural receptors to guarantee a near-constant level of perfusion. These receptors, located in the major arteries leading to the brain, are sensitive to variations in BP. When pressure increases, the receptors cause arterial constriction. This reflex action protects the brain's delicate capillaries from possible injury caused by a sudden rise in pressure. If BP drops, the arteries dilate, thus ensuring a consistent flow of blood through the brain despite a possible momentary decrease elsewhere (AHA, 2001a).

The coronary arteries that nourish the heart tissue are perfused primarily during the resting portion of the cardiac cycle (diastole). At increased heart rates, sufficient time may be unavailable for the coronary arteries to fill completely. Adequate coronary perfusion also depends on adequate CO.

Blood

The blood carries essential nutrients to the cells, but it can do so effectively only if its composition is normal and its volume is sufficient to fill the cardiovascular system. In women, fluctuating levels of estrogen and other hormones affect the blood composition (Wingate, 1997). The red blood cells are responsible for delivering oxygen, which is carried on the hemoglo-

bin portion of the cell. Plasma, which is the liquid portion of the blood, carries electrolytes, trace minerals, and nutrients (e.g., glucose) to the cells. To function optimally, the cardiovascular system must contain a relatively constant fluid volume. The thickness (or viscosity) of the blood is generally consistent.

Lifespan Considerations

Newborn and Infant

The newborn's heart rate is normally 130 to 160 beats/minute. Its rhythm is commonly irregular. A heart rate of less than 100 beats/minute in a newborn is cause for alarm. As babies mature, the heart rate becomes more rhythmic and slower, but it can easily increase during activity or when the baby cries. BP is lowest during the newborn period, with a systolic pressure in the mid-40s. By 1 month of age, average systolic pressure is 80 to 90 mm Hg, with diastolic pressure ranging from the mid-40s to 60 mm Hg. Between 1 and 7 years of age, the systolic pressure can be calculated by taking the age in years and adding 90; the diastolic pressure is around 60 mm Hg. The infant's heart rate varies widely whether awake or resting, between 80 and 150 beats/minute (Weber & Kelley, 1998).

Toddler and Preschooler

The heart rate slows somewhat as the infant becomes a toddler. Steady activity, however, is likely to keep it high throughout the daytime hours. By the end of this period, the heart rate has decreased to a resting rate of about 70 to 110 beats/minute. BP varies slightly within this age group but usually is equal to double the age in years plus 90 (Weber & Kelley, 1998).

Child and Adolescent

As the heart increases in size, its rate continues to decline (Fig. 35-5). BP changes are gradual and slight during this period. At any age during this time, boys generally have slightly higher BP and lower heart rate than girls. By the age of 19 years, heart rate and BP have stabilized at the adult values of 60 to 80 beats/minute and 120/80 mm Hg, respectively (Weber & Kelley, 1998).

Adult and Older Adult

As people mature throughout adulthood, changes in the cardiovascular system may lead to decreased activity tolerance and decreased endurance. Along with natural aging, diet, stress, smoking, and several other lifestyle factors may contribute to the processes of calcification, fatty degeneration, and diminished elasticity of the blood vessels. These processes are likely to account for increases in BP as adults grow older. Because of the added work higher BP places on the heart, the heart rate is often slightly higher in the older adult than in the younger adult.

FACTORS AFFECTING CARDIOVASCULAR FUNCTION

A host of factors can influence cardiovascular function. Lifestyle choices, such as nutritional status, exercise, and smoking,

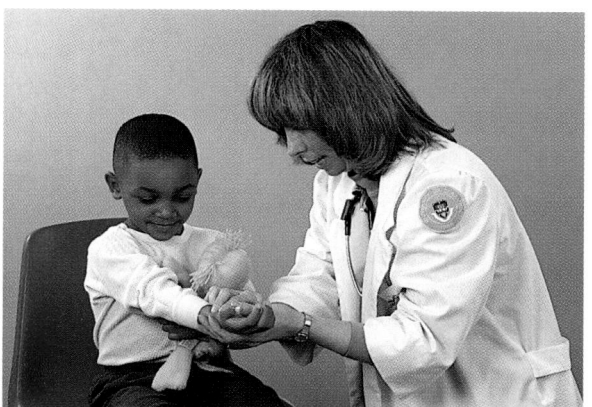

FIGURE 35-5 Measuring the radial pulse in a preschool-age boy.

⌂ CORONARY HEART DISEASE RISK FACTORS

Controllable Risk Factors
- High blood pressure
- Cigarette/tobacco use
- High blood cholesterol
- Physical inactivity

Uncontrollable Risk Factors
- Family history of heart disease
- Being male (women after menopause)
- Age (risk increases with age)
- Diabetes mellitus

Contributing Factors
- Diabetes
- Obesity
- Individual response to stress

can greatly affect the abilities of the heart and blood vessels. Air pollution has been implicated by possibly inflaming the airways, activating the immune system, and leading to hypercoagulability (Utell & Frampton, 2000; Levy et. al, 2001). Research has shown that reducing multiple risk factors provides the most substantial benefit. Reduced risk is associated with a decrease in cardiovascular-related hospital admissions and procedures and an improved quality of life (Zafari & Wenger, 1998).

Many risk factors contribute to the development of cardiovascular problems. Adequate knowledge of these risk factors (Display 35-1) and their impact on cardiovascular health can encourage lifestyle changes that help to promote cardiovascular function. Being male, older, or African American and having a positive family history are uncontrollable risk factors. Age is the single most important risk factor (AHA, 2001a).

Cigarette Smoking

Smoking has been called the most important modifiable risk factor for cardiovascular disease. Smoking has caused more deaths from cardiovascular disease than from lung cancer or chronic obstructive pulmonary disease. It increases the heart rate and BP, constricts arterioles, and may cause irregular cardiac rhythm. It enhances the process of atherosclerosis and is the major cause of peripheral vascular disease. Smoking also limits the blood's oxygen-carrying capacity by displacing oxygen with carbon monoxide (Emerson, 2000).

Smokers who stop reduce their risk of cardiovascular disease. Smoking risk increases in relation to the number of cigarettes smoked. Within 3 to 4 years, smoking cessation is associated with a significant reduction in cardiovascular risk (Gensini, Comeglio, & Colella, 1998).

High Blood Pressure

High BP is undoubtedly the most common manifestation of altered blood flow, affecting 25% of the adult population. It is the most common risk factor for cardiovascular disease in de-

veloped and developing countries (AHA, 2001a). Researchers have postulated that primary high BP results from an increased level of circulating vasoactive substances or increased sympathetic nervous system activity. Changes in sodium excretion in the kidneys or in arterial smooth muscle contractility caused by changes in calcium absorption also cause high BP.

High BP can affect anyone, but it occurs most often in men, those with a positive family history, and the elderly. Urban dwellers, particularly African Americans, are most susceptible. People who are overweight, use too much salt or alcohol, or are inactive are at risk for high BP. Women who take birth control pills or are pregnant are also at risk. High BP is unique in that it is a manifestation of cardiovascular dysfunction and, in turn, a cause of further dysfunction, resulting in severe tissue and organ damage.

Nutrition

The relationship between dietary factors and cardiovascular problems is complex, but a diet high in total fat and saturated fat is strongly associated with the risk of heart disease (Lichtenstein et al., 1998). Cholesterol is the primary component of the plaque (fatty lesion) that gradually occludes arteries. There are two primary types of cholesterol, high-density lipoprotein (HDL) or "good" cholesterol and low-density lipoprotein (LDL) or "bad" cholesterol. High levels of LDL cholesterol lead to peripheral vascular disease and hypertension, which greatly increases the chance of myocardial infarction (MI).

The role of salt in foods has received close scrutiny. A diet that is high in salt can increase blood volume and CO and therefore aggravate chronic hypertension or congestive heart failure (CHF). Convenience foods and preserved foods often contain a large amount of sodium. Increased sodium intake in sodium-sensitive people can increase the incidence of hypertension (Henshaw, 2000).

Lack of Exercise

Just as regular exercise strengthens leg and arm muscles, it can improve the heart's pumping efficiency. Increased blood circulation also helps prevent the formation of thrombi and atherosclerotic plaques by decreasing platelet stickiness, serum cholesterol, and triglyceride levels. Exercise protects the cardiovascular system and promotes weight reduction by raising the "good" (HDL) cholesterol and reducing triglycerides, BP, and resting heart rate. A well-conditioned person has a lower risk of heart or circulatory problems than a person who does not exercise regularly. The resting heart rate in the person who exercises regularly is usually lower than in the person who does not. All-cause mortality is lower among more fit women (Limacher, 1998). Occupations that require the worker to stand or sit for long periods promote venous pooling and predispose the person to varicose veins and possible hypercoagulation problems.

Diabetes

Diabetes is an independent risk factor for MI and stroke. People with diabetes often have other risk factors, such as high cholesterol and obesity, that further increase the risk. The risk of disease is three times greater in diabetic women and twice as great in diabetic men (AHA, 2001a).

Obesity

Being overweight places excessive demands on the cardiovascular system. The extra adipose tissue must be supplied with blood to meet its metabolic requirements. The extra cells are served by miles of blood vessels. To perform the additional work of pumping blood to these tissues, the heart may become enlarged. BP increases, but perfusion may decrease. Obesity also has been shown to correlate positively with cardiovascular disease (Al Suwaidi et al., 2001). Restricting caloric intake in obese people has been shown to reduce LDL cholesterol and triglyceride levels, as well as central abdominal fat (Markovic et al., 1998).

Medical and Family History

Although it is clear that many cardiovascular problems have no hereditary basis, genetics may play a role in certain disorders. For example, some clients may report that an unusually high number of close relatives have suffered strokes or heart attacks. Hypertension also is more prevalent in some families than in others. Therefore, a positive family history for cardiovascular disease must be considered carefully. Syndrome X is a genetic metabolic disorder involving diabetes, hypertension, atherosclerosis, centrally distributed obesity, and elevated blood lipids (Minchoff & Grandin, 1996). These factors together greatly increase the risk of disease.

Medications and Drug Use

Medications, either prescription or over-the-counter, may affect CO and BP. Asthma preparations and some cold remedies can substantially increase heart rate and BP. Diuretics (prescribed or "natural diuretics" from health stores) can decrease blood volume and alter electrolyte balance, causing potentially dangerous changes in heart rhythm. Birth control pills significantly enhance the process of blood clot formation and increase the risk of embolism. Use of hormone replacement therapy in postmenopausal women reduces LDL cholesterol and raises HDL cholesterol.

Some herbal remedies, such as garlic, are used by some to lower cholesterol and BP, but other herbs can have serious cardiovascular side effects. Ephedra can interact with BP medications or antidepressants to dangerously elevate BP and heart rate.

Drinkers of caffeinated coffee and cola usually have higher heart rates and BPs than those who drink decaffeinated beverages. Excessive alcohol intake has been associated with hypertension and increased cardiovascular risk, so prudent alcohol consumption of less than 1 oz/day is recommended. Some "natural" weight loss remedies contain ephedrine, which can cause arrhythmias.

The use of illicit drugs can have serious cardiovascular complications. Intravenous (IV) use of any drug provides a portal of entry for bacteria into the bloodstream and puts the user at high risk for infection. Impurities in the injected drug can cause cardiac inflammation and may form the nucleus of an embolism. Repeated IV injections in the same vessel can result in its eventual destruction. Cocaine use has been increasingly associated with sudden cardiac arrest, because it increases oxygen demand and reduces supply to the myocardium (Hahn & Hoffman, 2001). Overdoses of opiates (e.g., heroin, morphine) can cause severe hypotension and respiratory arrest. They also may induce pulmonary edema.

Stress

Stress is often mentioned as a cause of high BP, angina, and MI. Stress elevates serum lipids, increases blood coagulation, elevates BP, and can cause myocardial ischemia. People with preexisting cardiac problems who encounter extraordinary or protracted periods of business, family, or personal stress may be at added risk for exacerbations of these problems.

Much has been written about personality types and their predisposition toward heart disease. The hard-striving, competitive, highly assertive person with the "type A" personality is believed to suffer a higher incidence of heart attacks than the easygoing, relaxed, more cooperatively oriented "type B" person. Type A personality and hostility are related to greater BP reactivity in response to challenging activities (Fichera & Andreassi, 1998).

Aging

Diseases leading to problems with tissue perfusion are uncommon in early adulthood. Peripheral vascular disease and its resultant perfusion problems increase in frequency with age. Disorders such as diabetes mellitus, chronic hypertension, kidney disease, or problems with lipid metabolism cause peripheral vascular disease in the elderly. Although coronary heart disease is not considered part of the normal aging process, it has traditionally affected older adults.

ALTERED CARDIOVASCULAR FUNCTION

Tissue oxygenation requires that all portions of the cardiovascular system work properly. Alterations in the conduction system, improper opening or closing of the valves, or damage to cardiac muscle fibers can diminish the heart's effective pumping ability. Changes in the blood vessels and in the blood itself can create the potential for altered function.

Manifestations of Altered Cardiovascular Function

Altered cardiovascular function has a wide range of manifestations. Vital signs are typically affected. When cardiovascular changes cause tissue ischemia, common indicators of inadequate tissue perfusion include pain, changes in the skin, and changes in cognition. Edema and **thrombus** (clot) formation are manifestations and causes of alterations in blood flow. Finally, organ dysfunction and possible failure are manifestations of altered cardiovascular status.

Changes in Vital Signs
Blood Pressure. The BP may fluctuate with changes in CO and fluid volume. Decreased circulating volume or increased venous pooling may be indicated by orthostatic hypotension. High BP leads to complications over time and should be treated (Jarvis, 2000). Abnormally low BP (less than 90 mm Hg systolic), when accompanied by other indicators of diminished oxygenation, is a serious sign of decreased CO (AHA, 2001b).

Pulse Character. Diminished or absent pulses may indicate inadequate blood flow to an area. Although the pulse normally becomes fainter as the distance from the heart increases, absence of pulse may indicate vessel occlusion, especially when differences occur bilaterally. Complete vessel occlusion is most often associated with other signs, such as skin changes

and pain. In some people, the most distal peripheral pulses (the dorsalis pedis and posterior tibial) may not be palpable but can be confirmed with the use of a Doppler instrument (Jarvis, 2000).

Heart Rate. The heart rate increases in response to increased oxygen demand. It decreases at rest when oxygen demands are low. A heart rate of 100 beats/minute at rest may indicate problems with CO if known contributing factors (e.g., fever, pain, medications, anxiety) are absent. An increase in heart rate of more than 20 beats/minute during mild activity (e.g., walking, moving to the commode) may indicate that decreased CO is contributing to activity intolerance. Conversely, a heart rate that does not increase with exercise may indicate that the heart is unable to adjust to changing oxygen demands. The heart rate should return to baseline within 3 minutes after exercise.

Respiration. Respiratory rate and effort often increase in the person with cardiovascular dysfunction. Decreased CO or diminished blood flow limits the amount of oxygen available to the tissues. As activity increases and tissues demand more oxygen, respiration increases to supplement blood oxygenation. Shortness of breath can occur in a person with heart or circulatory problems with even slight activity, because the cardiovascular system is unable to meet the added oxygen demand. In extreme cases, the person may experience shortness of breath at rest or when lying down. Finally, a cough productive of frothy sputum is a common manifestation of heart failure (Jarvis, 2000).

Changes in the Skin
Skin color is an indicator of the level of blood oxygenation and adequacy of local blood flow. Because skin color varies so greatly among individuals, it is helpful to compare differences between sides of the body. The mucous membranes of most people are generally pink. Assess the inner linings of the lips and mouth and the inner lining of the eyelids.

In light-skinned people, sudden constriction of peripheral blood vessels (caused by fear, low CO, or trauma) causes the skin to be pale. Rubor is a bluish-red skin coloration caused by hyperemia, or increased blood flow. Temporary increases in skin perfusion cause flushing, as is evident during fever or times of embarrassment. Cyanosis occurs when hemoglobin is not carrying an adequate amount of oxygen, resulting in a bluish appearance. Peripheral cyanosis (of the fingers, toes, and earlobes) occurs when blood flow is restricted. Central cyanosis is a serious sign of decreased oxygenation. It appears around the lips and tissues of the oral cavity (Jarvis, 2000).

Skin temperature rises with increased blood flow to the skin; vascular constriction or poor perfusion cools the skin. If the sympathetic nervous system has caused the constriction (e.g., in shock), sweat glands may become activated, and the client will feel clammy to the touch.

Skin character changes occur with alterations in perfusion. Chronically poor perfusion may result in hair loss in the affected area, discolored skin, thickened nails, and shiny, dry skin indicative of inadequate tissue nutrition. Some people with chronic heart disease also have clubbed fingers and toes (Jarvis, 2000).

Skin lesions, dermatitis, and ulcerations can develop readily in clients with compromised skin perfusion. Chronically limited arterial flow to an area can cause skin breakdown, with possible tissue necrosis and gangrene.

Decreased Cardiac Output

Muscle damage, valve dysfunction, or conduction problems can decrease the heart's ability to pump blood effectively, resulting CHF or cardiogenic shock. The example of a Critical Pathway for a client with CHF summarizes collaborative care.

Muscle Damage.   The heart requires a constant supply of oxygen and nutrients. If blood flow decreases through the coronary arteries, the active muscle becomes hypoxic (without oxygen). Unless blood flow is restored, portions of the heart muscle can die. This is called a **myocardial infarction** (MI) or heart attack. The person who survives a heart attack may have areas of scar tissue replacing healthy muscle tissue.

A second cause of cardiac muscle damage or weakening is severe overwork of the heart. The normal heart responds to extra work by enlarging. Eventually, excessive demands stretch the heart to its limits. It finally weakens and fails. Increased vascular resistance (e.g., with high BP), excessive blood volume, and alterations in blood viscosity are common contributing factors in the development of heart failure. Other possible causes of heart muscle damage are infection, inflammatory or metabolic disease, nutritional deficiencies, trauma, and substance abuse.

Valve Dysfunction.   The four valves of the heart must be able to open fully and close tightly to guarantee forward blood flow. Any of the heart's valves may be damaged by inflammation, infection, or trauma, or they may be congenitally malformed. Generally, valve damage results in stenosis (narrowing) or regurgitation (not completely closing). These conditions can limit stroke volume and force the heart to work much harder than normal to maintain an adequate CO. With time, heart failure occurs.

Conduction Problems.   Proper function of the conduction system ensures the orderly contraction of myocardial muscle fibers. This results in a coordinated, concerted pumping action, with all muscle fibers operating as a unit. If the conduction system is damaged or malfunctions, the electrical impulses it generates do not spread sequentially through the muscle. The fibers that normally contract together may do so out of sequence or may contract independent of each other. This discordant fiber contraction affects the heart's inherent rhythm and may impair its ability to pump effectively.

A **dysrhythmia** is an abnormality in heart rhythm. Dysrhythmias range from minor, clinically insignificant abnormalities to life-threatening conditions. Dysrhythmias may be caused by damage to the heart muscle or conduction system, diminished coronary blood flow, decreased blood oxygen levels, medications, alterations in serum electrolytes (e.g., potassium, calcium), stress (e.g., from exercise, fever, emotional stress), or overstretching of the heart muscle.

Altered Blood Flow

Conditions that affect the blood and blood vessels can alter tissue perfusion and CO.

Alterations in the Blood.   Alterations in the red blood cells or plasma or changes in circulating blood volume or consistency can affect cardiovascular function. An insufficient number of red blood cells (as in anemia) or damage to the hemoglobin molecules results in tissue hypoxia. Hypoxia affects all tissues, but the brain and heart are particularly sensitive to oxygen deprivation. Changes in the normal levels of serum electrolytes or pH can cause alterations in cardiovascular function. For example, slight changes in serum potassium levels can cause serious irregularities in heart rhythm (dysrhythmias). Increased sodium intake can cause an increase in blood volume, which increases cardiac work. An acidotic blood pH can decrease the ability of hemoglobin to carry oxygen.

Dehydration or hemorrhage causes a decrease in circulating volume. Because tissue perfusion depends on a sufficient volume of circulating blood, any decrease in volume can lead to tissue hypoxia. This occurs in the condition commonly called **shock.**

Excessive fluid volume occurs in people with CHF, in those with kidney failure, and after overload from IV therapy. The heart must work harder than normal to pump the additional blood through the vascular system. The additional blood volume and pressure also overload capillaries, causing edema. In the peripheral tissues, overloading causes swelling and decreased perfusion. If fluid overload occurs in the lung, pulmonary edema fills the air sacs and decreases oxygenation.

Thinner, less viscous blood flows more quickly than normal blood through the vessels. Increased blood flow increases venous return to the heart. This usually forces the heart to pump faster to empty itself. The opposite condition, called polycythemia, results in thicker, more viscous blood. Polycythemic blood flows more slowly through the vessels. To pump this thicker blood through the system, the heart must work harder than usual (Emerson, 2000).

Arterial Dysfunction.   Atherosclerosis is by far the most common cause of arterial occlusion. It seriously compounds the problems of hypertension and is the most important factor in the majority of strokes and heart attacks. This condition is characterized by fatty deterioration of the arterial smooth muscle walls. With time, the lumen of the arteries narrows as the arterial walls absorb increasing amounts of circulating fat particles, or lipids. Affected vessels also become stiff and fibrinous and eventually may close completely. The resultant change in the walls of the vessel is called plaque formation.

(text continues on page 878)

COLLABORATIVE CARE PLAN
Critical Pathway

Congestive Heart Failure (CHF)

Client Name: _____

Case Type: _____   Admit Date: _____

DRG: _____   Date Path Initiated: _____

ICD-9: _____

Expected LOS: _____

Actual LOS: _____

Discharge Date: _____

Physician: _____

Case Manager: _____

Outcome Criteria

Client Problems	Day 1 CCU/MICU	D	E	N	Day 2 Telemetry	D	E	N	Day 3–6 Telemetry/Floor	D	E	N
Decreased cardiac output related to myocardial contractility, altered conduction, & valve defects	No life-threatening dysrhythmias HR <120—regular skin pink, warm, dry Capillary refill <3 sec. Palpable peripheral pulses bilaterally SBP >100 UO >30 mL/hr				Normal sinus rhythm—no ectopy Serum K 3.5–5 HR 60–100 regular Skin pink, warm, dry Cap. refill <3 sec. Palp. periph. pulses SBP >100 <140 DBP >50 <90				Normal sinus rhythm Serum K 3.5–5 HR 60–100 regular Skin pink, warm, dry Cap. refill <3 sec Palp. periph. pulses SBP >90 <140 DBP >50 <90 UO >30 mL/hr.			
Altered gas exchange related to pulmonary congestion, V/Q mismatching, ↓ diffusion	O₂ Saturation >90% Minimal crackles in lung bases Respirations <24 unlabored PO₂ >60 mm Hg Dyspnea on exertion				O₂ Sat >95% Decreased crackles heard in lungs R <20 unlabored PO₂ >80 mm Hg No dyspnea on exertion				O₂ Sat >95% HR <20 over baseline on ambulation Lungs clear Chest x-ray clear R <20 unlabored No dyspnea			
Activity intolerance related to imbalance between oxygen supply–demand, dyspnea, fatigue	Turns in bed, feeds self; performs self-toilet measures No dyspnea or fatigue				Tolerates commode or sits in chair t.i.d. without dyspnea, chest pain, fatigue Participates in activities of daily living (ADLs) without discomfort or fatigue				Performs ADLs without fatigue, dyspnea, or chest pain Ambulates with q.i.d. SBP ±10 mm Hg over baseline HR <20 BPM over baseline			

COLLABORATIVE CARE PLAN
Critical Pathway (Continued)

	Day 1				Day 2				Day 3–6			
Client Problems	**CCU/MICU**	D	E	N	**Telemetry**	D	E	N	**Telemetry/Floor**	D	E	N
Fluid volume excess related to pulmonary congestion, venous pooling	Resp <24 unlabored Lung sounds clear without crackles & diminished in bases No dependent edema Weight loss 1 lb/day until baseline				Resp 12–20 unlabored Lungs clear No edema No jugular venous distention (JVD) Weight loss 1 lb/day until baseline				Resp 12–20 unlabored Lungs clear No edema No JVD No weight gain			
Anxiety RT dyspnea, fear of death, & hospitalization	Verbalizes fears & concerns related to hospitalization & diagnosis, fear of death				Relaxed nonverbals & posture Identifies source of anxiety & possible coping mechanisms				Identifies appropriate coping mechanisms & sources of social support			
Interventions												
Consult/Referral	Cardiologist Pulmonologist Social Service				Assess need for dietary consult & RT				Assess need for Home Health Care Social Service referral			
Diagnostic Test	Chest radiography Electrocardiography Electrolytes, Chemistry Profile CBC, cardiac enzymes, BUN/Creatinine Urinalysis Arterial blood gases				Chest x-ray ECG Electrolytes BUN/Creatinine Possible echocardiography				Electrolytes BUN/Creatinine			
Assessment	VS q 15 min until stable then q hr; Cardiac monitor; Assess heart sounds S_3/S_4 Lungs (crackles) Edema, JVD Daily weight I&O q hr—Foley catheter Arterial line/Swan-Ganz catheter				VS q4h Focus on heart sounds (S_3 or S_4) & lungs (crackles or wheezes) Edema, JVD Daily weight I&O q8h—discontinue Foley Discontinue monitor/arterial line/Swan-Ganz catheter				VS q8h Assess heart & lung sounds q8h, crackles, wheezes Edema, JVD Daily weight I&O q8h			
Treatments	Insert IV—#18—20 gauge Incentive spirometer (IS) q2h O_2 4 L/NC or intubation/ventilator O_2 saturation (pulse oximetry) SVN q4h				Saline Lock IV when adequate PO IS q2–4h O_2 2 L/NC PRN O_2 Sat SVN q4h				Discontinue Saline Lock IS q4h Discontinue O_2 when O_2 sats >92%			

	Phase 1 (CCU)	Phase 2	Phase 3 (Discharge)
Activity	Bedrest with bedside commode Head of bed ↑ 45°–90° Conserve energy Balance rest c̄ activity	Bathroom privileges → chair ×3 Out of bed as tolerated Assist with all ADLs	Ambulate in hall ×3 → up ad lib Self ADLs Shower daily
Diet	Clear liquids as tolerated	Low Na, low cholesterol cardiac soft	Low Na, low cholesterol cardiac diet as tolerated
Medications	Diuretic IV Anti-anxiety Rx Assess need for nitrates (nitroglycerin drip, patch) or KCl replacement Morphine SO$_4$ Inotropes (Dobutamine, Dopamine) Digoxin	Diuretics PO Evaluate need for preload & afterload reducers— Discontinue → nitroglycerin Nitropaste ACE inhibitors Stool softener/laxative of choice KCl replacement	Diuretics PO Digoxin PO Nitroglycerin paste Stool softeners KCl replacement Discharge prescription written
Teaching	Explain CCU environment, routines, procedures Teach pain rating scale & mgt tech. Involve family in all teaching Give critical path to pt/family	Teach CHF disease process, treatment regimen. Give CHF teaching packet Instruct in need for frequent rest periods & conservation of energy Begin medication teaching	Reinforce CHF teaching & answer questions. Review medications & importance of smoking cessation. Activity progression Diet teaching, especially no added salt Daily record wt, edema Teach importance of weight control
Discharge/Transfer Planning	Assess home care situation, physical arrangements, social support, caregiver If stable, transfer to telemetry Case manager visit	Assess discharge needs Contact social worker, home health if needed	Review discharge orders/meds with pt/family. Arrange follow-up appointment & when to contact physician Cardiac rehab, smoking clinic nutrition referral if needed Emerg phone numbers

D = Day
E = Evening
N = Night

Write "V" for variance in box if expected outcome not met or staff intervention not performed as stated. Client variances need to be explained in progress notes.

Initials/Signatures:

_____

_____

_____

_____

This degenerative process occurs gradually, over a period of years. High BP, high serum lipid levels, and cigarette smoking are the most important contributing lifestyle factors. Other important causes of arterial occlusion include infection, inflammation, and trauma to the arteries. Arteries also can have increased smooth muscle tone as a result of increased sympathetic nervous system stimulation (Copsead & Banasik, 2000).

Capillary Dysfunction. Problems within the arteries, veins, and surrounding tissues affect the capillaries because they are passive structures. Capillaries can become leaky and can cause or contribute to tissue edema. Increased BP or venous congestion can excessively stretch the walls of the capillaries, allowing fluid to leak out into interstitial tissues. Toxins, trauma, and inflammation can increase capillary permeability, promoting fluid leakage. Capillaries can leak if plasma proteins are deficient, because these substances are responsible for exerting the osmotic pressure that retains fluid in the blood vessels.

More importantly, swollen tissues may compress capillaries and smaller arteries, limiting blood flow and causing ischemia. Possible causes of such swelling include edema, bruising, and tumors. Often, swelling results from venous pooling caused by heart failure or incompetent venous valves. The resultant edema can cause pain by compressing local nerves (Emerson, 2000).

Venous Dysfunction. Decreased venous blood flow can aggravate hypertension and cause ischemia. Unless blood moves steadily through the veins, tissue edema or clot formation may occur. Causes of venous pooling include right-sided heart failure and ineffective venous valves.

Trauma or vein inflammation (phlebitis) can cause venous valve incompetency. More often, however, gravity and muscle inactivity are responsible. In the upright person, gravity hinders venous return, thereby promoting the gradual collection of blood in the veins of the lower leg. A person who must stand or sit for long periods (or who is immobile, such as a client confined to bed) does not have the benefit of regular muscle compression against the veins. As more blood collects in the leg veins, the veins can become dilated and distorted varicosities develop. The valves become so overstretched that their edges cannot approximate, so blood moves backward and forward through the incompetent valves.

An additional effect of venous pooling is increased myocardial work. Because stroke volume depends on how much blood enters the heart, venous pooling limits venous return. To maintain normal output, the heart must beat faster. This added work is compounded because increased venous pressure causes increased vascular resistance (Emerson, 2000).

Decreased Tissue Perfusion

Decreased tissue perfusion causes tissue hypoxia because less oxygen is available for metabolism. The tissue also experiences starvation because compromised blood flow provides fewer nutrients and contributes to abnormalities resulting from the buildup of waste products. This condition of inadequate perfusion, along with its consequences, is called **ischemia.** The manifestations of ischemia depend on the organ that is targeted and include pain and organ dysfunction.

A thrombus is a solid mass or clot which can develop in veins and steadily increase in size until it occupies the entire lumen of the vein. The thrombus halts blood flow because the mass or clot becomes a barrier to incoming arterial blood. Wherever a clot blocks a vessel, ischemia, infarction, and tissue necrosis can occur.

Thrombi can form in any blood vessel, but they are particularly likely to form in the deep veins of the legs. The surgical client, the immobile client, and those with added risk for clot formation are the most susceptible to thrombus formation. Polycythemia, infection, malignancy, pregnancy, and oral contraceptives greatly increase the risk of clot formation (Emerson, 2000).

An embolus occurs when a thrombus breaks loose and travels in the circulation. Emboli can also be caused by other things, such as plaque or fat from bone. If an embolus or thrombus lodges in the pulmonary artery, it is called a pulmonary embolism. Pulmonary emboli disrupt blood flow to the affected portion of the lung, disrupt gas exchange, and, if large enough, can cause death. If the thrombus or embolus lodges in the brain, it can cause a stroke.

Pain. Pain occurs commonly with ischemia when tissues are deprived of oxygen. The exact mechanism by which it results is not fully understood, but theorists have hypothesized that peripheral nerve endings may be stimulated by pressure caused by cellular edema, or the nerves may release chemical pain mediators as a response to their own hypoxia (Fallon & Roques, 1997). Pain that is not lessened by rest or by measures to improve blood flow and oxygenation may signal tissue infarction. **Angina** is chest pain associated with decreased coronary blood flow (Fallon & Roques, 1997). **Intermittent claudication** is limb pain caused by poor blood flow.

🔲 SAFETY ALERT
Teach clients never to ignore chest pain or discomfort and to report such unrelieved symptoms to medical personnel immediately.

Organ Dysfunction and Failure. The vital organs require consistent, normal CO and perfusion for optimal function. High BP or ischemia can have serious consequences for the brain, the kidneys, and other vital organs. The greater the impairment of perfusion, the greater the possibility of permanent damage and possible organ failure. The kidneys are commonly affected. If the kidneys do not receive a good blood supply, they will be unable to filter the blood, causing waste products to accumulate. Urine will not be produced, and additional fluid will build up, causing heart failure (AHA, 2001a).

Cognitive Dysfunction. The brain is extremely sensitive to any alterations in blood flow. If cerebral blood supply diminishes even slightly, changes in cognition occur. Most commonly, the client becomes restless and anxious. Confusion, fatigue, listlessness, and slurred speech may occur with a prolonged decrease in cerebral blood flow, as in shock. Chronic brain ischemia limits cognitive function.

When the blood supply to the brain is acutely diminished or completely interrupted (as when the vessels to the brain are blocked or when CO is abnormally low), dizziness and loss of consciousness may result. A **transient ischemic attack** (TIA) is a temporary decrease in blood flow to the brain, with brief disturbances in speech, vision, and mobility; confusion; and numbness felt on one half of the body. TIAs are important warning signs of possibly impending stroke. Complete lack of blood flow to specific areas of the brain causes tissue infarction, resulting in **stroke** (cerebrovascular accident) (AHA, 2001a).

Impact on Activities of Daily Living

The functional range of activities for the client with cardiovascular problems varies widely. Some clients are severely disabled; others experience little change in their activity levels (Coyne & Allen, 1998). The ability to perform activities of daily living (ADLs) is determined by the extent to which the disease has affected oxygen delivery to tissues. Because all activity increases tissue oxygen demands, severe ischemia greatly limits activity. Conversely, minor alterations in blood flow or CO have less effect on ADLs.

Frequently, after an acute cardiovascular episode such as an MI or stroke, a person's ability to perform normal ADLs is severely restricted. Activity after an MI should slowly increase and be individualized to ensure balance between oxygen supply and demand. The client may continue to experience fatigue after discharge. The time needed before returning to work, normal social interaction, driving, and normal sexual activity varies but is ordinarily within 6 to 8 weeks of discharge.

The client with impaired circulation, especially those with severe peripheral vascular disease, may limit their activity because of pain. Time needed for walking from place to place must include adequate time for rest. The client who has had a stroke can initially have great difficulty accomplishing ADLs. As the condition improves, the ability to perform ADLs depends on the extent of resultant brain damage.

Any client who has limited activity tolerance will probably need help with normal tasks that require extensive movement or effort. Frequently, such a development changes role relationships; a family member may need to assume the role of caregiver or breadwinner if the client is no longer able to work. Many cardiovascular problems are chronic and progressive, so the burden of care continually increases (Smeltzer & Bare, 2000).

ASSESSMENT

The extent and timeliness of the cardiovascular assessment vary depending on the client's immediate condition. All clients require a thorough and methodical assessment, which is easi-est to perform in clients with stable or chronic cardiovascular conditions. Acutely ill clients who are experiencing severe chest pain or other acute symptoms must be assessed rapidly and on a moment-to-moment basis. In such cases, intervention begins immediately, and evaluation is ongoing (McGrath & Cox, 1998). Only after the client is stabilized can a thorough assessment be conducted. The method of assessment described here focuses on the client with stable cardiovascular problems.

Subjective Data

Normal Pattern Identification

Most people take normal cardiovascular function for granted; as a continuous process, the system's regularity is virtually unnoticeable. The nurse can gain information about the client's normal functional pattern by assessing activity tolerance. The ability to perform a normal range of ADLs and to tolerate a reasonable level of physical exertion strongly indicates good cardiovascular health. Most people experience no chest pain or other remarkable discomfort while at rest or while engaged in moderate activity.

Practically everyone is aware that strenuous work or exercise causes the heart to beat faster and more forcefully. Although these changes are noticeable, few people would describe them as "pain" or "discomfort." Consequently, complaints of chest pain with activity always warrant a full investigation. People with cardiovascular problems often experience discomfort, pain, or other symptoms at a lower level of activity than healthy persons do. This tendency usually leads to self-imposed activity restriction as the client adjusts to the condition.

Risk Identification

Many factors contribute to the development of cardiovascular problems. Question the client concerning past cardiovascular conditions, such as a previous MI, stroke, or circulatory difficulties. Determine any functional deficits that resulted from these conditions and the management program the client is using. Determine the extent of the client's smoking. The number of packs of cigarettes smoked daily and the number of years smoked (pack-per-year history) are important measures of the client's total exposure.

Assess dietary intake of saturated fats, cholesterol, and sodium. Ask clients directly about cooking habits and dietary patterns. Many people are unaware of the fat, cholesterol, and sodium content of specific foods. It may help to ask the client to describe a normal day's intake and ask for an estimate of specific high-risk foods ("How many fried foods do you eat per week?" "How often do you eat red meat or eggs?"). Despite an increased emphasis on health, many prepackaged supermarket foods and "fast foods" contain an extremely high percentage of fat and sodium. Because many people regularly eat these convenience foods, investigate the client's eating habits with this in mind. Also evaluate how often the client eats out, where, and what types of food are usually ordered.

Assess activity and exercise patterns to determine increased risk for cardiovascular dysfunction. Questions such as, "How often do you exercise each week, and what type of activities do you enjoy?" may be helpful. Determine how much of the client's work day is composed of sedentary activity.

Obtain information concerning any medications (prescription, over-the-counter, or herbal) the client is taking. Many medications have side effects that can have an impact on cardiovascular function. If the medication is specifically for a cardiovascular condition, assess the length of time the medication has been taken, the dose, the client's knowledge of the medication, and any side effects the client may have experienced. Also ask whether the client is taking the medications as prescribed, because many people take the medications when feeling poorly and reduce or stop taking the medications when feeling better. Determine the client's use of recreational drugs, especially alcohol, IV drugs, or cocaine. The nurse may introduce the questions about drug use by explaining that the information is important in determining healthcare advice and recommendations for treatment.

Dysfunction Identification

Finding out why the client has sought medical care is the first step in determining the nature of the client's health complaint. The client should explain reasons in his or her own words without interruption. After the client's initial explanation, seek specific clarification concerning the problem.

Pain is the most common reason people with cardiovascular dysfunction seek medical and nursing aid. Determine the specific nature of the pain: its location, its intensity, and the circumstances that cause it (Display 35-2). Additionally, elicit any other symptoms, such as indigestion, chest pressure, or numbness and tingling in the left arm, because they may also be symptoms of heart disease.

Activity restriction is an important subjective measure of cardiovascular dysfunction. Establish the level of activity the client associates with the onset of pain or discomfort. Some relevant questions to determine activity restriction include, "Do the symptoms occur only during strenuous exercise, such as running or playing basketball?" "Do they occur when walk-

DISPLAY 35-2

🔄 **INITIAL ASSESSMENT QUESTIONS FOR THE CLIENT EXPERIENCING CHEST DISCOMFORT**

- What does it feel like (pressure, weight on chest)?
- Does the pain go anywhere else (e.g., to the arms, neck, or back)?
- Does the pain increase with deep breathing or movement?
- How bad is it (0–10 scale, with 10 being the worst)?
- When did the pain start?
- What were you doing when it began?
- Does anything you do make it better/worse?
- Do you feel any other unusual symptoms (e.g., sweating, shortness of breath, nausea, dizziness, fear)?

ing at a normal pace? If so, how far can you walk before the symptoms begin?" "Does quiet household activity bring on the symptoms?" "Do you experience the symptoms during periods of rest?" "Do any other circumstances, such as weather or emotional stress, tend to cause or exaggerate the problem?" "Do the symptoms appear at particular times of the day?"

Other subjective complaints may occur with cardiovascular problems. Dizziness, "blackouts," swelling of hands or ankles, and changes in skin color or sensation are significant. Also ask about shortness of breath, difficulty lying flat, and cough.

Objective Data

Physical Assessment

Inspection. Observing the client's general behavior and appearance yields significant information about tissue perfusion and CO. Decreased CO, vascular disease, or both can change cognitive and perceptual function. Because the brain is extremely sensitive to any decrease in blood flow, assessment of cognition and level of consciousness provides clues about cerebral perfusion.

Cognition is often the first indicator of perfusion to be assessed because it is readily apparent in the nurse's first interactions with the client. People with normal cerebral perfusion usually speak in a normal cadence, answer questions quickly and appropriately, and are oriented to person, place, and time. They are able to follow directions. Note a client's slowness of speech or other overt difficulties with speaking. Inappropriate responses to questions or statements, confusion, apathy, decreased understanding, disorientation, restlessness, and anxiety are all possible signs of decreased cerebral perfusion. Level of consciousness is indicated by the client's arousability. The client who requires much stimulation to respond may have diminished cerebral blood flow.

Because skin color can roughly indicate blood flow adequacy, examine the client for central and peripheral cyanosis. In light-skinned persons, pallor or blanched skin is evidence of possible ischemia or anemia. Note localized skin discolorations, such as bruises, redness, or mottling. The presence of dependent edema (in the hands, sacrum, or ankles) indicates possible circulatory problems. Neck veins should be relatively flat; engorgement of these veins implies inefficient right-sided heart pumping.

Inspect the legs and arms for changes in hair distribution, skin color, shiny skin, ulcerations, edema, and venous distention (Walker, 1999). Note any varicosities. Toenails and fingernails should be smooth; ridged, thickened, hornlike nails indicate decreased peripheral perfusion. Digits are normally round in shape, but "clubbed" fingertips are associated with oxygenation problems, from lung or cardiovascular disease.

Palpation. The well-perfused client is warm and dry to the touch. Although cool extremities are normal in many people, chronically cold fingers and toes often indicate poor circulation.

Palpate the pulse for quality and rate. Note regularity of rhythm, pulse intensity, and the number of beats per minute.

Assess peripheral circulation by checking femoral (groin), popliteal (behind the knee), posterior tibial (ankle), and dorsalis pedis (foot) pulses for equal intensity in both legs. If you detect an irregular pulse, assess the apical and radial pulses simultaneously to determine whether all heartbeats are being perfused further away from the heart (Jarvis, 2000).

Capillary refill time, which reflects peripheral tissue perfusion and CO, is determined by pressing a nailbed until it blanches. Pressure is released, and the time it takes for the nail to return to its original color is noted. This "capillary refill time" is ordinarily less than 3 seconds. A longer refill time indicates narrowing of the blood vessels, decreased circulating blood volume, or otherwise decreased CO (Jarvis, 2000) (Fig. 35-6).

Palpate for edema and note its extent (Fig. 35-7). Edema has traditionally been described in terms of a scale ranging from 0 (no edema present) to 4 (severe, pitting edema). This scale offers a subjective but moderately useful means for indicating the amount of edema present (Jarvis, 2000).

More accurate means of measuring edema include serial girth measurements of affected extremities or abdomen (for ascites). Daily weight assessment also can indicate the extent of edema. A weight gain of 10 lb (indicative of 5 L of extracellular fluid volume) precedes visible edema in most clients.

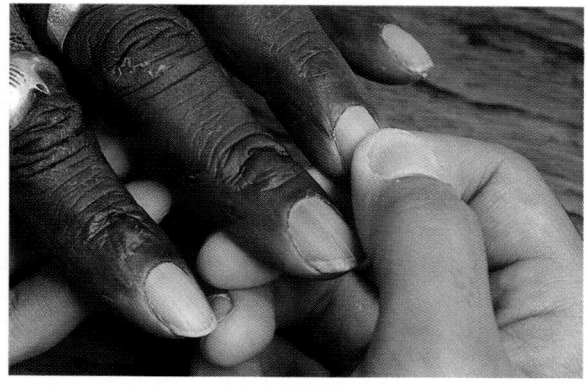

FIGURE 35-6   Test for capillary refill time. Pressure is applied to nail bed and then released. Time for nail to regain color is noted.

The Homan sign, performed by bending the client's foot upward toward the leg (dorsiflexion), was historically used to detect thrombophlebitis of the lower extremity. This is no longer recommended because of the increased risk of dislodging a clot and causing an embolus.

Auscultation. A stethoscope is used to determine BP, count the apical pulse, and identify normal and abnormal heart sounds.

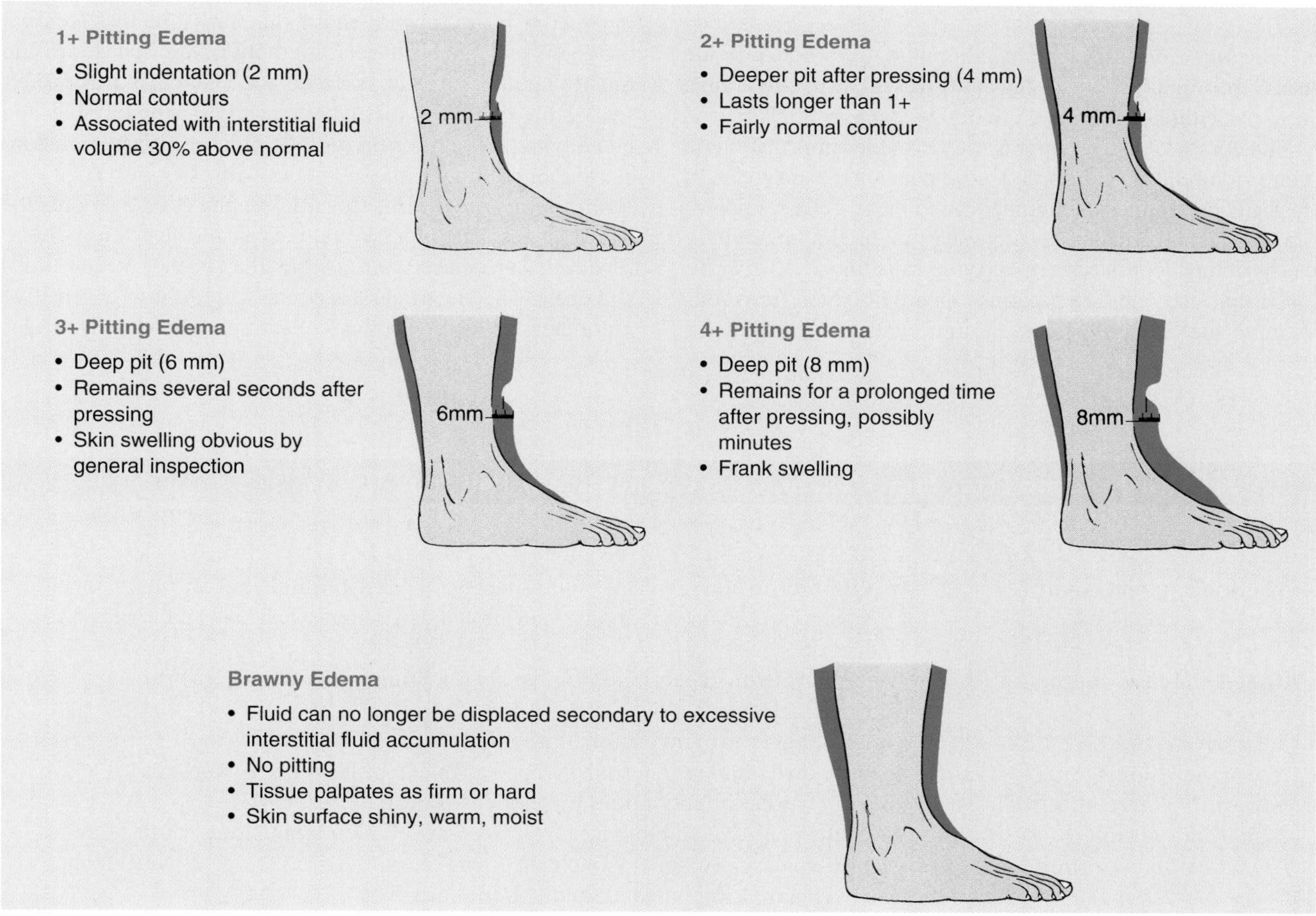

1+ Pitting Edema
- Slight indentation (2 mm)
- Normal contours
- Associated with interstitial fluid volume 30% above normal

2 mm

2+ Pitting Edema
- Deeper pit after pressing (4 mm)
- Lasts longer than 1+
- Fairly normal contour

4 mm

3+ Pitting Edema
- Deep pit (6 mm)
- Remains several seconds after pressing
- Skin swelling obvious by general inspection

6mm

4+ Pitting Edema
- Deep pit (8 mm)
- Remains for a prolonged time after pressing, possibly minutes
- Frank swelling

8mm

Brawny Edema
- Fluid can no longer be displaced secondary to excessive interstitial fluid accumulation
- No pitting
- Tissue palpates as firm or hard
- Skin surface shiny, warm, moist

FIGURE 35-7   Edema can be graded by gently pressing the edematous area with the fingers for up to 5 seconds.

Auscultate the apical pulse to establish its rate and character. This simple measurement is essential for complete assessment of the client who has a pulse that is difficult to palpate or an irregular heart rate. It also is necessary to auscultate the apical pulse for 1 full minute when administering certain medications, notably cardiac glycosides (e.g., digoxin).

Normal heart sounds, murmurs, and other abnormal sounds also are audible by stethoscope. S_1 and S_2 are the "lub" and "dub" that are normally heard as the heart valves close. They are discussed along with abnormal heart sounds, such as murmurs, gallops, or clicks, and normal heart sounds in Chapter 24. Interpretation of these sounds takes a considerable amount of practice and a strong understanding of their underlying physiology (Jarvis, 2000).

Assess BP to establish the presence of hypotension, high BP, and positional differences. (For a detailed discussion of pulse and BP assessment, see Chapter 25.)

Diagnostic Tests and Procedures
The most common tests and procedures are described briefly here. Table 35-1 lists selected tests and diagnostic procedures used to assess cardiovascular function. The diagnosis of MI should be made after interpreting the results of more than one test, because no single cardiac marker is totally specific and sensitive (Murphy & Berding, 1999).

Laboratory Studies. Several laboratory tests that provide useful information concerning cardiovascular function range from basic blood assessment to highly sophisticated assays.

The complete blood count (CBC) provides information on white blood cells, platelets, and sedimentation rate. In addition, the CBC determines the number of red blood cells, hemoglobin, and hematocrit. These latter measures are important indicators of the blood's oxygen-carrying capability.

Cardiac enzymes are proteins that are liberated from cells when tissue damage occurs. Serum levels of creatinine ki-

nase (CK), CK-MB, troponin, and lactic dehydrogenase are measured to confirm a suspected MI (Jaffe, 1997).

Kidney function studies can indicate problems with perfusion. Blood urea nitrogen (BUN) and creatinine may be elevated in clients with hypoperfusion of the kidneys.

Deviations from normal levels of serum electrolytes can adversely affect cardiovascular function. Dysrhythmias result from potassium, calcium, and magnesium imbalances. Serum sodium is a reflection of water balance. Diuretics and other medications that affect cardiac function influence serum electrolyte levels. Changes in kidney function, acid–base status, and fluid or water balance affect electrolyte levels.

Blood lipids include cholesterol and triglycerides. Lipids, linked to proteins known as lipoproteins, also are measured. Elevated blood levels of LDLs are strongly associated with peripheral vascular disease and coronary artery disease, and commonly called the "bad" cholesterol. Conversely, "good" cholesterol, or HDLs, have been associated with a reduced risk for cardiovascular diseases. Although this test does not confirm or rule out the presence of cardiovascular disease, it is a useful screening tool for identifying those who are at risk (Pagana & Pagana, 1997).

Diagnostic Procedures. Diagnostic procedures can yield information about cardiac function or blood flow. Tests relating to the heart include those that measure its electrical conductivity (e.g., electrocardiography, exercise testing) and those that measure its size and mechanical ability (e.g., echocardiography, cardiac catheterization). Angiography and hemodynamic monitoring provide precise information concerning blood flow.
Electrocardiography. Electrocardiography (ECG) records the heart's electrical impulse conduction in the resting client. Electrodes are placed on specific areas of the client's limbs and chest. The electrodes are connected to a highly sensitive voltmeter, which controls a delicate pen. As the electrodes

TABLE 35-1

Selected Tests and Procedures Used to Assess Cardiovascular Function	
Test/Procedure	**Purpose**
Complete blood count	Yields information on platelets, presence or absence of infection, oxygen-carrying capacity; to diagnose anemias, nutritional deficiencies, and selected metabolic disorders
Blood chemistry tests	Determine serum electrolytes, lipids; also creatinine and blood urea nitrogen to assess kidney function
Serum enzymes	Rule out or confirm myocardial infarction (MI)
Electrocardiography (ECG)	Identify arrhythmias, determine types and extent of heart damage from MI
Stress ECG (treadmill)	Identify cardiac abnormalities not evident on resting ECG
Echocardiography	Measure heart size and thickness; observe valve function; measure cardiac output
Heart catheterization	Measure pressure within heart chambers to determine heart strength, valve competency, cardiac output, and fluid volume status
Angiography	Outlines blood flow through vessels to identify blockages, aneurysms
Electrophysiology	Identifies arrhythmias and effectiveness of antiarrhythmic treatment

detect electrical impulses, the pen scribes a tracing on a moving strip of paper. The various deflections of the ECG tracing correspond to the individual events of the cardiac conduction cycle (Fig. 35-8).

Electrodes are placed on several areas of the limbs and chest to provide several "views" of cardiac impulses. Many views (called "leads") are needed to differentiate among the various conditions that can affect the heart, because abnormalities may not appear in all leads. Single-lead ECGs are useful for continuous monitoring of a client, but the standard 12-lead ECG is needed for a thorough evaluation of the heart's electrical conductivity. When properly interpreted, the ECG can detect myocardial damage, cardiac ischemia, alterations from normal heart rhythm, changes in heart position or size, or problems within the conduction system.

Exercise Testing. Exercise testing can assess a person's response to cardiovascular stress. In some people, problems of cardiac ischemia are not detectable with a conventional resting ECG because ischemia occurs only during periods of activity. The test involves the use of a treadmill with adjustable speed and slope. The client begins walking at a normal pace on the treadmill. The ECG and BP are monitored continually while the speed and slope of the treadmill are gradually increased. The test usually lasts about 15 minutes, unless it is terminated because of ECG or BP changes or by the client's fatigue, pain, or shortness of breath. Exercise testing allows practitioners to determine with some precision the degree of the person's functional ability.

Echocardiography. Echocardiography uses ultrasonic waves to diagnose structural heart defects. This technique evolved from the use of marine sonar equipment, in which sound is bounced off structures, forming identifiable patterns. A pen-like probe sends high-frequency sound waves through the chest wall. The waves produce "echoes" as they bounce off the heart, and the echo pattern is recorded. Using these patterns, cardiologists can obtain an accurate view of the heart without performing potentially dangerous invasive procedures, such as catheterization. Echocardiography can detect myocardial muscle thickness and motion, structure and motion of the valves, the size of the chambers, and the presence of fluid around the heart.

Blood flow studies determine the patency and shape of blood vessels and the direction and volume of blood flow through them. The simplest and least expensive test of this type is *Doppler examination.* It is commonly used to monitor blood flow in the extremities and the brain. Doppler instruments enhance the turbulent sounds the blood makes as it circulates through the heart or vessels. Using ultrasound technology, the Doppler instrument produces a graphic representation of the course of blood flow.

Radiography. Chest radiography can establish the size and shape of the heart and aorta and detect pulmonary congestion or edema. It is used to confirm correct placement of indwelling heart catheters and pacemakers.

Catheterization. Catheterization of the heart and large vessels is used to determine precise information concerning valve function and cardiac muscle strength. This type of procedure is more invasive than the previously discussed tests. Various types of catheters can be inserted through a vein or artery and directed (under fluoroscopy) into the heart's chambers. The catheter is able to measure the pressure generated within each chamber and to establish how efficiently the heart is pumping.

Some types of cardiac catheters also can measure CO and pressures within the pulmonary vascular system. Because they furnish information about vascular pressures, indwelling catheters are valuable tools in fluid and BP management. Pulmonary artery and central venous pressure catheters are used for this purpose. Arterial catheters allow the nurse to monitor arterial BP closely and to draw blood for evaluation of oxygenation and acid–base status. Arterial and other indwelling vascular catheters are used only where constant monitoring is possible, usually in an intensive care setting.

Angiography. Angiography uses a radiopaque dye to outline blood vessels and to confirm or rule out vessel blockage. This technique also is used to detect aneurysms. Radionuclide examinations use radioactive substances to detect MI and decreased myocardial blood flow.

Electrophysiology. Electrophysiology is a study done to determine whether problems exist with electrical conduction or automaticity in the heart. Specialized wires are threaded through large veins and arteries and attempts are made to stimulate the

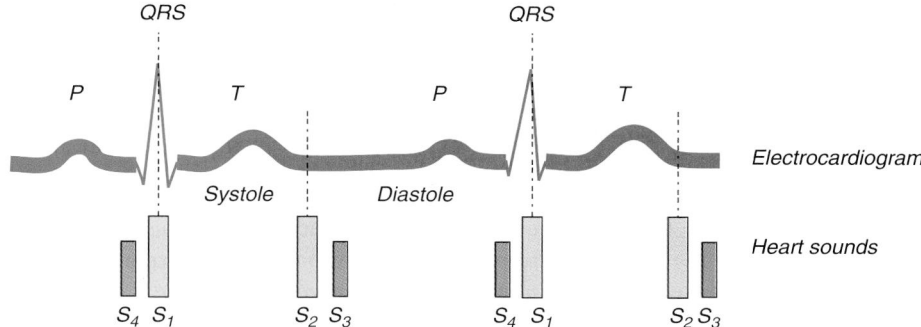

FIGURE 35-8 An electrocardiogram provides valuable information about the heart's ability to conduct impulses.

dysrhythmia. Clients are treated with medication or devices, and testing may be done to evaluate whether the treatment is effective (Lane, 1997).

NURSING DIAGNOSES

The two primary North American Nursing Diagnosis Association (NANDA) nursing diagnoses that specifically address problems of cardiovascular function are Decreased Cardiac Output and Ineffective Tissue Perfusion. Activity Intolerance also is a significant problem for many clients with cardiovascular dysfunction, although it is not exclusively a cardiovascular problem.

Diagnostic Statement: Decreased Cardiac Output

Definition. Decreased CO describes a person who is experiencing or is at high risk of experiencing inadequate blood pumped by the heart to meet the metabolic demands of the body (NANDA, 2000).

Defining Characteristics. Defining characteristics include assessment findings related to altered heart rate and rhythm, altered preload, altered afterload, altered contractility, behavioral and emotional status, and altered stroke volume (NANDA, 2000).

Related Factors. Etiologic factors include high BP, previous history of heart or blood vessel disease, smoking, high blood cholesterol or triglycerides, increased age, male gender, diabetes, sedentary lifestyle, obesity, stress, increased cardiac workload, and increased fluid volume.

Diagnostic Statement: Ineffective Tissue Perfusion (Renal, Cerebral, Cardiopulmonary, Gastrointestinal, Peripheral)

Definition. Ineffective tissue perfusion is the state in which a person experiences or is at risk of experiencing a decrease in oxygen resulting in failure to nourish the tissues at the capillary level (NANDA, 2000).

Defining Characteristics. The following are defining characteristics for ineffective peripheral tissue perfusion: edema, altered skin characteristics, weak or absent pulses, skin discoloration, skin temperature changes, altered sensation, claudication, bruits, delayed healing, and diminished arterial pulses (NANDA, 2000).

Related Factors. The following are known etiologic factors: hypovolemia, hypervolemia, interruption of arterial or venous flow, and mechanical reduction in arterial or venous flow.

Diagnostic Statement: Activity Intolerance

Definition. Decreased activity intolerance is insufficient physiologic or psychological energy to endure or complete required or desired daily activities (NANDA, 2000).

Defining Characteristics. Defining characteristics include verbal report of fatigue or weakness, abnormal heart rate or BP response to activity, ECG changes reflecting ischemia or arrhythmias, and exertional discomfort or dyspnea (NANDA, 2000).

Related Factors. The following are known etiologic factors: bed rest or immobility, generalized weakness, imbalance between oxygen supply and demand, sedentary lifestyle, presence of circulatory or respiratory problems, and deconditioned status.

Related Nursing Diagnoses

Other nursing diagnoses that are common for people with cardiovascular dysfunction include Excess Fluid Volume, Risk for Infection, Imbalanced Nutrition: Less than Body Requirements, Chronic or Acute Pain, and Disturbed Sleep Pattern. Circulatory problems and heart disease also affect the client's ability to carry out ADLs. Possible related nursing diagnoses include Self-Care Deficit and Impaired Home Maintenance. Anxiety, Ineffective Coping, and Disabled Family Coping are examples of possible psychosocial nursing diagnoses. Deficient Knowledge is common because clients often must learn about new medications, diet, or management strategies to cope with cardiovascular dysfunction.

OUTCOME IDENTIFICATION AND PLANNING

Specific outcomes for the healthy person focus on prevention of cardiovascular problems by increased awareness of risk factors associated with them. Outcomes pertinent to the client who is admitted with an acute problem focus on recovery from the cardiovascular problem without residual complications. Realistic outcomes for the client with chronic cardiovascular disease focus on helping the client to live within limitations imposed by the disease and to improve acceptance of changes in lifestyle and self-concept. Outcomes for the terminal cardiovascular client center on maintenance of adequate comfort and acceptance of impending death (Johnson et al., 2001).

Goals are individualized based on the client's health status. In general, the following are appropriate goals for the client with cardiovascular dysfunction:

- The client will demonstrate adequate knowledge concerning cardiovascular dysfunction, prevention, or care.
- The client will maintain adequate CO.

- The client will demonstrate adequate tissue perfusion with adequate oxygenation of body tissue.
- The client will cope effectively with resulting changes in self-concept and lifestyle.

Examples of nursing interventions commonly used in planning for clients with cardiovascular problems are summarized in the accompanying display (Johnson et al., 2001).

IMPLEMENTATION
Health Promotion
Modifying Risk Factors
Primary prevention of cardiovascular disease begins with understanding its causes. Healthcare providers teach in the areas of smoking cessation, nutrition, and activity. Presenting information concerning risk factors in an objective manner can help clients choose appropriate behavior modification measures.

Nurses can help clients who are seeking to modify their risk for cardiovascular disease by being knowledgeable about (and taking part in) local support groups and classes that focus on this goal. The recent proliferation of self-help programs, fitness clubs, and aggressively advertised diets has provided the public with many options. Offer guidance in program selection and help the client identify (and avoid) programs that promise overly simplistic or unrealistic means to cardiovascular health.

PLANNING: Example of NIC/NOC Interventions

Accepted Cardiac Function and Tissue Perfusion Nursing Interventions Classification (NIC)
Cardiac Care: Acute
Circulatory Care
Energy Management
Hemodynamic Regulation
Respiratory Monitoring

Accepted Cardiac Function and Tissue Perfusion Nursing Outcomes Classification (NOC)
Circulation Status
Electrolyte and Acid–Base Balance
Energy Conservation
Fluid Balance
Neurologic Status
Respiratory Status: Ventilation
Self-Care: Activities of Daily Living (ADL)
Tissue Integrity: Peripheral
Tissue Perfusion: Cardiac
Tissue Perfusion: Peripheral
Vital Sign Status

Refer to the following for specifics regarding NIC/NOC:
   McCloskey, J., & Bulechek, G. (2000). *Iowa Intervention Project: Nursing Interventions Classification (NIC)* (2nd ed.). St. Louis, MO: C. V. Mosby.
   Johnson, M., & Maas, M. (2000). *Iowa Outcomes Project: Nursing Outcomes Classification (NOC)* (2nd ed.). St. Louis, MO: C. V. Mosby.

The client may need to become aware of appropriate supervised physical activity programs. If the client has a known medical problem or is older than 35 years of age, recommend a complete physical examination before the client starts an intensive exercise regimen. Various classes or support groups may be available to help the client alter unhealthy lifestyle habits. Clinics, hospitals, and other local agencies often sponsor diet management, smoking cessation, and stress management programs. Group formats that offer an opportunity to share experiences are particularly important for women, who tend to be more social than men and receive support from others in the group setting (Arnold, 1997). Nurses can be instrumental in developing and implementing such programs in the private workplace.

Preventing Venous Stasis
Venous stasis in the client with limited mobility may result in edema and the formation of deep vein thrombosis. By taking measures to improve the return of blood to the heart, nurses help to reduce the risk of dangerous clot formation. Leg exercises, antiembolism stockings, sequential compression devices (SCDs), and avoidance of constriction help to prevent venous stasis.

Assisting with Leg Exercises. Nurses commonly teach leg exercises to preoperative clients to prevent postoperative circulatory complications. These simple exercises are helpful for any client with impaired mobility, especially those confined to bed rest.

Leg exercises alternately contract and relax the muscles of the lower extremity. Contraction of these muscles helps promote the flow of blood back to the heart. Three separate leg movements can be encouraged (Fig. 35-9). First, have the client perform calf-pumping exercises, which involve alternate dorsiflexion and plantar flexion of the feet. Second, have the client bend one knee, sliding the foot up as far as possible along the mattress and back again. The client should repeat this process with the other leg. Finally, have the client alternately raise and lower each straight leg off the mattress as far as comfort allows.

Leg exercises should begin as soon as the client returns from surgery or whenever the client is immobile. The client should perform exercises at least once every 1 to 2 hours while awake. If the client is not able to perform leg exercises independently because of decreased strength or neurologic impairment, assist with passive leg exercises, encouraging as much client participation as possible.

Applying Antiembolism Stockings. Immobility deprives the bedridden client of the circulatory benefit of muscular contraction against the veins. Venous engorgement can be offset in these clients by the use of antiembolism stockings. Antiembolism stockings are made of strong elastic material. They are not the same as support hose, because they provide varying degrees of compression at different areas of the leg. When correctly fitted and applied, they exert external pressure, decreasing venous blood from pooling in the extremities. The

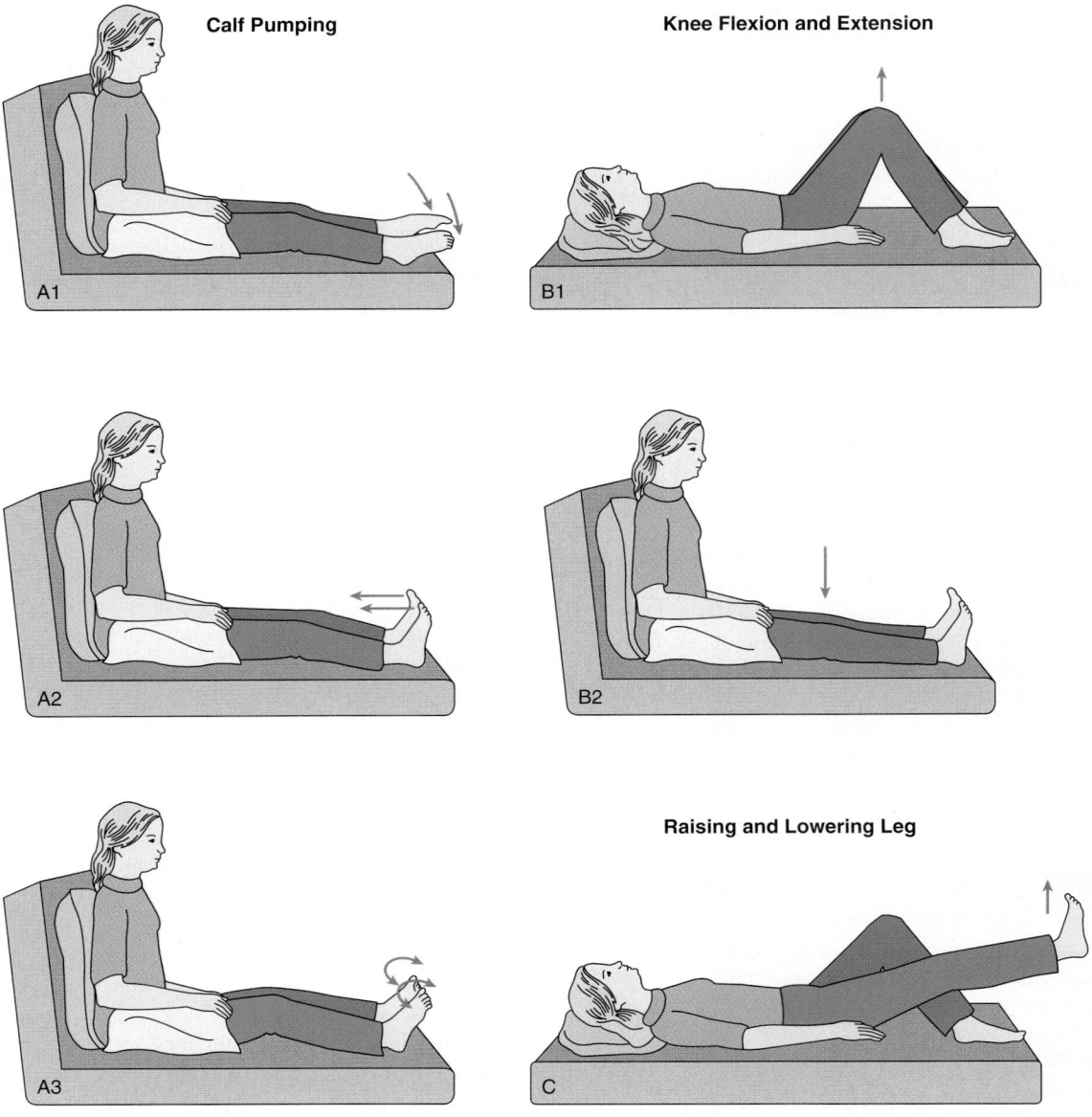

FIGURE 35-9   Leg exercises to improve circulation. **(A)** Calf pumping exercises: dorsiflexion and plantarflexion. Point toes of both feet toward the foot of the bed (A1); relax. Pull toes toward the chin (A2); relax. Make circles with both ankles (A3), in one direction and then in the other; repeat three times; relax. **(B)** Knee flexion and extension. With knees flexed and feet flat on the bed (B1), slide feet forward as far as possible (B2) and then back to flexed position (B1). **(C)** Raising and lowering leg. Raise and lower each straight leg alternatively while the other leg is flexed. Raise as far as comfort allows without straining.

stockings promote venous return in much the same manner as the leg muscles, using continuous instead of intermittent pressure.

To do their job effectively, antiembolism stockings must fit properly. Stockings that are too large for the client cannot provide sufficient vein compression, and stockings that are too tight obstruct blood flow to the legs. Guidelines for proper measurement and size selection of antiembolism stockings

are available from the manufacturer and should be followed instead of estimating stocking size by the height or weight. Wrinkles and poorly made seams can lead to pressure sores on the skin. Procedure 35-1 provides instructions on application of antiembolism stockings.

Inspect the client's legs and feet regularly to ensure that circulation is not impeded by the stockings. Antiembolism stockings are usually removed for 30 minutes once every 8 hours.

APPLYING ANTIEMBOLIC STOCKINGS

Purpose
1. Supplement the action of muscle contraction and aid venous return from the lower extremities
2. Prevent deep vein thrombosis in the immobile client.

Assessment
- Identify clients at high risk for deep vein thrombosis (e.g., long-term bed rest, cardiovascular disease).
- Obtain physician order.

Equipment
Stockings (available in knee-high and thigh-high lengths)
Baby powder or talcum powder

Procedure
1. Position client in supine position for one-half hour before applying stockings.
   Rationale: Veins should not be distended with blood when stockings are applied.
2. Provide for the client's privacy and explain the purpose of the antiembolic stockings.
   Rationale: Adequate knowledge increases client's participation and compliance.
3. Measure for proper fit before first application. Measure length (heel to groin) and width (calf and thigh) and compare to manufacturer's printed material to ensure proper fit.
   Rationale: Stockings that are too tight can lead to venous occlusion, and stockings that are too loose do not promote venous return.

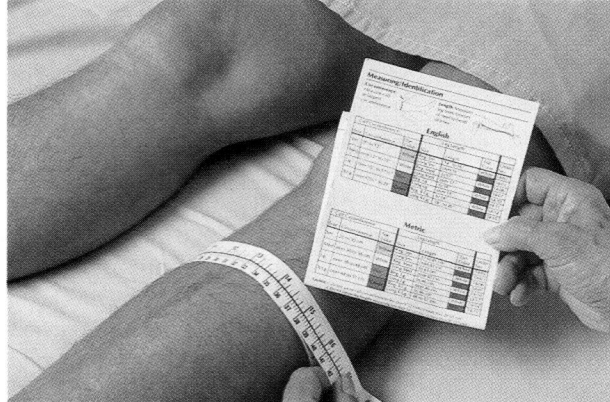

Step 3 Measure to ensure proper fit.

4. Make sure legs are dry or apply a light dusting of powder. Turn the stocking inside out, tucking the foot inside.
   Rationale: Dry legs ease application. Inside-out method allows for easier application of stocking, because stocking is not bunched up.

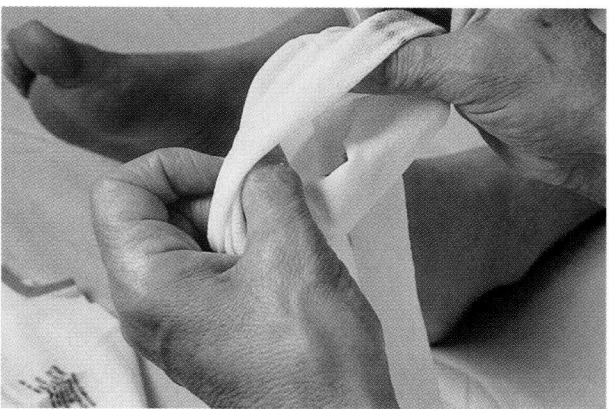

Step 4 Turn stocking inside out, tucking heel inside.

5. Ease foot section over the client's toe and heel, adjusting as necessary for proper smooth fit.
   Rationale: Wrinkles impede circulation.

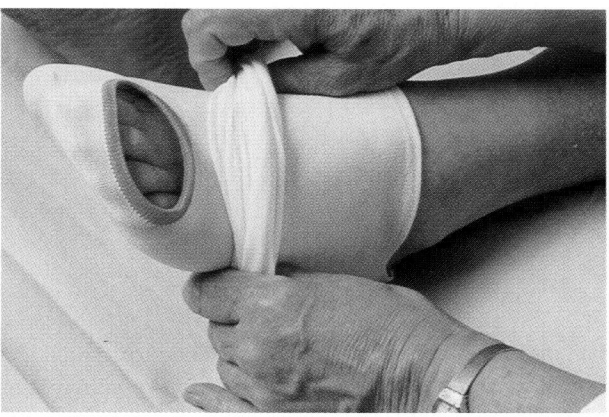

Step 5 Ease foot section over toe and heel.

6. Gently pull the stocking over the leg, removing all wrinkles.
   Rationale: Irregularities in fit may cause pressure areas.
7. Assess toes for circulation and warmth. Check area at top of stocking for binding.

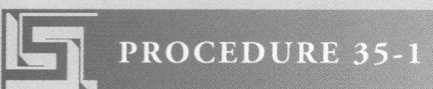

PROCEDURE 35-1 (Continued)

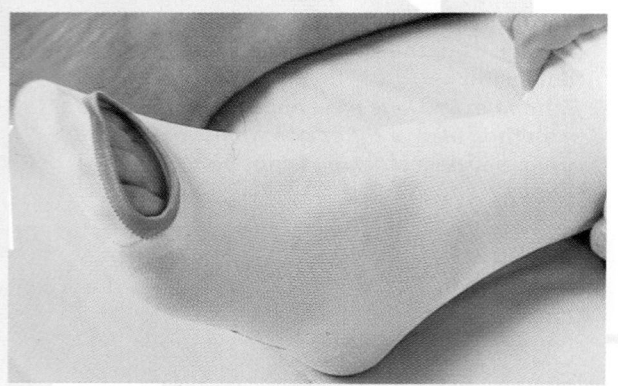

Step 6 Pull stocking over rest of leg.

> *Rationale: Constriction and rolling down of stockings during wear are the result of poor fit and can impede circulation and cause thrombosis.*

8. Antiembolic stockings should be removed at least twice daily.
   Rationale: Wash skin and assess for edema or irritation.

Lifespan Considerations
Child
- Antiembolic stockings are infrequently used in children.

Adult: The Obese Client
- Proper fitting of antiembolic stockings is difficult in the obese client and requires special attention for areas of constriction and binding.
- Elastic (Ace) bandages may be an alternative to provide antiembolic protection in clients for whom correct fit is impossible with standard stocking sizes.

Home Care Modifications
- Instruct clients to apply stockings before getting out of bed.
- Instruct clients to remove stockings regularly for skin inspection and cleansing.
- Be sure clients understand that commercial support stockings are not a substitute for medical antiembolic stockings.

Collaboration and Delegation
- Frequently, unlicensed assistive personnel remove and replace antiembolic stockings while performing hygiene care. Ensure that unlicensed assistive personnel do these procedures at least twice every day and that they report any signs of pressure or breakdown to you.

When the stockings are in place, the client's toes should remain warm, and the stockings should cause no obvious constriction or excoriation. The stockings should be applied in the morning, before the client has gotten out of bed, in order for them to be fitted while the client's legs are least edematous.

 SAFETY ALERT
Inspect the client's legs and feet regularly to ensure that the stockings do not impair circulation.

Using Pneumatic Compression Devices. Intermittent compression devices improve venous return by use of alternating pressure exerted against the extremity by inflation and deflation of plastic sleeves that are wrapped around the leg. The pneumatic compression device consists of an air pump, extremity sleeves, and connecting tubing. Pneumatic compression devices are of two types: intermittent and sequential. Intermittent devices turn chambers off and then on. SCDs sequentially compress various chambers within the extremity sleeve to promote venous return. A complete cycle can take 75 seconds to 5 minutes. Each of these devices is attached to an air pump that alternates inflation and deflation of the sleeve. Frequently, SCDs are ordered for the immobilized client and for surgical clients while on bed rest. Clients often wear antiembolism hose underneath the plastic sleeves to decrease irritation from the plastic and provide extra support. When the client gets up to ambulate, the devices are removed; once ambulation has resumed, use of the SCD is usually discontinued. Pneumatic compression devices should not be used for clients with arterial occlusive disease, severe edema, cellulitis, or infection of the extremity. Refer to Procedure 35-2 for application of SCDs.

Avoiding Constriction. Immobilized and inactive clients must be warned against venous constriction. Any article of clothing that exerts excessive pressure on the calves or thighs may constrict the veins, diminishing venous return and promoting the formation of clots and varicosities. Discourage the use of garters and the practice of wearing stockings knotted above the knee. Clients should avoid socks with tight elastic bands around the tops and short-legged pants with tight elastic or belted bottoms.

In addition to garments, orthopedic casts made of plaster or other materials can tighten and restrict blood flow. Warm fingers or toes indicate sufficient blood flow, but cool extremities, numbness or tingling, and limited capillary refill may indicate a need for altering the cast or recasting.

Point out to clients that crossing the legs creates pressure points against veins and should be avoided. Clients who must sit for extended periods (e.g., at work) should be careful not to create venous constriction by sitting too far back in chairs. The back of the calves should not rest against the edge of the chair because this compresses the veins. Teach these clients to flex their leg muscles periodically and to stand and walk frequently to encourage venous return.

Nursing Interventions for Altered Cardiovascular Function

Quality of life for the client with cardiovascular function often depends on teaching and support. Important areas for instruction include medication management, edema reduction, pain management, and energy conservation. The nurse also must be skilled at providing cardiopulmonary resuscitation (CPR) in an emergency.

Client Teaching
Teach the client with cardiovascular disorders to recognize warning signs of decreased CO or decreased perfusion. Signs and symptoms that indicate the need for medical help are listed in Display 35-3. Instruct the client in how to promote blood flow and reduce edema, promote skin integrity, and avoid fatigue.

Medications
The client with cardiovascular disease often must take numerous medications. The quality of the nurse's teaching can help promote client compliance with the medication regimen. Cardiovascular drugs are complex and may be confusing to the client. Therefore, it is beneficial to include the client's spouse or significant other in discussions concerning medications. Explain clearly the reasons for taking prescribed medications and provide written information. Explain drug effects, side effects, and special considerations to the client. Written information and schedules are also helpful so that clients have a reference if problems arise.

Simple yet accurate descriptions of each medication's action help the client appreciate and remember the importance of complying with the medication regimen. Also stress the importance of taking medications as ordered. Warn the client against missing doses or stopping a medication without consulting the physician. Be certain the client understands how and when to take medications, whether to avoid any foods or other substances (to prevent interactions), and what side effects to expect. Also teach the client to recognize signs of toxicity and when to contact the physician.

Often, multiple medications are necessary and regimens are complex and difficult to follow. To help with organizing, a small box with multiple compartments can be used to "load" in the day's or week's supply of medications. Side effects can be unpleasant and potentially serious, at times making compliance difficult. Many cardiovascular medications (e.g., antihypertensive agents, nitrates) can cause postural hypotension, potentially resulting in a fall or injury. Caution clients to get out of bed slowly and to avoid hot baths, which could increase vasodilation and syncope. Table 35-2 lists some drug classes that are commonly used to treat cardiovascular problems.

Edema Reduction
Peripheral edema can impede blood flow to the tissues. It is unsightly and often uncomfortable or painful for the client. Control of edema is an important nursing priority (Fig. 35-10).

Elevation of Limbs. One of the simplest measures for reducing edema is to elevate affected limbs. Limb elevation allows gravity to assist venous return to the heart and helps to decrease venous pressure, reducing fluid leakage from vessels and promoting its reabsorption. Vessels can reopen, and perfusion is improved.

Avoid causing venous constriction when elevating edematous limbs. The legs should be fully supported when elevated, and there must be no pressure points. Do not raise the client's leg so high that a constriction occurs at the groin. Do not elevate the hospital bed at the knees, because this restricts venous flow behind the knee.

Diet Teaching. The current dietary guidelines (AHA, 2001a) suggest restricting fat consumption to 30% of daily calorie intake. For most people, diets rich in saturated fats also increase the blood cholesterol level. The foods to be eaten in moderation are meat, animal fats, dairy products, and some vegetable oils (palm kernel oil, coconut oil, cocoa butter, and heavily hydrogenated margarine) (AHA, 2001a). Use lean cuts of meat, fish, and poultry, and eat small portions. The client should cook with small amounts of oil. Olive oil is a good choice because it is a monosaturated fat. The client should eat nonfat or skim milk products. Eat no more than three egg yolks per week, or use egg substitutes in place of eggs. The client should avoid eating fried foods.

The client with fluid retention problems usually benefits from a low-sodium diet. Because sodium molecules attract

(text continues on page 892)

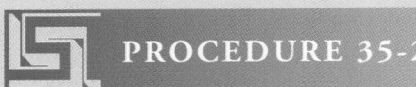

PROCEDURE 35-2

APPLYING A SEQUENTIAL COMPRESSION DEVICE (SCD)

Purpose
1. Promote venous return from legs to decrease the risk of deep vein thrombosis and pulmonary embolism in clients with reduced mobility.

Assessment
- Identify clients at increased risk for development of deep vein thrombosis.
- Assess skin integrity and identify any existing leg condition that would be exacerbated by use of the plastic sleeve or compression device. Clinical examples in which use of SCD is contraindicated are
  - Dermatitis, cellulitis
  - Postoperative vein ligation
  - Gangrene
  - Recent skin graft
  - Massive edema of legs
  - Extreme deformity of legs
  - Suspected or existing deep vein thrombus
- Verify physician order

Equipment
Antiembolism stockings
Measuring tape
Compression sleeves
Inflation unit

Procedure
1. Measure leg to ensure proper sleeve sizing.
   Note: Knee length—one size fits all; thigh length—measure length of leg from ankle to popliteal fossa. Measure circumference of thigh at the gluteal fold. Use the correct sleeve size, as follows: extra small (circumference, 22 inches; length, 16 inches); regular (circumference, 29 inches; length, 16 inches); extra large (circumference, 35 inches; length, 16 inches).
   Rationale: Proper sleeve size ensures proper fit and function of the sleeve.
2. Apply antiembolism stockings. Ensure that there are no wrinkles or folds (see Procedure 35-1).
   Note: Stockinette or Ace wraps are recommended options if client cannot be fitted with antiembolism stockings.
   Rationale: Wearing stockings decreases the risk of skin irritation and diaphoresis under the plastic sleeves.
3. Place client in supine position.
   Rationale: Proper positioning makes it easier to secure plastic sleeve.

4. Place a plastic sleeve under each leg so that the opening is at the knee. If only one sleeve is required, leave the other sleeve in package and connect to control unit.
   Rationale: Unit will not reach proper pressure if single sleeve is left to inflate in unconfined area.

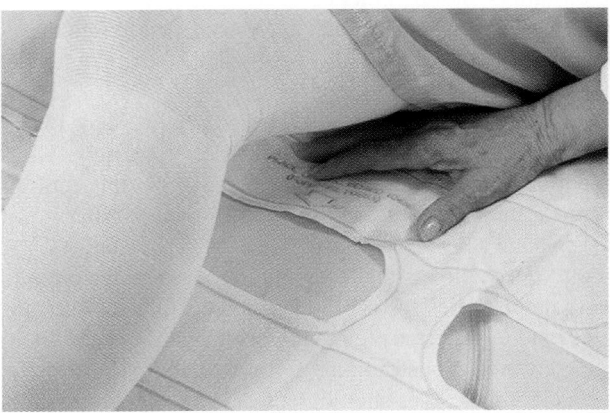

Step 4 Place plastic sleeve under leg.

5. Fold the outer section of the sleeve over the inner portion and secure with Velcro tabs. Check sleeve fit. Two fingers should fit between the sleeve and leg.
   Rationale: Proper fit prevents irritation to the leg and allows the unit to reach adequate inflation pressure.

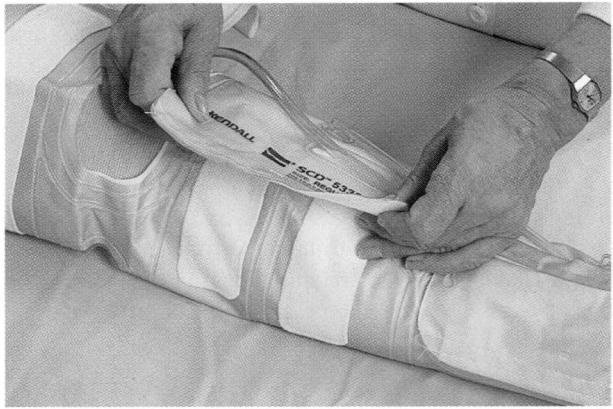

Step 5 Secure plastic sleeve around leg.

6. Connect tubing to control unit. The premarked arrows on the tubing from the sleeve and from the controller must be aligned to make adequate connection. Turn machine on.

PROCEDURE 35-2 (Continued)

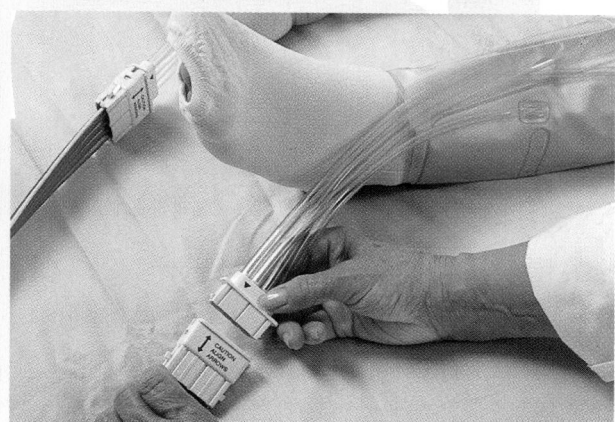

Step 6 Connect tubing to control unit.

> *Rationale: Control unit performs a system self-check.*

7. Adjust control unit settings as necessary. Unit control is preset with sleeve cooling in "off" position and audible alarm in "on" position. Sleeve cooling should be in "on" position at all times except during surgery. Ankle pressure should be set at 35–55 mm Hg.
   Rationale: Plastic sleeves can become warm and uncomfortable if cooling is in "off" position. Skin and stocking under sleeve can become wet with diaphoresis, which increases risk for impaired skin integrity. Cooling may be turned "off" during surgery to preserve warmth for the client.

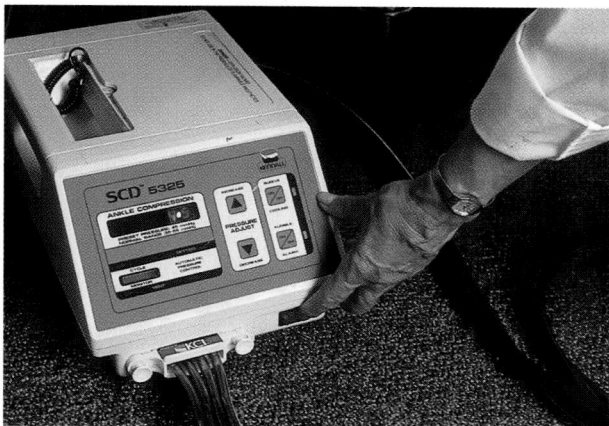

Step 7 Turn on control unit.

8. Recheck control unit settings whenever unit has been turned off.
   Rationale: The unit will convert to preset mode.
9. Respond to and promptly correct all "fault" indicator alarms. *Note:* The control unit will sense and indicate four pressure "fault" conditions: (a) pressure failed to drop to zero during the cycle; (b) the ankle pressure failed to reach 20 mm Hg for five consecutive cycles; (c) the ankle pressure exceeded 90 mm Hg; (d) internal diagnostics error has occurred.
   Rationale: Adequate functioning of unit is imperative to prevent complications.
10. Document time and date of application. If SCD is applied to only one leg, document reason.
11. Assess and document skin integrity every 8 hours.
    Rationale: Frequent assessment of skin integrity is necessary to prevent and provide early intervention in case of skin irritation.
12. Remove sleeves and notify physician if client experiences tingling, numbness, or leg pain.
    Rationale: These findings may indicate nerve compression.

Collaboration and Delegation

- Unlicensed assistive personnel frequently remove and then reapply SCDs as they help clients ambulate or shower. Check to ensure that SCDs are reapplied, so that clients do not experience long periods without SCD in place to promote circulation.

DISPLAY 35-3

□ SIGNS AND SYMPTOMS OF CARDIOVASCULAR DYSFUNCTION

Call Your Doctor When You Experience
- Unusual insomnia or extreme, prolonged fatigue after physical exercise
- Angina pain that does not subside with rest or after three nitroglycerin tablets taken 5 minutes apart (for clients who have documented chronic angina)
- Sudden confusion or incoordination
- Unusual fatigue

Call An Ambulance (911, If Available) When You Experience
- New discomfort in the chest, arms, neck, or jaw (if this is not a normal occurrence)
- Rapid, irregular, or unusually slow heart beat (if this is abnormal)
- Dizziness or fainting
- Severe pain and loss of normal color in an extremity (not caused by exposure to cold)

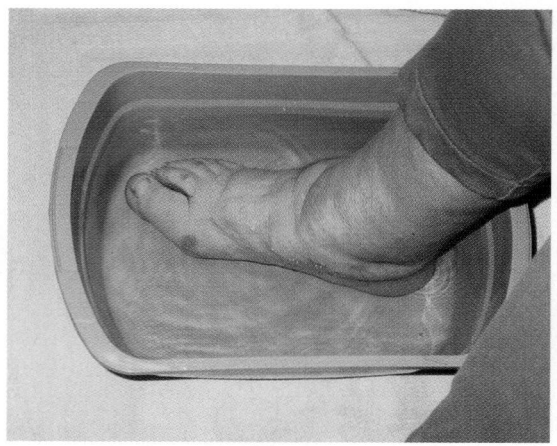

FIGURE 35-10 Foot care is very important for the client with edema or peripheral vascular disease. Note the edema and reddened areas that could easily break down.

water, limiting salt intake helps to control edema. Limiting use of table salt is a logical first step in a sodium-restricted diet, but the client also must understand "hidden" sodium content. Teach the client to look for sodium content on the labels of beverages, health products, over-the-counter medicines (es-pecially antacids), and foods. The client should avoid highly processed convenience foods. Spices and herbs can be used as a replacement for salt in cooking. Finally, encourage the client to discuss possible salt substitutes with the physician. Salt sub-stitutes contain potassium and should not be used by clients with renal failure.

Fluid Restriction. Clients who have fluid volume excess may restrict fluid intake until balance is restored. Monitor in-take and output carefully to assess fluid status. An intake

TABLE 35-2

Medications Affecting Cardiac Function and Tissue Perfusion			
Medications	**Example**	**Drug Action**	**Side Effects**
Cardiac glycoside	Digoxin	Increases cardiac contractility; decreases heart rate	Bradycardia, arrhythmias
Antihypertensive agents			
β-adrenergic blockers	Inderal	Decreases blood pressure	Low blood pressure, dizziness, syncope
Calcium channel blockers	Nifedipine		
Vasodilators	Apresoline		
Angiotensin-converting enzyme inhibitors	Captopril		
Vasopressor	Norepinephrine	Increases blood pressure	High blood pressure
Antiarrhythmic	Quinidine sulfate	Regulates heart rhythm	Hypotension, dizziness
Nitrates	Nitroglycerin	Relieves angina via peripheral vasodilation	Hypotension, headache
Antilipid agents	Lovastatin	Decreases cholesterol levels, reducing atherosclerosis risk	Nausea, bowel changes
Diuretics	Lasix	Reduces edema and fluid volume by increasing urinary output	Electrolyte imbalance (hypo-kalemia), volume depletion
Anticoagulants	Heparin Coumadin	Decreases potential for clot formation	Bleeding

more than 2 L (2,000 mL) greater than output suggests fluid retention. Weigh the client daily, preferably at the same time and ideally before breakfast. Weight should not vary by more than 1 kg (2.2 lb) per day.

Positioning

Body position affects cardiac work and tissue perfusion. The heart works harder in the supine position than in the upright position. Lying flat promotes venous return. Because all vessels are at the same level of the heart, gravity's effect on the blood is minimized. Blood can flow more freely into the venae cavae. The increased volume of blood entering the atria increases stroke volume.

Recommended positioning for a hypotensive client is with legs elevated 20 to 30 degrees (6 to 12 inches) to improve venous return and blood perfusion to vital organs. During this period, the hypotensive client also must receive specific treatment for the cause of the shock to ensure restoration of perfusion to all vital organs.

On a smaller scale, positioning can be used to improve perfusion to selected underperfused areas. Gravity enhances arterial flow. Allowing ischemic hands or feet to hang in dependent positions may improve perfusion; however, this measure is contraindicated in the edematous client.

Pain Management

Some clients with cardiovascular problems experience infrequent, relatively slight discomfort; others have constant debilitating pain. Some clients complain of chest tightness, pressure, or numbness and tingling in the neck and arm instead. Helping these clients to manage their ischemia is an essential nursing skill.

Chest Pain. When acute chest pain is evident, the client should stop all activity and rest, sitting comfortably; lying flat inhibits full chest expansion and limits gas exchange in the lung, so the client should avoid this position. The client should rest after an episode of pain. Document the pain's duration, activity during onset, and vital signs during the episode. Report this information to the physician.

🥛 SAFETY ALERT

Never ignore any client's complaints of chest pain or discomfort. Such feelings have many causes, but unless proven otherwise, chest pain in the cardiac client must be assumed to be a serious sign of cardiac hypoxia. As a student, chest pain is a situation in which you will want to get help right away.

Oxygen should be started as ordered. Administer sublingual nitroglycerin while the client is sitting or lying. Assess BP 5 minutes after giving this medication, because nitroglycerin is a vasodilator and the BP may fall. If the pain is not relieved after two repeat doses of nitroglycerin, notify the physician, or the family should call 911 or emergency services.

Clients with chronic angina can be helped primarily by assistance with activity management. They should learn to monitor their pulse rate and to pace activities to prevent increases of more than 20 beats/minute above the baseline rate. They should perform activities on an empty stomach whenever possible to avoid acute angina. Because blood is diverted to the gut after eating, less oxygen is available to the muscles, including the heart. For this reason, the nurse should not schedule procedures or activities, such as bathing or walking, immediately after meals. If sublingual nitroglycerin is ordered, the client may take a dose before performing an activity that has previously produced pain (Smeltzer & Bare, 2000).

Claudication and Peripheral Ischemic Pain. These categories of pain from peripheral vascular disorders are not life-threatening, but the discomfort they produce can be crippling. Cold surroundings, cigarette smoking, or activities that exceed individual tolerance may precipitate pain. Nursing measures to prevent such pain are directed at enhancing oxygen delivery to tissues by improving blood flow or decreasing oxygen demand. Exercise has been proven to reduce symptoms of claudication (Braun, Colucci, & Patterson, 1999) and can be an appropriate nursing intervention.

🥛 SAFETY ALERT

Chronically impaired perfusion of extremities can cause impaired perception of the sensation of heat. For this reason, the client with vascular disease is prone to burns. Exercise great care to avoid excessively hot soaks or compresses. Their temperature should not exceed 95° to 100°F (35°–38°C).

When a heating pad is used, it should be covered with a towel or pillowcase and not allowed to come into direct contact with the skin (Smeltzer & Bare, 2000).

Increased Activity

As part of rehabilitation after a heart attack or cardiovascular problem, activity begins slowly and progresses gradually. Initially, the client is sedentary with ambulation to the bathroom and up in the room. The client performs lower and upper range-of-motion exercises to maintain muscle tone and joint movement. He or she then progresses to sitting in the chair for meals and walking in the room. A sitting shower and short walking (100 to 250 feet) are then done if the client has tolerated previous activity. Finally, the client can perform independent activities; walking 100 to 250 feet three to four times daily is recommended. Monitor the client for ability to climb stairs without difficulty.

At home, healthcare providers and family members should encourage the client to start a walking program of 10 minutes/day at a slow, regular pace. Instruct the client to accommodate for hills, because they necessitate increased effort. Also, reinforce the concept that the client should plan to allow 5 minutes away and then 5 minutes back. He or she should increase time for walking as tolerated up to 1 hour. Within

THERAPEUTIC DIALOGUE
Cardiac Surgery

Scene for Thought
Jean Norman is a 77-year-old woman lying in her bed in the ICU with tubes and beeping monitors around her. She turns to the nurse, who approaches with an extra blanket that she had requested.

Less Effective

Client: Thank you for the blanket, dear. I'm so cold here. *(Speaks softly and weakly.)*

Nurse: How are you feeling otherwise, Ms. Norman? *(Arranges the blanket over her.)*

Client: Very tired and sore. I guess a bypass operation takes a lot out of you. *(Smiles weakly.)* But I'm sure it will turn out fine. *(Doesn't maintain eye contact.)*

Nurse: You seem to be doing just great—your vital signs are normal, your incisions are healing well, and everything else looks good. I don't think I've seen too many people recover from surgery this fast, honestly. Are you in much pain right now? *(Stands quietly by the bed and holds the client's hand.)*

Client: A little. If you have some time perhaps you could get me something? *(Still smiling.)*

Nurse: Right away, Ms. Norman. You only have to let me know. *(Smiles and gives her hand a warm squeeze.)*

Client: Thank you, dear. I appreciate it. *(Squeezes back.)*

More Effective

Client: Thank you for the blanket, dear. I'm so cold here. *(Speaks softly and weakly.)*

Nurse: How are you feeling otherwise, Ms. Norman? *(Arranges the blanket over her.)*

Client: Very tired and sore. I guess a bypass operation takes a lot out of you. *(Smiles weakly.)* But I'm sure it will turn out fine. *(Doesn't maintain eye contact.)*

Nurse: Tell me more about that. *(Stands at the bedside, looking at her.)*

Client: What do you mean, dear?

Nurse: You sound a little worried.

Client: *(Her eyes fill with tears, and she looks toward the hallway where her husband is sitting.)* Yes. I'm really worried if I'll be able to be as active as I was. *(Cries.)*

Nurse: *(Holds her hand, stands quietly by the bed.)*

Client: I know I'm being silly. People go through this operation all the time. *(Dries her eyes.)*

Nurse: It's usual for people to be worried. I'm glad you decided to share that worry with me.

Client: Do you think so? You don't think I'm being neurotic about this?

Nurse: I'm not sure what you mean by neurotic, but I know that you seem fearful, and sometimes talking about fears helps them become more manageable.

Client: That's true. *(She begins to talk about her fear of becoming an invalid and not being able to golf with her husband.)*

Critical Thinking Challenge
- Both nurses cared for Ms. Norman's needs. Compare and contrast the dialogues.
- What made the first dialogue less effective?
- Consider how the nursing assessment, diagnoses, and interventions differ between the first and second dialogues.
- Discuss which nursing outcome would be most effective in Ms. Norman's care.

---

2 to 3 weeks after the event, an outpatient cardiac rehabilitation program is recommended. Physical therapists and others progress and monitor more vigorous physical exertion and weight training.

Energy Conservation. Pain can occur when the client exceeds normal activity tolerance. Effective conservation of energy can promote activity tolerance and thus can help prevent pain.

Newly diagnosed clients with MI should avoid repeated movement of the upper arms. This movement increases the metabolic demands of the arm muscles, and forces the heart to pump harder for the blood to overcome gravity.

Warn the client against using the Valsalva maneuver, which occurs during bearing down. Air in the chest pushes against a closed glottis, raising intrathoracic pressure. This can suddenly increase BP while simultaneously hindering venous return. Activities involving lifting or pushing heavy objects and straining during bowel movements often involve the Valsalva maneuver. Instruct the cardiac client to avoid the stress this places on the heart by consciously maintaining a steady breathing pattern or exhaling slowly during such activities.

🗒 SAFETY ALERT
Remind cardiovascular clients to avoid isometric exercises, which tend to cause changes in blood pressure and heart rate.

The most important energy conservation measure for the client with acute cardiovascular problems is regular rest. Breathlessness or increased heart rate lasting for longer than

10 minutes after exercise indicates a need to go slower in the rehabilitation effort. Nocturnal insomnia or daytime fatigue also may mean that the previous day's exercise has been too strenuous. The client should rest undisturbed for 1 hour after meals. Encourage rest before and after activities such as bathing or when lengthy treatments are scheduled.

Space activities to avoid fatigue. Periods of work should alternate with rest or lighter activity. During activities, the client should sit whenever possible to avoid cardiovascular strain. When activities or tasks require gathering several materials, good planning is essential to eliminate unnecessary and inefficient or wasted effort. The client should immediately stop any activity that produces fatigue, breathlessness, pressure, or pain (Smeltzer & Bare, 2000).

Cardiopulmonary Resuscitation

Cardiac arrest is the most serious emergency that can occur. When a client's heart stops, acute hypoxia begins to destroy all tissues. Unless oxygenation is restored quickly, the victim will die. CPR is a means of artificially supporting circulation and oxygenation until the victim's heart begins beating on its own.

CPR is a systematic approach to life support that has been revised and refined over the years. Healthcare agencies usually require most or all personnel to be trained in basic life support (BLS). The ability to maintain a cardiac arrest victim's breathing and circulation with basic CPR skills is essential to the suc-

ETHICAL/LEGAL ISSUE
Client's Refusal of Treatment

Mrs. Chow, a competent 74-year-old client, lives in a retirement center. She has had congestive heart failure for the past 12 years. Her feet are swollen and painful when she walks on them. Difficult breathing from the heart failure limits her activity tolerance. When you enter her room to give her the "water pill," Lasix, she states, "I don't want to take it any more." You explain that the water pill is necessary to help her kidneys excrete the excess fluid. Her response is, "When I take it, I wet on myself. I would rather have my dignity than have that happen." Over the course of several days, her condition worsens to the point where she needs the Lasix to live. She continues to state that she would rather die with dignity than take the Lasix.

Reflection
- Identify the important issues in this case.
- Explore how your own feelings, values, and beliefs are the same or different from Mrs. Chow's.
- Consider your position. What is your role as a nurse in this situation?
- Target ways to work with the client to help her make choices about her healthcare and the outcomes.

cess of all resuscitation efforts. The Red Cross, American Heart Association, and other agencies offer classes for BLS certification. These courses can be completed in 1 day, often through the employing agency. Procedure 35-3 outlines basic CPR (AHA, 2001a).

Advanced cardiac life support (ACLS) requires extensive training and rigorous testing. People certified in ACLS are trained in ECG interpretation and advanced airway management. They are qualified to administer cardioactive drugs or electrical shock (defibrillation) as needed (AHA, 2001b).

Hospital resuscitation is often referred to as a "code" (e.g., cardiac arrests may be announced as "code 199" or "code blue"). The "code" team consists of physicians, nurses, pharmacists, and respiratory therapists. All members of the code team should be certified in ACLS.

The nurse may be the first person to discover a cardiac arrest victim. Knowing what to do before and after help arrives increases the chances for the victim's survival. Along with the techniques of CPR, nurses must be proficient in handling many duties at the scene of a cardiac arrest. The following discussion focuses on some important nursing aspects of CPR efforts in an agency with emergency equipment and trained responders. Each healthcare agency establishes specific cardiac arrest protocols, which usually are published in the nursing procedure manual. It is every nurse's responsibility to be familiar with these protocols.

Initial Management. After quickly establishing that an arrest has occurred, shout for help and press the emergency button (if available). If you are working alone in the home or community setting, establish unresponsiveness and then call the emergency response operator. Do not hang up until instructed by the operator. Continue CPR until the rescuers arrive. If a facility emergency response is available, alert the telephone operator. Dial the emergency number and announce to the operator, "There is a cardiac arrest on (location), room (number)." The operator can summon help using the paging system.

The nurse's first calls for help should bring other nurses to the room. They bring the emergency supplies ("crash cart"), while the first nurse begins preparations for CPR (Fig. 35-11). Whether or not assistance comes immediately, the discovering nurse must stay with the victim and continue to call for help until it arrives.

If the client has been sitting upright, lower the bed to a flat position. Move extra equipment away from the bed for easy access to the client. Remove the pillow from under the client's head. If the bed is elevated to stretcher level, lower it. Put the board or other hard surface under the client's chest. All these adjustments must be made as quickly as possible, and CPR must be initiated immediately. Other nurses can move the furniture from around the bed to make room for the crash cart, defibrillator, and ECG machine.

The Code Team. Management of a cardiac arrest usually requires no fewer than four people. The first team member is

(text continues on page 900)

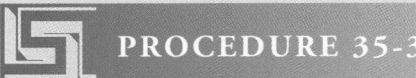

PROCEDURE 35-3

ADMINISTERING CARDIOPULMONARY RESUSCITATION (CPR)

Purpose
1. Restore cardiopulmonary functioning
2. Prevent irreversible brain damage from anoxia

Assessment
- Determine that the client is unconscious. Shake the client and shout at him or her to confirm unconsciousness rather than being asleep, intoxicated, or hearing impaired.
- Assess for presence of respirations.
- Assess carotid artery for pulse. *Note:* Presence of pulse *and* respiration contraindicates initiation of CPR.

Equipment
A hard surface: Client may be placed on floor, ground, or backboard.
No additional equipment is necessary, but in the hospital setting, an emergency (crash) cart with defibrillator and cardiac monitoring should be brought to the bedside. A crash cart usually contains:

- Airway equipment
- Suction equipment
- Intravenous equipment
- Laboratory tubes and syringes
- Prepackaged medications for advanced life support

Procedure
One Rescuer—Adult Client

1. Verbally ask, "Are you okay?" Assess to determine responsiveness. Shake gently.
   Rationale: Determine need for resuscitation.
2. Call for help or activate the emergency response system (911).
   Rationale: The majority of adults with sudden cardiac arrest are in ventricular fibrillation. Recent studies confirm that survival is linked to early access to defibrillation from emergency medical systems.
3. Turn client onto back while supporting head and neck. Place a cardiac board under the back or place client on the floor.
   Rationale: A firm surface is needed for adequate compression of the heart beneath the sternum.
4. Open the airway.
   a. Use a head tilt/chin lift maneuver.

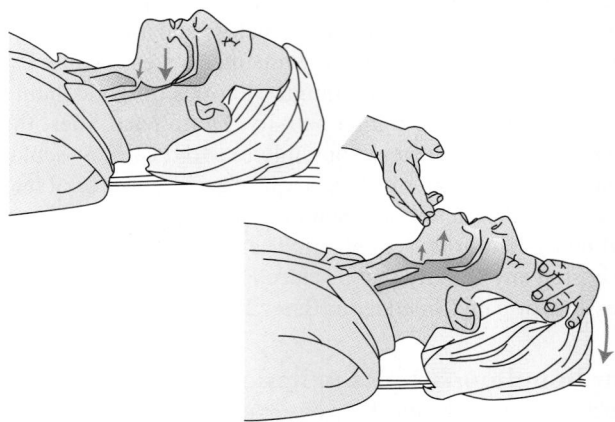

Step 4a Open the airway. Relieve airway obstruction by head tilt–chin lift maneuver.

   Rationale: Moving the jaw forward lifts the tongue away from the back of the throat and opens the airway.
   b. Use the modified jaw thrust if a neck injury is suspected.
   Rationale: Jaw thrust maneuver can be accomplished without extending the neck and exacerbating a potential neck injury.

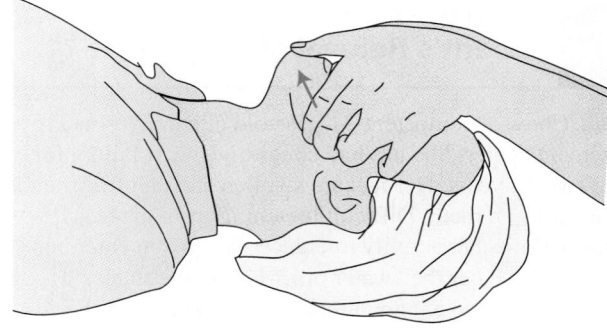

Step 4b Open the airway using jaw thrust maneuver.

5. Place your ear over client's mouth, and observe the chest for rising with respiration. Listen, look, and feel for breathing for 3 to 5 seconds.
6. Pinch the client's nostrils with thumb and index finger of hand holding the forehead.
   Rationale: Pinching the nostrils prevents air from escaping.
7. Take a deep breath, and place your mouth around the client's mouth with a tight seal. *Note:* If client wears dentures, they should remain in place to enable an airtight seal.

PROCEDURE 35-3 (Continued)

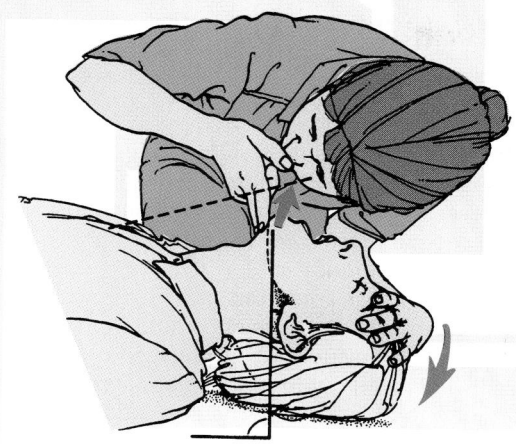

Step 5 Observe for breathlessness.

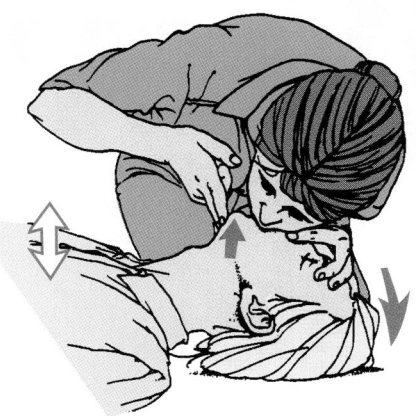

Step 7 Perform mouth-to-mouth breathing.

Rationale: Tight seal is required for effective ventilation.

8. Ventilate two slow breaths. Each breath should take 2 seconds to deliver. Pause between breaths to allow for lung deflation and to take another deep breath.
Rationale: Slow ventilations and complete exhalation between breaths decrease gastric distention, regurgitation, and aspiration.

9. If the victim is breathing but still unresponsive, turn on to side (recovery position).
Rationale: Modified lateral position maintains airway and spine alignment while allowing rescuer to observe victim.

10. Assess for carotid pulse for 5 to 10 seconds on the side next to which you are kneeling. Maintain head tilt with the other hand.

Rationale: The carotid is the most accessible, reliable, and easily learned location for checking the pulse in adults and children. The pulse area should be pressed gently to avoid compressing the artery. Serious medical complications may occur if chest compressions are performed on a person who has a pulse.

11. If client is pulseless, start chest compressions.
12. With the hand nearest client's legs, place middle and index fingers on lower ridge or near ribs, and move fingers up along ribs to the costalsternal notch (in center of lower chest).
13. Place middle finger on this notch and the index finger next to the middle finger on the lower end of the notch.

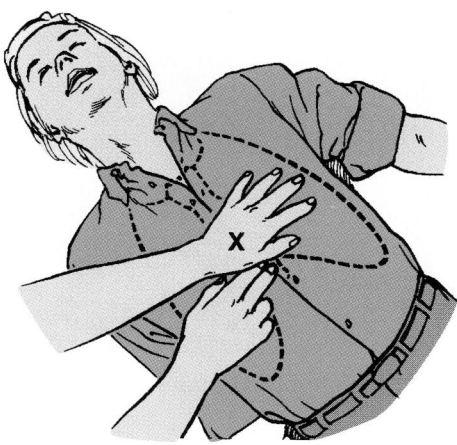

Steps 12 & 13 Find correct position for external chest compression.

14. Place heel of other hand along the lower half of the sternum, next to the index finger.
Rationale: Careful attention to hand placement during cardiac compression prevents fractured ribs and organ trauma.

15. Remove first hand from the notch and place heel of that hand parallel over the hand on the chest. Interlock fingers, keeping them off client's chest.
Rationale: This prevents trauma from pressure on the ribs.

16. Keeping your hands on sternum, extend your arms, locking the elbows, with your shoulders directly over the client's chest.
Rationale: Weight of your upper body and strength of both arms are needed for adequate cardiac compression. Placing your shoulders over client's chest provides additional muscle

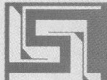

PROCEDURE 35-3 (Continued)

power and prevents hands from slipping off sternum and breaking ribs.

17. Press down on chest, depressing sternum 1.5 to 2 inches.

    Rationale: This depth is needed to compress the heart between sternum and vertebrae to pump blood out of heart.

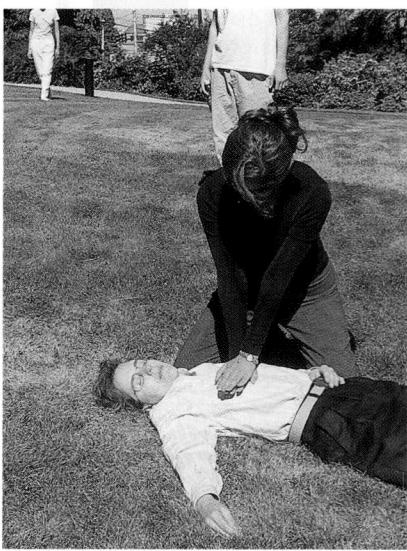

Step 17 Keeping shoulders over person's chest, depress sternum 1.5 to 2 inches.

18. Completely release compression while maintaining your hand position. Repeat in a smooth rhythm 100 times per minute. *Note:* Saying the mnemonic "one and two and . . . fifteen" may help maintain the rhythm.

    Rationale: Pressure on the sternum must be released between compressions to allow the heart to fill with blood. Leave your hands in position on the chest to prevent internal injury from malposition of the hands.

19. Ventilate with 2 full breaths after every 15 chest compressions.

20. Repeat 4 cycles of 15 chest compressions and 2 ventilations.

21. Reassess for carotid pulse. If client is pulseless, continue CPR. Reassess for carotid pulse every few minutes. *Note:* Never interrupt CPR for longer than 7 seconds.

Rationale: Stopping CPR can result in cerebral anoxia and brain damage.

Two Rescuers—Adult Client

1. When second rescuer arrives, the first rescuer stops CPR after completing two ventilations and assesses for a carotid pulse for 5 seconds.

2. The second rescuer moves into the chest compression position.

3. If pulselessness continues, the first rescuer states "no pulse" and delivers one ventilation.

4. The second rescuer begins chest compression while counting out loud, "one and two and three and four and five and." The compression rate is 100 per minute.

5. The first rescuer gives two slow ventilations after 15 chest compressions. The first rescuer also assesses carotid pulse during chest compressions to evaluate effectiveness.

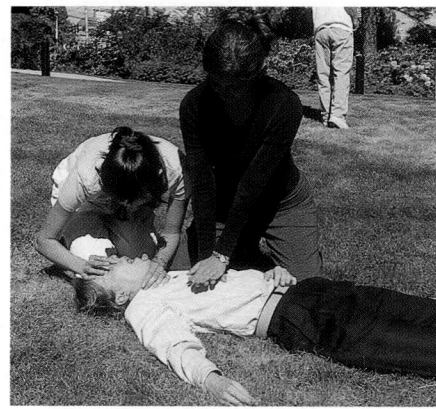

Steps 4 & 5 Two rescuers synchronize chest compression and ventilation.

6. If second rescuer wishes to change positions, he or she states, "Change, one and two and three and four and five and."

    Rationale: CPR can be tiring, and fatigue decreases effectiveness.

7. The first rescuer delivers the ventilation then moves into the chest compression position.

8. The second rescuer moves to the ventilator position and assesses for a carotid pulse for 5 seconds. If pulseless, resume CPR. *Note:* Do not interrupt CPR for more than 7 seconds.

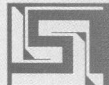

PROCEDURE 35-3 (Continued)

Rationale: Providing chest compressions is very fatiguing. Switching positions helps to ensure effective CPR efforts.

One Rescuer CPR—Infant or Child

1. Assess unresponsiveness.
2. If client is unresponsive, activate emergency response system (911) for children older than 8 years of age.
3. Place child on hard surface. Provide basic life support for 1 full minute before activating emergency medical system.
   Rationale: Airway obstruction and respiratory arrest are the most common causes of collapse in infants and young children. Early support is essential and should be attempted first.
4. Open the airway using head tilt/chin lift. Avoid overextension of head in infants.
   Rationale: Overextension of the head is thought to collapse the trachea in infants, causing an airway obstruction.
5. Place your ear over child's mouth, and observe chest for rise. Listen, look, and feel for breathing. *Note:* If airway obstruction from food or foreign object is suspected, perform Heimlich maneuver.
6. If breathlessness is determined, seal mouth and nose and ventilate twice (1 to 1.5 seconds for each breath). Observe for chest rise. *Note:* Infants and small children may require the rescuer to place mouth over the child's mouth and nose to establish an airtight seal.
7. Assess pulselessness by palpating for carotid artery on near side in children older than 1 year. In infants younger than 1 year, assess brachial or femoral pulse for 5 seconds.
   Rationale: Infants younger than 1 year have short, chubby necks, which make it difficult to assess the carotid pulse.
8. Begin chest compression if pulseless.
   a. For infant up to 1 year:
      (1) Visualize an imaginary line between the infant's nipples.
      (2) Place your index finger on the sternum just below this imaginary line.
      (3) Place your middle and fourth finger on sternum next to index finger. This is the location for cardiac compression.
   b. For child 1 to 8 years of age:
      (1) Placement of hand on sternum is the same as for adult CPR. Use heel of one hand to

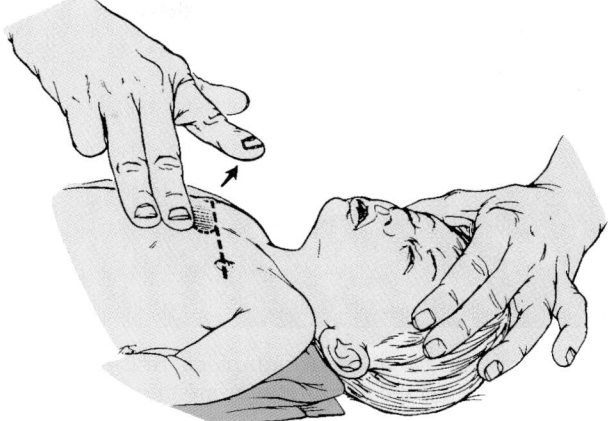

Step 8 Chest compression with fingers on infant up to 1 year old.

compress sternum 1 to 1.5 inches 100 times per minute.
      (2) Continue chest compressions, and ventilate at the rate of one breath to five compressions.
      (3) Continue CPR as for an adult.

Home Care Modifications

- Emphasize public education in the performance of CPR. CPR is a complex skill—be sure to address efforts to decrease the complexity for lay people.
- Place emphasis on teaching one-rescuer CPR, because lay people rarely use two-rescuer CPR.
- Nonphysicians who initiate CPR should continue resuscitation efforts until:
  – Spontaneous circulation and ventilation are effectively restored.
  – Another competent person is available to continue CPR.
  – A physician or physician-directed team assumes responsibility.
  – The rescuer is physically exhausted and unable to continue CPR.
- Automated external defibrillators (AED) are now available in highly populated areas such as malls, airplanes, and public gathering places. This device is easy to use with directions given. Usually designated personnel have been instructed in AED use. Prompt defibrillation decreases mortality and morbidity.

PROCEDURE 35-3 (Continued)

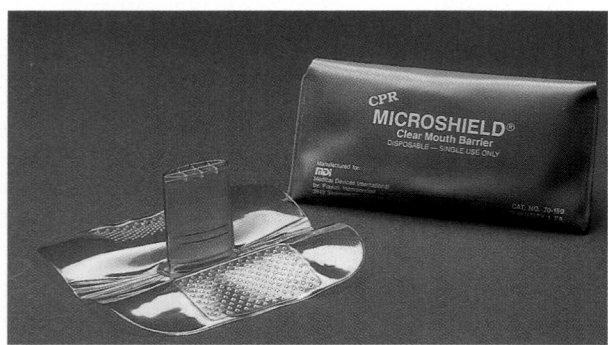

Home Care Modifications Mouthpiece for CPR, which people carry in the community for infection control purposes.

• A mouthpiece for CPR may be available for use in the community to promote infection control and decrease reluctance to perform mouth-to-mouth ventilation.

Collaboration and Delegation
• CPR, especially when performed in a healthcare facility, is a TEAM effort. Nurses often know clients the best and communicate information about them to other team members. Although the nurse is not always the team leader, he or she may be in a position to coordinate others, directing nursing assistants to obtain supplies or take samples to the laboratory.

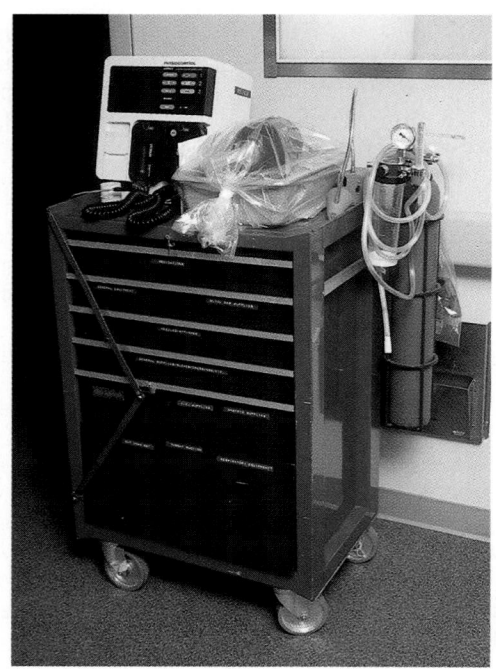

FIGURE 35-11   Crash cart contains emergency supplies and medications to manage a cardiac arrest.

responsible for establishing and managing the client's airway. This person is often a nurse anesthetist, anesthesiologist, or respiratory therapist. The second person performs chest compressions to maintain circulation. The third team member establishes IV lines and administers medications. The fourth member maintains an accurate record of medications and interventions and can help by retrieving needed supplies. Team members may switch roles during the resuscitation effort and take turns at compressions, which are especially fatiguing.

After Resuscitation Begins. Once the code team has taken charge, the nurse who discovered the person should remain with the team to provide essential information. The circumstances under which the person was found, the client's prearrest status, primary diagnoses, recent medications, and recent laboratory data are relevant. The nurse also may be needed to assist with procedures. The person in charge assigns specific duties to members of the code team. Those who are not actively participating in the resuscitation efforts should leave the room and care for other clients.

Consideration of privacy is important. If another client shares the room, he or she should be moved elsewhere if possible. If moving the roommate is not practical, the curtain should be drawn, and a nurse should stay with the roommate. This client may be anxious; answer his or her questions honestly.

Finally, one of the most difficult tasks for the nurse is dealing with the sorrow and fears of the victim's loved ones. These people need support during and after the resuscitation. Provide honest information, but do not speculate on the client's condition. Recent studies have demonstrated the benefit of having family members present during resuscitation efforts (Myer et al., 2000). Family presence during invasive procedures and resuscitation has been endorsed by the Emergency Nurses Association based on this research.

Healthcare Planning and Home or Community-Based Nursing

Most cases of cardiovascular dysfunction are managed in the community (Ludwig, 1998). Hospital stays for acute episodes, such as MI or open-heart surgery, have decreased dramatically in length during the last decade. Many other less acute problems are diagnosed in ambulatory settings and completely managed at home.

Community-based care often focuses on prevention, especially among high-risk people. On routine examination, if a client is found to be overweight, to be sedentary, to smoke, or to have high cholesterol levels, lifestyle modification education is appropriate. Often detection of elevated cholesterol or hypertension is significant motivation for making necessary changes. Follow-up is important for these clients (Goodwin, 1999) (Fig. 35-12).

Cardiac Rehabilitation

For many clients, cardiovascular problems need not permanently prevent them from enjoying a normal lifestyle. The purpose of rehabilitation is to help the cardiovascular client restore or improve lost function. This goal depends on physical endurance, which is improved by graded physical activity. Therefore, although rest is an essential part of the management of cardiovascular problems, activity also must play a part. Exercise may be a more important intervention for women, because it reduces BP and produces improvements in the lipid profile (Glassberg & Balady, 1999).

Promotion of activity tolerance starts after the medical problem has been identified and treated. Next, a functional

---

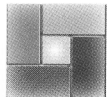

Nursing Research and Critical Thinking
When Someone is Assigned to Watch the Cardiac Monitors at All Times, Is the Mortality Rate Reduced?

A group of critical care nurses wanted to know if it is necessary to have someone watching the telemetry monitors at all times, or if it is sufficient for nurses to rely on alarms to alert them to the presence of dysrhythmias. These nurses conducted a quasi-experimental study in a 26-bed cardiac progressive care unit at an 875-bed university hospital. The nurses reviewed the medical records of 2,383 clients. For a 9-month period in 1993 when the unit had a dedicated monitor watcher, outcomes for 1,185 clients were evaluated. For a similar 9-month period in 1994 when no dedicated monitor watcher was present, outcomes for 1,198 clients were evaluated. Chi-square and *t*-test analyses were used to compare baseline characteristics between the clients in the unit when a monitor watcher was present and when no monitor watcher was present. Multivariate analysis with logistic regression was used to control for pertinent demographic and clinical variables if significant differences ($P < .05$) were found. The study showed that the presence of a monitor watcher was not associated with lower rates of most adverse outcomes evaluated. However, fewer episodes of sustained ventricular tachycardia occurred when a monitor watcher was present.

Critical Thinking Considerations. A randomized clinical trial would result in a monitor watcher group and a non-monitor watcher group that would have more similar baseline characteristics than was present in this study. Differences between the groups in this study are confounding variables and make the results less reliable. Implications relevant to nursing practice are as follows:

- In this sample of almost 2,400 acutely ill cardiac clients, there was an unexpectedly low frequency of adverse outcomes: 10 deaths, 7 instances of asystole, and 6 episodes of ventricular fibrillation. The small number of these outcomes provided insufficient statistical power to detect differences between the two groups.
- The decrease in the number of RNs, a decline in opportunities for inservice education, and increase in the proportion of unlicensed personnel and "float" nurses without cardiac experience working in progressive care units as a result of managed care may lead to very different findings if this study were to be repeated today.

From Funk, M., Parkosewich, J. A., Johnson, C. R., & Stukshis, I. (1997). Effect of dedicated monitor watchers on patients' outcomes. *American Journal of Critical Care, 6*(4), 318–323.

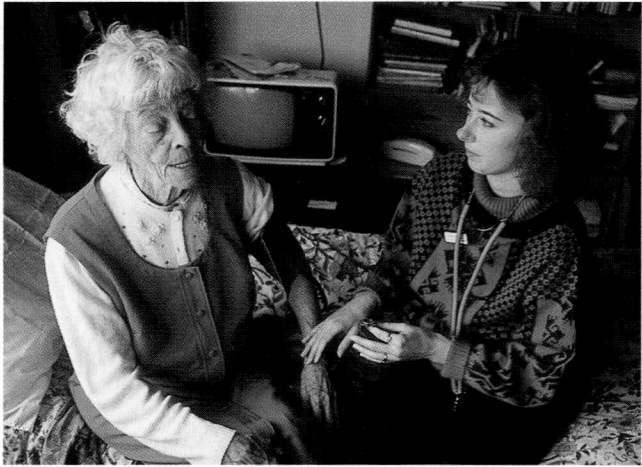

FIGURE 35-12   Monitoring blood pressure in the home may be necessary for some elderly clients. (Courtesy of Seattle University School of Nursing and Yesler Terrace.)

APPLY YOUR KNOWLEDGE

You are a home health nurse visiting Mr. Brown. He has recently had a heart attack, followed by emergency open heart surgery for blocked coronary arteries. He tells you that he has been feeling tired lately. He has been trying to eat right, remember his medications, and walk. Every time he tries to move, his chest is painful. His wife says that he has stopped buttering his bread and is taking naps frequently during the day. Explain what you will do next, and provide your rationale.
Check your answer in Appendix A.

assessment of the client is conducted. Only after the client's physical, mental, and emotional readiness for rehabilitative measures have been thoroughly assessed can appropriate measures be implemented.

Exercise should be part of a continuing rehabilitation program after the client's discharge from the hospital. A program of gradual progressive exercise is prescribed by the physician. The nurse should teach the client about safe exercise practices at home. Warm-up exercises prevent sudden demands on the heart; cool-down exercises help prevent pooling of blood in the legs. Clients should not exercise in extremes of weather, nor within 1 hour after a meal. They should avoid isometric exercises, because they involve the Valsalva maneuver.

Instruct the client to recognize untoward symptoms of overexertion, such as palpitations or fluttering in the chest, racing pulse, pain, and pressure. Teach the client how to take the pulse using the carotid or radial sites. The client should stop activity if the pulse rate exceeds the specific target zone prescribed by the physician. If the pulse lowers with activity, if it becomes irregular, or if the heart rate does not return to its resting level within 10 minutes after exercise, the client should contact the physician.

Patience is essential for the client and the nurse; neither should try to hurry the rehabilitation process. Exercise must be graduated, with more strenuous activities being added to the regimen only as client tolerance allows. Warn the client against thinking, "If this much exercise is good, twice as much will cure me in half the time." Exercise can provide several valuable physiologic and psychological benefits to the client with cardiovascular disease, but it is not a cure-all. Exercise is one facet of a holistic approach to regaining health. Adherence to prescribed medical therapies, reduction of stress, and modification of lifestyle risk factors are vital parts of any successful rehabilitation program.

A common area of concern for the client during rehabilitation is the possible impact such limitations will have on sexual function. After cardiac surgery or an MI, sexual activity

may be limited for about 6 to 8 weeks until recovery permits more strenuous activity. Another common concern is the fear that another serious cardiac episode may occur during sexual activity. This can create much stress for the client and his or her sexual partner. Instruct the client to use positions that require less energy expenditure (e.g., side-lying, supine), to participate when well rested, to avoid sexual activity after a large meal or heavy consumption of alcohol, and to stop and rest if any chest pain occurs (Smeltzer & Bare, 2000).

Emergencies
The client and family members need to be knowledgeable concerning emergency situations. In clients with a history of pain, nitroglycerin should always be available so that it can be quickly administered if chest pain occurs. Nitroglycerin breaks down over time and with exposure to light. The prescription should be refilled whenever it has passed the expiration date to ensure potency in case an emergency occurs. If after three doses, administered 5 minutes apart, the chest pain persists, the client or a family member should notify 911 or emergency community services. The client should not attempt to drive to the hospital. All family members should complete a BLS course and be able to administer CPR (AHA, 2001a).

EVALUATION

Clients with cardiovascular dysfunction show widely variable rates of progress. For this reason, specific goals for these clients must be individualized. Together, the nurse and client can establish realistic goals with appropriate outcome criteria for measuring goal attainment.

Goal

The client will demonstrate adequate knowledge concerning cardiovascular dysfunction prevention or care.

Possible Outcome Criteria

The following should occur by the end of the teaching session:

- The client demonstrates an understanding of cardiovascular risk factors by reciting those that apply and discussing their physiologic effects.

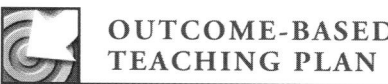

OUTCOME-BASED TEACHING PLAN

George Porter, a 54-year-old executive, is being discharged from the telemetry unit following a myocardial infarction. He and his wife have both expressed concern that an emergency could arise when they return home. They want to be prepared to handle such an emergency.

OUTCOME: Mr. and Mrs. Porter can verbalize how to recognize and treat anginal pain.
Strategies
- Provide handout explaining angina and its treatment.
- Review medications (names, dosages, when to take, special considerations) for each new medication that has been ordered.
- Provide above information about medications in writing and have client restate it.
- Stress the necessity for rest when Mr. Porter feels any pain or pressure to see if it subsides.
- Instruct Mr. Porter to space oxygen-consuming activities (e.g., don't exercise right after eating).
- Review specifics regarding PRN nitroglyceride. Have Mr. and Mrs. Porter reverbalize.

OUTCOME: Mrs. Porter can verbalize when to call 911 and develop a plan to become proficient in CPR.
Strategies
- Discuss with Mr. and Mrs. Porter their plan for handling a cardiac emergency (unrelieved chest pain and cardiac arrest).
- Explore Mrs. Porter's comfort with performing CPR on her husband if needed.
- Assess Mrs. Porter's specific plans for taking a community course to learn CPR.
- Provide a written list of when to call 911 (unrelieved chest pain; new onset of rapid, irregular, or very slow heart rate, especially if accompanied by severe fatigue or dizziness; fainting or loss of consciousness).
- Provide a sticker with emergency numbers for the Porters to keep on the phone.

- The client describes a specific plan and timetable for modifying his or her cardiovascular risk factors.
- The client states the following for any medication administered for cardiovascular problems: name, action, and side effects of the drug; dose to be taken; and any special considerations for administration.
- The client describes the rationales for prescribed therapies.
- The client lists and describes signs or symptoms of acute or emergency situations.

Goal

The client will demonstrate adequate tissue perfusion with adequate oxygenation of body tissue.

Possible Outcome Criteria

The following will occur within 48 hours after initiation of nursing interventions:

- The client reports absence of severe ischemic pain and improvement in comfort.
- The client demonstrates improved color and temperature of extremities.
- The client demonstrates improved activity tolerance by experiencing decreasing pain with ambulation.

Goal

The client will effectively cope with changes in self-concept and lifestyle.

Possible Outcome Criteria

The following will occur by the second home visit:

- The client verbalizes how his or her cardiovascular condition has caused life changes.
- The client identifies support people from whom he or she can derive emotional strength.
- The client demonstrates energy conservation measures, evidenced by sitting while dressing and planning rest periods.
- The client discusses realistic plans concerning return to work and other normal activities.

KEY CONCEPTS

- Good cardiovascular function depends on a healthy heart to pump blood, an adequate blood volume, and healthy blood vessels to distribute blood to tissues.
- Tissue perfusion, or the flow of blood through the tissues of the body, is essential for cell viability. Tissue perfusion depends on adequate functioning of the cardiovascular system to supply body tissues with oxygen and to remove waste products.
- Normal cardiovascular function usually produces a pulse rate between 60 and 100 beats/minute, a BP between 100/60 and 140/90 mm Hg, and an absence of pain on exertion.
- Cardiovascular function is affected by age, gender, race, exercise, high BP, smoking, nutrition, obesity, and medical and family history.
- Altered cardiovascular function can occur when the heart is less effective as a pump (e.g., dysrhythmias, muscle damage, valve dysfunction); when the blood vessels are not able to deliver blood adequately to the tissues (atherosclerosis, vein problems, clots, emboli); or when abnormalities occur within the blood (anemia, low blood volume).
- Manifestations of altered cardiovascular function include changes in vital signs, changes in the color or temperature of the skin, decreased CO, altered blood flow to vital organs, and decreased tissue perfusion.
- Cardiovascular dysfunction can have a great impact on a person's ability to perform ADLs and may necessitate lifestyle changes.
- The nurse is instrumental in promoting optimal cardiovascular health by teaching risk modification for the general public.
- Nursing measures that can help maximize cardiovascular health and prevent complications include risk factor modification,

NURSING PLAN OF CARE

THE CLIENT WITH ACTIVITY INTOLERANCE

Nursing Diagnosis

Activity Intolerance related to an imbalance between oxygen supply and demand manifested by verbal reports of fatigue or weakness; abnormal heart rate or blood pressure response to activity; exertional discomfort or dyspnea.

Client Goal

Client will balance activity with physical limitations.

Client Outcome Criteria

- Client's heart rate has regular rhythm and remains between 60 and 100 beats/min at rest. (Values may require adjustment for clients with chronic cardiovascular or pulmonary problems.)
- Client's heart rate rises in proportion to level of activity and does not exceed an increase of 20 beats/min.
- Client's blood pressure remains within normal limits for age group; fluctuations with position are minimal.

Nursing Intervention	Scientific Rationale
1. Limit activity 1 hr after meals.	1. Blood flow is directed to digestive tract to aid digestion; increases workload on the heart.
2. Plan heavy activities (e.g., morning hygiene, ambulation) to alternate with rest period of 1 to 2 hr.	2. Careful scheduling allows for uninterrupted rest period. Spacing activity conserves energy and avoids activity intolerance.
3. Offer prescribed nitroglycerin before activity or when pain develops with activity.	3. Nitrates vasodilate, decreasing venous return and decreasing cardiac workload.
4. Monitor pulse, blood pressure, and respiratory rate before, during, and after activity.	4. Sudden changes in vital signs indicate activity intolerance and provide a parameter for scheduling activity.
5. Gradually increase activity within physician's activity order.	5. Gradual increase in activity level helps client build endurance and better tolerate increased activity.

Client Goal

Client will effectively cope with necessary lifestyle and activity changes.

Client Outcome Criteria

- Client demonstrates energy-conserving measures, as evidenced by sitting while dressing and planning rest periods during hospital stay.
- Client discusses realistic plans concerning return to work and other normal activities by end of hospital stay.

Nursing Intervention	Scientific Rationale
1. With client, establish a plan for day's activity schedule.	1. Offering opportunity to plan activity periods increases client's feeling of control.
2. Educate client regarding signs of activity intolerance (e.g., shortness of breath, increased heart rate).	2. Knowledge of symptoms of activity intolerance helps client identify activity tolerance and manage own activity level.
3. Encourage goal-setting for future activity periods (i.e., "Next time, what would you hope to be able to do for yourself?").	3. The goal-directed client is in greater control of situation. Communicates confidence that progress will occur.
4. Explore with the client inventive ideas to conserve energy (e.g., doing tasks from a chair rather than standing; sitting in shower).	4. Conservation of energy increases energy available for other, more important activities and increases independence.

prevention of venous stasis, client teaching, edema reduction, positioning, pain management, increased activity, and energy conservation.

- Cardiac arrest is a medical emergency for which CPR must be quickly and effectively performed to prevent morbidity and mortality.

REFERENCES

Al Suwaidi, J., Higano, S. T., Holmes, D. R., Lennon, R., & Lerman, A. (2001). Obesity is independently associated with coronary endothelial dysfunction in patients with normal or mildly diseased coronary arteries. *Journal of American College of Cardiology, 37*(6), 1523–1528.

American Heart Association. (2001a). *BLS for Healthcare Providers.* Dallas, TX: Author.

American Heart Association. (2001b). *ACLS Provider Manual.* Dallas, TX: Author.

Arnold, E. (1997). The stress connection: Women and coronary disease. *Critical Care Nursing Clinics of North America, 9*(4), 565–575.

Braun, C. M., Colucci, A. M., & Patterson, R. B. (1999). Components of an optimal exercise program for the treatment of patients with claudication. *Journal of Vascular Nursing, 17*(2), 32–36.

Copsead, L. C., & Banasik, J. L. (2000). *Pathophysiology: Biological and behavioral perspectives* (2nd ed.). Philadelphia: W. B. Saunders.

Coyne, K. S., & Allen, J. K. (1998). Assessment of functional status in patients with cardiac disease. *Heart & Lung, 27*(4), 263–273.

Emerson, R. J. (2000). Alterations in blood pressure. In L. C. Copsead, & J. L. Banasik (Eds.). *Pathophysiology: Biological and behavioral perspectives,* (2nd ed.).

Fallon, E. M., & Roques, J. (1997). Acute chest pain. *AACN Clinical Issues, 8*(3), 383–397.

Fichera, L. V., & Andreassi, J. L. (1998). Stress and personality as factors in women's cardiovascular reactivity. *International Journal of Psychophysiology, 28*(2), 143–155.

Gensini, G. F., Comeglio, M., & Colella, A. (1998). Classical risk factors and emerging elements in the risk profile for coronary artery disease. *European Heart Journal, 19,* (Suppl. A), A53–A61.

Glassberg, H., & Balady, G. J. (1999). Exercise and heart disease in women: Why, how, how much? *Cardiology Review, 7*(5), 301–308.

Goodwin, B. A. (1999). Home cardiac rehabilitation for congestive heart failure: A nursing case management approach. *Rehabilitation Nursing, 24*(4), 143–147.

Hahn, I. H., & Hoffman, R. S. (2001). Cocaine use and acute myocardial infarction. *Emergency Medicine Clinics of North America, 19*(2), 493–510.

Henshaw, C. M. (2000). Alterations in blood pressure. In L. C. Copsead, & J. L. Banasik, *Pathophysiology: Biological and behavioral perspectives* (2nd ed.).

Jaffe, A. S. (1997). Troponin, where do we go from here? *Clinical and Laboratory Medicine, 17*(4), 737–752.

Jarvis, C. (2000). *Physical Examination and Health Assessment,* (3rd ed). Philadelphia: W.B. Saunders.

Johnson, P., Chaboyer, W., Foster, M., & van der Vooren, R. (2001). Caregivers of ICU patients discharged home: What burden do they face? *Intensive Critical Care Nursing, 17*(4), 219–227.

Lane, P. (1997). Cardiac electrophysiology studies and ablation procedures: A literature review. *Intensive Critical Care Nurse, 13*(4), 244–249.

Levy, D., Sheppard, L., Checkoway, H., Kaufman, J., Lumley, T., Koenig, J., & Siscovick, D. (2001). A case-crossover analysis of particulate matter air pollution and out of hospital primary cardiac arrest. *Epidemiology, 12* (2), 193–199.

Lichtenstein, A. H., et al. (1998). Dietary fat consumption and health. *Nutrition Review, 56*(5, Pt 2), S3–S9.

Limacher, M. C. (1998). Exercise and rehabilitation in women: Indications and outcomes. *Cardiology Clinics, 16*(1), 27–36.

Ludwig, L. M. (1998). Cardiovascular assessment for home healthcare nurses. Part 1: Initial cardiovascular assessment. *Home Healthcare Nurse, 16*(7), 450–456.

Markovic, T. P., et al. (1998). Beneficial effect on average lipid levels from energy restriction and fat loss in obese individuals with or without type 2 diabetes. *Diabetes Care, 21*(5), 695–700.

McGrath, A., & Cox, C. L. (1998). Cardiac and circulatory assessment in intensive care units. *Intensive and Critical Care Nursing, 14,* 283–287.

Meyers, T. A., Eichhorn, D. J., Guzzetta, C. E., et al. (2000). Family presence during invasive procedures and resuscitation. *American Journal of Nursing, 100*(2), 32–42.

Minchoff, L. E., & Grandin, J. A. (1996). Syndrome X: Recognition and management of this metabolic disorder in primary care. *Nurse Practitioner, 21*(6), 74–75, 79–80, 83–86.

Murphy, M. J., & Berding, C. B. (1999). Use of measurements of myoglobin and cardiac troponins in the diagnosis of acute myocardial infarction. *Critical Care Nurse, 19*(1), 58–66.

North American Nursing Diagnosis Association (NANDA). (2000). *Nursing diagnoses: Definitions and classification 2001–2001.* Philadelphia: Author.

Pagana, K. D., & Pagana, T. J. (1997). *Mosby's diagnostic and laboratory test reference* (3rd ed.). St. Louis: Mosby.

Smeltzer, S. C., & Bare, B. G. (2000). *Brunner and Suddarth's textbook of medical-surgical nursing.* Philadelphia: Lippincott.

Utell, J. J., & Frampton, M. W. (2000). Acute health effects of ambient air pollution: The ultrafine part hypothesis. *Journal of Aerosol Medicine, 13*(4), 355–359.

Walker, D. J. (1999, Sept/Oct). Venous stasis wounds. *Orthopaedic Nursing,* 65–95.

Weber, J., & Kelley, J. (1998). *Health assessment in nursing* (pp. 940–943). Philadelphia: Lippincott-Raven.

Wingate, S. (1997). Cardiovascular anatomy and physiology in the female. *Critical Care Nursing Clinics of North America, 9*(4), 447–452.

Zafari, A. M., & Wenger, N. K. (1998). Secondary prevention of coronary heart disease. *Archives of Physical Medicine Rehabilitation, 79*(8), 1006–1017.

BIBLIOGRAPHY

American Heart Association. (2001). *BLS for Healthcare Providers.* Dallas, TX: Author.

American Heart Association. (2001). *ACLS Provider Manual.* Dallas, TX: Author.

Arnstein, P. M., Buselli, E. F., & Rankin, S. H. (1997). Women and heart attacks: Prevention, diagnosis, and care. *Nurse Practitioner, 21*(5), 57–58, 61–64, 67–69.

Brennan, A. (1997). Efficacy of cardiac rehabilitation 2: Smoking and behaviour modification. *British Journal of Nursing, 6*(13), 737–740.

Dougherty, C. M. (1997). Reconceptualization of the nursing diagnosis Decreased Cardiac Output. *Nursing Diagnosis, 8*(1), 29–36.

Fagerberg, B., et al. (1998). Mortality rates in treated hypertensive men with additional risk factors are high but can be reduced: A randomized intervention study. *American Journal of Hypertension, 11*(1, Pt. 1), 14–22.

Fish, F. F., Smith, B. A., Frid, D. J., Christman, S. K., Post, D., & Montalto, N. J. (1997). Step treadmill exercise training and blood pressure reduction in women with mild hypertension. *Progress in Cardiovascular Nursing, 12*(1), 4–12.

Frantz, A. K. (1999). Exploring expert cardiac home care nurse competence and competencies. *Home Healthcare Nurse, 17* (11), 706–717.

Gay, S. (1999). Meeting cardiac patients' expectations of caring. *Dimensions in Critical Care Nursing, 18*(4), 46–50.

Ide, B., & Drew, B. J. (1998). Cardiac arrhythmias with aging. *Progress in Cardiovascular Nursing, 13*(4), 31.

Kernicki, J. G. (1997). A multicultural perspective of cardiovascular disease. *Journal of Cardiovascular Nursing, 11*(4), 31–40.

Lazzara, D., & Sellergren, C. (1996). Chest pain emergencies: Making the right call when the pressure is on. *Nursing '96, 26*(11), 42–53.

McAvoy, J. A. (2000). Cardiac pain: Discover the unexpected. *Nursing 2000, 30*(3), 34–39.

McCarron, D. A., et al. (1998). Comprehensive nutrition plan improves cardiovascular risk factors in essential hypertension. *American Journal of Hypertension, 11*(1, Pt. 1), 31–40.

McGrath, A., & Cox, C. L. (1998). Cardiac and circulatory assessments in intensive care units. *Intensive Critical Care Nurse, 14*(6), 283–287.

Pittman, K. P., & Hayman, L. L. (1997). Determinants of risk for cardiovascular disease during school-age/adolescent transition. *Progress in Cardiovascular Nursing, 12*(4), 12–22.

Roberts, C., & Banning, M. (1998). Risk factors for hypertension and cardiovascular disease. *Nursing Standard, 12*(22), 39–42.

Smeltzer, S. C., & Bare, B. G. (2000). *Brunner and Suddarth's textbook of medical-surgical nursing* (8th ed.). Philadelphia: Lippincott-Raven.

Stewart, J. J., Hirth, A. M., Klassen, G., Makrides, L., & Wolf, H. (1997). Stress, coping, and social support as psychosocial factors in readmissions for ischaemic heart disease. *International Journal of Nursing Studies, 34*(2), 151–163.

Thurau, R. (1997). Perceived gender bias in the treatment of cardiovascular disease. *Journal of Vascular Nursing, 15*(4), 124–127.

Vogele, C. (1998). Serum lipid concentrations, hostility, and cardiovascular reactions to mental stress. *Internal Journal of Psychophysiology, 28*(2), 167–179.

Woods, S. L., Froelicher, S. S., Motzer, S. U. (1999). *Cardiac nursing*. Philadelphia: Lippincott.

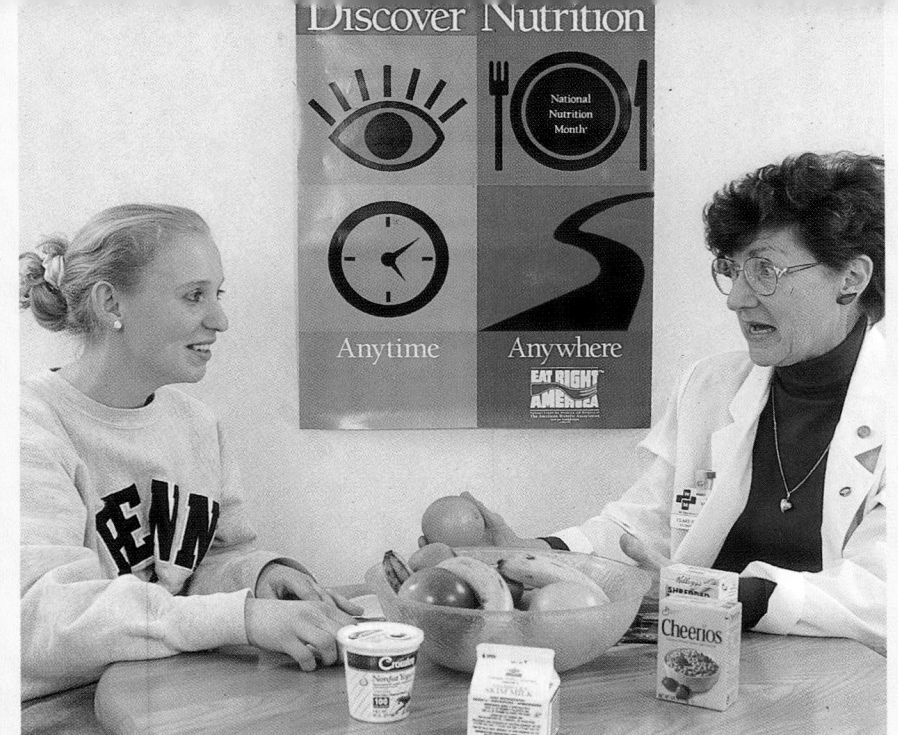

Discover Nutrition

National Nutrition Month*

Anytime   Anywhere

EAT RIGHT AMERICA

Cheerios

Unit 9

Nutrition and Metabolism

36 Fluid, Electrolyte, and Acid-Base Balance

⑤ Key Terms

acid
active transport
anion
baroreceptor
base (or alkali)
buffer
cation
diffusion
electrolyte
extracellular fluid
filtration
hyperosmolar
hypertonic

hypoosmolar
hypotonic
interstitial fluid
intracellular fluid
intravascular fluid
ion
milliequivalent
osmolality
osmolarity
osmosis
osmotic pressure
tonicity

⑤ Learning Objectives

Upon completion of this chapter, the student will be able to do the following:

1. Describe physiologic factors that affect fluid, electrolyte, and acid–base homeostasis.
2. Discuss common alterations in fluid, electrolyte, and acid–base balance.
3. Explain the impact of age on fluid and electrolyte status.
4. Describe assessment parameters for the client with potential or actual fluid and electrolyte imbalances.
5. Identify appropriate nursing diagnoses for clients with fluid imbalance.
6. Implement appropriate client teaching to prevent or to manage fluid and electrolyte imbalance.

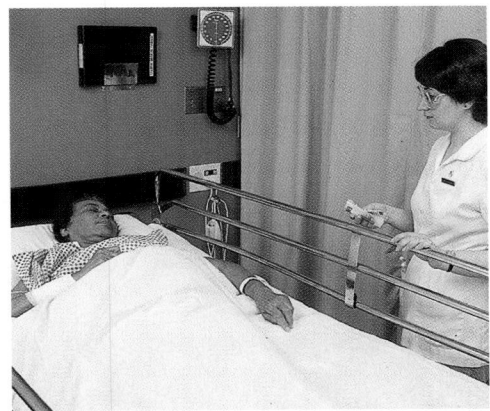

⑤ Critical Thinking Challenge

You are a student nurse working on a medical unit. One of your assigned clients has a diagnosis of pneumonia. During shift change, you are told that the client has had diarrhea for the last 4 days, accompanied by a 4-lb weight loss. She has been experiencing fever and chills, and she has had 150 mL of urine output during the last shift. The laboratory called with the following results: serum Na⁺, 128 mEq/L; serum K⁺, 4.1 mEq/L; blood urea nitrogen, 28 mg/dL; and blood glucose, 326 mg/dL. What is your client's fluid balance status? What tentative nursing diagnoses would you make? What further data should you collect to confirm or alter your tentative diagnoses? What nursing interventions may be indicated?

Once you have completed this chapter and have incorporated fluid, electrolyte, and acid–base balance into your knowledge base, review the above scenario and reflect on the following areas of Critical Thinking:

1. Summarize the information about this client's extracellular fluid (ECF) volume, water balance, and electrolyte balance.
2. Based on this information, make a tentative nursing diagnosis for each of the following: ECF volume status, water balance, and electrolyte balance. Describe what additional data for each you need to confirm or correct your nursing diagnoses.
3. Propose types of oral fluids you would offer this client to drink, and give your reasons.
4. Discuss your safety concerns for this client, and outline how you would plan her care to ensure safety.
5. Plan what teaching you would do today and before the client is discharged.

Health and normal body functioning depend on fluid, electrolyte, and acid–base balance. Vascular fluid is essential for the maintenance of adequate blood volume, blood pressure, and cardiovascular system functioning. Interstitial fluid, which surrounds the body's cells, is important for the transportation of oxygen, nutrients, hormones, and other essential chemicals between the blood and the cell cytoplasm. Both vascular and interstitial fluids also are important for waste removal. Intracellular fluid is critical for maintaining cell size and function. Optimal cell function depends on maintaining the volume and composition of body fluids within a narrow, normal range.

The balance of fluids, electrolytes, acids, and bases within the body is regulated by physiologic control mechanisms. Common activities, such as participating in vigorous exercise, can upset this precise balance if the body is not capable of making adjustments. Healthy adults and children are able to compensate for such physiologic challenges. For example, on a hot summer day, most people increase their fluid intake as a result of thirst, and their urine volume decreases. At the same time, changes in respiratory rate and urine composition play an important role in regulating acid–base balance.

Problems such as vomiting and diarrhea, or therapies such as surgery, can temporarily disrupt fluid, electrolyte, and acid–base homeostasis despite general good health. Sustained vomiting or diarrhea, for example, may require intervention by a healthcare professional to replace lost fluid and electrolytes. Diseases such as heart failure, kidney impairment, or liver dysfunction seriously disrupt the body's ability to maintain fluid, electrolyte, and acid–base balance. People with such medical problems are in constant danger of potentially life-threatening excesses or deficits.

Nurses play a vital role in promoting normal fluid, electrolyte, and acid–base balance and in preventing life-threatening imbalances. Client teaching about the importance of adequate food, fluid, and electrolyte intake and managing common problems such as fever, vomiting, and diarrhea can prevent imbalances. Nursing assessment of fluid, electrolyte, and acid–base balance is essential for early detection of imbalances so that appropriate interventions can begin promptly. Interventions such as promoting appropriate fluid intake, assisting with eating, monitoring intravenous (IV) infusions, and administering medications can all help to maintain fluid, electrolyte, and acid–base balance.

NORMAL FLUID AND ELECTROLYTE BALANCE

Body fluid is water containing chemical compounds called electrolytes plus blood cells and other soluble molecules. Within the body this fluid is contained within compartments or spaces. The body monitors and controls two aspects of body fluid balance:

- The volume of fluid in the extracellular space
- The water concentration (osmolarity) of all body fluids

People can experience an excess or deficit of either or both of these aspects of body fluid.

Fluid Compartments

Approximately 45% to 80% of body weight is fluid. This percentage varies depending on age, body fat, and gender (Table 36-1). Fat contains proportionately less fluid than muscle, so heavier people have relatively less fluid than leaner people. Women have a lower fluid content because they have more adipose tissue than men. Fluid accounts for 46% to 52% of body weight in adult women and 52% to 60% of body weight in adult men. Infants have a greater proportion of body fluid than adults do.

Body fluid is distributed into two major compartments: **intracellular fluid** (ICF), located within the cells, and **extracellular fluid** (ECF), comprising all the fluid outside the cells. Each compartment varies in electrolyte composition (see later discussion) and in location. The primary ICF electrolytes are potassium, phosphate, and sulfate. The primary ECF electrolytes are sodium, chloride, and bicarbonate. Adults have about two thirds of their total fluid within the ICF and one third in the ECF (Fig. 36-1). In contrast, newborns have more ECF than ICF; by 3 months of age, infants have equal amounts of ICF and ECF, and by 1 year they approach the same distribution as adults (Metheny, 2000).

The ECF is divided between **intravascular fluid,** the fluid inside the blood and lymphatic vessels, and **interstitial fluid,** the fluid between the cells. The maintenance of the proportional distribution of ECF between the vascular and interstitial spaces depends on three factors:

- Protein content of the blood (serum proteins, mainly albumin and globulin)
- Integrity of the vascular endothelium (the layer of cells lining blood vessels)
- Hydrostatic pressure inside the blood vessels

The protein content of the blood and vascular endothelium function to keep fluids within the blood vessels, whereas the

TABLE 36-1

Variations in Total Body Fluid According to Age and Sex	
Age	Total Body Fluid (% Body Weight)
Newborn (premature)	85%
Newborn (full-term)	70%–80%
Child (1–12 yr)	64%
Puberty to 39 yr	Male: 60%
	Female: 52%
40–60 yr	Male: 55%
	Female: 47%
Older than 60 yr	Male: 52%
	Female: 46%

From Metheny, N. (2000). *Fluid and electrolyte balance: Nursing considerations* (4th ed.). Philadelphia: Lippincott.

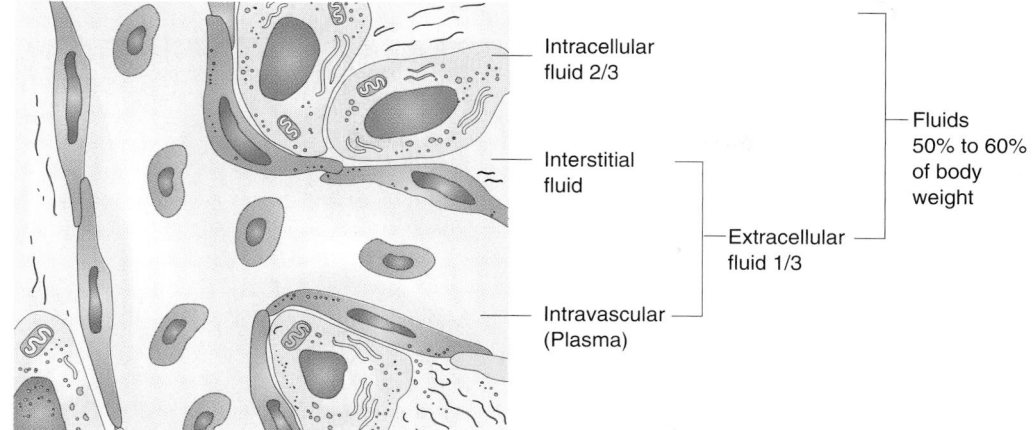

FIGURE 36-1 Fluid compartments, showing intracellular fluid and extracellular fluid (which contains intravascular and interstitial fluid). Total body fluid is 50% to 60% of body weight in adults.

hydrostatic pressure tends to force fluid out of the vessels. In healthy people, these forces are equally balanced so that approximately one third of the ECF volume is intravascular and two thirds is interstitial.

Extracellular Fluid Volume

The volume of ECF is the most important and regulated aspect of fluid balance. Without an adequate volume of ECF, blood pressure cannot be maintained. Prolonged periods of very low blood pressure are known as shock, a potentially lethal condition.

Stretch receptors, known as pressure receptors or **baroreceptors** and located in major arteries and veins, monitor ECF volume. The renin-angiotensin-aldosterone and natriuretic peptide hormone systems regulate ECF volume within narrow limits by adjusting fluid intake and the urinary excretion of sodium, chloride, and water.

Decreased arterial blood pressure, decreased renal blood flow, increased renal sympathetic nerve activity, and/or a low-salt diet can stimulate renin release. Renin, an enzyme secreted by juxtaglomerular cells in the kidney, splits angiotensinogen, produced by the liver and circulating in the blood, into angiotensin I. Converting enzymes in the lungs and other vascular beds convert angiotensin I into angiotensin II, a potent vasoconstrictor. Angiotensin II stimulates secretion of aldosterone. Aldosterone, produced by the adrenal cortex, regulates sodium reabsorption in the distal tubules and collecting ducts of the kidney. Chloride and water passively accompany the reabsorbed sodium, resulting in the reabsorption of saline, a 0.9% solution of sodium chloride, which is ECF.

Atrial natriuretic peptides (ANP) are produced by the cardiac atria, ventricles, and other body parts in response to changes in ECF volume. When atrial pressure is increased, ANP released by the atrial and ventricular myocytes acts on the nephron to increase sodium excretion. Low atrial pressures inhibit release of ANP (Levin, Gardner & Samson, 1998).

Water Concentration (Osmolarity) of Body Fluid

The second regulated aspect of body fluid balance is osmolarity. **Osmolarity** refers to the proportion of dissolved particles (solute) in a volume of fluid. **Osmolality** refers to the concentration of dissolved substances in a given weight of fluid (e.g., a kilogram), rather than in a given volume. Osmolarity is expressed in milliosmols per liter (mOsm/L), whereas osmolality is expressed in milliosmols per kilogram (mOsm/kg). Because body fluids are very dilute, these terms are often used interchangeably. The normal range for osmolarity is from 280 to 300 mOsm/L.

Hypothalamic osmoreceptor cells monitor changes in body fluid osmolarity and respond by varying the secretion of antidiuretic hormone (ADH) from the posterior pituitary. Some clinicians identify disorders of body osmolarity as disorders of body water balance, whereas others refer to these imbalances as hyponatremia or hypernatremia, because an excess or deficit of water directly influences the concentration of sodium. Sodium, its accompanying anions, and glucose are the predominant osmotically active particles in the ECF.

ADH is produced in the supraoptic and paraventricular nuclei of the hypothalamus. From these nuclei, ADH passes down axons into the posterior lobe of the pituitary, where it is stored. When plasma osmolarity increases and activates the hypothalamic osmoreceptors, ADH is released into the systemic circulation. ADH maintains the blood's osmolarity within normal limits by adjusting the amount of water excreted in the urine. The hormone acts by causing pore-like molecules called aquaporins to be inserted into the luminal membranes of the distal tubules and collecting tubules in the kidney, thus making them more permeable to water. This increased permeability allows more water reabsorption and serves to conserve water in the body. When ADH is increased, the urine becomes more concentrated. Conversely, if plasma osmolarity is decreased due to an excess of water in relation to solute, ADH release is inhibited. Water permeability of the distal tubules and collecting ducts is decreased. Less water is reabsorbed, causing the urine to be more dilute. Water is lost from the body, subsequently causing plasma osmolarity to increase.

When the ECF volume is normal, changes in plasma osmolarity control ADH release. However, when arterial blood pressure is markedly diminished (e.g., heart failure, shock), ADH is released regardless of plasma osmolarity in response to input from the vascular baroreceptors (Abraham & Schrier, 1994).

Electrolytes

Electrolytes are chemical compounds that partially dissociate (or separate) in solution into separate particles. These particles carry electrical charges and are known as **ions.** Positively charged ions are referred to as **cations,** and ions that have a negative charge are referred to as **anions.** Biologically important cations include sodium (Na^+), potassium (K^+), calcium (Ca^{++}), and magnesium (Mg^{++}). Chloride (Cl^-), phosphate ($HPO_4^=$ and $H_2PO_4^-$), sulfate ($SO_4^=$), and bicarbonate (HCO_3^-) are common anions. As previously mentioned, the concentration of each of these electrolytes is very different in the ICF and ECF compartments. The most common electrolytes in the ECF are sodium, chloride, and bicarbonate, whereas potassium, phosphate, and sulfate are the most common electrolytes in ICF.

Electrolytes are measured in terms of their combining power, or the ability of cations to combine with anions, rather than by their absolute weight in solution. The **milliequivalent** is the measure of this chemical activity. The amount of electrolyte in a solution is most commonly expressed in terms of milliequivalents per liter (mEq/L). For example, 1 mEq of Mg^{++} will combine with 2 mEq of Cl^-.

Maintaining electrolyte balance refers to keeping the concentration of each electrolyte in the serum within normal limits. Electrolyte imbalance refers to an increase or decrease of the concentration of ions within the serum. Because the concentration of cellular electrolytes cannot be measured clinically, the healthcare worker relies on changes in the serum levels to reflect body electrolyte imbalance. Normal serum electrolyte ranges for the adult are given in Table 36-2. Normal values vary slightly between laboratories. Whenever possible, monitoring of trends in electrolyte concentration over time provides more information about a client's status than a single laboratory value.

Sodium

Sodium is the most abundant cation in the ECF. Normal serum sodium levels range from 135 to 145 mEq/L. Changes in the serum sodium level reflect changes in body water balance or osmolarity and therefore do not reflect sodium intake and output directly. The kidneys excrete sodium from the body. Sodium, along with chloride, and a proportionate volume of water (normal saline) are regulated by the renin-angiotensin-aldosterone system and the natriuretic peptides.

Sodium is found in table salt (sodium chloride), dairy products, meat, eggs, and certain vegetables; food processing also

TABLE 36-2

Normal Serum Electrolyte Values	
Electrolyte	**Serum Value**
Cations	
Sodium (Na^+)	135–145 mEq/L
Potassium (K^+)	3.5–5.0 mEq/L
Calcium (Ca^{++})	4.3–5.3 mEq/L
	(8.9–10.1 mg/dL)
Magnesium (Mg^{++})	1.5–1.9 mEq/L
	(1.8–2.3 mg/dL)
Anions	
Chloride (Cl^-)	95–108 mEq/L
Bicarbonate (HCO_3^-)	22–26 mEq/L
Phosphate ($HPO_4^=$, $H_2PO_4^-$)	1.7–2.6 mEq/L
	(2.5–4.5 mg/dL)

Normal value ranges may vary slightly from laboratory to laboratory.

tends to add salt in the preserving process. Food labels list the number of milligrams of sodium in a serving of product. Some medications also contain significant amounts of sodium.

Potassium

Potassium is essential for normal cardiac, neural, and muscle function and contractility of all muscles. Potassium also plays an important role in cellular functions, such as protein and glycogen synthesis. Normal serum potassium ranges from 3.5 to 5.0 mEq/L (Tannen, 1996).

Two hormones exert major control over the extracellular concentration of potassium: insulin and aldosterone. Insulin, a pancreatic hormone, promotes the transfer of potassium (and also glucose) from the ECF into skeletal muscle and liver cells. Aldosterone enhances renal excretion of potassium. An increase in serum potassium stimulates the release of insulin and aldosterone to lower the concentration of the ion. Conversely, a decrease in serum potassium inhibits the release of aldosterone and insulin to reduce excretion of the ion.

A person loses approximately 30 mEq of potassium per day, while a typical Western diet contains 50 to 100 mEq/day (Tannen, 1996). The kidneys play the major role in the maintenance of potassium balance, varying excretion with daily intake. Potassium also is excreted from the body in stool and perspiration.

Calcium

Normal serum calcium levels range between 8.9 and 10.1 mg/dL (Kumar, 1996). Approximately 99% of the body's calcium is found within the bones and teeth. The remainder is in the serum. Calcium is present in the blood primarily in two states: ionized and bound to protein. Approximately 50% is ionized, with the remainder bound to proteins, mainly albumin, or complexed with other ions. The level of ionized calcium is most important for physiologic function. Because a large portion of the calcium is bound to albumin, the serum albumin levels should be checked when laboratory data are evaluated. If serum albumin levels are decreased, which may happen with liver disease or wasting, the total calcium level will probably also be decreased but the ionized calcium level may be within normal limits. Measurement of the ionized calcium level, which is normally 4.75 to 5.3 mg/dL, is required to determine whether calcium replacement is required (Kumar, 1996). Calcium usually has a reciprocal relationship with phosphorus.

Calcium is indispensable for healthy functioning. The cell membrane structure depends on calcium, which promotes cell-to-cell adhesion. Calcium also is important in wound healing, synaptic transmission in nervous tissue, membrane excitability, muscle contractility, and teeth and bone structure. Calcium is essential for blood clotting and is critical in metabolic reactions involved in energy production (glycolysis).

Parathyroid hormone (PTH), along with vitamin D and calcitonin, regulates calcium and phosphate balance. PTH causes serum calcium levels to increase by increasing intestinal and renal reabsorption of calcium and releasing calcium from bone. PTH increases calcium levels but decreases serum phosphate levels. Conversely, decreased secretion of PTH lowers serum calcium levels and increases the serum phosphate concentration.

The number of good dietary sources for calcium is limited. Dairy products (e.g., milk, cheese, yogurt) are excellent sources. Sardines, whole grains, and leafy green vegetables also contribute calcium. Food labels indicate the percentage of the daily value of calcium contained in a serving.

Magnesium

The normal serum magnesium level ranges from 1.5 to 1.9 mEq/L. Fifty to sixty percent of magnesium is in bone; much of the rest is in soft tissue and body fluids. Like potassium, magnesium is primarily an intracellular ion, with only 1% in the ECF (Rude, 1996). Magnesium is important in regulating neuromuscular function and cardiac activity. Alterations in magnesium are often paralleled by changes in potassium, and the signs and symptoms of a deficit of either ion are similar. In addition, a magnesium deficiency is often accompanied by hypocalcemia (Rude, 1996). The kidney regulates magnesium levels by reabsorbing the ion when serum levels are low and excreting it when serum levels are high. Good dietary sources of magnesium include green leafy vegetables, legumes, citrus fruit, peanut butter, and chocolate.

Phosphorus

The normal serum phosphorus level in adults ranges from 2.5 to 4.5 mg/dL. Serum levels are higher in children and even higher in infants. Approximately 85% of phosphorus is in bone, 14% is in the ICF, and only 1% is in the ECF (Cogan, 1991). In the plasma, phosphorus exists in the dibasic ($HPO_4^=$) and monobasic ($H_2PO_4^-$) forms. Blood levels of these phosphates are controlled by the regulation of renal excretion under the influence of vitamin D and PTH. Phosphorus is im-

portant in energy metabolism, structure of bones and membranes, and synthesis of nucleic acids (RNA and DNA). There is often, but not always, a reciprocal relation between body phosphorus and calcium levels. Good dietary sources of phosphorus include dairy products, meats, vegetables, fruits, and cereals.

Fluid and Electrolyte Distribution

Movement of fluid, electrolytes, nutrients, and waste products between compartments is constant. The membranes of individual cells, the vascular capillary walls, and the lymphatic capillary walls are semipermeable. Water and some electrolytes move easily across these semipermeable membranes. Larger molecules, such as proteins, are less able to move across capillary walls. Fluid movement occurs primarily by osmosis and filtration. Electrolytes and other dissolved particles move by means of diffusion, filtration, and active transport. Hydrostatic pressure and oncotic pressure are important determinants of fluid filtration between the ECF and ICF spaces.

Processes of Fluid and Electrolyte Movement

Diffusion. **Diffusion** is the movement of a solvent or solutes (molecules) from an area of higher solvent or solute concentration to an area of lower solvent or solute concentration. Molecules are in constant motion. If a drop of highly concentrated solution is placed in one side of a container of fluid, the molecules will bounce off each other until they are equally distributed throughout the solution.

Diffusion is an important process in maintaining electrical neutrality. *Electrical neutrality,* a state in which the numbers of anions and cations are balanced within each fluid compartment, is the normal condition within compartments. If any compartment contains an excess of cations, then an identical number of anions must diffuse into the compartment to balance the charge. The opposite is true if an excess of anions is present: a sufficient number of cations will diffuse into the compartment to balance the electrical charge and ensure neutrality.

Osmosis. **Osmosis** refers to the movement of a fluid through a semipermeable membrane. A semipermeable membrane allows some substances to travel through but not others. Osmosis can occur if a semipermeable membrane separating two fluid compartments is permeable to water, and if one compartment contains a greater concentration of a dissolved substance (**hyperosmolar**) than the other compartment (**hypoosmolar**). Water passes through the membrane to the area of greater concentration of the dissolved substance. The net effect of osmosis is to equalize solution concentrations on both sides of the membrane. The principle to remember is that, given a semipermeable membrane, water always moves in the direction of greater concentration of dissolved particles. Another way to think of water movement is that water moves down its concentration gradient from areas where there is more water (dilute or hypoosmolar fluids) to areas where there is less water (concentrated or hyperosmolar fluids). Capillary vessel walls and cell walls are semipermeable membranes.

Active Transport. **Active transport** is the process by which ions and other molecules move across membranes from an area of lesser concentration to an area of greater concentration. Energy is required to move ions against a concentration gradient. Enzymes, such as sodium–potassium adenosine triphosphatase (Na,K-ATPase), are involved in active transport. A specific carrier molecule binds with each ion transported against the concentration gradient. The carrier and the attached ion move across the semipermeable membrane and then separate. Decreasing the cell's temperature, decreasing the supply of glucose and nutrients available to the cell, and exposing the cell to medications or toxins can inhibit active transport.

The process of active transport can be illustrated by the functioning of the body's sodium–potassium pump (Fig. 36-2). A higher concentration of sodium ions is present in ECF (135 to 145 mEq/L), whereas the concentration of sodium in the ICF is lower (10 mEq/L). Sodium ions diffuse across the cell membrane into the cell down this concentration gradient. Without Na,K-ATPase, intracellular sodium would continue to rise and cell function would be disrupted. The sodium–potassium pump prevents sodium from accumulating inside cells by actively transporting sodium out. The difference in concentration between sodium and potassium in intracellular and extracellular compartments is essential for the resting membrane potential, action potential initiation, nerve impulse propagation, and muscle contraction.

Filtration. **Filtration** involves the transfer of water and dissolved substances through a permeable membrane from a region of high pressure to a region of low pressure. Hydrostatic pressure, or the pressure exerted by fluid against the walls of its container, promotes the flow of fluid out of the capillaries (Fig. 36-3). Filtration occurs within the kidney's glomerular capillaries and in blood capillaries.

Pressures Affecting Fluid and Electrolyte Movement

Osmotic Pressure and Tonicity. **Osmotic pressure,** the force of attraction for water by undissolved particles, helps to keep fluid within blood vessels, opposing net flow outward. Plasma proteins contribute to the osmotic pressure because they are hydrophilic, which means they attract water. The term for the osmotic pressure that is produced by plasma proteins is *colloid oncotic pressure.* Osmotic pressure depends on the solution's osmolarity.

Fluids can differ in osmolarity depending on the concentration of their solutes. The major extracellular substances that contribute to the movement of water between the ECF and cell cytoplasm are sodium, chloride, and glucose. A solution that has the same osmotic pressure or osmolarity as blood plasma is called isoosmotic.

Solutions are also categorized in relation to their **tonicity,** a term that refers to the fluid's effect on cell size. When an isotonic solution enters the circulation, there is no net movement of water across membranes, so cells retain their normal size. Normal saline (0.9%) is an isotonic solution. A **hypotonic** solution has a concentration of solute that is less than that of blood plasma. When a hypotonic solution (e.g., water) surrounds cells, water crosses the membrane into the cells, causing them to swell. The opposite is true for a hypertonic solution. In a **hypertonic** solution, the effective concentration of solute is greater than that of the blood plasma. When a hypertonic solution such as 3% sodium chloride (hypertonic saline) is infused, water leaves cells, causing them to decrease in size (Fig. 36-4).

All fluids that are hypoosmotic are also hypotonic, *but* not all fluids that are hyperosmotic are also hypertonic. Whether

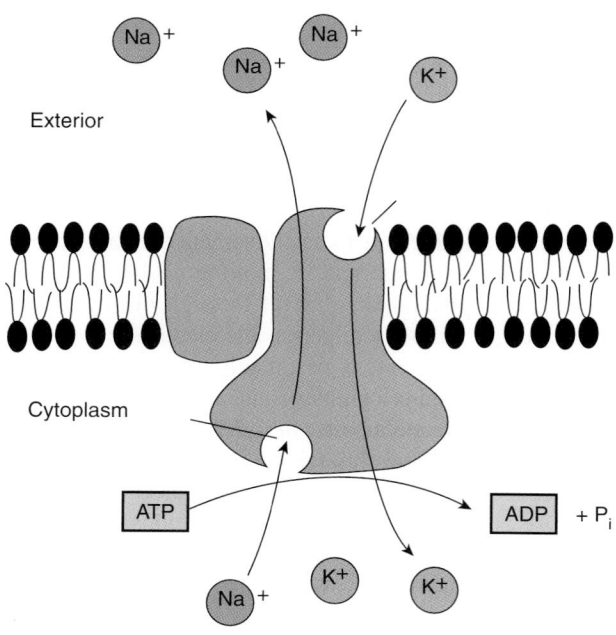

FIGURE 36-2   Sodium–potassium pump. Energy provided by ATP causes sodium to move to the outside of the cell and potassium to move to the inside of the cell. For every molecule of ATP, three molecules of sodium are transported out and two molecules of potassium move into the cell.

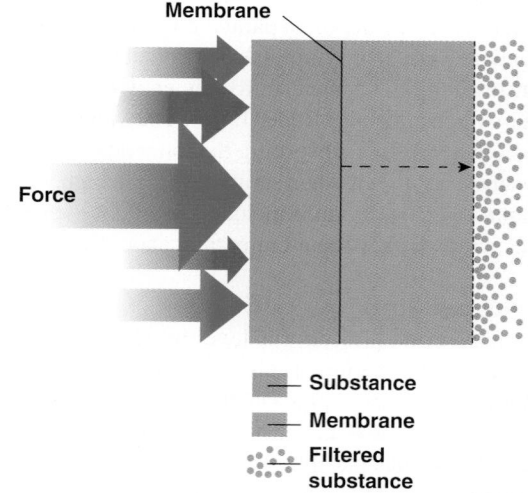

FIGURE 36-3   Filtration. A mechanical force pushes a substance through a membrane.

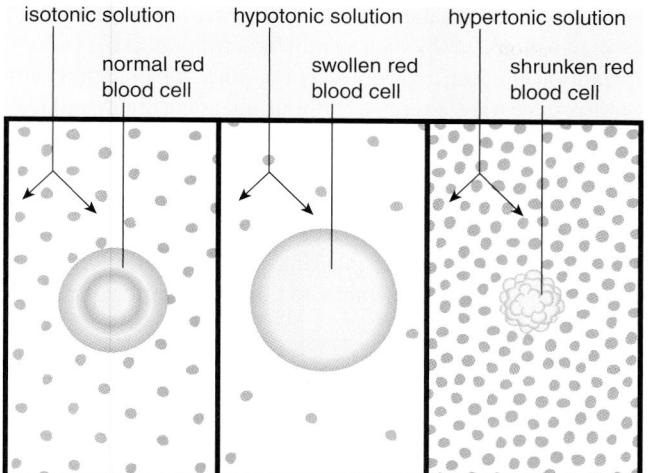

isotonic solution   hypotonic solution   hypertonic solution
normal red   swollen red   shrunken red
blood cell   blood cell   blood cell

FIGURE 36-4   Osmosis. Water molecules moving through a red blood cell membrane in three different concentrations of fluid. (*Left*) The normal saline solution has a concentration nearly the same as that inside the cell, and water molecules move into and out of the cell at the same rate. (*Center*) The dilute solution causes the cell to swell and eventually hemolyze (burst) because of the large number of water molecules moving into the cell. (*Right*) The concentrated solution causes the water molecules to move out of the cell, leaving it shrunken.

a hyperosmotic fluid is also hypertonic depends on the type of solute in the solution. If the solute can cross the cell membrane easily (a permeant solute), then that solute will distribute proportionately across cell membranes and not cause any change in cell size. If the solute in the hypertonic fluid cannot easily cross the cell membrane (an impermeant solute), then addition of that kind of hypertonic solution to body fluids will increase the solute concentration in the ECF and draw water from the cell down the concentration gradient for water. That is, the water moves from the area of higher concentration (inside the cell) to the area of lower concentration (outside the cell). Urea, which crosses cell membranes, is an example of a permeant solute; sodium and mannitol, which do not enter cells easily, are examples of impermeant solutes (Sterns, Spital & Clark, 1996).

Hydrostatic Pressure.   Hydrostatic pressure causes filtration of fluid from an area of higher pressure to an area of lower pressure, such as from the blood vessels into the interstitial fluid compartment. Factors that affect hydrostatic pressure include the arterial blood pressure (the force with which the heart pumps blood), the rate of blood flow, and the venous pressure.

Filtration Pressure.   Hydrostatic pressure minus osmotic pressure equals the filtration pressure. To illustrate what happens as blood circulates through the capillary bed, the filtration pressure needs to be examined (Fig. 36-5). In normal arterioles, the hydrostatic pressure of the blood is about 32 mm Hg, and the osmotic pressure is approximately 22 mm Hg. The filtration pressure of the arteriole is the difference between them, or approximately +10 mm Hg. Because this is a positive pressure, fluid filters out of the vessel into the interstitial fluid. In the venule, however, hydrostatic pressure is about 12 mm Hg, whereas the osmotic pressure remains 22 mm Hg. The filtration pressure is the difference, which is about -10 mm Hg. Because this pressure is negative, fluid filters from the interstitial fluid back into the venous capillaries and venules.

This process of fluid leaking out of the arterioles, only to be reabsorbed in the venules, is continuous. It also is the manner by which the body is able to transport oxygen and other nutrients to the cells and remove waste products. In the healthy person, this process is balanced so that almost all filtered fluid is returned to the vascular space. The lymphatic vessels return excess fluid to the circulation through the thoracic duct and, at the same time, carry cells and proteins from the periphery through the lymph nodes. Movement of fluid and white blood cells through the lymphatic vessels is a key aspect of the body's inflammatory and immune responses to injury and infection. If the hydrostatic pressure is greatly increased or the osmotic pressure is greatly reduced, some of the filtered fluid

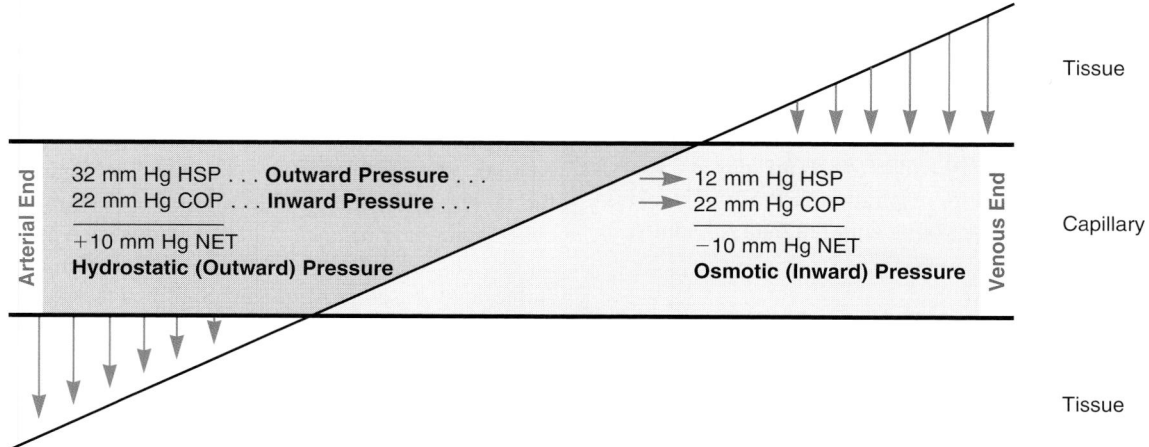

Tissue

Arterial End

32 mm Hg HSP . . . **Outward Pressure** . . .
22 mm Hg COP . . . **Inward Pressure** . . .
——————————
+10 mm Hg NET
Hydrostatic (Outward) Pressure

→ 12 mm Hg HSP
→ 22 mm Hg COP
——————————
−10 mm Hg NET
Osmotic (Inward) Pressure

Venous End

Capillary

Tissue

FIGURE 36-5   Filtration pressure in a capillary. In the arterial end of a capillary, fluid is pushed out into the tissues; in the venous end, fluid is absorbed back into the circulation.

remains in the interstitial space. This accumulation is called edema. Blockage of lymph drainage or removal of lymph nodes can also produce edema.

Lifespan Considerations

Age is a significant factor in fluid and electrolyte balance. The very young and older adults are at greatest risk for fluid or electrolyte imbalances. An understanding of age-related differences is important for the prevention, identification, and management of fluid and electrolyte problems.

Newborn and Infant

Infants have a proportionately larger percentage of total body weight as water (70% to 80%) than adults do (60%). Preterm infants have an even greater amount of body fluid, possibly up to 90% (Metheny, 2000). Compared with adults, a greater amount of the fluid is contained within the ECF compartment in infants. Because infants also have a greater surface area in relation to weight, they can lose a proportionately larger volume of fluid through the skin.

Fluid requirements vary according to age, as do normal urine outputs. Generally, infants have proportionately greater fluid requirements and greater fluid losses. The infant's kidneys are immature and lack the ability to concentrate urine fully (Robillard, Segar, Smith & Jose, 1992; Blackburn, 1994). Metabolic and respiratory rates are high in infants, contributing to increased insensible fluid loss. Fluid loss can occur very rapidly in this age group. The nurse should teach parents and caregivers about how serious vomiting or diarrhea can be for infants, urging them to contact their healthcare providers and to provide appropriate fluid replacement if these symptoms occur (Anonymous, 1994).

SAFETY ALERT

Carefully monitor infants when they are losing or being given fluid. Kidney immaturity and increased body surface area in relation to body size place infants at risk for fluid and electrolyte problems.

Toddler and Preschooler

Approximately 62% of the toddler's weight is water. Fluid requirements vary but are generally 1000 to 1200 mL for a 24-hour period. Urine output increases from approximately 500 to 700 mL/day at 2 years to 600 to 850 mL/day at 5 years. Water loss through the skin, respiration, urine, and stools is proportionately greater for young children than for adults.

Child and Adolescent

The ratio of total body water to total body weight decreases throughout childhood and adolescence. By the time a child is 12 years old, the percentage of body water to body weight is approximately the same as in adults. Children in this age group may drink soda or sugared beverages to supply their fluid needs. Research has shown that childhood obesity is linked with the intake of this type of sweetened drink (Ludwig,

Peterson, & Gortmaker, 2001). Encourage water and other, more nutritious fluids, such as milk and fruit juices.

Caution children and adolescents against the potential dangers of excessive exercise without adequate fluid replacement, especially in hot weather, because muscle damage (rhabdomyolysis) and fluid and electrolyte imbalances can occur (Anonymous, 1998). Balanced dietary intake is important to promote normal electrolyte balance. Dietary intake may be erratic in adolescents. Fad diets or purging to lose weight can cause severe fluid and electrolyte imbalances.

Adult and Older Adult

In middle age, adipose tissue tends to increase, resulting in a continual decline in the percentage of body weight that is fluid after 40 years of age. After age 25 years, the number of nephrons in the kidney begins to decrease. By the time a person is 85 years old, there are 30% to 40% fewer functioning nephrons. Consequently, the kidney has less ability to concentrate urine and conserve body fluids (Faull, Holmes & Baylis, 1993). When adults older than 65 years of age were compared with younger adults (mean age, 22 years), the plasma osmolarity at which the older group experienced thirst was increased, indicating an increased risk for development of a water deficit (Mack, Weseman, Langhans, Scherzer, Gillen & Nadek, 1994).

Adults most often develop fluid and electrolyte imbalances after an acute illness or elective surgery. Older adults commonly experience alterations in fluid and electrolyte status secondary to chronic disease (e.g., renal failure, heart failure). Diuretics, commonly given to treat high blood pressure and heart failure, can cause an ECF deficit or potassium deficit (hypokalemia). Excessive use of laxatives can reduce gastrointestinal absorption of potassium, promoting hypokalemia and loss of ECF. Some older people may restrict their fluid intake to prevent urinating in the middle of the night or while they are away from home. Although calcium levels are often normal in older adults, calcium leaves the bones, predisposing the person to osteoporosis and, consequently, to fractures when falls occur.

NORMAL ACID–BASE BALANCE

For cells to operate with maximum efficiency, they need oxygen, nutrients, electrolytes, a controlled temperature, and an otherwise predictably stable environment. An important component of cellular environment is the hydrogen ion concentration ($[H^+]$), which is regulated within extremely narrow limits. The maintenance of this narrow concentration range is called acid–base balance. Vital functions such as nerve conduction, hormonal activity, and cardiac rhythm depend on a stable acid–base environment. Significant deviations from normal blood $[H^+]$ are life threatening.

Acids, Bases, and pH

Any substance that can donate free H^+ ions to a solution is called an **acid.** By contrast, any substance that can decrease $[H^+]$ in a solution is a **base** (also called an alkali).

Acids and bases can be categorized as either strong or weak. Hydrochloric acid (HCl), which is secreted by cells in the stomach lining, is an example of a strong acid. When HCl goes into solution, it separates (or dissociates) almost completely into hydrogen and chloride ions. A strong acid in water can generate a large number of free H^+ ions. Sodium hydroxide (lye) is an example of a strong base. In solution, the hydroxyl group, OH^-, binds with some of the H^+ provided by water, greatly reducing the number of free H^+ ions. Weak acids and bases only partially dissociate in solution; they cause much smaller changes in the H^+ concentration than strong acids or bases do. Solutions that contain more acid than base are described as acidic, whereas solutions containing relatively more base are termed basic (or alkaline).

The number of H^+ ions in any solution is indicated indirectly by means of the pH scale (Fig. 36-6). The pH scale, which is the negative log of the hydrogen ion concentration, describes the degree of acidity or alkalinity of solutions. The pH scale ranges from 1 to 14, with 7 representing a neutral solution that is neither acidic nor alkaline. A solution with a pH between 1 and 7 is acidic. Weak acids have a pH only slightly below 7, whereas the strongest acids have pH values closer to 1. Similarly, bases have pH values above 7, with higher pH values indicating increasingly strong bases.

Acids and Bases in the Blood

The body's ECF has an average pH between 7.37 and 7.43 (Rose, 1994). This very narrow pH range is maintained by buffers that limit pH changes in the body fluids and by elimination of acids from the body through the lungs (carbon dioxide) and kidneys.

A very important acid in the body is carbonic acid. The body continually produces carbon dioxide, a cellular waste product, as it uses oxygen to metabolize glucose. When carbon dioxide enters the blood, it combines chemically with water to form carbonic acid. This weak, unstable acid partially dissociates to H^+ and HCO_3^- (bicarbonate) ions:

$$H_2O + CO_2 \leftarrow H_2CO_3 \leftarrow H^+ + HCO_3^-$$

Together, carbonic acid and bicarbonate ion form what is known as a *buffer pair* (a weak acid and its accompanying conjugate base). Although other buffer systems participate in maintaining acid–base balance, the bicarbonate–carbonic acid buffer system is the most important for two reasons. First, because all the buffer systems are in equilibrium, changes in the bicarbonate–carbonic acid system reflect changes in all other systems. Second, the body regulates the carbon dioxide level by changes in the respiratory rate (ventilation) and bicarbonate level by adjustments in the amount of bicarbonate lost in the urine or the amount regenerated by the kidneys.

Acid–Base Balance Regulation

Hydrogen ion balance is closely regulated. Compared with the electrolytes, which are present in the plasma in millimolar (10^{-3} M) concentrations, the concentration of H^+ in the blood is normally 1 million times smaller. That is, H+ is present in nanomolar (10^{-9} M) amounts. Death usually results if blood pH falls below 6.8 or increases above 7.8 (Rose, 1994). Because metabolism continually produces acids, maintenance of the pH within its incredibly narrow limits depends on two processes: buffering and compensation. Buffers allow acids or bases to be transported from where they are produced to where they are excreted, and the compensatory processes either excrete or retain acids or bases to compensate for losses. Acid–base balance is commonly evaluated by measuring arterial blood gases (Table 36-3).

Buffering

Buffers are substances that help prevent large changes in pH by absorbing or releasing H^+ ions. When the blood has excess acid, successful buffering prevents a large drop in pH, despite

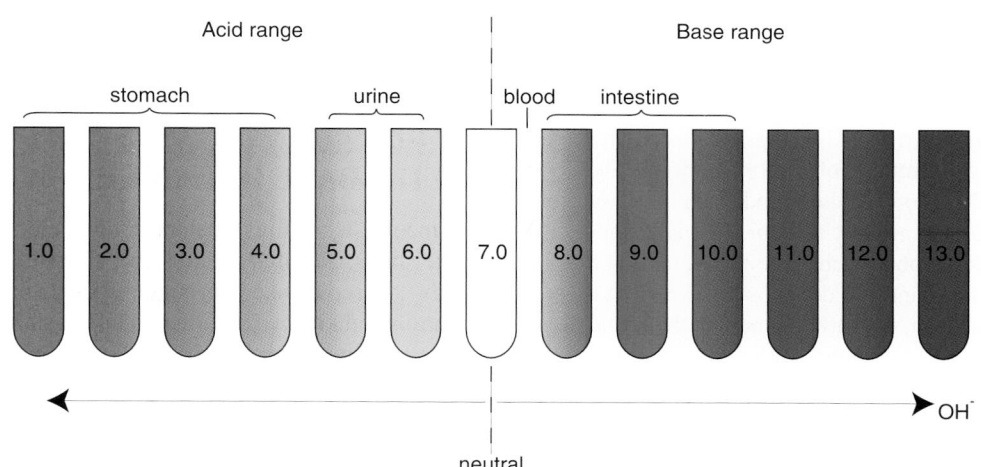

FIGURE 36-6   The pH scale measures degree of acidity or alkalinity.

TABLE 36-3

Normal Arterial Blood Gas Values		
Abbreviation	**Normal Range**	**Definition**
pH	7.37–7.43	Reflects the hydrogen ion concentration of arterial blood Acidosis: <7.37 Alkalosis: >7.43
$PaCO_2$	36–44 mm Hg	Reflects partial pressure of carbon dioxide in arterial blood Hypocapnia: low partial pressure of carbon dioxide in arterial blood, <35 mm Hg Hypercapnia: high partial pressure of carbon dioxide in arterial blood, >45 mm Hg
PaO_2	80–100 mm Hg	Partial pressure of O_2 in arterial blood
HCO_3^-	22–26 mEq/L	Amount of bicarbonate in arterial blood

the influx of extra H^+ ions into the blood. In such cases, buffers combine with additional H^+ ions the acid releases, minimizing the potentially damaging effect of extra free H^+ ions in the blood. Similarly, a deficit of blood acid or excess of base can result in a serious increase in pH. Successful buffering causes extra H^+ ions to be released into the blood.

The body relies on several buffers, including hemoglobin, carbonic acid–bicarbonate, and phosphate. The plasma proteins, such as albumin and globulins, along with hemoglobin in the red blood cell, have limited capacities for regulation of H^+ ion concentration. Compounds such as phosphate and ammonia bind H^+ ions in the urine and thus play a part in acid–base balance. Bone also participates in buffering.

Compensation

The respiratory and renal systems excrete acids and bases from the body and compensate for any imbalances. The lungs handle moment-to-moment maintenance of acid–base status because they can react almost instantly to minute changes in blood pH. The kidneys regulate more gradual or long-term changes in acid–base balance. They are slower than the lungs to react to changes, taking hours to days to respond. Failure or impairment of either system can lead to life-threatening acid–base imbalances. Therefore, preservation of optimal lung and renal function is crucial for any client at risk for acid–base disturbances.

Respiratory Compensation. The lungs are directly responsible for controlling the amount of carbon dioxide in the blood. Carbon dioxide diffuses into the blood from the tissues and is carried primarily as carbonic acid, bicarbonate, and hydrogen ions. When the blood reaches the lungs, carbon dioxide diffuses into the lung and is exhaled. As the carbon dioxide diffuses into the alveoli, the carbonic acid in the blood dissociates into more carbon dioxide and water so that more carbon dioxide can be exhaled. The lungs normally maintain the carbon dioxide level in the arterial blood ($PaCO_2$) at a pressure 36 to 44 mm Hg (Rose, 1994).

When the tissues produce large amounts of carbon dioxide, the lungs respond to input from the chemoreceptors and increase the rate and depth of ventilation, which increases the rate at which this acid is excreted and prevents any significant change in pH. The respiratory system reacts oppositely if carbon dioxide production decreases. Because breathing also is needed to supply oxygen to the blood and to regulate carbon dioxide, people are able to decrease ventilation only to a limited extent.

Renal Compensation. The kidneys influence the maintenance of the normal acid–base balance by changing the rate of excretion or retention of H^+ and HCO_3^- ions. The kidneys handle increases in blood acids in two ways: they increase excretion of H^+ ions into the urine and return HCO_3^- ions to the blood. Additional serum bicarbonate is thus made available to absorb more free H^+ ions, and normal pH can be reestablished. The kidneys balance a gradual loss of blood acid (or excess of blood base) by increasing retention of H^+ ions and increasing the excretion of HCO_3^- ions into the urine. In this way, they prevent any rise in pH by keeping the relative concentration of bases and acids in the correct ratio.

The kidneys' response takes several hours, and it may be as long as 2 days before it is fully functioning. For this reason, the kidneys are slower than the lungs to compensate for sudden changes in acid–base status.

FACTORS AFFECTING FLUID, ELECTROLYTE, AND ACID–BASE BALANCE

Homeostasis requires a balanced fluid, electrolyte, and acid–base status. Normally, fluids and electrolytes lost from the body are replenished through adequate intake. Hormonal controls and kidney function regulate this process; Table 36-4 shows a typical adult fluid intake and output pattern for a 24-hour period. Hormones also influence the movement of electrolytes in and out of cells. Many factors can increase the risk for fluid, electrolyte, or acid–base imbalances, including inadequate oral intake, excessive loss of fluid or electrolytes, stress, chronic illness, and surgery.

TABLE 36-4

Typical 24-Hour Intake and Output			
Intake		**Output**	
Oral fluids	1,300 mL	Urine	1,500 mL
Fluid in food	1,000 mL	Feces	200 mL
Oxidation of food	300 mL	Perspiration	100–200 mL
TOTAL	2,600 mL	Insensible loss	
		Skin	300–400 mL
		Respiration	300 mL
		TOTAL	2,400–2,600 mL

Fluid and Food Intake

Water is usually taken in orally, about two thirds in the form of water or other beverages and the remainder from foods. The body produces an additional small amount of water as it oxidizes hydrogen during food metabolism. An average daily intake for an adult is 1300 mL of water (about six glasses). An additional 1000 mL of water is obtained from foods, especially fruits and vegetables, which are 80% to 90% water. About 300 mL of water is obtained through food oxidation (Metheny, 2000).

The thirst mechanism helps to regulate fluid intake. The thirst center, located in the hypothalamus, is usually stimulated by an increase in plasma osmolarity; less frequently, it can be stimulated by a decrease in blood volume. Psychological factors or a dry mouth also may stimulate thirst. Adequate intake of fluids usually will satisfy thirst if osmolarity returns to normal or if there is an ECF deficit when blood volume is restored. The level of serum osmolarity at which people begin to experience thirst has been shown to be decreased in pregnancy and elevated in older adults (Paller & Ferris, 1996; Sterns, Spital, & Clark, 1996).

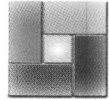
Nursing Research and Critical Thinking
Are Abnormal Preoperative Serum Potassium Levels Associated With Adverse Perioperative Events?

Abnormalities in the balance between intracellular and extracellular potassium concentrations can lead to serious arrhythmias. However, the association between an abnormal preoperative serum potassium level and perioperative adverse events such as arrhythmias had not been examined rigorously. A group of health care providers designed a prospective, observational, case-control study of data collected from 24 diverse U.S. medical centers to determine the frequency of abnormal preoperative serum potassium levels in patients undergoing elective coronary artery bypass grafting. The study also evaluated the association between abnormal preoperative serum potassium levels and adverse perioperative events in these patients. Participants were identified using systematic sampling of every nth patient, in which n was based on expected total number of procedures at that center during the study period. A total of 2402 persons (mean age, 65.1 ± 10.3 years; 24% female) were enrolled in the study. The main outcome measures were intraoperative and postoperative arrhythmias, need for cardiopulmonary resuscitation (CPR), cardiac death, and death due to any cause before discharge, by preoperative serum potassium level. For this study population, the incidence of adverse outcomes was 3.6% for death, 2.0% for cardiac death, and 3.5% for CPR. A serum potassium level of less than 3.5 mmol/L was a predictor of serious perioperative arrhythmia (odds ratio [OR], 2.2; 95% confidence interval [CI], 1.2–4.0), intraoperative arrhythmia (OR, 2.0; 95% CI, 1.0–3.6), and postoperative atrial fibrillation/flutter (OR, 1.7; 95% CI, 1.0–2.7). Adjusting for confounders did not change these relationships.

Critical Thinking Considerations. Because this was a multicenter study and clinical management was not prescribed by protocol, differences in clinical management between medical centers and demographic and clinical characteristics of patient populations were potential confounders. Implications of this study are as follows:

• Perioperative arrhythmia and the need for CPR increased as preoperative serum potassium levels decreased below 3.5 mmol/L.
• Further study is needed to evaluate whether preoperative intervention mitigates these adverse associations.
• Nurses need to assess preoperative serum potassium levels carefully.

From Wahr, J. A., Parks, R., Boisvert, D., Comunale, M., Fabian, J., Ramsay, J., & Mangano, D. T. (1999). Preoperative serum potassium levels and perioperative outcomes in cardiac surgery patients. *Journal of the American Medical Association 281*(23), 2201–2210.

Food also provides the body with electrolytes. Calcium is abundant in dairy products. Sodium is found in salt, processed meats and foods, bread products, and dairy products. Bananas, melons, oranges, apricots, broccoli, raisins, and dates are all good sources of potassium. A well-balanced diet contains all the necessary electrolytes.

Numerous circumstances can affect the ability to achieve adequate fluid intake. Fluids and food must be readily accessible. Older adults may be unable to shop for or prepare a well-balanced diet, and as a result they may decrease their intake of needed fluids and electrolytes. People in bed may be too weak to reach for and drink fluids or too fatigued to consume entire meals.

Psychological factors, such as depression or confusion, also may contribute to decreased oral food or fluid intake. Some people purposely limit oral intake to lose weight or decrease the number of times they must void. Lack of knowledge regarding the consequences of these actions may contribute to such behavior. Physiologic factors such as nausea can limit oral intake. In addition, the ability to swallow may be impaired after a stroke or by the discomfort of a sore throat.

Fluid and Electrolyte Output

Water and electrolytes can be lost from the body in four ways:

- From the kidneys as urine
- From the skin as perspiration
- From the gastrointestinal tract in stool or vomit
- From the lungs as insensible water loss

The kidney is the main organ regulating fluid balance. Glomerular filtration and tubular reabsorption permit the kidneys to conserve or excrete water and electrolytes as necessary to maintain homeostasis. The hormones discussed previously regulate these processes. Normal urine output for 24 hours is approximately 1500 mL if intake is normal (see Table 36-4). Loss of fluid through the skin as perspiration accounts for an average daily loss of 100 to 200 mL of fluid. In addition to perspiration, insensible fluid loss through the skin amounts to about 300 to 400 mL/day. Insensible water loss occurs when water molecules move from an area of higher concentration (the body) to an area of lower concentration (the atmosphere). Insensible water loss differs from perspiration, during which sweat glands actively expel water through the skin. Loss of fluid through the gastrointestinal system in the form of feces is usually minimal (approximately 200 mL) (Metheny, 2000). The final route for fluid loss is through the lungs during respiration. Exhalation contains not only carbon dioxide but also water vapor. The loss of water through respiration is approximately 300 mL/day (Metheny, 2000). As body temperature increases with fever, the amount of fluid lost as perspiration, as insensible water loss, and from the lungs with respiration increases proportionally.

Fluid, electrolyte, and acid–base imbalances can occur when a person experiences abnormal loss of fluid or electrolytes. Vomiting, diarrhea, diaphoresis, or increased urine output secondary to the administration of diuretics can cause such a loss. Not all losses result in imbalances; however, when losses do occur, be alert for any signs or symptoms of an imbalance.

Vomiting

If sufficient gastric juice is lost from the stomach, hydrogen, sodium, and chloride ions (ECF with additional acid) are depleted, increasing the risk for ECF volume deficit and/or metabolic alkalosis. Gastric fluid also is high in potassium, and excessive losses may contribute to hypokalemia. Vomiting compounds fluid and electrolyte problems because the ability to maintain adequate intake is reduced.

Diarrhea

Intestinal secretions contain bicarbonate. For this reason, diarrhea may result in metabolic acidosis. Intestinal contents also are rich in sodium, chloride, water, and potassium, possibly contributing to an ECF volume deficit and hypokalemia. The development and promotion of oral rehydration fluids, which replace the fluid and electrolytes lost in diarrhea, have significantly reduced worldwide death rates from diarrheal disease, particularly among infants (Avery & Snyder, 1990).

Diaphoresis

Diaphoresis, or excessive sweating, can occasionally increase the loss of fluid and electrolytes. Sweat is a hypotonic fluid containing sodium, potassium, and chloride. Diaphoresis can occur with increased physical activity, fever, or exposure to elevated environmental temperatures.

Use of Diuretics

Diuretics are prescribed to increase the excretion of sodium, chloride, and water in clients with high blood pressure or with chronic heart, renal, or liver problems. At times, the medications may remove too much ECF from the body, resulting in a deficit. Diuretics, except for the potassium-sparing diuretics, also promote the excretion of potassium and magnesium from the body, increasing the risk for electrolyte deficits as well.

Stress

Stress caused by many factors, such as physical trauma, anxiety, and pain, can affect fluid and electrolyte balance. When stress occurs, aldosterone production is increased, causing ECF retention. Stress also increases ADH production, resulting in decreased renal excretion of water.

Chronic Illness

Many chronic medical problems adversely affect a person's ability to maintain normal fluid, electrolyte, and acid–base homeostasis. Imbalances commonly accompany chronic renal problems, heart problems, and respiratory problems. Other problems, such as liver disorders, cancer, and diabetes mellitus, also result in fluid and electrolyte imbalances.

Renal Failure

As kidney function decreases due to damaged or lost nephrons, there may be an abnormal loss or accumulation of sodium, chloride, potassium, and fluid in the body, resulting in ECF volume and water excesses. The kidneys are less able to regulate electrolyte excretion, so abnormal levels may occur. Hyperkalemia and hypocalcemia are common. Because metabolism results in acidic byproducts, metabolic acidosis occurs when the kidneys fail.

Cardiac Failure

As the heart fails to pump effectively, blood pressure falls. The secretion of aldosterone and ADH is stimulated, often resulting in ECF volume and water excesses. This fluid collects in the lungs, increasing the risk of pulmonary edema, and in the rest of the body, where it appears as pitting or dependent edema. Fluid volume excess is complicated by the fact that as the heart pumps less effectively, blood flow to the kidneys decreases, resulting in decreased fluid excretion.

Respiratory Failure

Chronic respiratory problems affect acid–base balance. Progressive destruction of alveoli limits the lungs' functional ability to excrete carbon dioxide (carbonic acid). The pH of the blood falls, and chronic respiratory acidosis occurs.

Surgery

Many preoperative and postoperative factors influence the surgical client's fluid and electrolyte status. Preoperatively, the client may not be allowed food or fluids by mouth (NPO) and may receive enemas. During surgery, increased insensible water loss occurs as the internal body structures are exposed to air and blood is lost. The amount lost depends on the type of surgery. Potassium levels frequently fall after surgery owing to cellular trauma and inadequate intake. As cells are destroyed, potassium is released from inside the cell, which may cause a temporary increase in serum potassium. As this potassium is excreted in the urine, serum potassium can become reduced, and supplemental potassium may be necessary. Some postoperative clients are NPO or on a restricted diet for a period. Drainage from nasogastric tubes or surgical drains increases the potential for loss of fluids and electrolytes (Norris, 1993). Emotional stress, pain, nausea, and vomiting are common after surgery and can contribute to fluid and electrolyte imbalance.

Pregnancy

Physiologic changes occur during pregnancy that can alter fluid, electrolyte, and acid–base status. Fluid retention and edema occur frequently, although the exact underlying mechanism is not completely understood (Paller & Ferris, 1996). Aldosterone production increases during pregnancy, as does overall blood volume and total body fluid volume. Acid–base balance is altered. Higher progesterone levels cause hyperventilation and may result in alkalosis as $PaCO_2$ decreases.

ALTERED FLUID, ELECTROLYTE, AND ACID–BASE BALANCE

Disruptions in homeostasis and disease states can affect fluid, electrolyte, or acid–base balance. Fluid imbalances include ECF volume excess or deficit and water excess or deficit. Electrolyte imbalances include excesses or deficits of potassium, calcium, magnesium, or phosphate. Acid–base imbalances are referred to as respiratory acidosis, respiratory alkalosis, metabolic acidosis, or metabolic alkalosis.

Frequently, more than one imbalance occurs at a time. For simplicity, each imbalance is discussed separately here. Refer to a medical-surgical nursing text for more information on complex problems of fluid and electrolyte imbalance.

Fluid Imbalances

A state of fluid imbalance can occur if too much (excess) or too little (deficit) fluid is present in any fluid compartment. The two major categories of fluid balance problems are ECF volume balance problems and water or osmolar balance problems. A client may present with any of eight possible combinations of fluid balance problems: ECF volume excess or deficit, water excess or deficit, or a combination of an ECF and a water balance problem. To simplify and organize assessment and diagnosis, first assess ECF volume balance and then water balance. Once you have a diagnosis for both ECF and water balance (normal, excess, or deficit for each), then the information can be integrated to make management decisions.

Extracellular Fluid Volume Deficit

ECF volume deficit involves the loss of ECF, which contains primarily sodium, chloride, bicarbonate, and water in the same concentrations as plasma. Loss of this isotonic fluid results in a decrease in the volume of the ECF compartment. There are two subdivisions of the ECF: the vascular volume (fluid inside the blood and lymphatic vessels) and the interstitial volume (fluid between the cells). Other terms that are used for ECF volume deficit are *hypovolemia, saline deficit,* and *isotonic dehydration.* ECF volume deficit can occur because of inadequate intake and/or because of abnormal losses, such as vomiting or diarrhea.

A special type of ECF volume balance problem is sometimes called "third spacing." It occurs when fluid leaves the vascular volume and is trapped within the interstitial fluid in a given body area (Metheny, 2000). A "third space" is any area in which fluid accumulates and is physiologically unavailable to return to its appropriate compartment. For example, collection of fluid in the peritoneal cavity is known as ascites. There is no actual "third space," and the retained fluid is within the interstitial space.

Signs and symptoms of an ECF volume deficit reflect decreases in fluid volume in both the vascular and interstitial spaces. Weight loss (except in third spacing) and thirst result from the loss of fluid from both the vascular and interstitial spaces. The signs and symptoms of a decrease in *vascular volume* include orthostatic or postural changes in pulse rate

THERAPEUTIC DIALOGUE
Edema in Pregnancy

Scene for Thought

Eileen Watkins is 35 years old and happily pregnant for the second time. Her first child, Katie, is 4 years old.
Eileen and Katie are in the clinic for Eileen's 6-month checkup.

Less Effective

Nurse: Hello, ladies. How are you today?

Client: Hi, Cindy. We're doing just fine. Right, Katie?

Nurse: Let me get some weight and blood pressure readings on you, Eileen. *(Does so, and Katie gets her weight read, too.)* You know, I think your blood pressure is a little high this month, Eileen. Have you noticed anything different?

Client: *(Looks worried.)* What do you mean different?

Nurse: Have you had headaches, feet swelling, feeling extra tired? *(Good eye contact.)*

Client: *(Looks down at her feet.)* A little, right around the ankles and over the instep. *(Looks at the nurse.)* Is there a problem? *(Katie looks over at her mother.)*

Nurse: *(Reaches down to assess the edema—2+ pitting over the ankle.)* Nothing unusual for most pregnant women. If I remember, you had some swelling when you were pregnant with Katie, right?

Client: Yes, but not this early; it was in the eighth month, I think.

Nurse: Yes, it's a little earlier than last time, Eileen, but you're 4 years older, you're working harder now with Katie and your job, and besides, it's summertime! Edema is always worse in the summer. *(Pats Eileen's hand.)* Don't worry. You're fine. Let me give you some information on salt in food that might be hidden in stuff like biscuit mix. This is a really good pamphlet. . . . *(Continues to talk about hidden sodium and resting throughout the day in a reassuring tone.)*

Client: *(Listens carefully and anxiously, holds Katie close.)*

More Effective

Nurse: Hello, ladies. How are you today?

Client: Hi, Sarah. We're doing just fine. Right, Katie?

Nurse: Let me get some weight and blood pressure readings on you, Eileen. *(Does so, and Katie gets her weight read, too.)* You know, I think your blood pressure is a little high this month, Eileen. Have you noticed anything different?

Client: *(Looks worried.)* What do you mean different?

Nurse: Have you had headaches, feet swelling, feeling extra tired? *(Good eye contact.)*

Client: *(Looks down at her feet.)* A little, right around the ankles and over the instep. *(Looks at the nurse.)* Is there a problem? *(Katie looks over at her mother.)*

Nurse: *(Reaches down to assess the edema—2+ pitting over the ankle.)* Nothing unusual for most pregnant women. If I remember, you had some swelling when you were pregnant with Katie, right?

Client: Yes, but not this early; it was in the eighth month, I think.

Nurse: *(Checks the chart.)* That's right. This seems to worry you. *(Good eye contact.)*

Client: Yes. I guess I thought everything was going to be the same as last time—no problems. *(Smiles at Katie, a little sadly.)*

Nurse: Does something particularly worry you?

Client: I didn't tell you last time; my mother lost a baby after her blood pressure got really high and her legs swelled up. It happened when I was about 10, and it really scared me. I was so glad when my pregnancy was so easy.

Nurse: I understand your worry. You're scared that you'll swell up like your mom and have the same problems. *(Client nods; she looks scared. Katie keeps a close eye on her mom.)* Well, let's work on this together. There are a number of ways I can think of.

Client: You mean putting my feet up and staying off the chips? I do that already. What else should I do? *(Sounds a little frustrated.)*

Nurse: First, let's chat a little more. I want to find out about your daily routine and then talk about some salt hidden in foods that is not so obvious. Before all that, I just want to say that we can work on this together. Even Katie can help. *(Puts hand over Eileen's.)*

Client: Okay. I'm listening. *(Takes a breath and settles in.)*

Critical Thinking Challenge

- Relate anxiety to the ability to hear and learn.
- Detect what Cindy did to deal with Eileen's anxiety about the pedal edema.
- Analyze how you could tell one nurse was more effective than the other by observing body language.
- Determine what emotions you would assess on Eileen's next checkup.
- Describe how you would assess for them if you were Sarah and then if you were Cindy.

and blood pressure (i.e., an increase in pulse rate and decrease in blood pressure when the person moves from a lying to a standing position); weak, rapid pulse; decreased urine output; and slow-filling peripheral veins. The signs and symptoms of decreased *interstitial volume* include dry mucous membranes and poor skin turgor. Serum sodium values do not change noticeably, because the fluid that is lost has the same concentration of electrolytes as the serum.

Treatment of ECF volume deficit includes either oral or IV replacement of sodium, chloride, and water in the same concentrations that are found in body fluid. Either oral rehydration fluids or normal saline can be used. Protect the client from injury that could result from dizziness and weakness secondary to postural hypotension.

SAFETY ALERT
Monitor postural heart rate and blood pressure when getting clients with ECF deficit out of bed. Have them take several minutes to get up, going in slow steps from a lying to a sitting to a standing position. Be sure someone is present when they get out of bed.

Extracellular Fluid Volume Excess
ECF volume excess involves an increase of ECF, composed of a 0.9% solution of sodium, chloride, and water (normal saline). Increases in ECF volume often occur with cardiac failure, renal failure, or liver disease. When excess fluid cannot be eliminated, hydrostatic pressure forces some of it into the interstitial space, where it is observable as edema. A significant increase in ECF volume has to occur before edema is visible.

Rapid weight gain (>0.5 kg/day) is the most significant symptom indicating ECF volume excess. A weight gain of 1 kg reflects retention of 1 L of ECF. Other symptoms include increased blood pressure, bounding pulse, and fullness of neck veins. Although urine output might be expected to be increased when there is an ECF volume excess, it is often decreased because of the underlying cause (e.g., heart or renal failure). As venous pressures increase, excess ECF volume can filter across the alveoli into the lungs, causing pulmonary edema, manifested by dyspnea, orthopnea (difficulty breathing when supine), and crackles (rales). As with ECF volume deficit, serum sodium values are within normal limits unless the client also has a water balance problem.

Medical management of ECF volume excess involves restriction of sodium and saline intake (low-sodium diet) and administration of diuretics. The underlying pathology is identified and treated.

Water or Osmolar Imbalance
Water or osmolar balance problems occur when water intake is increased or decreased markedly or when water is retained or excreted excessively. To determine a water balance problem, the serum osmolarity must be either measured or estimated. Osmolarity is the number of dissolved particles in solution. Body fluid osmolarity can be approximately determined by estimating the number of particles per unit volume of body fluid. Making this estimate is simplified by the fact that the

most abundant osmotically active extracellular particles are the sodium ions, each one of which has an accompanying anion, either chloride or bicarbonate. Glucose is the only other molecule that makes a contribution to serum osmolarity that influences the distribution of body fluid. (Other molecules, such as urea, also contribute to serum osmolality, but, because they move easily across cell membranes, they have no net effect on body fluid volume distribution.) Use the following formula to estimate serum osmolarity:

$$\text{Estimated serum osmolarity} = (\text{serum sodium} \times 2) + (\text{serum glucose}/18)$$

where the osmolarity is given in units of mOsm/L, serum sodium in mEq/L or mmol/L, and glucose in mg/dL. The value for glucose is divided by 18 to transform the units from mg/dL to mOsm/L. The gram molecular weight of glucose (180) and the value for glucose must be multiplied by 10 to transform from dL to L; 10 divided by 180 simplifies to 1/18.

For example, if a client had a serum sodium concentration of 135 mEq/L and a glucose level of 90 mg/dL, his or her estimated serum osmolarity would be calculated as follows:

$$\text{Estimated serum osmolarity} = (135 \times 2) + (90/18) = 270 + 5.04 = 275 \text{ mOsm/L}$$

Because water moves freely across almost all cell membranes, the serum osmolarity indicates ICF osmolarity except for relatively brief periods when changes in one fluid compartment have not yet had time to equilibrate with the other.

Water moves down its concentration gradient from areas of higher concentration to areas of lower concentration. For example, if a client is given a hyperosmotic IV solution (e.g., 2× normal saline), the osmolarity of the ECF will increase, and water will move from the cells into the ECF until the osmolarity of both compartments is the same. Conversely, if a client takes in too much water, the osmolarity of the ECF will decrease, and water will move from the ECF into the cells. When clients receive an IV infusion of dextrose 5% in water, which initially has an osmolarity close to that of blood, the glucose is subsequently metabolized and actively transported into cells, leaving the water behind in the ECF. This water then distributes one third into the ECF and two thirds into the ICF, resulting in a decreased osmolarity of all the body fluids.

Water Deficit or Hyperosmolarity. A water deficit or serum hyperosmolarity occurs when there is a decrease in water intake, an increase in water loss, or an excess intake of solute. The estimated serum osmolarity is greater than 300 mOsm/L, and the serum sodium may be greater than 145 mEq/L, depending on the glucose level. As serum osmolarity increases, water is drawn from the ICF compartment, causing cellular shrinking. As fluid is pulled from the cells of the brain, confusion, agitation, convulsions, coma, and death may result. Other symptoms usually include decreased urine output with an increase in urine concentration, thirst, and dry mucous membranes (Takamata, Mack, Gillen, & Nadel, 1994). Other terms used for water deficit include *hypernatremia, hypertonic dehydration,* and *hypertonicity.*

Water Excess or Hypoosmolarity. A water excess or body fluid hypoosmolarity occurs when there is an increase in water intake, abnormal secretion of ADH, or decreased urinary output of water. The estimated serum osmolarity is less than 275 mOsm/L, and the serum sodium is less than 135 mEq/L, depending on the glucose level. As serum osmolarity decreases, water diffuses down its concentration gradient into cells. The major impact is on the cells of the central nervous system, because the swollen cells are encased with the rigid skull. The resulting symptoms include lethargy, irritability, confusion, personality changes, seizures, coma, and eventually death if there is no treatment or treatment is ineffective. Additional symptoms include anorexia, nausea, vomiting, weakness, and cramps. Other terms used for water excess include *hypotonic disorder, hyponatremia,* and *hypotonicity.*

SAFETY ALERT

If an unexplained change occurs in the client's level of consciousness, estimate serum osmolarity or request a serum osmolarity blood sample for analysis if current results are unavailable. Water excess or deficit can cause such changes.

Electrolyte Imbalance

Electrolyte balance is necessary for maintaining normal physiologic functioning. Table 36-5 summarizes the major imbalances.

Acid–Base Imbalance

An arterial pH between 7.37 and 7.43 is necessary for efficient cellular metabolism. Because the pH scale is actually the negative log of the hydrogen ion concentration, a person is said to be acidotic when the arterial pH is less than 7.37 and alkalotic when the pH is greater than 7.43 (Fig. 36-6). Acidosis and alkalosis can be categorized as either respiratory or metabolic, depending on the underlying cause. Disturbances in acid–base balance can influence blood oxygen transport, neurologic function, and cardiac rhythmicity. The degree of impairment varies with the severity, speed of onset, and type of acid–base imbalance.

Respiratory Acidosis

Respiratory acidosis is indicated by a low pH accompanied by an increased arterial concentration of carbon dioxide ($PaCO_2$, >44 mm Hg). The lungs normally maintain blood concentrations of carbon dioxide between 36 and 44 mm Hg (Rose, 1994). When lung disease (e.g., asthma, emphysema) or depressed neural or muscular function (as with narcotic overdose, head trauma, or polio) compromises breathing ability, carbon dioxide accumulates in the blood. As this acid increases, free $[H^+]$ increases, causing pH to drop. With time, the kidneys compensate for this acid buildup by increasing the excretion of H^+ ion into the urine and the return of HCO_3^- to the blood. Normal pH can be reestablished only if the orig-inal problem can be reversed. People with damaged lungs may have chronic respiratory acidosis.

Metabolic Acidosis

Metabolic acidosis occurs either when excess acid is ingested or created (diabetic ketoacidosis) or when the kidneys are unable to retain enough bicarbonate ion to buffer free hydrogen ions in the blood. Metabolic acidosis is characterized by a pH lower than 7.37 and a plasma HCO_3^- concentration lower than 22 mEq/L. It can occur with loss of bicarbonate, as may happen with severe diarrhea, or with acid accumulation (e.g., keto-acids formed in uncontrolled diabetes mellitus, lactic acids produced by oxygen deprivation).

The respiratory system compensates for metabolic acidosis by increasing ventilation, thus increasing the rate of carbonic acid excretion, resulting in a fall in $PaCO_2$. This respiratory compensation occurs relatively rapidly but cannot alone return the acid–base balance to normal limits. Renal compensation with the excretion of H^+ ion and retention of HCO_3^- takes hours to occur and can, in conjunction with respiratory compensation, return the pH to within normal limits. Renal compensation cannot occur if the kidneys are the cause of the metabolic acidosis.

Respiratory Alkalosis

Hyperventilation causes respiratory alkalosis, which is present when a high pH is accompanied by a blood carbon dioxide concentration lower than 36 mm Hg. Hyperventilation, commonly caused by anxiety or asthma, increases carbon dioxide (carbonic acid) excretion, leading to a relative excess of blood base and an increase in pH. To compensate, the kidneys increase the excretion of HCO_3^- to the urine, and pH returns toward normal. Intervention may be required to reduce the hyperventilation.

Metabolic Alkalosis

Metabolic alkalosis occurs when there is excessive loss of body acids or with unusual intake of alkaline substances. It can also occur with an ECF deficit (known as "contraction alkalosis"). Vomiting or vigorous nasogastric suction frequently causes metabolic alkalosis. Endocrine disorders and ingestion of large amounts of antacids are other causes. The loss of stomach acid or taking in of base causes H^+ shifts in the blood, and pH increases.

Compensation for this disorder includes a decrease in ventilation, which allows the blood carbon dioxide concentration to rise. The kidneys respond to metabolic alkalosis by retaining acid and excreting HCO_3^-. Renal compensation for metabolic alkalosis is impaired if the person has an ECF volume deficit or hypokalemia (Rose, 1994).

Manifestations of Fluid, Electrolyte, or Acid–Base Imbalances

Although each fluid, electrolyte, or acid–base imbalance has specific symptoms, groups of symptoms frequently accompany states of imbalance. The degree of the imbalance, the suddenness with which it occurs, and the client's age influence

TABLE 36-5

Electrolyte Imbalances

Imbalance	Causes	Signs and Symptoms	Treatment*
Hyperkalemia (serum potassium >5.0 mEq/L)	Most often accompanies kidney failure (renal impairment prevents proper excretion of excess potassium). Also associated with cellular damage (potassium released into ECF when cells are destroyed); insulin deficiency (less potassium moves into cells); adrenal deficiency (less aldosterone produced); and rapid IV infusion of potassium.	Resultant increase in cell membrane responsiveness to stimuli with changes in skeletal, smooth, and cardiac muscle activity: anxiety, irritability; gastrointestinal hyperactivity (diarrhea and intestinal cramping); characteristic electrocardiogram changes and cardiac dysrhythmias. Resultant decrease in cell membrane responsiveness if serum potassium is elevated (>8 mEq/L) with symptoms similar to those of hypokalemia: cardiac arrest (especially if serum levels increase rapidly).	Depends on severity of elevation and onset. *If levels very high:* Administer IV calcium gluconate to oppose potassium's effect on the membrane potential of excitable cells. Infuse insulin and glucose to move potassium into the cell. Remove potassium from body by dialysis or administration of ion exchange resins such as Kayexalate. *If levels moderately elevated:* Administer diuretics and potassium exchange resins. Identify and treat the underlying cause.
Hypokalemia (serum potassium <3.5 mEq/L)	Abnormal loss of potassium; inadequate replacement; increased movement into cells (possible when insulin given).	Resultant decreased responsiveness of cellular membranes to stimuli and lack of responsiveness to stimuli leading to characteristic skeletal muscle, smooth muscle, renal, and cardiac (symptoms usually appearing when serum potassium is below 3 mEq/L): muscle weakness (begins in lower extremities and moves up trunk to upper extremities); fatigue; impaired respiratory muscle function (if level severely low); abdominal distention, nausea, vomiting, constipation, and paralytic ileus (from decreased GI responsiveness); increased urination (polyuria) and thirst (polydipsia); dysrhythmias and characteristic electrocardiogram changes; elevated blood glucose levels (from suppression of insulin release).	Increase intake of potassium: encourage potassium-rich foods in diet; administer oral potassium supplements; use potassium-sparing diuretics; administer IV potassium (if level very low). Identify and treat underlying cause. Implement preventive teaching, if indicated.

(continues)

TABLE 36-5 (Continued)

Electrolyte Imbalances

Imbalance	Causes	Signs and Symptoms	Treatment*
Hypercalcemia (elevated serum calcium level >10.1 mg/dL)	Cancer; excessive intake of vitamin D; excessive intake of milk or alkaline "antacids"; hyperparathyroidism; immobilization; reduced renal function.	Resultant decreased neuromuscular excitability: muscle weakness; lack of coordination; confusion; lethargy; impaired memory; nausea, vomiting, and constipation; pruritus; kidney stones; bone pain.	Depends on underlying cause; administer IV normal saline and diuretics.
Hypocalcemia (serum calcium level <8.9 mg/dL)	Parathyroid deficiency; vitamin D deficiency; renal disease; some malignancies; pancreatitis; various treatments (e.g., massive blood transfusion); enema or laxative abuse.	Resultant spontaneous discharge of sensory and motor fibers of the peripheral nervous system: paresthesia (tingling in hands, fingers, feet, or around the mouth); tetany (manifested by grimacing, muscle twitching, cramping, hyperactive reflexes, and severe flexion of the wrist and ankle joints); laryngospasm, seizures, cardiac arrest (if untreated) leading to death.	Depends on serum level. *If mild deficit:* Administer oral calcium supplements. *If more severe deficit:* Give IV calcium slowly. Know that rapid IV replacement of calcium can result in cardiac dysrhythmias. Institute seizure precautions as necessary.
Hypermagnesemia (serum level >2.0 mEq/L)	Renal failure; diabetic ketoacidosis; magnesium sulfate therapy (Metheny, 2000); magnesium-based laxative use.	Resultant depression of muscular irritability: hypotension; weakness; depressed reflexes; paralysis; bradycardia; respiratory failure; cardiac arrest.	Depends on underlying cause; administer IV calcium or prepare for removal by peritoneal dialysis or hemodialysis.
Hypomagnesemia (serum level <1.4 mEq/L)	Impaired intake; impaired intestinal absorption; excessive urinary excretion (secondary to diuretics and chronic alcoholism).	Resultant neuromuscular irritability: tremors; cramps; difficulty swallowing; cardiovascular changes.	Identify and treat the underlying cause. Encourage intake of foods high in magnesium. Administer IV magnesium if indicated.
Hyperphosphatemia (serum level >5 mg/dL [rarely occurs])	Renal failure; rhabdomyolysis; tumor lysis syndrome; excess phosphate intake.	Resultant signs and symptoms from coexisting hypocalcemia.	Identify and treat the underlying cause. Possibly restrict phosphate intake (if renal failure present). Administer IV normal saline (if renal failure absent).

TABLE 36-5 (Continued)

Electrolyte Imbalances

Imbalance	Causes	Signs and Symptoms	Treatment*
Hypophosphatemia (serum level <2.5 mg/dL)	*Redistribution:* increased carbohydrate calories; respiratory alkalosis. *Depletion:* alcoholism; uncontrolled diabetes mellitus; renal phosphate wasting.	Neuromuscular dysfunction; weakness, especially respiratory muscles; fatigue; myocardial depression; ventricular dysrhythmias; rhabdomyolysis; confusion, coma; decreased oxygen delivery to tissues; renal loss of bicarbonate, calcium, magnesium, and glucose; bone changes (osteomalacia); endocrine changes (insulin resistance).	Identify and treat the underlying cause. Encourage foods high in phosphorus. Administer oral phosphate replacement if indicated.

* Most treatments require a physician's order.

symptom severity. When evaluating manifestations, check to see whether all of the data support the same conclusion. Suspect a fluid, electrolyte, or acid–base imbalance in any client who presents with the following signs or symptoms.

Imbalance of Intake and Output and Body Weight

Intake and output should be approximately equal for a 24-hour period. When output is significantly greater or less than intake, suspect a fluid balance problem. Because mistakes are common, make certain that the intake and output record is accurate. Comparison of daily body weights is the best way to confirm apparent discrepancies in intake and output. Normally, urine output is approximately 1500 mL in a 24-hour period, but a wide range of variation is normal, depending on many factors, particularly input. A decrease in body weight may indicate an ECF volume deficit or a water deficit; an increase may indicate an ECF volume excess or a water excess.

When evaluating trends in intake, output, and weight, consider at least the last 48 hours or longer for some chronic health problems. Look for a pattern of imbalance between intake and output or increases or decreases in weight.

Changes in Mental Status

Level of consciousness is a person's state of awareness and arousal. Changes in level of consciousness can occur with changes in serum osmolarity (water balance). At first, changes are minor and may not be apparent unless the nurse knows the client well. The client may simply report feeling fatigued, restless, or apprehensive. Confusion can occur as the imbalances become more severe. Changes in level of consciousness can vary from excessive excitability to lethargy. Lethargy can progress to coma and eventually death. Abruptness of onset of the imbalance results in increased severity of symptoms.

 SAFETY ALERT
Subtle changes in a person's ability to understand and relate to his or her environment can be the earliest indications of a fluid or electrolyte imbalance.

Changes in Vital Signs

Respiratory Rate and Depth. Deep, labored respirations may occur to compensate for metabolic acidosis, whereas shallow respirations may be present in alkalosis. In ECF volume excess, fluid can accumulate in the lungs, decrease oxygenation, and be accompanied by dyspnea. Lung auscultation can detect crackles (rales), a subtle sign of fluid excess, before dyspnea is observable.

Heart Rate and Rhythm. The quality of the pulse depends in part on vascular volume. With ECF volume excess, the pulse may be strong, full, and bounding, whereas with ECF volume deficit, the pulse is usually weak, thready, and rapid. Irregular heart rhythms are common with potassium, calcium, and magnesium imbalances.

Postural Pulse Rate and Blood Pressure. An increase in pulse rate and perhaps a decrease in blood pressure will occur in ECF volume deficit. To assess for an ECF volume deficit, determine the effect that position change has on pulse rate and blood pressure. The pulse and blood pressure are first measured in the supine position and then with the client standing (postural vital signs).

 SAFETY ALERT
Because clients who have a marked ECF volume deficit may become faint or dizzy when they stand, have help available and be vigilant to prevent client injury when taking postural vital signs.

ETHICAL/LEGAL ISSUE
Decisions Regarding Treatment

You have been assigned to care for Mr. Lane, 72 years old, who has heart failure and emphysema that are no longer responding to treatment. Earlier in the disease process, Mr. Lane participated in planning for end-of-life care, deciding to remain as comfortable as possible until his death. Mr. Lane's family seemed to agree with the physician's prognosis and the end-of-life treatment plan to discontinue further active treatment. Mr. Lane's youngest son, who lives at a distance, is disturbed by this decision. He believes that IV therapy should be started and that Mr. Lane should receive vitamins and fluids. He doesn't think they would hurt Mr. Lane and might even help him. Another nurse in the unit is protesting this treatment, expressing her view that it is utterly useless and offers false hope. The family at Mr. Lane's bedside are disturbed by this difference in opinion between their sibling and the healthcare provider.

Reflection
- Describe the feelings that you have after reading this situation. How would you feel if you were the youngest son? The nurse? Another family member?
- Identify any concerns you have regarding your nurse's role in this situation.
- Identify possible approaches to assisting the client's family in resolving the dilemma.
- Recognizing the client's rights, the family's rights, and the healthcare provider's advice, define what you see as your ethically appropriate behavior.

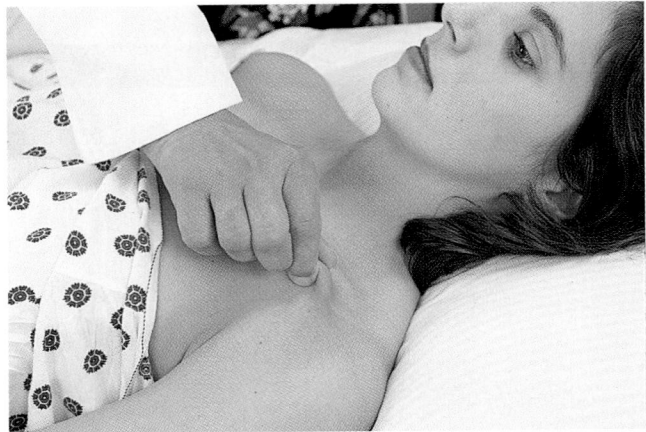

FIGURE 36-7   Normally the skin returns to its original shape rapidly after being pinched up, as in this photo. When there is fluid loss, however, the skin does not return to its normal shape as rapidly.

Edema is not observable in most clients until 2.5 to 3.0 L of fluid has been retained (Rose, 1994). Edema is most noticeable in dependent areas of the body (e.g., the legs when sitting or standing, the back and sacral area when supine in bed). When edema is severe, an indentation remains when a finger is pressed into edematous tissue ("pitting edema").

Abnormal Muscle Tone or Sensation

Changes in muscle tone and muscle irritability frequently accompany imbalances, as described in Table 36-5. Increased or decreased neuromuscular excitability manifests as increasing irritability, muscle weakness, twitching, or cramping. Changes in gastrointestinal neuromuscular tone result in anorexia, nausea, constipation, and vomiting. Clients with electrolyte imbalance may experience tingling and other paresthesias. Observe clients for seizure activity, which can occur with severe imbalances.

Impact on Activities of Daily Living

The ability of the client with a fluid, electrolyte, or acid–base imbalance to perform common activities of daily living (ADLs) may be impaired. Because the client may tire easily, activities may need to be limited, with frequent rest periods during energy-consuming activities. If a client assumes an upright posture and experiences any "lightheadedness" or dizziness, teach the client to change positions slowly, perhaps going from lying to sitting before standing up. Also encourage the client to wait until dizziness subsides before ambulating.

Families can be instrumental in assisting clients to avoid fluid and electrolyte imbalances by assisting them in basic ADLs. Some clients (especially older people) may not feel thirsty and would benefit from having family members remind them to drink adequate fluids. Confusion also may occur, so the nurse or family caregivers need to make sure that safety precautions are implemented, including orienting clients to person, place, and time; keeping side rails up; and assisting

An increase in pulse rate of more than 20 beats per minute is a more sensitive indicator of ECF volume deficit than is a decrease in blood pressure. A drop of more than 15 mm Hg in systolic pressure or 10 mm Hg in diastolic pressure with an increase in pulse rate frequently means the client is experiencing ECF volume depletion (Woods, Sivarajan-Froelicher, Halpenny, & Motzer, 1995). Postural pulse and blood pressure readings are a useful assessment tool with all clients at risk for ECF volume depletion (e.g., after surgery).

Abnormal Tissue Hydration

When ECF volume or water imbalances occur, tissues can retain excess fluid, appearing edematous (turgid), or lose fluid, appearing dry and shriveled. Tissue hydration can be noted in the mouth, where the mucous membranes and tongue can appear dry with ridges due to lack of moisture, or by pinching the skin. Fluid imbalance affects tissue turgor, or the skin's ability to return to normal position immediately after being pinched (Fig. 36-7). Poor tissue turgor occurs in ECF volume deficit or when elasticity is lost from the skin during normal aging.

clients with ADLs that they cannot perform independently. If mobility becomes a problem, standby assistance may be necessary to ensure safety. Aids such as ambulation belts, walkers, and canes can assist clients to ambulate more safely, thus supporting independent ADLs.

ASSESSMENT
Subjective Data
Normal Pattern Identification
Begin with obtaining or reviewing the client's history to gain an understanding of what the person's normal fluid status is and any factors that may predispose to imbalance. Question the client about normal intake and output, any recent changes that have occurred, and any past history of fluid, electrolyte, or acid–base problems. Note any special dietary restrictions, such as sodium restriction or use of salt substitutes. Reported increased thirst or a decrease in fluid intake also is significant. Assess the amount and pattern of urine output along with any changes.

Risk Identification
Collection of subjective data also can help identify risk factors that could contribute to dysfunction. Elicit information concerning recent acute illnesses. Nausea, vomiting, diarrhea, and severe diaphoresis are especially important to document. Be sure to document the severity and duration of these problems.

Certain chronic diseases also predispose a person to fluid and electrolyte imbalance. Question the client about any past or current history of renal failure, heart failure, respiratory dysfunction, diabetes mellitus, diabetes insipidus, Addison's disease, Cushing's disease, or thyroid disease. If any are present, question further regarding individualized management and any complications that may have occurred.

Also question the client about any prescription or nonprescription medications used. Medications such as insulin, diuretics, steroids, laxatives, and antacids can contribute to fluid and electrolyte disturbances. Also note the use of vitamin and mineral supplements or herbal remedies.

Finally, assess spiritual and sociocultural factors that may affect fluid and electrolyte balance. Religious beliefs, such as refusal to receive blood products, could increase the potential for fluid deficit problems if a client hemorrhages after surgery. A fixed income or lack of transportation may make it difficult for a person to buy medicine or special foods to comply with medical treatment.

Dysfunction Identification
Use the subjective data collected to help identify actual fluid and electrolyte problems. Actual fluid and electrolyte imbalances are most likely to cause altered cognitive functioning or imbalances of intake and output and weight. The client can provide information regarding significant differences from normal patterns of intake or output. Validate subjective data with objective information gained through physical assessment and evaluation of laboratory test results before making an actual diagnosis.

Objective Data
Objective data are obtained from all functional health patterns. Physical assessment data can be collected by assessing intake and output, body weight, vital signs, skin turgor and hydration, edema, and fullness of neck and hand veins. More invasive assessment techniques include monitoring central venous pressure and pulmonary artery pressure.

Physical Assessment
Intake and Output. Monitoring intake and output helps evaluate fluid and electrolyte status. The physician may order intake and output assessment after surgery or when evaluation of a medical problem such as heart failure is necessary. Nurses may decide to monitor a client's intake and output when

- Fluid intake or urinary output is less than normal
- Abnormal losses are occurring, such as from a surgical drain or vomiting
- IV therapy is being administered
- The client has medical problems that affect fluid or electrolyte status
- The client is not physiologically stable, such as after surgery or trauma

Intake measurements include oral and parenteral fluids. Oral fluids include any liquids ingested or any foods that become liquid at room temperature. Jello, sherbet, frozen treats, and ice cream are examples of solid foods to include in intake and output. Pureed food is not considered fluid intake. Other oral intake includes feedings delivered through any tube that enters the body (e.g., a nasogastric tube going into the stomach through the nose, a jejunostomy tube entering the jejunum through the abdomen, a gastrostomy tube entering the stomach through the abdomen). Parenteral intake includes any IV fluids, IV medications, and blood products administered.

Output measurements include urine, liquid stool, vomit, drainage from a wound or operative site (e.g., chest tube, Hemovac drain), and drainage from a nasogastric tube. Diaphoresis or drainage on a dressing cannot be precisely measured, but if they are excessive, their presence can be noted without an exact value for output. If greater precision is required, dressings or wet bedding can be weighed to estimate fluid loss.

Each agency has its own methods of recording intake and output. Most forms permit listing of intake and output with subtotals for each shift and then a total for the entire 24-hour period (Fig. 36-8). Some agencies also have worksheets that can be posted on the client's door or on the bathroom door to alert all staff that the client needs intake and output recorded. When clients are having their intake and output recorded, teach them and their families about the procedure so they can assist. The cubic centimeter (cc) or milliliter (mL) is the standard of measurement used, rather than household measures such as cups or ounces. One cubic centimeter is equal to 1 mL, with approximately 30 mL in a fluid ounce.

Intake measurements are often obtained by knowing the standard measurements of containers. Often what is normal

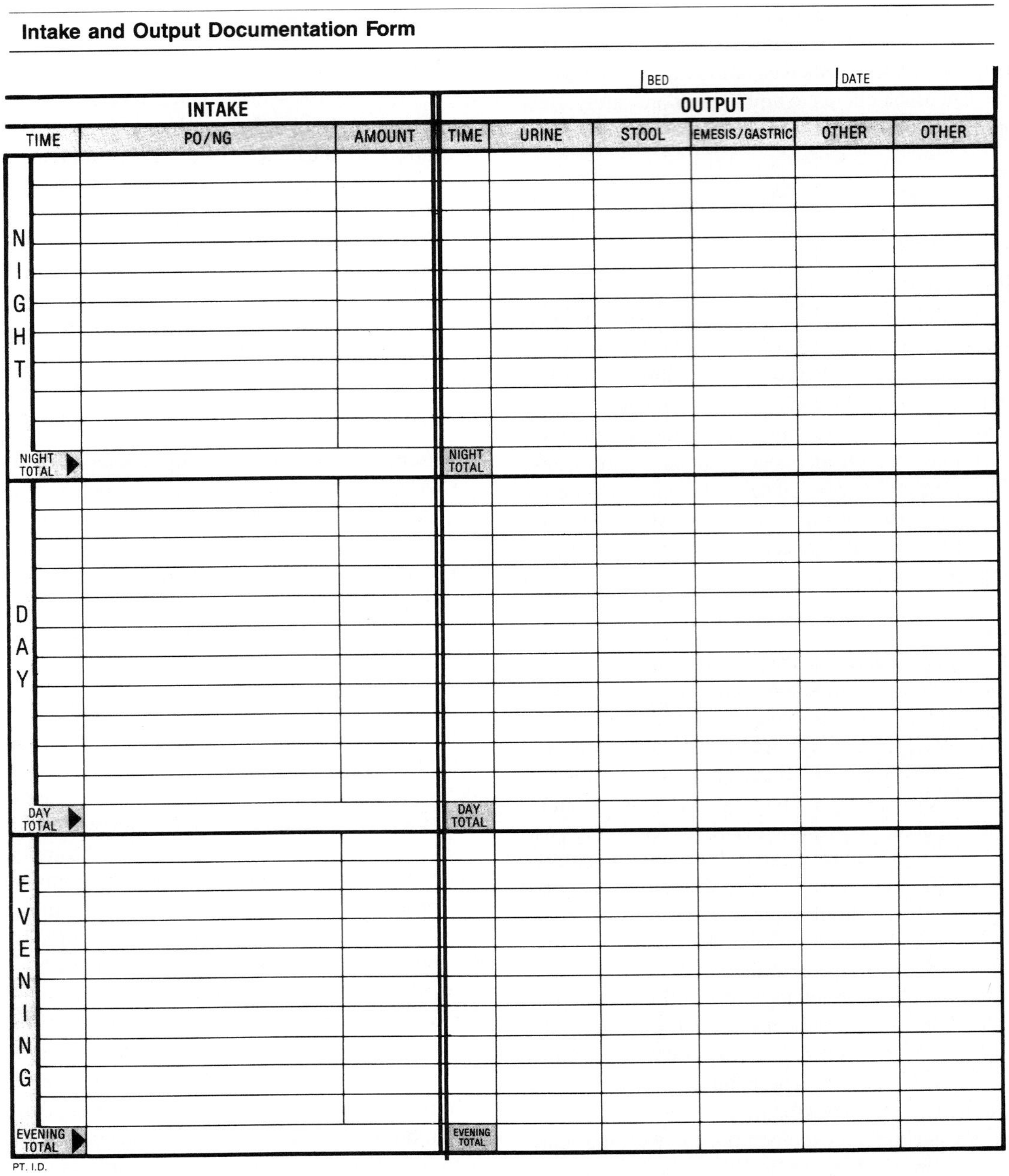

Intake and Output Documentation Form

			BED		DATE			
	INTAKE				**OUTPUT**			
TIME	PO/NG	AMOUNT	TIME	URINE	STOOL	EMESIS/GASTRIC	OTHER	OTHER
N I G H T								
NIGHT TOTAL ▶			NIGHT TOTAL					
D A Y								
DAY TOTAL ▶			DAY TOTAL					
E V E N I N G								
EVENING TOTAL ▶			EVENING TOTAL					

PT. I.D.

FIGURE 36-8   Example of an intake–output form.

for the agency may be printed on the intake and output sheet as a handy reference. For example, when a milk carton contains 240 mL and the client drinks half of the milk, 120 mL is recorded. All intake must be included. Sips of water taken during the day can add up to significant intake, as can oral medications (e.g., antacids) that are given frequently. Ice chips should be recorded as approximately half their volume.

Urine output is measured every time the client voids. To obtain an accurate measurement, keep toilet paper separate from the urine. If the client voids in a bedpan or a commode, transfer the urine into a calibrated container for measurement. If the client is able to use the toilet, place a measuring device (sometimes called a hat) between the toilet seat and the toilet

to collect the urine (Fig. 36-9). If a voiding cannot be measured, indicate it on the intake and output record (e.g., "320 mL plus incontinent ×1"). If the client has a Foley catheter, empty the collection bag and measure the urine at the end of each shift, unless the bag becomes full sooner. Other drainage also is usually emptied and measured at the end of each shift, or more frequently if indicated.

In addition to measuring and recording intake and output, also evaluate patterns and values that are outside the normal range. Intake and output should be roughly equal. When a person has significant other losses (e.g., vomiting, diarrhea), urinary output also may be affected. Urine output of less than 30 mL/hour indicates possible impending renal failure or

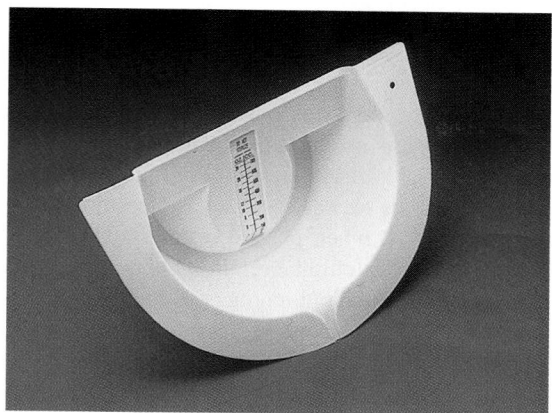

FIGURE 36-9 Urinary "hat" for measuring urine.

marked ECF deficit. If large discrepancies occur between intake and output, ascertain the accuracy of the data collected. Because many people may be responsible for recording intake and output, some values could have inadvertently not been recorded.

Body Weight. Assessing weight provides data concerning fluid balance. Rapid changes in weight indicate body fluid changes. Each kilogram of weight lost or gained equals approximately 1 L of fluid. A rapid loss of 2% of total body weight indicates a mild fluid deficit, whereas a rapid loss of 8% or more indicates a severe fluid deficit (Metheny, 2000).

Daily weights are often ordered for clients who are at risk for ECF volume problems. Obtain weights at the same time of day (preferably in the morning before breakfast), with the client wearing the same clothing, using the same scale to ensure accuracy. If a client is too ill or too weak to stand, use a bed scale, which is a portable scale on wheels onto which the client can be transferred and weighed.

Data from intake and output and daily weight are used together to evaluate for fluid imbalance. A decreasing output in conjunction with an increasing weight indicates ECF volume retention. A sudden weight loss with low urine output may indicate ECF volume deficit.

Integumentary Assessment. Changes in the skin and mucous membranes can indicate fluid imbalance. The skin's general appearance is important to note. Flushed, dry skin may signal a fluid volume deficit. Lack of tearing or perspiration also is important to note. Variations in hydration have already been discussed.

Edema, or excessive accumulation of interstitial fluid, also can be detected when examining the skin. Interstitial fluid can collect in various body parts, such as around the eyes, around the sacrum, and in the extremities. Pressing a finger into tissue over a bony prominence (e.g., lower tibia) best assesses edema. Pitting edema occurs when an indentation remains in the skin (often for 15 to 30 seconds) after a finger presses into edematous tissue. Pitting edema is not apparent until there is approximately a 10% increase in body weight. Edema is measured by the use of + signs; the range is + to ++++.

- A measurement of + indicates edema that is just perceptible (2 mm)
- A measurement of ++ or +++ indicates moderate edema (4 to 6 mm)
- A measurement of ++++ indicates severe edema (8 mm or more)

Edema may be more precisely evaluated by measuring the circumference of body parts (e.g., leg, abdomen). If the circumference is measured at the same location with the same technique, an increase in circumference indicates increased fluid in the interstitial space. Accumulation of fluid in the abdominal cavity (ascites) can be evaluated in this way.

Vital Signs. Vital signs are important parameters to monitor and detect potential fluid, electrolyte, and acid–base imbalances. Variations in vital signs have already been discussed.

Neck Veins. Distention of neck veins accompanies ECF excess. The jugular veins are visible in the neck. Changes in jugular vein distention can indicate alterations in ECF volume. To assess jugular vein distention, place the client in a sitting position with the head elevated to approximately 45 degrees (Fig. 36-10). The neck should be straight in alignment with the body. With the client in this position, the distention within the jugular vein should not extend more than 2 cm above the sternal angle. An increase in ECF volume may be indicated by distention of the neck veins from the top portion of the sternum to the angle of the jaw. Neck vein distention also occurs in people with heart failure.

Central Venous Pressure. Measurement of central venous pressure is a more accurate method of evaluating fluid status than visual inspection of neck vein distention. The central venous pressure is the pressure in the right atrium or vena

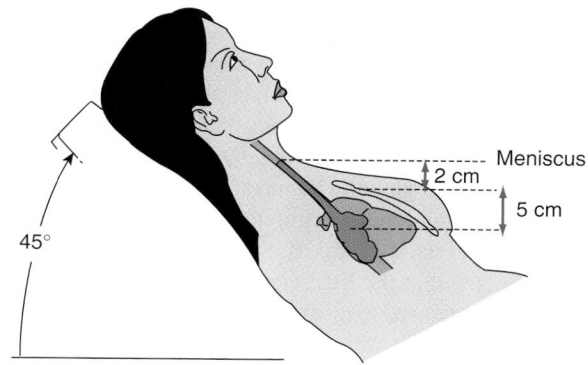

FIGURE 36-10 Measuring jugular venous distention. Place the client with the head of the bed elevated at approximately a 45-degree angle so that the sternal angle is approximately 5 cm above the right atrium. Then measure the vertical distance in centimeters from the sternal angle to the level at the highest point where you see visible pulsation of the neck veins. The distention should not extend more than 2 cm above the sternal angle.

cava. The normal pressure is approximately 4 to 11 cm H_2O. An increase in the pressure may indicate an ECF volume excess or heart failure. A decrease in pressure may indicate an ECF volume deficit.

Pulmonary Artery Pressure. Measurement of pulmonary artery pressure is a more precise method of evaluating fluid status than central venous pressure monitoring. Pulmonary artery pressure is measured by using a catheter placed through the right side of the heart into the pulmonary artery. The normal ranges for systolic and diastolic values are 20 to 30 mm Hg and 8 to 15 mm Hg, respectively. Low readings correspond to volume deficits, and high readings correspond to fluid excess. Monitoring of pulmonary artery pressure is an invasive procedure and is limited to critical care situations.

Bowel Assessment. Bowel elimination is important to consider when detecting fluid and electrolyte imbalances. Because diarrhea predisposes a person to ECF volume and electrolyte disorders, any diarrhea should be evaluated carefully. Bowel sounds should be assessed, with any hypoactivity or hyperactivity noted. Abdominal distention, hypoactive bowel sounds, or a paralytic ileus can accompany a potassium deficit, whereas constipation usually occurs with hypercalcemia.

Laboratory and Diagnostic Tests

Laboratory data assist in the early identification and continuous monitoring of fluid and electrolyte imbalances. Trends revealed in laboratory data are more significant than any single value. Be familiar with serum electrolyte, serum or urine osmolarity, urine specific gravity, and arterial blood gas values. Information from these laboratory tests can help the nurse individualize the client's plan of care.

Serum Electrolytes. Monitoring of serum electrolyte values provides information about trends and helps to evaluate whether electrolyte imbalances are developing, improving, or worsening. Electrolytes are usually obtained and evaluated in groups rather than singularly. Two standardized groupings are common. A profile including serum calcium, carbon dioxide, chloride, phosphate, magnesium, potassium, and sodium may be ordered to help screen electrolyte abnormalities. A more comprehensive profile also includes other blood components, such as glucose, blood urea nitrogen, creatinine, and protein (total, albumin and globulin values) and can be helpful when evaluating total fluid and electrolyte status. Normal reference values are found in Appendix B. Serum electrolyte values reflect amounts within the ECF compartment, because venous blood samples are used to measure the quantity of electrolytes.

Serum Osmolarity. Serum osmolarity can be obtained with a venous blood sample. Normal osmolarity is 280 to 300 mOsm/L. Serum osmolarity is decreased in water excess and elevated in water deficit.

Urine Osmolarity. Urine osmolarity measures the urine's solute concentration. Increased amounts of nitrogenous wastes

(e.g., urea, creatinine, uric acid) increase urinary osmolarity. Additionally, the circulating amount of ADH affects urine osmolarity. Normal urine osmolarity ranges from 50 to 1200 mOsm/L. The more concentrated the urine, the greater its osmolarity. Comparison of plasma and urine osmolarity can be informative. If the kidneys are functioning normally, urine osmolarity should be elevated when plasma osmolarity is elevated and decreased when plasma osmolarity is decreased. That is, the kidneys should be retaining water when plasma osmolarity is increased and losing water when the blood is hypoosmotic. If the urine concentration is not what one would predict from the plasma osmolarity, then the client may have a renal problem.

Urine Specific Gravity. Urine specific gravity measures the weight of a substance compared with an equal part of water. The specific gravity of water is 1.000. With normal fluid intake, urine specific gravity is usually 1.010 to 1.020. A higher specific gravity is obtained when the urine is concentrated, and a lower specific gravity is obtained when the urine is dilute. The urine specific gravity and osmolarity are correlated. A urine specific gravity of 1.010 is equivalent to an urine osmolarity of 300 mOsm/L.

Arterial Blood Gases. Arterial blood gases include the pH, partial pressure of carbon dioxide ($PaCO_2$), partial pressure of oxygen (PaO_2), bicarbonate (HCO_3^-), and oxygen saturation of hemoglobin (O_2 sat). These blood gases are used to evaluate acid–base balance and pulmonary function. A pH lower than 7.37 indicates acidosis, whereas a pH greater than 7.44 indicates alkalosis. Normal ranges for other blood gas values are given in Table 36-4.

NURSING DIAGNOSES

Information gathered in the assessment helps to identify actual or potential fluid and electrolyte problems. The North American Nursing Diagnosis Association (NANDA) has four diagnoses related to fluid disturbances: Deficient Fluid Volume, Excess Fluid Volume, Risk for Deficient Fluid Volume, and Risk for Imbalance of Fluid Volume. To make them more usable, these diagnoses have been expanded here to ECF Volume Excess or Deficit and Water Excess or Deficit. These fluid imbalances also can be actual or potential, and a client can present with both an ECF volume and a water balance problem. These diagnoses are more useful than those offered by NANDA because they reflect the ways in which the body monitors and regulates body fluid balance and, most importantly, how the problem should be managed.

Diagnostic Statement— Extracellular Fluid Volume Deficit

Definition. ECF volume deficit is the state in which a person experiences a deficit of vascular and interstitial fluid volume (ECF).

Defining Characteristics. Clients with an ECF volume deficit may have the following signs and symptoms:

- Decreased urine output
- Increased urine concentration
- Sudden weight loss
- Increased pulse rate and hypotension (especially on standing)
- Decreased venous filling
- Decreased pulmonary artery pressure
- Decreased central venous pressure
- Thirst
- Decreased skin turgor
- Decreased pulse volume or pressure
- Changes in mental state
- Increased body temperature
- Dry skin
- Dry mucous membranes

Related Factors. Related factors include prolonged or marked loss of body fluids, hypoaldosteronism, and a prolonged decrease in intake of fluids or food. Clients who use diuretics also have an increased probability of experiencing ECF volume deficit.

Diagnostic Statement—Extracellular Fluid Volume Excess

Definition. ECF volume excess is the state in which a person experiences an excess of vascular and interstitial fluid volume (ECF).

Defining Characteristics. The signs and symptoms of ECF volume excess include

- Edema
- Effusions
- Weight gain
- Shortness of breath
- Orthopnea
- Fluid intake greater than output
- Third heart sound
- Pulmonary congestion on chest radiograph
- Abnormal breath sounds and rales (crackles)
- Change in respiratory pattern
- Change in mental status
- Decreased hematocrit
- Increased central venous pressure and pulmonary artery pressure
- Jugular vein distention
- Oliguria
- Decreased specific gravity of the urine
- Azotemia

Related Factors. Factors that predispose to ECF volume excess include hyperaldosteronism, excess fluid intake, excess sodium intake, renal failure, heart failure, and liver failure.

Diagnostic Statement—Water Excess

Definition. Water excess, or serum hypoosmolarity, is the state in which the person has an excess of body water in relation to solute. It can result from an increase in water or a decrease in solute, and it is present when estimated serum osmolarity is less than 275 mOsm/L or measured serum osmolarity is less than 280 mOsm/L.

Defining Characteristics. In addition to the osmolarity values just described, the signs and symptoms of water excess include

- Low specific gravity of the urine
- Confusion
- Headache
- Anorexia or nausea or vomiting
- Weight gain
- Cramps
- Delirium
- Personality changes
- Convulsions
- Coma

Related Factors. Related factors include cardiac, hepatic, or renal failure; excess water intake (oral or intravenous); and the syndrome of inappropriate ADH secretion.

Diagnostic Statement—Water Deficit

Definition. Water deficit, or serum hyperosmolarity, is the state in which the person has a deficit of body water in relation to solute. It can result from a decrease in water or an increase in solute, and it is present when estimated serum osmolarity is greater than 300 mOsm/L.

Defining Characteristics. The signs and symptoms of a water deficit include

- Measured or estimated serum osmolarity greater than 300 mOsm/L
- Increased specific gravity of the urine
- Lethargy
- Disorientation
- Delusions
- Irritability
- Convulsions
- Coma
- Thirst
- Oliguria or anuria
- Tachycardia
- Fever (sometimes)

Related Factors. Inadequate water intake, particularly in the very young, very old, and those physically or mentally incapable of independently getting water, can contribute to the development of a water deficit. In addition, excess intake or production of solute, such as may occur with diabetes mellitus or overdoses, and excess water loss may be contributing factors.

Related Nursing Diagnoses

Many other nursing diagnoses may be present in clients with fluid and electrolyte imbalances. Related nursing diagnoses can be actual or potential, and early identification promotes successful intervention. Any of the Self-Care Deficits or Activity Intolerance diagnoses can occur if fatigue, weakness, or muscular irritability is present. Risk for Injury can occur if electrolyte or fluid imbalances cause postural hypotension, loss of consciousness, or impaired cognition. Impaired Skin Integrity is frequently associated with edema, and Constipation or Diarrhea is often associated with fluid or electrolyte imbalances. Deficient Knowledge or Noncompliance can occur when new treatment regimens are instituted without adequate client teaching.

OUTCOME IDENTIFICATION AND PLANNING

After nursing diagnoses and related factors have been identified, the nurse and client plan outcomes and interventions. In many situations, the nurse plans with the client's family or support people. Examples of some interventions that can be used in planning are listed in the accompanying display.

The nurse and client or client's family work together to set realistic, individualized goals. Goals of nursing intervention for a client with altered fluid, electrolyte, or acid–base balance focus on prevention, early recognition of the alteration, intervention in contributing factors, and provision of therapies to restore normal function. Goals must be individualized based on the client's history, risk factors, evidence of altered function, and related objective data. Examples of client goals include the following:

- The client will reestablish normal ECF volume, water, and/or electrolyte balance.
- The client will demonstrate knowledge regarding how to promote future ECF volume, water, and electrolyte balance.
- The client will remain free of complications from fluid or electrolyte imbalance.

The nurse and client together can determine specific outcome criteria to individualize the plan of care. Short-term goals (e.g., "The client will increase fluid intake to 2000 mL in 24 hours") may be easy to reach within a short period. Other goals may involve changes in long-established dietary patterns, which take longer to accomplish.

IMPLEMENTATION
Health Promotion

Teaching is an important nursing role to prevent fluid and electrolyte problems. Nurses can help people understand how fluid and electrolyte imbalances occur and how they can be prevented. The type of fluid replacement the client uses should be matched to the type of fluid that is being lost. If there is a deficit of ECF volume, consumption of mildly salty solutions (e.g., chicken broth) is appropriate. At particular risk for

---

PLANNING: Examples of NIC/NOC Interventions
Accepted Fluid, Electrolyte, and Acid-Base Balance Nursing Interventions Classification (NIC) Electrolyte Management Fluid Monitoring
Accepted Fluid, Electrolyte, and Acid-Base Balance Nursing Outcomes Classification (NOC) Bowel Elimination Electrolyte & Acid/Base Balance Hydration Nutritional Status: Food & Fluid Intake Urinary Elimination
Refer to the following for specifics regarding NIC/NOC: McCloskey, J., & Bulechek, G. (2000). *Iowa Intervention Project: Nursing Interventions Classification (NIC)* 2nd ed. St. Louis, MO: C.V. Mosby. Johnson, M., & Maas, M. (2000). *Iowa Outcomes Project: Nursing Outcomes Classification (NOC)* 2nd ed., St. Louis, MO: C.V. Mosby.

water excess are those who participate in athletic competitions or fund-raising walks or runs in hot weather and who drink only water. "Sports drinks" containing electrolytes are recommended instead in such situations; however, these drinks are relatively costly. One liter of boiled or clean water containing ½ teaspoon of salt and 8 teaspoons of sugar is an inexpensive substitute (Avery & Snyder, 1990). Fruit juices (except tomato juices), sodas, and other sugary drinks should be considered the equivalent of water.

Teaching can occur in various settings and with any age group. When interacting with new parents, stress the fluid needs of newborns; how quickly serious problems can develop if vomiting, diarrhea, or a fever occurs in an infant; and symptoms that warrant contacting a physician (Centers for Disease Control and Prevention, 1992; Anonymous, 1994). Follow-up teaching can occur as children grow, explaining normal fluid requirements and dietary patterns. When children are ill, explain measures to help parents adequately replace fluid that is lost. Balanced electrolyte solutions are available commercially. Ice pops and other frozen treats may be helpful to encourage fluid intake by reluctant children.

School nurses can reinforce teaching in health classes. Many school-age children are involved in sports activities. Encouraging adequate water and electrolyte intake before, during, and after strenuous exercise is important, particularly in hot weather. Discuss the dangers of fad diets, excessive training for sports, and eating disorders, especially with adolescents (Anonymous, 1998).

Nurses who work in industry should be aware of working conditions that could affect fluid and electrolyte balance. When employees must work in hot, humid environments and perform strenuous exercise, periodic breaks should be scheduled so that adequate fluid and electrolyte replacement is possible. Nurses can be influential in supporting policies and legislation to ensure such practices.

Health teaching is especially important among older adults. Classes can be offered through senior citizen centers or community agencies to reinforce good diet and fluid intake. Often, older people take medications, such as diuretics, that can increase the risk of fluid and electrolyte imbalance. Teaching is important to ensure client compliance and to help prevent any problems that can occur with treatment. Teach clients how to detect signs of fluid and electrolyte imbalance, such as rapid weight gain or loss, swelling, changes in normal urine output, muscle weakness, or abnormal skin sensation, and give them guidelines for when to notify a physician.

OUTCOME-BASED TEACHING PLAN

Mrs. Kern, a recent widow with a history of chronic bladder infections, comes to the clinic for a routine checkup. During your assessment, you discover she also has a problem with urinary frequency, which she controls by limiting her fluid intake. Mrs. Kern tells you that she drinks only one cup of tea at breakfast, lunch, and dinner, then nothing after dinner. That way she does not have to worry about her urinary urgency problem.

OUTCOME: Mrs. Kern will verbalize a realistic plan to increase fluid intake.

Strategies

- Discuss the reasons why an increased fluid intake is desirable (e.g., decreased risk of kidney stones, decreased risk of bladder cancer).
- Explore Mrs. Kern's feelings about her pattern of urinary urgency.
- Discuss possible evaluations and assessments that could help Mrs. Kern discover the cause and resulting treatment for her urinary urgency.
- Review her daily pattern of fluid intake. Discuss other sources of fluid in addition to water. Question Mrs. Kern about her likes and dislikes regarding fluids.
- Problem solve with Mrs. Kern a plan for increased fluid intake that she feels most inclined and motivated to follow.
- Encourage Mrs. Kern to increase her fluid intake with fluids she prefers throughout the day as a preventive measure for recurrent bladder infection.
- Have Mrs. Kern set up 6 to 8 glasses of water in her refrigerator. Remind her to drink them throughout the day and to consume them all before she goes to bed at night. Encourage her to place a reminder sheet and checklist on the refrigerator door to aid in monitoring and adhering to the plan.
- Provide phone call follow-up to assess and provide encouragement for increasing Mrs. Kern's daily fluid intake.

Nursing Interventions for Altered Fluid, Electrolyte, and Acid–Base Status

Oral Fluids

Depending on the client's current status, oral fluids may need to be regulated. If a potential or actual ECF volume or water deficit has been identified, institute a plan to increase oral intake of mildly salty fluids or water. If the nursing diagnosis involves potential or actual ECF volume or water excess, curtail oral intake of salt and salty fluids or water. Physicians also may order that fluids be either restricted or encouraged.

Increasing Oral Fluids. Instructions to *force fluids* or *push fluids* are general terms indicating that increased fluid intake is required. Individual goals should be set for each client, depending on current fluid status. To enhance compliance, explain why the increased fluid intake is desirable and involve the client in setting goals for fluid intake. Client teaching and goal setting may include the family if the client is unable or reluctant to drink fluids independently. Encourage the family members to offer fluids frequently during their visits, and teach them how to record intake and output.

Ensure that fluids are placed and kept within the client's reach. Determine what water temperature the client prefers, and change the water pitcher as often as needed to maintain that temperature. If the client is unable to drink independently, ensure that you and your support staff offer fluids and encouragement to drink during every client interaction. Some clients may verbally refuse fluids, but when the straw or glass is respectfully and gently placed in their mouth and encouragement is given, they may decide to drink. Providing fluids that the client especially likes may increase intake. Consider any dietary restrictions when providing clients with additional fluids. For example, a client on a potassium-restricted diet should not be offered fluids high in potassium, such as orange juice. You and your support staff can also encourage foods that have a high fluid content, such as custards, soups, and ice creams.

When a specific fluid order is given (e.g., "Increase fluids to 2000 mL per 24 hours"), plan how much the client should consume in each shift (or equivalent period for clients at home). Usually, the largest volume is consumed during the daytime and early evening. Large amounts taken near bedtime may necessitate having to go to the bathroom during the night, interrupting sleep.

Adequate fluid replacement also is necessary for clients who are receiving tube feedings. These clients may need additional water to prevent water deficit. They often cannot independently drink when they are thirsty or even notify a nurse or family member of their thirst. For this reason, carefully assess the fluid needs of clients receiving tube feedings, and administer water as needed.

Restricting Oral Fluids. Oral fluids may need to be restricted when ECF volume excess or water excess is present or when certain medical conditions, such as heart failure or renal fail-

Your client, Ms. Simpson, a 24-year-old woman requiring fluid restriction, has an IV line in her left arm and is allowed nothing by mouth. She has been irritable and impatient with the staff this morning, and now she has her call light on again. When you ask her what you can do for her, she says that she wants a drink. "I'm so thirsty, my mouth feels like cotton balls." How should you intervene?

Check your answer in Appendix A.

ure, occur. Assisting the client to comply with limited fluid intake despite thirst can be a challenge.

The physician's orders for fluid restriction will include the number of milliliters of fluid to be taken every 24 hours. Most fluid restrictions include all fluids ingested. When a free water restriction is ordered, mainly free water is restricted; other fluids, such as tomato juice or milk, which contain at least 150 mEq/L of sodium, can be given in moderate amounts because they would not contribute to a water excess (Sterns, Spital & Clark, 1996).

Plan with the client and family how best to allocate the allotted fluid during a 24-hour period. Some clients prefer to drink with their meals, whereas others prefer to save them and drink them between meals. Most fluids are designated for day and evening, with about 100 mL remaining for nighttime, in case the client has to take medication or wants a drink. Ice chips may help people on fluid restriction. Ice melts to one half its volume and should be noted as such on the intake and output record. If necessary, remove any water containers from the room and offer water in small cups to avoid the temptation of drinking too much at one time. Diversional activities also may help the client focus less on the thirst he or she is experiencing.

To minimize thirst for clients on fluid restriction, avoid salty or very sweet fluids. Gum and hard candy may temporarily relieve thirst by drawing fluid into the oral cavity, because the sugar content increases oral tonicity. Fifteen to 30 minutes later, however, oral membranes may be even drier than before. To avoid this rebound effect, sugar-free candy and gum may help. Dry foods, such as crackers and bread, also may increase the client's feeling of thirst. Allowing the client to rinse his or her mouth frequently may decrease thirst. The client takes a sip of water, swishes it around the oral cavity, and then spits it out before swallowing. Avoid giving mouthwashes that contain alcohol, because they have a drying effect. Frequent oral care is necessary for anyone on fluid restriction. Moisten the client's lips with a water-soluble gel to prevent drying and cracking.

Electrolyte Replacement
Diet Teaching.   After the potential for an electrolyte imbalance has been identified, an individualized diet teaching plan is needed. Provide the client with a list of foods that are high

or low in the identified electrolyte (Table 36-6). Give some guidelines for the amount to consume each day. For example, for the client who has recently been prescribed a potassium-depleting diuretic, indicate the importance of eating at least one banana or other potassium-rich food each day. Also teach the client about the signs and symptoms of hypokalemia so that he or she can monitor and report if any occur.

Electrolyte Supplements.   When normal dietary intake is insufficient, electrolyte supplements may be administered orally or intravenously. Liquid oral potassium supplements taste unpleasant and can be mixed with juice to promote compliance. IV administration is most commonly used for clients with severe electrolyte imbalances and for those who are unable to take anything orally. IV preparations of potassium must be administered carefully because a concentrated infusion can irritate the veins or cause rebound hyperkalemia, which is potentially lethal.

🔄   **SAFETY ALERT**
        Monitor clients receiving IV potassium carefully. Make sure the infusion rate does not exceed 10 to 20 mEq/hr, unless otherwise ordered.

Intravenous Therapy
IV therapy is used to prevent or treat fluid and electrolyte imbalances. In hospitals, nurses are responsible for initiating, monitoring, and discontinuing IV infusions. Physicians order the type and amount of IV fluid and electrolyte replacement. When IV fluid therapy is provided in the home, family members or visiting nurses assist with monitoring (see Chapter 28).

Healthcare Planning and Home- or Community-Based Nursing

Many clients continue treatment for fluid and electrolyte imbalances at home, which may require dietary changes. Certain restrictions may be enforced, or certain foods may need to be encouraged. Give clients appropriate lists of foods and work out a plan as to who will shop for and prepare meals. These tasks may tire clients who are weak from fluid or electrolyte imbalances.

Clients with fluid or electrolyte imbalances may take various medications. Emphasize, for each medication, its purpose, dosage, frequency, precautions, and potential side effects and complications. If the client has a prescription for a medication (e.g., diuretic), explain the signs and symptoms of potential electrolyte imbalance and methods for circumventing the problem. For example, if the client is taking a diuretic that enhances potassium excretion, reinforce the importance of the client's replacing potassium by taking ordered supplements and making necessary dietary changes (e.g., eating bananas, dried apricots, and other fruits daily).

Teach clients who are with restricted sodium intake how to read food labels. Be sure that the client understands that 1 g contains 1000 mg, because the food labels report sodium

TABLE 36-6

Selected Dietary Sources for Electrolytes	
Electrolyte	**Dietary Source**
Sodium	Salt (sodium chloride), monosodium glutamate (MSG), soy sauce, dairy products (milk, cheese), processed food (luncheon meats, bacon), snack foods (peanuts, chips, pretzels), bouillon, canned or packaged soup, pickles, olives, sauerkraut, tomato juice
Potassium	Fruits (banana, cantaloupe, apricots, peaches, dates, raisins), vegetables (avocado, navy beans, potatoes, squash, carrots, cauliflower), orange juice, tomato juice
Calcium	Dairy products (milk, cheese, yogurt, ice cream), dark green vegetables (broccoli, spinach, greens), sardines, salmon, oysters, tofu
Magnesium	Nuts and peanut butter, egg yolk, milk, whole grain cereals, bananas, citrus fruit, dark green vegetables, legumes, seafood, chocolate
Phosphorus	Dairy products, meats, fish, bran and wheat cereals, nuts

content in milligrams. Also, have the client or family member who does the cooking check the content of spices, because many spice mixtures contain sodium chloride.

Because fluid and electrolyte imbalances can cause poor coordination, weakness, confusion, and altered gait, emphasize the need for a safe home environment. Such teaching may include assistance with ambulation or suggestions for safety features in the home (e.g., installing nightlights, removing throw rugs).

Explaining signs and symptoms that need to be relayed to the physician is an important part of client teaching. For example, some physicians want to know if the client gains more than 5 pounds or has episodes of vomiting or diarrhea that lasts for more than 1 day. All client teaching is beneficial for preventing future occurrences of fluid and electrolyte imbalances.

EVALUATION

Evaluation is important to ensure that the goals of promoting optimum fluid and electrolyte balance, preventing complications of imbalance, and increasing the client's knowledge are achieved. Modifications or more realistic outcome criteria may be necessary if the goals are not attained.

Goal

The client will reestablish normal fluid and electrolyte balance.

Possible Outcome Criteria

- The client maintains equal intake and output within 300 mL in 24 hours.
- By discharge, the client demonstrates weight within 2 kg of baseline weight (give specific amount to be lost or gained).
- The client does not experience sudden changes in weight (i.e., an increase or decrease of more than 1 kg/day).
- By discharge, the client has reestablished electrolyte values within normal limits.

- The client experiences a decrease in postural pulse and blood pressure changes.
- By discharge, the client verbalizes that he or she does not have excessive thirst.
- By discharge, the client exhibits no signs or symptoms of edema.
- By discharge, the client does not have concentrated urine.

Goal

The client will demonstrate knowledge regarding how to promote future fluid and electrolyte balance.

Possible Outcome Criteria

- By the conclusion of the teaching session, the client verbalizes the importance of drinking eight glasses of water per day.
- By the conclusion of the teaching session, the client lists foods that are high in sodium and verbalizes needed modifications in diet.
- By the conclusion of the teaching session, the client demonstrates an ability to read and understand a food label.
- The client maintains a daily record of weight for the next month.
- The client notifies the physician of any significant weight gain.
- By the conclusion of the teaching session, the client verbalizes a plan to cope with temporary problems of diarrhea or vomiting.
- By the conclusion of the teaching session, the client lists foods high in potassium.

Goal

The client will remain free of complications from fluid or electrolyte imbalance.

NURSING PLAN OF CARE
THE CLIENT WITH ECF VOLUME DEFICIT

Nursing Diagnosis
ECF Volume Deficit related to inadequate oral intake as manifested by concentrated urine, decrease in urine output, dry mucous membranes, postural hypotension, and change in postural tachycardia.

Client Goal
Client will reestablish normal fluid and electrolyte balance.

Client Outcome Criteria
Client has increased urine output and no more postural tachycardia or hypertension.

Nursing Intervention	Scientific Rationale
1. Monitor intake and output.	1. Observation of trends in intake and output provides essential data regarding client's fluid and electrolyte status and guides interventions. Intake should approximately equal output, but observing for trends and significant increase or decrease is more important than specific numbers.
2. Monitor serum electrolytes, serum osmolality, and urine specific gravity.	2. Monitoring these common laboratory values provides essential data regarding client status and guides interventions.
3. Increase oral fluid intake to at least 2000 mL/24 hr of mildly salty solutions or as ordered by physician.	3. Increased intake of fluids (and high fluid-content foods) helps correct fluid volume deficit and maintain adequate hydration.
4. Monitor IV fluid therapy as prescribed.	4. Fluids must be provided when client cannot obtain adequate intake by oral intake alone. Monitoring ensures infusion at prescribed rate and allows early detection of complications.
5. Assess fluid preferences.	5. Client is more likely to increase fluid intake with fluids that are appealing.
6. Ensure optimal access to preferred fluids, and assist as needed.	6. Availability and assistance are necessary to ensure increased fluid intake.
7. Give positive reinforcement or verbal cuing as necessary.	7. Reinforcement helps to increase compliance for clients who may be forgetful or disinterested.

Possible Outcome Criteria

- The client stands and walks without dizziness or falling.
- The skin remains intact despite edema until edema is reduced.

KEY CONCEPTS

- Homeostasis of body fluids, electrolytes, and pH is necessary for cellular function and health maintenance. Processes such as diffusion, osmosis, active transport, and filtration that facilitate fluid or electrolyte movement maintain homeostasis.
- ICF refers to the fluid within the cells of the body; ECF refers to fluid outside the cell and includes the intravascular fluid and the interstitial fluid.

- Cations are positively charged electrolytes (sodium, potassium, calcium, and magnesium); anions are negatively charged electrolytes (chloride, phosphate, sulfate, and bicarbonate). Balance between anions and cations is a dynamic process that is necessary to maintain neutrality. The electrolyte composition of ICF and ECF is different although the osmolarity is the same in all body fluids.
- Inadequate intake; excessive loss through vomiting, diarrhea, diaphoresis, or use of diuretics; stress; chronic illness such as renal, cardiac, or respiratory failure; surgery; or pregnancy can increase the potential for altered fluid, electrolyte, and acid–base balance.
- States of altered fluid balance include ECF volume excess or deficit and water excess or deficit.
- States of electrolyte imbalance include hyperkalemia, hypokalemia, hypercalcemia, hypocalcemia, hypermagne-

semia, hypomagnesemia, hyperphosphatemia, and hypophosphatemia.

- States of altered acid–base balance include respiratory acidosis, metabolic acidosis, respiratory alkalosis, and metabolic alkalosis.
- Alterations in normal fluid, electrolyte, or acid–base balance are manifested by imbalances in intake and output, changes in mental status, changes in vital signs, abnormal states of tissue hydration, or abnormal neuromuscular status.
- Intake and output, weight, edema, tissue turgor, neck vein and hand vein engorgement, and vital signs are important objective data to collect to identify actual problems in fluid and electrolyte status. Laboratory data, such as serum electrolytes, serum osmolality, urine specific gravity, and arterial blood gases, also provide important information for identifying potential disruption in fluid and electrolyte status.
- Important nursing interventions include preventive health teaching; regulating oral fluids; assisting with electrolyte replacement; initiating, regulating, and monitoring intravenous therapy; and monitoring blood transfusions.

REFERENCES

Abraham, W. T., & Schrier, R. W. (1994). Body fluid volume regulation in health and disease. *Advances in Internal Medicine, 39,* 23–47.

Anonymous. (1994). Hyponatremic seizures among infants fed with commercial bottled drinking water—Wisconsin, 1993. *MMWR Morb Mortal Wkly Rep, 43*(35), 641–643.

Anonymous. (1998). Hyperthermia and dehydration-related deaths associated with intentional rapid weight loss in three collegiate wrestlers—North Carolina, Wisconsin, and Michigan, November–December 1997. *MMWR Morb Mortal Wkly Rep, 47*(6),105–108.

Avery, M. E., & Snyder, J. D. (1990). Oral therapy for acute diarrhea. The underused simple solution. *New England Journal of Medicine, 323,* 891–894.

Blackburn, S. T. (1994). Renal function in the neonate. *Journal of Perinatal and Neonatal Nursing, 8*(1), 37–47.

Centers for Disease Control and Prevention. (1992). The management of acute diarrhea in children: Oral rehydration, maintenance, and nutritional therapy. *MMWR Morb Mortal Wkly Rep, 41*(RR-16), 1–20.

Cogan, M. G. (1991). *Fluid and electrolytes: Physiology and pathophysiology.* Norwalk, CT: Appleton & Lange.

Faull, C. M., Holmes, C., & Baylis, P. H. (1993). Water balance in elderly people: Is there a deficiency of vasopressin? *Age and Aging, 22*(2), 114–120.

Kumar, R. (1996). Calcium disorders. In J. P. Kokko & R. Tannen (Eds.), *Fluid and electrolytes* (3rd ed., pp. 391–419). Philadelphia: W.B. Saunders.

Levin, E. R., Gardner, D. G., & Samson, W. K. (1998). Natriuretic peptides. *New England Journal of Medicine, 339*(5), 321–328.

Ludwig, D. S., Peterson, K. E., & Gortmaker, S. L. (2001). Relation between consumption of sugar-sweetened drinks and childhood obesity: A prospective, observational analysis. *Lancet, 357*(9255), 505–508.

Mack, G. W., Weseman, C. A., Langhans, G. W., Scherzer, H., Gillen, C. M., & Nadel, E. R. (1994). Body fluid balance in dehydrated healthy older men: Thirst and renal osmoregulation. *Journal of Applied Physiology, 76*(4), 1615–1623.

Metheny, N. M. (2000). *Fluid and electrolyte balance: Nursing considerations* (4th ed.). Philadelphia: Lippincott Williams & Wilkins.

Norris, S. O. (1993). Managing low cardiac output states: Maintaining volume after cardiac surgery. *AACN Clin Issues Crit Care Nurs, 4*(2), 309–319.

Paller, M. S., & Ferris, T. F. (1996). Fluid and electrolyte disorders of pregnancy. In J. P. Kokko & R. L. Tannen (Eds.), *Fluid and electrolytes* (3rd ed.; pp. 805–817). Philadelphia: W.B. Saunders.

Robillard, J. E., Segar, J. L., Smith, F. G., & Jose, P. A. (1992). Regulation of sodium metabolism and extracellular fluid volume during development. *Clinics in Perinatology, 19*(1), 15–31.

Rose, B. D. (1994). *Clinical physiology of acid–base and electrolyte disorders* (4th ed.). New York: McGraw-Hill.

Rude, R. K. (1996). Magnesium disorders. In J. P. Kokko & R. L. Tannen (Eds.), *Fluid and electrolytes* (3rd ed.; pp. 421–445). Philadelphia: W.B. Saunders.

Sterns, R. H., Spital, A., & Clark, E. C. (1996). Disorders of water balance. In J. P. Kokko & R. L. Tannen (Eds.), *Fluid and electrolytes* (3rd ed.; pp. 63–109). Philadelphia: W.B. Saunders.

Takamata, A., Mack, G. W., Gillen, C. M., & Nadel, E. R. (1994). Sodium appetite, thirst, and body fluid regulation in humans during rehydration without sodium replacement. *American Journal of Physiology, 266*(5, Part 2), R1493–R1502.

Tannen, R. L. (1996). Potassium disorders. In J. P. Kokko & R. L. Tannen (Eds.), *Fluid and electrolytes* (3rd ed.; pp. 111–199). Philadelphia: W.B. Saunders.

Woods, S., Sivarajan-Froelicher, E., Halpenny, J., & Motzer, S. U. (1999). *Cardiac nursing* (4th ed.). Philadelphia: Lippincott Williams & Wilkins.

BIBLIOGRAPHY

Brown, R. G. (1993). Disorders of water and sodium balance. *Postgraduate Medicine, 93*(4), 227–244.

CHOICE Study Group. (2001). Multicenter, randomized, double-blind clinical trial to evaluate the efficacy and safety of a reduced osmolarity oral rehydration salts solution in children with acute watery diarrhea. *Pediatrics, 107*(4), 613–618.

Convertino, V. A., Armstrong, L. E., Coule, E. F., Mack, G. W., Sawka, M. N., Senay, L. C., Jr., & Sherman, W. M. (1996). American College of Sports Medicine Position Stand: Exercise and fluid replacement. *Medical Science in Sports and Exercise, 28*(1), i–vii.

Fann, B. D. (1998). Fluid and electrolyte balance in the pediatric patient. *Journal of Intravenous Nursing, 21*(3), 153–159.

Faubel, S., & Topf, J. (1999). *The fluid, electrolyte and acid–base companion.* San Diego: Alert and Oriented Publishing Co.

Mange, K., Matsura, D., Cizman, B., Soto, H., Ziyadeh, F. N., Goldfarb, S., & Neilson, E. G. (1997). Language guiding therapy: The case of dehydration versus volume depletion. *Annals of Internal Medicine, 127*(9), 848–853.

Ozuna, L. A., & Adkins, A. T. (1993). Development of a vital-sign/fluid-balance flow sheet. *Oncology Nursing Forum, 20*(1), 113–115.

Phillips, P. A., Johnston, C. I., & Gray, L. (1993). Disturbed fluid and electrolyte homeostasis following dehydration in elderly people. *Age and Ageing, 22*(1), S26–S33.

Yucha, C., & Keen, M. (1996). Renal regulation of extracellular fluid volume and osmolality. *American Nephrology Nurses' Association Journal, 23*(5), 487–495.

37 Nutrition

⌐ Key Terms

absorption
anorexia
anorexia nervosa
basal metabolism
calorie (kilocalorie)
carbohydrates
complete proteins
digestion
disaccharides
fats
fiber
glycogenesis
incomplete protein

macronutrients
metabolism
micronutrients
monosaccharides
nutrients
obese
overweight
partially complete proteins
polysaccharides
proteins
trace elements
vitamins

⌐ Learning Objectives

Upon completion of this chapter, the student will be able to do the following:

1. Identify essential nutrients and examples of good dietary sources for each.
2. Describe normal digestion, absorption, and metabolism of carbohydrates, fats, and proteins.
3. Discuss nutritional considerations across the lifespan.
4. List factors that can affect dietary patterns.
5. Describe manifestations of altered nutrition.
6. Explain nursing interventions to promote optimal nutrition and health.
7. Discuss nursing responsibilities for interventions used to treat altered nutritional states.

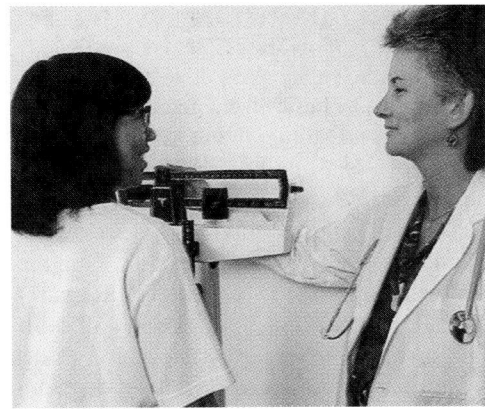

⌐ Critical Thinking Challenge

You are a nurse working in a wellness clinic where a number of men and women have expressed interest in losing weight. During this past week, 11 women and men, ages 42 to 63 years, have discussed with you how they lost weight but gained it back, plus more; or how they tried numerous diets or programs but were unable to maintain weight loss. You must decide how to respond to these people, addressing both nutritional needs and weight management.

Once you have completed this chapter and have added the many facets of nutrition to your knowledge base, return to the above scenario and reflect on the following areas of Critical Thinking:

1. Describe your immediate impressions, and identify the knowledge and values that led you to them.
2. Who and what would you focus on first for people beginning a weight loss program?
3. Describe how being overweight or obese can affect one's health.
4. Contrast and compare your assessments for possible biologic and psychological factors related to weight.
5. Describe the essential components of weight loss and weight maintenance programs for people at the wellness clinic.

As part of a holistic approach to good health, a nutritionally adequate diet is vital for promoting normal growth and development and preventing deficiency states. Optimal nutrition is essential to maintain health and to prevent disease. An adequate diet is necessary to maintain bodily functions, healthy tissues, and body temperature; to promote healing; and to build resistance to infection.

Nutrients are biochemical substances obtained from ingested food and fluids. Carbohydrates, proteins, and fats are nutrients that supply the body with energy. Vitamins, minerals, trace elements, and water are not sources of energy but are important in regulating body processes.

The body cannot synthesize essential nutrients in adequate amounts; therefore, the body must receive them through the diet. Dietary intake of nonessential nutrients is not required, because the body can synthesize such nutrients in adequate amounts or does not require them for body functioning.

Nurses are in key positions to access, monitor, and promote good nutrition. In many settings (e.g., health fairs, classes in schools and community centers, and interactions with families during health screening), they can teach principles of normal nutrition. Nurses also screen for altered nutritional states to detect obesity, overweight, malnutrition, and anorexia. Nutritional assessment is important for all preoperative clients. Nurses teach clients and family members how to adapt to dietary prescriptions or restrictions, especially when special diets are necessary. Nurses also are responsible for monitoring nutritional therapies, such as enteral tube feedings or total parenteral nutrition (TPN), which may be necessary to maintain optimal nutrition in clients with significant impairments.

NORMAL NUTRITION

The body uses nutrients to build and maintain body tissues, furnish energy, and regulate body processes (Mahan & Escott-Stump, 2000). Cellular composition is constantly changing. Cells need nutrients to supply building materials, such as calcium for teeth and bones and fat for padding and support of vital organs. Each cell requires energy to fulfill its daily tasks. Chemicals in the form of nutrients act and react to regulate body processes, which can be as basic as breathing or as circumstantial as wound healing. Water, which makes up one half to two thirds of adult weight, is an important regulator in body processes.

The body breaks down ingested nutrients into a form that it can absorb and use. Metabolism is the process by which cells use or store energy from nutrients. Anabolic processes build up substances and body tissues; catabolic processes break down substances or body stores. The body uses stored energy when the person is not eating, as in a serious illness, or when there is an increased need for nutrients, such as following trauma or during pregnancy.

Energy obtained from food is measured in large calories (kilocalories, abbreviated cal or kcal) or, in Canada, in kilojoules (kJ). The large **calorie (kilocalorie)** is the amount of heat required to raise 1 kilogram of water 1 degree Celsius.

NUTRIENTS

Nutrients, or food containing elements for normal body functioning, are divided into six categories: carbohydrates, proteins, fats, vitamins, minerals, and water. The first three are **micronutrients;** the next two are **macronutrients.** A subgroup of minerals is called **trace elements.** The metabolism of carbohydrates, fats, and protein provides energy. Water is essential to maintain normal fluid balance and promote normal digestion, absorption, and metabolism of food. Vitamins and minerals are organic and inorganic compounds important for normal body processes.

At one time, public health professionals were more concerned about people with nutrient deficiencies, and guidelines were written to help prevent these deficiencies. Current concerns, however, are related to avoiding excesses for possible prevention of chronic diet-related diseases. A discussion of normal nutrition and advice for healthy eating follows. Because no single food supplies all essential nutrients, people should eat a variety of foods (Variyam, Blaylock, Smallwood, & Basiotis, 1998).

Nutrient Guidelines

Recommended Dietary Allowances and Dietary Reference Intakes

The Food and Nutrition Board of the Institute of Medicine/National Academy of Sciences has developed Recommended Dietary Allowances (RDAs) for kilocalories, protein, and certain vitamins and minerals. These 1989 values are in the process of revision. In 1997, the first set of new recommendations was released, called Dietary Reference Intakes (DRIs). Presently, nutritional values include some recommendations from RDAs and others from DRIs (Committee on Dietary Reference Intakes, 1997; National Research Council, 1989; Trumbo, Yates et al., 2001). These values are recommendations for healthy people and do not consider factors that may significantly increase metabolic demands (e.g., exercise, hypermetabolic states). Because nutritional requirements vary with age (Trumbo, Yates et al., 2001), gender, pregnancy, and lactation, separate values are given for each category. Recommended levels include about 98% of the people in a given group, so a particular recommendation may be higher than a specific person in the group needs at a particular time. A common mistake is to think that the "D" in RDA and DRI stands for "daily" rather than "dietary."

World Nutrient Guidelines

Many countries other than the United States have developed nutrition guidelines. Canada's Department of National Health and Welfare developed recommended nutritional intakes. Great Britain also developed a nutrition guide. The World Health Organization (WHO), together with the United Nations Food and Agriculture Organization, developed nutritional guidelines for worldwide use. Factors within each country and the opinions of scientists vary, explaining the slight differences in recommendations.

Carbohydrates

Carbohydrates are simple sugars (monosaccharides and disaccharides) and complex sugars (polysaccharides). They are composed of carbon, hydrogen, and oxygen. Sugars, syrups, molasses, honey, fruit, and milk are excellent sources of simple carbohydrates. Bread, cereal, potatoes, rice, pasta, crackers, flour products, and legumes contain complex carbohydrates.

The main function of carbohydrates is to provide energy. Each gram of oxidized carbohydrate yields about 4 kcal. Carbohydrates also are important for oxidizing fats in normal fat metabolism; promoting desirable bacterial growth in the gastrointestinal (GI) tract, which contributes to the synthesis of vitamin K and small amounts of vitamin B12; producing the carbon component in the synthesis of nonessential amino acids; and producing other essential body acids and compounds.

Polysaccharides not digested in the GI tract are one of the main components of dietary fiber. Dietary **fiber** is a minimal source of energy but plays an essential role in stimulating peristalsis and maintaining normal bowel elimination. Another characteristic of carbohydrates is their protein-sparing action. Protein sparing occurs when the body uses carbohydrates rather than protein as a source of energy, thus sparing protein for the vital function of tissue building.

The circulation of blood supplies glucose to the cells as a source of energy and for the production of vital substances. The blood glucose level is maintained within relatively narrow limits (about 80 to 110 mg/dL). In the fasting state, the blood glucose level is about 60 to 80 mg/dL, but, if measured 2 hours after a meal, it can rise to 140 and 180 mg/dL, depending on the person's age. Hyperglycemia, in which the blood glucose level is higher than normal due to inadequate production or use of insulin, occurs in diabetes mellitus. Hypoglycemia, in which the blood glucose level is lower than normal, can be symptomatic of liver or pancreatic abnormalities.

Proteins

Proteins are organic compounds composed of polymers of amino acids connected by peptide bonds. They contain carbon, hydrogen, oxygen, and nitrogen. Depending on the specific amino acids of which they are composed, proteins also may contain trace elements such as iron or copper. The body synthesizes these proteins for specific functions, including hemoglobin for carrying oxygen to tissues, insulin for blood glucose regulations, and albumin for regulating osmotic pressure in the blood. These functions generally cannot be performed by another body protein.

Proteins are vital to growth, development, and normal functioning of almost all body systems. They are major constituents of most living cells and body fluids, including bones, skin, teeth, muscle, hair, blood, and serum. The main functions of proteins include growth, regulation of body functions and processes, replacement of cellular proteins, and energy. Protein catabolism supplies 4 kcal/g. Protein also plays an important role in regulatory functions and in the body's immune system. Catalytic enzymes derived from proteins function in the regulation of digestion, absorption, metabolism, and catabolism.

Dietary proteins can be classified as complete, partially complete, or incomplete. **Complete proteins** contain sufficient amounts of the essential amino acids to maintain body tissues and to promote growth. The diet must supply essential amino acids because the body cannot synthesize them at a rate sufficient to meet its needs. The body can synthesize nonessential amino acids from available sources. An adequate diet contains a good supply of essential and nonessential amino acids. Good sources of complete proteins are meat, fish, poultry, milk, cheese, and eggs.

Partially complete proteins contain sufficient amounts of amino acids to maintain life but do not promote growth. **Incomplete proteins** do not contain sufficient amounts of all essential amino acids to maintain life, build tissue, or promote growth. By themselves, incomplete proteins are not compatible with maintaining life. Sources of incomplete protein are dried peas and beans, peanut butter, seeds, fruits and vegetables, bread, cereal, rice, and pasta.

Protein requirements depend on a person's state of health, age, body weight, nutritional state, stress level, activity level, and other factors. One measure of the protein requirement is state of nitrogen balance. Nitrogen equilibrium, the normal state for a healthy adult, exists when the amount of nitrogen taken in equals the amount of nitrogen excreted. A state of positive nitrogen balance exists when the intake of nitrogen is greater than the amount excreted. This situation exists when new tissues are being synthesized, as in recovery from illness, athletic training, pregnancy, and childhood growth. A negative nitrogen balance exists when the excretion of nitrogen exceeds the intake. This undesirable condition may exist when a disease or treatment is causing excessive tissue breakdown or when the diet is inadequate in protein, calories, or both.

Fats

Fats, also called lipids, include neutral fats, oils, fatty acids, cholesterol, and phospholipids. Fats are organic substances composed of carbon, hydrogen, and oxygen. They are a significant component of the American diet.

Fat is a component of all body cells and ideally makes up approximately 20% of the body weight of healthy, nonobese people. Fat performs many important functions, including cellular transport, insulation, protection of vital organs in the form of padding, provision of energy, energy storage of adipose tissue, vitamin absorption, and transport of fat-soluble vitamins (vitamins A, D, E, and K).

The energy value of fats is significant; they supply 9 kcal/g of oxidized fat. This is more than twice as much energy per gram than is provided from oxidation of an equal amount of protein or carbohydrate. Fats also have a significant satiety value—they provide a feeling of fullness because they remain in the stomach longer than carbohydrates and proteins do.

Fats are classified as saturated or unsaturated, based on chemical differences. Saturated fats have two hydrogen atoms attached to each of the carbon atoms in the carbon atom chain. An unsaturated fat has a single hydrogen atom missing from each of two side-by-side carbon atoms; as a result, a double bond is formed between the two carbon atoms. This difference is significant in terms of the physical characteristics of the fats, including such factors as melting point, hardness, and the ability to form an emulsion.

Most sources of fat contain a combination of saturated and unsaturated fatty acids. Sources of animal fats, especially beef and lamb, generally contain a higher percentage of saturated fatty acids and are harder than vegetable sources of fatty acids. Coconut oil, palm oil, and palm kernel oil also are highly saturated. Chicken fat contains a significantly higher percentage of unsaturated fatty acids and is measurably softer than beef or lamb fat. Fish and vegetable sources are classified as unsaturated because they contain a higher percentage of unsaturated fatty acids and are generally softer than animal fats.

Vitamins

Vitamins are organic compounds that are essential to the body in small quantities for growth, development, maintenance, and reproduction (Table 37-1). They do not supply energy, but they assist in the use of energy nutrients. Most vitamins cannot be synthesized by the body and must, therefore, be supplied by the diet. The RDAs are the traditional standards for micronutrient intake. They specify the vitamins needed to prevent deficiencies. Groups are currently working on recommendations for various micronutrients; over the next few years, dietary reference standards will be a mixture of old and new values. Vitamins are present in small quantities in food. In varying degrees, exposure to light, air, heat, and some types of food preparation can destroy them. For this reason, fresh foods are usually the best source of vitamins. Some foods, such as fortified milk or cereals, have extra vitamins added. Vitamins are classified as fat-soluble or water-soluble.

Fat-Soluble Vitamins

Fat-soluble vitamins (A, D, E, K) are absorbed with fat into the circulation. A deficiency of fat-soluble vitamins can occur when fat digestion or absorption is altered. Excess fat-soluble vitamins are stored in the liver or adipose tissue; therefore, excessive intake of vitamins A and D can cause toxicity.

Vitamin A. Vitamin A is important in the following:

- Maintenance of normal vision, especially in dim light
- Maintenance of healthy epithelium
- Promotion of normal skeletal and tooth development
- Promotion of normal cellular proliferation

The effects of a vitamin A deficiency are significant, and, in many countries, vitamin A deficiency is the most prevalent vitamin deficiency. Signs of vitamin A deficiency are

- Night or total blindness
- Epithelial changes, such as keratinization (progressive degeneration of the cells that may lead to infections in the eyes, ears, or nasal passages)

- Follicular hyperkeratosis (skin changes leading to rough, dry, and scaly skin)
- Dryness of the eyes (xerophthalmia)
- Inadequate tooth and bone development

The RDA of vitamin A for adult men is 900 μg/day. For adult women, it is 700 μg/day; pregnant or lactating women need more (Trumbo, Yates et al., 2001). Vitamin A is stored in the liver, and excessive intake can be toxic.

Vitamin D. Vitamin D is changed to an active form by exposure of the skin to ultraviolet light. The liver and kidney also play a role in vitamin D metabolism. Vitamin D is important in the following:

- Intestinal absorption of calcium
- Mobilization of calcium and phosphorus from bone
- Renal reabsorption of calcium

These effects increase the blood levels of calcium and phosphorus, allowing for normal mineralization of bone and cartilage and maintenance of calcium extracellular fluid for normal muscle contraction.

A deficiency in vitamin D intake is significant because it leads to inadequate absorption of calcium and phosphorus and to a deficiency of mineralization in bones and teeth. The bones become soft and cannot bear weight, resulting in skeletal deformities. Signs of vitamin D deficiency are

- Rickets in children
- Poor dental health
- Tetany (muscle twitching and convulsions caused by low serum calcium)
- Osteomalacia (soft bones and a tendency toward spontaneous fractures secondary to vitamin D and calcium deficiency)

The DRI of vitamin D for adults is 5 μg; it is 10 μg for people 51 to 70 years of age (Committee on Dietary Reference Intakes, 1997). Excessive amounts can be toxic. Some older adults may exhibit poor vitamin D status.

Vitamin E. The physiologic effects of vitamin E are not well understood. A major function is its role as an antioxidant, in which vitamin E assists in maintaining the integrity of cellular membranes and protecting vitamin A from oxidation. Vitamin E deficiency is rare, but signs of severe deficiency are increased hemolysis of red blood cells, poor reflexes and impaired neuromuscular functioning, and anemia.

The RDA of vitamin E for adults is 1.5/day TE and more for pregnant or lactating women (Rock, 1998). The body does not store vitamin E to any appreciable extent, and toxicity is rare.

Vitamin K. An adequate intake of vitamin K is needed in the liver for the formation of prothrombin and other clotting factors. The major physiologic effect of vitamin K appears to be its role in blood coagulation.

TABLE 37-1

Summary of Vitamins			
Vitamin and RDA/DRI	**Functions**	**Signs and Symptoms of Deficiency**	**Food Sources**
Fat-Soluble Vitamins			
Vitamin A Men: 900 μg RE Women: 700 μg RE	Formation of visual pigments, which enables the eye to adapt to dim light; normal growth and development of bones and teeth; formation and of skin and mucous membranes	Night blindness; bone growth ceases and bone shape changes; skin becomes dry, scaly, rough, and cracked; eyes become dry; decreased saliva secretion; difficulty chewing, swallowing; anorexia; decreased mucous secretion of the stomach and intestines; impaired digestion and absorption; diarrhea, increased excretion of nutrients; susceptible to respiratory, urinary tract, and vaginal infections	Preformed retinol: liver, fish liver oils, whole + fortified milk and dairy products; fortified margarine, and fortified breakfast cereals. Carotenes: dark green and yellow vegetables (e.g., sweet potatoes, winter squash, carrots, broccoli, spinach, "greens," peaches, apricots, and cantaloupe)
Vitamin D 5 μg age 50 yr 10–15 μg age 51–70 yr	Maintenance of levels of calcium and phosphorus for normal bone mineralization	Rickets; osteomalacia (in adults)	Fortified milk, margarine, breakfast cereals; small amounts in butter, egg yolk, liver, salmon, sardines, and tuna
Vitamin E Men and Women: 15 mg α-TE	Protection of vitamins A and C and polyunsaturated fatty acids from being destroyed; protection of cell membranes	Increased RBC hemolysis; in infants, causes anemia, edema, and skin lesions	Vegetable oils, wheat germ, leafy vegetables, soybeans, corn, peanuts, pecans, walnuts, margarine, and salad dressings made with vegetable oils
Vitamin K Men: 120 μg Women: 90 μg	Essential for the formation of five proteins necessary for normal blood clotting	Delayed blood clotting → hemorrhage; hemorrhagic disease of the newborn	Green leafy vegetables, cabbage, cauliflower, spinach, cheese, egg yolk, and liver
Water-Soluble Vitamins			
Vitamin C (Ascorbic Acid) Men: 90 mg Women: 75 mg	Antioxidant; collagen formation; promotes iron absorption; protects against infection	Bleeding gums; pinpoint hemorrhages under skin; scurvy; poor wound healing	Guava, broccoli, brussels sprouts, green peppers, strawberries, "greens," citrus fruits, potatoes, tomatoes, and cabbage

(continues)

TABLE 37-1 (Continued)

Summary of Vitamins

Vitamin and RDA/DRI	Functions	Signs and Symptoms of Deficiency	Food Sources
Thiamine (Vitamin B₁) Men: 1.0 mg Women: 0.9 mg	Energy metabolism, especially the metabolism of CHO; normal nervous system functioning	Beriberi; fatigue; muscle weakness and wasting; anorexia; edema, enlarged heart	Pork, liver organ meats, whole and enriched grains, nuts, legumes, potatoes, eggs, and milk
Riboflavin (Vitamin B₂) Men: 1.1 mg Women: 0.9 mg	Carbohydrates (CHO), protein, and fat metabolism	Dermatitis; cheilosis; glossitis; photophobia; reddening of the cornea	Milk and dairy products, organ meats, eggs, enriched grains, and green leafy vegetables
Niacin (Vitamin B₃) Men: 12 mg Women: 11 mg	CHO, protein, and fat metabolism	Pellagra: (4 Ds) Dermatitis, diarrhea, dementia, death if untreated	Kidney, liver, poultry, lean meat, fish, yeast, peanut butter, enriched and whole grains, dried peas and beans, and nuts
Vitamin B₁₂ (Cobalamin) Men/Women: 2 µg	RNA and DNA synthesis; blood formation; maintenance of nervous tissue; CHO, protein, and fat metabolism; folate metabolism	GI changes; macrocytic anemia pallor, dyspnea, weakness, fatigue, and palpitations	Liver, kidney, shrimp and oysters, meats, milk, eggs, and cheese
Folacin (Folic acid) Men/Women: 300 µg	Amino acid metabolism; DNA and RNA synthesis; proliferation of cells; blood formation	Glossitis, diarrhea, macrocytic anemia, birth defects	Green leafy vegetables, asparagus, broccoli, liver, organ meats, milk, eggs, yeast, wheat germ, and kidney beans
Vitamin B₆ (Pyridoxine) Men: 2.0 mg Women: 1.6 mg	Amino acid metabolism; blood formation; maintenance of nervous tissue; conversion of tryptophan to niacin	Dermatitis, cheilosis, glossitis, abnormal brain wave pattern, convulsions, and anemia	Chicken, fish, peanuts, oats, yeast, wheat germ, pork, organ meats, egg yolk, whole grain cereals, corn, potatoes, and bananas
Pantothenic acid Men/Women: Safe and adequate intake, 4–7 mg	CHO, protein, and fat metabolism	Not observed in humans	Animal tissues, whole grain cereals, legumes, milk, vegetables, and fruit
Biotin Men/Women: Safe and adequate intake, 30–100 µg	Fat and CHO metabolism; glycogen formation	Observed only under experimental conditions	Liver, organ meats, egg yolk, milk, and yeast. Synthesized by GI flora

Adapted from Rolfes, S., DeBruyne, L., & Whitney, E. (1998). *Life span nutrition.* Belmont, CA: West/Wadsworth.

Vitamin K deficiencies are manifested in two ways: an increased tendency to hemorrhage (prolonged clotting time) and hemorrhagic disease of the newborn, which is most common in premature or anoxic newborns.

The Adequate Intake (AI) of vitamin K for adult men is 120 µg/day, and for adult women it is 90 µg/day (Trumbo, Yates et al., 2001). Approximately half of the body's requirement of vitamin K is synthesized by bacteria in the lower intestinal tract. The body does not store vitamin K to an appreciable extent. Large amounts are not usually toxic except in newborns.

Water-Soluble Vitamins

The water-soluble vitamins are vitamin C and the B-complex vitamins. Water-soluble vitamins are not stored in the body, although some body tissues can hold limited amounts. Adequate daily intake of water-soluble vitamins is recommended to prevent deficiencies. When the intake of water-soluble vitamins exceeds the amount absorbed by the tissues, the excess is excreted in the urine.

B-Complex Vitamins. Each B-complex vitamin has its own function and RDA. Vitamin B1 (thiamine) functions in carbohydrate metabolism, and adequate thiamine intake results in healthy nerve functioning and normal appetite and digestion. Deficiency symptoms include poor appetite, apathy, mental depression, fatigue, constipation, edema, cardiac failure, and neuritis. The disease associated with inadequate thiamine intake is beriberi. Acute beriberi adversely affects the cardiac, nervous, and GI systems. Death can result from cardiac failure. The Estimated Average Requirement (EAR) of thiamine is 1.0 mg/day for men and 0.9 mg/day for women, with additional amounts recommended for pregnant or lactating women (National Academy of Sciences, 1999).

Vitamin B2 (riboflavin) functions in protein and carbohydrate metabolism and contributes to healthy skin and normal vision. Deficiency symptoms are cheilosis (cracking and fissures at the corners of the mouth), dermatitis, increased vascularization of the cornea, and other vision irregularities. The EAR of riboflavin is 0.9 mg/day for men and 0.9 mg/day for women, with additional amounts recommended for pregnant or lactating women (National Academy of Sciences, 1999).

Vitamin B3 (niacin) is involved in glycogen metabolism, tissue regeneration, and fat synthesis. The niacin deficiency disease is pellagra; its symptoms are fatigue, headache, loss of appetite and weight loss, abdominal pain, diarrhea, dermatitis, and neurologic deterioration. The EAR of niacin is 12 mg/day for men and 11 mg/day for women, with additional amounts recommended for pregnant or lactating women (National Academy of Sciences, 1999).

Vitamin B12 (cyanocobalamin) functions in the formation of mature red blood cells and in the synthesis of DNA and RNA. It requires intrinsic factor for absorption. A vitamin B12 deficiency leads to pernicious anemia, other forms of anemia, and neurologic deterioration. The EAR of vitamin B12 is 2 µg/day for adults, with additional amounts recommended for pregnant or lactating women. This vitamin is found only in animal foods (meats, fish, poultry, milk, and eggs).

Folic acid functions as a coenzyme in protein metabolism and cell growth. Folic acid is necessary for red blood cell formation, and early in pregnancy it is essential for spine and spinal cord development in the fetus. Recently, folic acid has been suggested to prevent vascular clots in the hearts or brains of people with high circulating levels of homocysteine, an amino acid. Deficiency signs include glossitis, diarrhea, macrocytic anemia, and birth defects. Folic acid deficiency in pregnant women can lead to neural tube deficits (e.g., spina bifida) in the fetus. Because fetal neural development begins so early in pregnancy, women in their childbearing years must have adequate folic acid intake. The EAR for men and women is 300 µg/day (National Academy of Sciences, 1999). Typical American intake is 60 to 80 µg/day. Various investigators have recommended supplements of 100 to 1000 µg/day during pregnancy. Folic acid occurs in most foods, particularly dried beans, fresh vegetables, and fruits such as oranges and cantaloupe.

Other important B vitamins are vitamin B6, pantothenic acid, and biotin. Deficiencies are rare.

Vitamin C. Vitamin C is important in the following:

- Protection against infection
- Adequate wound healing
- Collagen formation
- Iron absorption
- Metabolism of several important amino acids

Vitamin C is an antioxidant that protects vitamins A and E from excessive oxidation. Signs of vitamin C deficiency are

- Inadequate formation of collagen (poor wound healing), increased susceptibility to infection, retardation of growth and development, joint pain, anemia
- Scurvy (now rare, but formerly common among sailors whose diets lacked fresh fruits and vegetables, particularly citrus fruits)

The RDA for vitamin C is 90 mg/day for adults and 75 mg/day for pregnant or lactating women (Rock, 1998). The body stores little vitamin C, so a daily supply is needed. Although large doses of vitamin C (30 to 100 times the recommended allowances) have not proved toxic, excessive doses are not advised because of the possibility of kidney stone formation and GI disturbances.

Minerals

Minerals are inorganic substances found in nearly all body tissues and fluids. When plant or animal tissue is burned, what remains is ash or mineral matter. Minerals help build body tissues and regulate metabolism. There are more than 25 known minerals in the adult body; the most notable are described here and in Table 37-2.

Calcium

Almost all of the calcium in the body is found in the bones and teeth. The bones provide the framework for the body and are a storage area that keeps the plasma concentration

TABLE 37-2

Summary of Several Minerals			
Mineral and DRI/RDA	**Functions**	**Signs and Symptoms of Deficiency**	**Food Sources**
Calcium AI: 1000–1200 mg	Bone and teeth formation and maintenance; blood clotting; nerve transmission; muscle function; cell membrane permeability	Stunted growth; rickets, osteomalacia; osteoporosis (porous bones); tetany (low serum calcium)	Milk and dairy products; green leafy vegetables; whole grains; nuts and legumes; seafood
Phosphorus 19 yr: 700 mg	Bone and teeth formation and maintenance; acid-base balance; energy metabolism; cell membrane structure; hormone and coenzyme regulation	Stunted growth; rickets (due to excessive excretion rather than dietary deficiency)	Meat; poultry; fish; eggs; legumes; milk and dairy products; soft drinks
Trace Elements *Magnesium* Men: 420 mg Women: 320 mg	Bone formation; smooth muscle relaxation; protein synthesis; CHO metabolism	Alcoholism or renal disease: tremors leading to convulsive seizures	Green leafy vegetables; nuts; legumes; whole grains; seafood
Iron Men: 8 mg Women: 18 mg; 8 mg age 51+ yr	Oxygen transport through hemoglobin and myoglobin; constituent of enzyme systems	Depletion of iron stores, anemia (microcytic, hypochromic), pallor, decreased work capacity	Liver; lean meat; dried beans; fortified cereals
Iodine 150 µg	Constituent of thyroid hormones that regulate basal metabolic rate	Goiter (not a problem in the United States)	Iodized salt; seafood; milk; eggs; bread
Zinc Men: 15 mg Women: 12 mg	Tissue growth, development and healing; sexual maturation and reproduction; constituent of many enzymes in energy and nucleic acid metabolism	Impaired growth, sexual maturation, and immune system functioning; skin lesions; acrodermatitis; enteropathica; decreased sense of taste and smell	Meat; oysters; seafood; milk; egg yolks; legumes; whole grains

AI: adequate intake.
Adapted from Rolfes, S., DeBruyne, L., & Whitney, E. (1998). *Life span nutrition.* Belmont, CA: West/Wadsworth.

of calcium relatively constant. Calcium, the most abundant mineral in the body, also is important in the following:

- Conversion of prothrombin to thrombin and other steps of the coagulation process
- Nerve impulse transmission by participating in the formation of acetylcholine
- Regulation of materials in and out of cells
- Contraction and relaxation of muscles, most notably the heart muscle

Calcium is absorbed mainly from the duodenum by active transport. Calcium also is passively diffused across the intestinal mucosa from the jejunum and the ileum. The amount of calcium absorbed is determined mainly by the body's need. About 30% to 40% of dietary calcium is absorbed in the healthy adult. Children, adolescents, and pregnant and lactating women absorb a greater percentage of their dietary calcium because of their increased need. Some ingested calcium forms insoluble salts, which cannot be absorbed.

Adequate amounts of vitamin D, parathyroid hormone, ascorbic acid, lactose, several other amino acids, and physical activity assist in calcium absorption. Inadequate amounts of vitamin D, insufficient exposure to sunlight, decreased amounts of ascorbic acid, decreased physical activity, and emotional stress may decrease calcium absorption. Other factors, such as a high consumption of dietary fiber and excessive phosphorus intake, impair the absorption of calcium. These factors are still being researched.

The effects of calcium deficiency can be profound. Rickets, a disease of infants and children caused by inadequate calcium and vitamin D, involves the inadequate deposition of calcium and phosphorus in the bone. Symptoms include soft bones, enlarged joints, enlarged skull secondary to delayed closure of the cranial fontanelles, bowed legs, and spinal and chest deformities. Osteomalacia, the adult form of rickets, results from inadequate intake of calcium, phosphorus, and vitamin D. The mineral content of the bone is reduced, but the bone stays the same size.

Osteoporosis involves a reduction in bone mass. It is commonly seen in postmenopausal women and in elderly men. Factors contributing to the development of osteoporosis may include a chronically insufficient calcium intake, decreased estrogens, heredity factors, smoking, race, and decreased physical activity. Symptoms vary in severity and may include reduced bone mass, leading to poor posture; increased fragility of bones, leading to an increase in bone fractures; and delayed healing of fractures. Malabsorption syndromes can lead to problems in calcium absorption, and osteoporosis can develop. Low dietary intake of calcium also has been associated with hypertension.

The AI for calcium is 1000 to 1200 mg for adults, with additional amounts recommended for adolescents, young women, and pregnant or lactating women (Committee on Dietary Reference Intakes, 1997). The estimated intake by women is less than 600 mg/day.

Iron

Most iron in the body is found in hemoglobin, the red-pigmented, iron-containing protein. Hemoglobin carries oxygen from the lungs to the tissues and helps transport carbon dioxide to the lungs. Iron also is found in the body's myoglobin, an iron-protein deficiency compound in the muscle that is an oxygen storage system for the muscles.

Iron deficiencies may manifest themselves in iron-deficiency anemia. This form of anemia is not uncommon, especially in infants, adolescents, and menstruating women. In anemia, circulating hemoglobin is reduced, and the blood cannot provide for the oxygen needs of the tissues. Iron-deficiency anemia may result from a diet chronically deficient in iron. Other factors that may lead to iron-deficiency anemia are blood loss, chronic disease, pregnancy and lactation, diarrhea, and other nutritional deficiencies (protein and calorie). Symptoms of iron-deficiency anemia are excessive fatigue, lethargy, and poor resistance to infection. Because obtaining sufficient iron to combat anemia by dietary measures alone is impractical, recommended treatment includes taking iron salts (ferrous sulfate or gluconate) along with a well-balanced diet.

The RDA of iron for adult men is 8 mg/day. The RDA for adult women is 18 mg/day, with additional amounts recommended for pregnant or lactating women. After age 51, it drops to 8 mg/day.

Sodium

Sodium is found primarily in the extracellular fluid in the body. As an ion, it helps maintain fluid and acid–base balance. RDAs for sodium intake have not been set, although the current guideline is a limit of 2.4 g/day. The average diet contains more sodium than the body requires, and sodium deficiencies (except rarely) have not been identified. Many people would benefit from eating less sodium, and sodium restriction is important for people with heart disease, hypertension, edema, renal disorders, liver disease, or pregnancy-induced hypertension. Only 10% of sodium intake is from natural sources, including salt, salt compounds, milk, meat, poultry, fish, and eggs; 75% of sodium comes from processed foods, and 15% comes from discretionary salt addition (in cooking and at the table) (Sanchez-Castillo, Warrender, Whitehead, & James, 1987).

Potassium

Potassium is found primarily in the body's intracellular fluid. It functions in protein synthesis, in fluid balance (as an ion), and in regulation of muscle contraction. RDAs have not been set, and deficiencies have not been identified, except in cases such as severe vomiting, diarrhea, use of non–potassium-sparing diuretics, and diabetic acidosis. Potassium restriction is indicated for clients with renal impairment or renal failure. Potassium is present in many foods, including protein-rich foods, bread, cereal, fruits, and vegetables.

Iodine

Although iodine is a trace element, it is an important mineral. The primary location of iodine in the body is the thyroid gland. Iodine is a component of the thyroid hormones, thyroxine and triiodothyronine. These hormones help regulate energy metabolism, nervous and muscle cell functioning, and mental and physical growth.

A chronic deficiency of iodine can lead to endemic goiter. The major initial symptom is an enlarged thyroid gland. This condition is especially significant in pregnant women because it can lead to physical and mental retardation in the fetus. In its severe form, this condition in the infant is known as cretinism. Cretinism is rare in the United States but remains a problem in certain areas of Central and South America, Africa, and Asia. Characteristics of cretinism are muscle flabbiness, weakness, dry skin, thick lips, skeletal retardation, and severe mental retardation. Thyroid hormone given early to infants can be of some value, but certain physical and mental deficiencies are irreversible. Everyone, especially pregnant women, should eat a diet sufficient in iodine. The RDA of iodine for adult men and women is 150 μg/day, with additional amounts recommended for pregnant or lactating women (Trumbo, Yates et al., 2001).

Fluoride

Fluoride, another trace element, is found primarily in the bones and teeth. It maintains bone structure and reduces tooth decay by strengthening tooth enamel. The DRI for adults is 3.8 mg for men and 3.1 mg for women (Committee on Dietary Reference Intakes, 1997). Fluoride is found in the diet, in water, and in soil in generally safe and adequate amounts. In many areas in the United States fluoride, a fluorine compound, has been added to the water in amounts equivalent to the normal soil concentration (1 part fluoride per 1 million parts water or soil).

Water

Water is necessary to maintain normal cell function. Water is obtained by drinking fluid and eating foods with a high water content (fresh fruits and vegetables) and by the oxidation of food. Generally, thirst signals the need for water and encourages a person to drink. This sensation often is diminished in the aged. Fluid balance is covered in Chapter 36.

The Food Guide Pyramid

The food guide pyramid, as revised by the U. S. Department of Agriculture (USDA), provides a general guide for planning nutritious, appetizing meals (USDA, 2000a). The pyramid emphasizes food from five major food groups: bread, cereal, rice, and pasta; vegetables; fruits; meat, poultry, dry beans, eggs, and nuts; milk, yogurt, and cheese. Fats, sugars, and alcohol are included in a sixth group. Guidelines suggest an appropriate daily number of servings from each group (Fig. 37-1).

Bread, Cereal, Rice, and Pasta Group

Bread, cereal, rice, and pasta are important food sources in many countries. Rice, wheat, and corn are worldwide dietary staples. This group includes whole grains, breads, cereals, rice, noodles, pasta, and products made with enriched flour and cereal. Six to 11 daily servings are recommended; one serving is equal to about ½ cup of a cooked product (pasta, rice, or cereal), one slice of bread, or 1 ounce of uncooked cereal (USDA, 2000a).

Breads and cereals are good sources of thiamine, iron, niacin, and riboflavin. Many breads and cereals are enriched, especially those processed and sold in the United States. Enrichment with vitamins and minerals adds to the nutritive value of these foods. Whole grains also are excellent sources of zinc, copper, B-complex vitamins, vitamin E, and fiber. These foods are a good source of carbohydrates, calories, and incomplete proteins, and they are low in fat.

Vegetable Group

The vegetable group includes cooked and uncooked parts of plants. Three to five servings of vegetables are recommended daily (USDA, 2000a). One serving is roughly equal to 1 cup of raw leafy vegetables or ½ cup of a cooked vegetable.

Vegetables provide vitamins A and C, folate, and minerals such as iron and magnesium. Because they are low in fat and provide fiber, they are excellent for human nutrition. Some vegetables are deep green or yellow in color and make meals more pleasing to look at. Legumes and other vegetables should be included.

Fruit Group

Fruit and fruit juices make up the fruit group. The food guide suggests two to four servings of fruit each day (USDA, 2000a). A medium apple, banana, or orange counts as one serving, as does ½ cup of chopped, cooked, or canned fruit or ¾ cup of fruit juice.

In addition to being important sources of vitamins A and C and potassium, fruits are low in fat and sodium. As a group, these foods have a high water content and are generally low in calories and protein. They contain no cholesterol.

Fresh whole fruit is the best source because of its high fiber content. Juice has little to no fiber content. People should avoid fruits canned in heavy syrups and sweetened fruit drinks.

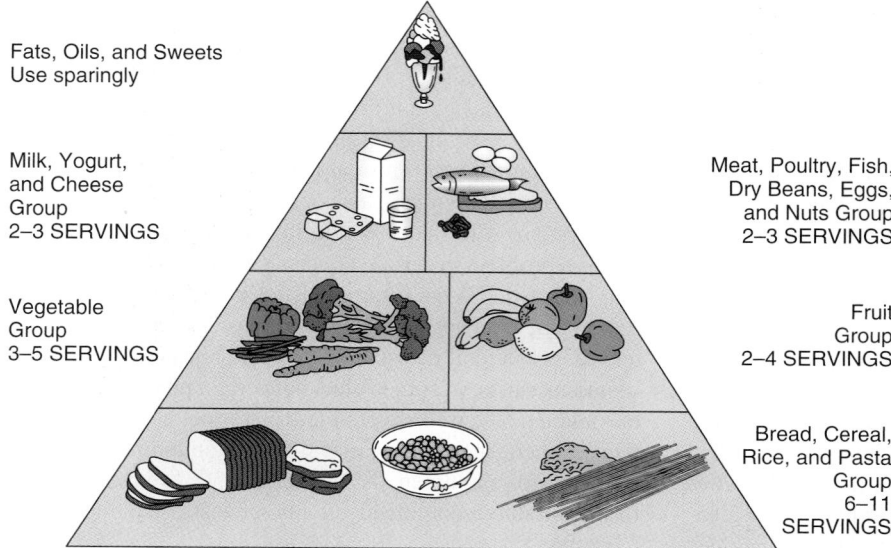

Fats, Oils, and Sweets
Use sparingly

Milk, Yogurt,
and Cheese
Group
2–3 SERVINGS

Meat, Poultry, Fish,
Dry Beans, Eggs,
and Nuts Group
2–3 SERVINGS

Vegetable
Group
3–5 SERVINGS

Fruit
Group
2–4 SERVINGS

Bread, Cereal,
Rice, and Pasta
Group
6–11
SERVINGS

FIGURE 37-1   The Food Guide Pyramid: A Guide to Daily Food Choices.

Meat, Poultry, Fish, Dry Beans, Eggs, and Nuts Group

Two to three servings from this group are recommended daily (USDA, 2000a). A serving is 2 to 3 ounces of the edible part of meat, fish, or poultry. Included in this group are eggs, dry beans or peas, lentils, soybeans, nuts, and peanut butter. One ounce of meat is roughly equal to one egg, $\frac{1}{2}$ cup of dry beans or peas, or 2 tablespoons of peanut butter.

The meat group is an excellent source of protein and a good source of B-complex vitamins and minerals (iron and zinc). Other foods in the group similarly provide protein and most vitamins and minerals. Some shellfish are good sources of calcium, and saltwater fish are a good source of iodine. This group can contain a large amount of fat, depending on the cut of the meat, the type of meat, and the method of processing and preparation. Animal foods can contain a significantly larger amount of cholesterol and saturated fat than plant foods do, but fish is generally lower in cholesterol and saturated fat. Egg yolks, in particular, contain a large amount of cholesterol.

Milk, Yogurt, and Cheese Group

The milk group is an important source of nutrition for all people but is especially important for infants, children, and pregnant or lactating women. The recommended number of daily servings depends on the person's physiologic needs, age, and developmental level. Children younger than 12 years of age need two or three servings; adolescents need four servings; adults need two or three servings; pregnant women need three or four servings; and lactating women need four servings. One serving equals 1 cup (8 ounces) of milk or yogurt, about 1.5 ounces of natural cheese, or about 2 ounces of processed cheese.

Milk is an excellent source of calcium, phosphorus, and riboflavin. It also is fairly rich in sodium, potassium, magnesium, vitamin A, thiamine, vitamin B6, vitamin B12, niacin, and vitamin D. Milk is an excellent source of protein, but it has little iron. The fat content of milk depends on the type of product. In recent years, many people have started drinking low-fat milk and eating low-fat cheese to decrease their fat intake.

The nutritional characteristics of cheese are similar to those of milk, depending on the type of cheese. One noteworthy difference (which could be important for people with lactose intolerance) is that cheese contains only a trace amount of lactose.

Fats, Oils, and Sweets Group

The foods in this group (e.g., sugar, jelly, jam, shortening, butter, margarine, salad dressings, soft drinks, alcoholic beverages) add flavor, variety, and interest to meals. There is no recommended number of daily servings. Most people should use them sparingly, to minimize their intake of sugar and fats, especially saturated fats. Foods in this group add to the energy value of diets but generally add little nutritive value. One noteworthy exception is fortified margarine, a fair source of vitamin A and vitamin E.

THE DIGESTIVE SYSTEM

Structure of the Digestive System

The digestive system consists of the organs of the GI tract (mouth, pharynx, esophagus, stomach, small intestine, and large intestine), through which food enters, travels, and exits the body, and accessory organs that play a role in the process of digestion (tongue, salivary glands, teeth, liver, pancreas, and gallbladder).

The mouth is lined with mucous membrane. The tongue is composed of skeletal muscle and is covered with mucous membrane. The papillae, which are the elevations on the tongue, contain the taste buds. The salivary glands are sublingual (the interior part of the mouth under the tongue), submandibular (the posterior part of the floor of the mouth), and parotid (near the temporomandibular joint). The salivary glands secrete saliva, which contains fluid and the salivary enzymes. Mastication includes chewing, reducing the size of food particles, and mixing the food with saliva. The pharynx extends from the base of the skull to the esophagus and is composed of muscle lined with mucous membrane. Food and air pass through this structure before reaching the appropriate outlet (the epiglottis for food and the trachea for air). The epiglottis closes off the airway during swallowing. The esophagus extends from the pharynx to the stomach and transports food from the mouth to the stomach. It is a long, collapsible tube composed of muscular walls lined with mucous membrane.

The stomach lies in the midline and left upper portion of the abdominal cavity. It is connected to the esophagus at the upper end and to the duodenum at the lower end. The stomach varies in size according to body size, sex, and distention. The stomach is lined with mucous membrane and has a muscle layer and an outer fibroserous layer.

The small intestine lies in the abdominal cavity and measures about 1 inch in diameter and 20 feet in length. It has a mucous lining, two muscle layers, and an outer visceral peritoneal layer. The small intestine consists of the duodenum, the jejunum, and the ileum.

The large intestine, located at the lower end of the GI tract, is about 2 to 3 inches in diameter and 6 feet long. It has a mucous lining, two muscle layers, and, over some sections, an outer visceral peritoneal layer. The large intestine consists of the cecum, the colon (ascending, transverse, descending, and sigmoid), and the rectum (see Chapter 41).

The accessory organs of digestion are located outside the GI tract, but their secretions are conveyed there by ducts. The liver, the largest gland in the body, lies in the right upper quadrant of the abdominal cavity. Bile produced in the liver is transported through the hepatic duct and the cystic duct to the gallbladder, where it is stored and concentrated. The common bile duct transports bile to the duodenum, where it participates in digestion. The pancreas is located behind the stomach and lies in the curvature of the duodenum. Pancreatic enzymes are transported to the duodenum through the pancreatic ducts.

Function of the Digestive System

The digestive system performs the vital function of converting food into substances that the body's cells can absorb and use. This conversion involves the processes of digestion, absorption, metabolism, and excretion.

Digestion

Digestion is the process by which foods are broken down for the body to use in growth, development, healing, and prevention of disease. Digestion includes the mechanical and chemical processes necessary to convert foods into their physically absorbable states.

Mechanical Process. The mechanical process of digestion consists of the following events:

1. Mastication takes place in the mouth. Food particles are reduced in size and mixed with enzymes in saliva.
2. Deglutition (swallowing) begins in the mouth and continues in the pharynx and the esophagus.
3. Churning movements and peristalsis mix and move the ingested material through the stomach and into the duodenum.
4. In the small intestine, the ingested material is further churned and mixed with many digestive enzymes. It comes in contact with the intestinal mucosa to allow for absorption.
5. Peristalsis moves the ingested material into the large intestine.
6. Further churning, peristalsis, and absorption help move the residual ingested mass along the full length of the large intestine, where it is stored until it is evacuated from the body.

Chemical Process. The chemical process of digestion changes the composition of ingested material. Most carbohydrates and all fats and proteins must be chemically reduced for absorption.

Carbohydrate digestion involves the hydrolysis of polysaccharides (with the exception of cellulose and other fibers) into disaccharides by the amylase enzymes found in saliva and pancreatic juices. Hydrolysis is a chemical process between a compound and water that results in the division of the compound into simpler components. A **polysaccharide** is a carbohydrate compound containing three or more saccharide groups; a **disaccharide** contains two saccharide groups; a **monosaccharide** contains only one saccharide group. Disaccharides are further hydrolyzed into monosaccharides by the enzymes sucrase, maltase, and lactase secreted by the intestines.

Fat digestion is accomplished by emulsification of fats, which is facilitated by bile. Emulsification involves breaking down fats into smaller fat droplets and dispersing these droplets into solution. The pancreatic enzyme lipase hydrolyzes the small fat droplets into fatty acids and glycerol.

Protein digestion involves the hydrolysis of the larger protein compounds into amino acids. This is done by the protease enzymes, which include pepsin from the gastric fluid, trypsin and other proteases from the pancreatic fluid, and peptidases from the intestinal fluid.

Absorption

Absorption is the process by which the digested proteins, fats, carbohydrates, vitamins, minerals, and water are actively and passively transported through the intestinal mucosa into the blood or lymphatic circulation. The proteins, such as amino acids, and the digested carbohydrates and simple sugars, in the form of monosaccharides, are absorbed into the bloodstream through the intestinal capillaries. The fats, in the form of glycerol and fatty acids, are absorbed into the lymphatic system through the lymphatic capillaries in the intestinal villi. Some finely emulsified neutral fats are absorbed undigested into the capillaries.

Metabolism

After ingested food is digested and absorbed, the products are ready to be metabolized. **Metabolism** is the complex chemical process that occurs in the cells to allow for energy use and for cellular growth and repair. Metabolism involves catabolic and anabolic processes: catabolic processes break down complex substances into simpler substances (e.g., tissue breakdown), and anabolic processes convert simple substances into more complex ones (e.g., tissue repair).

Carbohydrate Metabolism. The liver cells change short-term glucose excesses into glycogen in the presence of insulin; this anabolic process is called **glycogenesis.** Glycogen is stored in the liver and skeletal muscles until needed and is then converted back into glucose by a catabolic process called glycogenolysis.

Longer-term storage of glucose in the presence of insulin takes the form of fat deposits (adipose tissue). When the amount of glucose entering the cells is not enough to meet cellular demands, gluconeogenesis (the formation of glucose from protein and fat in the liver) occurs. This catabolic process yields about 4 kcal of energy per gram of oxidized carbohydrate.

Fat Metabolism. Fats are converted to adipose tissue and stored in the body's fat deposits if they are not immediately needed. Stored fat deposits make up the body's largest reserve energy source. The catabolism of fats involves the hydrolysis of fat into glycerol and fatty acids. The fatty acids are then converted by a series of chemical reactions known as ketogenesis into ketone bodies. In the tissue cells, ketones are converted by the citric acid cycle into energy, carbon dioxide, and water. Glycerol is converted by gluconeogenesis into glucose. Fats are a more concentrated source of energy than carbohydrates, yielding 9 kcal of energy per gram of catabolized fat.

Protein Metabolism. Protein anabolism builds tissues, produces antibodies, replaces blood cells, and repairs tissues. Temporary excesses of protein are stored in the liver and in skeletal muscle or converted to fat. Protein catabolism involves the hydrolysis of cellular proteins into amino acids in the tissue cell. It also involves the deamination process of amino acids, in which an amino group is split off from an amino acid to form ammonia and keto acid. This process takes place in the liver cell to form glucose and urea.

Excretion

The excretory organs (kidneys, sweat glands, skin, lungs, and intestines) remove waste products from the body. Water, toxins, salts, and nitrogen wastes are excreted through the kidneys, skin, and sweat glands. Carbon dioxide and water are excreted through the lungs. Digestive wastes are excreted through the intestines and rectum.

CHARACTERISTICS OF NORMAL NUTRITION

Normal nutrition involves a balanced intake of food to meet the energy requirements necessary for organ function, body movement, and work. Adequate food intake also provides raw materials for the production of enzymes and the production of cells necessary for growth, replacement of tissues, and tissue repair.

Nutrient Density

The concept of nutrient density can be used to evaluate the nutritional quality of foods. Foods that provide more nutrient value than just kilocalories are called "nutrient-dense" foods. Foods with low nutrient density (e.g., sugar, alcohol) provide energy but usually lack essential nutrients. Foods that are nutrient dense are preferred to promote optimal nutrition.

Dietary Guidelines for Americans

Because many Americans overeat and lead sedentary lives, the number of people with cardiovascular problems, diabetes, and cancer has risen significantly. To reverse this trend, the USDA and U. S. Department of Health and Human Services established dietary guidelines. The most current revision was published in 2000 (USDA, 2000b). These guidelines are outlined in Display 37-1. Additionally, a National Heart, Lung, and Blood Institute (NHLBI) and National Institutes of Health report outlined research-based clinical guidelines for adult obesity and overweight (NHLBI, 1998).

Energy Balance

Dietary patterns should be adjusted to maintain a balance between caloric intake and energy expenditure. **Basal metabolism** is the amount of energy required to carry out involuntary activities at rest (e.g., breathing, circulating blood, maintaining body temperature). Men usually have a higher basal metabolic rate (BMR) than women because of their proportionally greater muscle mass. Other factors, such as growth, infection, fever, stress, and extreme environmental temperatures, can increase BMR. Decreased BMR can occur as a result of aging, prolonged fasting, and sleeping. Increased physical exercise creates caloric demands above basal requirements.

To maintain body weight, dietary intake of calories must equal caloric expenditures. When caloric intake is greater

DISPLAY 37-1

> 🔄 **NUTRITION AND YOUR HEALTH: DIETARY GUIDELINES FOR AMERICANS (2000)**
>
> **Aim for Fitness**
> - Aim for a healthy weight
> - Be physically active each day
> - Let the Pyramid guide your food choices
>
> **Build a Healthy Base**
> - Choose a variety of grains daily, especially whole grains
> - Choose a variety of fruits and vegetables daily
> - Keep food safe to eat
>
> **Choose Sensibly**
> - Choose a diet that is low in saturated fat and cholesterol and moderate in total fat
> - Choose beverages and foods to moderate your intake of sugars
> - Choose and prepare foods with less salt
> - If you drink alcoholic beverages, do so in moderation.
>
> From Report of the Dietary Guidelines Advisory Committee on the Dietary Guidelines for Americans, 2000, to the Secretary of Health and Human Services and the Secretary of Agriculture.

than energy expanded, weight gain occurs, because energy is stored in body fat. When caloric intake is less than energy expended, weight loss occurs, because body stores of energy are depleted. For an average person, a daily deficit of 500 cal (3500 cal/wk) will result in the loss of 1 lb/week.

Caloric requirements can be calculated by estimating how much energy is required for basal activities and adding the calories needed for voluntary muscular activity. Display 37-2 shows one method for calculating kilocalorie energy output for BMR and voluntary muscular activity.

Nutritional Status

Body Mass Index

Body mass index (BMI) is the measure that describes a person's relative weight for height. BMI is calculated as weight (in kilograms) divided by the height (in meters) squared. If pounds and inches are being used, the formula is BMI = [(weight in pounds) ÷ (height in inches squared)] × 704.5. The BMI correlates with total body fat content and is recommended for use to assess overweight and obesity and to keep track of body weight changes (NHLBI, 1998).

Ideal Body Weight

Normal nutritional intake usually results in body weight appropriate for a person's height and frame. Ideal body weight (IBW) is the estimated optimal weight for body functioning and health. Ranges for IBW according to height and body frame are listed in standardized tables. Such information can

DISPLAY 37-2

🔄 CALCULATING ENERGY REQUIREMENTS

Shortcut for Estimating Energy Output:
Basal Metabolism
Use the factor 1.0 kcal/kg of body weight per hour for men or 0.9 for women. The following is an example for a 170-lb woman.

1. Change pounds to kilograms:

$$170 \text{ lb}/2.2 \text{ lb} \times 1.0 \text{ kg} = 77 \text{ kg}$$

2. Multiply weight in kilograms by the basal metabolic rate (BMR) factor:

$$77 \text{ kg} \times 1 \text{ kcal/kg/hr} = 77 \text{ kcal/hr}$$

3. Multiply the kilocalories used in 1 hr by the hours in a day:

$$77 \text{ kcal/hr} \times 24 \text{ hr/day} = 1848 \text{ kcal/day}$$

Energy for BMR equals 1848 kcal/day.

Shortcut for Estimating Energy Output:
Voluntary Muscular Activity
The figures to use are crude approximations based on the amount of muscular work a person typically performs in a day. To select the appropriate one, remember to think in terms of the amount of muscular work performed. Don't confuse being busy with being active.

- For sedentary (mostly sitting) activity (a typist), add 50% of the BMR.
- For light activity (a teacher), add 60%.
- For heavy work (a roofer), add 100% or more.

If the woman in the previous example were a typist, estimate the energy she needed for physical activities by multiplying her BMR kilocalories per day by 50%.

$$1848 \text{ kcal/day} \times 50\% = 924 \text{ kcal/day}$$

Her energy need for activities equals 924 kcal/day.

Adapted from Cataldo, C., Nyenhuis, J., & Whitney, E. (1987). *Nutritional and diet therapy: Principles and practice* (2nd ed., pp. 90–91). St. Paul, MN: West Publishing Co. All rights reserved.

be misleading, because it does not always reflect accurately the amount of body fat present. For example, a body builder may be heavier than the IBW listed but may have a less than average amount of body fat.

A rule of thumb for estimating IBW is that a woman who is 5 feet tall should weigh about 100 lb, and 5 lb should be added for each additional inch. The IBW for a 5-foot-tall man is 105 lb, to which 6 lb should be added for each additional inch.

Physical Status
Normal nutrition is apparent in the appearance of many parts of the body. General appearance should reflect alertness and responsiveness. The skin should have normal tone and good turgor. The mouth, gums, and lips should appear moist, pink, and free from cracks and lesions. Hair and nails should appear healthy. Bones should hold the body erect, and muscles should maintain good tone. Normal reflexes should be apparent. The abdomen should appear flat and undistended.

Normal Laboratory Values
Laboratory values are usually within normal ranges in healthy people. Normal hematocrit and hemoglobin values suggest adequate iron stores if hydration status is normal. Plasma protein values (e.g., serum prealbumin, albumin) are often used as a reflection of normal adequate protein intake.

Lifespan Considerations
Pregnancy and Lactation
The pregnant woman's diet should include a substantial increase in calories, protein, calcium, folic acid, and iron. Usually, a prenatal multivitamin and mineral supplement is prescribed. The pregnant woman should gain weight throughout her pregnancy, as prescribed and monitored by her healthcare professional. Pregnant women at particular risk for nutritional deficiencies are adolescents, underweight women, obese women, women with chronic nutritional problems, women who smoke or ingest alcohol or drugs, low-income women, and women with chronic illnesses such as diabetes or anemia.

The lactating woman also has special needs. Minor deficiencies in the lactating woman's diet are more likely to influence her nutritional state than the nutritional quality of her milk. Major deficiencies in the woman's diet may result in a decrease in the nutritional quality and quantity of her milk. Lactating women need to increase their intake of calcium, protein, fluid, and calories. These increases are important because the quality and quantity of breast milk produced directly affects the adequacy of the breast-feeding infant's diet (Dewey, 2001; Reitsneder & Gill, 2000).

Newborn and Infant
Adequate nutrition during infancy is important because the infant's growth and development are more rapid during the first year of life than at any other time. Birth weight usually doubles within the first 4 to 6 months and triples by 12 months of age. Newborns need more calories per pound of body weight because their BMR is so high. The infant's growth and development also are influenced by genetic characteristics and by the quality of prenatal nutrition and care.

Milk is the food of choice for newborns. Breast-feeding should begin as soon after birth as possible. For the first 3 days after birth, the mother's breasts produce colostrum, a thin, watery fluid. The breasts produce milk, which contains about 20 cal/ounce, after the third day. Weight gain may be less rapid in breast-fed infants. Feedings are usually frequent (e.g., every 2 to 3 hours), because breast milk is easily digested. Breast milk provides infants with immunity against some bacteria and viruses, results in different intestinal flora than with artificial formula, decreases the incidence of allergies, and provides a well-balanced, ideal source of nutrition. Breast-feeding mothers should avoid taking drugs, because small amounts can be transferred to the breast milk and ingested by the infant. Also, babies may not tolerate products from some foods.

Formula is a safe and nutritious substitute for mothers who prefer not to breast-feed or cannot do so. Iron-fortified commercial formulas should be used until the infant is at least 1 year old. Most formulas are modified cow's milk that has been heat-treated to aid digestion. Soy formulas and predigested formulas also are available. Foods (e.g., juices, fruits, vegetables, iron-fortified cereals) are gradually added to the diet to provide additional nutrition and to begin to accustom infants to foods of different textures, flavors, and consistencies. The age at which to introduce these foods varies according to the infant's need, the practices of the healthcare provider, and the influence of the infant's culture and environment. Cereals, fruits and vegetables, and egg yolk are added at about 4 to 6 months. When teeth begin to erupt at about 6 months, crackers and teething biscuits are often added. Parents and caregivers should introduce new foods one at a time so that any offending food can be identified if allergies develop. By the second half of the first year, motor development has improved so that the infant can begin to sit up, eat finger foods, and drink from a cup.

Toddler and Preschooler

Adequate nutritional intake is important between the ages of 1 and 5 years, because this is a period of rapid physical growth and development. Variations among toddlers necessitate some differences in their diets. During this period, the growth rate begins to decline, and the appetite decreases as children need less food to meet normal metabolic demands. Children's appetites may be erratic during these years. Teeth continue to erupt into the second and sometimes the third year. Muscle mass and bone density increase. These developments necessitate adequate protein, calcium, and phosphorus in the diet. Energy levels remain high, requiring adequate caloric intake.

Independence in feeding greatly increases as coordination and ability to use eating utensils develop. Many children can feed themselves by 2 years of age. Mental abilities and language development are increasing, so children are better able to communicate food likes and dislikes. Values and attitudes about eating develop during these stages. Parents and other caregivers must learn the importance of not using food to punish, reward, bribe, or convey love. Some children may become picky eaters, especially when refusal to eat gains them attention from their families.

Maintaining adequate dietary habits for toddlers and preschoolers is important because good habits are established at an early age. The most common dietary deficiency in this age group is iron deficiency, which leads to iron-deficiency anemia. A diet that includes iron-rich foods is indicated, and iron supplements may be necessary. Vitamins A and C also may be deficient in the diets of toddlers and preschoolers, so they must eat foods rich in these vitamins. Active children in this age group benefit from appropriately spaced, nutritious, between-meal snacks.

SAFETY ALERT

Remind parents and other caregivers to keep hot liquids away from toddlers or confused clients who may accidentally spill them or burn themselves.

Child and Adolescent

Children's growth rates vary greatly during the school years. The digestive system matures, and permanent teeth erupt. Children can eat larger meals less frequently, requiring fewer calories per unit of body weight. Adolescence is a period of rapid growth and sexual maturation. Macronutrients and micronutrients are needed to support body tissue growth during this time.

A diet that includes adequate carbohydrates and the recommended allowances of protein, vitamins, and minerals for the individual's age group, physical status, and developmental level is necessary for optimal health. Nutritional deficiencies that are most common during childhood and adolescence are those of iron, calcium, zinc, and vitamin A (Goodwin, Buchholz, et al., 1999). Adequate amounts of these minerals and vitamins must be included in the diet. Health problems that respond well to nutritional intervention during this age include dental caries, anemia, and obesity.

School lunch programs play an important role in providing nutritionally balanced, low-cost meals (Fig. 37-2). Some schools also have breakfast programs and snack programs. These programs usually are available free or at a reduced cost for needy children. In addition to providing a substantial part of the daily nutrition needs for children, these programs make

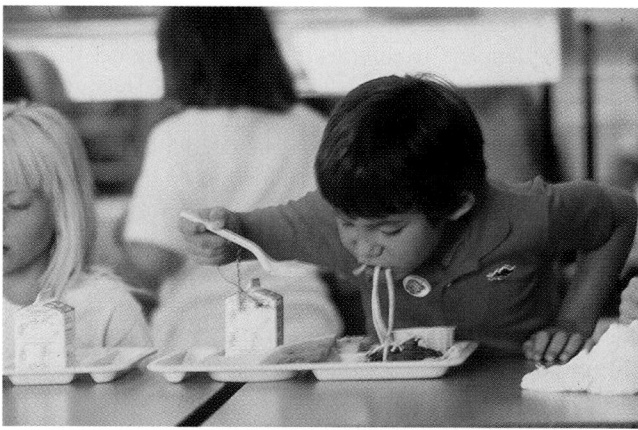

FIGURE 37-2 Children can receive well-balanced meals through a school lunch program. (USDA photo.)

a valuable contribution in terms of nutrition education and development of good nutrition habits.

Social pressure and emotional stress can have adverse effects on a young person's efforts to maintain a nutritionally adequate diet. Peers may dictate dietary choices (Emans, 2000; Strice, 1999). Children may eat fewer meals at home than in earlier years; fast food, soda, and candy are often favorites. Smoking, drinking, and substance abuse also can affect nutritional status. Children or adolescents may experience an unbalanced pattern of activity or rest. Increased participation in sports requires additional caloric intake. Weight gain is common during the preadolescent period as the body prepares for rapid growth. If the child leads a sedentary life and eats a high-calorie diet, weight gain can be excessive and can contribute to obesity. On the other hand, weight consciousness, especially among adolescent girls, can lead to fad diets, anorexia nervosa, and bulimia (Cash & Deagle, 1997).

Adult and Older Adult

Growth stops and metabolism declines during adulthood, so adults require fewer calories. Weight gain is common, especially if physical activity is limited. Calcium deficiency and osteoporosis can be concerns for adults, especially post-menopausal women. Adults should maintain a calcium intake of 1000 to 1200 mg/day throughout adulthood (Committee on Dietary Reference Intakes, 1997). Adequate intake of calcium is especially important before 30 years of age, when peak bone mass is being attained. Among adult Americans, nutritional excesses of fats, carbohydrates, and proteins are more common than deficiencies.

Inadequate nutritional intake during this time may result from increased daily demands that decrease the time and energy available for buying, cooking, and eating food. Dietary patterns can be affected when both parents in a family work. Some adults lack adequate resources or knowledge about good nutrition. Pregnancy and lactation, as discussed previously, greatly alter nutritional requirements.

Physiologic changes that have a major impact on nutrition occur in later years. The metabolic rate continues to decline. Although the need for calories decreases, the need for iron and vitamins remains high; however, a woman's need for iron decreases after menopause. The diets of many older adults are deficient in calories, fiber, calcium, zinc, vitamin C, vitamin D, and B-complex vitamins (Rolfes, DeBruyne, & Whitney, 1998). Adequate fiber intake is necessary to prevent constipation, a common problem in older adults. The senses of taste and smell diminish; this can affect enjoyment of eating and cause decreased intake of food. Digestion is affected by a change in the contents of bile and pancreatic secretions, decreased peristalsis, and decreased blood flow to the GI tract. Periodontal disease and ill-fitting dentures can make chewing difficult and painful.

For older adults, socioeconomic factors can contribute to inadequate nutrition (Fig. 37-3). Transportation for shopping and carrying of groceries can be problems for the older person with impaired mobility. Older adults may have trouble using cooking appliances because of failing eyesight and arthritis or

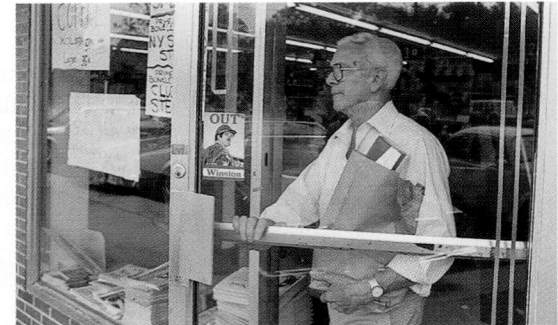

FIGURE 37-3   Learning proper food selection and preparation and ability to shop are significant to a person's health.

because of the complexity of modern appliances. Selecting economical, nutritious foods can be difficult for the older shopper because of the wide variety of products available.

Social isolation also can hinder nutrition. Those who have lost friends and live far from relatives may become lonely and depressed, making it more difficult to cook and eat.

Several community resources have been developed to help older adults continue living at home by combating the problems mentioned previously. Programs for home-delivered meals (e.g., Meals on Wheels) provide nutritious, low-cost meals for older, homebound people. This program is able to remain low in cost partly because of a volunteer staff. Food stamps and food banks are useful to older adults. Another excellent resource for older adults is local senior centers, which can provide meals, health screening and medication assistance, transportation assistance, dietary counseling, recreational activities, and assistance and referral for economic and legal problems.

FACTORS AFFECTING NUTRITION

Physiologic Factors

Healthy body functioning promotes normal digestion and absorption of food. Healthy teeth and gums or well-fitting dentures are important for chewing, which is necessary to break up food particles to facilitate digestion. The GI system must function properly for optimal use of ingested nutrients. Hormone production of insulin and pancreatic digestive enzymes also is important for food use.

Intake of Nutrients

Ability to Acquire and Prepare Food.   Physical factors can affect a person's ability to buy, transport, cook, and eat food. Physical mobility and energy are necessary for shopping, cooking, and eating. Being able to read and understand food labels can help with healthy food choices.

People who are unable to purchase, transport, and prepare food may have inadequate intake unless other people or agencies can be found to fulfill such needs. In Third World countries, starvation is common due to drought and famine. Starvation or malnutrition also can occur in developed nations when people lack the resources to obtain adequate food. Confused or disoriented persons may forget to eat or may be unable to organize the complex tasks of buying and cooking food independently.

Knowledge. Some people may not eat a balanced diet because they lack information about nutrition. People are likely to eat only what tastes good or what is convenient if they do not know or care that such eating patterns can be unhealthy. The consequences of poor nutrition are not immediately observable, so motivation to change poor eating patterns may be weak.

Swallowing Impairment. People who have difficulty swallowing may be unable to ingest sufficient nutrients to meet daily requirements. Swallowing impairment can occur when the gag reflex is absent due to neurologic dysfunction (e.g., cerebrovascular accident) or muscle weakness. Obstruction of the oropharyngeal cavity secondary to a tumor or edema also can impair swallowing.

ETHICAL/LEGAL ISSUE
Ending Tube Feeding

Mr. Camper (47 years old) was admitted to a long-term care facility 6 months ago, following a motorcycle accident. He experienced severe head injuries that left him comatose. He requires total physical care, including tube feedings for nutrition. Mr. Camper has started to develop increasing joint stiffness and contractures and has not shown any signs of responsiveness.
Mr. Camper's physician and family have been conferring on his prognosis and plans for care. They have decided together that it would be best to end the tube feedings and "let nature take its course." As the nurse on the unit, Ms. Goldmark has been asked to remove the gastrostomy tube and stop the feedings. Ms. Goldmark believes that removing the tube feedings will actually add to Mr. Camper's discomfort. She is reluctant to carry out this order and is also reluctant to require another nurse to do it, which would not erase her moral objection to the procedure.

Reflection
- Explore your feelings in this situation. Do you agree or disagree with Ms. Goldmark?
- Identify any concerns that Ms. Goldmark has not mentioned that you have about this situation.
- Identify possible approaches to seeking additional information and resolving the dilemma.
- Recognizing the client's rights, the family's rights, and the physician's order, define what you see as Ms. Goldmark's ethically appropriate behavior.

Discomfort during or after Eating. When people experience discomfort during or after eating, they may decrease their food intake. A sore throat, a tonsillectomy, a mouth lesion, and ill-fitting dentures are possible causes.

Anorexia. **Anorexia,** or loss of appetite, occurs for various reasons. Depression, GI dysfunction, infections, illnesses, malignancies, and side effects of many medications can cause anorexia, resulting in decreased food intake.

Nausea and Vomiting. Nausea and vomiting interfere with normal food intake. They may be caused by motion sickness, viral or bacterial infections of the GI tract, gallbladder disease, general anesthesia, disruption of inner ear function, side effects of various medications, or pregnancy. Some people may feel nauseated or vomit from unpleasant smells, sensations, or sights.

Excessive Intake of Calories and Fat. Caloric intake in excess of daily energy requirements results in storage of energy in the form of increased adipose tissue. As the percentage of stored fat increases, a person becomes overweight or obese. Approximately 97 million adults in the United States are considered to be obese or overweight, with a marked increase in the last decade (NHLBI, 1998). Excess weight increases stress on body organs and predisposes people to chronic health problems, such as diabetes mellitus and hypertension. Excessive caloric intake does not ensure adequate intake of essential nutrients: Obese persons may be malnourished in some areas due to a lack of elements such as essential vitamins or particular nutrients.

Americans have a higher percentage of fat in their diets than do people in many other countries. Fat makes up about 40% of the calories in the American diet (NHLBI, 1998). Excess fat intake has been related to obesity, increased risk of coronary artery disease (especially increased intake of saturated fats), and several forms of cancer, including breast, colon, and uterine cancer. Dietary modifications can lower fat and cholesterol intake.

Ability to Use Ingested Nutrients
Inflammation of the Gastrointestinal Tract. Inflammation of the lining of the GI tract causes discomfort and interferes with nutrient absorption. Esophagitis, an inflammation of the esophagus, can result from burns, poisons, infections, or chronic vomiting. It causes discomfort and impairs swallowing. Gastritis is characterized by inflammation of the mucosal layer of the stomach, which can proceed to ulceration if untreated.

Cholecystitis is an inflammation of the gallbladder; it is usually caused by the presence of gallstones. The presence of inflammation and stones causes pain after ingestion of a meal that is high in fat, because the gallbladder spasms as it attempts to release bile to assist with fat digestion.

Inflammatory bowel disease (i.e., Crohn's disease or ulcerative colitis) greatly affects absorption of nutrients and water from the intestine. The intestinal inflammation results in severe diarrhea. Treatment frequently requires removal of inflamed areas of the intestine, permanently decreasing the absorptive area.

Obstruction of the Gastrointestinal Tract.   Any obstruction caused by scar tissue, benign or cancerous growths, or structural abnormalities can alter nutritional status. Esophageal obstruction can severely limit intake or restrict oral intake to fluids. A hiatal hernia is a protrusion of part of the stomach through the diaphragm into the mediastinal cavity. It can cause esophageal reflux, or the backflow of stomach contents into the esophagus, resulting in heartburn. Intestinal obstruction usually necessitates withholding all oral intake until the obstruction has resolved or been surgically corrected.

Malabsorption of Nutrients.   The inability to tolerate certain foods can cause malabsorption syndromes. An intolerance to gluten, which is found in wheat, rye, oats, and barley, can cause mucosal villi to atrophy, decreasing their absorptive abilities. Lactose intolerance occurs when there is a deficiency of lactase, a digestive enzyme that breaks down the sugar found in milk.

A decrease in pancreatic enzyme production occurs in some pancreatic disorders, resulting in altered digestion of fats and protein. In cystic fibrosis, an inherited disorder, excessive mucus plugs pancreatic ducts, leading to altered protein, carbohydrate, and fat digestion.

Malabsorption also can occur secondary to surgical intervention. Gastric or intestinal resection removes large areas of the GI tract normally involved in absorption of nutrients. Decreased blood flow to the GI tract can decrease the rate of nutrient absorption.

Diabetes Mellitus.   Diabetes mellitus is a chronic condition in which the body produces insufficient amounts of insulin or cannot effectively use circulating insulin. Insulin is a hormone essential for proper metabolism of fats, proteins, and carbohydrates. When adequate insulin is unavailable, transfer of glucose into the cell is impaired, and the glucose level of the blood rises. Thus, cells cannot use glucose to produce energy. Procedure 37-1 discusses monitoring blood glucose.

Metabolic Demand

Certain conditions increase the body's nutritional requirements, potentially contributing to nutritional status:

- Periods of rapid growth (infancy, adolescence, pregnancy)
- Conditions that increase the BMR (infection, exercise, hyperthyroidism)
- Stress (from emotional distress, fear, trauma, surgery, or illness)
- Wasting diseases such as cancer and AIDS (from reduced energy and protein intake, malabsorption, and metabolic disturbances)

Lifestyle and Habits

Eating patterns are highly individualized and greatly determined by personal preference. Food patterns and eating habits are often set during childhood and may be passed from one generation to the next (NHLBI, 1998). Some families love trying new recipes; others prefer having specific meals prepared exactly the same way repeatedly. If children are raised in families that eat throughout the day, rather than at three distinct meals, this pattern will seem normal and will probably influence their lifelong eating patterns. Early experience also helps determine the amounts and types of food eaten. If children are fed large servings and rewarded with desserts, overeating may become a problem later. The atmosphere at mealtimes also subtly affects feelings about food and eating.

Peer pressure and sex-role stereotypes can affect eating patterns (Cash & Deagle, 1997). Many adolescents survive on hamburgers, french fries, pizza, and soda. Men may be less likely to order salad for lunch than women; likewise, women may feel less comfortable eating big steak sandwiches.

Food fads also can affect dietary patterns. Some foods and nutritional supplements can be linked with beliefs about health that are not grounded in scientific fact.

Professional persons who work long hours and are single may not have enough time to shop for and cook food. Families with two working parents may eat out often for the same reason. Some single older adults may have limited motivation or energy to cook and eat meals alone. People who lead active lives with strenuous physical exertion may need more frequent meals and more calories to meet their minimal nutritional requirements. On the other hand, sedentary people who spend hours in front of the television may gain weight from decreased physical activity and increased snacking.

Culture and Beliefs

Culture plays a significant role in the type of food eaten and feelings about diet and nutrition (Gard & Freeman, 1996). Staple products vary among cultural groups; for example, Asians may eat rice with most meals, and Italians may prefer pasta. Spices and methods of cooking also vary.

Some religions dictate when or whether certain foods can be eaten and how foods are to be prepared. An example of this is the Jewish dietary law, which restricts (among other things) eating dairy and meat products at the same time. Most religions have special foods that are traditional for specific observances. Listings of cultural and religious beliefs about nutrition have been published elsewhere (Williams, 1997; Westfall, 1999).

Economic Resources

An adequate diet may be related to a person's finances. Money is necessary to buy and transport food and to obtain and maintain the equipment needed to cook and store food safely. The lower a person's economic level, the less likely it is that the diet will be nutritionally adequate. Low-income areas usually have fewer grocery stores, with fewer selections and higher prices. People with low incomes may lack transportation to shop outside their neighborhoods. More affluent people can stock up when items are on sale, stretching their food budget.

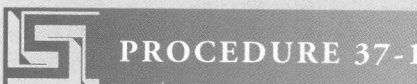

PROCEDURE 37-1

MEASURING BLOOD GLUCOSE BY SKIN PUNCTURE

Purpose
1. Monitor blood glucose levels for clients who are at risk for hypoglycemia or hyperglycemia.
2. Monitor the effectiveness of insulin administration.

Assessment
- Review the physician's order to determine the time and frequency of glucose monitoring. *Note:* The procedure should be performed before meals because carbohydrate ingestion alters blood glucose levels.
- Assess the client's medical history to determine risk for complications from skin punctures (e.g., bleeding disorders, anticoagulant therapy, low platelet count).
- Assess the skin area to be used for puncture (fingers, toes, heels). Avoid areas with open lesions or ecchymosis.
- Assess the client's understanding of the purpose of the procedure and his or her physical and emotional ability to learn and perform the procedure independently.

Equipment
Alcohol or povidone-iodine swab
Sterile lancet or autolet
Cotton balls
Blood glucose reagent strip
Glucose testing meter
Disposable gloves

Procedure
1. Have the client wash hands with soap and warm water.
   Rationale: The fingertips are the most common skin puncture sites in adults. Washing not only decreases the chances of infection but, due to the warm water, promotes vasodilation of the puncture site.
2. Position client comfortably.
3. Remove the reagent strip from the container and handle according to the manufacturer's instructions.
   Rationale: The glucose meter may need recalibration or "rezero-ing."
4. Place the reagent strip with test pad up on a dry surface.
   Rationale: Moisture on the test pad could alter the final test results.

5. Choose the finger to be punctured, massage gently, and hold in a dependent position.
   Rationale: The dependent position and stimulation will help increase circulation to the puncture site.
6. Wipe the puncture site with alcohol (or a povidone-iodine swab). Allow the site to dry completely.
   Rationale: If tracked into the puncture site, alcohol may cause stinging and could hemolyze or dilute the blood sample, giving an inaccurate reading.

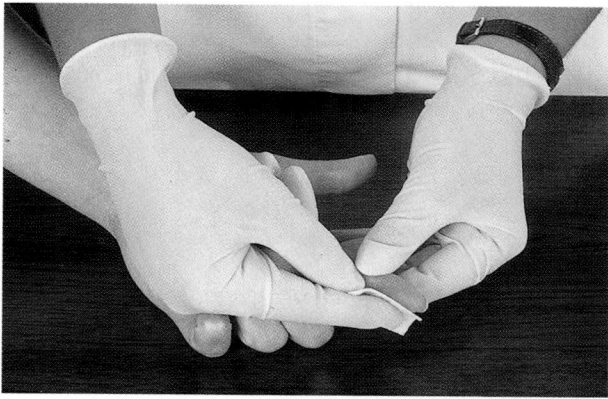

Step 6 Wipe puncture site with alcohol, allowing site to dry before puncture. (© B. Proud.)

7. Don gloves.
   Rationale: Observe Standard Precautions against transfer of microorganisms.
8. Remove the cover of the lancet or autolet. Place the autolet against the side of the finger and push the release button. If using a lancet, hold it perpendicular to the site and pierce the site quickly.
   Rationale: Quick brisk puncture of skin is less painful.
9. Wipe the initial drop of blood with a cotton ball.
   Rationale: The first drop of blood may contain more serous fluid than blood cells and lead to a false glucose reading.
10. Squeeze the puncture gently or massage the skin toward the site to obtain a large drop of blood. Hold the reagent strip next to the drop of blood and allow the blood to cover the test pad completely. Do not smear the blood. In some meters, bring the finger to the test site on the meter and allow blood to drop onto the appropriate area.
    Rationale: Smearing or incomplete coverage of the test pad will lead to false glucose readings.

PROCEDURE 37-1 (Continued)

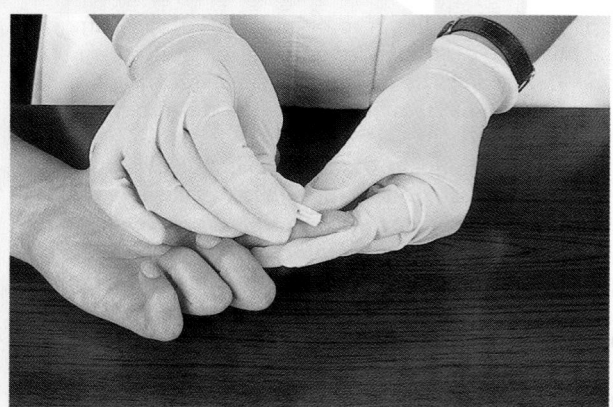

Step 8 Puncture site to obtain the blood sample. (© B. Proud.)

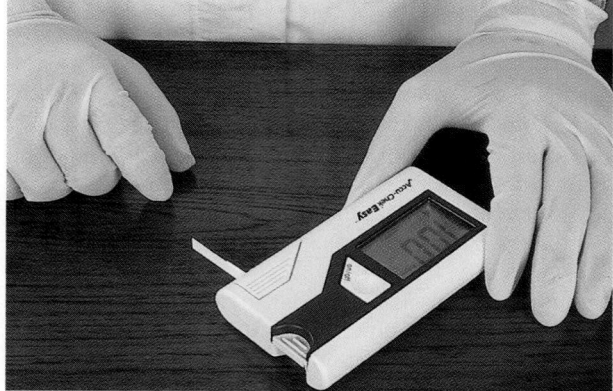

Step 13 Place reagent strip into the glucose meter and after appropriate time read the results. (© B. Proud.)

11. Start the timing (usually less than 60 seconds) using the glucose meter, or use a watch if the meter is not available.
    Rationale: Blood must be in contact with the test pad for the time required by the manufacturer to ensure accurate results.
12. Following the manufacturer's instruction, wipe the blood from the test pad with a cotton ball after the specified period. *Note:* Slight variations may occur in the procedure between different manufacturers.
13. Place the reagent strip into the glucose meter. After the recommended period, read the results. For meters on which blood is placed directly, read the results at the designated time. If a glucose meter is not available, compare the color of

the test pad with the color strip on the side of the reagent strip container.
    Rationale: Accurate timing of the test ensures a correct reading of the glucose level.
14. Turn off the glucose meter. Dispose of used equipment in the appropriate manner.
    Rationale: Dispose in a used-needle receptacle to avoid inadvertent punctures.
15. Share test results with client and record obtained values in the client's chart.
    Rationale: Encourage the client's participation and maintain appropriate documentation.

Lifespan Considerations
Infants
- The heel is the most common site for skin puncture. Use a heel-warming device or wrap a warm, moist towel around the foot before the skin puncture is done to promote vasodilation.

Children
- Children may be especially apprehensive about skin puncture. Use distraction techniques and allow parents to be present to increase the child's cooperation with the procedure.

Home Care Modifications
- Handwashing alone before skin puncture is sufficient to cleanse the skin when the test is performed at home.
- Instruct the client to keep a log of all blood glucose readings.

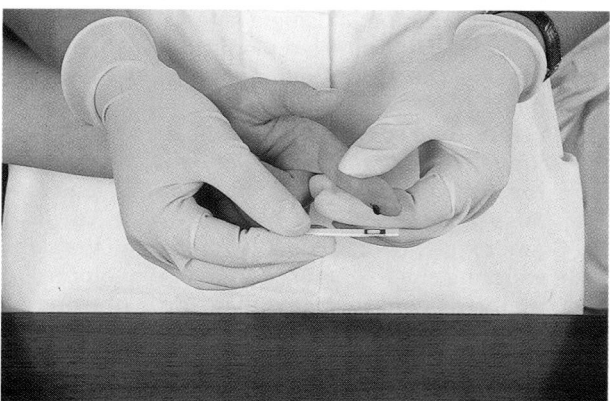

Step 10 Cover the test pad completely with a large drop of blood. (© B. Proud.)

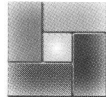

Low-income families may sacrifice their food budgets to leave enough money for other bills. The result may be less expensive meals that are low in protein and high in starch. Sources of protein, such as meat and dairy products, are usually expensive and require refrigeration.

Drug and Nutrient Interactions

Specific foods may interact with medications, altering the effectiveness of the drug. This consideration is particularly important with long-term drug treatments, use of multiple drugs, or declining nutritional status. For example, a high sodium intake decreases the effectiveness of lithium, a commonly used psychiatric medication. Vegetables high in vitamin K decrease the effectiveness of a commonly used anticoagulant, Coumadin. Specific drug–nutrition interactions can be found in the current USP-DI (United States Pharmacopoeia, 2001).

Gender

Nutritional requirements vary slightly between men and women. Men usually need more calories and protein to maintain a larger muscle mass. Women have proportionally more adipose tissue and need fewer calories to maintain body weight. To prevent anemia, women need more dietary iron to offset losses from menstruation.

Surgery

Surgery greatly increases the risk for nutritional deficits. Increased metabolic demands related to the stress of surgery and wound healing, along with inadequate postoperative intake, compound nutritional deficits. Many surgical clients are nutritionally depleted at the time of surgery due to chronic illness, GI problems, or prior medical procedures (Corish, 1999).

Cancer and Cancer Treatment

Cancer greatly increases the body's metabolic demands, and cancer cells compete with normal cells for nutrients. Clients with cancer may experience anorexia, nausea, vomiting, and depression, all of which can decrease food consumption. Radiation or chemotherapy also can alter nutrition, because loss of appetite, nausea, and vomiting are commonly associated with such treatments. Mouth lesions (known as stomatitis) may occur with chemotherapy, causing pain and difficulty in chewing. Chemotherapy and radiation cause fatigue, decreasing the amount of energy available for cooking and eating.

Nursing Research and Critical Thinking
What are the Effects of Race and Obesity on Health-Promotion Behaviors in Women?

One challenge the healthcare industry faces is finding ways to encourage better eating habits and more physical activity among the general public. These researchers found no previous studies that specifically addressed race, female gender, obesity, and health-promoting activities. Therefore, they designed this 2×2 comparative descriptive design study with two levels of body size (obese and nonobese) and two levels of race (African American and European American). Approximately equal numbers in each group ensured that the factors of body size and race remained independent of each other. The sample ($n = 86$) consisted of women purposefully selected by body mass index and race. Twenty were obese African American women, 22 were obese European American women, 20 were nonobese African American women, and 24 were nonobese European American women. The Health-Promoting Lifestyle Profile (HPLP) was used to measure health-promoting behaviors. Responses to the 48 items of the instrument were summed and averaged to obtain scores for the total HPLP and subscales, with higher scores denoting more positive health practices. Preliminary analysis indicated that all variables were approximately normally distributed. The nutrition subscale of the

HPLP was the only subscale for which African American women had significantly lower scores than European American women. For stress management, the difference between nonobese (M = 2.74) and obese (M = 2.20) women was significant ($P = .01$) for African Americans only. Obese women performed fewer health-promotion behaviors than did nonobese women. For the most part, no differences were seen between African American and European American women.

Critical Thinking Considerations. This study provided information about the associations among health-promotion lifestyles, body size, and race for women in a Southern city. Although these results may not be representative of other geographic locations or nonvolunteer samples, implications of the study are as follows:

- Because African American women have a greater propensity toward obesity, previous differences found between African American and European American women in health-promotion behaviors may be attributed more appropriately to obesity than to race.
- Health promotion counseling interventions are valuable for all obese women.

Nies, M. A., Buffington, C., Cowan, G., & Hepworth, J. T. (1998). Comparison of lifestyles among obese and nonobese African American and European American women in the community. *Nursing Research 47*(4), 251–257.

Alcohol and Drug Abuse

Excessive, chronic ingestion of alcohol can impair nutrition. Excessive alcohol intake may limit the necessary intake of calories and nutrients. People who abuse alcohol may use money normally spent on food to buy alcohol. Deficiencies of B-complex vitamins (thiamine, folate, niacin, and B6) are common because these vitamins are necessary to metabolize alcohol. Alcohol's toxic effect on the intestinal mucosa can impair the normal absorption of nutrients. Chronic alcohol use also can cause irreversible changes to liver cells, affecting the liver's role in metabolic pathways.

Drug abuse also can affect nutrition. Addiction to heroin or cocaine can decrease the user's desire for food, because preoccupation with buying drugs disrupts normal routines. Other drugs, such as amphetamines and barbiturates, can result in increased or decreased food intake.

Psychological State

Psychological state can affect a person's desire to eat. Anxiety causes some people to increase their food intake; others eat less when they feel anxious. Depression often decreases a person's appetite and depletes the energy available for cooking and eating. Some people willingly alter eating patterns to help achieve weight loss. Rather than changing eating patterns, some people seek rapid weight loss through crash diets. **Anorexia nervosa** is an eating disorder in which the person refuses to eat due to a fear of becoming overweight, even in the presence of normal or less than ideal body weight (Gard & Freeman, 1996; Cash & Deagle, 1997).

ALTERED NUTRITIONAL FUNCTION

The body undergoes constant renewal. If proper nutrition is not provided, body tissues will not be adequately maintained, energy will not be adequate for activities, and normal body processes will suffer.

Manifestations of Altered Nutrition

Indications of altered nutrition are overweight, obesity, underweight, recent significant weight loss or gain, decreased energy levels, altered bowel patterns, and altered appearance of the skin, hair, teeth, and mucous membranes (Table 37-3). If the client's weight varies significantly from IBW, a nutrition problem is likely.

Overweight

A person is said to be **overweight** if the BMI is between 25 and 29.9 kg/m^2. The National Center for Health Statistics estimates that 38.4% of men and 24.7% of women in the United States are overweight (NHLBI, 1998). A person gains weight when he or she takes in more calories than the body needs.

Obesity

A person is **obese** if the BMI is 30 kg/m^2 or more. Obesity is present in 19.9% of men and 24.9% of women in the United States (NHLBI, 1998). Morbid obesity is obesity that can interfere with normal functioning, such as mobility or breathing.

Underweight

A person is said to be underweight if he or she is at least 15% to 20% below weight standards. Greater mortality risk is linked with a BMI less than 18.5 kg/m^2 (NHLBI, 1998). This occurs when caloric intake is insufficient to meet the body's nutritional requirements.

Recent Significant Weight Gain or Loss

Minor fluctuations in weight occur on a day-to-day basis due to fluid losses and gains, but changing weight patterns over weeks or months may indicate altered nutrition. A significant weight gain (5% in 1 month or 10% in 6 months) can occur when a person eats more than the body needs for energy expenditure. This can happen when a person becomes less active or when the intake of food is increased from, for example, stress or boredom. Significant weight loss, especially when intake has remained constant, can indicate hypermetabolic states,

TABLE 37-3

Signs of Poor Nutrition and Possible Nutrient Deficiency	
Signs	**Possible Lacking Nutrient**
Hair: thin, coarse, lacking luster, breaks easily	Protein
Skin: excessive bruising, bleeding	Vitamin K
Skin: Pressure sores, poor wound healing	Vitamin C and protein
Gums: swollen, bleeding	Vitamin C
Muscles: wasting	Protein
Lack of growth	Protein, calories
Skeletal: poor posture, painful joints, bowed legs, increase in bone fractures	Calcium, vitamin D, vitamin C, protein
Mental: confusion, motor weakness	Thiamine, niacin, B complex

such as cancer or hyperthyroidism, or an inability to use ingested nutrients.

Decreased Energy

Food provides the body with energy to perform normal cellular processes and to carry out normal movement and activities. When nutritional deficits occur, adequate energy may be unavailable. Fatigue and activity intolerance are common manifestations of altered nutrition. The client may report feeling tired or weak.

Altered Bowel Patterns

Inadequate dietary intake may affect bowel function and regularity. Constipation can occur when fiber or fluid intake is inadequate. Diarrhea may result when clients eat large quantities of fresh fruits. With food intolerance (e.g., lactase deficiency) or malabsorption syndrome, GI distress occurs. When a client's bowel regularity changes, nutritional deficits must be ruled out as a causative factor.

Altered Skin, Teeth, Hair, and Mucous Membranes

Skin, nails, hair, and mucous membranes are rapidly growing tissues that continuously require adequate nutrition for growth. Protein is especially important in this process. Vitamin deficiencies are often manifested by altered development and growth of skin, teeth, hair, and mucous membranes. When protein is lacking, hair may become thin, lack luster, and break easily. Skin heals slowly and may appear thin and fragile when nutrition is inadequate. Mucous membranes may develop sores and bleed easily. Teeth and gums are more prone to disease.

Impact on Activities of Daily Living

Altered nutrition may marginally or seriously affect a person's activities of daily living (ADLs). Poor dietary habits can affect a person's ability to work or a child's performance in school. Poor nutrition reduces a person's energy to carry out ADLs and affects normal growth and development. Ingestion of alcohol impairs the person's intellectual and physical performance.

Increased susceptibility to common illnesses, chronic diseases, and complications is often a consequence of inadequate nutrition. For example, the person who has a long history of high fat intake may have chronic cardiovascular disease, which will affect all aspects of ADLs. If a man who has depended on his wife for meal preparation loses her, this may contribute to poor nutrition because he has not developed the skills for shopping and meal preparation.

Any illness, dietary deficiency, or other problem not prevented by healthy nutrition disrupts a family's usual level of functioning. Lack of transportation and low income limit the family's ability to obtain food for adequate nutrition. Some low-income families may need to use available money for housing or heat expenses, reducing the amount of money available for adequate nutrition.

If the person who is the primary food preparer is unable to fix meals, the entire family's nutritional status may decline as members resort to "fast foods" and foods that are high in calories and low in nutrients. If the nursing mother has poor nutrition, the infant who depends on her for nutrition also will become poorly nourished. Because so much family socialization centers around food and meals, disruption of those socialization opportunities may hinder development of social skills within the family.

ASSESSMENT

Subjective Data

Normal Pattern Identification

Ask questions to determine the client's normal eating patterns and food preferences. The client should describe his or her appetite as good, fair, or poor and discuss whether eating is usually pleasant.

Asking clients to describe food and fluid intake on a typical day provides a sense of what is normal for them. One of two surveying methods usually is used, the 24-hour recall or the food diary. In the 24-hour recall, the client recalls and records the type, quality, and method of preparation of all food eaten within a 24-hour period. In the food diary, the client keeps an ongoing log of the amount, time, and manner of preparation for all food consumed within a specific period. This time period can vary but is often 3 days to 1 week (Wold et al., 1998). The food diary ensures that the evaluation is affected less by "one time only" dietary indiscretions. Both surveying methods are subject to recall and recording errors.

Clients need to discuss food likes and dislikes, normal timing of meals, and routine snacks. Does the client follow a special diet for any reason, have food allergies, or limit the intake of certain foods? How do cultural or religious concerns or practices influence the diet? For some clients, it is important to inquire how stress affects eating patterns. Some people under stress limit their food intake, but others increase the amount and frequency of food consumption.

Find out who in the family is responsible for shopping and cooking, or whether family members share such responsibilities. Determine whether clients use prepackaged, prepared foods and how many times per week they eat out.

Risk Identification

Nutritional assessment helps to identify clients at risk for nutritional deficits. Determine a client's knowledge and values related to nutrition by asking questions such as, "Do you believe your diet helps promote health?" and "What (if any) changes in your diet do you believe might be beneficial?" If the client is following a specific diet, ask which foods are important to include or to avoid. Doing so can help assess the client's understanding of the dietary restrictions. Who prescribed the diet? Was it a neighbor or a nutritionist?

Identify the presence of anorexia, chewing problems, sore mouth, dysphagia, nausea and vomiting, and, if food intake has been affected, for how long. Note any chronic or acute health problems affecting the GI tract (e.g., ulcers, gallbladder disease, inflammatory bowel disease). Document chronic health conditions and their treatments (e.g., diabetes mellitus, cancer, renal disease, heart disease, lung disease), and assess their effect on appetite and food intake. Note any condition that impairs swallowing (e.g., a neurologic impairment) and its specific deficits.

Assessing socioeconomic factors helps to determine possible nutritional deficits. Does the client have money and transportation to buy nutritious food? Are safe storage and adequate cooking facilities available? Does the client or caregiver have the energy to shop for and prepare meals?

Document intake of over-the-counter drugs, alcohol, and illicit drugs, such as cocaine or heroin. Note the use of vitamin and mineral supplements and prescription medications, such as insulin, antacids, chemotherapeutic agents, and steroids. Assess any impact of such substances on nutrition.

Dysfunction Identification

Nutrition may be impaired when the client cannot buy and prepare food, is unwilling or unable to eat, eats excessively, or cannot use ingested nutrients. Such dysfunctions are often determined by asking questions. Nutritional alterations can be identified if the client's BMI is higher than 25 or lower than 20 kg/m².

Reports of significant recent weight loss without altered diet indicate an inability to meet normal nutritional requirements. A dietary intake that supplies significantly less than RDAs or DRIs also helps to identify deficits. Look for signs and symptoms of nutritional dysfunction, such as fatigue, muscle wasting, and obesity.

Objective Data

Physical Assessment

General Observations. General observation provides important information on nutritional status. An adequately nourished person appears robust, vital, and energetic and has erect posture. Skin, hair, and nails appear healthy (Display 37-3).

Anthropometric Measurements. Anthropometric measurements include height and weight, waist measurement, skinfold measurements, and arm circumference measurements. Skinfold and arm circumference measurements are reserved for nutritional screening (Ulijaszek & Kerr, 1999).

Height and weight are compared with findings in a table of standard measurements grouped by age, sex, and body frame. Estimate small, medium, or large body frame. Ask what the person thinks is his or her IBW; this may vary from standardized tables. BMI is calculated by height and weight values.

Waist measurement is taken just above the top of hip bones (iliac crest) and is a clinical measure of abdominal fat cells when the BMI is less than 35 kg/m². This measure provides information about relative risk and morbidity (NHLBI, 1998).

Skinfold measurements are used to help determine fat stores in the body. The triceps skinfold and the subscapular skinfold are most commonly used. A caliper measures the

DISPLAY 37-3

CHARACTERISTICS OF A WELL-NOURISHED PERSON

- Normal weight and height for age, body build, and developmental stage
- Adequate appetite
- Active, alert, and able to maintain adequate attention span
- Firm, healthy skin and mucous membranes
- Erect posture, with straight arms and legs
- Well-developed muscles without excess body fat
- Normal schedule of tooth eruption and healthy teeth and gums
- Normal urinary and bowel elimination patterns
- Normal sleep patterns
- Normal hemoglobin, hematocrit, and serum protein levels
- Absence of diet-related abnormalities

fold of skin, which includes the subcutaneous tissue but not the underlying muscle. Measurements are compared with a table of standards grouped by age and sex to detect excess fat.

Mid-arm circumference measurements are taken of the upper arm to provide information about the muscle mass. Because muscles are the major protein stores, measuring arm circumference helps evaluate protein status. Again, measurements are compared with a table of standards.

Calorie Count. When inadequate intake is suspected, calories can be counted. The percentage of calories eaten of each food served must be recorded. The dietitian uses this information to calculate the calories consumed and to evaluate whether the caloric intake is adequate. Computer programs are also available to aid in calculations.

Mouth Inspection. Observe the condition of the teeth, gums, and mucous membranes. Mucous membranes should be moist, and adequate saliva should be present. Note the presence of caries, excessive plaque, and gingivitis. If the client uses dentures, evaluate proper fit and condition. Detect any lesions of the oral cavity (canker sores, stomatitis, *Candida* infections) and treat them promptly. Discomfort associated with such lesions can alter food intake.

Swallowing Evaluation. A swallowing evaluation is necessary when potential difficulty in swallowing is suspected. Usually, clients are referred to speech therapists for swallowing evaluations, but nurses may need to evaluate swallowing abilities to determine whether feeding is safe. A swallowing evaluation includes assessment of motor function of the facial, oral, and tongue muscles; cough reflex; swallowing reflex; and gag reflex (McHale, Phipps, Horvath, & Schmelz, 1998).

Assess motor function by observing the face, jaw, and tongue for symmetry and strength during normal movements. Asking the client to cough permits evaluation of the briskness and strength of the cough reflex, which is necessary to clear aspirated food from the airway. Evaluate ability to swallow by placing the index finger and thumb on the client's laryngeal protuberance and asking the client to swallow. As the client with an intact swallowing reflex swallows, the nurse will feel the larynx elevate. Finally, evaluate the gag reflex by stroking the client's right or left pharyngeal wall with a tongue blade.

SAFETY ALERT
When ability to swallow is questionable, never give oral food or fluids until a complete evaluation is done.

Diagnostic Tests and Procedures

Biochemical data can help establish a diagnosis, determine the necessary dietary modifications, or identify specific nutritional deficiencies before clinical signs appear. Evaluation of blood and urine is most useful when analyzing a client's nutritional state. The most common laboratory data used are hematocrit, hemoglobin, serum albumin, prealbumin, serum transferrin, and total lymphocyte count. Anergy testing can be done to identify severe nutritional deficits.

Hematocrit and Hemoglobin. Hematocrit is the percentage of red blood cells found in 100 mL of blood. This measure of size and number of cells in the blood, combined with the hemoglobin value, aids in determining the presence and severity of anemia.

A hemoglobin count measures the blood's oxygen- and iron-carrying capacity. A decreased hemoglobin value indicates decreased iron intake or decreased iron reserves, conditions that often are present in anemia.

Serum Albumin and Prealbumin. Serum albumin accounts for more than half of the body's total serum protein. Serum albumin values reflect protein intake or absorption. Values of less than 3.5 g/dL may indicate nutritional deficits. Such protein changes take more than 2 weeks to appear in serum albumin values, because the half-life of albumin is about 18 days. A low albumin level also can be related to overhydration and may not necessarily indicate malnutrition. Prealbumin has a half-life of 2 days and therefore better reflects current nutritional status.

Serum Transferrin. Transferrin, a blood protein that binds with iron and is important in its transport, is considered a sensitive indicator of protein deficiency. Transferrin, which is synthesized in the liver, increases when iron stores are low and decreases when iron stores are high. Changes in protein intake or visceral protein stores are more rapidly reflected in serum transferrin levels than in serum albumin levels.

Creatinine Excretion. The rate of creatinine formation is proportional to total muscle mass. Creatinine is released during skeletal muscle metabolism and is excreted from the body through the kidneys. Creatinine excretion usually is measured by collecting and measuring creatinine in all voided urine during a 24-hour period. As muscles atrophy during malnutrition, creatinine excretion decreases.

Immunocompetence Testing. Nutritional status affects immunity. In severe nutritional depletion, clients may be unable to mount an immune response (anergy). Commonly, this is seen as the lymphocyte count decreases with protein depletion. Skin testing also may be performed to evaluate the impact of nutritional deficits on immune function. Antigen skin tests (e.g., tuberculosis, *Candida,* mumps) can be used to evaluate the client's response to antigens to which he or she has already been sensitized. If no skin response is observed after 48 hours, anergy is present. Anergy indicates the need for aggressive nutritional support.

NURSING DIAGNOSES

North American Nursing Diagnosis Association (NANDA) nursing diagnoses that have been identified for the area of nutrition include Imbalanced Nutrition: Less Than Body Requirements; Imbalanced Nutrition: More Than Body Requirements; Imbalanced Nutrition: Risk for More Than Body Requirements; and Impaired Swallowing.

Diagnostic Statement— Imbalanced Nutrition: Less Than Body Requirements

Definition. Imbalanced Nutrition: Less Than Body Requirements is the state in which a person's intake of nutrients is insufficient to meet metabolic needs (NANDA, 2001).

Defining Characteristics. One of the following defining characteristics or clinical cues that point to this nursing diagnosis must be present:

- Body weight of 20% or more under the ideal
- Reported food intake less than recommended
- Weight loss with adequate food intake
- Pale conjunctival and mucous membranes

Related Factors. These conditions may result from inability to ingest or digest food, inability to absorb nutrients, or increased body requirements because of biologic, psychological, or economic factors. Many etiologic or contributing factors may be associated with these changes in health status. Biologic factors that can cause weight loss include a painful, inflamed buccal cavity; weakness in the muscles required for swallowing; and abdominal pain with pathology, such as cramping, diarrhea, or steatorrhea (fatty stools). Psychological factors include lack of interest or aversion to eating, immediate sensation of satiety after ingestion of food, and perceived inability to digest food. Economic factors include evidence of or reported lack of food. Lack of information, misinformation, and misconceptions about nutrition also may be related to weight loss. Some conditions, such as cancer, thermal injuries, or sepsis, increase body requirements.

Diagnostic Statement— Imbalanced Nutrition: More Than Body Requirements

Definition. Imbalanced Nutrition: More Than Body Requirements is the state in which a person's intake of nutrients exceeds metabolic needs (NANDA, 2001).

Defining Characteristics. This nursing diagnosis is implicated when one of the following characteristics is present:

- Body weight of 20% or more than ideal for height and frame
- Triceps skinfold greater than 15 mm in men, 25 mm in women

Related Factors. Excessive intake in relation to metabolic need results in weight gain. Related factors include sedentary lifestyle, which decreases metabolic rate. Hypothyroidism also may decrease metabolic rate. Excessive intake may be related to a reported or observed dysfunctional eating pattern. Some eating patterns that contribute to weight gain include pairing food with other activities; concentrating food intake at the end of the day; eating in response to external cues, such as time of day or social situation; and eating in response to internal cues other than hunger, such as emotional distress.

Diagnostic Statement— Imbalanced Nutrition: Risk for More Than Body Requirements

Definition. Imbalanced Nutrition: Risk for More Than Body Requirements occurs when a person is at risk for experiencing an intake of nutrients that exceeds metabolic needs (NANDA, 2001).

Defining Characteristics. The major characteristics or clinical cues that point to this nursing diagnosis include at least one of the following:

- Obesity in one or both parents
- Rapid transition across growth percentiles in infants or children
- Reported or observed dysfunctional eating patterns

Related Factors. Contributing factors may include reported use of solid food before 4 to 6 months of age (Worthington-Roberts & Williams, 1996), use of food to comfort or reward, pairing food with other activities, concentrating intake at the end of the day, or eating in response to external or internal cues other than hunger. All these behaviors may result in excessive intake in relation to metabolic need.

Diagnostic Statement— Impaired Swallowing

Definition. Impaired Swallowing is abnormal functioning of the swallowing mechanism associated with deficits in oral, pharyngeal, or esophageal structure or function. (NANDA, 2001).

Defining Characteristics. The characteristics that point to this nursing diagnosis are as follows:

- Major: Observed evidence of difficulty swallowing (e.g., stasis of food in oral cavity, coughing, choking)
- Minor: Evidence of aspiration

Related Factors. Related factors include neuromuscular impairment (e.g., decreased or absent gag reflex, decreased strength or excursion of muscles involved in mastication, perceptual impairment, facial paralysis), mechanical obstruction (e.g., edema, tracheostomy tube, tumor), fatigue, limited awareness, and reddened, irritated oropharyngeal cavity (NANDA, 2001).

Related Nursing Diagnoses

Altered nutritional status affects many areas and can contribute to other problems. Alterations in normal elimination patterns (Diarrhea, Constipation) can stem from nutritional deficits or inability to use ingested nutrients. Feeding Self-Care Deficit can contribute to low nutrient intake. Decreased nutritional status greatly increases risk for infection and delays wound healing. Skin breakdown (Impaired Skin Integrity, Impaired Tissue Integrity) also is more common in poorly nourished persons. Fluid status alterations (Deficient Fluid Volume) can occur in severe malnutrition. Altered nutritional status often results in fatigue, because energy supply to the body cells is inadequate. When this occurs or when morbid obesity is present, clients may develop Activity Intolerance or Self-Care Deficit. If extreme, such limitations affect the ability to manage independently in the home (Impaired Home Maintenance).

Deficient Knowledge often occurs in clients who are prescribed new diets (e.g., clients with diabetes or heart problems) or new nutritional therapies (e.g., enteral or parenteral feedings) or who are experiencing growth and developmental changes. Noncompliance with diet orders or dietary restrictions can occur, particularly when the changes and lifestyle conflict. Altered nutritional status frequently affects appearance as clients gain or lose body weight. Extreme alterations in body weight can lead to Disturbed Body Image, Self-Esteem Disturbance, and Social Isolation.

OUTCOME IDENTIFICATION AND PLANNING

After the nursing diagnoses and related factors have been identified, client goals and nursing interventions are planned. Client goals for nutrition include ensuring adequate nutritional intake and understanding and complying with dietary modifi-cations. Common goals in nutrition include the following:

- The client will use nutritionally sound dietary intake to meet body requirements and to promote health.
- The client will maintain dietary intake adequate to meet the body's energy expenditures.
- The client will demonstrate adequate knowledge to adhere to dietary prescription or therapies to promote health.
- The client will achieve and maintain desired weight.

Cooperation from clients is necessary to plan and to set goals, because clients are responsible for their own nutrition (unless others plan meals for them). Planning revolves around each client's motivation and abilities. If the client is unable to shop or to prepare food, a support person must be included in the planning. Many nursing interventions for healthy nutri-tional balance are educational. Examples of nursing interven-tions commonly used in planning for nutritional education and support are listed in the accompanying display and are dis-cussed in the next section of this chapter.

IMPLEMENTATION

Health Promotion

Collaborating with the healthcare team, nurses are responsi-ble for promoting optimal nutrition through teaching. Pro-moting optimal nutrition, providing assistance, and creating an atmosphere that encourages healthy eating are important nursing roles.

Client Teaching

Nurses are active in promoting good nutrition in various set-tings: health fairs, schools, prenatal classes, health screening visits, and homes. The goal of such education is to encourage

---

PLANNING: Examples of NIC/NOC Interventions

Accepted Nutrition Nursing Interventions Classification (NIC)
Aspiration Precautions
Nutrition Management
Nutrition Therapy

Accepted Nutrition Nursing Outcomes Classification (NOC)
Nutritional Status
Nutritional Status: Food and Fluid Intake
Nutritional Status: Nutrient Intake
Self-Care: Eating

Refer to the following for specifics regarding NIC/NOC:
   McCloskey, J., & Bulechek, G. (2000). *Iowa Intervention Project: Nursing Interventions Classification (NIC)*, (2nd ed.). St. Louis, MO: C. V. Mosby.
Johnson, M., & Maas, M. (2000). *Iowa Outcomes Project: Nursing Outcomes Classification (NOC)*, (2nd ed.). St. Louis, MO: C. V. Mosby.

---

good nutrition by increasing understanding of the importance of a healthy diet (Display 37-1). Although knowledge about nutrients does not guarantee healthy eating, clients who have greater nutritional knowledge generally choose more healthful diets (USDA, 1998). In the early 1990s, new food labels were introduced to assist consumers in choosing healthier foods (Fig. 37-4) (USDA, 1994; Pennington & Hubbard, 1997; Pen-nington & Wilkening, 1997). Helping consumers and clients incorporate this information into their eating patterns can have lasting effects (Fletcher, Branen, & Lawrence, 1997). Nurses can refer at-risk persons to appropriate private and community resources, including USDA websites.

Some hospitalized clients are receptive to nutrition teach-ing. When working with such clients, direct your statements toward actions that the client can take immediately (e.g., "While your incision is healing, it's important to eat enough protein"). Informal diet instruction can occur when helping clients make menu selections. Praise food choices, empha-sizing the importance of each food in maintaining health. Gently encourage clients to improve diet selections (e.g., "Have you tried 1% milk rather than 2% milk? Many people don't notice the difference, and it's a good way to reduce your fat intake").

Clients often question nurses about nutrition or ask for sug-gestions for altering their diet. For example, an overweight client may ask the nurse's opinion of a new diet that a friend has recommended. Many magazines highlight food in each issue. Provide clients with accurate information, encourage-ment, praise, and referral to appropriate resources.

Promoting Optimal Intake

Illness often affects eating, and nurses play a role in en-couraging optimal nutrition for clients. Rooms where eating will take place should be clean, well ventilated, and free of strong odors. The atmosphere should be relaxing. Interrup-tions, such as treatments and procedures, should not occur during mealtimes. Oral care before eating promotes comfort and taste. Timing administration of medications to control nausea and pain will help clients achieve optimal relief at mealtimes.

Food should be served in an attractive, appetizing man-ner and at the right temperature. Microwave ovens can rewarm cooled food. Food preferences should be con-sidered. Small servings are preferable because they do not overwhelm clients. Family members can bring favorite foods from home, as long as such food is permitted in the client's diet.

Pleasant company can improve the incentive for eating for some clients, but conversation should not distract the client. Staff or relatives can provide verbal cues and encouragement during eating for confused or reluctant clients.

It is preferable for clients to be out of bed and sitting in chairs for meals. This position facilitates chewing and swal-lowing and prevents reflux of stomach contents. Some clients may need assistance in cutting food, opening packages, or eating. Procedure 37-2 suggests methods for assisting clients with feeding.

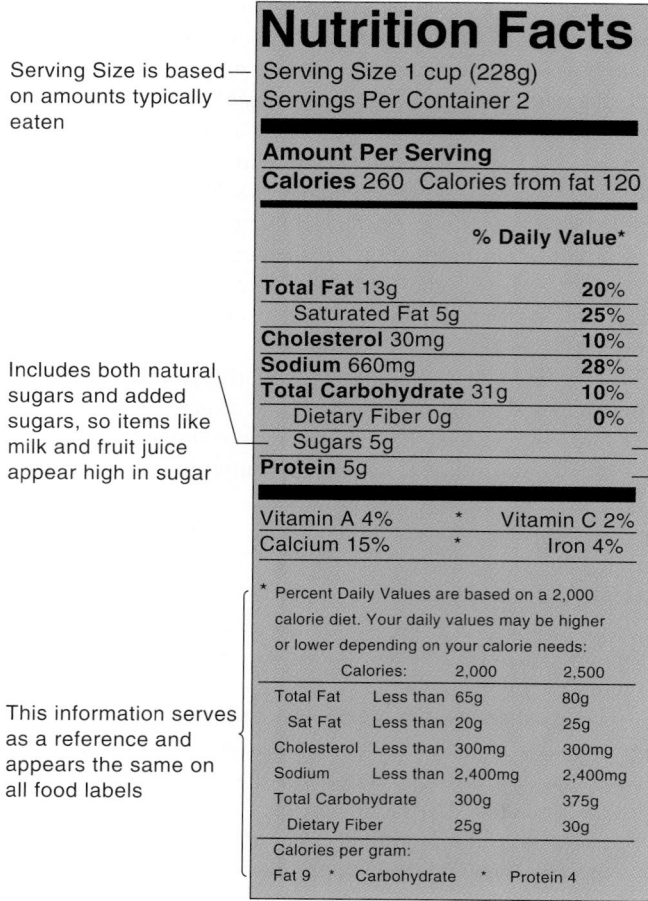

Serving Size is based on amounts typically eaten

Includes both natural sugars and added sugars, so items like milk and fruit juice appear high in sugar

This information serves as a reference and appears the same on all food labels

These percentages are based on 2000 calorie diet

No Daily Value has been set for added sugars

Companies can voluntarily list a percent Daily Value for protein based on 50g (10g of a 2000-calorie diet)

Nutrition Facts

Serving Size 1 cup (228g)
Servings Per Container 2

Amount Per Serving

Calories 260   Calories from fat 120

	% Daily Value*
Total Fat 13g	20%
Saturated Fat 5g	25%
Cholesterol 30mg	10%
Sodium 660mg	28%
Total Carbohydrate 31g	10%
Dietary Fiber 0g	0%
Sugars 5g	
Protein 5g	

Vitamin A 4%	*	Vitamin C 2%
Calcium 15%	*	Iron 4%

* Percent Daily Values are based on a 2,000 calorie diet. Your daily values may be higher or lower depending on your calorie needs:

	Calories:	2,000	2,500
Total Fat	Less than	65g	80g
Sat Fat	Less than	20g	25g
Cholesterol	Less than	300mg	300mg
Sodium	Less than	2,400mg	2,400mg
Total Carbohydrate		300g	375g
Dietary Fiber		25g	30g

Calories per gram:
Fat 9   *   Carbohydrate   *   Protein 4

FIGURE 37-4   Example of a food label and its nutritional information.

SAFETY ALERT

When feeding clients, maintain foods at proper temperature, including recommended temperature when cooking to minimize microbial contamination.

Nursing Interventions for Altered Nutritional Function

Withholding Food

The term "NPO," or nothing by mouth (Latin, *non per os*), is used when ingestion of food or fluids orally is contraindicated. Withholding food may be indicated in the following situations:

- To rest the GI tract to promote healing
- To clear the GI tract of contents before surgery or diagnostic procedures
- To prevent aspiration during surgery or in high-risk clients
- To give normal intestinal motility time to return
- To treat severe vomiting or diarrhea
- To treat medical problems, such as bowel obstruction or acute inflammation of the GI tract

Well-nourished clients can go without food for a few days, but they must receive fluids to prevent fluid and electrolyte disturbances. Some clients find being unable to eat difficult. The following nursing measures can promote comfort during this period:

- Provide frequent oral hygiene.
- Give ice chips, hard candy, and gum or mouth rinses if permitted.
- Avoid exposing clients to others who are eating, to food odors, or to advertisements for food.

If the NPO period is longer than a few days, alternative forms of nutritional support may be necessary.

Special Diets

When a client can eat any food, the diet is called general, regular, or house. A regular diet is well balanced and supplies the metabolic requirements for a sedentary person (about 2000 cal/day). Menus allow clients to select from a wide variety of choices, but all offerings are nutritionally planned to supply recommended daily allowances. In hospital or long-term care settings, special requests or preferences (e.g., vegetarian diet, kosher diet) and food allergies should be reported to the dietary department when the client is admitted.

Often, dietary intake must be altered to promote healing and to restore health. Some objectives of dietary treatment are to increase or decrease weight, to allow an organ to rest, to

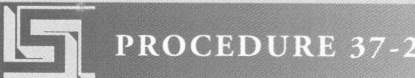

PROCEDURE 37-2

ASSISTING AN ADULT WITH FEEDING

Purpose
1. Maintain nutritional status.
2. Provide a time for socialization.

Assessment
- Assess client's physical and emotional ability to feed self (i.e., motor function, coordination, level of consciousness, vision, interest, depression).
- Assess client's eating habits and food preferences; cultural and religious beliefs may eliminate certain food from the diet.
- Review history for food allergies.
- Assess ability of gastrointestinal tract to absorb and digest oral nutrition (i.e., presence of bowel sounds, regular bowel movements, history of gastrointestinal disorders, Crohn's disease, duodenal ulcers, pancreatitis, cholecystitis, ulcerative colitis).
- Review physician's orders for type of diet.

Equipment
Personal hygiene supplies for client to wash hands
Glasses, if necessary
Special devices (splints, prostheses, spoons, cups)
Meal tray
Oral hygiene equipment

Procedure
1. Prepare client's environment for meal:
   a. Remove urinals, bedpans, dressings, trash.
   b. Ventilate or aerate room for unpleasant odors.
   c. Clean overbed table.
   Rationale: A clean, uncluttered environment enhances appetite.
2. Prepare client for meal:
   a. Help client urinate or defecate.
   b. Help client wash face and hands.
   c. Assist with oral hygiene.
   d. Help client apply dentures, glasses, or special appliances.
   e. Assist to upright position in bed or chair.
   Rationale: Comfort and optimal physical condition stimulate appetite and help client ingest meal.
3. Wash your hands before touching meal tray.
   Rationale: Clean hands help prevent transfer of microorganisms.
4. Check client's tray against diet order and with client's identification.
   Rationale: Diets are prepared for specific clients.

5. Place tray on overbed table and move in front of client.
6. Prepare tray. Open cartons, remove lids, season food, cut food into bite-size pieces.
   Rationale: Clients with impaired physical or cognitive function may be unable to prepare food for eating.
7. Place a napkin or towel under client's chin, and cover clothing.
8. If client can feed self, you may leave at this point. Return after 10 to 15 minutes to determine whether client is tolerating diet.
   Rationale: Self-care enhances feelings of independence and positive self-esteem. Note: Do not leave clients with overly hot liquids or food unless they are fully independent with feeding. Rationale: Decreased sensation or lack of motor coordination could result in burns from hot foods or liquid.
9. a. If client can sit in a chair but needs help to eat, sit in chair facing client.
   b. If client must remain in bed, nurse may stand to feed client.
   Rationale: Convey an unhurried social impression to client.

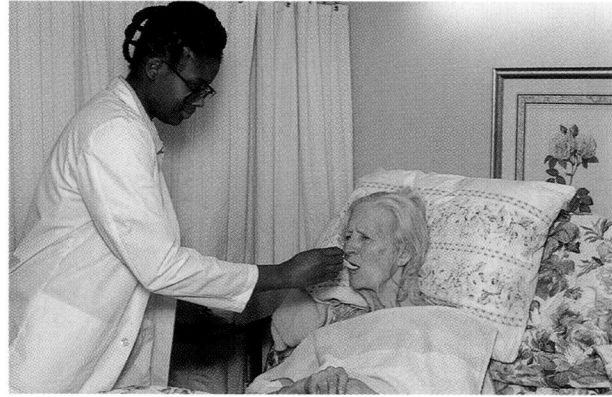

Step 9B The nurse assists the client in bed.

10. Allow client to choose the order he or she would like to eat. If client is visually impaired, identify the food on the tray.
11. Warn client if food is hot or cold.
12. Allow enough time between bites for adequate chewing and swallowing.
    Rationale: Allowing sufficient time to eat helps digestion.
13. Offer liquids as requested or between bites. Use a straw or special drinking cup if available.
    Rationale: Liquids assist in swallowing.

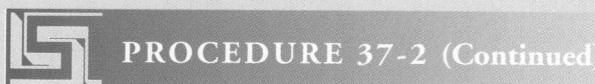

PROCEDURE 37-2 (Continued)

14. Provide conversation during meal. Choose topic of interest to client. Reorient to current events, or use meal as an opportunity to educate on nutrition or discharge plans. *Note:* Do not talk to clients who are relearning swallowing techniques; they need to concentrate.
15. Help client wash hands and face and perform oral hygiene after meal.
16. Assist to comfortable position, and allow rest period. *Note:* If at risk for aspiration, leave head of bed elevated for 30 minutes after eating.
17. Record fluids and amount of meal consumed, if ordered.
    Rationale: Documentation allows for monitoring of fluids and nutritional status.
18. Remove and dispose of tray.
19. Wash your hands.

Lifespan Considerations
Infant
- Infants do not usually need food other than breast milk or formula until 4 to 6 months of age. Strained or blended foods may be introduced at that time.
- Infant cereal is recommended as the first solid because of its iron content and low incidence of intolerance.
- At 6 months of age, infants are interested in self-feeding with a spoon or teething crackers.

Toddler
- Toddlers are often independent and insist on feeding themselves.
- Appropriate "finger foods" include meatballs, hard-boiled eggs, cooked carrots, fruit slices (without skins), cheese pieces, dry cereal, crackers. Avoid whole grapes, hard candy, and other foods that could cause choking.

Preschool
- This is a period of slow growth, so a decrease in appetite can be expected.

- Using foods in color games and allowing the child to help with food preparation (e.g., stirring gelatin and pudding, peeling oranges, washing vegetables) stimulate the child's interest and teach good eating habits.

Adolescent
- Ages 10 to 11 years in girls and 12 to 13 years in boys are periods of rapid growth. These children need larger consumption of nutrients and calories.
- Girls beginning menstruation need increased iron in their diets.
- Many adolescent diets are low in calcium, iron, vitamin A, and protein.

Older Adult
- Older adults may have diminished appetites from loss of taste and smell and decreased number of taste buds.
- Many older adults wear dentures. Poorly fitting dentures can impair their ability and desire to eat properly.
- People in this age group usually need fewer calories because of decreased activity and slowing metabolism.
- Calcium intake is often much lower than DRIs for both men and women.

Home Care Modifications
- Loneliness and poverty may decrease a client's ability or interest in eating balanced meals at home.
- Federal programs, such as food stamps and supplemental security income, can increase the food-buying power for clients at home.
- In 1972, a federally funded nutrition program for older adults was instituted that provides low-cost, nutritious meals served in community settings. These programs also provide socialization for lonely older adults.
- Meals on Wheels is available in many communities to deliver nutritious meals to clients in their homes.

OUTCOME-BASED TEACHING PLAN

When Mr. Lyman, a recent widower, comes to the clinic for a routine check-up, data reveal he has lost 15 lb since his wife's death 6 months ago. He is 6 feet tall and currently weighs 160 lb. During your assessment, you discover he usually eats cereal for breakfast, a sandwich for lunch, and skips dinner or has some soup. He states, "My wife always took care of the cooking. Since she died, nothing tastes good anymore." He has one son who lives 300 miles away and lots of friends in the area, but he doesn't feel comfortable hinting for dinner invitations. He asks you to help him develop a plan that he feels inclined and motivated to follow.

OUTCOME: Mr. Lyman will verbalize a realistic plan to increase food intake, which will permit him to maintain his present weight.

Strategies

- Explore Mr. Lyman's feelings about his recent weight loss and desire to reverse weight loss trend.
- If Mr. Lyman is motivated to maintain or gain weight, discuss his eating pattern before his wife's death, including food likes and dislikes.
- Have Mr. Lyman keep a food diary.
- Discuss possible community agencies that could support his efforts (e.g., Meals on Wheels; senior program at the community center).
- Discuss foods that are dense in calories and protein.
- Suggest protein supplements between meals to boost caloric intake.
- Discuss easy-to-prepare frozen dinners that can be microwaved.
- Provide home health follow-up to assess and provide encouragement for weight gain and good nutrition.
- Refer Mr. Lyman to a nutritionist if he continues to lose weight despite the above efforts.

remedy nutritional deficits, to promote healing, and to provide nutrients the body can metabolize.

Modifying a diet's texture, consistency, calories, or other nutrients may be necessary for clients who have had surgery or have a medical condition that requires an altered diet. Examples of diets with different textures and consistencies are clear liquid, full liquid, soft, and mechanical soft.

Clear Liquid. This diet includes only liquids that lack residue, such as juices without pulp (e.g., apple, cranberry), tea, gelatin, soda pop, and clear broth. The clear liquid diet is used as a first diet postoperatively, before some diagnostic tests, and after an acute episode of vomiting or diarrhea.

Full Liquid. A full liquid diet includes all fluids and foods that become liquid at room temperature (e.g., ice cream, sherbet). This diet may be ordered postoperatively after a clear liquid diet has been well tolerated or for clients who cannot chew food adequately.

Soft. Soft diets include soft foods and those with reduced fiber content, which require less energy for digestion. Soft diets are appropriate for clients who have difficulty chewing or no teeth. Mechanical soft diets include similar foods that are further chopped or pureed for those with difficulty chewing. They also may be used postoperatively as the diet progresses.

Diet As Tolerated. Diet as tolerated is ordered when a client's ability to tolerate certain foods will change, such as postoperatively or after GI distress. Nurses order such diets based on the client's appetite and ability to eat. For example, on the first postoperative day, a client may receive a clear liquid diet. If no nausea occurs, normal intestinal motility returns, and the client feels like eating, the diet may advance to a regular diet.

Restrictive Diets. Diets may be ordered to fulfill a special requirement in clients with chronic disease or altered metabolism. For example, clients with cardiac problems may need to limit sodium and types of dietary fat, obese clients may need to restrict calories, and diabetic clients may need to follow a prescribed American Diabetes Association diet. Any food or fluid given must fit the dietary restrictions. Examples of such dietary modifications are given in Table 37-4.

When clients are placed on restrictive diets, teaching must promote necessary dietary changes. Dietitians may do initial teaching, and nurses reinforce such teaching. Written materials are available to assist in such education. Changing long-established eating patterns is difficult for many clients, and goals should be realistic, mutually set, and individualized.

Nutritional Supplements

Nutritional supplements, in the form of formulas or vitamins and minerals, may be added to prescribed diets to provide necessary nutrients, especially during periods of increased metabolic demand. Nurses can request supplements, which physicians order. Supplements are typically milkshake-type drinks given between meals three or four times a day to increase calorie and/or protein intake. Malnourished clients and clients with excessive metabolic demands from trauma, fever, infection, surgery, or cancer benefit from such "power-packing" therapy.

Enteral Tube Feedings

Enteral nutrition is the direct delivery of nutrients into the GI system, bypassing the mouth. Tube feedings contain nutritionally balanced, commercial formulas given through a tube directly into the esophagus, stomach, duodenum, or jejunum. Access to the GI system can be achieved by inserting a tube through the nose into the stomach or intestine or directly into the system through the skin.

TABLE 37-4

Dietary Modifications for Diseases	
Disease	**Modification**
Renal disease	Restrict intake of sodium, potassium, protein, and possibly fluids.
Liver disease (cirrhosis)	Restrict intake of sodium; increase intake of protein, unless hepatic coma is pending; then protein is virtually eliminated.
Congestive heart failure	Restrict intake of sodium and calories.
Coronary artery disease	Restrict intake of sodium, calories, and fats (saturated fats and cholesterol).
Burns	Increase intake of calories, protein, vitamin C, and the B-complex vitamins.
Respiratory (emphysema)	A soft, high-calorie, high-protein diet is recommended.
Tuberculosis	Increase intake of protein, calories, calcium, and vitamin A.
Hypertension	Restrict sodium intake; lose weight, if appropriate.

Tube feedings provide nutrition to clients with functional GI systems who cannot swallow or who have an esophageal obstruction. Obstruction can occur secondary to edema from head or neck surgery, tumor, or trauma (e.g., swallowing caustic substances, inhaling smoke). Tube feedings are indicated when decreased level of consciousness prevents safe eating for clients. Tube feedings are used as adjunctive therapy for clients who can eat but who cannot consume adequate nutrients to meet the body's nutritional demands (e.g., clients who have cancer). Premature newborns who have an inadequate sucking reflex or lack of strength to feed also can be fed this way. Tube feedings are appropriate only when nutrients can be absorbed from the GI tract (Table 37-5).

Types of Tubes. The type of tube used to deliver enteral feedings depends on how long, where, and how the feeding is delivered. A nasogastric tube, such as a Levin tube, can be used for short-term tube feedings. Because some tubes are relatively rigid and have a large diameter compared with the nasal passage, discomfort and mucosal breakdown have been common with prolonged therapy. More recently, flexible, small-bore tubes have been developed when tube feeding is indicated. These tubes vary in size from 6 to 12 Fr and are composed of polyurethane, silicon, or polyvinyl chloride. Most have weighted distal tips and are placed with the use of a stylet. The tubes are radiopaque so that radiographic examination can confirm tube placement. Nasogastric tubes are attached to the nose with tape.

Tubes that are placed in the stomach or intestine through the skin usually are larger in diameter and are made of soft biocompatible material. Initially, some are sutured in place to prevent leakage and dislodgement. Aseptic care of the incision is important until healing has occurred. The tube can be clamped between feedings. After the incision has healed, the tube can be removed and then reinserted when feeding is required.

If long-term tube feedings are likely, a procedure can be performed to create an opening directly into the stomach or intestine through which feedings can be directly administered. A gastrostomy is an opening into the stomach. A newer procedure for gastrostomy placement is called percutaneous endoscopic gastrostomy (PEG). PEG involves endoscopic percutaneous insertion of a mushroom catheter into the stomach (Fig. 37-5). PEG is safer and less expensive because it does not require a general anesthetic and can often be done on an ambulatory basis (Rombeau & Rolandelli, 1997). Because surgery or anesthesia does not decrease GI

TABLE 37-5

Appropriate Formulas and Delivery Methods for Enteral Feeding Based on Feeding Tube and GI Function			
Tube (Caliber)	**Gastrointestinal Function**	**Diet**	**Preferred Administration Schedule**
Nasogastric (8–12 Fr) →	Normal → Abnormal →	Intact nutrient formula → Elemental formula →	Continuous or intermittent Continuous
Esophagostomy/ pharyngostomy/ gastrostomy (>10 Fr) →	Normal → Abnormal →	Intact nutrient formula Elemental formula →	Continuous or intermittent
Jejunostomy (>6 Fr) →	Normal → Abnormal →	Intact nutrient formula Elemental formula →	Continuous controlled by enteral pump

From Dudek, S. G. (2001). *Nutrition Essentials for Nursing Practice,* 4th ed. Philadelphia: Lippincott.

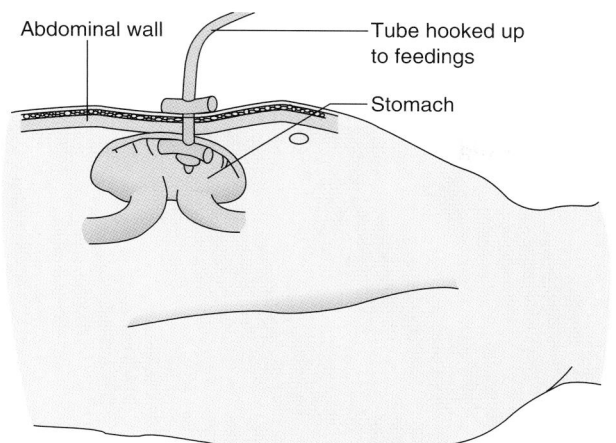

Abdominal wall — Tube hooked up to feedings — Stomach

A

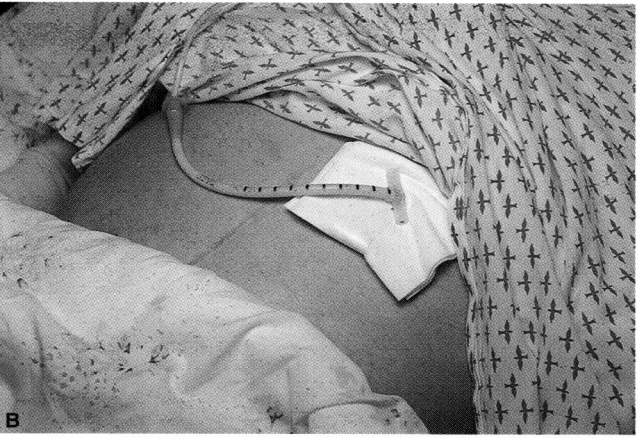

B

FIGURE 37-5 Percutaneous endoscopic gastrostomy (PEG). **(A)** Tube is placed in the stomach for feedings. A mushroom catheter prevents dislodgment. **(B)** Dressing over the tube on the abdomen protects the PEG tube site.

motility in this procedure, feedings can start within 24 hours. An opening into the jejunum (jejunostomy) is often used when aspiration has been a problem (Rombeau & Rolandelli, 1997). A dual gastrostomy/jejunostomy tube can be inserted if decompression is necessary along with feeding. A double-lumen tube allows feedings to enter the jejunum while a second lumen drains the stomach (Rombeau & Rolandelli, 1997).

Enteral Formulas. Enteral feedings consist of nutritionally balanced formulas. Many brands are available commercially; they vary in relative proportions of nutrients and calories, osmolarity, and ease of digestibility and absorption. Most formulas can be stored unrefrigerated until opened, but then they should be refrigerated to limit microbial growth. To minimize bacterial contamination, formula that remains in an open can after a set number of hours (usually 24 to 48) should be discarded.

Continuous Versus Intermittent Feedings. Enteral feedings may be given intermittently or continuously, as summarized in Procedure 37-3. The physician orders the rate of infusion and

the formula to use. Continuous feedings are permitted to flow in at the prescribed rate by the gravitational drip method, or they are monitored by an infusion pump. For clients who are eating, feedings may be ordered to infuse continuously during the night and may be discontinued a few hours before breakfast to stimulate the appetite.

Intermittent feedings are given at specific intervals, often corresponding to mealtimes (Forloines-Lynn, 1996). Intermittent feedings should be given slowly (e.g., over a 15-minute period) using a syringe or gravity flow. Such a schedule may also be called cyclic.

Hazards and Complications. Nursing responsibilities for clients receiving tube feedings include prevention and assessment of complications, such as nausea, vomiting, aspiration, fluid and electrolyte imbalance, diarrhea, intestinal cramping, tube occlusion, and hyperglycemia. Nausea and vomiting usually occur when the feeding is administered at a rate faster than the formula can be absorbed. To assess for this, check the residual volume left in the stomach before formula administration or at periodic intervals if tube feedings are continuous. This is usually done by inserting a syringe tip into the tube opening. If the suction used is so great that the tube collapses, the residual measure will be inaccurate. If residuals are greater than 100 mL or half of the previously administered volume for intermittent feedings, stop the feeding until the cause of the residual is determined because aspiration is likely if vomiting occurs.

Minimize the risk of aspiration by checking proper tube placement before initiating feedings and at frequent intervals and by keeping the client in Fowler's position at all times when feedings are infusing and for 30 minutes after an intermittent feeding. Food coloring can be added to the formula for clients at risk for aspiration. If color-tinged respiratory secretions are produced, aspiration has probably occurred.

SAFETY ALERT
Always check proper tube placement before beginning tube feedings to prevent accidental aspiration of feedings.

Diarrhea, intestinal cramping, and fluid loss can occur when high-osmolarity formulas are used. Diluting the formula by adding water or giving the client adequate free water may prevent severe osmotic shifts. Slow administration of room-temperature feedings helps limit GI intolerance.

Feeding tubes, especially those with small-bore lumens, clog easily. Tube occlusion, even for a short period, must be avoided. Prevent clogging by frequently flushing the tube with fluid such as water or carbonated beverage, especially after giving medications and before and after feedings (Mateo, 1996).

Hyperglycemia may occur in clients who cannot produce enough insulin to deal with the carbohydrate load in the formula. For clients with diabetes and others considered to be at high risk, blood glucose monitoring permits careful regulation of increased insulin need.

(*text continues on page 976*)

PROCEDURE 37-3

ADMINISTERING NUTRITION VIA NASOGASTRIC OR GASTROSTOMY TUBE

Purpose
1. Provide enteral nutrition for clients who cannot swallow or who have an esophageal obstruction.
2. Provide nutrition to comatose or semiconscious clients.
3. Provide additional nutrients for clients who cannot orally consume adequate calories.

Assessment
- Assess client's nutritional status and identify need for tube feedings:
  —Impaired swallowing
  —Decreased level of consciousness
  —Head, neck, or facial surgery or trauma
  —Extraordinary caloric requirements
- Review chart for food allergies and physician's order as to type, amount, rate, route, and frequency of feeding.
- Assess client's gastrointestinal system:
  —Observe and palpate for distention, tenderness.
  —Auscultate bowel sounds.
  —Determine time of last bowel movement.
  —Assess for presence of existing feeding tube.

Equipment
Formula
Blue food coloring (optional)
Disposable gavage bag and tubing
60-mL catheter tip irrigation syringe
pH strip
Infusion pump (optional)
Water
Measuring container

Procedure
1. Wash your hands.
2. Close room door or curtains around bed.
   Rationale: Privacy decreases embarrassment.
3. Explain procedure to client.
4. Help client to high-Fowler's position by elevating head of bed at least 60 degrees or assisting to a chair. If high-Fowler's position is contraindicated, help client to a right side-lying position with head slightly elevated.
   Rationale: Positions prevent aspiration of formula into lungs and facilitate flow of feeding into gut.

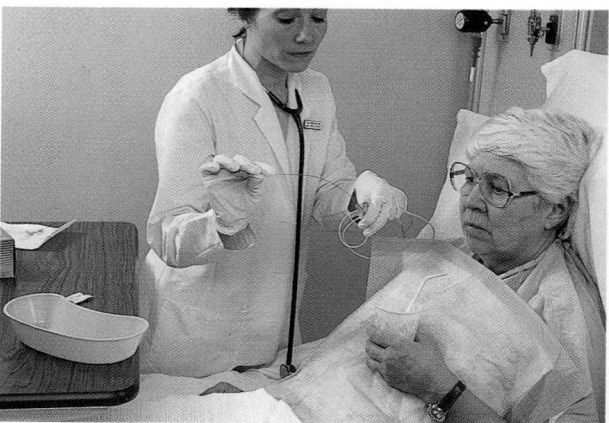

Step 4 The client is in a high-Fowler's position.

5. Confirm placement of tube in stomach:
   a. Withdraw sample of stomach contents and check for low pH level.
   Rationale: Gastric secretions have pH of 1 to 3.
   b. Attach 60-mL irrigation syringe to tube and inject 10 mL of air while auscultating over epigastrium.
   Rationale: Air can be heard entering stomach.
   Note: Auscultation of air is not always a reliable index of tube placement when a small-bore feeding tube is used.
   c. Aspirate all stomach contents, and measure for residual.
   Rationale: Presence of gastric fluid confirms tube placement in the stomach. Gastric residuals are checked to evaluate if gastric emptying is adequate.
   d. If 100 mL or more than half of the last feeding is aspirated, contact the physician before proceeding with tube feeding. The feeding is usually held.
   e. Reinstill the aspirated gastric contents through the tube and into the stomach.
   Rationale: Gastric content is rich in electrolytes. Electrolyte imbalance could occur if residuals are discarded.
6. Prepare correct amount and strength of formula. Formula should be room temperature. Add several drops of food coloring (optional).
   Rationale: Amount and strength of formula are gradually increased to prevent diarrhea and gastric intolerance. Formula should be at room temperature because it will not be warmed or cooled by the oral and esophageal mucosa as occurs in normal swallowing. Cold formula can

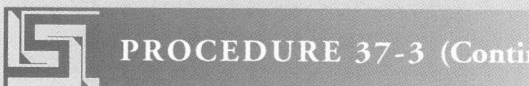

PROCEDURE 37-3 (Continued)

cause abdominal cramping and discomfort; hot formula can burn the stomach. Food coloring is frequently used when tube-feeding clients are at risk for aspiration. If formula is aspirated, nasotracheal suction reveals bluish secretions. Check agency policy.

Bolus of Intermittent Feeding

1. Remove plunger from irrigation syringe. Clamp gastric tubing and attach syringe. If using gavage bag, attach tubing to gastric tube.
   Rationale: Clamping tubing prevents air from entering stomach and prevents stomach contents from leaking out.
2. Fill syringe or gavage bag with formula.
3. Allow feeding to flow in slowly (10–15 minutes). If using syringe, raise or lower syringe to adjust flow rate by gravity. Refill syringe as needed without disconnecting, avoiding air spaces in tubing. If gavage bag is used, hang bag on IV pole, and adjust flow rate with clamp on tubing.
   Rationale: Feedings given too rapidly cause nausea, vomiting, flatus, and abdominal cramps.
4. Clamp tubing just as feeding is completing. Rinse tube with 30 to 60 mL tap water. Do not allow air to enter tubing.
   Rationale: Clamping tubing prevents air from entering stomach and thus reduces bloating or cramps. Rinsing with water clears the gastric tube to prevent blockage and bacterial growth.
5. Clamp gastric tube, and disconnect from syringe or gavage bag.
6. Have client remain in high-Fowler's or elevated side-lying position for 30 to 60 minutes after feeding.

Continuous Feeding

1. Connect gavage tubing to gastric tube.
2. Hang gavage bag on IV pole.
3. Pour in desired amount of formula. *Note:* Usually hang amount of formula to infuse in 3 hours. Check agency policy.
4. a. Connect tubing to infusion pump.
   b. Set rate.
   Rationale: If feeding is infused too rapidly, vomiting and cramps may result.
5. Clients receiving continuous feedings should have gastric residuals checked every 4 to 6 hours, according to agency policy. Then flush the tubing with 30 to 60 mL of water.
   Rationale: This assesses for adequate absorption of feeding and verifies correct placement of tube.
6. Have client remain in high-Fowler's or in slightly elevated side-lying position.

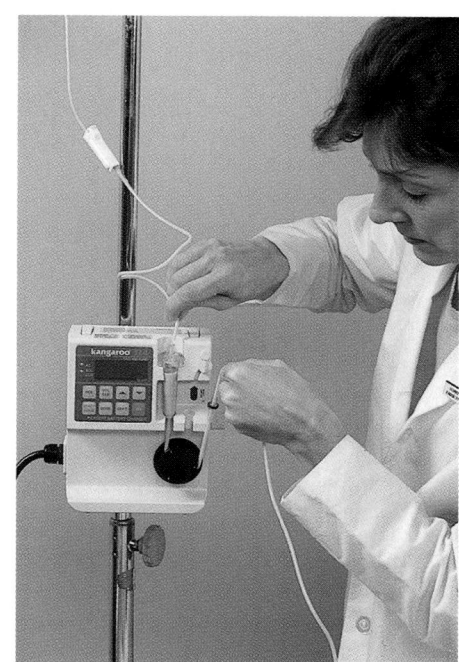

Step 4A Gavage tubing is placed in infusion pump.

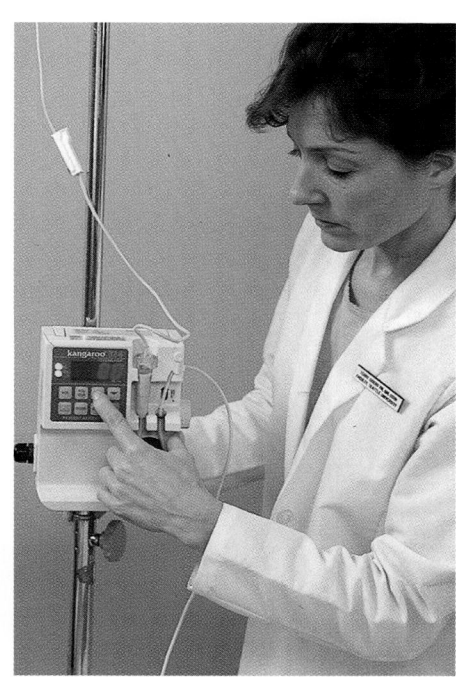

Step 4B The infusion rate is set.

PROCEDURE 37-3 (Continued)

7. Wash any reusable equipment with soap and water. Change equipment every 24 hours or according to agency policy.
   Rationale: Clean equipment prevents inadvertent administration of spoiled or contaminated feeding.
8. Wash hands.
9. Document appropriately.

Lifespan Considerations
Infant and Child
- Intermittent feeding and reinsertion of the nasogastric feeding tube at each feeding are recommended in children. There is significant risk of stomach perforation, nasal airway obstruction, and ulceration and irritation of the mucous membrane if a feeding tube is left in continuously.

Home Care Modifications
- Encourage clients to participate in the preparation and procedure of tube feeding if possible to increase their feelings of independence and self-esteem.
- Instruct client or caregiver in correct techniques and rationales as stated previously.

- Feedings can be provided from commercially prepared formulas or home-blended foods. Formulas may be thinned with juice, milk, or water.
- Teach caregiver proper storage of extra formula:
  —Seal and store commercially prepared formulas in refrigerator once the can is open. Use within 24 hours.
  —Tightly seal, date, and refrigerate home-blended feedings. Use within 24 hours after preparation.
- Tube-fed clients may feel isolated or may have altered self-esteem and body image from the loss of sensory and social stimulation associated with eating. Encourage caregivers to schedule feedings with family mealtimes.
- If medically permitted, the client can consume some favorite foods orally. If swallowing is contraindicated, it may be possible for the client to chew and taste a few favorite foods, then spit them out.
- Follow-up and consultation with a home health nurse often allow clients and caregivers to arrange creative solutions to problems or concerns that arise.

Healthcare Planning and Home- or Community-Based Care

Nutrition is an important consideration in independent home management. Clients must be able to buy, store, prepare, and eat food independently to function at home; many clients need assistance with shopping or cooking. Family and friends may be available to help. The nursing plan of care should reflect the client's needs and available support. Nurses can enlist the help of others to provide services if necessary.

Clients with chronic health problems may face great nutritional challenges. Many local and national agencies (e.g., American Cancer Society, American Heart Association, American Diabetes Association), as well as governmental agencies (e.g., U.S. Department of Agriculture, USDA Food and Nutrition Center, National Institutes of Health), publish pamphlets that provide dietary guidance and realistic suggestions. Malnourished clients and those at risk for nutritional deficits may be referred to community health agencies.

When new restrictive diets are ordered for clients, teaching should start as soon as possible. Dietitians sometimes begin such teaching. Clients should receive written materials outlining foods to include and those to exclude from the

APPLY YOUR KNOWLEDGE

Gina Round has a gastrostomy tube in place and is receiving full strength Isocal formula at 80 cc/h. Isocal comes in cans containing 240 cc. How would you prepare this tube feeding? What assessments and nursing considerations are important for clients who receive tube feedings?
Check your answer in Appendix A.

diet. Help clients determine how best to incorporate dietary changes into their lives. Including the persons who will actually prepare the food in these teaching sessions is essential.

Nutritional support technologies, such as tube feedings or TPN (see Chapter 28) are often managed at home. In many instances, nurses teach clients and their caregivers how to administer such therapies. Teaching should begin early in the hospitalization by explaining tube feedings and TPN as they are performed. Before discharge, the client or caregiver should be able to demonstrate necessary administration techniques and to solve problems that may arise. Arrangements for equipment and supplies should be made before discharge, and clients should receive the name of the vendor.

Governmental programs have been developed for people who need dietary enhancement and nutrition education. Nurses are actively involved in providing education and care through such programs. Community-based programs include the following:

- Senior center services
- Home-delivered meals
- Food stamps
- Missions and shelters
- Women, Infants, and Children (WIC), a nutrition and healthcare program for pregnant women, new mothers, infants, and children
- Child-care centers
- School lunch programs
- The M&I Program (maternal and infant nutritional supplementation and healthcare)

In addition to providing food for groups at risk, many of these services also provide education and counseling. The Nutrition Education and Training program has been developed to help public schools incorporate nutrition education in their curricula.

Community resources also include the nutritional services of public health nurses, nutritionists, home health caregivers, and welfare agency workers. These people teach, assist with meal planning and food buying, consult, make referrals, and conduct research.

International agencies promote health and nutritional adequacy on a worldwide level. Programs include the United Nations Food and Agriculture Organization, WHO, and the United Nations Children's Fund.

EVALUATION

Nursing interventions related to nutrition are helpful if nurse and client agree that progress has been made toward identified outcomes. Progress is measured by outcome criteria established in the planning phase. The following general goals were identified previously in this chapter with outcome criteria for clients, although goals and outcome criteria are always individualized. After reaching conclusions, the nurse

and client can decide whether to readjust previous goals, establish new goals, or terminate goals.

Goal

The client will use nutritionally sound dietary intake to meet body requirements and to promote health.

Possible Outcome Criteria

- Within 24 hours, the client describes a diet that provides his or her nutritional requirements using the Food Guide Pyramid.
- Within 3 days, the client verbalizes use of proper daily food selection from the Food Guide Pyramid.
- The client ingests healthful diet by limiting intake of saturated fats, refined sugar, and sodium, as witnessed by the caregiver at five meals during the next 5 days.
- The client's skin and nails demonstrate absence of clinical signs of nutritional deficiency or excess.
- During hospitalization, the client's blood glucose, albumin, and other values remain within normal limits as shown in laboratory tests.

Goal

The client will maintain dietary intake adequate to meet the body's energy expenditures.

Possible Outcome Criteria

- Within 24 hours, the client or caregiver describes dietary changes necessary to meet adequate caloric intake when demand is increased (e.g., pregnancy, lactation, adolescence, trauma, surgery).
- The client exercises daily for 30 minutes.
- For 1 month, the client uses nutritional supplements (e.g., protein supplement, vitamins) during periods of increased demand.

Goal

The client will demonstrate adequate knowledge to adhere to dietary prescription or therapies to promote health.

Possible Outcome Criteria

- After a teaching session, the client lists foods to avoid on the special diet (e.g., low sodium, low fat).
- Before discharge, the client describes how to alter his or her lifestyle (eating in restaurants, preparing food) to comply with dietary restrictions.
- Before discharge, the client discusses realistic use of family and community support groups to ensure adequate nutrition after discharge.
- Before discharge, the client or caregiver demonstrates how to safely administer tube feedings or TPN.

THERAPEUTIC DIALOGUE
Nutrition

Scene for Thought

Mr. Rose, an 83-year-old man with squamous cell cancer of the left jaw, had a radical left composite resection surgery and placement of tracheostomy and nasogastric tube. On admission, his weight was 150 lb (height 69 inches). Enteral feedings are to be his sole nutritional source for at least 3 weeks after discharge. His 80-year-old wife stays with him during the day and will care for him upon discharge, scheduled tomorrow.

Less Effective

Nurse: Good morning, Mr. Rose. I am Wilma Brown, your nurse. I understand you're going home tomorrow.

Mrs. Rose: That's what they said, but I don't know if I can manage, especially the tube feedings.

Nurse: *(Looks at Mrs. Rose.)* Did you care for him before he came into the hospital? *(Acknowledges wife; seeks some information.)*

Mrs. Rose: He was well until this surgery, and always cared for himself.

Nurse: I'm going to get his morning feeding ready now. Watch what I'm doing, and let me know if you have any questions. *(Requires wife to initiate questions.)*

Mrs. Rose: I'm so worried I won't be able to do all the things that you do. What happens if I do something wrong? *(Looks to Mr. Rose and asks him if he can remember the procedure used with his tube feeding. He responds by writing "yes" on a note pad.)*

Nurse: Between the two of you, this procedure should go fairly smoothly. *(Minimizes the complexity of a new skill that includes both knowledge and physical dexterity.)*

More Effective

Nurse: Good morning, Mr. Rose, Mrs. Rose. I am Jeff Wilcox. I will be your nurse today. How are you both feeling?

Mrs. Rose: He's getting better, but the doctors said he's going home tomorrow. Do you think he'll be ready? *(Mr. Rose is alert and follows the discussion, but cannot talk because tracheostomy has not yet been plugged.)*

Nurse: There are things you will need to know how to do. Can we talk about them? *(Acknowledges reality; gives choice.)*

Mrs. Rose: I don't know if I'm going to be able to do everything you do. *(Sounds anxious.)*

Nurse: What we can do is identify the most important things and have you help me with those today. Would you be willing? *(Looks at them both for affirmation; sets priorities, asks permission.)*

Mrs. Rose: I've sort of watched what happens when they start his feedings, but I don't know if I can remember everything. What if I do something wrong?

Nurse: Mrs. Rose, are you afraid you might hurt your husband? *(Seeks clarification.) (To Mr. Rose)* I'm going to start your feeding now. Let me get two copies of a paper that lists all the steps for the tube feedings. I'll tell you both what I'm doing and you can follow along with the list. *(Includes both client and his wife.)* Then, Mrs. Rose, you can help me flush the tube and disconnect the tubing when the feeding is finished.

Mrs. Rose: I do better when I have a checklist to follow. Will you stay while I work with the feeding tube?

Nurse: Yes, I will. I know this is new for you both. I want to be with you when you are learning what is safe, and not safe. *(Acknowledges unfamiliarity of situation and establishes boundaries.)*

Critical Thinking Challenge

- Discuss the factors affecting the amount and type of nutrients Mr. Rose needs.
- Identify questions this scenario raises about the concerns of Mrs. Rose.
- What success do you think each nurse will have in helping this couple successfully manage the tube feedings? Explain reasons for your feelings.
- What clues did Jeff notice that Wilma ignored?

Goal

The client will achieve and maintain desired weight.

Possible Outcome Criteria

- By mutual goal setting with the client, a specific weight to achieve is set.
- The client expresses satisfaction with meals.

- If overweight, the client achieves a 10% reduction in body weight by 6 months.
- The client loses weight at a rate of about 1 to 2 lb/week for 6 months.
- The client combines a lower-calorie healthy diet, increased physical activity, and behavior therapy into his or her lifestyle.
- If underweight, the client gains weight to a specific goal by a set time period.

NURSING PLAN OF CARE
THE CLIENT WITH IMBALANCED NUTRITION

Nursing Diagnosis
Imbalanced Nutrition: Less Than Body Requirements, as manifested by being underweight and having a low hematocrit and inadequate intake of calcium, iron, protein, vitamin A, and vitamin C

Client Goal
Client will construct a diet that meets the Food Guide Pyramid and RDA/DRI standards, is psychologically satisfying, can be readily understood, and is relatively easy to prepare or obtain.

Client Outcome Criteria
- Client obtains correct, useful information in which he or she expresses confidence.
- Client describes the basic function of nutrients.
- Client uses a diet that contains adequate amounts of all nutrients to meet the Food Guide Pyramid and RDA/DRI standards.
- Client reports satisfaction with the diet and an increased energy level.
- Client increases weight within the normal range for height, age, and sex.

Nursing Interventions	Scientific Rationale
1. Assess client laboratory values (hematocrit, hemoglobin, serum prealbumin) and physical parameters (height, weight, body mass index, skin-fold measurements).	1. Noting deviations from baseline and normal standards can help begin measures that correct deficiencies.
2. Assess the client's ability to obtain food.	2. Minimize or prevent financial or physical limitations from contributing to inadequate diet.
3. Assess the client's motivational level and ability to learn and follow the new diet prescription.	3. Prevent motivational or learning difficulties from interfering with obtaining a nutritionally adequate diet.
4. Instruct the client in the new diet prescription, and assess understanding (increased intake of protein, calcium, iron, vitamins A and C, and calories).	4. Encourage an improved intake of nutrients, especially those that had been determined to be low.
5. Provide the client with written information on the basic functions of the major nutrients; discuss this information and assess understanding.	5. Written format assists the client in retaining the information.
6. Answer client's questions; discuss areas of concern; provide the client with additional reference material as necessary.	6. Assist the client toward increased knowledge; relieve uncertainties; improve knowledge of self-care activities.
7. Assess the client's family history of diabetes and predisposing characteristics toward possible development of diabetes.	7. Establish a baseline of information to prevent potential problems or detect them early or treat promptly.

- The client is able to ingest food without pain or discomfort.

KEY CONCEPTS
- Adequate nutritional intake is important to maintain body functions, healthy tissues, and body temperature; to promote healing; and to build resistance to infection.

- Essential nutrients are carbohydrates, protein, fat, vitamins, minerals, and water.
- The complex processes of digestion, absorption, and metabolism permit the body to break down food and use it as energy.
- Great variations exist in dietary intake among people, but guidelines are useful when evaluating adequate intake.
- Manifestations of altered nutrition include body weight that is less or greater than the IBW, recent significant weight gain

or loss, decreased energy, altered bowel patterns, and altered skin, teeth, hair, or mucous membranes.

- A nutritional health assessment includes collecting subjective data about normal eating patterns, risk factors for nutritional deficits, and altered nutrition.
- Anthropometric measurements (height and weight, BMI, skinfold measurements, and arm circumference), calorie counts, and swallowing evaluation provide objective data to help assess a client's nutritional state.
- NANDA nursing diagnoses in the area of nutrition are Imbalanced Nutrition: Less Than Body Requirements; Imbalanced Nutrition: More Than Body Requirements; Imbalanced Nutrition: Risk for More Than Body Requirements; and Impaired Swallowing.
- Health promotion for optimal nutrition includes client teaching, measures to encourage healthy eating habits, and physical activity.
- Therapeutic diets are used to promote health, manage disease, or encourage healing.
- A variety of community programs are useful for clients who have nutritional needs.

REFERENCES

Beck, A., & Ovesen, L. (1998). At which body mass index and degree of weight loss should hospitalized elder patients be considered at nutritional risk? *Clinical Nutrition, 17*(5), 195–198.

Cash, T., & Deagle, E., III. (1997). The nature and extent of body-image disturbances in anorexia nervosa and bulimia nervosa: A meta-analysis. *International Journal of Eating Disorders, 22*(2), 107–125.

Committee on Dietary Reference Intakes. (1997). *Dietary reference intakes for calcium, phosphorus, magnesium, vitamin D, and fluoride.* Washington, DC: National Academy Press.

Corish, C. (1999). Pre-operative nutritional assessment. *Proceedings of the Nutrition Society, 58*(4), 821–829.

Dewey, K. (2001). Nutrition, growth, and complementary feeding of the breastfed infant. *Pediatric Clinics of North America, 48*(1), 87–104.

Edwards, S. (1998). Malnutrition in hospital patients: Where does it come from? *British Journal of Nursing, 7*(16), 954–958, 971–974.

Emans, S. (2000). Eating disorders in adolescent girls. *Pediatrics International, 42*(1), 1–7.

Fletcher, J., Branen, L., & Lawrence, A. (1997). Late adolescents' perceptions of their caregiver's feeding styles and practices and those they will use with their own children. *Adolescence, 32*(126), 287–298.

Goodwin, R., Bucholz, A., et al. (1999). Caregiving arrangement and nutrition: good news with some reservations. *Canadian Journal of Public Health, 90*(1), 41–45.

Kaplan, N. (2000). The dietary guideline for sodium: Should we shake it up? No. *American Journal of Clinical Nutrition, 71*(5), 1020–1026.

McGee, M. and Jensen, G. (2000). Nutrition in the elderly. *Journal of Clinical Gastroenterology, 30*(4), 372–380.

Mahan, L. K., & Escott-Stump, S. (1996). *Krause's food, nutrition, and diet therapy* (9th ed.). Philadelphia: W.B. Saunders.

McHale, J., Phipps, M., Horvath, K., & Schmelz, J. (1998). Expert nursing knowledge in the care of patients at risk of impaired swallowing. *Image: Journal of Nursing Scholarship, 30*(2), 137–142.

Metheny, N. and Titler, M. (2001). Assessing placement of feeding tubes. *American Journal of Nursing, 101*(5), 36–45; quiz 45–6.

National Academy of Sciences (1999). *Dietary reference intakes for thiamin, riboflavin, niacin, vitamin B_6, folate, vitamin B_{12},*

pantothenic acid, biotin, and choline. Washington, DC: National Academy Press.

National Heart, Lung, and Blood Institute, Obesity Education Initiative Expert Panel. (1998). *Clinical guidelines on the identification, evaluation, and treatment of overweight and obesity in adults.* Bethesda, MD: National Institutes of Health.

National Research Council. (1989). *Food and nutrition board recommended dietary allowances* (10th ed.). Washington, DC: National Academy Press.

North American Nursing Diagnosis Association (2001). *NANDA nursing diagnoses: Definitions and classification 2001–2002.* Philadelphia: Author.

Nourhashemi, F., Andries, S. et al. (1999). Nutritional support and aging in preoperative nutrition. *Current Opinion in Clinical Nutrition & Metabolic Care, 2*(1), 87–92.

Pennington, J., & Hubbard, V. (1997). Derivation of daily values used for nutrition labeling. *Journal of the American Dietetic Association, 97*(12), 1407–1412.

Pennington, J., & Wilkening, V. (1997). Final regulations for the nutrition labeling of raw fruits, vegetables, and fish. *Journal of the American Dietetic Association, 97*(11), 1299–1305.

Rader, J., Jones D., & Miller, L. (2000). The importance of individualized wheelchair seating for frail older adults. *Journal of Gerontological Nursing, 26*(11), 24–32.

Reifsnider, E. and Gill, S. (2000). Nutrition for the childbearing years [see comments]. *Journal of Obstetric, Gynecologic, & Neonatal Nursing, 29*(1), 43–55.

Rock, C. (1998). Dietary reference intakes, antioxidants, and beta carotene. *Journal of the American Dietetic Association,* 1410–1411.

Rolfes, S., DeBruyne, L., & Whitney, E. (1998). *Life span nutrition* (2nd ed.). Belmont, CA: West/Wadsworth.

Rombeau, J., & Rolandelli, R. (1997). *Clinical nutrition: Enteral and tube feeding* (3rd ed.). Philadelphia: W.B. Saunders.

Roubenoff, R., Heymsfield, S. et al. (1997). Standardization of nomenclature of body composition in weight loss. *American Journal of Clinical Nutrition, 66*, 192–196.

Ruibal-Mendieta, N. and Lints, R. (1998). Novel and transgenic food crops: Overview of scientific versus public perception. *Transgenic Research, 7*(5), 379–386.

Sanchez-Castillo, C., Warrender, S., Whitehead, T., & James, W. (1987). An assessment of dietary salt in a British population. *Clinical Science, 72*(1), 95–102.

Schmidt, D. (2000). Outlook for consumer acceptance of agricultural biotechnology. *Nutrition, 16*(7–8), 704–706.

Stice, E. (1999). Clinical implications of psychosocial research on bulimia nervosa and binge-eating disorder. *Journal of Clinical Psychology, 55*(6), 675–683.

Thompson, S., Corwin, S., & Sargent, R. (1997). Ideal body size beliefs and weight concerns of fourth-grade children. *International Journal of Eating Disorders, 21*(3), 279–284.

Trumbo, P., Yates, A. et al. (2001). Dietary reference intakes: Vitamin A, vitamin K, arsenic, boron, chromium, copper, iodine, iron, manganese, molybdenum, nickel, silicon, vanadium, and zinc. *Journal of the American Dietetic Association, 101*(3), 294–301.

Ulijaszek, S. and Kerr, D. (1999). Anthropometric measurement error and the assessment of nutritional status. *British Journal of Nutrition, 82*(3), 165–177.

U.S. Department of Agriculture. (2000a). USDA's food guide pyramid, revised. Available at: http://www.pueblo.gsa.gov/cic_text/food/food-pyramid/main.htm. Accessed November 19, 2001.

U.S. Department of Agriculture. (2000b). Nutrition and your health: Dietary guidelines for Americans, 2000 (5th ed.). Available at: http://www.health.gov/dietaryguidelines/.

United States Pharmacopoeia. (2001). *USP-DI: Drug information for the health professionals: Vol. I* (21st ed.). Rockville, MD: Author.

Variyam, J., Blaylock, J., Smallwood, D., & Basiotis, P. (1998). *USDA's healthy eating index and nutrition information.* U.S. Department of Agriculture, Economic Research Service. Technical Bulletin 1866. Washington, DC: USDA.

Westfall, U. (1999). Gastrointestinal assessment. In L. Bucher & S. Melander (Eds.). *Critical care nursing* (pp. 692–704). Philadelphia: W.B. Saunders.

Williams, S. (1997). *Nutrition and diet therapy* (8th ed.). St. Louis, MO: Mosby.

Wold, R., Lopez. S., Pareo-Tubbeh, S., Baumgartner, R., Romero, L., Garry, P., & Koehler, K. (1998). Helping elderly participants keep 3-day diet records in the New Mexico aging process study. *Journal of American Dietetic Association, 98*(3), 326–332.

BIBLIOGRAPHY

Altabe, M. (1998). Ethnicity and body image: Quantitative and qualitative analysis. *International Journal of Eating Disorders, 23*(2), 153–159.

American Society for Parenteral and Enteral Nutrition. (2001). Standards of practice for nutrition support nurses. *Nutrition in Clinical Practice, 16*(1), 56–62.

Baxter, J. P. (1999). Problems of nutritional assessment in the acute setting. *Proceedings of the Nutrition Society, 58*(1), 39–46.

Bloch, A. (2000). Nutrition support in cancer. *Seminars in Oncology Nursing, 16*(2), 122–127.

Caballero, B. (2001). Introduction. Symposium: Obesity in developing countries: Biological and ecological factors. *Journal of Nutrition, 131*(3), 866S–870S.

Caldwell, M., Brownell, K., & Wilfley, D. (1997). Relationship of weight, body dissatisfaction, and self-esteem in African American and white female dieters. *International Journal of Eating Disorders, 22*(2), 127–130.

Choban, P. S. and L. Flancbaum (2000). Nourishing the obese patient. *Clinical Nutrition, 19*(5), 305–311.

Compher, C., J. N. Kim, et al. (1998). Nutritional requirements of an aging population with emphasis on subacute care patients. *AACN Clinical Issues, 9*(3), 441–450.

Deitel, M. (1998). Overview of operations for morbid obesity. *World Journal of Surgery, 22*(9), 913–918.

Dudek, S. G. (2000). Malnutrition in hospitals. Who's assessing what patients eat? *American Journal of Nursing, 100*(4), 36–42; quiz 42–3.

Gladis, M., Wadden, T., Foster, G., Vogt, R., & Wingate, B. (1998). A comparison of two approaches to the assessment of binge eating in obesity. *International Journal of Eating Disorders, 23*(1), 17–26.

Goff, K. (1997). The nuts and bolts of enteral infusion pumps: CE series. *Medsurg Nursing, 6*(1), 9–16.

Goran, M. I. (2001). Metabolic precursors and effects of obesity in children: A decade of progress, 1990–1999. *American Journal of Clinical Nutrition, 73*(2), 158–171.

Harris, I. M. (2000). Regulatory and ethical issues with dietary supplements. *Pharmacotherapy, 20*(11), 1295–1302.

Johnson, A. M. (1999). Low levels of plasma proteins: Malnutrition or inflammation? *Clinical Chemistry & Laboratory Medicine, 37*(2), 91–96.

Kennedy, E., & Davis, C. (1998). US Department of Agriculture school breakfast program. *American Journal of Clinical Nutrition, 67,* (Suppl), 798S–803S.

Marian, M. J. and P. Allen (1998). Nutrition support for patients in long-term acute care and subacute care facilities. *AACN Clinical Issues, 9*(3), 427–440.

Murphy, L. and Bickford, V. (1999). Gastric residuals in tube feeding: How much is too much? *Nutrition in Clinical Practice, 14*(6), 304–306.

Nelson, K., Brown, M., & Lurie, N. (1998). Hunger in an adult patient population. *Journal of the American Medical Association, 279*(15), 1211–1214.

Noble, R. (1997). The incidence of parental obesity in overweight individuals. *International Journal of Eating Disorders, 22*(3), 265–271.

O'Neill, P. A. (2000). Swallowing and prevention of complications. *British Medical Bulletin, 56*(2), 457–465.

Osterholm, M. (2000). The changing epidemiology of food-borne disease. *International Journal of Clinical Practice, Supplement* (115), 60–64.

Pawluck, D., & Gorey, K. (1998). Secular trends in the incidence of anorexia nervosa: Integrative review of population-based studies. *International Journal of Eating Disorders, 23*(4), 347–352.

Refai, W. and D. L. Seidner (1999). Nutrition in the elderly. *Clinics in Geriatric Medicine, 15*(3), 607–625.

Rogers, L., Resnick, M., Mitchell, J., & Blum, R. (1997). The relationship between socioeconomic status and eating-disordered behaviors in a community sample of adolescent girls. *International Journal of Eating Disorders, 22*(1), 15–23.

Rose, D., & Oliveira, V. (1997). Nutrient intakes of individuals from food-insufficient households in the United States. *American Journal of Public Health, 87*(12), 1956–1961.

Scarbrough, F. (1997). Some Food and Drug Administration perspectives of fat and fatty acids. *American Journal of Clinical Nutrition, 65,* (Suppl), 1578S–1580S.

Scherbaum, V. and P. Furst (2000). New concepts on nutritional management of severe malnutrition: The role of protein. *Current Opinion in Clinical Nutrition & Metabolic Care, 3*(1), 31–38.

Schutz, Y., & Deurenberg, P. (1996). Energy metabolism: Overview of recent methods used in human studies. *Annals of Nutrition and Metabolism, 40*(4), 183–193.

Schwitzer, A., Bergholz, K., Dore, T., & Salimi, L. (1998). Eating disorders among college women: Prevention, education and treatment responses. *Journal of American College Health, 46*(5), 199–207.

Scott, E. (2000). Relationship between cross-contamination and the transmission of foodborne pathogens in the home. *Pediatric Infectious Disease Journal, 19*(10 Suppl), S111–S113.

Smith, J. L. (1998). Foodborne illness in the elderly. *Journal of Food Protection, 61*(9), 1229–1239.

Steen, B. (2000). Preventive nutrition in old age—a review. *Journal of Nutrition, Health & Aging, 4*(2), 114–119.

Tanco, S., Linden, W., & Earle, T. (1998). Well-being and morbid obesity in women: A controlled therapy evaluation. *International Journal of Eating Disorders, 23*(3), 325–339.

Wells, A., Garvin, V., Dohm, F., & Striegel-Moore, R. (1997). Telephone-based guided self-help for binge eating disorder: A feasibility study. *International Journal of Eating Disorders, 21*(4), 341–346.

Wilfley, D., & Cohen, L. (1997). Psychological treatment of bulimia nervosa and binge eating disorder. *Psychopharmacology Bulletin, 33*(3), 437–454.

38 Skin Integrity and Wound Healing

⑤ Key Terms

abrasion
approximated
binder
débridement
dehiscence
dermis
desquamation
epidermis
eschar
evisceration
fistula

granulation tissue
hematoma
laceration
macerated
pruritus
purulent
re-epithelialization
sanguineous
serosanguineous
serous
subcutaneous tissue

⑤ Learning Objectives

Upon completion of this chapter, the student will be able to do the following:
1. Discuss factors that affect integumentary function.
2. Identify manifestations of impaired integumentary function.
3. Describe normal wound healing and factors that affect it.
4. Discuss nursing assessment of skin integrity and wound healing.
5. List categories of support surfaces used to prevent pressure ulcers.
6. Discuss nursing interventions to promote skin integrity.
7. Explain scientific principles in the application of heat and cold to injured areas.
8. Describe categories of wound dressings and their indications.

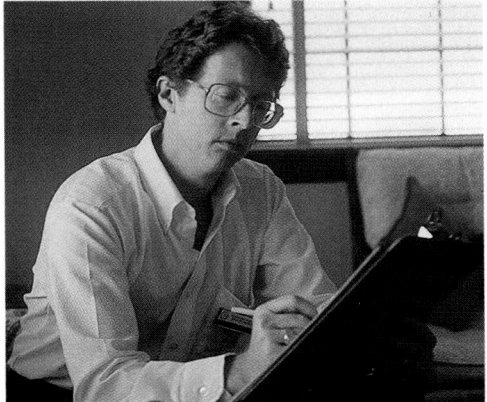

⑤ Critical Thinking Challenge

You are a home health nurse making visits twice a week to a client with a stage III pressure ulcer. The client is recovering from a stroke and receives daily visits from a physical therapist for mobility training. The client's wife is actively involved in his care. You are planning today's care.

The skin, which plays a major role in protecting the body from the environment, requires adequate blood flow, nutrient supply, and hygiene. If any of these factors are disrupted, a wound may develop. Once you have completed this chapter and have incorporated skin integrity and wound healing into your knowledge base, review the above scenario and reflect on the following areas of Critical Thinking:

1. Describe assessments you will make today and on subsequent visits.
2. Summarize factors that could affect the rate of wound healing in this client.
3. Outline teaching you will provide to help prevent further occurrence of pressure ulcers.
4. List the primary nursing diagnoses that will guide your care and related nursing diagnoses that might apply in this situation.
5. Explore how you would collaborate with the client, family, and other healthcare providers to promote effective wound healing.

S kin, also called integument, is the body's external covering. It is the body's largest organ, providing protective, sensory, and regulatory functions. Disruptions in skin integrity can interfere with these important functions.

A wound is a break in skin integrity. Acute wounds can occur when the skin is exposed to extremes in temperature or pH, caustic chemicals, excessive pressure, moisture, friction, trauma, or radiation. An incision is a type of acute wound created intentionally as part of surgical treatment. A chronic wound persists beyond the expected amount of time for usual wound closure. The body responds to an acute or chronic wound through a complex restorative process called wound healing.

Nurses play a significant role in preventing impaired skin integrity and promoting optimal healing when disruptions in the skin or underlying structures occur. They provide wound care and prevent pressure ulcers in clients at risk. Nurses also teach clients how to avoid accidental injury, maintain skin integrity, and promote optimal healing.

NORMAL INTEGUMENTARY FUNCTION

The body's ability to protect itself from the environment depends largely on the integrity of the integumentary system. The skin contributes to metabolic activities and is a key part of maintaining homeostasis. A review of the skin's structure and function provides a framework for understanding the importance of nursing care of skin and wounds.

Structure of the Skin

Skin Layers

The skin has two major tissue layers: epidermis and dermis (Fig. 38-1). The **epidermis,** the skin's outer layer, is avascular and relies on the dermis for its nutrition. The epidermis specializes to form the hair, nails, and glandular structures. The epidermis is composed of layers of stratified squamous epithelial cells. The thin, outermost layer of the epidermis (the stratum corneum or horny layer) is continuously shed in a process called **desquamation.** The major cell of the epidermis, the keratinocyte, produces keratin, the primary material in the shed layer of cells. Basal layers of the epidermis contain melanocytes, which produce melanin, the brown substance that colors the skin.

The **dermis,** which underlies the epidermis, is the thickest skin layer. It is composed of tough connective tissue and is well vascularized. The major cell of the dermis, the fibroblast, produces the proteins collagen and elastin. Lymphatic vessels and nerve tissues also are found in the dermis. This dermal matrix supports and nourishes the constantly changing epidermis.

Subcutaneous tissue underlies the skin. It consists primarily of fat and connective tissues that support the skin.

Skin Appendages

The skin appendages (hair, nails, eccrine sweat glands, apocrine sweat glands, and sebaceous glands) are formed by invagination of the epidermis into the underlying dermis. Hair consists of keratinous fibers; it grows on the entire skin surface except for the palms and soles. Nails are formed by rapidly dividing epidermal cells in the nailbed. Hair and nails have no nerve endings or blood supply. The eccrine and apocrine glands are sweat glands. Eccrine glands, which are widely distributed throughout the skin, help transport sweat to the outer skin surface. Apocrine sweat glands are found primarily in the axilla and the genital area. The apocrine duct empties into the hair follicle. Sweat produced by apocrine glands contributes to a characteristic body odor when bacteria decompose the secretions. Sebaceous glands secrete sebum, which lubricates the skin's outer layer. These glands are found in greatest concentration over the head and upper chest.

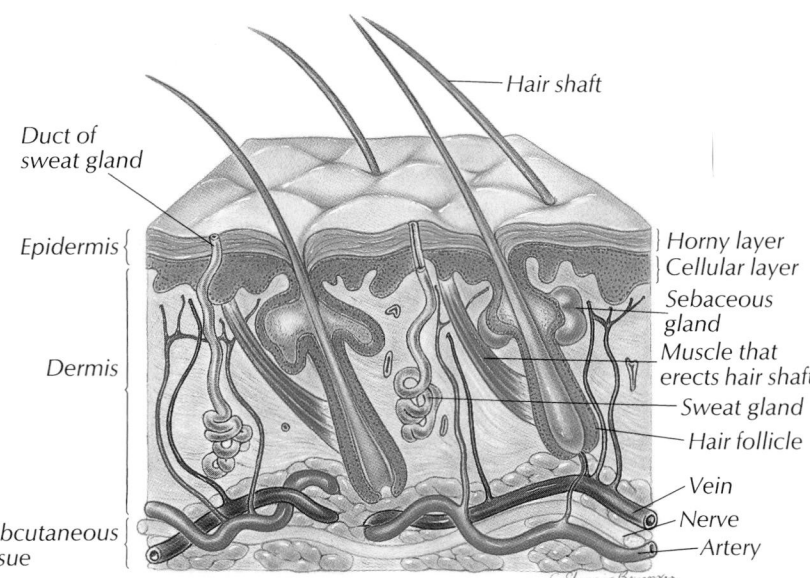

Duct of sweat gland

Hair shaft

Epidermis {

Horny layer
Cellular layer

Sebaceous gland

Dermis

Muscle that erects hair shaft

Sweat gland

Hair follicle

Vein

Nerve

Subcutaneous tissue {

Artery

FIGURE 38-1   Cross section of skin and underlying structures.

Function of the Skin

Protection

Intact skin protects the body from physical and chemical injury. Infection is less likely when intact skin provides a barrier to microorganisms. The cells that provide protection are the Langerhans cells and keratinocytes in the epidermis and the macrophages and mast cells beneath the epidermis' basal layer. Also, melanin protects against the sun's ultraviolet rays. Sebum, secreted by sebaceous glands, gives the skin an acidic pH, which retards the growth of microorganisms. Additionally, microorganisms that inhibit the growth of pathogens are present on the skin. These resident skin flora include *Staphylococcus, Streptococcus,* yeast, and others.

Thermoregulation

Through dilation and constriction of the blood vessels in the dermis, the skin helps to regulate body temperature and adjust to external temperature changes. Vasoconstriction produces shivering, which helps the body maintain its temperature in cool environments. Sweating cools the body through evaporation of fluid and dissipation of heat. Large volumes of fluid can be lost through profuse sweating during exercise or warm external temperatures. Loss of large areas of skin due to burns or other injury can significantly impair the body's ability to maintain temperature and retain fluid.

Sensation

The skin contains networks of nerves that are sensitive to pain, itch, vibration, heat, and cold. These nerve endings are contained within the dermis, and some extend into the epidermis. The fine hair on body surfaces also provides sensation because of the sensory nerves that surround the hair follicles.

Metabolism

From the sun's ultraviolet rays, the skin synthesizes vitamin D. Vitamin D is necessary for efficient absorption of calcium and phosphorus.

Communication

The skin provides a means of communication through facial expression and physical appearance. Facial skin and underlying muscles produce expressions, such as frowning, blinking, winking, and other nonverbal messages. The skin plays an important role in providing some aspects of body appearance and attractiveness. The skin, hair, and nails are often decorated and provide a basis for cultural sex differences.

Characteristics of Normal Skin

Color

Normal skin tones vary among races, depending on the production and accumulation of melanin. The greater the accumulation of melanin, the darker the skin tone. In races with darker skins, melanocytes produce more melanin when the skin is exposed to sunlight. Skin tones can range from tan to dark brown or black. The skin color of lighter-pigmented races also varies, ranging from ivory to pink. Areas of hyperpigmentation, such as freckles, normally occur in light-skinned people. Some races have yellow or olive undertones to their skin color. In all people, sun-exposed areas, such as the face or arms, can be darker.

Temperature

Skin is normally warm. However, peripheral areas, such as the feet or hands, may be cool if vasoconstriction in the skin has occurred.

Moisture

Normally, the skin is dry to the touch, but moisture can accumulate in skin folds. Moisture can be felt on the skin if the person is in a warm climate or has recently exercised. Anxiety can increase the moisture normally detected in the axillae or palms of the hands.

Texture and Thickness

The texture of unexposed skin usually is smooth. Areas exposed to friction (e.g., soles of the feet, palms of the hands) may become rough and hypertrophied. Sun exposure, aging, and smoking also make skin less smooth. Skin thickness varies depending on the body location. The skin on the soles of the feet may be 0.25 inch thick, but the skin covering the eyelids may be only 0.02 inch thick.

Normally, skin has good elasticity, rapidly returning to its normal shape when pinched between the thumb and forefinger. This quality is called skin turgor. As a person ages, skin turgor normally decreases. Another factor that decreases skin turgor is fluid loss caused by dehydration.

Odor

Skin is usually free from odor. A pungent aroma is normal with perspiration, especially in the axilla and groin.

Lifespan Considerations

Skin changes during the lifespan. The greatest variations occur in the very young and in older adults.

Newborn and Infant

The skin of newborns is thinner and more sensitive than that of older infants. Superficial blood vessels are so prominent that they give newborn skin a characteristic red color. Only the sebaceous glands are active during early infancy. Milia—sebaceous retention cysts seen as white, opalescent spots around the chin and nose—appear during the first few weeks of life and disappear spontaneously. Fine hair called lanugo covers the newborn's body. Lanugo is lost during the first weeks of life and is replaced by hair of a different color and texture. Infants characteristically have long, thin fingernails and toenails that often scratch their delicate skin.

Infant skin is susceptible to blistering, chafing, and rashes from friction or irritation. Exposure to a warm, humid environment can lead to prickly heat, and frequent bathing can cause dryness, leading to other skin problems. Exposure to cold environmental temperatures may produce hypothermia because infants have a decreased ability to thermoregulate. Contact dermatitis and bacterial infections can occur from exposure to soiled diapers.

Other common skin disorders of infancy are diaper rash and eczema. Parents and caregivers can prevent diaper rash by keeping infants clean and dry and by avoiding rubber pants or detergents to which babies are sensitive. Eczema may be an allergic response to foods, soaps, or other stimuli, so parents should introduce new foods one at a time into their babies' diets.

During the first year of life, the proportion of subcutaneous fat increases. Raw areas called intertrigo may develop in obese youngsters as skin rubs against skin. The proportion of subcutaneous fat decreases in the second year of life, and intertrigo is less common.

Toddler and Preschooler

After the first year of life, skin normally shows few changes until puberty. As motor skills develop, children are more prone to accidents, which may result in lacerations or abrasions. Many children spend extensive time outdoors, and sunscreen is necessary to protect against damage caused by ultraviolet rays.

Toddlers and preschoolers are susceptible to burns. Keeping hot liquids out of their reach and keeping children away from heaters, barbecue grills, stoves, and fires are necessary safety measures. Capping electrical outlets with protective covers helps prevent accidental electrical burns.

School-Age Child and Adolescent

Although the skin remains stable until adolescence, communicable illnesses, such as impetigo, scabies, and head lice commonly affect skin integrity and may necessitate absence from school. As children become older, they are more aware of their bodies and are concerned when rashes or scars affect their appearance. Therefore, identifying rashes and instituting measures to avoid spread of infectious diseases that impair skin integrity are important. Provide emotional support for parents and children when such conditions appear, so that the children are better able to cope with the stress and discomfort of skin disruptions.

During adolescence, pubic, axillary, and other body hair appears. The most common skin disorder of adolescence is acne vulgaris. As the sebaceous glands enlarge at puberty, production of sebum increases. Acne lesions result from plugging of pilosebaceous glands. Lesions form primarily on the face, neck, back, chest, and shoulders. Because adolescence is a time when physical appearance is important to self-concept, severe acne can be emotionally disturbing to an adolescent.

Adolescents engage in many leisure activities that involve sun exposure (e.g., swimming, outdoor sports, sunbathing). Because excessive sun exposure has been linked to skin cancer, teach teens to protect their skin by using effective sunscreen products.

Adult and Older Adult

Skin changes are part of normal aging. As skin ages, it generally becomes thinner because it loses dermal and subcutaneous mass. Because sebaceous and sweat glands are less active, dry skin is more common. Wrinkling and poor skin turgor result from loss of elastic fibers and collagen changes in the dermal connective tissue. Circulation to the skin is reduced, and healing is slower. The nails may become thicker and more brittle, and hair may lose pigment and turn gray. Pruritus (itching) commonly occurs in older adults and is caused mainly by dry, scaling skin.

The size and number of benign skin growths markedly increase in older adults. Skin tags, which are loose flaps of skin, occur mainly around the neck, eyelids, and axillae. Keratoses are horny, slow-growing proliferations of the keratinizing cells of the epidermis. They may itch and bleed if traumatized. Senile lentigines, also called age or liver spots, are pigmentation changes that occur on sun-exposed areas. Although many skin changes are benign, adults must self-examine their skin to enhance early detection of abnormalities such as melanoma, a type of skin cancer. These abnormalities frequently arise from preexisting moles (Jackson, 1998).

FACTORS AFFECTING INTEGUMENTARY FUNCTION

Circulation

Adequate blood flow to the skin is necessary for healthy, viable tissues. Adequate skin perfusion requires four factors:

- The heart must be able to pump adequately.
- The volume of circulating blood must be sufficient.
- Arteries and veins must be patent and functioning well.
- Local capillary pressure must be higher than external pressure.

Alterations in any of these factors can lead to skin that has abnormal color, texture, thickness, moisture, or temperature or that becomes ulcerated.

Leg Ulceration

Leg and foot ulcers occur from various causes, but the most common are venous disease, arterial disease, and diabetes mellitus. Impaired arterial or venous function in the lower extremities can produce ulcerations that are refractory to healing unless the underlying disorder is treated.

Stasis dermatitis results from impaired venous return secondary to venous disease or structural alterations in the legs. Pooling of blood leads to edema, vasodilatation, and plasma extravasation, all of which result in dermatitis by increasing the distance between the blood vessels and the skin they nourish (Pontiere-Lewis, 1995). A venous leg ulcer is illustrated in Figure 38-2.

Pressure Ulcers

Pressure ulcers, sometimes called decubitus ulcers or bedsores, result when capillary blood flow to the skin or underlying tissue is impeded. These ulcers primarily result from

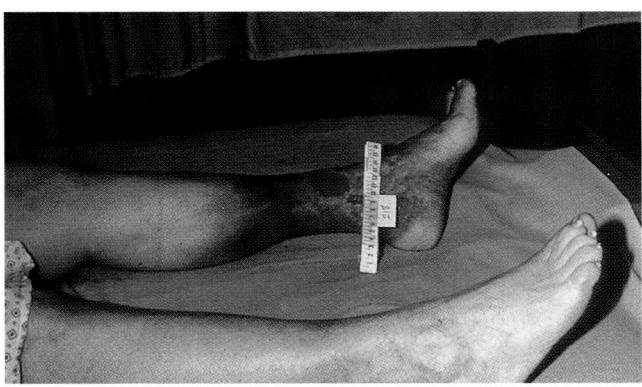

FIGURE 38-2   Stasis ulcer on lower leg.

unequal distribution of pressure over bony prominences. Because of decreased blood flow, the supply of nutrients and oxygen to the skin and underlying tissues is impaired. Cells die and decompose, and an ulcer forms.

Ulcers may be superficial, involving the epidermis and dermis, or deep, involving underlying tissue layers; they are classified according to their stage of development (Display 38-1). Ulcers may develop a dark black crust, called **eschar.** When eschar is present, accurate staging of the pressure ulcer is impossible until the wound has been débrided. Débridement is the removal of dead tissue from an area of injury.

Pressure ulcers most commonly develop over bony prominences, where body weight is distributed over a small area with inadequate padding (Fig. 38-3). Most pressure ulcers

DISPLAY 38-1

PRESSURE ULCER STAGING

Stage I
Nonblanchable erythema of the skin over a bony prominence or area of pressure. Most stage I ulcers are reversible if pressure is relieved. Assessment of stage I pressure ulcers may be difficult in dark-skinned individuals.

Stage III
Full-thickness skin loss involving damage or loss of subcutaneous tissue that may extend down to, but not through, underlying fascia. It manifests clinically as a deep crater with or without undermining of adjacent tissue. Stage III ulcers can require months to heal.

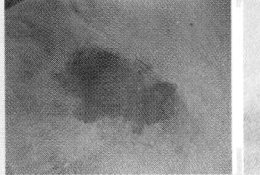 

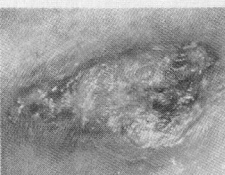 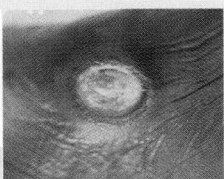

Stage II
Superficial ulcer that manifests as an abrasion, shallow crater, or blister. This partial-thickness skin loss involves the epidermis, dermis, or both. The ulcer is usually painful.

Stage IV
Full-thickness skin loss with extensive destruction, tissue necrosis, or damage to muscle, bone, or supporting structures (e.g., tendons, joint capsule); it may have undermining or sinus tracts.

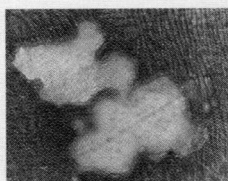 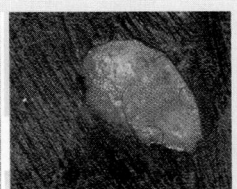

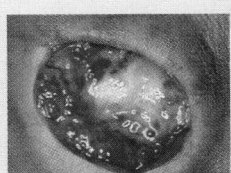 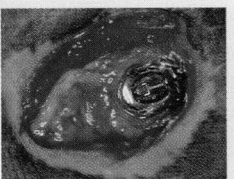

Photos from Calrenno, C. (2000). Assessing and preventing pressure ulcers. *Advances in Skin and Wound Care, 13*(5), 245.

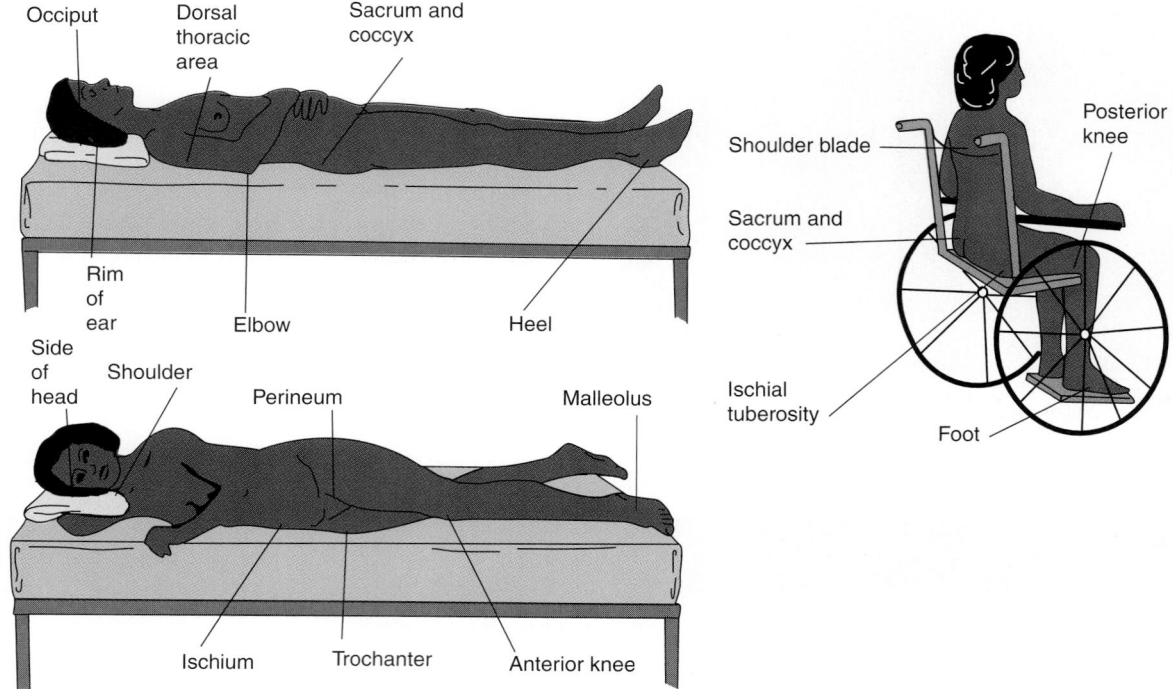

FIGURE 38-3   Common locations for pressure ulcers when supine and sitting.

develop in the pelvic area. When supine, the greatest points of pressure are the back of the skull, the elbows, the sacrum and coccyx, and the heels. When sitting, the greatest points of pressure are the ischial tuberosities and the sacrum.

Pressure ulcer formation commonly results from increased pressure and decreased tissue tolerance. Decreased mobility, decreased activity, and decreased sensory/perceptual ability increase the risk for pressure ulcers. Extrinsic factors that decrease tissue tolerance and increase the likelihood of pressure ulcer development are moisture, friction, and shearing force. Other contributing factors are malnutrition, age, and low arteriolar pressure. Often, the relationship among risk factors ultimately causes a pressure ulcer to develop.

Pressure. When pressure is unevenly distributed, it can exceed normal capillary pressure (32 mm Hg). The greater the pressure and the longer its duration, the more likely it is that a pressure ulcer will develop. Any rigid object (e.g., bed, chair) puts pressure on the skin. When the client is sitting or lying, gravity increases the pressure over bony prominences. Normally, a person unconsciously shifts his or her body weight to prevent the occlusion of capillaries due to increased pressure. Everyone has had the experience of numbness or prickly sensation in an area of the body to which blood flow was impeded due to pressure. However, people who cannot sense increased pressure (e.g., people with neuropathy) or who cannot independently reposition themselves because of reduced mobility or strength are at risk for the development of pressure ulcers.

Mental Status. Altered mental status can occur when clients are confused, comatose, or receiving medications that alter normal cognitive processes. Such clients may not reposition themselves as needed to prevent ulceration. Altered mental status also may contribute to incontinence and inadequate self-care, which can increase the potential for ulcer formation.

Moisture. Moisture can predispose skin to breakdown. Skin that is continually bathed in moisture softens, increasing its susceptibility to trauma and infection. Skin that is continually exposed to moisture becomes **macerated.** Macerated tissue is lighter in appearance than healthy tissue and is damaged more easily. Incontinence may cause clients to lie in urine or feces. Diaphoresis or inadequate drying after hygiene, especially in skin folds, can increase moisture and encourage the growth of yeast, leading to rashes.

Friction. Friction occurs when two surfaces rub together. When skin rubs against a firm surface, such as wrinkled bedding, small abrasions occur, increasing the possibility of ulcer formation. Adequate lubrication of the skin and care during handling, moving, and washing clients limit the negative effect of friction.

Shearing Force. Shearing force occurs when tissue layers move on each other, causing blood vessels to stretch as they pass through subcutaneous tissue (Fig. 38-4). Most commonly, this occurs when clients slide down in bed or are pulled up in bed. The client's skin remains relatively immobile because friction anchors it to the sheets, but deeper structures, such as fascia, move with the client, because they are attached to the bone. In the process, capillaries in the underlying tissue are stretched and often torn, increasing the risk of ulcer formation.

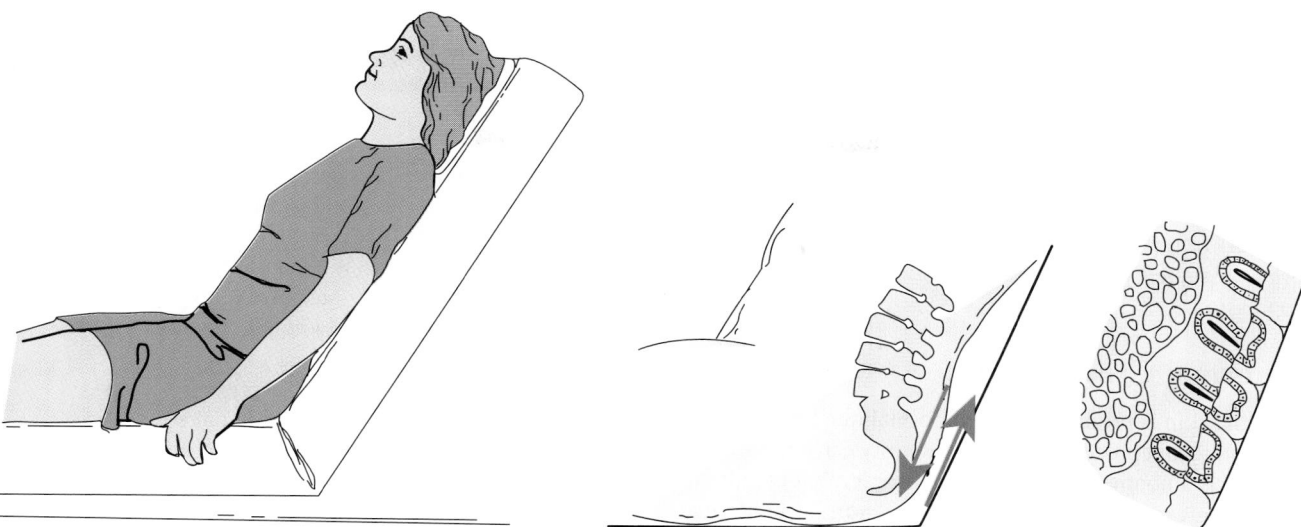

FIGURE 38-4 Shearing force contributes to pressure ulcer development when opposing forces cause capillaries to stretch and tear as the client slides down in bed.

SAFETY ALERT
Move and reposition immobile clients carefully to prevent injury to the skin as a result of shearing force.

Nutrition and Metabolism. Impaired nutritional status increases the risk of pressure ulcer development. In clients who are nutritionally depleted, capillaries become more fragile, and, as they break, blood flow to the skin can be impaired. Clients who are malnourished may have weight loss, decreased serum proteins, and reduced immune function. Loss of subcutaneous tissue and muscle mass affects the amount of protective padding between skin and bone and increases the risk of pressure ulcers.

Nutrition

A well-balanced diet promotes healthy skin. With a deficiency of protein or calories, hair becomes dull and dry and may fall out. Skin also becomes dry and flaky. Adequate intake of vitamins A, B6, C, K, niacin, and riboflavin is important to prevent abnormal skin changes. Adequate intake of iron, copper, and zinc is important to prevent abnormal pigmentation and changes in nails and hair.

Lifestyle and Habits

Hygiene practices vary widely among people and cultures. Lack of cleanliness can hinder skin health, because washing removes debris, bacteria, and sweat from the skin and keeps pores open and unclogged. Repeated exposure to ultraviolet radiation in the form of sunlight or artificial tanning lights produces characteristic changes, including wrinkling, altered texture, and laxity of the skin.

Condition of the Epidermis

To maintain its protective function against invading microorganisms, the epidermis must be free from any breaks. Maintenance of the skin's natural moisture is necessary because abnormal drying can cause microscopic cracks.

Allergy

Allergic reactions and skin inflammation are responses to injury mediated by histamine release. External or internal irritants can cause the reactions. The irritants may be chemical (e.g., skin creams, latex gloves, detergents, plants such as poison ivy or poison oak) or mechanical (e.g., rubbing against an irritant, such as wool). Foods and medications also may cause skin reactions. Dermatitis, an inflammation of the skin, most often produces epidermal and dermal damage or irritation possibly accompanied by pain, itching, redness, and blisters. Chronic dermatitis produces changes in the epidermis, including thickening, scaling, and increased pigmentation. Treatment focuses on eliminating exposure to the allergen and may include lubrication of the skin and application of topical medications (Denig et al., 1998).

Infections

Bacterial, viral, or fungal infections can affect skin integrity. Streptococcal and staphylococcal organisms are responsible for most bacterial skin infections. Impetigo, which usually is caused by beta-hemolytic streptococci, is the most common bacterial skin infection. Cutaneous warts caused by the papillomavirus are one of the most common diseases of the skin, with hands and feet most typically affected. Herpesvirus infection is another common viral cause of skin disruption. Common locations are the lips, face, mouth, and genitals.

Many communicable childhood illnesses of viral origin cause rashes. Pruritus usually accompanies these rashes and may lead to secondary infection.

Fungal infections can infect nonhairy skin (tinea corporis), scalp (tinea capitis), the genital region (tinea cruris or "jock itch"), nails (tinea unguium), and, most commonly, the feet (tinea pedis or "athlete's foot"). Candidal (formerly called monilial) fungal infections often occur when normal body flora is disrupted secondary to antibiotic therapy or immunosuppression.

Abnormal Growth Rate

When the skin is produced at an abnormal rate by malignant or nonmalignant processes, normal integrity can be disrupted. Psoriasis is a nonmalignant, chronic disorder that greatly increases the rate of skin production: the normal epidermal turnover rate of 14 to 20 days accelerates to 3 to 4 days. Certain forms of psoriasis characteristically occur in children and young adults. The elbows, knees, scalp, and soles of the feet are common sites for psoriasis. Periods of remission are followed by exacerbations, which can be triggered by stress, infection, or environmental factors.

Benign or malignant neoplasms also can affect skin integrity. Most benign neoplasms result from viral infections or normal aging. Most malignant lesions result from prolonged exposure to ultraviolet radiation.

Systemic Diseases

Many chronic diseases can produce skin abnormalities and ulceration. Inflammatory bowel disease, pemphigus, and peripheral vascular disease are examples of diseases that, during exacerbations, can produce impaired skin integrity. The skin problem is most appropriately addressed in these cases by treating and controlling the underlying disorder.

Trauma

Any trauma to the skin, such as a wound, creates a risk for altered skin function. Wounds can be divided into broad categories of accidental and surgical (Table 38-1).

Accidental Wounds

Common wounds include abrasions, lacerations, and puncture wounds. An **abrasion** results when skin rubs against a hard surface. Friction scrapes away the epithelial layer, exposing the epidermal or dermal layer. Falls onto hands, elbows, or knees cause most abrasions. A **laceration** is an open wound or cut. Most lacerations affect only the upper layers of skin and subcutaneous tissue underneath. Permanent damage may result, however, if injury occurs to internal structures such as muscles, tendons, blood vessels, or nerves. Accidents involving automobiles, machinery, or knives may result in lacerations. A puncture wound is made when a sharp, pointed object penetrates tissue. Damage to underlying structures or gross contamination with debris and pathogens may result. Nails, pins, tacks, and other sharp objects are common causes.

TABLE 38-1

Types of Wounds

Wound	Description
Broad Categories	
Acute	Injury, such as knife, gunshot, burn, or surgical incision
Chronic	Wound that persists beyond usual healing time or recurs without new injury to the area
Open	Break is present in the skin; tissue damage is present
Closed	No break is seen in the skin, but soft tissue damage is evident
Descriptors	
Abrasion	Wound involving friction of skin; superficial; dermatologic procedure for scar-tissue removal
Puncture	Intentional or unintentional penetrating trauma by sharp instrument that penetrates skin and underlying tissue
Laceration	Ragged wound edges with torn tissues; object possibly contaminated; infection risk
Contusion	Closed wound; bleeding in underlying tissues from blunt blow; bruising
Classifications of Surgical Wounds	
Clean	Closed surgical wound that did not enter gastrointestinal, respiratory, or genitourinary systems; low infection risk
Clean/contaminated	Wound entering gastrointestinal, respiratory, or genitourinary systems; infection risk
Contaminated	Open, traumatic wound, surgical wound with break in asepsis; high infection risk
Infected	Wound site with pathogens present; signs of infection

Surgical Wounds

Surgical wounds vary from simple and superficial (e.g., a thyroidectomy incision) to deep and contaminated (e.g., an abdominal incision done for septic peritonitis). They may be divided into several categories (see Table 38-1). The wound's severity influences healing time, degree of pain, probability of complications, and presence of any tubes, drains, or suction devices.

Ostomies are surgical openings in the abdominal wall that allow part of an organ to open onto the skin. Medical conditions, such as cancer of the intestine or urinary bladder or inflammatory bowel disease, may require an ostomy. Because the skin surrounding the opening (stoma) may be continuously exposed to feces, urine, or intestinal secretions, skin irritation may develop if appropriately fitted ostomy pouches and products are not used.

Excessive Exposure

Exposure to excessive heat, electricity, caustic chemicals, or radiation results in tissue damage and burns. Burns range from minor injuries, such as simple sunburn, to major insults that cause significant life disruptions. The degree of damage depends on the type of burn, its extent and depth, and the client's preburn state of health.

Partial-thickness burns may be superficial or moderate to deep. A superficial partial-thickness burn (first degree; epidermal) is pinkish or red with no blistering; a mild sunburn is a good example. Moderate to deep partial-thickness burns (second degree; dermal or deep dermal) may be pink, red, pale ivory, or light yellow-brown. They are usually moist with blisters. Exposure to steam can cause this type of burn.

A full-thickness burn (third degree) may vary from brown or black to cherry red or pearly white. Thrombosed vessels and blisters or bullae may be present. The full-thickness burn appears dry and leathery. Sometimes, when fascia, muscle, or bone is extensively damaged, the injury is called a fourth-degree burn.

Thermal burns, the most common type, are caused by contact with various heat sources, including flames, hot liquids, hot surfaces, and steam. Chemical burns are caused by contact with noxious substances. The amount of tissue damaged as a result of chemical injury depends on the concentration of the chemical and the length of exposure. The severity of an electrical burn depends on the current's type and voltage, the pathway the current takes through the body, and the duration of contact. Radiation burns can occur when a person is accidentally exposed to radiation or when radiation is used as a form of therapy.

ALTERED INTEGUMENTARY FUNCTION
Manifestations of Altered Integumentary Function

Disruption in normal skin integrity can manifest as pain, pruritus, rashes, lesions, or open wounds; usually more than one symptom is present. Any break in the skin's epidermal layer signifies that skin integrity is altered. Usually, the disruption to the epidermis is evident. However, the break may be smaller and less obvious. For example, microscopic breaks in the skin may manifest as redness due to inflammation.

Pain
When the nerves within the skin are stimulated, the person may feel pain. Alterations to normal skin integrity can increase the quantity of impulses propagated along these nerves. Destruction of the epidermis and dermis creates highly sensitive, sharp, intense pain, but it is not uncommon for clients to report less pain over time or with pressure ulcers that involve deeper tissues.

Pruritus
Pruritus, or itching, is a common symptom associated with many skin and systemic problems. The majority of diseases that cause itching are inflammatory or allergic. Pruritus is often the cause of secondary lesions, because scratching breaks the skin surface.

Rash
Many conditions, such as excessive heat, communicable disease, allergy, or emotional distress, can cause a *rash,* a general term for a temporary skin eruption. A rash is described according to its characteristics and distribution on the body's surface. A macular rash is level with the skin surface; a papular rash involves solid elevations above the skin surface. A generalized rash covers most body areas, whereas a localized rash is limited to specific areas. Pruritus may accompany a rash.

Lesions
A lesion involves the loss of structure or function of normal tissue. Lesions vary in size from a fraction of a millimeter to many centimeters in diameter. Lesions also are described by their characteristics and distribution (Table 38-2).

A wheal, which normally results from insect bites or allergic reactions, is an elevated, irregularly shaped area of cutaneous edema. Urticaria, more commonly called hives, is a linear wheal that forms in response to capillary dilatation and passive transudation of plasma. Vesicles, bullae, and pustules are superficial skin elevations formed by fluid. A vesicle is less than 1 cm in diameter and is filled with serous fluid. A bulla is a vesicle larger than 1 cm in diameter. A pustule is filled with pus rather than serous fluid.

Lesions also can be classified by shape, arrangement, and distribution. Primary lesions arise in previously normal skin, and secondary lesions develop from primary lesions. Examples of secondary lesions include scales, crusts, and fissures. In the acute form of dermatitis, vesicles develop, burst, and ooze, and crusts form.

Wound Healing

When a wound is present, a type of healing by replacement occurs. The nature of this healing process is similar for wounds of similar depth, but the time frame for healing depends on (*text continues on page 994*)

TABLE 38-2

Basic Types of Skin Lesions With Examples

Primary Lesions (May Arise From Previously Normal Skin)

Circumscribed, Flat, Nonpalpable Changes in Skin Color

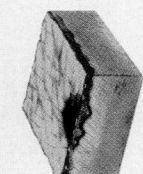

Macule—Small spot.
Examples: freckle, petechia

Patch—Larger than macule.
Example: vitiligo

Palpable Elevated Solid Masses

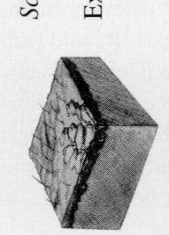

Papule—Up to 0.5 cm.
Example: an elevated nevus

Plaque—A flat, elevated surface larger than 0.5 cm, often formed by the coalescence of papules

Nodule—Larger than 0.5 cm; often deeper and firmer than a papule

Tumor—A large nodule

Wheal—A somewhat irregular, relatively transient, superficial area of localized skin edema.
Examples: mosquito bite, hive

Circumscribed Superficial Elevations of the Skin Formed by Free Fluid in a Cavity Within the Skin Layers

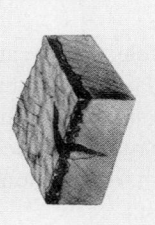

Vesicle—Up to 0.5 cm; filled with serous fluid.
Example: herpes simplex

Bulla—Greater than 0.5 cm; filled with serous fluid.
Example: second-degree burn

Pustule—Filled with pus.
Examples: acne, impetigo

Secondary Lesions (Result From Changes in Primary Lesions)

Loss of Skin Surface

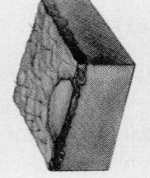

Erosion—Loss of the superficial epidermis; surface is moist but does not bleed.
Example: moist area after the rupture of a vesicle, as in chickenpox

Ulcer—A deeper loss of skin surface; may bleed and scar.
Examples: stasis ulcer of venous insufficiency, syphilitic chancre

Fissure—A linear crack in the skin.
Example: athlete's foot

Material on Skin Surface

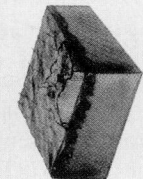

Crust—The dried residue of serum, pus, or blood.
Example: impetigo

Scale—A thin flake of exfoliated epidermis.
Examples: dandruff, dry skin, psoriasis

Miscellaneous Lesions

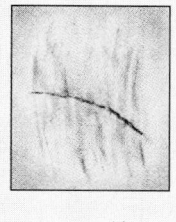

Lichenification—Thickening and roughening of the skin with increased visibility of the normal skin furrows. Example: atopic dermatitis

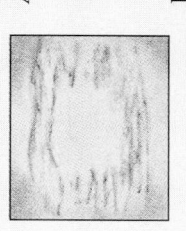

Scar—Replacement of destroyed tissue by fibrous tissue. May be thick and pink (hypertrophic) or thin and white (atrophic), but does not extend beyond the injured area

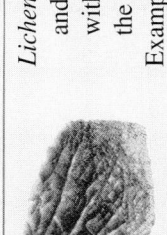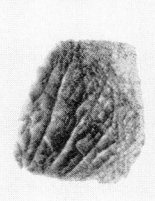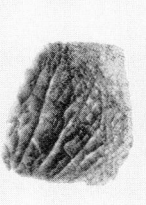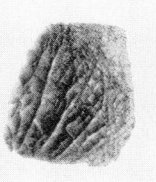

Atrophy—Thinning of the skin with loss of the normal skin furrows; the skin looks shinier and more translucent than normal. Example: arterial insufficiency

Excoriation—Abrasion or scratch mark. It may be linear, as illustrated, or rounded, as in a scratched insect bite.

Burrow of Scabies—A person with scabies has intense itching. Skin lesions include small papules, pustules, lichenified areas, and excoriations. With a magnifying lens, look for the *burrow* of the mite that causes it. A burrow is a minute, slightly raised tunnel in the epidermis that is commonly found on the finger webs and on the sides of the fingers. It looks like a short (5–15 mm), linear or curved, gray line and may end in a tiny vesicle.

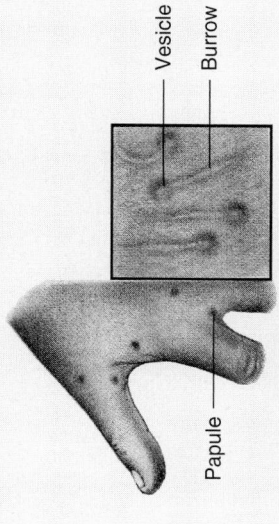

Vesicle

Burrow

Papule

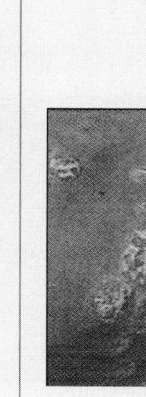

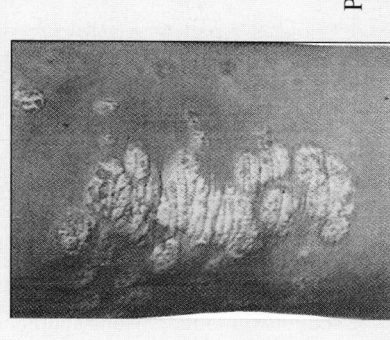

Plaques with scales on the front of a knee (in psoriasis)

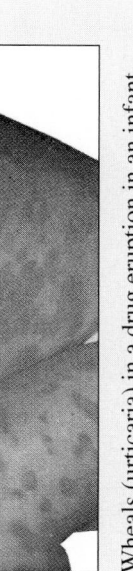

Wheals (urticaria) in a drug eruption in an infant

Color photographs from Sauer, G. C. (1996). *Manual of skin diseases* (6th ed). Philadelphia: Lippincott-Raven.

the wound's location and extent, the regenerative capacity of the injured cells, and the client's overall health.

Phases of Wound Healing

Wounded skin is repaired by regeneration or connective tissue repair. Many cells are involved in wound healing, a number of which produce and release chemical messengers called growth factors. Growth factors play an important role in the healing process and are being studied for possible use in optimizing wound repair (Martin, 1997).

The first phase of healing in partial and full-thickness wounds is *inflammation.* Injury to tissue prompts the responses of hemostasis, edema, and attraction of leukocytes to the wound bed. The inflammation phase lasts approximately 3 days.

Regeneration follows the inflammatory phase in the healing of partial-thickness wounds. Epidermal cells reproduce and migrate across the surface of the partial-thickness wound. This process is called **re-epithelialization.** When epithelial cells have covered the base of the wound, cells continue to replicate, increasing the number of cellular layers in the epidermis to assimilate the thickness of healthy epidermis.

In full-thickness wound healing, *proliferation* occurs after inflammation. Granulation tissue, consisting of a matrix of collagen embedded with macrophages, fibroblasts, and capillary buds, is produced and fills the wound with connective tissue. Open wounds (other than those primarily closed) undergo contracture during this phase of healing. Contracture can be identified by its effect of pulling the wound inward, leading to a decrease in depth and dimension of the wound. The proliferative phase lasts from day 4 after injury to about day 21 in a normally healing full-thickness wound.

Maturation is the final stage of full-thickness wound healing. It begins about 3 weeks after the injury and may last up to 2 years. The number of fibroblasts decreases, collagen synthesis stabilizes, and collagen fibrils become increasingly organized, resulting in greater tensile strength of the wound. The tissue usually reaches maximum strength in 10 to 12 weeks, but even after complete healing only 70% to 80% of the original strength can be expected.

Types of Wound Healing

Wounds heal differently depending on whether tissue loss has occurred. The major types of wound healing are classified as primary, secondary, and tertiary intention (Fig. 38-5).

Primary Intention. Wounds with minimal tissue loss, such as clean surgical incisions or shallow sutured wounds, heal by

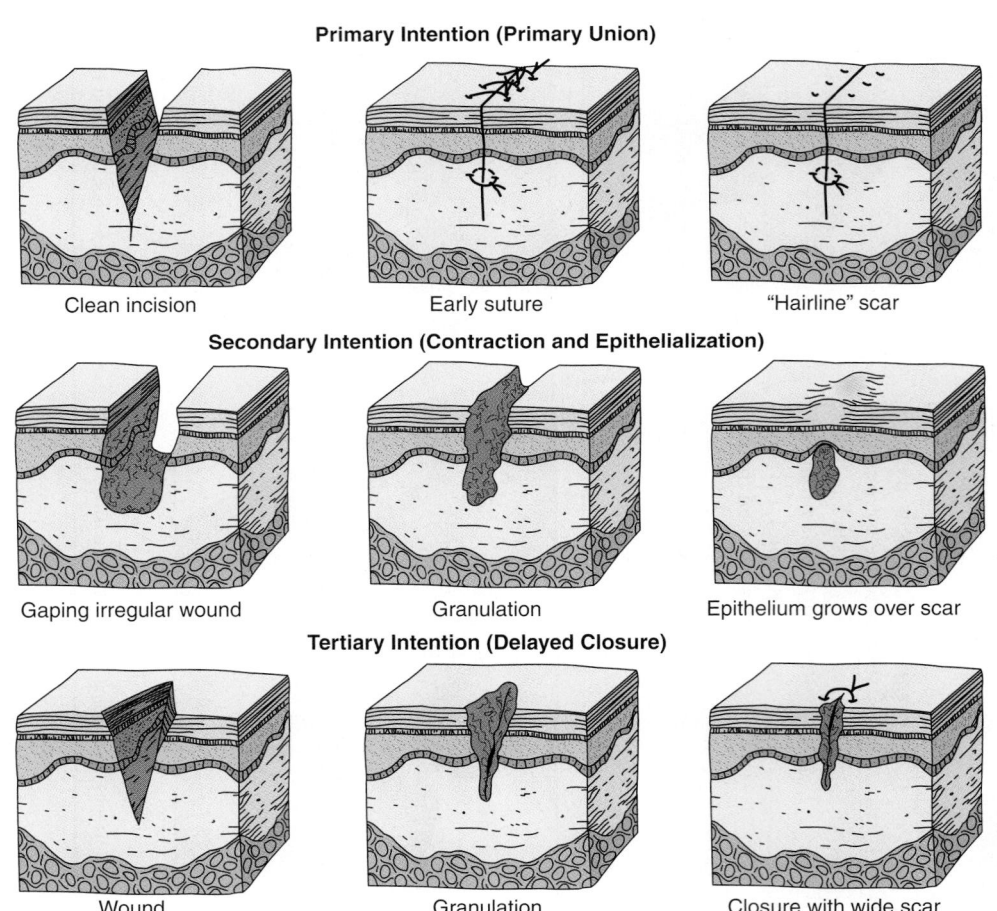

Primary Intention (Primary Union)

Clean incision   Early suture   "Hairline" scar

Secondary Intention (Contraction and Epithelialization)

Gaping irregular wound   Granulation   Epithelium grows over scar

Tertiary Intention (Delayed Closure)

Wound   Granulation   Closure with wide scar

FIGURE 38-5   Wound healing by primary, secondary, and tertiary methods.

primary intention. The edges of the primary wound are **approximated** or lightly pulled together. Granulation tissue is not visible, and scarring is usually minimal. Infection risk is lower when a clean, surgical wound heals by primary intention.

Secondary Intention. Wounds with full-thickness tissue loss, such as deep lacerations, burns, and pressure ulcers, have edges that do not readily approximate. They heal by secondary intention. The open wound gradually fills with soft, pinkish-red buds that bleed easily (**granulation tissue**). Eventually, epithelial cells grow over these granulations, completing the cycle. Scarring is more prevalent. Because the wound is open for a longer time, it becomes colonized with microorganisms that may lead to infection.

Tertiary Intention. Healing by tertiary intention occurs when a delay ensues between injury and wound closure. This type of healing also is referred to as delayed primary closure. It may happen when a deep wound is not sutured immediately or is purposely left open until there is no sign of infection and then closed with sutures. When a wound heals by secondary or tertiary intention, a deeper and wider scar is common.

Factors Affecting Wound Healing

Many variables can enhance or delay wound healing. Systemic factors include nutrition, circulation, oxygenation, and immune cellular function. Individual factors include age, obesity, smoking history, and drug therapy. Local factors include the nature and location of the injury, the presence of infection, and the type of wound dressing used.

Systemic Factors

Nutrition. Sound nutrition is essential for optimal wound healing. Nutritional deficiencies can retard wound healing by inhibiting collagen synthesis and epithelialization and by reducing the activity of cells that are important to the healing process. Nutritional requirements increase with physiologic stress, which may contribute to protein deficiencies. Clients with sepsis or burns and those undergoing surgery (especially major abdominal surgery) are susceptible to protein deficiency. Clients with protein deficiencies are most likely to develop wound infections because they have decreased leukocyte functions (e.g., phagocytosis, immunogenesis).

Vitamins A, C, and E, protein, arginine, zinc, and water are especially important in wound healing (Scholl & Langkamp-Henken, 2001). Carbohydrates, glucose, and fats also play key roles. Fats are essential because they are the building blocks for the cell membranes being formed. Many vitamins and minerals are important in wound healing, including the following:

- Vitamin A promotes epithelialization and enhances collagen synthesis and cross-linking.
- Vitamin B complex is a cofactor of enzyme systems.
- Vitamin C (ascorbic acid) is essential for collagen synthesis; with decreased amounts of vitamin C, the tensile strength of the wound decreases. Ascorbic acid also enhances capillary formation and decreases capillary fragility. It provides a defense to infection by playing a role in the immune response.
- Vitamin K is essential in the synthesis of prothrombin, which is important in coagulation.
- Minerals such as iron, zinc, and copper are involved in collagen synthesis.

Circulation and Oxygenation. Circulation to the involved wound and oxygenation of the tissues greatly influence wound healing. Wound healing slows whenever local blood flow is reduced, which is why venous stasis ulcers and pressure ulcers are so difficult to heal. Decreased arterial oxygen tension alters both collagen synthesis and formation of epithelial cells (Stotts & Wipke-Tevis, 1997). When hemoglobin levels are reduced by more than 15%, such as in severe anemia, oxygenation is reduced, and tissue repair is altered. Anemia may combine with preexisting states, such as diabetes or arteriosclerosis, to impair blood flow further and retard wound healing. Elevated blood glucose found in patients with uncontrolled diabetes has been associated with delayed wound closure and increased susceptibility to infection.

Immune Cellular Function. Drugs and therapies can affect immune cellular function and, subsequently, wound healing. Immunosuppressive drugs, such as corticosteroids, which may be given to prevent rejection of a transplanted organ, also depress the natural defenses against infection and mask the inflammatory response. Immunosuppressive agents also usually suppress protein synthesis, wound contraction, and epithelialization.

Clients with cancer are at risk for delayed wound healing and infection. Some clients have deficient or defective circulating antibodies. Chemotherapy and radiation treatments retard wound repair. Chemotherapeutic agents, such as 5-fluorouracil, inhibit fibroblast replication and collagen synthesis, whereas vincristine suppresses antibody production. Radiation therapy negatively affects fibroblastic activity.

Individual Factors

Age. Changes that are part of the normal aging process can hinder wound healing. Circulation slows slightly, compromising oxygen delivery to the wound. Changes occur in the clotting process, and the inflammatory response and phagocytosis are impaired, increasing the risk of infection. Fibroblastic activity and collagen synthesis decrease with age, so cell growth, differentiation, and reconstruction are slower.

Obesity. Wound healing may be retarded in obese clients. Because adipose tissue is relatively avascular, it provides only a weak defense against microbial invasion and impairs delivery of nutrients to the wound. Obese clients are at increased risk for complications and are often advised to lose weight before elective surgery. In general, surgery on an obese person takes longer, and suturing of adipose tissue can be difficult. The potential for wound dehiscence and infection also is greater in obese clients.

Smoking. Physiologic changes that hinder wound healing occur in smokers. Functional hemoglobin levels decrease, vasoconstriction occurs, and tissue oxygenation is impaired. Long-time smokers have an increased number of platelets, which are also more adhesive. This hypercoagulability leads to the formation of thrombi, which may block small vessels. *Medications.* Many drugs, in addition to those that directly affect the immune response, affect wound healing. Anticoagulants, given to decrease potential thrombus formation, increase the potential for bleeding into the wound. Even over-the-counter drugs, such as aspirin and nonsteroidal anti-inflammatory drugs, decrease platelet aggregation and prolong bleeding time. Antibiotics may be prescribed preoperatively for certain surgeries that carry a high risk for postoperative infection. The use of anti-inflammatory medications such as prednisone can contribute to delayed wound closure and increased risk for skin injury.

Stress. Physical and emotional stress triggers the release of catecholamines, causing vasoconstriction and ultimately decreasing blood flow to the wound. Trauma, pain, and acute or chronic illness can cause stress.

Local Factors

Nature of the Injury. Usually, a surgical incision made with strict aseptic technique heals faster than, for instance, a deep wound embedded with debris from a traumatic accident. The deeper the wound and the more extensive the tissue loss, the longer the wound will take to heal. Even the wound's shape has an effect: the greater the irregularity, the more prolonged the wound healing process. If trauma has caused hematomas (blood clots) to form, this also can impede healing.

Presence of Infection. Although most open wounds quickly become colonized with diverse microbial flora, healing usually progresses. When sufficient quantities of pathogens are present to produce clinical infection, wound healing is delayed. This is especially true with pressure and leg ulcers. Aerobic bacteria commonly found in pressure and leg ulcers include *Staphylococcus aureus, Pseudomonas aeruginosa,* and *Proteus mirabilis* (Colsky, Kirsner & Kerdel, 1998). Inadequate handwashing and poor dressing-change techniques may introduce infection. Infection may also result from surgery, especially if a contaminated area, such as the gastrointestinal or genitourinary tract, is the operative site. Infection is more likely to occur in wounds that contain foreign particles or necrotic tissue.

Local Wound Environment. Many factors in the local wound environment affect healing. The pH, which should be between 7.0 and 7.6, can be altered by drainage, which may need to be contained or siphoned away for proper healing.

Bacterial growth must be controlled, because infection slows the healing process. The elimination of all microorganisms is neither required nor desirable, because normal flora help to regulate some events that occur in wound healing. Although excess debris and drainage can slow the healing process, a moist surface is essential to the activity of the cells (platelets, leukocytes, fibroblasts, and epithelial cells) that work to heal the wound.

Tension or stress on the wound is a factor in healing. Any activity that puts tension on the wound during healing can cause stress. Vomiting, coughing without splinting, and abdominal distention can place tension on an abdominal incision, potentially interfering with wound healing.

Complications of Wound Healing

Hemorrhage and Interstitial Fluid Loss. After the initial trauma, bleeding is expected, but within several minutes hemostasis occurs as part of the first phase of wound healing. If large blood vessels are severed or the client has poor clotting ability, however, bleeding may continue. Hemorrhage can occur later in the postoperative period if a suture slips, a clot dislodges, erosion through a blood vessel occurs, or abnormal stress or trauma is applied to the wounded area.

Hemorrhage may occur internally or externally. External bleeding is obvious: bloody drainage, more than normally expected, is visible from the wound. Internal bleeding is less observable and may be indicated by swelling of the affected area, an abnormal amount of bloody drainage from a catheter or drain, an increase in pain, or abnormal vital signs.

Electrolyte-rich fluids may be lost in significant amounts in certain types of wounds, such as burns and other large open wounds. Clients with large draining wounds or loss of a large amount of skin require careful monitoring of fluid balance with appropriate fluid replacement as indicated.

Hematomas. A **hematoma** is a localized collection of blood. It appears as a swelling or mass underneath the skin surface, often with a bluish color. Small hematomas are readily absorbed into the systemic circulation as debris from the wound. Larger hematomas may take weeks to reabsorb, creating dead space and dead cells that inhibit healing. Large hematomas may require evacuation or surgical removal to promote optimal wound healing.

Infection. A break in skin integrity, whether caused by a surgical incision or by trauma, gives microorganisms a portal for entry into the body. Bacterial contamination of a wound can result in infection if the client's defenses are inadequate. The incidence of wound infection depends on the following:

- Local factors: Contamination, degree of closure, presence of foreign bodies
- Treatment factors: Surgical technique, environmental conditions
- Host factors: Client's age, nutritional status, chronic health problems
- Virulence of the organism

Symptoms of an infected wound are purulent drainage, an inflamed incisional area, fever, and an elevated leukocyte count. Wound infections greatly increase the cost of medical care and can substantially lengthen recovery time.

Dehiscence. **Dehiscence** is a total or partial disruption in wound edges (Fig. 38-6). Wound separation, synonymous with dehiscence, is most commonly used to describe surgical incisions in which the skin has separated but underlying subcutaneous tissue has not parted. As wound edges separate, an increase in drainage usually occurs. Dehiscence most commonly occurs before collagen formation is complete in high-risk clients (3 to 14 days after injury). Obesity, poor

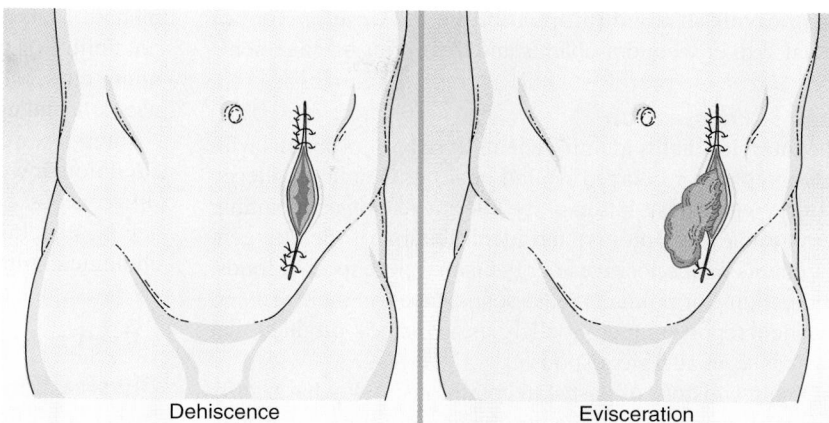

FIGURE 38-6 *Dehiscence* is the disruption of wound edges. *Evisceration* is the protrusion of viscera through that wound opening.

nutritional status, and increased stress on the incisional area increase the risk of dehiscence. Clients often report feeling that their incision has "given way" after activities, such as coughing or vomiting, that increase the pressure on the incision. Dehiscence also may occur if sutures or staples are removed before the wound is healed adequately.

SAFETY ALERT
Monitor postoperative wounds carefully and prevent undue stress to the wound by supporting the wound during coughing or vomiting.

Evisceration. **Evisceration** is the protrusion of viscera through an abdominal wound opening (see Fig. 38-6). Evisceration can follow dehiscence if the opening extends deeply enough to allow the abdominal fascia to separate and internal organs to protrude.

Fistula. A **fistula** is an abnormal tubelike passageway that forms between two organs or from one organ to outside the body. Fistula tracts can be the result of poor wound healing after tissue injury from surgery. Fistulas also may result from illness, such as inflammatory bowel disease. The name of the fistula designates the site of the abnormal communication. For example, a rectovaginal fistula is an abnormal opening between the rectum and the vagina that permits feces to enter the vagina.

Protection of surrounding skin is essential if the fistula output is caustic. Pouches, drainage tubes, and moist dressings may be used to manage output until the fistula is closed (Beitz & Caldwell, 1998). Fistulas may be managed conservatively with good nutrition and bowel rest, or they may require surgical closure.

Impact on Activities of Daily Living

Altered skin integrity can change a client's ability to perform activities of daily living (ADLs). Some skin conditions restrict clients to home because of treatment demands, discomfort, or limitations on their ability to return to work with open lesions or wounds.

Systemic responses to skin alterations, such as fever and malaise, may lower a client's activity tolerance. Nutritional needs are higher during healing, and clients may feel unable to prepare the meals necessary to provide adequate calories and nutrients. Clients who have activity restrictions due to wound and skin problems may be unable to spend time on their feet to cook, groom, and perform other ADLs. This may lead to social isolation, altering the client's ability and motivation to perform ADLs.

Adults with impaired skin integrity can often manage their own care if they receive adequate information. Clients with coexisting diseases or disabilities and those with wounds requiring complex management plans often require assistance from a healthcare professional or trained family member. Clients with wounds in difficult-to-reach areas require help with the use of topical products, such as ointments or dressings. A client with limited hip mobility and lower-extremity ulcers, for example, might require assistance to secure a dressing and apply a compression stocking to the leg.

Wound management can be a financial burden if medical insurance does not cover supplies, equipment, or healthcare visits. Obtaining special equipment and supplies usually becomes the family's responsibility if the client's mobility level prevents him or her from leaving home. Many clients rely on family members for transportation to medical follow-up appointments, which may affect the family's schedule and occupational demands.

Family members may be asked to learn how to provide wound care. Their ability and willingness to provide this care depends on cultural factors, prior relationships with the client, and personal health.

ASSESSMENT

Subjective Data

Interviewing the client allows the nurse to gather data about the client's normal skin status, history of skin problems, and presence of risk factors that can increase the potential for altered skin integrity or affect wound healing. Subjective data also provide detailed information on the development of actual skin or wound problems and their prior management.

Risk Identification

The interview helps identify clients at risk for problems with skin integrity or delayed wound healing. Obtain an allergy history, with a description of the allergic response (including dermatologic symptoms) and identification of the allergen. For clients with a positive allergy history, note specific foods, medications, or products (e.g., soaps, tape) on their records. If a client reports numerous allergies, avoid new products that may cause an allergic response.

Obtain a history of past skin conditions. Ask what factors triggered the problem, whether the condition was seasonal, and how the client handled the problem (e.g., prescribed medications, home remedies, over-the-counter preparations). When indicated, question the client about a family history of skin problems, because some dermatologic problems (e.g., eczema, psoriasis) commonly run in families.

Document any recent exposure to factors that can cause skin trauma, rash, or lesions. Note any contact with family members or others with infectious illnesses (e.g., measles, chickenpox, scabies, lice). Travel to foreign countries or activities such as hiking or camping can expose the client to parasites, insect bites, or poisonous plants. Exposure to caustic chemicals, excessive heat, or radiation also may be important in identifying the risk for skin alterations.

Before any surgery, assess for any possible factors that may delay wound healing, such as malnutrition, impaired circulation, immunosuppression, obesity, smoking, diabetes mellitus, or infection.

Determine the risk for pressure ulcer formation. A client who cannot move independently or who will be immobilized is at increased risk. Clients with diabetes and neuropathy and clients with paralysis are at increased risk due to impaired sensation. The risk for ulcer development is increased if the client is malnourished, is incontinent of urine or feces, is obese or very thin, or has altered cognitive functioning. Structured assessment tools are available to assist in the prediction of clients at increased risk for pressure ulcers. The two risk assessment tools that have been tested extensively are the Braden Scale (see Clinical Research box) and the Norton Scale. These scales provide a numeric score to rate the individual client's level of risk (Panel for the Prediction and Prevention of Pressure Ulcers in Adults, 1992).

Dysfunction Identification

If any skin problems (rashes, wounds, lesions) are present, obtain additional information about the problem, its duration, what it looked like when it first appeared, if and how it spread, and any associated symptoms. Also ask whether the client has used any treatments, including medical advice and therapies, home remedies, and over-the-counter preparations.

If an injury has resulted in a wound, burn, or other problem, evaluate the nature of the events leading to the trauma. Note any contamination of the area with dirt or debris. Ask parents about children's injuries. If they give vague or suspicious ex-

planations, obtain a follow-up evaluation to determine the possibility of child abuse. For all accidental wounds, even minor ones, ask about the status of the client's tetanus immunization, and update it if necessary.

Interview questions also can help assess the impact a skin condition or wound has on ADLs. Such conditions can affect self-concept, causing clients to withdraw from social interaction. Watching nonverbal cues helps nurses assess the psychological impact of the skin impairment.

Objective Data

Physical Examination

Inspection of the Skin. A general inspection of the skin is followed by a more detailed examination of any abnormalities noted. Examine the skin for color, vascularity, turgor and mobility, texture, and the presence or absence of lesions. A good source of light is essential. Compare for symmetry in contralateral areas throughout the examination.

Skin color varies from one person to another, from one body part to another, and according to race. Some pigment variations are normal. Pigment changes also normally occur during pregnancy. Other changes in skin color may be evidence of systemic disease. Cyanosis (bluish discoloration) in nailbeds may be caused by vasoconstriction, although cyanosis in the mouth or conjunctiva may indicate hypoxemia secondary to heart or lung dysfunction. The yellow hue of jaundice may indicate liver or biliary disease.

Skin texture refers to the palpable and visible surface structure, the fineness or coarseness of the skin, and whether it is scaly, crusted, or macerated. Skin may appear thick and tough or thin and friable. Note the presence of any edema and presence or absence of peripheral pulses when assessing clients with ulcers or wounds of the extremities.

If any skin abnormality is present, note its shape, pattern, distribution, and color. Note whether the abnormality is localized or generalized and whether distribution is symmetric. Lesions can occur in clusters, circles, or lines, or their placement may be irregular. Measure the size of the lesion so that changes in size can be detected.

Examine the client's hair and nails. Inspect the hair for distribution, quantity, and quality. Absence of hair growth on lower extremities can indicate decreased peripheral circulation. Nutritional deficits or impaired circulation may cause thin and brittle nails. Also assess for nail clubbing, a change in the angle of the fingernail and nail base associated with chronic respiratory and cardiac dysfunction, and capillary refill time, indicative of peripheral circulation.

Inspection of the Wound. Inspection permits nurses to evaluate wound healing and to detect possible complications. Appraise the wound's general appearance, type and amount of drainage, functioning of drainage systems, amount and characteristics of incisional pain, and signs of complications, such as infection.

General Appearance. Note and record the wound's size and shape, and compare it with previous measurements. Size is

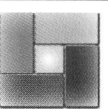

Clinical Research

Braden Scale for Predicting Pressure Sore Risk

Patient's Name _____	Evaluator's Name _____		Date of Assessment	/	/	/	/
Sensory perception Ability to respond meaningfully to pressure-related discomfort	**1. Completely limited:** Unresponsive (does not moan, flinch, or grasp) to painful stimuli, due to diminished level of consciousness or sedation OR limited ability to feel pain over most of body surface.	**2. Very limited:** Responds only to painful stimuli. Cannot communicate discomfort except by moaning or restlessness OR has a sensory impairment that limits the ability to feel pain or discomfort over half of body.	**3. Slightly limited:** Responds to verbal commands but cannot always communicate discomfort or need to be turned OR has some sensory impairment that limits ability to feel pain or discomfort in one or two extremities.	**4. No impairment:** Responds to verbal commands. Has no sensory deficit that would limit ability to feel or voice pain or discomfort.				
Moisture Degree to which skin is exposed to moisture	**1. Constantly moist:** Skin is kept moist almost constantly by perspiration, urine, etc. Dampness is detected every time patient is moved or turned.	**2. Moist:** Skin is often but not always moist. Linen must be changed at least once a shift.	**3. Occasionally moist:** Skin is occasionally moist, requiring an extra linen change approximately once a day.	**4. Rarely moist:** Skin is usually dry; linen requires changing only at routine intervals.				
Activity Degree of physical activity	**1. Bedfast:** Confined to bed.	**2. Chairfast:** Ability to walk severely limited or nonexistent. Cannot bear own weight and/or must be assisted into chair or wheelchair.	**3. Walks occasionally:** Walks occasionally during day but for very short distances, with or without assistance. Spends majority of each shift in bed or chair.	**4. Walks frequently:** Walks outside the room at least twice a day and inside room at least once every 2 hours during waking hours.				
Mobility Ability to change and control body position	**1. Completely immobile:** Does not make even slight changes in body or extremity position without assistance.	**2. Very limited:** Makes occasional slight changes in body or extremity position but unable to make frequent or significant changes independently.	**3. Slightly limited:** Makes frequent though slight changes in body or extremity position independently.	**4. No limitations:** Makes major and frequent changes in position without assistance.				

(continued)

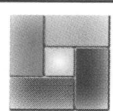

Clinical Research

Braden Scale for Predicting Pressure Sore Risk (*Continued*)

Patient's Name _____	Evaluator's Name _____		Date of Assessment	/	/	/	/
Nutrition Usual food intake pattern	**1. Very poor:** Never eats a complete meal. Rarely eats more than half of any food offered. Eats 2 servings or less of protein (meat or dairy products) per day. Takes fluids poorly. Does not take a liquid dietary supplement OR is NPO and/or maintained on clear liquids or IV for more than 5 days.	**2. Probably inadequate:** Rarely eats a complete meal and generally eats only about half of any food offered. Protein intake includes only 3 servings of meat or dairy products per day. Occasionally will take a dietary supplement OR receives less than optimum amount of liquid diet or tube feeding.	**3. Adequate:** Eats over half of most meals. Eats a total of 4 servings of protein (meat, dairy products) each day. Occasionally will refuse a meal, but will usually take a supplement if offered OR is on a tube feeding or TPN regimen, which probably meets most of nutritional needs.	**4. Excellent:** Eats most of every meal. Never refuses a meal. Usually eats a total of 4 or more servings of meat and dairy products. Occasionally eats between meals. Does not require supplementation.			
Friction and shear	**1. Problem:** Requires moderate to maximum assistance in moving. Complete lifting without sliding against sheets is impossible. Frequently slides down in bed or chair, requiring frequent repositioning with maximum assistance. Spasticity, contractures, or agitation leads to almost constant friction.	**2. Potential problem:** Moves feebly or requires minimum assistance. During a move, skin probably slides to some extent against sheets, chair, restraints, or other devices. Maintains relatively good position in chair or bed most of the time but occasionally slides down.	**3. No apparent problem:** Moves in bed and in chair independently and has sufficient muscle strength to lift up completely during move. Maintains good position in bed or chair at all times.				
		Total Score:					

NPO, nothing by mouth; IV, intravenously; TPN, total parenteral nutrition

From Braden, B., Bergstrom, N. Copyright, 1988. Reprinted with permission; Panel for Prediction and Prevention of Pressure Ulcers in Adults. (1992). Pressure ulcers in adults: Prediction and prevention. Clinical Practice Guideline No. 3. AHCPR Publication No. 92-0047. Rockville, MD: Agency for Health Care Policy and Research, Public Health Service, U.S. Department of Health and Human Services.

usually estimated in centimeters. When wound healing is watched carefully, size and shape may be measured weekly with concentric circle overlays, tracings, or photographic measures (Bergstrom et al., 1994).

Clean surgical incisions are usually closed with sutures, staples, or clips so that the skin edges are well approximated to promote healing. Initially, the incision may appear slightly swollen or red due to normal inflammation. Usually within 1 week after surgery, the wound edges heal together and swelling subsides. If staples have been in place for a prolonged period, they may rise and show signs of inflammation where they enter the skin.

If wound edges are not well approximated and healing does not occur by primary intention, granulation tissue or exposed tendon, bone, or subcutaneous tissue may be visible. Deep wounds should be checked for sinus tracts, undermining, and the presence of nonviable debris, which can delay healing and may require specific topical therapies.

Drainage Systems. Drainage devices are placed in the wound when the surgeon anticipates a large amount of fluid accumulation, which could inhibit wound healing. Closed drainage systems consist of a drain attached to a portable or external suction source. Open drainage systems, such as a Penrose drain, drain directly from the wound.

A *Penrose* drain is a hollow, fat rubber tube placed directly into the incision or into a stab wound in the incisional area. It allows fluid to drain through capillary action into absorbent dressings. Penrose drains may be advanced or shortened to drain different areas.

A *Hemovac* is placed into a vascular cavity where blood drainage is expected after surgery (Fig. 38-7). Suction is maintained by compressing a springlike device. When inspecting a Hemovac drain, expect bloody drainage and ensure that it remains in the compressed state. Suction can be interrupted if leaks are present in the system or if the Hemovac has filled with drainage.

A *Jackson-Pratt* or grenade drain permits drainage to collect in a bulblike device that can be compressed to create gentle suction. Suction is lost when the bulb is expanded because of too much drainage or a leak in the system.

With any drainage system, inspect the system to ensure that it is patent and functioning. Drains may or may not be sutured in place, so take care not to inadvertently remove them during inspection.

Wound Drainage. The type and amount of drainage vary depending on the wound's type, location, and depth. Note the amount, color, consistency, and odor of any drainage. Several terms are commonly used to describe wound drainage:

- **Serous** drainage is pale yellow, watery, and like the fluid from a blister.
- **Sanguineous** drainage is bloody, as from an acute laceration.

- **Serosanguineous** drainage is pale pinkish-yellow, thin, and contains plasma and red cells.
- **Purulent** drainage contains white cells and microorganisms and occurs when infection is present. It is thick and opaque and can vary from pale yellow to green or tan, depending on the offending organism.

Attempt to quantify the amount of drainage by noting the number of dressings that were saturated and the number of times the dressing required changing. If the dressing is not being changed (as in a fresh postoperative wound), drainage is sometimes circled on the dressing and marked with a date and time.

Inspection for Infection. Observe for symptoms that may indicate infection in the wound, such as pain, redness, swelling, induration, and purulent drainage. Systemic signs include fever and an elevated leukocyte count. Wound infection can occur at any time, but often such infections do not become apparent until late in the postoperative period or after débridement procedures. See Chapter 38 for a detailed discussion of wound infections.

Palpation. Palpation can be used along with inspection to gather objective data about wound status of skin. Palpation is helpful in assessing raised skin surfaces, texture, and temperature. If wound infection is suspected, gently palpate the incisional area to detect swelling or induration.

SAFETY ALERT
Use gloves when examining the skin when drainage is present to avoid exposure to infectious agents.

Diagnostic Tests and Procedures
Laboratory and diagnostic tests may be performed to confirm the cause of a skin or wound abnormality. Most commonly, culture and sensitivity testing is done to identify infectious organisms that can cause a skin lesion or infect a wound. A biopsy is sometimes performed to rule out malignant causes of skin abnormalities.

NURSING DIAGNOSES

Impaired Skin Integrity and Impaired Tissue Integrity are North American Nursing Diagnosis Association (NANDA) diagnoses used to identify problems with skin breakdown and healing. Impaired Skin Integrity is used to identify disruption of the skin's surface. Impaired Tissue Integrity is used when the damage involves mucous membrane, cornea, skin, or subcutaneous tissue. Risk for Impaired Skin Integrity and Risk for Trauma are used when the client's skin is at risk due to extremes in temperature, mechanical trauma, immobility, client behaviors, or other factors.

Impaired Skin Integrity

Definition. Impaired Skin Integrity is the state in which a person has altered epidermis and/or dermis (NANDA, 2000).

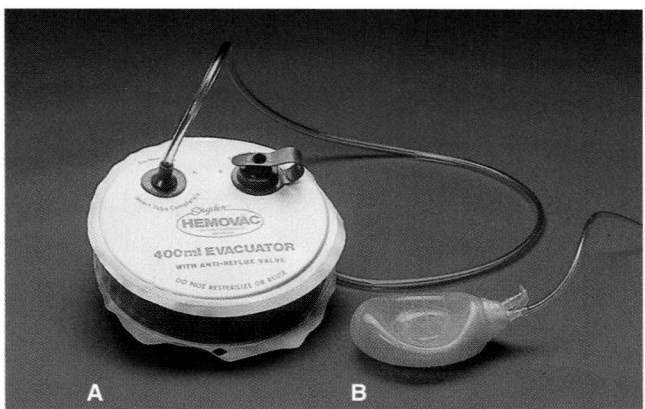

FIGURE 38-7 Closed drainage systems. **(A)** Hemovac. **(B)** Jackson-Pratt or grenade.

Defining Characteristics. Of the defining characteristics or clinical cues that point to this diagnosis, disruption of the skin surface (epidermis), destruction of the skin layers (dermis), or invasion of body structures must be present (NANDA, 2000).

Related Factors. Environmental factors may cause or contribute to Impaired Skin Integrity. These may include hyperthermia or hypothermia, which damage the skin, causing burns or frostbite; chemical substances, humidity, radiation, extremes in age, moisture, altered fluid status, medications, or mechanical factors, such as shear or friction, which destroy the epidermis; and physical immobility or immobilization leading to pressure ulcers or excessive moisture leading to macerated skin (Gordon, 1997).

Somatic factors contributing to Impaired Skin Integrity may include those that lower the tissue tolerance to pressure, such as altered nutrition, decreased skin turgor, altered metabolic states, and altered circulation or sensation.

Impaired Tissue Integrity

Definition. Impaired Tissue Integrity is the state in which a person experiences damage to mucous membrane, corneal, integumentary, or subcutaneous tissue (NANDA, 2000).

Defining Characteristics. Of the defining characteristics or clinical cues that point to this diagnosis, damaged or destroyed tissue (cornea, mucous membrane, integumentary, or subcutaneous tissue) must be present.

Related Factors. The etiologic or contributing factors that may have contributed to Impaired Tissue Integrity are similar to those listed for Impaired Skin Integrity.

Risk for Impaired Skin Integrity

Definition. Risk for Impaired Skin Integrity is present when a person's skin is at risk of being adversely altered (NANDA, 2000).

Related Factors. Risk factors include but are not limited to radiation, physical immobilization, mechanical factors, hypothermia/hyperthermia, humidity, chemical substances, moisture, extremes of age, medications, skeletal prominence, altered circulation, and nutritional deficits.

Related Nursing Diagnoses

Client problems that lead to injury to skin or tissue may be listed as nursing diagnoses. For example, a client with the diagnosis of Impaired Physical Mobility, Impaired Bed Mobility, or Total Self-Care Deficit can develop Impaired Skin Integrity. Clients with diagnoses of Imbalanced Nutrition: Less Than Body Requirements, Ineffective Tissue Perfusion, Disturbed Sensory Perception, Bowel Incontinence, or Urinary Incontinence also may develop the need for the

diagnoses of Impaired Skin Integrity or Impaired Tissue Integrity.

Factors affecting the client's ability to heal may be summarized in the nursing diagnosis. Nutrition or fluid intake may be inadequate. The effects of the wound can also be described in diagnostic terms. The client with skin and tissue injury effects may have the diagnosis Risk for Infection and, in the case of extensive burns, Ineffective Thermoregulation or Deficient Fluid Volume. Acute Pain, Disturbed Body Image, and Chronic Low Self-Esteem may accompany skin impairments. If impairment is severe, it can cause Anxiety, Ineffective Coping, or Social Isolation.

OUTCOME IDENTIFICATION AND PLANNING

Planning for nursing interventions to promote skin integrity is based on data gathered in the assessment and resulting nursing diagnoses and outcome identification. Interventions fall into the general categories of promoting skin integrity and providing an environment for optimal healing. Examples of nursing interventions commonly used in achieving these categories are listed in the accompanying display and are discussed in the following section.

Client-centered goals for skin and tissue integrity involve preventing damage and promoting optimal healing of damaged tissues:

- The client's skin will remain intact without areas of local inflammation.
- The client's wounds will demonstrate evidence of healing.
- The client will verbalize understanding of preventive skin care.

PLANNING: Examples of NIC/NOC Interventions

Accepted Skin Integrity and Wound Healing Nursing Interventions Classification (NIC)
Skin Care: Topical Treatment
Skin Surveillance
Wound Care

Accepted Skin Integrity and Wound Healing Nursing Outcomes Classification (NOC)
Fluid Balance
Immobility Consequences: Physiological
Nutritional Status
Self-Care: Hygiene
Tissue Integrity: Skin & Mucous Membranes
Tissue Perfusion: Peripheral
Wound Healing: Primary Intention
Wound Healing: Secondary Intention

Refer to the following for specifics regarding NIC/NOC:
  McCloskey, J., & Bulechek, G. (2000). *Iowa Intervention Project: Nursing Interventions Classification (NIC)* (3rd ed.). St. Louis, MO: C.V. Mosby.
Johnson, M., & Maas, M. (2000). *Iowa Outcomes Project: Nursing Outcomes Classification (NOC)* (2nd ed.). St. Louis, MO: C.V. Mosby.

- The client or family will demonstrate appropriate wound management techniques.

These goals must be individualized to reflect the needs of the person at risk. At that point, specific nursing interventions support goals.

IMPLEMENTATION
Health Promotion
Skin Care

There are several basic principles of skin care (Display 38-2). One of the most important involves maintaining intact skin, because skin is the body's first line of defense against trauma and infection. Measures to prevent irritation or injury are imperative. Avoiding mechanical irritation from rubbing or friction can prevent skin breakdown. Removing tape carefully and patting skin dry prevent traumatization of delicate skin. To minimize chemical irritation, use mild soap, plain water, or products that contain emollients. Clients who are very young, old, emaciated, or obese may have particularly sensitive skin that is more prone to chemical irritation and dryness.

Maintaining adequate hydration of the skin also contributes to healthy function. Because very dry skin is susceptible to breakdown, avoid drying agents, such as alcohol. Instead, use lotions or creams with lanolin. Clients with dry skin should bathe only once or twice a week. However, exposure to excessive moisture for prolonged periods can lead to bacterial growth and irritation. Clients who are incontinent of urine or stool or who perspire excessively need prompt, thorough, and frequent washing and drying. Areas where skin lies in folds, such as under the breasts and in the gluteal areas, can collect moisture and require special attention. A gauze pad or light dusting of powder may help prevent moisture buildup in skin folds. Many pH-balanced cleansing agents are available for frequent perineal cleansing. Repeated use of soap that has an alkaline pH decreases the skin's acidity and its protective function.

Adequate nutrition is essential for normal skin integrity. Adequately nourished cells are better able to resist injury and disease. A diet with appropriate vitamins, minerals, and protein is essential. A client who has poor absorption of nutri-

ents, excessive losses of protein, or inadequate food and fluid intake may need additional nutritional support (e.g., high-protein enteral or parenteral supplements) to prevent skin breakdown and to promote healing.

Adequate circulation also is needed to maintain cell life. Inadequate blood flow to the skin results in ischemia and tissue breakdown. Keeping clients warm prevents vasoconstriction. Treating underlying cardiac or circulatory problems helps ensure adequate blood flow to the skin. Clients with impaired venous circulation from the legs and feet require leg elevation and compression to heal venous ulcers (Pontiere-Lewis, 1995). Exercising adequately and avoiding constrictive clothing can help ensure optimal blood flow. Frequent turning and repositioning also can prevent localized obstruction of blood flow due to increased pressure.

Client Teaching

Hygiene teaching is important to maintain skin integrity. Because clients with impaired sensation from neuropathies or paralysis are less able to sense injury to the skin, teach them to inspect skin surfaces (especially the feet) routinely for signs of breakdown. When clients are wearing new shoes, advise them to avoid blisters and irritation. Prevention strategies can decrease the incidence of amputation in people with diabetes (Krasner, 1998). Because temperature discrimination also is affected, encourage clients to turn down the temperature of water heaters to avoid accidental burns.

Hygiene teaching is important for the parents of newborns. Teaching should include how to prevent skin trauma (e.g., clipping fingernails short and putting mittens on children if scratching is anticipated). Reassure parents about normal skin changes or congenital skin lesions. Parental bonding with infants can be hindered if the parents view the infant as deformed or scarred.

Education about trauma prevention is important. Many motor vehicle injuries (which can lead to skin and tissue injury) can be prevented by driving carefully, adhering to speed limits, using seatbelts, and driving cars with air bags. Bicycle injuries can be prevented or limited by observing safety rules and wearing helmets. Smoke detectors should be installed to prevent serious burns. See Chapter 30 for more information on safety.

Protection from the Sun

All clients should learn the importance of limiting exposure to ultraviolet radiation (sunlight and artificial tanning lights). The use of clothing, wide-brimmed hats, and sunglasses to protect frequently exposed areas is most practical. Discourage clients from using tanning machines for cosmetic purposes. Urge fair- and light-skinned people to use sunscreen with a minimum sun protection factor of 15 daily. Because sunscreen is not recommended for infants younger than 6 months of age, encourage parents to avoid exposing young babies to the sun.

Pressure Ulcer Prevention

Most pressure ulcers can be prevented, and many stage I ulcers disappear with pressure reduction. Prevention is less costly than treatment in terms of both money and the impact on the client. Once a client is determined to be at risk and the

DISPLAY 38-2

🔲 PRINCIPLES OF SKIN CARE

- Intact skin is the body's first line of defense against trauma and infection.
- Breakdown of the skin's integrity must be prevented.
- Skin must be adequately hydrated.
- The body's cells must be adequately nourished.
- Adequate circulation is needed to maintain cells.
- Skin hygiene is necessary.
- Skin sensitivity varies among people and according to their health status.

ETHICAL/LEGAL ISSUE

Judgment of Client's Self-Care

Jim Neal, a 35-year-old man, is paraplegic as a result of a motorcycle accident 7 years ago. He lives at home, and home care assistants help him sporadically. He is frequently readmitted to acute care for treatment of recurrent pressure ulcers. Health-care providers have repeatedly advised him about appropriate care for these lesions and the need to relieve pressure on his buttocks regularly. He is now an inpatient, with more problems with his pressure ulcers. You overhear two nurses talking:

"I'm so sick of taking care of this man over and over!"

"I agree. He won't help himself and keeps doing all the wrong things for his pressure ulcers. He should just have to live with the consequences of his choices!"

Reflection
- Identify your concerns about Mr. Neal and his situation.
- Describe your feelings in light of what you overheard the nurses say. How do their attitudes contribute to your reaction?
- Identify possible approaches to this situation.
- Recognizing the client's dysfunction, define what you see as your ethically appropriate behavior.

factors that produce that risk are identified, nursing measures are implemented. A synopsis of the interventions for prevention of pressure ulcers is provided in Display 38-3.

Pressure ulcers can often be prevented by the use of a pressure-reducing support surface, such as a pad, mattress, or product that distributes pressure more evenly across the body surface on the bed or chair used by the person at risk. A variety of such beds, mattresses, and cushions are available. Most manufacturers conduct research on the pressure-reducing effects of their products. However, more research is needed to compare the effects of products when used with at-risk clients, rather than with healthy, young volunteers.

Support surfaces may be purchased, rented, or leased for client use. The primary goal for any of these products is to prevent and/or manage pressure-related skin breakdown. Choosing a particular support surface for a client requires consideration of product efficacy, desired effect, anticipated duration of treatment, client preferences, cost, upkeep, and impact on client mobility.

The support surfaces used for pressure ulcer prevention and care can be broadly categorized as static and dynamic overlays, mattress replacements, and specialty beds, which include low-air-loss beds and air-fluidized beds. Kinetic therapy beds and bariatric (obese) beds may reduce pressure. However, their purposes are primarily to promote respiratory function (kinetic beds) and to provide a sleep surface for clients who weigh more than 300 lb (bariatric beds).

DISPLAY 38-3

 PRESSURE ULCER PREDICTION AND PREVENTION

Risk Prediction
- Identify clients at risk and the specific factors placing them at risk.

Skin Care
- Maintain and improve tissue tolerance to pressure to prevent injury. Inspect pressure points at least once a day; document all findings.
- Cleanse skin regularly and whenever soiled, using a mild cleansing agent and warm, not hot, water.
- Minimize factors that dry the skin. Treat dry skin with moisturizers.
- Do not massage bony prominences.
- Minimize exposure of skin to incontinence, perspiration, or wound drainage.
- Protect skin from friction and shear.
- Provide adequate calories and nutrients.
- Maintain or improve mobility, activity level, and range of motion.

Pressure Reduction for At-Risk Clients
- Reposition every 2 hours. Use a 30-degree side-lying position when the patient is lateral to avoid excessive pressure on the trochanter.

- Use pillows to keep bony prominences from rubbing against each other.
- Keep heels from pressing on the bed if the client is completely immobile.
- When the client is on his or her side, avoid positioning directly on the trochanter.
- Limit the time the head of the bed is elevated.
- Lift, do not drag, clients to move them up in bed. Use overbed trapeze.
- Place clients on a pressure-reducing device when in bed.
- Avoid prolonged sitting. Reposition or shift the client's weight every hour.
- For chair-bound clients, place a pressure-reducing device on the chair that maintains good postural alignment, balance, and stability.
- Use a written plan regarding the use of positioning devices and repositioning schedules.

Education
- Provide structured education about pressure ulcer prevention to healthcare providers, clients, and family or caregivers.

APPLY YOUR KNOWLEDGE

Gwen Nelson, 66, is in the clinic for a follow-up visit related to her diabetes mellitus. While she is there, she mentions to you that she has a discolored spot on her foot. She thought she would just soak it and use an emery board to remove it. She stated that it didn't have any feeling anyway so removing it in this fashion shouldn't hurt.

What assessment data do you need to collect at this point? Discuss how you will help to maintain skin integrity for this client.

Check your answer in Appendix A.

Given the wide variety of available support surfaces, deciding which product will best meet the needs of individual clients can be difficult. To narrow and to standardize the selection of support surfaces, many facilities create algorithms or guidelines. One such algorithm is displayed in Fig. 38-8.

Mattress Overlays. An overlay is a product that is placed on top of an existing bed mattress. Overlays can be made of foam or filled with air, gel, or water. Eggcrate foam, a loose, convoluted overlay, provides little pressure reduction unless the base of the foam is at least 4 inches high. It is most appropriately used as a comfort measure. Foam overlays with greater density and thickness provide pressure reduction when used with normal-weight clients. Air-filled overlays also reduce pressure when the product is correctly inflated. Air-filled overlays may be static (like an air mattress) or dynamic (attached to a motorized air blower or pump). Examples are given in Fig. 38-9.

Replacement Mattresses. Replacement mattresses are used on a standard bed frame after removal of the original mattress. Replacement mattresses reduce some pressure because of their design, which includes layers of dense foam or foam and gel combinations within a lightweight, bacteriostatic cover. Replacement mattresses are relatively new to the market of support surfaces, but early research has shown them to be of benefit (Rojas & Reynolds, 1996).

Specialty Beds. Specialty beds for use in pressure ulcer care include low-air-loss beds and air-fluidized beds (Fig. 38-10). Low-air-loss beds consist of multiple air-filled, horizontally positioned cushions within a traditional electrical bed frame. The cushions in the seat area contain a higher amount of air to support the increased weight required in this area when the head of the bed is elevated. Air-fluidized beds use a high flow rate of air to blow fine particles of silicone within a protective cover. The resulting support surface behaves like a liquid and feels similar to a waterbed. When the air flow is turned off, the beads settle to the bottom of the bed and become a firm, hard surface, holding the client in position until the air flow is resumed.

Nursing Interventions for Skin Impairment

Multidisciplinary care planning is necessary for clients with skin impairment. Nursing interventions to encourage independence, reinforce client accomplishments, and teach clients and families to achieve optimal self-care are important. Nurses can help clients with chronic wounds to learn ways to minimize factors that impair wound healing (Krasner, 1995). Heat and cold also can be used as therapeutic modalities to promote healing and provide pain relief. Nurses help select topical therapies that will cleanse, débride, and protect the wounded area during healing.

Pruritus Relief

Pruritus often accompanies skin problems. Nursing management aims at relieving the situations that cause pruritus, decreasing the associated discomfort, and preventing additional trauma to the skin.

Excessive drying of the skin often causes pruritus, especially in older clients. Applying lotions and moisturizing creams regularly promotes rehydration of dried areas. Limiting bathing prevents excessive drying of the skin. If clients use soap, instruct them to rinse it thoroughly from the skin. If appropriate, they may add oil to the bath water.

 SAFETY ALERT
Alert clients to take extra care when adding oil to tub bath water because oil makes the bathtub slippery and may contribute to falls.

Clients should use tepid (not hot) water and should gently pat the skin dry to decrease skin irritation. Explaining the importance of not scratching may increase compliance for adults, but such cautions rarely work for young children. Keeping children's fingernails cut short and having them wear cotton gloves may help to decrease skin trauma. Diversional activities also may help focus a child's attention away from unpleasant sensations.

Cool baths and moist, cool compresses promote vasoconstriction and provide relief. Baking soda or oatmeal baths are soothing. Prescriptive medications may also be required. Antihistamines and sedatives, although commonly used, have systemic side effects. Topical medications, such as corticosteroids or antibiotics, can decrease inflammation or treat infection.

First Aid for Minor Wounds

Basic principles in caring for minor wounds are to promote hemostasis, cleanse the wound, and protect it from further injury. Bleeding can be controlled by putting direct pressure on the wound or by elevating the affected part. Initial bleeding may help remove dirt and contaminants from the wound.

Cleansing the wound removes potential sources of infection. Try to remove foreign materials, such as dirt or cinders, unless the wound is extensive or the client complains of excessive pain. For most minor wounds, running water as an irrigating solution and mild soap as a cleansing agent are recommended.

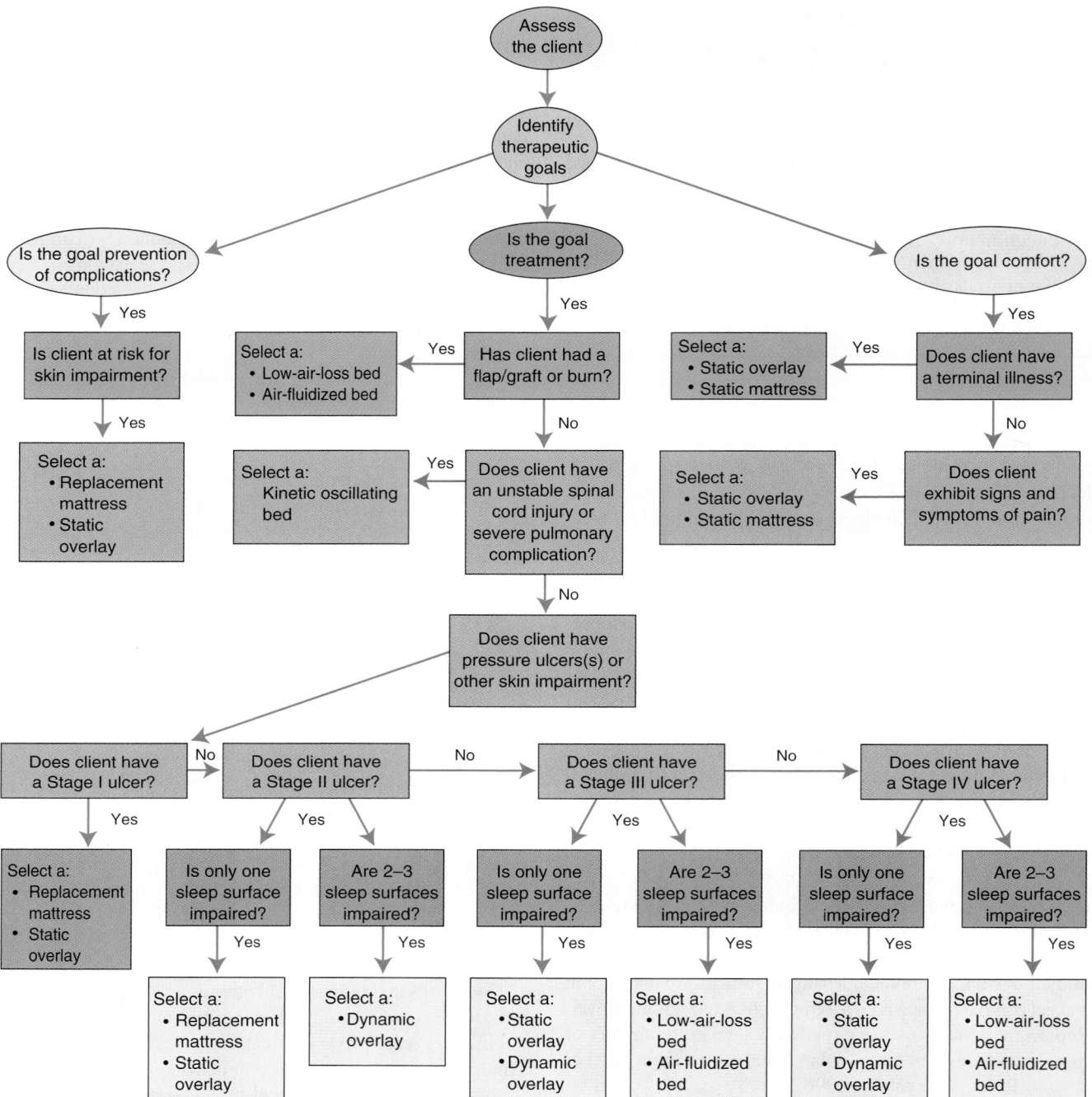

Note: If only one sleep surface is impaired, it is assumed the client will not be turned on the affected site. A device with pressure relief is indicated if two-to-three sleep surfaces are impaired.

FIGURE 38-8   Support surface algorithm. (From Thomason, S., Hawley, G. G., & Wurzel, J. [1993]. Specialty support surfaces: A cost containment perspective. *Decubitus* 6(6), 32–40. Modified and reprinted with permission of the author.)

After bleeding has subsided and the area has been cleansed, protect the wound with a sterile or clean dressing. Small cuts may be left open to the air. Extensive wounds may require a bulky dressing applied with pressure to minimize movement.

Assess the wound closely for potential complications. Any client with a wound that requires more extensive treat-ment should be referred for immediate care. Signs of in-fection usually take up to 24 hours to develop. Exudate, fever, or severe redness and swelling indicate that the wound needs medical attention. If excessive bleeding occurs, su-tures are usually necessary to ensure healing by primary intention.

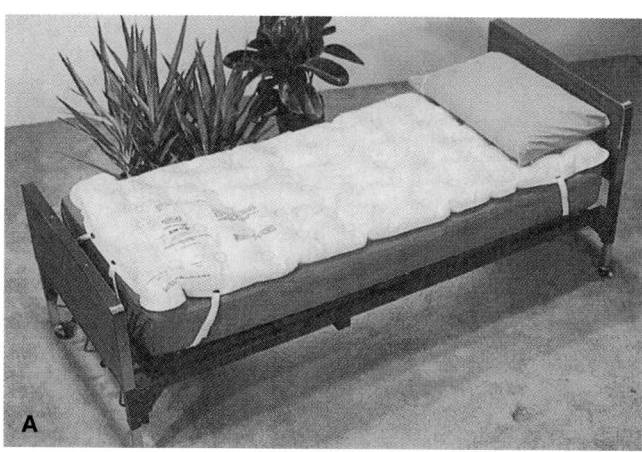
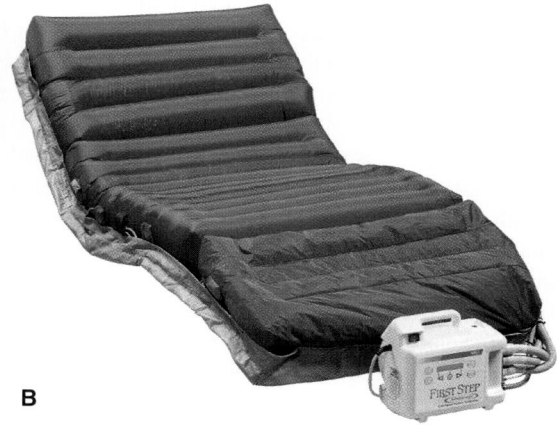

FIGURE 38-9   Examples of air-filled overlay mattresses. **(A)** Static air flotation mattress with corner straps gives 17 to 25 mm Hg interface pressure relief. (Photograph courtesy of Lotus Health Care Products, Naugatuck, CT.) **(B)** Dynamic air-filled overlay mattress. (Photograph of First Step® Advantage courtesy of Kinetiz Concepts Inc., San Antonio, TX.)

First Aid for Minor Burns

The type of burn dictates the appropriate first-aid measures. In all cases, it is important to halt the burning process, prevent further damage, and take emergency measures to promote adequate airway, breathing, and circulation. Burn-related complications can develop quickly and warrant medical evaluation in an emergency room or burn/trauma center.

In the case of thermal burns, first remove the heat source. If someone is on fire, immediate action should be to "stop, drop, and roll." After the heat source has been removed, immediately flush the burned area with copious amounts of cool water. If done quickly, this action halts the burning process by speeding heat dissipation. It also helps to relieve pain. Remove any of the client's clothing and jewelry in the affected area, because clothing and metal can retain heat. If clothing sticks to the burned area, cut around it rather than pulling it, which may traumatize underlying burned tissues. Avoid ointments and home remedies because they can complicate burn healing.

Treatment of chemical burns is similar to that of thermal burns. The first step is to remove the client's clothing and

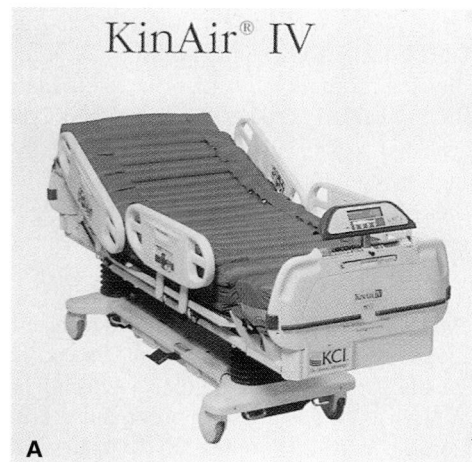
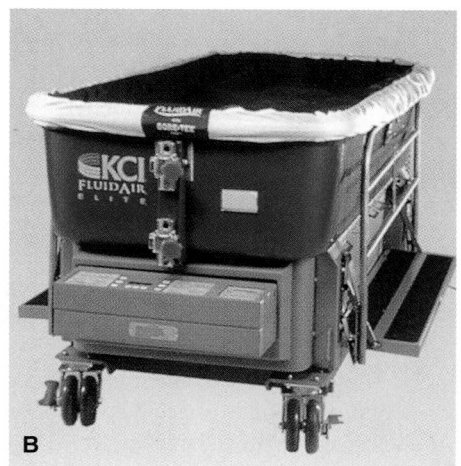

FIGURE 38-10   Examples of specialty beds. **(A)** KinAir® IV. **(B)** Fluidair Elite® (Photographs courtesy of Kinetic Concepts Inc., San Antonio, TX.)

flush the burned area with water, which dilutes the chemical and halts the burning process. If a large area has been exposed, placing the client in a shower may be the easiest way to flush the burned area. Brush powdered chemicals off the area before irrigating. Avoid splashing any of the irritant, because even dilute exposure to some chemicals can result in burns or irritation of mucous membranes. Some chemicals (e.g., alkali powders) react with water to produce heat, so industrial nurses should be knowledgeable about the chemicals used in their workplaces.

Before an electrical burn can be treated, the victim must be freed from the electrical source. If the person is still in contact with the electrical current, it must be turned off at its source. Removing the victim from the source of current requires special training and equipment. Once the victim has been freed from the current, if the injury site or clothing is smoldering, douse it with water to dissipate the heat. Cardiopulmonary resuscitation may be necessary, because ventricular fibrillation or cardiac arrest often occurs with electrical burns.

Treatment of Denuded Skin

Denuded skin can result from many causes. If it occurs on the buttocks or perineal area, it is often a result of urinary or fecal incontinence. The most important factor leading to skin healing in these cases is resolution of the underlying problem. The reasons for incontinence must be investigated and treated. A urinary catheter may be necessary temporarily to allow the skin's surface to re-epithelialize. Options for protecting skin from incontinent stool include adult briefs and protective ointments, rectal pouches, and rectal tubes. While the skin is protected, take measures to resolve the underlying cause of the incontinence.

Topical Wound Therapy

A dressing is a protective covering placed on a wound. Dressings may be used for the following reasons:

- To absorb drainage
- To prevent contamination
- To prevent mechanical injury to the wound
- To help maintain pressure so that excessive bleeding is avoided
- To provide a moist wound environment
- To provide comfort for the client

The type of dressing used depends on the type of wound, location, status, and personal preference.

Types of Dressings. More than 1300 products are available for the care of skin and wounds (Anonymous, 2000). These dressings can be broadly grouped into categories based on their characteristics and indications (Table 38-3). Of all the products listed, gauze dressings have been used in wound care the longest. They are versatile and easy to use. Because they do not keep the surface of open wounds moist, they are often moistened with saline before being packed into large cavities.

Polyurethane film, polyurethane foam, and hydrocolloid dressings are often selected for topical therapy of partial-thickness wounds and stage I or II pressure ulcers. These dressings provide protection for wounds and provide a moist wound environment. They can be left in place up to 1 week unless the wound requires more frequent visualization or the amount of drainage overwhelms the dressing's capacity.

Hydrogels are used to encourage granulation within full-thickness wounds and to provide comfort in tender, partial-thickness wounds. Alginate products, the newest of the listed dressings, are known for their capacity for absorption. Alginate is indicated for deep or moderately draining wounds.

Some of the newest products being placed on wounds are ointments and lotions containing platelet-derived growth factors. These products are being evaluated for their effects on stimulating and hastening healing in chronic wounds (Martin, 1997).

Methods of Securing Dressings. Tape, Montgomery straps, gauzes, Ace wraps, stretch nets, or binders can hold dressings in place. Tape is most commonly used as a securing device. Adhesive tape is not often used on the skin. Although it holds securely, its removal can be painful. If adhesive tape must be used, clip the hair before application and use an adhesive remover solution when the tape is gently pulled from the skin. Nonallergenic paper or plastic tape is preferred for dressings that adhere to the skin.

Older people and others with fragile skin require paper tape or nonadhesive products to secure dressings without tape. Microfoam tape is a pliable, foamlike tape used for compression or pressure dressings.

Montgomery straps or ties, used when dressings require frequent changing, are commercially prepared strips of nonallergenic tape (Fig. 38-11). Ties are inserted through the holes at one end. Montgomery straps help prevent skin breakdown because they eliminate the need to remove tape with every dressing change. Changing Montgomery straps is required only when they become loose or soiled.

Bandages, binders, and stretch nets also can be used to hold gauze dressings in place. They are discussed and illustrated later in this chapter.

Dressing Changes. The frequency of dressing changes is determined by wound status, type of dressing, amount of drainage, and frequency of wound assessment required. Sometimes, the physician orders the type of dressing and the frequency of dressing changes, but other times the nurse determines what type of dressing will best promote healing. Hydrocolloid dressings, for example, may be left in place for 1 week on clean, partial-thickness wounds. Procedures for changing a dry sterile dressing and applying a moist saline dressing are given in Procedures 38-1 and 38-2, respectively.

Packing. Sterile packing can be inserted into an infected wound or an open wound that has the potential for infection. Packing prevents the wound from closing prematurely, which could lead to growth of microorganisms and abscess formation. Packing is commercially prepared in long, thin strips. Usually, plain or saline-moistened gauze packing is used, but gauze impregnated with iodophor, petrolatum, or povidone–iodine also is available.

TABLE 38-3

Types of Dressings, Characteristics, and Indications

Category	Characteristics	Indications
Alginate dressings 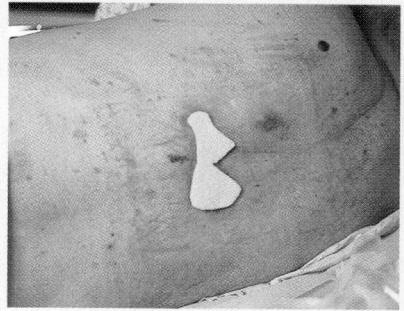	• Highly absorbent product designed to be placed inside the wound • Require a cover dressing • Available in sheet form or as packing strips	• Deep, moderately draining wounds
Gauzes 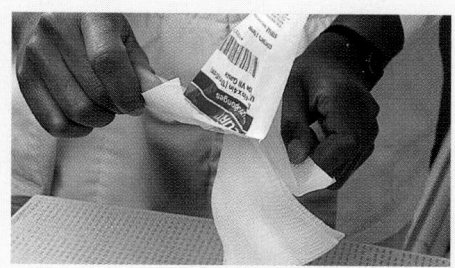	• Woven cotton material available in many sizes and thicknesses • Nonocclusive, allowing environmental oxygen to reach the wound surface • Highly absorbent • May be moistened with sterile saline to create a moist packing	• Newly created surgical incisions or wounds requiring pressure for hemostasis • Packing of deep wounds • Cover dressing over hydrogels and other primary dressings
Hydrocolloid wafer dressing 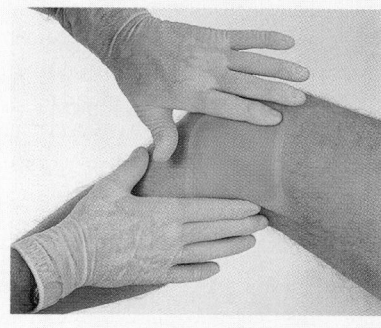	• Adhesive-backed pad, often tan in color, made of hydroactive materials • Pad absorbs excess exudate into its matrix, maintaining a moist wound surface • Most are occlusive, keeping environmental oxygen from reaching the wound • Moderate absorptive properties	• Partial-thickness wounds • Pressure ulcers • Venous leg ulcers
Hydrogel 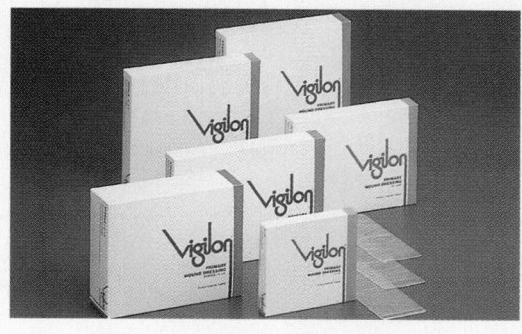	• Hydrophilic polymer product with a high percentage of water within the matrix • Available in transparent sheetlike wafer or as tube gel • Provide moderate absorption of drainage and a moist wound environment • Sheetlike wafer provides cooling sensation on the skin	• Partial-thickness wound • Pressure ulcers, stage II–IV (with a cover dressing, such as gauze) • Minor burns • Skin graft donor sites

(*continues*)

TABLE 38-3 (Continued)

Types of Dressings, Characteristics, and Indications		
Category	Characteristics	Indications
Polyurethane foam	• Pads of compressed foam (vary in thickness according to brand; sometimes have an adhesive backing) • Mild to moderate absorptive capacity, depending on thickness • Provide a moist wound surface	• Partial-thickness wounds • Absorbent covering for deep wounds that have been packed
Transparent adhesive dressings	• Clear, polyurethane film with adhesive backing • Different brands allow varying levels of moisture vapor to evaporate through the dressing • Maintain a moist wound surface • Multiple sizes and shapes • No absorptive properties	• Partial-thickness wounds • May be used instead of tape to secure a gauze pad or other type of absorbent dressing in place • Wounds with minimal exudate • Protective cover for areas exposed to friction (e.g., sacrum and heels in bed-bound clients)

Packing also may be used after surgery on body areas that are hard to suture (e.g., vagina, nasal septum) to apply pressure and to prevent blood loss from small capillaries. When packing has been inserted during surgery, it should be noted on the client's record so that the packing is not accidentally removed when the dressing is changed. Pressure packing usually remains in place for 2 or 3 days and is then removed by the surgeon or the nurse with a physician's order so that it does not become a reservoir for pathogenic growth.

Cleansing and Disinfection. Intact skin is prepared for surgical incisions or invasive procedures by a process called skin preparation. Skin preparation often involves the use of antiseptic solutions, such as iodine or chlorhexidine, to scrub the skin's surface. Skin preparation decreases the possibility of infection from breaking the intact skin barrier and is an appropriate use of disinfectants.

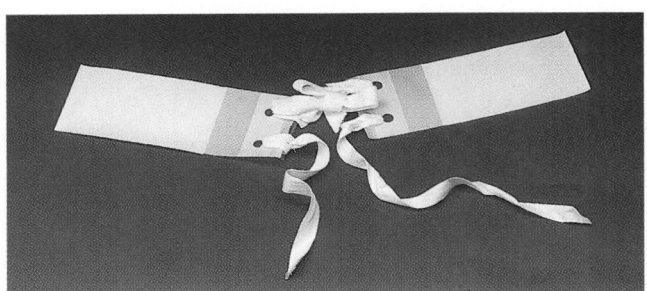

FIGURE 38-11 Montgomery straps or ties are used to prevent skin breakdown from frequent tape removal when dressings need to be changed often.

Wound cleansing is performed to remove debris, contaminants, and excess exudate. Wound cleansers should not contain agents that are harmful to the cells involved in wound healing. This is especially important in the care of chronic wounds, such as pressure ulcers. Sterile normal saline (0.9% NaCl) is the cleansing solution of choice for chronic wounds. Many commercial wound cleansers are available, with varying levels of toxicity to cells (Kirsner & Froelich, 1998). Commercial wound cleansers contain agents such as surfactant, which may facilitate the removal of wound debris. Procedure 38-3 describes how to irrigate a wound.

Débridement. **Débridement** is the removal of foreign material or dead tissue from a wound to discourage the growth of microorganisms and to promote wound healing. There are four main types of débridement: mechanical, surgical, enzymatic, and autolytic. Surgical débridement refers to the use of sharp instruments to débride the wound, as done during surgery or at the bedside. Physicians and other providers who specialize in wound care (e.g., wound, ostomy, and continence nurses [WOCN]; physical therapists) perform sharp débridement. Enzymatic débridement refers to the process of placing chemical products within the wound to help break down the necrotic debris. Autolytic débridement is the process of removing debris and necrotic tissue using the body's own fluids and cells. Autolytic débridement occurs when an occlusive dressing is applied over a wound and left in place while wound exudate and body fluids build up. The wound fluid softens the eschar, making it easier to remove, and, in some cases, totally dissolves

(text continues on page 1013)

PROCEDURE 38-1

CHANGING A DRY STERILE DRESSING

Purpose
1. Protect wound from trauma and external contamination.
2. Provide opportunity to assess the wound.
3. Provide an absorbent covering over the wound.

Assessment
- Assess location and degree of pain. Medicate if necessary.
- Assess for presence of generalized symptoms of infection (e.g., elevated temperature, leukocytosis, diaphoresis).
- Assess dressing for drainage. Observe linen for drainage.
- Review medical history and identify factors that may contribute to delayed wound healing (e.g., poor nutritional status, age, obesity, immunosuppressive therapy, disorders such as anemia or diabetes mellitus).
- Assess client's ability to cooperate during procedure. Arrange for assistance, if necessary, to ensure client's safety during procedure.
- Note client allergies to tape or dressing materials.

Equipment
Clean gloves, sterile gloves
Sterile, prepackaged dressings
Sterile towel
Sterile cup
Clean, flat work surface
Tape (micropore or paper)
Montgomery straps (optional)
Disposable suture-removal set for scissors and forceps (optional)
Cleansing solution as ordered, with applicator
Plastic bag

Procedure
1. Close client's door or curtains around bed. Explain procedure to client.
2. Position client comfortably. Expose only wound area.
   Rationale: Keep the client safe and comfortable.
3. Wash your hands.
   Rationale: Handwashing helps prevent spread of microorganisms.
4. Make a cuff on top of plastic bag and place within easy reach of dressing table.

Rationale: Cuff allows contaminated dressing to be easily contained without contaminating outside of bag.
5. Put on clean disposable gloves.
   Rationale: Gloves protect against contamination from wound drainage.
6. Remove dressing from wound, and discard into plastic bag. *Note:* If dressing adheres to wound, pour a small amount of sterile saline on the wound to loosen the dressing and prevent disruption of healing tissue.

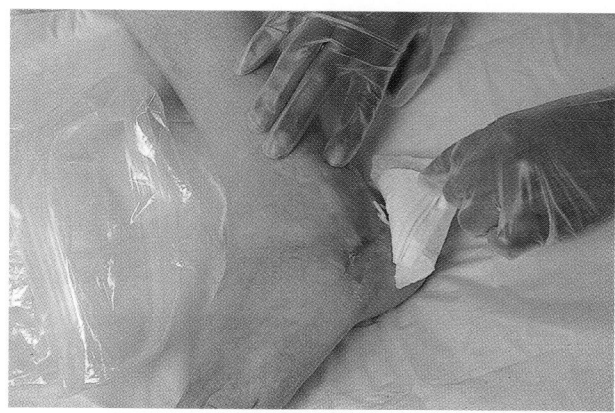

Step 6 Remove soiled dressing.

7. Dispose gloves. Wash your hands.
   Rationale: Gloves are contaminated. Handwashing helps prevent spread of microorganisms.
8. Set up sterile supplies.
   a. Open sterile towel, and hold it by the edges.
   b. Place it on a clean, flat surface without contaminating the center of the towel.
   c. Open dressing package (or packages) by peeling paper down to expose dressing. Let it fall onto the sterile field.
   d. Open cleansing solution container, and pour solution into sterile cup.
   e. Open any supplies for wound irrigation and set materials at the side of the sterile field.
   Rationale: Setting up sterile supplies after removing and discarding the soiled dressing permits assessment of what dressing materials are needed and whether changes are necessary without charging the client for unneeded supplies. Optional: Instead of using the sterile towel as a sterile field, the nurse may open the dressing packages and suture set carefully, allowing the inside of the packaging material to serve as the sterile field.

PROCEDURE 38-1 (Continued)

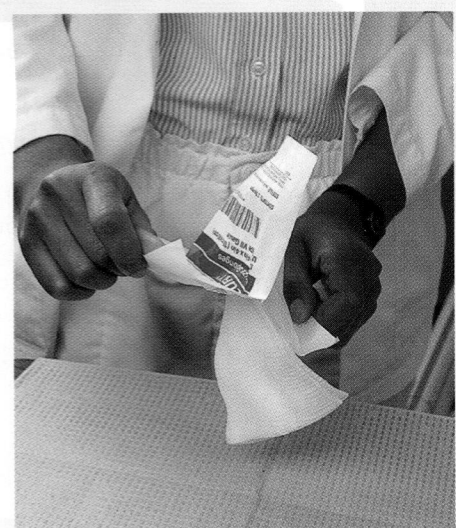

Step 8c Open sterile dressings and let fall onto sterile field.

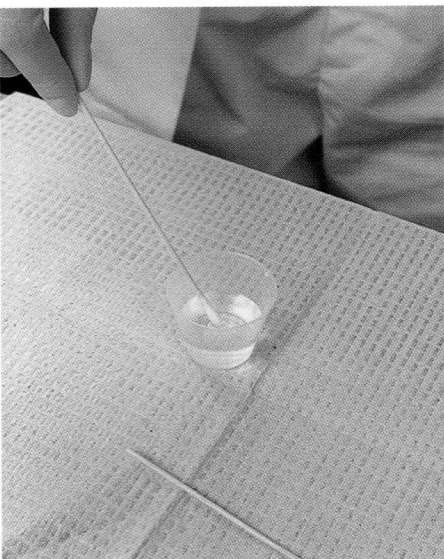

Step 9 Dip cotton-tipped applicators into cleansing solution.

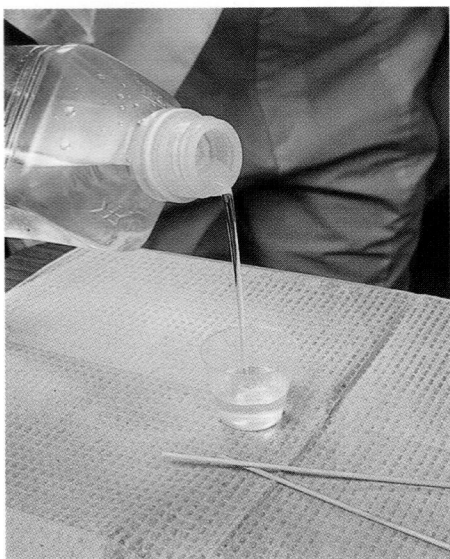

Step 8d Pour container of cleansing solution.

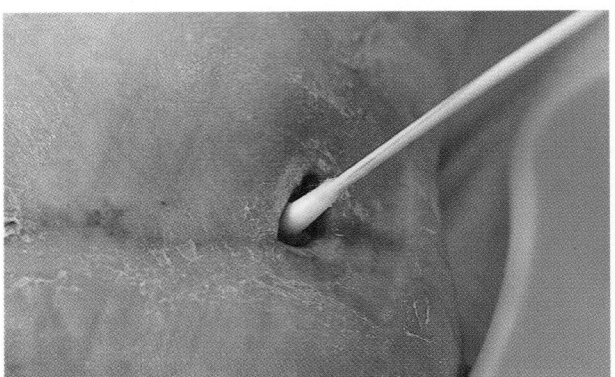

Step 10 Clean wound from the least contaminated area to most contaminated area.

9. Don sterile gloves. Grasp applicators at nonabsorbent end and dip them into the cleansing solution.
10. Clean drainage from the wound's center outward, using each applicator only once and discarding without placing the applicator back into the cleansing solution.
    Rationale: Cleansing from the center of the wound outward prevents introduction of

microorganisms into the wound. Using the applicator once prevents transfer of microbes into the cleansing solution container.
11. Dry the surrounding skin gently with gauze.
    Rationale: Microorganisms grow well in dark, moist environments.
12. Inspect the incision for bleeding, inflammation, drainage, and healing. Note any areas of dehiscence (opening or gaping of wound edges).
    Rationale: Note and treat inadequate healing or complications immediately.
13. Apply sterile dressings one at a time over the wound.

PROCEDURE 38-1 (Continued)

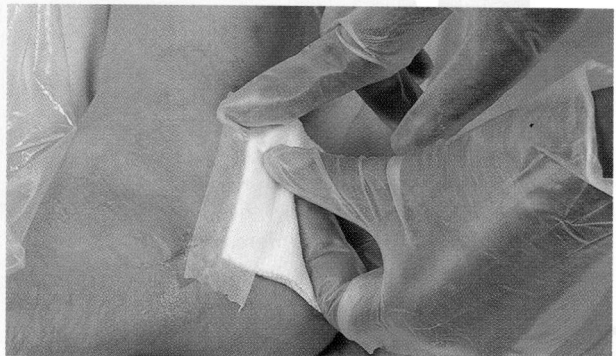

Step 13 Apply sterile dressing over the wound.

> **Rationale: Careful application of dressings prevents introduction of microorganisms into the wound.**

14. Wash your hands.
    > **Rationale: Handwashing helps prevent spread of microorganisms.**
15. Document procedure and observations.

Lifespan Considerations
Child

- Remind young children not to touch the incision when their dressing is removed. Enlist the aid of assistants to prevent children's moving and contaminating the wound or the sterile field.
- Preschool and young school-age children may think that the body part covered by a dressing is not there. Allow them to see their incision if they are interested. Seeing their body part will reassure them.

- Change the dressing immediately if a child is not toilet trained and the dressing becomes wet with urine or feces. Consider using wide plastic tape over the dressing to keep it dry.

Older Adult

- Remember that as skin ages, it loses its elasticity and becomes more sensitive. Adhesive tape may tear the skin. Use paper tape or Montgomery straps, which provide more protection.

Home Care Modifications

- When a client needs to change dressings at home, instruct him or her in the following points:
  - Handwashing before and after the dressing change is the most important aspect of maintaining asepsis. For some dressings, gloving is not required. Sterile dressing changes are rarely done at home.
  - Where to buy and how to open and use dressings.
  - How to clean the wound and which cleansing solution to use.
  - Signs of infection that indicate the need to call the nurse or physician.

Collaboration and Delegation

- Instruct ancillary staff to observe for excessive drainage that may overwhelm the dressing and to report when dressings become soiled or loosened from the skin.

---

debris so that it can be irrigated from the wound during a subsequent dressing change.

Wound Support

Butterflies and Steristrips. Butterflies and Steristrips can be applied to wounds to approximate wound edges and promote healing. A butterfly is a type of adhesive strip shaped like a butterfly. One edge is placed on the skin and pulled until wound approximation is achieved; then the other adhesive side is placed on the skin. On small wounds, a butterfly strip may eliminate the need for sutures. Steristrips are commercially prepared adhesive strips used for the same purpose. They come in various widths. Tincture of benzoin or other commercially available skin preparations (e.g., barrier films) may be applied to the skin before application to help them stick longer.

Sutures, Staples, and Clips. Support is provided in a surgical incision by use of sutures, surgical staples, or surgical clips to hold the incision together until healing occurs. The type of material used for wound closure affects wound healing.

PROCEDURE 38-2

APPLYING A SALINE-MOISTENED DRESSING

Purpose
1. Promote moist wound healing.
2. Protect the wound from contamination and mechanical trauma.

Assessment
- Review the physician's orders for frequency of dressing changes.
- Assess the wound's location and size to determine needed dressing supplies.
- Assess client's level of comfort. Give analgesics as needed before wound care.
- Review nursing notes for previous wound description and for presence of generalized symptoms of infection (e.g., elevated temperature, leukocytosis).

Equipment
Clean disposable gloves
Sterile gloves
Sterile dressing instrument set (forceps, scissors)
Sterile thin-mesh gauze dressing
Sterile gauze dressings
Absorbent secondary dressing
Sterile basin
Prescribed sterile solution
Sterile saline
Tape or ties
Waterproof disposal bag
Sterile cotton-tipped applicators (optional)
Sterile drape (optional for sterile field)

Procedure
1. Prepare client and remove dressing according to Steps 1 through 5 of Procedure 38-1. *Note:* Forceps may be used to remove a soiled dressing. If dressing adheres to underlying tissues, moisten with saline to loosen. Gently remove the dressing while assessing client's discomfort level.
   Rationale: Moistening the dressing prevents disruption of healing tissue.
2. Observe dressings for amount and characteristics of drainage. Note odor and color.
   Rationale: Changes in the type or amount of drainage may be signs of wound infection.
3. Observe wound for eschar (thick layer of dead cells and dried plasma), granulation tissue (reddish capillary loops that bleed easily), or epithelial skin buds. Measure and record wound depth, diameter, and length.
   Rationale: Assess wound for healing.
4. Prepare sterile supplies. Open sterile instruments, sterile basin, solution, and dressings.
5. Place fine-mesh gauze into basin, and pour the ordered solution over mesh to saturate.
   Rationale: Gauze touching the wound surface must be thoroughly moistened to increase its absorptive ability. Note: If the wound is very large, warm the ordered solution to body temperature to prevent excessive loss of body heat.
6. Don sterile gloves.
   Rationale: Gloves prevent contamination of wound or supplies and protect against contamination from body fluids.
7. Cleanse or irrigate wound as prescribed or with normal saline, moving from least to most contaminated areas.
   Rationale: When cleaning debris from wound, take steps to prevent spread of contamination.
8. Squeeze excess fluid from gauze dressing. Unfold and fluff out the dressing.
   Rationale: Doing so provides a thin, moist layer to contact all wound surfaces.
   a. Gently pack moistened gauze into the wound.

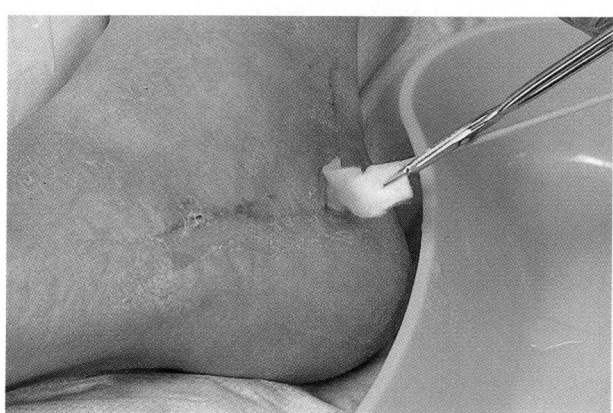

Step 8a Gently press gauze into wound.

   b. If wound is deep, use forceps or cotton-tipped applicators to press gauze into all wound surfaces.
   Rationale: Moist gauze absorbs drainage.
9. Apply several dry, sterile 4 × 4 pads over the wet gauze.

PROCEDURE 38-2 (Continued)

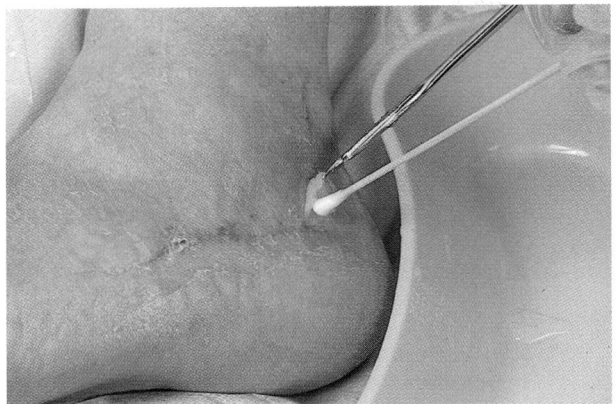

Step 8b Press gauze into all wound surfaces.

Rationale: Extra pads help absorb excess moisture from under dressings.

10. Place ABD pad over dry 4 × 4 pads.
    Rationale: Protect the wound from contamination.
11. Dispose of sterile gloves.
12. Secure dressings with tape, Kerlix gauze (for circumferential dressings), or Montgomery ties.
13. Assist client to a comfortable position.
14. Wash your hands.
15. Document procedure and observations.

Lifespan Considerations, Home Care Modifications, and Collaboration and Delegation

See Procedure 38-1.

A suture, the material used to sew an incision together, can be absorbable (e.g., catgut, chromic) or nonabsorbable (e.g., nylon, silk, polypropylene). The type of suture used depends on the wound's size and location, how strong the suture material needs to be, the desired cosmetic effect, and the surgeon's preference. Usually, the least amount and smallest size of suture result in optimal wound closure.

Skin staples are made of stainless steel and are minimally reactive to the body as a foreign substance. Usually when skin staples are used, absorbable sutures are used to close viscera and underlying tissue layers. Staples decrease the risk of infection and reduce tissue handling because they allow faster wound closure. Larger stainless-steel clips also may be used to approximate wound edges.

Inspect sutures, staples, or clips when dressings are changed and routinely if a transparent dressing is used. The physician determines how long they must remain in place. Sutures are usually removed 7 to 10 days after surgery if wound edges are well approximated and healing appears normal. Skin staples are usually removed in 5 to 7 days, but larger retention sutures may remain in place longer. Sometimes, the physician orders removal of every other staple or suture to ensure that adequate healing has occurred and to avoid dehiscence. Most surgical clients also have absorbable sutures in place holding deeper layers of tissue or fascia together.

Staples are removed with a staple remover (Fig. 38-12); it is inserted under each staple, and the handle is compressed.

The pressure causes the staple to bend in the middle, and the edges pop out of the skin. The client may experience minor discomfort as the staples are removed. Steristrips are usually applied after the staples are removed to keep skin edges approximated until healing is more complete.

Sutures are removed with a forceps and scissors. The suture is cut close to the skin, and the forceps is used to remove the suture. Care is essential to avoid pulling the visible portion of the suture through underlying tissue, because this can contaminate the incisional area and contribute to an infection. Sutures may be intermittent or continuous, and the nurse must discern the suturing technique before removing the sutures. As with staples, Steristrips are often applied after suture removal.

Cyanoacrylate Glue. An adhesive glue for human skin is available and may be used to close acute wounds in certain situations. The wound must be easily approximated and on a part of the body that will not be subject to tension or stretching. The adhesive material gradually sloughs away over a period of days and must be protected from scratching or rubbing during the first several days after application.

Ace Wraps and Bandages. Ace wraps are elastic bandages used to support an area and frequently to secure dressings (Fig. 38-13). Incorrectly applied, Ace wraps and gauze wraps can lead to edema and impaired circulation. An Ace bandage should be applied in a distal to proximal direction when used

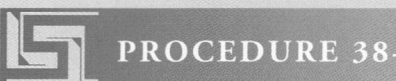

PROCEDURE 38-3

IRRIGATING A WOUND

Purpose
1. Cleanse the wound by removing debris and exudate.
2. Instill medication into the wound (if ordered).
3. Promote wound healing.

Assessment
- Review physician's orders for type and strength of solution to use for irrigation.
- Assess wound's location and size to determine needed dressing supplies.
- Assess client's comfort level. Give analgesics as needed before wound care.
- Assess for symptoms of anxiety.
- Review chart for presence of generalized symptoms of infection (e.g., elevated temperature, leukocytosis).

Equipment
Sterile dressing instrument set and dressing materials, as in Procedure 38-2
Sterile gloves
Sterile basin
Mask, goggles, and gown may be indicated to protect nurse's eyes, mouth, and clothes from splatter
Clean basin to collect contaminated irrigating solution
Prescribed irrigating solution warmed to body temperature
Sterile irrigating solution
Sterile latex or silicone catheter (optional for deep wounds)
Waterproof disposal bag
Waterproof underpad
35-ml syringe and 19-gauge needle

Procedure
1. Close door or curtains around bed. Explain procedure to client.
2. Position client comfortably to allow irrigating solution to flow by gravity across the wound and into a collection basin.
   Rationale: Solution must flow from least contaminated to most contaminated area. Gravity directs the flow.
3. Expose only the wound area. Place waterproof pad under client.
   Rationale: Protect linen from spill of irrigating solution.
4. Wash your hands.
   Rationale: Handwashing helps prevent transfer of microorganisms.

5. Don mask, goggles, and gown if needed.
   Rationale: Protect mucous membranes and clothing from accidental splashing of wound irrigation.
6. Remove dressing and inspect wound. See Steps 1 through 4 of Procedure 38-2.
7. Pour warmed irrigating solution into sterile basin.
   Rationale: Warmed solution is more comfortable for client and reduces risk of chilling.
8. Open irrigating syringe, and place into basin with solution.
9. Place second basin at distal end of wound.
   Rationale: Basin will catch contaminated irrigating solution.
10. Don sterile gloves.
    Rationale: Wearing gloves maintains surgical asepsis.
11. Fill irrigating syringe with solution. Holding syringe tip about 1 inch above the wound, gently flush all wound areas. Continue flushing until solution draining into basin is clear.
    Rationale: Holding syringe tip above tissue prevents trauma to granulation tissue and prevents risk of contaminating syringe tip. Irrigating until clear ensures removal of all debris and exudate.

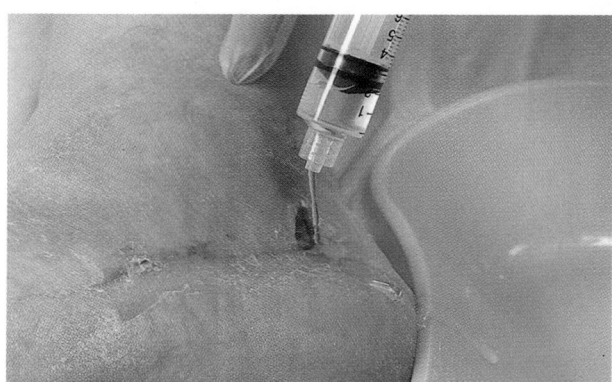

Step 11 Flush the wound with irrigating solution.

12. If wound is deep, attach a latex or silicone catheter to filled syringe with irrigating solution. Gently insert catheter into wound and flush until returning solution is clear.
    Rationale: Catheter introduces solution deeper into wound. Note: When refilling irrigation syringe with solution, disconnect catheter, fill syringe, and reconnect catheter. Doing so prevents contaminating the basin of solution with microorganisms from the catheter.

PROCEDURE 38-3 (Continued)

13. Dry surrounding skin thoroughly.
    Rationale: Excess moisture on skin promotes growth of microorganisms and skin breakdown.
14. Apply sterile dressing.
    Rationale: Sterile dressing provides protective barrier over wound.
15. Remove and discard gloves.
16. Secure dressing with tape or Montgomery straps.
17. Assist client to a comfortable position.
18. Dispose of equipment. *Note:* Retain remaining bottle of sterile solution for future irrigations.

Mark date and time of opening on bottle for reference. Dispose according to agency policy.
19. Wash your hands.
20. Document procedure and observations.

Lifespan Considerations, Home Care Modifications, and Collaboration and Delegation
Refer to Procedure 38-1.

---

on an extremity. Pressure, when applied circumferentially to an extremity, should be more snug at the distal end of the extremity to facilitate venous return.

Frequent assessment of body parts distal from the bandage site (e.g., fingers, toes) is necessary to detect impaired circulation promptly. Cyanosis, pallor, coolness, numbness, tingling, swelling, or absent or diminished pulse are signs that circulation may be decreased or that nerve function is impaired. Many bandages are routinely removed so that the area can be inspected and areas of pressure avoided.

Binders. **Binders** are used to support a specific body part or to hold dressings in place. The use of Velcro in binders has increased their ease of application and comfort. Velcro fas-

teners permit individualized adjustments and securely fasten the binder in place, while permitting quick and easy release. Binders come in different shapes and sizes depending on the area for use. The binders most commonly used for support are abdominal binders and slings.

An abdominal binder is applied to the lower abdomen but not over the ribs. It is used to support the torso, especially after abdominal surgery. It is usually a straight piece of elastic fabric, 15 to 20 cm wide and long enough to go around the torso.

Drainage Management
A large amount of wound drainage can inhibit wound healing and impair skin integrity around the wound. Nurses promote optimal wound healing by ensuring that closed drainage

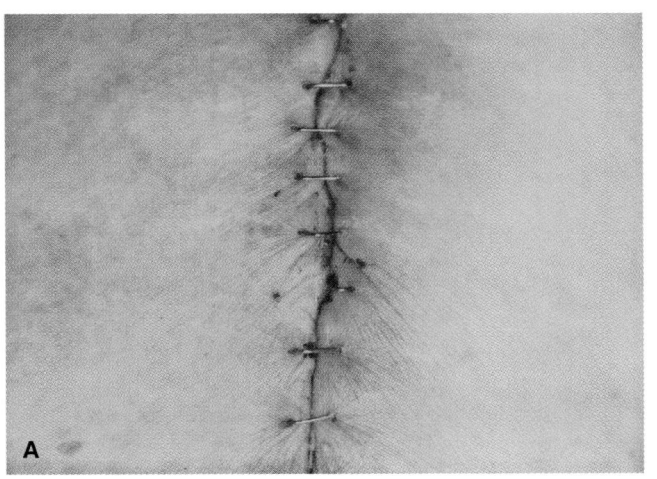
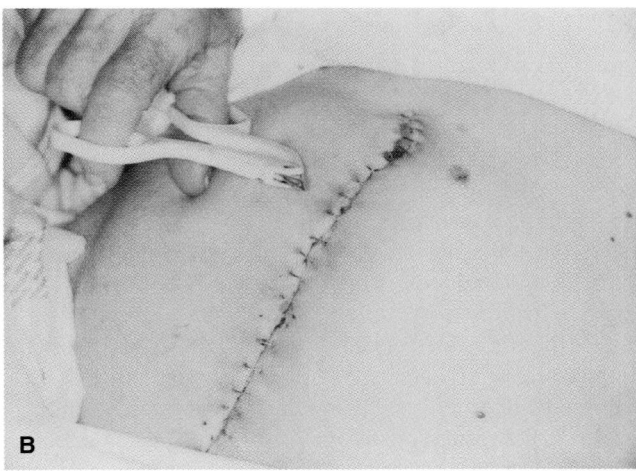

FIGURE 38-12   (A) Skin staples. (B) Skin staples and staple remover.

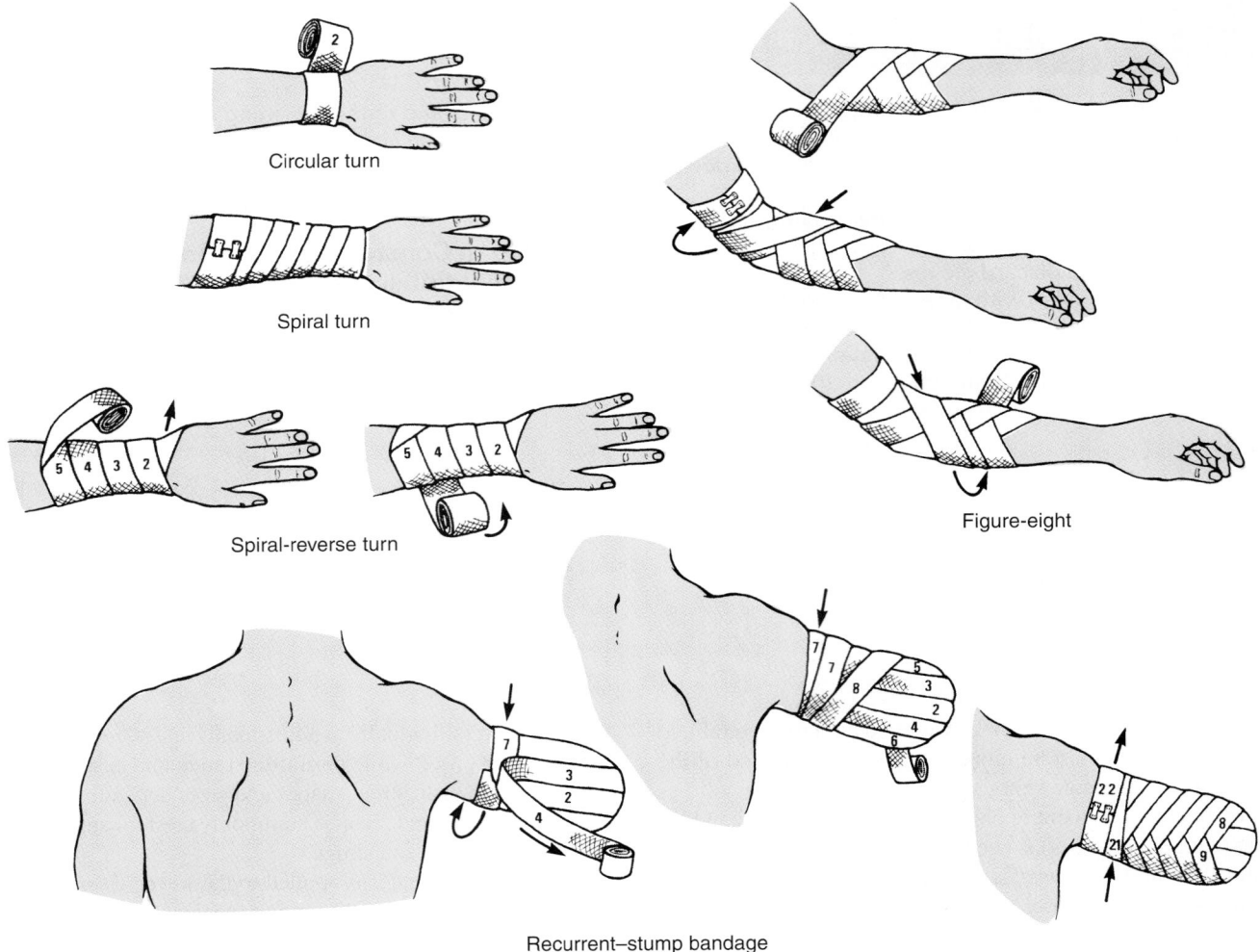

Circular turn

Spiral turn

Spiral-reverse turn

Figure-eight

Recurrent—stump bandage

FIGURE 38-13   Techniques for bandage application.

systems function properly and by selecting dressings that adequately absorb wound drainage. Nurses also protect skin from irritation by protecting surrounding skin from caustic drainage or constant moisture (Procedure 38-4).

Local Application of Heat and Cold

Therapeutic uses of heat and cold to promote healing and client comfort are summarized in Table 38-4. Cold therapies are usually used immediately after injury to control hemorrhage, edema, and pain. Cold is used to control local bleeding because it causes vasoconstriction, which decreases blood flow to the area and helps control swelling. Heat therapies are used to increase blood flow, resolve inflammation, improve healing of soft tissues, and relieve muscular pain and stiffness. Local heat causes vasodilation, increasing the supply of oxygen, nutrients, leukocytes, and antibodies to the tissues. The increased blood flow also promotes removal of metabolic wastes and dissipation of heat. Heat allows pus to consolidate in infected areas. Heat also promotes muscular relaxation and relieves muscle tension, spasms, and joint

stiffness. A disadvantage of local heat is that increased capillary permeability can increase edema formation.

Client safety is an important consideration when using heat or cold, because these therapies can damage tissues or alter thermoregulation. Table 38-5 lists precautions for the safe use of heat or cold.

The duration of application is important. Maximum vasodilation or vasoconstriction usually occurs in 30 minutes, and prolonged application may result in burns or freezing. Very young clients and older clients have a decreased ability to tolerate heat and cold and are more likely to suffer adverse effects. Impairments to circulation, sensation, or cognitive abilities also increase the incidence of injury. Body areas where heat or cold therapy is used can be more or less sensitive, depending on the skin's sensitivity or thickness. Impaired skin integrity increases the chance that heat or cold application could damage tissues. Extensive exposure to heat or cold can have systemic and local effects. Unexpected adverse effects can occur, especially in high-risk clients, such as the very young and the elderly.

PROCEDURE 38-4

MAINTAINING A PORTABLE (HEMOVAC) WOUND SUCTION

Purpose
1. Facilitate healing by removing drainage from the incisional area where granulation tissue is forming.

Assessment
- Assess client for generalized signs of infection (e.g., elevated temperature).
- Assess drainage for amount, color, clarity, and odor.
- Assess the client for inflammation or discomfort around the drain.

Equipment
Clean disposable gloves
Calibrated drainage receptacle

Procedure
1. Explain procedure; assist client to a comfortable position; pull curtains or close door.
2. Wash your hands. Don clean disposable gloves. *Rationale: Handwashing and gloves help prevent transfer of microorganisms.*
3. Expose Hemovac tubing and container while keeping client draped. *Rationale: Provide privacy and warmth for the client.*
4. Examine tubing and container for patency and suction seal. *Note:* If the system's seal is broken, the Hemovac reservoir will be expanded and not compressed.
5. Open the drainage plug (it is labeled).

6. Pour drainage into a calibrated receptacle without contaminating the drainage spout. *Rationale: This action prevents transfer of microorganisms to the wound. A closed drainage system is established.*
7. Reestablish suction by placing reservoir on a firm, flat surface. With drainage plug open, compress the unit and reinsert drainage plug.

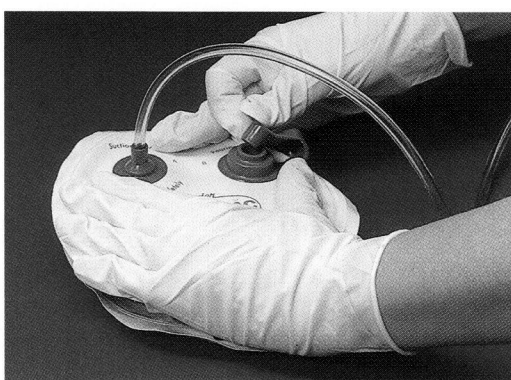

Step 7 Compress the reservoir and close the drainage plug.

8. Remove and discard gloves.
9. Return client to a comfortable position.
10. Measure drainage and record amount, color, and any other pertinent information.

Collaboration and Delegation
- Instruct ancillary staff to report if suction device becomes filled with drainage or tubing appears dislodged.

 SAFETY ALERT
During heating pad use, inspect the skin frequently, especially for clients with decreased sensation. Thermal burns may result.

Cold Packs and Ice Bags. Cold packs and ice bags are used to deliver local dry cold. Commercial cold packs contain an alcohol-based solution that is released inside the bag when it is squeezed or kneaded, creating a cold temperature. The outer covering is soft and pliable, so it can be molded to fit the body's contours and applied directly to the skin surface. These packs cannot be refrozen.

Ice bags come in a variety of sizes and can be used to control localized bleeding, reduce swelling, and reduce pain. Some ice bags are made of rubber and have screw-on caps for filling. Before applying a rubber bag, place a cloth cover over the rubber surface to avoid irritating the skin and to maintain

TABLE 38-4

Uses for Heat and Cold		
Effect	Physiologic Mechanism	Selected Uses
Heat Application		
Promotes healing and suppuration (consolidation of pus)	Results in vasodilation leading to increased blood flow, thus increasing oxygen and nutrients to the area and promoting removal of waste products	Surgical wounds, infected wounds, hemorrhoids, episiotomies
Decreases inflammation by accelerating inflammatory process	Increases capillary wall permeability, increases leukocyte and antibody flow to area, promotes action of phagocytes	Phlebitis, IV infiltration
Decreases musculoskeletal discomfort	Increases sensory nerve conduction, promotes muscle relaxation, decreases viscosity of synovial fluid	Low back pain, menstrual cramps, contractures, arthritis, muscle spasms
Cold Application		
Controls bleeding	Results in vasoconstriction, which decreases blood flow, and, in turn, decreases metabolic tissue demands and the supply of oxygen and nutrients	Fractures, trauma, superficial lacerations, puncture wounds
Decreases edema	Decreases capillary permeability; causes vasoconstriction	Sprains, muscle strains, sports injuries
Relieves pain	Decreases nerve conduction velocity; induces numbness or paresthesia	Arthritis, trauma, musculoskeletal injuries

TABLE 38-5

Precautions for the Safe Use of Heat and Cold	
Assessment Factor	Rationale
Acute sudden pain that may indicate abscessed tooth or appendicitis	Application of heat may cause rupture, with systemic spread of infection.
Broken skin or deep open wounds	Subcutaneous and visceral tissues are more sensitive to temperature extremes. Fewer pain and temperature receptors are available to warn of possible tissue damage.
Circulatory impairment (peripheral vascular disease, diabetes)	Cold application vasoconstricts, thus decreasing circulation to the already compromised area. Heat is not dissipated well from the area, making tissue damage more likely.
Sensory deficits (cerebrovascular accident, paraplegia, quadriplegia)	Alterations in nerve conduction limit the sensation of temperature or pain, thus increasing the likelihood of tissue damage.
Mental status impairment (confusion, decreased level of consciousness)	Decreased reliability of reporting pain and altered sensation increases the possibility of tissue damage.
Age extremes	Very young children have immature thermoregulation, cannot communicate pain or discomfort specifically, and cannot alter their environment. Elderly may have reduced sensation to pain and often have another impairment (e.g., circulatory, sensory) that compounds the risk. Heat should not be applied to the abdomen of a pregnant woman because fetal growth could be affected.
Metallic implants (pacemakers, total joint replacements)	Metal is a good conductor of heat, thus increasing the potential for burns because the implant cannot be readily removed.

medical asepsis. When administering cold therapy with children, using a plastic glove with a "face" marked on it may be helpful as a way of decreasing fear.

Cold Compresses. Cold compresses are used to relieve swelling and inflammation. Gauze pads are moistened with chilled saline or water and applied to the appropriate area. If cold compresses are applied to an open wound, asepsis must be maintained. Compresses easily conform to the contour of the intended area and can soften exudate. Because cold compresses quickly warm to the temperature of the client's skin, they need to be changed frequently. If they are left on a wound for a prolonged period, maceration can occur.

Warm Compresses. Warm compresses may be applied to improve circulation and to promote suppuration. If commercially prepared compresses are unavailable, solution can be warmed and applied to gauze pads. Avoid using temperatures that might cause burns.

The heat of a warm compress dissipates quickly but can be retained longer by applying a layer of plastic over the compress. If a constant warm temperature is desired, apply a heating mechanism over the compress (e.g., an aquathermia pad). But because moisture conducts heat, the temperature of the heating mechanism must set at low.

Warm Soaks. Warm soaks involve immersing a body part in a warm liquid (usually water) to promote relaxation, improve circulation, or soften wound exudate. They also can be used to apply a medicated solution. Warm soaks usually take about 20 minutes, and the solution may need to be changed because cooling commonly occurs.

Sitz Baths. A sitz bath provides moist heat to the pelvic and perineal areas. A sitz bath is used after rectal or perineal surgery or after vaginal delivery to decrease inflammation and discomfort. The client sits in a special tub or in a basin that fits onto the toilet seat, so the legs and feet remain out of the water. Using a bathtub does not serve the same purpose, because immersing the entire body in warm water nullifies the effect of local heat applied to the pelvic area. The client's feet and upper torso should remain covered to prevent chilling. The sitz bath is filled with warm water (105° to 110°F [40° to 43°C]). A plastic bag with attached tubing is filled with warm water and inserted into the portable sitz bath, where it slowly replenishes warm water during the procedure. Sitz baths usually last for about 20 minutes. Because heat is being applied to a large area, vasodilation can occur, causing the client to feel lightheaded and faint. If this occurs, assess the client for a rapid pulse, pale facial color, or complaints of nausea. If these signs and symptoms are present, discontinue the sitz bath.

Hot Packs. Dry local heat can be applied with hot-water bottles, commercially available packs, or electric heating pads. Local heat treatments are usually applied for 20 to 30 min-

utes at a time. Instruct the client not to lie on the heating pad, which increases the likelihood of a burn.

Aquathermia Pads. An aquathermia pad is a heating unit consisting of a waterproof pad through which water circulates. It is used to provide moist heat, treat muscle spasms, and reduce inflammation. Check the water level in the aquathermia unit periodically, because evaporation may occur. Refill it as necessary.

Heat Lamps. Heat lamps are used to increase circulation and to provide comfort to small areas, such as episiotomy incisions. The area to be treated must be free of moisture, which could conduct heat. The heat lamp is placed an appropriate distance away from the treatment area (at least 45 cm), and low-wattage bulbs (40 to 60 watts) are used. The treatment lasts about 20 minutes. During treatment, the client's skin should be assessed periodically to ensure that no burns occur. Heat lamps are contraindicated in pressure ulcer care.

Adjunctive Therapies

A number of modalities that complement traditional wound management are available (Papantonio, 1998). Although their effect on wound healing is unclear, their use is widespread among clients who seek both medical and alternative therapies. These modalities include practices such as tribal healing rituals, energy healing (therapeutic touch), magnet therapy, and acupuncture.

New treatment methods for the management of very large or chronic wounds are being developed as well, including vacuum-assisted closure devices, radiant heat bandages, and hyperbaric oxygen therapy. Further studies are indicated to show the effects of new treatment methods on wound healing.

Emotional Support

Skin conditions can cause low self-esteem and altered body image, especially if the face or other highly visible area is disfigured. Clients may choose isolation over appearing in public. Getting clients to express feelings about perceived or actual disfigurement is the first step in facing the problem. Nurses can help clients identify appropriate diversional activities. Support people can help clients work through the isolation. Referrals to appropriate community resources can help avoid isolation.

Healthcare Planning and Home or Community-Based Nursing

Skin disorders and wounds require regular care and assessment for complications. Some clients obtain their care at home, whereas others require temporary hospitalization. Regardless of where the care is provided, the following principles apply:

- The environment should be clean.
- Wound care supplies must be accessible and available.

THERAPEUTIC DIALOGUE
Skin Integrity and Wound Healing

Scene for Thought
Mrs. Cook is a 72-year-old woman, active in the retirement community where she lives. The community health nurse frequently visits the retirement community. Today, Mrs. Cook wants to see the nurse about "a rash."

Less Effective

Nurse: Hi, Mrs. Cook. What can I do for you?

Client: I need to show you this mole. It's been bleeding when it rubs against my collar *(Looks worried.)*

Nurse: *(Examines the mole carefully.)* I don't see any problem right now, Mrs. Cook, but I think you need to see your primary care provider. Shall I make the appointment for you? *(Looks up the physician's number in the card file.)*

Client: No, no. I'll do it myself. I'll use the one that removed my husband's skin cancer. *(Still looks worried.)*

Nurse: That sounds like a good plan. At least the physician will be familiar. Anything else?

Client: No, that's okay. Have a good week. *(Leaves the office with mouth set grimly.)*

More Effective

Nurse: Hi there, Mrs. Cook. How are you?

Client: Hi, Rhonda. I'm so glad to see you. I was worried you wouldn't be here today. *(Looks concerned and a little scared.)*

Nurse: Here I am. What can I help you with?

Client: I'm worried about this mole I have on the back of my neck. It rubs against my collar, and yesterday I found blood on the collar in the same place as the mole. Could you look at it? *(Shows the nurse who finds a small amount of dried blood on the mole.)*

Nurse: How long have you had the mole?

Client: Years and years. I never noticed anything about it until now, though. *(Continues to look worried.)*

Nurse: What worries you about this, Mrs. Cook?

Client: Cancer. My husband had a lot of these removed, and both my parents had skin cancer. Could it be cancer? *(Her body stiffens as she awaits the answer.)*

Nurse: It could be, but it may not. Your primary care provider needs to see it and will possibly remove it in the office. Then it'll go to the pathologist for examination of the cells. You should know if it's cancer or not within a week. What do you think?

Client: I think I'd better make the appointment today. I want to know as soon as possible. Thanks, Rhonda.

Critical Thinking Challenge
- Analyze what the second nurse did that the first didn't.
- Detect what clue the first nurse missed and what difference it made.
- In both instances, Mrs. Cook will call the primary care provider to be seen, evaluated, and helped. Compare and contrast the nursing care that each nurse supplied.
- Infer how Mrs. Cook would seek care in the future from both nurses.

- The client should receive adequate calories and nutrients to facilitate healing.
- The person providing wound or skin care should demonstrate the ability to perform the procedures and should know what symptoms to report to the healthcare provider.

Provide information about methods to prevent pressure ulcers: frequent turning and proper positioning, hygiene, and nutrition. Describe the topical wound care products and demonstrate the correct method of use. Encourage the use of pressure-reducing support surfaces. Assist clients to select an appropriate support surface for their use.

Clients who need dressing changes must demonstrate the ability to perform wound care or receive assistance from a caregiver or healthcare worker in that process. Clients and involved family members should learn how to detect infection and monitor the client's temperature. Instructions (written and verbal) that include information on where to buy supplies should be provided. Clients who are unable to afford the needed products should receive assistance in making the treatment plan workable, which may include referral for assistance with healthcare expenses. Family members' acceptance of the skin impairment and their willingness to assist with care boost the client's self-esteem.

Wound and skin problems can take an extended time to resolve. Instruct clients about the frequency of required follow-up medical appointments and symptoms of complications or recurrence. As indicated, teach about the disorder's etiology, control or risk factors, and the importance of maintaining healthy skin function.

EVALUATION

The evaluation of client-centered goals determines whether the outcome criteria have been met for the prevention of tissue damage and promotion of optimal wound healing.

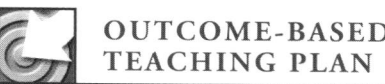

OUTCOME-BASED TEACHING PLAN

Sidney Smith, a 56-year-old engineer, is being seen in the clinic after a surgical procedure to repair a fracture in the foot. The site of the surgical incision has failed to heal. As a result, the incision site is open and requires daily dressing changes. He and his wife are here to learn the procedure.

OUTCOME: Client/spouse can demonstrate the correct procedure for the dressing change.
Strategies
- Describe the reasons for doing this dressing change with packing.
- Review the equipment necessary to perform the procedure.
- Demonstrate the correct way to remove the old dressing and cleanse the wound.
- Explain how to handle the new packing and dressing aseptically.
- Provide a written plan of the procedure for their reference.
- Review both the procedure and plan to determine any questions.
- Have client, and spouse if indicated, return demonstrate the procedure before leaving the clinic.
- Arrange for follow-up with home care as necessary to evaluate performance and continue teaching.

OUTCOME: Client/spouse can verbalize the signs and symptoms to watch for in the wound.
Strategies
- Discuss with Mr. and Mrs. Smith the changes in the wound site that might indicate infection or other aspects of poor healing.
- Provide a written list of warning signs that necessitate contacting their healthcare provider.
- Have Mr. and Mrs. Smith verbalize these factors back to you.
- Problem solve with Mr. and Mrs. Smith how they will record the progress of the wound closure and healing and bring the record to the next clinic visit.

Outcome criteria should be individualized for each client and revised as necessary.

Goal

The client's skin will remain intact without areas of local inflammation.

Possible Outcome Criteria

- The client develops no skin lesions or pressure ulcers.
- The client develops no redness or abrasions of the skin.
- The client has intact skin without excessive drying or flaking.

Goal

The client's wound will demonstrate evidence of healing.

Possible Outcome Criteria

- Within 24 hours, wound edges are well approximated.
- Within 48 hours, the wound shows evidence of increased granulation tissue.
- By discharge, the client's wound is free of redness, swelling, and purulent drainage.

Goal

The client will verbalize understanding of preventive skin care.

Possible Outcome Criteria

- After a teaching session, the client verbalizes interventions that can prevent pressure ulcer formation.
- The client identifies causes of mechanical or chemical tissue destruction.
- The client demonstrates routine skin care measures to prevent excessive drying or abrasions.

Goal

The client or family will demonstrate appropriate wound management technique.

Possible Outcome Criteria

- After a teaching session, the client states important measures to promote skin integrity and wound healing.
- The client maintains adequate nutritional intake.
- By discharge, the client or family members demonstrate wound care and dressing change.
- The client discusses signs of wound infection and when to contact a healthcare provider.
- The client or family members demonstrate proper use of special equipment needed to promote skin integrity.

KEY CONCEPTS

- The skin's physiologic functions are protection, thermoregulation, sensation, metabolism, and communication.
- The skin's health depends on sufficient blood flow, adequate nutrition, an intact epidermis, and proper hygiene.
- The very young and the very old are most susceptible to skin disruption.
- Altered skin integrity may be manifested by pruritus, rash, lesions, pain, and inadequate wound healing.
- Understanding the phases of wound healing is vital for proper wound assessment and management.
- Depth of injury affects the choice of topical treatment.
- Hemorrhage, infection, dehiscence, and fistula formation are potential complications of wounds.
- Factors affecting wound healing include oxygenation and nutrient supply, immune cellular function, age, obesity, smoking, drug intake, systemic disease, stress, nature of the injury, wound infection, and the environment.

NURSING PLAN OF CARE

THE CLIENT WITH IMPAIRED SKIN INTEGRITY

Nursing Diagnosis

Impaired Skin Integrity related to pressure, friction, and immobility manifested by 3-cm stage III sacral pressure ulcer

Client Goal

Client/family will comply with regimen to prevent and treat pressure ulcers.

Client Outcome Criteria

• Client discusses pressure ulcers in his or her own words.
• Client describes five contributing factors to pressure ulcer development.
• Client inspects skin daily.
• Before discharge, client demonstrates interventions to relieve pressure effectively.

Nursing Intervention	**Scientific Rationale**
1. Teach the client and family what pressure ulcers are; use photographs.	1. Knowledge is important in developing values to maintain preventive health practices.
2. Discuss factors that can increase incidence of pressure ulcer formation.	2. Specific knowledge allows client to develop interventions that help prevent pressure ulcers.
3. Teach client or family to inspect all pressure points daily and to use a mirror for hard to visualize areas.	3. Daily inspection helps to detect any evidence of skin abnormality promptly.
4. Elicit client's preference for equipment (e.g., support surfaces), skin treatment, turning schedules.	4. Client's active involvement in individualizing prevention plan helps ensure compliance.

Client Goal

Client's sacral pressure ulcer will heal.

Client Outcome Criteria

• Client demonstrates increased granulation tissues in healing wound.
• Client demonstrates absence of redness, swelling, and purulent drainage.

Nursing Intervention	**Scientific Rationale**
1. Reposition q2h, increasing frequency of positioning if redness or blanching does not disappear.	1. Repositioning relieves pressure, which can include capillary blood flow leading to tissue damage and ulcer formation.
2. Do not allow client to lie on healing pressure ulcer. Turn right to left, left to right, and right to prone.	2. Delicate healing tissues are more susceptible to trauma and impaired blood flow; pressure delays healing.
3. Use pillows to position and support pressure points.	3. Padding decreases pressure and friction, which can increase pressure sore development.
4. Instruct client to get up in chair at least 30 minutes twice a day.	4. Different body positions and movement improve overall circulation and relieve pressure from ulcer area.
5. Communicate turning schedule on wall at client's bedside.	5. Communication of specific times and positions helps promote compliance with turning schedule.
6. Avoid high Fowler or semi-Fowler position while client is in bed.	6. These positions increase shearing force, which impairs circulation as client slides down in bed.
7. Use turning sheet when moving client up in bed.	7. This action decreases shearing force and friction from bed when moving client.

NURSING PLAN OF CARE

THE CLIENT WITH IMPAIRED SKIN INTEGRITY (*Continued*)

8. Apply pressure-reducing or pressure-relieving overlay.

9. Keep skin clean and dry, especially after episodes of incontinence.
10. Apply hydrocolloid dressing to pressure ulcer; change every 7 days unless barrier is broken. Inspect each shift.
11. Encourage protein and vitamin-rich diet; assess dietary intake, and assist with menu choices.

8. Special mattress overlays decrease the chance of occlusion of capillary blood flow, which can increase pressure sore development and delay healing.
9. Moisture promotes maceration of tissues and delays healing.
10. Hydrocolloid dressing protects ulcer to promote healing and prevent infection.

11. Adequate nutrition is necessary for wound healing.

- In the nursing assessment, data are collected about normal skin status, risk for skin impairment, and identification of altered skin integrity.
- Planned nursing interventions are important to prevent pressure ulcer development and trauma to skin.
- Gauzes, transparent film, polyurethane foam, hydrocolloids, hydrogels, and alginates are categories of dressings used in topical care.
- Sutures, staples, clips, Steristrips, bandages, and binders can provide wound support.
- Effective management of drainage promotes optimal wound healing.
- Local application of heat and cold can decrease inflammation, improve healing, and reduce pain.
- Client teaching is important for long-range promotion and maintenance of skin integrity.

REFERENCES

Anonymous. (2000). The Wound Product Sourcebook (3rd ed.). Hinesburg, VT: Green Mountain Wellness Publishers.

Beitz, J. M., & Caldwell, D. (1998). Abdominal wound with enterocutaneous fistula: A case study. *Journal of Wound Ostomy, and Continence Nursing, 25*(2), 102–106.

Bergstrom, N., Bennett, M. A., Carlson, C. E., et al. (1994). *Treatment of pressure ulcers. Clinical Practice Guideline, No. 15.* AHCPR Pub. No. 95-0652. Rockville, MD: U.S. Department of Health and Human Services, Public Health Service, Agency for Health Care Policy and Research.

Colsky, A. S., Kirsner, R. S., & Kerdel, F. A. (1998). Microbiologic evaluation of cutaneous wounds in hospitalized dermatology patients. *Ostomy/Wound Management, 44*(3), 40–42, 44, 46.

Denig, N. I., et al. (1998). Irritant contact dermatitis: Clues to causes, clinical characteristics, and control. *Postgraduate Medicine, 103*(5), 199–200, 207–208, 212–213.

Gordon, M. (1997). *Manual of nursing diagnosis 1997–1998* (8th ed.). St. Louis, MO: Mosby–Year Book.

Jackson, A. (1998). The clinical signs of melanoma. *The Practitioner, 242*(1585), 254, 256, 260, 262, 264.

Kirsner, R. S., & Froelich, C. W. (1998). Soaps and detergents: Understanding their composition and effect. *Ostomy/Wound Management, 44*(3A Suppl.), 62S–69S.

Krasner, D. (1995). Minimizing factors that impair wound healing: A nursing approach. *Ostomy/Wound Management, 42*(1), 22–26, 28, 30–32.

Krasner, D. (1998). Diabetic ulcers of the lower extremity: A review of comprehensive management. *Ostomy/Wound Management, 44*(4), 56–58, 60–62, 64–66, 68, 70, 72.

Martin, P. (1997). Wound healing: Aiming for perfect skin regeneration. *Science, 276*(4), 75–81.

North American Nursing Diagnosis Association. (2000). *NANDA nursing diagnoses: Definitions and classification 2000–2001.* Philadelphia: Author.

Panel for the Prediction and Prevention of Pressure Ulcers in Adults. (1992). *Pressure ulcers in adults: Prediction and prevention. Clinical Practice Guideline, Number 3.* AHCPR Publication No. 92—0047. Rockville, MD: U.S. Department of Health and Human Services, Public Health Service, Agency for Health Care Policy and Research.

Papantonio, C. (1998). Alternative medicine and wound healing. *Ostomy/Wound Management, 44*(4), 44–55.

Pontiere-Lewis, V. (1995). Venous leg ulcers. *Medsurg Nursing, 4*(6), 492–493.

Rojas, M. G., & Reynolds, A. (1996). Pressure reducing capability of the Therarest hospital replacement mattress. *Journal of Wound, Ostomy and Continence Nursing, 23*(2), 100–104.

Scholl, D., & Langkamp-Henken, B. (2001). Nutrient recommendations for wound healing. *Journal of Intravenous Nursing 24*(2), 124–132.

Stotts, N. A., & Wipke-Tevis, D. (1997). Co-factors in impaired wound healing. In D. Krasner & D. Kane (Eds.), *Chronic wound care* (2nd ed.). Wayne, PA: Health Management Publications, pp. 64–72.

BIBLIOGRAPHY

Braden, B. J., & Bergstrom, N. (1987). A conceptual schema for the study of etiology of pressure sores. *Rehabilitation Nursing, 12*(1), 8–12.

Bryant, R. A. (2000). *Acute and chronic wounds* (2nd ed.). St. Louis, MO: Mosby.

Eager, C. A. (1997). Monitoring wound healing in the home health arena. *Advances in Wound Care, 10*(5), 54–57.

Faller, N. A., Kantorski, L., Morgan, B., & Keller, D. (1995). Using the nursing process to solve a problem: Post-op tape blisters. *Ostomy/Wound Management, 41*(1), 68–70.

Gleeson, C. A. (1995). Diabetic peripheral neuropathies. *Medsurg Nursing, 4*(2), 121–125.

Goldstein, B. G., & Goldstein, A. D. (1997). *Practical dermatology* (2nd ed.). St. Louis, MO: Mosby–Year Book.

Gordon, M., & Goodwin, C. W. (1997). Burns: Initial assessment, management, and stabilization. *Nursing Clinics of North America, 32*(2), 237–249.

Grindel, C. G., & Costello, M. C. (1996). Nutrition screening: An essential assessment parameter. *Medsurg Nursing, 5*(3), 145–156.

Knight, C. L. (1996). The chronic wound management decision tree: A tool for long-term care nurses. *Journal of Wound, Ostomy and Continence Nursing, 23*(2), 92–99.

Krouskop, T., & Van Rijswijk, L. (1995). Standardizing performance-based criteria for support surfaces. *Ostomy/Wound Management, 41*(1), 34–36, 38, 40–45.

Levin, M. E. (1998). Prevention and treatment of diabetic foot wounds. *Journal of Wound, Ostomy and Continence Nursing, 25*(3), 129–146.

Maklebust, J., & Sieggreen, M. (2001). *Pressure ulcers: Guidelines for prevention and management* (3rd ed.). Springhouse, PA: Springhouse Corporation.

McGough-Csarny, J., & Kopac, C. A. (1998). Skin tears in institutionalized elderly: An epidemiological study. *Ostomy/Wound Management, 44*(3A Suppl.), 14S–25S.

Morison, M., Moffatt, C., Bridel-Nixon, J., & Bale, S. (1997). A color guide to the nursing management of chronic wounds (2nd ed.). Barcelona, Spain: Mosby.

Phillips, J. K. (1998). Action stat: Wound dehiscence. *Nursing '98, 28*(3), 33.

Pieper, B. L., Sugrue, M., Weiland, M., et al. (1998). Risk factors, prevention methods, and wound care for patients with pressure ulcers. *Clinical Nurse Specialist, 12*(1), 7–14.

Robinson, J. K., et al. (1998). What promotes skin self-examination? *Journal of the American Academy of Dermatology, 38*(5) Part 1, 752–757.

Wikblad, K., & Anderson, B. (1995). A comparison of three wound dressings in patients undergoing heart surgery. *Nursing Research, 44,* 312–316.

39 The Body's Defense Against Infection

Key Terms

agranulocytes
anaerobes
antigen
bacteremia
colonization
communicable disease
complement system

granulocytes
interferon
leukocytosis
neutropenia
normal flora
nosocomial infection
opportunistic

Learning Objectives

Upon completion of this chapter, the student will be able to do the following:

1. Name the major components of the body's normal resistance to infection and the role of each.
2. Differentiate between cellular and humoral immunity and between active and passive immunity.
3. Identify possible risk factors for infection or infectious diseases.
4. Name four common nosocomial infections.
5. Recognize common manifestations of infection.
6. Identify common diagnostic and laboratory tests used to identify or confirm an infectious process.
7. Describe major consequences of an infectious process.
8. Describe nursing measures that strengthen defense mechanisms against infection.

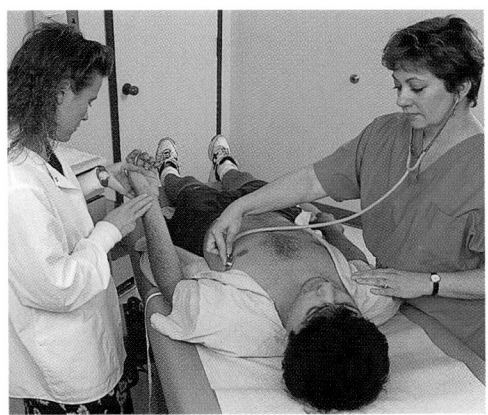

Critical Thinking Challenge

You are a nurse doing tuberculosis (TB) surveillance for the public health department. A new client is a 31-year-old man who had a positive purified protein derivative (PPD) test for TB last week when he was admitted to the hospital after a brawl in a local bar. Your client left the hospital AMA (against medical advice) before a definitive diagnosis of TB could be made. When you find your client, he is drinking in the same bar. After you introduce yourself, he swears at you, telling you to go away. He says he is not sick and does not need a nurse prying into his affairs.

Caring for people who are at risk for infection and protecting yourself and others who come in contact with clients with infections are nursing interventions of paramount importance. Once you have completed this chapter and incorporated information about infection into your knowledge base, review the above scenario and reflect on the following areas of Critical Thinking:

1. Analyze how you would feel personally after this verbal attack.
2. Propose possible factors contributing to your client's reluctance to talk to a nurse from the public health department.
3. Prioritize what is most important for your client at this time, and explain how you can help your client achieve these goals.
4. Weigh the rights of this client to refuse treatment with the rights of the general public to live in a safe environment.

Infectious diseases have changed history by wiping out large numbers of people, stopping industrial growth, causing migrations, and altering social structures. They continue to affect today's society significantly. Infections consume billions of dollars in healthcare costs and are a major cause of absenteeism from work and school. They are a common cause of significant morbidity and mortality throughout the world. In the past several decades, changing sexual practices have led to a dramatic and rapid spread of sexually transmitted diseases (STDs), including herpes, gonorrhea, and acquired immunodeficiency syndrome (AIDS). All of these diseases have had enormous social consequences. Tuberculosis, once thought to be a well-controlled communicable disease, is in some cases proving to be drug resistant. Increasing numbers of antibiotic-resistant infectious organisms are posing a very serious challenge to healthcare providers.

For infection to occur, an uninterrupted chain of conditions must allow microorganisms to grow, reproduce, be passed from place to place, and enter a susceptible host. This "chain of infection" is described in detail in Chapter 26 and illustrated in Fig. 26-1. When the chain of infection remains intact, people must rely on their bodily defenses to fight disease-causing microorganisms.

NORMAL RESISTANCE TO INFECTION

Microorganisms that live on the skin, in the nasopharynx, in the gastrointestinal (GI) tract, and on other body surfaces are referred to as **normal flora.** Normally, they pose no threat to the body. Sometimes, however, an agent can interact with a host that provides an environment for the agent's replication and growth. Infection results in such instances if the body's inflammatory and immune defenses fail.

Characteristics of Normal Resistance to Infection

The body's defenses against infection can be divided into two major groups: nonspecific natural defenses and specific acquired defenses. The types of human defenses against infection are outlined in Table 39-1.

Nonspecific Natural Defenses
Culture. Many ethnic groups have developed cultural habits that act as barriers to the spread of infection. Scientists are attempting to identify the roles of customs, genes, and religious rituals and practices in resisting infection.

A population can develop increased resistance to certain microorganisms over time or through other mechanisms. For example, Africans and African Americans living today who have inherited the genetic disease of sickle cell anemia do not contract malaria. This is presumably because the sickled shape of the RBC makes it difficult for the parasite causing malaria to enter. Because malaria kills more than 1 million people each year, this resistance provides an important form of immunity. But sickle cell anemia has other serious consequences.

Anatomic, Mechanical, and Chemical Barriers. The first line of defense against infection is intact skin and mucous membranes covering body cavities. They are the most important barriers to infection, and when they are intact, infection is rare. Chemical composition aids these physical barriers further. For example, the acidic nature of the skin and vagina helps to kill potential invaders before they enter the body. Some barriers, such as cells in the saliva, mucus, tears, and sweat, contain bactericidal enzymes.

Normal flora that grow on healthy tissues use local nutrients. Lack of nutrients and oxygen can inhibit the colonization and growth of pathogens. Mechanical forces, such as tears, saliva, and urine, wash bacteria from surfaces as they flow through the ducts and tracts. Peristalsis increases the mechanical cleansing of organ walls. Secretion of specific substances also defends against infection. **Interferon** is a nonspecific chemical inhibitor that is secreted by body cells in response to viral invasion.

White Blood Cells. Leukocytes, also called white blood cells (WBCs), and the inflammatory response make up the second line of defense to microbial invasion. Many leukocytes function as phagocytes, ingesting and thus destroying microbes. There are two categories of leukocytes:

- **Granulocytes** are polymorphonuclear cells that contain granules of digestive enzymes. Specific types of granulocytes include neutrophils, eosinophils, and basophils.
- **Agranulocytes** are mononuclear cells that lack digestive enzymes. Monocytes, which are immature macrophages and lymphocytes, are examples of agranulocytes.

Table 39-2 lists the actions of various WBCs.

Inflammatory Response. Inflammation is a nonspecific response to tissue injury that can be caused by microbial invasion or by mechanical, chemical, or heat injury. Inflammation attempts to limit an injury's extent. The blood vessels dilate, and plasma flows out of the capillaries into the irritated tissue. WBCs (typically neutrophils and then monocytes/macrophages) migrate into the area to attack and ingest the invaders by the process of phagocytosis. This activity leads to the four signs of inflammation at the injured area:

- *Redness* from blood accumulation in the dilated capillaries
- *Warmth* from the heat of the blood
- *Swelling* from fluid accumulation
- *Pain* from pressure or injury to the local nerves

The area becomes red, warm, swollen, and tender. It is inflamed but not necessarily infected.

Inflammation and phagocytosis work together to contain microorganisms. If these processes are successful, a collection of dead leukocytes, digested bacteria, dead tissue cells, and plasma may form into the material called pus.

Fever. Elevated body temperature also aids in the battle against infection. The hypothalamus raises the body's ther-

TABLE 39-1

Human Defenses Against Infection

Defense	Examples
Nonspecific Natural Defenses	
Individual factors	Heredity
	Good hygiene practices
	Good nutritional status
	Immunization history
Anatomic barriers	Intact skin
	Intact mucous membranes
Mechanical removal of microorganisms	Gastrointestinal motility
	Ciliary action in the respiratory tract
	Cleansing effect of urine's flow
	Expulsive effect of coughing and sneezing
	Lavaging effects of tears and saliva
	Shedding of uterine lining in menstruation
	Flow of organ secretions through ducts (e.g., bile)
Chemical factors*	Acidity of gastric secretions, vaginal secretions, and fatty acids of the skin
	Lysozyme enzymes in tears, nasal secretions, urine, and saliva
	Hormones secreted by the adrenal cortex and pancreas
	Indigenous microflora (competition)
Local tissue factors	Tissue surface receptor (occupancy)
	Inflammation
White blood cell function	Fever
	Phagocytosis
Acquired Specific Defenses[†]	Cellular immunity (T lymphocytes elaborate killer cells and helper cells)
	Humoral immunity (B lymphocytes produce antibodies to specific microorganisms)
	Memory of the organisms produces lasting immunity

* Factors that retard growth and provide less favorable media for growth.
[†] Person may acquire resistance naturally if he or she has had the infectious disease or has been immunized.

mostat in response to pyrogens released by some phagocytic cells (macrophages) after stimulation by microorganisms or endotoxins (Vander, Sherman, & Luciano, 2001). The rise in temperature increases cell metabolism.

Fever (defined as body temperature greater than 38.2°C [101°F]) helps combat infection by interrupting viral replication and slowing the rate of bacterial growth. Fever also increases the mobility of leukocytes and enhances their ability to phagocytize microorganisms. Also, the effects of endotoxins (toxins released by the immunogenic part of the bacterial cell wall of gram-negative bacteria, which triggers an immune response) decrease with elevated temperatures.

Fever is thought to have a beneficial effect on an infection's outcome if other body systems are not compromised. If fever is too high or prolonged, however, the person may become exhausted or suffer convulsions.

Specific Acquired Defenses: Immunity

Another important defense against infection is immunity. **Antigens** are foreign particles, such as microbes, that enter a host. In some cases, such as in autoimmune diseases, the immune system senses or recognizes the person's own cells as antigens.

The immune system response is stimulated when antigens enter the lymphatic and circulatory systems. The antigens are phagocytosed by macrophages, monocytes, or neutrophils, and the microbes are digested. Portions of the microbe, antigenic particles, stay with the phagocyte and are carried to the lymphoid tissue in the lymph node or the spleen. The phagocyte, usually a macrophage, presents this processed antigen to the lymphocytes, which then stimulate immune responses.

The two types of lymphocytes are T lymphocytes and B lymphocytes. Both originate from stem cells in the bone

TABLE 39-2

White Blood Cell Functions in Infection	
Cells	**Action**
Granulocytes	
Neutrophils	Phagocytes. They ingest and break down foreign particles, particularly bacteria and parasites. They are also an important link in generating fever to combat the proliferation of microorganisms.
Eosinophils	Allergic reaction. They increase in response to allergic and parasitic conditions when an antigen-antibody response occurs.
Basophils	Unknown. They contain heparin and histamine in their granules, which may be important in preventing blood clotting during an inflammatory response.
Agranulocytes	
T lymphocytes	Synthesis of immunoglobins. They produce cellular immunity. They are effective in destroying bacteria, viruses, and cancer cells. They recognize antigens and stimulate B lymphocytes and macrophages. Three types have been identified: helper cells, which stimulate other leukocytes; killer T cells, which recognize and destroy virus-infected cells; and suppressor cells, which tell the other cells to stop fighting after the antigenic substance is cleared.
B lymphocytes	Synthesis of antibodies. They produce humoral immunity. They are important in the immune response. They are stimulated by the T cells to divide and produce the plasma cells, which then produce specific antibodies to antigens. The memory cells carry the memory of the antigen and produce lasting immunity to the specific microorganism.
Monocytes (macrophages)	Scavenger cells. They dispose of cellular debris. Their numbers increase in the late stage of acute infections and during chronic infections. Levels also rise in response to viral, bacterial, and parasitic infections. They are considered important in activating the lymphocytes and are found in the reticuloendothelial system.

marrow and differentiate to become the lymphopoietic cells. Some pass through the thymus gland and become modified to form the thymus-dependent or T lymphocytes (also known as T cells). Others are modified by unknown mechanisms to become B lymphocytes.

The immune system conveys lasting resistance to infection by forming a "memory" of the antigen by means of specialized T and B lymphocytes and memory cells. T and B lymphocytes, the building blocks of the immune system, accumulate in lymph nodes along lymphatic vessels and are exposed to all antigens except those that enter the bloodstream directly. These lymphocytes are heavily concentrated in the tonsils and spleen, which are important tissues in children and young adults.

The immune system, if properly functioning, can produce resistance to disease recurrence. After an active infection, which may or may not be symptomatic, immunity to a specific pathogen usually results.

Cellular Immunity. Cellular immunity, consisting principally of T-lymphocyte activity, is stimulated by fungi, protozoa, bacteria, and some viruses. After T lymphocytes are stimulated, they enter the circulation from the lymphoid tissues and seek the site of the microbe. At the site, the lymphocytes produce proteins called lymphokines that draw more phagocytes to the area, keeping them there to fight the invader and increasing their killing power. Lymphokines disappear after the antigen has been eliminated. Some T cells, however, remain in the tissues and keep a memory of the antigen. Memory T lymphocytes are reactivated rapidly if the same antigen reappears.

Humoral Immunity. Humoral immunity takes place in the bloodstream. B lymphocytes provide humoral immunity by producing antibodies that convey specific resistance to many bacterial and viral infections. B lymphocytes, stimulated by the antigenic particles contained within the macrophages, produce plasma cells. The plasma cells then produce antibodies that are released into the bloodstream from the lymphoid tissue. **Antibodies,** also called *immunoglobulins,* circulate in the bloodstream and interact with antigens they encounter.

Antibodies are formed in response to substances found in bacterial cell walls, toxins, microbial enzymes, viruses, and other individual allergens. Antibodies act to make bacteria more susceptible to phagocytosis or to help in bacterial cell lysis. Antibodies formed in response to a virus neutralize the virus, act as antitoxins, or cause microbes to clump together or precipitate. Other antibodies make it easier for phagocytes to ingest microbes. Memory B lymphocytes remain in lymphoid tissue, where they can become reactivated if the pathogen appears again.

The **complement system,** a series of proteins found in the bloodstream, also aids in the antigen–antibody reaction. The complement system enhances phagocytosis of microbes, helps in lysis of bacterial cell walls, and encourages the inflammatory response.

Active Immunity. Active immunity is produced when the immune system is stimulated, either naturally or artificially, to produce antibodies. Natural immunity occurs after an infection has run its course. The client experiences a disease and produces an immune (antibody) response to the antigen. Active immunity can also be produced through vaccination. Vaccination is the process of injecting weakened or killed organisms into a person, stimulating antibody production. Vaccination produces an artificially acquired active immunity.

Passive Immunity. Passive immunity does not involve the host's immune response; rather, immunity is transferred to the recipient. This can be done in two ways. Antibodies can pass from a woman to her fetus by way of the placenta, or to her newborn through breast milk. Also, antibodies from a person or animal that has had a disease can be taken from the blood and given to another person for temporary passive protection. Passive immunity, which provides only temporary protection, is given in the form of immune globulins when there is not enough time for the person to acquire active immunization or when a vaccine does not exist for the disease.

Lifespan Considerations

Newborn and Infant
The immune system does not become fully operational until a baby reaches about 6 months of age. Before then, the infant's resistance to infection comes from the antibodies passed by way of the placenta and breast milk. Newborns have difficulty localizing infections (preventing the spread of organisms from the site of contact). Their phagocytes have difficulty trapping microbes, and they do not produce enough antibodies. At this time viral diseases such as chickenpox or herpes simplex, acquired from the birth canal or from an infected sibling, can cause severe widespread disease.

Newborns have immature thermoregulatory mechanisms and do not become febrile. Instead, they manifest infections more subtly, becoming lethargic or restless, or not feeding. After 2 to 4 months of age, infants begin producing antibodies. By 6 months, their lymphocytes are fully operational if they have had adequate nutrition (Tortora, Funke, & Case, 2001).

Toddler and Preschooler
Toddlers and preschoolers need supervision to prevent infections. Toddlers often play in dirt, are incontinent of urine and feces, and put things in their mouths. Although they are de-

veloping a mature immune system, they may not have been exposed to pathogens to give them immunity. By age 3 to 4 years, the immune system has matured to a level similar to that of adults in producing antibodies. Childhood vaccinations are timed to take advantage of this developing immunocompetence.

The most common infections in early childhood are respiratory tract infections. In children, the eustachian tubes are shorter and straighter than those of adults; middle ear infections (otitis media) are common because bacteria can easily pass from the nasopharynx to the ear canal. Children may suffer many colds each year, but by age 5 or 6 years their immune systems and body defenses have matured and the infections are more localized. The common communicable diseases are transmitted as children play with others.

Prevention of infections in early childhood requires the following:

- Good hygienic care of children and their food
- Adequate vaccinations
- Early infection treatment to prevent spread or prevent complications
- Isolation from infected people

Child and Adolescent
Communicable diseases are most prevalent as children enter school and organized play activities. They are most common during the winter, when children stay indoors. Children are also exposed to skin diseases, such as impetigo (from staphylococcal infections), roundworm infestations, and lice (from sharing combs, clothes, and sports equipment). A high incidence of streptococcal infections occurs in children age 6 to 12 years, resulting in pharyngitis, tonsillitis, and scarlet fever.

The person's immune system should be fully mature by adolescence but may be compromised by malnutrition or acquired disorders, such as chronic infections or illnesses. STDs, such as infectious mononucleosis, chlamydia, herpes simplex, syphilis, gonorrhea, and AIDS, are on the rise in adolescents. Those who contact STDs run an increased risk of serious consequences. For example, pelvic inflammatory disease in young women is a major cause of ectopic pregnancy and infertility, and inflammation and infection of the urethra and testes can lead to sterility in men (Braverman, 2000; Orr et al., 2001).

Adult and Older Adult
Immunity to many diseases is established by adulthood. Although adults have fewer respiratory tract infections, they have more chronic lung diseases, which can increase the risk for infection. Also, depending on the person's lifestyle, STDs continue to be a major problem in this age group. Infections during pregnancy can be transmitted across the placenta to the fetus. A minor or subclinical infection can be passed to the fetus, who may suffer either minor consequences, major congenital anomalies, or death.

As people age, their lifestyle begins to affect their ability to resist infection. The thymus begins to shrink in late adolescence and continues to diminish into middle age, leading to a decline in cell-mediated and humoral immunity. Cardiovascular disease, cancer, diabetes, obesity or malnutrition, alcoholism, anxiety, depression, and stress have all been shown to decrease defense mechanisms against infection. Medications and treatments used to combat these diseases may also impair immune system function. Adults with chronic diseases may require frequent hospitalizations, putting them at risk for **nosocomial infections** (infections acquired while receiving healthcare).

With the increase in air travel and the development of global economic ties, people are traveling more and living in foreign countries, where they may be exposed to infectious diseases that are not indigenous to their native area. They may then bring these infectious organisms home, contributing to the spread of infection. Because the initial exposure occurs during adulthood, symptoms and complications of such diseases may be severe (Long, Pickering, & Prober, 1997).

As a person ages, the skin becomes thinner and drier. It loses elasticity and fat and receives less circulation, leading to an increased susceptibility to injury and subsequent infection. The body's pH secretions change, peristalsis slows, and endogenous flora also change with age and use of medications. The cough and gag reflexes of older clients may be impaired after a stroke or from medications that cloud thinking. Loose-fitting dentures and impaired swallowing mechanisms may lead to aspiration, which can contribute to respiratory infection.

Older adults may have problems with urinary retention, possibly leading to bacterial growth in stagnant urine and decreased cleansing of the urethra by a brisk stream of urine. Adults who are incapacitated may be incontinent of urine and feces, leading to excoriation of the skin in the perineal and sacral regions and further contributing to infections. If confused or agitated, older clients may carry microorganisms from these areas to their nose or mouth if they are not given adequate help with hygiene.

The immune systems of older adults also may be impaired. Aging diminishes both nonspecific and specific defenses to microbial invasion. Metabolism, synthesis, and repair of body cells and tissues decrease. WBC counts do not always rise in response to infections, and phagocytosis is ineffective. There is a decreased inflammatory response, and body temperature may not be elevated in response to infection. The ability to wall off and limit the spread of infection is decreased. Cellular immune response is decreased, and old infections such as tuberculosis may be reactivated (Chin, 2000).

Infections as a cause of death in older adults are exceeded only by cancer and myocardial infarction. Urinary tract infections (UTIs) and respiratory tract infections are most common and most lethal. Infections use up energy that is necessary for other body processes. Older people have twice the incidence of influenza as young adults, and their mortality rate is higher. They are also vulnerable to postoperative infections, particularly when the chest or abdomen is the operative site.

FACTORS AFFECTING NORMAL RESISTANCE TO INFECTION

Presence of Infectious Agents

In the past, only a few organisms were thought to be pathogenic. It is now recognized that almost any microorganism can cause disease, given the right conditions for entry and growth in the body. Even normal flora can cause disease under the right circumstances. Such organisms are **opportunistic.** Although normally not considered pathogens, they take advantage of being in the right place at the right time and cause infection, especially in clients with compromised immune systems.

Bacteria, viruses, fungi, and parasites are pathogenic organisms. Common infectious diseases caused by bacteria and viruses are listed in Table 39-3.

Bacteria

Bacteria contain thousands of species, but only a few hundred cause human disease. They are what most people think of when they say "germs." *Gram-positive* bacteria, such as staphylococci, are commonly found in wound infections and in food poisoning. Streptococci contribute to skin, wound, and respiratory infections. *Gram-negative* rods, which comprise much of the bowel's normal flora, are often associated with nosocomial infections caused by self-contamination. The most common causes of UTIs are gram-negative organisms.

Anaerobes, or organisms requiring reduced oxygen for growth, are often associated with serious infections. Anaerobic microorganisms are often seen with infections involving a combination of organisms (polymicrobial infections). These organisms are part of the normal flora of the mouth, intestines, and female genital tract.

Bacteria liberate toxins called exotoxins and endotoxins. Exotoxins are liberated by the bacteria that cause tetanus, diphtheria, botulism, cholera, and staphylococcal food poisoning. Exotoxins of gram-positive bacteria are able to move easily across cell membranes into healthy tissue and cause tissue injury. Endotoxins are particularly potent poisons when they are released into the blood.

Viruses

A virus invades a living cell many times its size, uses the cell's metabolism, and replicates itself while either destroying the cell or changing the cell's genetic makeup. Viruses cause AIDS, chickenpox, colds, cold sores, encephalitis, hepatitis, herpes, influenza, measles, mononucleosis, mumps, polio, rabies, shingles, pneumonia, and many other diseases. They have been associated with some cancers and leukemias and with many autoimmune diseases, including multiple sclerosis, rheumatoid arthritis, and diabetes.

Fungi

Only a few fungal infections cause disease in humans, but fungi can be deadly if they disseminate through the body tissues. Unicellular fungi, called yeasts, are often normal flora

(*text continues on page 1039*)

TABLE 39-3

Common Infectious Diseases Caused by Bacteria and Viruses

Infection	Agent	Transmission	Symptoms	Possible Complications	Prevention
General Infections					
Common cold	Rhinovirus	Airborne droplet nuclei	Sneezing, nasal and sinus stuffiness, nasopharyngeal irritation, watery eyes, chills, malaise	Pneumonia, otitis media	Avoid direct contact with infected people. Keep body defenses strong through good nutrition and exercise.
Influenza	Virus	Large particle respiratory droplets	Coldlike symptoms, fever, body stiffness, and discomfort; gastrointestinal symptoms of vomiting and diarrhea with some strains	Pneumonia	Avoid direct contact with infected people. Keep body defenses strong. Obtain or give vaccine as available.
Childhood Infections					
Measles (rubeola)	Virus	Airborne droplet nuclei	Fever, malaise, anorexia, photophobia, coryza, cough, Koplik spots on lateral surface of mouth followed a few days later by red rash	Encephalitis	Administer measles vaccine. Avoid contact with infected people if not immunized. Wear a mask if contact with infected person is necessary.
German measles (rubella)	Virus	Large particle respiratory droplets	Malaise, headache, swollen lymph glands, anorexia, low-grade fever, and runny nose followed by maculopapular rash	Severe retardation and birth defects if contracted in utero	Obtain or give rubella vaccine. Avoid contact with infected people if not immunized. Wear mask if contact with infected person is necessary.
Mumps	Virus	Large particle respiratory droplets	Malaise, muscle aches, headache, anorexia, swollen and tender parotid glands, fever	Encephalitis, arthritis, deafness, sterility in adult men	Obtain or give mumps vaccine. Avoid contact with infected people if unimmunized. A mask may help decrease infection. *(continues)*

TABLE 39-3 (Continued)

Common Infectious Diseases Caused by Bacteria and Viruses

Infection	Agent	Transmission	Symptoms	Possible Complications	Prevention
Chickenpox	Varicella-zoster virus	Large particle respiratory droplets	Fever; malaise; anorexia; rash characterized by macules, papules, and vesicles that crust over; pruritus secondary to rash	Secondary skin infections due to scratching	Give vaccine. Isolate infected person until lesions crust over or disappear.
Scarlet fever	Streptococcal bacteria	Large particle respiratory droplets	Sore throat, bright red tongue, high fever, nausea, vomiting, rash	Rheumatic fever, glomerulonephritis, renal failure	Avoid contact with infected people. Isolate client until 24 hr after antibiotic treatment.
Pertussis (whooping cough)	Gram-negative bacillus (*Bordetella pertussis*)	Large particle respiratory droplets	Cold symptoms that progress to severe cough that includes a "whoop" as glottis closes during deep inspiration. Vomiting, epistaxis, and hemorrhaging can occur from severe coughing bouts.		Administer pertussis vaccine. Isolate client from non-immune people. Use a mask during acute infectious stage.
Neurologic Infections					
Encephalitis	Enterovirus, arbovirus, or as sequela of measles, rubella, chickenpox, or influenza	Large particle respiratory droplets	Fever; vomiting; aching head, neck, and back muscles; drowsiness; convulsions; paralysis; coma	Brain damage	Administer vaccinations for measles, rubella, chickenpox, and influenza.
Meningitis	Gram-negative bacteria or virus	Large particle respiratory droplets	Fever, anorexia, intense headache, intolerance to light and sound, delirium, convulsions, coma	Shock, respiratory distress, brain damage	

Disease	Causative Agent	Mode of Transmission	Signs and Symptoms	Complications	Prevention/Treatment
Polio	Virus	Ingesting contaminated food and water	Nausea; vomiting; cramps; paralysis of arms, legs, and body; if nerve supply is affected, impaired swallowing and breathing	Permanent paralysis	Administer Salk or oral Sabin vaccine. Take enteric precautions for infected clients.
Sexually Transmitted Diseases					
Syphilis	Spirochete (*Treponema pallidum*)	Sexual contact, woman to fetus via placenta, blood transfusion if donor is in early stage of disease and undiagnosed	*Primary stage:* Genital lesion, enlarged lymph nodes *Secondary stage (6 wk later):* Lesions of skin and mucous membrane, with generalized symptoms of headache and fever	*Tertiary stage:* Central nervous system and cardiovascular damage, paralysis, psychosis	Educate public on safe sex practices. Screen blood donors. Do serologic testing before and during pregnancy. Avoid contact with body secretions from infected clients.
Gonorrhea	Gonococcus (*Neisseria gonorrhoeae*)	Sexual contact; woman to fetus during delivery	Yellow mucopurulent discharge of genital area, painful or frequent urination, pain in genital area; may be asymptomatic	Sterility, cystitis, arthritis, endocarditis	Educate public on safe sex practices. Test woman before delivery. Treat newborn's eyes with silver nitrate. Treat all contacts with antibiotics.
Genital herpes	Virus Herpes simplex type 2	Sexual contact; woman to fetus during vaginal delivery	Genital soreness, pruritus; and erythema; vesicles appear that usually last for about 10 days, during which time transmission of virus is likely		Educate public on safe sex practices. Encourage avoidance of sexual contact when lesions are present. Anticipate cesarean delivery for infected pregnant women.

(*continues*)

TABLE 39-3 (Continued)

Common Infectious Diseases Caused by Bacteria and Viruses

Infection	Agent	Transmission	Symptoms	Possible Complications	Prevention
Chlamydia	Bacteria (*Chlamydia trachomatis*)	Sexual contact; woman to fetus during vaginal delivery	Mucopurulent genital discharge, genital pain, dysuria	Sterility	Educate public on safe sex practices. Encourage avoidance of sexual contact when lesions are present. Anticipate cesarean delivery for infected pregnant women.
Acquired immunodeficiency syndrome (AIDS)	Human immunodeficiency virus (HIV)	Sexual contact; exposure to blood or blood products; woman to fetus	*Active phase:* Rash, cough, malaise, night sweats, lymphadenopathy *Asymptomatic phase:* No symptoms but test is positive for HIV antigens *AIDS-related complex (ARC):* Lymphadenopathy, diarrhea, oral candidiasis, weight loss, fatigue, skin rash, recurrent infections, fever *AIDS:* Rare infections such as *Pneumocystis carinii* pneumonia or rare cancers such as Kaposi's sarcoma or B-cell lymphomas	Neurologic impairment	Educate public, especially high-risk groups, on safe sex practices. Screen blood or blood products used for transfusion carefully. Advise IV drug abusers not to share needles. Use Standard Precautions consistently in all healthcare settings. Institute measures to avoid needlesticks among healthcare workers.

Blood-Borne Infectious

AIDS (see above)

Hepatitis B	Hepatitis B virus (HBV)	Transfusion with infected blood or blood products (less common with other body fluid contact), punctures with HBV-contaminated sharps, woman to fetus in utero	Malaise, anorexia, nausea, vomiting, fever, headache, abdominal pain, jaundice, enlarged liver	Hepatic damage or failure, encephalopathy	Recommend hepatitis B vaccine for high-risk people who often come in contact with blood. If exposed, give immune globulin. Screen blood donors. Avoid needlesticks. Use Standard Precautions.
Hepatitis C	Hepatitis C virus (HCV)	Transfusion with infected blood or blood products (less common with other body fluid contact), punctures with HCV-contaminated sharps	Fatigue and malaise (mild clinical course); increased risk to progress to chronic infection	Hepatic damage or failure	Educate public on safe sex practices. Screen blood or blood products used for transfusion. Advise IV drug abusers not to share needles. Use Standard Precautions consistently. Avoid needlesticks in all healthcare settings.

Food- or Water-Borne

Hepatitis A	Hepatitis A virus (HAV)	Contaminated water or food or fecal–oral contamination	Malaise, anorexia, nausea, vomiting, fever, headache, abdominal pain, jaundice, enlarged liver	Hepatic damage or failure, encephalopathy	Educate public on good sanitation and personal hygiene, especially after using toilet and before handling food. Educate and monitor food handlers and day-care workers. Give immune globulin to travelers visiting endemic areas.

(continues)

TABLE 39-3 (Continued)

Common Infectious Diseases Caused by Bacteria and Viruses

Infection	Agent	Transmission	Symptoms	Possible Complications	Prevention
Typhoid fever	Bacteria (*Salmonella typhi*)	Contaminated water or food, contact with urine or feces of a carrier	Headache, weakness, fever, rash, abdominal tenderness, diarrhea, decreased level of consciousness (stupor, delirium, coma)	Intestinal hemorrhage or perforation	Assist with monitoring water sanitation, waste disposal, and fly control. Give vaccinations in regions with contaminated water supply. Encourage good handwashing after toilet use. Check to ensure milk and dairy products are pasteurized.
Salmonella	Bacteria (various species of *Salmonella*)	Contaminated food, especially inadequate refrigeration or sanitation; improperly cooked meat	Vomiting, diarrhea, abdominal cramps, fever	Dehydration, shock due to fluid volume deficit	Encourage proper handling, refrigeration, and cooking of food, especially eggs and poultry.
Shigella	Bacteria (*Shigella*)	Contaminated water or food; crowded environments such as jails or institutions	Vomiting, diarrhea, abdominal cramps, fever	Dehydration, possibly leading to shock	Properly store and prepare food.
Accident-Related Tetanus (lock-jaw)	Bacteria (*Clostridium tetani*)	Puncture wound from needle, nail, dog bite, or gunshot wound	Increased neuromuscular tone and irritability, twitching, convulsions	Respiratory arrest and death	Keep immunization current; after accident, give booster dose or tetanus to stimulate recall. If prolonged time has elapsed since booster, give combination of antitoxins (tetanus immune globin) and tetanus and diphtheria toxoids.

of the skin and mucous membranes. Yeasts do not injure the host until defenses are lowered, as with *Candida* in the mouth of infants (thrush) or in clients with cancer or AIDS. Antibiotics, which can destroy normal bacterial flora, can contribute to fungal infections. Infestations of yeast by inhalation of spores can cause coccidioidomycosis or histoplasmosis lung infections. The most common yeast infections affect the skin, hair, and nails (e.g., athlete's foot, ringworm, groin itch).

Parasites

Parasites that infect humans are either protozoa, helminths, or arthropods. Parasitic infections are associated with poor socioeconomic conditions, such as inadequate sanitation measures for water and sewage. When public health measures do not control these organisms, disease is prevalent.

Protozoal infections are common in underdeveloped countries and probably cause more suffering worldwide than any other group of diseases. Trichomoniasis, an STD, is one of the most common protozoal diseases in the United States, causing an estimated 3 to 6 million infections annually (Cates, 1999; McKinzie, 2000). Other diseases include African sleeping sickness, malaria, and giardiasis. Pneumocystosis, a disease of the alveolar sacs, is increasing in frequency in clients with immunosuppression (e.g., cancer, AIDS).

Helminths include pinworms, flatworms, and roundworms. Some invade the tissues; others live in the GI tract or in the blood. Pinworms, found worldwide, are one of the most common parasites in humans. Roundworms, also passed among humans, are common. Flatworms are best known from reports of intestinal tapeworms.

Arthropods include mites, ticks, fleas, lice, and fly larvae. They irritate the skin because of the toxins introduced with human skin bites. Bacterial superinfections often complicate the dermatitis. Arthropods also serve as vectors for some protozoal infections and for dreaded bacterial infections (Tortora, Funke, & Case, 2001).

Compromised Host

A few infections result directly from the virulence of the infectious agents or its byproducts. Most infections result from decreased host defenses. Before an infectious process becomes a disease, a breakdown or impairment must occur in the physical and chemical barriers to bacterial colonization, the inflammatory and febrile response, and the response of the WBCs, including those involved in immunity. Decreased resistance to infection may result from age, preexisting disease, medical therapy, malnutrition, or stress. Many conditions can compromise the body's anatomic barriers.

Breaks in Skin and Mucous Membranes

Breaks in skin and mucous membranes predispose a person to infection. Both natural and therapeutic processes can alter intact epithelial surfaces. Skin in infants and older adults is thin and more easily broken or penetrated by microorganisms. Some medications, such as steroids, cause thinning of the skin and increase the potential for breakdown.

Surgical intervention and many diagnostic procedures break normal skin integrity, greatly increasing the possibility of infection. Therapeutic procedures invade every epithelial surface. Nasogastric tubes, urinary catheters, suction catheters, and rectal thermometers can cause surface abrasions and also obstruct the natural flow of cleansing fluids.

Invasive Devices

Any invasive device that enters the body provides a portal of entry for microorganisms, thus increasing the chance for infection. Invasive devices are often used to treat illnesses. Tubes through the skin and body orifices provide microorganisms with direct access to internal organs and the bloodstream. Intravascular lines are inserted to give medications and fluids or to serve as monitoring devices. Urinary catheters or tubes placed in the GI tract for decompression or feeding also increase infection risk. Surgical drains placed postoperatively to promote adequate wound drainage provide an access route for microorganisms into the wound.

Stasis of Body Fluids

Stagnant secretions in the body provide a warm, moist environment that fosters bacterial growth. Normal defense mechanisms prevent stasis of body fluids, but these can be altered. Tubes inserted into the trachea and drugs that cause sedation can bypass or suppress the normal cough and sneezing clearance of respiratory secretions. Smoking, with the associated inhalation of toxic chemicals, inhibits normal nasopharyngeal ciliary action. Tumors or other obstructions in ducts of exocrine glands hinder the flow of normal secretions, providing a rich medium for microbial growth. Decreased fluid intake, immobility, and urinary tract obstruction foster urinary stasis, increasing the risk of UTI.

Inadequate Nutrition

Malnutrition depresses almost every normal defense to infection. Neutrophil and microphage function is defective, blood levels of complement are low, and both cellular and humoral immune reactions are diminished. When infection occurs, cellular metabolism increases as the body tries to fight it. Because increased metabolism requires increased calories and protein, inadequate protein stores decrease the body's ability to manufacture antibodies and WBCs. A vicious cycle occurs, with increased nutritional needs and decreased body reserves.

Stress

Stress increases greatly when a client is ill or hospitalized. Physical or emotional stress causes the body to release cortisol, which can increase the risk of infection by suppressing the immune response. Cortisol increases the level of serum glucose, providing a good medium for bacterial growth. The metabolic rate increases, depleting energy stores necessary for tissue healing and production of antibodies. Extreme

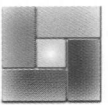

Nursing Research and Critical Thinking
Is Distress Associated with Immune Function Among Women with Suspected Breast Cancer?

The period between discovery of a breast lump and definitive treatment is extremely distressing for many women. An optimally functioning immune system is important to women newly diagnosed with breast cancer to combat the disease, heal surgical wounds, and protect against infections. Nurse researchers learned from the literature that women experiencing the diagnostic phase of breast cancer may be distressed and that this distress can alter immune function. They designed a prospective, descriptive, correlational study to determine the levels of cytokines and psychological and symptom distress and to investigate relationships among psychological distress, symptom distress, and immune function in women with suspected breast cancer. A convenience sample of women ($n = 35$) from a major teaching hospital who had either fine-needle aspiration or open breast biopsy for suspicion of breast cancer were asked to participate. Data were collected from each subject at three points: time 1, after the physician visit when the need for breast biopsy was ascertained; time 2, 10 days after biopsy; and time 3, 7 to 10 days after the second data collection point. Blood was drawn at each time for cytokine analysis; subjects also completed the Brief Symptoms Inventory (BSI) as a measure of psychological distress and the Adapted Symptom Distress Scale (ASDS) as a measure of symptom distress. The researchers used means and standard deviations to describe the levels of psychological distress, symptom distress, and cytokines of the sample. Significant correlations between psychological distress and symptom distress were found at time 2 and time 3. The only significant relationship between psychological distress and any immune function variable was between the BSI and TNF levels at T2 ($r = 0.44$, $P < .05$).

Critical Thinking Considerations. The researchers believe that the lack of other significant correlations is a result of the very high variability of cytokine levels between and among women. A larger sample size would help resolve this issue. Implications of this study are as follows:

- Distress levels of women with both benign and malignant tumors did not significantly decrease over time.
- Healthcare providers should be aware of the extremely stressful nature of the diagnostic phase and provide as much support as possible to these women.

From DeKeyser, F. G., Wainstock, J. M., Rose, L., Converse, P. J., & Dooley, W. (1998). Distress, symptom distress and immune function in women with suspected breast cancer. *Oncology Nursing Forum, 25*(8), 1415–1422.

continuous stress causes exhaustion, which limits a person's ability to resist infection.

Immune System Dysfunction

The immune system's ability to produce memory cells and antibodies (humoral immunity) or to activate T lymphocytes (cell-mediated immunity) can be impaired in several ways. AIDS can compromise immune function by destroying helper T cells. Cancer can overwhelm the immune or inflammatory components.

Coexisting Medical Problems

Cancer, especially if it affects bone marrow production of leukocytes, increases the risk of infection. Cancers such as leukemia may accelerate the rate of leukocyte production, but the cells are immature and ineffective in fighting infection. Treatment of many forms of cancer by chemotherapy or radiation may suppress bone marrow and WBC production, affecting the body's ability to resist infection.

Some diseases affect the factors that attract neutrophils and circulating macrophages to the site of infection. This attraction, called chemotaxis, is decreased in diabetes mellitus, cirrhosis, and uremia. Clients with burns have impaired neutrophils that do not ingest and destroy microorganisms efficiently. Because neutrophils release chemical mediators of inflammation, impairment of their number and effectiveness profoundly affects host defenses.

Medical problems that affect blood circulation and nutrient transport can impair host defenses. Cardiovascular conditions, such as peripheral vascular disease or heart failure, can limit the body's ability to supply leukocytes and antibodies to the site of an infection, thus decreasing the infection-fighting potential.

Inflammatory disorders can also increase the risk of infection. The inflammatory response normally helps destroy and contain microbes to prevent systemic infection. Inflammation can be destructive, however, if it impairs vascular control and if the tissue exudate is extensive enough to provide a medium for microbial growth.

Drug Therapy

Drug therapy can cause defects in the host's response to infection. Steroids, chemotherapy, antimetabolites, and inappropriate or prolonged use of antibiotics can increase the risk of infection. *Superinfection* (a new infection caused by an organism different from an initially infecting organism and usually resistant to treatment for the initial infection) can occur. For example, if the course of antibiotic administration is prolonged or an incorrect antibiotic is chosen, bacterial growth may be stimulated as normal flora in the gut, mouth, and skin are destroyed. Invading organisms can take advantage of the alteration in the normal flora, leading to serious infection in the host.

ALTERED RESISTANCE TO INFECTION

Type of Infection

Being infected and becoming ill are different. Illness results when the agent overcomes the body's defenses and the normal state of health changes. When an obvious complex of symptoms occurs, the infection is called a clinical disease. When the body successfully resists being overwhelmed by the infection, the condition is called subclinical. There may be few symptoms, and the host may be unaware of the exposure, but antigens form that can be recovered from the person's blood.

Colonization is the introduction of microorganisms onto a body surface where they grow and multiply but do not invade the body or cause an immune response or symptoms (Black, Hawks, & Keene, 2001). The host, if ill or in a vulnerable state, may become ill and develop an infection. Infection is described as primary when it occurs in an otherwise healthy person and secondary when it develops in a weakened client.

Local Versus Systemic

An infection may be localized to a single body area, or it may disseminate to deeper organs. When it spreads to other body systems, the infection is called systemic. If bacteria spread through the bloodstream, the term **bacteremia** is used. Another term, *septicemia,* is often used as a synonym, but it more accurately refers to the presence of microorganisms (or their toxic products) in the bloodstream that are disrupting normal body functions. *Blood poisoning* is a common term for the presence of infectious agents such as *Staphylococcus* or *Streptococcus* in the blood.

Acute Versus Chronic

An infection may be acute or chronic depending on the severity and duration of symptoms. An acute infection usually develops rapidly, causes symptoms, climaxes, and then fades fairly quickly. A chronic infection, on the other hand, can linger: symptoms usually develop more slowly, and convalescence may take months. An acute infection can become chronic when the body cannot rid itself of the organism.

Nosocomial Infections

A person's defenses may be compromised when exposed to the healthcare system. Nosocomial infections, or infections associated with healthcare delivery, can occur during visits to physicians who use poor aseptic practices, during home visits if nurses do not wash their hands after care of previous clients, or in ambulatory surgery centers that do not observe strict surgical asepsis. (For more information, see Chapter 26.) Nosocomial infections occur frequently in nursing homes, jails, and other residential facilities where auxiliary staff who may be overworked and poorly trained care for high-risk individuals.

Most nosocomial infections involve the urinary tract, surgical or traumatic wounds, the respiratory tract, or bacteremias in association with intravascular lines. Risk factors for common infections, some of which may be nosocomial, are presented in Display 39-1.

Progress of an Infection

The course of an infection that results in a disease state is a dynamic series of events that express competition between the host and the invading organism. Disease usually results from the organism's growth and multiplication inside the host. The exception is when the disease is caused by the release of toxins, as in food poisoning or botulism. The pattern for most diseases follows a predictable course that includes the incubation period, the prodromal period, acute illness with symptoms, and the convalescent period. The time frame during which a disease can be passed from one person to another is known as the *communicable period.*

Incubation Period. The incubation period is the time between the pathogen's entrance and the appearance of symptoms. The length of this period varies depending on the number of organisms absorbed, the time they require to grow and multiply, their virulence, and the host's resistance. The point of entry may also be a factor.

Prodromal Period. The prodromal period is characterized by nonspecific symptoms such as nausea, fever, general weakness, or aches and pains. Although prodromal symptoms are nonspecific, the cluster of symptoms and their order of appearance often help in the diagnosis of the disease.

Acute Phase of Illness. The acute phase of an illness occurs when specific symptoms appear. Depending on the pathogen, there is a cluster of symptoms, and often laboratory analysis can identify the disease. The period during which the symptoms subside is included in this phase.

Convalescent Period. Convalescence completes the progress of an infection. The body systems return to normal, and appetite and energy return. Antibodies begin to appear in the person's blood.

Communicable Disease

If the causative agent of the disease is transmissible between one person and another, the disease is said to be a **communicable disease.** If the agent passes with ease from one host to the next, it may be called contagious. Not all diseases are contagious. For example, tetanus can be contracted in an isolated event when a person sustains a puncture wound. Childhood diseases (e.g., measles, mumps, chickenpox) are classic examples of communicable diseases. Infections among clients in healthcare facilities are not necessarily contagious, but because of the large number of clients with lowered host defenses, such infections are more easily transmitted in the facility than they would be in the community.

DISPLAY 39-1

🔄 **FACTORS PREDISPOSING TO COMMON INFECTIONS**

Factors Predisposing to Urinary Tract Infection
Factors Increasing Contamination of Urethral Area
- Fecal incontinence
- Atrophic changes (senile vaginitis)
- Wiping back to front

Factors Facilitating Urethral Ascent of Organisms
- Catheterization
- Surgery
- Sexual intercourse
- Pelvic relaxation with aging
- Urethral incompetence (incontinence)
- Diapering incontinent clients

Factors Reducing Flow of Urine
- Outflow obstruction (urethral stricture, prostatic hypertrophy, fecal impaction)
- Neurogenic bladder
- Inadequate fluid intake (dehydration)

Factors Promoting Bacterial Colonization
- Foreign body (tumor, calculi)
- Aging (epithelial cell changes, reduced mucus production, waning immunity)
- Increased urinary glucose (diabetes)

Factors Predisposing to Wound Infection
Local Factors
- Degree of contamination of the wound
- Virulence of contaminating organisms
- Adequacy of local blood supply
- Amount of necrotic or injured tissue in the wound
- Degree of closure of the wound
- Presence of dead spaces, hematomas, and seromas
- Presence and type of foreign bodies
- Location of the wound
- Mechanism of injury

Treatment Factors
- Length of stay in an acute care facility
- Time, type, and thoroughness of treatment
- Duration of operative procedure(s)
- Timeliness and appropriateness of antibiotic administration
- Appropriate surgical closure
- Surgical technique
- Appropriateness of wound dressing
- Nutritional support
- Adequacy of oxygenation and tissue perfusion
- Use of invasive devices for monitoring, drainage, and fluid or nutritional support
- Adequate treatment of coexisting infections

Host Factors
- Age

- General immunologic competence
- Chronic health problems
- Preoperative nutritional status
- Obesity
- Remote infections
- Extent of injury (multiple wounds or extensive surgery)
- Corticosteroid use

Factors Predisposing to Respiratory Infection
Factors Increasing Secretion Production
- Smoking
- Intubation
- Chemical irritation (air pollution, allergies, inhalation anesthetics, aspiration of gastric contents, impaired cough or swallowing mechanisms)

Factors Decreasing Chest Wall Movement
- Pain (chest or abdominal injuries or incisions)
- Obesity
- Abdominal distention
- Tight casts or bandages
- Age
- Skeletal deformities (traumatic or congenital [e.g., scoliosis])

Factors Inhibiting Secretion Clearance
- Weak cough
- Dry, tenacious secretions
- Dehydration
- Chronic lung disease
- Decreased diaphragmatic movement (neurologic deficits, paralysis, muscle weakness)

Factors Depressing the Respiratory Center (Hypoventilation)
- Sedatives
- Narcotics
- Altered levels of consciousness (resulting from trauma or cerebrovascular events)
- Acid-base imbalance

Factors Increasing Risk of Microbial Colonization
- Extended hospital stay
- Residence in long-term care facility
- Endotracheal intubation
- Tracheostomy
- Superinfection after long-term use of antibiotics
- Malnutrition
- Primary or acquired immunodeficiency
- Contaminated respiratory equipment
- Steroids
- Immunosuppressive therapy
- Poor personal hygiene practices

An infected person may be contagious during the incubation period, prodromal period, acute phase, or convalescent period, depending on whether organisms are being shed into the environment. When the agent is not present in body secretions but is hidden within the host's cells, the infection is called *latent.* The latent period refers to the time between exposure to the organism and the appearance of signs and symptoms. When the agent is being shed from the host's body in respiratory secretions, feces, blood, or urine, or is cultured from body tissues, the infection is communicable. The period of communicability begins after the agent has multiplied sufficiently for shedding to begin and lasts as long as the level of shedding is sufficient for transmission. Diseases spread more rapidly if they have a short latent period. The latent period is almost always shorter than the incubation period; therefore, the infected person usually is shedding microorganisms before any signs and symptoms appear.

Periods of communicability vary with each disease and with the control of microorganisms within the infected person's tissues. Because of the uncertainty of the period of communicability and the lack of identifiable infection in some people, all body secretions should be considered as potentially infectious.

Manifestations of Infection

The human body has various internal sensors that signal when something is wrong. Often, this inner sense is the first warning of an impending infection. These early warnings include malaise (a general sense of feeling not completely well), listlessness, inability to concentrate, uneasiness, lightheadedness, weakness, muscle or joint discomfort, headache, and anorexia. As the person becomes more ill, symptoms change from subjective, vague complaints to objective findings. Common manifestations of infections are listed in Display 39-2.

Fever

Fever, a common manifestation of infection, should be considered a sign of infection until other causes are ruled out. Fever is the hypothalamic thermoregulatory center's response to circulating pyrogens. These pyrogens are released when phagocytic cells (macrophages) are stimulated by microorganisms or endotoxins (Vander, Sherman, & Luciano, 2001). A low-grade fever is a temperature that is slightly elevated (37.1°C to approximately 38.2°C [98.8°F to 100.6°F]). A temperature elevation above 38.2°C is considered a high-grade fever, and a temperature greater than 40.5°C (104.9°F) is referred to as hyperpyrexia. Very young children tend to produce high fevers with infection (up to 40°C [104°F]), but older people may not show a fever or may produce only a low-grade fever when infection is present.

After surgery, an elevated temperature may be normal initially, but if it continues, it may signal a possible infection. During the first postoperative day, an elevated temperature is most likely caused by the physiologic stress of surgery or by atelectasis. Fever during the second to fifth postoperative day most likely results from pneumonia. A fever on the second to eighth

DISPLAY 39-2

⬚ COMMON MANIFESTATIONS OF INFECTION

Wound Infection
- Redness, swelling, pain
- Localized heat
- Fever
- Purulent or malodorous drainage
- Bruising around incision or induration of area around wound

Urinary Tract Infection
- Urgency and increased frequency of urination
- Burning with urination (dysuria)
- Cloudy, bloody, or malodorous urine (pyuria, hematuria)
- Fever
- Flank pain

Respiratory Infection
- Productive cough
- Sputum color change (yellow, brown, or green)
- Fever, increased pulse and respiratory rate
- Abnormal breath sounds
- Painful breathing (pleuritic chest pain)
- Difficulty in breathing (dyspnea)

Gastrointestinal Infection (Gastroenteritis)
- Severe abdominal cramping and nausea after eating
- More than usual number of stools and/or loose, watery, or bloody stools

postoperative day suggests UTI. One occurring from the third to the eleventh postoperative day often suggests a wound infection. A fever developing weeks or months after surgery may suggest a deep operative infection or infected prosthetic device.

Phases of Febrile Episodes. A febrile episode has three distinct phases: the chill phase, the fever phase, and the flush phase or crisis. Each phase exhibits unique symptoms.

During the *chill phase,* the body's heat-producing mechanisms attempt to increase the core body temperature. The client experiences a feeling of being cold and may shiver. Gooseflesh, caused by contraction of the arrector pili muscles in an attempt to trap air around body hairs, may be evident. The client's skin appears pale and cool due to vasoconstriction.

The *fever phase* occurs when the fever reaches the new, higher set point. The client's skin feels warm to the touch and appears flushed because of vasodilation. During this phase of the fever, the client feels neither hot nor cold. The client may experience thirst if fluid volume deficit has occurred. Complaints of general malaise, weakness, and aching muscles (due to the increased rate of protein catabolism) may be present. In addition, the client may be either drowsy or restless. An unchecked fever can cause the client to become delirious and to suffer from convulsions secondary to cerebral nerve cell irritation.

The *flush* or *crisis phase* is the third phase in a febrile episode. During this phase, the client experiences profuse diaphoresis, decreased shivering, and possible fluid volume deficit. The client's skin appears flushed and warm to the touch because of vasodilation.

Increased Pulse and Respiratory Rate
Infection increases the body's metabolic rate, which increases the heart rate. The pulse may become bounding. The rate and depth of respiration also increase as the body attempts to rid itself of excess waste produced during increased metabolism.

Inflammatory Symptoms
Infection stimulates the inflammatory response to promote leukocyte migration to the area. The inflammatory response is discussed in detail in Chapter 38. As inflammation occurs, the area appears red, swollen, tender, and warm.

Pain
Most infections cause discomfort. Pain can occur when inflammation causes swelling within an enclosed area or when normal function is impeded. Examples of pain caused by infection include the following:

- Pleuritic pain when breathing, with a respiratory infection
- Burning on voiding, with a UTI
- Pain on swallowing, with a streptococcal throat infection

Purulent Drainage
As WBCs migrate to the infection, purulent (containing pus) drainage may be observed. Because of the increased numbers of WBCs, body fluids such as urine or sputum may become cloudy or whitish-yellow. Purulent drainage is usually thicker than normal, and it often is foul smelling because it contains a great deal of cellular debris from the inflammatory response.

Enlarged Lymph Nodes
During an infection, the lymph nodes that drain an infected area may become enlarged and easily palpable ("swollen glands"). As the swelling increases, the nodes may also become tender. During inflammation, the lymphatic capillaries dilate as excess interstitial fluid, proteins, and invading microorganisms enter the lymphatic system. The swelling indicates that lymphocytes and macrophages in the lymph node are fighting the infection and trying to limit its spread.

Rash
A rash may occur with primary infections of the skin (e.g., impetigo) but also may accompany some generalized infectious diseases. The diagnosis of many communicable childhood diseases is made on the specific characteristics of the rash. Many rashes cause pruritus (itching). Scratching may disrupt the skin's integrity, possibly resulting in secondary skin infections.

Gastrointestinal Symptoms
Viruses, bacteria, and toxins produced by certain bacteria and parasites may cause acute GI inflammation. Anorexia, nausea, and vomiting may occur when the stomach lining is inflamed; diarrhea is more common when the small or large intestine is inflamed.

"Traveler's diarrhea" may occur when tourists drink water or eat uncooked food that contains endemic bacteria or parasites. Travelers have little previous exposure to these microorganisms, so they have limited antibodies to fight the infectious agent.

Impact on Activities of Daily Living

Depending on the infection's severity and duration, the client's normal activities of daily living (ADLs) may be affected. The client may experience pain, other physical discomfort, or social isolation because of the possible stigma attached to the infection or others' lack of knowledge about it. The community may suffer from loss of the client's economic contribution and inability to participate in church, political, or charitable activities.

An infection saps the energy needed for normal ADLs. Clients with an infection may not have the necessary energy to perform normal grooming or to purchase, prepare, and eat meals. If the infection is located in a joint or necessitates bed rest, mobility is affected.

Whenever one family member has an infection, the risk of infection for all family members increases, especially if transmission occurs by way of the airborne route. When one family member is ill, hygienic practices (e.g., handwashing, not sharing eating utensils) must be followed. Separation of high-risk family members (e.g., newborns, immunocompromised family members) may be necessary.

Infectious illnesses can also pose financial hardship for the family. Parents may find it necessary to stay home from work or to pay someone to watch the sick child (if such a person can be found). Wage-earners may lose their salary if they do not have sick time as an employee benefit, and they may be forced to pay for medical care if they do not have medical insurance.

Families may need to shift routines so that other members can assume the ill person's responsibilities. Fatigue may hinder sexual and social relations. The family's food intake may be affected if the infected person is the one who buys and prepares food. If infection is acute and of short duration, the impact on the family is usually minimal and easily handled. If the infection is severe or prolonged, significant impact can occur.

ASSESSMENT
Subjective Data
Normal Pattern Identification
Information about the client's normal defense system against illness is important (Display 39-3). Ask the client or caregiver about measures that are normally taken to avoid illness, including the client's usual pattern of rest and exercise, nutrition,

ETHICAL/LEGAL ISSUE
Reaction to HIV/AIDS

Mabel is a nursing student who has just finished caring for her first HIV-infected client. The client is only 25 years old and very ill. When Mabel goes home, she relates to her family her sorrow concerning the client's poor prognosis. Mabel's father gets very angry and states. "Under no circumstances are you to be taking care of those AIDS patients!" Mabel has always been very respectful, obeying her parents' wishes (especially her father's). She believes he is being very unreasonable but is unsure how to proceed.

Reflection
- What factors could have contributed to the father's outburst?
- Identify the conflicting emotions that Mabel may be experiencing.
- Does any healthcare worker have the right to refuse to care for clients with HIV?
- What supports might Mabel use to provide necessary information to her family regarding HIV?

use of vitamins and folk remedies, and understanding of germ exposure. Obtain a history of immunizations and determine whether it is complete and current. A description of the client's usual experience of illness, including childhood diseases, provides valuable data to determine whether the pattern is normal.

Risk Identification

Closely screen the client for infection risk and document any recent exposure to infectious illness. Sometimes, this means asking questions such as, "Has anyone in your immediate family recently been infected with [specify disease]?" Consider school records and community documentation of infectious disease outbreaks in evaluating each client for risk. Include questions about the client's general health, such as normal sleep and exercise patterns; nutritional history; use of drugs, cigarettes, or alcohol; and sexual practices. Note any recent travel, especially to foreign counties. Explore any chronic health conditions, such as heart disease, lung disease, or diabetes, and their treatment. Determine whether the client has received chemotherapy or radiation, because such treatments often increase the risk of infection by suppressing the immune system. Also, obtain a medication history, focusing on immunosuppressive drugs (e.g., steroids) and current or previous use of antibiotics.

Dysfunction Identification

If infection was a reason the client sought medical assistance, questions should elicit more specific information:

- How long has the infection been present?
- What symptoms first occurred?

- Was the occurrence of infection associated with any change in routine?
- How does the infection affect the client's ability to perform ADLs?

If infection was not a reason the client sought advice but the client displays symptoms of infection, address the following:

- Do you have any pain, redness, swelling, or abnormal drainage? When did it start? How long has it lasted? What is its intensity?
- Do you have a fever? If so, when did it start? Describe the pattern.
- Are you experiencing any nausea, vomiting, diarrhea, malaise, or general aches and pains (symptoms that accompany many viral infections)?

The nursing history (as opposed to the medical history) focuses on how the infection has affected the client's ability to function normally and to carry out usual activities and routines.

Objective Data

Physical Assessment
General Inspection. Determine whether the client is comfortable or in obvious pain. Detect any signs of fatigue in the client's posture and movement. Look for abnormal skin color, presence of rashes or lesions, and any swelling and signs of inflammation.

Vital Signs. Assess vital signs frequently to detect the presence of infection or to monitor its progress. The accuracy of such assessment is important in determining the presence of infection. In a client with an infection, look for elevations in temperature (above 38.2°C [101°F]), pulse rate, and respiratory rate.

When evaluating the significance of vital signs that differ from baseline values, consider other factors that could be responsible. Look at the pattern of changes in vital signs. A consistently elevated and rising temperature is significant. Usually, the physician obtains cultures and begins to look for the source of a possible infection when the temperature rises above 38.2°C (101°F). However, some people, such as older adults and immunosuppressed clients, may not show a fever when infection is present.

Auscultation of Breath Sounds. Auscultation of breath sounds can help detect respiratory infections. Pneumonia can alter normal breath sounds, producing crackles (rales), rhonchi, and wheezes. Atelectasis, which can predispose a client to respiratory infection, is noted by diminished breath sounds.

Auscultation of Bowel Sounds. Auscultation of bowel sounds can help detect increased intestinal peristalsis. Increased peristalsis often accompanies microbial irritation of the gut, which can cause diarrhea.

Palpation of Lymph Nodes. Lymph nodes can enlarge and become tender because of localized or systemic infection.

THERAPEUTIC DIALOGUE
Family Illness

Scene for Thought
The community health nurse is responsible for visiting 20 families per week. Today, she will see the Holden family, which consists of Ann, age 38; John, age 39; Maureen, age 11; and John, Jr., age 9 years. As she drives up to the small, neat house, she notices that the family car is in the driveway, an unusual occurrence because John is usually at work when the nurse comes to see the family.

Less Effective

Nurse: *(Knocks on the door.)* Ann, it's Rosie Connors.
Client: Hello, Rosie, come on in. *(Looks tired and pale.)*
Nurse: *(Settles on couch with Ann beside her.)* How are things?
Client: Not wonderful. We're all sick with the stomach flu, and John and I have been up most of the night either with the kids or sick ourselves. It's just miserable.
Nurse: I know how that is! Especially when everyone gets it at once. No wonder you look tired. I'll bet a good night's sleep would feel just great! *(Smiles warmly and sympathetically.)*
Client: That's the truth. *(Smiles wearily.)* I suppose you need to see Maureen now. I know you're busy.
Nurse: Okay. How's she doing, by the way? *(Goes with Ann to see Maureen, chatting as they go.)*

More Effective

Nurse: *(Knocks on the door.)* Ann, it's Evelyn Mason.
Client: Hello, Evelyn, come on in. *(Looks tired and pale.)*
Nurse: *(Settles on couch with Ann beside her.)* How are things?
Client: Not wonderful. We're all sick with the stomach flu, and John and I have been up most of the night either with the kids or sick ourselves. It's just miserable.
Nurse: I noticed the car outside and wondered about John being home. What can I help you with while I'm here? *(Sits quietly and attentively.)*
Client: Well, I know you usually come to check on Maureen's diabetes, and I don't want to trouble you with the rest of it.
Nurse: It's no trouble. Maureen's health and the family's health are connected. I'll be happy to do what I can.
Client: *(Looks relieved.)* Well, could you maybe check us all over before you go, just to make sure it is the stomach flu and not something else? And then, I need some advice about what to eat. We're all thirsty but some things don't really agree with me, and John, Jr., won't drink juices. I'm not sure what to do.
Nurse: Sure, no problem. Shall I start with you since you're right here? *(Continues to sit with her without moving.)*
Client: I'd rather you start with Maureen. You know, these things hit her harder than the rest of us. *(Face is somewhat anxious.)*
Nurse: Okay. Let's go see her.

Critical Thinking Challenge
- Detect what the first and second nurses did differently.
- Infer how likely Ann is to ask the first nurse questions about the family's health in the future.
- Compare this with Ann's inclinations in the future to ask the second nurse questions about the family's health.
- Analyze at what point the first nurse could have picked up cues from Ann that indicated she might like some help.

Gently palpate, using the tips of the middle three fingers, to detect any enlargement in lymph nodes. Normally, cervical lymph nodes are smaller than 1 cm in diameter, soft, and mobile. Note any tenderness during palpation.

Diagnostic Tests and Procedures
Because clinical signs sometimes provide insufficient evidence to identify a pathogen, diagnostic procedures are used to detect and identify an infection's source. Laboratory analysis, culturing of body fluids, radiographic studies, and other imaging methods are used. Antibiotic sensitivities and therapeutic drug monitoring are used to identify optimal drug therapy. Common studies included in an initial workup for infection are

- Complete blood count including hemoglobin, hematocrit, and WBC count
- Urinalysis
- Erythrocyte sedimentation rate (ESR or sed rate)

If infection is strongly suspected, the physician may also order a series of WBC counts with differentials and body fluid cultures and sensitivities.

White Blood Cell Count. The number of WBCs, or leukocytes, rises in response to infection, tissue necrosis, stress, or neoplastic changes in bone marrow. A rise in circulating WBCs above the normal adult range of 5,000 to 10,000 cells/mm^3 is called **leukocytosis.** Infection processes may be discovered by examining the WBCs and differentiating the cell types. Each type is based on a percentage of the total number.

Neutrophils normally comprise about 50% to 70% of all WBCs. Their numbers increase during infection. If the in-

DISPLAY 39-3

🔲 HEALTH INTERVIEW INFORMATION

- Immunization history, history of exposure to communicable diseases, and any recent acute infections
- Chronic diseases that have been complicated by infections and the usual method of treatment; signs and symptoms experienced and medications used
- Medications or medical therapy the client is receiving (e.g., antibiotics, steroids, immunosuppression drugs, chemotherapy, or radiation therapy)
- Client's usual diet and its nutritional adequacy
- Client's patterns of sleep, exercise, and recreation to determine health beliefs and lifestyle factors that may contribute to the risk of infection
- History of nausea, vomiting, diarrhea, anorexia, general malaise, muscle aches, or headaches

fection is severe or prolonged, the body cannot manufacture neutrophils quickly enough, resulting in the release of immature granulocytes (also called bands) into the blood. This increase in the number of immature cells is called a *"shift to the left"* or leftward shift in the granulocytic differential count. A leftward shift is considered a strong indication of bacterial infection; the greater the leftward shift, the more worrisome the infection appears. When the proportion of neutrophils increases, the client's resistance is good and the body is considered to be fighting the infection well.

Very low neutrophil counts, often associated with cancer or chemotherapy, greatly increase infection risk. When the neutrophils fall below 500/mm^3, the client is said to be neutropenic (Black, Hawks, & Keene, 2001). Clients are instructed to institute measures to prevent possible lethal infections, including good personal hygiene and avoiding contact with infectious agents or individuals with infectious diseases (Black, Hawks, & Keene, 2001). Common signs of infection are often caused by the actions by neutrophils, so when neutrophil counts are very low, symptoms of infection may be absent.

Some clients, such as those who are malnourished, older, immunosuppressed, or taking steroids, cannot produce more WBCs in response to an infection. In such cases, the absence of an increase in total WBCs or a lack of clarity on the differential count does not rule out infection.

Erythrocyte Sedimentation Rate. The ESR measures, in millimeters per hour, the rate at which RBCs settle in unclotted blood. The result is elevated both in acute noninfectious inflammatory conditions and in infectious processes. Collagen disease, tissue necrosis, malignancy, or stress can also increase the rate of sedimentation. This test is most commonly used to provide a crude estimate of a disease process or of the response to therapy. Because drugs and other factors affect the ESR, all medications the client is taking should be brought to the laboratory's attention.

Serology Tests. Serology tests that detect antigen–antibody reactions are sometimes done as part of a diagnostic workup for a fever. Early in an infection's course, an acute-phase blood specimen is collected. If the infection's cause is not determined by the third week, a convalescent-phase specimen is obtained and both specimens are examined simultaneously for a change in antibody titer. The laboratory needs to know the client's clinical signs and symptoms and immunization history. By comparing antigen–antibody reactions between the two specimens, a diagnosis can be made.

Culture, Sensitivity, and Minimum Inhibitory Concentration. Cultures are obtained from body fluids to isolate the source of unknown fevers and to identify the microorganism causing signs of clinical infection. Culture specimens are obtained from blood, sputum, stool, throat, wound exudate, or urine, or from spinal, joint, pleural, or other body cavity fluids.

Specimens are sent to the laboratory for Gram's stain and culture and sensitivity results. Gram's stains, when properly prepared, broadly classify the microorganisms. This information may be used to order antibiotic therapy while waiting for specific culture results. Results of Gram's stains can be obtained from the laboratory in less than 30 minutes. Usually, 24 to 36 hours is required to grow good cultures, and 48 hours is needed to obtain growth and sensitivity results.

Sensitivity testing of microorganisms to antibiotics is a benefit of obtaining good culture specimens. After microorganisms are grown in culture media, various concentrations of antibiotics are used to test their ability to inhibit growth or to kill the organism. The laboratory reports the names of the organisms present and whether they are sensitive or resistant to specific antibiotics. A helpful way to report this information is the minimum inhibitory concentrations (MIC), which quantifies the minimal amount of the drug that is necessary to inhibit microbial growth in the laboratory. Use of the MIC permits primary healthcare providers to select antibiotics that can kill the organism with a concentration that will not be toxic to the client. The serum level of the drug is usually kept above the MIC value (Shirrell, Gibbar-Clements, Dooley, & Free, 1999).

The accuracy of laboratory analysis for all cultures is only as good as the specimen provided. Factors affecting the results of the analysis include the following:

- Contamination of the specimen
- Delay in sending the specimen to the laboratory (which increases the growth of contaminating organisms and causes deterioration of the constituents to be examined)
- Use of inappropriate containers and/or culture media
- Failure to identify the source of the specimen
- Failure to tell the laboratory about current client medications (e.g., antibiotics) that may affect the analysis

Elicit the client's cooperation by explaining why the specimen is being obtained. Obtain specimens before starting administration of antibiotics that could alter the results. Label the specimen with the time, date, and site of collection and send it to the laboratory immediately.

SAFETY ALERT

When obtaining cultures, use aseptic techniques and wear gloves to avoid potential transmission of pathogens.

Blood Cultures. Blood cultures are ordered when a high degree of suspicion exists that an infectious process is occurring in the bloodstream. Blood cultures are usually obtained from two separate venipuncture sites. Because indwelling intravascular lines may be contaminated with surface pathogens, blood is not usually drawn for culture from previously inserted lines. The ideal specimen is drawn just before or during the rise in temperature, because the pathogens are usually circulating in high concentrations at that time.

Obtaining a blood culture requires use of a set of culture bottles, a sterile syringe, two sterile needles, skin preparation equipment, and a tourniquet. The skin is cleaned according to the institution's procedure. Usually, a combination preparation of povidone-iodine (Betadine; Purdue Frederick, Norwalk, CT) and alcohol is recommended. Clean the tops of the culture bottles and allow them to dry. Apply gloves and then use the sterile needle and syringe to aspirate blood. Change the needle before inoculating the culture medium into special vacuum bottles. After ensuring hemostasis at the puncture site, remove the gloves and wash your hands before transporting the specimen to the laboratory.

Sputum Culture. Sputum cultures are obtained in a fever work-up when the client has a productive cough. Because infections may be located in either the upper or lower respiratory tract, a good culture specimen should not contain saliva (saliva and postnasal drip secretions contaminate the specimen). Sputum ideally should be obtained in the morning, before the client eats. Collect the specimen in a sterile container with a lid and transport it to the laboratory as soon as it is obtained (unless it is a 24-hour specimen, which usually is placed in a special fixative).

Occasionally, a client cannot cooperate with sputum specimen collection or a specimen must be obtained from a client who is endotracheally intubated. Obtain the specimen by suctioning with a sterile suction catheter by way of the nasotracheal or endotracheal route. The physician may also elect to perform a bronchoscopy or to insert a small catheter through a needle into the trachea to aspirate secretions transtracheally. Again, transport specimens to the laboratory immediately.

Throat Culture. Throat cultures are obtained with a sterile cotton swab that is touched to the back of the throat as the client says "Aaahh." Perform this procedure as quickly as possible, because it may trigger the gag reflex. Maintaining sterility, place the swab into a culture medium and transport it to the laboratory.

Wound Culture. Wound cultures are taken when signs of local inflammation or purulent drainage from the wound are noted (Procedure 39-1). Suitable culture media kits are used; they differ depending on whether the wound is being cultured for aerobic or anaerobic organisms. Use fresh exudate for culture specimens. After removing the dressing, gently wipe away any crusted drainage with sterile gauze before swabbing the area. Obtain the specimen from deep in the wound, if possible; swabs from the skin usually are of no value.

Body Cavity and Fluid Culture. Body cavity and fluid cultures are obtained with the use of aseptic technique when inflammation in the area is indicated. Spinal, joint, and pleural cavity fluids are commonly cultured for microorganisms based on clinical observations and a high index of suspicion for an infectious process. Special kits are available, and sterile technique is always used. Assist the physician in obtaining these specimens by ordering supplies, positioning and draping the client, and ensuring rapid transport of specimens to the laboratory.

Stool Culture. Stool cultures may be ordered to rule out infectious causes of diarrhea. Cultures are usually necessary to examine the stool for leukocytes and to identify enteric bacterial or fungal pathogens. Parasites, another common cause of diarrhea, lay eggs in the GI tract that can be detected on examination. Usually, when a client is being screened for parasitic infection, stool specimens are collected daily for 3 days. Moving organisms can easily be detected in fresh specimens.

Collect stool specimens in a sterile bedpan and transfer the specimens to a sterile container with a sterile tongue blade. On the laboratory form, identify the test required, the organism being screened, and whether the client has been traveling or backpacking in remote areas. Urine, toilet paper, soap, disinfectants, antibiotics, antacids, barium, laxatives, enemas, and cool temperatures can affect stool specimens.

Urinalysis. The urine is routinely examined to check for kidney and endocrine function and to identify the presence of UTI. Urinalysis provides information about the color, pH, specific gravity, and presence of protein, glucose, and ketones in the urine. Microscopic examinations search for casts, RBCs and WBCs, epithelial cells, and bacteria. Changes in color, concentration, or odor of the urine may indicate an infectious process. Alkaline urine (pH > 8) may indicate bacteriuria. High levels of glucose and protein may indicate systemic infection or UTI. The presence of erythrocytes (RBCs) or their cellular casts may indicate infection but also may be caused by noninfectious inflammatory conditions. Large numbers of WBCs usually indicate a UTI. A clean-catch or midstream urine specimen is requested if more than four WBCs are found or if bacteria are seen on the slide made from the urine sample. See Chapter 40 for more information on collecting urine samples. Report any abnormal results to the physician so that treatment can start.

Therapeutic Drug Monitoring. Drug monitoring is used to determine a drug's concentration in blood. Blood levels of antibiotics are tested to avoid possible toxic effects such as renal damage (nephrotoxicity) or eighth cranial nerve damage (ototoxicity). The timing of specimen collection is of critical importance. For the laboratory and physician to interpret the plasma drug level, they must know when the last dose of

PROCEDURE 39-1

OBTAINING A WOUND CULTURE

Purpose
1. Identify organisms colonized within a wound so that antibiotics sensitive to the microorganisms can be prescribed, as needed.

Assessment
- Frequently inspect surgical incisions and other wounds for signs of inflammation and infection (i.e., redness, swelling, warmth, drainage).
- Monitor vital signs for evidence of infection (i.e., increased temperature, pulse).
- Identify and document amount, color, and odor of any drainage from wounds.
- Assess client for level of discomfort associated with dressing changes and premedicate if necessary with analgesics.
- Identify factors that contribute to potential development of wound infections.

Equipment
Sterile culture swab (anaerobic or aerobic) and transport container
Disposable, clean gloves
Sterile dressing and tape
Name label and completed laboratory requisition

Procedure
1. Identify client and verify order for culture noting site and type of culture.
   Rationale: Prevents potential errors.
2. Wash hands and apply disposable gloves.
   Rationale: Prevent the transfer of microorganisms and protect hands from contact with drainage.
3. Remove soiled dressing. Observe drainage for amount, odor, and color.
   Rationale: Assess wound for signs of infection.
4. Clear and remove exudate from around wound with antiseptic swab.
   Rationale: Old drainage and microorganisms from wound could interfere with accurate culture and sensitivity report.

Obtaining Aerobic Culture
1. Perform Steps 1 to 4 above.
2. Using sterile swab from culture tube, insert swab deep into area of active drainage. Rotate swab to absorb as much drainage as possible.
   Rationale: Adequate sample is necessary for culture of organism.

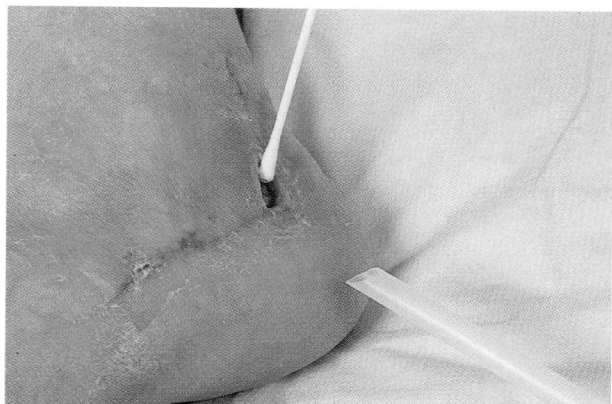

Step 2 Insert culture swab into wound to obtain sample.

3. Insert swab into culture tube, taking care not to touch the top or outside of the tube.
   Rationale: The outside of the culture tube must remain free of pathogenic microorganisms to prevent possible spread of infection to others.
4. Crush ampule of medium and close container securely.
   Rationale: Culture medium keeps bacteria alive until analysis is complete. Closing the container prevents transmission of microorganisms to other areas and also prevents introducing other microorganisms into the tube.
5. Continue with Step 4 below.

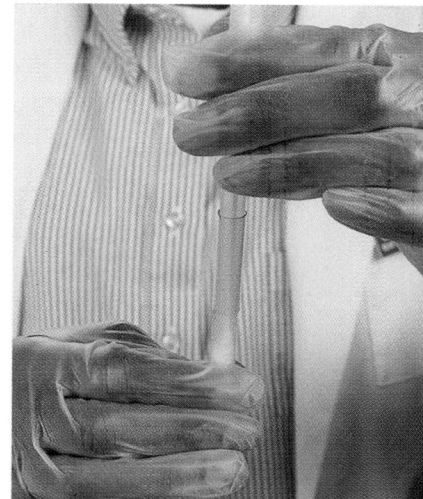

Step 4 Crush ampule of medium.

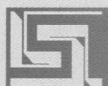

PROCEDURE 39-1 (Continued)

Obtaining Anaerobic Culture

1. Perform Steps 1 to 4 at beginning of procedure.
2. Using sterile swab from special anaerobic culture tube, insert swab deeply into draining body cavity.
   Rationale: Take drainage sample from deep cavity to identify organisms that may grow where oxygen is not present.
3. a. Rotate swab gently and remove. Quickly place swab into inner tube of collection container.
   b. *Alternative method:* Insert tip of syringe with needle removed into wound and aspirate 1 to 5 mL of exudate. Attach 21-gauge needle to syringe, expel all air, and inject exudate into inner tube of the culture container.
   Rationale: The inner tube of the culture container has either a carbon dioxide or a nitrogen environment to prevent potential contaminating organisms from growing until the laboratory analysis is complete. Note: Drainage is sampled from only one drainage site per culture swab. If a specimen is required from another site, repeat the above steps to identify accurately microbes present at each drainage site.
4. Label each culture tube and send specimens with appropriate requisition immediately to the laboratory. Some agencies require that specimens be transported in clean plastic bags to further prevent transfer of microorganisms.
   Rationale: Bacteria grow rapidly within culture media of specimen tubes. Prepare cultures quickly for accurate results.
5. Clean and apply sterile dressings to the wound, as ordered.
   Rationale: Protect the wound from environmental contamination; dressing contains further drainage to prevent spread of infection.
6. Remove and discard gloves. Wash hands.
   Rationale: Reduce the risk of transmission of microorganisms.
7. Assist client to comfortable position.
8. Document all relevant information on the client's chart. Include the location the specimen was taken from, and the date and time. Record the wound's appearance, and the color, odor, amount, and consistency of drainage. Record how the client tolerated the procedure and any discomfort that he or she experienced.
   Rationale: Documentation maintains accurate client records and provides a means of communication with other health team members.

Lifespan Considerations
Infants and Children

* Perform procedures that are uncomfortable or potentially fear-inducing in areas other than the child's room, so the child continues to regard his or her room as a safe place.

Home Care Considerations

* Teach client the signs and symptoms of infection and what to report to the healthcare provider.
* When obtaining cultures from the client at his or her home, transport the specimens as quickly as possible to the closest laboratory for analysis.

Collaboration and Delegation

* Notify healthcare provider promptly of positive culture results, noting if prescribed antibiotics are indicated for the identified infectious agent.
* Supervise all personnel to ensure appropriate infection control measures to prevent the possible transmission of pathogens.

---

antibiotic was given and when the specimen was obtained. The highest level of drug concentration (*peak level*) should occur shortly after the drug is given, and the lowest level (*trough level*) should occur just before a dose is due to be administered. Specimens must be labeled as to whether they are being analyzed as a peak or a trough specimen. Depending on the test results, the amount of the antibiotic and the frequency of dosing may be adjusted to match the client's rate of metabolism and drug clearance.

Diagnostic Imaging. Rapid advances are being made in the ability to visualize internal organs and to evaluate them for infection. After these tests are performed, monitor the client's vital signs. When contrast material is used, observe for any signs of allergic reaction.

Chest radiographs are used to diagnose pneumonia, lung abscesses, and tuberculosis. Endoscopic procedures are used to visualize the respiratory and GI tracts and to obtain specimens for microbiologic testing. Computed axial tomography (CT or CAT) is used to obtain multidimensional images of the body, which the computer interprets to construct images of internal structures. By visualizing the differences in density among organs and any organ deformities, the study can help locate abscesses or other areas of infection. The study can be done with the use of contrast medium, which enhances visualization of normal versus abnormal tissue.

Magnetic resonance imaging (MRI) is used with increasing frequency to detect infections of the nervous system. The procedure uses opaque contrast materials, injected intravenously, that have affinities for concentrations of WBCs in abscesses or other areas of infection.

NURSING DIAGNOSES

Risk for Infection is the only nursing diagnosis related to infection that is accepted by the North American Nursing Diagnosis Association (NANDA). If a client has an actual infection, the problem is collaborative, necessitating intervention from nurses, physicians, pharmacists, and other members of the healthcare team. Nurses can independently develop individualized plans to help prevent infection for clients at risk.

Risk for Infection

Definition. Risk for Infection is the state in which a person is at increased risk for being invaded by pathogenic organisms (NANDA, 2001).

Risk Factors. Risk factors for infection include
- Insufficient knowledge to avoid exposure to pathogens
- Invasive procedures, trauma, rupture of amniotic membranes, tissue destruction, and increased environmental exposure to pathogens
- Malnutrition, immunosuppression, pharmaceutical agents
- Inadequate primary defenses (broken skin, traumatized tissue, decrease in ciliary action, stasis of body fluids, change in pH secretions, altered peristalsis)
- Inadequate secondary defenses (decreased hemoglobin, leukopenia, suppressed inflammatory response) and immunosuppression
- Inadequate acquired immunity, tissue destruction, increased environmental exposure, chronic disease, invasive procedures, malnutrition, pharmaceutical agents, trauma, rupture of amniotic membranes, insufficient knowledge to avoid exposure to pathogens.

Related Nursing Diagnoses

Other nursing diagnoses are common in people with infection. Deficient Knowledge may occur, and inadequate knowledge of hygiene or infection control measures can contribute to increased incidence of infection. Many clients with infection are discharged to home with new treatments and protocols to master.

APPLY YOUR KNOWLEDGE

Mr. Foscarelli, a 76-year-old client with asthma, is recovering from abdominal surgery. He is having moderate incisional pain and is reluctant to move because of the pain. Your morning assessment reveals vital signs as follows: temperature 38°C, B/P 142/64, P 96, R 26 and shallow. He appears slightly confused and has developed a productive cough of thick, tan sputum. Lung auscultation reveals diminished breath sounds with rhonchi in the right middle lobe. His urine is clear, and the output is good.

What risk factors does Mr. Foscarelli have for infection? What data support the presence of infection? What type of infection seems most likely? What laboratory tests would you expect the primary care provider to order?

Check your answers in Appendix A.

Acute Pain, Hyperthermia, and Fatigue are other common nursing diagnoses associated with infection. The inflammation that accompanies infection causes discomfort. Discomfort also may occur secondary to fever. Disturbed Sleep Pattern can occur if discomfort is great.

Depending on its location, infection can affect the function of various body systems. Impaired Physical Mobility can occur if the infection is in an extremity or bed rest is needed to treat the infection. Impaired Urinary Elimination can occur with a UTI. Bowel Incontinence can occur if infection results in diarrhea or the client experiences it as an adverse effect of antibiotic therapy. Impaired Gas Exchange is common with lung infections. Impaired Skin Integrity can occur secondary to rashes that accompany many infections or because of impaired healing of surgical incisions in the presence of an infection.

Disturbed Self-Esteem can result when a client assumes the sick role or adjusts to a changing body image. Anxiety and Ineffective Coping can occur when clients and their families face severe infection. Ineffective Role Performance may be a consequence when an infection limits a person's ability to work, go to school, or carry out normal family responsibilities. Sexual Dysfunction can occur because of lowered energy reserves or as a direct consequence of an STD.

OUTCOME IDENTIFICATION AND PLANNING

Client goals and outcome criteria focus on preventing infections and minimizing potential complications. Examples of client goals related to infection include the following:

- The client or caregiver will demonstrate adequate knowledge to recognize and report signs of infection.
- The client or caregiver will demonstrate use of good health practices to prevent occurrence and spread of infection.
- The client will participate in treatment regimens to prevent infection and minimize complications.

Planning for nursing interventions is directed at the following:

- Controlling the spread of infection
- Providing education to modify risk behaviors
- Supporting normal defense mechanisms and behaviors that prevent infection
- Reducing or eliminating the adverse effects of infection on functional abilities
- Detecting behaviors that increase the potential for infection
- Participating in community planning and activities for infection prevention

Examples of nursing interventions are listed in the accompanying display and discussed in the next section of this chapter.

IMPLEMENTATION

Health Promotion

Personal Hygiene

Decreasing the number of microorganisms present on body surfaces can help prevent and fight infection. Encourage clients to wash their hands after using the toilet, before eating, and after coming in contact with articles likely to be contaminated. Regular bathing, shampooing, and general grooming help keep body surfaces clean. In some instances, such as before surgery, antimicrobial soap may be used to impede microbial growth.

> ### 🟦 SAFETY ALERT
> **Handwashing is the most significant measure to decrease the transient growth of microorganisms.**

Daily brushing and flossing of teeth remove microorganisms that collect in the oral cavity. Regular dental checkups are important to remove plaque and tartar, which provide good foci for bacterial growth.

Protection of Skin and Mucous Membranes

Intact skin and mucous membranes provide a physical barrier against invasion from possible pathogens. Encourage clients to prevent excessive drying of skin by ensuring adequate hydration and applying lubricants or cream. They should use a water-soluble lubricant applied to the nares or lips to prevent cracking. Avoiding trauma that could impair skin integrity is important. Remind clients to avoid harsh chemicals and excessive heat or friction that can abrade skin.

For bedridden clients, establish regular turning schedules to decrease the chance of skin breakdown and possible infection. Use specialized equipment such as kinetic beds or special mattresses for high-risk immobile clients.

Rest and Relaxation

Adequate rest and freedom from stress are important in fighting and preventing infection. Sleep disturbances can occur when clients must be awakened at night. Keep the environ-

---

PLANNING: Examples of NIC/NOC Interventions

Accepted Infection Nursing Interventions Classification (NIC)
Immunization/Vaccination Administration
Infection Control
Infection Protection

Accepted Infection Nursing Outcomes Classification (NOC)
Immune Status
Infection Status
Knowledge: Infection Control
Risk Control
Tissue Integrity: Skin and Mucous Membranes

Refer to the following for specifics regarding NIC/NOC:
   McCloskey, J., & Bulechek, G. (2000). *Iowa Intervention Project: Nursing Interventions Classification (NIC)*, 2nd ed. St. Louis, MO: C.V. Mosby.
   Johnson, M., & Maas, M. (2000). *Iowa Outcomes Project: Nursing Outcomes Classification (NOC)* (2nd ed.). St. Louis, MO: C.V. Mosby.

---

ment quiet and comfortable to induce sleep. Allow naps during the day as indicated. Encourage activities that promote relaxation and reduce stress.

Nutrition and Hydration

A well-balanced diet and adequate hydration are important to maintain adequate host defenses against infection. The body's ability to synthesize antibodies, which are proteins, becomes ineffective if protein stores are depleted. Encourage foods that are rich in vitamins and minerals, such as fruits and vegetables. Eight glasses of water per day ensure adequate hydration, which helps maintain healthy skin and urine flow.

Immunization Programs

Nurses participate in establishing programs for people to receive immunizations. They help to identify outbreaks of infectious disease in the community, give vaccinations, establish record-keeping mechanisms, and counsel people about precautions and possible complications of immunization. Many vaccination programs take place in clinics, schools, and industrial settings.

Immunizations may be given by injection, oral solution, or nasal spray. To avoid multiple injections, they are given in combination (when the compounds are stable and minimal danger exists of overwhelming the immune system). Booster injections of some vaccines are given throughout the lifespan to stimulate the memory cells. Table 39-4 provides guidelines for immunizations of healthy infants and children.

Because of frequent changes, new immunization guidelines must be obtained yearly. This information is available from the Advisory Committee on Immunization Practices of the U.S. Public Health Service and from the Committee on Infectious Diseases of the American Academy of Pediatrics.

TABLE 39-4

Recommended Childhood Immunization Schedule: United States, 2002

Vaccine ▼ / Age ▶	Birth	1 mo	2 mos	4 mos	6 mos	12 mos	15 mos	18 mos	24 mos	4-6 yrs	11-12 yrs	13-18 yrs
										range of recommended ages / catch-up vaccination / preadolescent assessment		
Hepatitis B[1]	Hep B #1	only if mother HBsAg (-)								Hep B series		
		Hep B #2				Hep B #3						
Diphtheria, Tetanus, Pertussis[2]			DTaP	DTaP	DTaP		DTaP			DTaP	Td	
Haemophilus influenzae Type b[3]			Hib	Hib	Hib	Hib						
Inactivated Polio[4]			IPV	IPV		IPV				IPV		
Measles, Mumps, Rubella[5]						MMR #1				MMR #2	MMR #2	
Varicella[6]						Varicella					Varicella	
Pneumococcal[7]			PCV	PCV	PCV	PCV				PCV	PPV	
Hepatitis A[8]										Hepatitis A series		
Influenza[9]						Influenza (yearly)						

Vaccines below this line are for selected populations

This schedule indicates the recommended ages for routine administration of currently licensed childhood vaccines, as of December 1, 2001, for children through age 18 years. Any dose not given at the recommended age should be given at any subsequent visit when indicated and feasible. ▓ Indicates age groups that warrant special effort to administer those vaccines not previously given. Additional vaccines may be licensed and recommended during the year. Licensed combination vaccines may be used whenever any components of the combination are indicated and the vaccine's other components are not contraindicated. Providers should consult the manufacturers' package inserts for detailed recommendations.

1. Hepatitis B vaccine (Hep B). All infants should receive the first dose of hepatitis B vaccine soon after birth and before hospital discharge; the first dose may also be given by age 2 months if the infant's mother is HBsAg-negative. Only monovalent hepatitis B vaccine can be used for the birth dose. Monovalent or combination vaccine containing Hep B may be used to complete the series; four doses of vaccine may be administered if combination vaccine is used. The second dose should be given at least 4 weeks after the first dose, except for Hib-containing vaccine which cannot be administered before age 6 weeks. The third dose should be given at least 16 weeks after the first dose and at least 8 weeks after the second dose. The last dose in the vaccination series (third or fourth dose) should not be administered before age 6 months.

Infants born to HBsAg-positive mothers should receive hepatitis B vaccine and 0.5 mL hepatitis B immune globulin (HBIG) within 12 hours of birth at separate sites. The second dose is recommended at age 1-2 months and the vaccination series should be completed (third or fourth dose) at age 6 months.

Infants born to mothers whose HBsAg status is unknown should receive the first dose of the hepatitis B vaccine series within 12 hours of birth. Maternal blood should be drawn at the time of delivery to determine the mother's HBsAg status; if the HBsAg test is positive, the infant should receive HBIG as soon as possible (no later than age 1 week).

2. Diphtheria and tetanus toxoids and acellular pertussis vaccine (DTaP). The fourth dose of DTaP may be administered as early as age 12 months, provided 6 months have elapsed since the third dose and the child is unlikely to return at age 15-18 months. **Tetanus and diphtheria toxoids (Td)** is recommended at age 11-12 years if at least 5 years have elapsed since the last dose of tetanus and diphtheria toxoid-containing vaccine. Subsequent routine Td boosters are recommended every 10 years.

3. Haemophilus influenzae type b (Hib) conjugate vaccine. Three Hib conjugate vaccines are licensed for infant use. If PRP-OMP (PedvaxHIB® or ComVax® [Merck]) is administered at ages 2 and 4 months, a dose at age 6 months is not required. DTaP/Hib combination products should not be used for primary immunization in infants at age 2, 4 or 6 months, but can be used as boosters following any Hib vaccine.

4. Inactivated poliovirus vaccine (IPV). An all-IPV schedule is recommended for routine childhood poliovirus vaccination in the United States. All children should receive four doses of IPV at age 2 months, 4 months, 6-18 months, and 4-6 years.

5. Measles, mumps, and rubella vaccine (MMR). The second dose of MMR is recommended routinely at age 4-6 years but may be administered during any visit, provided at least 4 weeks have elapsed since the first dose and that both doses are administered beginning at or after age 12 months. Those who have not previously received the second dose should complete the schedule by the visit at 11-12 years.

6. Varicella vaccine. Varicella vaccine is recommended at any visit at or after age 12 months for susceptible children (i.e. those who lack a reliable history of chickenpox). Susceptible persons aged $\geq$13 years should receive two doses, given at least 4 weeks apart.

7. Pneumococcal vaccine. The heptavalent **pneumococcal conjugate vaccine (PCV)** is recommended for all children aged 2-23 months and for certain children aged 24-59 months. **Pneumococcal polysaccharide vaccine (PPV)** is recommended in addition to PCV for certain high-risk groups. See MMWR 2000;49(RR-9);1-37.

8. Hepatitis A vaccine. Hepatitis A vaccine is recommended for use in selected states and regions, and for certain high-risk groups; consult your local public health authority. See MMWR 1999;48(RR-12);1-37.

9. Influenza vaccine. Influenza vaccine is recommended annually for children age $\geq$ 6 months with certain risk factors (including but not limited to asthma, cardiac disease, sickle cell disease, HIV, and diabetes; see MMWR 2001;50(RR-4);1-44), and can be administered to all others wishing to obtain immunity. Children aged $\leq$12 years should receive vaccine in a dosage appropriate for their age (0.25 mL if age 6-35 months or 0.5 mL if aged $\geq$ 3 years). Children aged $\leq$ 8 years who are receiving influenza vaccine for the first time should receive two doses separated by at least 4 weeks.

For additional information about vaccines, vaccine supply, and contraindications for immunization, please visit the National Immunization Program Website at www.cdc.gov/nip or call the National Immunization Hotline at 800-232-2522 (English) or 800-232-0233 (Spanish).

Approved by the Advisory Committee on Immunization Practices (www.cdc.gov/nip/acip), the American Academy of Pediatrics (www.aap.org), and the American Academy of Family Physicians (www.aafp.org).

Similar committees exist in Canada and through the World Health Organization (WHO).

Encourage parents to maintain immunization records for their children and to give them to their children when they move away from home. Physicians need to record this information and make clients aware of any unusual reaction. Commonly, families maintain excellent vaccination records for children through their first years of school but then neglect to update records as children grow older. Children may need this information if questions arise about whether immunizations are current (especially for tetanus after an injury).

Vaccinations are contraindicated in clients with immunodeficiency states, allergy to eggs, or previous allergic reactions. Clients should not receive live vaccines during pregnancy, acute debilitating disease, or periods of severe malnutrition.

In addition to routine childhood immunizations, certain people who are at increased risk need additional immunizations. All healthcare workers and people exposed to blood and body fluids should receive immunizations for hepatitis B virus. Older adults, the chronically ill, and people with respiratory dysfunction should receive annual influenza shots and pneumococcal vaccines. Table 39-5 provides a more complete list of adults at risk and specific recommended immunizations. A person may require additional vaccinations when traveling to a foreign area, where different diseases are endemic.

Nursing Interventions for Altered Function

When an infection becomes established, nursing measures aim at helping the client combat the illness and preventing the infection from spreading to others. Because nothing is more important in controlling infection than maintaining natural barriers against it, nurses devote much time to supporting these defenses. Enhancing host defenses is both preventive and supportive therapy.

Comfort Measures

Manifestations of infection (e.g., aches and pains, feelings of lethargy or malaise, fever, chills, nausea and vomiting, itching) cause generalized discomfort. This discomfort is most often managed by relieving the individual symptoms. Generally, comfort measures aim at relieving debilitating symptoms so as to conserve the client's energy for healing and fighting infection.

Analgesics are used to relieve aches and pains, based on their impact on rest, sleep, and ambulation. Warm broth, a cool cloth to the head, warm blankets, and rest may ease feelings of malaise. Prolonged or excessive fevers may be treated with tepid sponge baths, antipyretics, or cooling blankets. Warm blankets and warm fluids can relieve shaking chills; if they are prolonged, however, intravenous (IV) meperidine may be necessary. Removing objects with objectionable odors, offering carbonated beverages, and providing a darkened, quiet room

TABLE 39-5

Adult Immunizations for High-Risk Groups	
Vaccine	**High-Risk Groups**
Diphtheria–tetanus	All adults who have not been immunized during last 10 yr, especially after puncture wounds or trauma
Measles–mumps–rubella (MMR)	Adults who have never had the disease or been immunized, especially women of childbearing age
	All healthcare workers
	Adults who were born before 1956 and were immunized before 12 mo of age
Pneumococcal infections	Elderly older than 65 yr of age
	Residents of institutions (e.g., prisons, nursing homes)
	Adults with chronic medical problems, especially respiratory or cardiovascular disease
Influenza	Healthcare workers
	Elderly, especially those in nursing homes
	Adults with chronic health problems, especially diabetes, respiratory, and cardiovascular disease
Hepatitis B	All healthcare workers
	Intravenous drug users
	Hemodialysis clients
	Hemophiliac clients
	Immigrants from countries with endemic disease
	Sexually active people with multiple partners
	Adolescents

may relieve nausea and vomiting. In more severe cases, oral intake may need to be restricted and antiemetics administered. Itching may be treated with moist, cool cloths, calamine lotion, pastes made from baking soda, or prescribed antihistamines (e.g., diphenhydramine).

Pulmonary Toilet

Encouraging clients to cough, deep-breathe, blow their nose, and move promotes clearance of respiratory secretions, which may become infected if allowed to pool in the lower respiratory tract. Retained secretions prevent adequate gas exchange at the alveolar level and reduce oxygen available to the tissues to combat infection, heal injured tissues, and meet metabolic needs. Secondary infections are commonly associated with impaired respiratory tract function.

Teach clients to cover their mouths when they cough or sneeze, to prevent droplet transmission of microorganisms. When blowing their noses, clients should always keep one nostril open to avoid forcing secretions into ear canals. Caution youngsters not to pick their noses, because they can easily transmit infected organisms to other body parts and other people. Instruct everyone to dispose of tissues and respiratory secretions properly. See Chapter 34 for detailed information on pulmonary hygiene and care.

Fever Management

Because fever is thought to be an adaptive state that assists the body in fighting infection, interventions to reduce fever should be employed only when very high body temperatures exhaust body resources. Fever management focuses on comfort measures that differ for each fever phase (i.e., chill, fever, and flush). Appropriate nursing interventions are highlighted in Table 39-6.

Antipyretics. Drugs such as aspirin and acetaminophen are called antipyretics because they lower the setting of the hypothalamic thermostat so that body temperature falls. Antipyretics may be used to reduce temperature when fever threatens a client's well-being. Use of antipyretics has been questioned in routine fever treatment, because higher body temperatures help support the body's defenses to fight infection. Most authorities agree that antipyretics are advisable for fever greater than 40°C (104°F).

Aspirin is effective in lowering elevated temperature without reducing it to a lower than normal range. Aspirin promotes heat loss by dilating blood vessels and fostering diaphoresis, but does not affect the body's heat production. Usually, people take aspirin mainly to reduce aches and discomforts associated with fever.

🧴 SAFETY ALERT

Do not give aspirin to children with flulike illnesses. Use of aspirin in such cases has been associated with Reye's syndrome, a potentially fatal condition involving liver damage and encephalopathy (Saez-Llorens & McCracken, 1997).

TABLE 39-6

Caring for the Febrile Person		
Phase	**Signs/Symptoms**	**Nursing Interventions**
Chill phase	Client feels cold and shivers; skin is pale and cool to touch; "gooseflesh" appears; body temperature increases.	Apply extra blankets. Increase fluid intake. Restrict activity. Supply supplemental oxygen if client has pre-existing cardiac or respiratory problem.
Fever phase	Client feels neither hot nor cold; oral mucosa are dry; client is thirsty, possibly dehydrated; client experiences feelings of general malaise, weakness, aching muscles, drowsiness, or restlessness.	Cover with light, warm clothing to avoid chilling client. Encourage cool fluids. Promote rest. Apply lubricant to dry lips and nasal mucosa. Use tepid sponging if temperature becomes very high. Increase air circulation to encourage cooling. Implement safety precautions to protect client if restless or delirious.
Flush phase	Client sweats profusely, is possibly dehydrated. Shivering decreases. Skin is flushed and warm to touch.	Use tepid sponging. Avoid chilling client. Encourage cool fluids. Restrict activity. Cover client with light clothing or bed linens.

When administering an antipyretic to a febrile client, take the client's temperature immediately before giving the medication and approximately 1 hour later to determine whether the medication has had the desired effect.

Tepid Baths. Tepid baths and sponging are used for febrile clients when their temperature reaches seriously elevated levels. They should not be administered during a fever's chill phase. Use tepid, rather than cool, water to prevent chilling. Clients may find this procedure either soothing or uncomfortable, depending on skin temperature. Tepid baths or sponging is intended to replace artificially the body's sweating mechanism by cooling the skin's surface, thereby cooling the blood delivered to the body core. Also, this technique promotes cooling by the process of evaporation. Be careful to avoid chilling the client, which will trigger the shivering mechanism. Measure the client's temperature before and 30 minutes after the procedure to determine the intervention's effectiveness.

Hypothermia Blankets. These special blankets can be used to reduce the temperature of the hyperpyrexic client. Such blankets consist of rubber or vinyl coils through which distilled water or alcohol is pumped. The fluid's temperature can be programmed by a control device similar to a thermostat. When cooling is desired, the blanket is usually set slightly lower than normal body temperature (e.g., 35°C [96°F]). A rectal probe is inserted to continuously monitor core body temperature so that excessive cooling does not occur. During use of the hypothermia blanket, medication may be necessary to block the shivering mechanism.

Neutropenic Precautions

Neutropenia is present when the absolute neutrophil count (ANC) falls to fewer than 1000 cells/mm³. Serious bacterial infection is almost certain if the ANC is less than 500 cells/mm³ (Black, Hawks, & Keene, 2001). When there are fewer than 200 neutrophils per cubic millimeter, the inflammatory response is absent even in the presence of an infection (Black, Hawks, & Keene, 2001). When neutropenic precautions are indicated, place the client in a private room and limit visitors, especially children and people with any signs of infection. Handwashing is essential for all who enter the room. Keep the door closed to limit airborne exposure. Whenever it is necessary for the client to leave the hospital room, he or she should wear a mask. Take special care to prevent any breaks in mucous membranes. Provide gentle oral care, and avoid flossing. Avoid razors with blades and do not take rectal temperatures. Avoid injections whenever possible. Also, remove any sources of pathogens in the environment, such as stagnant water, fresh flowers, or potted plants. Low microbial diets, which eliminate fresh vegetables or fruits and undercooked or raw meat, are indicated (Johnson & Gross, 1998; Yarboro, Frogge, Goodman, and Groenwald, 2000).

Clients who are neutropenic after chemotherapy experience a predictable drop in neutrophils, which at its lowest point is referred to as *nadir*. Estimate when the client will experience nadir based on the specific chemotherapeutic drug adminis-

tered. Also teach clients that this is when they will be most susceptible to infection and that preventive measures at this time are essential. Encourage clients to avoid crowds and other likely sources of infection exposure.

Granulocyte colony-stimulating factors (G-CSF) have been developed with the use of DNA technology. These factors are administered to stimulate production of neutrophils in the bone marrow, thus decreasing the degree and duration of neutropenia (Yarboro et al., 2000).

Antimicrobial Therapy

Antimicrobial agents are used to combat the growth and replication of microorganisms. Administering and monitoring of these drugs are collaborative functions of nurses, physicians, pharmacists, and laboratory technicians.

Prescribed antibiotics are based on the presumed antibiotic sensitivity of the infecting species. A culture and sensitivity analysis is obtained to determine appropriate antibiotic therapy. Antibiotics should not be used routinely for all infections. Several species of organisms have mutated over the years since antibiotics were introduced and now are resistant to all but a few toxic drugs (see Chapter 26).

Remember what antibiotics can and cannot do. They cannot cure the client; at best, they slow the growth of or kill the infecting organism, which is necessary for clients to recover from infection. They control the size of the microbial population against which the client's immune system must contend. Antibiotics "buy time" during which the client's own immune system can mobilize. Eliminating the microbes may prevent further injury, but a return to normal depends on the body's healing capacity.

As a group, antibiotics have a wide range of safety, but they can produce severe allergic reactions and toxic effects. Renal and hepatic failure, interactions with other drugs, underlying disease, and extremes of age predispose clients to adverse reactions. Both the very young and the very old have impaired renal clearance of drugs. Anticipate the need for dosage adjustments in these age groups. Monitor blood levels of antibiotics to ensure safety and optimal effectiveness.

🥤 **SAFETY ALERT**
Always ask clients about allergies to foods or drugs and any drugs they currently use to prevent allergic reactions and incompatibilities.

Antibiotics may eradicate the endogenous flora of the skin and mucous membranes of the mouth, GI tract, and vaginal tract. This flora normally protects the host's mucous membranes; when it is eliminated, opportunistic organisms may invade the tissues. A *superinfection* is a secondary infection that occurs when antibiotics, immunosuppression, or cancer treatment destroys normal flora. These infections are more common when antimicrobials are given in large doses, several antimicrobials are given concurrently, or broad-spectrum antibiotics are used. Usually, superinfection appears 4 to 5 days after antimicrobial therapy begins. Superinfections commonly are fungal infections of the mouth or vagina.

Prevention of Infection Spread

Nurses perform interventions that prevent the spread of infection to others. Chapter 26 discusses aseptic practice: handwashing; cleaning, disinfection, and sterilization; use of barriers; isolation precautions; and surgical asepsis.

Handwashing and sterile technique are two significant measures to prevent the occurrence and transmission of infection in healthcare settings. Although experts say that proper handwashing can reduce nosocomial infection rates by 50%, studies have demonstrated that compliance rates by healthcare personnel are consistently substandard, frequently less than 50% (Pittet, Mourouga, and Perneger, 1999; Bischoff et al., 2000; Harbarth, 2000).

Often, nurses are the first to identify symptoms indicating infection in clients and to institute precautions to prevent transmission. Instruct clients and their families about proper methods for disposal of body secretions such as sputum, feces, urine, and wound drainage. Also, provide clients with tissues to cover the nose and mouth while coughing and sneezing. Place disposal bags within convenient reach, and empty any bags that become full. Replace them as necessary.

Healthcare Planning and Home- or Community-Based Nursing

Nurses work at various levels to plan, implement, and evaluate measures to prevent and control infection. Four levels are the person and family (household), the community, the nation, and the world.

Home Care Management

Many clients are discharged home with indwelling devices that increase the risk for infection. Whether such care is short or long term, avoiding infectious complications and supporting the family are important in helping clients maintain functional abilities.

The trend is toward keeping all but the most seriously ill clients at home for the delivery of healthcare. Hospitalization, once thought to protect clients who are severely immunosuppressed, is now controversial. During hospitalization, clients are more likely to become infected with virulent, sometimes drug-resistant, organisms.

Clients and their caregivers must learn how to evaluate vital signs, give medications, and observe for signs of toxicity. Stress the importance of basic hygiene measures such as bathing, toileting, and oral care, as well as basic aseptic practices. Educate about the importance of handwashing and proper disposal of contaminated supplies. Instruction in sterile technique is necessary for managing IV devices and medications.

Also teach caregivers to wear rubber gloves when caring for clients with known infections. Lightweight rubber gloves, the kind commonly used for dishwashing and household cleaning, are suitable for the home care of clients with diarrhea or wound infections. These gloves can be washed with mild soap and water and reused after drying. Caution caregivers to keep these gloves separate from those they use for food preparation or dishwashing.

If drug therapy is ordered, be sure to instruct clients and caregivers in the drug regimen, including signs and symptoms of infection that they should report to the healthcare provider.

Community, Nation, and World Infection Control

Community regulations controlling the quality of drinking water, food served in public places, and disposal of sewage and solid waste are important aspects of community infection control. Community or regional health authorities gather statistics

OUTCOME-BASED TEACHING PLAN

Mr. Petrenkov, a 76-year-old client with asthma, developed pneumonia after abdominal surgery. He is being discharged with an antibiotic to take for the next 7 days. He will return to his primary care provider (PCP) in 1 week to have staples removed from his incision and to be evaluated.

OUTCOME: Mr. Petrenkov will verbalize signs and symptoms of any wound or respiratory infection and when to notify PCP.
Strategies
- Review with Mr. Petrenkov a handout that lists the signs and symptoms of wound infection (elevated temperature, increased redness or pain in incision, drainage especially containing pus from the incision).
- Verbalize symptoms of respiratory infection (increased shortness of breath; increased sputum, change in tenacity or color of sputum) and add them to list.
- Instruct Mr. Petrenkov to take his temperature daily and to notify PCP of any elevation over 100.8°F.
- Teach Mr. Petrenkov how to inspect incision every morning and evening for signs of infection.
- Have Mr. Petrenkov verbalize symptoms of infection that require calling PCP.

OUTCOME: Mr. Petrenkov will verbalize how to take antibiotic medication safely.
Strategies
- Provide Mr. Petrenkov with a computerized handout about the prescribed antibiotic. Add the specific trade name, dose, and frequency.
- Review the handout with Mr. Petrenkov and reinforce plans for antibiotic regimen.
- Have Mr. Petrenkov explain how he will take his medication after discharge. Provide positive reinforcement of an appropriate plan.
- Review common side effects such as diarrhea and rash, explaining the importance of contacting his PCP should they occur.
- Stress the importance of finishing the entire prescription to prevent recurrence of infection and possible drug resistance.

on the incidence of infectious diseases in their areas. They decide which diseases pose a hazard to the community's well-being and must be reported. Many communities and states have passed laws forbidding unimmunized children from attending school. Some bar children with active infections from classrooms.

Some countries have public health agencies that gather statistics from regional reports and compile them for yearly comparisons. These agencies govern quality of air, water, food, and wastes that cross state, regional, or international boundaries, and they set standards for reduction of pollutants and microorganisms. They bar people with designated acute infections from immigrating into the country and prohibit the return of natives without proof of immunization against diseases endemic in the areas to which they have traveled.

Several international health organizations, such as WHO, gather statistics from national groups and have formed commissions for the education of healthcare providers. These organizations establish priorities for infection control and make recommendations about immunizations for international travelers. International commissions also provide supplies and personnel for some immunization programs.

EVALUATION

The success of a program to prevent or control infection requires cooperation from both the client and the healthcare team. Excellent communication is necessary, and trust must be established. People must assume responsibility for their own behaviors and healthcare practices. The healthcare system must educate the public and scrutinize its own infection prevention methods. Healthcare workers must diligently practice infection control.

The optimal outcome of efforts to control infection (which is not always attainable) is freedom from signs and symptoms of infection. Some outcome criteria for goals involving infection are listed here.

Goal

The client will demonstrate adequate knowledge to recognize and report signs of infection.

Possible Outcome Criteria

- After a teaching session, the client or caregiver lists four signs of infection.
- After a teaching session, the client or caregiver demonstrates accurate monitoring of body temperature.
- Before discharge, the client or caregiver verbalizes indications that would require contacting a healthcare professional.

Goal

The client will demonstrate use of good health practices to prevent the occurrence and spread of infection.

Possible Outcome Criteria

- After each teaching session, the client or caregiver demonstrates correct handwashing technique.
- Before discharge, the client or caregiver verbalizes proper methods of infection control to use at home.
- By the time of discharge, the client verbalizes selected strategies to minimize the risk of infection.

Goal

The client will participate in treatment regimens to prevent infection and minimize possible complications.

Possible Outcome Criteria

- The client uses recommended aseptic practices for dressing changes or manipulation of invasive devices, as evidenced by a return demonstration at the next home visit.
- The client takes prescribed medications to treat or prevent infections, as reported to the nurse at the next appointment.
- The client keeps the next three appointments with healthcare providers.

KEY CONCEPTS

- The body has an elaborate system of barriers to protect against infection.
- Most infections result from a breakdown of nonspecific and specific host defenses. Infections are responsible for most visits to healthcare facilities.
- Inflammation and fever are two nonspecific natural defenses. The four signs of inflammation are redness, warmth, swelling, and tenderness. Fever is an important mechanism in fighting infection, but it consumes a great deal of metabolic energy.
- The immune response, a specific defense, involves two methods: humoral and cellular immunity. T lymphocytes and B lymphocytes form memory cells that can be reactivated on reexposure to an antigen.
- Infection progresses through four stages: incubation, the prodromal period, the acute phase, and convalescence.
- Very young and very old people have decreased resistance to infection. Age affects both nonspecific and specific barriers to infection.
- The inflammatory response helps control the spread of infection, but if it goes on too long it can harm the client.
- Fever supports host defense mechanisms and is treated with antipyretics, tepid baths, or hypothermia blankets only when very high (i.e., greater than 40°C [104°F]).
- A culture and sensitivity analysis is necessary to identify the specific organism causing an infection and antibiotics that may be useful for treatment.
- Immunizations are given to children and adults to prevent some infectious diseases. Because communicable childhood diseases can result in severe complications, all children should be immunized.
- Preventing infection is an individual, community, national, and international responsibility.
- Increasing numbers of clients are being treated at home for chronic conditions or rehabilitation. Many of them have several risk factors for infection. Nurses must assume the responsibility for teaching these clients or their caregivers how to prevent and control infection.

NURSING PLAN OF CARE
THE CLIENT AT RISK FOR INFECTION

Nursing Diagnosis
Risk for infection related to delayed wound healing, immunosuppressive treatment for cancer of the bowel, and age.

Client Goal
Client/family will demonstrate knowledge about methods for preventing and detecting infection.

Client Outcome Criteria
- Client/family member describes methods to avoid infection after teaching session.
- Client/family member verbalizes signs and symptoms of infection after teaching session.
- Client/family member demonstrates acceptable technique in applying a dressing by next visit.
- Client/family member describes food and fluid that will meet nutritional needs by next visit.

Nursing Intervention
1. Begin instruction of wound care as early in the course of recovery as possible. Include family member.
2. Review principles of good handwashing before wound care.
3. Demonstrate the technique for dressing change. Allow time for practice and a return demonstration.
4. Demonstrate removal of old dressing, including how to discard in moisture-proof bag.
5. Review the causes of wound contamination.
6. Discuss activities that may cause trauma to the wound and how to avoid them.
7. Review signs and symptoms of infection, encouraging client and family to ask questions.
8. Instruct client in the importance of well-balanced diet high in protein calories. Discuss sources of vitamin C and vitamin supplements.
9. Provide the client with written instruction concerning how to change the dressing, signs and symptoms of infection, and when to call the physician.

Scientific Rationale
1. Prepare client and involve family in wound management before discharge.
2. Handwashing is the single most important mechanism in stopping the transmission of pathogenic organisms.
3. Clients can acquire technical skills better if they observe and practice them.
4. Proper waste disposal is important in preventing the spread of microorganisms.
5. Better understanding aids client compliance.
6. Trauma can prevent wound healing and increase the chance of infection.
7. Early detection and treatment of infection decrease incidence of serious complications.
8. Wound healing requires protein and calories for building new cells. The immune system depends on protein and calories to produce antibodies.
9. Client may forget instructions received in the hospital when at home. Written instructions provide a handy reference.

REFERENCES

Bischoff, W. E., et al. (2000). Handwashing compliance by health care workers: The impact of introducing an accessible, alcohol-based hand antiseptic. *Archives of Internal Medicine, 160*(7), 1017–1021.

Black, J. M., Hawks, J. H., & Keene, A. M. (2001). *Medical-surgical nursing: Clinical management for positive outcomes* (6th ed.). Philadelphia: W.B. Saunders.

Braverman, P. K. (2000). Sexually transmitted diseases in adolescents. *Medical Clinics of North America, 84*(4), 869–889.

Cates, W. (1999). Estimates of the incidence and prevalence of sexually transmitted disease in the United States. American Social Health Association Panel. *Sexually Transmitted Diseases, 26*(4 Suppl.), S2–S7.

Chin, A. P. (2000). Immunity in frail elderly: A randomized controlled trial of exercise and enriched foods. *Medicine and Science in Sports and Exercise, 32*(12), 2005–2011.

Harbarth, S. (2000). Handwashing: The Semmelweis lesson misunderstood. *Clinical Infectious Diseases, 30,* 990–991.

Johnson, B. L., & Gross, J. (1998). *Handbook of oncology nursing* (3rd ed.). Boston: Jones and Bartlett.

Long, S. S., Pickering, L. K., & Prober, C. G. (1997). *Principles and practice of pediatric infectious diseases.* New York: Churchill Livingstone.

McKinzie, J. (2001). Genitourinary emergencies: Sexually transmitted diseases. *Emergency Medicine Clinics of North America, 19*(3), 723–744.

North American Nursing Diagnosis Association. (2001). *Nursing diagnoses: Definitions and classification 2001–2002.* Philadelphia: Author.

Orr, D. P., et al. (2001). Subsequent sexually transmitted infection in urban adolescents and your adults. *Archives of Pediatrics and Adolescent Medicine, 155*(8), 947–953.

Pittet, D., Mourouga, P., & Perneger, T. V. (1999). Compliance with handwashing in a teaching hospital. *Annals of Internal Medicine, 130*(2), 126–130.

Saez-Llorens, X., & McCracken, G. (1997). Genesis of fevers and inflammatory response. In S. Long, L. Pickering, & C. Prober (Eds.). *Principles and practice of pediatric diseases.* New York: Churchill Livingstone.

Shirrell, D., Gibbar-Clements, T., Dooley, R., & Free, C. (1999). Understanding therapeutic drug monitoring. *American Journal of Nursing, 99*(1), 42–44.

Tortora, G. J., Funke, B. R., & Case, C. (2001). *Microbiology: An introduction.* San Francisco: Benjamin Cummings.

Vander, A., Sherman, J., & Luciano, D. (2001). *Human physiology: The mechanisms of body function* (8th ed.) Boston: McGraw-Hill.

Yarboro, C. H., Frogge, M. H., Goodman, M., & Groenwald, S. (2000). *Cancer nursing: Principles and practice* (5th ed.). Boston: Jones and Bartlett.

BIBLIOGRAPHY

Braunwald, E., et al. (Eds.). (2001). *Harrison's principles of internal medicine* (15th ed.). New York: McGraw-Hill.

Carpenito, L. J. (2001). *Handbook of Nursing Diagnoses* (9th ed.). Philadelphia: Lippincott Williams & Wilkins.

Carruthers, S. G., et al. (Eds.). (2000). *Melmon and Morrell's clinical pharmacology* (4th Ed.). New York: McGraw-Hill.

Centers for Disease Control and Prevention (CDC). (1998). Notice to readers: Recommended childhood immunization schedule—United States, 1998. *MMWR Morb Mortal Wkly Rep, 47*(1), 8–12.

Keusch, G. T. (1998). Nutrition and immunity: From A to Z. *Nutrition Reviews, 56*(1), 53–54.

Maas, M. L., et al. (2001). *Nursing care of older adults.* St. Louis: Mosby.

Mandell, G. L., Gennett, J. E., & Dolin, R. (Eds.). (2000). *Mandell: Principles and practice of infectious diseases* (5th Ed.). Philadelphia: Churchill Livingstone.

Mayhall, G. C. (Ed.). (1999). *Hospital epidemiology and infection control* (2nd Ed.). New York: Lippincott Williams & Wilkins.

McCance, K. L., & Huether, S. E. (1998). *Pathophysiology: The biologic basis for disease in adults and children* (3rd ed.). St. Louis: Mosby.

Yoshikawa, T. T. (2000). Epidemiology and unique aspects of aging and infectious diseases. *Clinical Infectious Diseases 30*(6), 931–933.

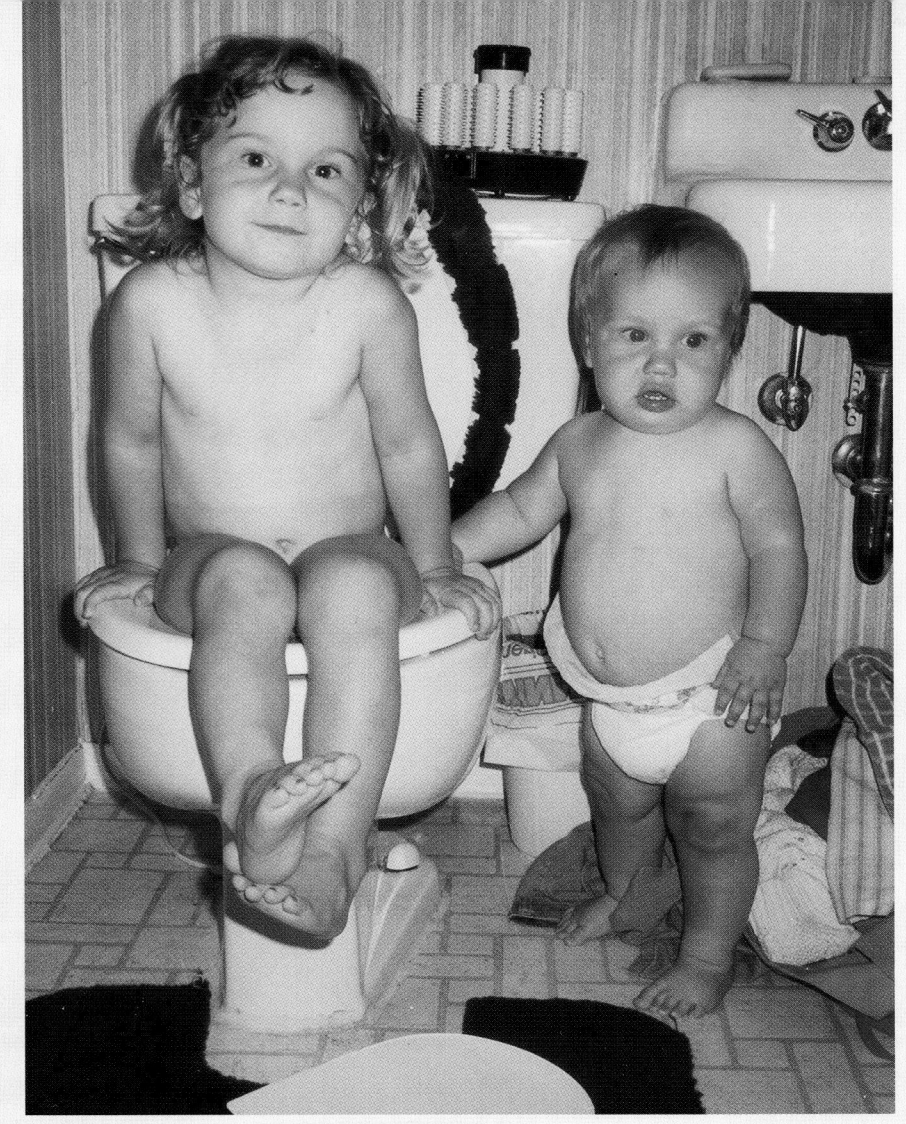

Elimination

40 Urinary Elimination

🔲 Key Terms

anuria

detrusor muscle

diuresis

dysuria

enuresis

hematuria

intermittent catheterization

micturition

nocturia

oliguria

polyuria

pyuria

urinary incontinence

urinary retention

🔲 Learning Objectives

Upon completion of this chapter, the student will be able to do the following:

1. Describe the structure and function of the urinary system.
2. Outline the process of micturition.
3. List and describe alterations in normal voiding patterns.
4. Recognize age-related differences in urinary elimination.
5. Describe factors that can alter urinary function.
6. Discuss nursing assessment of urinary function.
7. Identify nursing diagnoses related to urinary elimination.
8. Describe nursing interventions to promote normal urinary elimination.
9. Discuss interventions for altered urinary function.
10. Develop appropriate collaborative and community-based nursing interventions to manage problems with voiding.

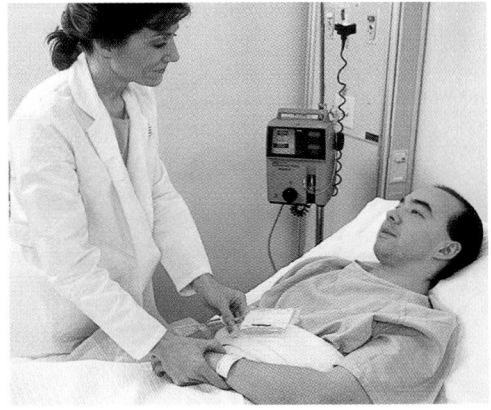

🔲 Critical Thinking Challenge

You are a nurse working with John, an 18-year-old boy who has been recovering for 2 weeks after a motor vehicle accident on the night of his senior prom. John has had a Foley catheter in place for 1 week, draining large amounts of urine. Yesterday, you noted that John's urine was cloudy and he had a temperature of 37.8°C. When you reported these findings to the physician, he discontinued John's catheter and ordered a urine sample for culture and sensitivity.

Once you have completed this chapter and incorporated urinary elimination into your knowledge base, review the above scenario and reflect on the following areas of Critical Thinking.

1. Identify risk factors that could alter John's urinary function.
2. Analyzing the information provided, determine what alteration in urinary function the data suggest.
3. Construct appropriate client teaching for when an indwelling catheter is removed. Plan how you will individualize this teaching for John.
4. Consider which data are essential to identify whether John is voiding adequately after the catheter removal.

The elimination of fluid waste is an essential function of the human body. Nurses are instrumental in promoting optimal urinary function and preventing urinary complications for all clients. Nurses individualize teaching and carry out specific interventions to help clients of all ages deal with problems of incontinence, urinary retention, and urinary tract infection (UTI). An understanding of the structure and function of the urinary system and factors that can affect normal urinary elimination is important for individualizing client care.

NORMAL URINARY FUNCTION

Structures of the Urinary Tract

Structures within the urinary tract include the kidneys, where urine forms; the ureters, which connect the kidneys with the bladder; the bladder, which stores urine; and the urethra, which enables urine to leave the body (Fig. 40-1).

Kidneys

The two kidneys are located on the posterior abdominal wall, in front of and on either side of the vertebral column between the twelfth thoracic and third lumbar vertebrae. Each kidney is enclosed by a fibrous capsule and supported by a mass of adipose tissue.

The functional unit of the kidney is called the nephron. Each kidney has more than 1,000,000 nephrons, and each nephron is capable of forming urine. The nephron consists of the glomerulus, Bowman's capsule, proximal convoluted tubules, loop of Henle, distal tubule, and collecting duct. The glomeru-lus is a network of blood vessels, surrounded by Bowman's capsule, where urine formation begins. The tubules, loop of Henle, and collecting ducts are passageways that permit urine to flow to the bladder. More importantly, they selectively reabsorb or secrete substances from the urine to maintain fluid and electrolyte balance.

Ureters

The ureters are narrow (1.25 cm), smooth muscle tubes that serve as passageways for urine to flow from the kidneys to the bladder. Peristaltic movement in the ureters propels urine toward the bladder. A flap of mucous membrane, which acts as a valve, covers the juncture between the ureters and the bladder. Under normal conditions, this valve prevents reflux of urine up through the ureter into the kidney.

Bladder

The bladder is the storage compartment for urine. It is a hollow, smooth muscle that lies behind the symphysis pubis when empty. In women, the bladder is located in front of the uterus and vagina (Fig. 40-2). In men, the bladder is located in front of the rectum and above the prostate gland.

The body of the bladder is composed of three layers of smooth muscle. The inner and outer layers are longitudinal, whereas the middle layer is circular. Collectively, these three layers are called the **detrusor muscle.** The bladder is hollow when empty but is capable of expanding to hold a considerable amount of urine.

The lower portion of the bladder, approximately 2 to 3 cm long, is called the bladder neck or internal urinary sphincter. Autonomic nervous innervation affects smooth muscle con-

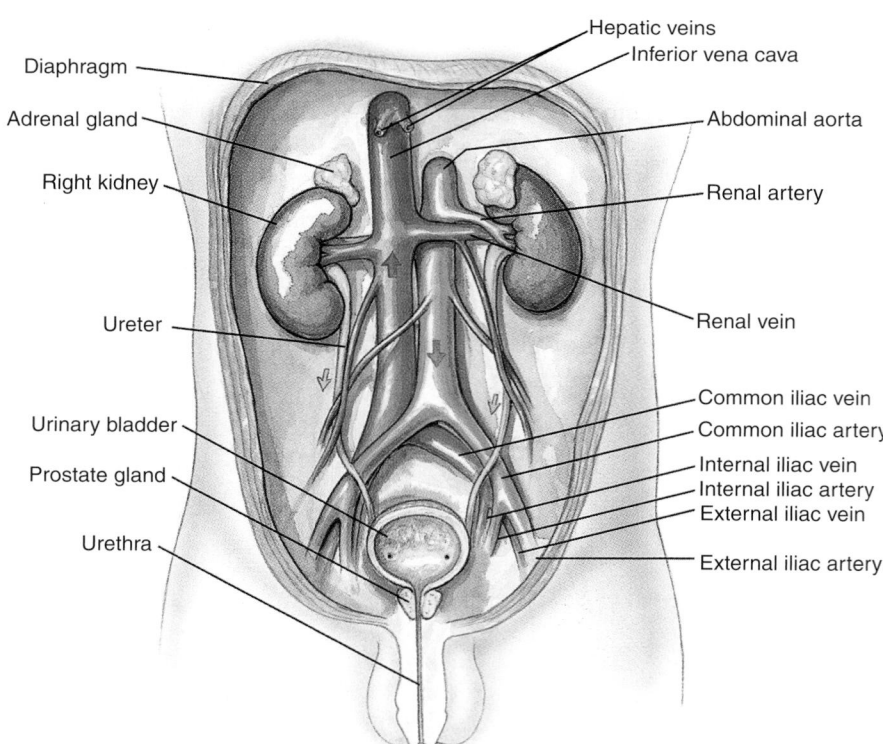

Diaphragm
Adrenal gland
Right kidney
Ureter
Urinary bladder
Prostate gland
Urethra

Hepatic veins
Inferior vena cava
Abdominal aorta
Renal artery
Renal vein
Common iliac vein
Common iliac artery
Internal iliac vein
Internal iliac artery
External iliac vein
External iliac artery

FIGURE 40-1   Anatomic structures of the urinary tract.

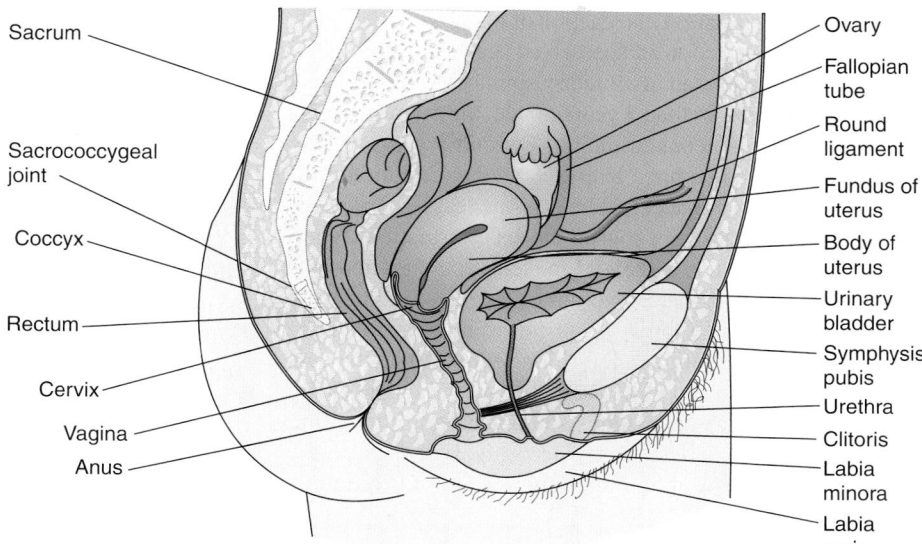

FIGURE 40-2 Female genitourinary tract showing the location of the urinary bladder and urethra.

trol of the internal sphincter. Sympathetic impulses cause the sphincter to contract, keeping the urine in the bladder. Parasympathetic nerve stimulation results in contraction of the detrusor muscle and relaxation of the internal sphincter, which causes urination.

Urethra

The urethra is the exit passageway for urine from the bladder. In women, the urethra is short, about 3 to 5 cm (1 to 2 inches), a factor that increases the opportunity for bacteria to enter the urinary system. In men, the urethra is longer, about 20 cm (8 inches), and serves to transport both semen and urine.

The external sphincter is located in the urethra. This band of skeletal muscle surrounds a section of the urethra and permits voluntary control of urination. The external sphincter is usually contracted to keep the urethra closed and to prevent urine from flowing constantly from the bladder. When the external sphincter relaxes, urine can flow from the bladder.

Function of the Urinary System

The elimination of fluid waste from the body is the function of the urinary system. This elimination process can be divided into two parts: urine formation and urine excretion.

Urine Formation

The kidney's major function is to regulate the volume and composition of the body's extracellular fluid (ECF). It performs this function by selectively retaining wanted water and other substances and excreting unwanted water and other substances in urine. Urine formation occurs by the processes of filtration, reabsorption, and secretion.

Filtration. The process of filtration begins at the glomerulus. The renal arteries bring blood to the kidneys; the smaller branches of these arteries bring blood to the glomerulus of each nephron. The capillaries of the glomerulus are porous,

and, as the blood passes through the glomerular capillaries, some constituents of the blood are actually filtered out. The red blood cells and the proteins are too large to be filtered and remain in the capillary, but most remaining plasma constituents can be filtered. The fluid that is filtered from the glomerulus into Bowman's capsule is called the glomerular filtrate.

Reabsorption. The glomerular filtrate then enters the second segment of the nephron, the tubule. The tubule actively and passively reabsorbs substances that the body wants to retain. These substances include varying amounts of water and electrolytes (Na^+, K^+, Cl^-, and HCO_3^-), as well as all glucose and amino acids. Reabsorption occurs mostly in the proximal convoluted tubule but also in the distal and collecting tubules. The tubules reabsorb almost 99% of the glomerular filtrate. The 1% that remains unabsorbed forms the fluid waste called urine.

Secretion. In addition to reabsorbing substances, the tubules secrete some substances to rid them from the body. They secrete varying amounts of H^+ and K^+ ions, as well as ammonia, creatinine, uric acid, and other metabolites.

Urine Excretion

Several words are used to describe the process of excreting urine from the body, including urination, voiding, and **micturition.** In adults, emptying of the bladder usually occurs when 250 to 400 mL of urine stretches or distends the bladder. Smaller amounts of urine trigger bladder emptying in children. When the volume of urine in the bladder reaches the range of 250 to 400 mL, the pressure of that amount stretches the detrusor sufficiently to begin to force the bladder neck to open. This sensation of stretch in the detrusor is transmitted to sacral segments of the spinal cord; reflex motor action is transmitted back to the detrusor muscle to cause it to contract. The detrusor contraction causes even more stretch and pressure; usually, at this point, the person perceives a full bladder and feels the need to urinate. This reaction of bladder stretch, leading to bladder contraction and perceived need to void, is called the micturition reflex, an involuntary spinal cord reflex.

In children younger than 3 years of age, the micturition reflex leads to spontaneous urination. Beyond 3 years of age, however, most people have learned to delay urination until the time and place are acceptable; this is because nerve centers in the brain ultimately control the act of urination. When the external sphincter, a skeletal muscle, is contracted in a closed position, a person can voluntarily delay voiding. This contraction effectively prevents urine from being released, even in the presence of the micturition reflex. When the person decides the time and place are right for voiding, he or she can consciously relax the external sphincter, permitting urine to flow from the bladder. Emptying of the bladder also involves contraction of abdominal muscles and relaxation of pelvic floor muscles.

Characteristics of Normal Urine

Common characteristics of urine include volume or amount, color, clarity, and odor. Many factors produce normal variations among different people and at different times for the same person.

Volume

In adults, the average amount of urine per void is approximately 250 to 400 mL. All but 5 to 10 mL of urine is typically emptied from the bladder. Urinary output can vary greatly, depending on intake and other fluid losses. Catheterized clients should drain a minimum of 30 mL of urine per hour. Urine output of less than 30 mL/hour may indicate inadequate blood flow to the kidneys.

Color

The color of urine ranges from a light yellow, to a darker yellow, to a dark yellow-brown, called amber. The client's state of hydration affects the color. Urine may be almost colorless if it is very dilute secondary to a high fluid intake. Urine may be dark amber or orange-brown if it is very concentrated secondary to a decreased fluid intake. Medications can also alter urine's color. Urine may appear cloudy, dark reddish-brown, or streaked with blood when a woman is menstruating.

Clarity

Urine is normally transparent. Freshly voided urine should appear clear, without sediment. Urine draining from a retention catheter should appear clear and without sediment in the tubing, but it may contain occasional mucus shreds. Urine that has been sitting unemptied in a urinal or collecting device for an hour or longer may normally appear cloudy secondary to separation or settling of urinary constituents.

Odor

The odor of freshly voided urine is typically described as aromatic. Generally, the more dilute the urine, the fainter the odor; the more concentrated the urine, the stronger the odor.

Collected urine that has been sitting unemptied for a long period may have a strong ammonia scent. Medications and certain foods can alter urine's odor. A strong, offensive odor is not normally present in urine that is free of infection.

Normal Pattern of Urinary Elimination

Many people have a routine pattern associated with urinary elimination. Most people void four to six times a day. Typically, people void soon after getting out of bed in the morning. Many people tend to void within an hour after mealtime and once again before bedtime. Variations in patterns of fluid intake directly affect routine patterns of voiding.

The total amount of urine voided during a 24-hour period usually ranges between 1200 and 1500 mL. Each void should contain a minimum of approximately 200 mL and a maximum of 500 mL.

Lifespan Considerations

Newborn and Infant

From about the third month after conception, the fetal kidneys begin functioning and the fetus voids urine in utero. Newborns, therefore, may have urine in their bladders at birth and should be able to void within the first 24 hours after birth. The first voiding may be of slightly pink-tinged urine, caused by an accumulation of uric acid crystals. Noting the first voiding after birth is important to verify that the infant's urine formation and excretion are adequate. At birth, the kidneys are still not fully developed; Bowman's capsule and the tubules are still refining their respective filtering and reabsorption abilities. Newborns usually void small amounts (15 to 30 mL, up to 30 to 40 times a day) of dilute, light yellow urine.

As infants grow, they are able to void slightly larger amounts at less frequent intervals. Urine's color remains pale yellow throughout infancy. The total amount of urine that infants void in a 24-hour period depends on total fluid intake and fluid losses from other sources. The average urine output for newborns and infants is about 500 to 600 mL in 24 hours. Table 40-1 gives the normal ranges of daily urine output across the lifespan.

TABLE 40-1

Normal Ranges for Daily Urine Output During Lifespan	
Age (years)	Output (mL)
Newborn–2	500–600
2–5	500–800
5–8	600–1,200
8–14	1,000–1,500
14 and over	1,500

Infants lack voluntary control of urinary elimination. The sacral spinal cord segments innervating the bladder are still immature. The bladder empties in reflex fashion after a degree of bladder stretch occurs.

Congenital malformations of the urinary tract or the central nervous system may cause serious alterations in urinary elimination. UTIs, which are more common in female than in male infants, can also disrupt normal urinary function.

Toddler and Preschooler

During the toddler and preschool years, children usually achieve voluntary urinary continence because they become physiologically and psychologically capable of this task. Sometime between 12 and 18 months, the myelinization of the sacral spinal segments that control the bladder becomes complete, and children can then perceive bladder fullness. A good indicator of the maturation of the spinal cord is when a toddler begins to walk independently (Fig. 40-3).

Beginning sometime between 2½ and 3 years of age, most children can perceive a full bladder and voluntarily delay voiding. Children also need a sufficient vocabulary to communicate the need to urinate, the ability to access toilet facilities, and sufficient fine motor control to loosen or remove necessary clothing. Signs that a child is ready to achieve bladder continence include less frequent voidings (longer periods of diaper dryness) and the abilities to feel bladder fullness and to verbalize the need to urinate. Sometimes, toddlers need to experience outdoor play time without diapers to see what happens when they experience bladder fullness followed by urethral relaxation and bladder emptying. They begin to understand the relationship between bladder fullness and voluntary bladder

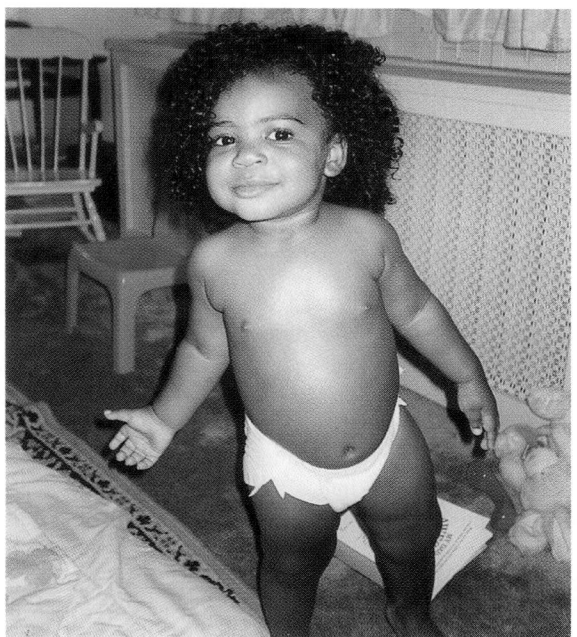

FIGURE 40-3 A sign of a toddler's readiness to begin "potty-training" is the ability to walk independently.

emptying and are ready for toilet training. Children in North American cultures usually achieve daytime urinary continence by 3 years of age; boys may take longer than girls. Nighttime continence may not occur until 4 or 5 years of age.

School-Age Child and Adolescent

School-age children and adolescents have achieved both daytime and nighttime urinary continence. They are forming urinary elimination habits similar to those of adults, voiding straw-colored urine six to seven times a day. The amount of oral fluid intake greatly influences the amount of urine output; Table 40-1 lists average ranges of urine output in a 24-hour period for children of various ages.

Some healthy school-age children continue to experience involuntary urinary incontinence, which is termed enuresis (Swithinbank et al., 1998). Many parents seek advice from healthcare providers when nocturnal enuresis occurs in their children older than 7 years of age. Specific nursing interventions for the management of nocturnal enuresis are discussed later in this chapter.

Adult and Older Adult

Incontinence is not usually identified as a significant health problem in the early to middle adult years. For those affected with adverse urinary symptoms, a significant correlation exists between urinary incontinence symptoms and their negative impact on travel, social, physical, and emotional activities. In late middle age, men may experience altered urinary elimination related to prostatic hypertrophy, and women may experience altered urinary elimination related to weakened perineal muscles (cystocele or rectocele).

As a result of cardiovascular changes that occur with aging, most older adults experience decreased perfusion to the kidneys. This decreased arterial flow to the renal arteries is a gradual change that results from decreased cardiac muscle strength, which reduces cardiac output to the periphery, and decreased elasticity of the peripheral blood vessels. Over time, owing to decreased arterial perfusion, kidney function progressively decreases; the kidneys become a less effective regulator of the body's ECF.

The ureters, bladder, and urethra lose some muscle tone with aging. The bladder becomes less able to hold large amounts of urine (decreased bladder capacity), and older persons may experience an urgency to empty the bladder more frequently of smaller amounts of urine. They may sense the urge to void only when the bladder is at the limit of its capacity, which diminishes the ability voluntarily to delay voiding. Uninhibited bladder contractions can further increase the sense of urgency. These factors place older people at risk for incontinence. Nocturia is a frequent complaint of older adults, and urinary retention is also more common. Urinary retention predisposes older adults to UTIs.

Women may experience incontinence as they age, related to decreased estrogen levels and weakened perineal muscles. Older men eventually experience urinary hesitancy and difficulty starting the urinary stream, related to prostatic hypertrophy.

FACTORS AFFECTING URINARY ELIMINATION

Fluid intake, loss of body fluid, dietary intake, body position, and psychological factors can affect urinary patterns. Many other factors can predispose a person to disruption of normal patterns of urinary elimination (Display 40-1). Obstruction of urine flow, UTIs, hypotension, neurologic injury, medications, surgery, and pregnancy are common causes.

Fluid Intake

The amount of fluid that a person ingests is the most influential factor in determining urine output. If a person increases his or her volume of fluid intake, an associated increase will occur in the volume of urine output. Conversely, a decrease in fluid intake will cause a corresponding decrease in urine output.

This relationship is hormonally controlled. Several hormones, the most important of which is antidiuretic hormone (ADH), play significant roles in the reabsorption of water in the tubules of the nephron. The name "antidiuretic" implies the function of ADH, which is to prevent **diuresis,** or water excretion. ADH is secreted by the hypothalamus and released by the posterior pituitary in the brain. Increased plasma osmolarity stimulates the release of ADH (discussed in detail in Chapter 36). When ADH is present, the distal tubule of the nephron becomes more permeable to water. Release of ADH causes the kidney to reabsorb more water, thus producing a more concentrated urine. When fluid intake increases, ADH release is suppressed. In the absence of ADH, the renal tubules become relatively impermeable to water, and little water is reabsorbed, producing an increased volume of dilute urine.

DISPLAY 40-1

🖑 FACTORS THAT INFLUENCE URINARY PATTERNS

- Fluid intake
- Loss of body fluid
- Nutrition
- Body position
- Psychological factors
- Obstruction of urine flow: renal calculi, prostatic enlargement, tumors, structural abnormalities
- Infection
- Hypotension
- Neurologic injury: spinal cord injury, cerebral vascular accident (stroke), brain tumor
- Decreased muscle tone: aging, multiple pregnancies, obesity
- Pregnancy
- Surgery: anesthesia, edema, immobility
- Medications
- Urinary diversions

The amount of fluid intake not only affects the amount of urine produced but also influences the frequency of urination. If fluid intake is greatly increased, frequency of voiding increases because the bladder fills more quickly. Conversely, if fluid intake is low, voiding frequency decreases.

Loss of Body Fluid

When a person loses a great deal of body fluid, the kidneys increase reabsorption of water from the glomerular filtrate to maintain the proper osmolarity of the ECF. This "water saving" to regulate the concentration of solutes in the ECF results in decreased urine output. Increased loss of body fluids can occur with vomiting, diarrhea, excessive diaphoresis secondary to fever or exercise, excessive wound drainage, extensive burns, or blood loss from trauma or surgery.

Nutrition

Diet may affect urinary elimination. If the diet contains a high percentage of foods with a high water content (e.g., soup, Jello, fruits, vegetables), urine volume will be greater than if intake of such foods is limited. If a person ingests large quantities of salty foods without increasing water intake, urine output will decrease and be more concentrated. Alcohol and foods that contain caffeine (e.g., coffee, tea, cola, chocolate) contain a diuretic and increase urine output.

Body Position

Body position plays an important role in the ability to empty the bladder completely with each voiding. The typical body position for urinary elimination in men is standing upright. Some men find it difficult to empty their bladders fully into a urinal while lying flat in bed. Commonly, this difficulty alters the voiding pattern, so voiding becomes more frequent, but with less volume. The normal position for voiding in women is sitting. If a woman must use a bedpan while flat in bed, she also may be unable completely to empty her bladder.

Psychological Factors

Because the release of urine from the bladder is ultimately under voluntary control, anything that causes a person to think about voiding can influence the process. If another person talks about the need to void, one may also feel the urge to void. If one reads a chapter about urinary elimination, one may need a bathroom break before finishing. If one hears running water, the need to void may be intensified. Pouring warm water over a client's inner thigh or perineal area may stimulate voiding; giving a client a cold bedpan may temporarily delay voiding.

Stress and anxiety can affect urinary elimination. In stressful situations, a person can experience a strong urge to urinate. Stress can also cause the reverse problem of urinary retention. A person's muscles may become so tense that relaxation of the perineal muscles does not occur, and voiding is inhibited.

Privacy for voiding is important psychologically. Many people are unable to relax their perineal muscles if they feel they have inadequate privacy. Women, in particular, have been culturally trained to require more privacy for voiding. Women's public restrooms always have private stalls for elimination, whereas men's public restrooms have open rows of receptacles for urinary elimination. People have varying needs for privacy during voiding.

Obstruction of Urine Flow

Obstruction of the normal flow of urine can lead to problems with urinary elimination, and, when severe, can cause kidney damage. Structural abnormalities within the urinary tract, urinary tumors or other tumors that press against the urinary tract, renal stones, and prostatic enlargement are possible causes of urinary obstruction. Obstruction can also occur when clients have catheters or tubes in place that become plugged or kinked.

One of the complications of obstruction within the urinary system is hydronephrosis, which is distention of the kidney pelvis with urine secondary to the increased resistance caused by obstruction to normal urine flow. Unrelieved hydronephrosis can cause renal cell atrophy and necrosis, which can cause permanent kidney damage.

Urinary stasis also occurs secondary to urinary obstruction. The stagnant urine proximal to the obstruction provides a good growth medium for microorganisms, fostering the development of UTIs.

Infections of the Urinary Tract

UTIs are usually caused by microorganisms normally found in the gastrointestinal tract. The species commonly responsible for UTIs are of the Enterobacteriaceae group and include *Escherichia coli, Klebsiella,* and *Proteus.* These microorganisms typically gain access to the urinary system by way of the urethral meatus. Hence, the most common UTIs are infections of the urethra (urethritis) or bladder (cystitis). Urethritis and cystitis are classified as lower UTIs, whereas infections of the ureters (ureteritis) and the kidney pelvis or tubule system are classified as upper UTIs. Upper UTIs occur less frequently than lower UTIs, but they are more serious, because kidney damage and renal failure may result.

Normally, the urinary tract is sterile, except at the urethral meatus. In the healthy person, the act of voiding tends to flush away bacteria. Infection occurs when microorganisms from the surrounding perineal skin or anal opening find their way to the urinary meatus and ascend the urethra. Women are more susceptible to lower UTIs because of the short length of their urethras and the proximity of the vagina and anus to the urinary meatus. Men are less susceptible to lower UTIs because of the longer length of the male urethra, and also because of the antibacterial properties of prostatic secretions.

Other factors that can increase the incidence of UTIs include incorrect wiping of the anal area after bowel movements; sexual intercourse, which can bring perineal microorganisms into closer contact with the urinary meatus; and any procedure that places an object in the urethra or bladder for diagnostic or therapeutic reasons. The longer a catheter remains in the bladder, the greater the chance of nosocomial infection. About one half of catheterized clients become infected within 1 week of catheterization (Marchiondo, 1998).

Infections of the urinary tract can disrupt the normal pattern of urinary elimination in many ways. Voiding becomes painful and more frequent. The person with a UTI often experiences urgency, a subjective feeling of being unable voluntarily to delay the urge to void. Urine becomes abnormal, containing pus (pyuria) and blood (hematuria). Ultimately, if the infection ascends to the kidney, renal damage can occur and possibly result in renal failure.

Hypotension

Adequate blood perfusion to the kidneys is necessary to ensure urine formation. When arterial blood pressure drops too low, the renal arteries do not have enough pressure to cause glomerular filtration. Inadequate circulating volume or inability of the heart to pump adequately can decrease blood flow to the kidneys. Decreased circulating volume can occur after surgery, after trauma, or when the client experiences severe fluid loss, such as from diarrhea or vomiting. If urine output is less than 30 mL/hour for two consecutive hours, decreased perfusion of blood to the kidneys and other vital organs must be suspected.

Neurologic Injury

Neurologic injury after a stroke or spinal cord injury can disrupt normal patterns of urinary elimination. Injury by trauma, hemorrhage, or tumor to the frontal lobes of the brain, which control the voluntary nature of voiding, can lead to incontinence.

The micturition reflex occurs at the sacral level of the spinal cord. If injury occurs to the spinal cord at the sacral level or above, the person will experience a change in control of urinary elimination. The person may experience reflex voiding, which results in incontinence. Reflex voiding occurs when the bladder, as soon as it is stretched to a certain degree, contracts reflexively, resulting in loss of urine. This condition is called reflex neurogenic bladder. If the reflex arc is injured, the bladder may fill without the bladder stretch contraction mechanism's working, resulting in urinary retention. This condition is called autonomous neurogenic bladder.

Decreased Muscle Tone

Weakened abdominal and perineal muscles can impair bladder contraction and control of the external urinary sphincter. Abdominal and perineal muscles can weaken because of obesity, multiple pregnancies, stretching during childbirth, menopausal atrophy due to decreased estrogen, and chronic constipation. A cystocele is the protrusion or herniation of the bladder into the vaginal canal; it produces symptoms of stress incontinence, frequency, dribbling, and inability to empty the bladder completely.

Continuous bladder drainage with a catheter can also decrease bladder tone. Continuous bladder drainage prevents the bladder from ever filling; therefore, stretch of the bladder musculature is limited, promoting bladder atrophy. After removal of a catheter, some clients experience dribbling and difficulty with urinary control. This problem is usually temporary, lasting until bladder tone returns.

Pregnancy

During pregnancy, the increasing size and weight of the growing uterus can exert pressure on the bladder, a common cause of urinary frequency in pregnant women. Compression of the bladder by the uterus may also lead to obstruction of urinary flow and incomplete emptying of the bladder. UTIs are more common during pregnancy owing to hormonally related changes in the urinary tract (Porth, 1998). Trauma from vaginal delivery causes swelling in the perineal area, which can obstruct the flow of urine and cause urinary retention during the early postpartum period.

Surgery

Postoperative clients should be able to void within 10 hours after surgery. Some clients have difficulty voiding postoperatively for various reasons. Many postoperative clients are volume depleted because of limited fluid intake and loss of blood and fluid during surgery. The stress of surgery triggers the release of ADH, which decreases urinary output. During the immediate postoperative period, clients usually cannot get up to use the bathroom. Using a bedpan or urinal in a supine position may impede normal urinary patterns. Many medications used to control postoperative pain have urinary retention as a side effect. This is especially true when opioids are administered epidurally for pain control.

Surgery involving the urinary system, intestines, or reproductive organs predisposes a client to urinary retention. Trauma to tissues may cause edema, which can potentially obstruct urine flow. The use of a retention catheter is indicated after any surgery on the urinary tract.

Anesthesia can also affect urinary elimination. Anesthetic agents slow the glomerular filtration rate, reducing urinary output. People who receive a spinal or regional block during surgery are at increased risk for postoperative urinary problems because these agents impair the sensory and motor impulses that control micturition. Until the anesthesia has worn off, the client will be unable to perceive bladder fullness and unable to initiate voiding.

Medications

Medications classified as diuretics are administered to increase urine output. They affect the reabsorption of sodium and water in the tubules of the nephron. Commonly used diuretics include chlorothiazide, hydrochlorothiazide, furosemide, spironolactone, and triamterene. People with edema or a propensity toward development of edema are candidates for diuretic therapy. Cholinergic medications (e.g., bethanechol) may be given to promote voiding, because they stimulate contraction of the detrusor muscle. Oxybutynin (an anticholinergic) may be used to treat urinary urgency and frequency caused by overactive detrusor muscle activity (Bemelmans, Kiemeney, & Debruyne, 2000).

Side effects of medications used to treat other health problems can adversely affect urinary elimination. The risk of urinary retention is increased with medications having anticholinergic effects. Belladonna alkaloids, phenothiazines, tricyclic antidepressants, and antihistamines are examples of such drugs. Narcotics can decrease the glomerular filtration rate and the sensation of bladder fullness.

Some medications change the color of urine. For example, phenazopyridine (Pyridium) causes urine to turn bright orange, and amitriptyline turns urine blue-green.

Urinary Diversion

A urinary diversion is a surgical procedure in which the normal pathway of urine elimination is altered. The ureters are rerouted from a diseased or damaged urinary system to a new outlet, called a stoma, created surgically on the client's abdomen. The diversion may be permanent, as with cancerous conditions that require removal of the bladder (cystectomy). In other conditions, such as trauma or severe chronic UTI, the diversion may be temporary to promote healing. Urinary diversions alter normal urinary elimination because the person no longer has control over voiding.

ALTERED URINARY FUNCTION

Manifestations of Altered Urinary Function

Dysuria

Dysuria means painful voiding. Pain is often associated with UTIs and is felt as a burning sensation during urination. Any bladder inflammation or trauma or inflammation of the urethra can cause dysuria. Painful voiding should be referred to a physician, because dysuria has many causes.

Polyuria

Polyuria is the formation and excretion of excessive amounts of urine in the absence of a concurrent increase in fluid intake. Urine output of more than 2500 to 3000 mL in 24 hours is considered polyuria. Untreated diabetes insipidus and diabetes mellitus can greatly increase urine output. Ingestion of diuretics, caffeine, and alcohol also results in polyuria.

Oliguria

Oliguria is the formation and excretion of decreased amounts of urine, or urinary output less than 500 mL in 24 hours. A severe decrease in fluid intake or any disease state or injury that leads to an excessive loss of body fluids can cause oliguria. For example, excessive vomiting, diarrhea, diaphoresis, burns, or bleeding can decrease urine output. People with renal disease may be oliguric. As the kidney approaches complete failure, the person may become anuric. **Anuria** is the formation and excretion of less than 100 mL of urine in 24 hours.

Urgency

Most adults can postpone emptying of the bladder until it contains 250 to 400 mL of urine. Urgency describes the subjective feeling of being unable voluntarily to delay the urge to void. Urgency implies a strong micturition reflex caused by inflammation or infection of the urethra or bladder, incompetent urethral sphincter, weak perineal muscle control, or psychological stress.

Frequency

Voiding at frequent intervals is known as frequency. Frequency occurs when a person voids more often than normal, without a significant increase in fluid intake. Each voiding usually contains less than 250 mL of urine. Frequency not associated with increased fluid intake can be related to other factors, such as UTI or pressure on the bladder from pregnancy. Frequency and urgency often occur together.

Nocturia

Voiding during normal sleeping hours is called **nocturia.** If a person voids before going to bed, it should be possible to sleep for 7 to 8 hours without feeling a strong micturition reflex. Ingestion of large amounts of fluids before bed, especially those containing alcohol or caffeine, may promote nocturia. People with medical conditions such as congestive heart failure may also experience nocturia. When lying supine, edema decreases as fluid enters the circulation. Blood flow to the kidneys increases, increasing glomerular filtration and urine output.

Hematuria

Hematuria indicates blood in the urine; it can be gross (visible on visual examination) or occult (not visible on visual examination). Occult blood may change the color of urine from normal clear yellow or amber to a cloudy or hazy yellow or amber. As the number of red blood cells increases, the urine may become bright red. Pathologic causes of hematuria include UTIs, urinary tract tumors, renal calculi, poisoning, and trauma to the urinary mucosa. Hematuria is expected and temporary after urinary tract or prostatic surgery.

Pyuria

Pyuria means that the urine contains pus, which is the accumulation of the end products of an inflammatory response. Pus containing microorganisms and white blood cells gives urine a cloudy color and, often, a strong, unpleasant odor. Pyuria occurs in the presence of any UTI.

Urinary Retention

Urinary retention is the inability to empty the bladder of urine. In urinary retention, the person is either unable to perceive the feeling of bladder fullness or unable to relax the bladder neck and external urethral sphincter to allow urine to pass from the body. Because the kidneys continue to form urine, the volume within the bladder grows until, in extreme cases, the bladder holds up to 2000 to 3000 mL of urine. Bladder distention of more than 600 mL can often be palpated in the suprapubic area of the abdomen.

Urinary retention with overflow is the loss of small amounts of urine from an overdistended bladder. As the bladder becomes overdistended, it no longer responds to bladder stretch as a stimulus to initiate detrusor contraction and voiding. The bladder can maintain only a certain degree of overdistention before excess urine is eliminated in small amounts at frequent intervals. The small amounts of urine that are voided are known as "overflow."

Complications of urinary retention include the loss of bladder tone secondary to excessive stretch of the detrusor muscle fibers. Even after the primary retention is relieved, it may take a period of weeks for the bladder stretch–bladder emptying response to return to normal. Accumulation of urine in the bladder also leads to stasis of urine, which predisposes the person to UTIs and calculi development. Bladder distention can also lead to hydronephrosis as the urine backs up into the ureters and kidney.

People at risk for development of urinary retention include those with neurologic impairment, such as spinal cord injury or brain lesions. Postoperative clients may experience temporary urinary retention until edema subsides and spinal anesthesia wears off. After vaginal delivery of a baby, swelling of the urinary meatus is common and may cause temporary obstruction to urine outflow.

Incontinence

Urinary incontinence is the involuntary loss of urine from the bladder. Five types of urinary incontinence are identified by patterns of uncontrolled voiding and related causative factors: stress, urge, reflex, functional, and total incontinence. The accompanying Therapeutic Dialogue discusses urinary incontinence.

Stress Incontinence. The sudden, involuntary loss of small amounts (less than 50 mL) of urine that accompanies a sudden increase in intra-abdominal pressure is called stress incontinence. Examples of activities that increase intra-abdominal pressure are coughing, sneezing, laughing, lifting, and jumping.

Factors associated with stress incontinence include weakening of the pelvic floor muscles, high intra-abdominal pressure, damage to the bladder neck, and side effects of medications. Stretching that occurs during childbirth can weaken the pelvic floor muscles. Women who have experienced a long and difficult labor and delivery or who have experienced multiple childbirths are most likely to have weakened pelvic muscles. Estrogen is necessary to maintain the normal tone of reproductive organs and associated musculature; therefore, postmenopausal women who have decreased estrogen levels may suffer from stress incontinence (Agency for Health Care Policy and Research, 1992). Obesity or pregnancy can cause high intra-abdominal pressure. Obese, postmenopausal women who have had multiple pregnancies are most likely to experience stress incontinence. Another cause of stress incontinence is

THERAPEUTIC DIALOGUE
Urinary Incontinence

Scene for Thought
Mrs. Clements is a 55-year-old woman who has been referred for complaints of incontinence of urine for 3 months. The nurse is scheduled to perform a history and physical.

Less Effective	More Effective

Less Effective

Nurse: Good morning, Mrs. Clements. How are you today? Please sit down so I can ask you about your history. *(Asks about age, address, number of children, and other items on assessment sheet.)*
Client: *(Answers all questions quietly.)*
Nurse: I understand that you have an incontinence problem. Many women your age have that kind of difficulty, and I'm sure we can fix you up so you'll be just fine.
Client: My mother's doctor told her that years ago, but she never got better. *(Looks down at her lap.)*
Nurse: Well, we'll just see what we can do for you here. Could you undress and put on this gown? I'll be back in a minute to do your physical. *(Leaves room, closing the door quietly.)*

More Effective

Nurse: Good morning, Mrs. Clements. Please sit down so we can talk a while before I do your physical. *(Acknowledges client, gives simple directions.)* What can I do for you this morning? *(Asks open-ended question.)*
Client: You can help me stop wetting myself. *(Looks down at her lap.)*
Nurse: You look worried about that. *(Observes behavior accurately.)*
Client: Yes, I am. *(Looks relieved.)* Before my mother died last year, she had to wear adult diapers; she always smelled and had bladder infections, and it was awful for her and for everyone else. I don't want to get that way.
Nurse: So what you would like is for me to help you figure out a way to deal with the wetting problem so you don't have to live the way your mother did. Is that right? *(States understanding of what the client wants and clarifies with her.)*
Client: Yes! That would be great.
Nurse: Okay. Why don't we start with some questions, and then I'll do a physical and we can go from there. *(Gives client some idea of planning.)*

Critical Thinking Challenge
- Critique what the nurse did that was effective in the second scene.
- Consider how you think the client felt.
- Determine what was less effective about the first scene.
- Consider how you think the client felt in both scenes.
- Although each nurse spent the same amount of time with the client, analyze how the first nurse could have been more effective.

---

direct trauma, which may result from a fractured pelvis or during genitourinary surgery.

Urge Incontinence. The involuntary loss of urine after a strong feeling of the need to urinate is termed urge incontinence. The person with urge incontinence is unable simultaneously to perceive a full bladder and to hold urine until reaching the bathroom. Frequency, dysuria, and nocturia commonly accompany urge incontinence.

Factors associated with urge incontinence include UTIs, use of diuretics, consumption of fluids that contain caffeine or alcohol, and increased fluid intake. An overdistended bladder can precipitate urge incontinence. Some clients experience urge incontinence for a short period after removal of an indwelling catheter. They have become accustomed to an empty bladder and need time to accommodate to the usual degree of bladder distention.

Reflex Incontinence. An involuntary loss of urine that occurs at somewhat predictable intervals when a specific bladder volume is reached is called reflex incontinence. The person is unable to sense bladder fullness because of neurologic impairment, and the bladder simply empties when a certain degree of bladder stretch occurs. Bladder emptying occurs at the sacral reflex level, because of impairment of the connection to the cerebrum that allows voluntary inhibition of voiding. Reflex incontinence is seen in clients with neurologic impairment, such as spinal cord lesion, cerebrovascular accident, or brain tumor.

Functional Incontinence. Functional incontinence involves the inability or unwillingness of a person with normal bladder and sphincter control to reach the bathroom in time to void. Environmental barriers, disorientation, or physical limitations may contribute. The amount of urine that the person loses is typically large.

Many factors can interfere with the ability to reach the toilet in time. A poorly lit, cluttered room may obstruct easy access to the bathroom. Raised side rails or a call bell that is out of reach can contribute to functional incontinence in a hospitalized client. Sensory and cognitive factors are also associated with functional incontinence, because confusion, disorientation, and sedatives or side effects of medications can impair cognitive functioning. Motor deficits, such as impaired gait and loss of fine motor control needed to release necessary clothing, can also contribute.

Total Incontinence. The continuous, involuntary, unpredictable loss of urine from a nondistended bladder is termed total incontinence. The designation is sometimes used when the observed incontinence does not fit any other category and does not respond to usual treatment methods. Factors associated with total incontinence include a specific neurologic lesion in the brain or spinal cord, traumatic or surgical injury to the genitourinary area or spinal cord, and a congenital malformation within the urinary tract or spinal cord.

Enuresis

Enuresis is involuntary voiding, with no underlying pathophysiologic origin, after the age at which bladder control is usually achieved. By the time most children are 4 or 5 years of age, they can control urinary elimination during both day and night. Enuresis beyond age 5 years is typically nocturnal. Nocturnal enuresis is commonly called "bed-wetting." Involuntary voiding during sleep can also occur during daytime naps, but it is more common during longer periods of sleep at night. Factors associated with nocturnal enuresis include small bladder capacity, sound sleeping, stress and anxiety at home or school, UTIs, and family history of nocturnal enuresis. Enuresis can occur in older people too. In one study, nocturnal enuresis was found to be present in 17.3% of the women older than 80 years of age (Swithinbank et al., 2000).

Impact on Activities of Daily Living

The loss of control over urinary function can create feelings of anxiety or fear, whether in the 8-year-old child with enuresis, the 45-year-old person with stress incontinence, or the 80-year-old person with urge incontinence. Incontinence can lead to social isolation and other depressive symptoms because many people fear that bladder incontinence will prove embarrassing in social situations (Dugan et al., 2000). Sometimes, affected people limit trips outside the home or enjoy social encounters only with close friends who will understand if incontinence occurs.

Planning should assist clients in maintaining normal urinary elimination whenever possible. Clients should choose clothing that is easy to remove and does not require dry cleaning. Some people may need to choose styles that will hide protective pants. If the location of the bathroom is upstairs or difficult to access, a urinal or bedside commode can help promote urinary continence. Adequate bathing after incontinence decreases odor and prevents skin breakdown. Adequate washing may be difficult for older adults, those who are cognitively impaired, or children.

Alterations in urinary elimination may place extra financial burdens and care responsibilities on family members or designated caregivers. Protective pants and special equipment (e.g., ostomy supplies) can be financially burdensome, especially if insurance does not cover the cost of such products. Frequent trips to the primary care provider and required medications can add to financial and caregiving responsibilities (Vernarec, 1998). Frequently, extra energy and time must be spent washing clothing and bedding. If a child is experiencing nocturnal enuresis, sleep is usually disrupted for parents or other caregivers who get up to help the child.

Frequent uncontrolled incontinence in the older person often contributes to a family's decision to seek institutional care. For many people, a move to an extended care facility drastically affects independence in the tasks of daily living.

ASSESSMENT

Subjective Data

Normal Pattern Identification

Clients may find it easier to describe alterations in urinary elimination than to describe normal urinary elimination. Many factors in daily living can affect normal elimination patterns, so some people have difficulty recognizing their own normal pattern within daily variations.

Specific questions regarding when the last voiding occurred; how many times per day urination usually occurs; whether each void contains a small, medium, or large amount of urine; and whether the client often wakes during the night to void help identify normal patterns of urinary elimination. Ensure privacy, and be sensitive to feelings of embarrassment that clients may experience during discussion of urinary function. Clarify the term *urinating* by using other words that clients may be more familiar with, such as voiding, "peeing," passing water, or "going potty." Analyze data gathered from such questions to evaluate whether a client's typical pattern falls within expected parameters.

Risk Identification

A nursing history also helps to identify factors that could potentially alter urinary elimination. Elicit information concerning previous renal or urinary tract problems, such as UTIs, renal calculi, or renal failure. If one of these conditions is present, obtain a history of the condition and how it was treated and resolved. Question the client about any previous genitourinary surgery, such as prostatic surgery or repair of a cystocele. Evaluate other acute or chronic medical problems, such as congestive heart failure or neurologic injury, in terms of their impact on urinary function.

Elicit data about recent changes in daily routines: exercise, diet, or fluid intake. Note any significant change in oral intake or consumption of beverages that contain alcohol or caffeine. Medications that can alter urinary output or function, such as diuretics or anticholinergics, should also be identified.

Assess motor or cognitive dysfunction that could impede successfully getting to a bathroom. Visual impairment or communication difficulties could also affect the ability to reach the bathroom in time, especially in a new environment.

Assess the client's ability to understand and follow directions to individualize teaching.

Dysfunction Identification

An open-ended question, such as, "Have you noticed any problems with voiding lately?" is a good way to begin. If the client responds by indicating no urinary difficulties, clarify the meaning of his or her answer by asking more specific questions, such as:

- Do you have any pain or burning with urination?
- Have you noticed any pink or reddish color in your urine?
- Do you feel you are able to empty your bladder completely every time you urinate?
- Do you accidentally lose any urine when you sneeze or cough?
- Do you have any difficulty stopping or starting your urinary stream?

Such questions are useful because alterations in urinary function are usually gradual and clients may perceive them as normal. For example, an older man may have had difficulty starting his urinary stream for the past 10 years as a result of prostatic enlargement yet not view this as a urinary problem.

Abnormal patterns of voiding such as polyuria, oliguria, or anuria are important to document, as well as hematuria, dysuria, frequency, or urgency. When any of these are present, question the client as to the length of time the problem has persisted and when it first began.

If the client indicates a chronic problem with urinary function, such as stress incontinence or a urinary diversion, question the client regarding individual management of the problem. When a problem in urinary elimination is identified, assess the client's support systems. Because urinary elimination problems are stressful, support from family and friends is helpful and necessary for the client.

Objective Data

Assessment of Urine

Assessment of urine is best done when the client does not void directly into the toilet, but rather into a urine collection device (urinal for men, bedpan for women) or when a retention catheter is in place. If assessment of the urine is important, request that the client void into one of these devices. A "hat" is a device that can be placed between the toilet and the toilet seat to catch urine (Fig. 36-8). Use of the hat permits the client to void normally in the toilet, but still allows for visual inspection or measurement of urine.

Assessment of urine includes visual inspection for color, clarity, presence of blood or mucus, and odor. Assess the amount of urine for each void and the total urine output over a 24-hour period.

Intake and Output

When a client's intake and output is being monitored on a flowsheet, urine output should be within approximately 200 to 300 mL of intake for any 24-hour period. Urine output that

ETHICAL/LEGAL ISSUE
Possible Neglect of a Client

You are a home health nurse supervising nursing assistants who provide basic care for clients in their homes. A nursing assistant comes to you expressing concern regarding the care that family is providing for one of her clients. She states, "I believe Mrs. James (an 86-year-old client with dementia who is confined to bed because of medical problems) is being neglected and abused by her family. The last few times I arrived to bathe her, she was incontinent. She smelled strongly of urine, and it appeared that she had been sitting in urine for a long time. She even has a small area that is beginning to break down."

Reflection
- Is there a difference between neglect and abuse? Outline what the nursing responsibility would be if neglect occurred. If abuse occurred.
- How might Mrs. James' dementia and immobility contribute to this problem?
- Do you need to collect any additional information before drawing any conclusion concerning the neglect and/or abuse of this client?
- Outline possible ways to collaborate with the family to improve the care that they provide for Mrs. James.

exceeds fluid intake may indicate diuresis. Urine output less than fluid intake may indicate decreased kidney perfusion, loss of body fluids from other sources (vomiting, diarrhea, bleeding, excessive perspiration), or physiologic conservation of body fluids. Trends of increasing or decreasing output require further evaluation.

The absence of voiding during any 8- to 12-hour period, or frequent voiding of small amounts of urine (50 to 100 mL) per void, suggests acute urinary retention or urinary retention with overflow voiding. Consider risk factors such as anticholinergic medications, surgery, vaginal delivery, and prostatic hypertrophy. If urinary retention is suspected, physical assessment of the lower abdomen is indicated. Bladder ultrasound can also assist in determining the amount of urine in the bladder.

Noninvasive Urine Volume Monitoring. Bladder ultrasound is a noninvasive technology by which the volume of urine in the bladder can be estimated. The portable device consists of an ultrasound probe connected to a screen capable of visualizing the bladder. Lubricating jelly is placed on the lower abdomen, and the probe is moved until a clear outline of the bladder is present on the screen. Two separate readings are taken, from which the machine computes the volume of urine.

Portable bladder ultrasound allows the nurse to obtain measurements at the bedside, in the clinic, or in the home. Bladder ultrasound can also be used to measure postvoid residual (the amount of urine remaining in the bladder immediately after voiding, usually 50 mL or less), thus avoiding the necessity of in-and-out catheterization for assessment purposes only. If acute urinary retention is present, catheterization to relieve bladder distention is necessary.

Physical Assessment

Inspection. Inspect the client's lower abdomen. When the client is lying in a supine position, a bulge in the central lower abdomen just above the symphysis pubis can be noted if the bladder is distended. If the bladder contains less than 500 mL, no bulge will be present. If the bladder holds more than 700 mL, the bulge may be observed extending in the direction of the umbilicus. It may not be easy to observe a distended bladder in an obese person.

It is not necessary to inspect the client's perineal area routinely, unless the client complains of severe dysuria and the presence of purulent drainage. When a client has no specific complaints, examine the urinary meatus while performing perineal hygiene for the client unable to meet his or her own hygiene needs. Always inspect the urinary meatus when inserting or removing a urinary catheter. If healthy, the skin surrounding the urinary meatus is nonreddened, moist, and without discharge. Smegma, an accumulation of white, odorous secretions from sebaceous glands found under the labia minora in women and under the foreskin in men, is normal and is not discharge from the urinary meatus. Abnormal findings on inspection of the perineum are reddened, inflamed skin surrounding the urinary meatus and purulent discharge.

Percussion. Percussion of the lower abdomen follows inspection to determine the presence of a distended bladder. Percussion should begin at the umbilicus and proceed downward toward the symphysis pubis. If the bladder is empty or contains less than 150 mL of fluid, a hollow note will be heard—the normal sound expected over the abdomen. Percussion over a distended bladder produces a duller sound. Urine, being liquid, is denser than the mixture of air and fluid in the small intestines and therefore produces a duller sound. The closer the dull sound is to the umbilicus, the greater the degree of bladder distention. Percussion is more reliable than palpation in evaluating the degree of bladder distention.

Palpation. As with percussion, palpation should start at the level of the umbilicus and move in a downward direction toward the symphysis pubis to detect bladder distention. Use the fingertips of both hands to palpate in an attempt to feel the top edge of the bladder. If the bladder contains more than 150 mL of urine, the edge of the bladder will feel smooth and rounded. The top edge of the distended bladder should be at the same level of the abdomen where percussion changed from a hollow to a dull sound. Although palpation of the bladder must be deep to feel the edge of the bladder, be sure to perform it gently. Palpation can cause discomfort and stimulate voiding. Palpation of the bladder is sometimes omitted because it is less reliable than percussion. Table 40-2 gives a comparison

TABLE 40-2

Comparison of Normal and Abnormal Findings on Physical Examination of Lower Abdomen for Bladder Distention	
Normal	**Abnormal**
Inspection	
No distention	Bulging above symphysis pubis
Percussion	
Hollow	Dull
Palpation	
Bladder not palpable	Smooth, round edge of bladder can be felt

of normal and abnormal findings during physical assessment of the lower abdomen.

Diagnostic Tests and Procedures

Nurses are responsible for collecting or supervising the collection of urine specimens for laboratory examination. Nurses perform some urine tests independently, but some tests require nurses to send urine to a laboratory for more sophisticated examination. Nurses are also involved in preparing clients for diagnostic procedures that help identify pathologic urinary conditions. They are responsible for client teaching and preparation before such procedures, assisting with procedures, and providing postprocedure care.

Collection of Urine Specimens. Different tests require different collection procedures. Special considerations may be required during collection of urine from infants or small children. Guidelines are given in Procedure 40-1.

Random Specimen. Random urine specimen collection is used when sterile urine is not required. The clean specimen may be collected in a urinal, bedpan, hat, or directly into a specimen cup. The urine should not be contaminated with feces or toilet paper. If a woman is menstruating, note this finding on the specimen. Properly label the specimen and promptly send it to the laboratory, or use it for tests to be made at the bedside.

Clean-Catch or Midstream Specimen. A clean-catch or midstream-voided specimen is used when a specimen relatively free of microorganisms is required. A sterile specimen cup or sterile bedpan or urinal is used to collect the urine specimen. The urinary meatus should be free of microorganisms normally found on the skin that surrounds the meatus. Instructions for obtaining a clean-catch urine specimen are provided in Procedure 40-1.

24-Hour Specimen. A 24-hour urine specimen is required to measure accurately kidney excretion of substances (e.g., urine protein, creatinine, urobilinogen, uric acid, certain hormones) that the kidney does not excrete at the same rate throughout the day. Nurses are responsible for explaining

(text continues on page 1078)

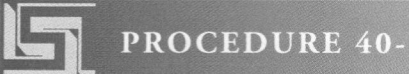

PROCEDURE 40-1

COLLECTING URINE SPECIMENS

Purpose
1. Obtain a noncontaminated urine specimen for routine analysis or culture and sensitivity.

Assessment
• Determine client's ability to understand directions and to obtain specimen independently.
• Identify purpose for obtaining specimen to guide selection of best method for obtaining specimen.

Equipment
Disposable gloves
Container, label, specimen biohazard bag
For collecting sterile urine specimen from indwelling catheter: Betadine or alcohol swab, 10-mL syringe
For collecting midstream urine specimen: cleansing solution, towel, specimen container
For collecting a specimen from a child without urinary control: cleansing solution, towel, pediatric urine collection bag, diaper

Procedure
Collecting Sterile Specimen from an Indwelling Catheter
1. Confirm the physician's order and verify the client.
2. Explain procedure to client.
   Rationale: Prevents potential errors.
3. Wash hands. Put on disposable gloves.
   Rationale: Handwashing and gloves prevent transmission of microorganisms.
4. Position client so that catheter is accessible.

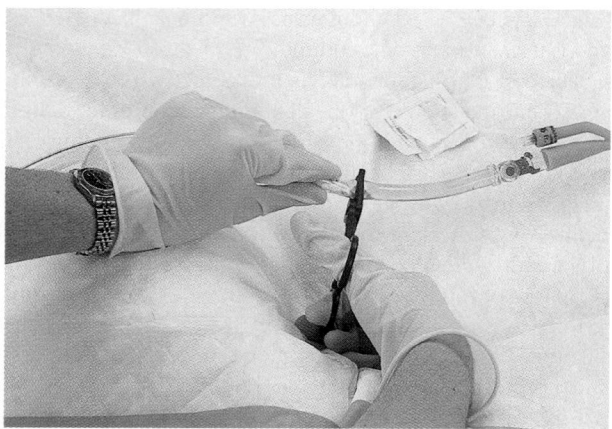

Step 4 Clamp tubing to allow urine to collect.
(Photo © B. Proud.)

5. Drain urine from tubing into collection bag. Allow fresh urine to collect in tubing by clamping or bending tubing (2 mL of urine is sufficient for a culture and sensitivity specimen, 30 mL for urinalysis).
   Rationale: Fresh urine is needed for accurate test results.
6. Cleanse the aspiration port of the drainage tubing with alcohol or Povidone-iodine (Betadine) swab.
   Rationale: Alcohol or Betadine prevents microorganisms from entering the drainage tubing.

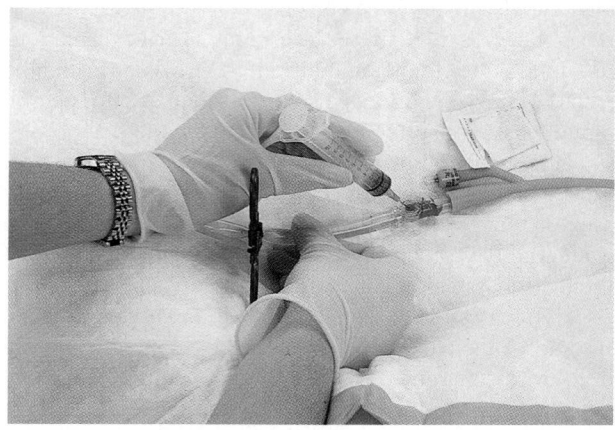

Step 6 Aspirate urine sample into syringe.
(Photo © B. Proud.)

7. Insert syringe into aspiration port. Draw urine sample into syringe by gentle aspiration. Remove needle.
   Rationale: Sterile equipment prevents contamination of the specimen.
8. Transfer urine from syringe into a sterile specimen container. Note: Agency policy may allow transport of specimen to laboratory in syringe with a sterile cap in place of needle.
9. Label the container. Date and time laboratory requisition. Place in plastic biohazard bag for delivery to the laboratory.
   Rationale: Incorrect identification of specimen could cause diagnostic or therapeutic error; bagging prevents spread of microorganisms.
10. Send specimen to laboratory within 15 minutes or place in specimen refrigerator. If specimen is for microbiology testing, it must be sent immediately and not refrigerated. Rationale: Microorganisms grow quickly in urine, especially at room temperature. Refrigeration retards bacterial growth.
11. Dispose all contaminated supplies. Wash hands.
12. Document procedure and observations.

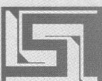
PROCEDURE 40-1 (Continued)

Self-Collecting Midstream Urine Specimen for a Woman

1. Confirm the order and identify the client.
   Rationale: Prevents potential errors.
2. Instruct client how to cleanse urinary meatus and obtain urine specimen.
   a. (Client) Wash hands.
   b. Separate labia minora and cleanse perineum with commercially prepared aseptic swabs, starting in front of the urethral meatus and moving swab toward the rectum.
      Rationale: Cleansing in this manner prevents spread of microorganisms from the rectum to the urinary meatus.
   c. Repeat this cleansing process three times with different cotton balls or swabs.
   d. Begin to urinate while continuing to hold labia apart. Allow first urine to flow into toilet.
      Rationale: First urine washes microorganisms and cellular debris out of meatus.
   e. Hold specimen container under the urine stream and collect sample.
   f. Remove specimen container, release hand from labia, seal container tightly, and finish voiding; wash hands.
3. (Nurse) Put on disposable gloves to receive specimen container from the client. Dry outside of container with a paper towel.
   Rationale: Take steps to prevent transfer of microorganisms to other healthcare workers from possible urine spillage outside container.
4. Date and time laboratory specimen. Label the container and place specimen container in biohazard bag.
   Rationale: Incorrect identification of specimen could cause diagnostic or therapeutic error. Bagging prevents possible transfer of microorganisms to other healthcare workers.
5. Send specimen to laboratory within 15 minutes or place in specimen refrigerator. *Note:* If specimen is for microbiology testing, it must be sent immediately and not refrigerated.
   Rationale: Microorganisms grow quickly in urine, especially at room temperature. Refrigeration retards bacterial growth.
6. Dispose of all contaminated supplies. Wash hands. Multiplying bacteria may split urea, which produces a more alcoholic urine.
   Rationale: Maintains good infection control practices.

Self-Collecting Midstream Urine Specimen for a Man

1. Confirm the physician's orders and identify the client.

2. Instruct client how to cleanse urinary meatus and obtain urine specimen.
   a. (Client) Wash hands, starting at the top in a circular motion.
   b. Cleanse end of penis with cotton balls and soap or commercially prepared antiseptic swabs. If man is not circumcised, instruct him to retract foreskin to expose urinary meatus before cleansing and throughout specimen collection.
      Rationale: Retraction of the foreskin is necessary to ensure adequate cleansing of the urethral opening.
   c. Repeat cleansing three times with three separate cotton balls or aseptic swabs.
   d. Begin to urinate, allowing urine to flow into toilet.
      Rationale: First urine washes microorganisms and secretions from urethra before collecting specimen.
   e. Pass specimen container into urine stream and collect sample.
   f. Remove container, seal tightly, and finish voiding.
3. Follow steps 2 to 5 above.

Collecting a Specimen from a Child without Urinary Control

1. Confirm the physician's order and identify the client.
2. If parents are present, explain procedure to them.
   Rationale: Increase parents' understanding and support of child during the procedure.
3. Position child gently on the back. Put on disposable gloves. Remove diaper.
   Rationale: Prevent the spread of microorganisms.
4. Clean perineal–genital area gently with soap and water, followed by antiseptic.
5. For a girl: Separate labia and cleanse from front of urethral meatus toward the rectum. Rinse with water and dry with cotton balls.
   Rationale: Cleansing removes lotions, powders, and fecal matter and decreases the numbers of microorganisms present on the skin. Drying the area thoroughly facilitates adhesion of the urine collection bag.
6. For a boy: Cleanse the penis and scrotum. If boy is not circumcised, retract the foreskin and cleanse. Rinse with water and dry with gauze or cotton balls.
   Rationale: Same as for girl.
7. Remove paper backing from adhesive of collection bag.
8. Spread the child's legs widely apart.

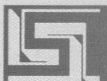

PROCEDURE 40-1 (Continued)

Rationale: Separate and flatten skin folds to increase adhesion of bag and decrease chances of leaking.

9. Apply collection bag over child's perineum, covering penis and scrotum of boy, urinary meatus and vagina of girl. Press adhesive to secure, starting at the perineum and working outward.
    Rationale: Securing adhesive from the center toward the outside decreases wrinkling and subsequent leaking of urine.
10. Place a diaper on the child loosely.
    Rationale: Diaper helps hold urine collection bag in place.
11. Remove gloves, wash hands.
12. Check the collector for urine every 15 minutes. *Note:* Parents can check child for urine specimen.
13. When urine specimen is obtained, glove again, gently remove collection bag from the skin, and empty urine into specimen container.
14. Tighten lid, cleanse outside of container if contaminated with urine, and place in plastic biohazard bag for transfer to the laboratory.
    Rationale: Cleansing outside of container and bagging prevent spread of microorganisms.

15. Label the container. Record date and time on laboratory requisition.
    Rationale: Incorrect identification of specimen could cause diagnostic or therapeutic error.
16. Send specimen to laboratory within 15 minutes or place in specimen refrigerator. *Note:* If specimen is for microbiology testing, it must be sent immediately and not refrigerated.
    Rationale: Microorganisms grow quickly in urine, especially at room temperature. Refrigeration retards bacterial growth.
17. Dispose all contaminated supplies. Wash hands.
18. Document that specimen was collected and sent.

Collaboration and Delegation

- Specimen collection is often delegated to unlicensed assistive personnel. Validate their technique and understanding, because accurate collection method prevents specimen contamination.
- Communicate clearly with laboratory personnel. Transport may need to be notified to ensure prompt delivery of the specimen to the laboratory.

---

the procedure to the client and for taking steps to ensure the collection of all urine that the client excretes during the 24-hour period. Inadvertently discarding even a small amount of urine invalidates the test results, and urine collection must start all over again. A sign over the client's bed and on the bathroom door helps alert all healthcare personnel and family members to save all urine. The laboratory will usually provide a large container for urine collection. A preservative may be added to the container to prevent the breakdown of certain urinary constituents.

Usually a 24-hour sample is started early in the morning, after the client's first void. Instruct the client to void until the bladder is completely empty. Discard this voided urine and note the time as the beginning of the 24-hour period during which all urine will be saved. The client may void into any clean urinary container (bedpan, hat, urinal) but must take care to avoid contaminating the urine with stool or toilet paper. All voided urine is emptied into the 24-hour collection container, taking care not to splash, because the added preservative can be caustic. The large container should be refriger-

ated or placed in a bucket of ice during the 24 hours of collection. At the end of the 24 hours, ask the client to empty his or her bladder, and add this urine to the collection container. Label the container and send it to the laboratory.

Specimen from a Catheter. Obtaining a specimen from a catheter may be necessary if a client is unable to void or already has a catheter in place. Urine collected in this manner is sterile. When obtaining urine from a catheter, always maintain strict asepsis to prevent microorganisms from entering the bladder.

If catheterization is necessary to obtain urine, an in-and-out catheterization is performed. This means the catheter remains in place just long enough to obtain the specimen (see later discussion and Procedure 40-3). The sterile urine is permitted to flow into the specimen container, and then the container is properly labeled, placed in a plastic bag, and sent to the laboratory.

If the client already has a retention catheter in place, the specimen is obtained by using a syringe to draw urine from a self-sealing port in the catheter, as outlined in Procedure 40-1.

It may be necessary to clamp the catheter tubing, just below the specimen port for 20 to 30 minutes with a rubber band or screw clamp, to allow enough urine to collect in the tubing so that a specimen can be obtained. This is especially true if more than a few milliliters of urine is needed in the specimen.

Urine should never be collected from the catheter drainage bag. This urine is not considered sterile because the collection system has been opened to drain urine at various intervals. Also, as the urine sits for long periods in the drainage bag, growth of bacteria can occur.

Collecting Urine from Children. Collecting urine from an infant or a child may necessitate special attention if the child has not yet achieved control of voiding. Catheterization is often difficult and is not recommended because of the small meatal opening and the trauma to the young child. Plastic collection devices are a more acceptable method of collecting urine. Clear plastic bags with adhesive material can be attached over the child's urethral meatus (Procedure 40-1). Wash the child's perineal area and dry it thoroughly before application of the bag. Apply bags according to the manufacturer's instructions, and take care to avoid trauma to the delicate meatus.

Collecting specimens from children who have achieved bladder control can also be challenging. Many children find it difficult to start their stream on command. Giving the child a glass of water, running a faucet, and permitting the parent to help the child obtain the urine specimen may increase the chances of success.

Urine Tests. Common tests that nurses routinely perform on urine include specific gravity, pH determination, and assessing for the presence of glucose, protein, ketone bodies, or occult blood. The most common laboratory tests of urine include the urinalysis, culture and sensitivity, and 24-hour assays for various urinary constituents.

Specific Gravity. Specific gravity is the weight or concentration of urine as compared to water. Specific gravity can be measured with the use of a urinometer. The urinometer is calibrated to float at the 1.000 mark in distilled water. To test for specific gravity, urine is placed in a test tube and the urinometer is gently spun and allowed to float in the urine. The specific gravity is read where the meniscus of the urine hits the urinometer marking (Fig. 40-4). The more concentrated the urine, the higher the float will rise in the tube, and the higher the specific gravity reading. Normal specific gravity of urine is 1.010 to 1.025 g/mL. A low specific gravity usually is caused by overhydration or a pathologic condition that affects the kidneys' ability to concentrate urine. A high specific gravity occurs because of fluid volume deficit.

Reagent Strips. Reagent strips (dipsticks) are available to measure the amounts of certain substances such as glucose, protein, or ketones in the urine. Such strips can also be used to determine urinary pH or the presence of occult blood. The instructions for proper use of the various reagent strips are clearly printed on the container. Follow these instructions precisely to ensure accurate results. The procedure usually involves dipping the reagent strip into the urine sample and comparing any color changes to the color chart provided on the container. Timing is crucial for the accurate interpretation of results for some tests (e.g., glucose, ketones). Assessment of the urine by reagent strips is ordered by the physician when he or she wants to monitor closely certain parameters in high-risk clients (e.g., assessing a pregnant woman for protein in her urine). Nurses may independently decide to use reagent

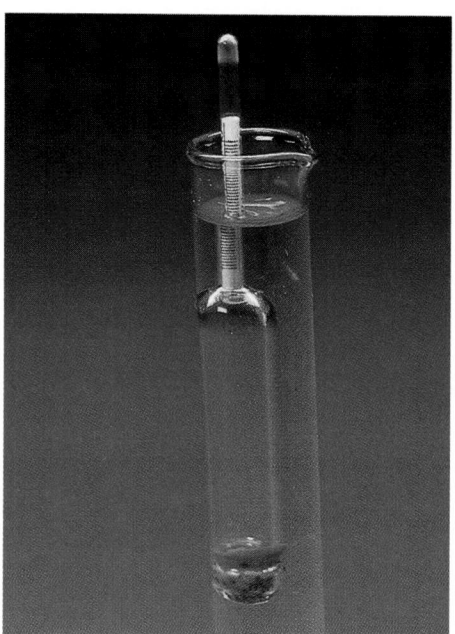
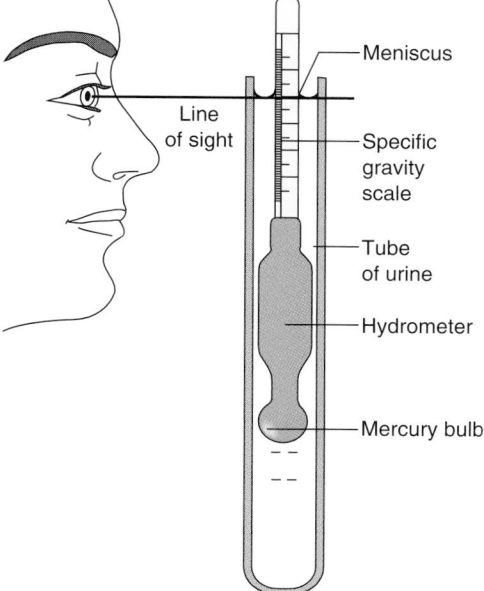

FIGURE 40-4 To read specific gravity, place a urinometer into a cylinder and read measurement where the meniscus meets the calibrated urometer.

strips when necessary for comprehensive assessment of high-risk clients.

Urinalysis. Urinalysis is one of the most common screening tests performed on urine. A urinalysis provides data about the color, turbidity, pH, and specific gravity of the urine and indicates the presence of protein, glucose, ketones, red blood cells, white blood cells, bacteria, or casts. The collection of a specimen for urinalysis is routine for all hospitalized clients. The test can be performed on any random specimen of 20 to 30 mL of urine. Although the specimen can be collected at any time during the day, the first voided morning specimen is preferred. The first urine voided in the morning is ordinarily more concentrated because the client usually consumes no fluids during the night and the influences of diet and activity are minimized. These factors make the first voided specimen most

likely to reveal the presence of any abnormalities. Table 40-3 presents a concise summary of the parameters tested in a urinalysis, the range of acceptable normal values, and the clinical significance of abnormal values.

Urine Culture and Sensitivity. Culture and sensitivity tests can be performed on urine to identify any microorganism causing a UTI and to determine which antibiotics can effectively kill the organism. The culture allows bacteria to grow and multiply over a period of at least 48 hours. The laboratory is able to make a preliminary identification of the organism within 24 hours, but another 24 to 48 hours may be necessary to conduct the definitive analytic tests that identify the exact microorganism responsible for the infection. After identification of the organism, the laboratory can test to see which antibiotics will inhibit its growth. If an antibiotic inhibits bac-

TABLE 40-3

Urinalysis Parameters

Parameter	Normal Values	Clinical Significance of Variations
Color	Light yellow-amber	Almost colorless: ↑ fluid intake; Dark color: ↓ fluid intake; Pink, red, dark brown: red blood cells in urine; pink, orange, red, brown, blue-green: medications or foods
Turbidity	Clear	Hazy, cloudy, smoky: urine specimen allowed to stand at room temperature; red blood cells, white blood cells, bacteria, mucus threads: mucosal irritation secondary to indwelling catheter
pH	Normal: 6 Range: 4.6–8	<6: Diet high in meat or some fruits (cranberries); metabolic acidosis (diabetes mellitus, starvation); respiratory acidosis (emphysema) >6: Diet high in vegetables and citrus fruits; urinary tract infections; metabolic alkalosis (vomiting, prolonged diuretic therapy); respiratory alkalosis (hyperventilation)
Specific gravity	Range: 1.015–1.025	<1.015: ↑ Fluid intake; diuretic therapy, diabetes insipidus, renal diseases >1.025: ↓ Fluid intake; ↑ fluid loss (vomiting, diarrhea, fever); antidiuretic hormone secretion (trauma, stress)
Protein	None-trace	Present in severe stress, renal disease, preeclampsia of pregnancy
Glucose	None	Present in diabetes mellitus
Ketones	None	Present in diabetes mellitus, ketoacidosis, starvation
Microscopic examination: high-power field		
Red blood cells	0–3	>3: Urinary tract infection, bleeding, urinary tract trauma, anticoagulant therapy
White blood cells	0–5	>5: Urinary tract infection
Bacteria/yeast	None-few	Few: contamination from perineal skin Many: urinary tract infection
Casts (precipitation or clumping of protein substances)	None-occasional	Many: possible renal diseases

terial growth, the bacteria is said to be sensitive to the antibiotic. If the antibiotic does not inhibit bacterial growth, the organism is considered resistant. The purpose of performing a culture and sensitivity test is to ensure effective antibiotic therapy in the treatment of UTIs.

Blood Test. Small samples of blood can be analyzed in the laboratory to screen for kidney disease. Two commonly performed tests are blood urea nitrogen (BUN) and serum creatinine.

The BUN test measures the amount of urea nitrogen in the blood. Urea, the major nitrogenous end waste product of metabolism, is formed in the liver. The bloodstream carries urea from the liver to the kidneys for excretion. When the kidneys are diseased, they are unable to excrete urea adequately, and urea begins to accumulate in the blood, causing BUN to rise. Normal BUN is 8 to 25 mg/100 mL. Because other factors, such as high dietary intake of protein, fluid deficit, infection, gout, or excessive breakdown of protein stores, can also elevate BUN, it is not a highly sensitive indicator of impaired renal function.

Serum creatinine is a more sensitive indicator of renal function. Creatinine is the waste product formed from the breakdown of skeletal muscle tissue; diet and other factors do not influence its formation. As creatinine forms, the bloodstream carries it to the kidneys for filtration and excretion. Damage to a large number of nephrons prevents efficient excretion of creatinine and causes it to accumulate in the blood. An elevated serum creatinine concentration is indicative of impaired renal function.

Creatinine clearance is a combination blood and urine test that measures the rate at which the kidneys clear creatinine from the blood. Creatinine is excreted in the urine by the process of glomerular filtration. Creatinine is not secreted by the kidney tubule, nor is it reabsorbed anywhere in the kidney tubule. Therefore, its excretion is an accurate measure of the kidney's glomerular filtration ability. To compute the creatinine clearance, a measurement of the creatinine level in the blood, the creatinine level in the urine, and the amount of urine produced in a set period (usually 24 hours) is needed. A decreased creatinine clearance value indicates renal impairment.

Diagnostic Procedures. The physician can order many diagnostic urologic procedures to understand better the functioning of the client's urinary system and to identify any abnormalities. The nurse prepares the client physically and psychologically for these tests, monitors the client during and after the procedure, and uses information obtained to individualize the plan of care.

Radiologic Examination. The two most commonly performed radiologic examinations to visualize the urinary system are the flat plate of the abdomen to visualize the kidneys, ureters, and bladder (KUB) and the intravenous pyelogram (IVP).

KUB is helpful for detecting malformations in the size or shape of the kidneys, ureters, or bladder and the presence of any stones that could obstruct urine flow. This procedure is painless and requires no special care before or after it is performed.

An IVP is a radiologic procedure that visualizes the urinary system with the use of a radiopaque (contrast) dye that is injected intravenously. X-ray films are taken at set intervals to permit visualization of the dye as the kidneys excrete it, empty it into the ureters, and finally deposit it in the bladder. A radiograph is also taken immediately after the client voids to check whether the bladder is completely empty. The procedure takes about 1 hour to complete. Special preparations before the procedure include clear liquids or a light meal the evening before the test; nothing by mouth (NPO) after midnight (although sometimes clear fluids are permitted); and enemas and laxatives to clear the colon of feces, because fecal contents can interfere with visualization. Also check for any history of allergy to iodine (radiopaque dye) before beginning preparation for the test.

Computed axial tomographic scanning (CT), magnetic resonance imaging (MRI), renal scanning, and abdominal ultrasound are also helpful in visualizing the urinary system and detecting abnormalities of the kidney or bladder. During these procedures, various types of energy are directed over the abdomen. Computer technology converts the information into visual pictures of the kidney. Client preparation varies with each test. Some discomfort may be associated with maintaining body position during the procedures, but the procedures themselves are not painful.

Cystoscopy. Cystoscopy involves insertion of a tube into the bladder for the purpose of direct visualization. A cystoscope is a flexible tube that can be inserted into the urethra and guided into the bladder. A light at the end of the cystoscope allows the physician to look for abnormalities such as tumors, stones, or structural problems. Specialized instruments can be passed through the cystoscope to remove small stones or to take tissue biopsies. Radiopaque dye may be injected for subsequent kidney radiographic studies; this is known as a retrograde pyelogram. The client needs to sign a consent form before the cystoscopy. After the procedure, assess for hematuria, urinary retention, dysuria or bladder spasms, and any signs or symptoms of UTI. A retention catheter may remain in place for a short period after the cystoscopy.

Urodynamic Studies. Urodynamic studies are used to detect abnormalities in bladder function or voiding. These procedures (uroflowmetry, cystometrograms, and urethral pressure profile) measure pressure (in the bladder and urethra and within the abdomen), urinary flow, and striated muscle activity. The procedures require no special preparation before testing. Urodynamic studies usually are not painful, but the client may experience some intermittent discomfort.

NURSING DIAGNOSES

Accepted North American Nursing Diagnosis Association (NANDA) nursing diagnoses involving alterations in urinary elimination include (a) Urinary Incontinence: Stress, Urge, Reflex, Functional, and Total, and (b) Urinary Retention.

Diagnostic Statement: Stress Urinary Incontinence

Definition. Stress Urinary Incontinence is the state in which a person experiences a loss of urine of less than 50 mL occurring with increased abdominal pressure (NANDA, 2001).

Defining Characteristics. Defining characteristics are reported or observed dribbling with increased abdominal pressure, urinary urgency, or urinary frequency (more often than every 2 hours) (NANDA, 2001).

Related Factors. Related factors are degenerative changes in pelvic muscles and structural supports associated with increased age; high intra-abdominal pressure (e.g., obesity, gravid uterus); incompetent bladder outlet; overdistention between voidings; and weak pelvic muscles and structural supports (NANDA, 2001).

Diagnostic Statement: Urge Urinary Incontinence

Definition. Urge Urinary Incontinence is the state in which a person experiences involuntary passage of urine occurring soon after a strong sense of urgency to void (NANDA, 2001).

Defining Characteristics. Defining characteristics are urinary urgency, frequency (voiding more often than every 2 hours), bladder contracture or spasm, nocturia (more than twice per night), voiding in small amounts (less than 100 mL) or in large amounts (more than 550 mL), and inability to reach the toilet in time (NANDA, 2001).

Related Factors. Related factors are decreased bladder capacity (e.g., history of pelvic inflammatory disease, abdominal surgeries, indwelling urinary catheter); irritation of bladder stretch receptors causing spasm (e.g., bladder infection); consumption of alcohol, caffeine, or increased fluids; increased urine concentration; and overdistention of bladder (NANDA, 2001).

Diagnostic Statement: Reflex Urinary Incontinence

Definition. Reflex Urinary Incontinence is the state in which a person experiences an involuntary loss of urine, occurring at somewhat predictable intervals when a specific bladder volume is reached (NANDA, 2001).

Defining Characteristics. Defining characteristics are no sensation of urge to void; no sensation of bladder fullness; sensations associated with full bladder, such as sweating, restlessness, and abdominal discomfort; inability to voluntarily inhibit or initiate voiding; no sensation of voiding; and a predictable pattern of voiding (NANDA, 2001).

Related Factors. Related factors are neurologic impairments, such as a spinal cord lesion that interferes with conduction of messages above the level of the sacral reflex arc; tissue damage from radiation cystitis, inflammatory bladder conditions, or radical pelvic surgery (NANDA, 2001).

Diagnostic Statement: Functional Urinary Incontinence

Definition. Functional Urinary Incontinence is the inability of a usually continent person to reach the toilet in time to avoid unintentional loss of urine (NANDA, 2001).

Defining Characteristics. Defining characteristics are an amount of time required to reach the toilet that exceeds the length of time between sensing the urge to void and uncontrolled voiding; loss of urine before reaching the toilet; sensation of need to void; ability to completely empty the bladder; and possibly incontinence only in the morning (NANDA, 2001).

Related Factors. Related factors are altered environment and sensory, cognitive, or mobility deficits (NANDA, 2001).

Diagnostic Statement: Total Urinary Incontinence

Definition. Total Urinary Incontinence is the state in which a person experiences a continuous and unpredictable loss of urine (NANDA, 2001).

Defining Characteristics. Defining characteristics are a constant flow of urine occurring at unpredictable times without distention or uninhibited bladder contractions or spasm; unsuccessful incontinence-refractory treatments; nocturia; lack of perineal or bladder-filling awareness; and unawareness of incontinence (NANDA, 2001).

Related Factors. Related factors are neuropathy preventing transmission of reflex indicating bladder fullness; neurologic dysfunction causing triggering of micturition at unpredictable times; independent contraction of detrusor reflex due to surgery; trauma or disease affecting spinal cord nerves; and anatomic fistula (NANDA, 2001).

Diagnostic Statement: Urinary Retention

Definition. Urinary Retention is the state in which a person experiences incomplete emptying of the bladder (NANDA, 2001).

Defining Characteristics. Defining characteristics are bladder distention; small, frequent voids or absence of urine output; sensation of bladder fullness; dribbling; residual urine; dysuria; and overflow incontinence (NANDA, 2001).

Related Factors. Related factors are high urethral pressure caused by weak detrusor muscle, inhibition of reflex arc, strong sphincter, and blockage (NANDA, 2001).

Related Nursing Diagnoses

Clients with alterations in urinary elimination can experience other problems, such as Impaired Skin Integrity and Deficient Fluid Volume. Psychological stress due to problems with urinary elimination can result in Anxiety or Ineffective Coping. Disturbed Sleep Pattern and Sexual Dysfunction also can result. Deficient Knowledge may occur when new treatment regimens are needed to prevent or cope with problems with urination.

OUTCOME IDENTIFICATION AND PLANNING

Outcomes for clients with urinary dysfunction should be individualized depending on assessment data. General client goals might encompass the following:

- The client will reestablish control over voiding.
- The client will strengthen or maintain adequate perineal muscle control.
- The client will verbalize understanding of procedures necessary to promote optimal urinary function.

Examples of some nursing interventions to meet these outcomes are listed in the accompanying display and discussed in the following section.

PLANNING: Examples of NIC/NOC Interventions and Outcomes

Accepted Urinary Elimination Nursing Interventions Classification (NIC)
Urinary Bladder Training
Urinary Catheterization
Urinary Catheterization: Intermittent
Urinary Habit Training
Urinary Incontinence Care
Urinary Retention Care

Accepted Urinary Elimination Nursing Outcomes Classification (NOC)
Neurologic Status
Self-Care: Toileting
Tissue Integrity: Skin & Mucous Membranes
Urinary Continence
Urinary Elimination

Refer to the following for specifics regarding NIC/NOC:
McCloskey, J., & Bulechek, G. (1996). *Iowa Intervention Project: Nursing Interventions Classification (NIC)*. St. Louis, MO: C.V. Mosby.
Johnson, M., & Maas, M. (1997). *Iowa Outcomes Project: Nursing Outcomes Classification (NOC)*. St. Louis, MO: C.V. Mosby. *Nursing Outcomes Classification (NOC) (2nd ed.)*. St. Louis, MO: C.V. Mosby.

IMPLEMENTATION

Health Promotion

Client Teaching

Client teaching is important in promoting optimal urinary health and function. Teach all clients the importance of adequate fluid intake, ways to avoid UTIs, and measures to maintain adequate perineal muscle tone.

Promoting Water Intake. Educating people regarding the importance of adequate water intake is a significant nursing intervention. Normally, adults should drink between six and eight glasses (1500 to 2000 mL) of fluid, preferably water, each day. Water intake may have to increase proportionally with any excessive loss of body fluid.

People should their space water intake throughout the waking hours to prevent transitory dehydration. They may need to restrict fluid intake before bed to avoid waking during the night. Water is the preferred fluid because excessive intake of caffeine (e.g., coffee, tea, cola), glucose (juices), or sodium (soda) can alter elimination patterns.

Adequate water intake serves two functions. First, adequate urine production flushes microorganisms out of the urinary system, thus decreasing the chance of infection or obstruction caused by stones. Second, production of large amounts of urine helps to distend and stretch the detrusor muscle, preventing atrophy. For these reasons, adequate fluid intake is helpful in preventing UTIs and maintaining bladder tone.

Preventing Urinary Tract Infections. In addition to maintaining adequate water intake, other measures can prevent UTIs. Encourage people to void every 4 hours to avoid stagnant urine remaining in the bladder. Adequate perineal hygiene is important to prevent pathogens from the anus or vagina from entering the urethra. Instruct women always to wipe from front to back after urinary or fecal elimination. Voiding immediately after engaging in sexual intercourse also helps to prevent bacteria from entering the woman's urinary tract. Adequate perineal care is essential during menstruation and during the postpartum period. Instruct women to avoid tight-fitting pants, harsh soaps, bubble baths, and powders because they can irritate the urethra. Cranberry or blueberry juice can prevent bacteria from adhering to the bladder wall, and therefore can be helpful in preventing chronic UTIs (Marchiondo, 1998). Remind men and women of the importance of washing their hands carefully with soap and water whenever they touch their perineal areas or body fluids.

Also teach the signs and symptoms of UTIs, namely fever, flank pain, dysuria, frequency, urgency, pyuria, or hematuria. Teaching is especially important after any instrumentation of the bladder. Some people may be embarrassed to contact their physician about urinary problems, so stress the importance of prompt treatment for potential UTIs. See the Outcome-Based Teaching Plan for more information.

Promoting Optimal Muscle Tone. Loss of perineal and abdominal muscle tone can contribute to urinary retention and incontinence. Promoting regular exercise of these structures

OUTCOME-BASED TEACHING PLAN

Jean Stedman, a young married woman, comes to the clinic with her third urinary tract infection (UTI) since her wedding 18 months ago. Each time, she has received antibiotics as treatment. Today, you both decide to review methods to prevent recurrent UTIs.

OUTCOME: By the end of the teaching session, Jean will be able to identify personal factors that might contribute to her recurrent UTIs.
Strategies
- Give Jean a list of factors that can contribute to UTIs (e.g., inadequate fluid intake; contamination from endogenous bacteria after sexual intercourse or defecation; delayed urination; tight, restrictive pants; urinary calculi).
- Ask Jean to select those factors that might apply to her situation, and develop a plan with Jean to reduce her risk. (She selects inadequate fluid intake, newly sexually active since wedding, and delaying urination.)

OUTCOME: On a return visit in 1 month, Jean's log will document compliance with prevention plan and no recurrent UTIs.
Strategies
- Determine goal for daily fluid intake (3,000 mL/day).
- Brainstorm strategies for increasing fluid intake without caffeine (keep sports bottle at side, drink a full glass of water with meals, drink after every voiding).
- Increase intake during periods of increased fluid loss (e.g., exercise).
- Explain how contamination can occur after sexual activity. Encourage Jean to get up immediately after intercourse to void and to wash area from front to back.
- Explain the importance of frequent voiding to avoid stagnant urine in the bladder for long periods.
- Keep a log of fluid intake and voiding until next visit.
- Praise Jean for compliance with preventive measures.

can prevent loss of tone. Kegel exercises involve tightening of the perineal and anal muscles. Clients should perform this activity several times per hour, incorporating it into their activities of daily living. Kegel exercises are discussed in Chapter 50. Another muscle-strengthening exercise involves voluntary stopping and starting of the stream of urine when voiding. Exercise instruction is especially important during the postpartum period. Client teaching concerning weight reduction for obese persons is also helpful in achieving improved muscle tone.

Measures to Promote Voiding
Illness and hospitalization can disrupt usual routines of urinary elimination. Unfamiliar and sometimes uncomfortable medical procedures, loss of privacy, strange surroundings, and anxiety concerning medical diagnosis or prognosis are just a few factors that can disrupt usual habits. In addition to promoting adequate fluid intake, a number of comfort measures promote urinary elimination and assist clients in maintaining their usual patterns:

- Provide a private setting for voiding.
- Allow adequate, unhurried, and uninterrupted time for voiding.
- If nursing assistance is needed for voiding, assess the client's usual voiding times (e.g., when awakening, before meals, at bedtime), offer assistance at those times in particular, and be available for assistance between those times.
- Encourage voiding every 4 hours.
- Promote relief of physical discomfort and anxiety-producing situations. Discomfort and anxiety may increase muscle tension and inhibit the relaxation needed for urination.
- Provide medications for pain as ordered, and give emotional support and reassurance.
- Aid clients in assuming a comfortable and, if at all possible, physiologic position for voiding (i.e., a sitting or squatting position for women and a standing position for men).
- If a client has difficulty initiating urination, nurses can help by providing sensory stimuli that either promote relaxation or act as unconscious suggestions. Examples of such stimuli include pouring warm water over the perineum, running water from the faucet, having the client relax in a warm bath, placing the client's hands in warm water, stroking the inner thighs, providing music or reading material, and offering a beverage.

Nursing Interventions for Altered Function

Nurses can use many therapeutic nursing interventions to assist clients who are experiencing altered urinary function. External catheters, protective pants, or indwelling catheters can be used for incontinent clients if bladder training is unsuccessful.

Bladder Training
Bladder training is the major independent nursing intervention used to treat urinary incontinence. Bladder training involves regulating fluid intake and establishing regular voiding times; these measures assist clients to postpone voiding despite a sensation of urgency. Additional techniques such as biofeedback, electrical stimulation, and pelvic muscle exercises may also be used to retrain the bladder.

Sufficient water intake is important for the success of a bladder training program. The bladder requires at least 200 mL volume to initiate the micturition reflex. A fluid intake of at least 2000 mL daily is recommended to provide sufficient hydration to allow the normal bladder stretch–contraction reflex to occur. Help clients to decide on their daily fluid volume goal. Clients should ingest most fluids during daytime hours, decreasing fluid intake as bedtime approaches. Clients will find it best to avoid fluids with a diuretic effect (e.g., coffee, tea, cola, alcohol) during bladder retraining.

Establishing and maintaining a voiding schedule is the most challenging aspect of bladder training. Several options are available; if one is unsuccessful, another may be tried.

- *Traditional bladder retraining* starts with scheduled voidings. Clients void at scheduled times (usually every 2 hours) and suppress the urge to void before scheduled times. The interval between voidings is gradually increased to 4 hours.
- *Habit retraining* schedules voiding times in an attempt to approximate the client's usual voiding pattern.
- *Timed voiding* is the continuous use of an unchanged, fixed voiding schedule (usually every 2 hours).
- *Prompted voiding* involves the use of regular checks to see whether the client perceives the urge to void. Sometimes, just the reminder or suggestion of the need to void is sufficient stimulus to initiate the process. Prompted voiding can prevent incontinence in clients who have difficulty perceiving bladder fullness.

Clients and all those responsible for their care must be aware of the method of bladder retraining and the schedule. Posting the schedule above a client's bed or at the bedside and recording data there are helpful measures. Success of bladder retraining depends on consistency over time, because the bladder is being retrained to respond to a normal micturition reflex. Refer to the Nursing Plan of Care near the end of this chapter for an example of a bladder retraining schedule.

Muscle-strengthening exercises are the third part of a bladder retraining program. Kegel exercises to strengthen the pubococcygeal muscles and exercises such as situps to strengthen the abdominal muscles are helpful in promoting optimal urinary control (Dougherty, 1998).

Habit Training

Habit training does not actually retrain the bladder but may be helpful in preventing episodes of incontinence. Verbal cues or prompts are given to the client to encourage voiding, usually at scheduled intervals (e.g., every 2 hours). Clients receive positive reinforcement when voiding occurs after verbal cuing. Habit training is especially helpful for cognitively impaired clients who may delay voiding until incontinence results. The success of habit retraining may depend on how willing and diligent caregivers are in providing prompts to clients on schedule.

Bladder Credé

Bladder credé involves manual compression of the bladder walls with the hands. This technique is helpful to promote complete emptying of the bladder, especially for clients who have neurologic impairment that contributes to urinary retention. The hands are placed on the abdomen below the umbilicus and above the symphysis pubis, with the fingers pointed toward the bladder. As the hands are pressed into the bladder, the client tightens the perineal muscles and performs the Valsalva maneuver (holds breath while bearing down) to assist voiding.

External Catheters and Protective Pants

For some clients, bladder or habit training may be unsatisfactory because of an inability to control voiding. Examples include older clients with some form of cognitive dysfunc-

tion, unconscious clients, and other clients who are extremely weak. Clients who are unable to control urination need assistance with urine collection. They also need frequent cleansing or bathing to remove odors and to maintain clean, dry, and intact perineal tissues.

Condom Catheter. An external catheter (condom catheter) is sometimes used for male clients who are unable to control voiding. External catheters have a much lower risk of promoting UTIs than indwelling catheters do, and they may decrease the risk of fecal contamination for incontinent clients. Condom catheters have also been shown to effectively control odor associated with incontinence. The external catheter is composed of a condom that is placed on the penis and attached to tubing that inserts into a closed collection bag. The collection bag may be similar to the type used for indwelling catheters; for clients who are more mobile, it may be a bag that attaches securely to the leg. Although condom catheters are preferred for patient comfort and decreased incidence of UTI, dislodgment and leaking are the major drawbacks of the external condom catheter (Saint et al., 1999). When applying or removing an external catheter, follow carefully the specific directions of the manufacturer or of the healthcare agency. For general guidelines on applying and removing an external catheter, see Procedure 40-2. Be sure to empty the client's leg bag or larger urine collection bag at least every 8 hours or more frequently as needed.

SAFETY ALERT

Remove the external catheter daily to cleanse the penis and surrounding tissues and to assess the skin for any edema or areas of excoriation.

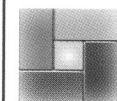

Clinical Research
AHCPR Guidelines for Urinary Incontinence

Behavioral Techniques
- Bladder training (retraining)
- Habit training (timed voiding)
- Prompted voiding
- Pelvic muscle exercises

Techniques that may be used in conjunction with above behavioral methods:

- Biofeedback
- Vaginal cone retention
- Electrical stimulation

Pharmacologic Treatment

Surgical Treatment

From Agency for Health Care Policy and Research. (1992). *Clinical practice guidelines for urinary incontinence in adults.* (AHCPR 92-0038). Rockville, MD: U.S. Department of Health and Human Services.

APPLYING A CONDOM CATHETER

Purpose
1. Provide a means of collecting urine and controlling incontinence without the risk of infection that an indwelling urinary catheter imposes.

Assessment
- Identify male clients who require control of incontinence.
- Assess client's mental status to determine ability to cooperate with procedure.
- Inspect penis for irritation or areas of skin breakdown from previous incontinence.
- Determine client's activity level and need for leg bag or continuous drainage system for urine collection.

Equipment
Soap, warm water, towel, prepackaged skin protector
Commercially packaged condom catheter with adhesive strip
Disposable gloves
Urine collection bag with drainage tubing or leg bag with straps

Procedure
1. Close room door or bedside curtain. Explain procedure to client.
   Rationale: Provide privacy and encourage cooperation.
2. Wash hands.
   Rationale: Handwashing prevents the transfer of microorganisms.
3. Assist client to supine position with only genitalia exposed.
   Rationale: Provide client with comfort and privacy.
4. Put on disposable gloves. Wash client's genitals with soap and water. Towel dry.
   Rationale: Remove secretions to prevent skin breakdown. Catheter adheres best if skin is thoroughly dry.
5. Trim or shave excess pubic hair from base of penis, if necessary.
   Rationale: Excess hair adheres to the condom adhesive, interferes with a good seal, and is uncomfortable when condom is removed.
6. Apply thin film of skin protector on penis shaft (usually found in commercially packaged condom catheter kits). Allow to dry for 30 seconds.
   Rationale: Protect sensitive penile skin from irritation and provide better adherence to the adhesive liner.
7. Peel paper backing from both sides of adhesive liner and wrap spirally around penis shaft.
   Rationale: Spiral wrap prevents a constricting tourniquet effect of the adhesive strip on the penis that could impede circulation.
8. Place funnel end of prerolled condom against the glans of penis. Unroll the sheath the length of the penis, over the adhesive liner. Some brands of condom catheters are held in place with a Velcro strap over the condom catheter.
   Rationale: Proper placement of condom sheath allows for urine collection.

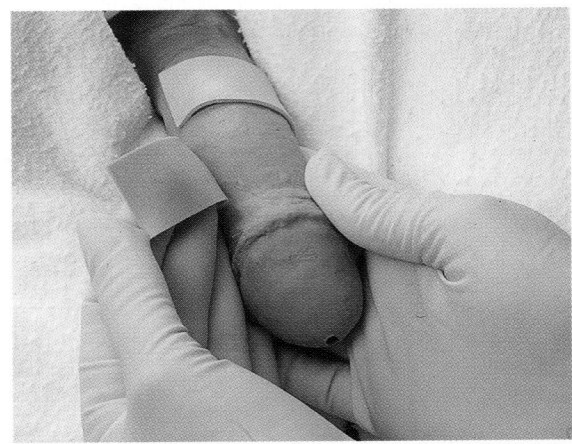
Step 7 Wrap adhesive spirally around penis.

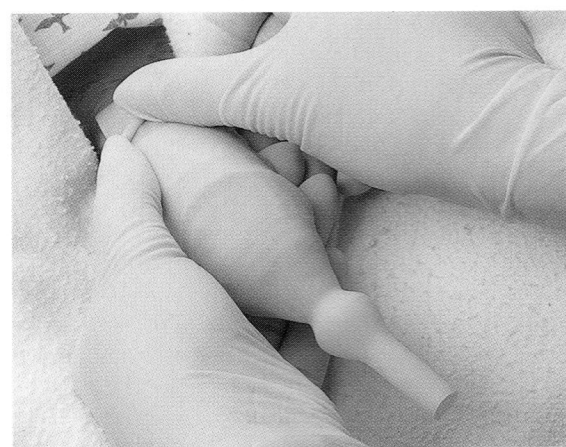
Step 8 Unroll condom sheath over adhesive liner.

PROCEDURE 40-2 (Continued)

9. Attach funnel end of condom to collection system. Tape may be used to secure the connection below level of condom. Avoid kinks or loops in the tubing.
   Rationale: Tape reinforcement prevents disconnection of tubing as client turns and moves. Tubing system allows free drainage and observation of color and quantity of urine.
10. Discard used supplies and wash hands.
11. Observe penis, 15 to 30 minutes after application of condom, for swelling or changes in skin color.
    Rationale: Swelling or discoloration of penis indicates condom is too tight and should be removed and reapplied in a larger size.
12. Document procedure and observations.
    Rationale: Keeps legal record and communicates with other health team members.

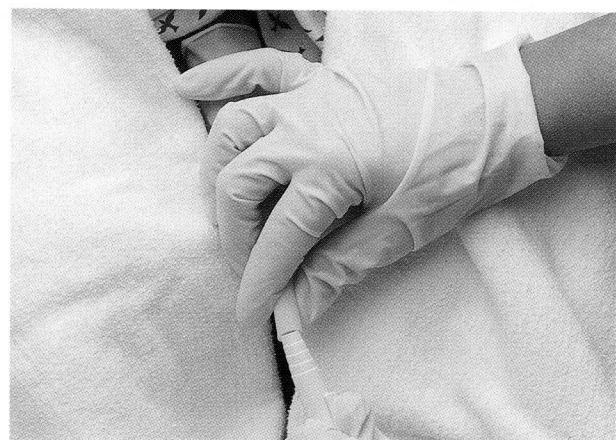

Step 9 Attach funnel end of condom to collection system.

Lifespan Considerations
- Condom catheters are not indicated for use in children.
- Young men might experience an erection as the penis is grasped for condom application.
- When penis is grasped in older men, it may retract into lower abdominal skinfolds, making application difficult.

Home Care Modifications
- Teach clients using condom catheters at home how to empty and care for their drainage collecting bag. In addition, instruct clients how to attach the condom to a leg bag to allow physical activity without fear of embarrassment from urine incontinence.
- Remind clients to change condom catheters daily to permit assessment of skin and to promptly detect skin breakdown.

Collaboration and Delegation
- Unlicensed assistive personnel frequently apply condom catheters. Make sure they apply catheters properly and check clients frequently for signs of constriction or skin breakdown.

Protective Pants. For female clients who are unable to control urination, a device such as an external catheter has not been developed. As an alternative to indwelling catheterization, some female clients (and some male clients) use protective pants. Also known as incontinent briefs, protective pants typically are disposable, waterproof briefs lined with soft, absorbent material. The briefs open at the sides, with tape or Velcro closures that facilitate application for clients who have difficulty moving, turning, or pulling on clothes. Clients need to change the protective pants frequently to avoid odor and to prevent skin irritation from prolonged exposure to moisture. Protective pants are not recommended for clients with total urinary incontinence because of the high risk of impaired perineal skin integrity.

Clients wearing protective pants should bathe at least daily. Each time the protective pants are changed, the perineal area should be cleansed and examined for any areas of irritation.

Urinary Catheterization

Urinary catheterization involves inserting a small tube, called a catheter, through the urethra into the bladder, to allow urine to drain. The most frequently used method is urethral catheterization, but urine can also be removed through a suprapubic catheter. When catheters remain in place to drain urine over an extended period, they are referred to as indwelling (or retention) catheters. When a urethral catheter is inserted temporarily to empty urine from the bladder and then is removed, it is referred to as in-and-out catheterization. If in-and-out catheterization is performed on a routine, scheduled basis for a particular client, it is called **intermittent catheterization.**

Indications for Catheterization. A urethral catheter may be inserted when a client is experiencing incontinence or urinary retention. A catheter may also be inserted when accurate assessment of urinary output is necessary, such as after trauma, burns, or surgery. Surgical clients may have a catheter in place for a few days to permit tissues to heal and edema to subside. For clients undergoing urologic surgery, catheters provide a means to irrigate the bladder or instill bladder medications. Catheterization may also be necessary to collect urine specimens or to assess how much urine remains in the bladder after a person has voided.

Types of Catheters. Urinary catheters are usually made of rubber, plastic, or nylon. A straight catheter with only one lumen is used for in-and-out and intermittent catheterization procedures. When an indwelling catheter is required, a double-lumen catheter known as a Foley is used. A Foley catheter contains one lumen to remove urine and a second, smaller lumen to inflate a balloon that keeps the catheter from falling out of the bladder. The balloon is located near the insertion tip of the catheter and can be inflated and deflated with a syringe. A third type of catheter, the triple-lumen indwelling catheter, is inserted when urine must be removed from the bladder and irrigation of the bladder with fluid or medications must also be performed. A triple-lumen catheter is usually used after urologic or prostatic surgery (Fig. 40-5). A catheter coudé has a curved tip that permits easier insertion, especially as the catheter passes an area of urethral narrowing, such as that caused by prostatic hyperplasia. Silver-impregnated or coated catheters have been developed to delay the incidence of bacteriuria and prevent ureteral entry of microorganisms (Marchiondo, 1998).

Urinary catheters are available in various sizes. Selection of the proper size is important to help prevent trauma to urethral tissues. A catheter smaller than the external meatus should be used to minimize trauma. Catheters are sized on the French scale of numbers, according to the diameter of the lumen. According to this scale, the larger the lumen size, the larger the French number. Available adult sizes range from 14 to 22 Fr, with sizes 18 and 20 Fr commonly used for men and sizes 16 and 18 Fr commonly used for women.

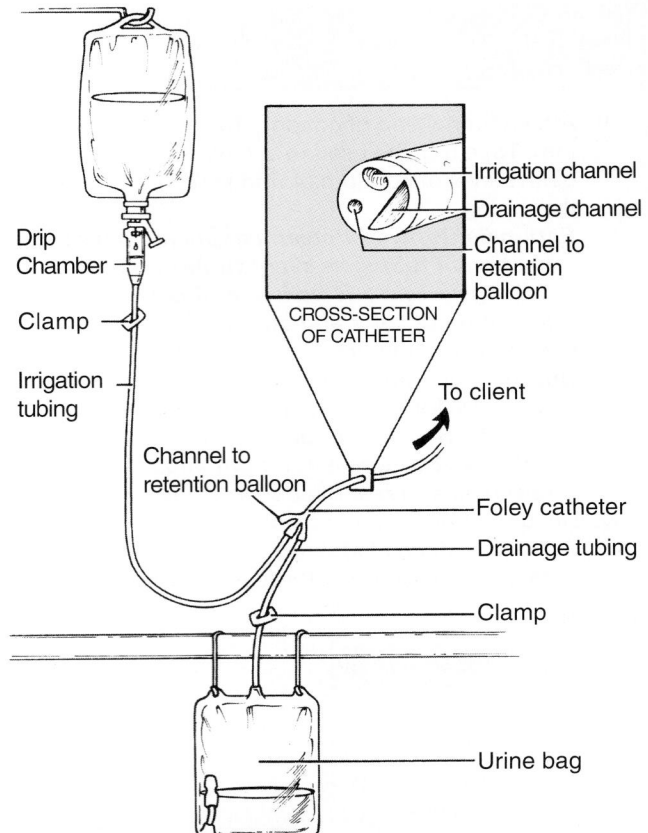

FIGURE 40-5 Closed irrigation system showing the triple-lumen catheter.

Catheterization. To avoid introducing microorganisms into the urinary system, which is sterile, aseptic technique is necessary for insertion of urinary catheters. Procedure 40-3 outlines the correct technique for catheterization.

Male clients can be positioned in a supine or semi-Fowler's position. Female clients usually are placed in a dorsal recumbent position (supine with knees flexed) for catheterization. An alternative, especially for clients who have limited hip mobility, is the side-lying position (Procedure 40-3). This position is more comfortable for weak clients who may have difficulty keeping their legs flexed and spread apart to permit visualization. The side-lying position also permits excellent visualization of the urinary meatus.

Risks of Catheterization. Any break in sterile technique during catheter insertion carries the risk of infection to the bladder, the ureters, and, eventually, the kidneys. In addition, with an indwelling catheter, risk of infection continues and increases as long as the catheter remains in place. The risk of infection is especially significant if the catheter remains in place longer than 72 hours, and 50% of clients develop infections within 1 week of catheterization (Marchiondo, 1998). The indwelling catheter must be connected to a closed drainage bag to prevent the migration of microorganisms up the in-

(text continues on page 1094)

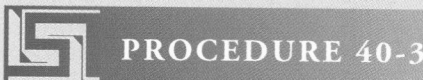

PROCEDURE 40-3

INSERTING A STRAIGHT OR INDWELLING URINARY CATHETER

Purpose
1. Monitor urinary function, prevent or relieve bladder distention.
2. Provide continuous bladder drainage.
3. Obtain sterile urine specimens.
4. Measure residual urine.
5. Provide a means for irrigating the bladder with fluids or medication.

Assessment
- Assess why catheterization has been ordered.
- Assess client for bladder distention.
- Assess client's physical ability to tolerate positioning.
- Assess client for allergy to iodine solution.

Equipment
A light source
Prepackaged, sterile catheterization kits that usually include the catheter (the most commonly used adult indwelling catheter is the Foley catheter, size 16 Fr with a 5-mL balloon), cotton balls, lubricant, disposable forceps, cleansing Betadine solution, specimen cup, gloves and drapes, drainage bag, and 2% lidocaine gel
Extra catheter and sterile gloves

Procedure
1. Verify the physician's orders and identify the client.
   Rationale: Prevents potential errors.
2. Explain the procedure and rationale to client.
   Rationale: Clients who understand the procedure are more apt to relax, which facilitates the procedure and is more comfortable for clients.
3. Provide the client with opportunity to perform personal perineal/penile hygiene. Assist as necessary.
   Rationale: Strict asepsis must be maintained to reduce the possibility of introducing a urinary tract infection. Initial cleansing rids body of gross contamination.
4. Wash your hands.
   Rationale: Handwashing prevents transfer of microorganisms.

Inserting Catheter for a Woman
1. Position client in dorsal recumbent position (supine with knees flexed). Externally rotate thighs. Side lying is an alternative position.

Rationale: Allow for visualization of the urinary meatus.
2. Set up light source.
   Rationale: Adequate lighting and correct positioning are crucial for clear visualization of the urinary meatus.
3. Open the catheterization tray maintaining asepsis.
4. Slide sterile drape under client's buttocks, grasping corners of drape. Ask client to lift hips so drape can be slid under.
   Rationale: The drape provides a large sterile field.
5. Don sterile gloves.
   Rationale: This is a sterile procedure. Once gloves are on all equipment in kit can be touched yet remain sterile.
6. Open sterile lubricant and lubricate catheter tip. Open cleansing solution and pour over half of the sterile balls. Open the sterile specimen container. Inflate balloon with prefilled syringe to check for defective balloon. Aspirate fluid back into syringe and leave attached.
   Rationale: Attention to preparation of tray decreases chances of contaminating sterile hands or equipment before completing procedure.
7. Place nondominant hand on labia minora and gently spread to expose urinary meatus. Visualize exact location of meatus. During cleansing and catheter insertion, do not allow labia to close over meatus until after the catheter is inserted. (This hand is now considered contaminated.)
   Rationale: If the labia closes over the meatus before catheter insertion, the meatus is considered contaminated and must be recleansed.
8. Using sterile hand, pick up antiseptic solution–saturated cotton ball with sterile forceps.
   Rationale: Using forceps during cleaning protects sterile hand from contamination.
9. Cleanse the urinary meatus with one downward stroke. Discard the cotton ball. Repeat this step three to four times.
   Rationale: Cleansing from front to back avoids introducing microorganisms from the rectum to the urinary meatus.
10. Use forceps and dry cotton balls to absorb excess antiseptic solution.
    Rationale: Absorbing excess antiseptic solution decreases slipperiness of tissues, aids visualization of the meatus, and prevents introducing antiseptic into urethra, which could cause discomfort.
11. With sterile hand, pick up the catheter approximately 3 inches from the tip and dip into sterile

PROCEDURE 40-3 (Continued)

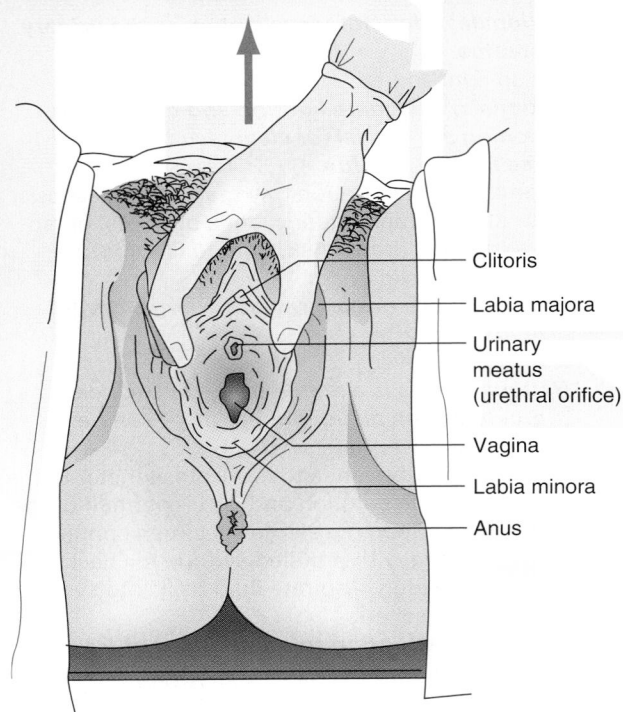

- Clitoris
- Labia majora
- Urinary meatus (urethral orifice)
- Vagina
- Labia minora
- Anus

Step 7 Spread labia to expose urinary meatus.

lubricant (2% lidocaine gel may also be used). Place distal catheter end into sterile basin.
Rationale: Lubricant facilitates catheter insertion and reduces urethral trauma. Lidocaine decreases discomfort on insertion.

12. Gently insert catheter into urethra (approximately 2 inches) until urine begins to drain. If no urine appears, have client cough or reposition catheter by rotating. Have client take slow, deep breaths during catheter insertion.
Rationale: Coughing increases intra-abdominal pressure and may assist urine flow. When the client takes slow, deep breaths, the external sphincter relaxes.

13. Insert the catheter an additional 1 inch (2.5 cm).
Rationale: Ensures that the balloon inflates inside the bladder and not inside the urethra, where it would cause trauma. If the catheter enters the vagina by mistake, leave it there as a landmark and insert a second catheter into the meatus.

14. Obtain urine specimen in sterile container, if ordered.

15. If using a straight catheter, allow the bladder to empty, then remove the straight catheter. Measure urine volume.

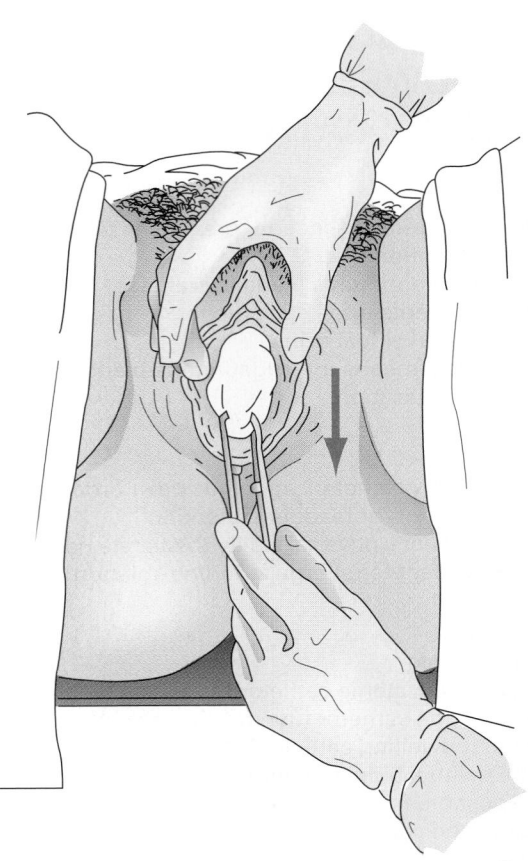

Step 9 Cleanse urinary meatus with downward strokes.

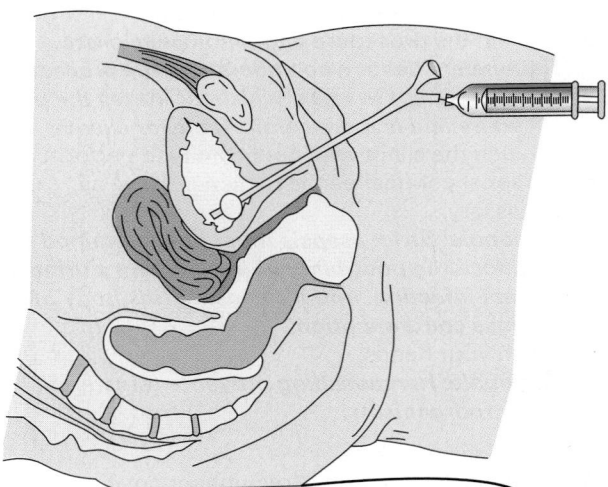

Step 16 Inflate retention balloon with prefilled syringe.

PROCEDURE 40-3 (Continued)

16. If using an indwelling catheter, inflate the retention balloon with the prefilled syringe. Check to ensure placement by gently pulling on catheter.
    Rationale: If resistance is felt, the catheter balloon is properly inflated in the bladder.
17. Connect distal end of catheter to drainage bag. In some kits, the catheter is already connected to the drainage unit. Some nurses prefer to connect equipment before catheter insertion.
    Rationale: Maintains sterility of the system.
18. Tape the catheter securely with 1-inch tape to inner thigh, with enough give so it will not pull when the legs move.
    Rationale: Securing the tape reduces urethral friction and irritation during client movement.
19. Attach drainage bag to bed frame, ensuring that tubing does not fall into dependent loops and that side rails do not interfere with drainage system.
    Rationale: Dependent loops fill with urine and can prevent free drainage of urine.
20. Remove gloves and wash hands.
21. Record the time of completion of the procedure, size of catheter inserted, amount and color of urine, and any adverse client responses.
    Rationale: Maintains legal record and communicates with health care team.

Inserting Catheter for a Man

1. Position client in supine position with only genitalia exposed.
   Rationale: Provide for comfort and privacy.
2. Drape legs to midthigh with bath blanket or sheet.
   Rationale: Prevent chilling, to increase comfort and aid client relaxation.
3. Open the catheterization tray.
4. Put on sterile gloves. Open sterile lubricant and lubricate catheter liberally. Open cleansing solution and pour over half of the sterile cotton balls. Open the sterile specimen container. Inflate balloon with prefilled syringe to check for defective balloon. Aspirate fluid back into syringe and leave attached.
   Rationale: Attention to preparation of tray decreases chance of contaminating sterile hands or equipment before procedure is completed.
5. Place the fenestrated drape over the client's genitalia.
   Rationale: Maintains asepsis during sterile procedure.
6. With your nondominant hand, hold the penis at a 90-degree angle to the body. If the client is not circumcised, pull back the foreskin with this hand to visualize the urethral meatus. (This hand is now considered unsterile.)

Rationale: Holding the penis at a 90-degree angle is important to straighten the urethra and allow for nontraumatic catheter insertion.
7. Using the sterile hand, pick up an antiseptic solution–soaked cotton ball with sterile forceps.
   Rationale: Using forceps during cleaning protects sterile hand from contamination.
8. Cleanse the urinary meatus with one downward stroke or use a circular motion from meatus to base of penis. Discard the cotton ball. Repeat this step at least three to four times.
   Rationale: Cleaning from meatus outward helps keep insertion site as clean as possible.
9. Use forceps to pick up one dry cotton ball to dry the meatus.
   Rationale: Drying the meatus prevents introduction of cleansing solution into meatus, which could cause discomfort.
10. With sterile hand, pick up the catheter approximately 3 inches from the tip and lubricate catheter generously (2% lidocaine gel can also be applied). Place distal catheter end into sterile basin.
    Rationale: Lubricant facilitates catheter insertion and reduces urethral trauma. Lidocaine gel reduces discomfort on insertion.
11. Gently insert catheter into urethra (approximately 8 inches) until urine begins to drain.
12. Insert catheter an additional 1 inch (2.5 cm).
    Rationale: Ensures that the balloon inflates inside the bladder and not inside the urethra, where it would cause trauma.
13. If using an indwelling catheter, inflate the retention balloon with the prefilled syringe.
    Rationale: Inflation prevents the catheter from slipping out of the bladder.

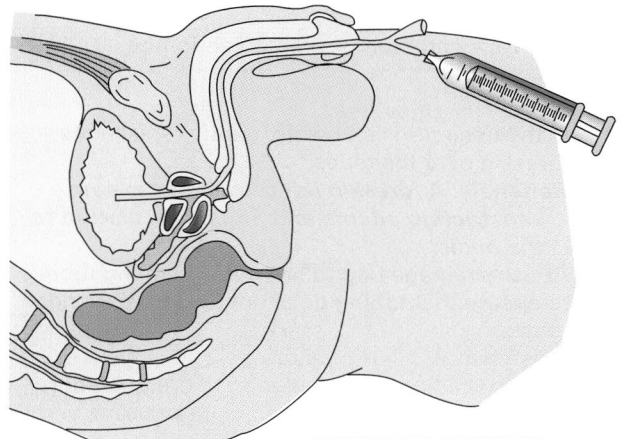

Step 13 Inflate retention balloon with prefilled syringe.

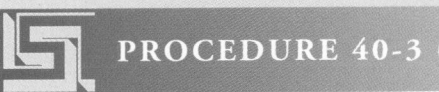

PROCEDURE 40-3 (Continued)

14. Check for placement by gently pulling on catheter.
    Rationale: If resistance is felt, the catheter balloon is properly inflated in the bladder.
15. Connect distal end of catheter to drainage bag if necessary.
16. Tape the catheter securely with 1-inch tape to the abdomen.
    Rationale: Securely taping the catheter prevents trauma to the penis–scrotum junction and reduces friction and irritation of the urethra from catheter movement.

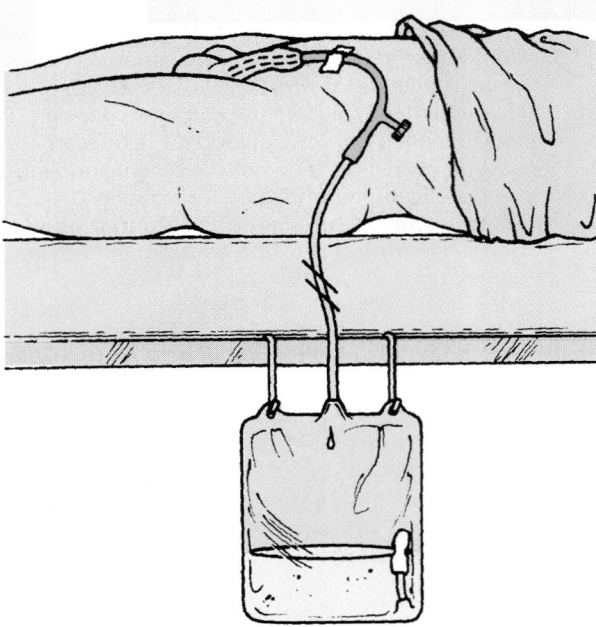

Step 16 Tape catheter securely to abdomen.

17. In the uncircumcised male, gently replace the foreskin over the glans.
    Rationale: A foreskin left retracted can cause constricting edema and impair circulation to the penis.
18. Attach drainage bag to bed frame, coiling tubing to ensure that tubing does not fall into dependent loops.
19. Wash hands.
20. Record the time of completion of the procedure, size of catheter, amount and color of urine, and any adverse client responses.
    Rationale: Maintains a legal record and communicates with health team members.

Removing an Indwelling Catheter

1. Wash your hands.
2. Don clean, disposable gloves.
   Rationale: Handwashing and use of gloves prevent transfer of microorganisms.
3. Clamp the catheter (optional).
   Rationale: Clamping prevents urine collected in the catheter from leaking onto the bed after removal.
4. Insert hub of syringe into balloon inflation tube of catheter and draw out all liquid. Size of balloon is indicated on catheter; most commonly, sizes smaller than 10 mL are used. Larger balloons (30 mL) may be used after prostatic or urologic surgery.
   Rationale: The balloon must be completely deflated to prevent trauma to the urethra as catheter is removed.
5. Ask client to breathe in and out deeply. Pinch gently and remove catheter as client exhales.
   Rationale: Breathing provides distraction and exhalation prevents tightening of abdominal and perineal muscles as catheter is withdrawn. Pinching catheter prevents leakage of urine.

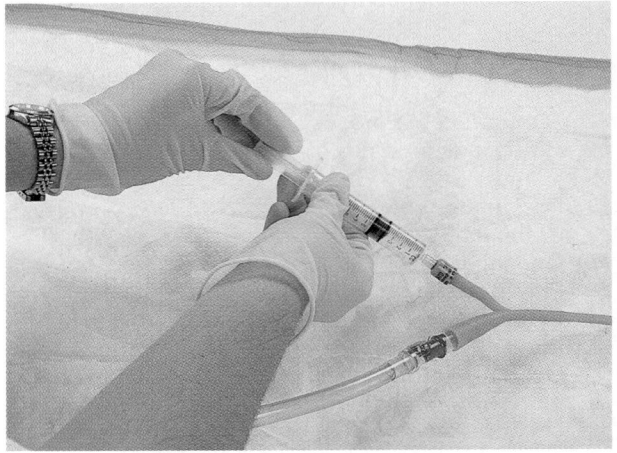

Step 4 Insert hub of syringe into balloon inflation tube. (Photo © B. Proud.)

6. Assist client to cleanse and dry genitals.
   Rationale: Provides for client comfort.
7. Measure and document urine in drainage bag and time of catheter removal. Estimate when client should void (within 8 hours).
   Rationale: Maintains legal record and communicates with members of health care team.
8. Wash hands.

PROCEDURE 40-3 (Continued)

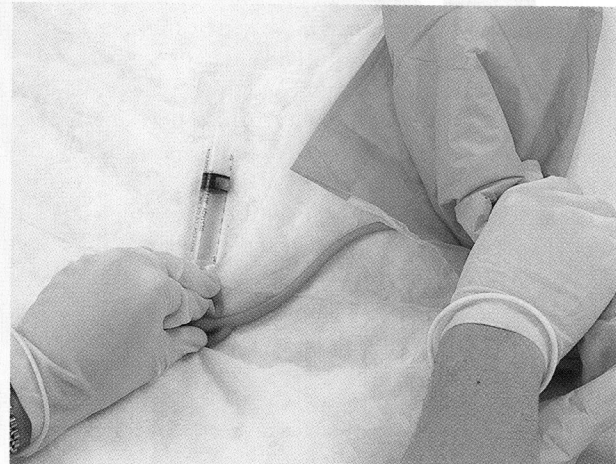

Step 5 Gently remove catheter as client exhales. (Photo © B. Proud.)

Safety Alert

- Strict adherence to sterile technique is necessary to prevent introduction of microorganisms into the urinary tract.
- Minimize trauma and pain by teaching the client before the procedure to gain cooperation. Ensure adequate lighting for visualization of the urethral meatus, and select the proper size of catheter. Distraction techniques are useful during insertion to reduce catheter resistance by relaxing the bladder sphincter.
- Always return the foreskin in the uncircumcised man to the normal (unretracted) position. Swelling can occur, which will impede circulation, if the foreskin is left in the retracted position.

Lifespan Considerations
Child

- Catheterization can be a frightening, painful procedure for a small child. It should be done in the treatment room so that the child's bed remains a "safe" area.
- An assistant may be necessary to help the child remain still during the procedure.
- Locating the urethral meatus on young girls takes extra care because the vaginal opening is more anterior than in grown women.
- A variety of sizes of catheters are available for use in children.

Older Woman

- The labia of women atrophy after menopause. The skinfolds can feel loose and slippery when they are being held before catheter insertion.

- Arthritis and other age-related musculoskeletal conditions may make it difficult for the older woman to maintain the position for insertion without an assistant. A side-lying position often is more comfortable.

Older Man

- The prostate gland often hypertrophies with aging, pressing in at the urethra–bladder junction. Always catheterize gently; if resistance is met, change the angle of the penis and advance the catheter again, or use a condom catheter. If resistance continues, stop the procedure and notify the client's physician.

Home Care Modifications

- Clients may return home with an indwelling catheter. Home health nurse follow-up is recommended.

Infection

- Instruct clients in signs and symptoms of urinary tract infection, and give directions about whom to notify. Symptoms include fever; chills; cloudy, foul-smelling urine; and possibly a burning sensation around the catheter.
- Instruct clients to wash their hands before and after touching any part of their urinary drainage system.
- Clients or caregivers should cleanse the urinary meatus and catheter with warm water and soap at least twice a day. The uncircumcised man should retract the foreskin and cleanse the entire glans well.
- Intermittent self-catheterization in the home is usually done using clean technique.

Urinary Drainage Bags

- Leg bags (see Fig. 40-9) are available to increase independence in the ambulating client.
- Bed-hanging, larger-volume collection bags are used at night.
- Check and follow home agency guidelines for changing the catheter and collecting tubing and drainage bags.

Collaboration and Delegation

- Nurses usually perform catheterization. In some acute care facilities, male nursing assistants perform male catheterization.
- In rehabilitation units, where many clients are intermittently catheterized, often a cath team of technicians have been trained to perform catheterizations.
- If catheter insertion is very difficult or impossible, consult a urologist.

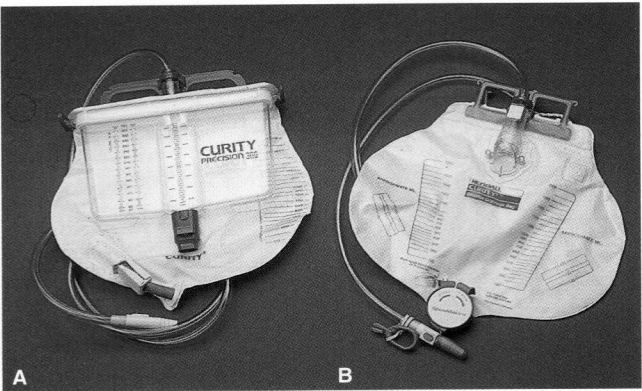

FIGURE 40-6   Foley catheter drainage systems. **(A)** Contains a urimeter for hourly urine measurements. **(B)** Standard drainage bag.

side of the catheter lumen to the bladder (Fig. 40-6). What still can occur, even with the use of a closed drainage system, is the migration of microorganisms from the meatus up the outside of the catheter and drainage tubing toward the bladder. Manipulation of the catheter, especially advancing the catheter into the bladder after it has been originally placed, can increase risk of infection.

Another risk of urethral catheterization is trauma to the urethral tissues, which can also contribute to eventual infection. Men are particularly at risk for tissue trauma because of the length and the curvature of the male urethra. Particular care is essential to insert the catheter along the normal contour of the urethra to avoid trauma to the tissues. The normal curve of the male urethra can be straightened somewhat by elevating the penis to a position perpendicular to the body. The use of small amounts of 2% lidocaine gel coating the catheter and also rubbed over the urethral meatus (for women) or injected into the urethra (for men) is sometimes recommended to reduce the discomfort of catheter insertion (Gray, 2000).

Care of Indwelling Catheters. Because the presence of an indwelling urethral catheter increases the risk of acquiring a UTI, nursing personnel must take special care to minimize

> ### 🔄 APPLY YOUR KNOWLEDGE
>
> Mr. Sanchez, age 90, has been on the rehabilitation unit for 3 weeks. When you go to perform your morning assessment, Mr. Sanchez appears very confused and is mumbling incoherently (a significant change from the previous day when he was oriented to person, place, and time). His vital signs are T 37.5, B/P 142/86, P 92, R 18. He has a catheter in place with an output of 250 to 300 mL of dark amber urine with much cloudy sediment. What do you suspect is happening? How should you proceed?
> Check your answers in Appendix A.

that risk. The catheter, drainage collection tubing, and bag make up a closed drainage system that preferably should not be disconnected except to change to a new closed system. Change the retention catheter and collection bag and tubing as frequently as necessary, as indicated by the presence of increasing sediment in the urine and along the catheter tubing. Empty the drainage collection bag through the outlet port at the bottom of the bag at least every 8 hours, and more frequently if necessary, because pooled urine is an excellent growth medium for microorganisms.

To prevent the catheter from pulling or kinking, tape it securely to the client's body in a fashion that keeps the catheter securely in place but with enough slack to allow the client to move freely. Tape the catheter to the inner aspect of the thigh for women or to the lower abdomen for men. Taping the catheter to men's abdomens rather than their legs helps prevent irritation at the penile-scrotal angle. In addition, sometimes a water-soluble lubricant is applied to the meatus to decrease irritation of the urethra.

The drainage collection bag and tubing should remain below the level of the bladder to maintain proper drainage and to prevent pooling or backflow. Most collection bags have a one-way valve at the insertion of the tubing into the collection bag that also prevents backflow. Attach the collection bag to the frame of the bed. Do not attach it to the side rail or rest it on the floor. Coil the tubing on the bed and attach it to the bed linens in such a way that there are no dependent loops. The collection bag and tubing come equipped with means to attach both the collection bag to the bed frame and the tubing to the bed linens.

Cleanse the client's perineal area and the catheter at least twice daily to remove normal secretions and to help prevent infection. Because specific directions for catheter care vary among agencies, be sure to check the relevant policy before performing these procedures. Most agencies suggest using soap and water for cleansing. Cleanse the perineal area thoroughly, wash the meatus carefully, and rinse and dry the area thoroughly. To avoid introducing microorganisms from the rectum forward toward the meatus, cleanse the woman's perineal area from front to back. During catheter care, assess clients for any complaints of perineal irritation or burning, and inspect the area for redness or excoriation. Note the color of urine in the tubing and the presence or absence of mucus. When caring for clients with indwelling catheters, monitor input and output to ensure a fluid intake adequate to produce 30 mL of urine per hour or 250 mL/8 hours.

Urinary Catheter Irrigation. The purpose of catheter irrigation is to cleanse the lumen of the catheter to promote patency of the tube. The purposes of irrigation of the urinary bladder include the instillation of solutions to help remove mucus, blood clots, or other tissue in the bladder (particularly after genitourinary surgery), and the application of medications to the bladder wall. A physician's order is required before either procedure is performed. In addition, the physician will prescribe the type and amount of solution to administer and whether irrigation should be closed or open.

The closed method of irrigation is performed without disruption of the closed drainage system using a triple-lumen indwelling urethral catheter (Fig. 40-5). One lumen is used to inflate the balloon of the catheter to keep it securely inside the bladder, one lumen is used for the removal of urine into a closed drainage system, and the third lumen is connected to a container of sterile irrigating solution. The specified type and amount of irrigating solution is administered by continuous drip at a rate prescribed by the physician or by written protocol. The catheter lumen used for removal of urine can be clamped until the prescribed solution has been instilled, and then opened to allow drainage. Or it can be left open to allow outflow of urine throughout the procedure (Fig. 40-7). Throughout the closed method of irrigation, the catheter and drainage tube remain connected to decrease the risk of entry of microorganisms into the system, which could cause infection.

The open method of irrigation is performed with the double-lumen indwelling catheter. It is rarely performed in acute care settings and is associated with an increased risk of UTI related to disconnection of the catheter and drainage tubing. After cleansing the junction between the urethral catheter and the drainage tubing and using sterile technique, disconnect the catheter and the drainage tubing. Using a sterile syringe, usually an Asepto syringe, administer the prescribed type and quantity of solution slowly, either by gravity or with gentle pressure, into the catheter tubing. Allow the irrigating solution to drain by gravity from the catheter. This procedure may be repeated depending on the amount of solution to be instilled and the physician's order. After completion of the irrigation, connect the catheter and drainage tubing again. Take care through-

out the procedure to maintain sterile technique because of the increased risk of UTI associated with this procedure.

When carrying out either the closed or the open method of catheter and bladder irrigation, assess the client's response to the procedure. Note any complaints of pain or discomfort, along with the quantity, color, and characteristics of the fluid draining from the bladder. In addition, note whether the amounts of solution entering and flowing from the bladder seem to be in appropriate proportions. In most circumstances, irrigation procedures are painless.

Removal of Indwelling Catheter. Removal of the indwelling urethral catheter is a simple procedure performed with clean technique (see Procedure 40-3). Care is necessary to avoid trauma to the urethra and discomfort for the client. Inform the client about what to expect after catheter removal (delay in voiding for a few hours because the bladder is empty, the need to save first voided urine for measurement, the need to increase fluid intake). After assembling the necessary equipment (an absorbent pad, disposable gloves, a 10- or 30-mL syringe depending on the size of the catheter balloon, and a washcloth, soap, and towels for perineal care), explain the procedure and position the client to allow visualization of the perineum. Remove the tape that has secured the catheter tubing to the client's body. Put on gloves. Insert the syringe into the entry port of the lumen of the catheter that was used to fill the balloon, and then aspirate all fluid from the balloon.

After aspirating the fluid from the balloon, instruct the client to inhale, and then remove the catheter slowly and carefully as the client exhales. As the catheter is removed, pinch the tubing to prevent urine from dribbling onto the bed linens, and then allow the urine to drain into the collection bag. Wrap the catheter in towels, then measure and record the amount of urine remaining in the collection bag at the time of catheter removal.

After removal of the catheter, assess the client's perineum and meatus for any signs of redness or irritation, and then provide perineal care. Inform the client that it is not uncommon to experience some dribbling of urine after catheter removal, particularly if the catheter was in place for several days.

Encourage the client to drink plenty of liquids to distend the bladder. Voiding should be expected within the next 6 to 8 hours. Continue to assess the client's input and output. Note the time of catheter removal, and also the time 8 hours later when the client is due to void. If the client has not voided in 8 hours, assess for urinary retention using a bladder scanner, if available. If the client has difficulty reestablishing voluntary control of urination, notify the physician. It may become necessary to reinsert the catheter or to perform an in-and-out catheterization.

Suprapubic Catheter. A suprapubic catheter (Fig. 40-8), designed exclusively for suprapubic catheterization, is a narrow-lumen tube with a curl at the distal end that helps prevent the bladder from expelling the catheter. A physician inserts the suprapubic catheter into the client's urinary bladder from an abdominal entry point just above the symphysis

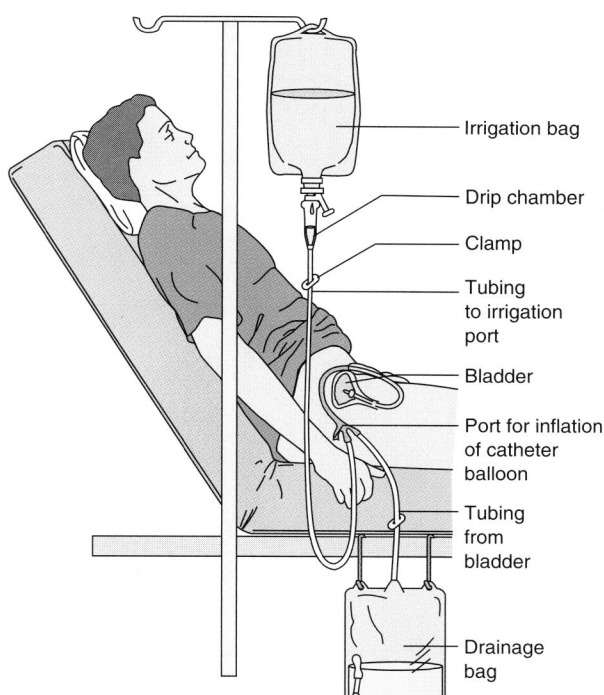

- Irrigation bag
- Drip chamber
- Clamp
- Tubing to irrigation port
- Bladder
- Port for inflation of catheter balloon
- Tubing from bladder
- Drainage bag

FIGURE 40-7 Irrigating an indwelling catheter using continuous bladder irrigation (CBI).

🔄 APPLY YOUR KNOWLEDGE

You remove Mr. Phillips's Foley catheter, which had been in place for 10 days. You provide him with a urinal and ask him to let you know when he voids. Six hours later, he voids 100 mL of clear, light yellow urine. How would you assess his voiding after catheter removal?
    Check your answer in Appendix A.

pubis. Suprapubic catheterization can be performed with the client in his or her hospital bed under local anesthesia, or in the operating room under general anesthesia and in conjunction with bladder or vaginal surgery.

The suprapubic catheter is kept in place by sutures at the abdominal entry point or by a form of body retention seal, which is a part of each catheter. The catheter tubing is then connected to a closed urinary drainage system. When the suprapubic catheter is to be removed, the sutures or body retention seal is removed and, as the catheter is guided out of the bladder, the bladder muscles contract over the entry site and seal off the opening made into the bladder. The abdominal entry point is then cleansed, and a sterile dressing is applied according to agency policy.

Advantages of suprapubic catheterization include association with a lower rate of UTIs than with urethral catheterization and potentially increased comfort for the client. In addition, they can make it easier to evaluate bladder emptying and residual urine (urine remaining in the bladder after voiding). The catheter is first clamped, and the client voids normally. After voiding, the catheter is unclamped and the amount of residual urine is assessed. Doing so avoids the need for catheterization to assess residual urine volumes after the indwelling catheter is removed.

Complications that can occur with suprapubic catheters include obstruction of urine flow from the bladder due to accumulation of sediment or clots, and closing of the bladder wall over the catheter tip. The small lumen size of the suprapubic catheter also increases the incidence of tube kinking and obstruction. The catheter can become dislodged or trauma to the bladder wall can occur during suprapubic catheter insertion. Nursing assessment of a client with a suprapubic catheter includes frequent observations of the client's urine for color, clarity, and quantity. In addition, assess the client's fluid intake, temperature status, and level of comfort and the condition of the abdominal insertion site.

Intermittent Catheterization. Intermittent catheterization involves the introduction and removal of a catheter into the bladder to permit drainage of urine at routine intervals, usually every 6 to 8 hours. Spinal cord–injured and neurologically impaired clients who are not able to void most commonly use intermittent catheterization. The incidence of UTI is less with intermittent catheterization than with a retention catheter. Intermittent catheterization also permits the client with chronic neurogenic bladder greater control and independence in self-care. Intermittent catheterization can be performed with clean or sterile technique, but when done in the home setting it is almost always performed using clean technique, which enables the client to self-catheterize. A mirror helps the female client visualize the meatal opening. To locate the meatus without a mirror, instruct the client to place the index finger of her nondominant hand on the clitoris and the third and fourth fingers at the vagina, directing insertion of the catheter between these two landmarks. For the quadriplegic client, a caregiver learns the procedure.

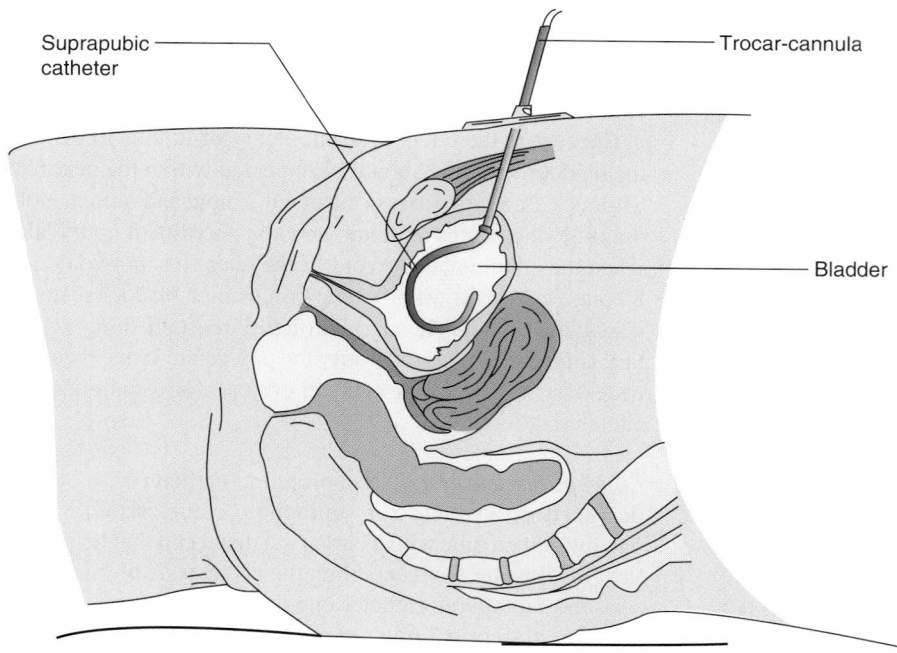

Suprapubic catheter

Trocar-cannula

Bladder

FIGURE 40-8 A suprapubic catheter is placed into the bladder through the abdomen to drain urine.

Leg Bags. Leg bags are smaller drainage units that can be attached to the leg and worn under clothing. Leg bags are helpful when the client must return home with a catheter or urinary drainage system (e.g., condom catheter, nephrostomy tube, suprapubic catheter) in place. Often, the leg bag is used during daytime hours, enabling the client to participate in normal daily activities without having to carry a large urinary drainage bag. The leg bag contains a smaller volume of urine, so it must be emptied often. This is done by opening a clamp on the system and allowing urine to flow into the toilet or appropriate container.

Teach clients how to change from one drainage system to another, as illustrated in Figure 40-9. First, have the client gather equipment and wash his or her hands. If doing this for the client, wear clean gloves. Wipe the connecting area with an alcohol wipe, using friction, before disconnecting tubing from the collection system. Recap the old drainage system and connect the leg bag, keeping all ends sterile. Once connected, the bag can be attached to the leg using the rubber straps provided with the drainage unit.

Renal Dialysis

Renal dialysis involves use of a semipermeable membrane to remove fluid, electrolytes, and other waste products from the body that healthy kidneys normally remove. It is used in acute renal failure to allow the kidneys time to heal and to help prevent further complications of the disease process. In instances of irreversible renal failure, dialysis is necessary to sustain life. Dialysis may be performed as a temporary or permanent measure, depending on the renal impairment. Hemodialysis (Fig. 40-10) and peritoneal dialysis are two types of renal dialysis.

Healthcare Planning and Home or Community-Based Nursing

Clients manage urinary dysfunction, especially chronic conditions, in the home with assistance and support from their family. The nurse's role changes from that of direct care provider to teacher, promoting and enabling clients to be successful in self-care and management. Teach all clients to recognize the symptoms of infection, and give clear guidelines regarding when to contact a healthcare provider.

Clients and their families may need to learn the correct methods to care for indwelling urethral or suprapubic catheters, to manage urinary diversion devices, or to perform intermittent straight catheterization. Standardized teaching plans are often prepared for common procedures with appropriate audiovisual aids to assist in teaching the care of complex home care equipment. Urinary procedures in the home, such as self-catheterization, are performed with clean technique. When clients are sent home with an indwelling catheter, instruct them on how to use a leg bag for drainage, changing back to a drainage unit at night. Vinyl drainage bags and leg bags can be decontaminated with household bleach. A 10% bleach solution can be used for daily cleaning of the interior of the drainage bag. The drainage bag should be agitated twice with the bleach solution, rinsed well between cleanings, and then hung to air-dry.

Sometimes adjustments in the home environment are necessary to promote optimal self-management. Clients can rent bedside commodes if ambulating or easy access to the bathroom is difficult, or a family may install a raised toilet seat for a client with mobility limitations. Bathroom remodeling may be necessary in some situations (e.g., doorways too narrow to accommodate wheelchair entry).

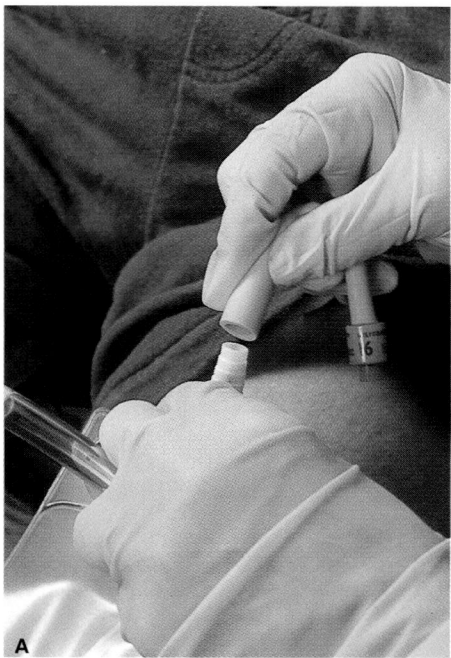
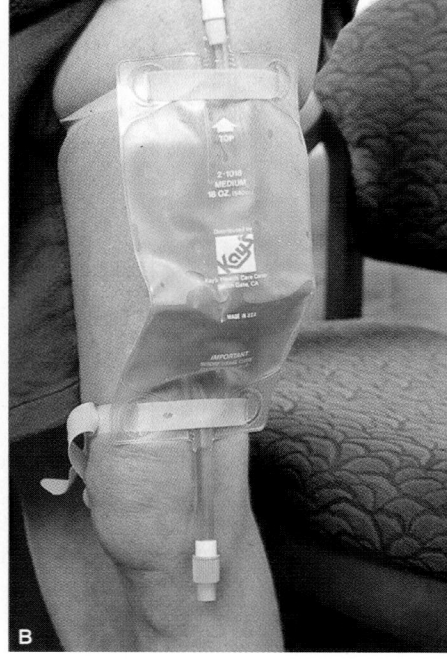

FIGURE 40-9 Changing from one drainage system to another when a leg bag is worn. **(A)** Connect new drainage system keeping ends sterile. **(B)** Attach to leg with rubber straps.

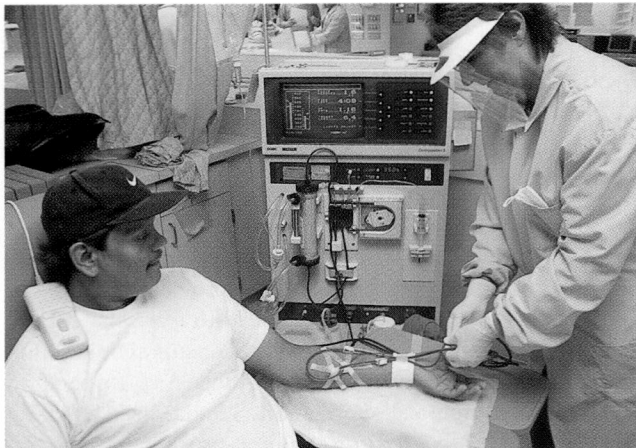

FIGURE 40-10   During hemodialysis a machine filters the client's blood when the kidney is no longer able to rid the body of waste products.

Contacts with resource people in the community for follow-up and home management may be necessary, especially if a client is experiencing urinary incontinence, has recently learned self-catheterization, has a new urinary diversion, or will have dialysis in the home. Nurses can visit clients in their homes routinely to assess progress in the management of their healthcare needs. These nurses may be associated with the discharging hospital, but they are more likely to be associated with a city or county health agency or with an independent home healthcare agency. The hospital-based nurse should be involved in the decision to make referrals to community agencies.

EVALUATION

Some examples of goals and outcome criteria for people with urinary dysfunction are listed in this section. Some criteria may be appropriate for more than one goal. Identify specific outcome criteria that will uniquely measure the attainment of the client's goal.

Goal

The client will re-establish control over voiding.

Possible Outcome Criteria

- The client remains continent for 2-hour intervals over the next 48 hours.
- The client voids four to five times a day, remaining continent for 48 hours before discharge from rehabilitation.

- By the next home visit, the caregiver reports that the client recognizes the urge to void in time to use the toilet or commode.

Goal

The client will demonstrate understanding of procedures necessary to promote optimal urinary function.

Possible Outcome Criteria

- The client verbalizes steps in intermittent self-catheterization by the end of the teaching session.
- The client practices proper self-catheterization technique during teaching sessions and twice in the next 48 hours.
- The client demonstrates proper application of the stoma appliance before discharge.
- The client demonstrates use of the leg bag before discharge.

KEY CONCEPTS

- The voluntary process of micturition is stimulated by stretch of the detrusor muscle as the bladder fills with urine.
- Between 250 and 400 mL of clear, yellow, aromatic urine per void is considered normal.
- As children approach 3 to 4 years of age, their kidneys mature and they achieve voluntary control over urinary elimination; kidney function declines in older adults owing to normal age-related changes.
- Many factors, such as fluid intake, loss of body fluid, dietary intake, body position, psychological state, obstruction, infection, hypotension, neurologic injury, decreased muscle tone, pregnancy, surgery, and medications, can affect urinary elimination.
- Manifestations of altered urinary function include dysuria, polyuria, oliguria, urgency, frequency, nocturia, hematuria, pyuria, urinary retention, urinary incontinence, and enuresis.
- Physical assessment of urinary function includes inspection of urine and percussion and palpation of the bladder for residual urine.
- Diagnostic tests and procedures that are helpful in identifying urinary dysfunction include urinalysis, urine culture and sensitivity, specific gravity, BUN, creatinine, cystoscopy, and urodynamic studies.
- Six approved NANDA nursing diagnoses identify problems in urinary function.
- Nursing measures to promote normal urinary function include ensuring adequate fluid intake, preventing UTIs, and promoting optimal perineal muscle tone. Nursing interventions for urinary retention include bladder credé, in-and-out catheterization, and intermittent catheterization.
- Nursing interventions for urinary incontinence include bladder training, use of external and internal catheters, and use of protective pants.
- Self-management of many urologic problems occurs in the home setting with adequate support from the family, the community, and the healthcare provider.

NURSING PLAN OF CARE
THE CLIENT WITH URGE INCONTINENCE

Nursing Diagnosis

Urge incontinence related to decreased bladder capacity and tone secondary to indwelling catheter postoperatively as manifested by strong urinary urge with incontinence, frequency, dribbling, and nocturia.

Client Goal

Client will reestablish control over voiding.

Client Outcome Criteria

- Client remains continent for 2-hour intervals over next 48 hours.
- Client verbalizes the importance of fluid intake and complies with prescribed intake.
- Client will demonstrate Kegel exercises after teaching session.

Nursing Interventions

1. Measure and record input and output.

2. Percuss and palpate lower abdomen after an incontinent episode. Straight catheterize for postvoid residual volume (PVR), if necessary.
3. Teach client perineal muscle-strengthening exercises and tell him or her to perform them 10 times every 2 to 3 hours during the day.
4. Work with client to develop acceptable regimen. Increase fluid intake to 1500 to 2000 mL/day, concentrating most fluid intake during day.
5. Post fluid intake schedule by the bedside.

6. Begin bladder training routine:
   6a. Assist client, as necessary, to the bathroom to void every 2 hr during daytime, every 4 hr at night. Decrease between-voiding interval to 1.5 hr if client is initially unable to consistently remain continent for the longer intervals.
   6b. Encourage the client to "hold" his or her urine if he or she experiences the urge to void before the next scheduled voiding time.
   6c. Increase between-voiding intervals by 0.5 hr after client has successfully remained continent for 24 hr.
7. Post voiding schedule in client's room. Change prn. Include details of current voiding schedule at change of shift report.

Scientific Rationale

1. Use data to assess for pattern of urinary output, relationship of intake to episodes of incontinence, relative overall fluid balance, success of bladder training.
2. Assessment is made to rule out urinary retention and overflow incontinence as the primary urinary alteration.
3. These exercises strengthen skeletal perineal muscles and increase voluntary contraction of urethral sphincter.
4. Adequate hydration is necessary to cause bladder filling and trigger the normal stretch/contraction response.
5. Concentration of most fluids during daytime hours will decrease nocturia.

6a. This regimen allows bladder to refill between voidings and gradually retrains the normal bladder stretch/contraction response.

6b. Suppressing the urge to void assists in retraining of voluntary contraction of external urethral muscles.
6c. Gradual retraining aims at achieving fewer voids with larger amounts, a more normal pattern.

7. Communication increases client and staff compliance.

REFERENCES

Agency for Health Care Policy and Research. (1992). *Clinical practice guidelines for urinary incontinence in adults* (AHCPR 92-0038). Rockville, MD: U.S. Department of Health and Human Services.

Bemelmans, B. L. H., Kiemeney, L. A. L. M., & Debruyne, F. M. J. (2000). Low-dose oxybutynin for the treatment of urge incontinence: Good efficacy and few side effects. *European Urology, 37,* 709–713.

Dougherty, M. C. (1998). Current status of research on pelvic muscle strengthening techniques. *Journal of Wound Ostomy Continence Nursing, 25*(2), 75–83.

Dugan, E., Cohen, S. J., Bland, D. R., et al. (2000). The association of depressive symptoms and urinary incontinence among older persons. *Journal of the American Geriatric Society, 48,* 413–416.

Gray, M. (2000). Urinary retention: Management in the acute care setting. Part 2. *American Journal of Nursing, 100*(8), 36–44.

Marchiondo, K. (1998). A new look at urinary tract infection. *American Journal of Nursing, 98*(3), 34–38.

North American Nursing Diagnosis Association (NANDA). (2001). *NANDA nursing diagnoses: Definitions and classifications 2001–2002.* Philadelphia: Author.

Porth, C. (1998). *Pathophysiology: Concepts of altered health states* (5th ed.). Philadelphia: Lippincott-Raven.

Saint, S., Lipsky, B. A., Baker, P. D., et al. (1999). Urinary catheters: What type do men and their nurses prefer? *Journal of the American Geriatric Society, 47,* 1453–1457.

Swithinbank, L. V., Brookes, S. T., Shepard, A. M., et al. (1998). The natural history of urinary symptoms during adolescence. *British Journal of Urology, 81,* (Suppl 3), 90–93.

Swithinbank, L. V., Donovan, J. L., Rogers, C. A., et al. (2000). Nocturnal incontinence in women: A hidden problem. *The Journal of Urology, 164,* 764–766.

Vernarec, E. (1998). The high costs of hidden conditions . . . the most sensitive conditions for patients to talk about. *Business & Health, 16*(1), 19–23.

BIBLIOGRAPHY

Addison, R., (1999). Changing a suprapubic catheter, 1–3. *Nursing Times, (42–44),* S1–S2.

Bergstrom, K., Carlsson, C. P. O., Lindholm, C., et al. (2000). Improvement of urge- and mixed-type incontinence after acupuncture treatment among elderly women: A pilot study. *Journal of the Autonomic Nervous System, 79,* 173–180.

Bickley, L. (1999). *Bates' guide to physical examination* (7th ed.). Philadelphia: Lippincott-Raven.

Button, D., Roe, B., Webb, C., et al. (1998). Consensus guidelines for the promotion and management of continence by primary health care teams: Development, implementation, and evaluation. *Journal of Advanced Nursing, 27*(1), 91–99.

Doherty, W. (1999). Indications for and principles of intermittent self-catheterization. *British Journal of Nursing, 8*(2), 73–80.

Gray, M. (2000). Urinary retention: Management in the acute care setting. Part 1. *American Journal of Nursing, 100*(7), 40–47.

Johnson, T. M., Kincade, J. E., Bernard, S. L., et al. (2000). Self-care practices used by older men and women to manage urinary incontinence: Results from the national follow-up survey on self-care and aging. *Journal of the American Geriatric Society, 48,* 894–902.

Lekan-Rutledge, D., Palmer, M. H., & Belyea, M. (1998). In their own words: Nursing assistants' perceptions of barriers to implementation of prompted voiding in long-term care. *Gerontologist, 38*(3), 370–378.

Miller, J. M., Ashton-Miller, J. A., & DeLancey, J. O. (1998). A pelvic muscle precontraction can reduce cough-related urine loss in selected women with mild SUI. *Journal of the American Geriatric Society, 46*(7), 870–874.

Roberts, R. O., Jacobsen, S. J., Rhodes, T., et al. (1998). Urinary incontinence in a community-based cohort: Prevalence and healthcare seeking. *Journal of the American Geriatric Society, 46*(4), 467–472.

Sampselle, C. M., & DeLancey, J. O. L. (1998). Anatomy of female incontinence. *Journal of Wound Ostomy Continence Nursing, 25*(2), 63–74.

Schnelle, J. F., Cruise, P. A., Alessi, C. A., et al. (1998). Individualizing nighttime incontinence care in nursing home residents. *Nursing Research, 47*(4), 197–204.

Scura, K. W., & Whipple, B. (1997). How to provide better care for the postmenopausal woman. *American Journal of Nursing, 97*(4), 36–44.

Smith, A. B., & Adams, L. L. (1998). Insertion of indwelling urethral catheters in infants and children: A survey of current nursing practice. *Pediatric Nursing, 24*(3), 229–234.

Winn, C. (1998). Complications with urinary catheters. *Professional Nurse Study Supplement, 13*(5), S7–S10.

41 Bowel Elimination

Key Terms

borborygmi
colostomy
constipation
defecation reflex
diarrhea
distention
enema
flatus
gastric lavage
gavage

guaiac
ileostomy
impaction
meconium
ostomate
paralytic ileus
peristalsis
sigmoidoscopy
stoma
suppository

Learning Objectives

Upon completion of this chapter, the student will be able to do the following:

1. Explain the process of defecation.
2. Recognize age-related differences in bowel elimination.
3. Identify factors that affect bowel elimination.
4. Describe the manifestations of altered bowel elimination.
5. Describe appropriate subjective and objective data to collect to assess bowel function.
6. Identify nursing diagnoses relating to altered bowel elimination.
7. Describe independent and collaborative nursing interventions to promote normal bowel function.
8. Discuss appropriate community-based care for clients with altered bowel function.

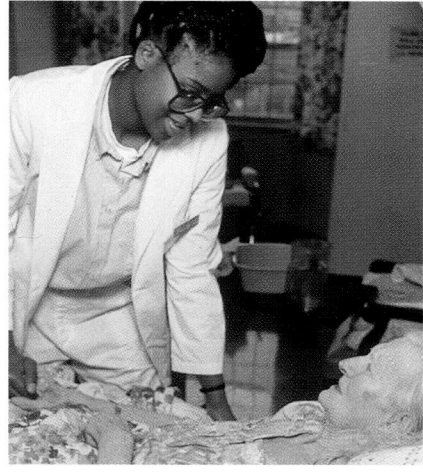

Critical Thinking Challenge

You are working in a nursing home, caring for a 76-year-old woman with metastatic cancer. For the last few weeks, she has been receiving increasing doses of morphine to control her back pain. Her appetite is poor, and she spends most of the day in bed. At change of shift report, you learn that she has not had a bowel movement for 7 days and she has an order for an enema. When you go in to assess her and explain that she needs an enema, she replies, "Please leave me alone. Can't you see how tired I am and how much I hurt?"

What might be considered normal bowel function for one person may be considered abnormal for another. Once you have completed this chapter, review the above scenario and reflect on the following areas of Critical Thinking.

1. Examine factors that could contribute to the client's constipation.
2. Reflect on how you feel when you must ask clients questions about elimination or perform procedures such as enemas.
3. Appraise possible factors that may have influenced the woman's refusal to have an enema.
4. Consider ethical and legal factors in determining how to respond to the client.
5. Critique the use of therapeutic communication in responding to this client.

The elimination of waste from the bowel is an essential body function. Defecation is the process by which the solid waste products of digestion, known as feces or stool, are eliminated from the bowel. The major nursing responsibilities associated with bowel elimination include assessing bowel function, promoting normal bowel health, and intervening to manage alterations in bowel function.

Such responsibilities span many age groups and different health settings. For example, nurses might teach new parents about the color and consistency of stool to expect from their newborns, or they might help families cope with older parents in whom fecal incontinence has recently developed. Nurses who work in the community might develop an education program to alert workers to the symptoms of colorectal cancer. In acute care settings, nurses might assess the resumption of bowel motility during the postoperative period for clients who have had colon surgery; individualize bowel management programs for clients who have had strokes; and teach clients how to manage and adjust to a new colostomy.

NORMAL BOWEL FUNCTION

Structures of the Gastrointestinal Tract

Although the final formation of feces occurs in the large intestine (the lower portion of the gastrointestinal tract), the type and amount of food and fluids ingested have a definite effect on the amount and consistency of the waste produced. As food and fluids enter the mouth, the food is mixed with salivary enzymes, and the process of digestion begins (Fig. 41-1). The bolus of food is propelled to the pharynx, down the esophagus, and into the stomach, where secretions from the stomach further break down and digest the food.

From the stomach, the food enters the small intestine, which has three anatomic divisions: the duodenum, the jejunum, and the ileum. After about 3 to 10 hours, the contents leave the small intestine and enter the large intestine, which comprises the cecum, colon, rectum, and anus. Here, muscle fibers, both circular and longitudinal, permit circumferential and lengthwise changes in size and shape that promote intestinal motility.

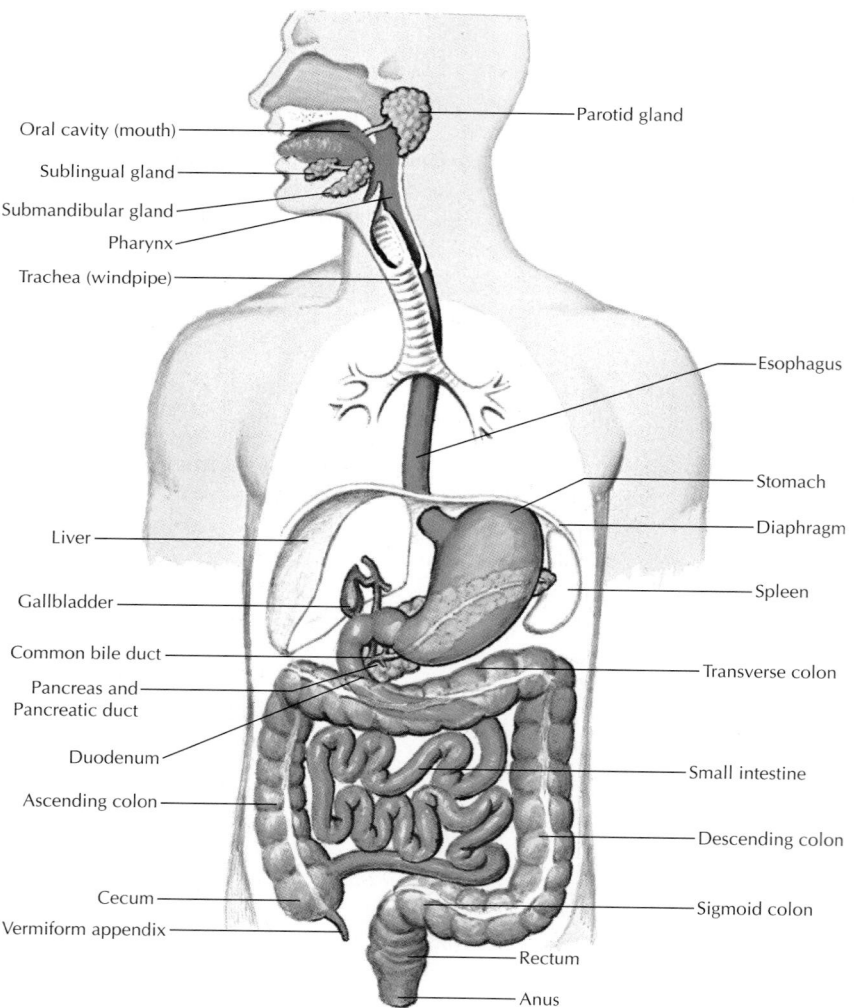

FIGURE 41-1   Anatomic structures of the gastrointestinal tract.

At the junction of the ileum and the cecum is the ileocecal valve, which serves (a) to retard movement of semidigested food into the large intestine, allowing more time for the small intestine to absorb nutrients, and (b) to prevent the backflow of fecal contents from the large intestine into the small intestine.

The colon, the major portion of the large intestine, has four parts: ascending, transverse, descending, and sigmoid colons (see Fig. 41-1). The rectum is the portion of the large intestine that immediately follows the sigmoid colon. The rectum, normally empty, is capable of considerable expansion to accommodate stool. The anus, the last portion of the large intestine, has two sphincters: the internal sphincter (smooth muscle that is under involuntary neural control) and the external sphincter (striated muscle under voluntary neural control). Both sphincters are normally in a contracted (closed) position.

Function of the Intestine

Motility

Two types of movements, segmentation and peristalsis, occur within the intestine and are responsible for assisting with absorption and transportation of waste products over the full length of the intestines. During segmentation, alternating contraction and relaxation of the intestinal smooth muscle occur. This type of movement slows the passage of intestinal contents to permit more complete digestion and absorption of nutrients.

The second type of movement, **peristalsis,** propels the intestinal contents along the entire length of the small and large intestines. The walls of the intestine reflexively induce peristalsis, but peristalsis is particularly stimulated when partially digested food enters the duodenum from the stomach. This duodenocolic reflex is especially strong when food or fluids enter the duodenum after several hours of not eating.

Autonomic nervous system input affects the rate of intestinal motility. Sympathetic stimulation slows down peristalsis and delays passage through the intestine, whereas parasympathetic stimulation increases bowel motility and emptying.

Absorption

Partially digested food (also known as chyme) empties from the stomach into the small intestine, where the digestive process is completed and the absorption of nutrients and fluids begins. Most nutrient and electrolyte absorption occurs in the duodenum and jejunum. Some vitamins, iron, and fluid are absorbed in the ileum.

Final absorption of nutrients, especially the absorption of fluid and electrolytes, occurs in the large intestine. The amount of absorption that occurs depends on the speed at which the intestinal contents move through the colon: The longer that intestinal contents remain in the colon, the greater the absorption of fluid and electrolytes. The intestinal contents that enter the ascending colon are liquid. When the contents leave the transverse colon, they are semisolid and mushy and can be called feces. Although the distal colon's principal function is storage of feces, some sodium, chloride, and water continue to be absorbed during storage.

Defecation

The process of defecation begins when peristalsis propels feces into the rectum and causes rectal distention. This rectal distention begins a series of smooth muscle responses that can trigger bowel evacuation. When stool distends the rectum, parasympathetic afferent nerve fibers in the sacral segment of the spinal cord are stimulated, causing contraction of the descending and sigmoid colon, rectum, and anus and relaxation of the internal anal sphincter. This stimulus–response sequence is a sacral reflex, not under voluntary control. It is called the **defecation reflex.**

Defecation will automatically follow unless the external anal sphincter (a striated muscle under voluntary control) remains contracted. In the presence of the defecation reflex, the external anal sphincter can remain contracted until the person decides that the time and place for defecation are appropriate. At that time, the person can voluntarily relax the external anal sphincter. Defecation is assisted by taking a deep breath against a closed glottis (to move the diaphragm down), contracting the abdominal muscles (to increase intra-abdominal pressure), and contracting the pelvic floor muscles (to push the feces downward). These actions are called the Valsalva maneuver.

Characteristics of Normal Feces

The feces consist of 75% water and 25% solids. The solids include bacteria, undigested fiber, fat, inorganic matter, and some protein. Cellulose is the major undigested fiber left in the feces after digestion and absorption have occurred. If dietary fiber intake is small, less stool is produced daily.

The normal color of feces is brown, resulting from the chemical conversion of bilirubin, an orange or dark yellow bile pigment, into urobilin and stercobilin (brown pigments) by intestinal bacteria and enzymes. The food ingested can affect the color (e.g., beets may give stool a reddish color). Ingestion of certain medications can also affect the stool's color and consistency.

The characteristic odor of feces comes from solids produced by bacterial decomposition of proteins in the intestine. The feces normally have a soft consistency and a cylindrical form that approximates the shape of the rectum. Between 150 and 300 g of feces is produced daily. Table 41-1 compares normal and abnormal feces.

Normal Bowel Pattern

The normal bowel elimination pattern is highly individualized. The frequency of defecation can normally range from one or two bowel movements per day to one bowel movement every 2 to 3 days.

Lifespan Considerations

Newborn and Infant

Newborns usually evacuate stool within 24 to 48 hours after birth. This stool, which is softly formed and dark greenish, is called **meconium.** Meconium is the partially dried intestinal

TABLE 41-1

Characteristics of Normal and Abnormal Feces		
Characteristic	Normal	Abnormal
Frequency	Variable Usual range: 1–2 per day to 1 every 2–3 days	Dependent on usual pattern Guideline: >3 per day; <1 every 3 days
Color	Brown	Black, tarry Reddish-brown, maroon Clay-colored Yellow-green
Consistency	Soft, formed	Hard Loose, liquid High mucus content
Shape	Cylindrical	Narrow, pencil-thin
Amount	100–300 g/day	<100 g/day >300 g/day
Odor	Aromatic; pungent	Foul, objectionable

secretions that accumulated in the large intestine before birth.

By about the third day after birth, the stool's characteristics begin to reflect the type of milk in the diet. If newborns are fed breast milk, the stools will be bright yellow, soft, and unformed with an unobjectionable odor. If newborns are fed formula, which is usually cow's milk, the stools will be dark yellow or tan, slightly more formed than the stools associated with breast milk, with a strong, somewhat objectionable odor. Because the digestive and absorptive capacities of the gastrointestinal system are not mature at birth, intestinal contents pass through the system more quickly than in older children and adults, producing less firm stool. Stools become firmer as the gastrointestinal system matures and as the infant ingests more solid foods.

Frequency of bowel elimination varies among newborns and infants, as it does in adults. They may pass stool with every feeding, just once a day, or even only once every 3 days. As infants become older, they may seem to have bowel movements in more regular or identifiable patterns. Infants cannot control bowel elimination until their central nervous systems become more mature.

Toddler and Preschooler

The duodenocolic reflex is strong in toddlers and preschoolers. Any ingestion of food may stimulate a bowel movement, and toddlers and preschoolers may normally have more than one bowel movement per day. Toddlers are curious about the products their bodies produce. It is not unusual that, at some time during toddlerhood, smearing or playing with feces will occur. In a matter-of-fact manner that does not threaten the child's self-esteem, parents and caregivers should let the toddler know that smearing feces is unacceptable. They should encourage play with alternative substances, such as modeling clay or finger paints.

Privacy for bowel movements is a value learned early in one's culture. Young toddlers who are not yet toilet trained will sense the urge to defecate and then may hurry to another room or hide behind a couch to squat down for a bowel movement. Older preschoolers who have mastered the voluntary control of bowel movements usually prefer the privacy of their own bathrooms at home, rather than public restrooms.

During toddlerhood, usually between 22 and 36 months, children are ready to learn voluntary control of bowel elimination. By this time, the central nervous system has matured enough to allow voluntary control. Myelinization of the sacral spinal cord segments, which control the anus, becomes complete between 12 and 18 months. When this occurs, toddlers can recognize that stool is present in the rectum. A good indicator of spinal cord maturation is the ability to walk independently.

Bowel training is easier when the number of daily bowel movements decreases to one or two. Successful bowel training usually does not occur before the age of 22 months. Until that age, a toddler's rectum and colon cannot hold large amounts of feces. Also, before that age, many toddlers do not have sufficient vocabulary to communicate the need to defecate and would not remember to do so before actually defecating. Children are seldom ready for bowel training until they can sense rectal distention, are able and willing momentarily to defer defecation, and can communicate the need to defecate. In the U.S. culture, most parents believe that children are emotionally, socially, and physically mature enough to begin toilet training for bowel movements somewhere between the age of 22 and 36 months. Most children attain bowel control before 4 years of age. They usually achieve bowel control before bladder control.

School-Age Child and Adolescent

School-age children are bowel trained and are approaching the bowel elimination habits of adults. Stools are brown and softly formed. Consistency and frequency of bowel movements depend on intake of sufficient fluids and dietary fiber and the amount of daily exercise. School-age children and adolescents may choose to defer defecation until they are in the privacy of their own bathrooms at home. Often, children delay elimination because they are enjoying an activity such as playing with friends. Continuous practice of this habit puts children at risk for decreased bowel responsiveness to rectal distention and may contribute to constipation.

Adult and Older Adult

By the time individuals reach adulthood, they have developed bowel elimination patterns that are normal or typical. Because gastrointestinal motility slows with aging, frequency of bowel movements commonly decreases. Older adults need to increase the amount of fluids and high-fiber foods in the diet to prevent the formation of a harder stool. Weakened pelvic muscles and decreased activity level also contribute to constipation in older adults.

Because of physiologic changes that occur in the gastrointestinal tract with aging, older adults are at risk for thinking they are constipated when, in fact, they are experiencing symptoms associated with normal aging. More research is needed to document specific changes in gut transit times and to distinguish between an actual increase in constipation among the elderly versus an increase in perceived constipation (Abyad & Mourad, 1996).

Some people have a strong belief that a daily bowel movement is essential to health. Therefore, when normal age-related bowel changes occur, older persons may resort to a laxative to restore the "normal" daily pattern of bowel evacuation. Unfortunately, this type of laxative abuse is common among older adults. Educating older persons to recognize that decreased frequency of bowel movements is usually a normal result of aging and encouraging a change in dietary habits and an increase in activity to prevent a change in stool consistency are important. With aging, the strength of the striated external sphincter muscles decreases, leading to decreased sphincter control, which increases the possibility of fecal incontinence.

FACTORS AFFECTING BOWEL ELIMINATION

Nutrition

The 25% of feces that is solid comes chiefly from the intake of food that has a high cellulose or fiber content. Cellulose or fiber is contained in plant foods. Foods in the high-fiber category include fresh fruits and vegetables with the skins and intact outer coverings and cereal grains with the outer covering of bran in place. A person who consumes approximately 20 to 30 g of dietary fiber from fruits, vegetables, and grains will most likely have sufficient bulk in the stools to allow for easy defecation (Hinrichs & Huseboe, 2001).

A person whose diet is deficient in fiber usually has less frequent bowel movements and stools with less bulk and may experience some difficulty in bowel elimination. On the other hand, ingestion of large amounts of certain foods, such as fresh fruits, may produce loose stools.

Food intolerances also may alter bowel function. Many people have difficulty digesting lactose (the sugar contained in milk products). The breakdown of lactose into its component sugars, glucose and galactose, requires a sufficient quantity of the enzyme lactase in the small intestine. If a person is lactase-deficient, alterations of bowel elimination, including the formation of gas, abdominal cramping, and diarrhea, can occur after ingestion of milk products.

Some people cannot digest gluten, a protein found in wheat, rye, barley, and buckwheat. For these people, ingestion of gluten-containing food results in the retention of carbohydrates and fats, which cannot be digested and absorbed through the intestine. The person experiences abdominal distention and a bloated feeling, along with a diarrhea of bulky, greasy stools.

Fluid Intake

Because 75% of the feces is water, fluid intake also has a great deal of influence on stool consistency. The need of body cells for water is a higher priority than stool consistency. When the body needs to conserve fluid, it will absorb more water from the large intestine to meet its needs.

A fluid intake of approximately 2000 mL/day is necessary to meet cellular needs and have enough left over to promote a soft stool consistency. Clients should exclude fluids that cause diuresis (e.g., coffee, tea, soft drinks, beer) from the 2000-mL goal, because these fluids do not help hydration (Hinrichs & Huseboe, 2001). When a person loses excessive water, such as from a high fever, profuse diaphoresis, or other abnormal drainage, the usual fluid intake may be insufficient. When fluid intake is inadequate, stools become harder and more difficult to pass.

Storage time in the large intestine also affects stool consistency. The longer feces remain in the large intestine, the more water will be absorbed; the result is a harder, drier stool. Conversely, feces that do not spend sufficient time in the large intestine will be watery and a source of fluid loss for the person.

Activity and Exercise

Physical activity and regular physical exercise promote muscle tone and facilitate peristalsis. Strong abdominal and perineal muscles are needed to increase intra-abdominal pressure during defecation. Muscle tone is lost when activity decreases or neurologic impairment results in loss of neurologic control. Any limitation of normal or usual physical activity can increase the risk of constipation.

Body Position

A sitting or semisquatting position is the most advantageous position for defecation. This position allows gravity to assist the elimination of feces and also makes it easier for the client to contract the abdominal and pelvic muscles, thereby applying external pressure to the large intestine and encouraging evacuation. Some people find it very difficult to defecate using a bedpan in a reclined position.

Ignoring the Urge to Defecate

Most people require a certain degree of privacy to feel psychologically comfortable defecating. Although part of the defecation reflex is involuntary, the external anal sphincter is under voluntary control, allowing one to ignore the urge to defecate until the time and place for defecation are appropriate.

The defecation reflex and the urge to defecate subside after a few minutes if the initial urge is ignored. The feces then remain in the rectum until another mass colonic movement propels more stool into the rectum, which may not be for several hours or longer. While the feces remain in the colon and rectum, the intestinal mucosa continue to absorb water from the feces, resulting in a harder and drier stool that may be more difficult to evacuate. Eventually, if the person continually denies the defecation reflex, recognition of the urge to defecate becomes more difficult and the defecation reflex weakens and subsides. Rather than relying on inherent body signals to initiate defecation, a person in this situation may have to depend on alternative methods, such as the persistent use of laxatives or enemas or manual disimpaction of stool.

People who experience pain during defecation may choose to deny the urge to defecate, which can lead to constipation. People at risk for delaying defecation because of pain include those with chronic constipation and those with rectal or anal abnormalities, such as hemorrhoids or fissures. Hemorrhoids are enlarged or varicose veins in the anal canal (Fig. 41-2).

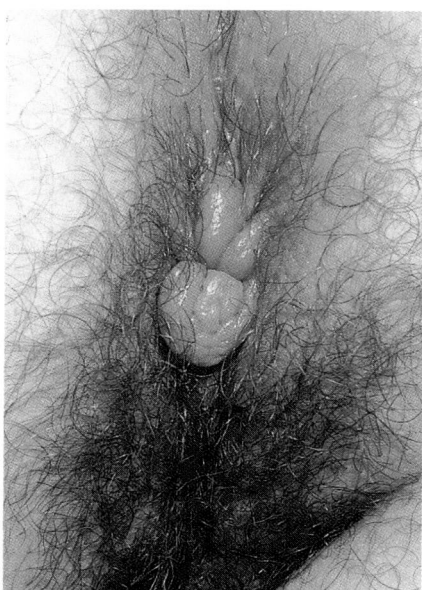

FIGURE 41-2   Hemorrhoids. An external hemorrhoid that has become thrombosed. It contains clotted blood, is very painful and swollen, and itches and bleeds with bowel movements. (Courtesy of Dr. P. Marazzi/Science Photo Library/CMSP.)

Pain and rectal bleeding are sometimes associated with hemorrhoids, and these may lead to frequent denial of the defecation reflex to avoid pain. An anal fissure is an ulcerous crack or split in the anal mucosa. Bleeding and pain occur as the stool passes the fissure. In addition, clients may delay defecation after anal or perineal surgery because of the pain.

Lifestyle

Many people develop a pattern with respect to the timing of bowel elimination. For some people, ingestion of food or fluid first thing in the morning stimulates an urge to defecate. Over time, a pattern of bowel elimination every morning can be established and is considered a normal pattern for that person. Some people are ritualistic, using the same method to promote a regular pattern of bowel elimination, whereas others have no set pattern except to respond to the defecation urge whenever it occurs.

Alterations in a person's lifestyle or pattern of daily living can have an effect on bowel elimination. Vacations and travel often change daily routine enough to cause alterations in bowel elimination. Lifestyle changes that cause either acute or chronic feelings of anxiety, anger, fear, depression, excitement, or other strong emotions can lead to an altered bowel elimination pattern. Any acute stress or change in a person's lifestyle can increase bowel motility and mucus secretion. The result may be a sudden increase in frequency of bowel movements, with the stool containing large amounts of mucus. Hospitalization, a career change, a disruption in personal or family relationships, and anticipation of final examinations are just a few examples of situations that can stimulate acute stress. Chronic exposure to stress can slow bowel activity, resulting in decreased frequency of bowel movements. Long-term depression is an example of a chronic stressor that may slow bowel activity.

Pregnancy

Constipation frequently occurs during pregnancy because hormonal changes relax muscles of the gastrointestinal tract (Murray, 2002). Also, the growing fetus puts pressure on the intestines, possibly affecting normal bowel function. In addition, most pregnant women take iron supplements, which are very constipating.

Medications

Side effects of many medications can increase a person's risk for bowel elimination problems. For example, narcotics and iron preparations can cause constipation, antibiotics can cause diarrhea, and antacids can lead to either constipation or diarrhea. Laxatives, stool softeners, and enemas are medications that are administered to promote stool evacuation. Antidiarrheal medications may be given to decrease stool frequency.

Diagnostic Procedures

Some radiologic and endoscopic procedures require cleansing fecal material from the large bowel before the procedure. The thorough cleansing of the large bowel alters the normal pattern of elimination for 2 or 3 days after the test. When the person resumes his or her usual diet, the normal bowel elimination pattern usually reemerges.

Bowel elimination also may be affected after a diagnostic test. For example, if barium is administered as a test agent, the stools after the procedure will appear chalky white or tan until all of the barium has been eliminated from the gastrointestinal tract. If barium remains in the colon, it hardens and can cause impaction of stool. Therefore, laxatives are commonly ordered after the diagnostic test to facilitate barium removal.

Surgery

Surgical intervention can place the client at risk for altered patterns of bowel elimination. General anesthetics may slow gastrointestinal motility, causing the surgical client to experience a period of decreased bowel functioning for 1 to 2 days postoperatively.

Clients who have had abdominal surgery, especially surgery on a portion of the gastrointestinal tract, will require 3 or 4 days for bowel activity to return to normal. These clients are usually given preoperative laxatives or enemas to cleanse the large intestine of feces. During surgery, the bowel is exposed to air and manipulation, leading to further decreased bowel motility.

Postoperative use of narcotic analgesics, reduced activity, and fear of pain further inhibit normal bowel motility. Postoperative clients are not allowed food and fluids orally until there is evidence of the return of active bowel motility.

Fecal Diversion

The presence of all or part of the large intestine is not necessary to maintain life. In some clients, cancer or other conditions, such as inflammatory bowel disease, necessitate surgical removal of all or part of the colon, rectum, and anus. In such

cases, the proximal portion of the remaining bowel may be redirected through the abdominal wall to the abdominal skin surface. The portion of intestine brought through the abdominal wall is known as a **stoma.** When this surgery is performed, it is referred to as a fecal diversion, because the normal route for feces is altered.

Fecal diversions can be permanent or temporary. The bowel segment used to form the stoma depends on the location of the bowel abnormality. For example, if the person has rectal cancer, the segment of bowel removed will be the cancerous rectum. The healthy, noncancerous sigmoid colon, which is the segment of the bowel just proximal to the rectum, can be used to form the stoma. A bowel diversion surgery that brings a segment of the large colon out to the abdominal skin is called a **colostomy.** It is also possible that the entire length of the large colon is so diseased that the next healthy proximal segment of intestine is the ileum. When a portion of the ileum is used to make the stoma on the abdomen, the procedure is called an **ileostomy.** Figure 41-3 illustrates fecal diversions.

People with colostomies or ileostomies evacuate feces through a stoma. The consistency of the stool is affected by the length of functioning intestine that remains after the surgery. When an ileostomy is created, the large intestine is no longer available to absorb water from the stool. Therefore, stool produced from an ileostomy is liquid and contains large quantities of electrolytes. In a person with a descending colostomy, in which only the rectum has been removed, stool is soft in consistency, and elimination may be controlled with daily colostomy irrigations. This may permit a pattern of bowel evacuation similar to that experienced before surgery.

Continent Fecal Diversions

Modern surgical methods aim for as little disruption of normal bowel patterns as possible despite fecal diversion. The ileoanal reservoir, sometimes referred to as a J pouch, involves construction of an internal pouch by removal of the colon and attachment of a limb of the ileum to the anus. Fecal material goes directly from the small intestine out the anus. A Kock pouch or continent ileostomy is another development in fecal diversions. A pouch is made from 30 cm of ileum and

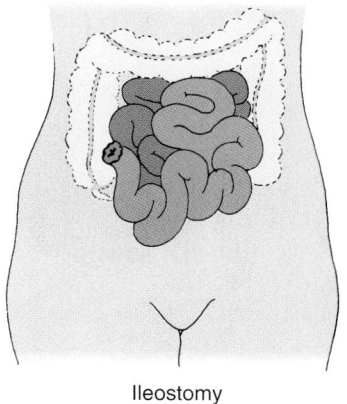
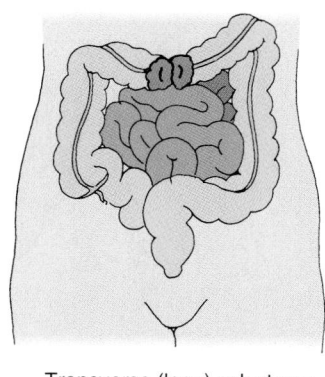
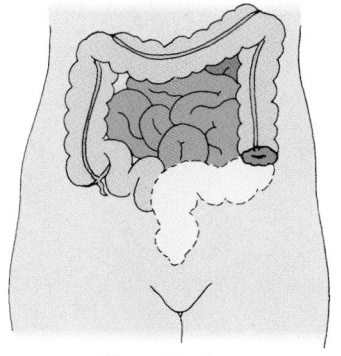

Ileostomy   Transverse (loop) colostomy   Sigmoid colostomy

FIGURE 41-3 Intestinal diversions: Ileostomy, transverse colostomy, and sigmoid colostomy.

an outlet valve is constructed. Although this procedure requires a stoma, feces can be drained at the client's convenience rather than having it continually draining into an external pouch, as occurs in the traditional ileostomy. Figure 41-4 illustrates one type of continent ostomy.

ALTERED BOWEL FUNCTION

Manifestations of Altered Bowel Function

Constipation

Constipation is the infrequent, sometimes painful passage of hard, dry stool. It occurs when stool moves through the large intestine too slowly or remains in the large intestine too long. Constipation is defined in relation to the person's normal defecation pattern and involves a change in stool consistency (harder and drier than usual) and a change in defecation frequency (less often than usual). Look for the following contributory factors:

- Inadequate dietary fiber intake
- Large intake of refined foods or other low-residue foods
- Diet low in natural fiber
- Fluid intake less than 1500 mL/day
- Consistent delay of bowel evacuation (e.g., lack of access to facilities, unreasonable privacy requirements, unwillingness to interrupt other activities, embarrassment about using a bedpan)
- Decreased physical activity
- Chronic stress
- Continual use of laxatives
- Medications used for other purposes with possible side effects that decrease gastrointestinal activity
- Slower motility of the gastrointestinal tract associated with aging

Fecal Impaction

A fecal **impaction** is the accumulation of hardened feces in the rectum. The word "impaction" implies that the stool is lodged or stuck in the rectum; the person is unable to voluntarily evacuate the stool. A fecal impaction is usually the result of untreated and unrelieved constipation.

Suspect fecal impaction when there is a history of absence of a regular bowel movement for several days (3 to 5 days or more), followed by the passage of liquid or semiliquid stool. The person is typically incontinent of the liquid stool, complaining of an inability to perceive urge. The passage of liquid stool usually does not relieve the reported rectal and abdominal fullness. The passage of semiliquid stool results from seepage of unformed fecal contents around the impacted stool in the rectum; the pressure from the large volume of accumulated fecal contents forces liquid feces to the anus (Fig. 41-5). This liquid or semiliquid stool is not diarrhea but is sometimes confused with it. Fecal impaction is confirmed by the detection of hardened stool in the rectum on digital examination.

Symptoms similar to those experienced with constipation are also present—a subjective feeling of rectal and abdominal fullness or bloating, an urge to defecate but an inability to pass stool, and a generalized feeling of malaise. Loss of appetite and nausea or vomiting are typical as well. Abdominal distention is usually apparent.

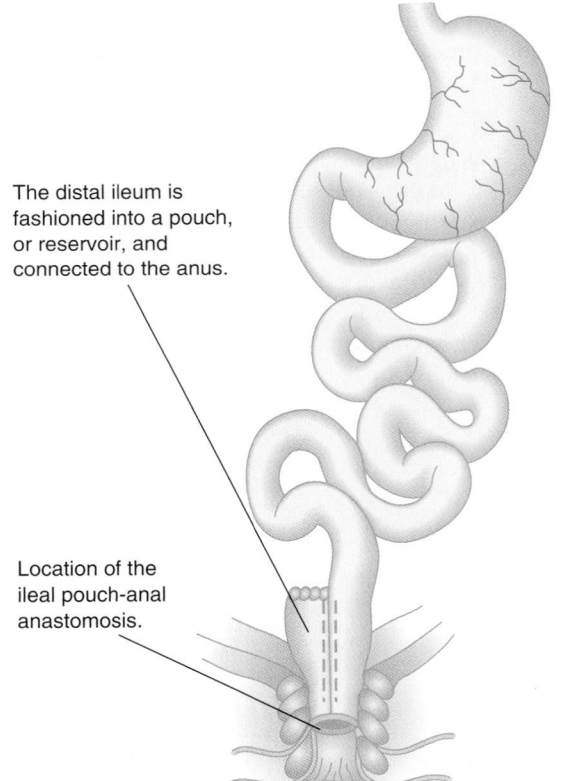

The distal ileum is fashioned into a pouch, or reservoir, and connected to the anus.

Location of the ileal pouch-anal anastomosis.

FIGURE 41-4 Ileoanal reservoir. The distal ileum is fashioned into a pouch and connected to the anus to create a continent fecal diversion.

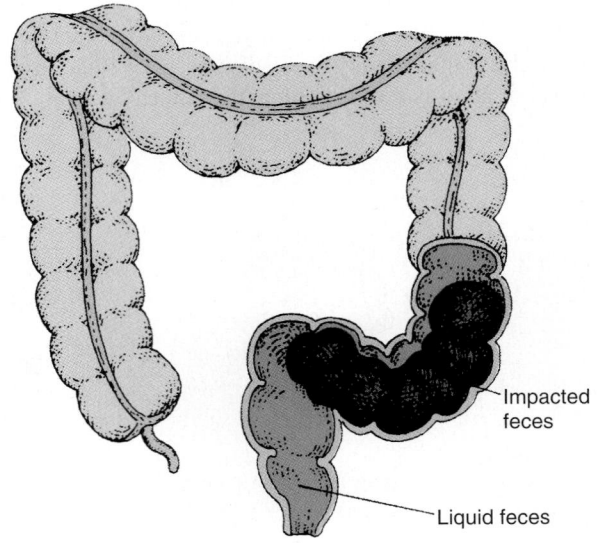

Impacted feces

Liquid feces

FIGURE 41-5 Fecal impaction in the sigmoid colon. Liquid stool may pass around hard fecal plug.

Fecal impaction usually results from the same conditions as those associated with constipation. Fecal impaction also may result from the hardening of barium used in radiologic examination of the gastrointestinal tract. Clients who have swallowed barium or have received a barium enema should be monitored for complete evacuation of barium after the radiologic procedure. Some healthcare protocols require use of laxatives for 1 or 2 days after the procedure to ensure complete evacuation of the barium.

People with fecal impactions need medications or special treatments to remove the impacted stool. Laxatives, enemas, and manual removal of the stool are possible measures.

Diarrhea

Diarrhea is manifested by frequent evacuation of watery stools. Diarrhea is usually associated with increased gastrointestinal motility and, therefore, a rapid passage of fecal contents through the lower gastrointestinal tract. It is the consistency of the stool (less formed and more watery than normal) that is more definitive of diarrhea than the increased frequency of defecation. In addition to having a high water content, diarrheal stools may also have increased mucus; both of these factors contribute to increased volume. The extra volume and the rapidity with which it reaches the rectum cause rectal distention, resulting in an intense urge to defecate. Diarrheal stools may vary in color from light brown to yellow to green.

Diarrhea is often accompanied by abdominal cramping, an intense urge to evacuate fecal contents, nausea (with or without vomiting), and a painful burning sensation at the anus. Diarrheal stool is usually highly acidic. Frequent passage of acidic stools can cause anal soreness and inflammation of the skin surrounding the anus, resulting in bleeding and breakdown of the perianal tissue.

The causes of diarrhea are many and varied. Any disease that inflames the intestinal tract can lead to diarrhea. Specific microorganisms or the toxins they produce can cause intestinal inflammation and diarrhea. The inflammation irritates the intestinal mucosa to increase its secretions and motility.

Medications, such as the overuse of laxatives, can cause diarrhea. Antacids taken to decrease stomach acidity, especially those containing magnesium, also can lead to diarrhea. Antibiotics can promote diarrhea by irritating the gastrointestinal mucosa or by inhibiting the growth of normal intestinal flora. Normal intestinal flora inhibit the growth of *Clostridium difficile*. When broad-spectrum antibiotics are administered and normal flora is altered, *C. difficile* can proliferate and release toxins that cause antibiotic-associated diarrhea (Bliss, Johnson, Savik, Clabots, & Gerding, 2000).

Lifestyle changes causing acute stress and anxiety can result in episodes of diarrhea. Acute stress may increase stimulation of the large intestine, increasing the transit time of the feces through the intestines.

While traveling, some people experience diarrhea after ingesting food or water from an unfamiliar locale. Often, a waterborne foreign strain of *Escherichia coli* causes the intestinal inflammation and consequent symptoms known as traveler's diarrhea.

Additional diarrheal responses may be precipitated by lactase deficiency, gluten intolerance, or a specific food allergy. For example, apple juice can cause chronic diarrhea in some children. The hyperosmolality of parenteral tube feedings may precipitate a diarrheal response.

Fecal Incontinence

Fecal incontinence is the involuntary elimination of bowel contents; it is often associated with neurologic, mental, or emotional impairments. Clients with injury to the cerebral cortex may have difficulty perceiving a distended rectum or initiating the motor responses required to inhibit defecation voluntarily. People who have sustained sacral spinal cord injury or who have neurologic diseases that impair the nerve supply to the rectum and anal sphincters (e.g., multiple sclerosis) also may be unable to inhibit voluntary anal sphincters to postpone defecation.

Clients who are disoriented or confused may have lost the social inhibition that prevents immediate fecal evacuation. In the absence of voluntary contraction of the external anal sphincter, the immediate evacuation of the rectum follows rectal distention.

Diarrhea predisposes a person to fecal incontinence. Sometimes, the volume of feces is so large and the defecation urge so intense that the person cannot maintain sphincter contraction long enough to access toilet facilities and remove the necessary clothing.

Flatulence

Flatus is the accumulation of gas in the gastrointestinal tract. Gas enters the gastrointestinal tract from three sources: swallowed air, bacterial action in the large intestine, and diffusion from the blood.

Excessive swallowing of air sometimes occurs with anxiety, rapid food or fluid ingestion, improper use of drinking straws, ingestion of large amounts of carbonated beverages, gum chewing, candy sucking, and smoking. Swallowed air is usually eliminated by burping or belching.

Gases produced by bacterial activity in the large intestine are eliminated through the anus. When larger than usual quantities of flatus are expelled, it is most often a result of increased colonic motility secondary to intestinal irritation. The colonic activity propels the gases toward the anus before they have time to be absorbed by the intestinal mucosa.

Certain foods (e.g., cabbage, onions, legumes) often increase the amount of flatus produced in the intestine. Many other high-fiber foods that are recommended to promote normal bowel elimination can cause excess flatus production when they are not introduced into the diet gradually.

Distention

An accumulation of excessive amounts of flatus or liquid or solid intestinal contents causes abdominal **distention.** Subjectively, the person complains of abdominal fullness and discomfort and the inability to pass flatus or stool. Visual inspection of the abdomen reveals a distended or a convexly stretched abdomen. Depending on the amount of flatus and feces in the intestines, the abdomen can appear only slightly distended or taut and stretched.

An obstruction that blocks the passage of flatus and intestinal chyme or feces is a primary cause of abdominal distention. Paralytic ileus and abdominal tumors are types of bowel obstruction that produce distention. Long periods of bed rest or relative inactivity can slow peristalsis and lead to accumulated flatus in the large intestine. Peristalsis also slows after surgery with general anesthesia. In particular, surgery involving bowel manipulation, especially bowel surgery, causes decreased peristalsis postoperatively, with abdominal distention as a possible consequence. Constipation and fecal impaction also may lead to abdominal distention.

Impact on Activities of Daily Living

Energy is required for normal daily tasks such as hygiene, grooming, feeding, and managing home and work activities. Available energy for activities of daily living decreases when a person has an acute or chronic bowel problem. Blood loss associated with frequent diarrhea can further deplete energy levels. Interference with restful sleep, such as with frequent night wakings or pain and discomfort, also can contribute to exhaustion.

Nutritional status is affected by altered bowel function. For example, constipation causes bloating, which decreases ap-petite. Diarrhea often necessitates resting the gastrointestinal tract by eliminating all oral intake or limiting intake to clear fluids. In addition, the person with altered bowel function may be unable or unwilling to shop for or prepare food.

Altered bowel function can potentially alter social relationships. For some, the fear of sudden episodes of loose stool necessitates staying close to bathroom facilities, calling in sick to work, or avoiding social obligations outside the home. For others, related hospitalizations and decreased work efficiency can cause financial strain and family stress.

Alteration in bowel function can affect sexual function. The fear of loose stool or flatus during sexual activity can cause anxiety and decrease sexual spontaneity. The changes caused by ostomy surgery require adjustment by both partners. Decreased energy reserves related to bowel dysfunction can also negatively affect sexual function.

ASSESSMENT

Asking questions about a person's bowel habits is potentially an embarrassing situation for the client and the beginning nursing student. Bowel elimination is considered a private function. For optimal care, obtain factual information both from the client's perspective and through direct observation. Use of a matter-of-fact approach often eases the client's embarrassment.

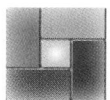

Nursing Research and Critical Thinking
Does a Relationship Exist Between Psychological Distress and Gastrointestinal Symptoms in Women With Irritable Bowel Syndrome?

Nurses working with women with irritable bowel syndrome (IBS) are aware that people with IBS have been reported to experience significantly more symptoms compatible with psychopathologic disorders, abnormal personality traits, and psychological distress. It has also been reported that people with psychiatric disorders, such as panic and anxiety disorders, report higher levels of gastrointestinal (GI) symptoms compatible with IBS. Nurse researchers designed a study to examine psychological distress in women with IBS, women with similar GI symptoms but not diagnosed with IBS (IBS-NP), and a control group of asymptomatic women. The women ($N = 97$) were interviewed, completed questionnaires, and maintained daily diaries for 2 months. Across-women and within-woman analyses were used to calculate the results of the study. The IBS and IBS-NP groups had a significantly higher percentage of lifetime psychopathology ($P < .03$) and recalled psychological distress ($P < .001$). At least 40% of the women in the IBS and IBS-NP groups had positive relationships between daily psychological distress and daily GI symptoms.

The researchers concluded that psychological distress is an important component of the IBS symptom experience and should be considered when designing treatment strategies.

Critical Thinking Considerations. The original sample for this study was 124. Twenty-six women discontinued participation in the study after the initial interview, and two women were excluded from the study because of prolonged menstrual cycles. Evaluation of the demographic characteristics of those that did not complete the study showed that they did not differ from the group that completed the study. Implications applicable to nursing practice are as follows:

• This study cannot answer the question of whether psychological distress precipitated the GI symptoms or the opposite relationship exists.
• Psychological distress should be assessed as a contributing factor in both the onset and exacerbation of GI symptoms when assessing clients with IBS and in designing treatment strategies for them.

From Jarrett, M., Heitkemper, M., Cain, K. C., Tuftin, M., Walker, E. A., Bond, E. F., & Levy, R. L. (1998). The relationship between psychological distress and gastrointestinal symptoms in women with irritable bowel syndrome. *Nursing Research, 47*(3), 154–161.

Subjective Data

Normal Pattern Identification

To determine the client's current bowel elimination pattern, obtain the following information from current medical records, the client, or significant others:

- What is the client's usual pattern of bowel elimination?
- What are the usual characteristics of the client's stool?
- Which aids, if any, does the client routinely use for defecation?
- When was the client's last bowel movement?
- What are any recent changes in the client's normal bowel pattern?

Risk Identification

Areas of risk to assess include dietary factors, such as adequacy of fiber and fluid intake; ignoring the urge to defecate; factors or conditions that may alter the client's mobility pattern; diagnostic procedures, especially those involving the use of radiographic contrast material such as barium; surgical procedures; fear of pain on defecation; and lifestyle changes.

A client needs good teeth to chew high-fiber foods such as fresh fruits and vegetables. Poor dentition with concomitant chewing difficulty may lead to an insufficient intake of such foods and place the client at risk for constipation.

Dysfunction Identification

Assessing a client's beliefs about "normal" bowel function is necessary to determine the existence of a problem. Some people believe that a normal pattern is a bowel movement every day; they may further believe that a laxative or enema is necessary to correct any deviations from this pattern. People's concept of whether they have a bowel elimination problem usually depends on their beliefs about "normal" bowel elimination and whether their current pattern fits these beliefs. Many clients claim to be constipated despite having a daily bowel movement (Abyad & Mourad, 1996). Although a client may believe he or she has an altered bowel elimination pattern, analysis of the data may differ. Understanding the client's beliefs about normal bowel patterns helps direct subsequent nursing interventions.

Bowel problems can be identified as significant deviations from the client's normal pattern or a pattern that is outside the standards for bowel function. For instance, if a person usually has a bowel movement each day and states the absence of stool for the last 3 days, the nurse may identify constipation as a bowel problem. Also, a bowel problem may be identified if a client states he or she normally has a bowel movement every 3 weeks, because this does not fall within the range of normal bowel function.

Objective Data

Physical Assessment

Visual inspection of the feces and physical assessment of the abdomen and perirectal area provide objective data on the client's bowel elimination status. Inspection, auscultation, percussion, palpation, and measurement of abdominal girth are used. Table 41-2 compares normal and abnormal findings on physical examination of the abdomen and perirectal area.

TABLE 41-2

Normal and Abnormal Findings on Physical Examination of the Abdomen and Perirectal Area		
Examination	**Normal**	**Abnormal**
Abdomen		
Inspection		
Contour	Convex or flat	Hollow or scaphoid; distended
Symmetry	Symmetric	Asymmetric
Auscultation	Bowel sounds in all quadrants every 5–15 sec	Bowel sounds absent in all quadrants
		Hypoactive bowel sounds—every 15–30 sec
		Hyperactive bowel sounds—continuous or more than every 5 sec
		Absent bowel sounds—no sounds in 1–2 min
Percussion	Hollow, tympany in LUQ (stomach)	Dull, tympany in quadrants other than LUQ
Palpation	Soft	Firm distention
		Presence of mass
Perirectal		
Inspection	Intact, nonreddened skin	Excoriated, reddened skin
		Hemorrhoids
		Bleeding
Palpation	No stool or only soft, brown stool present in rectum	Presence of hard stool
		Bleeding

LUQ, left upper quadrant.

Inspection. The abdominal examination begins with inspection. Observe the abdomen for contour and symmetry. Normally, the abdomen is convex (i.e., slightly rounded). It may be flat in a muscular or athletic person. An abdomen that appears hollow or scaphoid is not normal and may be associated with malnutrition. An abdomen that appears more than slightly rounded is called protuberant or distended; an abdomen may be protuberant because of excess subcutaneous fat, pregnancy, or accumulated fluid or gas. Note any signs of obvious asymmetry, comparing the contour of the right side of the abdomen with that of the left side, and the upper quadrants with the lower quadrants. The normal abdomen shows no obvious asymmetry.

Auscultation. Auscultation of the abdomen must be performed before percussion or palpation. Percussion or palpation of the abdomen may stimulate intestinal activity and therefore change the quality or frequency of bowel sounds. If the client has a nasogastric or intestinal tube connected to suction, shut off the suction temporarily so that the sound of suction is not misinterpreted as bowel sounds. Bowel sounds, which are a result of peristalsis throughout the intestine, are heard through the stethoscope as a bubbling or gurgling noise. Everyone has heard his or her stomach "growl" without the benefit of a stethoscope. These loud bowel sounds are termed **borborygmi.** Bowel sounds heard through the stethoscope sound similar, only quieter.

Place the diaphragm of the stethoscope on the client's abdomen, starting at the right lower quadrant, because bowel sounds are heard best at the ileocecal junction (Jarvis, 2000). If the client complains of pain in the abdomen, auscultate that quadrant last. Normally, bowel sounds are heard in each of the quadrants within 5 to 15 seconds after the diaphragm is placed on the abdomen; infrequent bowel sounds suggest decreased gastrointestinal peristalsis and motility. Hypoactive bowel sounds in a client previously without bowel sounds suggest the return of intestinal peristalsis.

An absence of bowel sounds means that the nurse has listened in each of the four quadrants for at least 1 to 2 minutes and heard no bowel sounds; it is the rare clinical nurse who has the time to listen to a client's abdomen for 8 minutes. Clinically, most nurses define absent bowel sounds as no sounds heard within 30 seconds for each quadrant; this requires auscultation for only 2 minutes to document absent bowel sounds. A client who has undergone abdominal surgery may have hypoactive or absent bowel sounds for 1 to 3 days postoperatively. Bowel sounds should gradually resume, indicating that normal peristalsis has begun. A continued absence of bowel sounds beyond 72 hours may signal **paralytic ileus,** a condition in which the bowel is temporarily paralyzed and distention occurs.

Abnormal bowel sounds also include hyperactive sounds. Continuous bowel sounds or sounds heard more frequently than every 5 seconds can be termed *hyperactive.* Clients with diarrhea usually have hyperactive, high-pitched bowel sounds, indicating hypermotility in the intestines. A client with a bowel obstruction may have a combination of hypoactive and hyperactive bowel sounds, with hypoactive sounds below the level of the obstruction and hyperactive sounds above that level.

Percussion. Percussion is used to identify air, fluid, or solid masses in the abdomen, usually when an abnormality has been identified during inspection or auscultation. Begin percussion in the quadrant that was first auscultated. It is normal to hear a high-pitched, hollow sound, called tympany, over the left upper quadrant (LUQ). The stomach is in the LUQ and contains more air than the small or large intestine. The normal percussion sound heard in the other three quadrants is a hollow sound that is not quite as high-pitched as tympany, reflecting a mixture of air and fluid in the intestines. When an abdomen is abnormally distended with air (or gas), tympanic percussion notes may be heard throughout the abdomen. When an abdomen contains an excess fluid accumulation, duller, lower-pitched sounds are heard over the fluid-filled areas. A mass or feces in the large intestine produces a dull sound.

Palpation. Palpation is the last physical assessment technique used in examining the abdomen. If the history indicates problems in bowel elimination, or if abnormal findings have been observed during inspection, auscultation, or percussion, the nurse may wish to use light palpation. In light palpation, the examiner uses the warmed fingertips of one hand to press on the abdomen firmly yet gently enough to prevent causing discomfort. Palpate all quadrants of the abdomen in a systematic manner, saving the area that is thought to contain abnormalities for last (Jarvis, 2000). Instructing the client to flex the knees during this part of the examination often helps the client to relax abdominal muscles, resulting in less discomfort. From light palpation, the nurse can determine the firmness or softness of the abdominal muscles, the relative degree of abdominal distention, and possibly abdominal masses.

A special method called deep palpation is also part of the abdominal physical examination. During deep palpation, the examiner uses both hands and special techniques to assess deep abdominal masses and specific abdominal organs such as the liver and spleen. It is recommended that beginning nursing students not perform deep palpation independently. If possible, they should take the opportunity to observe the technique performed by a more experienced practitioner.

Measurement of Abdominal Girth. An assessment technique that nurses can perform independently is the measurement of abdominal girth. A plastic tape measure marked in inches or centimeters is wrapped around the client's abdomen and the measurement is taken. Comparison of abdominal girth measurements over time is an objective way of determining whether abdominal distention is increasing, decreasing, or remaining unchanged. For the comparison of abdominal girth measurements to be valid, measure the same abdominal circumference each time. Mark an "X" with a marking pen on the client's abdomen at the point of greatest distention, ensuring that any subsequent measurement will be made from the same location.

Perirectal Examination. Examination of the perirectal area completes the physical assessment. Place the client in a side-lying position with one or both knees flexed forward. Gather disposable examination gloves and a packet of water-soluble lubricant. On inspection, perianal skin should appear intact.

Abnormal inspection findings include any of the following:

- Excoriation (red, bleeding, tender skin), often caused by the frequent evacuation of diarrheal stools
- Hemorrhoids, possibly resulting from the evacuation of hard, constipated stools over time
- Bleeding, such as from recent evacuation of a constipated stool past hemorrhoids

Palpation of the rectal area is next. To perform a digital examination of the rectum, separate the client's buttocks and insert the lubricated index finger of a gloved hand into the client's anus and rectum. Direct the finger toward the client's umbilicus, feeling the sides of the rectal wall and for stool in the rectum at the tip of the finger. If any stool is felt, determine whether it is hard or soft. To help the client relax the anal sphincter, employ distraction by directing the client to inhale deeply at insertion and then to exhale while the rectum is quickly assessed.

Sometimes, as the nurse's finger enters the rectum, the client may exhibit a temporary loss of sphincter control and involuntarily release stool from the rectum. This is especially true for weak clients, older clients, and infants and small children. For these clients, place a disposable pad under the client's buttocks before performing the digital examination. Normally, no hard stool is present in the rectum.

Diagnostic Tests and Procedures

Two laboratory tests are commonly performed on stool specimens for diagnostic purposes: the guaiac, or Hemoccult, test and the stool culture. Other diagnostic procedures include radiologic examinations and endoscopic examinations.

Collecting Stool Specimens. Regardless of who tests a stool specimen, it is commonly the nurse's responsibility to collect it. First, explain to the client the need for a stool sample. If the client can walk to the bathroom, place a container (hat) used for obtaining specimens in the toilet. If the client cannot ambulate to the bathroom, ensure that a bedpan or bedside commode is readily available in the client's room. When obtaining a specimen for stool culture, inform the client that it is best if urine is not mixed with the stool in the bedpan. The male client can easily use a urinal to prevent this from occurring, but it is more difficult for the female client. Having two bedpans ready in the room, one to be used for urine and the second to be used for the stool specimen, may be necessary.

Hemoccult Test. "Heme" refers to blood, and "occult" means hidden or not visible on inspection. The test for hidden blood in the stool is called a **guaiac** (Hemoccult) test. A small amount of stool is placed on a card or slide made especially for this purpose, and a few drops of a chemical developer are then placed on the slide. The nurse then observes the specimen for a color change. Blue is a positive diagnostic finding, indicating the presence of blood in the stool sample. No color change or any color other than blue is a negative diagnostic finding, indicating the absence of blood in the stool sample. Guaiac testing is a simple procedure, as explained in Procedure 41-1, but the nurse should be sure to read the instructions that accompany the test slide and to follow them every time for accurate results.

Stool is tested for occult blood to check for pathologic sources of bleeding from the gastrointestinal tract. Gastrointestinal bleeding could be caused by ulcers or tumors of the gastrointestinal tract. If blood is on the surface of the stool, it is likely to be caused by bleeding from hemorrhoids and is not occult. If blood is mixed in the stool mass itself, its likely source is intestinal. When collecting a stool specimen for occult blood, a stool sample obviously contaminated by hemorrhoidal or menstrual blood should not be used.

A false-positive result on a Hemoccult test can occur if the client has recently taken medications known to irritate the gastric mucosa. People who routinely take aspirin or other nonsteroidal anti-inflammatory drugs (NSAIDs) or steroidal medications should avoid taking these medications for 3 days before a stool specimen is collected. The ingestion of rare red meat in large quantities for 3 days before guaiac testing can also cause a false-positive result. False-negative results can occur if the client has eaten horseradish, radishes, beets, or melons or has taken more than 250 mg/day of vitamin C in the 3 days before the test (Dammel, 1997).

Stool Culture. A culture for specific infectious organisms can be obtained from a stool specimen. The stool normally has a high bacteria count as a result of normal intestinal flora. A stool culture is performed to distinguish atypical intestinal organisms present in the stool sample. Examples of atypical infectious organisms that might be cultured from a stool sample include *Salmonella* and *Shigella* species. When these organisms are present in the intestine, they usually cause diarrhea. Specific antibiotics are necessary to kill the offending organism and stop the diarrhea. Stool is often cultured for *C. difficile,* another potential cause of diarrhea.

A special kind of stool culture that is sometimes necessary is the testing of the stool for ova (eggs) and parasites. When collecting a stool specimen for specific parasitic organisms or their eggs, such as *Giardia lamblia* or *Entamoeba histolytica,* send it to the laboratory soon after the client defecates (i.e., while the stool is still warm).

Radiologic Procedures. The small and large intestines can be visualized by x-ray imaging if a radiopaque substance, such as barium, is swallowed or instilled in the rectum. The small bowel radiologic procedure is usually done in conjunction with a radiograph of the upper gastrointestinal tract. The client must swallow barium, which aids visualization of the soft tissues of the gastrointestinal tract. The radiologist then monitors the progress of the barium from the esophagus through the ileum. The lower gastrointestinal

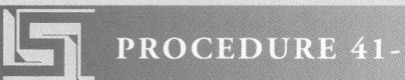

PROCEDURE 41-1

ASSESSING STOOL FOR OCCULT BLOOD

Purpose
1. Screen clients who have or who are at risk for gastrointestinal bleeding.
2. Screen for early-stage colon cancer.

Assessment
- Review client's medical and drug history for risk factors for gastrointestinal bleeding.
- Assess client's understanding of need for the procedure and his or her ability to cooperate.
- Note client's dietary history and need for any modifications before the test. Rare meats, beets, radishes, melons, and vitamin C can cause false-positive test results for occult blood. Some physicians may restrict ingestion of these substances for 72 hours before the test.
- Note use of medications such as aspirin, ibuprofen, or steroids, which can cause gastrointestinal irritation.

Equipment
Bedpan, bedside commode, or toilet hat to catch stool
Disposable examination gloves
Tongue blade or wooden applicator stick
Prepackaged Hemoccult cardboard slide, developing solution or Hematest tablets, guaiac filter paper, and several drops of water

Procedure
1. Identify client. Ask the client to void before collecting the stool specimen.
   Rationale: Urine mixed with stool sample could dilute stool sample and prevent detection of occult blood. If urine has red blood cells, the test results might be positive, but the source would be masked.
2. Assist client onto bedpan, commode, or to bathroom. Provide privacy; leave call bell handy.
   Rationale: Provides for client safety and dignity.
3. Once the client has passed stool and is clean and comfortable, don disposable gloves and obtain small amount of stool with a tongue blade or wooden applicator.

Hemoccult Slide Test
1. Open flap of slide and apply a very thin smear of stool taken from the center of the specimen onto first window.
   Rationale: Samples obtained from the edges are likely to be contaminated. The guaiac filter

paper is very sensitive to blood content, so only a small sample is needed.
2. Using second applicator, obtain a second sample from a different area of the stool. Smear thinly on second window of slide.
   Rationale: Blood may not be equally distributed throughout stool sample. Testing findings from one area may not reveal blood in another area. In acute care agencies, physicians typically order samples to be tested on three different occasions.
3. Close slide cover. Open flap on reverse side and apply two drops of Hemoccult developing solution onto each window.
   Rationale: The developing solution penetrates the stool sample to react chemically with the blood.
4. Wait 30 to 60 seconds. Read test results.
   Rationale: Test results are positive, indicating the presence of blood, if the filter paper has a bluish tint. Test findings are negative if there is no color change.

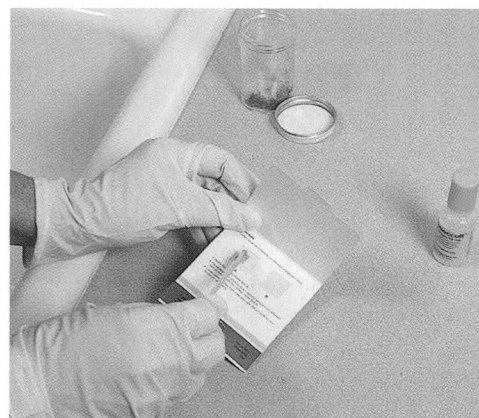

Step 1 Apply a thin smear of stool on Hemoccult slide.

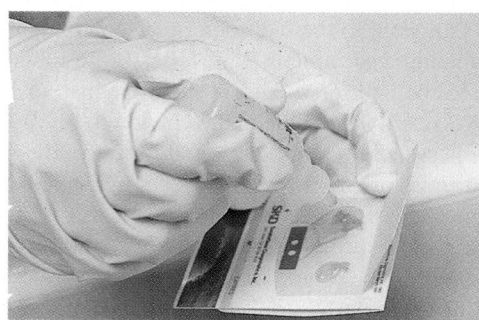

Step 3 Apply Hemoccult developing solution on slide window.

PROCEDURE 41-1 (Continued)

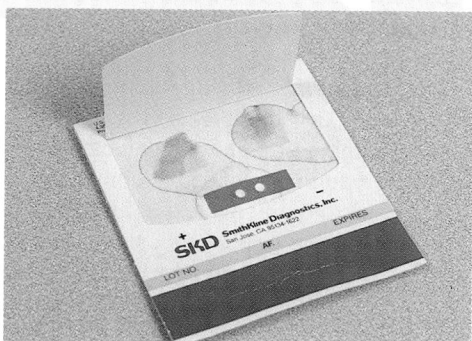

Step 4 Blue discoloration indicates the presence of occult blood.

Test With Hematest Tablets

1. Apply small smear of stool onto guaiac filter paper.
   Rationale: Guaiac paper is highly sensitive to blood, so only a thin smear is needed.
2. Place Hematest tablet on stool sample. Apply two to three drops of water onto Hematest tablet. Hold paper so that water runs onto it.
   Rationale: Hematest tablet contains a solid developing solution that dissolves with addition of water.
3. Read test results within 2 min by observing color of guaiac paper.
   Rationale: Test is positive if filter paper has a bluish tint. Test is not valid after 2 min.

4. Remove gloves, wash hands, and document findings.
   Rationale: Maintains infection control and legal client record.

Lifespan Considerations
- Remember that a child who is not toilet trained cannot cooperate with stool specimen collection. Obtain the specimen from a diaper if it is not contaminated with urine.
- If the child has watery diarrhea, place a plastic liner inside the diaper and use a cotton swab to obtain the specimen.

Home Care Modifications
- If client will collect stool sample at home, instruct client to prepare slide with sample, close cardboard flap, write name on slide, and mail or return to the office or clinic for specimen developing.

Collaboration and Delegation
- Because the client, the caregiver, or unlicensed assistive personnel frequently are responsible for assessing stool for occult blood, allow practice first with hamburger juice to see if technique has been mastered.
- Encourage validation of test results if color change is minimal.

---

tract can be radiologically visualized by instilling the barium through the rectum. The term *barium enema* is often used for this procedure.

The purpose of these two radiologic procedures is to visualize the segments of the small and large bowel and detect abnormalities in shape, motility, and functioning. Examples of abnormal findings include tumors, diverticula, obstructions, and filling defects.

For best results and maximum visualization, the bowel must be as free as possible from fecal contents. Clients need to take a combination of oral and rectal laxatives the day before and the morning of the procedure; tap water enemas can sometimes be substituted for the laxative regimen. The client's oral intake is also restricted, usually beginning at midnight on the day of the test. The client is NPO (allowed no food or fluids by mouth) until the procedure is finished; oral medications are also withheld until the procedure is completed if doing so will not pose an adverse risk for the client. The nurse is responsible for informing the client about the preparatory regimen and the purpose of the procedure, and the nurse may also be responsible for administering the laxatives or enemas and maintaining the client's NPO status.

When the client returns from the procedure, he or she may again eat and drink. Barium left in the bowel after the procedure can harden and become extremely difficult to eliminate. Therefore, administer a laxative until the client passes no more white-colored, barium-containing stool.

Endoscopic Examination. Various endoscopic procedures permit visualization of internal structures of the gastro-intestinal tract with the use of a flexible, fiberoptic instrument. Endoscopic procedures are helpful in diagnosing inflammation, ulceration, or tumors when less invasive tests, such as the barium enema, do not provide definitive results. Tissue can be extracted during endoscopic procedures and biopsied.

Proctoscopy or **sigmoidoscopy** examines the rectum and sigmoid colon. Colonoscopy can visualize the colon up to the ileocecal valve. During the sigmoidoscopy or colonoscopy, the endoscope is inserted into the rectum. The client is placed in a knee-to-chest position, which is an uncomfortable and somewhat embarrassing position for most people. Clients also feel the urge to defecate when the fiberoptic probe is inserted into the rectum, another embarrassing feeling for most people. For clients who are too weak to be examined in the knee-to-chest position, a side-lying position with the upper leg flexed (Sims' position) can be used, although this position makes visualization of the sigmoid colon more difficult. Colonoscopy takes longer and produces more discomfort than sigmoidoscopy or proctoscopy; therefore, the client is given intravenous medications to control pain, to reduce bowel spasm, and to produce light anesthesia.

The esophagogastroduodenoscopy is a newer endoscopic procedure that visualizes the esophagus, stomach, and duodenum. During the esophagogastroduodenoscopy, the endoscope is passed through the mouth while the client is in a left lateral position with the head bent forward.

The client must sign a consent form before an endoscopic procedure. A biopsy (retrieval of a small piece of mucosa or tumor for analysis) or polypectomy (complete surgical removal of a colonic lesion) can be done during endoscopy.

Before the procedure, nursing responsibilities focus on educating the client. Explain the purpose of the examination, the position necessary for the procedure, and sensations likely to be felt during the procedure. Also, discuss any dietary restrictions and test preparations. For example, the client may be allowed only clear liquids the evening before and the morning of the test. Laxatives, a rectal suppository, or a small-volume enema may also be required to clean the lower colon of stool before the procedure begins.

Afterward, the client needs rest but must be closely monitored for signs of rectal bleeding or the onset of continuous, dull abdominal pain, possibly indicating colonic perforation. The client will probably be tired and perhaps hungry and thirsty. Provide rest and offer food and fluids as allowed.

NURSING DIAGNOSES

North American Nursing Diagnosis Association (NANDA) nursing diagnoses concerning bowel elimination include Perceived Constipation, Risk for Constipation, Diarrhea, and Bowel Incontinence. Before 1988, Altered Bowel Elimination was an accepted nursing diagnosis, but it was found to be too broad for clinical use.

Diagnostic Statement: Constipation

Definition. Decrease in normal frequency of defecation accompanied by difficult or incomplete passage of stool and/or passage of excessively hard, dry stool (NANDA, 2001).

Defining Characteristics. Change in bowel pattern or inability to pass stool; dry, hard, formed stool; decreased volume of stool; straining or pain with defecation; soft, paste-like stool in the rectum; distended abdomen and increased abdominal pressure or pain; percussed abdominal dullness; feeling of rectal fullness or pressure; anorexia, indigestion, nausea, vomiting; hypoactive or hyperactive bowel sounds; severe flatus (NANDA, 2001). Atypical presentation in the older adult may include changes in mental status, urinary incontinence, unexplained falls, or elevated temperature (NANDA, 2001).

Related Factors. Factors include functional, psychological, pharmacologic, mechanical, and physiologic conditions (NANDA, 2001) that have been outlined throughout this chapter.

Diagnostic Statement: Perceived Constipation

Definition. Perceived Constipation is the state in which a person makes a self-diagnosis of constipation and ensures a daily bowel movement through abuse of laxatives, enemas, and suppositories (NANDA, 2001).

Defining Characteristics. Characteristics are expectation of a daily bowel movement with resulting overuse of laxatives, enemas, and suppositories; expected passage of stool at the same time every day (NANDA, 2001).

Related Factors. Related factors are cultural—family health beliefs, faulty appraisal, and impaired thought processes (NANDA, 2001). Note that a sudden change in normal bowel status, together with inadequate knowledge, can motivate a person to overuse medical therapies to ensure a daily evacuation of stool. This is more likely to occur if the person tends to be obsessive-compulsive in behavior or has a long-held belief that deviation from a stool every day is unhealthy (Carpenito, 2001).

Diagnostic Statement: Diarrhea

Definition. Diarrhea is a state in which a person experiences passage of loose, unformed stools (NANDA, 2001).

Defining Characteristics. At least three loose, liquid stools per day; abdominal pain; cramping; hyperactive bowel sounds; urgency (NANDA, 2001).

Related Factors. Related factors are inflammation or infection; parasites; malabsorption; treatments such as medications, radiation, or tube feedings; and altered situations such as stress, travel, or ingestion of certain foods (NANDA 2001).

Diagnostic Statement: Bowel Incontinence

Definition. Bowel Incontinence is the state in which a person experiences a change in normal bowel habits characterized by involuntary passage of stool (NANDA, 2001).

Defining Characteristics. The defining characteristics include involuntary passage of stool, urgency and inability to delay the urge to defecate, fecal straining, inability to recognize or inattention to the urge to defecate, fecal odor, and constant dribbling of soft stool (NANDA, 2001).

Related Factors. Decreased muscle tone of sphincter control, impaction, chronic diarrhea, toileting self-care deficit, laxative abuse, upper or lower motor nerve damage, dietary

habits, medications, stress, immobility, and inaccessible bathroom facilities are related factors (NANDA, 2001).

Related Nursing Diagnoses

Altered bowel status can contribute to or cause many potential or actual problems for the client. Emotionally, altered bowel function can result in the following nursing diagnostic statements: Anxiety, Situational Low Self-Esteem, or Ineffective Coping. Deficient Knowledge is often present as a person learns to cope with new treatment modalities. Pain can result from constipation, diarrhea, or abdominal distention. Alteration in bowel status can disrupt physiologic homeostasis by contributing to Deficient Fluid Volume; Imbalanced Nutrition, Less Than Body Requirements; Decreased Cardiac Output; Impaired Skin Integrity; and Risk for Infection. Disturbed Sleep Pattern and Ineffective Sexuality Patterns can also occur.

OUTCOME IDENTIFICATION AND PLANNING

The overall goals for clients with bowel elimination pattern disturbances may include the following.

- The client will demonstrate a normal pattern of bowel elimination without evidence of constipation, diarrhea, fecal incontinence, or distention.
- The client will remain free of preventable complications or adverse consequences from altered bowel elimination.
- The client will participate in a program to maintain and promote an acceptable pattern of bowel elimination.

The time frame for the client to achieve a normal pattern of bowel elimination depends on the particular alteration involved. For example, constipation can usually be relieved in 1 or 2 days, whereas relief of diarrhea or incontinence is not always achievable in this time frame. The etiologic factors associated with the dysfunction also dictate the realistic time frame in which an outcome can be accomplished.

Promoting an acceptable bowel elimination pattern is, realistically, a long-term goal; in actual clinical practice, however, it is often subject to short-term management. Client teaching is a major management tool for achieving this goal. Examples of nursing interventions for various bowel problems are listed in the accompanying display and discussed in the following section.

IMPLEMENTATION
Health Promotion
Client Teaching

Diet. The nurse should assist the client with planning a diet that contains sufficient daily intake of high-fiber foods, because dietary fiber is necessary to provide bulk to the stool. High-fiber foods include fresh or cooked fruits and vegetables

THERAPEUTIC DIALOGUE
Constipation

Scene for Thought

Helen Palumbo is a 73-year-old woman who comes to the clinic for a check-up about every 6 months. She is busy, active, pleasant, and committed to staying healthy so she can continue to enjoy life.

Less Effective

Nurse: Hi, Mrs. Palumbo. Glad to see you. How are you feeling?

Client: Hi, Barbara. I'm doing fine except I think I'm a little constipated. *(Whispers this last word.)*

Nurse: Tell me a little more. *(Listens attentively.)*

Client: Well, I usually go every morning, but over the last few months I only go every 2 days, and I'm worried. *(Looks worried.)*

Nurse: You certainly look worried. But, a woman your age is bound to slow down in some areas, even though you're still active and busy. Your bowel is slowing down and so you don't need to evacuate every single day.

Client: *(Looks doubtful.)* Really?

Nurse: Absolutely. Many senior clients are perfectly fine even though they don't have a movement every day. They drink enough fluids, eat enough fruits and vegetables, exercise, and do just fine. I know from our last visit that you're doing all those things. Tell you what, if you have any questions, give me a call. But I think you're doing great, Mrs. Palumbo.

Client: Well, okay. I guess I'm just being silly. I'll call you if anything new comes up. *(Smiles and says goodbye.)*

Nurse: Great! I'll talk to you then. *(Smiles.)*

More Effective

Nurse: Hi, Mrs. Palumbo. Glad to see you. How are you feeling?

Client: Hi, MaryJo. I'm doing fine except I think I'm a little constipated. *(Whispers this last word.)*

Nurse: Tell me a little more. *(Listens attentively.)*

Client: Well, I usually go every morning, but over the last few months I only go every 2 days, and I'm worried. *(Looks worried.)*

Nurse: What worries you about that?

Client: Well, when I was in my 20s, I had a fistula. I put off having my first baby because of it. Then, 5 years ago, I had diverticulitis that put me in the hospital for a week with antibiotics. It wasn't fun, I'll tell you. If I get constipated, I'm worried about putting strain on my fistula scars or going back to the hospital. You see?

Nurse: I understand why you're concerned. Let me ask you a few questions about nutrition and fluids. I'll examine your abdomen, then we can talk more about some things you might do. Is that okay with you?

Client: Whatever you say, I always learn something new when I come here. *(Big smile.)*

Nurse: *(After the assessment.)* Well, you seem to be drinking lots of fluids, which is wonderful. You tell me you go every 2 days and have no gas or pain in the abdomen. I wonder if maybe our definitions of constipation are different.

Client: What do you mean?

Nurse: My definition of constipation is hard, dry stool that passes after 3 days or more and is accompanied by gas, bloating, and pain, maybe even nausea.

Client: *(Looks surprised.)* No, I don't get that!

Nurse: Lots of people believe that they're constipated if they don't go every day. They use laxatives and enemas, which can make it worse. From your description, it sounds as though your bowel function is fine for a healthy woman your age. You have none of the symptoms of constipation. *(Smiles.)*

Client: *(Smiles back.)* Good, I'm glad.

Nurse: Call me if you have any questions. You know I'm happy to talk to you anytime.

Client: Thank you so much. I will. *(Looks relieved and beams happily as she briskly leaves the office.)*

Critical Thinking Challenges

- Compare and contrast the different determinations Barbara and MaryJo made, as shown by their different responses to Mrs. Palumbo.
- Infer what Mrs. Palumbo needed from her nurse.
- If you were the nurse, what changes would you have made in MaryJo's conversation with Mrs. Palumbo?
- In Barbara's?

with their skins, whole-grain breads and cereals, and fruit and vegetable juices. The nurse can assist the client in selecting foods from a list, identifying those foods that the client will most likely incorporate into his or her lifestyle. A dietitian can be consulted for a more extensive list of high-fiber foods and recipes using these ingredients. For example, unprocessed bran flakes can be added to cooked or processed cereals. The client should start with small amounts (1 or 2 teaspoons) to determine whether bran causes any intestinal irritation or flatulence. Unprocessed bran can absorb eight times its weight

PLANNING: Examples of NIC/NOC Interventions and Outcomes

Accepted Bowel Elimination Nursing Interventions Classification (NIC)
Bowel Incontinence Care
Bowel Incontinence Care: Encopresis
Bowel Irrigation
Bowel Management
Bowel Training
Constipation/Impaction Management
Diarrhea Management
Flatulence Reduction
Gastrointestinal Intubation
Tube Care: Gastrointestinal

Accepted Bowel Elimination Nursing Outcomes Classification (NOC)
Bowel Continence
Bowel Elimination
Hydration
Infection Status
Mobility Level
Neurological Status
Nutritional Status: Food & Fluid Intake
Treatment Behavior: Illness or Injury

Refer to the following for specifics regarding NIC/NOC:
McCloskey, J., & Bulechek, G. (2000). *Iowa Intervention Project: Nursing Interventions Classification (NIC)*, 3rd ed. St. Louis, MO: C.V. Mosby.
Johnson, M., & Maas, M. (2000). *Iowa Outcomes Project: Nursing Outcomes Classification (NOC)*. St. Louis, MO: C.V. Mosby.

OUTCOME-BASED TEACHING PLAN

Mrs. Chin is being discharged from the acute care facility on Tylenol #3 for pain (a narcotic analgesic), ferrous sulfate to improve her anemia, and Colace as a stool softener after hip replacement surgery. Mrs. Chin uses a walker, and her mobility is very restricted. After surgery, she required a suppository to have a bowel movement. Mrs. Chin states she is very worried that she will be constipated after she is discharged home.

OUTCOME: At the end of the teaching session, Mrs. Chin can verbalize factors that could contribute to constipation during the surgical recovery period.
Strategies
- Evaluate Mrs. Chin's normal bowel routine including her knowledge of factors contributing to constipation, and her usual treatment for constipation.
- Discuss factors that slow bowel motility and increase risk for constipation (decreased motility, altered diet and fluid intake, pain medication, iron supplements) during the postoperative period.
- Have Mrs. Chin verbalize factors back to you.
- Provide Mrs. Chin with a written list of factors for her reference.

OUTCOME: Before discharge, Mrs. Chin will verbalize a plan to decrease constipation risk and treat constipation if it should occur.
Strategies
- Provide Mrs. Chin with a handout on Promoting Regular Bowel Function.
- From a list of foods high in fiber, have Mrs. Chin select those foods she likes and can easily incorporate into her diet.
- Problem solve together how to increase fluid intake (e.g., large sports bottle filled with water at side, fruit juices (e.g., prune) that are also high in fiber).
- Review prescribed medications and their effect on bowel function.
- Review medications (prescribed and over the counter) to prevent and treat constipation.
- Have Mrs. Chin verbalize how and when she will take laxative medications (e.g., Colace every day to keep my stool soft, milk of magnesia if no bowel movement for 3 days).

in water. An acceptable amount of bran is added gradually to the diet to achieve an acceptable bowel elimination pattern. The daily intake of about 800 g of high-fiber foods (e.g., any combination of five or six servings of fruit or vegetables, and whole-grain bread or cereal) is encouraged. A sandwich with two slices of whole-grain bread, served with a large fresh vegetable salad and two pieces of fruit, would provide about five servings of fiber. A nursing study demonstrated that men who received bran fiber in their diet every day had 80% reduction in the need for medications to promote bowel function (Howard, West, & Ossip-Klein, 2000).

Fluids. Fluid intake between 1500 and 2000 mL/day promotes a normal bowel elimination pattern. The nurse should discuss with the client his or her fluid preferences and find a way to encourage the intake of eight to ten glasses of fluid per day.

Some fruit and vegetable juices provide not only fluid but bulk because of their high pulp or fiber content. A glass of prune juice is equivalent to more than one serving of the dried fruit, has high magnesium content, and is an excellent source of fluid to promote bowel elimination. Hot fluids, such as coffee, tea, or hot water with lemon juice, may also increase intestinal motility. However, caffeinated fluids, such as soft drinks, tea, coffee, or beer, should be used in moderation because they have a diuretic effect (Addison, 2000).

Activity and Exercise. A sufficient amount of daily exercise is necessary to promote general muscle tone. Exercise also encourages normal smooth muscle functioning, which is important for normal intestinal functioning. Walking is an excellent exercise in which most people can participate. Isotonic or isometric exercises also help to increase abdominal muscle tone. An example of these exercises is the alternate contraction and relaxation of the abdominal muscles for eight to ten repetitions. The many variations of sit-up exercises isometrically tone and strengthen the abdominal muscles. Assist the client who is on bed rest to perform range-of-motion exercises until he or she can perform more independent activities.

Bowel Habits. Many people recognize that their bodies have a regular time for bowel elimination. Some people have a bowel movement at the same time of day or after a certain regular stimulus. The duodenocolic reflex is a strong reflex, especially when food or hot liquid is ingested after a period of fasting, such as after a night's sleep. For some people, ingestion of breakfast or a cup of coffee, tea, or any liquid is stimulus enough to activate the duodenocolic reflex. Teach clients to heed their body signals and stress that ignoring the urge to defecate can lead to constipation.

SAFETY ALERT
Never leave a client sitting on a toileting device without a ready access for summoning assistance. Teach clients to exhale slowly during defecation to avoid straining and the Valsalva maneuver, which for high-risk clients, can lead to cardiac dysrhythmias, increased intracranial pressure, and syncope.

Colorectal Screening. Colorectal cancer is the third most common cause of cancer among men and women in the United States (American Cancer Society, 2001). Risk for colorectal cancer increases significantly after 50 years of age and for people who have a positive family history; previous colorectal cancer, ulcerative colitis, or Crohn's disease; or a history of benign adenoma (polyps). Teaching about annual screening after the age of 50, including digital rectal examination, occult blood testing, and flexible endoscopic examination every 3 to 5 years, is an important nursing responsibility.

Nursing Interventions for Altered Bowel Function

Nursing interventions are individualized to reestablish optimal bowel function and treat common bowel alterations such as constipation, diarrhea, flatulence, abdominal distention, and related problems. Fecal impaction, neurologic impairment (requiring bowel training), fecal incontinence, and stoma care and irrigation required by fecal diversion surgery are more complex bowel problems that nurses independently or collaboratively manage. Constipation is treated with laxatives, suppositories, enemas, and, if chronic, a bowel management program. Diarrhea is managed by treating the underlying cause, resting the bowel, and administering antidiarrheal medications. Fecal incontinence is managed by instituting a bowel-training program and using fecal collection devices. Flatulence is treated by increasing activity, administering medications, using rectal tubes, and administering

return-flow enemas. Persistent abdominal distention may require decompression by nasogastric intubation. Other nursing interventions may involve measures to relieve fecal impaction, to facilitate bowel training, and to care for the stoma and client after fecal diversion surgery.

Medication Use
Almost all medications used to manage altered bowel function are available over the counter without prescription. People self-medicate to treat bowel problems, frequently seeking the advice of a healthcare professional only when symptoms become severe or extend over a long period. Teaching regarding normal bowel function and nonpharmacologic methods to regain normal bowel regularity is important to avoid overuse of laxatives. Also, inappropriate use of over-the-counter bowel medications can worsen some serious medical problems, such as bowel obstruction or appendicitis. Nurses are often in an ideal position to teach individuals or groups about appropriate use of bowel medications.

Laxatives. Usually, oral laxatives are the treatment of choice for constipation because these medications promote evacuation of hardened stool from the bowel. Table 41-3 presents some common agents, such as oral laxatives and stool softeners, that are used to relieve constipation. Oral laxatives take longer to evacuate stool than do laxatives given rectally. However, oral laxatives are preferred by most clients for their ease of administration and the more gradual effect on intestinal motility.

Laxatives may be given in the form of a rectal suppository. A **suppository** is a medication prepared in a base (e.g., glycerin) that, when inserted into the rectum, melts and can be absorbed for systemic or local effects. Many suppositories are used to promote bowel evacuation, but other drugs that do not affect bowel status (e.g., aspirin) can be administered in suppository form. A suppository is administered when a quick effect (15 to 60 minutes) is desired.

To administer a rectal suppository, gather the medication, a packet of water-soluble lubricant, and a pair of disposable gloves. If the client cannot ambulate independently to the bathroom, place a bedside commode or bedpan nearby before administering the suppository. Placement of disposable underpads on the bed may be advisable if the client's motor or mental abilities are compromised.

The client should assume a side-lying position. With gloved hands, remove the outer wrapper from the suppository and cover the suppository with lubricant. While separating the client's buttocks, locate the anus and insert the suppository, pointed or rounded end first, past the internal sphincter. For the adult, the internal sphincter is at approximately 4 inches, or at the end of the nurse's index finger. Guide the suppository with your index finger, aiming in a slightly upward direction toward the umbilicus. Typically, you will feel the client's sphincter close around your finger. A suppository melts at body temperature and releases its medication as it rests against the rectal mucosa. Be sure the suppository is not inadvertently deposited into stool that

TABLE 41-3

Common Agents Used to Relieve Constipation			
Laxative Type	Examples	Mechanism of Action	Nursing Considerations
Bulk	Fibercon, Metamucil	Hydrophilic Nonabsorbable fibers attract water into large intestine	Usually well tolerated and used to regulate stool in constipation and diarrhea. Concurrent administration with other medications avoided. Contraindicated in bowel obstruction
Emollient (stool softeners)	Colace, Surfak, Dialose, DOSS	Decrease surface tension of stool allowing water to enter stool more readily	Short-term treatment when risk for constipation is high (e.g., when client is less mobile or is taking narcotics)
Saline	Milk of magnesia (MOM), magnesium citrate, Fleet enema	Hyperosmolar Increase colon motility through release of cholecystokinin (a hormone)	Possible resultant electrolyte imbalances, especially hypermagnesemia. Not for chronic use or use in renal failure. Frequently used to prepare bowel for diagnostic testing
Stimulant	Castor oil, Dulcolax (bisacodyl), Pericolace (casanthranol), Ex-Lax, Correctol (phenolphthalein), Senokot (senna)	Direct stimulation of intestinal mucosa	Chronic use avoided. Possible resultant electrolyte imbalances. Use during pregnancy and lactation avoided

might be present in the rectum, because this prevents absorption by the rectal mucosa.

Antidiarrheal Agents. Medications that act directly on the intestine to slow bowel motility or to absorb excess fluid in the bowel are called antidiarrheals. Table 41-4 lists the antidiarrheal agents that are most commonly administered. Absorbents and bulk-forming agents change the consistency of the stool to relieve diarrhea; they cause few adverse systemic effects and are considered safe for general use. Opiates and antispasmodics act systemically to decrease intestinal motility. Antidiarrheal agents are contraindicated when viral or bacterial infections cause diarrhea, because diarrhea is a protective mechanism to shed the microorganisms from the body.

Medications may also be used to relieve the underlying problem causing diarrhea. For example, antibiotics are administered when an infectious microorganism causes diarrhea. Steroids may be given to decrease inflammation in the exacerbation of a chronic inflammatory bowel disease.

Antiflatulence Agents. Antiflatulence agents, such as simethicone, are used to relieve gas. Simethicone coalesces gas bubbles in the intestine, allowing gas to pass from the gastrointestinal tract either by belching or by anal expulsion. It does not prevent the formation of gas. Antiflatulence medication is usually given in combination with an antacid. Suppositories that increase intestinal motility can also relieve accumulated intestinal flatus.

Enemas

An **enema** is the cleansing of a portion of the large bowel by insertion of fluid rectally. Enemas can be small volume, containing a laxative medication (approximately 150 mL), or large volume, containing only ordinary tap water or saline solution (up to 1000 mL for the adult). Procedure 41-2 gives the steps in administering an enema.

Small-Volume Enemas. Small-volume enemas are commercially prepared and usually are administered after an oral laxative fails to produce sufficient stool return or if a rapid evacuation is preferred. The laxative solution is hypertonic, osmotically drawing water from colonic mucosa to cause water retention in the lower colon. It also increases peristalsis. The volume of fluid itself distends the rectum to trigger a defecation reflex.

An oil retention enema is a small-volume enema containing a quantity of mineral oil. The mineral oil softens any hardened stool that is present, making the stool easier to pass. An oil retention enema usually is given only when a fecal impaction is suspected.

Small-volume enemas come from the manufacturer in disposable containers with prelubricated tips. The client usually

TABLE 41-4

Medications Used to Relieve Diarrhea	
Agent	**Action**
Absorbents Kaolin/pectin (Donnagel) Attapulgite (Kaopectate) Bismuth subsalicylate (Pepto-Bismol)	Absorbs excess fluid and bowel irritants; provides soothing effect to irritated bowel
Bulk-Forming Agents Psyllium (Metamucil, Effer-syllium)	Attracts water to absorb excess fluid
Opiates Paregoric Codeine	↓ Intestinal motility ↑ Intestinal water and electrolyte absorption
Synthetic Opiates Lopermide (Imodium) Diphenoxylate/atropine (Lomotil)	↓ Intestinal motility ↑ Intestinal water and electrolyte absorption
Antispasmodics Atropine Tincture of belladonna	↓ Intestinal motility

experiences the urge to defecate within 5 to 10 minutes after administration of the enema.

Large-Volume Enemas. Large-volume enemas cleanse the bowel of stool by distending the bowel with up to 1000 mL of fluid for the adult (15 to 60 mL is recommended for an infant, 240 to 360 mL for a child). Warm tap water or saline solution is used as the cleansing agent. However, saline solution is the only fluid recommended for infants and children. The large volume of fluid instilled into the bowel causes distention and stimulates the defecation reflex. The large-volume enema can be used as a treatment for constipation or as a method of cleansing the bowel before bowel radiologic studies or surgery.

After gathering the equipment, position the client as for administration of a suppository or small-volume enema. Most authorities recommend positioning on the left side, but some favor the right side (Addison, Ness, Abulafi & Swift, 2000). Once the tubing has been flushed or primed, insert the lubricated tip of the tubing approximately 4 inches, aiming toward the umbilicus, and slowly instill the solution into the client's rectum.

SAFETY ALERT
Care must be taken not to insert the tubing too far or to advance the tubing forcefully, because doing so could injure mucosal tissue or, in extreme situations, perforate the intestine.

Control the amount and speed of the fluid instillation by opening and closing the tubing clamp and by adjusting the height of the solution container. Opening the clamp or raising the container increases the rate of flow of the solution into the rectum. Conversely, closing the clamp or lowering the enema bucket decreases the rate of flow. If the client complains of abdominal discomfort or cramping, the nurse momentarily stops the flow of solution. To cleanse the bowel successfully of stool, the average adult needs to tolerate approximately 350 to 500 mL of solution instilled before expelling the enema. When the client cannot tolerate any more solution per rectum, the nurse stops the enema and assists the client as necessary to the bedpan, commode, or toilet.

A large-volume enema can be repeated up to three times in succession.

SAFETY ALERT
Never administer more than three large-volume tap water enemas in succession. Excess absorption of the hypotonic solution by colonic mucosa leads to fluid and electrolyte imbalances.

Guidelines for repeating an enema include the statement that the client feels there is more stool in the bowel that needs to be evacuated, evidence of large pieces of stool in the enema returns, and the presence of heavily stool-colored water in the enema returns. A step-by-step guide is given in Procedure 41-2.

(text continues on page 1125)

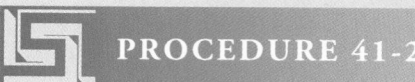

PROCEDURE 41-2

ADMINISTERING AN ENEMA

Purpose
1. Relieves gas, constipation, or fecal impaction.
2. Cleanses the bowel in preparation for diagnostic tests or surgical procedures.
3. Evacuates feces in clients with hemiplegia, quadriplegia, or paraplegia.
4. Delivers medication.

Assessment
- Assess client's past and present elimination history: presence of hemorrhoids, external and internal.
- Review healthcare provider's order, and determine the purpose for the enema to guide selection of the solution.
- If constipation or impaction is suspected, palpate abdomen for distention, and perform digital rectal examination.
- Determine client's understanding of purpose of enema, what to expect during the procedure, and how he or she can help.

Equipment
Enema container with appropriately sized tubing (adults—size 22–32 Fr, children—size 14–18 Fr, infants—size 12 Fr, or a bulb syringe)
Possible solutions: Normal saline, tap water, soap solution, medications, commercially prepared small-volume enema
Disposable gloves and water-soluble lubricant
Personal hygiene items: soap, towel, water
Waterproof bed protector
Clean bedpan or commode, and toilet paper. Children may use potty chair or diaper.

Procedure
1. Assemble the needed equipment in one place; then provide privacy by closing curtains or room door.
   Rationale: Adequate preparation of equipment speeds the procedure. Providing privacy reduces embarrassment for the client, and increases his or her ability to relax.
2. Identify client. Position client on left side (Sims' position) with right knee flexed.
   Rationale: Sims' position improves retention of enema by allowing solution to flow along the natural sigmoid colon curve.
3. Put on disposable gloves. Place waterproof towel under client's buttocks.
   Rationale: Prevent soiling of linen and maintain infection control.

4. Cover client with bath blanket, exposing only the rectum.
   Rationale: Blanket provides privacy and warmth and increases ability to relax.

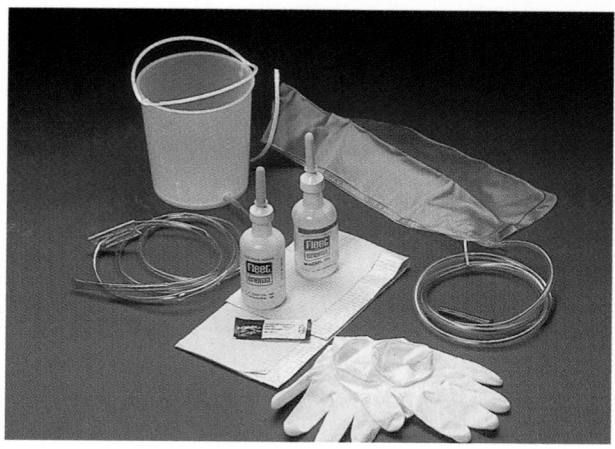

Step 1 Assemble equipment.

Large-Volume Enema
1. See steps 1 to 4.
2. Fill enema bag with 750 to 1000 mL lukewarm solution (105° to 110°F; for child, 500 mL or less, 100°F). Check temperature of solution by pouring some over your inner wrist.
   Rationale: Intestinal mucosa can be damaged if solution is too warm. Cold solutions are difficult to retain and can cause abdominal cramping.
3. Open clamp on tubing and allow solution to flow through tubing to remove the air. Reclamp tubing.
   Rationale: Air in the rectum causes discomfort.
4. Lubricate 2 to 3 inches of the tip of the rectal tube with water-soluble lubricant.
   Rationale: Insertion is smoother and trauma is minimized with lubrication.
5. Separate the buttocks to visualize the anus. Observe for external hemorrhoids. Ask client to take a slow, deep breath. Gently insert the rectal tube, directing the tip toward the umbilicus (adult: 3–4 inches).
   Rationale: Prevent injury to the intestinal mucosa by directing the tube along the natural bowel curve.
6. Continue holding the tube in the rectum. With other hand, open the clamp and allow solution to slowly enter the client. Raise container 18 inches above the anus, allowing solution to flow slowly

PROCEDURE 41-2 (Continued)

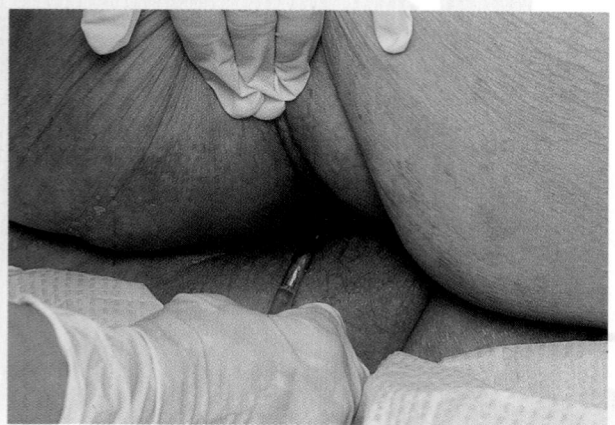

Step 5 Raise buttocks and insert tubing into anus.

over 5 to 10 minutes. If client complains of cramping or pain, have client breathe deeply and lower bag until the sensation stops.
Rationale: Slow instillation reduces client discomfort from bowel distention and cramping, thereby allowing a greater volume of solution to be retained.

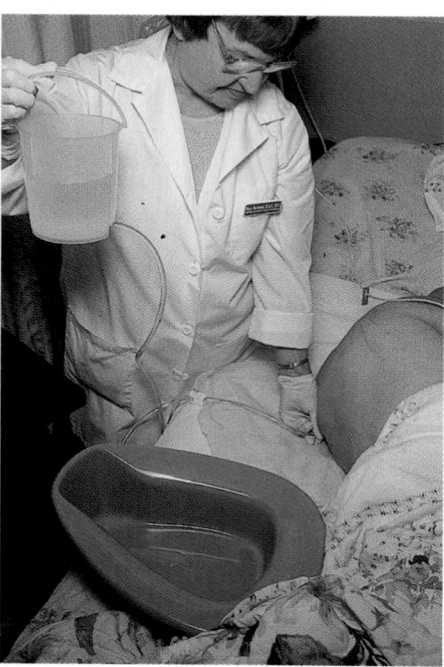

Step 6 Raise enema solution about 18 inches above rectum and instill slowly.

7. Reclamp tubing when desired amount of solution has infused.
   Rationale: Clamping prevents air from entering the rectum.
8. Remove tube gently and have client squeeze buttocks together firmly for several minutes.
   Rationale: The urge to defecate caused by tube removal will decrease if sphincters are contracted.
9. Have client retain solution as long as possible.
   Rationale: Longer retention enhances peristalsis and evacuation of bowel contents.
10. Assist client to bathroom, commode, or bedpan. Place call bell with reach. Provide privacy until all of the solution has been expelled.
    Rationale: Increases client comfort and safety.
11. Visually inspect character of the feces and solution.
    Rationale: If enemas are ordered "until clear" as preparation for diagnostic testing, it is essential to assess expelled solution for fecal material. Allow client to rest, then repeat as necessary.
12. Assist client into comfortable position. Assist with cleansing as needed. Provide materials for client to wash hands. Open windows or provide air freshener if needed. Clean and dispose of equipment as necessary. Remove gloves and wash hands.
    Rationale: Spread of microorganisms is prevented, and client comfort is increased.

Small-Volume Enema
1. See Steps 1 to 4 at beginning of Procedure.
2. Remove protective cap from prelubricated catheter tip. You may add more lubricant if necessary.
   Rationale: Allow smooth insertion of the rectal tip and minimize trauma to the mucosa.
3. Separate the buttocks to visualize the anus. Observe for hemorrhoids and gently insert rectal tip into rectum, directing the tip toward the umbilicus.
   Rationale: Prevent injury to the intestinal mucosa by following the natural curve of the bowel.
4. Squeeze bottle to empty contents into the rectum and colon (approximately 240 mL of solution).
   Rationale: Prepackaged solutions are usually hypertonic and require only small volumes to stimulate defecation. They are not to be used in children!
5. Maintain pressure on the enema container until you withdraw it from the rectum.
   Rationale: Releasing the pressure while the container is still in the rectum will cause the liquid to be drawn back into the container.
6. Continue same as with large-volume enema.

PROCEDURE 41-2 (Continued)

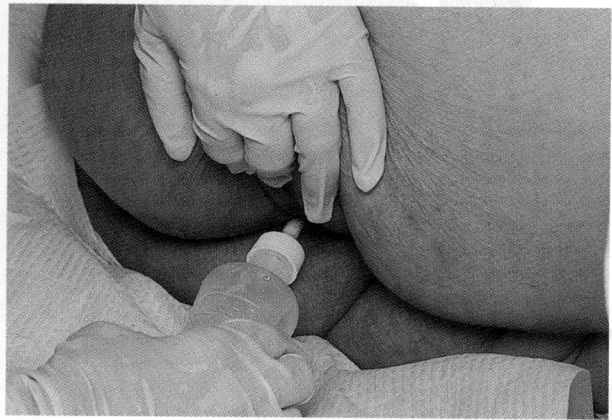

Step 4 Squeeze small enema container to insert fluid into rectum.

Lifespan Considerations
Infants and Children
- Administer an enema with the child in the dorsal recumbent position. Children who are not toilet trained are incontinent, and other children may be unable to control their rectal sphincter sufficiently to retain enema solutions.
- Ensure that the healthcare provider orders the amount of solution to be administered for children under 2 years of age.
- Children and infants do not usually receive tap water or prepackaged hypertonic enemas because fatal water intoxication or circulatory depletion could occur.
- Insert the rectal tube 1 to 1.5 inches in an infant and 2 to 3 inches for a child.

Older Adults
- If adult is incontinent, place clean dry, waterproof linen under his or her buttocks until enema solution has been expelled and buttocks are cleaned.
- Because the skin of older adults macerates easily from prolonged contact with moisture, check frequently for newly expelled stool and clean as necessary.
- If the older adult has poor sphincter control, administer the enema with the client in the dorsal recumbent position on a bedpan.

Home Care Modifications
- Teach clients not to rely on enemas to maintain bowel regularity. Enemas do not treat the cause of irregularity and, if used frequently, can result in dependence on enemas for defecation because they can disrupt normal elimination reflexes.

Collaboration and Delegation
- Be sure to give clear instructions when delegating the enema procedure to clients, caregivers, or unlicensed assistive personnel.
- Reinforce the need to avoid inserting the enema tubing too far into the rectum, which could result in intestinal irritation or perforation.
- Mark the appropriate length on the tubing for the client, caregiver, or personnel as necessary.
- When high colonic irrigations are ordered or in cases of severe impaction, consult a nurse who has extensive experience in gastroenterology.

Return-Flow Enemas. The return-flow enema is used to relieve accumulated flatus. Use the same equipment and proceed in the same fashion as for the large-volume enema. However, only 300 to 500 mL of warm tap water is necessary. When the client indicates he or she feels abdominal discomfort or cramping, lower the enema solution container and allow the water to return through the tubing into the container. Flatus will also return, as evidenced by the bubbling of the water in the container. Continue to repeat the procedure until there is no more evidence of expelled flatus, or the client reports relief. This procedure may take 15 to 20 minutes to be effective. The return-flow enema can be repeated as necessary.

Rectal Tubes
A rectal tube, which is a short piece of plastic tubing similar to the tubing used for large-volume enemas, may be used if increased activity or medication does not relieve flatulence. The nurse inserts the lubricated tip of the tube about 4 inches into

the client's rectum and leaves it in place for 15 to 20 minutes or until the client reports relief. The gas in the rectum can pass from the rectum through the tube and into a collecting device, such as a bag. Abdominal pain is the predominant adverse consequence of flatulence. It is wiser to relieve the cause of the pain by using antiflatulence agents or rectal tubes than to administer pain medications. Narcotic analgesics, in particular, slow intestinal motility and compound the problem.

Nasogastric Intubation

A nasogastric tube is a thin, pliable plastic tube that can be inserted into a client's nose and advanced into the stomach (Fig. 41-6). Nasogastric intubation may be ordered by the healthcare provider for gastric decompression, gastric lavage, or gastric feeding.

Gastric Decompression.   Decompression drains stomach contents, relieving the stomach and intestines of pressure caused by accumulated gastrointestinal air and fluid. The nasogastric tube is connected to suction to facilitate decompression of the stomach contents. Gastric decompression is indicated for a bowel obstruction, for paralytic ileus, and when surgery is performed on the stomach or intestine. In each situation, potential or actual accumulation of fluid and gas in the intestine can cause abdominal distention, discomfort for the client, and potentially serious physiologic alterations. The tube usually re-

mains in place until normal bowel function resumes, as evidenced by active bowel sounds on auscultation.

Gastric Lavage.   **Gastric lavage** is the irrigation of the stomach. In cases of accidental poisoning or accidental or intentional drug overdose, swift removal of stomach contents is required. If the client cannot swallow an emetic medication, gastric lavage is necessary. In this situation, a nasogastric tube is inserted both to aspirate gastric contents and to instill a rinsing solution (usually normal saline) into the stomach to dilute the toxic substances. Clients with gastric bleeding are sometimes treated with an iced saline lavage, which involves instillation and aspiration of iced saline solution through the nasogastric tube to empty the stomach of blood and slow the bleeding at its source.

Gastric Feeding.   For clients who cannot obtain adequate nourishment orally, liquid food can be instilled into the stomach through the nasogastric tube. This type of feeding is also called enteral nutrition or gastric **gavage.** Nasogastric tubes for feeding are intended to be used for a longer time than are nasogastric tubes used for decompression or lavage. They are narrower and are made of a more pliable material. Nasogastric feeding tubes and the nursing care associated with enteral nutrition are discussed in Chapter 37.

Equipment
Nasogastric Tubes.   The most commonly used nasogastric tube is the double-lumen (two channels) gastric sump tube (Fig. 41-7). The double-lumen gastric sump tube is clear plastic and is sized according to the French method. Sizes 14 to 18 Fr are typical adult sizes, with a length of 120 cm (48 inches). The larger lumen is connected to suction and a drainage container to collect the aspirated gastric contents; the smaller second lumen terminates in a blue vent, often called the tube's "pigtail." The blue vent is always open to the air, providing continuous atmospheric air irrigation. Markings along the length of the tube serve as guides for depth of insertion. Both lumens have openings at the tip end to allow for fluid or air flow in and out of the tube.
Nasointestinal Tubes.   When intestinal decompression for mechanical or nonmechanical bowel obstruction is the desired outcome, a longer tube capable of advancing the length of the intestine is used. These tubes may be single- or double-lumen. Some newer tubes permit stomach decompression as well as intestinal feedings.

The Harris tube (6 feet) and the Cantor tube (10 feet) are single-lumen tubes intended for intestinal decompression. Both tubes have mercury-weighted bags attached to the tip of the tube. The weight of the mercury assists the tube in passing from the pylorus of the stomach into the duodenum. The weighted tip and the natural peristalsis of the intestine keep the tube advancing through the intestine.

The Miller-Abbot tube is a double-lumen, 10-foot tube. One lumen drains or decompresses the intestine; the second lumen is used to inflate the balloon at the tip of the tube with mercury. The double-lumen tube allows for insertion of the

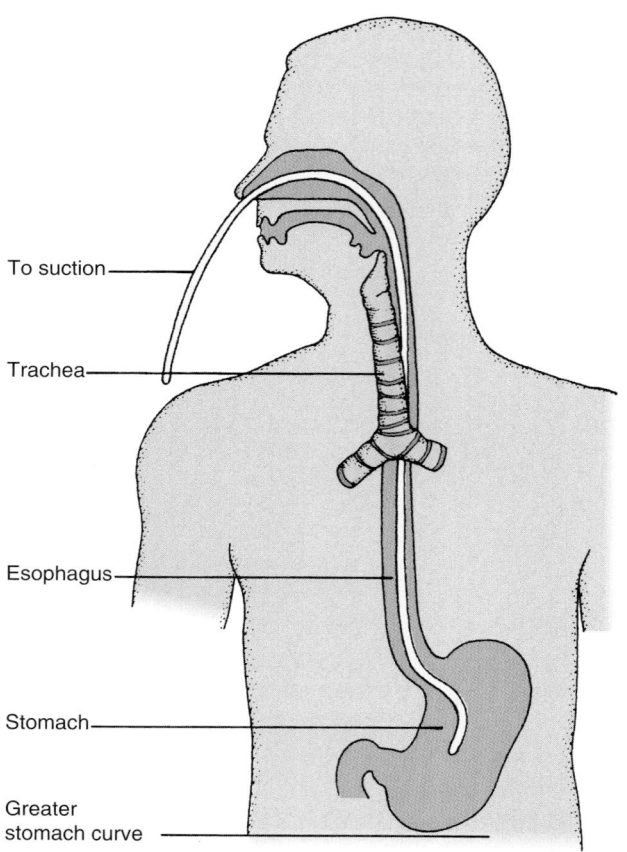

To suction

Trachea

Esophagus

Stomach

Greater
stomach curve

FIGURE 41-6   Proper placement of the nasogastric tube.

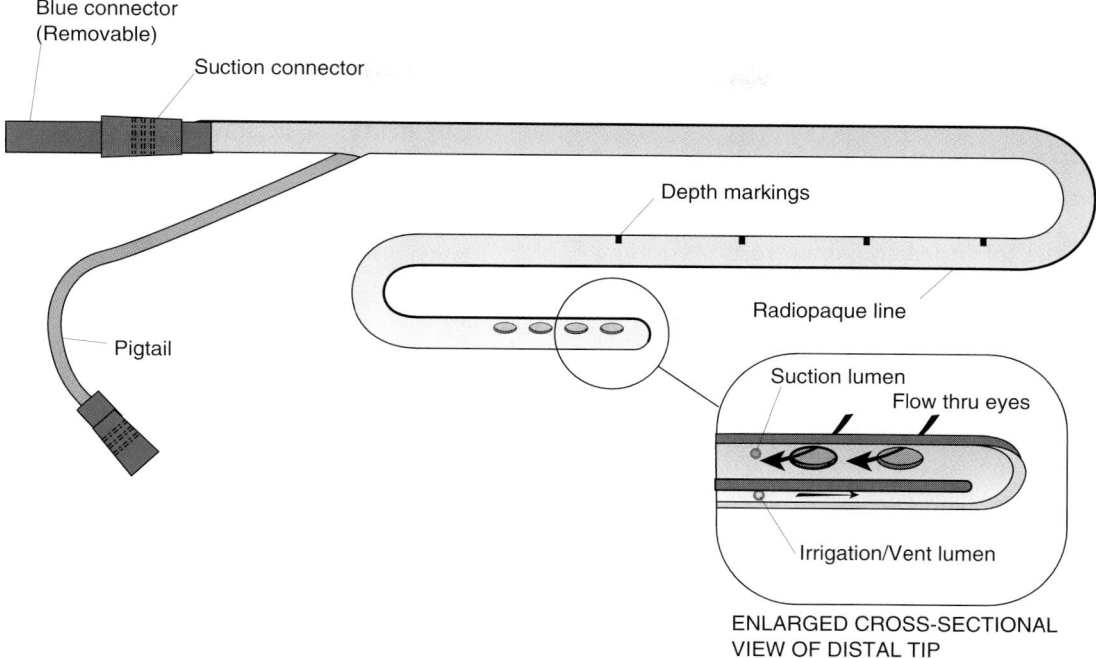

Blue connector
(Removable)

Suction connector

Depth markings

Radiopaque line

Pigtail

Suction lumen
Flow thru eyes

Irrigation/Vent lumen

ENLARGED CROSS-SECTIONAL
VIEW OF DISTAL TIP

FIGURE 41-7 Double-lumen gastric sump tube. (Courtesy of National Catheter Co., Argyle, NY.)

mercury after the tip of the tube has passed through the nose and into the stomach.

Nasointestinal tubes are inserted in the same manner as nasogastric tubes. When the tip of the tube has reached the stomach, the tubing is not taped to the client's nose. The client can be positioned on the right side, allowing gravity and the mercury bag to enhance passage of the tube into the duodenum. In a few hours, passage of the tube into the small intestine should be verified by radiography. If the tube has not advanced on its own, it can be advanced manually from the stomach into the duodenum under fluoroscopy by the healthcare provider or radiologist. Client activity, position changes in bed, and ambulation encourage increased intestinal peristalsis and self-advancement of the tube along the length of the intestine. Markings along the length of the tube help to estimate progress of the tube through the intestine.

Nasointestinal tubes can be attached to a bag positioned below the client's torso to achieve drainage of intestinal contents by gravity. Suction, either continuous or intermittent, can also be applied, and contents can be emptied into a collecting device.

Suction. Subatmospheric or negative pressure is applied to nasogastric tubes to pull air or fluid out of the stomach. Most healthcare facilities have wall outlet suction at the client's bedside. A suction regulator is inserted into the wall unit. The suction gauge can be set at a specific pressure: 20 to 40 mm Hg is low suction; 80 to 120 mm Hg is high suction. Suction can be regulated as continuous or intermittent.

Intermittent suction provides for suction at preset time intervals—up to 60 seconds—followed by set intervals of no suction. In the home or healthcare facilities without wall outlet suction, portable suction units are available. These portable units usually provide only for intermittent suction at a "low" or "high" setting.

Continuous suction greater than 25 mm Hg can lead to irritation of the gastric mucosa if the mucosa are inadvertently "sucked" against one of the openings at the tip of the nasogastric tube. The blue air vent of a double-lumen sump tube is designed to minimize gastric irritation associated with suction pressure; the blue air vent is left open to the air, allowing air under atmospheric pressure to flow continually into the stomach. As long as the air vent is patent, air will continuously irrigate the distal tip of the tube, keeping the gastric mucosa from tightly adhering to the larger outlets of the suction lumen. To be effective as an air vent, the pigtail must be kept at a level above the client's stomach; otherwise, gravity allows gastric contents to flow out of the air vent. Whenever gastric contents or the irrigation fluid enters the air vent, it must be cleared with 5 to 10 mL of air to reestablish air irrigation. Some gastric sump tubes come with an antireflux valve. When the antireflux valve is firmly in place in the blue air vent of the double-lumen sump tube, spillage of gastric contents from the blue pigtail is prevented regardless of pigtail position. Low continuous suction (30 to 40 mm Hg) is recommended for double-lumen tubes, but it may be increased as needed to stimulate flow of gastric contents.

Nursing Considerations

Ensuring Accurate Placement. Accurate placement of the tube is important for client safety. Before inserting the tube, explain its purpose and let the client know that discomfort may be felt as the tube passes along the back of the throat (initiating the gag reflex). Clients usually experience transient nausea, and some clients vomit at this point. Once the tip of the tube passes the gag reflex, the client can assist in advancing the tube down the esophagus by swallowing. With each client swallow, gently guide the tube to the predetermined mark (Procedure 41-3).

🥛 SAFETY ALERT
Accurate placement is verified by performing a radiography study, aspirating gastric contents, and auscultating the left upper quadrant with a stethoscope for a "burp" as 10 to 20 mL of air is instilled by syringe into the tube.

Research by Metheny and colleagues (1994) indicates that visualization and pH testing of the stomach aspirate are the preferred method to ascertain accurate placement. Radiographic confirmation is used when a feeding tube is placed.

Maintaining Suction. Maintaining suction is important when nasogastric tubes are used for gastric decompression. Use the least suction pressure that will achieve successful drainage, check the suction gauges every 4 hours for proper setting, and observe the drainage tubing every hour to make sure that gastrointestinal contents are flowing in the direction of the collection container. To test suction, temporarily disconnect the tubing at the junction between the nasogastric and drainage tubing to hear the "whoosh" of suction and feel the suction at your fingertip. Replace any nonfunctioning suction units.

Maintaining Tube Patency. Tube patency is important to ensure proper functioning of the inserted tube. Occasionally, thick or solid particles of gastrointestinal contents plug the holes of a nasogastric or nasointestinal tube. The tube then ceases to drain gastrointestinal contents, even with properly functioning suction. When a tube clogs, minimal drainage appears in the tubing or collecting receptacle. The client may begin to complain of nausea, which does not occur with a properly functioning system. The abdomen may appear distended.

The nurse can irrigate the tube with about 20 mL of water to dislodge particles or viscous gastrointestinal contents from the tip of the tube. When large volumes of irrigant are instilled, such as during gastric lavage, normal saline solution should be used to prevent fluid and electrolyte shifts that can occur when a hypotonic solution is used.

Nasogastric irrigation is a clean rather than a sterile procedure, because the gastrointestinal tract is not sterile. A physician's order is required for irrigation after gastric surgery. When irrigating a double-lumen nasogastric tube, the nurse can instill irrigant in either lumen. If using the blue air vent, do not disconnect suction during irrigation, but *always* remember to clear the air vent with 10 mL of air after the procedure. Air clears the blue lumen of fluid and restores continuous air irrigation.

If a tube does not appear to be draining well even after irrigation, its placement may need to be checked. To do this, the nurse slightly advances or, alternatively, pulls back on the tube and assesses for any increase in drainage. Changing the client's position sometimes improves nasogastric drainage.

Monitoring Intake and Output. Intake and output (including the volume, color, and type of gastrointestinal drainage) are assessed and recorded every 8 hours. Gastrointestinal contents contain essential body fluids and electrolytes, including water, hydrogen (H^+), potassium (K^+), sodium (Na^+), chloride (Cl^-), bicarbonate (HCO_3^-), and magnesium (Mg^{++}). Losing too many fluids and electrolytes can lead to fluid volume deficit and metabolic acid–base imbalances. In addition, a client with a nasogastric or nasointestinal tube for decompression is usually NPO. Any fluids swallowed would be immediately returned by way of the tube; any food swallowed would eventually clog the tube. Clients with nasogastric or nasointestinal tubes will receive intravenous therapy to supply needed fluids and electrolytes. It is the responsibility of the nurse to measure and record all intake and output and to monitor fluid and electrolyte status.

Some protocols require testing the pH of the stomach aspirate. Very acidic stomach contents (pH < 3.5) can be very corrosive to the stomach lining and to the esophagus if aspiration occurs (Burrell, Gerlach & Pless, 1997). An antacid or histamine blocker can be administered to make the stomach contents less acidic.

Providing Nasal and Oral Care. Nasal and oral care is an important nursing concern during a client's intubation. Skin irritation and breakdown at the nares (nostrils) can be prevented by appropriately taping the tube and providing frequent skin care. Applying a water-soluble lubricant to the nostrils provides moisturizing relief to dry skin.

🥛 SAFETY ALERT
Use of an oil-based lubricant (e.g., petroleum jelly) can inadvertently result in aspiration of oil particles into the lungs, leading to lipid pneumonia.

To prevent constant tension and pulling on the tube, secure the tube to the client's gown (channeling it through tape and securing with a safety pin). Ensure enough slack so the client can turn the head from side to side without pulling on the tubing.

Frequent oral hygiene can prevent the consequence of dry mouth associated with nasogastric intubation. Clients usually become mouth breathers with a tube in the nose. Sucking on ice chips or hard candies, if approved by the healthcare provider, can also provide some relief.

Encourage clients who can brush their teeth to do so frequently. An oral swab soaked in a solution of one-half water and one-half mouthwash is refreshing to many clients. Use of lemon-glycerin oral swabs or swabs soaked in full-strength mouthwash should be avoided. The immediate relief provided by the swab is sometimes followed by rebound dryness. Offer lubricant for the lips to prevent drying and cracking.

Administering Medication. Although usually clients with gastric decompression receive parenteral medications, medication intended for oral consumption may be administered through a nasogastric tube. A liquid form of the medication is preferred, but many tablets can be crushed, mixed with water, and safely administered through the tube. All nasogastric medication administration should be followed with water to clear the tube

(text continues on page 1131)

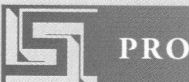

PROCEDURE 41-3

INSERTING A NASOGASTRIC TUBE

Purpose
1. Decompresses the stomach to relieve pressure and prevent vomiting.
2. Provides a means for irrigating the stomach (lavage).
3. Provides access to gastric specimens for laboratory analysis.
4. Provides a route for delivering liquid enteral feedings (gavage) in clients who can't swallow or ingest adequate calorie intake.

Assessment
- Identify client's need for nasogastric intubation and type of tube to be placed.
- Assess client's mental status and ability to understand and cooperate with procedure.
- Review medical history for nosebleeds, deviated septum, nasal surgery.
- Assess nostrils for size, lesions, obstructions, or deformities. *Note:* Have client breathe through one nostril while occluding the other. The tube should be inserted through the most patent nostril.

Equipment
Nasogastric tube of appropriate size (Adult: 14–18 Fr, Infant/child: 5–10 Fr)
Small-bore feeding tube with guide wire if used for enteral feedings
Water-soluble lubricant
20- to 50-mL syringe with catheter tip or adapter
Glass of tap water with straw
Towel, stethoscope, disposable gloves
Hypoallergenic tape

Procedure
1. Identify client and explain procedure. Insertion is not painful, but it is uncomfortable because the gag reflex is usually stimulated.
   Rationale: Client is more cooperative when the procedure is understood.
2. Provide privacy by closing curtains or room door. Raise bed to high-Fowler's position, cover chest with towel, and place emesis basin nearby.
   Rationale: Elevated head protects against aspiration.

3. Wash hands, and put on gloves. Determine length of tubing to be inserted by measuring nasogastric tube from tip of ear lobe to tip of nose, then to tip of xyphoid process. Mark tubing with adhesive tape or note striped markings already on the tube.
   Rationale: This measure determines approximate length of esophagus from nares to stomach, which varies among clients.

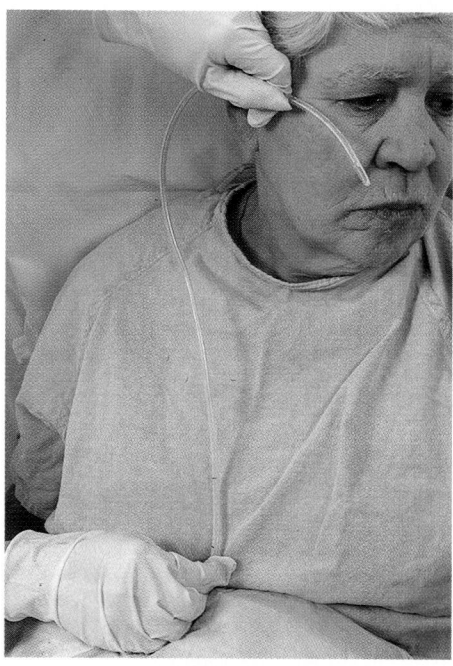

Step 3 Measure proper tube length to insert.

4. Lubricate tip of tube with water-soluble lubricant.
   Rationale: A water-soluble lubricant will be reabsorbed if tube inadvertently enters the lung. Do not use an oil-based lubricant because respiratory complications may occur if aspirated.
5. Gently insert tube into nostril. Advance toward posterior pharynx.
   Rationale: Following natural contour prevents trauma to nasal mucosa.
6. Have client tilt head forward and encourage client to drink water slowly. Advance tube without using force as client swallows. Advance tube until desired insertion length is reached.

PROCEDURE 41-3 (Continued)

Rationale: Forward tilt of head facilitates passage of tube into esophagus and not the larynx. Swallowing moves epiglottis over the larynx and facilitates tube passage.

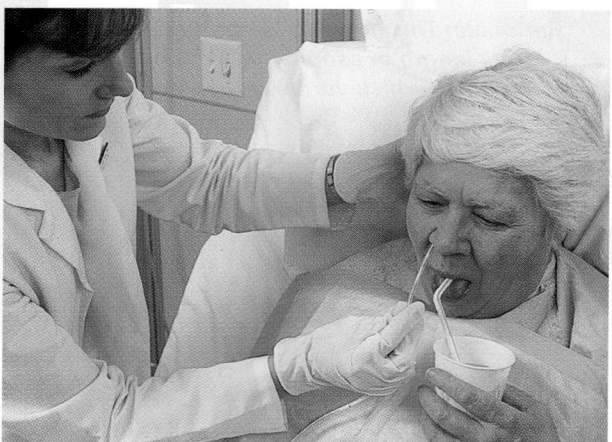

Step 6 Advance tube as client swallows water.

7. Temporarily tape the tube to the client's nose; then assess placement of the tube:
   a. Aspirate gastric content with 20- to 50-mL syringe and test pH.
      Rationale: Gastric content is yellow to green and usually present in amounts greater than 10 mL; pH is acidic.
   b. Auscultate over epigastrium while injecting 10 to 20 mL air into nasogastric tube.

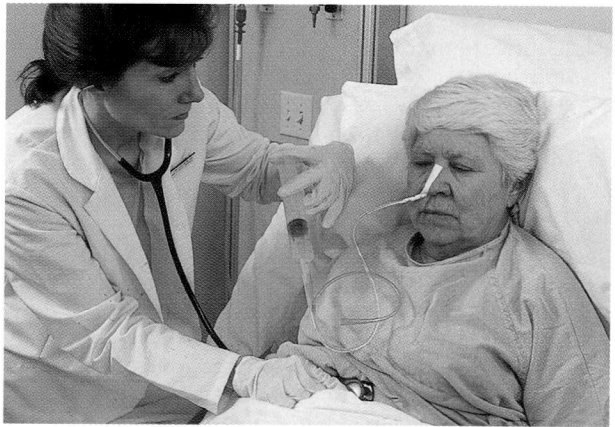

Step 7 Check proper tube placement.

Rationale: Bubbling is heard if tube is in stomach.
   c. If feeding tube is placed, x-ray confirmation of placement is required before day feeding is administered.
8. If placement in stomach is not verified, untape tube, advance tube 5 cm, and repeat assessment in Step 7.
9. Secure tube by taping to bridge of client's nose. Anchor tubing to client's gown.
   Rationale: Correct taping prevents the tube from dislodging or pulling and traumatizing the nostril.

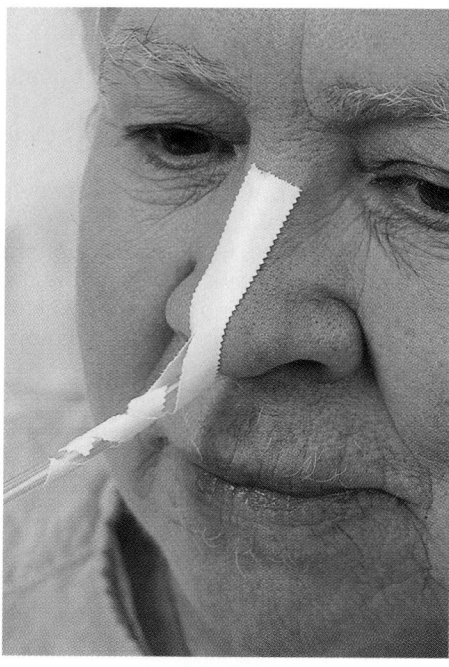

Step 9 Securely fasten tube to nose.

10. Clamp end of tubing or attach to suction, as ordered by healthcare provider.
    Rationale: Suction facilitates drainage.
11. Wash hands, provide for client's comfort, and remove equipment.
12. Establish and document a nursing plan for daily care of the nasogastric tube:
    a. Inspect nostril for irritation.
    b. Cleanse nostril frequently.
    c. Change adhesive as required to prevent skin irritation or pressure sores on nostril from the tube.

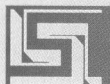

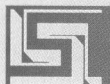

PROCEDURE 41-3 (Continued)

d. Increase frequency of oral care because clients with nasogastric tubes often mouth breathe and may be NPO.

Lifespan Considerations
• Measure tube length from the tip of the nose to the ear lobe, then to point halfway between xyphoid process and umbilicus.

Collaboration and Delegation
• Know that in some healthcare facilities, physicians insert nasogastric tubes. Teach unlicensed assistive personnel how to provide oral and nasal care and empty the suction catheter.

and ensure that the medication has reached the stomach. This is especially important when small-bore feeding tubes are used, because they can clog easily. During gastric decompression, discontinue suction before administering the medication, and keep the tube clamped for 30 minutes afterward to permit absorption by way of the gastric mucosa.

Fecal Impaction Removal

Removal of fecal impactions is a nursing responsibility. Manual removal of an impaction can be embarrassing for the client. Explain the purpose and necessity of the procedure, telling the client before beginning what will be done. Proceed in a matter-of-fact manner to reduce anxiety and embarrassment for the client.

The equipment necessary for manual removal of fecal impaction includes plenty of disposable gloves, a gown, packets of water-soluble lubricant, several disposable underpads to protect the bed and floor, two bedpans, and a commode if the client is capable of transferring to it. It is possible for the large intestine to distend to hold a large amount of stool. Because the nurse cannot accurately predict the volume before beginning the procedure, it is best to be prepared to remove a large quantity of stool. Also, wear an impermeable or disposable gown, because some stool is likely to spill or splash during the procedure. The odor of the stool can be strong, and an open window or other form of ventilation should be provided.

Begin the procedure with the client in the side-lying position. Then insert a double-gloved, lubricated index finger into the rectum. With a gentle hooking motion of the index finger, remove some of the stool from the rectum.

SAFETY ALERT
Be careful when using the hooking motion during normal disimpaction. Perforation of the rectum can occur.

The removal of stool begins slowly, but as the hardened stool that is blocking the lumen of the rectum is removed, the remaining stool may pass more quickly. The bedpan should be ready to place under the client so that he or she can evacuate stool into it if possible; the stool may come so quickly that the client is unable to control its evacuation. Weak clients with poor muscle tone may require assistance. Continue to remove stool manually until you can no longer feel stool at the fingertip and the client is not voluntarily evacuating any more stool. Remove and dispose of collected stool and soiled linens, and provide hygiene care for the client. Removal of a fecal impaction is a tiring procedure for the client, so provide the client with some uninterrupted time and a restful environment

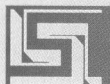

APPLY YOUR KNOWLEDGE

You are caring for a postoperative client who had colon surgery 2 days ago. During report, you are told that he has a nasogastric tube, which drained 350 cc of thick, green, mucus-filled liquid during the last shift. When you obtain your morning assessment, it reveals the following: vital signs stable, pain 6 on a 1–10 scale (client frequently using patient-controlled analgesia), absent bowel sounds, no abdominal distention, some complaint of nausea, NG to low suction, no drainage in the suction container. What, if any, actions are indicated at this time, based on your assessment?

Check your answer in Appendix A.

after the procedure. Reassessment and redisimpaction may be necessary for some clients.

Nursing interventions to prevent complications in the management of fecal impaction include effective yet gentle insertion of the gloved index finger into the client's rectum when performing digital examination and manual removal of stool.

SAFETY ALERT

Excess vagal stimulation during digital rectal examination and removal of stool can precipitate cardiac dysrhythmias in weak clients or those with cardiovascular disease. Forceful pressure against the rectal mucosa can damage the bowel tissue.

Bowel Training

A long-term approach to control of bowel elimination may be necessary, especially for clients who are in the rehabilitation phase of a neurologic impairment (e.g., paralysis, stroke, head injury). These clients are at high risk for constipation or fecal incontinence, or both. Bowel training is not appropriate for clients with inflammatory bowel disease, infection, or lactose intolerance.

A standard bowel-training program aims to maintain a soft stool consistency and develop a routine method of stool evacuation. The routine is repeated at the same time each day with the same techniques, to train and control the bowel's evacuation time. An example of a standard bowel-training program for neurologically impaired clients appears in Fig. 41-8.

A common bowel-training program includes use of a stool softener twice a day, a bulking agent daily, and a suppository

(glycerin or bisacodyl [Dulcolax]), usually given after breakfast, followed by toileting and digital stimulation. Bowel training may require weeks to months of persistence before success is attained. Reassurance and verbal expressions of confidence in the client contribute to success of the program. Client teaching about normal bowel function and factors to promote a soft stool is helpful.

For clients with anal sphincter control that is weak but not lost, a variation of the classic bowel-training program is implemented. Stool softeners and an increase in dietary fiber are used to maintain a soft stool, but instead of relying on the routine use of suppositories and digital stimulation, emphasis is placed on the client's recognizing the body's own defecation signals. Careful assessment and documentation of incontinent episodes are performed for several days. From then on, the client is assisted to the toilet at a time that has been identified as "routine." The time often coincides with a duodenocolic mass movement after eating. The intent is to establish a regular defecation time in synchrony with the client's natural physiologic function.

Pelvic floor exercises, biofeedback, and abdominal massage have been used by some healthcare providers to promote regular stool evacuation. When performing pelvic floor exercises, the client alternately contracts and relaxes anal sphincter and puborectal muscles 25 to 30 times three times a day for a brief period (3 or 4 seconds).

Biofeedback is used to help clients recognize rectal distention and to provide a visual cue as to the effectiveness of pelvic muscle contraction. Abdominal massage stimulates peristalsis. The abdomen is massaged starting at the right iliac fossa, moving along the large colon and proceeding from the ascending to the transverse and descending colon.

Date	Time	Related Meal or Fluid	Time and Type of Suppository	Comments: How, Where, Level of Independence
8/10	0800	Breakfast containing fiber	0830 Suppository with digital stimulation	Can transfer independently to bedside commode

1. Time bowel movement to occur 20 to 30 minutes after eating a meal or at least drinking some warm fluid.
2. Begin program by inserting a well-lubricated suppository past the external and internal anal sphincters.
3. 0 to 20 minutes after inserting suppository, transfer patient to commode or toilet (unless the program is to be done in bed).
4. At 15-minute intervals starting approximately 30 minutes after suppository insertion, perform rectal massage or digital stimulation. This is done by gently inserting a well-lubricated, gloved finger into the anal canal. Then, using a gentle circular motion, the rectal wall is stretched to help stimulate the defecation reflex. The rectal stretching must be done gently and slowly to prevent trauma and to allow enough stimuli for the reflex emptying to occur.

FIGURE 41-8   Classic bowel-training program.

Sensory retraining is a new method to help clients achieve control over fecal incontinence. This training, often done in an outpatient setting, involves three stages: increased recognition of the stimulus, exercises to increase maximal voluntary squeeze in the perianal area, and ability to coordinate external sphincter control (Bentsen & Braun, 1996). A Foley catheter is inserted into the rectum so that balloon inflation can mimic rectal distention from stool. Nurse practitioners are frequently involved in providing sensory retraining to incontinent clients.

Fecal Collection During Incontinence

If bowel training is unsuccessful or fecal incontinence is considered intractable, a drainable fecal collector may be used. The drainable fecal collector is similar to an ostomy appliance. It consists of a collecting pouch and a skin-protective barrier designed to adhere firmly to the perineum, anal cleft, and inner surfaces of the buttocks. If a formed stool collects in the pouch, the drainage outlet can be cut off with scissors, the stool emptied, and the end of the pouch resealed with a plastic clamp.

Just as diapers are considered appropriate management for the infant or child who is not toilet trained, protective pants, called incontinence briefs, are sometimes used for intractable fecal incontinence in the adult. Such absorbent pads wick liquid stool away from the skin better than plastic-coated underpads do (Haugen, 1997). Shear force and trauma when cleansing the area should be avoided.

Stoma Management

Stoma management consists of a group of nursing interventions that may be necessary after fecal diversion surgery. Nursing responsibilities for clients with stomas include stoma assessment and management of feces collection by way of an ostomy appliance or through stoma irrigation. Many healthcare facilities have enterostomal therapists, nurses with specialized training, to assist clients and to support other nurses in the care of clients with fecal diversions.

Stoma Assessment. After surgery, the stoma and abdominal incision may be covered with a sterile dressing. When removing the dressing or when changing appliances over the stoma, the nurse should assess the stoma for color and position. Ideally, the stoma should be a healthy pink; a dusky pink or bluish tint (cyanosis) suggests inadequate circulation to the stoma. The stomal mucosa must remain on the abdominal surface. If the stoma retracts, feces may potentially enter the abdominal cavity and cause peritonitis. Prolapse can also occur and should be reported to the surgeon (Erwin-Toth, 2001). The stoma should also be inspected for bleeding and drainage. Some bleeding may occur, because the stoma tissues are fragile.

Fecal Collection. Clients with ileostomies or colostomies that continuously drain liquid stool need an ostomy appliance (pouch or bag) over the stoma at all times. A large selection of ostomy appliances is commercially available; a common type of ostomy pouch is featured in Fig. 41-9. Usually when the enterostomal therapist (ET) visits a new ostomy client, he

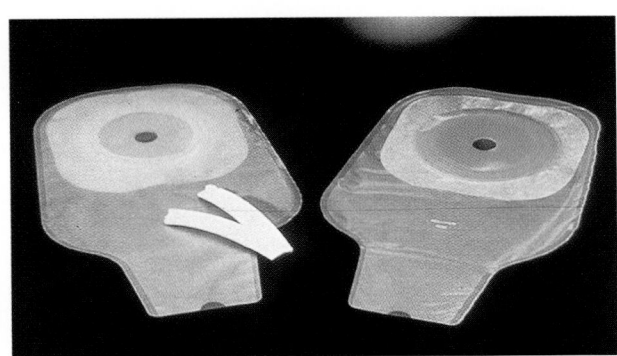

FIGURE 41-9   One-piece drainable ostomy pouch with clamp. (Courtesy of Hollister, Inc., Libertyville, IL.)

or she inspects the condition of the stoma and discusses the methods for feces collection. The diameter of the stoma must be measured accurately for an appliance with the correctly sized opening to obtain proper fit.

🥛 SAFETY ALERT

An opening that is too small may constrict the stoma and restrict circulation, whereas an opening that is too large will allow stool to leak onto the abdominal skin.

The enzymatic juices contained in the liquid stool will cause maceration and eventual skin breakdown. The back surface of the ostomy appliance contains a sticky substance that adheres to the abdominal skin. Also, the appliance is usually taped for extra security.

The ostomy pouch should be emptied of fecal contents when it is about one-fourth to one-third full. If the pouch becomes too full, the weight of fecal contents will disrupt the pouch seal, causing the stool to leak. The odor of the stool may be strong and offensive, especially to the client with a new stoma. In such cases, the nurse can open the window or spray a deodorant in the room before emptying the pouch. The bottom of the pouch has an opening secured by a clip, which is removed to empty the pouch into the toilet. The appliance can also be emptied into a bedpan if the client cannot get out of bed. As with all procedures in which the nurse handles feces or other bodily fluids, disposable gloves are worn.

Emptying an ostomy pouch is a clean, not a sterile, procedure. The pouch should be rinsed with clean, warm tap water after emptying. A large (60-mL) syringe works well for this purpose. Air is eliminated by compressing the pouch and reapplying the clip to close the pouch. Then, the pouch is checked for leaks from the stomal area, and the condition of the stoma is assessed. If the ostomy appliance leaks fecal contents where it is attached to the skin, the entire bag needs to be removed and replaced. The nurse or client cleanses the abdominal skin surrounding the stoma, inspects the stoma's appearance, gently dries the abdominal skin, and applies a new ostomy pouch. The latter process is described in Procedure 41-4.

(text continues on page 1136)

⑤ PROCEDURE 41-4

APPLYING A FECAL OSTOMY POUCH

Purpose
1. Contains drainage and odors for the comfort of the client and allows accurate assessment of output.
2. Protects the peristomal skin from excoriation.
3. Provides visualization of the stoma and sutures during the postoperative period.

Assessment
- Observe color and amount of drainage from stoma.
- Assess existing pouch for leakage, and note appearance of stoma and incision to determine need to change pouch. A pouch does not have to be changed if it is not leaking and if the skin barrier is intact.
- Inspect condition of peristomal skin for erythema, excoriation, ulceration, or fistulas before selecting type of skin barrier to apply.
- Note presence of skinfolds, creases, scars, and abdominal softness or firmness before selecting pouch.

Equipment
A clean, drainable pouch and clamp, skin barrier, and disposable gloves
Warm water, wash cloth and towel, mild soap
Plastic disposal bag for old pouch
Hypoallergenic paper tape

Procedure
1. Identify client and provide privacy.
   Don disposable gloves. The client may perform the procedure without gloves, as shown in the photos accompanying this procedure.
   Rationale: Prevents transmission of microorganisms to others.
2. Gently remove old appliance. If disposable, discard. If reusable, set aside for washing.
   Rationale: Maintains skin integrity.
3. Wash skin thoroughly around stoma with skin cleanser or soap and water.
   Rationale: Bacteria in the fecal secretions can cause infection in the incisional area and irritate the skin.
4. Rinse skin thoroughly and blot dry.
   Rationale: Soap residue or dampness can interfere with pouch adhesion, resulting in leakage. Blotting the area dry minimizes trauma to the stoma.

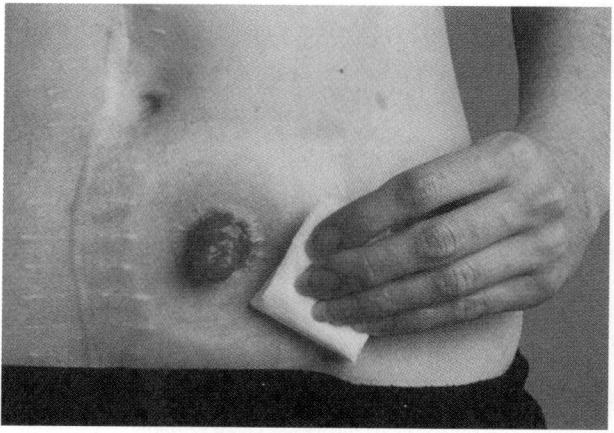

Step 4 Wash area around stoma and pat dry.

5. Observe condition of peristomal skin, the stoma, and the sutures. Teach the client to make these observations daily.
   Rationale: Observation allows monitoring for complications. The stoma is at risk for necrosis during the first postoperative week, as evidenced by dark color and lack of bleeding. The peristomal skin is at risk for breakdown from irritating fecal secretions. Infection is more easily corrected if detected early.
6. Prepare clean pouch: measure stoma and trace circle ⅛ inch larger than stoma on the adhesive paper backing. Cut the stoma pattern.

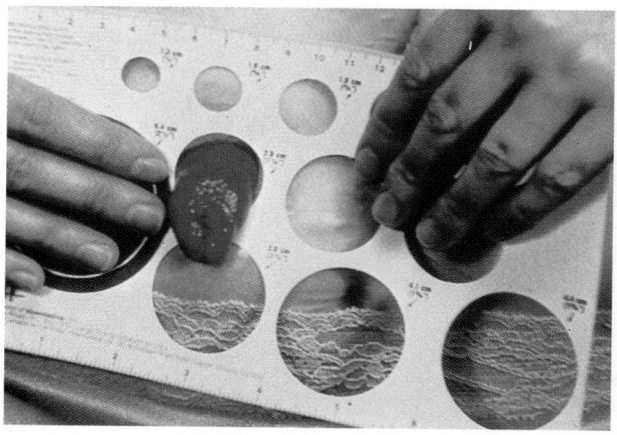

Step 6 Measure stoma size to ensure proper fit. *Note:* Prolapsed stoma is not normal, and should be reported to the surgeon. (Courtesy of Hollister, Inc., Libertyville, IL.)

PROCEDURE 41-4 (Continued)

Rationale: Pattern cut slightly larger than barrier avoids risk of paper cuts to stoma and ensures a tight seal with the barrier.

7. Prepare skin barrier: measure stoma and cut hole in barrier the same size as the stoma. Be sure edges are rounded.
Rationale: Close fit of barrier around stoma prevents fecal secretions from contacting and irritating the skin.

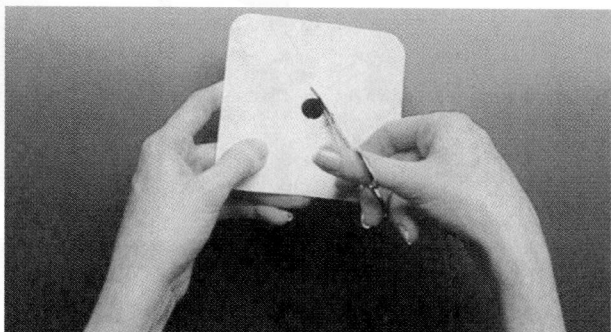

Step 7 Cut wafer to proper size.

8. If stoma is located in an abdominal crease or the skin is irregular, use a paste barrier to fill the irregularity.
Rationale: Minimizes leakage by providing a smooth surface for applying the skin barrier.
9. Apply protective skin barrier.
   a. Peel paper backing off wafer and center stoma in hole.
   b. Place on abdomen, pressing lightly over all areas of the barrier to promote adhesion with skin surfaces.
   Rationale: A tight fit will prevent leaking and protect the skin underlying the appliance.

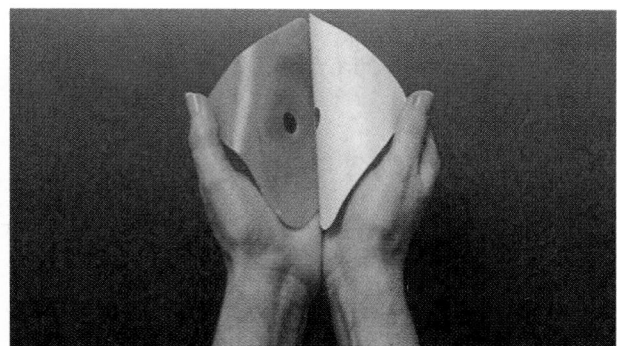

Step 9A Remove backing from skin barrier.

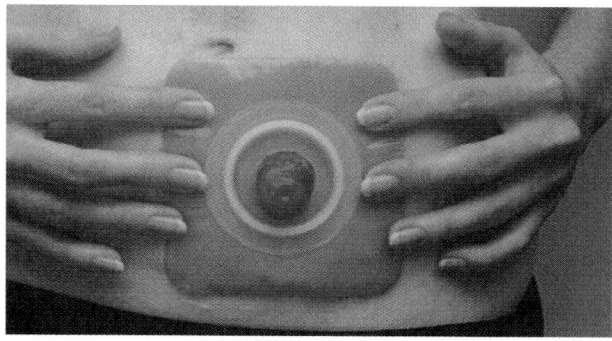

Step 9B Center hole over stoma and apply light pressure to ensure adherence to skin.

10. Attach drainable pouch to skin barrier. Some equipment attaches by means of a plastic flange that snaps in place; other models adhere through self-adherent tape that is exposed after protective paper backing is removed. Tug gently or inspect for secure fit.
Rationale: If pouch is not securely attached to protective barrier, leakage could occur, especially as weight from collected feces increases.

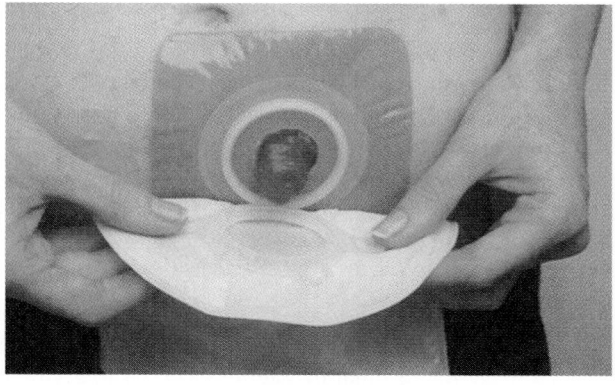

Step 10 Apply drainable pouch to skin barrier.

11. Frame every edge of the faceplate with hypoallergenic tape. This is called "picture framing."
Rationale: Provides reinforcement so bag will not separate.
12. Fold over bottom edge of pouch and clamp.
Rationale: Prevents stool from leaking.
13. Dispose of old appliance. Clean and store any reusable supplies. Wash hands. Document noted observations.

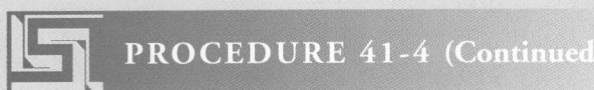

PROCEDURE 41-4 (Continued)

Rationale: Maintains infection control standards and communicates with health team members.

Lifespan Considerations

• Keep in mind that the very young and the elderly often are not able to perform their own ostomy care. Any client who is not able to change his or her pouch independently should have a caregiver instructed in this procedure.
• Assess for postoperative necrosis of the stoma, which occurs more commonly in obese clients. Notify the healthcare provider immediately if this is seen.
• New ostomy clients often experience the stages of grief as they try to adjust to their new body image.
• Young children and infants adjust more readily to lifestyle changes from ostomies than do adolescents and adults.

Home Care Modifications

• Teach spouses or other family members to assist with ostomy management, especially if the client is elderly, weak, or has poor fine motor skills.
• Provide good nurse–client communication to help the client develop a positive attitude about living with an ostomy.
• Provide the client with the name and phone number of an enterostomal therapist, community support groups, supply vendor, and other resource people to call if they have questions or problems after discharge.

Collaboration and Delegation

• Enterostomal therapist (ET) provides initial instruction and often follows client on an outpatient basis.
• Consult with ET so you can reinforce teaching and coordinate the plan.

If the ostomy is continuously draining fecal material, the pouch change will need to be quick and well planned. A sterile or clean gauze 4- × 4-inch pad may be placed temporarily over the stoma to collect a small amount of fecal contents as the skin is dried and the new pouch is secured.

Stomal Irrigation. Bowel training to achieve a predictable evacuation of stool from a sigmoid colostomy can be assisted by stomal irrigation. Stomal irrigation is similar to giving a large-volume enema through the stomal opening instead of through the anus. More specialized equipment is necessary, but the principle of instilling fluid into the colon to cause distention and resultant elimination is the same. Because stomal irrigation is essentially an enema, it can be administered to relieve constipation or to cleanse the bowel before diagnostic procedures or tests.

Figure 41-10 shows typical irrigation equipment, including an irrigating sleeve with belt and a water container connected to an irrigating catheter with cone and lubricant. The evacuation of the colon at predictable times allows the client a sense of control over his or her body and environment. Clients who have sigmoid ostomies and who have achieved reliable bowel training may not need to wear a fecal collection pouch at all times. Some can wear a specialized covering over the stoma between bowel evacuations. The covering protects the stoma from irritation by clothing.

Continent Fecal Diversion Management. The client with an ileoanal reservoir is taught Kegel exercises before surgery to strengthen the perineal muscles. When the ileoanal reservoir begins to function, the client may have 10 to 20 loose stools

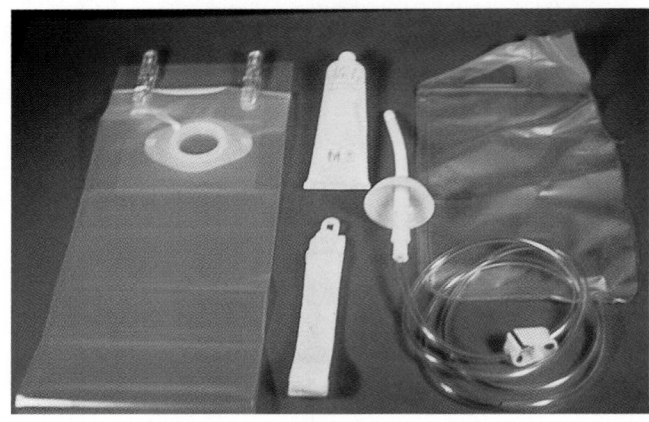

FIGURE 41-10   Colostomy irrigation equipment. (Courtesy of Hollister, Inc., Libertyville, IL.)

per day, but the number will decrease as the reservoir builds up capacity and the sphincter muscles strengthen.

The client with a Kock pouch will need to learn how to drain the pouch of feces by passing a catheter through the surgically created one-way valve. Scheduled evacuation of the pouch should be planned to avoid overdistention.

Healthcare Planning and Home or Community-Based Care

To develop a teaching plan that meets the client's unique needs, consider features of the client's home environment that could affect optimal bowel management. For example,

- Does the client have adequate access to toilet facilities?
- If the client has to use a walker or wheelchair for mobility, will these devices fit through the bathroom doorway?
- Are there any steps that need to be negotiated to get to the bathroom?
- Is there someone available to assist the person to the bathroom or with special interventions such as enema administration?
- Would the use of a bedside commode at home help a person with mobility or access problems prevent fecal incontinence?
- Are there any financial constraints?
- Does the client have health insurance, and does it cover the necessary medications or special equipment?

If the assessment data disclose potential problems with financial or social support resources, a social worker should be consulted as soon as possible. The social worker is knowledgeable about the many community agencies available for assistance and can begin contacting the community agencies that will best meet the client's unique needs.

Clients or their families may need assistance and advice in managing specialized equipment and techniques. The clients with a recent ostomy (known as an **ostomate**) and the client at high risk for fecal incontinence particularly need assistance in home management of their bowel alterations. ETs are often responsible for most client education about ostomy care; however, the home health nurse must reinforce the concepts of stoma management and be available to answer questions.

The client can be referred to ostomy organizations within the community. Usually, a member of an ostomy organization who also has an ostomy, and who has satisfactorily adjusted to the necessary lifestyle changes, visits with the new ostomate. The first visit can be arranged before hospital discharge, or it can occur when the client is at home. The "old" ostomate can be a source of support and advice for the "new" ostomate.

Diarrhea is still a leading cause of death worldwide among children younger than 4 years of age (World Health Organization, 2001). However, it and many other acute and chronic bowel problems can be managed in the home setting under the supervision of a healthcare provider. The viral and bacterial infections that cause severe diarrhea and that predispose the person to severe fluid volume deficit can be controlled as well. In such cases, adequate fluid replacement with rehydrating solutions containing electrolytes is important. Fortunately, various world relief organizations provide rehydrating solutions to decrease mortality from diarrhea. In developed countries, solutions such as Pedialyte or Gatorade can be purchased and used in the home during acute episodes of diarrhea. Hygiene teaching, especially good handwashing practice, is important in preventing transmission of microorganisms that cause diarrhea.

EVALUATION

Evaluation includes assessing the client and comparing the client's current condition with established outcomes as a measure of attainment. Continuation, modification, or termination of the plan of care is implemented based on the systematic evaluation of client progress.

Examples of outcome criteria are listed here. Note that some are appropriate for more than one goal. It is important to identify specific outcomes that will most uniquely measure the attainment of the individual client's goal.

Goal

The client will demonstrate a normal pattern of bowel elimination without evidence of constipation, diarrhea, fecal incontinence, or abdominal distention.

Possible Outcome Criteria

- The client experiences a bowel movement within 24 hours and then every other day during rehabilitation.
- The client has a decrease in loose stools from four to five per day to one to two per day within 2 days.
- The client demonstrates a stool consistency changing from liquid to semisoft within 24 hours.
- The client experiences a bowel movement every morning after suppository and digital stimulation during rehabilitation.
- The client has no evidence of hardened stool in the rectum on digital examination during each home visit.

Goal

The client will exhibit no preventable complications or adverse consequences from altered bowel elimination.

Possible Outcome Criteria

- The client's perianal skin remains intact throughout the hospital stay.
- After a teaching session, the client verbalizes the importance of exhaling during defecation.
- Throughout hospitalization, the client washes his or her hands after bowel movements.

Goal

The client will participate in a program to maintain and promote an acceptable pattern of bowel elimination.

NURSING PLAN OF CARE
THE CLIENT WITH CONSTIPATION

Nursing Diagnosis
Constipation related to immobility manifested by straining and inability to pass stool for 3 days.

Client Goal
Client will demonstrate a normal pattern of bowel elimination.

Client Outcome Criteria
Client has a formed brown stool within 24 hours and every 1 to 2 days during rehabilitation.

Nursing Interventions	Scientific Rationale
1. Notify dietitian to increase high-fiber foods in client's meals.	1. High-fiber foods increase the amount of bulk in the lower gastrointestinal tract and result in softer, easier-to-eliminate stools.
2. Increase fluid intake to 2,000 mL/day.	2. A fluid intake of 2,000 mL in 24 hours is necessary to promote the formation of soft stools.
3. Assist client to ambulate (within medically prescribed guidelines) at least three times daily.	3. Increased physical activity promotes increased gastrointestinal motility.
4. Assist client to bedside commode or toilet. Fit commode or toilet with raised seat if needed.	4. The sitting position enlists gravity to promote bowel elimination. A raised seat may be necessary to increase client comfort in sitting.
5. Provide privacy but do not compromise client safety.	5. Many people require a degree of privacy during bowel elimination.
6. Inspect client's abdomen and auscultate for bowel sounds every shift.	6. Inspection and auscultation provide essential data about bowel elimination status.
7. Administer stool softeners and laxatives as necessary per bowel management program.	7. Daily administration of stool softeners can prevent constipation for clients in high-risk groups. Laxatives can stimulate the evacuation of bowel contents on an as-needed basis.
8. Record client's bowel movements in the client's record.	8. Documentation provides essential data about client's current bowel elimination pattern.

Possible Outcome Criteria

- At the next appointment, the client identifies methods to increase dietary fiber.
- The client requests assistance to toilet at scheduled times during the day.
- The client drinks 2000 mL of fluid per day, as evidenced on a chart.
- The client demonstrates correct ostomy bag application by the time of discharge.

KEY CONCEPTS

- Defecation, the process of eliminating feces from the body, is initiated by reflexes in response to intestinal distention.
- Defecation is under voluntary neural control.
- Many lifestyle habits affect stool consistency and the pattern of bowel elimination. Physiologic alterations of the intestines also can adversely affect bowel elimination.
- The characteristics of feces and bowel elimination patterns change during the lifespan.
- Altered bowel elimination can be a source of physiologic, psychological, and social distress.
- The manifestations of altered bowel elimination are constipation, fecal impaction, diarrhea, incontinence, flatulence, and abdominal distention.
- A focused nursing assessment of bowel elimination includes client history, inspection of stool characteristics, and physical examination of the abdomen and perirectal area.
- The nurse has collaborative responsibilities in laboratory analysis of the feces and other diagnostic procedures.
- The nurse can diagnose and collaboratively treat altered bowel elimination. Treatment measures include medications, enemas, rectal tubes, nasogastric intubation, fecal impaction removal, bowel training, fecal collection during incontinence, and stoma care.
- Discharge planning considers the home environment, such as access to facilities, finances, and use of specialized equipment, and the unique learning needs of the client and family.

- Continuation, modification, and termination of nursing strategies are based on systematic evaluation of client response to therapy.

REFERENCES

Abyad, A., & Mourad, F. (1996). Constipation: Common-sense care of the older patient. *Geriatrics, 51*(12), 28–36.

Addison, R. (2000 Oct 5). Fluid intake: How coffee and caffeine affect incontinence. *Nursing Times, 96*(40), 7–8.

Addison, R., Ness W., Abulafi, M., & Swift, I. (2000). How to administer enemas and suppositories. *Nursing Times, 96*(6), 3–4.

American Cancer Society. (2001). Statistics related to colon and rectal cancers. [On-line]. Available at: www.cancer.org. Accessed 1/1/02.

Bentsen, D., & Braun, J. (1996). Controlling fecal incontinence with sensory retraining managed by advanced nurse practice nurses. *Clinical Nurse Specialist, 10*(4), 171–176.

Bliss, D. Z., Johnson, S., Savik, K., Clabots, C. R., & Gerding, D. N. (2000). Fecal incontinence in hospitalized patients who are acutely ill. *Nursing Research, 49*(2), 101–108.

Burrell, L., Gerlach, M. J., & Pless, B. (1997). *Adult nursing: Acute and community care* (2nd ed.). Stamford, CT: Appleton & Lange.

Carpenito, L. J. (2001). *Nursing diagnosis: Application to clinical practice* (9th ed.). Philadelphia: Lippincott-Raven.

Dammel, T. (1997). Fecal occult blood testing. *Nursing 97, 27*(7), 44–45.

Erwin-Toth, P. (2001). Caring for a stoma. *Nursing 2001, 31*(5), 36–40.

Haugen, V. (1997). Perineal skin care for patients with frequent diarrhea or fecal incontinence. *Gastroenterology Nursing, 20*(3), 87–90.

Hinrichs, M. D., & Huseboe, J. (2001). Research-based protocol: Management of constipation. *Journal of Gerontological Nursing, 27*(2), 17–28.

Howard, L. V., West, D., & Ossip-Klein, D. J. (2000 March-Apr.). Chronic constipation management for institutionalized older adults. *Geriatric Nursing, 21*(2), 78–83.

Jarvis, C. (2000). *Physical examination and health assessment* (3rd ed). Philadelphia: Lippincott.

Metcalf, C. (2001, May 10–16). Practical procedures for nurses. Stoma care 5(a): problem solving. *Nursing Times, 97*(19), 43–44.

Metheny, N., Reed, L., & Wehrle, M. (1994). Visual characteristics of aspirates from feeding tubes as a method for predicting tube location. *Nursing Research, 43*(5), 282–287.

Murray, S. (2002). *Foundations of maternal-newborn nursing* (3rd ed.). Philadelphia: Saunders.

North American Nursing Diagnosis Association (NANDA). (2001). *NANDA nursing diagnoses: Definitions and classification, 2001–2002.* Philadelphia: Author.

World Health Organization (2001). Diarrheal diseases and dysentery. [On-line]. Available at: www.who.int. Accessed 1/1/02.

BIBLIOGRAPHY

Ball, E. (2000). A teaching guide for continent ileostomy. *RN 63*(12), 35–40.

Eckes, L., & Norton, B. (1997). Ulcerative colitis: From medical management to ileal pouch anal anastomosis. *Gastroenterology Nursing, 20*(3), 91–100.

Heslin, J. (1997). Peptic ulcer disease: Making a case against the prime suspect. *Nursing '97, 27*(1), 34–39.

Jarrett, M. E., Lustyk, M. K., Cain, K. C. (2000). Exercise across the health continuum. A paradigm shift: Exercise as a therapeutic for women with IBS. *Communicating Nursing Research, 33,* 113.

Martin, F. (1997). Ulcerative colitis: How to manage this chronic inflammatory disease and prevent systemic complication. *American Journal of Nursing, 97*(8), 38–39.

Pontieri-Lewis (2000). Colorectal cancer: Prevention and screening. *MedSurg Nursing 9*(1), 9–13.

Schmieding, N., Waldman, R., & Desaulles, C. (1997). Nasogastric tubes: Insertion placement, and removal in adult patients. *Gastroenterology Nursing, 20*(1), 15–19.

Surratt, S., Ryan, A. B., Hallenbeck, P., et al. (1993). Trouble shooting a sump tube. *American Journal of Nursing, 93*(1), 41–47.

Thompson, J. (2000). A Practical ostomy guide. *RN 63*(11), 61–68.

Wald, A. (1997). Fecal incontinence: Three steps to successful management. *Geriatrics, 52*(7), 44–54.

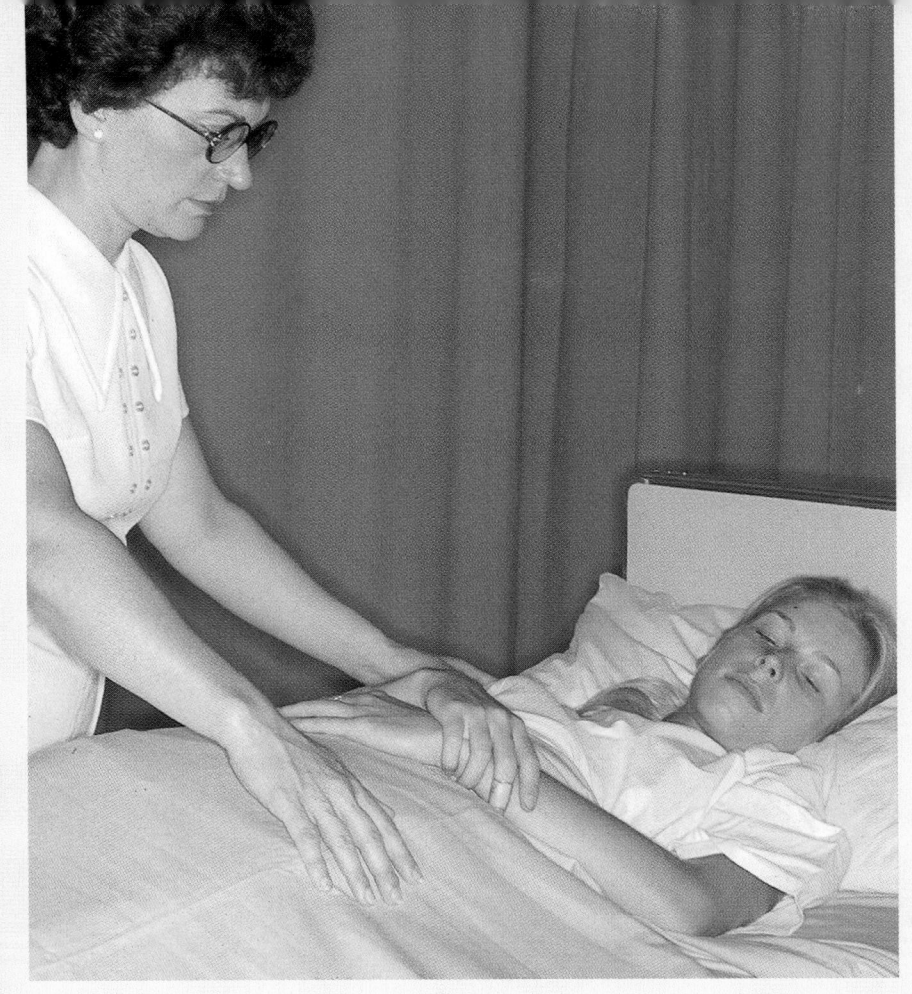

Sleep and Rest

42 Sleep and Rest

⌐ Key Terms

circadian rhythms
enuresis
fatigue
hormonal dysynchrony
hypnotics
hypopnea
insomnia
narcolepsy

parasomnias
rest
sleep
sleep apnea
sleep latency
sleepiness
somnambulism

⌐ Learning Objectives

Upon completion of this chapter, the student will be able to do the following:
1. Describe the five stages of sleep.
2. Describe normal patterns of sleep and rest throughout the lifespan.
3. Identify factors that affect sleep and rest.
4. Conduct an assessment interview regarding normal sleep patterns, risk for disturbance, and actual sleep problems.
5. Develop a daily schedule with a client, incorporating his or her unique needs and patterns for sleep and rest.
6. Discuss interventions to promote rest and sleep.
7. Develop a nursing plan of care for a client with sleep pattern disturbance.

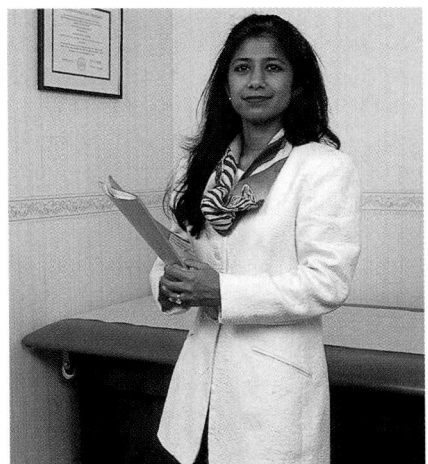

⌐ Critical Thinking Challenge

You are the invited speaker to a high school biology class. When given a choice of health-related topics, the students chose sleep. The teacher has asked you, as a community health nurse, to lead a class discussion on this topic. He tells you that questions they submitted include the following: Why do we sleep? How much is enough? Why do parents think it is so important to get up early? I get so uptight when I can't get to sleep, is there anything I can do? How come I sometimes walk in my sleep? The teacher also confides in you that he is worried about a couple of students: one who always seems to be dozing off in class although she claims to get 9 to 10 hours of sleep most nights; and several high achievers who stay up late at night studying, then come dragging into class the next morning. He asks you to include some discussion of different kinds of sleep problems like those he has observed among the students.

You have acquired a broad base of knowledge about the nursing profession and nursing care. In this chapter, you will learn about sleep and rest as a normal body function, and how nurses can promote adequate sleep. This chapter will expand your knowledge about the necessity of sleep and rest in relation to other body functions. Once you have completed this chapter and incorporated sleep and rest into your knowledge base, review the above scenario and reflect on the following areas of Critical Thinking.

1. Recall the thoughts that came to your mind when you initially read the situation.
2. Spend a few moments imagining yourself in high school. Reflect on the quality and quantity of sleep you used to get and what you believed about sleep.
3. Develop your priorities for teaching this class.
4. Discuss ways in which their developmental stage may affect the sleep needs and experiences of high school students. Consider these needs from a holistic perspective.

One third of human life is spent sleeping. Periods of rest may account for another major portion of the lifespan. The significance and mechanisms of sleep and rest, however, remain largely a mystery. Sleep has long been assumed to have a restorative function, and until recently many people believed sleep to be a passive state of decreased stimulation. It is now known that active physiologic processes are involved.

Sleep and rest are important concerns in health and illness. Sleepiness has been shown to influence health status, including a person's perceived levels of energy and fatigue (Briones et al., 1996). People use phrases like "feeling well rested" and "energetic" to describe good sleep and good health. Sleep deprivation may exacerbate some health problems. For example, risk of seizures in people who have epilepsy is higher when they are sleep deprived. Many health problems affect sleep, either directly through shared pathophysiologic mechanisms (e.g., depression) or indirectly through symptoms (e.g., pain, impaired mobility) or treatment (e.g., medication side effects).

NORMAL SLEEP AND REST

Sleep is a naturally occurring altered state of consciousness characterized by decreases in awareness and responsiveness to stimuli. Sleep is distinguished from abnormal states of consciousness (e.g., coma) by being readily reversible. With **rest,** awareness of the environment is maintained, but motor or cognitive response is decreased. Whereas sleep is a total body phenomenon, rest may involve the total system or only a part. The person sunbathing on a beach during summer vacation may be experiencing a generalized state of rest associated with decreased mental and physical activity, whereas a person with an injured arm in a sling is resting that body part but otherwise may be relatively active mentally and physically.

Physiologic Function

The physiology of sleep can be discussed in relation to two basic research approaches, each of which has provided building blocks for developing concepts relating to mechanisms and functions of sleep. The approaches are the electrophysiologic approach and neurotransmitter balance.

Electrophysiologic Approach

Polygraph recordings of electrophysiologic changes in brain waves (electroencephalogram [EEG]), eye movements (electrooculogram [EOG]), and muscles (electromyogram [EMG]) show five sleep stages. The first four stages are classified as non–rapid eye movement (NREM) sleep. The other stage is called REM or paradoxical sleep, because rapid eye movements are characteristic (Table 42-1).

Non–Rapid Eye Movement Sleep
Stage 1. Stage 1 is the transitional stage between drowsiness and sleep, indicated by a shift from alpha waves to low-voltage, fast theta waves on the EEG. Muscles relax, respirations become even, and pulse rate decreases. This stage usually lasts only a few minutes, and, if awakened, the person may say he or she was not asleep.

Stage 2. Stage 2 is still a relatively light sleep from which the person is easily wakened. Bursts of sleep spindles appear on the EEG (Fig. 42-1). Rolling eye movements continue, and snoring may occur.

Stages 3 and 4. Stages 3 and 4 constitute "deep" sleep, sometimes termed slow-wave sleep or delta sleep after characteristic waves seen on the EEG (Fig. 42-1). These two stages are differentiated primarily by the amount of delta waves, and they are usually discussed together. During slow-wave sleep, the muscles are relaxed, but muscle tone is maintained; respirations are even; and blood pressure, pulse, temperature, urine formation, and oxygen consumption by muscle decrease. These are the stages during which snoring, sleepwalking (**somnambulism**), and bed-wetting (**enuresis**) are most likely to occur. Strong stimuli are necessary to awaken people during these stages. Dream content tends to be realistic and may be without plot. Examples are a dream of driving to work or phoning a friend that causes the client to wonder, when awakening, whether it really happened!

Rapid Eye Movement Sleep. REM sleep closely resembles wakefulness except for very low muscle tone, indicated by a reduction in amplitude of the EMG (Fig. 42-2). The rapid eye movements from which REM sleep receives its name are documented through EOG recording but may also be noted by careful observation of tiny eye movements detectable through closed lids. The brain waves as recorded on the EEG are similar to those during the awake state (Fig. 42-1). Blood pressure and pulse rate show wide variations and may fluctuate rapidly. Respirations are irregular, and oxygen consumption increases. Thermoregulation is lost. Vaginal secretions increase in women, and erections may occur in men. Dreams occurring during REM sleep tend to be vivid and implausible, sometimes including a sense of being unable to move.

Sleep Rhythm. Electrophysiologic recordings of nocturnal sleep show a rhythmic pattern of approximately 90-minute cycles during which people progress in sequence through the sleep stages. The usual pattern is fairly rapid progression through stages 1 to 4 and then back through stages 3 and 2, from which the person then enters REM sleep (Fig. 42-3). During the early part of the night, periods of slow-wave sleep (stages 3 and 4) are longer. In contrast, the time spent in REM sleep during the first cycle may be only 3 to 4 minutes, whereas toward morning it may be as much as 45 minutes, balanced with shorter periods of slow-wave sleep in which stage 4 may not be present. If awakening occurs, the cycle begins again with stage 1. If the awakening was brief, the tendency is to reenter the type of cycle from which the person was aroused. Thus, an early morning awakening may be followed by return to one or more cycles in which a high percentage of REM sleep is present. In situations where REM sleep deficiency is sus-

TABLE 42-1

Characteristics of the Sleep Stages				
Stage	**Physiologic and Biochemical Correlates**	**Electroencephalogram**	**Dreaming and Subjective Awareness**	**Rebound**
1—Light	Muscles are relaxed; eyes display rolling movements; respirations are even; pulse rate is decreased.	Gradual loss of alpha waves	Person may feel a sense of floating or see idle images; if person is awakened, may say he or she was not asleep.	No
2—Transition to REM	Eyes may appear to roll.	Bursts of sleep spindles; sharp, slow waves	Person awakens easily and may report that he or she was thinking or daydreaming.	No
3—Deep, slow wave	Muscles are very relaxed but tone is maintained; respirations are even; growth hormone and serotonin are released.	Delta (slow wave); person may respond to outside stimuli but is unaware; spindles are present	Dreams are less dramatic, more realistic, and may lack plot; person requires stronger stimuli to awaken.	No
4—Deep, slow wave	Blood pressure, temperature, pulse rate, urine secretion, and oxygen consumption of muscle are decreased; snoring may occur.			Yes, priority
REM sleep	Muscles are at lowest tone; blood pressure, pulse, vaginal secretions, cerebral blood flow, and oxygen consumption are increased; respirations fluctuate; episodic cortisol and ACTH and catecholamine are released.	Desynchronized; extremely active; similar to wakefulness	Dreams have vivid content, full-color, sounds, implausible settings, and may involve a sense of paralysis; person is difficult to awaken except with significant stimuli.	Yes

pected, it is therefore more helpful to encourage clients to return to sleep immediately after an early awakening than to plan on napping in the afternoon.

Neurotransmitter Balance

Sleep is an active process involving the reticular activating system (RAS) and a dynamic interaction of neurotransmitters. The RAS consists of a network of interconnecting neurons in the medulla, pons, and midbrain, with projections to the spinal cord, hypothalamus, cerebellum, and cerebral cortex. The RAS literally fills in the spaces in the brain stem among the major tracts, bringing in sensory messages and relaying motor ones. Thus, it is in a strategic location for stimulation from a wide variety of inputs. The RAS includes the ascending facilitatory area, which is intrinsically active, and a less well understood bulbar inhibitory area, which appears to be particularly involved in decreasing muscle tone during REM sleep (Porth, 2002).

As with other parts of the nervous system, communication between neurons in the RAS primarily involves the re-

lease of specific neurotransmitters from axon terminals and their attachment to specific receptors on other cells. Serotonin is a major neurotransmitter associated with sleep. Produced in the raphe nuclei in the brain stem, serotonin is derived from its precursor, tryptophan, a naturally occurring amino acid. Serotonin is thought to decrease the activity of the RAS, thereby inducing and sustaining sleep. Other neurotransmitters—acetylcholine, primarily from the hippocampus, and norepinephrine, from the locus ceruleus (also in the brain stem)—appear to be required for the REM sleep cycle (Robinson, 1993).

Psychological Function

Psychological functions of sleep are thought to include the following:

- Sorting and discarding of neurophysiologic data. Much short-term memory is filled with inconsequential detail that the brain sifts through and discards. A person can

Awake:
low-voltage, fast

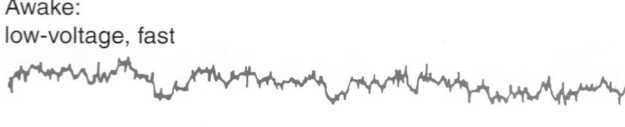

Awake eyes closed:
alpha-waves, 8–12 cps

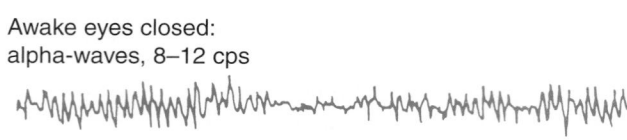

Stage 1:
theta-waves, 3–7 cps

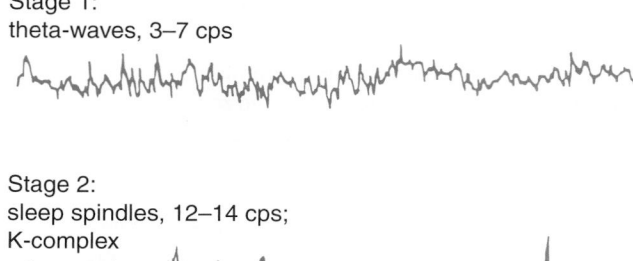

Stage 2:
sleep spindles, 12–14 cps;
K-complex

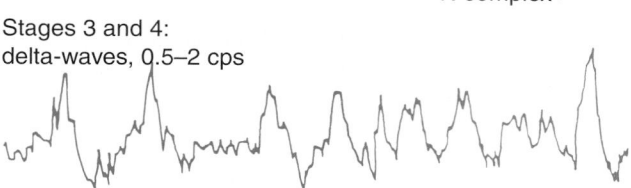

sleep spindle

K-complex

Stages 3 and 4:
delta-waves, 0.5–2 cps

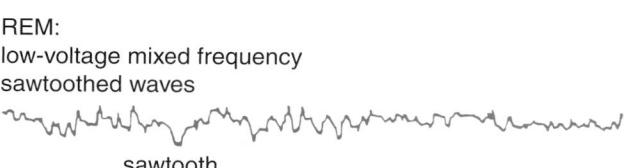

REM:
low-voltage mixed frequency
sawtoothed waves

sawtooth

FIGURE 42-1   Characteristic electroencephalogram wave forms by sleep stage. (Courtesy University of Washington School of Nursing, Sleep Laboratory, Seattle, WA.)

usually remember what he or she ate for breakfast that day or how long the bus took to come, but a month later those data will probably be beyond recall (unless something special happened that day).

- Character reinforcement and adaptation. The REM stage of sleep, in particular, appears to be important for mental and emotional stability. Through REM dreaming, a reprocessing of knowledge and memories is thought to occur. An increased need for REM sleep has been found in people experiencing stress, worry, or new learning situations.

Characteristics of Normal Sleep and Rest

Awareness of Need

Awareness of the need for sleep and rest is most commonly associated with the states of sleepiness and fatigue. These states usually overlap. **Sleepiness** refers to an urge of varying intensity to go to sleep. It may occur in response to too little or too much sleep or to lack of adequate sensory stimulation. **Fatigue** is a subjective state of weariness in which intense or rapid tiring accompanies physical activity. It is a common human response to illness, suggesting the need to conserve energy through rest and sleep.

Restoration and Protection

Sleep and rest are believed to be restorative and protective (Hodgson, 1991; Mornhinweg & Voignier, 1996). Oswald (1987), the leading proponent of the restorative theory, provided evidence that shifts in hormonal balance facilitate physical restoration through the processes of anabolism (synthesis of cell constituents) during sleep. Horne (1988), on the other hand, suggested that the main purpose of sleep may be energy conservation for parts of the body other than the brain. Periods of physical and mental rest are known to reduce the metabolic rate and the sense of fatigue.

Normal Sleep and Rest Patterns

The well-rested person is mentally alert, energetic, and spontaneous. Daytime activity, even that of a monotonous nature, is maintained with a minimum of drowsiness.

The range of "normal" sleep duration is great. Short sleepers (those who sleep for less than 6 hours in 24) tend to be efficient, hard-working people. Winston Churchill required little nighttime sleep, relying instead on his ability to take brief but renewing naps. Long sleepers (those who sleep for more than 9 hours in 24) have a higher percentage of REM sleep, and there is some suggestion that as a group they are more creative. Albert Einstein was a long sleeper.

The range of normality with respect to sleep patterns is also broad. Most people require 10 to 30 minutes to fall asleep; this period is called **sleep latency.** A regular sleep latency of less than 5 minutes suggests excessive sleepiness. Sleep latency of longer than 30 minutes may be accompanied by some sense of frustration with the time taken to get to sleep.

Changes of position during sleep typically occur 20 to 40 times during the night in all but older adults (Lorrain & De Koninck, 1998). For people with impaired physical mobility, the normally unconscious act of changing positions during sleep may require awakening, conscious planning and effort, or the assistance of the bed partner or care provider. The institutional norm of turning clients every 2 hours scarcely meets the physiologic norm of natural position changes during sleep. Such simple interventions as the use of satin sheets have been found to help people with impaired physical mobility turn more easily.

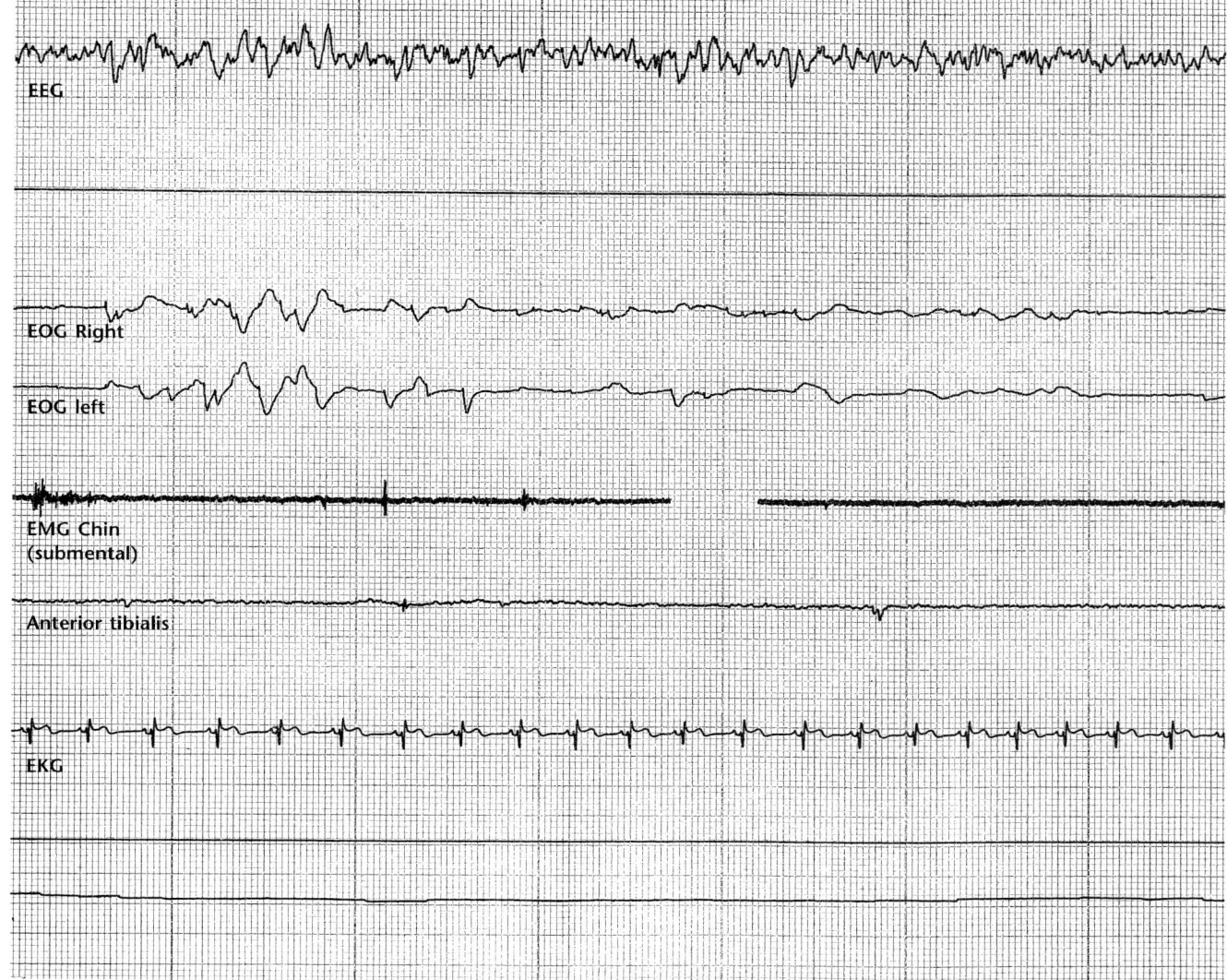

FIGURE 42-2   REM sleep on polygraph recording. Note the rapid, low-amplitude waves on the EEG, eye movements on EOG, and minimal muscle activity on EMG. (Courtesy of Alberta Lung Association Sleep Center, Calgary, Alberta, Canada.)

One to two awakenings per night are common for young adults; the frequency and duration of awakenings tend to increase with age. The final awakening is often spontaneous, even in North American society, where alarm clocks symbolize the precision of occupational and educational schedules. The well-rested person usually awakens feeling refreshed and energized.

Daytime naps and rest periods are infrequent among North American adults and older children, except when associated with illness, pregnancy, or "catching up" on a day off. In warmer climates, however, the midday rest period is a cultural expectation. Rest breaks in the more industrialized nations have tended to be associated with the use of stimulants such as caffeine in coffee or nicotine in cigarettes. The value of mini-rests in the form of stretching exercises, focusing thoughts or vision on a pleasant scene away from the work station, or going for a walk can be incorporated into client teaching.

Circadian Rhythms

Biologic rhythms that follow a cycle of about 24 hours are termed **circadian rhythms,** from the Latin words *circa,* "about," and *dies,* "day" (Porth, 2002). The sleep–wake cycle is an example. The sleep–wake cycle is closely linked with other circadian rhythms, such as body temperature and gastric acid and hormone secretion.

Sleep–wake patterns appear to be affected by and to affect certain hormone levels. Melatonin, synthesized in the pineal gland during the hours of darkness, has an apparent rhythm-setting function closely related to light conditions. The superchiasmatic nucleus (SCN), located above the optic chiasm in

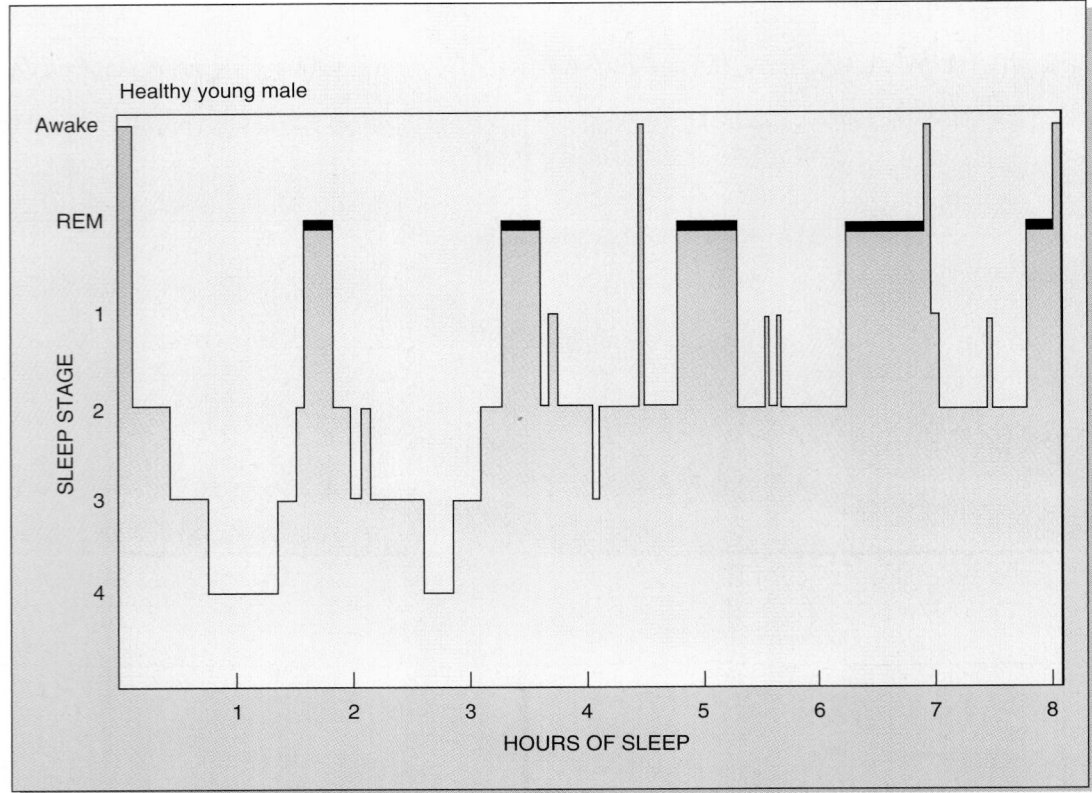

FIGURE 42-3   Typical sequence of sleep stages in a young, healthy, adult man. Progression occurs through a sequence of 1–2–3–4–3–2 and into REM. Note increased amount of REM sleep and absence of stage 4 toward end of sleep period. (Courtesy of University of Washington School of Nursing, Sleep Laboratory, Seattle, WA.)

the anterior hypothalamus, functions essentially as the "clock" for most circadian rhythms by relaying information from the retina to the pineal gland. Growth hormone and prolactin levels are closely tied to actual sleep time, changing immediately in relation to variations in the sleep period, irrespective of light–dark conditions. Secretion of both hormones increases early in the sleep period. Adrenocorticotropic hormone secretion from the pituitary is high during the early part of the sleep period, and levels of cortisol, its target hormone from the adrenal cortex, rise toward the end of the nocturnal sleep period. This pattern remains stable in relation to clock time despite variations in sleep time (e.g., shift work), unless such changes are sustained for up to 2 weeks. The significance of this **hormonal dysynchrony,** in which hormonal levels adjust at different rates to alterations in the timing of the sleep period, is not clearly understood but is an important research area, particularly in relation to shift work and jet travel.

In situations where environmental cues to time are largely removed, circadian rhythms are maintained, but the duration may extend to 25 or more hours and may become less synchronized. Experimental conditions typically involve controlled artificial light and removal of all indicators of time. Nurses are sometimes involved with people who have established life patterns in which environmental cues to time are decreased to the point at which erratic sleep and temperature

cycles develop (Robinson, 1993). People living alone without regular occupational or social contact are among those at risk.

Lifespan Considerations

Developmental variations in sleep patterns are evident. Circadian rhythms develop in the first few months of life, are well established throughout childhood and adulthood, and gradually decrease with advancing age. The polyphasic two-to-one ratio of sleep to wakefulness characteristic of infants gradually shifts to the biphasic one-to-two ratio of adulthood.

Newborn and Infant

Two major sleep states can be observed in newborns. Closed eyes, regular respirations, and absence of eye and body movements characterize quiet sleep. Eye movements observable through the closed lids, other body movements, and irregular respirations characterize active sleep. Of the three waking states—quiet awake, active awake, and crying—quiet awake would seem to correspond to a state of rest in adults. Newborns sleep an average of 16 to 17 hours per day, divided into about seven sleep periods distributed fairly evenly throughout the day and night (Renaud, 1996).

Infants' sleep patterns differ from those of adults in that the sleep cycle is shorter (50 to 60 minutes), the proportion of active or REM sleep is higher (approximately 50%), and the initial stage is active rather than NREM. Between 1 and 2 months of age, NREM sleep becomes differentiated into stages 1 through 4 (Robinson, 1993).

One of the infant's major adaptive tasks is to establish sleep–wake patterns compatible with the environment (Fig. 42-4). Most infants sleep through the night by 3 months of age, but nocturnal awakenings continue to be frequent during the latter half of the first year.

The number of sleep periods continue to drop, from four to five per 24-hour day at 3 months to one nighttime period and two naps at 6 months. Total sleep time averages 14 to 15 hours, but there is wide variability among infants.

Toddler and Preschooler

By 1 year of age, napping has usually been reduced to once or twice a day. Some sleep disturbance is observed in almost all children between 1 and 2.5 years of age, which is believed to relate to children's rapidly developing mental abilities. Getting the child to fall asleep is the most commonly reported problem, but frequent awakenings and occasional night terrors may also occur. Total sleep time drops from an average of 13 to 14 hours at age 2 years to 12 hours by the end of the fifth year, mainly because of elimination of the afternoon nap. REM sleep drops to about 30%, which is still higher than for adults. The percentage of slow-wave sleep is also higher through childhood, whereas the amount of stage 1 sleep is lower.

School-Age Child and Adolescent

Sleep and rest needs fluctuate somewhat for school-age children and adolescents in relation to growth spurts and activity patterns. REM content gradually drops to about 20% at puberty. Adolescents actually require slightly more rest than they did before puberty. The cardiovascular and respiratory systems mature less rapidly than other systems, contributing to fatigue from inadequate oxygenation.

Adult and Older Adult

Adults vary widely in the number of hours of sleep that they require and in their preferred portion of the 24-hour period for sleeping. By middle age, the frequency of nocturnal awakenings tends to increase, and satisfaction with the quality of sleep tends to decrease. Situational variables such as job-related stress, parenting responsibilities, and illness probably account for much of the variation seen among early and middle adults.

As people age, the amount of stage 4 sleep decreases significantly (Fig. 42-5). The intranight distribution of REM sleep becomes more even, and the percentage decreases (Ancoli-Israel, 1997). Older men tend to have decreased stage 3 sleep as well, and they have more difficulty remaining asleep toward the end of the sleep period. Circadian rhythms become less prominent with increasing age. There is a tendency to "phase advance"—that is, to go to bed earlier but also waken earlier (Phillips & Ancoli-Israel, 2001). Sleeping patterns may become polyphasic, with a shorter nocturnal period plus daytime naps. Core body temperature may no longer show the usual circadian changes. If external cues to time also decrease, as with institutionalization, cognitively impaired older adults may develop "sundowner's syndrome," characterized by nocturnal wakefulness and agitation. The syndrome may be related to a drop in stimulation level to the point at which the cognitively compromised client can no longer maintain contact with reality.

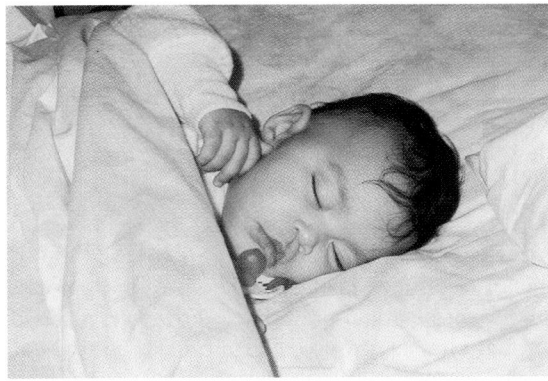

FIGURE 42-4 Infants establish sleep–wake cycles that fit their environment.

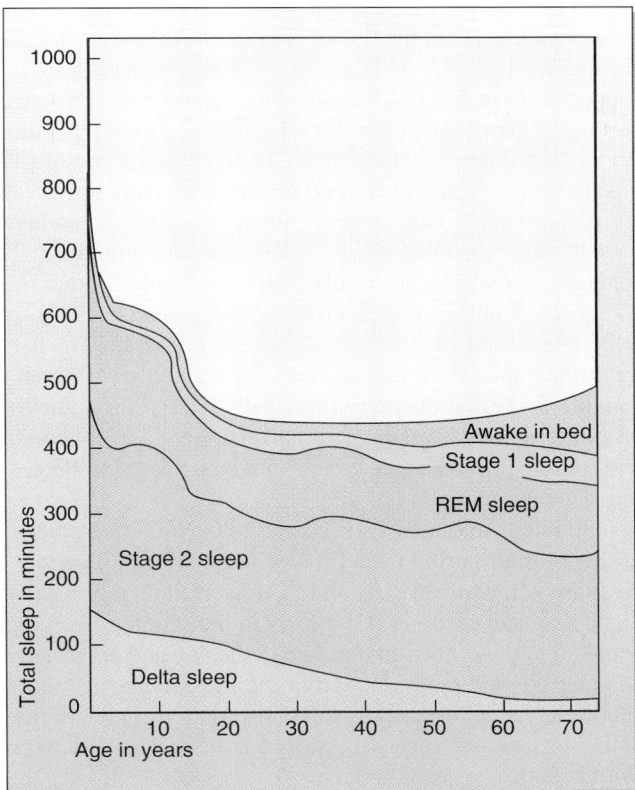

FIGURE 42-5 Schematic representation of the changes in sleep stages by age. Note that older adults spend more time in bed than younger adults but have less deep sleep. (Adapted with permission from Williams, R. L., Karacen, I., & Hursch, C. J. [1994]. *Electroencephalography [EEG] of human sleep: Clinical applications.* New York: Wiley.)

Time spent napping and in bed increases with advancing age. Daytime napping does not appear to interfere with night-time sleep for older adults. Total time in bed gradually increases because of napping, longer sleep latency, increases in the number and length of awakenings, and general fatigue.

Older adults frequently express concern about taking longer to fall asleep, awakening more frequently, feeling sleepy during the daytime, and needing longer to adjust to changes in schedule. Help them to recognize that these changes are a natural part of aging and to establish or maintain a schedule of rest and activity that meets their individual needs and preferences.

FACTORS AFFECTING SLEEP AND REST

Need

Need for sleep and rest fluctuates according to developmental, individual, and situational variables. Developmental variables are discussed in the section on Lifespan Considerations. Individual variations occur in relation to total sleep need and preferred schedule.

Horne (1988, p. 312) suggested two forms of sleepiness: "core sleepiness, associated with the loss of core sleep and reflected in impaired cerebral functioning, and optional sleepiness, associated with the loss of optional sleep and mostly affecting motivation." This concept of lower sleep need is supported by studies that have shown that students in the latter part of the 20th century averaged 1.5 hours less sleep per day than their counterparts did in 1910. The unresolved question is whether this represents less need for sleep or a chronic state of sleep deprivation (lack of sleep). More recently, researchers have hypothesized that much of the population in industrialized nations may be chronically sleep deprived (Report of the National Commission on Sleep Disorders Research, 1993).

People should attune themselves to their own specific patterns rather than aiming for the traditional standard of 8 hours a night. Generally, the person who falls asleep fairly quickly on going to bed, awakens feeling refreshed, and functions with minimal daytime sleepiness can be assumed to be getting adequate sleep.

Individual variations also occur as to the preferred portion of the 24-hour period used for sleeping. "Morning people" are those who awaken early and easily, feel at their best early in the day, and prefer to retire early in the evening. Evening people find they function best late in the day and are usually wide awake and ready for activity in the evening. Evening people seem to more readily tolerate variations in the timing of the sleep period, such as those that as occur with shift work (Monk, 2000).

Environment

Generally, in a new environment, sleep latency increases, whereas total sleep time and the proportion of REM sleep decrease. Those who have chronic difficulties sleeping may associate certain objects in the environment, such as their bed, with poor sleep. These people report sleeping better away from home. In the hospital setting, certain objects in the room may be associated with pain. If a sleeping room doubles as a work area, the individual may associate the room with work rather than sleep. Objects of play in a child's room may disturb the child's sleep and rest.

Reduction of environmental stimuli, particularly light and noise, facilitates sleep. People vary in their sensitivity to different stimuli and appear to vary in the intensity and degree of fluctuation of sensory input they require. Some people seem to require a slight elevation of sensory input, sleeping better when surrounded by low-level noise such as a radio, after drinking coffee, or after exercising.

Awakening or a lightening of sleep pattern may occur when the bed partner changes position or snores. Presence of the habitual partner may provide a sense of security, and absence of the habitual partner may be disturbing. As discussed in the next section, the nature, quality, and present state of the relationship are factors that contribute to the effect of the partner's presence or absence. For those who habitually sleep alone, the presence of another person may be disturbing.

Noise

People who are chronically exposed to high noise levels have less slow-wave and REM sleep with more stage 1 sleep and more awakenings than their counterparts who live in quieter neighborhoods (Roehrs, Zorick & Roth, 2000). Noise is more likely to awaken women and older people. As might be expected, the awakening threshold varies with the stage of sleep, with stage 1 being most vulnerable.

Noise levels recorded in critical care units have ranged from 60 to 80 decibels, the equivalent of a noisy office (Evans & French, 1995). Nurses can modify the noise level in such settings by keeping equipment noise to a minimum, avoiding unnecessary conversation, and closing doors when possible. Suggest to clients that they use ear plugs in home environments if noises in the same room (e.g., partner snoring) or outside (e.g., traffic) are disturbing sleep.

Light

Control of light is usually adequate in most homes. Outdoor brightness for night workers and people who live in northern latitudes during summer months may disrupt sleep. In acute care environments, control of light becomes a nursing responsibility often overlooked in the complexity of meeting other client needs.

Temperature

The benefits of cool versus moderate room temperatures are matters of personal preference; however, research has shown that either excessive warmth or excessive cold increases restlessness (Roehrs et al., 2000). During REM sleep, thermoregulation is impaired and shivering does not occur.

Relationships

The frequent awakenings associated with parenting may contribute to chronic sleep pattern disturbance. It is not unusual to hear mothers speak of never getting more than an hour's sleep at a time over a period of 1 week or longer when caring for a sick child or colicky baby. The associated REM sleep deprivation may make coping even more difficult. Likewise, caregivers of people with advanced disease may become chronically sleep deprived (Smith, Ellgring, & Oertel, 1997).

Disruptions in primary relationships are commonly associated with sleep pattern disturbance. Bereaved people often report nights as the most difficult time. Children who are away from home are frequently homesick at bedtime. Marital discord may contribute to sleep disturbance in children as well as in the involved adults. Security needs are heightened at bedtime for people of all ages.

Healthcare providers are among the most frequent disturbers of sleep in institutional settings. In critical care environments, they must awaken clients frequently for various assessments and treatments. Where possible, nurses should cluster these activities to provide periods of 90 to 120 minutes of undisturbed sleep. They may have to assume an advocacy role by coordinating interruptions from the many disciplines involved in client care.

Shift Work

Frequent changes in the sleep–wake schedule, such as those that occur with shift work, contribute to shorter and more fragmented sleep and a high incidence of fatigue (Roehrs et al., 2000). The dysynchrony of trying to sleep at times when the body's circadian rhythm is set for wakefulness is thought to be the main reason for the disturbed sleep. Fatigue is secondary. Nurses are among the 20% of the population in industrialized countries who are involved in shift work, as are many of the people for whom they care (Monk, 2000). Research on the effectiveness of various shift schedules has been inconclusive, suggesting the need for further investigation.

Research has shown that clockwise rotation of shifts is preferable and that short naps during breaks may temporarily enhance work performance. Attention to the sleeping environment is particularly important for nurses and others who work shifts. Simple strategies such as blacking out windows with dark curtains or tinfoil, shutting off or moving the telephone into another room, and allowing adequate time for sleep are helpful.

Nutrition and Metabolism

Hunger disturbs the sleep of some people, whereas others have difficulty sleeping after large meals. Ingestion of L-tryptophan, a precursor of serotonin found in foods such as milk, beef, eggs, wheat flour, turkey, and corn, has been found to decrease sleep latency and increase stage 4 sleep (Robinson, 1993). Synthesis is enhanced by eating complex carbohydrates, preferably without proteins that compete with L-tryptophan to cross the blood–brain barrier. Sleep patterns tend to be disturbed during periods of either rapid weight loss or rapid gain.

Elimination Patterns

The need to void is one of the most frequent internal stimuli to disturb sleep among the general population. Parents and other caregivers can assist children in establishing the habit of voiding as part of preparing for bedtime. Limiting fluid intake after supper may decrease this nocturnal stimulus.

Exercise and Thermoregulation

Habitual exercise contributes to deeper and longer sleep. In physically fit people, light-intensity exercise seems to decrease sleep latency and intensive exercise increases the proportion of slow-wave sleep (Driver & Taylor, 2000). The basis for increased slow-wave sleep after vigorous exercise may be related to an increase in core body temperature. Passive heating, as in a sauna or tub of warm water, especially in the early evening, has been shown to produce effects similar to those of vigorous exercise on the amount of slow-wave sleep (Bunnell et al., 1988). These findings suggest a promising area for nursing research regarding the value of a warm bath for enhancing the quality of sleep. The relationships between exercise and sleep are more complex than they may first appear, however. Contrary to what might be expected from the previous discussion, bed rest also increases slow-wave sleep by mechanisms not understood. Given that sleep onset occurs most readily as body temperature drops, it is preferable to schedule exercise or a hot bath a few hours before bedtime.

Vigilance

Another factor affecting sleep is the perceived need to maintain vigilance. Parents and others in protective roles seem able to establish a variable noise threshold in which they may respond to the faintest sound of a toddler changing position in the next room, and yet sleep through a thunderstorm. Hospital clients, such as those recently disconnected from cardiac monitoring equipment, may deliberately prevent themselves from entering the deeper stages of sleep for fear of succumbing to a complication that might go unnoticed by nursing staff.

Lifestyle and Habits

Certain bedtime rituals become such habits that to interfere with them is to interfere with sleep itself. Some rituals, such as a warm bath or a snack, may have a physiologic basis. The effectiveness of bedtime habits is also linked with decreasing arousal. Participation in a routine such as putting out the dog, winding the clock, and changing into night attire becomes associated with the expectation of sleep.

Lifestyle patterns influencing the sleep–wake schedule, such as time of rising, are closely linked with societal and occupational expectations. A regular time of rising is one of the

THERAPEUTIC DIALOGUE
Sleep and Rest

Scene for Thought

Joanna and Paco Estevez are parents of two small children: Enrique, who is 3 weeks old, and Theresa, who is 3 years old. Paco works nights, and Joanna has recently returned to work at her day job as a nurse's aide in a large nursing home. Emily Arana, a community health nurse, is at their home for a follow-up visit.

Less Effective

Client: I'm glad you came early, Ms. Arana. The kids are both asleep and so is Paco. We can talk in peace for a little while. *(Sits on sofa and motions Emily to sit down.)*

Nurse: Sounds like it's been busy around here lately. *(Settles onto sofa and sits attentively.)*

Client: You got that right! Enrique isn't sleeping through the night yet, and Theresa wakes up, too. Plus she has a cold so she isn't feeling too good. And Paco isn't around to help much since he's working nights. It gets pretty hairy around here at 2 AM. *(Smiles tightly.)*

Nurse: And I understand you're working, too. Day shift?

Client: Yes. *(Wearily.)* I had to go back or lose the job. I leave the kids with my mother all day until I get off at 3 PM. She lives close by. *(Yawns.)* Sorry! I didn't mean to yawn in your face!

Nurse: No problem. And is your husband able to help or is he too tired? *(Begins to open bag and take out assessment equipment.)*

Client: He helps on his days off. He's really good with both of them. *(Sounds a little defensive.)*

Nurse: I'm sure he is, having had three brothers and sisters of his own to take care of. Maybe I could see the baby now and how he's doing. Do you think Theresa will be up soon? I can look at her, too, and see what we can do for her cold. What do you think?

Client: Sure, you start on the baby, and I'll see if Theresa's about to wake up. *(Pauses to get a clean towel for the baby to lie on and goes in to the bedroom. Yawns again.)*

More Effective

Client: I'm glad you came early, Ms. Arana. The kids are both asleep and so is Paco. We can talk in peace for a little while. *(Sits on sofa and motions Emily to sit down.)*

Nurse: Sounds like it's been busy around here lately. *(Settles onto sofa and sits attentively.)*

Client: You got that right! Enrique isn't sleeping through the night yet, and Theresa wakes up, too. Plus she has a cold so she isn't feeling too good. And Paco isn't around to help much since he's working nights. It gets pretty hairy around here at 2 AM. *(Smiles tightly.)*

Nurse: How about you? *(Good eye contact.)*

Client: I do what I can. *(Shrugs wearily.)* I had to return to work after the baby came home or lose my job. I get up at 5 to get the kids ready to take to my mother's while I work. So I don't get much rest. Or much time with Paco. I really hate this night shift he's on. But it's extra money and it won't be forever. He's put in for a shift change so we can have some sort of normal life, but it won't come through for a while. *(Yawns.)* Sorry! I didn't mean to yawn in your face!

Nurse: No problem. You have reason to be tired. What are you doing to try and get more rest? *(Looks concerned, asking an open-ended question.)*

Client: I try to nap here and there. Paco takes the night feedings on his nights off so I can sleep through at least 2 nights a week. Other than that, I wait for the baby to grow so he'll sleep through and for Theresa's cold to get better. *(Shrugs again with a resigned look.)*

Nurse: Would you be willing to discuss things that might help both kids move along faster?

Client: *(Looks surprised.)* Sure! I didn't know there was anything else I could do for them. *(Baby begins to cry. Joanna rushes to get him so Paco won't wake. She returns.)* Let me just change him and get a bottle and then we can talk! *(Looks eager.)*

Critical Thinking Challenge

- Determine the factors affecting this family's sleep and rest patterns.
- Explain how the nurse in the second dialogue elicited additional information from the client.
- Explain what information the nurse in the first dialogue missed.
- Formulate your ideas of what consequences further sleep deprivation may have for this family.

---

most effective means of improving sleep quality and synchronizing circadian rhythms with clock time. Caregivers can help toddlers who are having difficulty settling into a bedtime routine by maintaining an early and consistent rising time and allowing them to stay up in the evening until they are sleepy enough to settle with quieting activities. Nurses can encourage adults who have difficulty getting to sleep to maintain a consistent rising time and to go to bed later if necessary, rather than lying awake for long periods.

Illness

During acute and chronic illness, clients are particularly vulnerable to loss of stage 3 sleep. Conditions involving pain have long been known to disturb sleep. Current research indicates that body system disturbances also affect sleep, and vice versa. For example, ventilatory responses to hypoxia and hypercapnia decrease during REM sleep. Although diaphragmatic function is essentially unchanged

ETHICAL/LEGAL ISSUE
Impact of Night Shift
on Healthcare Workers

Two months ago, you were hired for your first full-time position since graduating from your nursing program. You work the night shift permanently on a busy surgical unit. At first, you enjoyed the flexibility of having your days and evenings free and tended to sacrifice your sleep time. Lately, however, you have been having trouble sleeping during the day and staying alert during the night. Twice in the last week, you almost made medication errors. Tonight is the last night of this stretch, and you are experiencing difficulty concentrating on even the simplest procedures. You have asked your supervisor for a different shift rotation, but he says your schedule cannot be changed.

Reflection
- What alternatives might you consider in the above situation?
- Is self-care an ethical issue? Explain why or why not.
- Reread the Code for Nurses in Chapter 6. List the statements in the code that apply to this situation. Give rationales for your choices.
- Identify the legal and ethical responsibilities of the supervisor in this context.

during REM sleep, the intercostals and other accessory muscles lose substantial activity. Therefore, the pattern of frequent arousals seen in people with chronic obstructive lung disease may result from the body's adaptation to maintain adequate oxygenation. Hypnotics should be used cautiously, if at all, in people experiencing ineffective breathing patterns or impaired gas exchange. Usually, these clients require low doses of oxygen at night.

The pain and discomfort of angina or dyspnea that occurs during the night can disrupt sleep. Circadian variations in blood pressure, heart rate, and platelet aggregation around the time of wakening may be associated with the observed frequency of myocardial infarction and stroke from cerebral thrombus formation that occur in the latter part of the nighttime sleep period or within the first hours after wakening (George, 2000).

People with a history of seizure activity are at risk for increased occurrence of seizures after sleep deprivation or with variable sleep habits. Seizure activity may disturb sleep; some epileptic clients have seizures only at night. The recording of brain waves during sleep is an important method for diagnosing the site of abnormal electrical activity.

Hormonal changes contribute to many sleep pattern disturbances. Hyperthyroidism causes fragmented, short sleep with excessive slow-wave stages, whereas hypothyroidism seems to cause excessive sleepiness and a lack of slow-wave

sleep. The tremendous fatigue many women report after hysterectomy may be related to estrogen loss. Administration of estrogen to postmenopausal women has been shown to decrease sleep latency (Driver, 1996). In contrast, progesterone enhances ventilatory responses.

Skin conditions such as eczema have been shown to contribute to delay of sleep onset, frequent awakenings, and reduction of stages 3, 4, and REM sleep during the first part of the night. Itching and discomfort associated with hives, insect bites, and other skin lesions also disturb sleep.

Hospitalization as a result of illness increases the number of factors that may disturb sleep. In a survey of 143 adult clients on medical-surgical units, "difficulty finding a comfortable position" and "pain" were identified as the most common stimuli disturbing sleep in the hospital (Reimer, 1985). Anxieties arising from illness and hospitalization, such as those related to tests, surgery, diagnosis, and impact on family and job, were other frequently identified reasons for disturbed sleep (Fig. 42-6).

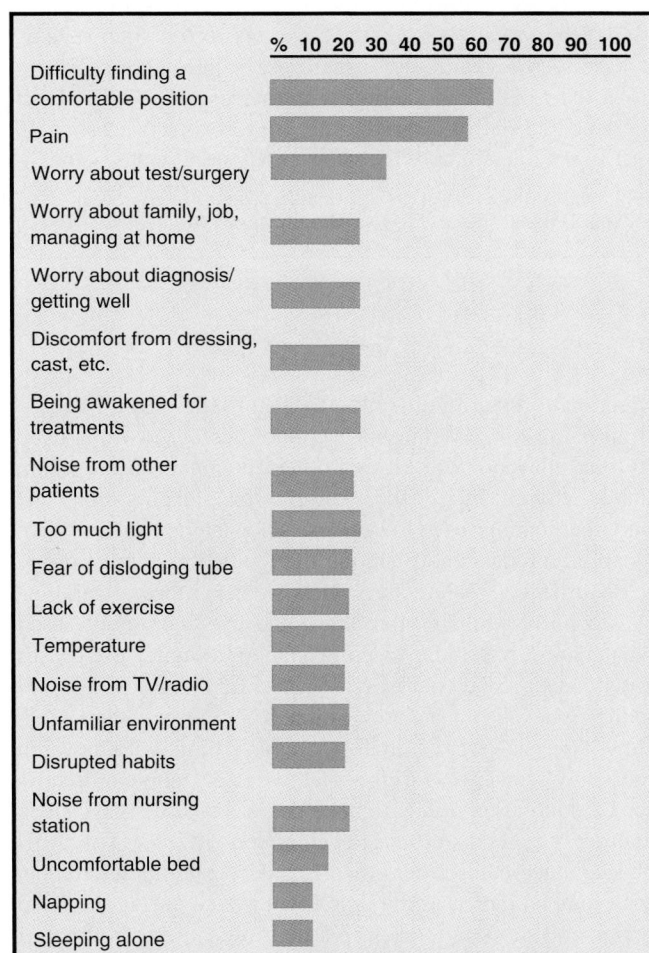

FIGURE 42-6 Percentage of clients identifying selected stimuli as disturbing to sleep in hospital. (From Reimer, M. A. (1985). *Nursing interventions perceived by patients and their nurses as facilitating nocturnal sleep in hospital.* Unpublished manuscript.)

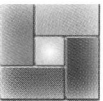

Nursing Research and Critical Thinking

What is the Role of Sleep in the Development of Acute Confusion Among Elderly People Undergoing Orthopedic Hip Surgery?

Sleep is a core human function that nursing intervention can effectively facilitate. This nurse researcher hypothesized that sleep satisfaction among elderly people who develop delirium after orthopedic hip surgery might differ from the sleep satisfaction recorded by those who do not experience delirium. She designed a study to compare sleep satisfaction, perceived pain, and acute confusion in elderly clients undergoing orthopedic procedures. Forty-three consecutively admitted subjects (29 female, 14 male) participated in the study. Subjects' mental status was tested with Folstein's Mini Mental Status Exam (MMS); subjects with known dementia or mental status test scores <23 were excluded from the study. Pain was assessed by means of a visual analog pain scale. An assessment of previous night's sleep satisfaction was recorded every morning for 5 days postoperatively. Subjects were considered to have experienced delirium upon meeting DSM-III criteria for delirium as evidenced at nurse's reports, on chart review, on interview with on-duty nurses, or through assessment at the time of interaction with the researcher. The incidence of delirium among all study subjects was 15/43 (34.9%). The study revealed client stability to be nega-

tively affected by disruptions of core sleep patterns, by pain, and by psychological concerns associated with perceived changes in health status and function. Sleep satisfaction was found to be poor among subjects who experienced delirium, and likely to play more of a role in pathogenesis of delirium than previously believed.

Critical Thinking Considerations. In this study, a higher incidence of delirium was found among people experiencing emergency surgery than among those having planned surgery. Those undergoing emergency procedures were also found to be older than those having planned surgery. Nursing implications of this study are as follows:

- Because advanced age is associated with an increased incidence of delirium, age might explain at least some of the difference between the planned and emergency groups.
- Nurses can have considerable impact on health outcomes of clients both by remaining focused on identifying stressors such as pain and anxiety and giving reduction of these stressors high priority.

From Bowman, A. M. (1997). Sleep satisfaction, perceived pain and acute confusion in elderly clients undergoing orthopaedic procedures. *Journal of Advanced Nursing, 28*(3), 550–564.

Medications and Chemicals

Sleep patterns are vulnerable to disturbance from medications taken to facilitate sleep, alcohol, medications used to treat other conditions, and other chemicals (Mendelson, 2000; Schweitzer, 2000). **Hypnotics,** or "sleeping pills," the very medications used to decrease sleep latency and improve sleep maintenance, are among the medications most prone to disturb sleep architecture. REM sleep is most vulnerable.

Alcohol is probably the oldest and most commonly used chemical for promoting sleep. A moderate single dose causes early onset of sleep but increases wakefulness in the last half of the night. With acute intoxication, REM sleep is suppressed; slow-wave sleep may initially increase. Abrupt withdrawal in the heavy drinker may trigger massive REM rebound. Recovered alcoholics continue to have decreased slow-wave sleep and gross cycle disturbance even after 1 or 2 years of abstinence. Other medications also affect sleep patterns. Morphine, for example, increases the time spent awake during the sleep period and shortens total sleep time by decreasing both REM sleep and stages 3 and 4. Antidepressants suppress REM sleep also. Phenytoin (Dilantin), used in the treatment of epilepsy, may contribute to insomnia.

The effects of caffeine on the central nervous system (CNS) may last up to 14 hours, delaying sleep onset and affecting sleep

patterns even in those who believe that they are not affected (Zarcone, 2000). The half-life of caffeine in older adults is even longer, making them particularly vulnerable to its effects. Nicotine, another mild CNS stimulant, accounts for the poorer sleep observed in heavy smokers compared with nonsmokers.

Mood States

Anxiety frequently delays the onset of sleep. Tension associated with psychological stress may also contribute to maintenance or early-awakening insomnia. Depression usually results in disturbed sleep. Both depression and sleep pattern disturbance may be linked to neurotransmitter imbalance. Poor sleep is likely to further distress depressed people.

ALTERED SLEEP AND REST

Manifestations of Altered Sleep

Signs and symptoms associated with sleep deprivation are fatigue, headache, nausea, increased sensitivity to pain, decreased neuromuscular coordination, general irritability, and inability to concentrate. Eventually, disorientation and hallucinations may occur with the breakthrough of "micro-sleeps," which further interfere with functioning.

Selective disruption of specific stages of sleep results in distinct symptom patterns. Those deprived of REM sleep become agitated and impulsive, whereas deprivation of slow-wave sleep results in withdrawal and vague physical complaints. In particular, tolerance of musculoskeletal pain significantly decreases after deprivation of slow-wave sleep. When deprived of stage 1, 2, or 3 sleep, the body makes no effort to recover those specific stages, but it seems to have a mechanism that gives priority to recovering stage 4 sleep and REM sleep as soon as it has the opportunity.

Insomnia

Insomnia is a perceived difficulty in sleeping. Persistent insomnia reflects a pattern of perceived difficulty with sleeping over months to years. Patterns of insomnia can also be classified as onset insomnia (prolonged sleep latency), maintenance insomnia (multiple awakenings), and early-awakening insomnia. When polygraph recordings of insomniacs have been compared with those of self-defined good sleepers, both have been found to be within normal range. Insomniacs consistently underestimated total sleep time but were accurate in identifying the pattern of insomnia and actually underestimated the number of awakenings. Therefore, the problem of insomnia appears to be more a lack of quality than of quantity (Edinger et al., 2000). *Psychophysiologic insomnia* is the diagnostic term used to refer to persistent insomnia associated with somatized tension and learned sleep-preventing associations (American Sleep Disorders Association [ASDA], 1997). Concern with the inability to sleep further interferes with sleep, contributing to a vicious cycle.

Narcolepsy

Narcolepsy is a disorder of excessive daytime sleepiness characterized by short, almost irresistible daytime sleep attacks, usually lasting 10 to 15 minutes, and abnormal manifestations of REM sleep (Cohen, Nehring & Cloninger, 1996). Onset usually occurs in adolescence. Narcolepsy is thought to be a disturbance between REM sleep and wakefulness-triggering systems, in which REM sleep intrudes into wakefulness. People who have narcolepsy typically experience REM sleep within the first 20 minutes after falling asleep. Episodes of profound weakness during intense emotion, called cataplexy, are reported by 70% of narcoleptics. Other common signs related to disturbed REM mechanisms include episodes of feeling paralyzed (sleep paralysis) and vivid hallucinations when falling asleep or awakening.

Sleep Apnea

Sleep apnea refers to recurrent periods of absence of breathing for 10 seconds or longer, occurring at least five times per hour (Flemons & McNicholas, 1997). Three types of sleep apnea are recognized: obstructive, central, and mixed (Robinson, 1993).

Use of hypnotics, alcohol, or antihistamines by clients with sleep apnea can be dangerous. Duration of apneic spells may increase because responsiveness to change in oxygen desaturation is already reduced. Drugs that induce drowsiness are more likely to do so in people who are already chronically sleep deprived. Sleep apnea essentially results in chronic sleep deprivation because of the frequency of mini-arousals and the lack of slow-wave and REM sleep.

SAFETY ALERT
Caution clients with impaired gas exchange or sleep apnea to use hypnotics and alcohol cautiously, if at all.

Obstructive Sleep Apnea. Obstructive sleep apnea involves collapse of the upper airway despite respiratory effort. With sleep, the muscles of the upper airway relax, occluding an airway that may already be narrowed because of obesity, jaw structure, or enlarged soft tissue structures. With arousal, voluntary control of the upper airway muscles is restored, relieving the obstruction. Some people do not become completely apneic, but recurrent periods of very shallow breathing (**hypopnea**) have a similar effect.

The person, who is usually a heavy-set man, may be partially roused hundreds of times each night. Symptoms include excessive daytime sleepiness and reports from the bed partner of apneic periods, heavy snoring, and restless sleep. Common treatments include continuous positive airway pressure applied through a nose mask and surgical reconstruction of the upper airway with removal of most of the uvula, posterior portion of the soft palate, and tonsils. Current developments include laser-assisted pharyngoplasty and various dental splints. Weight control, relief of nasal congestion, and avoidance of sleeping on the back may be effective in milder cases.

Obstructive sleep apnea is a common condition, affecting about 4% of adult males and 2% of adult females (ASDA, 1997). Occasional apneic periods occur normally during sleep stage transitions. Such apneas are not of concern. Encourage people who have frequent apneas that exceed 20 seconds at a time and occur most nights (with or without snoring or excessive daytime sleepiness) to seek assessment for possible obstructive sleep apnea.

Central Apnea. Central apnea during sleep occurs because of neurogenic failure to trigger respiratory effort. It is most

APPLY YOUR KNOWLEDGE

Mrs. Wilson, a 45-year-old executive, comes in for a yearly physical examination. She reports her only complaint is difficulty sleeping. She says that she wakes six to eight times each night from her husband's loud snoring. She is so tired some mornings that her productivity at work is beginning to suffer. She asks you if you think sleeping pills might help solve her problem. How will you respond to Mrs. Wilson?

Check your answer in Appendix A.

commonly seen with neurologic conditions such as stroke or brain stem involvement. Severely affected clients may require ventilatory support at night.

Mixed Apnea. Mixed apnea, a combination of the two preceding types of sleep apnea, is especially common in older adults. Manifestations and treatment are similar to those for obstructive sleep apnea.

Periodic Limb Movements

Periodic limb movements disorder is characterized by repetitive dorsiflexion of the foot and flexion of the knee during sleep at a rate up to once every 15 to 20 seconds. The resultant mini-arousals disrupt sleep, leading to excessive daytime sleepiness, or in some cases insomnia. Frequency tends to increase with age. Up to 45% of community-living people older than 65 years of age report having periodic leg movements (Bliwise, 1994). Many of these people also have a condition called "restless legs syndrome" in which they experience crawling, itching sensations in the legs at rest, often worst just before the onset of sleep.

Circadian-Rhythm Sleep Disorders

Circadian-rhythm disorders include transient disruptions, such as "jet lag" syndrome, and persistent disorders, such as delayed sleep phase syndrome. Jet lag tends to be worst after west-to-east travel across time zones, and it affects poor sleepers and older adults most intensely (ASDA, 1997; Arendt, Stone, & Skene, 2000). Delayed sleep phase syndrome is a less common but more problematic mismatch of personal circadian rhythm against societal expectations. Some people who function best by going to bed in the early hours of the morning and sleeping into the afternoon find occupations and partners to match. Other people with this disorder find that the continued struggle to awaken hours earlier than their internal clock dictates is not helped by simple treatments, such as establishing a consistent rising time. Exposure to bright light therapy, however, combined with good sleep habits such as consistent rising time and adequate total sleep time, can effectively alter circadian rhythms.

Parasomnias

Parasomnias are activities that are normal during waking but abnormal during sleep, such as sleepwalking (somnambulism), talking, and bed-wetting (enuresis). Parasomnias usually occur during slow-wave sleep and are most common in children. Usually, a family history of similar behaviors is present.

Occasional episodes of sleepwalking in children are fairly common, usually beginning before age 10 and stopping by age 15 years. Behavior during a sleepwalking episode may be semipurposeful, such as dressing or going to the bathroom, but lacking in coordination and appropriateness, such as voiding in the closet. Occurrence in adults is frequently associated with stress and anxiety. Parents and family members may need assistance in providing a safe environment to decrease the potential for injury.

Enuresis is not limited to slow-wave sleep, although almost two thirds of all episodes occur in the first third of the night. The prevalence decreases from 30% at age 4 to 10% at age 6 and 3% at age 12 years (ASDA, 1997). Enuresis is less common and tends to disappear earlier in girls than in boys.

Night terrors, another type of parasomnia, are repeated, sudden awakenings accompanied by screaming, acute anxiety, and disorientation. They occur mainly among children and are associated with incomplete arousal from slow-wave sleep early in the night. They are different from nightmares, or bad dreams that occur during REM sleep.

Discourage attempts to awaken people from the parasomnias of slow-wave sleep. Others should give help in the event of night terrors or somnambulism only to the extent that the person accepts, and they should encourage the person to return to sleep as the event subsides.

Impact on Activities of Daily Living

Sleep pattern dysfunction affects most activities of daily living (ADLs) to varying degrees. Closely linked to quality of life is the sense of feeling well rested and refreshed, with energy available for activity. Adequacy of sleep and rest directly affects and is affected by activity and exercise. Lack of sleep impairs coping and cognitive responses.

Role performance and social interactions may become disrupted in the presence of sleep pattern dysfunction. Irritability and impaired concentration accompany sleep deprivation. Snoring often disturbs the bed partner, who frequently seeks the refuge of another bedroom. The excessive sleepiness associated with disorders such as sleep apnea pose serious safety risks for those driving and operating hazardous machinery. Spouses of clients with chronic health problems (e.g., Parkinson's disease) that affect sleep are also vulnerable to sleep pattern disturbance (Smith et al., 1997).

ASSESSMENT

Sleep pattern disturbances in health and illness are frequent sources of concern to people. It is easy in the hospital setting for nurses to become preoccupied with assessments and treatments associated with the presenting illness. Likewise, in community practice, the diabetic's foot care or the new mother's ability to breast-feed may overshadow the concerns those people have regarding unsatisfactory sleep or inadequate rest. Professional nurses, however, can play a pivotal role in helping people to assess and to meet their needs for sleep and rest.

Subjective Data

The single most important criterion for adequacy of sleep and rest is the client's statement. The state of feeling rested is highly subjective. As discussed earlier, individual requirements for sleep vary widely. Besides the sense of feeling rested, people usually consider the congruency between their expectations and experience in relation to total sleep time, time in bed before sleep onset, number of awakenings, and time of final awakening. The history is the most important component of assessment of sleep and rest.

Normal Pattern Identification
Determine the person's usual sleep and rest patterns through questions such as the following:

- How many hours of sleep do you usually get?
- What time do you usually go to bed? Get up?
- What helps you get to sleep?
- What makes it hard for you to sleep?
- How do you feel when you awaken?
- How much sleep do you believe you should be getting?
- What helps you relax?
- How often do you nap? take rest periods?

Risk Identification
When assessing a person's risk for sleep problems, look for developmental and situational changes (environmental, physical, social) that may increase the need for or interfere with sleep and rest. Assess caffeine, nicotine, and alcohol intake and involvement in shift work.

Dysfunction Identification
Validate with the client whether he or she perceives that getting adequate sleep and rest is a problem. If a problem is identified, determine whether it is chronic or situational, what has helped, and what has made it worse. In situations of chronic disturbance, it may be useful to interview the sleep partner as well. Direct questions toward elaboration of the presenting concern. For example, if the person is concerned about daytime sleepiness, inquire about a history of snoring, awakenings accompanied by gasping, apneic periods that the partner may have observed, restlessness, and impact on activities associated with work, driving, and social interactions.

Having clients keep a sleep diary may be useful as an assessment and as an intervention. Giving clients responsibility for monitoring their own sleep pattern may help them recognize related factors. Young and middle-aged adults who are in the habit of sleeping late on days off sometimes express concern about sleep disturbances at the beginning of their work week, which they may attribute to job stress. Reviewing a sleep diary maintained for a couple of weeks may help them realize that when they consider their overall sleep time they are meeting their perceived requirements. It may also help them to recognize erratic sleep patterns or chronic sleep debts.

Objective Data

Physical Assessment
Observe for circles under the eyes, yawning, nodding, and slowness of response. Irritability, impaired concentration, and word-finding difficulties may indicate sleep pattern disturbances but may also indicate other problems.

Adequacy of rest after activity is often measured through return of heart rate and other physiologic parameters to baseline levels. Monitor vital signs after client- or caregiver-initiated activity for return to baseline resting levels in severely compromised clients.

Diagnostic Tests
People with severe sleep problems or excessive daytime sleepiness should be referred to a sleep laboratory for more thorough investigation. Polygraph recordings can be made, including evaluation of other parameters, such as oxygen saturation and periodic leg movements. Home monitoring has the advantage of familiar surroundings and is being used more for screening. It is important that a qualified sleep specialist interpret the results of home monitoring.

NURSING DIAGNOSIS
To formulate the nursing diagnosis, cluster the data, sifting out the incidental from the significant. For example, in an investigation of presleep rituals, 72% of respondents reported habitually watching television before going to bed, yet only 26% of them considered this activity important in getting to sleep (Reimer, 1985). Therefore, the absence of a television in a client's hospital environment may be of little significance. However, a client's seemingly casual comment regarding how the children at home are managing "without a disciplinarian around" may be a significant clue to sleep-disturbing anxiety. Diagnostic statements should be as specific as possible. Two diagnoses relate specifically to sleep problems.

Diagnostic Statement: Disturbed Sleep Pattern

Definition. Disturbed Sleep Pattern is "time-limited disruption of sleep amount and quality" (North American Nursing Diagnoses Association [NANDA], 2001).

Defining Characteristics. Of the defining characteristics for Disturbed Sleep Pattern, the following four are particularly important:

- Verbal complaints of difficulty falling asleep
- Awakening earlier or later than desired
- Dissatisfaction with sleep
- Verbal complaints of not feeling well rested

In other words, the length of time it takes to fall asleep, the time of awakening, and the number of arousals during the night are not sufficient to make the diagnosis. The person must express difficulty with these aspects of sleep and identify not feeling refreshed after sleep.

Related Factors. Sensory alterations may have caused or contributed to this change in functional health status. Internal sensory alterations, such as illness or psychological stress, may be affecting the client's state of arousal, ability to relax, or even balance of neurotransmitters that contribute to changing sleep stages.

Diagnostic Statement: Sleep Deprivation

Definition. Sleep Deprivation is "prolonged periods of time without sleep" (NANDA, 2001).

Defining Characteristics. This diagnosis is appropriate for many of the common types of sleep problems that nurses see in clinical situations. The most important defining characteristics are as follows:

- Daytime drowsiness
- Decreased ability to function
- Irritability
- Inability to concentrate

With more severe sleep deprivation clients may have hallucinations, transient paranoia, tremors and disturbed perception.

Related Factors. External sensory alterations from environmental changes or social cues may affect sleep patterns by modifying sensory input from changes in levels of light, noise, or social stimulation.

Related Nursing Diagnoses

Fatigue, in the NANDA classification, is defined as "an overwhelming sustained sense of exhaustion and decreased capacity for physical and mental work at usual level" (NANDA, 2001, p. 79). Some defining characteristics, such as tiredness and compromised concentration, are similar to Disturbed Sleep Pattern, but Fatigue persists despite an apparently adequate amount of sleep. Ineffective Coping may be the more appropriate nursing diagnosis if evidence shows that the client has a normal sleep pattern but wants to sleep more as a way of trying to avoid or cope with stress. Activity Intolerance can also be confused with Disturbed Sleep Pattern unless one listens carefully to the cues. The person with Activity Intolerance may describe fatigue or lack of energy but not inadequate sleep.

OUTCOME IDENTIFICATION AND PLANNING

After the nursing diagnoses and related factors are identified, client goals and interventions are planned. Client goals for Disturbed Sleep Pattern or Sleep Deprivation are specifically stated in terms such as minutes before sleep onset, hours of unbroken sleep, or verbal statement of feeling re-

freshed on wakening. Examples of specific client goals are as follows:

- The client will report fewer problems falling asleep.
- The client will report feeling more rested.
- The client will demonstrate physical signs of being rested.

Involving people in setting their own goals for sleep and rest is a useful way of helping them explore what is realistic for their developmental stage, lifestyle, and state of health.

Counseling may be high on the priority list of nurses in helping clients establish periods of adequate sleep and rest. Nurses may need to meet with family members and caregivers to address environmental needs and to teach caregiving practices for comfort. Examples of nursing interventions commonly used in promoting sleep and rest are listed in the accompanying display and discussed in the next section.

IMPLEMENTATION

Health Promotion

Environment Modification

Encourage clients to reserve the sleeping room for sleep whenever possible. Children should learn to play in other areas. Opportunities should be provided for home care, hospitalized, and residential clients to leave their rooms during the day when feasible. Objects associated with work, conflict, pain, or sleeplessness should be removed.

Encourage clients to establish a quiet, darkened environment modified according to their preferred level (e.g., low light may be a source of comfort for children or those in a strange environment). Instruct parents to remind children to use the bathroom before going to bed. Clients may need to restrict fluids in the evening. Clients can learn simple relaxation exercises for use at bedtime. People with impaired physical mobility should be assisted with voiding before retiring and made comfortable in the bed. Some older male clients appreciate having a urinal within reach.

SAFETY ALERT
Encourage clients to seek assistance when getting up, especially at night, if they are at risk for dizziness (e.g., postoperatively, after sedation) or have impaired mobility.

Provision of Intimacy and Security
A bedtime hug for a child, the shared bed with a marriage partner, and an enjoyable evening with friends are some ways in which people enhance sleep quality for one another. If social isolation is suspected as a related factor in Disturbed Sleep Pattern, assist the person to make or to improve social

contacts. A favorite blanket or stuffed animal is a way of enhancing security for children.

In the institutional setting, a backrub provides the warmth of human touch as well as physical relaxation. Arranging for family members to sit at a client's bedside may be helpful. Assurance of frequent checks by nursing staff, prompt responses to call bells, and a caring manner can do much to allay the fears of anxious clients. Prayer and reading scripture may facilitate a sense of peacefulness and subsequent sleep. Other people find meditation helpful. A sensitive assessment of the person's values and beliefs (see Chapter 51) helps nurses to maximize the client's strengths.

Sleep Rituals

Rituals play an important role in facilitating sleep. Whether it is a bedtime story for the toddler or a cup of tea for the older couple, the regular association of certain activities with the end of the waking period is one of the most effective ways to create the expectation of sleep.

A routine of "settling" clients in institutional settings can provide a similar marking of the end of the day. Assisting with washing of hands and face, giving a gentle massage, plumping pillows, and providing extra blankets may be incorporated. Use this time as an opportunity to help clients focus on small goals they accomplished during the day, visits from loved ones, or whatever else is helpful to settle their minds as well as their bodies.

Managing Individual Sleep Needs

Help clients to assess their individual sleep needs and to anticipate developmental changes. Remind middle-aged and older people that shorter unbroken sleep periods are normal. Likewise, insomniacs (and potential ones) may benefit from reassurance that they can function on relatively little sleep. Parents and other caregivers may need anticipatory guidance regarding the wide variability in sleep needs of individual children.

Nursing Interventions for Altered Function

Despite major advances in medical therapeutics, rest remains one of the most common symptomatic treatments for a wide variety of disease conditions. "Rest the affected part" is a standard intervention for almost any condition.

Rest

Clients who have suffered myocardial ischemia as a result of a blood clot are placed on a strict regimen of restricted activity. Helping these clients to maintain a resting state for the heart once the initial period of pain has subsided is a challenge to the nurse's creativity. Help these clients to realize that, although they may "feel great," the damaged heart needs further rest. Assist such clients to make lasting lifestyle changes that incorporate more rest and relaxation.

Research on the amount of rest required after various activities provides a basis for nurses to make decisions in implementing care. Alteri (1984) studied 10 male clients 8 to 20 days after myocardial infarction to determine the length of time required for vital signs to return to the preactivity baseline. Climbing one flight of stairs required 7 minutes to recover, a 10-minute walk on a level surface required 10 minutes to recover, and showering required 30.5 minutes to reach the preactivity baseline. She also found that participants consistently expressed the feeling that they had recovered long before their vital signs returned to normal.

Maintaining traction to "rest" a client's fractured femur or instilling eyedrops temporarily to paralyze and thus rest the eye after surgery are ways in which nurses help clients meet situationally induced changes in rest requirements.

Use of Medications

Hypnotics may be useful as a short-term intervention during situationally induced sleep pattern disturbance. Other interventions should be tried first, however. In making decisions and teaching clients regarding the use of hypnotics, consider the following principles:

- All hypnotics require judicious use because they interfere with normal sleep architecture to some degree. REM sleep is most vulnerable. Therefore, signs of selective stage deficit may be evident even though total sleep time has increased through hypnotic use. Teach clients that a night or two of increased dreaming (REM rebound) after the drug is discontinued is not unusual. Tapering withdrawal in long-term users can prevent REM rebound.
- All hypnotics impair waking function as long as they are pharmacologically active. Perception of daytime drowsiness and impairment of psychomotor skills fades more rapidly than do the actual effects. Therefore, teach people in the community environment who

are taking hypnotics about the half-life of the drugs and warn them to avoid driving or handling machinery while the drug is in their system. Also, take safety precautions in home and hospital when those who have taken a hypnotic need to get to the bathroom at night.

- The effectiveness of hypnotics decreases over a 4-week period, so long-term users are probably being affected more by the expectation of sleep associated with taking a pill than by the active drug. Teach these people alternative sleep-promoting strategies and prepare them for the possible short-term rebound effects that may follow withdrawal.
- Hypnotics are most appropriately used for insomnia of recent origin, such as after a situational crisis. Clients should take the smallest effective dose, and then only for a few nights or intermittently as required.
- Certain people are at increased risk from the use of hypnotics. The time required for older adults to metabolize long-acting benzodiazepines is increased. Arousal because of decreased oxygen levels is depressed after the administration of hypnotics. Therefore, use particular caution in administering ordered hypnotics to older adults and those whose pulmonary function is compromised.

Table 42-2 shows how knowledge of the specific properties of each hypnotic can help nurses determine implications for assessment and teaching. The chart is not intended to be exhaustive, but rather to highlight the need for nurses to be knowledgeable about the hypnotics that clients may take.

Sleep pattern disturbance is often associated with periods of high anxiety or depression. Therefore, nurses will also encounter clients who are taking anxiolytic or sedative antidepressants that improve sleep. Most anxiolytics are also benzodiazepines, but of the long-acting type, such as lorazepam (Ativan). The action of antidepressants on sleep may be direct,

through modulation of neurotransmission, especially serotonin, as well as indirect, through treating the underlying depression. Melatonin is not a hypnotic but rather acts on the sleep–wake cycle. Its use is promising, but large-scale systematic studies of its safety and efficacy are as yet unavailable.

Use of Consistent Routine

The single most important intervention for chronic sleep pattern disturbance is to establish a consistent rising time. Getting up is subject to voluntary control, whereas falling asleep usually is not. Slightly decreasing the time in bed solidifies sleep and, along with a consistent rising time, will finally lead to more regular times of sleep onset.

Counseling regarding the maintenance of routines may be required for socially and occupationally isolated clients. For acutely ill clients, enhance cuing by turning lights down at night, keeping window drapes open during the day when possible, and providing verbal cuing regarding time of day.

Healthcare Planning and Home or Community-Based Care

Clients often underestimate their need for rest when recovering from illness or surgery. Nurses may need to help them plan for periods of rest and for energy conservation. Assessment of and suggestions for correction or adaptation to environmental conditions may be necessary. Remember to consider the sleep and rest needs of home caregivers when ill or immobile clients need assistance during the night. Respite care may be an option, or caregivers may need counseling about their sleep and rest needs.

EVALUATION

Evaluate the degree to which disturbed sleep pattern, sleep deprivation, or inadequate rest has been resolved according to the client goals initially established. Particularly for this func-

TABLE 42-2

Selected Hypnotics: Their Properties and Nursing Implications		
Hypnotic	Properties	Nursing Implications
Benzodiazepines		
Flurazepam (Dalmane)	Onset: Rapid (17 min) Half life: 74–160 hr	Good for onset and maintenance insomnia; maximum effectiveness not until third night; less rebound effect because of a long half-life but more of a hangover
Temazepam (Restoril)	Onset: 1–2 hr Half-life: 9–12 hr	Poor for onset insomnia; most effective for maintenance or early wakening insomnia; hangover effect; safer for older adults
Other		
Zolpidem (Ambien)	Short-acting Half-life: 2.5 hr	Good for onset insomnia
Zopiclone (Imovane)	Short-acting Half-life: 4–6.5 hr	Good for onset and maintenance insomnia; less suppression of slow-wave sleep than the benzodiazepines

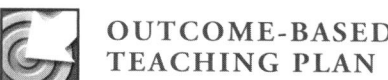

OUTCOME-BASED TEACHING PLAN

Ms. Song is an accountant with a heavy work schedule at the beginning of every calendar year. She finds that she has great difficulty getting to sleep and staying asleep at night. Yet she is drowsy during the day and worries that she may make accounting errors. She has come to the clinic to have her sleep problem assessed and to seek some advice.

OUTCOME: At the end of the teaching session, Ms. Song states factors that could contribute to her difficulty in falling asleep and maintaining sleep at night.
Strategies
- Evaluate Ms. Song's normal sleep routine, her knowledge of factors that contribute to sleep disturbance, and her usual approach to managing her sleep problem.
- Discuss factors that interfere with sleep onset and maintenance, such as use of alcohol or caffeine, lack of relaxation before bedtime.
- Have Ms. Song discuss these and related factors with you.

OUTCOME: Ms. Song will state a plan to decrease sleep disruption.
Strategies
- Suggest that Ms. Song employ the following approaches, and state how she will determine their effectiveness.
- Remind Ms. Song to get up at the same time each day and to avoid sleeping in on days off.
- Instruct Ms. Song to eat sensibly and regularly. If used to a bedtime snack, she should keep up the habit.
- Teach Ms. Song to avoid alcohol and caffeine. Their effects linger to disturb sleep.
- Plan for Ms. Song to exercise daily but not too late in the day. Enjoyable activities will enhance the benefits for sleep and rest.
- Help Ms. Song determine ways to set her mind at rest before going to bed with relaxing music, a good book, or valued companionship. If she cannot sleep, Ms. Song will get up and do something relaxing until feeling sleepy.

tional health pattern, validate findings with clients because of the subjectivity and individual variations in what people require for adequate rest and satisfying sleep. Examples of possible outcome criteria are listed below.

Goal

The client will report fewer problems falling asleep.

Possible Outcome Criteria

- Within 7 days, the client reports decrease in sleep latency to 10 to 15 minutes.

- Within 7 days, the client reports less anxiety regarding falling asleep.

Goal

The client will report feeling more rested.

Possible Outcome Criteria

- Within 10 days, the client verbalizes feeling less fatigued.
- As observed by nurse by the tenth day, the client non-verbally demonstrates increased restfulness (less dozing, greater animation in activity).

Goal

The client will demonstrate physical signs of being rested.

Possible Outcome Criteria

- By the seventh day, the client has decreases in circles under the eyes, excessive yawning, or slowness of response.
- Within 10 days, the client reports to nurse that he or she feels rested after activity.

KEY CONCEPTS

- Sleep is a naturally occurring, altered state of consciousness characterized by awareness and responsiveness to stimuli and by being readily reversible.
- Rest is a physical and emotional state of decreased muscle and cognitive activity.
- Sleep and rest have restorative, protective, and energy-conserving functions.
- The two main types of sleep are NREM (quiet sleep) and REM (rapid eye movement) sleep.
- NREM sleep consists of four stages: stage 1, transitional; stage 2, light; stages 3 and 4, deep and slow-wave sleep.
- REM sleep is similar to wakefulness in terms of brain activity, but muscle tone is lower and vital signs fluctuate widely.
- Adults progress through stages 1–2–3–4–3–2–REM in cycles of approximately 90 minutes.
- Sleep patterns change throughout the lifespan; the very young and the very old require the most sleep.
- Infants have sleep cycles that last about 50 minutes.
- Guidelines for evaluating adequacy of sleep are waking with a feeling of being refreshed and absence of daytime sleepiness.
- Factors affecting sleep and rest include environmental stimuli, nutrition, exercise, illness, and hospitalization.
- Common sleep problems include disorders of initiating and maintaining sleep (insomnia), excessive daytime sleepiness, disorders of the sleep–wake cycle, and parasomnias.
- Anticipating changes in sleep patterns and needs for rest can contribute to promotion of a healthy balance between rest and activity and a recognition that sleep pattern changes are developmentally normal.

NURSING PLAN OF CARE
THE CLIENT WITH DISTURBED SLEEP PATTERN

Nursing Diagnosis
Disturbed Sleep Pattern related to lack of cues for day–night schedule; manifested by erratic sleep schedule, frequent naps, nocturnal wandering, asking for breakfast at 0100 or 0200.

Client Goal
Client will sleep more at night and less during the day.

Client Outcome Criteria
- Client increases nocturnal sleep time by 20% over next 2 weeks.
- Client verbalizes more appropriate orientation to time of day.

Nursing Intervention
1. Offer meals at regular times, corresponding to client's previous pattern.

2. Provide active, meaningful activities during day-time hours, including exposure to natural light and an outdoor environment when possible.
3. Monitor frequency and duration of naps.

4. Create an individualized bedtime ritual that includes a quieting activity, a light carbohydrate snack, going to the bathroom, and a settling routine.
5. Do not waken even if incontinent. Change and assist the client to the bathroom when he or she spontaneously awakens.

6. If turning or other care is necessary, try to provide for periods of up to 2 hours of undisturbed sleep time whenever possible.

Scientific Rationale
1. Mealtimes are important social cues that reinforce circadian rhythms, which tend to weaken with advancing age.
2. Light exposure is communicated through the retina to the suprachiasmatic nucleus, helping to set the circadian "clock."
3. Napping is not contraindicated but is best at the time of day opposite to the midpoint of the nocturnal sleep period. Short naps (30 min or less) are preferable to avoid deep sleep.
4. Reduced stimulation and rituals associated with sleep enhance sleep onset.

5. Older adults who can turn themselves generally do better to have their sleep undisturbed and tend to waken spontaneously if wet when their sleep cycle lightens.
6. Sleep cycles average 90 minutes. A sleep latency of 20 to 30 minutes means it would take about 2 hours to experience a full sleep cycle.

REFERENCES

Alteri, C. A. (1984). The patient with myocardial infarction: Rest prescriptions for activities of daily living. *Heart and Lung, 13,* 355–359.

American Sleep Disorders Association (ASDA). (1997). *The international classification of sleep disorders: Diagnostic and coding manual* (2nd ed.). Rochester, NY: Author.

Ancoli-Israel, S. (1997). Sleep problems in older adults: Putting myths to bed. *Geriatrics, 52*(1), 20–30.

Arendt, J., Stone, B., & Skene, D. (2000). Jet lag and sleep disruption. In M. H. Kryger, T. Roth, & W. C. Dement (Eds.), *Principles and practice of sleep medicine* (3rd ed., pp. 591–599). Philadelphia: W. B. Saunders.

Bliwise, D. L. (2000). Normal aging. In M. H. Kryger, T. Roth, & W. C. Dement (Eds.), *Principles and practice of sleep medicine* (3rd ed., pp. 26–42). Philadelphia: W. B. Saunders.

Briones, B., Adams, N., Strauss, M., Rosenberg, C., Whalen, C., Carskadon, M., Roebuck, T., Winters, M., & Redline, S. (1996). Relationship between sleepiness and general health status. *Sleep, 19*(7), 583–588.

Bunnell, D. E. (1988). Passive body heating and sleep: Influence of proximity to sleep. *Sleep, 11*(2), 210–219.

Cohen, F. L., Nehring, W. M., & Cloninger, L. (1996). Symptom description and management in narcolepsy. *Holistic Nursing Practice, 10*(4), 44–53.

Driver, H. S. (1996). Sleep in women. *Journal of Psychosomatic Research, 40*(3), 227–230.

Driver, H. S. & Taylor, S. R. (2001). Exercise and sleep. *Sleep Medicine Reviews, 4*(4), 387–402.

Edinger, J. D., Sullivan, R. J., Bastian, L. A., Hope, T. V., Young, M., Fins, A. I., Glenn, D. M., Marsh, G. R., Dailey, D., Shaw, E., & Vasilas, D. (2000). Insomnia and the eye of the beholder: Are there clinical markers of objective sleep disturbances among adults with and without insomnia complaints? *Journal of Consulting and Clinical Psychology, 68*(4), 586–593.

Evans, J. C., & French, D. G. (1995). Sleep and healing in intensive care settings. *Dimensions of Critical Care Nursing, 14*(4), 189–199.

Flemons, W. W., & McNicholas, W. T. (1997). Clinical prediction of the sleep apnea syndrome. *Sleep Medicine Reviews, 1*(1), 19–32.

George, C. F. (2000). Hypertension, ischemic heart disease, and stroke. In M. H. Kryger, T. Roth, & W. C. Dement (Eds.), *Principles and practice of sleep medicine* (3rd ed., pp. 1030–1039). Philadelphia: W. B. Saunders.

Hodgson, L. A. (1991). Why do we need sleep? Relating theory to nursing practice. *Journal of Advanced Nursing, 16,* 1503–1510.

Horne, J. A. (1988). *Why we sleep.* New York: Oxford University Press.

Lorrain, D., & De Koninck, J. (1998). Sleep position and sleep stages: Evidence of their independence. *Sleep, 21*(4), 335–340.

Mendelson, W. B. (2000). Hypnotics: Basic mechanisms and pharmacology. In M. H. Kryger, T. Roth, & W. C. Dement (Eds.), *Principles and practice of sleep medicine* (3rd ed., pp. 407–413). Philadelphia: W. B. Saunders.

Monk, T. H. (2000). Shift work. In M. H. Kryger, T. Roth, & W. C. Dement (Eds.), *Principles and practice of sleep medicine* (3rd ed., pp. 600–605). Philadelphia: W. B. Saunders.

Mornhinweg, G. C., & Voignier, R. R. (1996). Rest. *Holistic Nursing Practice, 10*(4), 54–60.

North American Nursing Diagnoses Association. (2001). *NANDA nursing diagnoses: Definitions and classification 2001–2002.* Philadelphia: Author.

Oswald, I. (1987). The benefit of sleep. *Holistic Medicine, 2,* 137–139.

Phillips, B., & Ancoli-Israel, S. (2001). Sleep disorders in the elderly. *Sleep Medicine, 2,* 99–114.

Porth, C. (1998). *Pathophysiology: Concepts of altered health states* (6th ed.). Philadelphia: Lippincott Williams & Wilkins.

Reimer, M. (1985). Nursing interventions perceived by patients and their nurses as facilitating nocturnal sleep in hospital. Unpublished manuscript. Calgary, Canda: University of Calgary.

Renaud, M. T. (1996). Neonatal sleep patterns: Implications for nursing. *Holistic Nursing Practice, 10*(4), 27–32.

Report of the National Commission on Sleep Disorders Research. (1993). *Wake up America: A national sleep alert.* Washington, D.C.

Robinson, C. (1993). Impaired sleep. In V. K. Carrieri, A. M. Lindsey, & C. M. West (Eds.), *Pathophysiological phenomena in nursing* (2nd ed., pp. 390–417). Philadelphia: W. B. Saunders.

Roehrs, T., Zorick, F., & Roth, T. (2000). Transient and short-term insomnias. In M. H. Kryger, T. Roth, & W. C. Dement (Eds.), *Principles and practice of sleep medicine* (3rd ed., pp. 624–632). Philadelphia: W. B. Saunders.

Schwitzer, P. K. (2000). Drugs that disturb sleep and wakefulness. In M. H. Kryger, T. Roth, & W. C. Dement (Eds.), *Principles and practice of sleep medicine* (3rd ed., pp. 442–461). Philadelphia: W. B. Saunders.

Smith, M. C., Ellgring, H., & Oertel, W. H. (1997). Sleep disturbances in Parkinson's disease patients and spouses. *Journal of the American Geriatric Society, 45,* 194–199.

Zarcone, V. P. (2000). Sleep hygiene. In M. H. Kryger, T. Roth, & W. C. Dement (Eds.), *Principles and practice of sleep medicine* (3rd ed., pp. 657–661). Philadelphia: W. B. Saunders.

BIBLIOGRAPHY

Ancoli-Israel, S. (1997). Sleep problems in older adults: Putting myths to bed. *Geriatrics, 52*(1), 20–22, 25–26, 28, 30.

Beck-Little, R., & Weinrich, S. P. (1998). Assessment and management of sleep disorders in the elderly. *Journal of Gerontological Nursing, 24*(4), 21–29.

Cohen, F. L., Nehring, W. M., & Cloninger, L. (1996). Symptom description and management in narcolepsy. *Holistic Nursing Practice, 10*(4), 44–53.

Driver, H. S., & Taylor, S. R. (1996, Jan. 21). Sleep disturbance and exercise. *Sports Medicine, 21*(1), 1–6.

Epstein, R., Chillag, N., & Lavie, P. (1998). Starting times of school: Effects on daytime functioning of fifth-grade children in Israel. *Sleep, 21*(3), 250–256.

Evans, B. D., & Rogers, A. E. (1994). 24-Hour sleep/wake patterns in healthy elderly persons. *Applied Nursing Research, 7*(2), 75–83.

Evans, J. C., & French, D. G. (1995). Sleep and healing in intensive care settings. *Dimensions of Critical Care Nursing, 14*(4), 189–199.

Grossman, V. G. (1997). Defying circadian rhythm: The emergency nurse and the night shift. *Journal of Emergency Nursing, 23*(6), 602–607.

Kerr, S. M., Jowett, S. A., & Smith, L. N. (1996). Preventing sleep problems in infants: A randomized controlled trial. *Journal of Advanced Nursing, 24,* 938–942.

Landis, C. A., & Whitney, J. D. (1997). Effects of 72 hours sleep deprivation on wound healing in the rat. *Research in Nursing and Health, 20,* 259–267.

Matthews, E. A., Farrell, G. A., & Blackmore, A. M. (1996). Preventing sleep problems in infants: A randomized controlled trial. *Journal of Advanced Nursing, 24,* 938–942.

Mornhinweg, G. C., & Voignier, R. A. (1996). Rest. *Holistic Nursing Practice, 10*(4), 54–60.

Mosko, S., Richard, C., & McKenna, J. (1997). Maternal sleep and arousals during bedsharing with infants. *Sleep, 20*(2), 142–150.

Ouslander, J. G., Buxton, W. G., Al-Samarrai, N. R., Cruise, P. A., Alessi, C., & Schnelle, J. F. (1998). Nighttime urinary incontinence and sleep disruption among nursing home residents. *Journal of the American Geriatrics Society, 46,* 463–466.

Redeker, N. S., Mason, D. J., Wykpisz, E., & Glica, B. (1996). Sleep patterns in women after coronary artery bypass surgery. *Applied Nursing Research, 9*(3), 115–122.

Renaud, M. T. (1996). Neonatal sleep patterns: Implications for nursing. *Holistic Nursing Practice, 10*(4), 27–32.

Richardson, P. (1996). Sleep in pregnancy. *Holistic Nursing Practice, 10*(4), 20–26.

Shaver, J. L., Lentz, M., Landis, C., Heitkemper, M. M., Buchwald, D. S., & Woods, N. F. (1997). Sleep, psychological distress, and stress arousal in women with fibromyalgia. *Research in Nursing and Health, 20,* 247–257.

Smith, M. C., Ellgring, H., & Oertel, W. H. (1997). Sleep disturbances in Parkinson's disease patients and spouses. *Journal of the American Geriatrics Society, 45,* 194–199.

Stansberry, T. T. (2001). Narcolepsy: Unveiling a mystery. *American Journal of Nursing, 101*(8), 50–63.

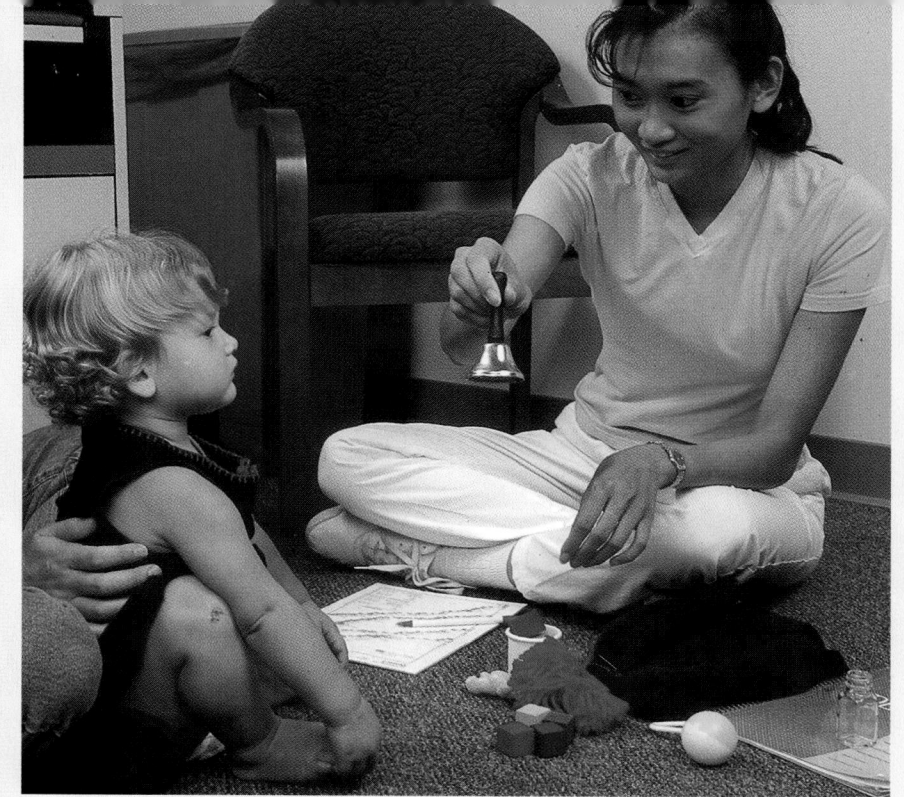

Cognition and Perception

43 Pain Perception and Management

Learning Objectives

Upon completion of this chapter, the student will be able to do the following:

1. Explain the transmission of pain sensation.
2. Outline how pain transmission is facilitated or inhibited.
3. Describe the four sensory pain components that must be included in the nursing database.
4. Examine nonpharmacologic methods of pain relief based on individual needs.
5. Describe the types, actions, and adverse effects of analgesics.
6. List nursing implications for various classes of drugs used for pain management.
7. Develop a nursing plan of care for a client experiencing pain.

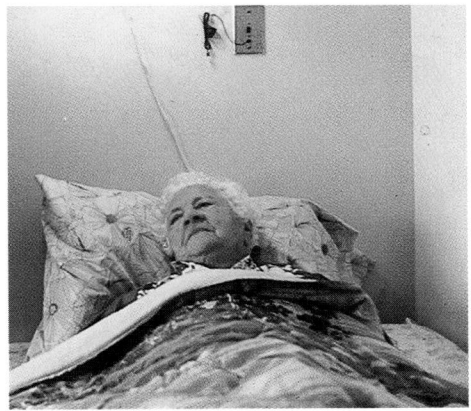

Critical Thinking Challenge

You are a home hospice nurse caring for an older client who was diagnosed 3 months ago with lung cancer. The client's history is positive for lung cancer (father died from it) and for smoking one to two packs of cigarettes per day for 50 years. Staging revealed metastases in the right lung, both kidneys, and the sixth cervical vertebra. Currently the client reports pain in the left shoulder, upper arm, and right upper thigh. The client rates the pain as 6 on a scale of 0 to 10. The client describes it as dull and aching but is unable to provide further description of its quality. She reports that the shoulder pain is constant and increases with particular movements. Her right leg pain is present only when ambulating and when turning onto her left side when in bed. The client's ability to tolerate activity has diminished since radiation treat-ments began. Before treatment, the client was out of bed 14 to 16 hours per day but now is out of bed 3 to 5 hours per day.

Once you have completed this chapter and have incorporated pain perception and management into your knowledge base, review the above scenario and reflect on the following areas of Critical Thinking.

1. Give your interpretation of the client's reports of pain and activity intolerance.
2. Reflect on your feelings about the client's health history and present condition. Infer what the client's thoughts and feelings may be.
3. Outline additional assessment data you need to develop a plan for relieving this person's pain.
4. Explain the rationale for using pharmacologic and nonpharmacologic methods of pain relief for this client.
5. Plan at least two health-promotion activities that may help this client.

Pain, one of the most complex human experiences, is an invisible phenomenon influenced by the interaction of affective (emotional), behavioral, cognitive, and physiologic-sensory factors. Because pain is a highly individual experience, the basis for pain management is simply the client's description of pain. Pain exists whenever the person says it does (McCaffery & Pasero, 1999).

PAIN PERCEPTION

Although pain is a great source of misery, initially it serves an important biologic purpose. It helps to minimize injury and is often a protective injury-prevention mechanism. For instance, pain makes a person pull his or her hand away from a hot stove, and right lower abdominal pain warns the person of a possibly diseased appendix, prompting early medical intervention. People who are born without the ability to feel pain usually do not survive past early childhood. Death occurs because of the lack of warning of injury or disease and the delay of prompt treatment. Persistent, unrelieved pain, however, serves no biologic function for most people. Conversely, it compromises quality of life and is an unnecessary stressor with pathophysiologic consequences on most body systems (Cousins, Power, & Smith, 2000).

Pain is one of the most common and compelling reasons that people seek healthcare. Understanding the structures and mechanisms related to pain and its perception aids in effective management.

Structures Related to the Pain Process

The brain perceives pain as a result of complex processing of stimuli from a site of actual or potential injury. The perception of the pain sensation is the result of many different inputs.

Peripheral Structures

Sensory pain receptors (**nociceptors**) are free nerve endings in the tissue that respond to tissue-injuring stimuli (noxious stimuli). Receptors that respond to noxious temperature changes (thermoreceptors), chemicals (chemoreceptors), or pressure (mechanical receptors) transmit a pain signal if the noxious stimuli are sufficiently strong.

Nociceptors or neurons responding to noxious stimuli are found in the skin, blood vessels, subcutaneous tissue, muscle, fascia, periosteum, viscera, joints, and other structures (Besson, 1999). Nociceptors are located on two types of peripheral nerve cells (A-delta fibers and C-fibers) that are responsible for transmitting pain sensations from the tissues to the central nervous system (CNS). A-delta fibers give rise to bright, sharp, well-localized pain that is immediately associated with the injury. Slow-conducting C-fibers cause a second pain sensation that is dull, poorly localized, and persistent after injury.

The difference between pain from A-delta and C-fiber activation can best be described as first versus second pain. For example, if a sharp object falls on your foot, a fast, sharp pain alerts you to the injury. This pain is caused by stimulation of the A-delta fibers. After removing the object from the foot, a burning, dull, aching sensation persists and is caused by stimulation of the C-fibers.

Central Structures

Ascending Pathways. Signal transmission from the peripheral nociceptive fibers to the brain is complex. Signals carried by A-delta fibers and C-fibers travel along the fibers from peripheral tissues through the dorsal root of the spinal cord and terminate in the dorsal horn of the spinal cord. Signals communicate with local interneurons (excitatory and inhibitory) and neurons with long axons (projection cells) that ascend to the brain by way of several crossed and uncrossed pathways. The spinothalamic tract appears to be the most important pathway for pain sensation. This crossed pathway is located in the white matter of the anterolateral quadrant of the spinal cord (Fig. 43-1). The spinothalamic tract transmits sensations of pain and temperature and crudely localized touch. The spinothalamic tract enters the brain stem and terminates principally in the thalamus, where other neurons convey the information to the sensory cortex (Besson, 1999).

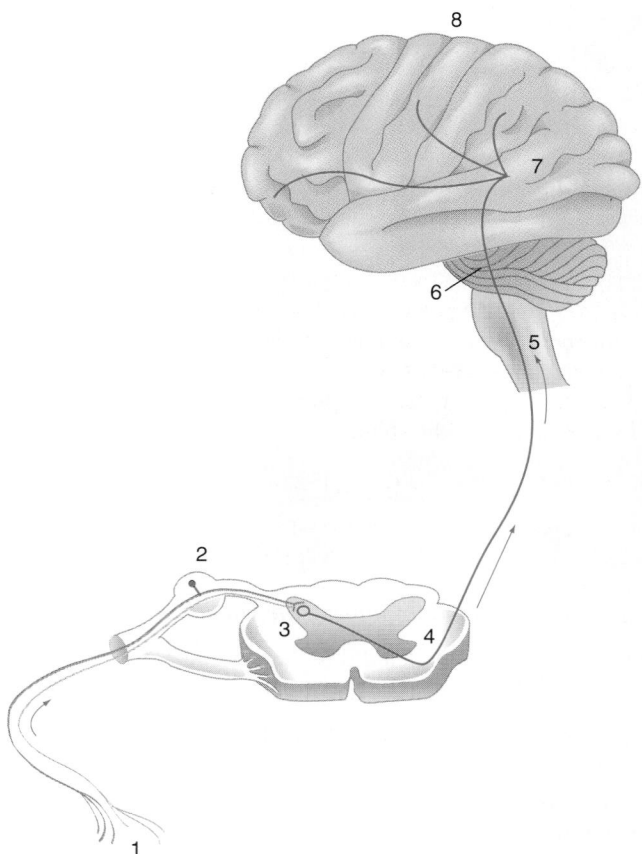

FIGURE 43-1   Pain stimuli are transmitted from pain receptors (1) by way of sensory nerves into the dorsal root ganglia (2). The impulse enters the spinal cord, and synapses terminate on neuron cells in the substantia gelatinosa (3). Signals then cross the cord and ascend in the spinothalamic tract (4), through the reticular formation (5) and areas of the midbrain (6) to the thalamus (7) and cortex (8). Pain is perceived somewhere in the brain.

Descending Pathways. Several pathways convey information from the brain in the dorsolateral white columns to the spinal dorsal horn (Besson, 1999). Descending in the lateral white columns, a third of corticospinal tract neurons terminate on neurons in the spinal dorsal horn and modify afferent nociceptive information (i.e., allow the brain to pay selective attention to certain stimuli and to ignore other painful stimuli). This information from the brain can modulate pain perception.

Pain Modulation

The afferent nociceptive message is subject to modulation (both enhancement and inhibition) at all levels of the nervous system. Modulation at the peripheral nerve, spinal cord, and several brain sites influences pain perception. The capacity for modulation helps to explain the tremendous variability in pain that people with similar injuries experience.

Peripheral Modulation

Mechanical, chemical, or thermal events that injure tissue usually stimulate nociceptors. Injured cells and tissue-repair mechanisms release one or more chemical substances that bind to peripheral nociceptors and activate the nerve fiber (cause an action potential). Some chemicals activate the nerve fiber, whereas others sensitize the nerve for activation with a smaller stimulus than usually required (Basbaum, 1999). These chemicals cause A-delta and C-fibers to become excited and transmit an action potential toward the spinal cord. Presence of these chemicals increases the amount of pain a person perceives. Blocking release or production of these chemicals, some of which are part of the inflammatory response, is one peripheral mechanism to inhibit pain perception. Another way to inhibit pain is by blocking the sodium channels on the A-delta or C-fibers, such as through use of local anesthetic agents, thus preventing transmission of the action potential to the spinal cord.

Spinal Cord Modulation

The **spinal dorsal horn,** where complex processing of messages occurs, is one of the most important areas for pain modulation. Input to dorsal horn excitatory interneurons releases substance P and glutamate, both of which have the potential to facilitate pain sensation (Basbaum, 1999). Input to inhibitory interneurons and from descending neurons releases a number of neurochemicals that have inhibitory effects on pain sensations. These neurochemicals bind to several types of receptors. For example, the opioid receptors, important for the inhibition of pain perception, are sites where **endogenous** (produced by the body) opioids and **exogenous** (administered to the person) opioids bind. Three groups of endogenous opioids relieve pain: enkephalin, endorphin, and dynorphin.

Spinal Reflexes

Some sensory impulses that enter the spinal cord produce a reflex response through motor neurons in the spinal ventral horn with fibers to a muscle near the pain site. The muscle then con-

tracts in a protective action (e.g., a pinprick causes immediate withdrawal of the extremity). These spinal reflexes may enhance pain through an effect on the injured tissue. For example, trauma may provoke an efferent (motor) reflex that produces muscle spasm in the injured area and causes more pain.

Pain Theories

Many theories have been developed to describe the complex phenomenon of pain. The gate control theory, developed by Melzack and Wall (1965), was the first to incorporate some aspects from other theories and to present the notion of pain modulation at the spinal cord and brain levels. According to this theory, dorsal horn cells act as a gate, closing to prevent nociceptive impulses from reaching the brain or opening to allow impulses to be transmitted to the brain. In simple terms, when the gate is open, pain impulses flow through and the person feels pain. When the gate is closed, pain impulses stop. Opening the gate is influenced by the A-delta and C-fibers, and closing the gate is influenced by the activity of the large A-alpha and A-beta fibers, the reticular formation in the brain stem, other brain sites, and the cerebral cortex (Fields, 2000; Melzack & Wall, 1965).

The gate control theory emphasizes sensory, emotional, behavioral, and cognitive dimensions of pain as playing a role in modulation of the physiologic dimension. The theory stimulated much research to understand what is now known about normal processing of nociceptive information and the altered processing that occurs in persistent, unrelieved pain states. Many mechanisms suggested by the gate control theory are specifically known today; others are still under investigation. The theory, however, provided ideas about pain relief therapies that act in different parts of the nervous system.

Characteristics of Pain

Typically people describe pain by its location, intensity, quality, and temporal pattern (Display 43-1). Sensory components of the pain experience are subjective but can be measured using standardized tools. One person's description of pain intensity may differ from another's, even though the pain stimuli are the same. This difference emphasizes the role of pain modulation in the unique personal experience. There are, however, some commonalities in location, quality, and temporal pattern when people experience similar types of pain.

Location

Superficial pain that emanates from the skin or from tissues close to the surface is usually localized, and the client's pain location report matches the location of tissue damage. When pain originates from internal organs, however, the location the person reports may not be localized in the area of tissue damage. For example, pain from the abdominal or pelvic organs (liver, spleen, kidney, bladder) may be referred to areas far distant from the site of tissue damage (Fig. 43-2). If referred pain is not considered when evaluating the client's reported pain location, therapy could be misdirected.

DESCRIPTIONS OF PAIN

Location

Localized vs diffuse	Right vs left
Proximal vs distal	Upper vs lower
Medial vs lateral	Phantom
Anterior vs posterior	Referred

Intensity

Mild	Severe
Slight	Excruciating
Moderate	

Quality

Aching	Sickening
Annoying	Stabbing
Burning	Tender
Exhausting	Terrifying
Gnawing	Throbbing
Heavy	Tight
Intense	Tiring
Nagging	Torturing
Sharp	Unbearable
Shooting	

Temporal Pattern

Acute	Intermittent
Chronic	Spasmodic
Constant	Transient

Associated Characteristics

Anger and aggression	Muscle spasms
Anorexia	Nausea and vomiting
Anxiety	Regression
Depression	Visual disturbance
Fatigue	Withdrawal
Fear	

Intensity

Pain intensity indicates the magnitude or amount of pain perceived. Terms used to describe pain intensity include none, mild, slight, moderate, severe, and excruciating. Pain intensity also may be described on a numeric scale (e.g., on a scale of 0 to 10, with 0 indicating no pain and 10 indicating pain as bad as it could be).

Pain intensity may vary among clients, depending on their previous experience with pain, personal expectations, ability to be distracted or to concentrate on other things, level of consciousness, and activity level. Fear of the consequences of reporting pain intensity may cause clients to minimize their reported pain. Level of activity also influences pain intensity. A person may have no pain at rest or when lying still but have severe pain with the slightest movement such as shifting positions, taking deep breaths, or coughing.

Pain Threshold.   The amount of pain stimulation a person requires before feeling it is that person's **pain threshold.** Under normal conditions, the pain threshold is remarkably uniform throughout a person's life and among different people, regardless of race. In the presence of tissue damage, however, the same stimulus that once caused no or little pain can produce intense pain. The person's state of consciousness (i.e., under anesthesia) can dramatically change his or her pain threshold.

Pain Tolerance.   **Pain tolerance** is the highest intensity of pain that the person is willing to tolerate. Pain tolerance varies markedly in the same person over time and among different people. Some people can tolerate severe pain without intervention; others can tolerate only minimal discomfort. Endogenous pain modulation systems (facilitating or inhibiting the pain) may account for these differences.

Quality

Pain quality refers to how the pain feels to the client or words that describe the pain's nature. When presented with a list of verbal descriptors, clients frequently use words such as those listed in Display 43-1. Without a list of descriptors, many clients find it easier to use an analogy. For example, a headache may be "pounding like a hammer" or chest pain may be "like an elephant sitting on my chest."

Temporal Pattern

Onset (when it starts) and duration (how long it lasts) are components of temporal pain pattern. Clients may have pain all the time, incident pain (with movement or specific procedures), or breakthrough pain (returns before a regularly scheduled dose of analgesic). Pain pattern can be used to determine the appropriate dosing schedule and medication preparation. Return of pain before the end of analgesic duration suggests the need for an increase in the drug's amount or frequency.

The terms acute and chronic often are used to designate the two main types of pain onset and duration. **Acute pain** occurs abruptly after an injury or disease and persists until healing occurs. Acute pain also may be associated with anxiety and fear. Acute pain consistently increases at night and during wound care, ambulation, coughing, and deep breathing. If acute pain is not effectively managed, it may progress to a chronic state.

Chronic pain lasts for a prolonged period, and its cause is not amenable to specific treatment tissue (Merskey & Bogduk, 1994). It is associated with prolonged tissue pathology or pain that persists beyond the normal healing period for an acute injury or disease. It also increases at night. Depression related to chronic pain is not uncommon. Frustration and fear also are common feelings that clients experience when no identifiable cause for their chronic pain can be determined.

Malignant pain is a third type, with recurrent, acute pain episodes, persistent chronic pain, or both associated with a progressive malignant-type process. The etiology for malignant pain is resistant to cure, and the pain may be described as intractable. Clients with malignant pain often describe it as all-consuming and interfering with their quality of life. Examples of causes of malignant pain are arthritis or cancer. Like chronic and acute pain, malignant pain often increases at night.

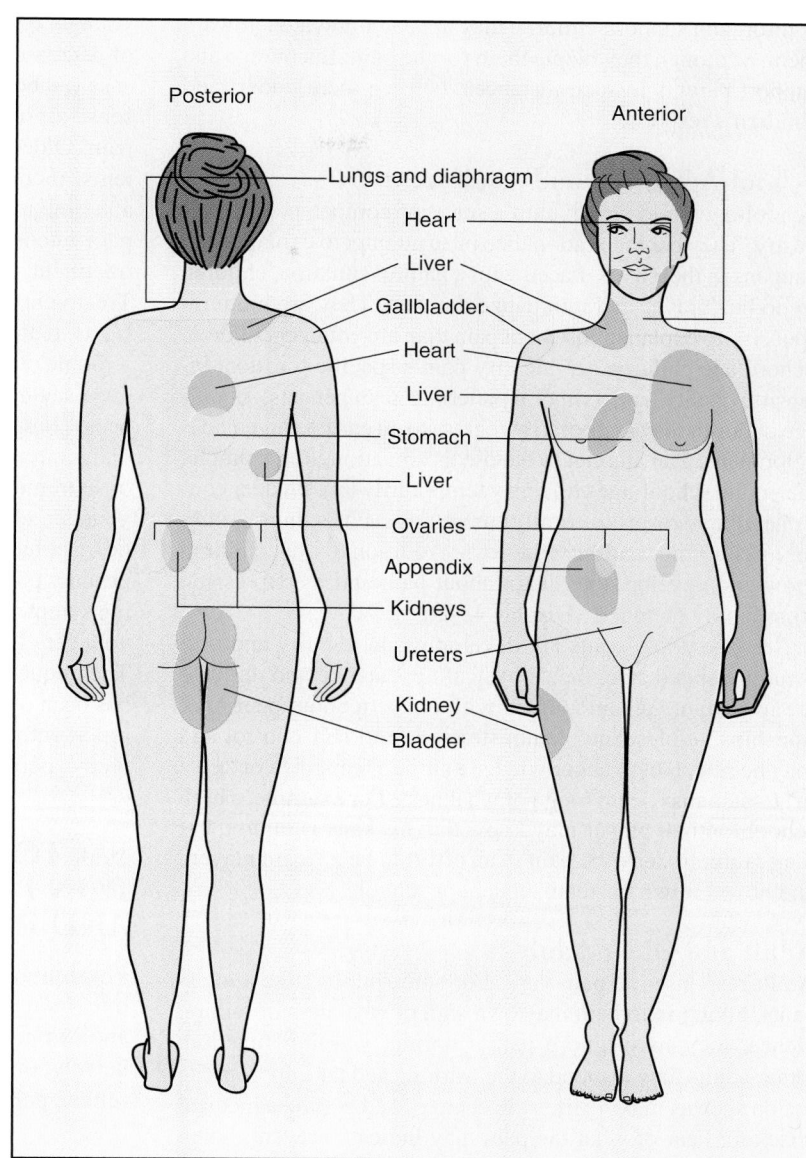

FIGURE 43-2   Common referred pain sites. These anterior and posterior views of the body show where a client might feel pain referred from various visceral organs.

Lifespan Considerations

Newborn and Infant

A newborn or infant cannot verbally report pain. Although theorists formerly believed that newborns' neurophysiologic systems were too immature to transport pain impulses, researchers have learned that newborns do perceive pain (Rahman, Dashwood, Fitzgerald, Aynsley-Green, & Dickenson, 1998). Newborns respond to pain with increased sensitivity at birth with whole body movement (Marsh, Hatch, & Fitzgerald, 1997). Within 3 seconds of a heel lance, the newborn begins to cry and cries for several minutes with a heart rate of about 50 beats/min over baseline (Stevens & Koren, 1998).

After birth, as large fibers become myelinated, endogenous pain inhibition develops (Jennings & Fitzgerald, 1998). As infants develop more motor control, they try to pull or roll away from the pain and show general physical resistance (Stevens, Johnston, Petryshen, & Taddio, 1996). Overall, the

infant's responses may be influenced by behavioral or emotional reactions of parents or healthcare providers.

Toddler and Preschooler

Young toddlers cannot identify the pain they are experiencing or its source. Older toddlers and preschoolers develop the ability to describe, identify, and locate sources of pain and can begin to use terms to define intensity and severity. Characteristics commonly associated with pain, such as lethargy, fatigue, anorexia, and regression, are important in these age groups.

During the toddler and preschool years, children are achieving a sense of autonomy. Because pain can be a source of fear and a threat to security, children respond with crying, anger, physical resistance, or withdrawal. Reasoning with these children about pain and its cause or management is difficult. Thus, children may withdraw from attachments for fear of being hurt again. Although parents are children's greatest source of comfort and support, children may appear ambivalent toward them, as though they blame them for the pain. Encourage and support parents in such instances, helping them understand children's response.

School-Age Child and Adolescent

School-age children develop a sense of competence and industry. They begin to rationalize in an attempt to explain what happens in their lives. Faced with a painful situation, children try to be "brave" and rationalize the pain. They are more responsive to explanations about pain than are younger children. School-age children can identify pain's specific location, intensity, quality, and temporal pattern. If pain persists, school-age children may temporarily regress to an earlier stage of development in an attempt to handle the situation. For example, the young school-age child may temporarily lose bladder control and may revert to comfort measures such as thumb sucking, nail biting, and favorite toys. Additionally, as children grow and develop, they learn about pain and its expression from family members (Display 43-2).

Because adolescents are developing an identity and personal independence, their physical appearance and abilities are important. When coupled with concern about peer relationships, adolescents demonstrate careful self-control and may be reluctant to acknowledge pain. To recognize or "give in" to pain may seem a sign of weakness. For example, a high school football player may know that his knee is injured but may prefer to deny the pain in an effort to be a "team player" and not let down his team, coach, or school.

Adult and Older Adult

Adult responses to pain vary. For some adults, like adolescents, giving in to pain may be a sign of weakness or failure. Hence, they may ignore pain's normal warning function. Other adults may respond to the warning and take appropriate action such as making lifestyle changes and getting a medical checkup. Fear of what the pain may indicate prevents some adults from taking action.

Older adults present other problems, often because of misconceptions about the effects of aging on pain perception. Older persons who are well instructed in the use of pain measurement tools and free of diseases (e.g., diabetes) that affect the nervous system tend to report pain intensity similar to

DISPLAY 43-2

> ⑤ **CHILDREN LEARN BY FAMILIAL ROLE MODELING**
>
> - What pains are and are not appropriate to talk about
> - Appropriate and inappropriate behavior when in pain
> - What circumstances cause pain and should be avoided
> - Methods to avoid or relieve pain
> - Reasons we experience pain (e.g., punishment, testing, bad thoughts)
> - Possible consequences of pain

younger people (Gagliese & Melzack, 1997). In the presence of decreased sensation associated with peripheral nerve disease (diabetic neuropathy), however, older persons may not sense a pinprick as painful yet may report chronic burning pain. Older age also is associated with chronic health problems, increased risk for musculoskeletal pain, depression, and limitations in activities of daily living (ADLs). Increased pain intensity has been noted, particularly when adequate treatment is not provided for chronic and recurrent pain. Treatment of pain in older persons is likely to be as successful as treatment in younger persons.

Some older people fail to notice conditions that would produce acute pain in some younger people until complications occur. For example, an older person experiencing a myocardial infarction may complain of excess gas, an upset stomach, or extreme fatigue rather than the crushing chest pain that younger adults identify. In this situation, the complication of heart failure may be the first indicator of the older person's primary problem. However pain is the most frequent presenting symptom of acute myocardial infarction in both older and younger clients, about two-thirds to three-quarters of clients. The frequency of silent myocardial infarctions in older people has been overestimated. Compared to younger people, elders report similar pain intensity scores but lower sensory and affective pain scores after surgery (Gagliese & Melzack, 1997).

FACTORS AFFECTING PAIN PERCEPTION AND PAIN RESPONSE

Physiologic, affective (emotional), behavioral, and cognitive (thoughts or attitudes) factors influence pain perception and can make it more intense, as shown in Fig. 43-3. Conversely, other emotions, behaviors, and cognitions can help relieve pain.

Physiologic Factors

Persistent, unrelieved pain serves no useful purpose. Unrelieved pain can be harmful to recovery, lead to abnormal anatomic and genetic changes, and interfere with quality of life. Pain even can kill (Page & Ben-Eliyahu, 1997). Recent findings indicate that chronic pain can lead to early death and decreases in natural killer cell activity (an immune response). **Neural plasticity** (nervous system adaptation after pain) involving processes such as peripheral and central sensitization and regenerative neuronal growth produce pathophysiologic pain that leads to some of pain's detrimental effects (Basbaum, 1999).

Neural Plasticity

Allodynia and **hyperalgesia** are two types of dynamic nervous system plasticity (nervous system adaptation after pain). These abnormal sensations occur with tissue injury that leads to inflammation. Allodynia is a pain sensation produced by an innocuous stimulus such as light touch. Hyperalgesia is an enhanced pain sensation produced by a noxious stimulus. For

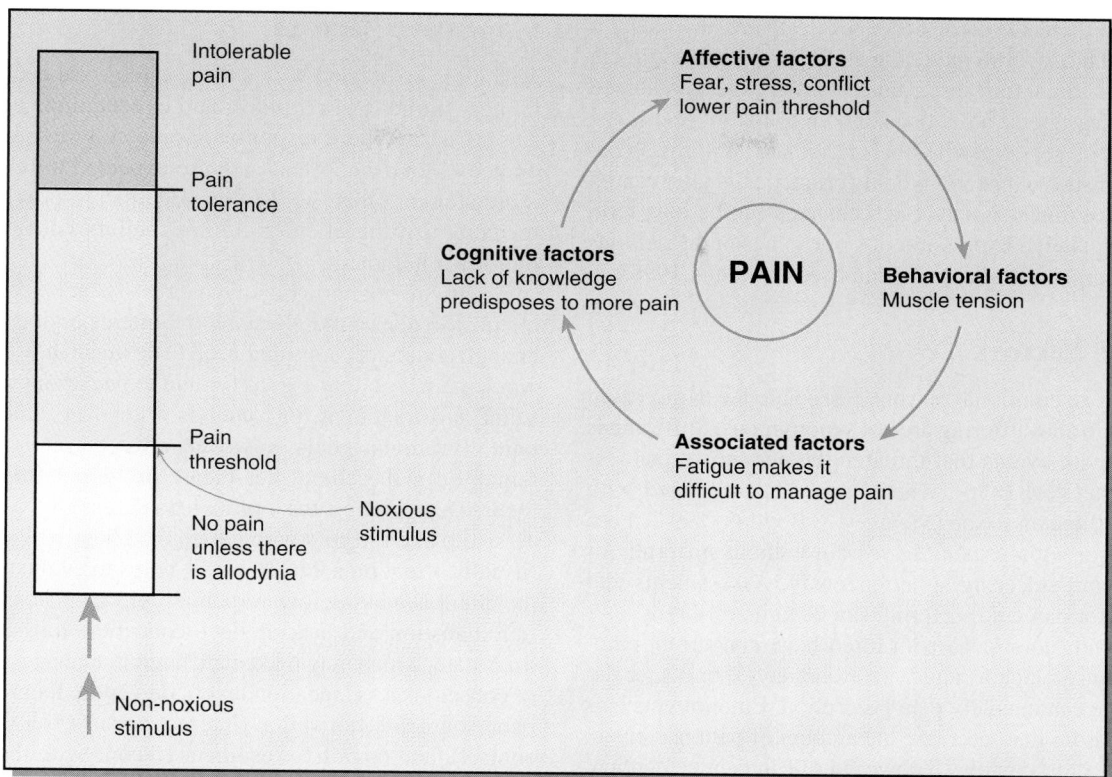

FIGURE 43-3   Factors affecting pain perception and response. Pain is a normal function of the body. It warns the body of injury and disease. Factors can lower the pain threshold and pain tolerance, and a cycle of pain can follow.

example, inflamed pharyngeal tissue produces allodynia type pain on swallowing, and micturition produces allodynia type pain when a person has a urinary tract infection. Swallowing very hot fluid would produce hyperalgesic pain in inflamed pharyngeal tissue. Plasticity in the peripheral and central nervous systems is involved with these types of pain.

Peripheral Sensitization. Allodynia and primary hyperalgesia result from adaptation in the peripheral nervous system (peripheral sensitization). Three characteristics of sensitization are a decrease in the threshold at which the nerve is activated, an enlarged response to noxious thermal or chemical stimuli, and ongoing spontaneous activity in the A-delta and C-fibers. Additionally, a decreased response to non-noxious mechanical stimuli by A-beta fibers (e.g., touch) is a characteristic of sensitization (Garrett & McShane, 1999; Willis & Westlund, 1997). An example of peripheral sensitization is pain produced by the weight of bed linens or clothing (light pressure) in a person with a sunburn.

Central Sensitization. Allodynia and secondary hyperalgesia result from adaptation in the CNS (central sensitization). This type of sensitization is important not only in pain from tissue injury (inflammation) but also in chronic pain. It is characterized by enhanced pain to non-noxious mechanical stimuli (touching) but not thermal stimuli (Ali, Meyer & Campbell, 1996). Touch causes pain because continuous or

very frequent C-fiber input to the dorsal horn enables dorsal horn receptors (N-methyl-D-aspartate [NMDA] and neurokinin, which are normally inactive) to become hyperexcitable and project the pain signal to the brain (Siddall & Cousins, 1997). Although this sensitization may promote healing by encouraging immobilization of an injured body part, it may continue after the injury is healed which helps explain some chronic pain states.

Regenerative Neuronal Growth. Injured peripheral nerve axons produce pathophysiologic pain by generating impulses at abnormal sites (ectopic) along their course, such as at sites of injury. Cut nerves produce pathophysiologic pain by growing a neuroma (tumor-like growth on the nerve) at the cut end. Nearby intact afferent nerves are triggered to sprout when nerves are injured. Neuromas and nerve sprouts are other sources of ectopic impulses. Nerve fibers that have lost some of their myelin due to injury or disease processes (diabetic neuropathies, heavy metal neuropathies, multiple sclerosis) also produce spontaneous neural discharge. These ways for nerves to send messages to the spinal cord without ongoing tissue injury may help to explain pain reported by people whose injuries have appeared to heal (i.e., people with chronic pain). Recent evidence indicates that norepinephrine released by the sympathetic nervous system, which normally does not excite nociceptors, can do so if the nociceptors have been injured (Perl, 1996).

Injuries sufficient to cause nerve cell death produce changes in the spinal dorsal horn including attempts at regeneration in other cells to maintain lost connections. Large myelinated fibers (A-beta fibers) have been shown to sprout and make connections in areas where C-fibers terminate (Willis & Westlund, 1997). Such connections could dramatically alter central processing of touch signals. Such changes can be long term and result in altered expression of some genes in the nervous tissue (Hammond, Wang, Nakashima, & Basbaum, 1998).

Affective Factors

Suffering is an emotional response associated with increased pain, but pain and suffering are not synonymous. Suffering is associated with events that threaten the person's intactness (Kahn & Steeves, 1996), whereas pain is associated with events that threaten tissue (Merskey & Bogduk, 1994). People can suffer without pain, have pain without suffering, or have pain and suffering simultaneously. Assessments and treatments for pain and suffering can be quite different.

Clients with unrelieved pain often have concurrent emotional responses such as anger, fear, anxiety, sadness, or depression that can intensify pain perception. Emotions such as joy and pleasure may decrease the amount of pain perceived. Emotional factors can play a powerful role in pain perception. Helping clients understand the link between emotions and pain perception is an important role for nurses in all care settings.

Behavioral Factors

Many different behaviors are associated with pain; some aggravate it and others alleviate it. Clients with pain notice that certain activities can cause pain to be noticed or increased. Clients often avoid such activities, but this avoidance may not be in their best long-term interest. Pain may interfere with usual behaviors that bring joy and satisfaction. When pain prevents many activities, clients may experience increased emotional distress such as anxiety. Clients also engage in a number of behaviors to control their pain (reduce pain, prevent pain onset, reduce pain duration, and tolerate the pain). For example, watching television or talking with friends, staff, or family members helps to distract clients from their pain and can be effective in helping to control it. How clients comply with or adjust analgesic therapy plans also is an important aspect of pain behavior.

Emotional responses to pain, such as fear and anxiety, increase muscle tension, which increases perception of pain intensity. Fear of the unknown also may worsen pain because of tension and anxiety the client brings to the situation. For instance, a toddler who fears an injection will cry and tense the muscles, thus intensifying pain. Aggressive behavior is not an uncommon way of "fighting back" against the pain. At the other extreme, the person in pain may withdraw from it by minimizing interaction with the environment and other people. Regression to earlier developmental stages may occur.

Pain can be fatiguing, possibly predisposing the client to more pain. What might be tolerable to a well-rested person may be intolerable to one who is fatigued.

Cognitive Factors

Meanings associated with a disease (e.g., cancer) and pain, along with beliefs, attitudes, and expectations about them can influence client responses. Some cultures see pain tolerance as a virtue; often, men are expected to tolerate pain more stoically than women do. Healthcare providers need to recognize the client's cultural beliefs and not impose their own judgments.

A sense of not knowing may increase a person's pain. The client who does not understand treatments or does not know enough about decisions that need to be made may experience worse pain. A client's goal for and expectations about pain relief and treatment outcomes is crucial in understanding pain. Treatment goals, however, must be realistic and attainable for the client, healthcare providers, and environment. Determining the optimal goal (usually 0 on a 0 to 10 scale) and the goal with which the client will be satisfied (usually 1 to 4 on a 0 to 10 scale) helps to evaluate progress the client is making toward pain relief.

Exhaustion and lack of sleep contribute to a chronically tired state, which may make it difficult to manage pain. Level of consciousness (sedation level), dementia, memory of past pain, source of motivation (internal versus external locus of control), and cognitive resources to cope with the pain can dramatically influence the pain experienced.

Clients may use cognitive and behavioral activities to cope with pain. In general, when clients actively engage in behaviors to cope with the pain, they are less likely to be debilitated by it. Clients who focus on how terrible the pain is (coping by catastrophizing) are more likely to have functional and emotional problems related to the pain. Display 43-3 lists examples of coping strategies.

ALTERED FUNCTION RESULTING IN PAIN

Manifestations of Pain

Physiologic and behavioral responses occur in the person in pain. Observers consider these responses indicators of pain; but for the person with pain, some responses represent dangerous effects of pain. Absence of these responses does not indicate a client has no pain or has less intense pain than he or she reports.

Physiologic Responses

Observable physiologic signs of acute pain include changes in blood pressure, heart rate, respiratory rate, and metabolic responses. Commonly observed responses in acute pain are usually absent in persistent and chronic pain because adaptation occurs. It is unclear how long it takes for adaptation to occur. Therefore, lack of elevation in vital signs cannot be used as a reliable indicator of the presence or magnitude of persistent pain. Furthermore, other reasons for alterations in physiologic responses must be considered (e.g., effects of drug therapy lowering blood pressure in the presence of severe pain).

DISPLAY 43-3

🔲 EXAMPLES OF PAIN COPING STRATEGIES

Active Cognitive Coping Strategies

Reinterpreting the Pain Sensation
I don't think of it as pain but rather as a dull or warm feeling.
I try not to think of it as my body but rather as something separate from me.
I pretend it's not a part of me.

Diverting Attention From the Pain
I try to think of something pleasant.
I count numbers in my mind or run a song through my mind.
I play mental games with myself to keep my mind off the pain.
I replay in my mind pleasant experiences in the past.

Ignoring the Pain
I don't think about the pain.
I tell myself it doesn't hurt.
I pretend it's not there.
I just go on as if nothing happened.

Coping Self-Statements
I tell myself to be brave and carry on despite the pain.
I tell myself that I can overcome the pain.
I tell myself I can't let the pain stand in the way of what I have to do.
No matter how bad it gets, I know I can handle it.

Passive Cognitive Coping Strategies

Praying/Hoping
I know someday someone will be here to help me, and it will go away for awhile.
I pray to God it won't last long.
I try to think what everything will be like after I've gotten rid of the pain.
I have faith in doctors that someday there will be a cure for my pain.

Catastrophizing (associated with emotional distress and functional status)
It's terrible, and I feel it's never going to get any better.
I worry all the time about whether it will end.
I feel my life isn't worth living.
I feel I can't stand it anymore.

Behavioral Coping Strategies
I do anything to get my mind off the pain.
I do something active, like household chores or projects.
I try to be around other people.
I leave the house and do something, such as going to the movies or shopping.

From Rosenstiel, A. K., & Keefe, F. J. (1983). The use of coping strategies in low back pain patients: Relationship to patient characteristics and current adjustments. *Pain, 17,* 33–44.

Increased Blood Pressure. The increase in blood pressure that may accompany acute pain is believed to be due to overactivity of the sympathetic nervous system. Peripheral vasoconstriction is an adaptive response as the blood shifts away from the periphery (skin, extremities) to the heart and lungs when the body perceives a threat. The increased blood pressure also increases the heart's work, possibly leading to coronary artery vasoconstriction and potential myocardial ischemia. Also the decreased peripheral circulation can be dangerous to people undergoing vascular grafting procedures by diminishing blood flow needed to promote healing.

Increased Heart Rate. Increased heart rate reflects the body's attempt to increase available oxygen and circulating fluid volume to promote healing of damaged tissues. The shunting of blood from the periphery to the vital organs (brain, heart, liver, kidney) is an effort to preserve the body's life-support systems.

Increased Respiratory Rate. An increase in the respiratory rate is an effort to increase the amount of oxygen available to the heart and circulation. Unrelieved pain classically includes rapid and shallow breathing that is inefficient to meet oxygen needs, which results in hypoxemia. The rapid, shallow breathing is corrected with effective pain relief.

Neuroendocrine and Metabolic Responses. Unrelieved pain produces a catabolic state. That is, stored energy is consumed to provide energy to vital organs and injured tissue. This response also is known as the stress response, which is capable of producing widespread metabolic effects. Some of these effects include generalized increase in metabolism, oxygen consumption, blood glucose, free fatty acids, blood lactate, and ketones. These effects related to the degree and duration of tissue damage can last for days.

Behavioral Responses

Observable behavioral signs of acute and chronic pain include verbal, vocal, and/or nonverbal responses. As with physiologic signs, behavioral responses often adapt with time (Table 43-1).

Verbal Responses. Verbal behavioral responses to pain, although subjective, are the most dependable indicators of pain in people who are able to communicate verbally. Therefore, healthcare providers should believe these reports and not dismiss them even if they vary from other objective information. In people without verbal abilities (e.g., preverbal children, cognitively impaired clients), vocal responses may provide important clues about pain's presence but do little to indicate

TABLE 43-1

Objective Behavioral Indicators of Pain	
Type of Indicator	**Examples**
Verbal Behavior	
Vocalization	Moaning, groaning, grunting, sighing, gasping, crying, screaming
Verbalization	Praying, counting, swearing or cursing, repeating nonsensical phrases
Nonverbal Behavior	
Facial expression	Grimacing, clenching teeth, tightly shutting lips, gazing/staring, wrinkling forehead, tearing
Body actions	Thrashing, pounding, biting, rocking, rubbing, stretching, shrugging, rotating body part, shifting weight
Behaviors	Massaging; immobilizing; guarding; bracing; eating or drinking; applying pressure, heat, cold; assuming special position or posture; reading; watching television; listening to music; crossing legs

These behaviors may signal presence of pain, but absence of behavior does not signal lack of pain.

where, what kind, or how much pain there is, or how it changes with time.

Nonverbal Responses. Nonverbal behaviors often give a clue about pain location, but verbal reports indicate more clearly its location, intensity, quality, and temporal pattern. Common nonverbal behavioral responses include rubbing painful areas, frowns and grimaces, and increased muscle tension that occurs with guarding and immobilization. Increased muscle tension shown by guarding, which is part of the body's fight-or-flight response, is a reaction to protect against further pain. Prolonged muscle tension, however, contributes to impaired muscle metabolism, muscle atrophy, and significantly delayed normal muscle function.

Impact on Activities of Daily Living

Unrelieved pain generally causes decreased energy, which affects all aspects of living. Clients in pain often find it difficult to perform basic ADLs. People who have difficulty with independent living may experience anxiety or alterations in self-concept. Basic ADLs (bathing, dressing, eating, grooming) may be mildly or severely affected depending on the pain's location and degree. Household activities also may be difficult to perform. Persistent pain can interfere with the person's ability to concentrate on work or school. Physical activity may increase pain, possibly impacting leisure activities, walking, and/or driving.

A person with pain may find it difficult to fall or stay asleep. The resulting lack of sleep contributes to fatigue, predisposing the client to more pain. Pain also can be fatiguing. Sleep, however, does not indicate pain relief. After experiencing pain for an extended time, the client may become too tired to talk or cry and then falls asleep. Clients in pain may close their eyes and appear to be asleep but actually may be conserving energy or focusing on something else to make the pain bearable.

Clients with pain may focus on finding pain relief and thus be unable to explore outside interests and relationships. This may alter family and social relationships. Persistent, unrelieved pain can lead to family conflict. Decreased energy also hinders sexual functioning.

Often, family members assume tremendous responsibilities in assisting clients with pain, an important consideration for family health and well being. Many decisions and ethical conflicts may arise involving family members and their participation in dealing with the client's unrelieved pain.

ASSESSMENT

An accurate assessment focusing on pain's cause is essential for determining the proper therapy. Ongoing assessment also is important for implementing an effective pain management plan. Question the client about specific factual information and directly observe the client for nonverbal indicators of pain. Remain objective and nonjudgmental. Keep in mind that pain occurs whenever the client says it does. The client is the expert about how the pain feels. Direct observation may corroborate the client's report but must not be used to dismiss that report.

Document pain assessment information in an accessible location. Even the best pain assessment conducted by one nurse is of limited value unless he or she shares the information with other healthcare professionals responsible for the client's care.

Subjective Data

Normal Pattern Identification

In an attempt to assess the client's pain, obtain answers to the following questions:

- Where is the pain located?
- What is the magnitude or intensity (level) of the pain?
- What level of pain would the client like to have?

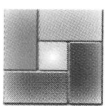

Nursing Research and Critical Thinking
Would the Use of Pain Assessment Tools Enable Nurses to Improve Pain Management?

This nurse researcher was concerned that, despite dramatic advances in pain control over the past 20 years, many clients continue to suffer unrelieved pain. A small group of professionals met to discuss how they might facilitate improved pain management for the clients in their care. The results of an initial hospital pain audit revealed an absence of formal pain assessment tools and a high incidence of pain. The nurse devised this study to evaluate a pain assessment tool and care plan. The pain assessment tool incorporated drawings of the front and back of the body, which allowed the client to locate the pain's source. It also included the pain ruler (numerical rating scale) developed by Bourbonnais. The reverse of the pain assessment chart had a blank care plan and asked for the problem, goal, interventions, and evaluation to be documented. Nurses completed the tool on a 28-bed mixed rehabilitation ward for older adults. The nurses used the document with any client they identified as having pain. A total of 18 assessment charts and care plans were completed. All the nurses were able to use the tool. It is suggested, however, that the introduction of a tool alone may only partially improve pain management because, no matter how well pain assessment might be documented, the pain experience for the client will not improve unless this is linked to effective interventions. On the care plans, the problem was clearly stated and a cause was identified, but there was no indication of how this affected the client. None of the goals were measurable, although one care plan stated that the client should "say they have less pain," which might be considered to be partly measurable.

Critical Thinking Considerations. This pilot study was to test the use of this pain assessment tool and care plan by nurses caring for clients with pain. It was not a study to test the instrument's validity and reliability. Implications of this study are as follows:

- The care plans reflected interventions related to the pain's physical cause and meandered away from the problem of pain.
- The nurses used none of the psychosocial interventions related to pain management (e.g., distraction, touch, massage, music, and client information).

From Carr, E. C. J. (1997). Evaluating the use of a pain assessment tool and care plan: A pilot study. *Journal of Advanced Nursing, 26*(6), 1073–1079.

- What level of pain would the client be willing to tolerate?
- How does the pain feel to the client; how is it described (its quality)?
- How does the pain change with rest, activity, or time (its temporal pattern)?

In critical care areas, pain location and intensity are the most important aspects to assess. Other aspects can be assessed when the client's condition is stable. For an ongoing assessment, assess pain intensity routinely and assess other aspects such as quality and pattern, if the pain has changed.

When asked about pain, some clients deny it unless it is severe. These same clients will report that they hurt a lot or have a great deal of discomfort. For this reason, inquire about the client's meaning of hurt, discomfort, and soreness to determine if a person has pain. Using tools to measure the pain experience helps simplify and standardize a pain assessment.

Location. Because clients initially are inclined to describe where the pain or discomfort is located, it is logical and efficient to start with measurement of pain location. Pain location can be measured objectively by using a drawing of a body outline and asking the client to mark all the places where he or she perceives pain (Fig. 43-4). Clients should make marks as big as or small as they perceive pain in those places. Body outlines have been used successfully with children as young as 8 years and adults older than 85 years. Alternatively, the nurse may ask a client to point to the places where he or she feels the pain, but pointing may be inconvenient or embarrassing.

Intensity. Pain intensity is measured with the use of a scale. Evaluate pain intensity at rest, with various activities, and when painful procedures are performed. The following script can be used when giving the client directions on use of such a numbered scale:

> "I need to know how much pain you have so I can help relieve it. Because I can't feel your pain, I want you to use a scale to let me know how much pain you have right now. The numbers between 0 and 10 represent all the pain a person could have. Zero means no pain and 10 means pain as bad as it could be. You can use any number between 0 and 10 to let me know how much pain you have right now. *Call your pain* a number between 0 and 10 so I will know the intensity of the pain you feel now."
>
> *Note:* Use the phrase "call your pain" rather than "rate your pain" because clients have difficulty knowing what is expected of them when asked to rate their pain. They easily "call" their pain a number.*

Record the number the client gives for comparison with the number representing the amount of pain the person wants and is able to tolerate and with future pain intensity measurements. These numbers provide a perspective on how pain intensity

* Copyright © 1990, Wilkie, D. J.; reprinted with permission.

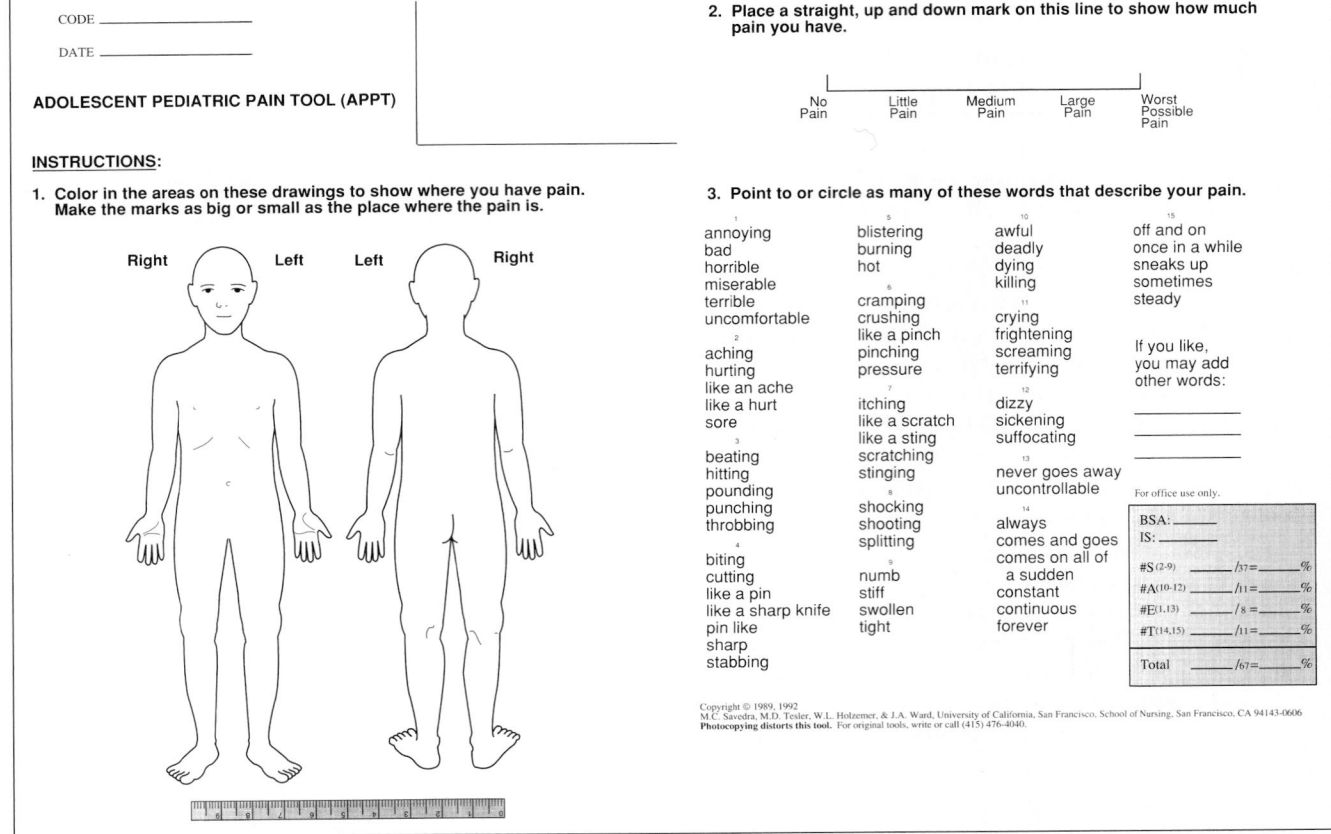

FIGURE 43-4 Adolescent Pediatric Pain Tool. (Courtesy of Savedra, Tesler, Holzemer, and Ward © 1992)

fluctuates with time (they also show a temporal pattern). If clients are unable to call their pain a number, they can select an intensity word from one of the tools to report pain intensity.

Children as young as 8 years can use a 0 to 10 number scale, although most children prefer to use a graphic rating scale, as shown in Fig. 43-4, to report pain intensity (Tesler, Savedra, Holzemer, Wilkie, Ward, & Paul, 1991). Alternatively, children can be asked to select the number of poker chips (Hester, Foster, & Kristensen, 1990) or faces of children in pain (Beyer & Aradine, 1987) that reflect their pain.

Quality. The most widely used measure of pain quality is the McGill-Melzack Pain Questionnaire (Melzack, 1975; Fig. 43-5). It includes a list of verbal descriptors from which the client selects the one word per group that best describes the pain. Supplying the list makes the task easy for clients who do not know how to describe the quality of the sensation. Clients who would use other words will supply that information as they select words from the list. If clients have pain in more than one site, they often will select two words per group and indicate that one word describes one site and the other word another site. Words in groups 1 to 10 represent sensory qualities of pain. Words in groups 11 to 15 represent affective qualities of pain. Group 16 words are evaluative qualities, and words from groups 17 to 20 are miscellaneous words (sensory, affective, and evaluative). A total pain quality score

is obtained by counting the number of words selected. Children also are able to use descriptors to describe their pain (Savedra, Holzemer, Tesler, Ward, & Wilkie, 1993). Complex pain quality, as reflected by a large number of words, is associated with increased client attempts to engage in behaviors intended to control the pain.

Temporal Pattern. The duration of pain is described by terms such as brief, momentary, transient, rhythmic, periodic, intermittent, continuous, steady, or constant. To measure onset, ask the client the date or time the pain started and how long it lasted. Assessing when the pain began (onset) is important in determining whether the client's pain is acute, recurrent, or chronic.

Risk Identification

Pain management is often suboptimal (Agency for Health Care Policy and Research [AHCPR], 1992; 1994). Together, healthcare professionals, the healthcare system, and client-related barriers to pain management add to the risk of poor pain control.

Healthcare Professionals. Inadequate or poor pain assessment is a leading factor in poor pain control because the healthcare professional may not know a client has pain. The healthcare professional's attitude toward pain may contribute to a poor assessment. For example, assuming that a client will

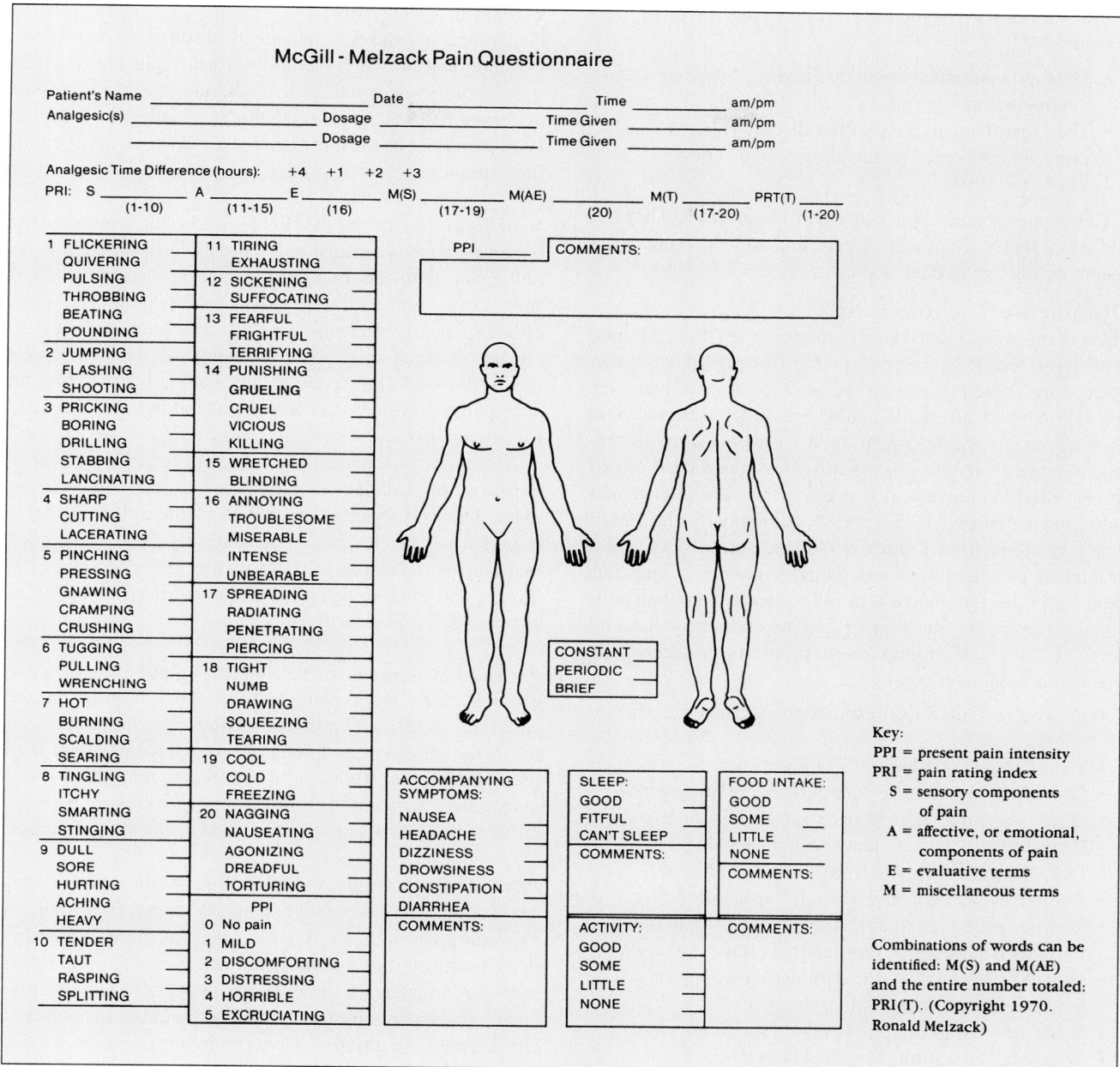

FIGURE 43-5 The McGill-Melzack Pain Questionnaire.

always report pain further interferes with the healthcare professional's awareness of the client's actual discomfort level. If the nurse and client perceive pain differently, major conflicts may arise, adding to the client's anxiety level and possibly increasing the pain. Inadequate knowledge of pain management, concerns about regulation of controlled substances, fear of client addiction, and concerns about clients becoming tolerant to analgesics or about their side effects also pose barriers to adequate pain management.

Healthcare System. Some institutions do not provide all types of pain management therapies that a person may need. For example, an extended care nursing facility may not allow admin-istration of continuous intravenous (IV) infusions of opioids, a treatment that a terminally ill person with pain might require. Access to treatment also is a barrier that puts clients at risk for poor pain relief. For example, inadequate reimbursement for pain therapies and restrictive regulation of controlled substances interfere with a person receiving adequate pain relief.

Clients. Often, clients do not realize they are the experts about their pain. Clients assume that health professionals are the experts because they have provided care to so many people with similar types of pain. About half the clients say that they try not to let others know they have pain and the other half say they tell others about their pain.

Many clients are reluctant to report pain for three main reasons:

- They are concerned about distracting physicians from treating the pain's cause.
- They fear the pain means their disease is worse.
- They are concerned about being "good" clients (AHCPR, 1994).

Clients also are reluctant to take pain medications. They fear addiction, worry about side effects, and are concerned about becoming tolerant to pain medications (AHCPR, 1994).

Dysfunction Identification

Many of the client-related barriers to pain relief are emotional, behavioral, and cognitive and can dramatically influence pain perception. These factors must be assessed if initial pain therapies do not provide the degree of pain relief expected. Two clinically useful measurement tools for these factors include the Memorial Pain Assessment Card (measures general mood), and the Brief Pain Inventory (measures pain interference with mood and activities; AHCPR, 1994). Additionally, the McGill Pain Questionnaire (Melzack, 1975) measures affective and evaluative pain qualities and includes interview questions about activities that increase or relieve pain. To obtain additional information, interview questions and active listening skills are key. Use the following questions to gain access to the client's personal pain experience:

- Do you feel anxious, upset, depressed, sad, fearful, or angry?
- What brings you pleasure and joy?
- Does the pain interfere with personal relationships?
- Does the pain affect self-care, job, or leisure activities?
- How do you let others know you have pain?
- Does the pain keep you from sleeping at night?
- Does it awaken you and, if so, for how long?
- Do you relate pain to alterations in other body functions such as appetite, elimination, menses, or sex?
- How do you usually cope with pain (medications, home remedies, rest, or other therapies)?
- What are your expectations in relation to the pain?
- What are your cultural beliefs about pain?
- What are your experiences with pain?
- What are your beliefs about pain medications and non-drug therapies for pain, such as distraction or imagery?
- What are your beliefs about the disease, illness, or injury causing the pain?
- Are you concerned about addiction, tolerance, dependence, and side effects?
- Do you believe you have the ability to control the pain, or do you leave control of pain to other means (health professionals, deity, chance)?

Objective Data

Objective data about the client's pain are gathered through ongoing physical assessment. Diagnostic or screening tests cannot quantify the degree of pain. Objective data are used to supplement, not replace, subjective data.

Physical Assessment

Physiologic responses to pain are the result of the activation of the autonomic nervous system. With acute pain, the general responses observed include tachycardia, elevated blood pressure, increased respiratory rate, diaphoresis, and gastric distress. With persistent or chronic pain, these responses may be modified or absent.

Vital Signs. Assessing the client's vital signs is important for obtaining baseline information, particularly before a potentially painful procedure. The sympathetic nervous system responses to acute pain are evident with diaphoresis and increases in heart rate, respiratory rate, and blood pressure. For clients who have difficulty expressing pain or are unable to do so, the vital sign readings and comparisons before and after pain relief measures may be useful but not conclusive for acute pain evaluation.

A common misconception about pain and vital signs is that objective, physiologic responses are less likely to be manipulated than self-reports. This belief is unfounded. Do not interpret a lack of elevation in the vital signs as an indication that pain is not present. Many factors influence heart rate, blood pressure, and respiratory rate and may obscure these physiologic responses to pain.

Associated Characteristics. Related symptoms may give additional clues about pain. Nausea and vomiting, fatigue, anorexia, and/or withdrawal are common with pain. Assess for these symptoms as a potential source for pain and in the presence of pain. Relieving the pain also may relieve these associated characteristics. For example, relieving pain may allow the client to relax and rest, thus diminishing fatigue.

Physical Expressions of Pain. Observe the client's facial expressions and body movements. Wincing, frowning, and grimacing can indicate pain, but lack of these expressions does not mean that a client is not experiencing pain. People with chronic pain are likely not to show these facial expressions. The most common facial expression associated with chronic pain in a group of clients with lung cancer was movement of the lower eyelid to make a squinting appearance (Wilkie, 1995). In general, these clients with chronic pain had a mask-like appearance and little spontaneous movement of facial muscles. Expecting to see wincing, frowning, and grimacing when a person has pain may lead to a misdiagnosis.

Body movements may represent protective actions to decrease the pain. Body movements such as rubbing, splinting, guarding, immobilizing, elevating the painful extremity, or changing positions frequently may increase with pain. For example, a woman in labor rhythmically rubs her abdomen. As pain increases, total body activity decreases, and eventually the client lies still and is quiet if pain is not relieved. Splinting, guarding, and immobilization by a person in pain protects the client from pain but can be harmful. This decrease in activity may delay recovery (e.g., when the postoperative client refuses to ambulate, turn, cough, or deep breathe and subsequently develops atelectasis, thrombophlebitis, or a pulmonary embolus).

Pain evokes emotional responses that may be expressed as depression, anger, fear, anxiety, sadness, excitement, denial, or regression. A wide range of verbal responses (moaning, sighing, screaming, crying, and repetition of words or phrases) can be a result of pain. However, such restlessness, moaning, and grimacing can be misleading. The client may not be in pain but may be disoriented, hypoxic, febrile, or having a medication reaction. Unrelieved pain also leads to disorientation or confusion that clears with appropriate pain management. Any of these expressions of pain may be absent in clients who are stoic or have prolonged chronic pain.

SAFETY ALERT
Remember that lack of pain expression does not mean lack of pain because clients adapt physically and psychologically to pain. Therefore, actively solicit information about pain. Observe accurately, listen, and never judge or jump to conclusions.

Diagnostic Tests and Procedures
Although tests cannot quantify the degree of pain, procedures can validate painful events (e.g., an electrocardiogram shows a myocardial infarction after chest pain). Other diagnostic tests relate to the specific pain source. For example, a bone scan may be used to diagnose that cancer has spread to the bone, a frequent cause of pain in the person with cancer.

NURSING DIAGNOSES
Diagnostic Statement: Acute Pain

Definition. Pain is "an unpleasant sensory and emotional experience associated with actual or potential tissue damage, or described in terms of such damage" (Merskey & Bogduk, 1994, p. 210; North American Nursing Diagnosis Association [NANDA], 2001); "sudden or slow onset of any intensity from mild to severe with an anticipated or predictable end and duration of less than 6 months" (NANDA, 2001, p. 129).

Defining Characteristics. Several clinical cues point to the nursing diagnosis of Acute Pain. There is communication (verbal or coded) of pain descriptors (NANDA, 2001). The client reports the location, intensity, quality, and temporal pattern of the experienced pain. There may be guarding behavior that protects the injured area from movement. The client appears to have a narrow focus within himself or herself. The client has an altered perception of time, has impaired thought processes, or withdraws from social contact. The client engages in distraction behavior (moaning, crying, pacing, seeking out other people or activities). The client appears restless (fixed or scattered movement) with a facial mask of pain in which the eyes lack luster; there is a "beaten look" or a grimace. The client's muscle tone may alter from listless to rigid. Autonomic responses may be present including diaphoresis, blood pressure and pulse change, pupillary dilation, and increased or decreased respiratory rate (NANDA, 2001).

Presence of these behaviors may confirm but cannot rule out the possibility that the client has pain. Similarly, absence of these behaviors must not negate the client's report that pain is present or its intensity, quality, or pattern. Many clients do not look like they have pain when their pain is quite severe.

Related Factors. Biologic, chemical, physical, and psychological agents of injury are related factors (NANDA, 2001).

Diagnostic Statement: Chronic Pain

Definition. Chronic Pain also is "an unpleasant sensory and emotional experience associated with actual or potential tissue damage, or described in terms of such damage; sudden or slow onset of any intensity from mild to severe with an anticipated or predictable end and duration of greater than 6 months" (NANDA, 2001, p. 130). Many pain experts, however, argue that 6 months is an arbitrary time frame and recently have defined Chronic Pain "as a persistent pain that is not amenable, as a rule, to treatments based upon specific remedies, or to the routine methods of pain control such as non-opioid analgesics" (Merskey & Bodguk, 1994).

Defining Characteristics. According to NANDA (2001), the nurse makes this diagnosis when the client reports pain that has existed for more than 6 months. Chronic Pain is defined by weight changes, verbal or coded report, or observed evidence of protective or guarding behavior. Facial mask, irritability, self-focusing, restlessness, depression, atrophy of muscles, and changes in sleep may occur. Fatigue, fear or reinjury, reduced interactions with people, altered ability to continue previous activities, responses mediated by the sympathetic nervous system including skin temperature, tropic changes, and hypersensitivity, and anorexia also define Chronic Pain (NANDA, 2001).

Related Factors. Chronic physical or psychosocial disability increases Chronic Pain (NANDA, 2001). Many neural changes (neural plasticity) are likely to be factors in continued pain (Basbaum, 1999; Willis & Westlund, 1997), but other affective, behavioral, and cognitive factors contribute to chronic pain the person experiences.

Related Nursing Diagnoses

Although Acute Pain and Chronic Pain are the obvious nursing diagnoses for the person in pain, assessment may indicate that the client has other related problems. For instance, Anxiety, Ineffective Coping, Disabled Family Coping, Ineffective Health Maintenance, Impaired Home Maintenance, and Disturbed Sleep Pattern may be related to pain. If the client suffers from Chronic Pain, additional nursing diagnoses may include Self-Care Deficit, Chronic Low Self-Esteem, Hopelessness, Impaired Physical Mobility, Sexual Dysfunction, and Spiritual Distress. If the client is taking medications for pain, other nursing diagnoses may be evident such as Constipation and Disturbed Thought Processes.

OUTCOME IDENTIFICATION AND PLANNING

The overall goal in pain management is for the client to seek interventions that maximize his or her pain relief and quality of life. Specific goals for the client in pain may include the following:

- Client will report no new pain sites and reduced pain intensity and pain quality complexity.
- Client will monitor and report changes in pain location, intensity, quality, and pattern.
- Client will identify and avoid emotional, behavioral, and cognitive factors that precipitate pain.
- Client will identify and use cognitive and behavioral techniques to decrease or cope with pain.

Care of the person in pain involves a four-step process:

1. Assess sensory pain.
2. Provide pain therapy.
3. If relief is not as expected, assess emotional, behavioral, cognitive, and physiologic aspects of pain.
4. Revise plans for therapy to meet needs.

The accompanying display outlines some nursing interventions used in planning individualized care for the client with pain. A realistic goal for the client in acute and/or chronic pain is to reduce pain to the level the client indicates he or she desires or is able to tolerate. Complete elimination of acute pain is possible during recovery and healing. The client with chronic pain needs to learn that no interventions will cure the cause of the pain, pain may not be eliminated entirely, pain may recur, and pain intensity can be reduced through use of pharmacologic and nonpharmacologic therapies. Adapting daily activities to control the pain effectively is often necessary as part of the overall goal for clients with persistent or recurrent pain.

PLANNING: Examples of NIC/NOC Interventions

Accepted Pain Perception and Management Nursing Interventions Classification (NIC)
Analgesic Administration
Environmental Management: Comfort
Pain Management

Accepted Pain Perception and Management Nursing Outcomes Classification (NOC)
Comfort Level
Pain: Disruptive Effects
Pain Control Behavior
Pain Level

Refer to the following for specifics regarding NIC/NOC:
McCloskey, J., & Bulechek, G. (2000). *Iowa Intervention Project: Nursing Interventions Classification (NIC)* 2nd ed. St. Louis, MO: C.V. Mosby.
Johnson, M., & Maas, M. (2000). *Iowa Outcomes Project: Nursing Outcomes Classification (NOC)* 2nd ed. St. Louis, MO: C.V. Mosby.

Because results are not always predictable, the nurse's confidence and enthusiasm increase the chances that a pain-relief measure will be successful. If the client knows that numerous methods are available, he or she will not be devastated if one is less than totally effective.

IMPLEMENTATION

Although physicians prescribe many pain management techniques, the nurse is responsible for assessing, administering, monitoring, and evaluating the effectiveness of these techniques and initiating independent nursing measures for pain relief. Using the four-step process allows collaborative planning for optimal pain relief before or soon after pain is experienced or to control persistent pain.

Based on the client's assessment, the healthcare team provides appropriate therapies (pharmacologic and nonpharmacologic). One key area is monitoring the client's response to the therapy. If treatment eliminates the pain's cause, the pain disappears. If the pain's cause cannot be eliminated, the pain intensity should decrease to the level the client desires or at least to the level the client indicates he or she is willing to tolerate. Pain quality often diminishes, and the pain pattern may change. It is not unusual for some therapy adjustments to be needed before these improvements are seen. If the degree of pain relief expected is not achieved, however, then an in-depth assessment of all the factors that contribute to the pain is needed.

Health Promotion

Teaching clients ways of anticipating and managing painful procedures or situations helps to decrease anxiety and fear and allows clients to become active participants in preventing pain and promoting recovery. Recognizing pain-inducing situations and factors is the first step in preventing pain. For instance, many procedures performed routinely, such as blood pressure, needlestick for blood tests, and inserting an IV or urinary catheter, produce pain. Preparation, including premedication, is indicated for all painful procedures even if they produce only mild pain. If a client is scheduled for a potentially painful procedure, discuss techniques such as relaxation exercises, deep breathing, and distraction that will add to the effect of analgesic therapies to decrease the pain and improve coping mechanisms.

Chronic pain can be prevented or minimized. For example, someone who gets migraine headaches may be aware that certain foods, such as chocolate, induce migraines. Increased knowledge about the ways that sports or other recreational activities can aggravate pain allows the person to modify activities to prevent pain and promote function. Adequate warm-up activities to stretch muscles and loosen joints before sports help prevent pain during and after the activity. Using appropriate posture and body mechanics at work can help preserve function and prevent pain by avoiding strained muscles and other injuries.

Clients with chronic pain can learn lifestyle changes to avoid precipitating pain and dysfunction. For instance, teaching about proper lifting and bending techniques and exercises to decrease muscle contraction and increase back muscle strength may help the client with chronic low back pain (see Chapter 33). Using analgesics effectively and alternating pain-relief measures also are important areas of client teaching.

Nursing Interventions for the Client Experiencing Pain

Nursing management of pain includes physical, cognitive (focuses on client's beliefs, attitudes, expectations, control, and cognitive coping), behavioral (targets actions under the client's control), and pharmacologic therapies. Being familiar with these techniques and the types of pain for which they are effective helps the nurse decide which ones to use, when to initiate them, what outcomes to expect, and how to teach them to clients.

Physical Pain Relief Techniques

Positioning and Hygiene. For clients who spend many hours in bed, the bed and the client's position may contribute directly to pain. Sheets tend to bunch up, creating pressure and discomfort. Tightening sheets regularly or changing them, if needed, can make the client more comfortable. Repositioning the client on a regular schedule also can help promote comfort. Pressure areas created by lying in one position too long can be painful. If not contraindicated, backrubs can contribute to relaxation and comfort. Giving a backrub also allows the nurse to spend a few minutes with the client, listening attentively and continuing the ongoing pain assessment.

Any constrictive item including gowns that twist or bind, support hose, and wrist restraints contributes to pain. Gowns must be the correct size for the client and should be checked for comfort whenever the client's position is changed. Restraints and support hose must be removed regularly to assess pressure on the skin and other problems that may cause pain.

Areas of irritation or excoriation may be sources of pain. Clients who require a bedpan or who are incontinent of urine or stool are at risk for skin impairment and pain if perineal hygiene is not carefully managed. Skin that may be exposed to secretions from gastrostomy sites, ileostomies, or colostomies also is at risk for irritation, breakdown, and, subsequently, pain.

Cutaneous Stimulation. Cutaneous stimulation relieves acute or chronic pain. Techniques such as pressure, massage, vibration, heat, cold, and plain or menthol ointments are safe and effective. All these methods have the added benefit of distracting and relaxing the client and helping to establish or extend the nurse–client relationship. Cutaneous stimulation should be moderate in frequency and duration, and its use should be determined by the extent of pain relief. Areas that can be used include the skin over or near the pain site, trigger or acupuncture points, and peripheral nerves.

The analgesic effects of these therapies are thought to be caused by activation of large A-beta fibers and inhibition of smaller A-delta and C-fibers, thus closing the gate to pain impulses. The exact mechanism by which this gating occurs has not been established but it may be through endorphin release. If a person has allodynia, these types of therapies may be inappropriate because they would dramatically increase pain sensation.

The effects of cutaneous stimulation are variable and unpredictable. So be patient when trying various methods, and adjust them as necessary. For some clients, the pain is relieved for a long period after stimulation. Others find that their pain returns to pretreatment levels immediately after therapy. In others, stimulation may not relieve pain or may actually cause further pain when the therapy is abandoned. Try using a technique more than once before deciding that it does not work.

Massage. Massage (rubbing a painful area) may relax muscles and reduce tension (Wilkie et al., 2000). It is contraindicated, however, over broken skin, mucous membranes, and/or rashes. Massage can be performed alone or with counterirritants such as mustard plasters, poultices, and liniments. Menthol products are the most common over-the-counter irritants, but the smell of menthol may offend some clients. Most menthol products contain methyl salicylate, which is absorbed through the skin to cause the analgesic effect. The immediate sensation of warmth or coolness may last for hours. Increasing the strength of the menthol, prolonging the massage, and ensuring that pores are open may intensify the sensation. If the ointment relieves the pain, wrapping the painful area in plastic will prolong relief.

Heat and Cold. Heat and cold may be used to reduce muscle spasm and decrease pain. Except for decreasing muscle spasm and reducing pain, heat and cold have opposite effects on the body. Do not use heat (from a hot water bottle, heating pad, moist pad, warm bath, or the sun) within 24 hours of an injury because it increases blood flow, edema, and bleeding at a site. However, after 24 hours, heat is especially effective for joint and muscle pain. Cold (from crushed ice in a towel, ice bag, reusable gel pack, frozen paper cup of ice, bag of frozen peas, and Popsicles) decreases the inflammatory response, blood flow, and edema and relieves chronic migraines and back pain.

 SAFETY ALERT

When using heat or cold, take these precautions:
- **Do not use heat for pain before medical diagnosis of its cause.**
- **Do not use heat over areas of impaired circulation.**
- **Avoid extremes of temperature, which can cause burns or frostbite.**
- **Do not use heat over a new injury; it may cause increased bleeding and edema.**
- **Discontinue use of heat if stimulation increases pain.**

Contralateral Stimulation. In **contralateral stimulation,** the opposite area is stimulated with pressure, massage, cold, heat, or menthol to relieve pain. For instance, the left hand is stimulated when the right hand is painful. This therapy is effective when the painful area cannot be reached because of a cast or bandages, the affected skin is too sensitive to touch, or phantom pain is present. Contralateral massage may be useful for muscle cramps, spasms, or itching. The precautions are the same as for heat and cold and for massage.

Transcutaneous Electrical Nerve Stimulation (TENS). **Transcutaneous electrical nerve stimulation** (TENS) is used as an adjunct in the overall management of acute and chronic pain. The TENS unit consists of a palm-sized, lightweight, battery-operated stimulator that generates a mild electrical impulse. Two to four electrodes are taped to the skin near or over a pain zone, and the client controls the electrode output to produce a pleasant sensation that relieves pain. TENS is thought to produce analgesia by stimulating A-beta fibers to block A-delta and unmyelinated C-fibers, thus blocking noxious stimuli from the periphery by stimulating endorphins in the dorsal horn.

The location of the electrodes and the voltage, frequency, and duration of the stimulus are determined by the spinal dermatomes most likely affected by the pain and the client's response. Initially, the client may feel a tingling, buzzing, or vibrating sensation. Although usually mild, some clients find it unpleasant or intolerable. TENS is advantageous because it

- Appears to increase blood flow
- May allow the client to decrease or eliminate pain medications
- Does not produce dependence
- Does not interfere with the client's daily activities

Correct electrode placement and precise output adjustment are essential for this method's success. Skin problems are the major adverse effect. Skin irritation can be caused by tape irritation or an allergy to the tape or the gel. Using hypoallergenic tape, a stockinette-type dressing, or a belt may help. Rashes from the gel may be remedied by changing to another gel, using cortisone cream by itself or mixed with the gel, rotating the electrode sites, and cleaning the electrodes daily with soap and water.

The client must use TENS only as the physician has prescribed. Using TENS for new pain could lead to a delay in diagnosis and treatment. Clients who have pacemakers should not use TENS because it may interfere with or inhibit the output of some demand-type pacemakers. Electrodes should not be placed over the eyes, over the carotid sinus (could precipitate a vasovagal reaction), and over the anterior neck or mouth areas (could cause spasms and the danger of airway closure). Safety has not been proven for the first trimester of pregnancy, but TENS has been used on the lower back during childbirth.

Cognitive Pain Relief Techniques

Anticipatory Guidance. Fear and dread may enhance or precipitate pain. Provide an honest explanation of what the client can expect. Sharing information about what the client will feel (sensory) and about the procedure is more effective than procedure information alone. Even if the nurse says that there probably will be pain, the client can usually manage the pain better knowing what to expect and how to manage it. Anticipatory guidance can be used along with analgesics to prevent pain as much as possible.

Because early ambulation and pulmonary hygiene are important after surgery, teach the preoperative client how to cope with postsurgical pain and how to improve mobility. Be aware and inform the client that most of these activities increase pain. Some techniques to relieve pain associated with these activities include the following:

- Premedicating with an analgesic before painful activity; amount of time before the activity depends on the drug's peak action
- Splinting the incision with pillows to provide external immobilization and decrease muscle tension at the site
- Positioning techniques such as moving side to side, transferring to the side of the bed and to the chair, and proper walking posture

Distraction. Distraction is useful when clients are undergoing brief periods of sharp, intense pain such as dressing changes, wound debridement, biopsy, or incident pain from shifting positions. The pain relief tends to be temporary, lasting only through the distraction exercise (i.e., the Lamaze method for the woman in labor). Use complex stimuli that include multiple senses or high levels of concentration for mild to moderate pain. As the intensity of pain increases, use simple stimuli that involve one sense or limited concentration.

Distraction may be visual (reading [a complex stimulus]; looking at pictures [a simple stimulus]), auditory (playing an instrument [a complex stimulus]; listening to music [a simple stimulus]), or tactile (stroking a pet or rocking [a simple stimulus]). The distraction is most effective if it is something the client enjoys doing. Listening to music has been shown in many studies to be an effective way to reduce the intensity of many types of pain including cancer pain.

Guided Imagery. Guided imagery is a technique in which the person focuses on a pleasant, relaxed mental image as a way to decrease the intensity of pain or as a substitute for pain. The image of a healing ball of energy that reduces pain is sometimes used.

Hypnosis. Hypnosis heightens a person's susceptibility to suggestion and alters the subject's state of consciousness. It blocks the awareness of pain through suggestions or by substituting another feeling for pain, altering the pain's meaning, increasing pain tolerance, and, in extreme cases, dissociating the perception of the body from the person's awareness. In general, about 20% of clients with moderate to severe pain achieve total relief with hypnosis. Clients with cancer and severe mucositis pain in the mouth and throat from bone marrow transplant therapy obtained excellent analgesia with hypnosis and required less pain medication than clients not using hypnosis (Sellick & Zaza, 1998; Syrjala, Cummings & Donaldson, 1992). Common myths about hypnosis, however, limit its acceptance. Plus, it can be expensive and time consuming, requiring practitioners to have advanced training.

Behavioral Pain Relief Techniques

Relaxation. Relaxation techniques, which can be useful pain-relief measures, usually involve a combination of a quiet environment, a comfortable position, a passive attitude, and

OUTCOME-BASED TEACHING PLAN

Dean Norman, 53 years old, has chronic back pain. He is in the clinic where he receives pain medication. He seems a little unsure how to best manage the medication and asks you to help him figure it out.

OUTCOME: *The client will verbalize a plan to monitor and report his pain.*
Strategies
- Discuss with Dean the way to describe his pain. Provide him with a body outline and a list of words that he can use as descriptors and review the list periodically.
- Work with him to develop a plan about how to monitor his pain and record it in a journal including the following points:
  - Where he has pain
  - How much pain he has at rest and with activity (using a 0–10 scale)
  - How his pain feels (descriptive terms)
  - How his pain changes with activity and time
- Ask him to practice reporting the information to you.
- Instruct Dean to write down any events that he thinks may be related to the occurrence of pain.
- Suggest that he anticipate possible painful events and alter his behavior to prevent or minimize pain.
- Advise Dean to take his journal with him to the healthcare provider and encourage him to report this information to the provider.

OUTCOME: *The client will demonstrate appropriate measures to manage his pain.*
Strategies
- Review his medication prescription including:

- Drug name, dosage, and frequency
- Analgesic action
- Adverse effects and ways to minimize them, especially constipation
- Discuss the nature of his pain and prescribed time intervals for taking his medication including:
  - Keeping the pain intensity level as close as possible to his goal for pain relief
  - Taking the medication regularly for constant pain, before pain begins for intermittent pain
  - Taking the medication before the pain becomes more intense than he would like to tolerate
- Discuss his plan to report inadequate pain relief to his healthcare provider.
- Urge him to obtain another prescription before the pain medications are all used.
- Discuss his concerns about using the pain medication, provide clarification for any misconceptions he may have.
- Review with Dean a plan of response in the event of a drug interaction.
- Give Dean the phone number of his healthcare provider and encourage him to keep it readily available.
- Advise him to always take a list of all medications with him to his healthcare provider appointments.
- Discuss his plans to use nonpharmacologic methods for pain control. Provide written and verbal instructions in the methods chosen.
- Have him practice the methods to determine the most effective ones. Instruct him to use alternate methods if one seems ineffective.

---

a focus of concentration such as a word, sound, or breathing pattern. Relaxation techniques usually are initiated independently by a nurse with additional training in their use. Relaxation can counteract the effects of the fight-or-flight response and promote mental and physical freedom from tension and stress. Physical and mental tension can aggravate any pain. They may actually cause conditions such as headaches and back pain. Relaxation therapies promote a sense of detachment. The client feels a sense of control over the pain in a particular body part. Other benefits of relaxation include the following:

- Enabling the client to fight fatigue and sleep restfully, thus increasing energy
- Complementing other pain-relief techniques
- Allowing the client to cope more effectively with the same intensity of pain
- Improving the client's mood and flexibility

- Producing physiologic changes (decreased muscle tension, increased blood flow, decreased heart and respiratory rate)

Relaxation training is not without problems. Many clients require booster sessions to refamiliarize themselves with procedures they may have forgotten. Some clients with chronic pain may resort to excessive use of relaxation procedures to escape from normal stresses of daily living. Hence the technique itself becomes a debilitating pain behavior.

Meditation. Meditation is a technique in which the person focuses on a single thought or sound. Transcendental meditation is a popular form. Yoga is a combination of meditation and stretching exercises. Progressive relaxation is a technique of discriminating between tension and relaxation of specific muscles from head to toe. In autogenics (passive progressive relaxation) the person repeats certain phrases silently to induce relaxation without discriminating between tension and relaxation. Autogenics can be useful for a client with a cardiac condition because tensing the muscles might increase the heart's workload. Visualizing relaxation of muscles could decrease pain.

Biofeedback. In **biofeedback,** the client learns voluntary control over autonomic functions such as heart rate, hand temperature, and muscle tension. Electrodes are placed on the client's body, and auditory or visual feedback (i.e., lights, sounds, digital or graphic readings) provides the client with information about muscle relaxation, heart rate, blood pressure, and skin temperature. After baseline data are obtained, the client learns relaxation and deep-breathing exercises. The relaxation decreases pain by decreasing anxiety and increasing the client's sense of control over pain. With practice, the client learns to call on the skills at will. This technique is helpful in clients with hypertension, muscle tension, tension headaches, migraines, temporomandibular joint syndrome, insomnia, chronic pain, and stress-related disorders. Motivation is an important component in its success because the technique requires extensive training.

Pharmacologic Management

Analgesic medication is the most common approach to pain management. Although the physician orders analgesics, the nurse is responsible for giving the drugs, evaluating and documenting their effectiveness, and notifying the physician if the relief obtained is inadequate.

Analgesics may be separated into three major groups: nonopioid, opioid, and adjuvant. Their actions and nursing implications are given in Table 43-2.

Nonopioid Analgesics. Nonopioid analgesics include aspirin, nonsteroidal antiinflammatory drugs (NSAIDs), and acetaminophen. Aspirin and the NSAIDs have strong antiinflammatory actions in peripheral tissue. Aspirin and other NSAIDs are generally effective for pain related to tissue damage. Also, these drugs have antiprostaglandin effects in both the peripheral and central nervous systems. The analgesic action of acetaminophen is unclear, but it also appears to act through CNS mechanisms. These drugs are used as single-agent therapy principally for mild pain but can be combined with opioids to improve pain control for mild, moderate, and severe pain. Because aspirin, several NSAIDs, and acetaminophen are so readily available without prescription, their effectiveness is often underestimated. New NSAIDs target a specific receptor associated with pain (Cox2) and may decrease gastrointestinal and renal side effects common with other NSAIDs. Examples of these new NSAIDs include Celebrex (celecoxib) and Vioxx (rofecoxib), both of which are effective for arthritis and other painful conditions.

Opioid Analgesics. The opioid analgesics are a group of naturally occurring and synthetic agents for relief of moderate to severe pain in the conscious state. Opioids are used for postoperative or trauma analgesia and are the mainstay of pain management for cancer. Opioids also can be used for long-term management of chronic nonmalignant pain (Dickinson, Altman, Nielsen, & Williams, 2000).

Opioid agonists are drugs that bind to specific opioid receptors to produce analgesia. Morphine is the prototype. Opioid antagonists block the opioid receptors or displace the agonists from these sites. Naloxone is the prototype. Opioid antagonists can reverse the depressant effects of opioids and are used to treat acute opioid overdoses. Opioid agonist-antagonists are drugs that bind to opioid receptors but exert effects only at certain receptors. Use of an opioid agonist-antagonist drug in a person dependent on an opioid agonist can precipitate acute withdrawal syndrome.

Combining opioid and nonopioid analgesics is logical and effective because pain is attacked by two different mechanisms. This approach allows better pain control without increasing the opioid dose. When the drugs are combined into one tablet, however, caution is needed to avoid excessive doses of the nonopioid analgesic. For example, total daily acetaminophen dosage should not exceed 2,700 to 4,000 mg or liver damage is possible (American Pain Society, 1999). The opioid in most of the combination products (Percodan [oxycodone with aspirin] or Percocet [oxycodone with acetaminophen]), however, can be increased to as high a dose as is needed to provide pain relief.

Generally, intramuscular or subcutaneous administration of an opioid is appropriate for only a few days because subcutaneous and muscle tissue can quickly become irritated. Oral opioids are useful for the client in prolonged pain and with a functioning gastrointestinal tract. The transdermal fentanyl (a synthetic opioid) patch is now available for clients with chronic pain or cancer pain who cannot tolerate oral analgesics. This method of opioid delivery through the skin has an analgesic action with a slow onset (12 to 18 hours) and long duration (48 to 72 hours). Clients with a stable temporal pattern to their pain are most likely to benefit from the patch. In cancer pain management, continuous subcutaneous infusion of opioids has been effective for months.

Epidural and Intrathecal Analgesia. Injecting opioids or combinations of opioids and local anesthetics directly into the epidural or intrathecal spaces also can control severe cancer pain, postoperative pain, and chronic nonmalignant pain. Epidural catheters may be temporary or permanent. Permanent catheters may be surgically implanted or placed percutaneously (through a needle). Although the lumbar region is the most common site of placement, epidural catheters may be placed in the cervical, thoracic, lumbar, or caudal regions. Elderly clients may be more sensitive to epidural opioids due to slowed or altered metabolism and excretion.

The American Nurses Association (ANA) (1990) established practice guidelines for the role of the registered nurse in management of clients receiving the analgesia by catheter techniques. Timing, frequency, and type of nursing assessment (e.g., sensory and motor effects) depend on the epidural drug(s). Opioids with diluted concentrations (0.125% or less) of local anesthetics, such as bupivacaine, are examples of

(text continues on page 1189)

TABLE 43-2

Drug Actions and Nursing Implications

Category/Drug	Action	Nursing Implications
Nonopioids		
Acetylsalicylic acid (ASA)	Analgesic: Blocks prostaglandin synthesis, thus decreasing sensitivity of peripheral pain receptors to mechanical or chemical activation. Antipyretic: Decreases outflow of vasoconstrictor impulses from hypothalamus, thus promoting vasodilation, sweating, and heat loss. Antiinflammatory: Decreases capillary permeability and fluid leakage into surrounding tissues; interferes with release of enzymes. Other actions decrease platelet aggregation.	Because gastric irritation is the major side effect of ASA, give on a full stomach (although this delays absorption and pain relief). Also, avoid stomach upset by using enteric-coated ASA, which isn't absorbed until it reaches the intestine. Over several days or after several doses, be alert for ringing in the ears (tinnitus), which reflects damage to the auditory nerve. Reduce dose immediately. Never give ASA with oral anticoagulants, methotrexate, probenecid, or sulfinpyrazone because significant drug interactions will occur. Know that chronic use is associated with analgesic nephropathy.
Acetaminophen	Analgesic and antipyretic: Elevates the pain threshold and reduces sympathetic outflow from hypothalamic temperature-regulating center. Weak antidiuretic action. Exerts no significant antiinflammatory effect and does not produce gastric erosion, inhibition of platelet aggregation, or prothrombin depression.	Use with caution in people with known liver disease because it may cause liver toxicity. Do not exceed daily dosage of 4,000 mg.
Corticosteroids (e.g., hydrocortisone, prednisone, dexamethasone)	Antiinflammatory: Stabilize tissue membranes and inhibit capillary dilation and permeability. Block synthesis of leukotrienes and prostaglandins.	Give with food or milk and urge clients to advise physician if gastric irritation persists because drug can cause gastric ulceration. Anticipate using supplemental antacids, which may alleviate the distress. Inform clients to notify physician if excessive weight gain, edema, hypertension, muscle weakness, bone pain, sore throat, fever, cold, infection, mood changes, or visual disturbances occur.
Nonsteroidal antiinflammatory drugs (NSAIDs; e.g., ibuprofen, naproxen, tolmetin, indomethacin)	Analgesic, antiinflammatory, and antipyretic effects: Block synthesis and possibly release of prostaglandins. The principal advantage of these drugs is a somewhat lower incidence of the milder forms of GI distress that commonly occur with high-dose salicylate use (excluding indomethacin).	Observe diabetics closely during steroid therapy because hyperglycemia or loss of blood sugar control could occur. Observe clients with a history of GI problems for signs of gastric pain, nausea, cramping. Stop drug if symptoms persist. Know that reversible and preventable renal insufficiency is associated with most NSAIDs. Clients most at risk for this problem are those with heart failure, renal disease, cirrhosis with ascites, and those over age 60. Keep in mind that some clients may respond to only one of the several available nonsteroidal agents. Try different derivatives at 2- to 3-week intervals before concluding that this type of drug is ineffective.

(continues)

TABLE 43-2 (Continued)

Drug Actions and Nursing Implications		
Category/Drug	**Action**	**Nursing Implications**
Opioid Antagonist Naloxone	Binds to all the opioid receptors but does not produce any effect on them. If an opioid agonist is bound to the receptor, this drug will displace the agonist and thereby counteract the agonist effect.	Administer as the drug of choice to counteract respiratory depression induced by opioids. Know that large doses will reverse the analgesic effects of opioids as well as the respiratory depression and could cause seizures.
Opioid Agonist-Antagonists Pentazocine, nalbuphine, butorphanol, dezocine	Bind to several types of opioid receptors, but produce a morphine-like action only at certain receptors (e.g., agonist pain relief effect at kappa receptors). No morphinelike action is produced by binding at the mu or delta receptors (antagonist-like effect). If the receptor is dependent on agonist binding, withdrawal effects may be produced.	Observe for possible withdrawal in people who have been receiving agonist opioids. Antagonize the analgesic effects, and provide poor pain relief. Adverse effects include hallucinations.
Opioid Agonist Naturally occurring opium alkaloids (morphine, codeine) Semisynthetic derivates (hydromorphone, oxycodone, oxymorphone) Entirely synthetic derivates (meperidine, fentanyl, methadone)	Bind to opioid receptors in the peripheral and central nervous systems and produce pain-relieving effects at mu, delta, and kappa receptors. Agonist drugs alter perception and response to pain, may produce CNS depression (sedation and respiratory depression), and usually decrease gastric motility.	Know that morphine provides satisfactory pain relief in about 70% of clients with moderate to severe pain. However, if morphine fails to relieve pain or produces side effects (i.e., nausea), anticipate better pain relief with fewer side effects by changing to another opioid. Use meperidine cautiously (although effective in many clients with acute pain) because of possible CNS toxicity, hallucinations, seizures, and disorientation, especially in clients with renal or hepatic dysfunction. Poor oral absorption and short duration of action preclude its use in chronic pain. Remember that methadone is useful in managing severe chronic pain, such as cancer pain, because it is only mildly sedating after the initial 2–5 days, has a long duration of action, and is absorbed well from the GI tract. Observe for possible adverse effects including drowsiness, nausea, respiratory depression, CNS depression, and constipation.

drugs used epidurally. When epidural opioids are administered, the nurse monitors the levels of pain and sedation, respiratory rate and depth, and blood pressure. When local anesthetics are administered, the nurse also monitors the client's motor function and the spinal dermatome level at which the client has sensation. The nurse routinely assesses the skin condition. The nurse also assists the client to change positions frequently to prevent skin breakdown in the client with potentially altered sensation due to the numbing effect of an epidural local anesthetic, which is an undesired effect of the local anesthetic on the fibers that mediate sensation. The nurse also checks the epidural catheter position at the exit site routinely (e.g., every 8 hours) and if the client suddenly complains of inadequate pain relief. Also the nurse checks the epidural catheter placement prior to any bolus injection. The nurse does not administer the injection and calls the physician if greater than 1 cc of fluid or any blood is aspirated from the catheter. This finding may indicate that the epidural catheter is not in the correct position and continued injection could have severe consequences.

Intrathecal (into the cerebral spinal fluid) administration and monitoring guidelines are similar to epidural administration. Doses administered, however, are much lower because the entire dose reaches the spinal cord (i.e., is not influenced by the dura and high vascularity of the epidural space).

The frequency with which a client receives an opioid for pain is often left largely to the nurse's discretion within the parameters of the prescription. This approach, however, should not preclude preventive pain relief. Because clients may not request an analgesic, assess the pain and determine if the client could benefit from one. With constant pain, opioids are given at fixed intervals before the pain returns (i.e., before the analgesia wears off). Thus the client's anticipation of pain is eliminated, and the client's anxiety decreases thereby controlling the vicious cycle of increasing pain with anxiety. This method may contribute to decreased pain and a decreased need for analgesia.

Respiratory Depression. Respiratory depression with opioid use is uncommon, is easily observed, and is treated with an opioid antagonist such as naloxone. The rare case of respiratory depression occurs most often after acute administration of an opioid and is associated with other signs of CNS depression. Maximal respiratory depression occurs within 7 to 20 minutes of IV administration, 30 minutes of intramuscular administration, 60 minutes of oral administration, or 24 hours of epidural or intrathecal administration.

When giving the initial opioid dose to a sleeping person, closely observe the client for pain relief and respiratory depression (rate and depth). Clients who are awake do not succumb to respiratory depression (American Pain Society, 1999). The nurse also should monitor clients with a decreased respiratory reserve of effort (e.g., those who have undergone thoracic or upper abdominal surgery). Because breathing causes considerable pain in these clients, they often do not breathe deeply, possibly leading to atelectasis and pneumonia. In these clients, opioids may actually increase respiratory activity by relieving the pain associated with breathing (Siddall & Cousins, 1997).

Clients in respiratory depression, usually defined as less than 8 breaths/min, can initially be treated by directing the client to "breathe now" and "breathe deep" (American Pain Society, 1999). If the client cannot follow instructions or is apneic, artificial ventilation is needed until naloxone, the opioid antagonist of choice for treating respiratory depression, is given. Small doses of naloxone can be given safely without causing withdrawal symptoms or counteracting all the analgesic effect of the opioid.

Addiction. Opioids can produce addiction, a psychological condition characterized by a drive to obtain and take substances for other than the prescribed value (AHCPR, 1994). Despite recent studies clearly indicating that medical use of opioids rarely leads to drug abuse or addiction, fear of addiction is still a major barrier to effective use of opioids in clients with pain. Less than 0.1% of clients who receive opioids as part of their medical treatment regimen become addicted. That is, 4 out of nearly 12,000 clients became addicted (Porter & Jick, 1980). Share these numbers with clients to help reduce their concerns about addiction.

Dependence. Dependence develops in most clients who receive opioids regularly for more than 10 days. It is an expected physiologic response to ongoing exposure to opioids (AHCPR, 1994). A person who is dependent on opioids responds to abrupt discontinuation or to administration of an opioid antagonist with characteristic withdrawal symptoms: anxiety, nervousness, irritability, diarrhea, and alternating chills and hot flashes. A prominent withdrawal sign is "wetness," including salivation, lacrimation, rhinorrhea, profuse perspiration, and gooseflesh. At the peak of withdrawal, clients may experience nausea and vomiting, abdominal cramps, insomnia, and, rarely, multifocal myoclonus. Abstinence symptoms usually occur within 6 to 12 hours and peak at 24 to 72 hours after cessation of morphine. A delayed onset is seen with drugs with long half-lives such as methadone.

To prevent withdrawal syndrome, the preferred practice is to discontinue the opioid by reducing the dose with a taper schedule. For example, to withdraw from morphine, calculate the 24-hour dose, decrease it by 50%, and give 25% of it every 6 hours. After 2 days, reduce the daily dose by an additional 25% every 2 days until the 24-hour oral dose is 30 mg/d, then discontinue the morphine (American Pain Society, 1999). Clonidine hydrochloride is useful for counteracting the side effects of withdrawal.

Tolerance. Tolerance develops when a dose of an opioid becomes less effective on repeated administration. Hence, larger doses are needed to produce the original effect. Tolerance is not addiction, but it does involve physiologic changes related to drug metabolism, the nervous system's adaptation to the drug action, or other factors. Intermittent use of opioids does not usually lead to significant tolerance and not all clients experience tolerance. The need for an increase in the analgesic dose may reflect other factors such as disease progression (e.g., cancer progression) or new pathology (e.g., pulmonary embolus). Do not ignore the client's reports of increased pain. Pain should be treated while the cause is pursued.

THERAPEUTIC DIALOGUE
Pain Medication

Scene for Thought
While walking down the hall, the nurse hears quiet moaning. She enters the room and sees Kathy Goodman lying on her side, facing the wall. Her body is restless, and she is breathing erratically. Her roommate says (a little irritably) that she's been that way for the last 10 minutes. The client had varicose vein surgery earlier today and is 42 years old.

Less Effective

Nurse: Ms. Goodman, I'm Liz Newman, the charge nurse. Can you tell me what's happening? *(Stands by the bed.)*
Client: My leg hurts. *(Grimaces and gasps as she turns over.)*
Nurse: Has it gotten worse recently?
Client: No, it's just constant unless I move. So I don't move.
Nurse: I'll just run and get your chart so I can see when you had your last pain medication. *(Does so.)* Okay, you're about due for more medication, but maybe we can get you an increase until your pain decreases and you start to heal a little.
Client: No! I don't want to take more.
Nurse: But you seem to be in such pain! Besides *(whispers)* I think your roommate is really concerned for you and may be a bit annoyed.
Client: *(Looks embarrassed.)* Oh, I didn't know I was bothering her. Are the pills safe to take? Someone told me I could become, you know, addicted. *(Body is tense.)*
Nurse: As long as you're in such pain, you won't become addicted. We're careful about that. I'll bet they'll help.
Client: *(Reluctantly.)* Okay.
Nurse: Great! I'll get them to you right away. *(Leaves in a hurry.)*
Client: *(Glances at roommate as if to speak, but then remains silent. Roommate doesn't make eye contact. Kathy's body remains tense.)*

More Effective

Nurse: Ms. Goodman, I'm Linda Norman, the charge nurse. Can you tell me what's happening? *(Stands by the bed.)*
Client: My leg hurts. *(Grimaces and gasps as she turns over.)*
Nurse: Has it gotten worse recently?
Client: No, it's just constant unless I move. So I don't move.
Nurse: I'll just run and get your chart so I can see when you had your last pain medication. *(Does so.)* Okay, you're about due for more medication, but maybe we can get you an increase until your pain decreases and you start to heal a little.
Client: No! I don't want to take more.
Nurse: I'm surprised to hear you say that. Could you explain?
Client: *(Looks down.)* I don't want to get too dependent on the pain pills.
Nurse: *(Pays silent attention.)*
Client: The last time I had my veins stripped, the nurses would give the pain pills only every 4 hours and no more. They said it wasn't allowed because I'd get addicted. So I don't want any more. *(Looks down.)* I'll just have to deal with it. *(Begins to close her eyes and settle her body stiffly into position.)*
Nurse: Can I help in any way?
Client: *(Opens her eyes wearily.)* How?
Nurse: Well, first, I need to examine your leg and ask you a few questions. Then we might be able to add a nonnarcotic pain pill to the ones you have to provide some overlap. When narcotics are used for medical purposes, such as your surgery pain, very few people become addicted—actually only 4 in 12,000 according to several studies. I also can teach you some relaxation techniques that might help relax you and reduce the pain. How do those options sound?
Client: *(Thinking about it.)* They might work. Worth a try, anyway.
Nurse: I thought you might be interested. Let's get started.

Critical Thinking Challenge
- Relate Kathy's body language to her pain.
- Explain the relationship between pain and stress.
- Detect what the first nurse taught Kathy. Compare and contrast what the second nurse taught her.
- Propose other ways to help Kathy handle her pain.
- Explain what happened by the end of the first dialogue to contribute to Kathy's tension.
- Describe each nurse's manner in talking to Kathy.

One way to manage tolerance is by adjusting the drug dosage based on the client's response (**titration**) to balance desired effects and adverse effects to maintain client comfort. This type of dose adjustment is known as titrating the dose. Other approaches include changing to another drug in the same class or adding a nonopioid drug such as ibuprofen. There is no ceiling effect or maximum dose for opioid agonist drugs. As tolerance or need for more pain relief increases, doses can be increased. Doses as large as 1,654 mg IV morphine per hour (37,536 mg/d) have been administered (Miser, Moore, Green, Gracely, & Miser, 1986).

Adverse Effects. Other adverse effects of opioids are constipation, nausea and vomiting, and sedation. Constipation is the most common and most problematic. Opioids act at multiple

ETHICAL/LEGAL ISSUE
Possible Dependence on Pain Medication

Mr. Stuart, 34 years old, has experienced first- and second-degree burns over 40% of his body. He was in good physical health before this accident but requires extensive treatment. Clearly, Mr. Stuart is going to survive his injuries, but the treatment process will be long-term and painful. He is anxious about the treatment. He requests you be sure that he experiences as little pain as possible and that you give him all the pain medication that he can have. You discuss this with the healthcare team, advocating for your client regarding his concerns about pain relief. Another team member responds by saying that Mr. Stuart is probably exhibiting "drug-seeking" behavior, and the amount of pain medication has to be limited to prevent Mr. Stuart from becoming addicted.

Reflection

- Identify your concerns about Mr. Stuart, his request for pain relief, and the other team member's response.
- For what reasons could the healthcare team member be responding as he is? What are your feelings in light of that opinion? What are ethical and legal consequences of complying with Mr. Stuart's request? Of withholding medication?
- Identify possible approaches to advocating for your client in this situation.
- Recognizing the client's injuries, his anxiety about pain, and the team member's opinion, define what you see as your ethically appropriate behavior.

sites in the gastrointestinal tract and spinal cord to reduce intestinal secretions and decrease peristalsis. Tolerance to constipation does not develop at the same rate as tolerance to the other adverse effects. Encourage clients taking routine doses of an opioid to drink at least 2 liters of fluid daily, get daily exercise, eat a high-fiber diet, and take daily stimulant laxatives; a stool softener is insufficient.

Nausea and vomiting are caused by delayed gastric emptying, stimulation of the medullary chemoreceptor zone and resultant stimulation of the nearby vomiting center, and stimulation of the vestibular part of the ear. Substituting an equianalgesic dose of another opioid may reduce or stop nausea and vomiting. Or an antiemetic may be given with the opioid. Metoclopramide is an effective antiemetic for opioid-induced nausea because it increases gastric emptying. Many clients become tolerant to this adverse effect in a few days if it is not severe.

Sedation and drowsiness, which occur in most clients receiving opioids, are useful in some clinical situations such as before anesthesia. When excessive, sedation may be countered by reducing the dose and increasing the interval between doses. In addition, discontinuing other CNS depressants, such as sedative-hypnotics and antianxiety agents that potentiate the sedative effects of opioids, can reduce the sedating effects. However, fatigue and insomnia may result from the pain itself. An opioid dose may allow the client to sleep. In the client taking regular opioids, drowsiness is usually temporary, occurring for the first 2 or 3 days (AHCPR, 1992; 1994). Psychostimulants, particularly methylphenidate, dramatically improve opioid-induced sedation (AHCPR, 1994).

Older clients are more susceptible to drug effects and may more readily experience confusion, excessive sedation, or respiratory depression from opioids. With age, the liver and kidneys become less efficient at metabolizing and clearing drugs from the body, which can lead to accumulation of the drug in older clients. Because older clients tend to take more drugs, there is an increased risk of drug interactions. Therefore, titration is mandatory.

Precipitous Death. Some people believe that administering large doses of morphine constitutes assisted suicide or euthanasia. It is not uncommon for health professionals, clients, and family members to be concerned about the effect of sufficient pain relief on precipitating the death of a person with a terminal illness. Relieving pain, even if it hastens death in a person facing the end of life, is the ethical and moral obligation of the professional nurse; it is not euthanasia or assisted suicide (ANA, 1992). When consistent with the client's wishes, the ANA's position is, "Nurses should not hesitate to use full and effective doses of pain medication for the proper management of pain in the dying client. The increasing titration of medication to achieve adequate symptom control, even at the expense of life, thus hastening death, is ethically justified" (ANA, 1992, p. 14). Titrating pain medications for pain relief is not euthanasia or assisted suicide; rather it allows the client and family to experience a peaceful death (American Association of Colleges of Nursing (AACN), 1997).

Patient-Controlled Analgesia. Patient-controlled analgesia (PCA), in which clients give themselves doses of opioid analgesics, allows clients to become more involved in their own care (AHCPR, 1992). Clinical studies show that it is safe and effective and that selected clients tend to take only as much drug as they need for pain control (AHCPR, 1992). The small, frequent IV doses given in PCA systems relieve pain without excessive sedation because they do not produce the wide variations in blood levels of analgesics with conventional therapy (Fig. 43-6).

The PCA system has a safety feature to prevent accidental overdoses. Even if the client pushes the button for another dose, the device cannot deliver another full dose until the correct amount of time, as preset, has elapsed. This lockout time should not be so long that the client must wait in pain between doses, however. In clients with severe acute or prolonged pain that cannot be controlled by any other route, a continuous IV or subcutaneous infusion may be used in addition to the PCA approach. This method provides a steady blood level of the analgesic.

Postoperative Pain. The Clinical Research display lists guidelines for managing acute postoperative pain. Unfortunately,

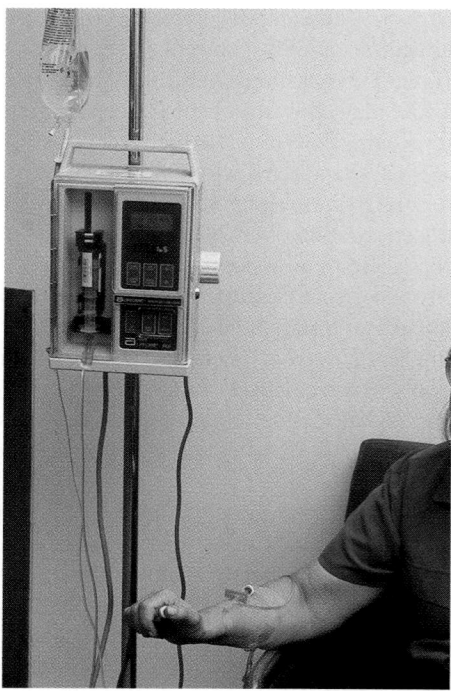

FIGURE 43-6   Patient-controlled analgesia (PCA) allows the client to self-administer only as much medication as needed to control pain.

too often these guidelines are not used in the treatment of pain in adults or children (AHCPR, 1992).

Adjuvant Analgesics. Several medications are analgesic when used alone or as adjuvants to opioid analgesia, or they counteract the side effects of analgesics. Adjuvant drugs include corticosteroids, tricyclic antidepressants, antihistamines, benzodi-

---

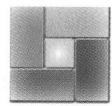

Clinical Research

Managing Acute Postoperative Pain

- Assess the client's physiologic, affective, behavioral, and cognitive response to pain, both verbal and nonverbal.
- Give narcotics around the clock, not prn, for the first 36 hr after surgery.
- Give analgesics before or as soon as pain returns.
- Give analgesics before activities, such as ambulation or incentive spirometer use.
- Individualize the drug and dosage.
- Monitor and record the client's response using a pain scale routinely.

From Agency for Health Care Policy and Research. (1992). *Acute pain management: Operative or medical procedures and trauma.* (Clinical practice guideline). Rockville, MD: U.S. Department of Health and Human Services.

---

azepines, caffeine, anticonvulsants, local anesthetics, and psychostimulants (AHCPR, 1994; American Pain Society, 1999).

Corticosteroids, useful for inflammation-related pain, are used for short-term treatment in young, otherwise healthy clients with sports-related pain that does not respond to NSAIDs. Corticosteroids also can be useful for various inflammatory conditions (such as active rheumatoid arthritis and ulcerative colitis) and can be injected at the inflammation site or given by other routes. Corticosteroids provide a range of other effects that are useful in the treatment of cancer pain, such as mood elevation, antiemetic activity, and appetite stimulation (AHCPR, 1994). In clients with cancer, corticosteroids, particularly those with mineralocorticoid-sparing activity (dexamethasone), have been used for more than 6 months without adverse effects outweighing their useful effects.

Antidepressant drugs are effective analgesics especially in clients with pain from nerve damage (**neuropathic pain**). These drugs potentiate the analgesic effect of opioids and have innate analgesic properties. They provide analgesia in people who are not depressed and in those who are depressed. In addition to pain relief, which occurs within 1 to 2 weeks, these drugs elevate mood and improve sleep. The most widely reported experience has been with amitriptyline, the tricyclic antidepressant of choice, even though it produces adverse effects (dry mouth, constipation, urinary retention, and orthostatic hypotension) related to its anticholinergic activity. To minimize adverse effects, small (10 to 25 mg) doses at bedtime are recommended (AHCPR, 1994).

SAFETY ALERT

When administering amitriptyline, ensure the client's safety to reduce the risk of falling from orthostatic hypotension. Encourage adequate hydration and resting in a sitting position before shifting from a reclining to a standing position.

Other adjuvant drugs interfere with nerve conduction (anticonvulsants and local anesthetics), block histamine effects on nociceptors (antihistamines), or reduce anxiety (benzodiazepines, antihistamines). Caffeine increases analgesia when given with aspirin-like drugs (American Pain Society, 1999). Psychostimulants, such as dextroamphetamine or methylphenidate, improve opioid analgesia and decrease sedation (AHCPR, 1994).

Use of Placebos. Placebos historically have been used in selected situations to differentiate psychological pain from nociceptive or neuropathic pain. Pain relieved by a placebo was considered to be psychogenic. Now it is clearly known that a positive placebo response does not prove that a client's pain is psychogenic. Placebos act through endogenous opioids and are reversed by naloxone, just like morphine's effects are reversed by naloxone (Levine, Gordon, & Fields, 1978). Use of a placebo without the client's knowledge is considered unethical nursing practice. A placebo, however, can be used with client consent to determine if a particular therapy is effective. When placebos are used in this manner, the client must have access to other analgesics if he or she requests additional pain relief.

The nurse who explains the drug's effects optimistically to the client may find that the drug works more effectively. This approach is thought to maximize the placebo response and minimize emotional and cognitive factors that influence pain perception.

Invasive Medical Management of Pain

When analgesics and other nonpharmacologic approaches cannot control intractable pain, as in advanced cancer or excessive pain with tic douloureux (trigeminal neuralgia), surgical intervention to interrupt pain pathways may be necessary. Table 43-3 summarizes common invasive interventions. Proper client and family teaching is essential before any

TABLE 43-3

Invasive Pain Management Interventions

Technique	Advantage	Limitations/Precautions	When Used
Nerve roots or pathway interrupted or destroyed: Neurectomy— peripheral sensory nerves Sympathectomy— sympathetic ganglia Rhizotomy— dorsal root ganglia Cordotomy— anterolateral spinothalamic tract	May decrease or eliminate pain	May leave permanent damage (i.e., paralysis, loss of control of the elimination process and sensation) or more severe pain	Intractable pain (i.e., advanced cancer or tic douloureux [trigeminal neuralgia])
Nerve blocks (injected with anesthetic to interrupt nerve pathway)	May decrease or eliminate pain	Pain relief variable	Intractable pain (i.e., celiac block for gastrointestinal malignancy)
Alcohol injections through transnasal or transphenoid approach of pituitary gland	Nontraumatic, easily performed, inexpensive	Pain relief variable; complications are signs of pituitary inactivation: hypopituitarism, steroid deficiency, decreased libido	Intractable pain from bony metastases from breast and prostate that are estrogen-sensitive
Injections of opioids, local anesthetics, or clonodine into central nervous system through a catheter placed in either the epidural space (space just outside dura mater; analgesic must filter through dura throughout the cerebrospinal fluid [CSF] and spinal cord) or subarachnoid space (contains the CSF)	Catheters can be left in place for months or years. Client or caregiver can give injections or have intermittent or continuous pump placed to deliver drugs. This allows independence and allows client to go home and into community. May decrease or eliminate pain.	Preservative-free opioid is used to avoid damage to spinal cord or nerve roots. A pump increases the cost of therapy. Preservative-free opioids are costly. Complications may include nausea/vomiting, urinary retention, pruritus, myoclonus, and respiratory depression, which naloxone can reverse. Close nursing monitoring for somnolence and respiratory depression for the first 24 hr is imperative.	Acute pain (i.e., postoperative thoracic or abdominal surgery, postcesarean section, phantom pain), chronic intractable pain

surgical procedure. Be sure that the client and family understand the procedure, risks, possible complications, and possible duration of pain relief.

Healthcare Planning and Home/Community-Based Nursing

Increasingly, pain management is occurring across a variety of healthcare settings. Economic trends suggest that even clients with pain from cancer will soon be managed without hospitalization. Pain experts agree that a combination of pharmacologic and nonpharmacologic strategies provides the best management in all healthcare settings (AHCPR, 1994).

Pain management in the home is critical in determining the functional ability and quality of life of clients with chronic pain. Chronic pain may immobilize clients and hinder their daily activities, relationships, sleep, and appetite. Family members often provide complex symptom management. Ambulatory and home-health nurses assess the interventions and test new interventions.

The nurse is responsible for anticipating the length of time pain will be experienced and, as early as possible in the course of care, teaching the client and family about pain management and their roles and expectations. The postoperative client needs information on the healing process with encouragement to maintain his or her pain at the lowest level possible, to get adequate rest and nutrition, to avoid fatigue, and to increase mobility. These factors affect client comfort and enhance recovery. The client should know how long recovery should take so he or she can seek medical intervention if complications occur.

Instruct clients taking analgesics about the correct dosage and ways to avoid or manage common adverse effects. Warn them that analgesics initially may produce changes in judgment, perception, and coordination when doses are increased, but these effects clear in a few days. Caution them not to drive or operate machinery until these cognitive effects have cleared. Clients with cancer often drive safely when they require huge doses of morphine (more than 1000 mg/d) to control their pain because they are adjusted to the adverse effects. Inform breast-feeding mothers if the drug is present in their milk and whether it may affect infants. At home, urge clients and family members to keep analgesics in safe, childproof bottles away from children or others.

EVALUATION

An important part of the nurse's role in pain management is accurately evaluating the effectiveness of pain-relief measures by questioning and observing the client. Never assume that nursing interventions have been successful. Depending on the results, the pain assessment measures may be modified or an alternate therapy tried. Although some examples of outcome criteria are presented below, develop individualized outcome criteria for each client.

Goal

The client will report a reduced pain intensity level that is at or less than he or she states is tolerable (e.g., 2 on a scale of 0 to 10).

Possible Outcome Criteria

- At the time of therapy onset, the client calls the pain intensity a lower number (0 to 10) than that reported when the therapy was administered (e.g., at 5 minutes for IV morphine).
- Client states that the pain intensity level is 0 to 2 on a scale of 0 to 10 at the time of peak effect for the therapy (e.g., at 20 minutes for IV morphine).
- Within the duration of effect for the therapy administered, the client will perform self-care activities to the extent of his or her ability (e.g., within 20 minutes and 2 to 4 hours of the IV morphine dose).

Goal

The client will identify factors that precipitate pain.

Possible Outcome Criteria

- At the next appointment, client describes factors that precipitate pain.
- At the next appointment, client describes thoughts and feelings that aggravate pain.
- On the next home visit, client reports behaviors that aggravate the pain.

Goal

The client will use techniques that decrease pain.

Possible Outcome Criteria

- Within 24 hours, client describes at least one behavioral intervention that helps to control pain.
- At the next appointment, client identifies the medication regimen that optimally controls pain.

KEY CONCEPTS

- Pain is a subjective experience that occurs whenever the client says it occurs.
- Initially, pain minimizes injury and warns of disease. Persistent pain has no purpose.
- Sedation does not always indicate pain relief.
- All pain-relief measures are based on a thorough ongoing assessment. Because clients may not always report pain, the nurse must assess for pain regularly. Lack of pain expression does not mean a lack of pain.
- Pain may be expressed in physiologic, verbal, and nonverbal ways.
- Clients of all ages experience pain, but the way they express it differs with age, the type of pain, and their ability to cope with the pain.

NURSING PLAN OF CARE
THE CLIENT EXPERIENCING PAIN

Nursing Diagnosis
Pain related to abdominal surgical incision manifested by verbal report of pain (9 on a 0–10 scale) and nonverbal communication of pain.

Client Goal
Client will experience pain level no greater than 2 (on a 0–10 scale) (number able to tolerate).

Client Outcome Criteria
- Client reports location, intensity, quality, and temporal pattern of pain and appropriate relief measures for pain.
- Client reports pain immediately at each occurrence.
- Client states pain is minimized at onset of analgesic effect and relieved at peak effect of analgesic therapy.

Nursing Intervention
1. Evaluate preoperative comprehensive pain assessment.

2. Assess level of pain every 2 hr for first 24 hr using a self-rating scale of 0 to 10. Also assess location, quality, and temporal pattern if they have changed since initial assessment.
3. Provide optimal pain relief with prescribed analgesics.

   a. Individualize medication regimen. Collaborate with physician to prescribe opioid around the clock instead of prn in the first 36 hr to maintain opioid blood levels and provide good pain relief.
   b. Assess response to medications.
   c. Monitor for and minimize common adverse effects of medications (specify).
4. Solicit techniques that have previously been helpful.

5. Establish a trusting relationship.

6. Instruct client to report pain promptly so relief measures can be instituted before severe pain occurs. Use therapeutic approaches for the prevention, not the relief, of severe pain.

7. Allow rest periods during day and periods of uninterrupted sleep at night when possible. Keep environment quiet.
8. Collaborate with client to initiate the appropriate noninvasive pain relief measure(s).
   a. Instruct in distraction technique (specify). Example: Engage in conversation or turn radio to favorite station during abdominal dressing change.
   b. Instruct in cutaneous stimulation (specify). Example: Give backrub after turning and before bedtime.
   c. Instruct in relaxation techniques (specify). Example: Relax muscles when turning.

Scientific Rationale
1. The most important component of pain is an ongoing, accurate, thorough pain assessment.
2. Frequent assessment provides data about how this person reports pain intensity and helps determine effectiveness of therapy.

3. Optimal pain relief decreases anxiety and fear, both of which increase pain. Goal is to use a preventive approach to avoid severe pain.
   a. Ongoing assessment of severity of pain before and pain relief after medication is important. This identifies if the drug or dose is sufficient for the client's pain.
   b. Opioids can cause respiratory depression, constipation, nausea, vomiting, and dry mouth.

4. Individual techniques that a client has used in the past enhance pain relief.
5. An effective nurse–client relationship enhances all pain-relief measures because it conveys caring and trust.
6. Relief measures are instituted based on client's verbal report of pain and regular client assessments. This also informs client of the expectation to communicate when in pain, because many ethnic and cultural influences often discourage or prohibit expression of pain.
7. Rest facilitates comfort and sleep, reduces stress, relieves muscle tension, and increases relaxation. Fatigue may enhance pain by lowering pain tolerance.
8. Focus attention away from pain, and increased pain tolerance results.
   a. Distraction may stimulate endorphins.

   b. Change of position and back rub increase circulation and decreases muscle tension.
   c. Relaxation reduces sympathetic nervous system effects.

- Cognitive and behavioral pain-relief measures can augment the effectiveness of pharmacologic or invasive methods.
- All routes of opioid administration are effective for mild, moderate, and severe pain but the IV route acts faster.
- Combining nonopioid, opioid, and adjuvant drugs with non-pharmacologic methods produces excellent analgesia because pain is relieved through different methods.
- The nurse's optimistic attitude about expected pain relief helps produce a positive result.
- Educating the client and family about pain reduces anticipatory fear and anxiety, thereby decreasing the client's pain.
- Using a preventive approach for pain relief is more beneficial than waiting until pain becomes severe.

REFERENCES

Agency for Health Care Policy and Research. (1994). *Management of cancer pain* (Clinical Practice Guideline). Rockville, MD: U.S. Department of Health and Human Services.

Agency for Health Care Policy and Research. (1992). *Acute pain management: Operative or medical procedures and trauma* (Clinical Practice Guideline). Rockville, MD: U.S. Department of Health and Human Services.

Ali, Z., Meyer, R. A., & Campbell, J. N. (1996). Secondary hyperalgesia to mechanical but not heat stimuli following a capsaicin injection in hairy skin. *Pain, 68*(2–3), 401–411.

American Association of Colleges of Nursing (AACN) Roundtable Participants. (1997). *Peaceful death: Recommended competencies and curricular guidelines for end-of-life nursing care*. Available at: *http://www. aacn.nche.edu/Publications/deathfin.htm.*

American Nurses Association (ANA). (1992). *Compendium of position statements on the nurse's role in end-of-life decisions (M-30)*. Washington, DC: Author.

American Nurses Association (ANA). (1990). *Position statement on the role of the registered nurse (RN) in the management of analgesia by catheter techniques (epidural, intrathecal, intrapleural, or peripheral nerve catheters)*. Washington, DC: Author.

American Pain Society. (1999). *Principles of analgesic use in the treatment of acute pain and chronic cancer pain: A concise guide to medical practice* (4th ed.). Skokie, IL: Author.

Basbaum, A. I. (1999). Spinal mechanisms of acute and persistent pain. *Regional Anesthesia and Pain Medicine, 24*, 59–67.

Besson, J. M. (1999). The neurobiology of pain. *Lancet, 353*, 1610–1615.

Beyer, J. E., & Aradine, C. R. (1987). Patterns of pediatric pain intensity: A methodological investigation of a self-report scale. *The Clinical Journal of Pain, 3*, 130–141.

Cousins, M. J., Power, I., & Smith, G. (2000). 1996 Labat lecture: Pain—a persistent problem. *Regional Anesthesia and Pain Medicine, 25*, 6–21.

Dickinson, B. D., Altman, R. D., Nielsen, N. H., & Williams, M. A. (2000). Use of opioids to treat chronic, noncancer pain. *Western Journal of Medicine, 172*, 107–115.

Fields, H. L. (2000). Pain modulation: Expectation, opioid analgesia and virtual pain. *Progress in Brain Research, 122*, 245–253.

Gagliese, L., & Melzack, R. (1997). Chronic pain in elderly people. *Pain, 70*(1), 3–14.

Garrett, N., & McShane, F. (1999). The pathophysiology of pain. *AANA Journal, 67*(4), 349–357.

Hammond, D. L., Wang, H., Nakashima, N., & Basbaum, A. I. (1998). Differential effects of intrathecally administered delta and mu opioid receptor agonists on formalin-evoked nociception and on the expression of Fos-like immunoreactivity in the spinal cord of the rat. *Journal of Pharmacology & Experimental Therapeutics, 284*(1), 378–387.

Hester, N. O., Foster, R., & Kristensen, K. (1990). Measurement of pain in children: Generalizability and validity of the Pain Ladder and the Poker Chip Tool. In D. C. Tyler & E. J. Krane (Eds.), *Pediatric pain. Advances in pain research and therapy* (Vol. 15; pp. 79–84). New York: Raven Press.

Jennings, E., & Fitzgerald, M. (1998). Postnatal changes in responses of rat dorsal horn cells to afferent stimulation: A fibre-induced sensitization. *Journal of Physiology London, 509*(Pt 3), 859–868.

Kahn, D. L., & Steeves, R. H. (1996). An understanding of suffering grounded in clinical practice and research. In B. R. Ferrell (Ed.), *Suffering*. Boston: Jones & Bartlett.

Levine, J. D., Gordon, N. C., & Fields, H. L. (1978). The mechanism of placebo analgesia. *Lancet, 2*, 654–657.

Marsh, D. F., Hatch, D. J., & Fitzgerald, M. (1997). Opioid systems and the newborn. *British Journal of Anaesthesia, 79*(6), 787–795.

McCaffery, M., & Pasero, C. (1999). *Pain: Clinical manual for nursing practice* (2nd ed.). St. Louis, MO: C. V. Mosby.

Melzack, R. (1975). The McGill Pain Questionnaire: Major properties and scoring methods. *Pain, 1*, 277–299.

Melzack, R., & Wall, P. (1965). Pain mechanisms: A new theory. *Science, 150*, 971–979.

Merskey, H., & Bogduk, N. (1994). *Classification of chronic pain: Descriptions of chronic pain syndromes and definitions of pain terms*. Seattle, WA: IASP Press.

Miser, A. W., Moore, L., Green, R., Gracely, R. H., & Miser, J. S. (1986). Prospective study of continuous intravenous and subcutaneous morphine infusion for therapy-related or cancer-related pain in children and young adults with cancer. *Clinical Journal of Pain, 2*, 101–106.

North American Nursing Diagnosis Association (NANDA). (2001). *Nursing diagnoses: Definitions & classification 2001–2002*. Philadelphia: Author.

Page, G. G., & Ben-Eliyahu, S. (1997). Increased surgery-induced metastasis and suppressed natural killer cell activity during proestrus/estrus in rats. *Breast Cancer Research and Treatment, 45*(2), 159–167.

Perl, E. R. (1996). Cutaneous polymodal receptors: Characteristics and plasticity. *Progress in Brain Research, 113*, 21–37.

Porter, J., & Jick, H. (1980). Addiction rare in clients treated with narcotics. *New England Journal of Medicine, 302*, 123.

Rahman, W., Dashwood, M. R., Fitzgerald, M., Aynsley-Green, A., & Dickenson, A. H. (1998). Postnatal development of multiple opioid receptors in the spinal cord and development of spinal morphine analgesia. *Brain Research. Developmental Brain Research, 108*(1–2), 239–254.

Savedra, M. C., Holzemer, W. L., Tesler, M. D., Ward, J. A., & Wilkie, D. J. (1993). Assessment of postoperative pain in children and adolescents using the adolescent pediatric pain tool. *Nursing Research, 42*, 5–9.

Sellick, S. M., & Zaza, C. (1998). Critical review of 5 nonpharmacologic strategies for managing cancer pain. *Cancer Prevention & Control, 2*(1), 7–14.

Siddall, P. J., & Cousins, M. J. (1997). Neurobiology of pain. *International Anesthesiology Clinics, 35*(2), 1–26.

Stevens, B., Johnston, C., Petryshen, P., & Taddio, A. (1996). Premature Infant Pain Profile: Development and initial validation. *Clinical Journal of Pain, 12*(1), 13–22.

Stevens, B., & Koren, G. (1998). Evidence-based pain management for infants. *Current Opinion in Pediatrics, 10*(2), 203–207.

Syrjala, K. L., Cummings, C., & Donaldson, G. W. (1992). Hypnosis or cognitive behavioral training for the reduction of pain and nausea during cancer treatment: A controlled clinical trial. *Pain, 48*, 137–146.

Tesler, M. D., Savedra, M. C., Holzemer, W. L., Wilkie, D. J., Ward, J. A., & Paul, S. M. (1991). The word-graphic rating scale as a measure of children's and adolescents' pain intensity. *Research in Nursing and Health, 14*, 361–371.

Wilkie, D. J. (1995). Facial expressions of pain in lung cancer. *Analgesia, 1,* 91–99.

Wilkie, D. J., Kampbell, J., Cutshall, S., Halabisky, H., Harmon, H., Johnson, L. P., Weinacht, L., & Rake-Marona, M. (2000). Effects of massage on pain intensity, analgesics and quality of life in patients with cancer pain: A pilot study of a randomized clinical trial conducted within hospice care delivery. *Hospice Journal, 15*(3), 31–53.

Willis, W. D., & Westlund, K. N. (1997). Neuroanatomy of the pain system and of the pathways that modulate pain. *Journal of Clinical Neurophysiology, 14*(1), 2–31.

BIBLIOGRAPHY

Casey, K. L. (2000). Concepts of pain mechanisms: the contribution of functional imaging of the human brain. *Progress in Brain Research, 129,* 277–287.

Davies, J., & McVicar, A. (2000). Issues in effective pain control. 2: From assessment to management. *International Journal of Palliative Nursing, 6*(4), 162–169.

Fagerlund, T. H., & Braaten, O. (2001). No pain relief from codeine . . . ? An introduction to pharmacogenomics. *Acta Anaesthesiologica Scandinavica, 45*(2), 140–149.

Farber S., et al. (1998). Improving cancer pain management through a system wide commitment. *Journal of Palliative Medicine, 1*(4) 377–385.

Fields, H. L. (1999). Pain: an unpleasant topic. *Pain* (Suppl. 6). S61–69.

Hudinski, D. M. (1995). An algorithmic approach to cancer pain management. *Nursing Clinics of North America, 30,* 711–723.

Kleiber, C., & Harper, D. C. (1999). Effects of distraction on children's pain and distress during medical procedures: A meta-analysis. *Nursing Research, 48*(1), 44–49.

McGuire, D. B., Yarbro, C. H., & Ferrell, B. R. (1995). *Cancer pain management* (2nd ed.). Boston: Jones & Bartlett.

Mercadante, S., & Portenoy, R. K. (2001). Opioid poorly-responsive cancer pain. Part 2: Basic mechanisms that could shift dose response for analgesia. *Journal of Pain Symptom & Management, 21*(3), 255–264.

Morley S, Eccleston C, Williams A. (1999). Systematic review and meta-analysis of randomized controlled trials of cognitive behaviour therapy and behaviour therapy for chronic pain in adults, excluding headache. *Pain, 80*(1–2), 1–13.

Payne, R. (1998). Practice guidelines for cancer pain therapy. Issues pertinent to the revision of national guidelines. *Oncology (Huntington), 12*(11A), 169–175.

Sandlin, D. (2000). The new Joint Commission Accreditation of Healthcare Organizations' requirements for pain assessment and treatment: a pain in the assessment? *Journal of Perianesthesia Nursing, 15*(3), 182–184.

Van Fleet, S. (2000). Relaxation and imagery for symptom management: Improving patient assessment and individualizing treatment. *Oncology Nursing Forum, 27*(3), 501–510.

Wall, P. D., & Melzack, R. (Eds.). (1994). *Textbook of pain* (3rd ed.). New York: Churchill Livingstone.

Woolf, C. J., & Decosterd, I. (1999). Implications of recent advances in the understanding of pain pathology for the assessment of pain in patients. *Pain, 6,* S141.

44 Sensory Perception

Key Terms

delusion
hallucination
perception
reticular activating system

sensation information
sensoristasis
sensory deprivation
sensory overload

Learning Objectives

Upon completion of this chapter, the student will be able to do the following:
1. Associate stress and sensoristasis with the sensory/perceptual process.
2. Describe the five senses and their role in sensory perception.
3. Summarize factors affecting sensory perception.
4. Specify how sensory overload, deprivation, and deficit can occur, with interventions for each.
5. Relate manifestations of altered sensory function to their causes.
6. Identify clients who are at risk for altered sensory function in healthcare settings and in the home.
7. Discuss the relationship of safety to sensory dysfunction.

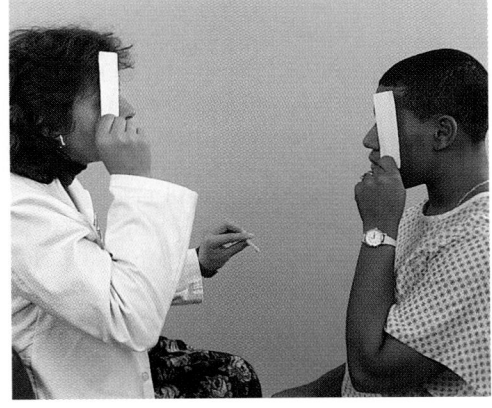

Critical Thinking Challenge

Patrick Matthews, an active and popular college baseball star, was treated in your emergency department after being hit in the face with a baseball. He talked a great deal to the staff about his concerns, and the staff all commented on how likable he was. Patrick's eyes needed to be patched, and he received instructions to stay in an environment with minimal activity. His father has brought Patrick back to the hospital today. Patrick has refused to engage in conversation and has cut off contact with his friends. On the second night after the injury, Patrick showed signs of hallucinations that a roommate was talking to him, and delusions that he was being poisoned through his meals. You have been assigned to give nursing care to Patrick the next morning.

Once you have completed this chapter and incorporated sensory perception into your knowledge base, review the above scenario and reflect on the following areas of Critical Thinking:

1. Determine what additional information you might need.
2. Identify any specific concerns that you have about communicating with Patrick.
3. Considering the information and your concerns, describe how you feel about being assigned to Patrick.
4. Examine the possible sources for disturbances in sensory perception that you believe are critical for Patrick.
5. Prioritize the areas you need to address in determining your nursing care.

In today's fast-paced society, many people believe they lack the time to deal fully with one demand before the next one is nipping at their heels. The average American is exposed to 65,000 more stimuli (demands) daily than his or her ancestors were 100 years ago (Schafer, 1995). Human beings uniquely deal with these demands through senses and higher cognitive processes (the latter are discussed in Chapter 45).

Sensing stimuli is basic to human functioning, growth, and development. Persons with permanent sensory alterations, such as blindness, deafness, or paralysis, typically learn to make adaptations necessary to lead full and productive lives. Therefore, their risk for problems is no greater than that for persons with full sensory function. However, when any new or temporary alteration in sensory function occurs, the person's risk for more serious mental and physical health deficits increases unless coping takes place.

Nurses encounter clients with preexisting sensory alterations and those with new alterations because of the stress of illness. This stress affects the person's ability to adapt and may alter sensory perception. Assessment of sensory function and risk factors for sensory alterations is necessary for all clients, especially when the alteration is a new or temporary one. Older adults require close assessment because they experience age-related sensory changes and subsequent underlying visual and hearing impairments.

NORMAL SENSORY PERCEPTION

Sensory perception depends on the sensory receptors, reticular activating system, and functioning nervous pathways to the brain. The RAS influences awareness of stimuli, which are received through the five senses: sight, hearing, touch, smell, and taste. Kinesthetic and visceral senses are stimulated internally.

Structure and Function of Sensory Perception

Sensory Awareness

The **reticular activating system** (RAS) is responsible for bringing together information from the cerebellum and other parts of the brain with that obtained from the sense organs. Awareness of the world depends on the RAS, which is located between the nerve centers of the medulla oblongata in the brain stem. Sensory, visceral, kinesthetic, and cognitive input (Lee, 1991) stimulate the RAS. Multiple stimuli received by the senses reach the RAS. Here, certain selected impulses are conducted to the cerebral cortex of the brain to be perceived.

When the nervous system is oriented to a stimulus and receptive toward it, the neurons of the RAS arouse the brain, facilitating information reception (Vander, Sherman, & Luciano, 2000). The RAS is highly selective. For example, a parent may be awakened in the middle of the night by the slightest murmur of an infant in a bedroom down the hall but may sleep through the sound of loud traffic noises outside the bedroom window. Destruction of the RAS produces coma and an electroencephalograph pattern characteristic of sleep (Vander, Sherman, & Luciano, 2000).

Input by Senses

Sensory function begins with reception of stimuli by the senses. Externally, the senses receiving stimuli are vision, hearing, smell, taste, and touch. Their respective receptor organs are the eyes, ears, olfactory receptors in the nose, taste buds of the tongue, and nerve endings in the skin. Internally, the kinesthetic and visceral senses receive stimuli. Their receptors are nerve endings in the skin and body tissues. The kinesthetic sense influences awareness of the placement and action of body parts. The visceral sense receives stimuli that affect awareness related to the body's large interior organs. Vision, hearing, smell, and taste are termed *special senses*. Touch, kinesthetic (or proprioceptive) sensation, and visceral sensation are termed *somatic senses* (Vander, Sherman, & Luciano, 2000).

After stimuli are received, they are perceived with the help of the RAS. **Sensory perception** is a conscious process of selecting, organizing, and interpreting sensory stimuli that requires intact and functioning sense organs, nervous pathways, and the brain. (Chapter 45 provides more information on cognitive function.)

Characteristics of Normal Sensory Perception

Characteristics of normal sensory perception are the normal measures in quality and quantity of the special and somatic senses. Normal vision is associated with visual acuity at or near 20/20, full field of vision, and tricolor vision (red, green, blue). Normal hearing is associated with auditory acuity of sounds at an intensity of 0 to 25 dB (decibels), at frequencies of 125 to 8000 cycles per second. Normal taste involves the ability to discriminate sour, salty, sweet, and bitter. Normal smell involves the discrimination of primary odors, such as camphoraceous, musky, floral, pepperminty, ethereal, pungent, and putrid. The characteristics of somatic senses include discrimination of touch, pressure, vibration, position, tickling, temperature, and pain (Vander, Sherman, & Luciano, 2000).

Normal Sensory Pattern

Sensoristasis

Each person has his or her own comfort zone or zone of optimum arousal (Schafer, 1995). This comfort zone varies from person to person and is the range at which a person performs at his or her peak. **Sensoristasis** is a state of optimum arousal—not too much and not too little. The RAS is viewed by some theorists as a monitor for sensoristatic balance.

Adaptation

Beyond the point of sensoristasis, sensory adaptation occurs. Sensory receptors adapt to repeated stimulation by responding less and less. Eventually, the brain will not perceive constant stimulation, such as background traffic noise. Varied and irregular stimuli will still be perceived, however.

Lead time and afterburn are two necessary time periods crucial to helping a person deal with new stimuli (Schafer,

1995). *Lead time* is the time each person needs to prepare for an event emotionally and physically. *Afterburn* is the time needed to think about, evaluate, and come to terms with the activity after it happens. The necessary amount of lead time and afterburn is different for each person. Lead time and afterburn help a person process stimuli so that he or she can respond appropriately without becoming overwhelmed.

Lifespan Considerations

Newborn and Infant

At birth, sensory perception is rudimentary. Newborns require repeated stimulation for the nervous system to mature and discrimination within the senses to develop (Mueller, 1996). Newborns and infants receive most stimulation by touch, needing to feel objects in the environment and learning to feel comfortable with their own bodies in space. They respond to holding, cuddling, soothing, rocking, and changing position. Newborns see only gross patterns of light and dark or bright colors. As they grow, vision becomes more discriminating.

Toddler and Preschooler

Children's growth, development, and attachment are directly linked with sensory stimulation (Fig. 44-1). Full acquaintance with the world includes exploration with the senses. As children grow, they react to a world of people and things. Lack of meaningful stimulation can lead to developmental and motor delays (Gesell & Ilg, 1949). Successful adaptation to change occurs when stimulation is not too much or too little.

Toddlers are explorers; they investigate and learn about the environment by seeing, hearing, touching, tasting, and smelling. Preschoolers seek out information using more organized play, such as singing and story telling, to perceive and respond to stimuli through the senses.

Child and Adolescent

Children and adolescents experience rapid changes in their world, and learning occurs at an accelerated pace. Reading and listening to school lessons dominate a child's day. School-age children and adolescents are learning to make independent responses based on what is perceived through the senses, such as crossing the street when the light turns green or reporting a fire when smelling smoke.

Adult and Older Adult

An adult's sensory perception function is at its peak. However, as people reach middle age, they begin to notice certain changes in their sensory system. Eyesight diminishes, sounds become more muffled, and the other sensory systems deteriorate. As a person approaches 60 to 70 years of age, marked decrements in sensory/perceptual behaviors begin. This reduction in efficiency means that older people cannot process sensory input as rapidly as they did when they were young. Because of this slowing, they need more time to deal with stimulating events (Hampton, Craven, & Heitkemper, 1997; DiGiovanna, 2000).

FACTORS AFFECTING SENSORY PERCEPTION

Environment

Sensory stimuli in the environment affect sensory perception. For example, a teacher may not notice the noise in a consistently noisy environment, such as the school cafeteria. But the same teacher may perceive a loud television set very differently in his or her own home, which is usually quiet.

Previous Experience

Previous experience affects sensory perception in that people become more alert to stimuli that evoke a strong response. For example, a person may drive to work by the same route each day, noticing little along the way. A person may listen to the radio inattentively until a favorite song is played, then listen to every word. A new experience, such as hospitalization, may cause a client to perceive a barrage of threatening new stimuli.

Lifestyle and Habits

Lifestyle affects sensory perception. One person may enjoy a lifestyle of abundant stimulation, surrounded by many people, frequent changes, bright lights, and noise. Another person may prefer less contact with crowds, less noise, and a slow-paced routine. People with different lifestyles perceive stimuli differently.

Cigarette smoking causes atrophy of the taste buds, decreasing the sensory perception of taste. Chronic alcohol abuse may lead to peripheral neuropathy, a functional disorder of the peripheral nervous system that results in sensory impairment.

Illness

Certain illnesses affect sensory perception. Diabetes and hypertension cause changes in tiny blood vessels and nerves, leading to visual deficits and decreased sensation of touch in

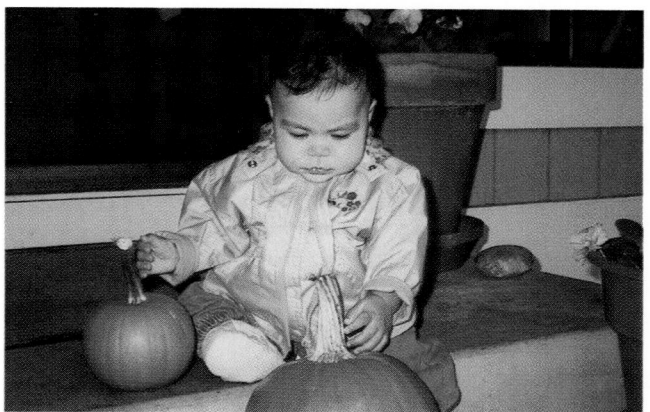

FIGURE 44-1 Young children explore using the senses, including sight and touch. Such exploration facilitates learning and knowledge of the world.

the extremities. Cerebrovascular disorders impair blood flow to the brain, possibly blocking sensory perception. Pain, fatigue, and stress caused by illness also affect perception of stimuli.

Medications

Some antibiotics, including streptomycin and gentamicin, can damage the auditory nerve, impairing hearing. Central nervous system (CNS) depressants, such as narcotic analgesics, decrease awareness and impair perception of stimuli.

Variations in Stimulation

If a person experiences more sensory stimulation than he or she is used to or can make sense of, distress and sensory overload may occur. On the other hand, if a person experiences less than the usual stimulation, that person is below his or her optimum state of arousal and may be at risk for sensory deprivation.

Reactions to sensory overload or sensory deprivation are special challenges that nurses frequently encounter in themselves and clients. Sensory overload or sensory deprivation can lead to perceptual, cognitive, and decisional problems. Separating where one area begins and another ends is often difficult. For example, when a person's senses are bombarded with seeing, feeling, and hearing too much information at one time, it may be difficult to perceive accurately, think clearly, or make a good decision.

When the RAS is overwhelmed with input, a person may experience sensory overload and feel confused, anxious, and unable to take constructive action. When the RAS fails to recognize a stimulus because it is below the threshold level or lacks relevant meaning to the person, **sensory deprivation** may occur, and the person experiences boredom, depression, restlessness, and vivid sensual imagery, including hallucinations (Lee, 1991; Paquette & Rodemich, 1997).

Sensory Overload

Sensory overload occurs when a person is unable to process or manage the intensity or quantity of incoming sensory stimuli. The person feels out of control and overwhelmed by the excessive input from the environment (Lee, 1991; Bostwick, 2000). Routine activity in the healthcare setting can contribute to sensory overload in clients. Conversation about the client's condition in the client's presence but without participation of the client may become problematic.

These activities fall into three main categories: internal factors, information, and environment.

Internal Factors. Internal factors, such as thinking about impending surgery or the meaning of a medical diagnosis, can contribute to anxiety and cognitive overload so that the person cannot process additional stimuli (Fig. 44-2). Pain, medication, lack of sleep, worry, hypoxemia, electrolyte disturbances, and brain injury also can contribute to a person's vulnerability to sensory overload.

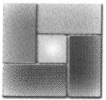

Nursing Research and Critical Thinking
What Sensory Responses Do People Experience Before, During, and After Chemotherapy?

Previous studies had shown that clients who receive preparatory sensory information before various healthcare procedures experience less discomfort. Literature describing subjects' sensory experience before, during, and after antineoplastic chemotherapy (ANCT), however, was lacking. These researchers designed an exploratory study to elicit sensory responses from subjects before, during, and after one of six cycles of their initial course of treatment on one of two emetogenic ANCT protocols. A convenience sample of 54 subjects was accrued from three Midwestern hospitals and one physician's office. All study subjects had to be starting their initial course of ANCT. Ten subjects either could not be reached by telephone or were unable to answer the questions in the scheduled time, leaving a final sample of 44 subjects. The researchers developed the Sensory Information Questionnaire (SIQ) to document the sensory perceptions of participants receiving ANCT. The questionnaire contained questions related to each of the five senses. Detailed descriptions and definitions were developed for each sense, along with descriptors that included a range of

suggestions, in an effort to avoid influencing responses. The SIQ was administered during a telephone interview with each subject within 24 hours after ANCT. The senses about which most of the subjects provided descriptors were taste, smell, and touch. The first thing subjects responded to when asked about the experience was the uncertainty and lack of information regarding cancer and chemotherapy.

Critical Thinking Considerations. The researchers recommended further validation of the SIQ with other populations and a larger sample with a balanced age distribution. Implications of this study are as follows:

* The actual descriptions from clients about what they can expect to hear, feel, taste, touch, or smell may decrease fear and anxiety and promote self-care and coping strategies for those receiving ANCT.
* The use of printed materials was helpful for some subjects, and several subjects continued to search for information about sensory perception during the course of their treatment.

From Rhodes, V. A., McDaniel, R. W., Hanson, B., Markway, E., & Johnson, M. (1994). Sensory perception of patients on selected antineoplastic chemotherapy protocols. *Cancer Nursing, 17*(1), 45–51.

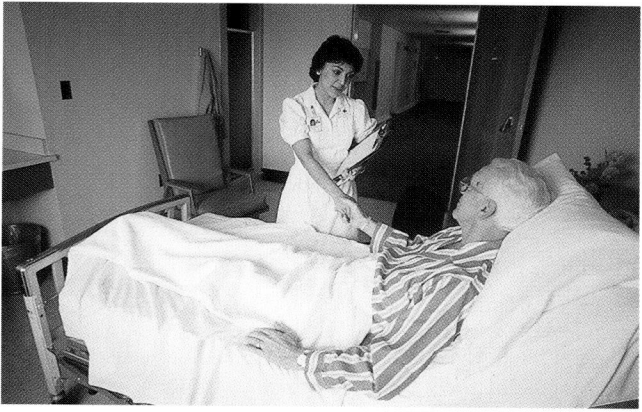

FIGURE 44-2 Anxiety related to medical diagnosis, prognosis, and treatment can contribute to sensory overload.

Information. Imparting information to a client may lead to sensory overload. Some examples include teaching a client about a procedure, informing a client about a diagnosis, making requests of a client, or helping the client solve a problem.

Environment. The environment of the healthcare agency provides a higher than usual amount of sensory stimulation. A client newly admitted, for example, may have to cope with adjusting to a new roommate, having the television on more than usual, bright lights, paging systems, unexpected intrusions, meeting many staff members, having the bed move up and down at someone else's bidding, waiting for someone to answer the call light, uncontrolled pain, and having strangers touch and probe private body areas. Clients in intensive care units often exhibit symptoms of sensory overload because of the high degree of light, noise, and activity around the clock (Fig. 44-3). Disorientation can occur when expected day/night differences in levels of general activity are lost. To reduce such disorientation, provide a clock displaying a clear distinction of AM/PM time, day, and date (Casey, DeFazio, Vansickle, & Lippmann, 1996; Dyer, 1995a, 1995b; Geary, 1994).

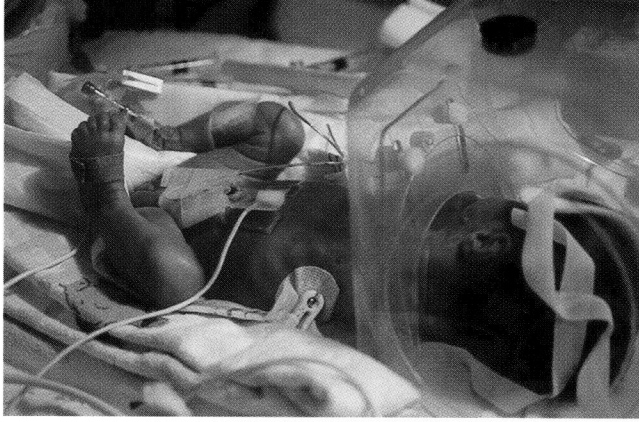

FIGURE 44-3 Lights and frequent activity can cause sensory overload in a premature newborn in the neonatal intensive care unit.

Sensory Deprivation

Although **sensory deprivation** can be thought of as the opposite of sensory overload, they share many elements. Think about the paradoxical statement, "The silence was deafening." Sensory deprivation generally means a lessening or lack of meaningful sensory stimuli, monotonous sensory input, or an interference with the processing of information (Lee, 1991; Bostwick, 2000).

Sensory deprivation (understimulation) can be just as disruptive as sensory overload. Cognitive and emotional deterioration can occur when stimuli are reduced below a person's optimum level of stimulation (Schafer, 1995). One common source of sensory deprivation is a sudden decrease in stimuli when a person moves from a fast- to a slow-paced environment (Schafer, 1995). Each person's tolerance of and reaction to a lessening or lack of meaningful sensory stimuli differs, but clients with extreme cases experience a gross misperception of events and personality changes (Ryan, 1998).

Any time a client experiences an interference with or a diminution of sensory input, that person may be at risk for sensory deprivation. In a healthcare agency, such occurrences fall into two general categories: altered sensory reception and deprived environments.

Altered Sensory Reception. Altered sensory reception occurs in such conditions as spinal cord injury, brain damage, changes in receptor organs, sleep deprivation, and chronic illness. The person does not receive adequate sensory input because of an interference with the nervous system's ability to receive and process stimuli. This inability also can lead to secondary problems, as in the following example: A client who suffered a spinal cord injury in an automobile accident was left paraplegic with loss of motion and sensation in the lower extremities. One day, he decided to sneak a cigarette while no one was looking. He accidentally dropped the lighted match on his knitted slipper and burned his foot because he could not feel the heat when his slipper began to smolder.

Older people are especially susceptible to sensory deficit, as shown in the following example: An elderly client stopped attending her senior citizen group. She began to spend most of her time sitting alone. She became more depressed, ate less, and began to show signs of confusion. Nurses who observed these actions were able to intervene to assist her to increase her socialization and communication with others.

Deprived Environments. Deprived environments can have negative effects on a person's sensoristasis. A person who is immobilized or isolated for any reason is deprived of the usual amount of stimulation and may show manifestations of sensory deprivation (Fig. 44-4). Consider Patrick Matthews' circumstances as presented in the situation at the beginning of this chapter. His verbal communication diminished dramatically after his injury. Because he could not see, he did not have visual senses and therefore experienced perceptual distortions. He misinterpreted sounds outside his room. He changed from being a likable, open person to being angry and suspicious.

Patrick was showing signs of sensory deprivation. Used to being active, Patrick suddenly needed to change his environ-

THERAPEUTIC DIALOGUE
Sensory Dysfunction

Scene for Thought

Charlie Brisco is 62 years old and in the ICU after a car accident. He sustained internal injuries and many lacerations on his face and arms. He has an IV, urinary catheter, heart monitor, and nasogastric (NG) tube. The pumps and monitors give off soft beeps. The ICU has been busy and noisy since Charlie was admitted.

Less Effective

Nurse: Hi, Charlie. How're you doing? (*Checks the IV and NG tube pumps.*)
Client: Who are you?! What are you doing with those machines?! (*Sits up in bed abruptly, wincing with pain, looking frightened.*)
Nurse: (*Turns to look at him, then continues to check the equipment.*) I'm Gigi, Charlie, your nurse.
Client: Gigi? I don't know you! Where's my wife? What did you do with her? (*Looks frightened.*)
Nurse: She's right over there, Charlie, at the desk. See her? Sounds like you need a little sedative to calm you down. I'll go get it right now.
Client: Betty! Betty! Where are you?! (*Struggles to sit up in bed.*)
Nurse: (*Gets sedative and calls for help to restrain Charlie so he won't dislodge his tubes.*)

More Effective

Nurse: Hi, Charlie. How're you doing? (*Checks the IV and NG tube pumps.*)
Client: Who are you?! What are you doing with those machines?! (*Sits up in bed abruptly, wincing with pain, looking frightened.*)
Nurse: (*Turns to look at him, stands still with arms at side and hands open.*) I'm Georgia. I'm your nurse.
Client: Georgia? I don't know you! Where's my wife? What did you do with her? (*Looks frightened.*)
Nurse: She's right there, Charlie. Do you see her standing at the desk?
Client: Oh. Yeah. (*Focuses on his wife. Slumps back on the pillows.*) Sorry. (*Starts to cry but tries to hide it.*) I get confused.
Nurse: I can see that.
Client: Yeah. (*Closes his eyes wearily.*) And I can't sleep too good.
Nurse: I know. I was wondering if you had a portable cassette player at home.
Client: Yeah. Why?
Nurse: Well, how about using it to shut out noise with some music. Not loud music, something mellow.
Client: Yeah, that would be good. (*Shifts and winces.*)
Nurse: You look uncomfortable.
Client: I am.
Nurse: I'll get you some more pain pills, and I'll talk to your wife about the cassette player, too. You can tell her what tapes to bring later.
Client: Okay. Thanks. (*Closes his eyes and lies still.*)

Critical Thinking Challenge

- Name and explain some factors that contributed to Charlie's sensory dysfunction.
- Decide whether this dysfunction was sensory overload or deprivation. Give your reasons.
- Describe the relationship between traumatic events and pain and sensory dysfunction.
- Appraise how each nurse related to Charlie and summarize the outcomes.

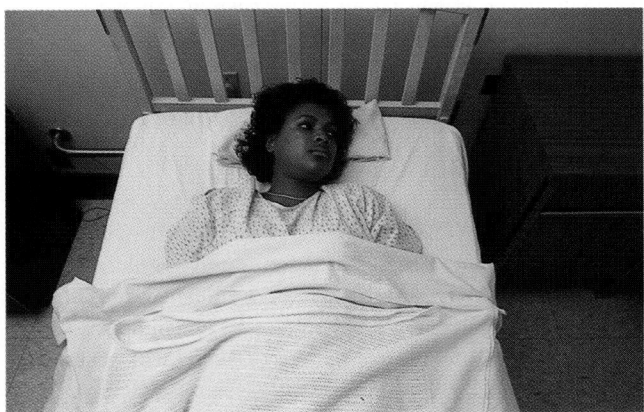

FIGURE 44-4 Isolation and lack of mobility may contribute to sensory deprivation.

ment to nonstimulating and quiet. To compensate for temporary loss of sight, his senses of hearing and taste became more acute, leading to misinterpretations of sounds and taste of food. His personality changed drastically.

ALTERED SENSORY PERCEPTION FUNCTION

Manifestations of Altered Sensory Perception Function

Anxiety

Altered sensory perception frequently leads to anxiety, and anxiety can further compound altered sensory perception. For example, an older woman with poor hearing who lives alone may be anxious about going to bed at night because she believes that she might not hear a smoke alarm, the telephone ringing, or someone trying to break into the house. Anxiety stems from not being able to interact fully with the environment due to sensory deficit, fear of embarrassment when trying to communicate with others, or misinterpretation of information perceived through the senses.

Cognitive Dysfunction

Disturbances in remembering, reasoning, and problem solving can occur with sensory overload. Decision making may be irrational or dysfunctional. Other common behaviors indicative of cognitive dysfunction include disorientation; verbalizing disconnected thoughts; complaining of too much going on, sleeplessness, and fatigue; inability to think; and poor work performance (Gordon, 1994). Sensory deprivation also reduces mental capabilities. Mind wandering occurs, along with fantasy activity. The person may have difficulty concentrating and thinking logically.

Hallucinations and Delusions

Hallucinations, sensory impressions that are based on internal stimulations, have no basis in reality. Hearing voices when no one is there is a typical auditory hallucination. **Delusions,** beliefs not based in reality, reflect an unconscious need or fear (e.g., believing that the hospital food is poisoned). Both hallucinations and delusions have been documented in cases of sensory deprivation, sensory overload, and sensory deficits, such as hearing or vision loss (Lee, 1991). For example, an older woman with glasses and a hearing aid is suddenly hospitalized. Her glasses are misplaced, and the battery is weak in her hearing aid. She may not understand why strange people come into her room at night. She has difficulty ambulating and locating the call light to ask for assistance with toileting, so she soils her bed. Her sensory deficits cause her to misinterpret stimuli and distort reality. She has delusions that she is in a prison, the nurses are guards, and other prisoners are trying to take advantage of her. She hallucinates that her dead sister is telling her to join her in heaven.

Sensory Deficit

Sensory deficit is impaired function in sensory reception or perception. The deficit may be blindness due to disease of the eyes, such as glaucoma. In this case, reception is affected. Spinal cord injuries and strokes that cause loss of tactile sensation affect perception because of disruption in nerve pathways or the brain.

A sudden loss of sensory perception through a sensory deficit can cause total disorientation because compensation does not occur immediately. Compensation for a deficit usually occurs when loss of function is gradual. The client may change his or her behavior to adapt to the sensory deficit, such as turning a functioning ear toward a speaker to hear, or measuring the temperature of bathwater with a thermometer (if there is decreased sensation of the extremities). Physiologic compensation also occurs, with the remaining senses becoming more acute. For example, a blind person may develop a more acute sense of smell or hearing.

A sensory deficit may be temporary or permanent because of illness or treatment (Glide, 1994). Temporary bandaging after eye surgery may render a client totally unable to care for himself or herself. Nasal packing that temporarily eliminates the sense of smell affects taste, possibly leading to anorexia. The client with sudden loss of lower extremity sensation from a spinal cord injury is at risk for injury to the lower extremities.

Depression and Withdrawal

Depression may result from sensory deficits or sensory deprivation. Helplessness and loss of self-esteem lead to depression and withdrawal. The client who is placed on isolation precautions may show signs of poor appetite, sleeplessness, and loss of interest in activities or interaction with others as he or she becomes depressed, leading to further sensory deprivation.

Impact on Activities of Daily Living

Sensory perception dysfunction can have profound effects on activities of daily living (ADLs). Visual deficits cause problems with self-care activities as basic as dressing, toileting, and preparing meals. Hearing deficits may restrict people from watching television, listening to the radio, and answering the

ETHICAL/LEGAL ISSUE
Client Decision Making

Jane Nelson, 24 years old, was admitted to intensive care after a motor vehicle accident. She had multiple injuries to the chest and abdomen, leg fractures, and facial lacerations. She has improved sufficiently now to be transferred to a hospital unit. Her face is still bandaged, and the damage to her eyes is unknown at this time. Although she is expected to fully recover from her other injuries, a strong possibility exists that she may lose her sight in one or both eyes. She has said that if she is going to lose her vision, she doesn't want to know. You have heard her say, "I don't know what I might do to myself if I thought I was going to be blind the rest of my life." You have overheard the physicians say that Jane will, in all likelihood, be blind. One of the other nurses believes that Jane should know and start preparing for the possibility.

Reflection
- Explore your own feelings about these interactions.
- Identify your personal values and beliefs in this situation.
- Think about ways in which you can respond to Jane about her situation.
- Think about ways in which you can respond to the other nurse about her beliefs.
- Identify possible approaches that might be needed in this situation.

telephone. Safety hazards also exist for pedestrians who are hearing impaired. People with taste or smell deficits may lose interest in eating. Those with sensory deficits involving touch are at risk for burns and injuries to the extremities (St. Pierre, 1998).

Moving around outside the home may be impossible without special aids or help. Many jobs are prohibited for people with sensory deficits, and driving may not be allowed. This further restricts the environments in which these clients may move about safely, making them dependent on others. If the affected person is the major wage earner, reduction or loss of income may occur.

People with cognitive dysfunction from sensory overload or deprivation may exhibit poor judgment and problem solving during everyday activities, increasing the necessity for family members to monitor activities and decisions. All of these concerns place more stress on the family to cope with the client's sensory dysfunctions.

ASSESSMENT

Explore the client's sensory perception through subjective and objective data collection, focusing on the client, environment, and the client's interaction with others. Family and friends may provide helpful data about changes in the client's behavior that indicate problems in sensory perception. Objective data are collected by physical examination and diagnostic tests of the neurologic system and special senses.

Subjective Data

Normal Pattern Identification

To determine a client's normal pattern of sensory perception, start with a general question, such as "How do you spend a typical day?" This question can provide information about the level of stimulation the client usually experiences daily and the client's response to that stimulation.

Next, assess how the client responds to change. Because change and stress can affect perception, find out how the client handles them. Asking, "Have there been any recent changes in your life?" can lead to an informative discussion of the degree of complexity of the changes and the client's responses.

Next, investigate the client's living and social situation and available modes of transportation to get a better idea of how complex the client's life is and his or her level of independence. Use the following questions to determine important information about the client's daily functioning: "With whom do you live?" "Do you prepare your own (or your family's) meals?" "When you want to go someplace, how do you get there?"

Finally, focus questions on the person's lifestyle and habits. If the client's usual diet consists of highly spiced foods, a change in menu may seem dull and uninteresting, possibly affecting the client's appetite because it does not meet his or her usual need for gustatory stimulation. Determine how much alcohol the person drinks daily or weekly, how much sleep he or she is used to, and the usual time for sleeping and waking. Also, determine the client's educational level, hobbies and interests, and previous or present employment. Table 44-1 gives examples of general and specific questions to elicit information about the client's interaction with his or her environment.

Risk Identification

Elicit information about the client's age, culture, language, activity level, medical history, and medications. If the person is hospitalized, assess the degree of stimulation in the environment in light of the client's experiences. Some risk factors in the hospital environment are listed in Display 44-1.

Older clients are more at risk for sensory deficits because of normal physiologic changes of aging, especially in hear-

TABLE 44-1

General and Specific Questions About the Client and Environment	
General Questions	**Specific Questions**
How do you spend a typical day?	Do you go to school? Do you work outside the home? Do you watch TV, listen to the radio, read the newspaper? How often do you talk to friends and family?
Have there been any recent changes in your life?	Have you experienced any changes, such as loss of a loved one, change of a job, a friend moving away, new baby in the house? How are you adjusting to the change?
What are your living arrangements like?	With whom do you live? What is the size of your home? Do you cook and care for family members? Do you live in a neighborhood? How convenient is shopping? Do you have transportation?
What are your interests and habits?	What are your hobbies? Are you involved in sports? Do you smoke, and, if so, how much? Do you drink alcohol, and, if so, how much? Do you use any recreational drugs? How much sleep do you need; how much do you get? Do you like to go out? What types of food do you eat?

DISPLAY 44-1

🖪 **RISK FACTORS FOR SENSORY PERCEPTION DYSFUNCTION IN THE HEALTHCARE ENVIRONMENT**

Sensory Overload
Lengthy verbal explanations before procedures
Room close to nurse's station
Intensive Care Unit or intermediate unit
Bright lights
Use of mechanical ventilator
Use of electrocardiographic monitor
Use of oxygen
Use of intravenous tubes
Other equipment
Roommate
Frequent treatments

Sensory Deprivation
Private room
Eyes bandaged
Bedrest
Sensory aid not available (hearing aid, glasses)
Isolation precautions
Few visitors

ing and vision. Clients with cultural and language barriers may be at risk for sensory deprivation.

Question the client about his or her usual level of activity. For example, immobilization due to physical disability restricts clients from their usual amount of stimulation. Also, review the client's history including present illness, any chronic illnesses, past hospitalizations, accidents, and surgeries. A history of sensory deficits, such as visual or hearing impairments, places the client at risk for sensory deprivation. A history of illnesses such as diabetes, hypertension, stroke, or spinal cord injury also increases the client's risk for sensory deficits.

The client's experience with the healthcare environment determines the effect of stimulation on the client. Lack of experience with an intensive care unit or isolation precautions may place the client at risk for sensory overload or deprivation during hospitalization (Dyer, 1995a, 1995b). Also, evaluate the client's medication history including CNS depressants, such as narcotic analgesics and sedatives that affect sensory perception, and large doses of antibiotics that may affect hearing.

Dysfunction Identification

During the nursing assessment, collect data about any actual sensory perception problems, determining whether the client has difficulty with vision, hearing, smell, taste, and touch. If problems are identified, find out when the problem started, its severity, what actions the client has taken, and the effectiveness of those actions. This information is useful in helping the client adapt to his or her environment.

Also determine whether the client is anxious, depressed, withdrawing from social contact, or having difficulty concentrating, making decisions, or remembering. Has the client ever experienced hallucinations or delusions? This information will uncover any manifestations the sensory dysfunction may have caused.

Objective Data

Physical Assessment

The focus of the physical assessment is to determine whether the senses are impaired. The following must be assessed: hearing, vision, taste, smell, touch, somatic senses, and mental status. Mental status data, including level of consciousness, orientation, attention span, memory, and cognitive skills, can be collected during the client history. See Chapter 24 for more information on assessment.

To collect objective data about the sensory system systematically, first inspect, then perform simple tests. Inspect the head for any abnormalities of the eyes, ears, nose, or mouth and the extremities for any burns or injuries. Table 44-2 lists tests used to assess sensation.

Diagnostic Tests and Procedures

Electrolyte imbalances, alterations in blood chemistry (e.g., elevated ammonia, elevated blood urea nitrogen), and toxic levels of drugs that affect the CNS can alter sensoristasis (McFarland, 1996). Special visual and auditory acuity tests also may be ordered. Neurologic tests, such as nerve conduction studies, computed tomographic scanning of the brain, and cerebral angiography, may be performed to determine the cause of sensory deficits.

NURSING DIAGNOSES

The accepted North American Nursing Diagnosis Association (NANDA) nursing diagnosis for sensory overload, deprivation, and deficit is Disturbed Sensory Perception. These may include visual, auditory, kinesthetic, gustatory, tactile, or olfactory alterations. Assessment data are used to determine the presence or risk of any of these disruptions in normal sensory/perception function.

Diagnostic Statement: Disturbed Sensory Perception

Definition. Change in the amount or patterning of oncoming stimuli, accompanied by a diminished, exaggerated, distorted, or impaired response to such stimuli (NANDA, 2000).

Defining Characteristics. Defining characteristics include poor concentration; auditory distortions; change in usual response to stimuli; restlessness; reported or measured change in sensory acuity, such as vision or hearing; irritability; disorientation to time, to place, or with people; change in problem-solving abilities; and change in behavior pattern. Altered communication patterns also characterize this nursing

TABLE 44-2

Physical Assessment of Sensory Function	
Sense	**Technique for Assessment**
Vision	Use Snellen chart to measure visual acuity (or have client read newspaper, menu, or whatever is available). Test visual fields.
Hearing	Whisper numbers in each ear, while occluding the other; ask client to repeat.
	Perform Weber and Rinne tuning fork tests.
	Observe client's conversation with others.
Smell	With eyes closed, have client identify three odors, such as coffee, tobacco, and cloves, one nostril at a time, while occluding the other nostril.
Taste	With eyes closed, have client identify three tastes, such as lemon, salt, and sugar, waiting 1 minute and giving sips of water in between. Have client close eyes for all tests.
Somatic sensation	Test light touch of extremities with a wisp of cotton.
	Test sharp and dull sensation using the point and blunt end of a pin.
	Test two-point discrimination using two pins held close together.
	Test hot and cold sensation using test tubes filled with warm and cold water.
	Test vibration sense using a tuning fork over joints.
	Test position sense by moving the client's fingers or toes.
	Test stereognosis by giving the client a common object (quarter, paperclip) to identify by feel.

diagnosis, as do hallucinations and visual distortions (NANDA, 2000).

Related Factors. Altered sensory perception; excessive or insufficient environmental stimuli; psychological stress; altered sensory reception, transmission, and/or integration; biochemical imbalances; and electrolyte imbalance are related factors (NANDA, 2000).

Related Nursing Diagnoses

Other nursing diagnoses identified for the client with sensory alterations may include the following: Impaired Environmental Interpretation Syndrome, Disturbed Body Image, Chronic or Situational Low Self-Esteem, Deficient Diversional Activity, Fatigue, Delayed Growth and Development, Risk for Injury, Risk for Poisoning, Self-Care Deficits, and Disturbed Sleep Pattern. If the sensory alterations are the result of spinal injury, additional nursing diagnoses may include Dysreflexia, Impaired Home Maintenance, Ineffective Role Performance, or Impaired Skin Integrity.

OUTCOME IDENTIFICATION AND PLANNING

Client goals are individualized but focus on achieving optimal sensory function. The client goals for Disturbed Sensory Perceptions may include the following:

- The client will demonstrate an understanding of contributing factors by reducing or eliminating them.
- The client will demonstrate an understanding of interventions and rationale by using this information as foresight in maintaining sensoristasis.

- The client will achieve sensoristasis through a decrease in the symptoms of sensory overload or deprivation.
- The client will demonstrate achievement or maintenance of self-care.
- The client will remain safe.

Planning centers on the client's ability to function on a perceptual level. Client teaching, procedure preparation, provision of stimulation or stimulation reduction, and safety are major issues. Examples of nursing interventions commonly used in problems with sensory overload and deprivations are listed in the accompanying display and discussed in the following section.

PLANNING: Examples of NIC/NOC Interventions

Accepted Sensory Perception Nursing Interventions Classification (NIC)
Environmental Management
Reality Orientation

Accepted Sensory Perception Nursing Outcomes Classification (NOC)
Anxiety Control
Cognitive Orientation
Distorted Thought Process
Rest
Sleep

Refer to the following for specifics regarding NIC/NOC:
McCloskey, J., & Bulechek, G. (2000). *Iowa Intervention Project: Nursing Interventions Classification (NIC),* 2nd ed. St. Louis, MO: C. V. Mosby.
Johnson, M., & Maas, M. (2000). *Iowa Outcomes Project: Nursing Outcomes Classification (NOC),* 2nd ed. St. Louis, MO: C. V. Mosby.

IMPLEMENTATION

Health Promotion

Client Teaching

Client teaching to promote sensory health and function focuses on ways to prevent sensory loss and to maintain general health. Teaching topics include the importance of frequent eye examinations and close control of chronic illnesses such as diabetes.

Teaching healthcare consumers the importance of sensory function and the roles of sensory receptors and the CNS in receiving and perceiving stimuli is important. Preventing sensory dysfunction enables clients to interact with the environment optimally. Yearly eye examinations (or more frequently if problems arise) help promote optimal visual function. Other measures to prevent visual dysfunction include avoiding eye strain, infection, and injury. Prompt recognition and treatment of ear infections and childhood immunization against illnesses such as rubella may prevent hearing loss.

People should wear protective eyewear whenever there is a risk of injury or contamination to the eyes. Plain glasses without side shields are not effective protection. Protective earwear is essential to avoiding hearing loss, particularly that related to occupational noises.

OUTCOME-BASED TEACHING PLAN

When Nicole Travis, mother of an 11-month-old child named Jessie, comes to the clinic for a routine well-child visit, you learn that Jessie is not paying attention when spoken to. Her mother reports that Jessie frequently ignores her when she tries to get her attention. Nicole states, "I'm not sure what kind of discipline or punishment I should use."

OUTCOME: *Nicole Travis will verbalize a realistic plan to determine whether Jessie is ignoring her on purpose or is truly not hearing her.*
Strategies

- Discuss with Nicole the common methods of determining adequate hearing in an infant.
- Suggest a referral to an audiologist.
- Have Nicole observe Jessie's response to sounds that are out of her vision.
- Instruct Nicole to record Jessie's reactions to sounds and her facial expressions.
- Encourage Nicole to record and describe the verbal sounds and words that Jessie says, including listening for inflections in Jessie's voice.
- Urge Nicole to bring these observations to the next appointment and to the audiologist for a more detailed discussion.
- Encourage Nicole to avoid discipline about not responding until Jessie's hearing is thoroughly evaluated.

Teach older adults who are at risk for sensory loss due to physiologic changes of aging about the need for routine checkups. Encourage these clients to seek attention for any developing problems. They may delay medical attention, fearing that hearing loss is inevitable, when simple ear irrigation might dislodge impacted cerumen and restore hearing. Instruct clients with chronic illnesses such as diabetes or hypertension about the importance of closely controlling blood sugar and blood pressure, respectively. Control can help prevent pathophysiologic changes that might lead to tactile and visual dysfunction. Self-monitoring of blood sugar or blood pressure, compliance with medications, diet control, and medical follow-up are essential.

Procedure Preparation

A primary nursing concern is to prevent symptoms of sensory overload for clients. Risk for sensory overload greatly increases when unfamiliar procedures are taking place. Overstimulation can be prevented by preparing clients before procedures, using a technique called **sensation (sensory) information.** The purpose of this intervention is to alleviate a client's distress responses to threatening stimuli and to improve the client's coping through stimulation of the cognitive processes. The technique involves objectively and specifically describing to the client, in serial order, what he or she typically will see, hear, smell, taste, or feel (tactile) in a particular situation (rare or atypical events are not to be included). This preparation must be from the client's point of view, not the observer's.

A solid understanding of this technique is necessary before it can be used. In general, sensation information is useful when a client feels threatened by a procedure. The client, not the nurse, must make that appraisal. Clients who indicate a high level of anxiety before a procedure seem to benefit from sensation information more than those with low levels of anxiety. Finally, determine what client outcomes are desired. Sensation information does not help clients achieve new coping skills, but it may enhance their current coping mechanisms.

Other interventions to help prevent sensory overload include educating clients about why a procedure will be done, who will do it, and how long it will take. Helping clients gain a sense of control through interventions, such as establishing a schedule for routine care, providing a calendar and clock, and allowing choices whenever possible, also can reduce the risk of sensory overload (Dyer, 1995a, 1995b; Lee, 1991).

Nurse–Client Interaction

Individualized nurse–client interaction promotes sensory health function. Clients at risk for sensory deprivation may need frequent interaction initiated by the nurse, whereas others may not. In any case, provide appropriate stimuli, such as addressing the client by name, introducing and reintroducing yourself as necessary, explaining all activities, and, when leaving, acknowledging when you will return. Length, frequency, and content of interactions should be based on individual needs. Talking to the client, showing the client equipment or articles used in care, encouraging the client to smell and taste food that is served, and touching the client are appropriate stimuli during interactions (Fig. 44-5).

Nursing Interventions for Altered Sensory Perception Function

Stimulation Provision

Providing meaningful external stimuli can help a client overcome sensory deprivation or sensory deficit. Measures to provide stimulation include playing the television or the radio occasionally, playing music for brief periods, encouraging use of a clock and calendar, encouraging the client to dress for the day's activities, putting up colorful pictures, encouraging visitors, opening the drapes, and turning on lights. Place the bed or chair so the client can see or hear activities in the area and when someone enters the room.

Frequent interaction with the client also may help. Discussing scheduling of care and placement of equipment, encouraging self-care activities, providing tactile stimulation through back rubs, combing and brushing the client's hair (or encouraging the client to do so), reading to the client, speaking slowly and clearly, and identifying yourself verbally and with a name tag are meaningful interactions. Reorienting the client frequently to person, place, and time may be necessary. Because the client may be having difficulties concentrating, he or she may need repeated direction to accomplish even simple tasks.

> ### ⬛ SAFETY ALERT
> **Add stimulation slowly so clients are not overwhelmed. Include a variety of stimuli and keep the amount of sensory input at a moderate level.**

Orienting the client to the environment can help avoid misinterpretations. Visiting the client often and letting him or her know when to expect another visit helps the client overcome a feeling of isolation. Providing a calendar and a clock to assist in keeping track of time helps keep the client in touch with activities in the environment. A roommate for a client experiencing sensory deprivation can help a great deal. Preparation for any procedure that may add to the sensory deprivation, such as being restricted to bed rest, gives the client time to think of alternatives to sensory stimulation (Bostwick, 2000).

Also encourage clients to provide self-stimulation, such as singing, reading, and talking into a tape recorder and playing it back. Self-care activities also are forms of self-stimulation. Provide a variety of different types of stimulation to encourage maximum use of the client's available senses. Doing so also helps the person adapt to any changes.

A client can use up restless energy and prevent symptoms of sensory deprivation by using physical movement. Encouraging the client to move around in the bed or walk around the room, sit in a chair, do ADLs as independently as possible, and do exercises in the room or in bed to provide stimulation to the client's senses.

Stimulation Reduction

If the client is experiencing sensory overload, interventions should focus on reducing stimulation, involving information, the environment, and internal factors. Limiting extraneous noise, lights, room clutter, interruptions, pain, and stress reduces stimulation.

Clients with sensory overload may neglect their ADLs to the point that they need assistance. Such assistance can be problematic because it can add to sensory overload. With this in mind, assist the client only with the immediately essential ADLs (moving, eating, toileting, and resting). Additional tasks may be added as the client is able to cope.

Sensory Aids

If a client is experiencing a sensory deficit, sensory aids help promote optimal function of that sense and other available senses (e.g., hearing aids in good working order, clean eyeglasses, good oral hygiene). In addition to providing actual physical and situational sensory aids, enlist significant others whenever possible to assist the client in dealing with the deficit. Suggestions for sensory aids are listed in Display 44-2.

Sensory aids can be used in the healthcare environment and taught to clients for use at home. When one sense is lost, sensory aids can be used for other senses to enhance general stimulation. For example, a blind client should be encouraged to savor the aroma, taste, and texture of food.

At times the nurse may be called upon to assist clients with sensory aids such as contact lenses and hearing aids. See Procedure 44-1, Removing Contact Lenses, and Procedure 44-2, Assisting an Adult With Inserting a Hearing Aid.

Safety

Implementation of safety precautions is essential for clients with sensory perception dysfunction. Sensory deficits and the cognitive effects of sensory deprivation or sensory overload place the client at risk for injury from the environment. Implement actions such as assisting clients with ambulation; use of bed side rails, night lights, and a call system; and frequent or continuous observation as necessary.

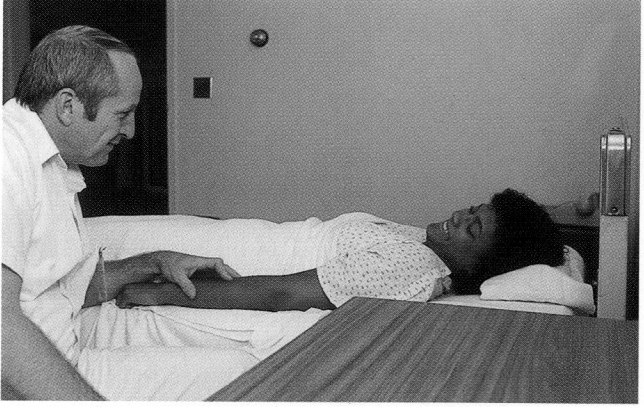

FIGURE 44-5   The simple act of touching a client, or talking, or listening may provide sensory stimulation.

DISPLAY 44-2

🖫 SENSORY AIDS

Vision
- Eyeglasses with the proper prescription, clean and in good repair
- Adequate room lighting, drapes open
- Sunglasses or window shades to reduce glare
- Literature with large print
- Uncluttered environment, no furniture rearranging
- Clock with large numbers
- Telephone dial with large numbers
- Magnifying glass
- Bright, contrasting colors in environment
- Color-coded dials on appliances, medication bottles, and so forth
- Braille, recorded books, seeing-eye dog, and so forth, as necessary

Hearing
- Hearing aid in good repair with working battery
- Speaking slowly and distinctly in client's full view, no mouth covering or gum chewing
- Avoidance of background noise
- Amplified phone ringer, doorbell, smoke alarm, and so forth
- Head set for telephone communication
- Closed-caption television

Smell
- Fresh food served for meals
- Fresh flowers or fragrance in the room
- Others wearing light perfume or fragrance
- Notice of environmental smells

Taste
- Fresh food, seasoned, appropriately, not overcooked or overprocessed to preserve texture
- Foods served at appropriate temperature and time of day
- Note smell and taste of food
- Sips of water between foods
- No mixing of foods

Touch
- Therapeutic touch
- Massage (self or nurse)
- Turning and repositioning
- Hairbrushing and grooming (self or nurse)
- Activity around environment
- Amount of pressure individualized to client's comfort level
- Clothing of various textures

SAFETY ALERT
When assisting a visually impaired client with ambulation, stand on the client's non-dominant side, about one foot in front of him or her. Have the client grasp your arm with the nondominant hand and use the dominant hand to feel around for barriers or landmarks. And always maintain an uncluttered environment.

Teach clients with sensory deficits how to ensure safety at home. For example, advise clients with decreased sensation to temperature in the extremities to adjust their hot water heater to a lower temperature and to test water temperature with a thermometer before bathing. If the client is unable to check the temperature, encourage a family member to help. Also instruct clients to inspect their legs and feet for any injuries or pressure sores they cannot feel.

Teach clients with a decreased sense of smell about the dangers of using gas and chemicals. For example, cleaning with ammonia in a confined space such as a bathroom may cause the client to be overcome by fumes before he or she can smell them. A client may not smell a gas leak in the home, but if a stove or gas heater is not working properly, it should be reported promptly. Urge the client to inspect food for freshness, looking for color and texture and checking the expiration date,

because the client may not smell spoiled meat or dairy products. Clients with hearing and visual deficits need to take additional safety precautions as well. See Chapter 30 for more information on safety.

Healthcare Planning and Home or Community-Based Nursing

With rising costs and shorter hospital stays, a client may be discharged while still adjusting to his or her condition. This can be a new or worsening sensory deficit or an illness or treatment that causes sensory deprivation or sensory overload. Initiate planning as soon as possible to help the client adjust to sensory dysfunction. Include client teaching, enlisting the help and cooperation of family and friends, assembling sensory aids and equipment, contacting home-health services, and locating additional support groups as needed.

Assess the client's home environment as necessary to determine what will be needed to help the client adapt to his or her sensory dysfunction. Teach the client and family how to interact in the home environment, using other senses and sensory aids to adapt and remain safe. The client may need much help during the adaptation process, but eventually he or she

(text continues on page 1214)

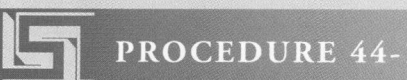

PROCEDURE 44-1

REMOVING CONTACT LENSES

Purpose
1. Remove contact lenses in the event that the client is unable to do so.

Assessment
- Review the physician's order to determine the need for contact lens removal.
- Assess the client's medical history to determine risk for complications from contact lens removal.
- Assess the eye area for open lesions or ecchymosis.
- Assess the client's understanding of the purpose of the procedure and his or her physical and emotional ability to learn and perform the procedure independently, if possible.

Equipment
Wetting/cleaning and soaking solution for hard contact lenses
Sterile lens disinfecting and/or enzyme solution for soft contact lens
Contact lens storage container
Lens suction cup
Clean disposable gloves

Procedure
Removing Hard Contact Lenses

1. Wash hands with soap and warm water.
   Rationale: The fingers are the most common source of skin bacteria and debris. Washing not only decreases the chances of infection but helps protect lenses from damage.
2. Position client comfortably in a sitting position, if possible.
3. Pull the client's upper and lower lid apart and pull tautly toward the lateral side.
4. Ask the client to blink and the lens should pop out into your hand.
5. An alternative method for removing hard contact lenses is the use of a lens suction cup. This is particularly useful for a client who cannot consciously assist with the removal.

Removing Soft Contact Lenses

1. Wash hands with soap and warm water.
   Rationale: The fingers are the most common source of skin bacteria and debris. Washing not only decreases the chances of infection but helps protect lenses from damage.
2. Position client comfortably in a sitting position, if possible.

3. Ask the client to look upward and inward. Pull down on the lower lid and place your index finger on the lower edge of the lens, moving it onto the white part of the eye.

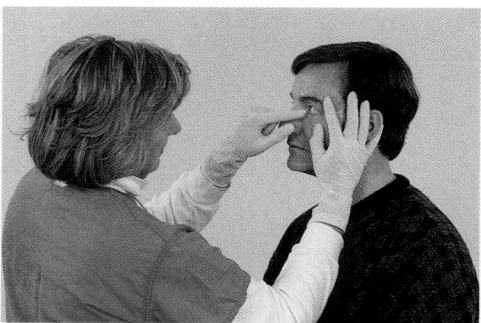

Step 3 As the client looks upward and inward, pull down on the lower lid.

4. Gently grasp lens between your thumb and index finger to release the suction of the lens. The lens will fold over and can easily be removed. Gently roll the lens, using normal saline as needed, to separate it and return it to its normal form.

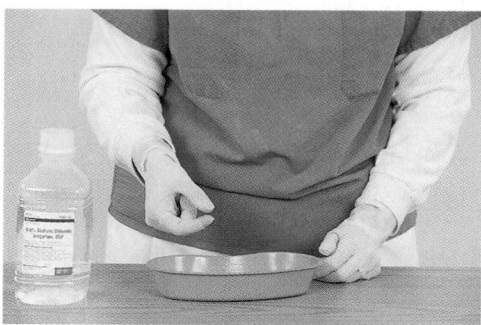

Step 4 Use normal saline to separate the lens.

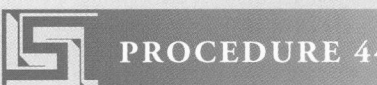

PROCEDURE 44-2

ASSISTING AN ADULT WITH INSERTING A HEARING AID

Purpose
1. Maintain hearing status.
2. Provide assistance with insertion.

Assessment
- Assess client's physical ability to manage the hearing aid unaided (i.e., motor function, coordination, level of consciousness, vision, interest, depression).
- Review history for adaptations to hearing impairment (i.e., lip-reading).

Equipment
Personal hygiene supplies for cleaning the ear mold as recommended by the manufacturer

Cotton tips, mild soap, and water to cleanse the outer ear canal

Special devices (fresh battery, if needed; other equipment that the hearing aid style may have)

Procedure
1. Check to be sure the battery is functional. Hold hearing aid in your hand and turn up the volume until you hear a "feedback" whistle. The feedback results from sound leaking around and back into the microphone and being amplified.
2. Inspect the hearing aid to be sure that tubing and ear mold are intact and not cracked or broken. The opening in the ear mold should be free of cerumen.
3. With the volume turned down, insert the ear mold into the ear canal, twisting slightly for a snug fit.
4. Secure the battery behind the ear, if of that type. There are other styles of hearing aids that may fit in other ways.
5. Turn the volume up slowly while speaking to the client in a normal voice tone. Ask the client to let you know when the sound level is comfortable.
   Rationale: Assisting the client to participate in the environment through improved hearing aids in the sensory function of communication.

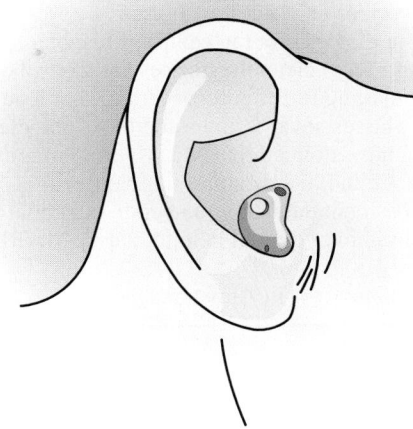

Step 2 Placement of an inserted in-the-ear hearing aid.

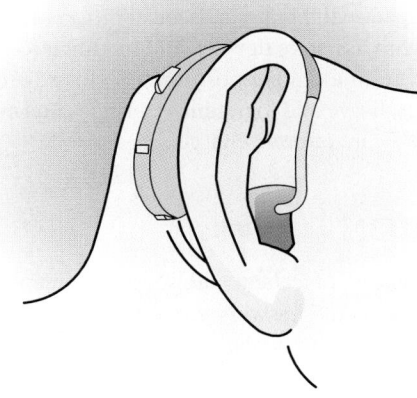

Step 3 Placement of a behind-the-ear hearing aid.

APPLY YOUR KNOWLEDGE

Stan Myer, 76, lives in an assisted living facility and occasionally has some confusion. He has been telling you that his new glasses are worthless. The glasses seemed to work at first, but now he says he sees something wavy or distorted in the center of his vision. He keeps asking you to clean the glasses and get rid of whatever is making it difficult for him to see. You have cleaned his glasses several times and they look clear to you, yet you have noticed that Mr. Myer no longer reads the paper and his signature has changed.

What assessment data do you need to collect at this point? Discuss how you will help to clarify Mr. Myer's sensory perception.

Check your answers in Appendix A.

may become independent. At first, the client may need help with basic care and hygiene; ongoing nursing assessment will determine the need for further interventions.

Because family roles can be changed suddenly (e.g., if the breadwinner becomes the care receiver), family members may need as much help and support as the client for their own issues and concerns. Enlist the aid of social services to help with financial problems related to the client's sensory dysfunction. Occupational therapy may be appropriate for helping the client with assistive devices and modifications in the home. Nurses are in a unique position to assess the client's needs before discharge and to organize services that can continue the client's care after discharge.

EVALUATION

Evaluation of the care of a client with sensory/perceptual dysfunction is based on the answers to the following questions developed from the client goals.

- Was sensoristasis achieved?
- Were contributing factors to sensory dysfunction reduced or eliminated?
- Can the client describe the interventions and rationale so that this information can be used in the future to deal with sensory dysfunction?
- Was self-care maintained?
- Was safety maintained?

Examples of positive outcome criteria for a client at risk for sensory overload are described below.

Goal

The client will demonstrate an understanding of contributing factors by reducing or eliminating them.

Possible Outcome Criteria

- The client uses ear plugs and eye shades during sleep for the next 3 nights.
- The client limits television and radio use to 1 to 3 hours per 8-hour period for next 48 hours.
- The client asks appropriate questions about care before and during treatment during next 24 hours.

Goal

The client will demonstrate an understanding of interventions and rationales by using this information as foresight.

Possible Outcome Criteria

- During next 24 hours, the client describes procedures to the nurse before they are done, including what he or she might see, hear, feel, smell, or taste.
- The client gives the rationale for a procedure and asks questions.

Goal

The client will achieve sensoristasis through a decrease in the symptoms of sensory overload or deprivation.

Possible Outcome Criteria

- The client demonstrates the ability to concentrate by listening to an explanation of medications, asking appropriate questions, and repeating the medication schedule every time medication is given during next 24 hours.
- The client sleeps 5 to 7 hours each night without awakening every night.
- The client is oriented to person, place, and time during visiting hours for the remainder of the day as reported by the nurse.
- The client listens to a relaxation tape with earphones when housekeeping personnel are cleaning the client's room.

Goal

The client will maintain self-care.

Possible Outcome Criteria

- The client bathes and performs adequate oral care daily.
- The client performs toileting independently and safely.
- The client ambulates in the hall three times a day.
- The client feeds himself or herself food and liquid for next three meals.

Goal

The client will remain safe.

NURSING PLAN OF CARE
THE CLIENT WITH DISTURBED SENSORY PERCEPTION

Nursing Diagnosis

Disturbed Visual Sensory/Perception related to temporary decrease in visual sensory input manifested by fear of body-image alteration, irritability, withdrawal, and misinterpretation of sensory stimuli

Client Goal

Client will demonstrate an understanding of the sensory deprivation experience.

Client Outcome Criteria

• Within 8 hours, client accurately describes this eye injury and expected medical outcome (i.e., full visual recovery).
• During hospitalization, client freely discusses problems with the staff, asking appropriate questions.
• Before discharge, client describes his or her behavioral changes and relates them to temporary deficit.
  Before discharge, client explains his or her behavior changes to family.

Nursing Intervention	Scientific Rationale
1. Introduce self from doorway before entering room and explain reason for being there.	1. Avoid startling the client and prevent misperceptions.
2. Post schedule for day on wall for all staff, visitors, and family to follow. Review schedule with client for input.	2. A schedule assists others to know and to inform the client about what is going to happen, reducing anxiety.
3. As rapport and trust build, invite the client to share his or her concerns about recovery; answer questions and correct misconceptions.	3. By focusing on concerns, the nurse can help the client separate fears from reality.
4. Encourage client to identify his or her frustrations and feelings related to being temporarily "blind" and to ask questions about his or her environment.	4. Expression of feelings helps to allay anxiety while also providing reassurance and a variety of sensory stimulation.
5. Hold a conference with the client's family to promote mutual discussion of the experience. Encourage client to teach the family what he or she understands about sensory deprivation.	5. Mutual discussion and sharing provide outlets for the client and family, aid in understanding of sensory deprivation, and provide opportunities for additional teaching related to the family's concerns about home management.

Client Goal

Client will demonstrate achievement of sensoristasis through a decrease in the symptoms of sensory deprivation.

Client Outcome Criteria

• Before discharge, client uses various sensory pathways to increase sensory variation.
• Before discharge, client reports no difficulty related to misperceiving sensory stimuli.
• During hospitalization, client visits with family and friends for a minimum of 15 minutes per visit.

Nursing Intervention	Scientific Rationale
1. Schedule 5-minute conversations every hour on the hour while client is awake for the first 24 hours.	1. Regular conversations provide gradual cognitive and sensory stimulation at a time the client can count on, so he or she is not overwhelmed.
2. Orient client to any noises that can be misinterpreted (e.g., air-conditioner thermostat on the wall, chimes indicating a fire drill, sound of the food cart being wheeled in at meal times).	2. Awareness of specific sounds helps the client stay focused in reality.

NURSING PLAN OF CARE

THE CLIENT WITH DISTURBED SENSORY PERCEPTION (*Continued*)

3. After the first 24 hours, on day and evening shifts, provide a minimum of two and maximum of four staff per shift, other than assigned caretakers, to talk with the client for a minimum of 10 minutes. Post a schedule in the front of the client's chart to sign up for these social visits.
4. Teach the client the importance of gradually increasing input from other sensory pathways when vision is temporarily unavailable; include teaching about self-stimulation, such as counting, singing, and using a tape recorder to talk into; isometric exercises; tactile stimulation; auditory variation, gustatory and olfactory stimulation.

3. Help build trust, reduce anxiety, and provide cognitive stimulation and sensory variation.

4. The client needs information about management of sensory deficit, how to increase stimulation gradually, and prevention of further sensory deprivation or overload.

Possible Outcome Criteria

- The client accurately and consistently uses safety devices such as side rails, night lights, and a call system.
- The client reports absence of injuries.

KEY CONCEPTS

- The senses are vision, hearing, taste, smell, and touch. Senses related to touch are the somatic senses of kinesthesia, or position sense, and visceral, or deep sensation.
- The RAS controls arousal and awareness to stimuli.
- Sensoristasis refers to a person's optimum state of arousal through stimulation. When stimulation is constant, adaptation occurs.
- Sensory perception generally decreases as a person approaches 60 to 70 years of age.
- Sensory overload occurs when a person is unable to process the intensity or quantity of incoming stimuli. Sensory deprivation is a lack of meaningful stimuli.
- Sensory deficits, impaired function in sensory reception or perception, that occur gradually may bring about behavior changes and sharpening of other senses to help the person adapt.
- Anxiety, cognitive dysfunction, depression, hallucinations, and delusions are manifestations of sensory perception dysfunction.
- Nursing assessment of sensory perception function includes subjective information about the client and his or her usual environment and physical examination for vision, hearing, taste, smell, and the somatic senses of touch, pressure, position, vibration, pain, and temperature.
- Goals for the client with altered sensory perception function include achieving sensoristasis, reducing contributing factors, describing intervention and rationales, achieving self-care, and maintaining safety.
- Client teaching about the importance of regular eye examinations and prompt treatment of ear infections may help promote sensory function. Preparing clients for procedures and their associated sensory experiences is another crucial nursing intervention.

- Nurses must provide appropriate stimulation for clients with sensory deprivation while reducing excess stimulation for those with sensory overload.
- Sensory aids may be physical (e.g., glasses, hearing aids, large-print books, sound amplifiers) or situational (e.g., speaking directly in front of a hearing-impaired client, encouraging a client to smell and taste food).
- Safety precautions, crucial for clients with altered sensory perception function, include assisting with ambulation and care; encouraging use of side rails, night lights, and call systems; and frequently observing the client.

REFERENCES

Bostwick, J. M. (2000). The many faces of confusion: Timing and collateral history often hold the key to diagnosis. *Postgraduate Medicine, 108*(6), 60–62.

Casey, D. A., DeFazio, J. V., Jr., Vansickle, K., & Lippmann, S. B. (1996). Delirium: Quick recognition, careful evaluation, and appropriate treatment. *Postgraduate Medicine, 100*(1), 121–124, 128, 133–134.

DiGiovanna, A. G. (2000). *Human aging: Biological perspectives.* New York: McGraw-Hill.

Dyer, I. (1995a). Preventing the ITU syndrome or how not to torture an ITU patient! Part 1. *Intensive and Critical Care Nursing, 11*(3), 130–139.

Dyer, I. (1995b). Preventing the ITU syndrome or how not to torture an ITU patient! Part 2. *Intensive and Critical Care Nursing, 11*(4), 231–232.

Geary, S. M. (1994). Intensive care unit psychosis revisited: Understanding and managing delirium in the critical care setting. *Critical Care Nursing Quarterly, 17*(1), 51–63.

Gesell, A., & Ilg, F. (1949). *Child development.* New York: Harper Brothers.

Glide, S. (1994). Maintaining sensory balance. *Nursing Times, 90*(17), 33–34.

Gordon, M. (1994). *Nursing diagnosis: Process and application* (3rd ed.). St. Louis, MO: C. V. Mosby.

Hampton, J., Craven, R. F., & Heitkemper, M. M. (1997). *The biology of human aging* (2nd ed.). Dubuque, IA: Wm. C. Brown.

Lee, K. A. (1991). Sensory overload, sensory deprivation, and sleep deprivation. In M. L. Patrick, S. L. Woods, R. F. Craven, et al. (Eds.), *Medical–surgical nursing: Pathophysiological concepts* (2nd ed.). Philadelphia: J. B. Lippincott.

McFarland, G. K. (1996). *Nursing diagnoses and process in psychiatric mental health nursing.* Philadelphia: Lippincott-Raven.

Mueller, C. R. (1996). Multidisciplinary research of multimodal stimulation of premature infants: An integrated review of the literature. *Maternal Child Nursing Journal, 24*(1), 18–31.

North American Nursing Diagnosis Association. (2000). *NANDA nursing diagnoses: Definitions and classification 2001–2002.* Philadelphia: Author.

Paquette, M., & Rodemich, C. (1997). *Psychiatric nursing diagnosis care plans DSM IV.* Sudbury: Jones and Bartlett Publishers.

Ryan, M. C. (1998). The relationship between loneliness, social support, and decline in cognitive function in the hospitalized elderly. *Journal of Gerontological Nursing, 24*(3), 19–27.

Schafer, W. (1995). *Stress management for wellness* (3rd ed.). New York: HB College Publications.

St. Pierre, J. (1998). Functional decline in hospitalized elders: Preventive nursing measures. *AACN Clinical Issues, 9*(1), 109–118.

Vander, A. J., Sherman, J. H., & Luciano, D. S. (2000). *Human physiology: The mechanisms of body function* (8th ed.). New York: McGraw-Hill.

BIBLIOGRAPHY

Barnason, S., Zimmerman, L., & Nieveen, J. (1995). The effects of music interventions on anxiety in the patient after coronary artery bypass grafting. *Heart and Lung: Journal of Critical Care, 24*(2), 124–132.

Barry, P. D. (1998). *Mental health and mental illness* (6th ed.). Philadelphia: Lippincott-Raven.

Black, P., McKenna, H., & Deeny, P. (1997). A concept analysis of the sensoristrain experienced by intensive care patients. *Intensive and Critical Care Nursing, 13*(4), 209–215.

Coble P., & Davis J. (2001). Restraint reduction in a large tertiary medical center. *Journal of Nursing Administration, 31*(7–8), 344–345.

Ely, E. W., Margolin, R., Francis, J., May, L., Truman, B., Dittus, R., Speroff, T., Gautam, S., Bernard, G. R., Inouye, S. K. (2001). Evaluation of delirium in critically ill patients: Validation of the Confusion Assessment Method for the Intensive Care Unit (CAM-ICU). *Critical Care Medicine, 29*(7), 1370–1379.

Hoskins, C. C. (1996). Altered sensory perception. In M. K. Elkin, et al. (Eds.), *Nursing interventions and clinical skills.* St. Louis, MO: Mosby–Year Book, pp. 648–663.

Johnson, L. H., & Roberts, S. L. (1996). A cognitive model for assessing depression and providing nursing interventions in cardiac intensive care. *Intensive and Critical Care Nursing, 12*(3), 138–146.

Levanen, S., & Hamdorf, D. (2001). Feeling vibrations: Enhanced tactile sensitivity in congenitally deaf humans. *Neuroscience Letter, 301*(1), 75–77.

McGuire, B. E., Basten, C. J., Ryan, C. J., & Gallagher, J. (2000). Intensive care unit syndrome: A dangerous misnomer. *Archives of Internal Medicine, 160*(7), 906–909.

Meehan, T., Vermeer, C., Windsor, C. (2000). Patients' perceptions of seclusion: A qualitative investigation. *Journal of Advances in Nursing, 31*(2), 370–377.

Ruiz-Bueno, J. (1998). Sensation information. In M. Snyder, et al. (Eds.), *Complementary/alternative therapies in nursing* (3rd ed.). New York: Springer, pp. 191–201.

Schofield, P. (1996). Sensory delights. *Nursing Times, 92*(6), 40–41.

45 Cognitive Processes

⑤ Key Terms

anomia
aphasia
articulation
attention
cognition
coma
communication
comprehension
consciousness
delirium
delusions
dementia

dysarthria
hallucinations
judgment
learning
memory
perceiving
phonation
reality orientation
resonance
schizophrenia
sundown syndrome

⑤ Learning Objectives

Upon completion of this chapter, the student will be able to do the following:

1. Identify key components of cognition and communication.
2. Describe characteristics of normal cognition.
3. Describe influences on cognitive function related to the life-span.
4. Explain factors that can affect cognitive processes.
5. Identify manifestations of altered cognitive processes.
6. Apply the nursing process to the care of persons experiencing altered cognitive processes.
7. Discuss socialization needs of people with altered cognition and their families.
8. List resources available to families of people with altered cognitive processes.

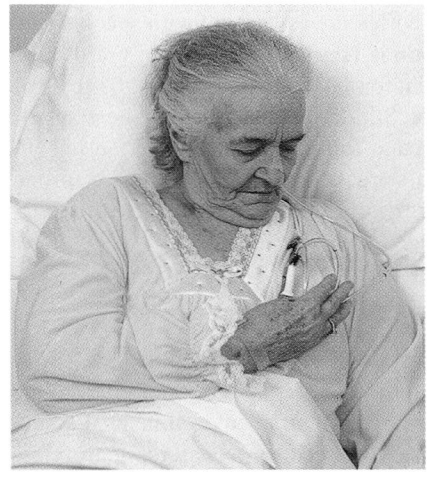

⑤ Critical Thinking Challenge

You are a nurse working on a general surgical unit of a hospital. A client returns to the unit after repair of a broken hip. She appears agitated and confused despite a pain control regimen of morphine. The client's daughter, Donna, comes to visit and looks acutely anxious. Donna tells you that her mother lived in a nursing home for 16 months before falling two nights ago after getting up to go to the bathroom. Donna says she thinks that the nurses at the home ignored her mother's call light because "Mom would never get up at night without calling a nurse." While you are talking with Donna, the client moans, pulls at intravenous tubing, and calls for "Dorothy."

Once you have completed this chapter and have added cognitive processes to your knowledge base, return to the above scenario and reflect on the following areas of Critical Thinking:

1. Describe your immediate impressions of this situation.
2. Determine how the information in the scenario and your own knowledge and values contributed to these impressions.
3. Given the situation as presented, formulate and prioritize your plans for nursing interventions.
4. Organize your plans for assessing the client's cognitive function.

In all practice settings, nurses work with people experiencing temporary or irreversible impairment of cognitive function. Nurses play a central role in identifying people at risk for and experiencing cognitive impairment and in the ongoing assessment of the impairment's impact on self-care and safety. Nursing interventions focus on promoting optimal function by preventing, minimizing, or restoring factors affecting function and by compensating for deficits. Planning and evaluating nursing care require an understanding of normal cognition, factors that place a person at risk for cognitive impairment, and effective interventions to be individualized as appropriate.

NORMAL COGNITIVE PROCESSES

Cognition is the systematic way in which a person thinks, reasons, and uses language. Each instant of awareness can be defined as a thought, and awareness itself can be defined as **consciousness. Attention** is the ability to concentrate on and take in specific sensory stimuli. **Memory** is the ability to recall a thought at least once and usually again. **Learning** is the capability of the nervous system to store memories. **Communication** is the exchange of information between at least two people and involves the use of language to store, process, and transmit thought content. The cerebral cortex coordinates consciousness, thought, memory, learning, and communication.

Anatomic Structures Involved in Cognition

For information to be processed, the person must be able to perceive it. Perception of information begins when the information enters the person's awareness through the senses; consciousness, thought, memory, learning, and language all play roles in further processing that information. Intact structure and functioning of the sensory receptors, the afferent nervous pathways, and the cerebral cortex are necessary for a person to take in information through the senses and to assimilate and interpret that information in the cerebral cortex. Additionally, the efferent nervous pathways, major reflexes, and muscles are needed to communicate information to others.

The eyes and ears are the major means of sensory input. The eyeball (Fig. 45-1A) is a mobile, spherical structure located in the orbit of the skull. It is composed of the sclera (the white, outer, fibrous layer), the choroid (the vascular layer), and the retina (the neural layer). The eyeball's interior chambers are filled with clear media (the aqueous and vitreous humors) through which light is transmitted to the retina. The rods and cones of the retina convert light energy to nerve impulses; the optic nerve and optic tract carry these impulses to the brain's visual receiving area (Fig. 45-2). The nearby visual interpretation area and previous learning give meaning to visual images.

The ear (see Fig. 45-1B) consists of the external ear (the auricle and the external acoustic meatus or ear canal), the tympanic membrane, the middle ear (the ossicles and the eu-

stachian tube), and the inner ear (the cochlea, vestibule, and semicircular canals). Sound is transmitted through the auricle and ear canal to the tympanic membrane, which vibrates freely. The vibration is transmitted to the ossicles (malleus, incus, and stapes) that continue transmission to the labyrinth or inner ear. The vibration moves through the fluid of the inner ear to the apex of the cochlea and the organ of Corti. In response to vibration, hair cells of the organ of Corti generate nerve impulses that the cochlear nerve, in company with the vestibular nerve, carries to the central auditory pathway. Nerve impulses travel over the central auditory pathway to the receiving and integrating areas of the brain's temporal lobes (see Fig. 45-2). These areas of the brain are necessary for sound to be meaningful and to integrate past experience with current auditory information.

The reticular formation, also referred to as the reticular activating system (RAS), is a diffuse cluster of neurons that extends from the brain stem and projects upward and throughout the cerebral cortex and downward into the spinal cord (McCance & Heuther, 1998). The RAS is essential for maintaining wakefulness and controls portions of vital cardiovascular and respiratory reflexes (McCance & Heuther, 1998). The nervous system, including the cranial nerves (see Chapter 16), must be intact for full cognition and speech.

The cerebral cortex is composed of a thin layer of neurons covering the surface of all the convolutions of the brain. Areas of the cerebral cortex are associated with specific sensory and motor functions (see Fig. 45-2). The brain's left hemisphere is dominant for language function in 90% to 99% of right-handed people. Similarly, the brain's left hemisphere is dominant for language function in 50% to 75% of left-handed people. Broca's area is associated with word formation and speech; Wernicke's area is associated with the interpretation of language and understanding.

Normal Cognitive Function
Perception of Information
Perception of information includes sensing and interpreting stimuli from the external and internal environments. Perception depends on functioning sensory receptors, neurotransmission, and central processing.

Sensory receptors can be classified into three groups: exteroceptors (external sensors), proprioceptors (position sensors), and interoceptors (internal sensors). Neurotransmission occurs when the stimuli to the sensory receptors are converted to neural impulses and transmitted to the appropriate area of the brain for central processing and interpretation.

Exteroceptors. The exteroceptors respond to stimuli from the external environment. They include the receptors for vision (rods and cones) and hearing (hair cells in the organ of Corti) and the somatic receptors for pain, touch, and pressure in the skin. Assuming vision remains intact throughout a lifetime, this sense allows people to perceive and to learn about the world from birth onward. Vision permits people to link abstract concepts with concrete objects, thus contributing to

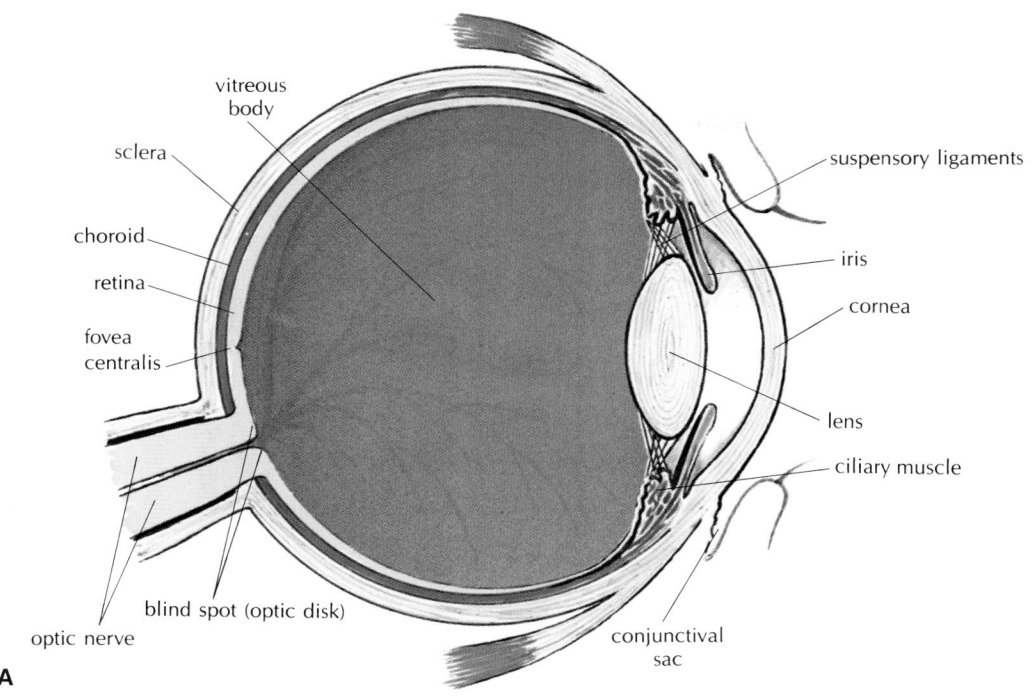

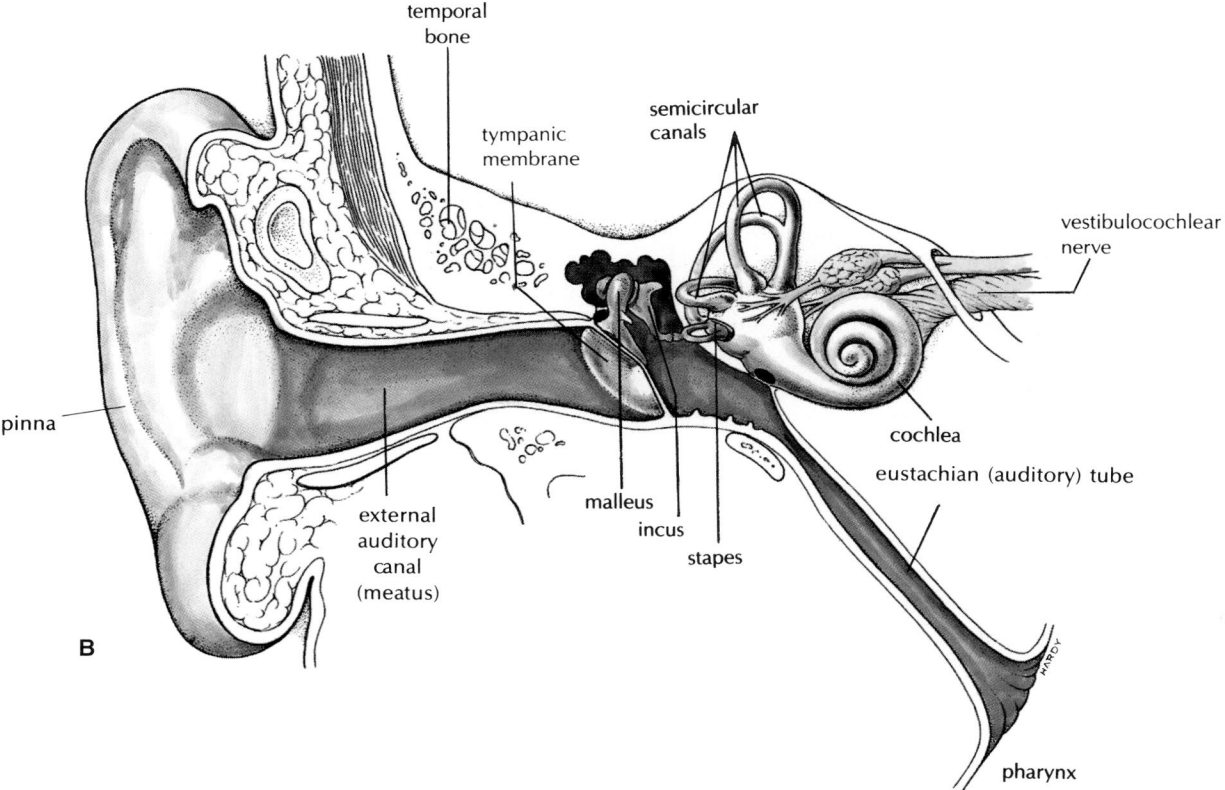

FIGURE 45-1   The major means of sensory input is through the eyes and ears. (**A**) Cross section of the eye. (**B**) Cross section of the ear, showing external, middle, and internal subdivisions.

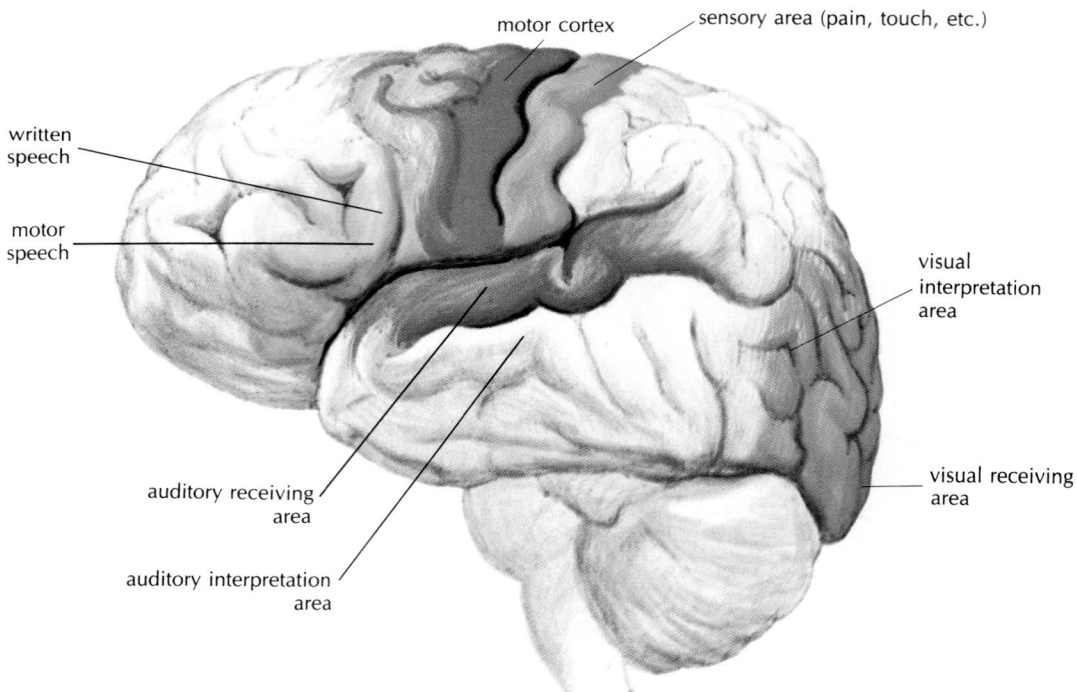

written speech

motor speech

auditory receiving area

auditory interpretation area

motor cortex

sensory area (pain, touch, etc.)

visual interpretation area

visual receiving area

FIGURE 45-2   Lateral view of left brain showing functional areas of the cerebral cortex.

learning and memory. Hearing, also present from birth, links concepts with the frequency, intensity, and duration of sounds. Both vision and hearing enhance environmental awareness and facilitate experiences that amplify cognitive development.

Touch, pressure, heat, cold, or chemicals in the tissue activate somatic sensors in the skin. Resulting nerve impulses enter the spinal cord through the posterior roots. Depending on the sensation, the impulse is transmitted to the brain through either the dorsal column system or the spinothalamic system. The dorsal column transmits sensory information that must be sent rapidly, incorporates fine gradations of intensity, and is discretely localized. The spinothalamic system carries information that lacks fine gradations, has less exact localization, or does not need rapid transmission. From the spinal cord, sensory information is transmitted through the thalamus to the somatosensory cortex in the brain's parietal lobes.

Taste is a function of the taste buds of the tongue and includes sweet, sour, salty, and bitter components. A taste bud is a group of 50 to 150 chemoreceptors. The sensation of taste is transmitted via the seventh and ninth cranial nerves to the brain stem. Ascending fibers carry the impulses to the taste center of the sensory area. Smell is a function of the olfactory cells located in the upper nose and is the least understood of the special senses. The olfactory cells are actually projections from the brain. Taste and smell seem to be closely related because diminished function in one usually affects the function of the other (McCance & Heuther, 1998).

Proprioceptors.   Proprioceptors are located in the inner ear, muscles, tendons, and joints. Proprioceptive sensations relate to the body's physical state including the relative position of

different body parts and the sensation of movement. The proprioceptive function of the inner ear is discussed in Chapter 33.

Interoceptors.   Interoceptors are located in and respond to stimuli from the body's viscera and deeper tissues such as bone. Sensations relate to changes in the internal environment. With the exception of visceral pain receptors, the interoceptors operate at a reflex level. That is, sensory signals elicit reflex responses that enable the visceral organs to control their activities without conscious involvement (Berne, Levy, Koeppen & Stanton, 1998).

Consciousness

Consciousness, a state of awareness and full responsiveness to stimuli, relies on an intact RAS and cerebral cortex. The RAS mediates level of arousal, and the cerebral cortex mediates perception and interpretation of stimuli. The RAS is divided into facilitatory and inhibitory areas. The facilitatory area is intrinsically active, provides arousal to the cerebral hemispheres, and produces an increase in the body's muscle tone. The inhibitory area causes a decrease in muscle tone and permits decreased activity and sleep after prolonged wakefulness. When the facilitatory and inhibitory areas are balanced, the person is conscious but neither excited nor inhibited.

Thoughts

Each thought results from a momentary pattern of stimulation of many parts of the nervous system at the same time. This stimulation involves, most importantly, the cerebral cortex, thalamus, limbic system, and upper reticular formation of the brain stem. The stimulated areas of the limbic system, thalamus, and reticular formation give thought its crude nature such as pleasure, displeasure, pain, and comfort. The stimulated area of the cortex determines discrete characteristics of thought (what is seen in the visual field), discrete patterns of sensation (texture of objects), and other specific characteristics (Guyton & Hall, 1996).

Memory

Memory is the process by which information and experiences are stored and retrieved. Physiologically, changes in nerve transmission from one neuron to the next due to previous neural activity (learning) result in memories. Plasticity, the tendency of synapses and neural circuits to change as a result of activity, allows new synaptic pathways to form. These new pathways are called memory traces and, once established, can be activated to reproduce the memories (Guyton & Hall, 1996).

Memory is subdivided into three basic types based on the time span between stimulus presentation and memory retrieval. Immediate memories last for a few seconds to a few minutes and may be caused by local reverberating neural impulses. Intermediate memories may last for minutes or weeks but will be lost unless converted to long-term memories. Physiologically, intermediate memories involve changes in the strength of the synaptic connections, which may be attributed to changes in neurotransmitter or intracellular chemicals. Long-term memories, those that can be recalled indefinitely, are stored at the same site as intermediate memories but require the activation of previously inactive genes and the expression of new proteins (e.g., the number of cell membrane channels may increase; Kandel, 1997).

The hippocampi, part of the limbic system located within both temporal lobes, play a role in determining which memories are committed long term. The ability to retain some things and forget others is essential to intelligent behavior. Assimilating experiences and new information is a process involving memory. The hippocampi play a vital role in retaining new knowledge and preventing dissipation of the information.

Speech

Speech production is a motor activity that requires the integrated function of the laryngeal and respiratory structures with the language areas in the cerebral cortex. Speech consists of phonation (achieved by the larynx) and articulation (achieved by the mouth). Phonation, the process of creating vocal sounds, occurs when air from the lungs moves through the oral or nasal cavity during exhalation. As air moves past the vocal folds in the larynx, the vocal folds vibrate.

Laryngeal structures produce the pitch, volume, and quality or timbre of phonation. Vocal pitch can be changed by stretching or relaxing the vocal folds or by changing the mass of the vocal folds' edges by contracting the thyroarytenoid muscles. Vocal volume is partly controlled by the amount of air moving through the larynx. Exhalation is normally passive: The intercostal muscles and diaphragm relax, the lungs recoil, and air moves out through the larynx. Contracting the abdominal muscles can increase air flow through the vocal cords, thus increasing vocal volume. The lips, tongue, and

soft palate affect **articulation,** the enunciation of words and sentences. The tongue's position against the palate, the teeth, and the mouth's muscles influence the sound made. The mouth, nose, nasal sinuses, pharynx, and chest cavity all affect the voice's resonance (tone and timbre). **Resonance** is demonstrated by the change in voice quality that occurs when a person has a head cold with severe congestion.

In addition to vocalization, speech involves the formation of thoughts, words, and meanings. Thought formation and word selection occur in functional areas of the cerebral cortex. The patterns for control of the larynx, lips, mouth, respiratory system, and other muscles of articulation are controlled by Broca's area of the motor cortex (see Fig. 45-2).

Characteristics of Normal Cognition

Intelligence

Intelligence is the measurable product of intellectual functioning, which consists of memory (discussed earlier), comprehension, and concentration. **Comprehension,** a part of learning, involves grasping the meaning of stimuli (see below discussion on learning). Concentration is the ability to filter extraneous stimuli to focus on a task. People depend on intellectual functioning to learn in school settings, vocational surroundings, and living environments.

Reality Perception

Perception of reality, or reality orientation, includes awareness of time, place, situation, and self. It is the knowledge of how self and environment interact over time and transform sensory information into meaning. Reality perception is complex and depends on functioning sensory receptors, neurotransmission, and intact central processing. People with affective disorders, such as schizophrenia, experience alterations in reality perception.

Orientation

Orientation is the basic process by which people know their location in the dimensions of time and place. Orientation also includes the ability to know who one is as a person and in relation to others. People tend to take orientation for granted until they experience confusion. On a simple level, one can experience disorientation upon awakening in a new setting (e.g., on vacation) and momentarily forgetting where one is.

Judgment

Judgment, or insight, is the process of reasoning. It is the ability to process incoming stimuli and to determine the complex meanings associated with many aspects of a situation. For example, a person driving down the street may see a truck blocking the road ahead. The person determines that the truck is an obstacle and that evasive action is required to prevent a crash. The term insight is often used to express perceptions people make about behavior or feelings. For example, recognizing that a craving for chocolate while studying for exams is an indicator of stress is an insight.

Recall and Recognition

Recall and recognition are abilities used to retrieve information from long- and short-term memory. Recall involves the ability to retrieve information directly or by relating it to other information (e.g., seeing a person and "recalling" his or her name accurately). Recognition is the ability to relate accurately something in the current environment with what is stored in memory (e.g., seeing a rose and "recognizing" it as a type of flower). People depend on these abilities to perform in school, on the job, and in everyday life. Recall and recognition are cognitive characteristics that can be developed and need practice to remain actively useful.

Language

Language is the ability to convey needs, ideas, and feelings through the systematic use of symbols. Humans are unique in being able to use symbolic codes to communicate abstract ideas through a highly refined verbal language. The biophysical interaction and integration of the brain, neural system, and organs of speech permit humans not only to produce sounds but also to remember what they said in the past and to speak about the future.

Language enables people to relate to others in their families and communities. It helps people identify and express their roles in relationships. For instance, a father may discipline a child, an instructor may give an assignment, or a student may ask questions for clarification. In each example, people use language to communicate a relationship.

Normal Cognitive Patterns

Cognition is the sum of the various thinking processes through which a person gains, stores, manipulates, and expresses knowledge. Cognition enables the person to interact with the environment meaningfully and purposefully. Normal cognitive patterns integrate the processes of attending, perceiving, thinking, learning, remembering, and communicating.

Attending

Attending is the process of concentrating on a specific stimulus without being distracted by other, irrelevant stimuli (Wiebers, Dale, Kokmen & Swanson, 1998). Ability to concentrate is a cortical function of the brain's frontal lobe. Attending is different from alertness; an alert but inattentive person will be attracted to any environmental stimulus.

Perceiving

Perceiving is the process of receiving and interpreting sensory stimuli that function as a basis for understanding, knowing, or learning. In perceiving, a person integrates information obtained through vision, hearing, touching, taste, and/or smell with past experiences to understand or make sense of the environment. An example of perceiving is hearing a phone ring, seeing the phone, touching and holding the receiver, listening to the person speaking, interpreting the meaning, and responding appropriately. The integration of motor activities involved in handling the phone, sensory activities of seeing and hearing, and central perceptual activities of interpretation results in a meaningful interaction.

Thinking

Thinking is the process of sorting, organizing, and categorizing information to form mental concepts or perceptions. "Thinking" is forming ideas or arriving at conclusions; "reasoning" is following a logical thought sequence, starting with what is known and proceeding to a conclusion. A person is capable of different types of thinking. Concrete thinking involves objects that can be perceived by the senses. An example of concrete thinking is proving the arithmetic proposition that $1 + 1 = 2$ by attaching the numbers to objects such as apples. Abstract thinking is a higher-level process that involves a thought or idea apart from any material object. For example, the idea of beauty is a value. Beauty can be attributed to a flower but is not a concrete object in itself. Abstract thinking is required for people to interpret a veiled or abstract truth from the use of concrete objects and terms. Creativity is an innate human attribute that enables us to bring something new into existence.

Learning

Learning is the multidimensional process of acquiring knowledge that depends on abstract functions such as symbols, language, classifications, concepts, as well as concrete operations. Comprehension is the capacity for understanding and reasoning. For learning to be useful, the person needs to develop strategies for organizing information in memory so he or she can recall it as needed (for more discussion on learning, see Chapter 24).

Remembering

Memory is a complex biochemical storage system that is not yet completely understood. Experiences, ideas, and images are chemically coded and integrated for later retrieval (Berne et al., 1998; Kandel, 1997). The content of long-term memory, which is the storehouse of a person's knowledge, depends on the perceived value and significance of the past event. Specific significant life events, such as weddings or the birth of a child, hold great value and memory potential. The reason some items move from short- to long-term memory is not clear but is probably related to the perceived value of the information and its relation to other memories.

Communicating

Communication brings people together while differentiating them from one another. Communication allows people to be unique. People may communicate thoughts and ideas verbally through spoken or written language or nonverbally through facial expressions, body posture, movements, gestures, and touch (see Chapter 23). Touch, a very effective means of nonverbal communication, has many different meanings; understanding the true meaning may be difficult because of its personal nature. Familial, regional, class, and cultural influences shape tactile expressions. Age and gender also shape meanings that are associated with touch.

Lifespan Considerations

Physiologic health and the quality of the social and physical environments affect the complex process of cognitive development. Environment can strongly influence the rate at which a person proceeds through the usual stages of cognitive development. Each developmental phase has unique aspects related to language and communication. People need emotional security, human interaction, and a variety of sensory experiences to develop optimally. Jean Piaget (1969) is the most widely recognized theorist in cognitive development, although the work of other theorists, such as Erikson (1963) and Havighurst (1972), contributes to the understanding of cognitive development throughout the lifespan.

Newborn and Infant

Newborns and infants are in the "sensorimotor period" in which sensory experience is the major developmental task (Piaget, 1969). Infants interact with the environment through the five senses and learn to modify behavior in response to stimuli. Language skills are not developed, and infants express thoughts or needs through behavior. Bonding is essential to the development of basic trust. Primary caregivers are lifelines for infants. Through consistent relationships, infants learn to differentiate self from others, to communicate, and to relate to others.

Babies perform the cognitive developmental work of infancy by exploring the environment and playing. Infants learn to connect some behaviors with expected responses. For example, moving a toy in a certain way may cause a pleasing sound; that process is play. With repetition and maturity though, infants may begin to remember and repeat the action at will. Similarly, infants begin to assimilate language, linking specific words and sounds with objects of meaning such as "Mama" or "bottle." Providing stimulation through varied objects, different sounds, and face-to-face communication and interaction enhances cognitive development (Santrock, 1995).

Crying, smiling, pointing, and tugging are kinds of non-verbal communication that babies use. Language skills begin with cooing and progress to vocalizations that express various emotional states (Santrock, 1995). During the babbling period, infants produce sounds that form the basis of language. As they mature, babies begin to understand language and use words to communicate. Most babies speak their first words by the end of the first year.

Toddler and Preschooler

During these stages, young children develop the concept of object permanence and begin to label familiar items. Object permanence means that children learn that objects have constancy; they give objects names and use those names to communicate with others (Piaget, 1969). Vision and hearing are necessary to understand the environment as a basis of thinking. Language and thinking develop side by side. Preschoolers have concrete thinking patterns and demonstrate pronounced egocentrism, or self-concern. These children view the world only from their point of view.

By the time infants become toddlers, they have transformed vocalizations and gestures into words to express themselves. At 2 years of age, most children understand more than 300 words and can speak about 200 words (Santrock, 1995). Although children vary in their rate of language acquisition, uniformity exists in the way all children acquire language. Language is acquired not only in terms of learning principles but also through biologic, environmental, and cognitive factors. Any serious change or interruption in these factors can affect a child's acquisition of language (Harrison, 1990). Children who are abandoned, abused, or not exposed to language rarely learn to speak normally.

The process of reasoning begins as young children try to make sense of the world. When two events occur simultaneously, children think one caused the other (transductive reasoning). Thus preschoolers believe their thoughts to be all powerful. For example, if a child spilled her milk and later fell and scraped a knee, she might interpret the pain associated with the abrasion as punishment for spilling the milk. More significantly, a child may interpret parental divorce as punishment for "bad" thoughts or behavior. Because adults find this thinking so absurd, they may underestimate its seriousness to children.

As part of cognitive development, young children develop confidence in abilities and gain independence through parental encouragement in each new area of learning (Erikson, 1963). Positive, nurturing environments that encourage imaginative play, interaction, questioning, and use of language and symbols, while reinforcing earlier knowledge, will foster the preschooler's cognitive development (Fig. 45-3).

School-Age Child and Adolescent

School-age children can carry out complex mental operations such as addition, subtraction, grouping, classifying, and ordering (Piaget, 1969). They understand and can mentally represent multiple dimensions of objects and symbols

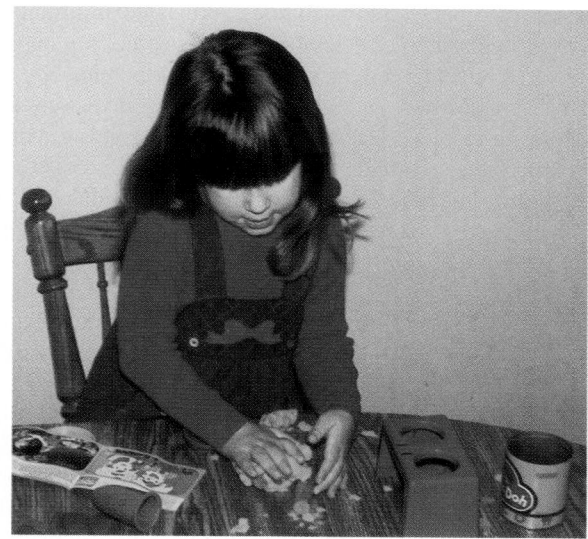

FIGURE 45-3 Play activities that incorporate imagination and creativity help to develop cognitive abilities in preschoolers.

and can encode stimuli for later retrieval. School-age children understand conservation, which is the idea that the properties of an object stay the same even if the object is altered in certain ways. For example, if an equal volume of fluid is poured into two differently shaped containers, a preschooler will perceive that the volume of water has changed, whereas the school-age child will recognize that there's a change in shape but the water volume is constant. This shift in comprehension indicates the ability to incorporate abstract thinking with concrete processes. At this stage, children derive great pleasure in accomplishments resulting from new learning and thinking skills (Erikson, 1963). Learning and play environments that reward children's achievements contribute positively.

Adolescence is a particularly difficult time for the development of thinking processes because of enormous emotional stress from many sources, including the struggle for separateness from family and a strong need to identify with the peer group (Erikson, 1963). Fluctuating hormonal levels add to the emotional stress. Abstract reasoning and logical judgment are two functions that emerge with increasing maturity.

During adolescence, teenagers become able to think abstractly and to perform complex mental processes. They are able to hypothesize situations and solutions as well as to conceptualize abstract ideas (Piaget, 1969). Teenagers develop the cognitive capacities of classification, serialization, spatial abilities, verbal skills, and abstract relationships. Communication with peers takes priority over communication with adults. At the same time, adolescents need adult guidance and protection. During illness, peer relationships provide support and companionship. Providing opportunities for independent thinking and decision making encourages increased maturity.

Adult and Older Adult

Throughout young and middle adulthood, people make steady progress in rational thinking abilities, formal and informal educational opportunities, career development, and life experiences. As adults feel progressively more competent, they become less rigid and more flexible. Making decisions and adjusting to changes usually creates less disruption during adulthood than in teenage years. Creativity and productivity in work contribute to continual cognitive development and to innovative use of integrated abstract and concrete thinking. Adults depend on communication for dealing instrumentally with the world, managing careers and vocations, maintaining relationships, and carrying out various roles. Communication conveys thoughts, feelings, and the innermost aspects of the human experience.

As aging progresses in the adult years, cognitive function remains relatively unchanged although processing information may require more time. Problems with thought processes and communication are more common among older adults than younger groups, but they usually relate to a decrease in coping reserves, trauma, or a specific condition. They are not a normal part of aging. Age-associated memory impairment

is a mild memory impairment that does not significantly interfere with activities of daily living (ADLs). Items forgotten are usually unimportant. People can use memory enhancement techniques to compensate for benign forgetfulness. Although the brain undergoes some degenerative changes as the ventricles enlarge slightly and brain weight decreases, significant cognitive impairment in older persons is never normal but is indicative of a disorder.

Diminished vision and hearing are common among older adults and can interfere with effective communication. Because these senses usually diminish gradually, older adults develop compensatory mechanisms for adapting to the changes and their effects on communication.

FACTORS AFFECTING COGNITIVE FUNCTION

The interaction of personal (physiologic and emotional) and environmental factors can affect cognitive processes. Culture, values, and beliefs are contextual factors that influence meaning and understanding.

Personal Factors

Any physiologic abnormality that affects the body's cellular environment can interfere with brain function and affect cognition. Disturbances range from mild mental clouding to disorientation and acute confusion to coma and death (Francis, 1997). Physiologic abnormalities contribute to schizophrenia, depression, and some kinds of dementia. Similarly, physiologic abnormalities that cloud the senses or interfere with usual cortical functioning may alter communication.

Communication may be altered by the functional impairment of the speech apparatus of the larynx, the ability to move air, the use of the tongue and the oral pharynx, and/or the innervation to each of these structures. Cancer of the throat is the major risk for impaired phonation. Neurologic impairment and muscular dysfunction also have the potential for affecting communication.

Muscular dysfunction can be related to cortical, cerebellar, or cranial neurologic impairment or from effects of drugs (e.g., alcohol, sedatives, or other medications). People who have a high cervical (C2, C3 quadriplegia) injury also have a permanent tracheostomy (and ventilatory support). They cannot speak because no air will be forced through the vocal cords. Other neurologic conditions, such as amyotrophic lateral sclerosis, multiple sclerosis, and myasthenia gravis, may lead to inability to speak because of loss of muscle function. These conditions may also necessitate a tracheostomy or ventilatory assistance, depending on the disease's severity.

Blood Flow

To function optimally, all cells need a continuous oxygen supply. Oxygenation depends on respiratory and circulatory function and hemoglobin production. During respiration, oxygen enters the alveoli, diffuses across capillary membranes to enter the pulmonary venous system, and binds with hemoglobin. Then the hemoglobin-bound oxygen is transported to brain cells. The brain accounts for 20% of the body's total oxygen uptake and requires a constant oxygen supply to support brain cell life.

Any interruption in blood flow to the brain cells causes cellular hypoxia, resulting in changes in function. A chronically inadequate blood supply causes cellular dysfunction and deterioration of mental processes (Porth, 1998). Any disease process that interferes with alveolar ventilation, pulmonary circulation, cardiac function, cerebral blood flow, or production of normal hemoglobin can result in hypoxia and altered cognition. A cerebrovascular accident (CVA) or stroke usually occurs because a thrombus occludes a cerebral blood vessel, resulting in inadequate blood flow. Approximately 20% of all stroke survivors require the specialized services of a speech pathologist to help them regain communication skills. The other 80% have only minor or temporary damage to the brain's language centers (Gresham & Weiss, 1993). The location of the insult and the extent of damage affect the pattern and severity of speech impairment.

Nutrition and Metabolism

The brain cells need glucose for metabolic energy and other nutrients for optimal functioning. The brain consumes 25% of the glucose the body uses. The efficiency with which oxygen is delivered to the cells is related to hemoglobin production, which requires an adequate dietary intake of iron. Vitamins and minerals are essential for effective neurologic functioning and neurotransmitter activity.

People with inadequate nutrition usually have low hemoglobin levels (anemia). Abnormal hemoglobin can be produced in people with specific genetic disorders such as sickle cell anemia. Disorders that impair metabolic processes and oxygen use, such as hypothermia and hypothyroidism, can also alter cognition (Porth, 1998). The body's inadequate intake or impaired use of glucose will limit the quantity available for the brain's metabolic demands.

Fluid and Electrolyte Balance

The brain cells require a constant extracellular environment of fluid and electrolytes for optimal function. The brain's cellular processes depend on the active and passive movement of water and charged particles across cell membranes (see Chapter 36). The brain is protected by the blood–brain barrier, a shield that prevents or delays the entry of certain substances from the blood into the cerebrospinal fluid or interstitial spaces. The blood–brain barrier protects the brain cells from substances (other than normal fluid and electrolytes) that could damage sensitive nerve cells. Maintenance of a dynamic state of fluid balance and electrolyte levels provides the ideal internal environment for neurologic function.

Disturbance in the concentration and balance of intracellular and extracellular fluid and electrolytes can cause cellular dysfunction and accompanying cognitive changes. Such disturbances have various causes including abnormal loss of body fluids, dietary deficiencies, acute and chronic disease,

and effects of medications. Although any disturbance in fluid or electrolyte balance can impair cognitive processes, a few common disturbances are hyponatremia and hypernatremia (variations in the serum sodium level), hypokalemia (reduced serum potassium level), hypercalcemia (elevated serum calcium level), and hypoglycemia and hyperglycemia (abnormal serum glucose levels; Porth, 1998).

Accumulated metabolic byproducts (metabolic end products) that are not eliminated from the body can be toxic to central nervous system (CNS) function. Impaired function of the kidney, liver, or both can impair the ability to break down and excrete such potential toxins. The liver converts ammonia, a byproduct of protein metabolism, into urea that the kidneys excrete. Liver or kidney dysfunction can interfere with this process, resulting in elevated ammonia levels and a delirium known as hepatic encephalopathy.

Sleep and Rest

Sleep's restorative function allows people to regain energy for cognitive functions (see Chapter 42). Sleep is necessary for consolidating learning and moving information from short-term to long-term memory. Rapid eye movement (REM) sleep seems to be particularly important to efficient cognitive functioning. Lack of sleep (sleep deprivation) can cause irritability, decreased calculation and problem-solving skills, poor concentration, and/or impaired memory. Everyone has experienced feeling dull and slow after a sleepless night or staying up too late. Rotating shifts can cause similar problems particularly if a person changes shifts frequently with inadequate time to adjust to new sleep patterns. Inadequate REM sleep may impair both learning and memory and decrease the subjective feeling of being rested.

Self-Concept

The way a person feels about himself or herself is called self-concept (see Chapter 46). Communication conveys the way a person feels about himself or herself in relation to the world. If a person feels competent, successful, and in control, the quality of his or her communication will reflect that confidence and security.

People who feel disadvantaged or less competent are likely to believe they have little control over their lives. Their self-concept is apt to be correspondingly less confident. If a person sees the self as unable to compete in a given arena (e.g., school, work, or play), the person's communication reflects that lack of confidence.

Others usually reflect the manner in which a person communicates. If a person communicates confidence and security, he or she will usually receive that response from others. Conversely if the person communicates insecurity, lack of control, or inadequacy, responses from others will mirror this communication.

The relationship between self-concept and communication is susceptible to change. People vary in personal skills and one can compensate for weaknesses in some areas with strengths in others. This adaptation and adjustment help create a balanced self-concept and more confident communication.

Infectious Processes

Infectious processes of the CNS, including encephalitis and brain abscesses, and the subsequent inflammatory response of nerve cells are obvious causes of altered cognition. The human immunodeficiency virus (HIV) can invade the CNS, causing acute infection or progressing to acquired immuno-deficiency syndrome (AIDS). Infections elsewhere in the body can also cause changes in mental status. Any person with a severe infection in the circulation (e.g., bacteremia, septicemia) may experience CNS effects including lethargy and confusion. Common sources for bacteremia or septicemia include the urinary tract, respiratory system, and any open wounds (Dunne, 1998). Altered cognitive function in an older adult may be the earliest indication of an infectious process anywhere in the body.

Degenerative Processes

Any process contributing to degeneration of the brain cells may ultimately affect cognitive function. Causes of degeneration may be related to an organism (viral or bacterial infection), aging, or unknown sources. Degeneration can impair judgment, insight, planning, memory, problem solving, and communication. Potential impairments range from mild disability to severe dysfunction that may be incompatible with normal cognition.

Clarifying the terms used to describe degenerative processes related to cognition is important. *Senility,* which literally means the process of aging, is a term used to describe cognitive impairments that are mistakenly thought to be a normal part of aging. Actually, significant memory and problem-solving impairment is never normal but rather indicates a pathologic process (Cummings, Arsland, & Jarvik, 1997). The terms senile dementia and organic brain syndrome have no place in current nursing practice.

Dementia is a clinical syndrome involving progressive impairment of intellectual function and memory. It is not associated with disturbance in level of consciousness, but it does interfere with social or occupational functioning. People with dementia experience a gradual decline in all cognitive processes, as contrasted to acute confusion in which dysfunctions may be reversible (Table 45-1). Potential causes for dementia include trauma, circulatory interferences, genetic predisposition, alterations in neurotransmitters, and infectious agents. The most common form of dementia is Alzheimer's type, which is a primary neuronal degeneration of unknown cause. Alzheimer's can occur at any age of adulthood but increases in incidence with aging, affecting 5% to 10% of people older than 65 years of age and 20% of people older than 75 years (Fratiglioni, 1996; Hendrie, 1998).

Pharmacologic Agents

Medications that primarily act on the CNS (e.g., anticonvulsants, antidepressants, antianxiety agents, antipsychotics, narcotics, and hypnotics) can impair thinking and cause confusion. In the early stages of use or with moderate to heavy dosages, the person may experience impairment in speech motor control (slowness and slurring) and in comprehension and expression (inability to think of the correct word or response). Discontinuing or decreasing the dosage of these medications will often improve cognitive function within a few days. Medications commonly prescribed to manage agitated or confused behavior, such as haloperidol and the benzodiazepines, may cause a paradoxical increase in confusion in some people, especially older adults.

Medications that do not have primary pharmacologic effects on the CNS can also cause confusion, either alone or in

TABLE 45-1

Differences Between Confusion and Dementia		
Feature	**Acute Confusion**	**Dementia**
Onset	Rapid, often at night	Insidious
Duration	Hours to weeks	Months to years
Course	Fluctuates over 24 hours; worse at night; lucid intervals	Relatively stable
Awareness	Impaired	Usually normal
Alertness	Reduced or increased; tends to fluctuate	Usually normal
Orientation	Always impaired, at least for time	Variable, often impaired
Memory	Immediate and recent impaired	Recent and remote impaired
Thinking	Disorganized; may be dreamlike	Impoverished; poor in abstraction
Perception	Illusions and hallucinations (especially visual) common	Misperceptions uncommon; usually normal
Sleep–wake cycle	Always disrupted; daytime drowsiness and nighttime agitation and restlessness	Fragmented sleep
Physical illness or drug toxicity	Either or both always present	Often absent

From Lipowski, Z. J. (1992). Delirium and impaired consciousness. In J. G. Evans & T. F. Williams (Eds.), *Oxford Textbook of Geriatric Medicine.* Oxford, England: Oxford University Press.

combination (Francis, 1997). The mechanism varies and is not well understood. In some cases such as with strong diuretics, the drug predisposes the person to another physiologic cause of confusion—hyponatremia. In practice, it is wise to consider almost any medication as a possible contributing factor to altered cognition.

Toxicity states can occur with overdose of a medication or alcohol and can cause confusion. Overdosage of drugs that normally have no CNS effects can potentially cause significant mental status changes. Overuse of drugs affecting the CNS alone or combined with alcohol will also impair thinking.

Head Trauma

People of all ages sustain head trauma but the greatest incidence occurs in adolescents and older adults (Jennett, 1996). Most seriously injured clients have major disabilities. Because specific injury sites are rare, classification of brain injury and prediction of outcome are difficult. The more severe the head injury, the more likely communication will be interrupted. Communication problems in head-injured clients are usually compounded by impairments in cognitive function such as behavior, memory, orientation, and attention.

Environmental Factors

The basic cognitive processes of perceiving, thinking, learning, and remembering depend on the ability to receive and to organize stimuli. The amount of stimuli in the environment, either increased or decreased, can influence cognition. For example, one student preparing for exams in an environment of noisy students, television, and loud music may find it difficult to study effectively. Another student may find that some background noise, depending on the level of distraction, assists with concentration.

As people age, perceptual ability, which contributes to cognitive functioning, declines as sense organ functions diminish. For example, older adults need more light to see objects, have more problems with light glare, and experience loss of accommodation for near objects (presbyopia). Hearing diminishes especially in the high-frequency range and acuity of sense of touch declines. These normal changes affect the ability to organize incoming stimuli.

Emotional stress or physical discomfort can lead to disorganized thinking, memory impairment, and poor judgment. A person learning of an injury to a loved one, finding out about a failed exam, or planning a wedding may have difficulty maintaining the usual level of cognitive performance. Concentration and problem solving are also difficult when a person is in pain, has a full bladder, or experiences other discomfort. Sometimes such everyday problems combine and accumulate, creating enough stress to impair thinking.

Psychological disorders, such as depression, interfere with cognitive function and can contribute to altered thought processes. Psychological and emotional disorders can interfere with sleep, rest, and nutrition and can affect cognitive functions directly.

Environmental Stress

The stress of an unfamiliar environment can affect the basic cognitive processes of orientation and arousal, which depend on the ability of the cerebral cortex to receive and to organize incoming stimuli (Haskell, Frankel, & Rotondo, 1997). Numerous stimuli are found in any environment, some of which are attended to and some ignored. Through a complex perceptual process, habituation or familiarization occurs to routine background stimuli such as the feel of clothing and the tick of a clock. As a result, the person is not "overloaded" with meaningless input. The brain can also conjure up input when none is available. People experiencing inadequate sensory input are at risk for cognitive dysfunction as the brain attempts to stimulate itself (see Chapter 44).

Hospitalization removes people from familiar surroundings and daily activities that provide orienting cues and places them in an environment of strange noises, sights, feelings, and procedures (Fig. 45-4). All these unfamiliar stimuli demand attention because the person has not had time to habituate to the new surroundings. This state of sensory overload can overwhelm the person's ability to find meaning, and a state of perceptual dysfunction occurs. Plenty of stimuli are present but none makes any sense.

Culture, Values, and Beliefs

Comprehension and meaning vary among cultures, and communication is often inhibited or blocked as a result. Words and their meanings carry different nuances and significance depending on a person's culture, values, and beliefs.

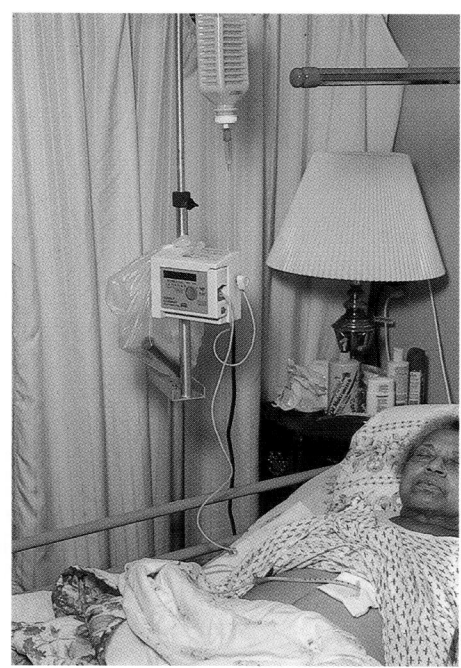

FIGURE 45-4 Older adults may be at risk for cognitive dysfunction related to unfamiliar environments and procedures.

ETHICAL/LEGAL ISSUE
Mistreatment of Client by Staff

Mr. Schooner, 80 years old, has entered a long-term care facility because of his forgetfulness, wandering behavior, and inability to care for himself. He is in good physical health but has a history of progressive dementia. Although his family members were reluctant to admit him, they were exhausted from the constant care that Mr. Schooner required.

At the long-term care facility, Mr. Schooner becomes agitated, has increased wandering, and talks loudly, which disturbs the staff and the other residents. You overhear a staff member saying to him, "If you don't sit still and be quiet, I'm going to tie you to your bed and put tape on your mouth!" You are aware that such behavior on the part of healthcare staff is not reflective of nursing philosophy, but you have to work closely with this staff member.

Reflection
- Identify your concerns about Mr. Schooner. How could the move to this facility and his cognitive dysfunction be contributing to his behavior?
- Describe your feelings about the staff member. What ethical concerns do you face in this situation?
- Identify possible approaches to this state of affairs.
- Recognizing the client's dependence and the staff member's behavior, define what you feel is your ethically appropriate behavior.

Although these differences may be particularly noticeable among immigrant groups, they also hold true for groups from different regions within the same country. For example, the same language and some of its meanings may sound different to and be comprehended differently by a person from the southeastern United States than by a person from northeastern states (Ahmann, 1994; Gropper, 1996).

Language barriers can result in anxiety, fear, and frustration for people who need to communicate daily and especially those who require healthcare. Because communication involves nonverbal and verbal language, the meaning of body position and expression can further facilitate or impede communication. Although putting an arm around the shoulder of a person from one culture indicates caring and concern, for a person of another culture it may be an intrusion that blocks rather than facilitates communication.

Values regarding thoughts and feelings that are appropriate to share with others also affect communication. In Western cultures, women tend to be more comfortable communicating feelings than men are. Western cultures value stoicism and emotional reserve in men, who are less likely to communicate personal thoughts and responses. This reluctance to communicate may actually interfere with effective communication if actual understandings and needs are not shared.

ALTERED COGNITIVE FUNCTION

Cognition is a complex process; the normal outcome is an appropriate, adaptive behavioral or emotional response. Anything that interrupts this complex process can result in impaired thinking and abnormal behavioral or emotional responses.

Manifestations of Altered Cognitive Function

Clinical manifestations of altered cognitive function include acute confusion (**delirium**), chronic irreversible confusion (dementia), sensory perceptual alterations, and impaired language skills. Dysfunctions can be either temporary or permanent depending on the cause.

Disorganized Thinking

A person experiencing disturbed thought processes or disorganized thinking interacts inappropriately with others or the environment and may have an altered perception of reality. Thinking, learning, reasoning, and remembering occur in a disorderly fashion. Manifestations of disorganized thinking may include inappropriately interacting and conversing with others, talking or gesturing to oneself, performing inappropriate activities, or exhibiting bizarre behavior. Withdrawal from others, hallucinations, and delusions are other common manifestations especially in schizophrenia and affective disorders. They may also occur in acute confusion and, less commonly, in Alzheimer's.

Cognitive impairment frequently interferes with perception of reality, which is based on life experience, personal relationships, and environment. When thought processes become altered, the person may find it difficult to separate accurately altered perceptions from reality. **Delusions** (fixed false beliefs) and **hallucinations** (perceptions arising from the person's own thoughts) are examples of altered perceptions of reality. Both responses are attempts to cope with or to manage stress or physiologic dysfunctions that impair cognition.

In disorganized thinking, the content of the person's speech may make no sense in the context of the conversation or a sentence may contain multiple unrelated ideas. Interactions with people with disorganized thinking are difficult because they are unable to follow a logical sequence or to respond rationally or predictably. The client who ignores the meal tray but tries to eat the tissue box with a spoon or who asks to go to the bathroom but resists assistance to get out of bed displays impaired reasoning processes.

Impaired Thought Processes

Abnormal levels of arousal, attention span deficits, and memory impairments can affect judgment, insight, planning, and problem solving. Most people with impaired thought processes have aspects of all three elements and severity can fluctuate.

Altered Level of Arousal. Arousal is a person's level of reactivity to incoming stimuli. Levels of arousal may be categorized as hypervigilant, alert, lethargic, obtunded, and comatose

(Williams & Salisbury, 1999). Hypervigilant means the person is acutely aware of environmental stimuli and may startle at unexpected noise; hypervigilance is often accompanied by a decreased ability to concentrate. Alert means the person is awake and fully aware of incoming stimuli. Lethargic describes the client who is not fully awake and tends to drift off to sleep when not actively stimulated. Obtunded describes the client who is difficult to arouse and when aroused is confused. **Coma** describes the client who is completely unresponsive to incoming stimuli. Arousal does not imply the ability to focus attention.

Altered Attention. Stress and illness can easily impair attention span and concentration. People with a short attention span are highly distractible and cannot filter competing stimuli. These people will be unable to focus on a conversational topic or will stop in mid-sentence to look out the window. This distractibility interferes with the ability to learn and to perform ADLs.

Disorders of arousal and attention are major features of acute confusion. Clients, particularly older adults with chronic cognitive impairment or reduced physiologic reserve, are at risk for acute confusion during acute illness or hospitalization or after surgical intervention (Davies, 1999). Acute confusion impairs abilities to reason, follow directions, concentrate, and remember. The sleep–wake cycle is often disrupted, and inappropriate behavior may be evident.

Delirium. Delirium is an acute organic mental syndrome characterized by global cognitive impairment, disturbance of attention, reduced level of consciousness, increased or reduced psychomotor activities, and disturbed sleep–wake cycle (American Psychiatric Association, 2000). Delirium results from one or more organic factors; medications and metabolic disorders are the most common causes. Predisposing factors include aging, dementia, systemic illness and infection, sensory impairment, and addiction to alcohol or other drugs. Delirium has an acute onset, is often unrecognized, and can lead to death if the underlying defect is not corrected.

Sundown Syndrome. Sundown (or Sundowner's) syndrome is defined as an increase in confusion and agitation that occurs at the end of the day. Sundown syndrome is thought to result from several factors including alteration in diurnal rhythms, sensory deprivation related to decreased ambient light, fatigue, disrupted sleep–rest cycles, and a decreased stress threshold (Hall & Gerdner, 1999). At night, there is less light, less activity, and fewer caregivers resulting in less available orienting stimuli. Although not limited to clients with dementia of the Alzheimer's type, sundown syndrome occurs most frequently in those with significant cognitive impairment.

Schizophrenia. Schizophrenia is a serious, persistent brain disease characterized by distortion of reality and difficulty processing information. People with schizophrenia experience problems with memory, attention, communication, and decision making. The cause of schizophrenia is unknown but current research implicates chemical and structural changes in the brain. Abnormalities found in the brains of people with schizophrenia include an excess of the neurotransmitter dopamine, a decrease in number of dopamine receptors in some brain areas, an imbalance between dopamine and serotonin (another neurotransmitter), and an alteration in gamma-aminobutyric acid (GABA) neurons (Weickert & Kleinman, 1998).

Memory Impairment. Memory impairment is a concern for old and young alike. Situational and emotional stress usually has few effects on long-term memory. Significant impairment of long-term memory usually indicates a CNS disorder or a severe confusional state. Short-term memory is much more sensitive to stress. For example, hospitalized clients may have little recall of conversations with healthcare professionals because the stress of illness interferes with usual memory functioning.

Impaired Communication. **Aphasia** is the complete or partial loss of language abilities including understanding speech (auditory comprehension), reading, speaking, writing, arithmetic, and expression through pantomime. This acquired communication dysfunction results from brain damage but does not affect intelligence. Aphasias are produced mostly through damage to the cortical language areas of the dominant left hemisphere (see Fig. 45-2). Rarely, an injury affects one isolated area of speech but injury usually affects all speech and language functions. The most common cause of aphasia is related to an interruption in circulation as a result of a cerebral vascular accident (stroke). Significant improvement in speech and communication occurs in the first 6 months and can continue up to 18 months after the onset of aphasia (Nicholas, Helm-Estabrooks & Ward-Lonergan, 1993).

The manifestation of speech impairment depends on location and extent of damage. It can range from slight slurring of speech to total loss of communication. Aphasia has been described and categorized based on lesion location and linguistic deficit (Kistler, Ropper, & Martin, 1994). The four most common types of aphasia are expressive (Broca's), receptive (Wernicke's), anomic, and global (Table 45-2).

Expressive Aphasia. Expressive aphasia (also called Broca's, motor, or nonfluent aphasia) is characterized by limited speech that is slow and halting with great effort, reduced grammar, and poor articulation. Because intellect is not necessarily impaired, the person knows what he or she wants to say but cannot find the needed words. Anomia refers to problems with word retrieval. In expressive aphasia, the person's speech often sounds like a telegraph message consisting of isolated or small groups of words and lacking tone or inflection. Writing is also affected and can be as severely or more severely impaired than speech.

Expressive aphasia can cause extreme frustration and anger. Sometimes the anger shows in physical behaviors such as pushing objects or people away and shouting. Often, clients direct anger at people who care the most about them. Such behavior makes it difficult for spouses or significant others to understand what is happening.

Receptive Aphasia. Receptive aphasia (also called Wernicke's, sensory, or fluent aphasia) is characterized by speech that is well articulated and has good melody and normal or slightly faster rate. The major manifestations are impaired auditory

TABLE 45-2

Expression and Comprehension With Major Types of Aphasia			
Types of Aphasia	**Oral Expression**	**Written Expression**	**Comprehension**
Expressive (Broca's or motor)	Nonfluent, telegraphic	Limited	Usually good
Receptive (Wernicke's or sensory)	Fluent, speech well articulated, disorganized content	Impaired	Impaired
Anomic	Speech fluent, talks around the subject	Variable, mild to severe impairment	Variable, mild to severe impairment
Global	Speech very poor, meaningless recurrent sounds	Severely impaired	Severely impaired

comprehension and feedback. People with receptive aphasia have difficulty understanding spoken and written words. They talk a great deal but may not make sense. Their speech lacks specific content. Their ability to read, write, listen, concentrate, or follow instructions is impaired; the severity level is usually consistent with or worse than the speech impairment. The affected person is unaware of the language impairment and appears euphoric in relation to his or her language problems.

A person with receptive aphasia also has a pattern of symptoms referred to as right hemisphere syndrome. He or she neglects the paralyzed side of the body, even to the point of not knowing that the left arm or leg is really his or hers. Behaviorally, these clients are impulsive, lack insight into their deficits, and have poor judgment. They are said to display inappropriate behavior when actually their behavior is a result of their injury. The combination of these symptoms and behaviors makes rehabilitation difficult.

Anomic Aphasia. Anomic or amnesic aphasia is characterized predominantly by word-finding problems of a milder nature than expressive aphasia. The speech is fluent and grammatically correct. The communication difficulties arise in using the correct names for particular objects, people, places, or events. If the person cannot remember the correct name, he or she talks about the subject until the listener understands what is meant. Auditory comprehension is generally good although levels of reading and writing impairment vary from mild to severe. Behaviorally these clients display anger, frustration, and depression in ways similar to those with expressive aphasia.

Global Aphasia. Global aphasia results from severe and extensive damage to all language areas (Broca's and Wernicke's). These clients have no consistent functional skills in any language modality. They cannot speak or understand speech nor can they read or write. Some clients' speech consists of meaningless, recurrent sounds.

Dysarthria

Dysarthria refers to a group of speech disorders that result from a disturbance of motor control, weakness, paralysis, or incoordination of the oral musculature. It results from damage to the central or peripheral nervous system. Clients with dysarthria usually have normal auditory comprehension and can select and order words correctly. They have a motor

speech disorder that causes them difficulty in saying words and sounds precisely, using appropriate stress, loudness, pitch, and control. The result is speech described as "slurred," "heavy," or unclear. There are numerous types of dysarthria. The specific type depends on the site of the neurologic lesion.

Impact on Activities of Daily Living

Memory, judgment, problem solving, and the ability to process sensory stimuli appropriately are essential to the performance of any activity. For example, brushing one's teeth requires remembering where the supplies are, knowing how to do the procedure, and deciding when. Mild cognitive impairment can be compensated for with written reminders, posted schedules, occasional supervision, and change in occupation or living situation. When cognitive impairment interferes with the ability to perform essential activities safely and appropriately, continued independent living is threatened. The critical outcomes of impaired cognitive function are loss of independence, altered self-concept, and impaired role performance.

Everyone has a lifestyle that requires a unique set of skills. For instance, the daily life of a mother juggling child care and a career in a large city requires skills that are different from those of a single migrant worker. Social support networks are also individual and may mitigate the impact of cognitive impairment on daily living. For example, the mild memory impairment of an older woman living with her husband in a retirement community may have little impact on daily living, whereas the same degree of memory loss may have major lifestyle implications for a single person employed at a low-income job.

Impairment to communication affects the ability to participate in usual roles, relationships, and activities. For example, a person whose career depends on speech production and written expression will find that role impaired if he or she has aphasia. People with altered communication may become frustrated with trying to express what they need in relation to hygiene, nutrition, and activities. The affected person may experience problems with continence as a direct result of the difficulty of communicating the need to urinate or defecate.

With Wernicke's aphasia, the person may also neglect one side of the body. He or she may need reminders and assistance in grooming the neglected side and in communicating needs related to that side. Eating may be a problem if the person is unable to see half the food presented.

Because communication is inseparably integrated with perceptual processes, many people with cognitive dysfunction cannot remain independent. Activities such as banking, food shopping, paying bills, and meal preparation are difficult, if not impossible, because these activities require arithmetic, reading, writing, and spelling. Impaired communication may necessitate a structured environment and around-the-clock assistance.

Relationships depend on exchange of ideas, thoughts, and feelings. The person with altered communication is unable to convey these things clearly, resulting in less intimacy and clarity. Friends and acquaintances sometimes find it easier to end the relationship or to distance themselves than to bridge the communication problem. Families usually work hard to maintain communication and relationships although they feel the strain as well.

ASSESSMENT

Assessment is essential to nursing care for clients with actual or potential alterations in cognitive function. Assessment identifies clients with alterations in cognitive processes and describes the client's ability to function safely within his or her environment. Determining how a person functions and the quality of the social and physical environment guides the establishment of client goals and nursing interventions. When assessing a client with communication difficulties, remain attentive and be patient when the person is attempting to communicate (Dzurec & Coleman, 1997). Doing so places the person at ease and encourages him or her to initiate communication.

Subjective Data

Collection of subjective information helps to identify patterns of cognitive function; risk factors that may predispose clients to alterations in roles, relationships, or functional patterns; and actual cognitive or communication dysfunction. Gathering subjective data about cognitive abilities is a time-consuming process that usually involves multiple, brief, planned interactions with many people. Keep a general assessment framework in mind to remember all key areas (Display 45-1). The situation can be especially complex when the client is hospitalized and unknown to the staff. Nurses, physicians, and social workers may individually gather then collaboratively share information from many sources. Nurses are in the best position to gather data related to the client's normal pattern of function, areas of risk, and areas of actual dysfunction. All healthcare team members must document essential subjective data for consistency and collaboration.

Normal Pattern Identification

When assessing thought processes, gather information about the client's usual cognitive function and its impact on daily living. The client's ability to communicate usually will be apparent in the assessment interview. Systematic assessment can determine the nature and extent of the impairment and its affects on the client and family. Changes in other cognitive functions are often nonspecific and most obvious to those who know the affected person well. For this reason, elicit information from family and friends as well as from the client.

To determine the type of communication disorder the client is experiencing, assess verbal expression, written expression, comprehension, and nonverbal expression. Table 45-2 defines the expected comprehension and verbal and written expression for the four major types of aphasia. Display 45-2 also delineates communication abilities to assess for in the major types of aphasia. Answers to these questions assist in determining the degree of the client's communication dysfunction.

Information about other cognitive functions is best obtained systematically. Assess consciousness, the most basic cognitive process, first. Describe it in terms of the intensity of the stimulus used and the nature of the client's response. Next, evaluate ability to pay attention. Then, assess abilities to use language and memory because they are basic to reasoning and problem solving.

The significance of any cognitive impairment lies in its relationship to function in daily living, not in the impairment itself. For example, an older woman may tell the nurse she does not remember the names, dosages, and purposes of her medications. On the surface, it seems that she has a problem with medication management. Upon further questioning, the nurse learns that the client identifies her pills by color and uses a medication management system that groups pills in daily dosage units. The client's granddaughter, a registered nurse, oversees the medication management. This woman and her family have developed an effective system to compensate for a mild cognitive deficit.

Detecting mild to moderate cognitive impairment during an interview or casual conversation can be difficult. People who are aware of and embarrassed by their poor memory can become experts at giving vague answers and steering conversations into "safe" territory. Using a formalized approach to cognitive testing (such as the Folstein or Pfeiffer mental status examinations) is advisable if cognitive impairment is suspected. A nonjudgmental, warm, and friendly demeanor is important to put the person at ease.

Assessing perception of reality includes determining the person's orientation to time, place, and person (sometimes referred to as "orientation times 3"). Determine orientation to time by asking questions pertaining to time: year, day, date, and approximate time of day. Determine orientation to place by asking questions related to city or location. Assess orientation to person by asking the client his or her name. Orientation to time will usually show deficits first, with deficits in orientation as to identity being the last and most severe form of dysfunction.

Levels of consciousness and orientation are not by themselves adequate assessments of cognitive function. Comprehensive assessment includes the use of a mental status questionnaire (such as Folstein's Mini–Mental Status Examination) and a behavioral rating scale (such as the Clinical Assessment of Confusion—A or the NEECHAM Confusion Scale; Vermeersch & Henly, 1997).

DISPLAY 45-1

NURSING ASSESSMENT: COGNITION

Current Cognitive Function
A. Objective tool—Mini-Mental Status or Pfeiffer
B. Subjective evaluation
   1. Attention
   2. Ability to answer questions
   3. Appropriateness of affect

History and Time Course of Cognitive Impairment
A. Previous difficulties with thinking, perception, or communication
B. Previous head trauma—details of accidents or periods of unconsciousness
C. Previous stroke, hypertension, elevated blood cholesterol
D. When current symptoms began and how they evolved; include information from family and friends

Presence of Contributing Factors
A. Chronic or acute illness
   1. Laboratory abnormalities
   2. CNS disorders
   3. Multisystem disease
B. Use/abuse of medications
   1. Drugs with CNS effects
   2. Drugs with CNS side effects
   3. Drugs with potential for toxicity
   4. Use of recreational drugs or alcohol
C. Sensory impairment
   1. Vision
   2. Hearing
D. Quality of environment
   1. Family support
   2. Frequency and number of social contacts
   3. Availability of transportation
   4. Adequacy of financial resources
   5. Nutritional status
   6. Living situation
E. Presence of psychological stressors
   1. Bereavement
   2. Major life change
   3. Lack of financial resources
   4. Family crisis
   5. Loss of independence
   6. Serious illness
F. Family history of dementia, schizophrenia, or affective disorders

Current Functional Status
A. Ability to communicate verbally or nonverbally
B. Ability to understand spoken and written word
C. Literacy
D. Ability to perform activities of daily living
E. Amount of assistance currently available in the home
F. Ability to exercise good judgment
G. Safety of home environment
H. Nutrition adequacy
   1. Protein, iron, sodium, and calcium intake
   2. Adequacy of fluid intake
   Previously identified nutritional disorder
I. Sleep and rest
   1. Restfulness after a night's sleep
   2. Changes in life events, patterns, or current environment
J. Motor activity
   1. Agitation or withdrawal from activity
   2. Recent patterns of increased or decreased mobility
K. Activities of daily living
   1. Level of independence in hygiene and home maintenance
   2. Problem-solving abilities, such as money management, use of telephone, and interactions with needed services

Physical Assessment
A. Respiratory function
   1. Rate, rhythm, depth of normal respirations
   2. Lung and breath sounds
B. Cardiovascular function
   1. Rate, rhythm, and quality of heartbeat
   2. Carotid pulses and presence of bruits
C. Nutrition and metabolism
D. Height, weight, skin turgor
E. Musculoskeletal function
   1. Muscle tone and strength
   2. Gait
F. Sensory function
   1. Vision
   2. Hearing
G. Neurologic function
   1. Cranial nerves
   2. Involuntary movements
   3. Deep tendon reflexes

In assessing reality, clarify how the environment may be contributing to disorganized thinking. For example, an older woman in a nursing home calls for her son and does not understand why he will not stop to see her when she saw him pass by her door. In exploring the environment, the nurse realizes that the woman is not wearing her glasses and that the man who walked by had a build and clothes similar to the son's. As a result, the client misperceived the information. Failure to be thorough in assessment might lead to a wrong conclusion that results in attaching a label of "confused" to a

DISPLAY 45-2

🔲 INITIAL ASSESSMENT CONCERNS ABOUT COMMUNICATION

Is the person able to speak at all?

If so, is the speech intelligible and appropriate to the situation?

Does the person use gestures or point in an effort to communicate?

Is the person literate?

How much formal education does the person have?

Is the person able to speak another language?

Can the person understand and follow simple one-step commands?

Did the person have a speech difficulty before this most recent difficulty?

Was the person previously an active conversationalist, or did he or she prefer to listen?

Assessment for Major Types of Aphasia
Verbal Expression

Does the person speak easily, fluently?

Is the content appropriate in context?

Does the person initiate speech on his or her own?

Is the speech telegraphic (short, choppy)?

Is the speech organized?

Does the verbal output contain recurrent sounds?

Does the person name objects correctly?

Does the person repeat words and phrases easily?

Written Expression

Can the person write own name and address correctly?

Can the person produce a short narrative written paragraph?

Does the written product have appropriate meaning?

Comprehension

Does the person give any indication of hearing impairment?

Does the person answer simple, open-ended questions appropriately?

Does the person answer yes/no questions in appropriate context?

Can the person correctly point to an object that has been named?

Does the person respond appropriately to simple commands?

Nonverbal Expression

Observe for the type of affect (sign of emotion):
  Flat—no sign of emotion
  Labile—wide fluctuation in emotions

Observe gestures for appropriateness to the situation.

Observe for the integrated context of voice tone, emotional expression, body movement.

---

client who is actually having difficulty with perception. Do not allow personal perceptions of reality to overshadow the ability to monitor another person's perception of reality.

Risk Identification

Risk identification assesses for physiologic, psychological, and environmental factors that increase the likelihood of impaired cognitive processes. The degree of risk from each category will depend on the individual client and setting.

Clients with brain damage from stroke or head injury, impaired speech apparatus (e.g., laryngectomy or tracheotomy), and other temporary dysfunctions are at greatest risk for communication impairment. The presence of pathophysiologic factors such as cerebral, neurologic, respiratory, or auditory impairments, and laryngeal infection or edema places the person at high risk for altered communication. A community health nurse making a home visit to an older client will include a detailed assessment of social and psychological support systems as well as physiologic assessment.

Medications can be a primary risk factor for altered thought processes, either alone or in combination with other substances. Clients and families need to know the expected actions of medications, potential side effects, potential interactions, and indications of toxicity. Many instances of altered cognitive function can be traced directly to the addition of a new

medication, toxic levels of a usual medication, or unexpected interactions with other substances. Clients and families need to be alert to subtle changes in cognition and mental status in relation to their pharmacologic therapies. As part of the assessment process, obtain a detailed medication history from primary or secondary sources. Include all medications (prescribed, over-the-counter preparations, herbal remedies, and others) that the client takes. Note medications recently added and stopped. Be sure to obtain information about the amount of alcohol the client consumes.

The presence of multiple risk factors does not always lead to dysfunction. Individual strengths and resources can enable a person to withstand multiple stressors. An important part of a nursing assessment is identifying existing and potential coping resources. Interventions can then be designed to support and to develop these resources.

Dysfunction Identification

Analyze information to determine if dysfunction is present for a specific client. When identifying the presence of dysfunction, document assessed data in clear terms that others can easily understand. Instead of using vague terms like "slightly confused" or "poor attention span," describe the behaviors associated with the deficits precisely, using anecdotes when appropriate. Phrases like "oriented to self only," "needs verbal cuing to wash face," and "when given toothbrush, combed hair with it" provide clear information for identifying dysfunction.

Objective Data

Physical Assessment

Assessment of physiologic function provides clues as to the source of altered cognitive processes. Because the earliest clinical signs of changes in the levels of oxygen, electrolytes, and metabolic byproducts are lethargy, mild confusion, and impaired thinking, assess those components. Assessing these functions requires skill in the physical examination and laboratory evaluation. Physical functions to be assessed are listed in Display 45-1. The mouth, tongue, and facial muscles must be intact to form and to articulate words correctly. Clients with altered communication related to impaired motor functioning or brain damage need a thorough examination of the muscles and organs of speech. Chapter 16 discusses assessment methods for cranial nerves.

Observation is useful for identifying clues to impaired thinking and to defining possible causes of impaired communication. Disheveled appearance, disorganized speech, and abnormal movements are obvious indicators of dysfunction, especially when they represent a change in status. Difficulty maintaining eye contact, a tendency to repeat the same story, inappropriate responses to stress or stimuli, and emotional lability can also indicate difficulty with thought processes. At times these behavior changes are subtle; repeated observation of behaviors is necessary.

The tongue receives its motor innervation from the 12th cranial nerve (hypoglossal). Assess motor control of the tongue by instructing the client to protrude the tongue. If there is damage to the hypoglossal nerve, the tongue will deviate to the side of the weakness as the strong side pushes it forward unopposed.

The facial muscles are innervated by the fifth (trigeminal) and seventh (facial) cranial nerves. Assess the motor function of these nerves by noting the symmetry of facial movement when asking the client to show teeth, purse lips, and frown. When the client's face is at rest, note any asymmetry of the forehead or cheeks along with facial drooping or drooling.

The muscles of swallowing and the gag reflex are supplied by the 9th (glossopharyngeal), 10th (vagus), and 11th (accessory) cranial nerves. The larynx is supplied by the 10th cranial nerve alone. Motor weakness of the soft palate contributes to difficulty swallowing (dysphagia). To test swallowing, ask the client to swallow chips of ice. The ice gives some substance for the client to manipulate in the mouth yet only introduces water if he or she is unable to swallow successfully.

Impairment in the use of the larynx is immediately obvious in the presence of an endotracheal tube or tracheostomy or a ventilator. Because the movement of air bypasses the laryngeal function, the client is unable to communicate verbally. Assess if the client is able to use other modes of communication such as gestures, codes using eye blinks or hands, or written notes.

Many factors complicate the assessment of cognitive function in infants and young children. Because their language skills are not fully developed and they have difficulty expressing thoughts, observation of behavior becomes the primary data source.

Diagnostic Tests and Procedures

Clients with altered communication are evaluated by speech pathologists, who perform detailed assessments of speech, expression, comprehension, and swallowing. Results from this assessment contribute to the plan of care and help to establish communication with clients. Clients with altered thought processes may require extensive testing to determine contributing (and possibly reversible) factors.

Physiologic Tests. Physiologic causes of confusion can result from disorders of multiple systems. Their diagnoses and management require multiple tests and procedures, from simple urinalysis to highly technical scans. Nurses use tests such as weight, vital signs, serum electrolytes, complete blood count, cultures, and measures of oxygen saturation to identify potential contributors. Monitoring these parameters helps to identify imbalances and to target early interventions to prevent complications.

Arterial Oxygen. Arterial oxygen level is best determined by measuring arterial blood gases. An oxygen partial pressure greater than 60 mm Hg reflects adequate oxygenation. A noninvasive technique for assessing oxygenation is pulse oximetry, which measures oxygen saturation (percentage of hemoglobin that is bound to oxygen). A saturation of 90% correlates with a partial pressure of 60 mm Hg, given a normal level of hemoglobin. If a low (less than 90%) value is determined, oxygen therapy and further evaluation may be indicated.

Electrolytes. A serum sodium level less than 135 mEq/L or greater than 145 mEq/L may result in cognitive impairment. Mild confusion can progress to agitation or severe confusion with hallucinations or delusions followed by stupor and coma if the condition is untreated. Because brain cells can adapt to slow changes, severity of symptoms is related to how rapidly the sodium level drops.

An elevated level of serum calcium can cause severe defects in neuromuscular activity with cognitive manifestations of lethargy or decreased level of consciousness. When the total serum calcium exceeds 14 mg/dL (normal level is 8.5 to 10.5 mg/dL), confusion is common and further increases in calcium concentration may result in coma or death.

Serum Glucose. Serum glucose levels below 70 mg/dL typically cause shakiness or nervousness but can progress to cause altered cognition. Although the determination of serum glucose from venipuncture is the most accurate method of measurement, the widespread availability of capillary blood glucose monitoring has promoted more reliable self-assessment of serum glucose.

Ammonia and Urea. Ammonia and urea are potentially toxic byproducts of protein metabolism. Liver failure can cause elevated ammonia levels; high blood ammonia levels are toxic to brain cells. Kidney failure can cause an elevated blood urea nitrogen level and produce confusion.

Toxic Levels of Drugs. Toxic levels of drugs can result from impaired ability to metabolize or excrete them. Serum concentration of many drugs can be measured to determine therapeutic and toxic levels. People with impaired hepatic or renal function are at risk for drug toxicity and require dosage reduction and regular monitoring. Drug and toxicologic screening is indicated for drug overdose or toxic exposure.

Tests of Cognitive Function. Intellectual function consists of short- and long-term memory, comprehension, and concentration. These straightforward abilities are easily tested and converted to objective measurements with standardized tools. Intelligence or IQ tests attempt to measure intellectual function. These tests rely on measuring verbal ability and vocabulary within a structured questioning format. They are standardized to the vocabulary and cultural experience of white, middle-class Americans and have questionable validity when administered to other ethnic and socioeconomic groups. Remember that standardized tests of verbal ability are not sensitive to sociocultural differences and so should not be used to assess "normality" for all groups. The primary usefulness of standardized tests is that each person using them encounters the same information, thus providing a common base of information and quantification for comparison.

Because of their limited attention span, children find it difficult to cooperate with tedious assessment procedures. Assessment tools for children focus on the observation of behavior, especially behavior elicited by a standard set of stimuli.

Standardized tools are available for the objective assessment of mental status. Two examples are the Pfeiffer Short Portable Mental Status Questionnaire (Pfeiffer, 1975) and the Mini–Mental Status Exam (Folstein, Folstein, & McHugh, 1975; Displays 45-3 and 45-4). A score of 7 or less on the Pfeiffer or 20 or less on the Mini–Mental Status Exam indicates significant cognitive impairment. These tools are most useful when given on an ambulatory basis to healthy people repeatedly, which allows identification of changes from baseline. Administering these tools during an acute confusional state can help quantify daily changes. Without a premorbid baseline and in the presence of physiologic imbalance though, little can be determined about the client's change from baseline function. There is a specific battery of tests used to diagnose dementia.

Behavioral Observation Scales. Two instruments have been designed to measure behavioral aspects of acute confusion in hospitalized clients. The NEECHAM Confusion Scale is an observational scale designed to detect unobtrusively cues to the onset of acute confusion and to monitor recovery (Neelon, Champagne, McConnell, Carlson, & Fink, 1992). The Clinical Assessment of Confusion–A scale is a 25-item observational scale that assesses cognition, general behavior, motor

DISPLAY 45-3

🖫 **PFEIFFER MENTAL STATUS QUESTIONNAIRE**

1. What is today's date? _____
2. What day of the week is it? _____
3. What is the name of this place? _____
4. What is your telephone number? _____
   If none, what is your address?
   _____
5. How old are you? _____
6. When were you born? _____
7. Who is the President of the U.S. now? _____
8. Who was the President before him? _____
9. What is your mother's maiden name? _____
10. Subtract 3 from 20 and keep going down to 0.
    _____

Total numbers of errors _____

From Pfeiffer, E. (1975). A short portable mental status questionnaire for the assessment of organic brain deficit in elderly patients. *Journal of the American Geriatric Society, 23,* 433–443.

activity, orientation, and psychotic or neurotic behaviors (Vermeersch & Henly, 1997).

NURSING DIAGNOSES

The accepted North American Nursing Diagnosis Association (NANDA) nursing diagnoses for clients with cognitive impairment are Acute Confusion, Chronic Confusion, Impaired Memory, Disturbed Thought Processes, and Impaired Verbal Communication. Each diagnosis describes alterations in cognitive function that interfere with daily living. These nursing diagnoses are classified by NANDA within the taxonomic domain of Perception and Cognition (NANDA, 2001).

Diagnostic Statement: Acute Confusion

Definition. Acute Confusion is the abrupt onset of a cluster of global, transient changes and disturbances in attention, cognition, psychomotor activity, level of consciousness, and/or sleep–wake cycle (NANDA, 2001).

Defining Characteristics. Of the defining characteristics or clinical cues that point to this nursing diagnosis, one of the following major characteristics must be present:

- Fluctuation in cognition
- Fluctuation in sleep–wake cycle

DISPLAY 45-4

MINI–MENTAL STATE EXAMINATION

Orientation
What is the (year) (season) (date) (day) (month)?
                                                    5 _____

Where are we: (state) (county) (town) (hospital)
    (floor)?   5 _____

Registration
Name 3 objects: 1 second to say each. Then ask the
client all 3 after you have said them. Give 1 point for
each correct answer. Then repeat them until he learns
all 3. Count trials and record. (trials _____).
                                                    3 _____

Attention and Calculation
Serial 7s (begin with 100 and count backwards by 7).
1 point for each correct answer. Stop after 5 answers.
Alternatively, spell "world" backwards.   5 _____

Recall
Ask for the 3 objects repeated above. Give 1 point for
each correct answer.   5 _____

Language
Name a pencil, and watch. (2 points)
Repeat the following: "No, ifs, ands, or buts."
    (1 point)
Follow a 3-stage command: "Take a paper in your
    right hand, fold it in half, and put it on the floor."
    (3 points)
Read and obey the following: Close your eyes.
    (1 point)
Write a sentence. (1 point)
Copy design. (1 point)   9 _____
                              Total Score **30** _____

Assess level of consciousness along a continuum:

_____

Alert   Drowsy   Stupor   Coma

Adapted from Folstein, M. F., Folstein, S. E., & McHugh, P. R.
(1975). "Mini-Mental state": A practical method of grading the
cognitive state of patients for the clinician. *Journal of Psychiatric
Research, 12,* 189–198. Copyright 1975. Pergamon Press, Ltd.

- Fluctuation in level of consciousness
- Fluctuation in psychomotor activity
- Increased agitation or restlessness
- Misperceptions
- Hallucination
- Lack of motivation to initiate and/or follow through with
  goal-directed or purposeful behavior (NANDA, 2001)

Related Factors. Related factors show a patterned relationship with the nursing diagnosis and may be described as an-

APPLY YOUR KNOWLEDGE

Joe Moran, 52, is admitted to the neurologic unit after
a brawl in a bar where he fell and hit his head. When
you enter his room to do the morning assessment, he
is very agitated and starts yelling, "I don't belong
here!" He has an IV infusion and he is trying to get
out of bed.
    What additional assessment data do you need to col-
lect at this time? How can you help maintain safety for
Mr. Moran?
    Check your answer in Appendix A.

tecedent to, associated with, related to, contributing to, or
abetting the diagnosed condition (NANDA, 2001). Factors
NANDA has identified as related to Acute Confusion include
age older than 60 years, dementia, alcohol abuse, drug abuse,
and delirium (NANDA, 2001).
    Etiologic factors for Acute Confusion can be physiologic,
environmental, and emotional in nature. Physiologic factors
include alterations in oxygenation and biochemical components, genetic disorders, and dementias. Environmental factors include change in surroundings or routine, loss of significant others, altered sensory input (too much or too little),
abuse or misuse of alcohol or drugs, and fear of the unknown.
Emotional factors include anxiety, depression, grief, family
conflict, or separation. Most often, the etiology of acute confusion is multifactorial (i.e., the presence of more than one
etiologic factor is common).

Diagnostic Statement: Chronic Confusion

Definition. Chronic Confusion is an irreversible, long-
standing and/or progressive deterioration of intellect and personality characterized by decreased ability to interpret environmental stimuli; decreased capacity for intellectual thought
processes; and manifested by disturbances of memory, orientation, and behavior (NANDA, 2001).

Defining Characteristics. Defining characteristics or clinical
clues that point to this nursing diagnosis include the following:

- Clinical evidence of organic impairment
- Altered interpretation/response to stimuli
- Progressive/long-standing cognitive impairment
- Altered personality
- Impaired memory (short- and long-term)
- Impaired socialization
- No change in level of consciousness (NANDA, 2001)

Related Factors. Factors NANDA has identified as related to
Chronic Confusion include Alzheimer's disease, Korsakoff's
psychosis, multi-infarct dementia, head injury, and cerebral
vascular accident (NANDA, 2001).

Diagnostic Statement: Impaired Memory

Definition. Impaired Memory is the state in which a person experiences the inability to remember or recall bits of information or behavioral skills. Impaired memory may be attributed to pathophysiologic or situational causes that are either temporary or permanent (NANDA, 2001).

Defining Characteristics. Defining characteristics or clinical clues that point to this nursing diagnosis include the following:

- Observed or reported experiences of forgetting
- Inability to determine if a behavior was performed
- Inability to learn or retain new skills or information
- Inability to perform a previously learned skill
- Inability to recall factual information
- Forgets to perform a behavior at a scheduled time
- Inability to recall recent or past events (NANDA, 2001)

Related Factors. Factors NANDA has identified as related to Impaired Memory include acute or chronic hypoxia, anemia, decreased cardiac output, fluid and electrolyte imbalance, neurologic disturbances, and excessive environmental disturbances (NANDA, 20001).

Diagnostic Statement: Disturbed Thought Processes

Definition. Disturbed Thought Processes is a state in which a person experiences a disruption in cognitive operations and activities (NANDA, 2001).

Defining Characteristics. Defining characteristics or clinical clues that point to this nursing diagnosis include the following:

- Inaccurate interpretation of environment
- Cognitive dissonance (disorganized thinking)
- Distractibility
- Memory deficit or problems
- Egocentricity (self-centered or existing only as created in the mind)
- Hypervigilance or hypovigilance (attention dysfunction)
- Inappropriate nonreality-based thinking (NANDA, 2001)

Related Factors. NANDA is developing related factors (NANDA, 2001).

Diagnostic Statement: Impaired Verbal Communication

Definition. Impaired Verbal Communication is the state in which a person experiences a decreased, delayed, or absent ability to receive, process, transmit, and use a system of symbols (NANDA, 2001).

Defining Characteristics. Defining characteristics or clinical clues that point to this nursing diagnosis include the following:

- Willful refusal to speak
- Disorientation in time, space, person
- Inability to speak dominant language that is the person's first language (e.g., English, Spanish)
- Does not or cannot speak
- Verbalizes with difficulty (e.g., dysarthria)
- Difficulty expressing thought verbally (e.g., aphasia)
- Inappropriate verbalization
- Difficulty forming words or sentences
- Stuttering
- Slurring words
- Absence of eye contact or difficulty attending
- Difficulty in comprehending and maintaining the usual communication pattern
- Partial or total visual deficit
- Inability or difficulty in the use of facial or body expressions (NANDA, 2001)

Related Factors. Related factors that may contribute to a client's diagnosis include physiologic factors such as decrease in circulation to the brain from interference to vascular circulation or brain tumor. Communication problems may be related to physical barriers (tracheostomy, intubation) that prevent normal air movement through the vocal folds; an anatomic defect such as cleft palate that mechanically interferes with speech; or psychological barriers (psychosis, lack of stimuli, absence of significant others, altered perceptions, lack of information, stress, alteration of self-concept). In addition, cultural differences in which culture defines the meaning of the communication and developmental or age-related factors may limit communication (NANDA, 1999).

Related Nursing Diagnoses

Related diagnoses, such as Impaired Environmental Interpretation Syndrome, may be antecedent to the presenting diagnosis. Other factors that can affect cognition encompass many nursing diagnoses. For example, Imbalanced Nutrition: Less Than Body Requirements, Hypothermia, Hyperthermia, Ineffective Tissue Perfusion (Cerebral), Excess Fluid Volume, Deficient Fluid Volume, Decreased Cardiac Output, Impaired Gas Exchange, Fatigue, Disturbed Sleep Pattern, and Pain are nursing diagnoses that can have direct pathophysiologic effects on cognition. Social Isolation, Dysfunctional Grieving, Anxiety, and Fear are nursing diagnoses related to environmental or emotional factors that may adversely affect cognition.

Consequences of altered cognitive function may include the following nursing diagnoses: Self-Care Deficits, Ineffective Role Performance, and Impaired Home Maintenance. Nursing care extends to the family of the client with altered thought processes. Nursing diagnoses that might be relevant for families include Deficient Knowledge, Ineffective Denial,

Anticipatory Grieving, Compromised Family Coping, and Caregiver Role Strain.

Because communication alterations may interfere with roles and relationships, related nursing diagnoses include Interrupted Family Processes, Impaired Parenting, Ineffective Role Performance, Impaired Social Interaction, Social Isolation, and Grieving. The specific disturbances in roles and relationships determine which, if any, of these related diagnoses are appropriate to consider.

OUTCOME IDENTIFICATION AND PLANNING

After nursing diagnoses and related factors are identified, nurses plan with clients and/or family outcomes and interventions. The goals of nursing intervention for clients with impaired cognition focus on prevention and early recognition of the disturbance, reversal of contributing factors, and provision of an environment that compensates for existing impairments, does not predispose to new impairments, and protects clients from harm. For clients with impaired verbal communication, the goals of nursing intervention focus on establishing alternate communication methods and preventing sequelae such as loneliness and role alterations. Goals need to be individualized and take into consideration each client's history, areas of risk, evidence of dysfunction, and related objective data. Examples of goals for the client with Acute Confusion include the following:

- The client will express a realistic perception of reality.
- The client will have absence of injury related to the confusion.

Examples of goals for the client with Chronic Confusion include the following:

- The client will experience adequate support to compensate for deficits.
- The client will participate in a safe, protected environment.

Examples of goals for the client with Impaired Memory include the following:

- The client will use memory aids to compensate for deficits.
- The client will participate safely in his or her home environment.

Examples of goals for the client with Disturbed Thought Processes include the following:

- The client will initiate conversation with at least one person.
- The client will verbalize intent to comply with prescribed medication regimen.

Examples of goals for the client with Impaired Verbal Communication include the following:

- The client will communicate basic needs.
- The client will verbalize experiencing less frustration with communication.

PLANNING: Examples of NIC/NOC Interventions

Accepted Cognitive Processes Nursing Interventions Classification (NIC)
Communication Enhancement: Hearing Deficit
Communication Enhancement: Speech Deficit
Delirium Management
Delusion Management
Dementia Management
Memory Training

Accepted Cognitive Processes Nursing Outcomes Classification (NOC)
Cognitive Ability
Cognitive Orientation
Communication Ability
Communication: Expressive Ability
Communication: Receptive Ability
Distorted Thought Control
Electrolyte & Acid/Base Balance
Information Processing
Memory
Neurological Status: Consciousness
Sleep

Refer to the following for specifics regarding NIC/NOC:
McCloskey, J., & Bulechek, G. (2000). *Iowa Intervention Project: Nursing Interventions Classification (NIC)* 2nd Ed. St. Louis, MO: C.V. Mosby.
Johnson, M., & Maas, M. (2000). *Iowa Outcomes Project: Nursing Outcomes Classification (NOC)* 2nd Ed. St. Louis, MO: C.V. Mosby.

Examples of some nursing interventions useful in planning are outlined in the accompanying display and discussed in the next section of the chapter.

IMPLEMENTATION

Appropriate nursing interventions vary with the specific nursing diagnosis. Preventing, reversing, or slowing the progression of dysfunction along with providing for safety and dignity are central goals of nursing care. For clients with impaired cognition, preventing alterations in roles and relationships and supporting effective relationships are central focuses of nursing intervention. Relationships are affected by the ability to communicate thoughts, feelings, needs, and other intimate aspects. Nursing interventions need to recognize those relationships and their importance to clients.

Health Promotion

Encouraging Healthy Lifestyles
Primary prevention of cognitive impairment involves maximizing brain reserve and minimizing brain damage across the lifespan (Nolan & Blass, 1992). Maximizing brain reserve begins with adequate prenatal and early childhood nutrition and educational experiences. Preventing brain damage means preventing unintentional injuries and toxic exposures. Prevention of cardiovascular disease, which can lead to cere-

brovascular disease and stroke, will prevent the major cause of impaired verbal communication.

Maintaining a lifestyle that includes adequate nutrition, rest, regular exercise, stress management, and social activity is essential. A balanced diet with sufficient protein, iron, and other nutrients is required for cells to function optimally. Serum imbalances of water, sodium, calcium, and glucose can be prevented through adequate fluid intake throughout the day in conjunction with a balanced diet. For people with known dysfunctions that place them at risk for some serum imbalances (e.g., diabetes mellitus), teach the importance of regulating the dysfunction, recognizing early indications of imbalances, and initiating preventive dietary or fluid therapy. Chapters 36 and 37 present complete discussions of ways to promote fluid and electrolyte balance and good nutrition.

Oxygen perfusion to brain cells is enhanced through the practice of regular exercise. Regular exercise also enhances cardiovascular conditioning, improves circulation throughout the body, and contributes to a sense of well-being and refreshment. Encourage clients to develop the habit of regular, vigorous exercise. Depending on the client, exercise may range from energetic walking to active sports.

Consult a dietitian to help clients plan menus, change recipes, and learn to read food labels. Clients should monitor their serum cholesterol regularly to determine the effects of a low-fat diet and an exercise program. Encourage clients who have high blood pressure to maintain their prescribed medication regimen, to check their blood pressure routinely, and to follow up with their physicians.

Smoking increases the risk of cardiovascular disease and throat cancer. Encourage clients to quit. Early warning signs of throat cancer are nagging cough and chronic hoarseness. Awareness of the warning signals can be helpful for early detection or prevention.

Equally important as sufficient exercise is adequate sleep and rest. Inadequate or interrupted sleep cycles usually result in loss of REM sleep. Manifestations are fatigue and, if prolonged, forgetfulness, confusion, and disorientation. Encourage people to maintain regular sleep patterns so they obtain sufficient sleep and feel rested when awake. Counsel clients to create an environment that is conducive to rest and sleep.

Stress management can contribute to healthy cognition by minimizing distractions, improving rest, and enhancing concentration. Effective coping skills allow clients to channel stress productively and to dissipate resulting tension. Exercise, as previously discussed, is one type of coping skill to encourage.

Cognitive skills developed throughout life need to be practiced regularly to be maintained. Social interaction is one such skill in which clients need to participate regularly for enjoyment of human contact, stimulation of conversation, and confirmation of personhood. Use social interaction on a one-on-one basis with clients and encourage opportunities for interaction with others in informal groups. These interactions can provide client feedback related to reality orientation, self-concept, and sensory perception.

For people with sensory impairments, a number of assistive devices can help maintain and promote cognitive function. People who have hearing difficulties can often be fitted with hearing aids. Telephone companies can provide equipment to assist with communication, and television offers programs with printed captions that permit hearing-impaired people access to cognitive stimulation. Talking books and other services from public libraries help supplement cognitive input for the visually impaired.

Improving Memory

Fatigue, stress, and illness may temporarily reduce the efficiency with which clients are able to store information or retrieve it from memory. Reassure clients that, in most situations, no organic basis exists for simple, occasional forgetfulness. Reducing stress, relieving fatigue, or recovering from illness should eliminate the temporary difficulty.

For people with minimal memory problems, memory training programs and devices may be beneficial. Memory training programs focus on personal and compensatory capabilities to stimulate cognitive function. Encourage such clients to participate in memory training or to use principles of memory enhancement. Focusing attention deliberately on the information to be remembered helps to reduce stress and to minimize distractions. Using both visual and auditory senses provides two important sources of perceptual input for cognition. Making lists, using mnemonic devices (formulas or patterns of letters to aid in remembering), and developing other association techniques can assist with remembering tasks or information. The regular practice or rehearsal of retrieving information from the memory helps maintain the skill. For example, doing crossword puzzles regularly helps many people rehearse the skill of knowledge and information retrieval from the long-term memory.

Maintaining Learning Skills

Developing learning skills is nearly as important as the actual knowledge gained. These learning skills, developed in childhood, need to be practiced, reinforced, and used throughout life. Strengthen these skills when teaching. People learn better when the relevance of the information is apparent; for example, if a person has experienced side effects of a medication, the learning related to potential effects of other medications has increased relevance because of the desire to prevent problems in the future.

Learning improves when it is meaningful and linked with previous learning. To illustrate, if the nurse wants to teach an automobile mechanic about the importance of exercise, associating various body parts with analogous parts of an automobile may increase meaningfulness. As another example, for a person needing to learn about medications, the classifications and generic names of drugs will be less meaningful than the color, shape, size, and frequency of the medication.

Nursing Interventions for Impaired Cognitive Function

When a diagnosis of impaired cognitive function is made, nurses can intervene to help identify causative factors, to restore or improve cognitive function, to protect the client from

OUTCOME-BASED TEACHING PLAN

Mrs. Harold has come to the clinic with concerns about her husband. Mr. Harold has had increasing problems with memory as evidenced by repeatedly asking the same questions, telling his wife the same things repeatedly, and forgetting where he puts things. Mrs. Harold thinks that he is beginning to realize this too. She wants some guidance on how to help him.

OUTCOME: Mrs. Harold will assist Mr. Harold to maintain orientation as to time and place.

Strategies

- Explore with Mr. Harold his concerns about his memory.
- If Mr. Harold is motivated to improve his memory, use cues for reality data such as clocks, calendars, and verbal reminders.
- Encourage Mrs. Harold to speak clearly and in short, simple statements.
- Discuss the need to maintain a predictable routine or schedule for Mr. Harold.
- Promote the use of lists and of stability of familiar objects in the home so he can develop habits of always placing things in the same location.
- Encourage activities, visits, and meaningful interaction with family and friends.
- Positively reinforce small changes in behavior that indicate increasing orientation to reality.
- Encourage Mrs. Harold to focus Mr. Harold's attention deliberately (with little stress and distractions) on information he needs to remember.
- Suggest the use of both vision and hearing to provide input from two perceptual sources.
- Discuss the usefulness of making lists and using other association techniques to help Mr. Harold remember tasks and information.
- Encourage the regular practice or rehearsal of retrieving information from memory such as doing crossword puzzles.

injury, and to help the family cope. Nurses have both an independent and a collaborative role in identifying clients at risk for acute confusion, modifying or structuring the environment, and initiating appropriate teaching. Nurses, as the healthcare professionals with the most client contact, are in the best position to monitor changes in cognitive function, to communicate these to the healthcare team, and to intervene as appropriate.

Cognitive deficits may be acute and reversible or chronic and irreversible, or an acute insult may exacerbate a chronic deficit. Nursing interventions designed to improve function include similar measures and activities for clients with each of these deficits. The major focus of nursing care is restoring

physiologic balance while creating an environment that provides appropriate sensory stimulation, adequate assistance with ADLs, and protection from physical injury.

Orientation to Surroundings

Clients who have difficulty with understanding require special considerations. Clients who are experiencing receptive (Wernicke's) aphasia may also be suffering from confusion related to this unfamiliar state. Maintaining a structured environment assists clients in adapting to cognitive alteration and in reestablishing communication. Structured routines minimize the number of factors on which clients must focus. Sequenced events, consistent daily schedules, calendars, and frequent reminders contribute to structure. To assist with orientation, ask clients why they are in the healthcare facility or where they are; gently correct false answers. Supportive environmental cues, such as the presence of a current calendar and a large, visible clock, assist clients with orientation to time.

SAFETY ALERT
Provide structure and predictable routines whenever possible to minimize distractions and potential injuries.

Alternative Communication Methods

A plan of care that provides clients with Broca's or nonfluent aphasia with an effective, efficient means to communicate is essential. Encourage clients to use any means available to express themselves. Methods of communication that may be helpful include offering clients pictures at which to point, having clients use gestures, or letting them show what they want. Writing and reading skills may be impaired along with speech, therefore, these skills may not be useful alternatives.

If it is difficult to understand what a client has said, be honest and let the client know. Ask the client to try again and perhaps use gestures to assist with understanding. If the client tries again and you still do not understand, take a rest, and come back in a few minutes. Do not pressure the client; some symptoms worsen if clients are fatigued, upset, or anxious. Be alert to the client's daily schedule, and allow for adequate rest at night and naps during the day.

For clients who have lost the ability to produce sound because of a laryngectomy, communication may be restored through the use of sophisticated electronic or computer communication devices or an electronic larynx. In these cases, nurses should know how to use these devices. Clients with disabilities, such as visual, mobility, hearing, learning, and communication disorders, may benefit from computer adaptations (Merrow & Corbett, 1994).

The Client With Dysarthria. To facilitate communication with a dysarthric client, face the client to read his or her lips. Augment communication by gestures, written messages, a communication board, or flash cards. Encourage the client to use slow speech, to speak loudly, and to take breaths between sentences. Ask the client to repeat unclear words. If the client appears tired, ask questions that require short answers. Establish a specific care plan and a routine for delivering care to reduce the time the client would otherwise need to explain his or her care to others.

Environmental Restrictions

The number of visitors with whom clients have to communicate may increase frustration for clients with impaired verbal communication. Many people and noises in the environment can interfere with cognitive functioning and understanding. Quiet environments allow clients to focus on understanding, speaking, or communicating.

Nurses may find that environmental restrictions are advantageous in assisting communication with clients. Be aware of excessive noise levels caused by equipment, loudspeaker systems, and/or other people. Limit the number of visitors present at any given time. Teach visitors how to communicate effectively with clients by using thoughtful methods such as one person speaking at a time and not carrying on simultaneous conversations.

Fluid Intake and Nutrition

Because shifts in nutrients, electrolytes, and fluids contribute to cognitive changes, monitor the food and fluid intake of clients. People who are ill may not feel like eating or may not find food appealing. Allow clients to choose foods they particularly like. Give supportive encouragement and monitoring so that diets are reasonably balanced.

Similarly, clients may not experience thirst even when increased fluid intake is needed. Keep fluids within easy reach of clients and give reminders to drink. Fluid intake and output records are useful to observe for patterns of fluid intake. The most accurate guideline for the adequacy of food and fluid intake is regular measurement of body weight. For clients at risk for fluid imbalances, a regular schedule of weighing will need to be established.

Clients and families will need health teaching regarding the factors that place them at risk for food and fluid imbalances. Diabetic clients who may have fluctuations in serum glucose must understand appropriate diet and medication management. Persons taking diuretics must understand the effects and side effects and know not to withhold water unless specifically prescribed by the physician or nurse practitioner. Clients who have any identified risk factors for the development of cognitive dysfunction should receive health teaching related to the problem, along with supportive nursing care.

Clients with chronic confusion need particularly close monitoring of food and fluid intake. With loss of judgment, some clients fail to respond to normal signals of appetite, thirst, or satiety. They may not eat or drink unless reminded, may overeat, may eat inappropriate things, or forget how to eat. Sitting with these clients while they eat, reminding them to eat, and assisting them with the mechanics of eating may be useful. For some clients, socialization opportunities when eating at a table with others may help to reinforce desired behaviors and activities. For others, a quiet environment free of distractions is best.

Clients with dysarthria need to be evaluated and treated by a speech therapist to ensure safe swallowing. Their intake should be monitored to ensure adequate caloric intake. Clients with difficulty swallowing should be placed in a full upright position when eating. They will usually tolerate foods with texture and consistency and thickened liquids better than thin, clear fluids. If clients are unable to consume an adequate number of calories safely, tube feeding may be required.

Mobility

Encourage isolated or withdrawn clients to move around. Physical activity improves ventilation, cardiovascular function, and oxygenation of the brain. It also helps people feel better physically and personally. Improved socialization is an important aspect of increased mobility. As clients move around more, even on hospital units, they increase contact with other people. Contact with others and exposure to more environments provide increased stimulation and reinforcement of reality.

> ### 🥛 SAFETY ALERT
> **Supervise clients with confusion during ambulation and other activities. They may have altered judgment as to where they are. To prevent potential falls, be sure the environment is free from unnecessary obstructions. Provide adequate lighting.**

Selectively providing sensory stimulation for all the senses is an important consideration, particularly for those clients with chronic confusion. In addition to hearing and seeing, make use of touch through personal contact and varied fabric textures, taste through varieties of food and beverages, and smell through food and flowers (Fig. 45-5). While providing stimulation, be sure to avoid overstimulating clients who have chronic confusion. Overstimulation can result in apparently purposeless behaviors such as wandering, agitation, and aggression. Recognize signs of overstimulation (i.e., inability to maintain eye contact, increased or decreased verbalizations,

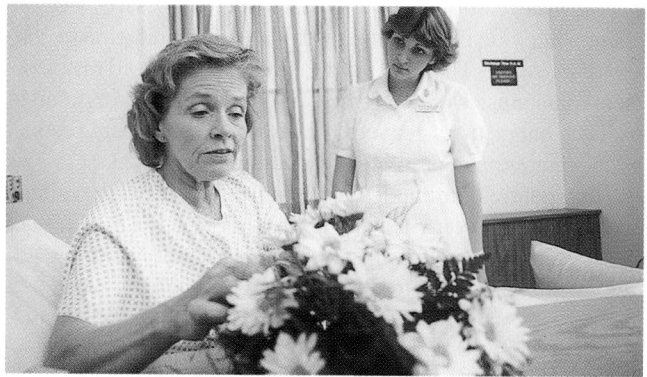

FIGURE 45-5 Vision, smell, and touch stimulate the client's cognitive processes and help the client maintain touch with reality.

or attempts to avoid or retreat from the situation) and reduce the level of stimulation to prevent these behaviors.

Safety

Persons with altered cognitive function are at risk for injury and require nursing interventions to ensure safety. For example, when clients are hospitalized or ill elsewhere, are in an unfamiliar location, and/or are subject to strange routines, they may temporarily lose orientation and think they are at home. They may be at risk for falling while trying to get out of bed or while going to the bathroom. Safety measures such as orienting clients to the room, the nurse call system, and lights help to prevent accidents and injuries.

Safety becomes a primary concern for clients with progressively impaired judgment. In institutional settings, safety measures for clients with chronic confusion involve keeping the bed at the lowest level; frequently assisting clients to get in and out of bed; supervising wandering behavior; and providing secured locks or alerting systems for elevators and doors. Monitoring behavior may identify relationships and temporal patterns that can be used to understand the nonverbal client's needs.

Physical or chemical restraints generally are not useful in maintaining safety. Studies have demonstrated that agitated behaviors tend to increase after the application of restraints (Werner, Cohen-Mansfield, Braun, et al., 1989). The desire for wandering behaviors intensifies, falls are not prevented, and risk of serious injury from falls increases (Capezuti, Evans, Strumpf, & Maislin, 1996; Capezuti, Strumpf, Evans, Grisso & Maislin, 1998). Many long-term care facilities are becoming more creative in their safety management. Innovations such as enclosed courtyards provide unlimited access for clients with dementia to wander within a protected confine.

Changes in routine and environment may upset and distress clients with chronic confusion. For this reason, the care environment should be as predictable as possible. Meals, baths, treatments, and other activities should be at regular times with familiar staff people. If changes are necessary, remember that clients with chronic confusion will need additional support and reassurance.

Therapeutic Communication

Therapeutic communication means that nurses respect the clients' individuality and use modes of communication to convey that respect. Therapeutic communication is used in assessment to obtain accurate information but is equally important in ongoing interactions between nurses and clients. Communication techniques are presented in detail in Chapter 23.

Therapeutic communication enables nurses to reevaluate and to intervene consistently by using information that's as accurate as possible. Regular use of these communication techniques allows nurses to detect cognitive changes whenever they occur; so the interventions are free from personal bias.

Understanding verbal and nonverbal responses is important in caring for people with chronic confusion. For example, clients who repeatedly call for "Mama" may be expressing needs for nurturing and affection. Clients who take food from the plates of others may be communicating that they are still hungry (Hall & Gerdner, 1999). Nonverbal communication can express positive regard through touch, facial expression, and eye contact. Finally, clients without other means of communication may express distress or dislike through behaviors such as spitting, turning away, or striking out. The importance of nonverbal communication may increase as other cognitive abilities decline.

Therapeutic communication with clients who have Chronic Confusion may be enhanced by assuming a nonthreatening posture (e.g., sitting at eye level with the client). Explain what you are going to do in a calm, friendly tone of voice. Avoid using commands or asking "why" questions. Do not try logically to convince a resistive client to comply with your requests; leaving the area for a few minutes and returning is usually more successful.

Reality Orientation

Reality orientation is a nursing technique used to assist clients in restoring awareness of reality. A hallmark in reinforcing reality for hospitalized clients is to provide those environmental cues on which people depend for orientation to time and place. Having the change in lighting match the usual day and night cuing is helpful. Clients who are in specialized units with few windows and lights have greater difficulty relying on environmental cues.

Clocks and calendars that allow clients to know the date, day of the week, and time of day are important sources of input for reality orientation. Additional interventions include allowing uninterrupted sleep periods when possible and encouraging visits from family and friends. Contact with familiar objects, such as photographs, favorite chairs, or special books, is also useful.

Allowing clients the maximal advantage in relation to sensory–perceptual data is equally important in reinforcing reality. If clients normally wear glasses or hearing aids, ensure these are available. Glasses must be clean and hearing aids adjusted correctly. If information that clients take in is as accurate as possible, interpreting and responding to reality are easier.

Although clients with irreversible changes such as dementia will not return to previous levels of cognitive functioning, nurses need to assist them in maintaining existing levels of function for as long as possible. Nonconfrontational reality orientation is an appropriate intervention, and a variety of modalities can be used such as clocks, calendars, lighting cycles, or personal contact. However, verbal attempts to orient a client with dementia to time, place, or person are often futile and may exacerbate behavioral problems. Attempts to understand and respond to the covert meaning of the client's utterances are more effective. Assist the family in understanding how to work with the client through teaching.

Socialization Therapies

Socialization therapies can take many forms such as music, recreation, and reminiscence. The purpose of these therapies is to encourage clients to expand contact with others in social settings in an effort to increase cognitive stimuli. For some

THERAPEUTIC DIALOGUE
Memory Loss

Scene for Thought

Carmen Morales has come in for a regular blood pressure check and has brought her grandmother, Rosa Gomez, to be checked too. Mrs. Gomez, age 84, smiles and affectionately pats the nurse's hand as they meet. Carmen tells the nurse that "Abuelita" is having some trouble with her memory, and the family is worried that she might be unsafe at home. She forgot to turn off the stove, has trouble with the household appliances, and is getting irritable when the children make noise after school. This problem has been occurring over the last 2 months. Mrs. Gomez has no physical problems except controlled high blood pressure and occasional constipation.

Less Effective

Nurse: Mrs. Gomez, you've heard what Carmen and I have been talking about? *(Mrs. Gomez nods, smiling brightly.)* What do you think?

Client: I lose my memory sometimes, but it's nothing to worry about. I'm old, I'm supposed to lose my memory sometimes. *(Continues to smile.)*

Nurse: It's true that as we get older our memories get a little worn out *(pats her hand)*, but Carmen is worried about your safety while you're taking care of the cooking, cleaning, and so on. I think that it would be a good idea for you to see one of the geriatric nurse specialists here in the clinic. He could talk with you, maybe run some tests, work with you on your memory. He's very good, caring, and has lots of experience with people your age. What do you think?

Client: Am I sick or something? Why do I need a specialist? *(Looks at Carmen anxiously.)*

Carmen: It's okay, Abuelita, we'll go see what this other nurse has to say. I'm sure he can help us with your memory. *(Rises to leave.)* Come on Abuelita, let's go and make the appointment.

Client: Okay, querida, if you say so. But I don't understand all this fuss over a little memory loss. *(Grumbles on her way out.)*

More Effective

Nurse: Mrs. Gomez, you've heard what Carmen and I have been talking about? *(Mrs. Gomez nods, smiling brightly.)* What do you think about that?

Client: I lose my memory sometimes, but it's nothing to worry about. I'm old. I'm supposed to lose my memory sometimes. *(Continues to smile.)*

Nurse: You expect that you will lose your memory as you grow older?

Client: Sure. My parents didn't live to be very old, but I remember my grandmother not remembering things very well by the time she was 70! So I'm doing fine. *(Gives a little laugh.)*

Nurse: I'm wondering if you can think of times that you have more trouble remembering than others.

Client: *(Concentrates for a minute.)* I think it's when there's too much commotion in the house or when I don't get enough sleep. Then I can't remember things very well. *(Turns to Carmen.)* That's when I forgot to turn off the stove, querida mia, and it was only once. Yes, it's when there's a lot to distract me from my work.

Nurse: I understand. You said you don't get enough sleep sometimes? Tell me a little more, please.

Client: Certainly. I sometimes have to go to the bathroom in the middle of the night. Then it's hard for me to get back to sleep all alone in that big bed. My husband died 2 years ago, and it's still hard for me to sleep in that big bed. *(She doesn't smile now.)*

Nurse: You're still missing him, I can see that. I guess it helps to take care of the family the way you do.

Client: Yes, it does help. And I want to do the best I can for them. I don't want them to worry about me, or send me away. *(Looks at Carmen with tears in her eyes.)*

Carmen: No, Abuelita, we don't want to send you away; we just want you to be safe and comfortable. Don't cry, don't cry. *(Puts her arm around her grandmother.)*

Nurse: I think if we three talk together we can come up with some ways to help you get better sleep, Mrs. Gomez. And there are some tricks I can think of to help you remember things better. Let's work together on this. What do you say?

Client: I would be happy to! Thank you very much! *(Squeezes the nurse's hand and smiles.)*

Critical Thinking Challenge

- Although Mrs. Gomez ultimately received effective care in both dialogues, detect what made the second dialogue "more effective" from the client's point of view.
- Explain what factors the first nurse never found out about.
- Describe the relationship between anxiety and cognitive processes.

people, contact within usual social groups, such as senior citizen centers, volunteer groups, church groups, or recreation groups, may provide beneficial stimulation.

For clients who are at risk for being isolated or who require more protected environments, reality orientation groups or day-care centers provide the same type of human contact and stimulation. Developing an ongoing relationship with people who staff these groups or centers provides continuity of care and consistent support for cognitive function.

In reminiscence therapy, clients use recall of the past to assist in clarifying meaning in the present or reconciling conflict. This therapy is particularly useful for older clients because it contributes to successful aging by maintaining self-esteem and reinforcing cognitive function. It requires facilitation by a nurse or other health professional skilled in group process and in reminiscence therapy.

Recreation therapy involves using recreation or hobbies to increase meaningful experiences and contact with others. It is another way of using familiar objects or past abilities to help clients ascribe meaning. Although recreation therapy may be prescribed and directed by another health professional, nurses also may use recreation or hobbies appropriate to the individual client to stimulate cognitive function. Activities that elicit pleasant memories may be used to engage chronically confused or withdrawn clients. Examples are the review of a personal scrapbook or photograph album.

Music therapy enhances cognitive contact through the familiarity of music. The music may be in the background or used for exercise or in group sings. Both the music and the socialization and recreation inherent in musical group opportunities are stimulating. Some therapists may use music in a specific, prescriptive fashion; however, nurses can use music as a part of nursing care as deemed appropriate. Although selected music may provide therapeutic cognitive stimulation, it must be individualized to the client's preferences and the risk of overstimulation must be kept in mind.

Family Support

Families of clients with acute confusion are often anxious and fear a progression to chronic confusion. Reassure clients and families that, in most cases, cognitive function will improve with time. Encourage families to participate actively in the planning and care of clients; the collaborative intervention goal will be to prevent or minimize the clients' altered thought processes.

Many clients with chronic confusion live at home and receive care from family members. Family caregivers usually receive inadequate training for this difficult task (Hall, Buckwalter, Stolley, Gerdner, Garand, Ridgeway, & Crump, 1995). Teaching family caregivers about the nature and progression of chronic confusion, along with techniques for managing the behavioral manifestations, may reduce exhaustion and delay institutionalization.

Nurses may also provide direct care and support to family members. Families have a difficult time adjusting to the fact that their loved ones are losing or have lost all memory of them and their lives together. The grief process begins before the death of clients with dementia. In essence, the person whom the family members once knew and interacted with is no longer present mentally but is still present physically. Use nursing interventions that aid the family in its grief, as discussed in Chapter 48.

Healthcare Planning and Home/Community-Based Nursing

Because of shorter hospital stays, clients may be discharged before cognitive function has returned to normal. Careful discharge planning is imperative. Planning may need to include teaching family caregivers effective techniques in communicating with and caring for clients. Community self-help groups, such as stroke clubs, the Alzheimer's Disease and Related Disorders Association, the Multiple Sclerosis Society, the National Spinal Cord Injury Society, and the International Association of Laryngectomies, can be beneficial. These groups offer support and provide clients and families with tips to make role adjustment easier and to improve the quality of relationships.

Home Care

Home-care services, which include nurses; occupational, physical and speech therapists; and home health aides, should be arranged as necessary before clients are discharged. Going home may help reverse the dysfunction of mildly cognitively impaired clients as they return to a familiar environment and routines. Clients who have more severe impairments may need frequent home visits for nursing care and homemaking.

If impaired cognitive function interferes with the ability to perform higher-level skills (e.g., managing medications and maintaining the home), support systems usually can be created to promote safety and independence. For people with minor memory impairment, ways to support and compensate include making lists of medications to take, things to do, or appliances to turn off. Maintaining organization in the home and in routines creates a predictable environment with few distractions, so that memory functions more effectively. Resources like chore service, volunteers, subsidized van service, Meals on Wheels, and grocery delivery can be arranged.

Day and Respite Care

Day care and respite care are two useful support services for irreversibly cognitively impaired people and their family caregivers. Fatigue is constant for caregivers of progressively impaired family members. One means of managing fatigue is access to services that allow some time away from caregiving, while providing impaired persons with health and rehabilitative services. Caregivers are assured that impaired family members are benefiting from the alternative care and simultaneously having much-needed rest and personal time.

Long-Term Care

Many times, people with progressive cognitive impairment or dementia need consistent support from long-term care settings with 24-hour supervision, structured environments, and

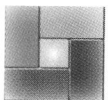

Nursing Research and Critical Thinking

Is There a Relationship Between Cognitive Status of Elderly Long-Term Care Residents and Pain Medication Orders or Administration?

These nurses were concerned that pain older adults experience is frequently undetected. Consequently, older clients who experience pain may not receive needed medications. Reports suggest that some older adults are unable to articulate the pain's nature and source, and their attempts at expressing pain may be ignored as not meaningful. The nurses designed a descriptive, exploratory study to examine the relationship between nurses' ratings of pain and corresponding administration of pain medication to older adults, and the cognitive status of elderly long-term care residents and pain medication orders/administration. Data were collected at a long-term care facility for 238 residents. Twenty-five nurses completed a visual analog scale for pain to measure residents' present pain levels. A review of the medication administration records was completed for all subjects in the study. The nurses' pain ratings for resident's pain were not significantly related with pain medications administered. The Mini-Mental State Examination (MMSE) was used to measure cognitive status of the subjects. For the study's purposes, two groups were developed from the original sample using the MMSE. Nineteen cognitively intact older adults were matched with 19 cognitively impaired older adults to form two equal groups. All cognitively intact subjects had a pain medication order, whereas 6% of the cognitively impaired subjects did not have a pain medication order. The cognitively impaired subjects were prescribed significantly less (Chi-square = 6.64, $P < .01$) scheduled pain medication and were given significantly less (Chi-square = 8.23, $P < .01$) pain medication than the cognitively intact subjects.

Critical Thinking Considerations. Data collected for this study came from one long-term care facility. The findings are not generalizable to other facilities or populations. Implications of this study are as follows:

- This study indicated that nurses did not give analgesics consistently when they rated residents as having pain. As a consequence, some elderly residents continued to suffer with pain unnecessarily.
- Pain is undertreated for cognitively impaired older adults. As the ability to communicate declines for these older adults, nurses will find it difficult to discern when these clients are having a painful experience.

From Kaasalainen, S., Middleton, J., Knezacek, S., Hartley, T., Stewart, N., Ife, C., & Robinson, L. (1998). Pain & cognitive status in the institutionalized elderly: Perceptions & interventions. *Journal of Gerontological Nursing*, *24*(8), 24–31.

extended health services. Caregivers need the support and reinforcement from healthcare providers as they make the decision to admit loved ones to long-term care. They need assurance that they have made the right decision, whatever that decision ultimately is.

Admission to long-term care can be very positive for clients, who will have contact with people, objects, and situations that provide increased stimulation. Full-time care allows the environment to be structured and predictable, which may actually increase a client's level of cognitive functioning even temporarily. The actual process of relocation can be stressful, but clients can be helped to cope through diligent orientation and unhurried repetition. A caring attitude on the part of healthcare professionals is essential.

EVALUATION

Evaluation of the effect of nursing interventions toward client goals includes a client assessment related to the outcome criteria. Continuation, modification, or termination of nursing interventions depends on the assessment. This process may be ongoing. Some examples of the relationship between goals and outcome criteria for clients with alterations in thinking and communicating are listed below.

Goal

The client will have absence of injury related to confusion.

Possible Outcome Criteria

- At discharge, there are no reports of injury (e.g., falls, abrasions, burns) related to cognitive dysfunction.

Goal

The client will experience adequate support to compensate for deficits.

Possible Outcome Criteria

- Before discharge, client demonstrates adequate nutrition, safety, and mobility.
- Before discharge, client receives support services as needed to offset needs presented by cognitive deficits.

Goal

The client will participate in a safe, protected environment.

NURSING PLAN OF CARE
THE CLIENT WITH DISTURBED THOUGHT PROCESSES

Nursing Diagnosis
Disturbed Thought Processes related to biochemical imbalances and sensory deprivation manifested by lack of orientation to place and time and inability to manage activities of daily living (ADLs).

Client Goal
Client will regain baseline cognitive function.

Client Outcome Criteria
- Client will be oriented to self, place, and time during course of care.
- Client's family will state that client's mental status has returned to pre-illness level.

Nursing Interventions	Scientific Rationale
1. Assess and record mental status every shift.	1. Regular assessment promotes recognition of changes in condition and allows determination of effectiveness of interventions.
2. Reorient as necessary. Provide orientation cues such as a clock, calendar, and a sign with room number.	2. Frequent reorientation and use of cues compensates for the short-term memory loss that occurs with cognitive impairment.
3. Encourage client to be out of bed for meals when possible. Establish a consistent bedtime routine.	3. Providing an ADL routine similar to that followed at home can help minimize the strangeness of health-care environment.
4. Assign consistent caregivers when possible.	4. Minimizing the number of caregivers allows the client to recognize staff and feel comfortable with their care.
5. Encourage family and friends to visit; put cards and flowers where client can see them.	5. The ability to recognize family and friends persists even in a state of severe confusion. Presence of loved ones can be reassuring and can minimize the negative effects of the illness experience.
6. Encourage client to participate in ADLs as much as possible.	6. Performing ADLs helps the client regain a sense of control and gives the nurse an opportunity to assess functional ability.

Possible Outcome Criteria

- The client demonstrates the absence of injury from environmental hazards.
- The client demonstrates relaxed behavior and other indications of comfort with the environment.

Goal

The client will communicate basic needs.

Possible Outcome Criteria

- By discharge, client demonstrates ability to express needs using a new method (gestures, writing, blinking, or electronic device) with nurse.

Goal

The client will verbalize experiencing less frustration with communication.

Possible Outcome Criteria

- Client verbalizes to nurse a decrease in frustration with communication problems.
- Client expresses a decrease in feelings of isolation and depression.

KEY CONCEPTS

- Cognition is the process of knowing, thinking, learning, and communicating; it is the complex processing of information by which sensory input, past experiences, awareness, and emotions are integrated and made meaningful, thereby enabling the person to interact with the environment in a purposeful way.

- To provide comprehensive nursing care, nurses need to be aware of factors affecting cognitive function such as physiologic state, infectious processes, medications, personal and environmental stressors, and affective states.
- Manifestations of impaired cognition include disorganized thinking, attention deficits, memory impairment, impaired thought processes, and impaired communication.
- For the person with disturbed thought processes, activities of daily living are disrupted, and the amount of support in the living situation must be assessed.
- Disorders in cognition can markedly disrupt the quality of life for the person affected and the person's family.
- To guide the development of the nursing process, the nurse needs to determine how a person functions along with assessing the quality of the social and physical environment.
- Identifying risk factors for disturbed thought processes will assist the nurse in defining the actual dysfunction and the appropriate interventions.
- Thorough assessment of physiologic and psychosocial function is essential in identifying causes of impaired cognitive processes.
- In adults, the main cause of impaired communication is brain damage. Other major causes are cancer and neurologic disorders.
- The plan of care involves collaboration of nursing, speech therapy, and other disciplines, as needed.
- Nursing goals should focus on restoring physiologic balance while providing an environment that supports function, does not cause new impairments, and protects the client from harm.
- If the nurse is aware of potential risk for dysfunction, preventive interventions will concentrate on minimizing those factors and supporting the client and caregivers.
- Among many supportive interventions for the impaired client is reality orientation, which is used to reinforce and restore awareness of reality.
- People with altered cognitive processes require careful discharge planning and home care along with referral for families to long-term care, day care, or respite care, as appropriate.

REFERENCES

Ahmann, E. (1994). "Chunky stew": Appreciating cultural diversity while providing health care for children. *Pediatric Nursing, 20,* 320–324.

American Psychiatric Association. (2000). *Diagnostic criteria from DSM-IV-TR.* Washington, DC: Author.

Berne, R. M., Levy, M. N., Koeppen, B. M., & Stanton, B. A. (1998). *Physiology* (4th ed.). St. Louis, MO: Mosby.

Capezuti, E., Evans, L., Strumpf, N., & Maislin, G. (1996). Physical restraint use and falls in nursing home residents. *Journal of the American Geriatrics Society, 44,* 627–633.

Capezuti, E., Strumpf, N., Evans, L. K., Grisso, J. A., & Maislin, G. (1998). The relationship between physical restraint removal and falls and injuries among nursing home residents. *Journal of Gerontology: Biological Sciences and Medical Sciences, 53A*(1), M47–M52.

Cummings, J. L., Arsland, D., & Jarvik, L. (1997). Dementia. In C. K. Cassel, H. J. Cohen, E. B. Larson, et al. (Eds.), *Geriatric medicine* (3rd ed.). New York: Springer.

Davies, H. D. (1999). Delirium and dementia. In J. T. Stone, J. F. Wyman, & S. A. Salisbury (Eds.), *Clinical gerontological nurs-*
ing: A guide to advanced practice (2nd ed.). Philadelphia: W. B. Saunders.

Dunne, W. M. (1998). Mechanisms of infectious disease. In C. M. Porth, *Pathophysiology: Concepts of altered health states* (5th ed.). Philadelphia: Lippincott-Raven.

Dzurec, L. C., & Coleman, P. (1997). "What happens after you say hello?" A hermaneutic analysis of the process of conducting clinical interviews. *Journal of Psychosocial Nursing, 35*(8), 31–36.

Erikson, E. H. (1963). *Childhood and society* (2nd ed.). New York: Norton.

Folstein, M., Folstein, S., & McHugh, P. (1975). Mini–mental status. *Journal of Psychiatric Research, 12,* 189–198.

Francis, J. (1997). Delirium. In C. K. Cassel, H. J. Cohen, E. B. Larson, et al. (Eds), *Geriatric medicine* (3rd ed.). New York: Springer.

Fratiglioni, L. (1996). Epidemiology of Alzheimer's disease and current possibilities for prevention. *Acta Neurologica Scandinavica. Supplementum, 165,* 33–40.

Gresham, G. E., & Weiss, C. J. (1993). The role of speech therapy in stroke rehabilitation. *Heart Disease and Stroke, 2,* 49–52.

Gropper, R. C. (1996). *Culture and the clinical encounter: An intercultural sensitizer for the health professions.* Yarmouth, ME: Intercultural Press.

Guyton, A. C., & Hall, J. E. (1996). *Textbook of medical physiology* (9th ed.). Philadelphia: W. B. Saunders.

Hall, G. R., Buckwalter, K. C., Stolley, J. M., Gerdner, L. A., Garand, L., Ridgeway, S., & Crump, S. (1995). Standardized care plan: Managing Alzheimer's patients at home. *Journal of Gerontological Nursing, 21,* 37–47.

Hall, G. R., & Gerdner, L. A. (1999). Managing problem behaviors. In J. T. Stone, J. F. Wyman, & S. A. Salisbury (Eds.), *Clinical gerontological nursing: A guide to advanced practice* (2nd ed.). Philadelphia: W. B. Saunders.

Harrison, L. L. (1990). Minimizing barriers when teaching hearing-impaired clients. *American Journal of Maternal Child Nursing, 15,* 113.

Haskell, R. M., Frankel, H. L., & Rotondo, M. F. (1997). Agitation. *AACN Clinical Issues, 8*(3), 335–350.

Havighurst, R. J. (1972). *Developmental tasks and education* (3rd ed.). New York: David McKay.

Hendrie, H. C. (1998). Epidemiology of dementia and Alzheimer's disease. *American Journal of Geriatric Psychiatry, 6*(2, Suppl. 1), 53–58.

Jennett, B. (1996). Epidemiology of head injury. *Journal of Neurology, Neurosurgery, and Psychiatry, 60*(4), 362–369.

Kandel, E. R. (1997). Genes, synapses, and long-term memory. *Journal of Cellular Physiology, 173*(2), 124–125.

Kistler, J. P., Ropper, A. H., & Martin, J. B. (1994). Cerebrovascular diseases. In K. J. Isselbacher, J. B. Martin, E. Braunwald, A. S. Fauci, J. D. Wilson, & D. L. Kasper (Eds.), *Harrison's principles of internal medicine* (13th ed.). New York: McGraw-Hill.

McCance, K. L., & Heuther, S. E. (1998). *Pathophysiology: The biologic basis for disease in adults and children* (3rd ed.). St. Louis, MO: Mosby.

Merrow, S. L., & Corbett, C. D. (1994). Adaptive computing for people with disabilities. *Computers in Nursing, 12,* 201–209.

Neelon, V. J., Champagne, M. T., McConnell, E., Carlson, J., & Fink, S. G. (1992). Use of the NEECHAM Confusion Scale to assess acute confusional states of hospitalized older patients. In S. G. Fink, E. M. Tornquist, M. T. Champagne, & R. A. Wise (Eds.), *Key aspects of eldercare: Managing falls, incontinence, and cognitive impairment.* New York: Springer.

Nicholas, M. L., Helm-Estabrooks, N., & Ward-Lonergan, J. (1993). Evolution of severe aphasia in the first two years post onset. *Archives of Physical Medicine and Rehabilitation, 74,* 830–836.

Nolan, K. A., & Blass, J. P. (1992). Preventing cognitive decline. *Clinics in Geriatric Medicine, 8*(1), 19–34.

North American Nursing Diagnosis Association. (2001). *NANDA Nursing diagnoses: Definitions & classification 2001–2002.* Philadelphia: Author.

Pfeiffer, E. (1975). A short, portable mental status questionnaire for the assessment of organic brain deficit in elderly clients. *Journal of the American Geriatric Society, 23,* 433–443.

Piaget, J. (1969). *The psychology of the child.* New York: Basic Books.

Porth, C. (1998). *Pathophysiology: Concepts of altered health states* (5th ed.). Philadelphia: Lippincott-Raven.

Santrock, J. W. (1995). *Life-span development* (5th ed.). Madison, WI: Brown & Benchmark.

Vermeersch, P. E. H., & Henly S. J. (1997). Validation of the structure for the "Clinical Assessment of Confusion—A." *Nursing Research, 46*(4), 208–213.

Wiebers, D. O., Dale, A. J. D., Kokmen, E., & Swanson, J. W. (Eds.) (1998). *Mayo Clinic examinations in neurology* (7th ed.). Rochester, MN: Mayo Foundation.

Werner, P., Cohen-Mansfield, J., Braun, J., et al. (1989). Physical restraints and agitation in nursing home residents. *Journal of the American Geriatric Society, 37,* 1122–1126.

Wieckert, C. S., & Kleinman, J. E. (1998). The neuroanatomy and neurochemistry of schizophrenia. *Psychiatric Clinics of North America, 21*(1), 57–75.

Williams, M. P., & Salisbury, S. A. (1999). Cognitive assessment. In J. T. Stone, J. F. Wyman, & S. A. Salisbury (Eds.), *Clinical gerontological nursing: A guide to advanced practice* (2nd ed.). Philadelphia: W. B. Saunders.

BIBLIOGRAPHY

Divela, A. L., Kongas, S. P., Saviaro, P., Pahkala, K., Kesti, E., et al. (1993). Five year prognosis for dysthymic disorder in old age. *International Journal of Geriatric Psychiatry, 8*(11), 939–947.

Holden, U. (1994). Dementia in acute units: Aggression. *Nursing Standard, 9*(11), 37–39.

Miziniak, H. (1994). Persons with Alzheimer's: Effects of nutrition and exercise. *Journal of Gerontological Nursing, 20*(10), 27–32, 46–47.

Moller, M. D., & Murphy, M. F. (1998). Neurobiological responses and schizophrenia and psychotic disorders. In C. W. Stuart & M. T. Laraia (Eds.). *Stuart & Sundeen's principles and practice of psychiatric nursing.* St. Louis, MO: Mosby.

Rader, J. (1991). Modifying the environment to decrease use of restraints. *Journal of Gerontological Nursing, 17*(2), 9–13.

Rantz, M. J., & McShane, R. E. (1994). Nursing home staff perception of behavior disturbance and management of confused residents. *Applied Nursing Research, 7*(3), 132–140.

Sullivan-Marx, E. M. (1994). Delirium and physical restraint in the hospitalized elderly. *Image: The Journal of Nursing Scholarship, 26*(4), 295–300.

Weinrich, S., & Sarna, L. (1994). Delirium in the older person with cancer. *Cancer, 74*(Suppl.), 2079–2091.

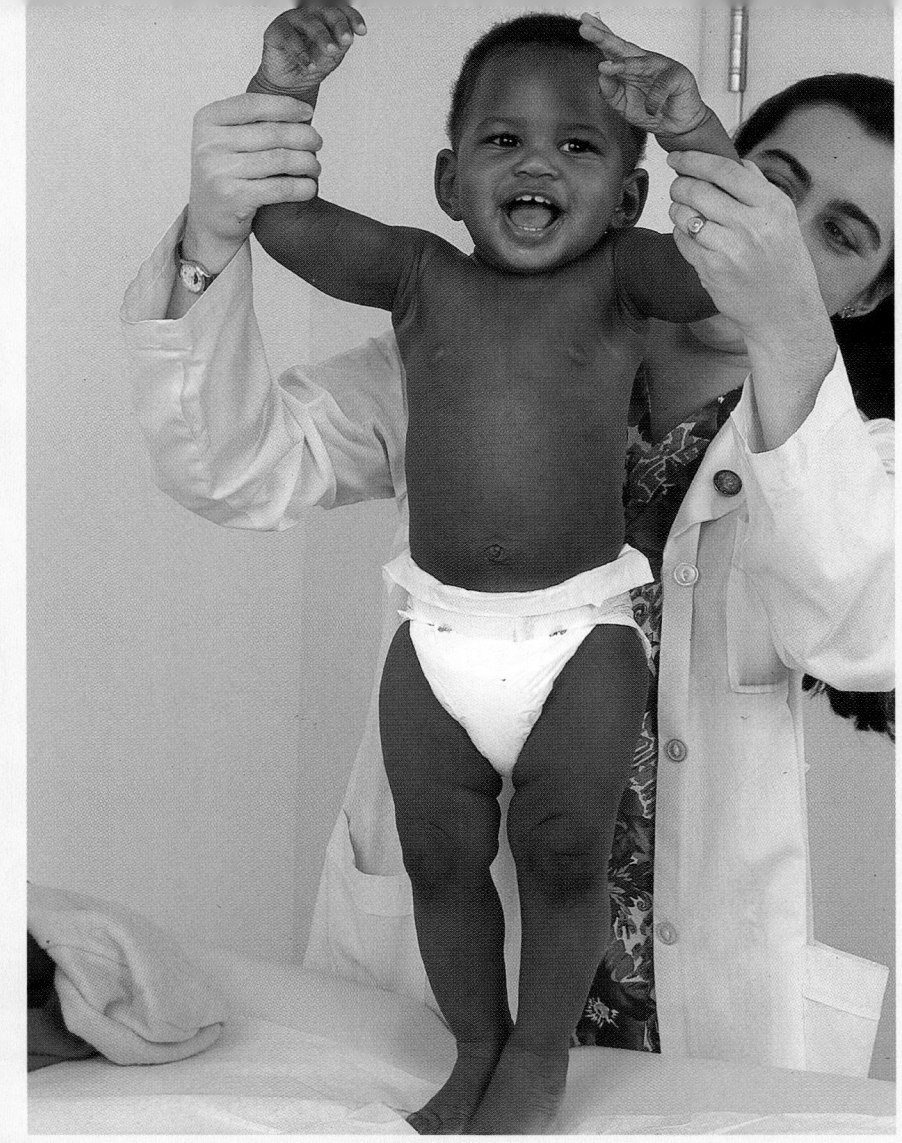

Self-Perception and Self-Concept

Chapter

46 Self-Concept

Key Terms

body image
identity
role
role ambiguity
role conflict
role strain
self
self-concept

self-efficacy
self-esteem
self-evaluation
self-expectation
self-knowledge
self-perception
social self

Learning Objectives

Upon completion of this chapter, the student will be able to do the following:

1. Describe the functions of self and self-concept.
2. Define self-concept, self-perception, self-knowledge, self-expectation, social self, and self-evaluation.
3. Identify the four patterns of self-concept.
4. Discuss how self-concept develops throughout the lifespan.
5. Discuss factors that can affect self-concept.
6. Identify possible manifestations of altered self-concept.
7. Apply theory to assess for self-concept functioning.
8. Plan care for a person with an altered self-concept.

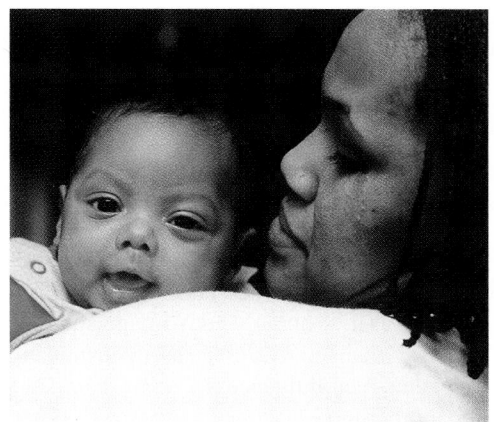

Critical Thinking Challenge

You are a nurse working in a well-baby clinic. A 31-year-old married woman brings in her 3-month-old child for a scheduled appointment. While you are weighing the baby, the mother talks about feeling tired and fat and says, "These breasts are too big." She tells you she misses the baby when she goes to her part-time job but feels better now that she is back to aerobics class. When you ask about the baby, she smiles and tells you how happy she and her husband are to have him. She describes how much more rewarding caring for her own child is than baby-sitting her nieces and nephews. She wonders if she'll ever feel rested again.

Experiences and expectations across the lifespan affect a person's view of himself or herself. Once you have completed this chapter and have incorporated self-concept into your knowledge base, review the above scenario and reflect on the following areas of Critical Thinking:

1. Describe your immediate impressions of the woman and her situation.
2. Reflect on the information provided as well as your own experience, knowledge, and beliefs. Consider how these might influence your impressions.
3. Analyze how the mother and infant may feel.
4. Consider additional assessment data that you might need to collect; develop appropriate questions to ask to obtain this data.
5. State possible nursing diagnoses for this family and identify some desired outcomes.
6. Given your assessment, nursing diagnoses, and outcome identification, plan interventions that may be appropriate.

As people adapt to changes in life, body image, role performance, self-esteem, and personal identity evolve. Self-concept is dynamic, influenced by experiences and expectations. A sound self-concept is a prerequisite for mental health. Nursing responsibilities associated with self-concept include self-knowledge, assessment of self-concept, promotion of adequate self-concept functioning, and interventions when self-concept is at risk or altered. The nurse who possesses a healthy self-concept will be better equipped to deal with the unique and varied needs of clients. Conversely, if a nurse's self-concept is dysfunctional, he or she will be unable to meet the needs of clients. In fact, coping with such a nurse may actually add to a client's work.

NORMAL FUNCTION OF SELF

Because of its importance in understanding human behavior, the concept of self has been examined by many disciplines and defined in various ways. **Self** may be defined as a person's unique dimensions, potentials, and purposes (Rogers, 1961). **Self-concept** is the mental image a person has of oneself. It is the person's meaning when stated as "I" or "me." Self-concept is the frame of reference that influences how a person handles situations and relationships. It is crucial to esteem and self-actualization, the highest needs in Abraham Maslow's hierarchy of needs.

Characteristics of Self-Concept

People who have a healthy self-concept exhibit a clear sense of self and others. They understand who they are in the world. They can and do distinguish themselves as separate individuals with strengths and weaknesses. These people acknowledge their emotions and find constructive ways to bring meaning into life. The person with a healthy self-concept views others realistically and is able to relate to them in a satisfying manner, which includes the capacity for intimacy and love. The person with a healthy self-concept handles life's realities and problems with appropriate coping behaviors.

Self-Concept and Self-Perception
According to Brown (1998), self-concept is the way a person thinks about himself or herself (p. 3), whereas **self-perception** is how a person explains behavior (p. 60) based on self-observation. How one perceives oneself has several dimensions: self-knowledge, self-expectations, social self, and self-evaluation.

Self-Knowledge. **Self-knowledge** or self-awareness involves a basic understanding of oneself, a cognitive perception. It is consciousness of one's abilities: cognitive, affective, and physical. Self-knowledge involves basic facts (age, weight, sex) and qualities (sincere, athletic, intelligent) related to oneself.

Self-Expectation. **Self-expectation** involves the "ideal" self—the self a person wants to be. It is the setting of present and future goals. If goals are realistic, the person may attain them.

Unrealistic goals, however, can be defeating. Self-expectation is based on the limits of a person's awareness. For instance, the goals of the person who watches glamorous shows on television may be to be thin, beautiful, popular with the opposite sex, and wealthy. The person who spends time reading may have increased knowledge as a goal. Significant others influence a person's self-expectation. If a mother pushes her son to be a physician, the son may share this goal or may feel like a failure if he lacks interest.

Social Self. **Social self** is how a person sees himself or herself in relation to social situations including behavior and interaction with others. One never fully knows how others see him or her. One can only guess, and the guess may be far from reality. Conversely, people tend to wear masks in their social obligations, trying to hide their true selves. The "religious" self that a person displays in church may differ from the self shown at parties. A person may hide aggressive feelings when being interviewed but display aggression later on the job.

Self-Evaluation. **Self-evaluation** is the conscious assessment of the self, leading to self-respect or self-worth. "Have I met my expectations? Do I like whom I see in the mirror? Do I like how I behave?" Self-evaluation involves the aforementioned dimensions plus self-esteem (discussed below).

Normal Self-Concept Patterns

Body image, self-esteem, personal identity, and role performance comprise the mental image of the self. The whole of self represents more than the sum of these four components. To clarify the dynamic of these components, consider the mother and 3-month-old child described in the opening Critical Thinking Challenge. The woman's body image and role performance have clearly changed with pregnancy and motherhood. These components then influence her self-esteem and identity into which motherhood must be incorporated. If her self-concept is healthy, she will be able to make the necessary changes to cope with and adapt to the dynamics of self.

Positive Body Image
The human body is the self's physical manifestation. How a person pictures and feels about his or her body describes **body image.** Body image includes the total conscious and unconscious disposition toward one's body. It is the unifying concept behind feelings about one's size, sex, and sexuality; the way one looks; the way one's body functions; and whether one's body can help one accomplish goals.

Culture and social experience influence body image. Western cultures, influenced by the media, value beauty, health, and youth. Other cultures value weight or old age. Most people have a picture of how they hope they look, an *idealized body image.* In addition, people have an awareness of how they really look, a *mirrored image.* When the real image is close to the ideal image, the person experiences positive regard for self. These positive feelings about body image are part of self-esteem.

A study of body image perceptions of diabetic African-American women and men (Anderson, Janes, Ziemer, & Phillips, 1997, p. 301) found that, "regardless of sex or weight category, perceived current body size was significantly related to BMI (body mass index)." Both men and women classified as overweight desired a body size smaller than their perceived current size and both expected their dietitian to favor a smaller size. These discrepancies between self-image and the perceived perceptions of others support that body image may affect dietary counseling.

Self-Esteem

While self-concept refers to the way people think about themselves, **self-esteem** refers to how people feel about themselves (Brown, 1998). Two sources for esteem are self and others (Fig. 46-1). Self-esteem develops throughout childhood and adolescence and becomes more stable in adulthood.

Early in life, children accept their parents' evaluations as their own. Then children incorporate others' appraisals and expectations to form a self-ideal. They then slowly begin self-evaluation, emerging into adulthood with a basic or core self-esteem. Coopersmith (1967) identified antecedents of high self-esteem: parental acceptance, clear expectations, limitations, and freedom to express opinions. From these four antecedents, fundamental criteria by which people's self-appraisals are made have been proposed:

- *Power:* The ability to influence people and events—the sense that one's opinion counts and will be heard
- *Meaning:* The sense of being valued and worthwhile—one's existence matters to others
- *Competence:* The ability to achieve personal goals—personal success
- *Virtue:* Behaving in a manner consistent with personal values—adherence to a moral or ethical standard

Core self-esteem is the person's consistent, overall appraisal of self. The person acts or perceives events in ways that tend to support his or her level of self-esteem. Although core self-esteem is relatively stable, people do change their perceptions

of self based on current experience. (Huitt, 1998). Such an example is the woman described at the beginning of this chapter.

The person with adequate self-esteem has learned to cope with personal deficiencies and to maximize strengths. This person is self-accepting. The person with high self-esteem accepts others, experiences less anxiety, and functions effectively in social situations.

Strong Personal Identity

Identity is an organizing principle of the self, the awareness that one is a distinct individual separate from others. The person with a strong sense of personal identity has integrated self-esteem, body image, and various roles into a whole self-concept. This whole or "I" is not associated with any one aspect. Identity provides the person with a sense of continuity through time. "I am not the person I was yesterday, but similarities and consistency provide links for today and the future."

The concept of boundaries is central to identity. Actual body boundaries (this is my hand; that is your hand) and ego boundaries (this is my thought or feeling, not your thought or feeling) must be intact for a person to maintain identity. To maintain mental health, the person must be able to differentiate self from others.

Role Performance

A person fills many roles in a lifetime. **Role** is defined as a person's expected characteristic behavior in a social position. Roles are ascribed or assumed. An ascribed role is one in which the person has no choice (e.g., being a daughter). Because the person is born female, she becomes a daughter. An assumed role is one that the person selects (e.g., career and relationship roles). Choosing to be a nurse is an assumed role. Roles overlap often; the person combines the roles to achieve a unified pattern for functioning. When the person perceives self as adequate in various roles, self-esteem is enhanced. Roles are discussed in Chapter 46.

Lifespan Considerations

Each developmental stage requires the completion of specific tasks that foster the development of positive self-concept. Prominent theories regarding development of self-concept are those of Freud (1920/1966), Piaget (1969), Erikson (1963), Havighurst (1972), and Kohlberg (1969). Sullivan (1953) discussed an interpersonal theory. Freud's, Sullivan's, Erikson's, and Havighurst's theories related to development of self-concept are listed in Table 46-1.

Newborn and Infant

Newborns have undifferentiated selves; they do not experience a separate existence from others. Parents and other caregivers transmit their self-concepts, sense of competence in new roles, and amount and intensity of anxiety they feel to newborns. When parents are reasonably calm and communicate warmth and acceptance to newborns, they help their babies establish the basis for positive self-concept.

Both family and newborn experience dramatic changes that can potentially affect the baby's self-concept. The mother

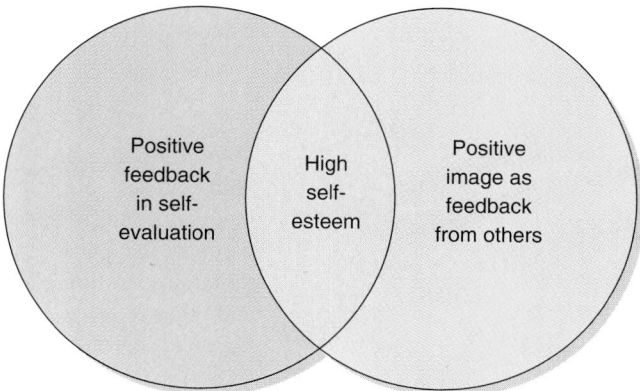

FIGURE 46-1 A person develops high self-esteem when he or she receives positive feedback from both self and others.

TABLE 46-1

Theories of Self-Concept Development				
	Freud: Psychodynamic (1920/1966)	**Sullivan: Interpersonal (1953)**	**Erikson Ego (1963)**	**Havighurst: Tasks (1972)**
Newborn/ Infant	Oral stage, 0–3 mo; child is undifferentiated from mother	Infancy: beginning self-concept formed; security = good me; anxiety = bad me; overwhelming anxiety or deprivation = not me	Trust vs mistrust; adequate mothering helps infant establish trust in self and others	Task: establishes physiologic stability
Infant	3 mo to 1.5 yr; child begins to distinguish his or her body from objects (people and things) in the environment	Infant has no separateness from caretaker		
Toddler	Anal stage; personal identity pronounced "I"; role performance learned in family	Early childhood: beginning differentiation; if relationship adequate, child begins to integrate good me, bad me, and not me into self-concept	Autonomy vs shame; personal identity: body image and self-esteem develop as child experiences self-control through exploration in the world	Tasks: learns body image through walking, talking, control of waste
Preschooler	Phallic stage; sex role, body image, and personal identity become more clearly differentiated		Initiative vs guilt; beginning role established through sexual identity development and family relationships	Learns own sex role and identity through above tasks
School-age child	Latency; role performance is primary work of this stage; body image problems may manifest if previous stages not resolved successfully	Juvenile: process of individuation occurs as peer relationships develop. Individual learns competition, compromise, and collaboration	Industry vs inferiority; socialization and competence are developing, helping continued growth of self-concept	Tasks: learns physical skills for games; roles (i.e., sex, student, and friend); values
Adolescent	Genital stage; body image is altered as the individual establishes self as sexual being; separation from parents leads to enhanced sense of identity; role choices are made	Identity, body image, and role continue to develop or be redefined as individuation progresses	Identity vs role confusion; search for self	Tasks: acceptance of body and sex role; independence from parents; occupational preparation and other roles learned (i.e., marriage, citizen)

TABLE 46-1 (Continued)

	Freud: Psychodynamic (1920/1966)	Sullivan: Interpersonal (1953)	Erikson Ego (1963)	Havighurst: Tasks (1972)
Adult	Individual works on conflicts/deficits from previous developmental stages		Intimacy vs isolation; primary task role related: acquisition of love, sexual fulfillment and closeness	Tasks: marriage, parenting, occupation
			Generativity vs self-absorption; as person concerns self with next generation(s), new sense of identity develops, increasing self-comfort and integration of varied roles	Tasks: adjusting to physiologic changes; role with aging parents
Older Adult			Integrity vs despair; individual accepts personal accomplishments or feels decreased worth; body image changes as the person experiences physical alterations associated with old age (e.g., decreased sensory acuity)	Tasks: adjusts to decreased physical strength, retirement, possible death of self or spouse, decreased income

shifts from being pregnant with a pregnant body to not being pregnant. If the mother chooses to breast-feed, she experiences further body image changes and has concerns about milk production, sexuality, and competence. If she chooses not to breast-feed, she may experience guilt or doubt concerning the mothering role. During this same time, the mother is shifting in existing roles and developing new roles. The father also experiences shifts in and development of new roles. He must integrate new relationships into his identity. The family's relationships with others change during this time. Extended family may either help or confuse role transition. Friends may treat the couple differently after a child is born. Any siblings of the newborn experience shifts in roles also. Healthy acceptance and working through changes during this period set the stage for positive self-concept development.

Infants begin to understand self as separate and that feelings (e.g., hunger) are their own. As an infant begins to distinguish self from others, self-concept starts to develop. As an infant interacts with meaningful others, he or she begins to read the wants of others.

For example when mom smiles and plays patty-cake, mom smiles even more when the infant smiles and makes noises.

Thus, the infant begins to learn social role expectations. During infancy, children learn to sit, stand, and possibly walk. This managing of the body allows infants to experience the world in different ways and teaches children body boundaries. Bodily control helps to establish a beginning sense of separateness from others. Through play, infants learn to control aspects of the environment. For instance, early during this stage infants bat objects such as colorful items on a mobile. Later they grasp items and, toward the end of infancy, may be able to stack two blocks. This play helps children during the earliest stages of acquiring identity, just as social control (e.g., smiles) helps children with beginning roles.

In addition, infants begin to communicate through symbols. For example, smiles mean good, cries mean bad, "mama" is associated with mothering persons, and infants begin to respond to their names. Infants accomplish these developmental tasks by interacting with caregivers and exploring.

Toddler and Preschooler

Toddlers have a rudimentary body image. Although they know the self as separate from others, they have no clear definition of where the body ends. For example, some toddlers may not want to flush the toilet after defecating because they see the stools as part of them. Toddlers are not aware of specific influences, only general feelings or thoughts. They do, however, understand others' responses to behavior. Thus excessive punishment leads to bad feelings and praise leads to good feelings. Gradually toddlers incorporate these feelings into self-concept.

Self-concept continues to develop actively during preschool years. Preschoolers' sense of self becomes more defined as they realize that they are separate and unique. During this stage of development, children exhibit great sexual curiosity. They are aware that they are different from others. In addition to this sense of sexual self, preschoolers are incorporating both spatial relationships and increased coordination into their body image.

Sense of how one relates to others is more defined in the preschool stage than in previous stages. Children's roles in the family and the world are beginning to take shape. Preschoolers often imitate adult roles (Fig. 46-2). During this stage, children may share in older siblings' accomplishments or perceive themselves as not as good because they cannot achieve the same things. If a new baby is added to the family, preschoolers may respond with anger, jealousy, or regression. The family's response to the child's reaction influences his or her role performance and self-esteem.

Because of curiosity, preschoolers learn body parts and names as well as attitudes about body and self. If questions are discounted, met with great anxiety, or answered with misinformation, children may develop a negative self-concept or poor body image.

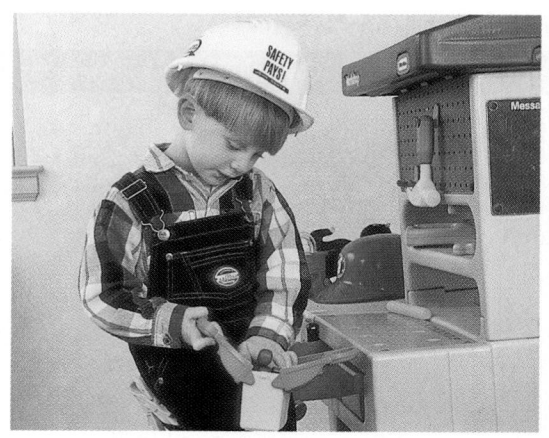

FIGURE 46-2   Preschoolers like to imitate adult roles as they learn about the world around them.

School-Age Child and Adolescent

The school experience can strongly reinforce or alter a child's body image, sense of self, and identity. Teachers and peers become important influences on self-concept. Basically children compare self to peers and measure looks, abilities, and social self against them. Because of rapid change and growth during school-age years, self-concept remains quite flexible, and changes are very individual. Figure 46-3 illustrates the flow of a child's self-concept development from 6 to 12 years of age.

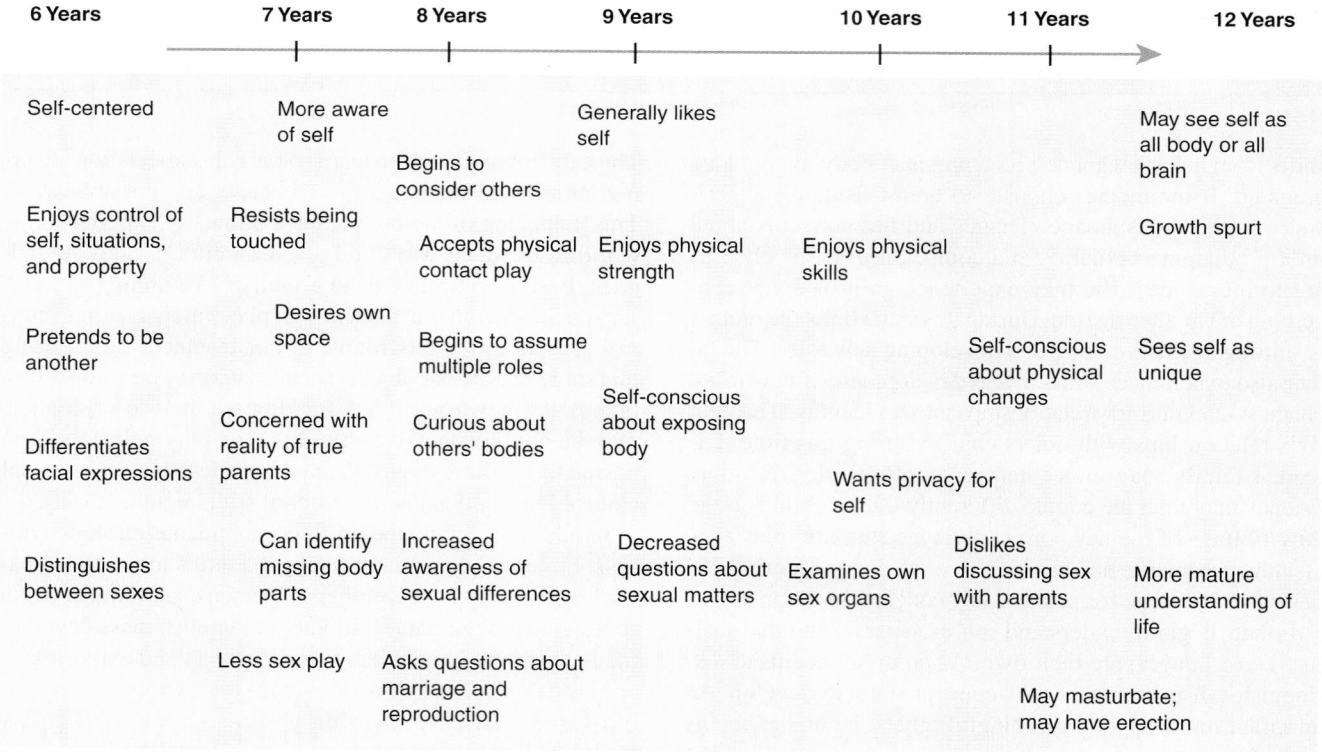

6 Years	7 Years	8 Years	9 Years	10 Years	11 Years	12 Years
Self-centered	More aware of self	Begins to consider others	Generally likes self			May see self as all body or all brain
Enjoys control of self, situations, and property	Resists being touched	Accepts physical contact play	Enjoys physical strength	Enjoys physical skills		Growth spurt
Pretends to be another	Desires own space	Begins to assume multiple roles			Self-conscious about physical changes	Sees self as unique
Differentiates facial expressions	Concerned with reality of true parents	Curious about others' bodies	Self-conscious about exposing body	Wants privacy for self		
Distinguishes between sexes	Can identify missing body parts	Increased awareness of sexual differences	Decreased questions about sexual matters	Examines own sex organs	Dislikes discussing sex with parents	More mature understanding of life
	Less sex play	Asks questions about marriage and reproduction			May masturbate; may have erection	

FIGURE 46-3   Self-concept development as shown on a continuum from age 6 to 12 years. Attributes are approximate. Although there is general consistency in development, each child is unique.

Through life experiences as children "place values on feelings and on themselves as individuals, they make decisions about how to behave. When significant others accept a person's expression of feelings, the self grows and thrives, and the individual feels valued and loved simply for existing. This acceptance is particularly important to the adolescent who is concerned with self-understanding of inner emotions and psychological characteristics" (Brown, 1998).

Adolescents experience remarkable changes. Their bodies grow rapidly, secondary sex characteristics appear, and hormone secretion increases—all of which necessitate rapid changes in view of self. Adolescents must incorporate these changes to establish a coherent body image. Peers and role models, such as sports or media stars, strongly influence self-concept. Clothes, hairstyles, and movement are extensions of body image influenced by peers. Sexual changes and peer group expectations regarding sexual behavior may lead to a sexually active role.

As adolescents seek added responsibility, parents need to learn new methods of parenting. All family members can perceive an adolescent's striving for independence as a conflict. Adolescents may act in ways that seem to directly oppose the family's values and expectations. This behavior occurs because the chief developmental task of adolescence is to develop and to define personal identity.

Adult and Older Adult

Adults continue to modify self-concept. Young adults move away from the conforming peer group with a struggled-for personal identity modified through life experiences. Much of assumed role formation happens early in the adult stage. Common life experiences for early adulthood include forming intimate relationships, choosing a career, establishing a home base, and starting a family.

During the fourth and into the fifth decade, adults may question the fit of their chosen identity and experiences. They may examine the meaning of self and contemplate the parts of self not previously explored. They examine roles and options taken and discarded as they look for more meaning in life. Sheehy (1974) has called this process an "authenticity crisis." The outcome of this authenticity crisis is renewal or resignation. With renewal, the person emerges with an expanded sense of self. With resignation, the person's self remains defined by the narrow constraints of his or her roles.

Retirement requires extraordinary changes in role performance and self-esteem. Because career roles have much to say about who a person is, retired persons are often described by who they were, which implies that they no longer have value; this greatly affects self-esteem.

Most older Americans live independently in their own homes. Independence and self-care have been correlated with higher self-esteem and life satisfaction (National Institute on Aging, 1988). Physical changes such as decreased strength, skin turgor, and sensory acuity affect body image in later life. Because of the valuation of youth in the media and popular culture, some older adults experience lowered self-esteem with

the changed body image. Sensory changes also affect personal identity. If the environment does not provide feedback, a person may have difficulty determining what is part of self.

When older persons accept self, they have found meaning in life. If others accept their contributions, especially younger people, self-esteem is enhanced. If older persons are treated as if they have no more to contribute, self-esteem is damaged.

FACTORS AFFECTING SELF-CONCEPT

Biologic Makeup

Biologic makeup comprises many characteristics that affect self-concept. Sex, height, weight, skin color, and appearance are characteristics that self and others perceive to help form self-concept (Fig. 46-4). These factors also influence what a person experiences. For example, men often have more opportunities to play competitive sports, which enhances self-concept, whereas in some cases, women are restricted from playing certain sports. Women who are athletically inclined may perceive their abilities as inferior, a perception damaging to self-concept. Recently opportunities for athletics and competitive sports for women have increased, thus helping to promote positive self-concepts. Likewise, someone who is black in a predominantly white society may have difficulty securing a positive self-concept if others' perceptions are discriminatory. People who are tall, slender, and attractive may easily develop positive self-concepts because these qualities are favorably perceived.

In recent years, the debate over nature (biology) versus nurture (environment) has fallen in favor of biology because of the results of studies of twins (Segal, 1998). Attributes such as assertiveness, happiness, and even vulnerability to stress have been found to be heritable (Colt, 1998). Although genes are not exclusive causes of such attributes, they are increasingly important to understanding nature's power and influence on nurture. Knowledge of biology offers hope for clearer understanding of therapeutic nursing interventions that build on inherent traits while simultaneously shaping environmental conditions to promote self-esteem and self-concept.

Culture, Values, and Beliefs

Children grow up internalizing the culture, values, and beliefs to which they are exposed. The degree to which they subscribe to those norms affects self-concept. The media provide daily lessons on cultural norms in Western societies. Dietary, childbearing, health, and religious practices are norms that vary among ethnic groups in the United States and Canada. Integration of cultural practices and mainstream beliefs can lead to a healthy self-concept. For example, an adolescent who cultivates an interest in ethnic music and dance but still shares a love of rock music with his peers will have a strong identity and self-esteem.

THERAPEUTIC DIALOGUE
Self-Concept

Scene for Thought
Gwen Jacobs is 12 years old. She comes to the clinic for her school sports physical, accompanied by her mother.

Less Effective

Nurse: Hi, Gwen, I'm Barbara Thompson, the nurse practitioner who will do your physical today. What sport are you trying out for this year?

Client: All of them. *(Looks at the nurse curiously.)* I thought only doctors did physicals.

Nurse: Actually, nurses do physicals, too. What sports do you particularly like? *(Checks head, eyes, ears, nose, and throat [HEENT].)*

Client: I like soccer and softball best. I want to play them in high school too.

Nurse: Good for you. *(Asks mom a question and continues to do exam, taking out stethoscope.)*

Client: Are you going to listen to my heart with that? *(Looks at stethoscope.)*

Nurse: Sure am. *(Opens client's gown and listens to heart sounds.)*

Client: *(Hunches shoulders as if to hide chest from view.)*

Nurse: Okay, now I'll listen to your lungs from the back. Breathe in for me. *(Completes exam. Gwen is silent.)* I can see you look pretty healthy, Gwen. All the normal milestones are being reached, Mrs. Jacobs, including some breast development. If you need any information about menstruation or anything like that, the clinic has some terrific pamphlets I could give you. Otherwise, we'll see her for her next exam next year. Hope you have a good year, Gwen. Win a lot of games! *(Smiles and leaves the room.)*

Client: *(Blushing.)* I hope we don't get her again! Let's go, Mom, I'm going to be late for practice.

More Effective

Nurse: Hi, Gwen, I'm Becky Thomas, the nurse practitioner who will do your physical today. What sport are you trying out for this year?

Client: All of them. *(Looks at the nurse curiously.)* I thought only doctors did physicals.

Nurse: Actually, nurses do physicals, too. What sports do you particularly like? *(Checks HEENT.)*

Client: I like soccer and softball best. I want to play them in high school too.

Nurse: Good for you. You really look strong, especially your leg muscles. Been playing sports a long time? *(Warms up the stethoscope for heart and lung assessment.)*

Client: Yes, since I was little. *(Looks at the stethoscope.)* Are you going to listen to my heart with that?

Nurse: *(Stops to look at her.)* Yes. And your lungs, too. Any problems?

Client: *(Looks down at the floor.)* Do I have to take my gown off?

Nurse: No. I can examine your heart this way *(shows her how the drape will continue to cover her chest)* and listen to your lungs through your back. Does something worry you about being examined?

Client: No. *(Blushes.)*

Nurse: I wonder if you're a little embarrassed about being examined. *(Listens to heart sounds under the gown.)*

Client: Yeah. *(Looks guilty.)*

Nurse: I understand. I have a daughter your age. She's also pretty shy about people seeing her body. She says it's because it's changing so fast, and she doesn't understand it all. *(Listens to lung sounds.)*

Client: Yeah. *(Looks interested.)* Does she play sports too? The hardest part is taking a shower after gym. Everybody always looks. I hate it.

Nurse: Not an easy time, I imagine. Could you lie down, please? *(Examines abdomen.)*

Client: *(Big sigh.)* Yeah. Are you almost done? *(Giggles.)* That tickles!

Nurse: Almost. *(Finishes exam.)* I'm going to leave the room so you can get dressed, and then you, your mom, and I can sit and talk for a bit. If you or your mom have any questions you want to ask, I can answer them then. Okay?

Critical Thinking Challenge
- Explain the relationship between body image and self-concept.
- Interpret how you think Gwen would describe herself.
- Compare and contrast how each nurse talked to Gwen and her response to each.
- Describe how Becky used self-disclosure to help Gwen.
- Identify to whom Barbara was primarily talking and why she was less effective.

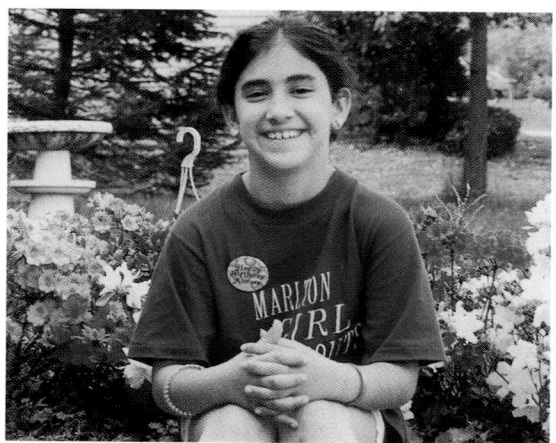

FIGURE 46-4   Sex, skin color, hair color, and eye color affect self-perception.

Coping and Stress Tolerance

Coping and stress tolerance influence self-concept. People who are able to adapt to stress and resolve conflicts through coping tend to develop healthy self-concepts. Internal resources, such as a sense of humor and productivity under pressure, and external resources, such as strong support groups, enhance coping. A single mother who has strong family support may master the roles of parenthood, financial provider, and activist for women's rights, while enhancing self-esteem and likewise strengthening performance in these roles. Poor stress tolerance may lead to crisis, however, and a damaged self-concept.

Stressful Life Events

Most people face numerous daily stressors, many of which occur simultaneously. Common stressors include financial difficulties, job problems, change or loss of employment, relationship concerns, sexuality concerns, divorce, moving, making new friends, loss of loved ones, competition, and making important decisions. Stressful events often challenge the person's identity and self-esteem. One stressor may be so intense that it paralyzes the person and damages self-concept. More often, however, cumulative stress wears away at self-concept (see Chapter 49). For example, a young couple marries and must move to another city where the husband found a job. They have difficulty buying a house because of the high cost of living in the new area and immediately have financial difficulties. The wife would like to start a family but must take a job for which she feels overqualified. They have difficulty making new friends and are overwhelmed by the numerous decisions that have to be made while starting their life together. The husband begins to feel that he is not a good provider and cannot afford the lifestyle he would like. The couple experiences stress in their relationship, and both may feel that self-esteem and identity are damaged.

Inadequate Coping

Inadequate coping can lead to problems with self-concept. In the previous example, the young couple needs strong coping skills to maintain intact self-concepts. Lack of support systems and inability to prioritize and problem solve, however, contribute to further problems. Some people with inadequate coping develop defensive self-esteem. Defensive self-esteem is a protective mechanism in which the person reports high self-esteem to deny negative personal information. The person has a high need for social approval while defending the self against hurt, failure, or anxiety through denial, grandiosity, or projection.

Self-Efficacy

Self-efficacy theory (Bandura, 1977) suggests a link between perceived self and coping behaviors. **Self-efficacy** is the degree of confidence a person has about ability to perform specific activities (*Manuscripts,* 2001). "The greater one's perceptions of self-efficacy are regarding the successful performance of specific activities, the less likely one is to develop depressive symptoms" (Kurlowicz, 1998). Self-efficacy offers nurses a tool for use in health promotion, client teaching for smoking cessation, dietary modification, and compliance with many therapeutic regimens (Beraducci & Lengacher, 1998).

Previous Experience

Self-concept is the individual's complex, ever-changing personal perspective on his or her relationship with the world. It is affected by one's previous experiences with the world. Experiences include opportunities for success and failure. If the person meets with success, he or she builds self-esteem and role satisfaction and begins to expect success. The person also learns what and whom he or she can influence. These experiences teach the person expectancies (Rotter, 1966).

An *expectancy* is a belief that one's behavior will lead to a given response. Two expectancies incorporated into the self are expectancy for success and locus of control, which can be external or internal. Expectancy for success means the person has a belief that personal behavior will lead to something desired. A person with *external locus of control* perceives that outcomes happen because of luck, chance, or the influence of powerful others. A person with *internal locus of control* believes that personal behavior influences outcome, and that he or she can achieve desired results. These expectancies develop from life experiences and influence the self. For instance, if a person believes that luck brought about an outcome, that person would not feel increased esteem because of the outcome, whereas a person with internal locus of control would have increased esteem. Illness may threaten a person with strong internal locus of control; however, self-concept can be preserved by the person's belief that subsequent health-seeking behavior will bring about wellness.

Experience also allows the person to develop and use coping strategies. As the person experiences stress in life, he or she uses the coping skills that fit with his or her views of self and the world. The person who is able to use health-coping mechanisms that worked in the past will reinforce self-esteem with future successful coping.

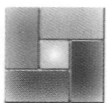

Nursing Research and Critical Thinking
What is the Impact of Self-Efficacy–Enhancing Interventions on Self-Efficacy Beliefs and Functional Outcomes?

Research with older adults demonstrates that efficacy beliefs predict recovery after a cardiac or orthopedic event, short-term memory ability, and physical competence and exercise activities. This nurse believed that because of normal age changes, as well as older adults' vulnerability to the maladaptive effects of self-doubting and failure, consideration of efficacy beliefs in older adults is especially important. She designed an experimental pretest–posttest study to assess the impact of self-efficacy–enhancing interventions on self-efficacy beliefs and functional outcomes of participants in a geriatric rehabilitation program. At the time of admission into the rehabilitation program, clients were randomly assigned to a hospital room, and all the rehabilitation rooms were randomly assigned to one of two treatment groups. The control group (n = 37) received the usual care, which consisted of 90 minutes of physical therapy and 90 minutes of occupational therapy 5 days per week. In addition to usual care, the efficacy–intervention treatment group (n = 40) received three self-efficacy–enhancing interventions: role modeling, verbal persuasion,

and physiologic feedback. Based on repeated measures analysis, with the exception of amount of analgesic used, there was a statistically significant effect of time for all study variables. At discharge, those in the treatment group had stronger efficacy beliefs related to participation, greater participation, and less pain than those in the control group.

Critical Thinking Considerations. Interventions were all completed privately, and the rehabilitation staff were blind to the participants' treatment group status. This helped to control confounding variables. Implications of the study are as follows:

- Self-efficacy and outcome expectancy beliefs are related to performance of the older adult, and efficacy-enhancing interventions strengthen efficacy beliefs and performance with regard to participation in rehabilitation.
- For older adults, the outcomes of performing an activity may be more important than a belief in their ability to perform the activity.

From Resnick, B. (1998). Efficacy beliefs in geriatric rehabilitation. *Journal of Gerontological Nursing, 24*(7), 34–44.

Developmental Level

Developmental level influences self-concept from birth through older adulthood. Whereas newborns have no separate sense of self and young children are learning that their identities are separate from others, adolescents must deal with body image changes. Each developmental level brings unique experiences that can reinforce or alter self-concept. If developmental tasks are not completed, problems with self-concept occur, possibly leading to uncompleted tasks at a later developmental level. Accomplishment of key tasks at each level enhances self-concept.

Incomplete Developmental Tasks

Incomplete developmental tasks can lead to problems with self-concept. Adolescence is a particularly difficult time because many physical, emotional, and sexual changes occur during this period. Adolescents make decisions about the future, seek independence from their parents, and feel pressure from peer groups. Body image and identity are not secure but depend on others' perceptions. Self-esteem is fragile.

Changes in role or body image can affect personal identity during developmental transitions. If personal identity is disturbed, the person has difficulty stating who he or she is. This person may be unable to differentiate personal thoughts and feelings from those of others. Decreases in amount or quality of social interaction may affect relationships.

Role Transition

People make multiple role transitions in a lifetime. Two types of role transition are developmental and situational. *Developmental role transitions* are commonly associated with aging and growth, such as the transition from student to wage earner. *Situational transitions* are associated with change in relationships, such as the death of a spouse or changing one's status from married to widowed. Either type of role transition can prompt role problems including role ambiguity, role strain, and role conflicts. **Role ambiguity** occurs when the person lacks knowledge of role expectations, which fosters anxiety and confusion. For example, a person assumes a new job without an orientation to expected performance and responsibilities. **Role strain** occurs when the person perceives himself or herself as inadequate or unsuited for a role. This can occur in any role or because of numerous roles. One example is a contemporary woman fulfilling roles of wife, lover, mother, employee, and professional with the feeling that she is not fulfilling any role the way she believes that she should.

Role conflict is related to expectations concerning the role. Role conflict can be described as intrapersonal, interpersonal, or interrole. *Intrapersonal role conflict* exists when role expectations conflict with the person's values, such as a nurse being asked to assist with an abortion when she believes it is immoral. *Interpersonal role conflict* exists when the person's expectations differ from that of some significant other. For example, an adolescent might want to play in a rock band but his or her parents value intellectual pursuits. *Interrole conflict* exists when a person is expected to fulfill two or more roles simultaneously. In the case of a spouse's death, the surviving spouse may become sole wage earner for the family, single parent, and caretaker of the house. He or she may be unsure what is expected in a new job. The role as wage earner may conflict with parenting responsibilities, and the combination of roles may be overwhelming. Self-concept can be damaged by such role transitions.

Illness, Trauma, and Surgery

Positive self-concept is usually based on a healthy self. Acute and chronic illness, trauma, or surgery can adversely affect self-esteem and body image, thereby producing stress and role strain, reducing self-esteem, and altering body image. Even physical changes associated with normal aging may alter self-concept. Successful coping during illness, however, may enhance self-esteem. For example, a person with cancer who tolerates chemotherapy, can hold down a job, and becomes closer to the family may emerge feeling emotionally stronger, more resourceful, and with a more positive self-concept than before the illness.

Altered body image occurs when the person experiences a disruption in the perception of the body image. Obviously if the person has an actual loss of a body part or function, he or she will have a disrupted body image until the change is incorporated. Feelings associated with disturbed body image include helplessness, hopelessness, powerlessness, fear of others' reactions, and anger.

Amputation, mastectomy, burns, and facial trauma cause significant change in body structure and appearance. Cardiac disease that limits activities, renal disease requiring dialysis, and a colostomy all impact the body's function. The ability to retain an intact self-concept in the face of illness, trauma, and surgery varies among people. The person's perception of the alteration and the importance he or she places on the body part or function affected influence body image dysfunction. For example, an athlete who places great importance on his or her long, strong legs for running would be devastated by a neurologic illness that produces weakness, placing him or her in a wheelchair. The athlete experiences decreased self-esteem and change in body image.

ALTERED SELF-CONCEPT

Manifestations of Altered Function

Manifestations of self-concept dysfunction range from subtle emotional and behavioral changes to full-blown, self-destructive behaviors. These manifestations also may reflect other problems such as anxiety, depression, or substance abuse. Accurate identification of the underlying problem is essential. Manifestations may occur as immediate reactions to self-concept dysfunction or may be revealed years after self-concept development has been altered.

Self-Care Deficit

People with dysfunctional self-concept may exhibit self-care deficit. For example, people with chronic disease may disregard special diet instructions, not take medications, and miss follow-up appointments. Hospitalized clients may avoid participation in medical and nursing treatment. Self-care deficit may also be characterized by poor personal hygiene, disregard for health maintenance activities, inappropriate exposure or concealment of body parts affected by disease, and lack of health-seeking behaviors. The person may refuse to acknowledge health concerns or express feelings of not being worth special care or concern. For example, a middle-aged diabetic woman with an amputated leg keeps her lower body covered by a blanket, even in warm weather. She rarely combs her hair or puts on makeup, frequently misses appointments, and eats sweets because she feels she is "not worth it."

Emotional and Behavioral Changes

Emotional changes with self-concept dysfunction include feelings of depersonalization, hopelessness, helplessness, alienation, fear of rejection, anger, sadness, shame, guilt, inadequacy, worthlessness, and suspicion of others. Emotional responses may be blunted or inappropriately intense.

Behavioral changes indicating self-concept dysfunction include lack of interest in activities, inability to make decisions, withdrawal from social situations, isolation, refusal to look in the mirror, refusal to look at an affected body part or

ETHICAL/LEGAL ISSUE
Anorexia

Angela Jackson, 14, comes to the clinic with her mother. Angela is reluctant but her mother is insistent and worried. Mrs. Jackson states that Angela has lost weight regularly over the past 6 months and seems to just pick at her food. She wants you to "do something" and make Angela eat, even if it means force-feeding her. Angela, who is 5 feet, 6 inches and weighs 98 lb, says she just isn't hungry. She doesn't understand her mother's worry. Angela states that she thinks she is "fat" and has to watch her weight. You recognize that Angela may have an eating disorder that may be a source of conflict between mother and daughter.

Reflection
- Identify additional information that you may want to obtain.
- Examine the relationship between mother and daughter and the potential ethical dilemmas that may involve you.
- Consider additional resources that you need to manage this situation.
- Determine your ethical and legal responsibilities in this situation.

discuss a limitation, avoidance of responsibility, show of hostility toward others, refusal to make eye contact, and negative verbalizations about self.

Behavior may become more dependent on or independent of others including healthcare providers. A woman who has undergone cancer chemotherapy, lost her hair, and undergone significant weight loss may show emotional and behavioral manifestations of self-concept dysfunction. She may refuse to look in the mirror, assume independence in bathing and dressing to prevent others from seeing her body, avoid eye contact with the staff, refuse visitors by saying she is tired, and seem emotionally apathetic.

Anxiety and Depression

Anxiety and depression are two common psychological disturbances that are manifestations of self-concept dysfunction. Whenever there is a change in body image, problems with roles or identity, and low self-esteem, the person is threatened. This threat is often the cause of great anxiety and is frequently followed by the grieving process. The decline of physical health among older women has been found to be related to increased depression (Heidrich, 1998). Low self-esteem is frequently evident in major psychiatric disorders such as depression (Tucker-Ladd, 2000). An older man who has recently experienced loss of a job, loss of a wife, and loss of good health may show signs of depression.

Self-Destructive Behavior

Substance abuse (drugs, alcohol), sexual promiscuity, gambling, and overeating can be manifestations of self-concept dysfunction. Brown (1998) described the intoxicated person's progression from becoming less self-aware to failing to use good judgment and subsequently behaving atypically. These self-destructive behaviors are addictive, giving immediate gratification only. Persons with low self-esteem and negative self-image find it difficult to change self-destructive behaviors because they have difficulty seeing themselves more positively. A 40-year-old male alcoholic who attributes loss of a job, financial insecurity, and injuries in a car accident to bad luck is an example of a person with self-destructive behavior and a self-concept dysfunction.

Impact on Activities of Daily Living

Alteration of self-concept may affect the simplest activities of daily living (ADLs). People with low self-esteem or altered body image may try to avoid social situations and minimize interactions with others. They may not attend to hygiene needs or keep up their appearances. They may show little interest in recreational activities. Those people with altered body image often have difficulty moving in the environment until they incorporate the change psychologically. Despite physical rehabilitation, they may not maneuver well if the body image change involves a disfigured, amputated, or dysfunctional limb.

People with identity dysfunction also lose interest in self-care activities and often cannot make personal decisions.

People with role dysfunction often place excessive demands on themselves to perform daily activities, becoming self-deprecating when they cannot meet these demands. In persons with self-concept dysfunction, the quality of ADLs is affected, often with a concurrent loss of enjoyment and productivity.

When a person suffers from an illness or exhibits a self-concept dysfunction, family members also may be affected. Family members may need to assist the individual to perform ADLs or have to change the living situation to accommodate adaptive equipment or other assistive devices. Members may also need to fulfill new role responsibilities. Often family members will feel helpless or guilty for an emotional response to the changes in the family or to the "sick" member. All these changes require integration in each family member's self-concept.

ASSESSMENT

The nurse who assesses the client's self-concept is better equipped to implement the nursing process, thus assisting the person in strengthening self-concept. At times, the client's self-concept will be an identified strength that the nurse uses to enhance interventions for other nursing diagnoses.

Subjective Data

Normal Pattern Identification

Gordon (1997) suggests asking clients the following questions about self-concept during a nursing history:

- How would you describe yourself?
- Most of the time, how do you feel about yourself?
- Are you experiencing changes in your body or the things you can do?
- Is this a problem for you?
- Have you or are you experiencing changes in the way you feel about yourself or your body?
- Do you find things frequently make you feel angry, anxious, frustrated, afraid, sad, or annoyed?
- If so, what helps?
- Do you ever feel as though you have lost hope?
- Do you ever feel that you are not able to control things in your life?
- What helps you when you feel hopeless, or out of control of your life?

Further assessment of roles and relationships is discussed in Chapter 47.

Risk Identification

When assessing a person at risk of self-concept dysfunction, consider the client's developmental stage, previous experience, intensity of a stressor or threat, and self-expectations. Certain developmental stages pose a greater risk than others do. If the client is an infant, what are the self-concepts of the parents? Is the client an adolescent who has had a body image change? Does the change affect sexuality? Assessment of previous experience should include past problems with self-concept, history of unsuccessful coping mechanisms, and lack of resources and support. Intensity of a stressor may help identify risk. Is the client threatened by a role? By an illness or body image change? How important is good health or performance of a role? How serious is an illness or change in body function?

Assessment of the difference between the real self and the ideal self can also identify risk. What are the client's expectations? How far is he or she from meeting these expectations? Are expectations unrealistic?

Dysfunction Identification

Dysfunction identification also involves assessment of the client's thoughts and feelings. People who do not possess a healthy self-concept are less able to cope with life, often expressing feelings of inferiority, self-doubt, and self-dislike. Does the client verbalize negative feelings, such as "I don't like myself;" "I'm so ugly now;" "I'm worthless;" or "I'm a terrible mother?" Why does the person feel this way? In what area is the person having a problem—self-esteem, role function, personal identity, or body image?

Objective Data

Objective data about the client's self-concept are gathered through direct observation. These data include behavioral manifestations such as lack of eye contact, and physical observations such as a missing body part or function. The person may try to conceal a body part, for example, by bandaging an arm scarred by burns after the burns have healed. The person may exhibit anxious behavior such as hand wringing and shallow breathing or grief behavior such as weeping.

Although some behaviors may be easily observed, assessing the meaning of these behaviors may be more difficult. For instance, if the person hides a body part, does this manifest body image disturbance or extreme need for privacy? These data are clues and must be judged with the subjective data to determine risk for or actual disturbances in self-concept. Ongoing observation of the client's behavior helps identify changes in the self-concept.

NURSING DIAGNOSES

Diagnostic Statement: Disturbed Body Image

Definition. Disturbed Body Image is confusion in the mental picture of one's physical self (North American Nursing Diagnosis Association [NANDA], 2001).

Defining Characteristics. The following are major defining characteristics or clinical cues that point to the diagnosis of Disturbed Body Image:

- Nonverbal response to actual or perceived change in structure and/or function

- Verbalization of feelings that reflect an altered view of one's body in appearance, structure, or function
- Verbalization of perceptions that reflect an altered view of one's body in appearance, structure, or function
- Behaviors of avoidance, monitoring, or acknowledgment of one's body

Related Factors. A variety of etiologic or contributing factors may affect this change in functional health status. They include amputation of a body part; brain injury with the effect of altering body perception; surgery; colostomy; urinary diversion; congenital deformity; eating disorders; morbid obesity; trauma with altered body part—structure or function; chronic illness resulting in structural or functional change; body scheme/perceptual disorders; lifestyle change; depression; trauma (e.g., rape); cultural or spiritual differences; developmental or age-related factors (NANDA, 2001).

Diagnostic Statement: Chronic Low Self-Esteem

Definition. Chronic Low Self-Esteem is a state in which a person has long-standing negative self-evaluation/feeling about self or self-capabilities (NANDA, 2001).

Defining Characteristics. Of the defining characteristics or clinical cues that point to this diagnosis, one of the following major characteristics must be present: long-standing or chronic self-negating verbalizations (the person discounts, minimizes, or criticizes self, personal ideas, or accomplishments), expressions of shame or guilt, evaluation of self as unable to deal with events, rejection of positive feedback or exaggeration of negative feedback, or hesitancy to try new things or situations (the person says "I can't" in relation to new experiences).

The following minor characteristics may be present but are not required for this diagnosis: frequent lack of success in work or other life events (the person may not excel or may quit or fail at school or work or in relationships), overly conforming behavior or dependency on others' opinions, lack of eye contact, passivity or nonassertiveness, indecisiveness, seeks excessive reassurance (NANDA, 2001).

Related Factors. NANDA has yet to develop related factors.

Diagnostic Statement: Situational Low Self-Esteem

Definition. Situational Low Self-Esteem is negative self-evaluation/feelings about self that develop in response to a loss or change in a person who previously had a positive self-evaluation (NANDA, 2001).

Defining Characteristics. Of the defining characteristics or clinical cues that point to this diagnosis, one of the following characteristics must be present: episodic occurrence of negative self-appraisal in response to life events in a person with a previous positive self-evaluation or verbalization of negative feelings about the self (the person expresses feelings of helplessness, uselessness, or extreme self-doubt).

The following minor characteristics may also be present but are not required for this diagnosis: self-negating verbalizations (the person makes statements such as "I can't" or "I'm no good" when describing self), expressions of shame or guilt, evaluation of self as unable to handle situations or events (the person expresses feelings of fear of failure or inability when discussing situations or events), or difficulty making decisions (NANDA, 2001).

Related Factors. A number of developmental, family, and school situations may result in negative self-perception. For example, a boy may feel negative about himself at the time of puberty, or experience a disturbed body image in relation to the growth of facial hair. The arrival of a new baby in a family can require a role change for a toddler or school-age child from being the only child to being a sibling. This can affect self-esteem as the child observes, "Baby gets all of Mom's attention. Who cares about me anymore?" School can be another source of Situational Low Self-Esteem for the child or adolescent who is doing poorly in learning a new language or failing to be selected for a sports team. Furthermore, individuals with a history of abuse or neglect, or those who have a physical illness, are at risk for developing Situational Low Self-Esteem (NANDA, 2001).

Diagnostic Statement: Ineffective Role Performance

Definition. Ineffective Role Performance means that patterns of behavior and self-expression do not match the environmental context, norms, and expectations (NANDA, 2001).

Defining Characteristics. Defining characteristics include change in self-perception of role (the person perceives the role or his or her ability to perform it has changed); role denial (the person denies that he or she has taken on or been assigned a role [e.g., a child denies that he is a brother after a new sibling is born]); inadequate external support for role enactment; inadequate adaptation to change or transition; system conflict; change in usual patterns of responsibility; discrimination; domestic violence; harassment; uncertainty; altered role perceptions; role strain; inadequate self-management; role ambivalence; pessimism; inadequate motivation; inadequate confidence; inadequate role competency or skills; inadequate knowledge; inappropriate developmental expectations; role conflict; role confusion; powerlessness; inadequate coping; anxiety or depression; role overload; change in others' perceptions of role; change in capacity to resume role; role dissatisfaction; inadequate opportunities for role enactment (NANDA, 2001).

Related Factors. Related factors fall into three different categories: social, knowledge, and physiologic. Some social factors include inadequate or inappropriate linkage with the healthcare system, job schedule demands, poverty, and inadequate support systems. Some knowledge factors include inadequate role preparation, education attainment level, lack of knowledge about role, and unrealistic role expectations. Some physiologic factors include substance abuse, mental illness, pain, and cognitive defects (NANDA, 2001).

Related Nursing Diagnoses

When making a diagnosis related to disturbed self-concept, the nurse must also consider diagnoses with common defining characteristics. Often these are inherent in dysfunctional self-concept. Among these diagnoses are Anxiety, Ineffective Coping, Compromised Family Coping, Defensive Coping, Fear, Interrupted Family Process, Anticipatory Grieving, Hopelessness, Powerlessness, Social Isolation, and Disturbed Thought Processes.

OUTCOME IDENTIFICATION AND PLANNING

Outcome identification and planning focus on either promotion of a healthy self-concept or change of altered self-concept. The following general areas may be included in the formulation of client goals:

- Client will integrate a realistic body image.
- Client will express positive feelings about self or self-capabilities.
- Client will distinguish between self and nonself.
- Client will perform capably.

Client goals will differ according to the defining characteristics that apply to each client. The client and nurse plan together to identify goals and interventions. Some interventions used in planning are listed in the accompanying display and discussed in the following section.

IMPLEMENTATION

Health Promotion

Identification of Strengths

Nurses can promote positive self-concept in their clients by assisting them in identifying strengths. The continued use of internal and external resources helps strengthen identity, role performance, self-esteem, and body image. Various personal strengths include good sense of humor, good communication skills, good problem-solving ability, a nice smile, strong health maintenance patterns, strong values, hobbies, strong social support systems (e.g., family relationships), a stable marriage, enjoyment in work, and a good education (Fig. 46-5). When presented with stressors such as illness or loss of a loved one, point out these strengths to clients to reinforce self-concept. Encourage clients to cultivate these strengths and use them in the coping process whenever the self is threatened.

Sense of Self

Always treat clients respectfully and personally to help them maintain a sense of self. By respecting each client's individ-

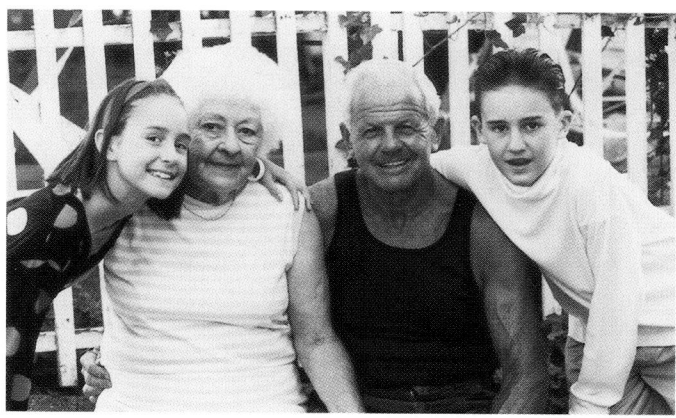 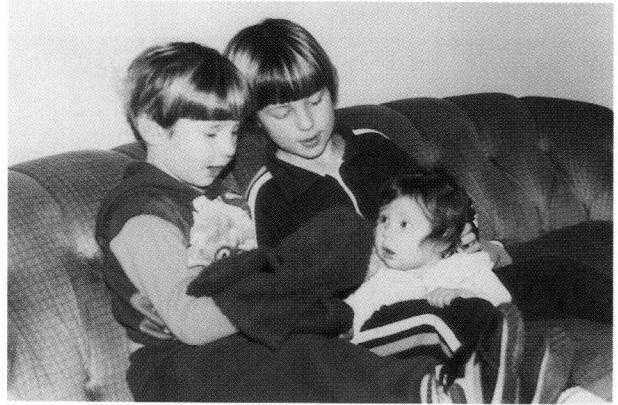

FIGURE 46-5 Families can provide stability and strength during changes. Strength may come from intergenerational relationships and/or sibling relationships.

uality, nurses promote positive self-concepts. Pay special attention to verbal and nonverbal interactions with all clients. Introduce yourself to clients, address clients by name, speak respectfully, and maintain the privacy of clients at all times. Explain all procedures and nursing activities, and pay attention to emotional responses of clients.

Development of Self-Concept

Helping clients to develop self-concept is related to developmental period. Table 46-2 lists nursing interventions for development of self-concept as specific to age group.

Newborn. During the neonatal period, anticipatory guidance assists family members to adapt to their new roles and the self-concept related to these roles. Most often, this is accomplished through a therapeutic relationship that allows for exploration of expectations and provides support to deal with

---

PLANNING:　Examples of NIC/NOC Interventions

Accepted Self-Concept Nursing Interventions Classification (NIC)
Body Image Enhancement
Decision-Making Support
Self-Esteem Enhancement

Accepted Self-Concept Nursing Outcomes Classification (NOC)
Body Image
Coping
Decision Making
Grief Resolution
Mood Equilibrium
Self-Esteem

Refer to the following for specifics regarding NIC/NOC:
McCloskey, J., & Bulechek, G. (2000). *Iowa Intervention Project: Nursing Interventions Classification (NIC)* 2nd ed. St. Louis, MO: C. V. Mosby.
Johnson, M., & Maas, M. (2000). *Iowa Outcomes Project: Nursing Outcomes Classification (NOC)* 2nd ed. St. Louis, MO: C. V. Mosby.

---

anxiety. Educate the family about parental roles, body changes, emotional changes, and family role expectations. When done early, care provided minimizes disturbances in self-concept for all family members, including the newborn.

Infant. Teach parents about the infant's need for movement, stimulation, and safety. If a child has an acute or chronic illness during this period, an environment that facilitates continued development is crucial. Activities should be age- and health-appropriate, providing safety and security. Parents need to provide as much care as possible for hospitalized infants. Assist parents to decrease their anxiety (to cope with the hospitalization). Doing so helps infants to feel more secure, fosters trust, and promotes continued self-concept development.

Toddler. Toddlers need an environment that allows practice of newly developing skills, especially movement-related skills, for body image and esteem to develop positively. Educate families that repetitive positive input and allowing toddlers to explore support the development of a favorable self-concept. Hospitalization or illness during toddlerhood affects the development of self-concept. Support toddler and family by helping the toddler maintain self-control.

Preschooler. During the preschool years, educate the family about normal development and support the family's establishment of an effective environment that facilitates growth. Because children have increased sexual feelings, preschoolers fear damage to their bodies. Therefore they need support and education concerning health maintenance behaviors such as personal hygiene and healthcare visits. This can be accomplished through visits to healthcare providers with other family members or through supportive treatment during routine examinations. Hospitalization or serious illness in preschoolers is especially difficult. Preschoolers have many fantasies about punishment, abandonment, or physical harm. Combat these fantasies by including preschoolers in decisions as much as possible. In addition, encourage families of hospitalized preschoolers to stay with their children as much as

TABLE 46-2

Developmental Interventions to Promote Self-Concept	
Developmental Level	**Interventions**
Newborn	Assist family in adapting to new roles by establishing therapeutic relationship and educating members.
Infant	Teach family about infant's need for movement, stimulation, and safety. Encourage parents to help provide physical care and security for hospitalized infants.
Toddler	Allow toddler to develop skills through exploration. Support family and help toddler maintain self-control.
Preschooler	Teach preschooler and family health maintenance behaviors. Encourage family to stay with the child if hospitalized, and let the child make some decisions about care.
School-age child	Allow privacy. Teach parents of need for socialization and belonging. Allow liberal visitation and age-appropriate activities if hospitalized.
Adolescent	Educate adolescent about sexual health, drug and alcohol use. Educate family about identity and body image changes. If adolescent is hospitalized, offer choices in care to maintain autonomy.
Adult	Use therapeutic relationship to support adult and significant other. Support decisions adult makes in relationships and work roles.
Older adult	Treat older adult with respect and allow independence and individuality. Help older adult integrate loss of spouse, job, social support network, health, and the like.

possible. Remember that a family may respond to a child's hospitalization with guilt, helplessness, and anxiety. To aid the child, assist the family in dealing with these feelings.

School-Age Child. Continue to teach and help parents understand their children's need for socialization and belonging. Frequently school nurses teach reproduction and health in school settings. If a child is hospitalized during this period, be cognizant of changing needs for privacy, and the child's need to know that he or she still belongs to the family and peer group. In addition, school-age children need information about their illnesses and treatments. Parents again need support and help dealing with their fear and anxiety.

Adolescent. Support adolescents and families through the process of assuming roles and establishing independence. The need for privacy is a major concern of teenagers. Teach the family about the developmental process and why individual family members may have intense feelings during this period. Adolescents experiment as they make choices to establish identity. Provide health teaching including information concerning birth control, AIDS, and sexually transmitted diseases. A further concern is drug use and alcohol abuse. Adolescents need to know the ramifications of choosing drugs or alcohol as a coping style. They may need assistance to learn and practice alternate coping behaviors.

Many adolescents are hospitalized on pediatric units, which may contradict a teen's view of himself or herself as an independent, grown-up person. Offering adolescents choices regarding care helps them maintain some autonomy. Provide feedback about the adolescent's strengths and weaknesses to help him or her establish a realistic self-concept.

Adult. Assist adults with role satisfaction primarily in intimate relationships and occupation through use of a therapeutic relationship. Structure the environment to provide for successes, and allow adults time and support while exploring the meaning of life. A feeling of generativity enhances self-concept. Continue to offer support to significant others.

Older Adult. Older people do not seek care as "old" people but as people with needs. Loss of independence associated with aging may bring loss of self-esteem. Support appropriate independence and self-care for older adults, which enhances self-concept. In working with older people, assist them in integrating changes, most often loss, into their self-concept. Also, enhance their self-concept by using respect and allowing individuality. Interventions aimed at older adults include allowing them to keep personal belongings in their settings for healthcare, listening to their stories, respecting privacy, explaining procedures, and allowing them extra time to accomplish tasks (Fig. 46-6).

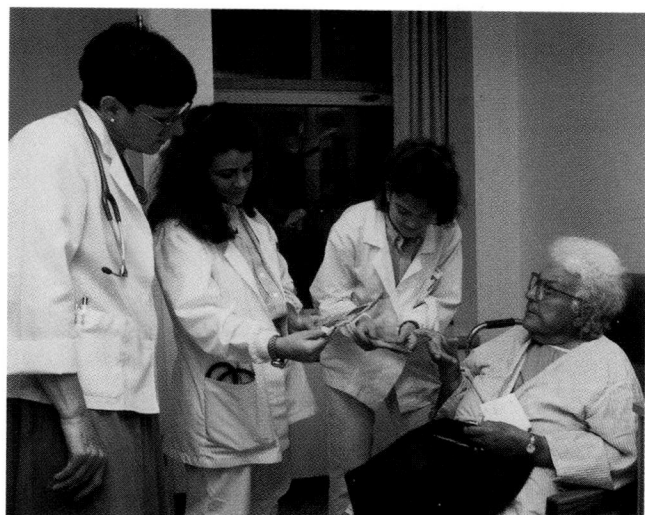

FIGURE 46-6 An older client tells her story through family pictures and mementos. (Courtesy of Seattle University School of Nursing.)

Nursing Interventions for Altered Self-Concept

Therapeutic Relationship

Nurses intervene with clients with altered self-concept through therapeutic relationships. To develop therapeutic relationships, nurses must demonstrate great self-awareness and effective communication. Conveying a sense of friendship and trust helps establish rapport with clients. When empathy is shown, clients believe that nurses understand their feelings and will care for their needs. Once the relationship is established, use therapeutic communication techniques such as active listening, reflection, and reality-based feedback. Therapeutic communication assists clients with defining self-concept problems and attempting to problem solve.

Self-Evaluation

Nursing interventions that assist clients with positive self-evaluation can help change poor self-concept. People with low self-esteem frequently put themselves down and act in ways that perpetuate negative self-evaluation. To break this cycle, clients need help in realistically evaluating the self and developing more positive thoughts and feelings about the self. Emphasize positive attributes rather than negative behaviors. Assist clients to point out tasks or accomplishments that deserve positive feedback. Offer praise honestly and encourage clients to make positive self-statements. Also, be a model for clients by acting confident, making positive statements, and accepting compliments.

Behavioral Change

Nursing interventions aimed at changing behavior also assist clients with self-concept problems. General measures that bring about behavioral changes include accepting responsi-bility for self, defining realistic goals, using resources to enact change, and rewarding positive outcomes. Help clients accept responsibility for self by suggesting they make "I" statements that reflect thoughts and feelings. For example, for a client with role performance problems, instead of saying, "nothing ever goes right," a more active statement might be "I can't get the hang of my new job." This is the first step in realizing that the client may have the power to change behavior.

In helping clients define realistic goals, assist them in evaluating expectations. If expectations are unrealistic or the discrepancy between the real self and the ideal self is too great, behavior will not change. Goals should be specific, such as "I will ask my boss for a 2-week training period on the new computer system." Help clients identify resources to accomplish goals including, for example, a computer training department at the office, night school courses, or someone to help around the house so the client can temporarily devote more time to work.

Clients will be more likely to change behavior if they believe they will be rewarded for more positive behavior. Point out rewards such as a feeling of greater competence, less time spent at the office, greater productivity, and praise by others. By assisting clients with problem solving, role performance should improve, which strengthens self-concept.

OUTCOME-BASED TEACHING PLAN

Maria Benet, 16, comes to the high school clinic for a "sore throat." Assessment reveals that her throat is not inflamed, and she does not have a fever. As you explore the situation, Maria states, "I'm too sick to go to class today. Besides, I'm no good at math and never will be. I think I'll just drop out of school." You realize that Maria may have some self-concept problems. You decide to try to help her overcome them.

OUTCOME: Maria will express more confidence in her ability to learn new things.
Strategies
- Explore Maria's feelings about her performance in math class.
- If Maria is motivated to try to change:
  - Have Maria discuss her performance privately with her teacher and/or counselor.
  - Discuss possible support mechanisms (e.g., peer tutors, special study sessions).
  - Discuss ways she uses math every day (e.g., memorizing phone numbers, figuring "percent off" at sales, making change when she shops).
  - Suggest she practice math activities and realize that she can handle them.
- Problem solve with Maria a plan that she feels most inclined and motivated to follow.
- Provide regular opportunities for follow-up to assess and provide encouragement from you and others.

Healthcare Planning and Home/Community-Based Nursing

Clients with self-concept disturbance usually require psychosocial assistance beyond the scope of routine nursing. Assist such clients to recognize difficulties and to accept additional therapy. Afterward, work with these clients to initiate plans for additional care. The goals of discharge planning are effective teaching and referral.

The teaching plan may include where and how to use community resources such as support groups or individual teaching concerning stages of loss. Referral may be to a specialized support group, such as for mastectomy clients, or may be for therapy through a psychiatric nurse specialist, psychologist, or psychiatrist. Consult the healthcare provider about ambulatory referrals. If the client is to receive home-health services, communicate with the home care nurse about the plan of care. For example, home care for the client after mastectomy should include interventions to help incorporate a change in body image and to strengthen self-esteem, if those problem areas were identified while the client was hospitalized. Describe interventions that have worked for continuity of care.

EVALUATION

Specific outcome criteria are used to measure the attainment of goals in self-concept. If the nurse asks what the client hopes to see or hear if the interventions chosen are effective, goals will be behavioral in nature. The nurse then asks under what circumstances the client will exhibit that behavior and by when. Such goals are measurable. Because the nurse and

---

NURSING PLAN OF CARE

THE CLIENT WITH DISTURBED BODY IMAGE

Nursing Diagnosis
Disturbed Body Image related to change in physical appearance manifested by client's refusal to look at body.

Client Goal
Client will express improved perception of physical appearance.

Client Outcome Criteria
- Client discusses his or her physical changes within 2 days of surgery.
- Client demonstrates participation in ADLs within 3 days.
- Client uses coping skills to prepare for changes in physical appearance within 3 days.
- Client views affected body part within 1 week of surgery.

Nursing Intervention	Scientific Rationale
1. Assess client's strengths that will positively affect body image, such as family relationships.	1. Assessment of factors that can contribute to improved body image builds on client's strengths.
2. Provide opportunities to discuss altered appearance and self-worth.	2. Stating feelings verbally often helps client to clarify and achieve perspective.
3. Assist with grooming.	3. When client is unable physically or emotionally to groom self, the nurse's care activities indicate concern for the client's welfare and help to establish rapport.
4. Encourage the client to participate in self-grooming and to strive for independence.	4. Encouraging participation in self-care provides client with a sense of control.
5. Encourage identification and use of positive coping strategies.	5. Use of coping strategies that have worked effectively for the client aids in successful coping with body image.
6. Encourage client to cultivate positive coping strategies.	6. Use of internal and external resources helps strengthen self-esteem and body image.
7. Provide a mirror for the client to view self. The client may want to do so in privacy.	7. Client must view physical changes before integrating them into a realistic body image.
8. Provide information and education regarding altered appearance, support groups, and other resources.	8. Individualized education and information meet the client's unique needs.

client (in most cases) establish goals and outcome criteria, they can discuss whether or not these criteria have been met. Outcome criteria for client goals discussed earlier in the chapter may include the following

Goal

Client will integrate a realistic body image.

Possible Outcome Criteria

- Client speaks about his or her body within 2 days after surgery.
- Client views self in mirror within 3 days after surgery.
- Client assists with dressing changes within 4 days after surgery.

Goal

Client will express positive feelings about self or self-capabilities.

Possible Outcome Criteria

- Client establishes eye contact with nurse during conversation within 2 days.
- Client lists negative attitudes and their effects on self by discharge.
- Client verbalizes feelings of success with self-care activities by discharge.
- Client verbalizes strategies to support self-care and positive feelings related to self at home.

Goal

Client will distinguish between self and nonself.

Possible Outcome Criteria

- Client identifies feelings of depersonalization as related to illness within 2 days.
- Client states realistic expectations for discharge within 5 days.
- Client expresses feelings of hope and power over own life within 7 days.

Goal

Client will perform capably.

Possible Outcome Criteria

- Client expresses interest in caring for newborn within 1 day.
- Client identifies three coping strategies to help assume new role within 2 weeks.

- Client performs basic care of newborn successfully within 24 hours and more complex care within 2 weeks.
- Before discharge, client verbalizes whom the client will contact for social support when home.

KEY CONCEPTS

- Self-concept is the mental image a person holds of the self.
- Characteristics of normal self-concept include the dimensions of self-perception: self-knowledge, self-expectation, social self, and self-evaluation.
- Positive body image, self-esteem, strong personal identity, and role performance are normal patterns of self-concept.
- Factors that affect self-concept include biologic makeup; culture, values and beliefs; coping and stress tolerance; self-efficacy; previous experience; developmental level and completion of developmental tasks; and illness including trauma and surgery.
- Manifestations of altered self-concept include self-care deficit, emotional and behavioral changes, anxiety and depression, and self-destructive behavior (e.g., alcoholism, drug abuse, and sexual promiscuity).
- Personal strengths that nurses can encourage clients to cultivate to promote positive self-concept include sense of humor, communication skills, strong health maintenance patterns, hobbies, social support systems, enjoyment in work, and education.
- Nurses help clients with low self-esteem by assisting them with realistic self-evaluation and development of more positive thoughts and feelings about themselves including emphasizing positive attributes rather than negative ones.
- Nurses can also help bring about behavioral change in clients with altered self-concept by assisting them to accept responsibility for themselves, define realistic goals, use resources to enact change, and reward positive outcomes.

REFERENCES

Anderson, L., Janes, G., Ziemer, D., & Phillips, L. (1997). Diabetes in urban African Americans: Body image, satisfaction with size, and weight change attempts. *The Diabetes Educator, 23*(3), 301–308.

Bandura, A. (1977). Self-efficacy: Toward a unifying theory of behavior change. *Psychological Review, 84,* 191–215.

Beraducci, A., & Lengacher, C. (1998). Self-efficacy: An essential component of advanced practice nursing. *Nursing Connections, 11*(1), 55–65.

Brown, J. (1998). *The self.* Boston, MA: McGraw-Hill.

Colt, G. (1998). Were you born that way? *Life, 21*(4), 39–42, 44, 46, 48, 50.

Coopersmith, S. (1967). *Antecedents of self esteem.* San Francisco, CA: Freeman.

Erikson, E. (1963). *Childhood and society* (2nd ed.). New York, NY: W. W. Norton.

Freud, S. (1920/1966). *Lectures on psychoanalysis.* (J. Strachey, Ed. and Trans.). New York, NY: W. W. Norton.

Gordon, M. (1997). *Manual of nursing diagnosis* (2nd ed.). New York, NY: McGraw-Hill.

Havighurst, R. (1972). *Developmental tasks and education* (3rd ed.). New York, NY: David McKay.

Heidrich, S. (1998). Older women's lives through time. *Advances in Nursing Science, 20*(3), 65–75.

Huitt, W. (1998, May). Self-concept and self-esteem. Retrieved August 21, 2001, from Valdosta State University: *http://chiron.valdosta.edu/whuitt/col/regsys/self.html*

Kohlberg, L. (1969). Stage and sequence: The cognitive developmental approach to socialization. In D. A. Goslin (Ed.), *Handbook of socialization: Theory and research.* Chicago, IL: Rand McNally.

Kurlowicz, L. (1998, July/August). Perceived self-efficacy, functional ability, and depressive symptoms in older elective surgery patients. *Nursing Research, 47*(4), 219–226.

Manuscripts on self-efficacy: Self-efficacy and health behaviors. (n.d.). Retrieved August 21, 2001, from Emory University: *http://www.emory.eu/EDUCATION/mfp/effms.html.*

National Institute on Aging. (1998). *Personnel for health needs of the elderly: through the year 2020.* Bethesda, MD: National Institutes of Health, Public Health Services, U.S. Department of Health and Human Services. (WT 30 P43)

North American Nursing Diagnosis Association (NANDA). (2001). *Nursing diagnoses: Definitions and classification 2001–2002.* Philadelphia: Author.

Piaget, J. (1969). *The psychology of the child.* New York, NY: Basic Books.

Rogers, C. R. (1961). *On becoming a person.* Boston, MA: Houghton Mifflin.

Rotter, J. B. (1966). Generalized expectancies for internal versus external locus of control reinforcement. *Psychology Monographs, 80,* 1–28.

Segal, N. (1998). Twin research perspective on human development. In N. L. Weisfeld & C. C. Weisfeld (Eds.), *Uniting psychology and biology.* Washington, DC: American Psychological Association.

Sheehy, G. (1974). *Passages.* New York, NY: E. P. Dutton.

Sullivan, H. (1953). *The interpersonal theory of psychiatry.* New York, NY: W. W. Norton.

Tucker-Ladd, C. E. (2000). Depression and self concept [electronic version]. Psychological Self-Help. Retrieved August 21, 2001, from *http://mentalhelp.net/psyhelp/chap6/*

BIBLIOGRAPHY

Alpers, R. (1998). The changing self-concept of pregnant and parenting teens. *Journal of Professional Nursing, 14*(2), 111–118.

Arthur, D., & Thorne, S. (1997). Professional self-concept of nurses: A comparative study of four strata of nursing students in a Canadian university. *Nurse Education Today, 18,* 380–388.

Bandura, A. (1986). *Social foundations of thought and action: A social cognitive theory.* Englewood Cliffs, NJ: Prentice Hall.

Burr, S., & Gradwell, C. (1996). The psychosocial effects of skin diseases: Need for support groups. *British Journal of Nursing, 5*(19), 1177–1178, 1180–1182.

DiBiase, R., & Waddell, S. (1995). Some effects of homelessness on the psychological functioning of preschoolers. *Journal of Abnormal Child Psychology, 23*(6), 783–785.

Doswell, W., Millor, G., Thompson, H., & Braxter, B. (1998). Self image and self esteem in African-American preteen girls: Implications for mental health. *Issues in Mental Health Nursing, 19*(1), 71–94.

Falk, R., & Miller, N. (1998). The reflexive self: A sociological perspective. *Roeper Review, 20*(3), 150–153.

Hanna, B. (1996). Sexuality, body image, and self-esteem: The future after trauma. *Journal of Trauma Nursing, 3*(1), 13–17, 19–20.

Huurre, T., & Aro, H. (1998). Psychosocial development among adolescents with visual impairment. *European Child and Adolescent Psychiatry, 7*(2), 73–78.

Jacelon, C. (1997). The trait and process of resilience. *Journal of Advanced Nursing, 25,* 123–129.

Muscari, M. (1998). Coping with chronic Illness. *American Journal of Nursing, 98*(9), 20.

Roberts, C., Turney, M., & Knowles, A. (1998). Psychosocial issues of adolescents with cancer. *Social Working Health Care, 27*(4), 3–18.

Robinson, B., & Kelley, L. (1998). Adult children of workaholics: Self-concept, anxiety, depression, and locus of control. *American Journal of Family Therapy, 26*(3), 223–238.

Robinson, L., & Mahon, M. (1997). Sibling bereavement: A concept analysis. *Death Studies, 21*(5), 474–499.

Segal, N. (1997). Same age unrelated siblings: A unique test of within-family environmental influences on I.Q. similarity. *Journal of Educational Psychology, 89,* 381–390.

Showers, C., Abramson, L., & Hogan, M. (1998). The dynamic self: How the content and structure of the self-concept change with mood. *Journal of Personality and Social Psychology, 75*(2), 478–493.

Stein, K., Roeser, R., & Markus, H. (1998). Self-schemas and possible selves as predictors and outcomes of risky behaviors in adolescents. *Nursing Research, 47*(2), 96–106.

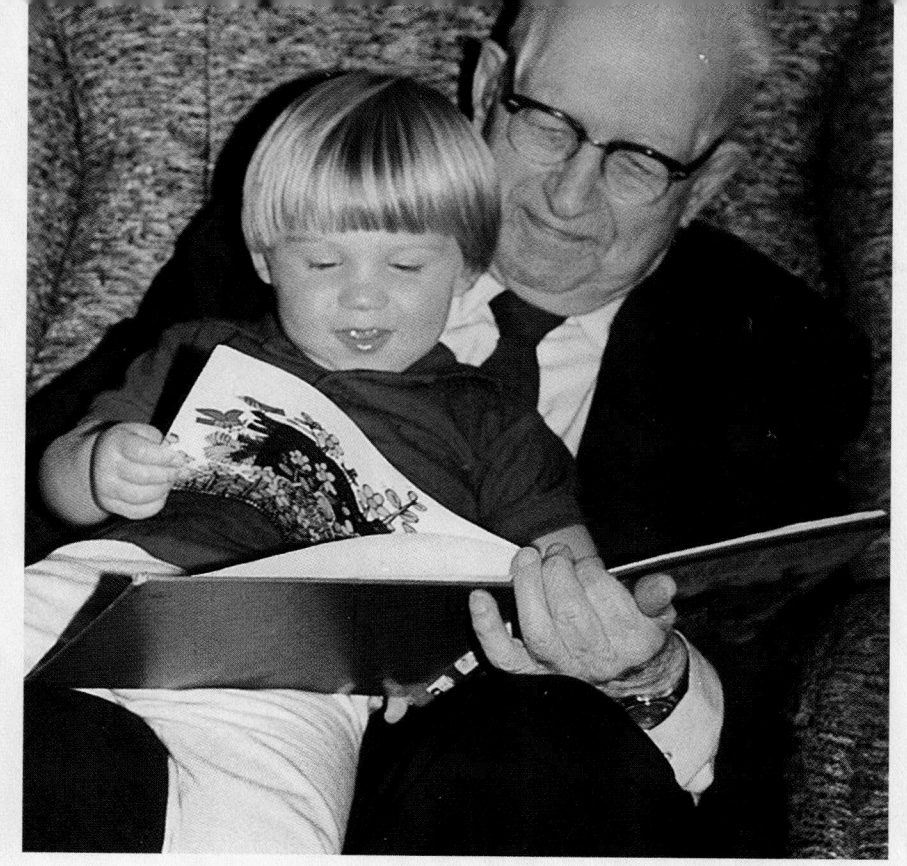

Roles and Relationships

47 Families and Their Relationships

Key Terms

altered family function
anticipatory guidance
blended family
cohabitated family
communal family
extended family

family-centered care
nuclear family
role strain
sandwich generation
single-parent families
social isolation

Learning Objectives

Upon completion of this chapter, the student will be able to do the following:
1. Describe variations in family structure and function.
2. Identify demographic, sociocultural, and economic factors that affect normal family relationships.
3. Describe manifestations of altered family function.
4. Evaluate the possible impact of altered family function on activities of daily living.
5. Differentiate subjective and objective data needed to assess family function.
6. Identify nursing diagnoses and related factors associated with altered family function.
7. Discuss nursing interventions to promote family health and function.
8. Discuss nursing interventions for altered family function.
9. List family-centered healthcare services in the community.

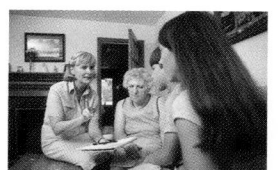

Critical Thinking Challenge

You are the home care nurse coordinator meeting for the first time with Jeffery and Sarah Jones and their 23-year-old granddaughter, Marissa. Their family nurse practitioner has referred them for home care after consultation with a neurologist. Mrs. Jones, 78 years old, has noted that her husband, 82 years old, has become increasingly forgetful, "getting lost" if he walks even a block away from home. Mr. Jones has recently begun several inappropriate behaviors such as "using the flower pot as a toilet." She suspects that he is "getting senile" just like his father before he died. She has asked Marissa to live with them for a while to help her handle Mr. Jones, especially during the nights when he is restless and wanders. Marissa sits quietly and does not look at her grandmother. When you ask if she has been able to stay full-time, the grandmother immediately replies that she has. "But," she continues, "I don't think she can do it much longer—it really interferes with her sleeping and makes it hard for her to keep her job. Besides she should get married before it's too late!" You find out that Marissa's mother, a 56-year-old social worker, is struggling to maintain her own career while caring for Marissa's younger brother, who has limited functioning due to a heart condition. Marissa does not know her father. The family members seem very concerned about each other but they don't know how they can continue to cope if things get any worse.

Once you have completed this chapter and have added families and their relationships to your knowledge base, review the above scenario and reflect on the following areas of Critical Thinking:

1. Analyze your initial feelings about this family's ability to care for the older male (Mr. Jones).
2. Plan how you will elicit the family's perception of needs, goals, and outcomes.
3. Describe what you think are the perceptions of the wife, daughter, and granddaughter in this situation. Compare and contrast them with your own feelings.
4. Summarize key areas to assess when you visit the family within 48 hours after referral.
5. Recommend ways to facilitate family-centered care, particularly if disagreements arise about the home care plan.

Two hundred years ago, children were raised in extended families that consisted of several generations of family members living in close proximity to one another. Large families were desired, members were interdependent, and socialization was accomplished by passing traditions from one generation to the next. Dynamic public policy and social changes, together with demographic trends including expanded opportunities for higher education, diverse avenues of employment, and women's economic independence, have changed family life (Bomar, 1996). At the beginning of the 21st century, family structures are more varied than in the past. The small, traditional family unit known as the **nuclear family** remains prominent; however, more than one fourth of family units now consist of children who live with a single parent (Fig. 47-1). One-sixth of the 11.9 million single parents in the United States are men (U.S. Census Bureau, 1998). Blended families, extended families, cohabitated families, and communal families are among the many other variations. Increased lifestyle options have established new family norms with a concurrent need for nurses to focus on helping individuals and families to adapt to these changes.

Although nurses deal with individuals, those individuals are integral parts of families. Consider the older couple, their career-focused daughter, and their granddaughter in the Critical Thinking Challenge. You can see from this example how the entire family influences the health perceptions and practices of its members. Nurses must understand the importance of family functioning to affect positively each person's health status. Nurses who practice **family-centered care,** which means caring for the client and family as a unit, recognize the positive aspects of diversity and facilitate client/caregiver/professional collaboration (Gedaly-Duff & Heims, 1996).

NORMAL FAMILY RELATIONSHIPS

A family is a social group whose members share common values, occupy specific positions, interact over time, and have diverse strengths and needs. Family members bear and rear children, cooperate economically and politically, and care for the ill and infirm of all ages.

Family Structure

Family structure means who the members are and what their relationships are to one another. Structure varies among families as well as within each family over time. Although the traditional structure of the family in the United States is the nuclear family, many other family structures are common today. Family members do not always live together in one household but remain connected by their relationships.

Nuclear Family

The nuclear family includes a married adult man and woman and their children (Fig. 47-2). Members live in the same house usually until the children leave home to support themselves or to attend college. In 1998, 27% of the nation's 102.5 million households were composed of a married couple with children younger than 18 years (U.S. Census Bureau, 1998). Variations in the nuclear family include couples who remain childless or whose older children return home after a period of independence (e.g., after college). More than 22 million adult children (over age 18) live with their parent(s), an increase from 15 million in 1970 (U.S. Census Bureau, 1998). Traditional roles in the nuclear family have been the man as breadwinner outside the home and the woman as responsible for physical provision of the home and children. The number of

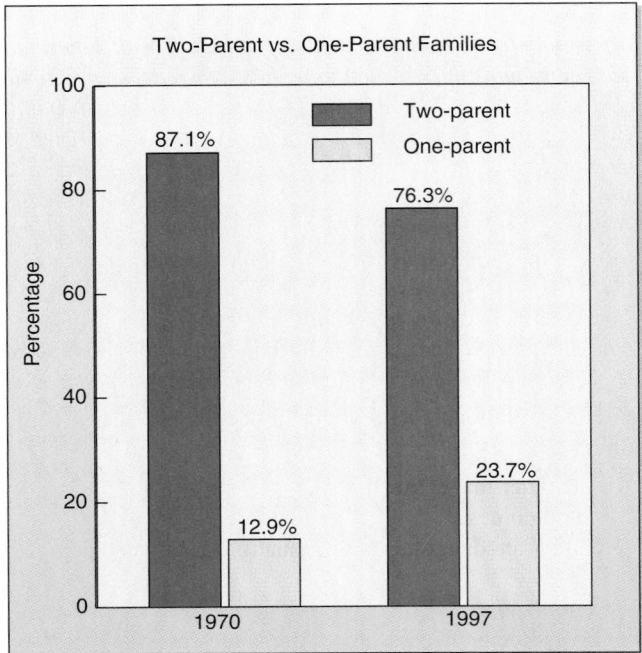

FIGURE 47-1   The percentage of single-parent families increased by 10% from 1970 to 1998.

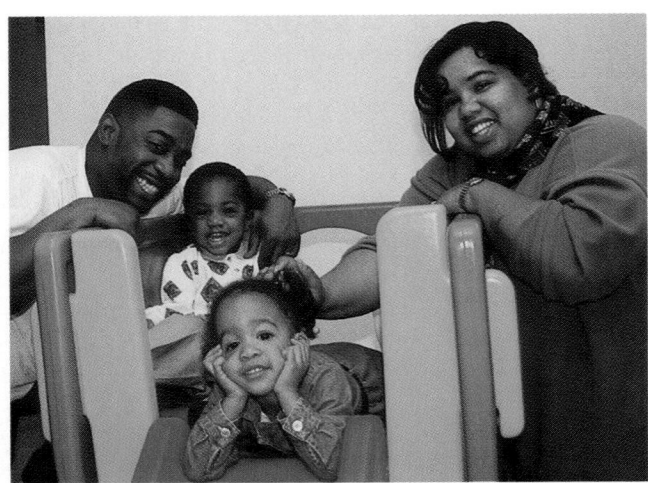

FIGURE 47-2   The nuclear family consists of a married man and woman with one or more children living together in one household.

traditional families remained stable over the last 30 years, ranging from 24.2 million to 26 million (U.S. Census Bureau, 1998). But in 68% of nuclear families with children younger than 18 years, both parents work outside the home (U.S. Census Bureau, 1998).

Single-Parent Families

Single-parent families, composed of one parent and one or more children, more than doubled from 11% in 1970, because of increasing rates of separation and divorce, to 24% in 1990 followed by a slower increase to 27% by 1998. (See Fig. 47-1). There were 11.9 million single parents in the United States in 1998, 49%% more than 10 years earlier (U.S. Census Bureau, 1998). Death of a spouse, desertion, adoption, or unwed pregnancy also result in single-parent families. Single-parent families may experience financial strain and an overburdened parent because of inadequate support systems. Women head more single-parent families than men by a margin of 4.6:1 (U.S. Census Bureau, 1998).

Blended Family

Members of a **blended family** (stepfamily) include children who live with one birth parent and one parent as well as any offspring of the non-birth parent. Each member faces the challenge of forming relationships with the new members while possibly maintaining ties and loyalties to biologic family members who are not part of the new unit.

Cohabitated Family

Cohabitated family structure means people living together without the formal or legal bond of marriage. Such couples include men and women who live together as a trial or an alternative to marriage as well as gay and lesbian couples. Cohabitated families may include children.

Extended Family

The **extended family** structure expands the previously listed family types by adding grandparents, aunts, uncles, and cousins (Fig. 47-3). Members may or may not live under the same roof and exert varying influence on each person. Extended families often consist of three or more generations.

Communal Family

A **communal family** includes a number of members who share a common bond such as religious affiliation, ideology, or economic need. Another example is when young adults share living quarters while attending college. Membership in this type of situation may be short-term, creating instability in the unit.

Other Families

Still other variations in family structure exist, including commuter marriages, in which one member lives away from the rest of the family part time to work or to attend school. Caring for foster or adopted children is another way to include children in a family. Many families have adopted children of a race different from their own, including orphans from Southeast Asia, South America, and Eastern Europe. A single adult living alone who has never married or has been widowed, separated, or divorced is described in census data as a "nonfamily household" but may still belong to a larger extended family. Information on the changing demographics of the U.S. population can be found through the web site of the U.S. Census Bureau (*http://www.census.gov*).

Family Function

Function is what the family does. Although family functions differ in each family, all families exist to meet some common goals. Hanson (1996) describes six support functions of the family and social groups. The usual functions of families involve physical and economic provisions of care, sexual intimacy, reproduction, education, socialization (including communication), and nurturing and support for problem solving and goal setting. Besides the physical bonds of family relationships, members experience emotional bonds that provide support and security for members, thereby fostering growth and development. Like family structures, family functions evolve over time within individual families.

Physical Provision

Physical provision of care is a common need for all family members but is greater for those who are dependent because of age or illness. Physical provision includes food, clothing, shelter, and healthcare. In most families, some members provide comfort and safety for others. Certain members cook, clean, shop for food and clothing, and possibly feed and bathe other members. Those being cared for and those providing the care may change owing to situations such as maturation or illness.

Economic Provision

One or more family members contribute monetary funds to provide basic necessities, such as food and clothing, as well as luxuries and provisions for the future such as college tuition.

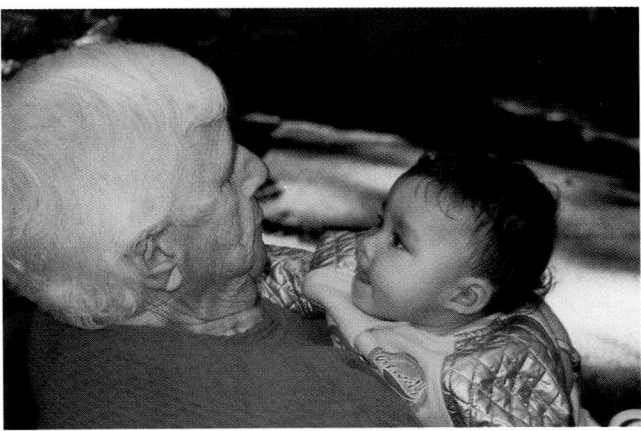

FIGURE 47-3   As part of the extended family, grandparents contribute to nurturing young children.

Families usually share the funds that some members earn. Dual-career families are increasingly common because of today's economic climate and increased standard of living. Over 60% of American women are in the labor force, constituting nearly half of today's total workforce (U.S. Bureau of Labor Statistics, 2001). Policy and legislation in the past 15 years, particularly the Family Medical Leave Act that guarantees up to 12 weeks of "job-protected" leave annually, have advanced the issues of workforce equality (Smith & Bachu, 1999).

Sexual Intimacy

Most couples in families need sexual intimacy. This basic human need and developmental concern can be met within a family. In a supportive family, partners play an active role in meeting each other's sexual needs. Human sexuality is discussed in Chapter 50. The development of dependable methods of family planning has influenced the couple's ability to express sexuality with less concern over unplanned pregnancies.

Reproduction

Reproduction is not a function of all families; it is more often a choice rather than a given in family life. Couples may postpone or be unable to accomplish childbearing or may choose to eliminate it as an option. Alternative methods of having children, such as adoption, foster parenthood, use of donor sperm, and surrogate mother programs, exist to fulfill a family's desire for children.

Education

Education, whether formal or informal, is a function of all families. Parents and other adults discipline children, teach them how to care for themselves and maneuver in the world, and send them to school for formal learning. Older members share with younger members information that they have learned through experience; younger members, in turn, teach older members about the changing world. Education not only involves communicating information but also techniques for problem solving, coping, attitudes, and values. Education is ongoing and lifelong in most families.

Socialization

Socialization is a function in all families, especially in close extended families. Gathering together at the dinner table and converging for holiday celebrations are prime opportunities for socialization. Through such events, family members learn to get along, behave appropriately in various situations, and express culture, tradition, and religious beliefs.

Nurturing and Support

Families provide nurturing and support to their members from initial bonding at birth through old age and death. Nurturing and support may be provided through the emotional tasks of love, belonging, and affection, as well as safety and security for growth.

Normal Functional Family Pattern

A normal functional family meets its developmental tasks and guides members to accomplish individual tasks appropriate for age and developmental level. Family development is discussed in Chapter 19, and Table 19-1 presents the developmental cycle of stages and tasks.

Lifespan Considerations

An understanding of lifespan developmental transitions serves as a reference for understanding families. Critical transitions can be grouped into three types of events: changes in the number of family members, changes in the ages and compositions of members, and changes in status such as retirement (Smith, 1997). The background for understanding these lifespan transitions can be found in Erik Erikson's (1963) classic theory of development from infancy through adulthood.

Newborn and Infant

The process of infant–parent attachment or bonding after birth is critical to family development. Factors that affect bonding include availability of both parents after birth, flexibility of schedules, feelings about the birth, comfort in parenting roles, emotional responsiveness of baby and parents, financial security, other demands such as care of another child, and presence of supportive others.

By 8 months of age, most infants have become attached to their primary caregivers and are developing "trust" (Erikson, 1963). An interactive family environment can support the socialization process. Changes in the infant's environment that necessitate separation (such as hospitalization of a primary caregiver or of the infant) may impede the infant's development. A study of mothers and preterm infants hospitalized in the neonatal intensive care unit reinforced the need for family-centered care and supported the important role nurses play in family growth and positive development during this stressful experience (Van Riper, 2001).

Toddler and Preschooler

In toddlerhood, learning to walk imparts mobility, and increasing cognitive ability stimulates curiosity. Protection from harm is an important focus for caregivers of toddlers and preschoolers. At the same time, the child's need to develop self-control can strain familial interactions as power struggles, frequently accompanied by temper tantrums, become the norm. Encourage caregivers to promote children's independence within established limits for children to develop "autonomy" (Erikson, 1963). Sibling rivalry may escalate as egocentric toddlers resent the dominance of older children and the attention given to younger children. Despite power struggles, toddlers remain attached to their caregivers, and severe separation anxiety may be noted when primary caregivers leave these children who are from 18 to 24 months of age. Hospitalization or other types of separation at this time may be especially traumatic. Role changes necessitated by the need to care for a disabled family member in the home may decrease a parent's contact time with the toddler, who may then regress into an earlier developmental stage.

Psychosocial development escalates during the preschool years. Preschoolers identify with the role of man or woman as they interact differently with parents or primary caregivers. The caregiver of the opposite sex becomes the focus of the child's love, whereas the child may direct aggression toward adults of the same sex. Consistent involvement with people of both sexes enhances preschoolers' development.

Associative play, with interaction but little organization, evolves into cooperative play as children approach school age. Cooperative play and generally increasing social skills help preschoolers to develop mutually supportive roles with siblings, although rivalry continues (Fig. 47-4).

The preschool years are crucial for the development of "initiative," which is the ability to begin actions independently (Erikson, 1963). Stable family relationships can enhance the development of creativity. Adults can prepare preschoolers for changes such as surgery by playing out feelings and focusing attention on the event one part at a time. Family members should assure children that changes such as death are not their fault.

Significant others can expand the socialization process as preschoolers develop an ability to separate from home and family. Preschoolers need both independence and security. Fear of separation remains and may be reinforced by parental anxiety.

School-Age Child and Adolescent

The school years are a time of change for both children and their adult caregivers. A need for association with peers, usually of the same sex, is enhanced. The role of "best friend" assumes importance. Family atmosphere continues to provide a sense of security as children move away from obvious signs of dependence on parents. Sibling rivalry is still present but continues to resolve unless adults compare children for differing levels of ability.

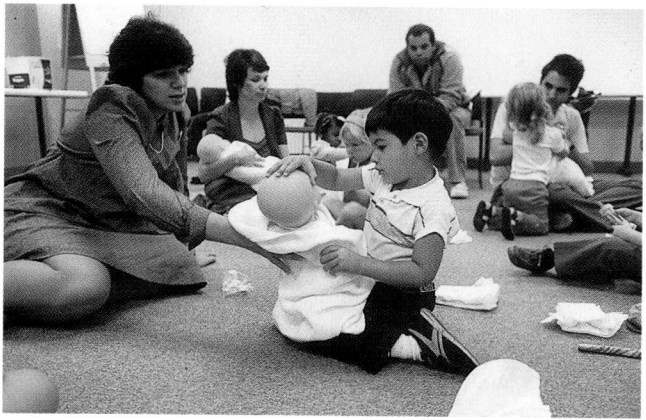

FIGURE 47-4 Sibling rivalry can be a problem throughout the lifespan. Toddlers and preschoolers who are preparing for younger siblings to join their families may benefit from sibling preparation classes.

Children's perceptions of their own abilities are significant as they seek to accomplish the task of "industry" (Erikson, 1963) and to avoid feeling inferior. Fears of illness, injury, punishment, and death of self or significant others are evidenced during this developmental stage. Children may use phobias and ritualistic "good luck" behaviors as adaptive mechanisms. Understanding of such behaviors, rather than denial, is important on the part of significant adults.

In some cultures, puberty, after the completion of identifiable "rites of passage," signals the assumption of adult roles. The family plays an important role in preventing emotional and behavioral problems and promoting resilience in adolescents (Steinberg, 2001). Western culture is less clear in defining the steps for transition into adulthood. To the extent that independence is desirable, alterations in family and social relationships are normal and inevitable in adolescence. Psychosocial development is closely related to changes in physical development. Peer group identity is strongly desired; adolescents strive to look and act like each other. Stability in the home and supportive relationships with others can help adolescents avoid "role confusion" (Erikson, 1963).

Adult and Older Adult

According to Erikson (1963), the chief developmental tasks of the adult period are "intimacy," which involves commitment to others and "generativity," which focuses on productivity. Both social and job-related concerns strongly influence development in adulthood. Critical life junctures (e.g., cohabitation, marriage, childbirth, career advancement, and mobility) influence development of intimacy and generativity.

A decision to remain single does not exclude the development of intimate relationships. Many young adults leave their families of origin usually to form families of procreation. Social relationships with peers remain important for feelings of identity. The need for peer group support may be intertwined with such serious problems as substance abuse, sexually transmitted diseases, unwanted pregnancies, and abortion. The family's acceptance is necessary to help deal with these serious health problems.

In the middle years, adults' relationships with children gradually change as children gain independence, and relationships with partners change as each person matures. Menopause in the woman and climacteric in the man can precipitate family crises that require role adjustments. Relationships with aging parents may result in conflict, frustration, and/or anger as older adults become more dependent. Caring for parents who are dying at home presents challenging legal and ethical issues that can affect the individual/family/nurse relationships (Ladd, Pasquerella, & Smith, 2000).

Demographic trends document the increased numbers of adults over age 65; the group over age 85 is growing fastest. Nearly all families are concerned about at least one older adult member. Formidable tasks face the family with aging adults as members try to balance personal and work obligations (Grasso, 1996). Support from family is essential to help older adults achieve "ego integrity" and to avoid "despair" (Erikson, 1963). Changes in family structure occur as children leave home (and sometimes return), as family members die, and as new relationships develop. Another substantial change has been noted in the increasing role that grandparents today play in raising and providing care for grandchildren. From 1970 to 1997 the number of children living in a home maintained by their grandparent(s) increased from 2.2 million to 3.9 million (Casper & Bryson, 1998). Changes related to caring for grandchildren and spouses, retirement, death, and decreasing social contacts alter family and social structure because members must redefine their usual roles.

FACTORS AFFECTING FAMILY FUNCTION

In addition to age, factors that may affect family relationships include cultural beliefs, economic status, lifestyle, and previous life experience. Acute and chronic illness, traumatic experiences, and substance abuse are other factors that influence family function. Evidence has shown that a family's socioeconomic status and marital discord are predictors of behavior problems in preschoolers (Benzies, Harrison, & Magill-Evans, 1998). Such influences may be mild, affecting only some members or lasting only briefly, or they may throw the entire family into prolonged crisis. Crisis may actually strengthen family bonds, however, if members become more committed to the family's common goals. Table 47-1 lists common family stressors.

Culture, Values, and Beliefs

Cultural traditions impact the family as it functions in Western society. Components of a sociocultural dimension include ethnic patterns, language, food customs, patterns of communication, role expectations, healthcare beliefs, childrearing practices, availability of extended family support, and religious beliefs and practices. Nurses may encounter many variations in family structure and function among different cultures; each variation can relate to the client's health status. For example, the extended family that is basic to Native American society values children and older adults, and childrearing is a group en-

deavor (Seiderman, Jacobson, Primeaux, Burns, & Weatherby, 1996). Other research has helped to define the role of family members in adopting healthy eating patterns within a different ethnic group (de Bourdeaudhuij & van Oost, 1998). The extended family acts as an essential support system to help families cope when stressors such as illness occur.

When extended family support is unavailable, parents employed outside the home may express concerns over the amount of time they spend separated from their children. Research has shown that children of employed mothers are able to develop well and have their needs met as long as adequate child care is available (La Montagne, Engle & Zeitlin, 1998). Inadequate child care remains a concern for dominant as well as minority cultures in the United States due to public policy's lack of response to social change.

Religious customs and expressions of spirituality also influence how children grow up in families. The Jewish religion considers the bar or bat mitzvah as the "rite of passage" (Leininger, 1995) (Fig. 47-5). Mormons emphasize self-discipline and strong family ties (Cramer & Cramer, 1995). Spirituality, behaviors that give life meaning and purpose, may or may not be connected to a specific religious group. In some Latino cultures, the belief that death extends life can provide a positive aspect to grieving, and the nurse's role in allowing Latino clients to respond in their own culturally appropriate way can enhance the family relationship (Munet-Vilaro, 1998).

In addition to spiritual influences, families pass down attitudes about male and female roles and childrearing through the generations; they also pass on beliefs and practices about health, illness, and healthcare. Even those people born and raised in traditional "American" culture may exhibit behavior arising from various cultural beliefs.

Economic Resources

A clear economic influence on family and social relationships can be observed as people with marginal incomes struggle to survive. Economic constraints often create problems in main-

TABLE 47-1

Sources of Family Conflict	
Source	**Problem Areas**
Finances	Lower socioeconomic status; income inadequate to meet needs; disagreement on money management
Occupation	Unemployment; semiskilled status, task sharing when both adults working
Culture/religion	Mixed religious or cultural background; in-laws; disagreement on childrearing practices
Education	Incongruent levels of education, especially if school dropout
Residence	Mixed rural/urban background; relocation for benefit of only one family member; isolation
Sexual	Dissatisfaction with intimacy level; disagreement on family planning
Substance abuse	Difference in values; physical/psychological changes due to chemical addiction
Social ties	Dissimilar selection of friends; single versus couple focus in friendships
Situational	Fatigue; loss; illness; separation, trauma, disaster
Developmental	Change in number, age composition, or status of family members

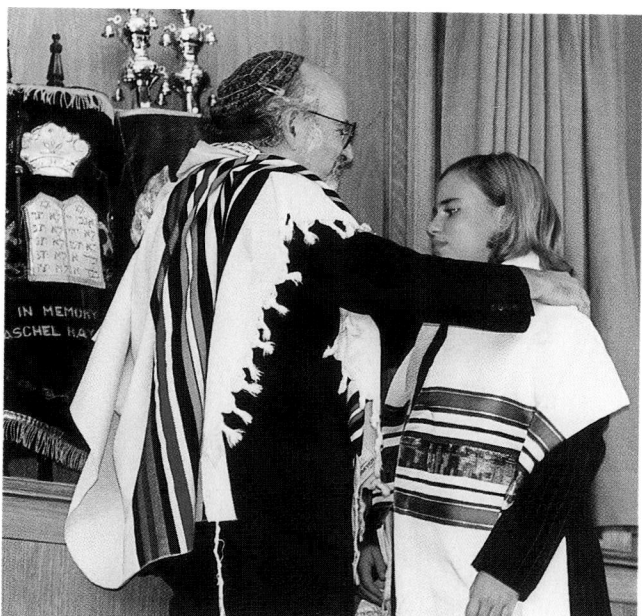

FIGURE 47-5 Cultural and religious traditions like the Bat Mitzvah can serve as "rites of passage" for members and can promote further family bonding.

taining a family's lifestyle after a divorce or change in employment or with a change from two wage-earners to one. Resentment toward society or other family members for forcing a below-standard lifestyle may arise. According to Ford-Gilboe (1997), functioning in single-parent families is difficult given chronic problems of limited economic support and role stress but can be balanced by positive aspects, such as decreased psychological stress, increased family cohesiveness, family resilience, and use of creative coping strategies.

Lifestyle

The mobility of families can affect relationships as adults change jobs or retire and children change schools. Support people and friendships also change. The family's lifestyle in terms of rest and relaxation, nutrition, smoking, drug and alcohol use, and exercise influences the health status of all members. Lack of support from extended family due to geographic distance can increase the strain on individuals and families after relocation. The need for two incomes has created the "latch-key" practice in childrearing in which children are responsible for their own care and supervision after school. The difficulty families may have in providing care to infirm older adults has also created a need for more nursing homes and community-based services.

Previous Life Experience

Previous life experience greatly affects a family's functioning. Children learn about relationships almost exclusively from their families of origin. They carry beliefs to their fam-

ilies of procreation about forming relationships, making decisions and solving problems, carrying out roles, raising children, using resources, and showing affection. Some coping strategies, such as using alcoholic beverages to numb mental pain and stress, may have been accepted in a person's previous life experience and yet destroy present relationships. Problem-focused coping behaviors have been associated with positive outcomes and emotion-focused approaches with problematic adjustment to chronic illness (Degotardi, Revenson, & Ilowite, 1999; Narsavage, 1997).

Coping and Stress Tolerance

Any stress on an individual can affect the entire family's functioning. For example, the term **sandwich generation** has been used to describe adult children facing the dilemma of meeting their own generativity needs while assisting the older generation (their parents) and the younger generation (their children). Other stresses, such as the loss of a family member, involvement in a natural or man-made disaster, or loss of employment can also alter a family's relationships.

Acute Illness

Acute illness may place sudden demands on a family. The ill member often looks to the others for validation that he or she is sick; with such validation the ill member can seek healthcare. Roles may change as the ill member depends on others for physical care, nurturing, and economic security. The ill member's self-esteem may decrease if he or she feels less valued.

Other members may temporarily sacrifice their own needs to provide for the ill person's needs. In a family with a seriously ill older female, the older male may become her primary caregiver and neglect his own health (Richards, 1996). Needs such as sexual intimacy may go unmet. Problems arise when members cannot adjust to new roles or as needs remain unmet. In some situations, the caregiver role adds an unprecedented and unequally distributed burden of care (Douglass, 1997). One member in particular may feel overburdened. For example, when a construction worker is unemployed while receiving treatment for fractured vertebrae, his spouse may work additional hours to provide for the family economically. Children may have to assume more responsibility for meeting their own needs, and housework may be left undone. The family tries to fit in support of the ill member, meal preparation, and chauffeuring the children around varied work schedules. Anxiety increases about the illness as well as about how the children are managing with decreased support. Consequently the caregiver's own physical needs for sleep and nutrition, as well as the family's need for nurturing, may go unmet. Depending on the severity of the illness and how suddenly it occurred, the family might need increased attention at this time. Stability of the family structure is essential when one or more members are absent or incapacitated. Some flexibility is necessary to share roles and still meet needs such as economic provision and physical care.

> **SAFETY ALERT**
> Assist families with finding resources for child care, finances, and other basic needs while a parent or primary caregiver is hospitalized.

Chronic Illness

Because chronic illness lasts longer than acute illness, it can influence the family to a greater extent. The course of chronic illness may require both individual and family adaptation to changes in lifestyle and roles and may result in the ill person's increased dependence on others. In caring for children with chronic illness, family functioning can be influenced by both the caregiver's role adaptation as well as by support provided by healthcare professionals (Shapiro, Perez & Warden, 1998). Actions by family or significant others can be supportive, but behaviors such as overprotection are problematic.

Because of the inherent dependency of children and frail older adults, their illnesses provoke yet other family adjustments. A newborn who has a congenital defect or the diagnosis of a chronic illness or an older adult with a traumatic disability may result in severe stressors to family relationships. The ability of a family to function will influence the affected person's ability to develop and to cope and will affect the course of the illness or disability (Sparks, 1997). A congenital birth defect that is initially stressful but ultimately correctable is likely to have less impact on family function than would a chronic illness or developmental disability that requires lengthy treatment.

Common stressors with regard to chronic illness include exhaustion, anxiety, needing help from relatives and friends, alterations in social contacts or travel abilities, concern about sibling needs, and financial concerns (Turnbull & Turnbull, 1997). Family roles, responsibilities, and social relationships change to meet the needs of the family system as well as the ill child or adult.

People with chronically ill children, parents, or other family members may express negative feelings about themselves such as guilt, inadequacy, failure, rejection, and helplessness (Santelli, Turnbull, & Higgins, 1997). The family may be in denial initially as members struggle with the shock of the illness, but after acknowledging the problem, the family will strive toward the goal of simply functioning as close to "normal" as possible.

Traumatic Experiences

Trauma, because it entails stress and disruption of normal interactions, can alter family relationships. Traumatic experiences can be physical (e.g., a gunshot wound) or emotional (e.g., robbery). They can involve one person or many and can be caused by humans (e.g., surgery) or nature (e.g., flood).

Personal involvement or involvement of a family member or significant other in a disaster (e.g., severe fire; flood; hurricane; or car, train, or plane accident) is associated with loss of control and role change. The role of "survivor" is fraught with conflicts. A family member may experience guilt that she or he was responsible or should have been the victim. One family member may blame another for contributing to the event. The victim may experience difficulty concentrating as he or she relives the event or may move from numbness to awareness.

Substance Abuse

The consequences of coping with substance abuse in a family are many. For each person afflicted with alcoholism, there are family members who also suffer social and emotional problems. Alcoholics and possibly family members will deny that alcoholism is a problem. A spouse or child usually becomes the alcoholic's "enabler," the person who keeps the family functioning even at an altered level. The enabler assumes tasks that the alcoholic cannot accomplish and cares and makes excuses for the alcoholic. These behaviors enable the alcoholic to continue drinking, which contributes to the deterioration of the family unit.

Drug abuse also alters family function. Economic destruction may play a greater role in the family of a drug abuser than in that of an alcoholic, owing to the higher cost of illegal drugs. Because drug use is less socially acceptable than alcohol use, the drug abuser and family may be isolated from the community. The threat of drug testing in the workplace may prevent the drug abuser from holding a job, which further compromises the family's economic security. Arrest and incarceration may completely disrupt the family unit. Legal drugs can also be abused, especially by those who suffer from chronic illness or use multiple medications. Both alcohol and drug abuse may lead to physical problems from the effects of the substance as well as injury incurred while intoxicated. Chronic liver disease, poor nutrition, and eventual heart failure are common in alcoholics. Intravenous drug abusers suffer from frequent infections, hepatitis, and possibly acquired immunodeficiency syndrome (AIDS). These illnesses further alter family dynamics.

> **SAFETY ALERT**
> Discuss the deleterious effects of alcohol or drug abuse with the abuser and his or her family, and refer the person to a substance abuse treatment program.

ALTERED FAMILY RELATIONSHIPS
Manifestations of Altered Family Function

Manifestations of **altered family function** include structural, functional, developmental, and systems changes (Hanson, 1996). Examples of structural changes are separation and

THERAPEUTIC DIALOGUE
Families

Scene for Thought

The Loeman family (Ronald and Marilyn, both age 50; Jeff, age 18; and Stefanie, age 14) are in the hospital visiting Mr. Loeman, Ronald's father, who lives with them. Mr. Loeman, otherwise healthy, was admitted for replacement of his pacemaker and is doing well at this time, 2 days postoperatively. He, his family, and his nurse are sitting in the unit's solarium chatting.

Less Effective

Ronald: Dad looks great, doesn't he, Mr. Boren? *(Beams at his father and pats his shoulder.)*

Nurse: He does seem to be recovering well after the surgery. How do you feel today, Mr. Loeman? *(Sits next to the wheelchair.)*

Mr. L: Wonderful, wonderful! Why do all of you keep treating me like I'm a baby? *(Grumpily.)*

Nurse: Now, now, Mr. Loeman, your family are all here to see you because they love you. You were looking forward to seeing them this morning, remember? *(Gives his hand a reassuring pat.)*

Jeff: Mom, Stef and I are going to the cafeteria for a soda. *(Starts to leave with his sister.)*

Ronald: Not now, Jeff. Stay and visit with Opa for a little while. We've only been here 5 minutes. *(Sternly.)*

Mr. L: Never mind, Ronald. Let them go. I'll see them later. Here, Jeff, have a soda on me. *(Hands Jeff a few dollars. The children quickly leave.)*

Nurse: That's sweet, Mr. Loeman. I'll bet they really appreciate you. *(Smiles at Ronald and Marilyn. They smile back weakly.)*

Mr. L: Mr. Boren, wheel me back to my room. I'm tired.

Nurse: Sure, Mr. Loeman. *(To Ronald and Marilyn.)* I'll be right back. I'll just get him settled.

Mr. L: What are you going to talk to them about? *(Suspiciously.)*

Nurse: Just about how to help you recover when you go home tomorrow. Don't worry, we'll take good care of you. *(Wheels Mr. L. into his room. Marilyn and Ronald silently watch them go.)*

More Effective

Ronald: Dad looks great, doesn't he, Mr. Ballard? *(Beams at his father and pats his shoulder.)*

Nurse: He does seem to be recovering well after the surgery. How do you feel today, Mr. Loeman? *(Sits next to the wheelchair.)*

Mr. L: Wonderful, wonderful! Why do all of you keep treating me like I'm a baby? *(Grumpily.)*

Marilyn: Now, Dad, don't start that. We're just concerned about you. *(Smiles tightly and throws a significant look at Ronald.)*

Jeff: Mom, Stef and I are going to the cafeteria for a soda. *(Starts to leave with his sister.)*

Ronald: Not now, Jeff. Visit with Opa for a little while. We've only been here 5 minutes. *(Sternly.)*

Mr. L: Never mind, Ronald. Let them go. I'll see them later. Here, Jeff, have a soda on me. *(Hands him a few dollars. The children quickly leave.)*

Ronald: You spoil them, Dad. *(Exasperated.)*

Mr. L: Why not? They're my only grandchildren. When I go, they won't get much but they'll think of me fondly. *(Looks sad, defiant, and angry.)* Mr. Ballard, wheel me back to my room. I'm tired.

Nurse: Sure, Mr. Loeman. Is it okay with you if I talk to Ronald and Marilyn while you rest? *(Continues to sit next to him.)*

Mr. L: What are you going to talk to them about? *(Suspiciously.)*

Nurse: What they need to do to help you recover when you're discharged tomorrow. Would you rather stay and participate? Or would you like to rest in bed and participate there?

Mr. L: *(Thinks about it.)* I'd rather rest in bed and listen to you in my room. I'm tired.

Nurse: Good idea. Let's go. I'll get us all some juice on the way. *(Wheels Mr. L. to his room. Mr. L. looks tired but more relaxed. Ronald and Marilyn are surprised at how easily the decision was accomplished. They make a mental note to try it at home with Mr. L.)*

Critical Thinking Challenge

- Analyze the effect Mr. Loeman's illness has had on his family (individually and collectively).
- Detect and examine how the stress appeared in the dialogues.
- Construct what the family must be like at home together.
- Evaluate indications of dysfunctional patterns in this family.
- Compare and contrast how the two nurses hindered or facilitated family coping.

divorce. Functional changes include role strain and abuse. Developmental changes may be manifested as social isolation and emotional problems. Systems changes reflect societal changes such as health insurance and disability regulations. Assessment of the impact of these changes is important in identifying problems. Some alterations, such as separation and divorce, may be solutions as well as problems.

Separation and Divorce

Separation or divorce may be a positive solution to altered family function or a manifestation of the family's difficulty in adjusting to change. Intervention may be needed if a family is unable to create and to maintain a system to nurture and support its members. A major family transition occurs when separation or divorce breaks the family unit. An increasing number of families are being thus affected. Most commonly, the mother and children form a new unit while the father moves into a separate environment. A problem that can lead to further altered family function is role overload for the custodial parent. Shared custody may help to reduce the strain on a single parent, but no single solution is best for all families.

Remarriage after divorce accounts for one third of all marriages in the United States (U.S. Census Bureau, 1990). Blended families that form are also at risk for altered family function as members maintain or break ties to previous marriages and question extended family relationships.

Role Strain

Role strain is a manifestation of altered family function when events and family developments force changes in roles. For example when a husband becomes chronically ill and unable to work, the wife may become the family's primary economic provider. She may experience role strain because she must combine the role of caregiver with the roles of wife, mother, and employee. The husband may experience stress as he gives up his role as economic provider and spends more time at home. Children may be assigned additional tasks including some physical care for the father.

Giving up familiar roles and assuming new ones may be by choice, as in the case of a two-career family who decides to suspend or to temporarily give up one parent's career for child-rearing. Family developmental stages call for changing roles periodically; however role strain develops when family members cannot adapt and meet their needs. Inherent decision-making power influences role strain. Altered roles and resultant role strain can further impede interactions within the family and between the family and society.

Abuse

Family abuse and violence are social problems of increasing significance. Abuse may be physical, sexual, emotional, or economic. It may be aimed at the spouse or partner, children, older parents, or grandparents. Factors that contribute to abuse in families include unemployment, substance abuse, chronic illness, inadequate housing, and lack of education and other resources (Parker, 1995; Plichta & Weisman, 1995). Abuse is not limited to lower socioeconomic levels and frequently is passed down through the generations. Many abused children grow up to abuse family members (Maker, Kemmelmeier, & Peterson, 1998). Almost two million child maltreatment cases were reported in the United States in 1998 (U.S. Census Bureau, 2000).

Domestic violence or spouse abuse has been reported by 25% of women and 1% of men; the abuser is usually a family member in a long-standing relationship (Parker, 1995).

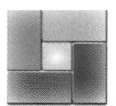

Nursing Research and Critical Thinking
What are the Effects of Critical Care Hospitalization on Family Roles of Adult Family Members?

Within the context of the family system, illness of a family member disrupts role function and may lead to role insufficiency. A group of nurses designed this study to explore the effects of critical care hospitalization on family roles and responsibilities of adult family members and how these effects changed over time. The self-reported changes that caused life to be more stressful, as well as description of the changes resulting from a hospitalization, were defined as changes in family roles and responsibilities. Subjects for the study were recruited from the adult family members who visited clients in critical care units in a large midwestern medical center. A total of 52 family members were enrolled in the study. Subjects completed the Iowa ICU Family Scale (IIFS), a 25-item scale designed to explore changes in family roles and responsibilities and to measure behavioral and emotional responses including sleep patterns, eating patterns, activity patterns, and support systems. Family members completed the scale each day during the first week and weekly for as long as the client remained in the critical care unit. Subjects were asked to describe any changes in family roles and responsibilities they had experienced as a result of this critical care hospitalization. The majority of the subjects reported the occurrence of changes in family roles and responsibilities. The top three themes derived from the data, "Change in feelings," "Increased responsibilities," and "Change in routine," reflected the physical and emotional burdens of having a family member in a critical care unit.

Critical Thinking Considerations. Most subjects in the study were women (N = 41; men N = 11). It is possible that support structures vary between men and women, and responses varied based on the roles held by each subject. Nursing care implications from this study are as follows:

- The researchers recommend that nurses implement family-centered interventions to decrease role strain and role overload in families during a crisis.
- Often, family research is related to families with children. Research is needed that looks at interventions targeted at families at various points and members in varying roles.

From Johnson, S. K., Craft, M., Titler, M., Halm, M., Kleiber, C., Montgomery, L. A., Megivern, K., Nicholson, A., & Buckwalter, K. (1995). Perceived changes in adult family members' roles and responsibilities during critical illness. *Image: Journal of Nursing Scholarship, 27*(3), 238–243.

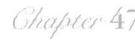

Changing abusive patterns of behavior is difficult. The nurse's ability to detect subtle behavioral cues is crucial when abuse is suspected because victims frequently attempt to hide their suffering. Violence increases during pregnancy and with the birth of children as relationships change (Parker, 1995).

Abuse in families is often manifested in parenting behaviors. A lack of attachment (bonding) may be evidenced by an adult's failure to care for the child's physical or emotional needs or by verbalized resentment or indifference toward the parenting role. Evidence of neglect or physical abuse may be noted as well as "failure to thrive." Rigidity in role expectations may be present in either or both parents; the consequence may be inhibited flexibility in meeting children's needs.

Sexual abuse, especially of children, is another area of concern. Emotional turmoil escalates when family members fail to report such abuse or ignore it to avoid shaming the family. The child is often confused about the appropriateness of the abuser's behavior and may feel that he or she is to blame.

With over two million victims annually, abuse of older adults is a growing problem (Lynch, 1997). In addition to physical abuse as they become physically dependent, older adults may be neglected or verbally and financially abused by their own children or other caregivers. Immobility or sensory disabilities may prevent them from seeking help. They may also be reluctant to prosecute because of family loyalty.

Social Isolation

Social isolation may result when family members are separated, communication within families is poor, or others do not accept a family or its members. Isolation can be physical or psychological. Separation may result from hospitalization, job commitments, or going away to college. Today many nuclear families, single adults, and older adults are separated from their extended families because the young have sought employment elsewhere. People without the usual family support may feel isolated in a new town. Daily demands of a job, parenting, home maintenance, college studies, finances, and illness may overburden the persons involved. They may not know where to turn for support if they have depended on family in the past. Geographic distance or desire to be independent may make family contact difficult and increase isolation.

APPLY YOUR KNOWLEDGE

You are working in a medical walk-in clinic when a woman, accompanied by her boyfriend, brings in her 3-year-old child who has fallen and injured his arm. The boy appears very stoic and emotionless: although he is in obvious pain, he does not cry. When you try to talk with him, he avoids eye contact. When you undress him to examine his injury, you notice old and new bruises on his arm, which he is unable to move. What might your assessment findings reveal? How should you proceed?
Check your answers in Appendix A.

The nurse-family relationship becomes extremely important in helping families adjust to stress and illness both in hospital and home settings (Hupcey, 1998; Houde, 1998). Older adults are facing their final years away from their children and grandchildren and may be living alone after their spouses die. They may feel isolated by a society that values youth.

Poor communication within a family can isolate individual members. Another form of isolation occurs when a family is not accepted socially or fears such rejection. Members may be discriminated against because of race, color, religion, ethnic origin, or stigma associated with illnesses such as AIDS. Fear of isolation by the community, in the workplace, or from others adds to tension within the family.

Emotional Problems

Emotional and developmental problems can be manifestations of altered family functioning. Parenting may suffer whenever family function is altered. Problems with bonding and attachment may arise, and children may have difficulty with emotional development. When family conflict arises, psychosocial development may be arrested. Family relationship patterns are associated with optimal and problematic adolescent adjustment (O'Connor, Hetherington, & Reiss, 1998). For example, if tension arises while a person is in adolescence and the family responds poorly, the adolescent may be left confused, indecisive, and unable to plan for the future.

The family's ability to teach, nurture, educate, and socialize offspring is important, according to many developmental models (Hanson & Boyd, 1996). Children usually display emotional problems by behaving inappropriately for age or situation. Acting out may occur in the form of temper tantrums, poor school performance, or sexual promiscuity. See Chapter 17 for more information on lifespan development.

As older adults face retirement, depression may become evident especially if the family has not actively planned for this change. Without communication of worth from other family members, maladaption in retirees has been found (Smith, 1997). Depression leading to suicide in older adults is an increasing societal problem.

Impact on Activities of Daily Living

Altered family function can affect both the person's and the family's activities of daily living (ADLs). Accomplishing routine ADLs, such as preparing meals, eating, sleeping, taking medications, and so on, may become problematic during illness. Issues center around required assistance with tasks as well as changing roles and lifestyles. To examine changes in a person's ADLs related to illness, consider the following example. A 62-year-old widow is diagnosed with lung cancer after repeated colds and a bout with pneumonia. The client will have to decide what kind of treatment (i.e., surgery, radiation, chemotherapy) to choose, then adjust to the side effects of the treatment (e.g., dressing changes, nausea, fatigue, hair loss). The consequences of the client's decision will determine whether she can continue to live independently or must move in with a married son and his family. Most care will be provided on an outpatient basis. Changes in ADLs are inevitable.

Continuation of family functioning in ADLs becomes a significant focus as members alter their normal patterns to meet the client's needs and altered roles. In the immediate crisis after the diagnosis of lung cancer, the woman will need to decide how to share the diagnosis with her 15- and 11-year-old granddaughters and whether or not to ask neighbors or other friends to come and "keep house" during the treatment period. Family relationships will change as members adjust usual roles. Someone must continue cooking, cleaning, driving to the hospital and medical appointments, and so forth. Who in the family will make decisions about spending money and organizing the home? What will be the financial impact of an extended illness? As the illness moves from an acute to a chronic stage, what options are available for extended care? The middle-aged children may need to return to their own jobs. Will friends be available to support the family? Will they feel comfortable continuing to interact with a person with cancer? Nurses must be able to identify the effects of illness on both the individual and the family. Assessing the family's strengths as well as limitations can help its members to develop a realistic perspective for coping with problems (Carpenito, 1997).

ASSESSMENT

Family functional assessment can be accomplished in terms of structure, function, development, communication, and support. Subjective and objective data are both important. Gather subjective data by interviewing clients and family members to explore their strengths and needs; gather objective data by observing family interactions and performing the physical examination. Nursing assessment helps to identify functional patterns, risks, and dysfunction. Assessment findings serve as a basis for making nursing diagnoses and formulating interventions.

Subjective Assessment

Normal Pattern Identification

A structural and functional assessment will incorporate data about the family's composition, ability to meet daily living needs (i.e., food, shelter, health maintenance, and so forth), patterns of communication, and support. Examine areas such as love and belonging, emotional stability, and sociocultural needs or interactions within the family and community. The developmental assessment considers the ways in which a family changes within its own life cycle (Hanson & Boyd, 1996).

Note function, communication, and support in family interactions in terms of the roles that each member assumes. Assessment would include but not be limited to a study of the relationships between husband and wife or parent and child; role relationships of cohabiting members could also be included in an interactional study of family structure and function in meeting individual and group needs. Communication patterns are considered the key to an interactional approach.

Work roles and responsibilities in current situations are subjective assessment factors related to the actual and perceived roles of family members. Assess client identification of satisfaction or disturbances in family, work, or social relationships, and responsibilities related to these roles. Refer to Chapter 19, Display 19-2, for a summary of assessment guidelines for family function.

Risk Identification

History taking to identify areas of risk or potential problems requires both open-ended and focused questioning. Questions related to potential sources of stress in the areas of roles, finances, lifestyle, previous experience, and general health are crucial. Follow a general question, such as "What are the potential sources of stress in your family?" with specific questions such as those given in Display 47-1.

Consider the family's developmental stage when assessing its risk for altered function. As the number, ages, and status of family members change, stressors are introduced.

Characteristic risk factors for potential alterations in family processes include unrealistic expectations of self or others; lack of appropriate role models; history of abuse; inability to bond with others; inadequate support systems; presence of stress; skill or knowledge deficit; acute or chronic illness; and unmet psychosocial needs of children or adults.

Dysfunction Identification

Altered family functioning can be identified when there is a significant difference from an effective pattern of functioning. Inability to express or accept emotions, lack of respect or support for other family members, and inability to adapt to change are contributing factors.

As an ill family member experiences change, the caregiver's role changes as well. This may be evidenced by verbalization of feelings of inadequacy, guilt, anxiety, failure, helplessness, and powerlessness. Parents may express concerns about the effects of a child's illness on siblings and finances. Noncompliance with treatment may be a manifestation of denial or refusal to acknowledge a problem's existence. Denial may serve as a mechanism to maintain or to restore "normality" in family life but it can indicate dysfunction if it prevents a family from dealing with the situation.

Objective Data

Objective data for assessing family function include observation of family interactions and the behavior of members as well as physical examination. Behavioral signs of family dysfunction include labile emotions, withdrawal, irritability, poor sleeping and eating, inability to concentrate, and dependency. Observe family communication patterns. How do members relate to one another, and how effectively do they communicate? Observe who does the talking, who remains silent, whether members listen to one another, how they handle disagreements, how they make decisions, and what they communicate nonverbally. Observation of which family members visit the ill person, how often, and how the client responds can also provide clues in family assessment.

DISPLAY 47-1

ASSESSMENT OF FAMILY SOCIAL RELATIONSHIPS

Family Structure and Function
- Description of client's family unit—age, sex, and so forth
- Client's responsibilities in the household
- Persons responsible for decision within client's household
- Management of finances
- Ways in which family responsibilities are distributed
- Pattern of eating, sleeping, and health practices

Family/Social Interaction
- Most significant person in client's life
- Availability of significant others to client
- Any other people whom client can turn to if necessary
- Number of friends
- Client's socialization with friends, neighbors, relatives
- Description of client's neighborhood, neighbors

Indicators of Change
- Any major change in client's role(s) or responsibilities (explain)
- Client's anticipated future changes in the coming years
- Preparations made for these changes
- Any family stressors—how are they being handled

Parental Role Function (If Person Is a Parent)
- Client's relationship with his or her children? Parents? Friends?
- Any plans to expand his or her family?
- Comparison of parenting patterns to those of client's parents (e.g., discipline). Explain.

Occupational Role Factors
- Client's occupation (include work role and responsibilities)
- Hours worked per week; work interfering with other aspects of client's lifestyle?
- Ability of client's income to maintain client's lifestyle

Leisure Time Management
- Usual activity pattern? Joint activities?
- Vacations taken and frequency
- Client's plans for retirement; if retired, is client enjoying it

Cultural Factors
- Ethnic/religious background
- Similarity of family values
- Family childrearing practices

Adapted from *University of Scranton Guide to Care Plan Assessment* (1994). Scranton, PA, Department of Nursing.

Physical assessment includes inspection, palpation, auscultation, and percussion performed systematically. While assessing physical health, look for clues of family dysfunction. Pay special attention to injuries or bruises that may indicate physical abuse; enlarged liver and other signs of chronic alcoholism; track marks indicating IV drug injection; nasal inflammatory symptoms of cocaine abuse; signs of stress (e.g., weight loss, fatigue, and impaired cognitive function); and multiple acute and chronic physical problems.

NURSING DIAGNOSES

Careful assessment of individual members and the family as a whole is needed to identify actual or potential problems. As suggested in the Critical Thinking Challenge at the beginning of the chapter, nurses work with families to formulate a diagnosis by eliciting each member's perceptions of needs, goals, and expectations. The North American Nursing Diagnosis Association (NANDA) has identified the following accepted nursing diagnoses in family problems: two diagnoses of Caregiver Role Strain (Actual and Risk for); Interrupted Family Processes, Dysfunctional Family Processes: Alcoholism; Compromised Family Coping; Disabled Family Coping; Readiness for Enhanced Family Coping, Ineffective Family Therapeutic Regimen Management as well as diagnoses for Impaired Parenting (Actual and Risk for); Parental Role Conflict, and Risk for Impaired Parent/Infant/Child Attachment.

Diagnostic Statement: Caregiver Role Strain

Definition. Caregiver Role Strain is a caregiver's felt or exhibited difficulty in performing the caregiver role (NANDA, 2001).

Defining Characteristics. Of the defining characteristics or clinical cues that denote this nursing diagnosis, one of the following major characteristics must be present and must be reported by the caregiver:

- Caregiver has difficulty in doing specific caregiving activities. (The caregiver lacks the needed knowledge, strength, developmental readiness, or confidence in ability to provide care such as bathing, toileting, and managing pain.)
- Caregiver health status is compromised with physical, emotional, or socioeconomic difficulty in caring for the client. (The caregiver has physical signs and symptoms of illness or worries about uncertain needs and ongoing care; may feel loss, stress, nervousness, anger, or depression owing to the client's previous relationship or present dependency; or may experiences changes in work or leisure activities.)
- Caregiver–care-receiver relationship is changed. (The caregiver experiences grief or uncertainty in relationship

with care receiver or difficulty watching care recipient experience illness.)

- Family processes are changed. (The family experiences conflict or expresses concerns about family member's care. NANDA 2001)

Related Factors. Numerous related or contributing factors may lead to or place a caregiver at risk for role strain. These include pathophysiologic/physiologic, developmental, psychosocial, and situational factors.

Pathophysiologic/physiologic factors include illness severity, addiction or codependency, premature birth or congenital defect, discharge with significant home care needs, caregiver's health, unpredictable course or instability in the care receiver's health, or the caregiver is female. Developmental factors include the caregiver not being developmentally ready for the caregiver role and/or developmental delay or retardation of the care receiver or caregiver. Psychosocial factors include psychological or cognitive problems in care receiver, marginal family adaptation or altered family function, caregiver's marginal coping patterns, past history of poor relationship between caregiver and care receiver, caregiver as spouse, or care receiver exhibiting deviant, bizarre behavior. Situational factors include abuse or violence, situational stressors that normally affect families, duration of time required for caregiving, inadequate physical environment for providing care, family/caregiver isolation, lack of respite for caregiver, inexperience with caregiving, caregiver's competing commitments, socioeconomic problems, or complexity/amount of caregiving tasks. Situational factors also include problems with resources as the caregiver desires to care for the client; because of other responsibilities or lack of support from other family members, caregiving requires more time, money, emotional strength, and/or physical energy than are available (NANDA, 2001).

Diagnostic Statement: Risk for Caregiver Role Strain

Definition. Risk for Caregiver Role Strain is a caregiver's vulnerability for perceiving difficulty in performing a family caregiver role (NANDA, 2001).

Defining Characteristics. The presence of risk factors such as those listed under Caregiver Role Strain are indications that the caregiver is at risk for significant emotional, physical, and financial stress. Especially critical are isolation and lack of respite for the caregiver.

Related Factors. Related factors are the same as those discussed under Caregiver Role Strain.

Diagnostic Statement: Interrupted Family Processes

Definition. Interrupted Family Processes is the state in which a family experiences a change in family relationships and/or functioning (NANDA, 2001).

Defining Characteristics. Of the defining characteristics or clinical cues that denote this nursing diagnosis, one of the following major characteristics must be present:

- Family system is unable to meet physical, emotional, security, or spiritual needs of its members. (Although the family continues to meet most of its requirements, for some reason such as lack of resources or poor communication, at least one area of need—physical, emotional, security, or spiritual—is not satisfied.)
- Family is unable to adapt to situational or developmental change. (The family may be unable to understand the change, to alter roles, or to express need or accept help from others or the community to adapt to the change.)
- Expressions of family conflict surface. (The family may be unable to communicate or make decisions, may not demonstrate respect or acceptance of individual members' ideas, feelings, and actions, or may inappropriately direct their energy; NANDA, 2001.)

Related Factors. Several related or contributing factors may be associated with interruptions in the process of family functioning: situation transition or crisis (such as job loss, surgery, or trauma) that requires families to deal with unexpected events and developmental transition or crisis (such as birth of a preterm infant or need to care for an aging parent) that increases the complexity of the family's normal pattern of functioning (NANDA, 2001).

Diagnostic Statement: Dysfunctional Family Processes: Alcoholism

Definition. Dysfunctional Family Processes occurs when the physiological, psychosocial, and spiritual family functions become disorganized related to abuse of alcohol, which often results in conflict, denial, resistance to changing behavior, ineffective problem solving, and ongoing crises (NANDA, 2001).

Defining Characteristics. Of the defining characteristics or clinical cues that denote this nursing diagnosis, one of the following major characteristics is required to be present and must be reported by the caregiver:

- Alcoholic family member is unable to function in family and occupational roles and relationships are altered.
- The family experiences anger, hostility, anxiety, depression, or other negative feelings; family relationships deteriorate; conflict ensues.
- Poor self-esteem manifests; the family is unable to meet its members' physical and emotional needs.
- Behavioral changes such as ineffective problem-solving, refusal to accept help, and manipulation are evidenced (NANDA, 2001.)

Related Factors. Related or contributing factors include family history of alcoholism, psychological disorders, stressful situations, depression due to death, loss of job, or other illness that perpetuates inadequate coping in response to stressful situations (NANDA, 2001).

Diagnostic Statement: Compromised Family Coping

Definition. Compromised Family Coping is the state in which a usually supportive primary person (family member or close friend) is providing insufficient, ineffective, or modified support, comfort, assistance, or encouragement that the client may need to manage or to master adaptive tasks related to his or her health challenge (NANDA, 2001).

Defining Characteristics. Defining characteristics or clinical cues that point to this diagnosis include both subjective and objective factors. One characteristic from the lists noted below must be present.

Subjective characteristics are the following:

- Client expresses or confirms a concern or complaint about significant other's response to his or her health problem. (The client has knowledge of the effectiveness of care that others provide.)
- Significant person describes preoccupation with personal reaction to client's illness, disability, or other situational or developmental crises. (The significant person may be experiencing fear, anticipatory grief, guilt, or anxiety.)
- Significant person describes or confirms an inadequate understanding or knowledge base. (A knowledge deficit interferes with effective assistive or supportive behaviors; NANDA, 2001.)

Objective characteristics include the following:

- Significant person attempts assistive or supportive behaviors with less than satisfactory results. (The effectiveness of care can be determined from observation of the client's physical or emotional condition.)
- Significant person withdraws or enters into limited or temporary personal communication with the client at the time of need. (Altered communication may indicate the personal discomfort that the significant person is experiencing.)
- Significant person displays protective behavior disproportionate to the client's abilities or need for autonomy. (Either overprotective behavior or neglect of the client can interfere with effective care; NANDA, 2001.)

Related Factors. Several related or contributing factors may result in compromised family coping behaviors. The factors include inadequate or incorrect information or understanding on the part of a significant person, which may result in incompetent care or temporary preoccupation by a significant person who is trying to manage his or her own emotional conflicts and personal suffering. The result can be the family member's inability to perceive or to act effectively regarding the client's needs. Also the significant person may be facing temporary family disorganization, role changes, or other situational or developmental crises or situations that can limit the resources available for helping the client. In turn, the client's diminished support for a significant person may inhibit that person's motivation to provide care. Also prolonged disease or disability progression may exhaust the significant person's supportive capacities (NANDA, 2001).

Diagnostic Statement: Disabled Family Coping

Definition. Disabled Family Coping is the behavior of a significant person (family member or other primary person) that disables his or her own and the client's capacities effectively to address tasks essential to either person's adaptation to the health challenge (NANDA, 2001).

Defining Characteristics. Of the defining characteristics or clinical cues that identify Disabled Family Coping, one of the following must be present:

- Neglectful care of the client with regard to illness treatment or physical, emotional, or spiritual needs (Neglect can be present even if the client's appearance is clean and orderly.)
- Distortion of reality regarding the client's health problem (This may be noted as denial of its existence or severity; intolerance, rejection, abandonment, or desertion of the client; or carrying on usual routines that disregard the client's needs.)
- Psychosomaticism (The significant person may take on illness signs of the client or show prolonged overconcern for client.)
- Impaired individualization (The significant other may limit meaningful life for client or self or neglect relationships with other family members; eventually agitation, depression, aggression, or hostility may result.)
- Decisions and actions by family that are detrimental to economic or social well-being (This may be seen as the client develops feelings of isolation, helplessness, and inactive dependence; NANDA, 2001.)

Related Factors. Related or associated factors may have contributed to the family's inability to cope. They may include a significant person who has chronically unexpressed feelings of guilt, anxiety, hostility, or despair that inhibit development of a trusting relationship and effective problem solving; incompatible coping styles of the significant person and client or among significant people, which limits their ability to deal with adaptive tasks; highly ambivalent family relationships, which have the effect of inhibiting ability to function supportively; and inconsistent handling of family's resistance to treatment, which tends to solidify defensiveness as it fails to deal adequately with underlying anxiety (NANDA, 2001).

Diagnostic Statement: Readiness for Enhanced Family Coping

Definition. Readiness for Enhanced Family Coping is the family member's desire and readiness to use adaptive behaviors in response to the client's health challenge (NANDA, 2001).

Defining Characteristics. Of the defining characteristics or clinical cues that denote this nursing diagnosis, one of the following major characteristics is required to be present and must be reported by a family member:

- Family member attempts to describe impact of crisis on life and relationships.
- Family expresses interest in being in contact with others who have dealt with similar situations.
- Family member moves in direction of health-promoting lifestyle and chooses activities that optimize wellness (NANDA, 2001).

Related Factors. Related factors for Compromised or Disabled Family Coping, listed earlier, become risk factors in this diagnostic statement.

Diagnostic Statement: Ineffective Family Therapeutic Regimen Management

Definition. Ineffective Family Therapeutic Regimen Management is defined as difficulty integrating a program for treatment of illness and its sequelae into a family's daily routine (NANDA, 2001).

Defining Characteristics. Of the defining characteristics or clinical cues that denote this nursing diagnosis, one of the following major characteristics must be present:

- Accelerated illness of family member
- Expressed difficulty in managing treatment
- Difficulty with regulating or including treatment in daily routine
- Family activities that inhibit meeting goals of treatment
- Lack of attention to illness

Related Factors. This diagnosis may be associated with several related or contributing factors. Factors include complexity of healthcare system; chronic, progressive illness such as HIV/AIDS; drug or alcohol addiction; eating disorders such as anorexia; prolonged hospitalization; intimidation with invasive or restrictive treatments; feelings of inadequacy; and interruptions of family life caused by the home care regimen.

Diagnostic Statement: Impaired Parenting

Definition. Impaired Parenting is the state in which a nurturing figure(s) experiences an inability to create, continue, or regain an environment that promotes the optimum growth and development of another human being (NANDA, 2001).

Defining Characteristics. Of the defining characteristics or cues, one of the following major characteristics must be present to define "Actual" Altered Parenting:

- Physical, psychological, or social trauma to child (This may be noted as obvious signs of abuse or other inappropriate behaviors such as inadequate feeding or failure to thrive or may be suggested by a history of child abuse, frequent injuries/illnesses, or repeated "runaway" behavior.)
- Lack of appropriate parental behaviors (Inappropriate visual, tactile, or auditory stimulation may be noted; the parent may have the child call him or her by the first name instead of by a traditional title like "dad" or "mom;" or the parent may verbalize resentment or negative perception of the child's gender, physical characteristics, and body functions. Abandonment may result.)
- Neglect and inattention to infant/child needs (This may be revealed in noncompliance with health appointments for self or child, a lag in growth and development, or the child receiving care from multiple caregivers without consideration for the child's needs.)
- Observed or verbalized role inadequacy (The parent may be using inappropriate or inconsistent discipline practices, may verbalize that he or she cannot control the child, or may compulsively seek role approval from others; NANDA, 2001.)

Related Factors. There are several etiologic or contributing factors that may result in Impaired Parenting. They include lack of knowledge and social, physiologic, or psychological difficulties. Not having an available role model or having ineffective role models can limit the person's parenting skill development. Factors include: physical or emotional abuse of the parent that may threaten the parent's survival; lack of support between/from significant other(s) that limits coping ability; unmet social, emotional, or maturational needs that may result in parental role inadequacy; interruption in the bonding process that may occur with the child's mental or physical illness so that the parent and child do not have an opportunity to develop a trusting relationship and may lack role identities; lack of knowledge or limited cognitive functioning resulting in unrealistic expectations; unrealistic expectations for self, infant, or partner resulting in frustration and inappropriate parenting behaviors; presence of stress (financial, legal, recent crisis, multiple pregnancies, cultural move) that may be expressed as child abuse or neglect; and a child showing no response or responding inappropriately to parents, which may discourage positive relationships (NANDA, 2001).

Diagnostic Statement: Risk for Impaired Parenting

Definition. Risk for Impaired Parenting is the state in which a nurturing figure(s) is at risk of experiencing an inability to create, continue, or regain an environment that promotes the optimum growth and development of another human being (NANDA, 2001).

Defining Characteristics. The presence of risk factors such as those listed earlier under Impaired Parenting are indications that the family is at risk for altered parenting. Especially critical are inattention to the infant's or child's needs and inappropriate caregiving behaviors.

Related Factors. Related factors are the same as those discussed earlier for Impaired Parenting.

Diagnostic Statement: Parental Role Conflict

Definition. Parental Role Conflict is the state in which a parent experiences role confusion and conflict in response to crisis (NANDA, 2001).

Defining Characteristics. Of the defining characteristics or clinical cues that indicate this nursing diagnosis, one of the following major characteristics must be present:

- Parent(s) verbalizes concerns or feelings of inadequacy, guilt, anger, frustration, or anger about providing for the child's physical or emotional needs. (This occurs in response to a crisis such as hospitalization or the need to care for an ill child at home.)
- There is demonstrated disruption in caregiving routines. (The family is not able to maintain its normal pattern of behavior during a crisis situation.)
- Parent expresses concern about changes in family. (These changes can include alterations in parental role, family functioning, family communication, or family health related to the crisis situation.)
- Parent expresses concern about perceived loss of control over decisions relating to the child.
- There is reluctance to participate in usual caregiving activities even with encouragement and support.
- Parent(s) verbalizes or demonstrates feelings of guilt, anger, fear, anxiety, or frustration about effect of child's illness on family process (NANDA, 2001).

Related Factors. Parental role conflict may be associated with several etiologic or contributing factors. The factors include separation from the child due to parent or child illness, specialized care center policies, or change in marital status; intimidation with invasive or restrictive treatments, such as isolation or intubation, that provoke anxiety in the parent; home care of a child with special needs, such as apnea monitoring, that causes parental feelings of inadequacy; and interruptions of family life caused by the home care regimen that may result in limited time for caring for other children and lack of respite for caregivers (NANDA, 2001).

Diagnostic Statement: Risk for Impaired Parent/Infant/Child Attachment

Definition. Risk for Impaired Parent/Infant/Child Attachment is a disruption in the interaction between parent and infant/child that inhibits developing a protective and nurturing relationship (NANDA, 2001).

Defining Characteristics. The presence of risk factors include:

- Anxiety with the parenting role, especially with a premature infant or ill infant/child
- Physical barriers to parenting
- Substance abuse
- Inability of parents to meet personal needs, separation, lack of privacy (NANDA, 2001)

Related Nursing Diagnoses

When a family has altered family functioning, other problems may arise for its members. Related nursing diagnoses include Anxiety; Decisional Conflict; Fear; Anticipatory or Dysfunctional Grieving; Chronic, Situational, or Risk for Situational Low Self-Esteem; Powerlessness; Ineffective Role Performance; Impaired Verbal Communication; Impaired Social Interaction; Social Isolation; Relocation Stress Syndrome; Spiritual Distress; and Risk for Other-Directed, or Self-Directed Violence.

OUTCOME IDENTIFICATION AND PLANNING

After the nursing diagnoses and related factors are identified, client goals and nursing interventions are planned. Goals are designed to identify the general and specific changes that the client and family think will demonstrate that the situation has improved. Client- and family-centered care goals are often derived from identifying the contributing factors and are designed to indicate specific, discernible behaviors. General goals can be identified for family functioning then individualized for each situation. Common client- and family-centered goals for families experiencing problems include the following:

- Client and family will identify instances in which they have achieved intrafamily communication.
- Client and family will demonstrate awareness of other members' needs for physical care, economic security, education, and nurturing.
- Client and family will demonstrate knowledge of effective coping mechanisms.
- Client and family will demonstrate achievement of individual and family development.

When using family-centered care, the nurse in the Critical Thinking Challenge at the beginning of the chapter will need to review and to clarify expectations with both the caregivers and extended family before proceeding to interventions. Implementation is most effective when the client, family, and nurse have collaboratively set goals and developed interventions.

Nurses plan with the client, the family, or both to promote healthy family patterns and function or to assist directly in meeting the needs of the family with altered function. Motivation and educational needs will influence planning. Examples of nursing interventions commonly used in family care are listed in the accompanying display and discussed in the following section.

IMPLEMENTATION

To promote family function, nurses support, reinforce, and teach. Interventions for altered family functioning include referral, counseling, and assistance with problem solving. The more family members the nurses can involve, the more family-centered the care will be, and the greater its potential impact.

Health Promotion

Identifying strengths, reinforcing positive behaviors, and providing anticipatory guidance and resources can support the family. These strengths and resources are key areas to assess that you can include in your first visit with the family.

Reinforcement of Family Strengths
From information obtained during assessment, help the client and family to identify their own areas of strength (Fig. 47-6). Strengths may include effective communication, mutual support of members, flexible roles, general stability, healthy coping mechanisms, and presence of good support systems. Identification of strengths will help the family to target resources to draw from for daily functioning as well as when crises develop. Focus on the family's strengths rather than

weaknesses. Point out examples of strengths such as a family member's ability to take a leave of absence to care for the ill person to relieve the primary caregiver or the spiritual support that the family's clergy or spiritual consultant provides. Encourage the client and family to think of examples of strengths they have used when faced with problems in the past and how they can draw on these strengths if needed. Identify both individual and family strengths.

Support and Teaching
Support the client and family in actions that promote family functioning by listening to and educating them. During serious or chronic illnesses, many nurses form close bonds with clients and their families. Families come to look to nurses for emotional support. Help families identify other sources of support as well such as extended family, religious affiliations, work groups, peers, and community groups. Then the family can strengthen contact with support groups. Assure the family that using support systems is a strength, not a weakness. **Anticipatory guidance** is a technique combining teaching and support. Instead of focusing on what has happened during the course of an illness, using anticipatory guidance prepares the client and family for what will happen next and why.

Nursing Interventions for Altered Family Function

If altered family functioning has been identified, interventions focus on behaviors that will return the family to positive outcomes, improve the problem, and support family relationships (Altschuler, 1997). Assist with problem solving, offer referrals, and facilitate family counseling if necessary.

Problem Solving
Families who are experiencing altered family function attain goals with assistance in problem solving. Aim interventions at resolving family conflicts by first identifying the participants' willingness to acknowledge a problem and to work on their ability to communicate. Stress effective communication practices: Allow each member to speak, listen, and express feelings as well as facts (Sparks, 1997). Nursing interventions to foster problem solving are as follows:

- Clarify the conflict with participants.
- Help participants identify contributing factors.
- Correct misconceptions.
- Provide concrete feedback based on nursing observations.
- Assist participants to develop solutions.
- Support decision making among participants.

Focus on helping the participants develop self-awareness and identify a working method to solve problems. Lead the family through problem solving while teaching them how to conduct the process themselves. Guide the family in solving a small problem first, providing reassurance that they can deal with larger problems as well.

Along with improving communication and problem solving, nurses must help the family strengthen its coping mechanisms (see Chapter 49). Assist the family in identifying what

---

PLANNING: Examples of NIC/NOC Interventions

Accepted Families and Relationships Nursing Interventions Classification (NIC)
Abuse Protection: Child
Caregiver Role Strain

Accepted Families and Relationships Nursing Outcomes Classification (NOC)
Abuse Cessation
Abuse Protection
Caregiver Stressors
Caregiver Well-Being
Parent–Infant Attachment
Parenting
Role Performance

Refer to the following for specifics regarding NIC/NOC:
McCloskey, J., & Bulechek, G. (2000). *Iowa Intervention Project: Nursing Interventions Classification (NIC)*. St. Louis, MO: C. V. Mosby.
Johnson, M., & Maas, M. (2000). *Iowa Outcomes Project: Nursing Outcomes Classification (NOC)*, 2nd ed. St. Louis, MO: C. V. Mosby.

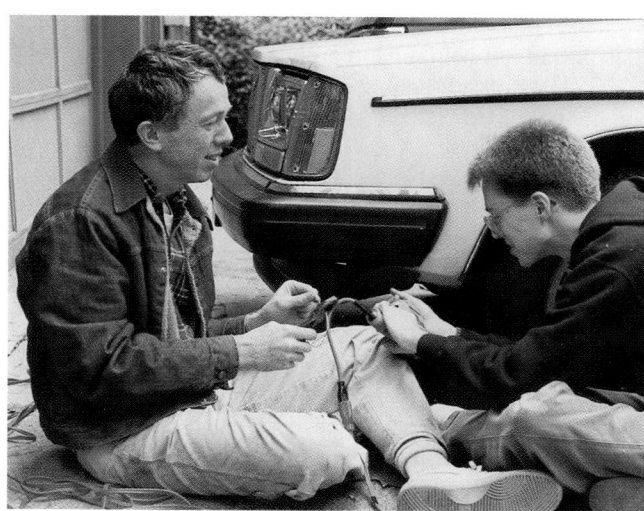

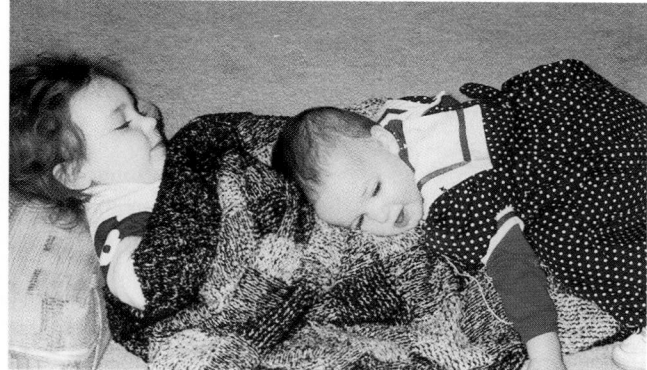

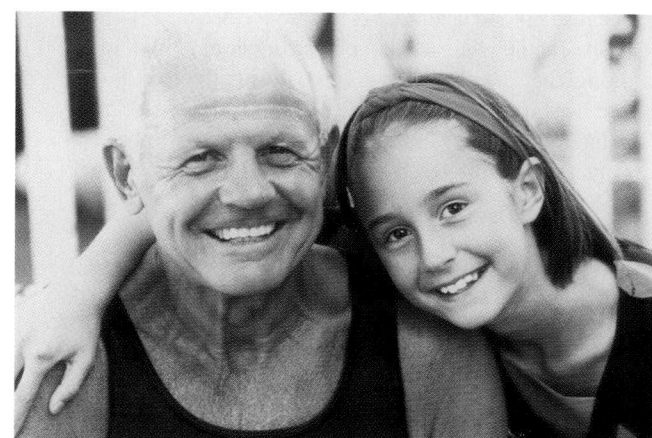

FIGURE 47-6 Sources of strength and support are found in various family relationships such as between father and son, siblings, and grandparent and grandchild.

coping mechanisms worked in the past and what coping mechanisms were detrimental.

Referral and Family Counseling

Nurses may be able to refer families with altered function to other resources. Members of the social service department or spiritual ministry may assist families with unmet financial or spiritual needs. Clinical nurse specialists, nutritionists, and physical and occupational therapists may provide information and training for clients and family members who have physical care needs.

Professional referrals and peer support groups may be sources of help to those experiencing difficulty with parenting roles. Self-help groups for parents include Parents Without Partners, La Leche League International, and Parent Effectiveness Training. Numerous support groups listed in the blue pages of phone books are valuable resources for referrals. The Association for the Care of Children's Health, an international organization located in Bethesda, Maryland, can provide information and a comprehensive list of support groups, their activities, and resources. The Area Agency on Aging and the American Association of Retired Persons (AARP) are excellent resources for older adults.

Other possible referrals are to psychiatric programs, police, drug and alcohol treatment programs, social workers, protective services, and shelters for battered women. When dealing with families in crisis, nurses are obligated to ensure the safety of individual members through notification and referral to the appropriate groups. Evidence of suspected child abuse necessitates notification of the police and referral to appropriate agencies.

🥤 SAFETY ALERT

If you suspect child abuse, notify the police or local child protective services agency. Tell the family that you are acting as an advocate for the child, and you are legally responsible to report your suspicions.

Ongoing counseling may be necessary for families with chronic stressors such as chronic illness, substance abuse, loss of a family member, role strain, separation, or divorce. Family or marital counseling focuses on the interaction of the members, not on counseling any one person. Roles and relationships are examined, communication and problem solving are fostered, and bonds are strengthened. Nurses can be instrumental in leading families to counseling if members are unable to overcome altered function without outside help.

Healthcare Planning and Home/Community-Based Nursing

Altered family relationships usually must be dealt with in the home environment, placing stress and additional responsibility on family members. When illness is the causative factor

ETHICAL/LEGAL ISSUE
Placement of an Elder in a Nursing Home

Janine Sanders was an independent, 75-year-old woman in spite of multiple illnesses including chronic lung disease, osteoporosis, and diabetes. She had been able to remain in her own apartment with visits and help from home care nurses and neighbors. Her family lives over 300 miles away and visits only occasionally. Recently, Janine was hospitalized for a fractured hip. Her doctor cannot recommend discharge to the home; he says the most reasonable option is to admit her to a nursing home because no one is available to care for her on a 24-hour basis. Janine wants to move in with her daughter, although her daughter is not home during the day. Janine and her family ask you what you think about placement in a nursing home and if you can suggest any other options. The hospital will discharge Janine within a week.

Reflection

- Reflect on your feelings as the family asks you to help them consider moving the previously independent woman to a nursing home. Try to identify any areas that you are uncomfortable discussing.
- Identify your underlying assumptions about the ethics of hospital discharge into facilities such as nursing homes.
- Reflect on how the Patient Bill of Rights in Chapter 6 applies to this situation. What information does the family need to make an informed decision?
- Think of at least three different ways to respond to the family's request for help. Identify a possible approach that could help Janine's family feel that they have supported Janine's right to independence along with her need for continuous support. How could her quality of life be maintained?

of alteration, assess the home for supports and barriers to providing appropriate care and quality of life. Family members can differ in their willingness to assume new or additional responsibilities. Referral to social agencies, such as home healthcare providers, may be necessary to ensure adequate support.

Healthcare planning should address specific needs, types of assistance and equipment needed, learning needs, and availability of alternative support. Teach family members techniques of care to meet the client's physical needs to assist in their adaptation to the caregiver's role. Teach signs of risk factors for complications to promote confidence in caring for the client at home. Provide the family with the name and phone number of someone to contact with questions to ease anxiety. An interdisciplinary approach should include referrals to social

workers, counselors, spiritual advisors, community resource centers, and self-help support groups as needed.

Examples of self-help and support groups that are often community-based include Alcoholics Anonymous, Al-Anon, Al-Ateen, Narcotics Anonymous, cancer support groups, Compassionate Friends, stroke support groups, and Alzheimer support groups. These groups can help the family solve problems by providing information and emotional support.

Case management, a means of coordination and ongoing evaluation of care, is used to help the client and family deal with the complex healthcare system. Case management includes identifying, coordinating, and evaluating the provision of services including cost, quality, and continuity. People must be connected to outside resources and support systems and assisted to maximize their own strengths in caring for clients at home. Family members, neighbors, and community organizations can form a "family-centered" network of care (Turnbull & Turnbull, 1997). Their goal is to provide as "normal" a lifestyle as possible with the client and family acting in partnership with the nurse case manager and other professional healthcare providers. If the caregivers, client, and family members disagree, the case manager needs to remain nonjudgmental and show acceptance of the differences. Encouraging everyone's active involvement facilitates family-centered care; asking questions about each family member's knowledge and understanding of past and present situations as well as expectations for the future should help to define problems and suggest solutions. In the Critical Thinking Challenge, questions addressed to the spouse, daughter, and granddaughter could facilitate optimal home care for the client.

EVALUATION

Evaluation is an ongoing process of determining progress toward the stated goals in the outcome identification phase. For alterations in family function, expected outcome criteria focus on client and family communication, family needs, use of coping mechanisms, and family development. The following are examples of possible outcome criteria for general goals.

Goal

Client will identify instances in which intrafamily communication has been achieved.

Possible Outcome Criteria

- By home care discharge, each family member engages in conversation during visit, as observed by nurse.
- By home care discharge, other members listen while family member is talking, as observed by nurse.
- Family member relates that content of conversations includes feelings within 48 hours.

NURSING PLAN OF CARE
THE FAMILY WITH CAREGIVER ROLE STRAIN

Nursing Diagnosis

Caregiver Role Strain related to anxiety, lack of knowledge, money, and emotional support manifested by altered sleep patterns; frequent crying; verbalized inadequacy of knowledge, finances, and husband.

Family Goal

Caregiver will develop a realistic care plan that includes support from the family and community.

Family Outcome Criteria

- Caregiver demonstrates decreased anxiety with increased confidence in caretaking behaviors within 1 month.
- Caregiver receives and accepts support from family and community within 1 month.
- Family seeks external resources within 2 weeks.

Nursing Intervention	Scientific Rationale
1. Assess caregiver's knowledge of dementia disease characteristics by questioning and observation. Be nonjudgmental. Encourage expression of feelings.	1. Objective data can validate verbal responses. Need to identify knowledge without provoking resentment.
2. Reinforce positive caregiving, accept expressions of negative emotions, and focus on positive behaviors.	2. Reinforcement encourages caregiver and decreases anxiety.
3. Role-model effective communication techniques: talk directly to older adult and maintain eye contact.	3. Communication is important for developing coping techniques.
4. Explore with caregiver ways to involve all family members in meeting the older adult's needs consistently and securely.	4. By decreasing denial, realistic planning can occur. Likelihood of compliance increases if all members are involved.
5. Initiate a plan to develop caregiving skills by providing information and opportunities for wife–family interaction with feedback.	5. Information about realistic expectations and solutions can promote effective coping. Practice reinforces these measures.
6. Explore possible sources of support. Offer to make initial contacts. Fear of authorities may inhibit initiating action.	6. Support needs to be ongoing for change to be maintained.
7. Refer to Area Agency on Aging for caregiver relief assistance; refer to Alzheimer support groups for respite care planning.	7. Continuity of care includes assessment and support.

- Caregiver expresses use of alternatives such as telephone and letter writing when personal visits are impossible due to distance or other time constraints.

Goal

Family members will demonstrate awareness of other members' physical care, economic security, educational needs, and nurturing.

Possible Outcome Criteria

- Within 48 hours, family states that bills are being paid and family members are attending social functions.

- Within 48 hours, family members display affection toward one another, as observed by nurse.

Goal

Client will demonstrate knowledge of effective coping mechanisms.

Possible Outcome Criteria

- During first counseling sessions, caregiver discusses family coping mechanisms that worked in past.
- During first counseling session, caregiver states coping mechanisms that were detrimental in past.

- By discharge, client verbalizes coping mechanisms that he or she will use in future.

KEY CONCEPTS

- Many family structures exist, including nuclear families, single-parent families, blended families, and extended families.
- Each family functions uniquely but all families share some common goals. Needs that families provide for their members include physical and economic provision of care, sexual intimacy, reproduction, education, socialization (including communication), and nurturing and support for problem solving and goal setting.
- Factors that affect family function include culture, values and beliefs, economics, lifestyle, previous life experience, stress, and illness.
- Families and their relationships change in reaction to daily and situational stress as well as acute and chronic illness. Roles may be redefined to meet individual and family needs.
- Common manifestations of altered family function include separation, divorce, role strain, abuse, social isolation, and emotional problems.
- Both subjective and objective data are useful for assessment of altered family function. Assessment seeks to identify normal patterns, families at risk for altered family function, and actual altered family function.
- Outcome identification and planning focus on the family members and the family unit. Goals, which involve applying family-centered care, include improved communication and coping mechanisms, fulfilled family needs, and accomplished development.
- A multidisciplinary approach is useful in interventions for altered family function. Interventions to promote family functioning include reinforcement of family strengths, support, and use of anticipatory guidance. Interventions for families with altered function include referral, problem solving, and counseling.
- Evaluation of nursing care is accomplished by comparing outcomes with criteria established during the planning stage.

REFERENCES

Altschuler, J. (1997). Family relationships during serious illness. *Nursing Times, 93*(7), 48–49.

Benzies, K. M., Harrison, M. J., & Magill-Evans, J. (1998). Impact of marital quality and parent–infant interaction on preschool behavior problems. *Public Health Nursing, 15,* 35–43.

Bomar, P. J. (1996). *Nurses and family health promotion* (2nd ed.). Philadelphia: W. B. Saunders.

Carpenito, L. J. (2002). *Nursing diagnosis: Application to clinical practice* (9th ed.). Philadelphia: Lippincott Williams & Wilkins.

Casper, L. M. & Bryson, K. B. (1998). Co-resident grandparents and their grandchildren: Grandparent maintained families. *U.S. Census Bureau, Population Division, Fertility & Family Statistics Branch,* Population Division Working Paper No. 26 (*http://www.census.gov/population/www/documentation/twps0026/twps0026.html*)

Cramer, C., & Cramer, A. (1995). Caring for the Latter-Day Saint patient. *Journal of Emergency Nursing, 21,* 503–504.

de Bourdeaudhuij, I. & van Oost, P. (1998). Family members' influence on decision making about food: Differences in perception and relationship with healthy eating. *American Journal of Health Promotion, 13* (2), 73–81.

Degotardi, P. J., Revenson, T. A., & Ilowite, N. T. (1999). Family-level coping in juvenile rheumatoid arthritis: Assessing the utility of a quantitative family interview. *Arthritis Care and Research, 12,* 314–324.

Douglass, L. G. (1997). Reciprocal support in the context of cancer: Perspectives of the patient and spouse. *Oncology Nursing Forum, 24,* 1529–1536.

Erikson, E. (1963). *Childhood and Society.* New York: Norton.

Ford-Gilboe, M. (1997). Family strengths, motivation, and resources as predictors of health promotion behavior in single-parent and two-parent families. *Research in Nursing and Health, 20,* 205–217.

Gedaly-Duff, V., & Heims, M. L. (1996). Family child health nursing. In S. M. Hanson & S. T. Boyd (Eds.), *Family health care nursing: Theory, practice, and research.* Philadelphia: F. A. Davis, 238–265.

Grasso, S. E. (1996). Perspectives. Rehabilitation nursing extends to oncology patients: A new challenge for rehabilitation nurses. *Rehabilitation Nursing, 21,* 327–328.

Hanson, S. M. H. (1996). Family assessment and intervention. In S. M. Hanson & S. T. Boyd (Eds.), *Family health care nursing: Theory, practice, and research* (pp. 146–172). Philadelphia: F. A. Davis.

Hanson, S. M., & Boyd, S. T. (Eds.) (1996). *Family health care nursing: Theory, practice, and research.* Philadelphia: F. A. Davis.

Houde, S. C. (1998). Predictors of elders' and family caregivers' use of formal home services. *Research in Nursing & Health, 21,* 533–543.

Hupcey, J. E. (1998). Establishing the nurse-family relationship in the intensive care unit. *Western Journal of Nursing Research, 20,* 180–194.

La Montagne, J. F., Engle, P. L., & Zeitlin, M. F. (1998). Maternal employment, child care, and nutritional status of 12–18 month old children in Managua, Nicaragua. *Social Science & Medicine, 46,* 403–414.

Ladd, R. E., Pasquerella, L., & Smith, S. (2000). What to do when the end is near: Ethical issues in home health care nursing. *Public Health Nursing, 17,* 103–110.

Leininger, M. (1995). *Transcultural nursing: Concepts, theories, research and practice.* Columbus, OH: McGraw-Hill.

Lynch, S. H. (1997). Elder abuse: What to look for, how to intervene. *American Journal of Nursing, 97,* 26–33.

Maker, A. H., Kemmelmeier, M., & Peterson, C. (1998). Long-term psychological consequences in women of witnessing parental physical conflict and experiencing abuse in childhood. *Journal of Interpersonal Violence, 13,* 574–589.

Munet-Vilaro, F. (1998). Forum focus: Grieving and death rituals of Latinos. *Oncology Nursing Forum, 25,* 1761–1763.

Narsavage, G. L. (1997). Promoting function in clients with chronic lung disease by increasing their perception of control. *Holistic Nursing Practice, 12* (1): 17–26.

North American Nursing Diagnosis Association. (2001). *NANDA Nursing diagnoses: Definitions and classification 2001–2002.* Philadelphia: Author.

O'Connor, T. G., Hetherington, E. M., & Reiss, D. (1998). Family systems and adolescent development: shared and nonshared risk and protective factors in nondivorced and remarried families. *Development and Psychopathology, 10,* 353–375.

Parker, V. (1995). Battered. *RN, 58*(1), 26–29.

Plichta, S. B., & Weisman, C. S. (1995). Spouse or partner abuse, use of health services, and unmet needs for medical care in U.S. women. *Journal of Women's Health, 4*(1), 45–53.

Richards, B. S. (1996). Gerontological family nursing. In S. M. Hanson & S. T. Boyd (Eds.), *Family health care nursing: Theory, practice, and research* (pp. 328–348). Philadelphia: F. A. Davis.

Santelli, B., Turnbull, A., & Higgins, C. (1997). Family matters. Parent to parent support and health care. *Pediatric Nursing, 23,* 303–306.

Seiderman, R. Y., Jacobson, S., Primeaux, M., Burns, P., & Weatherby, F. (1996). Assessing American Indian families.

MCN: American Journal of Maternal/Child Nursing, 21, 274–279.

Shapiro, J., Perez, M., & Warden, M. J. (1998). The importance of family functioning to caregiver adaptation in mothers of child cancer patients. *Journal of Pediatric Oncology Nursing, 15,* 47–54.

Smith, K. E. & Bachu, A. (1999). Women's labor force attachment patterns and maternity leave: A review of the literature. *U.S. Census Bureau, Population Division, Fertility & Family Statistics Branch,* Population Division Working Paper No. 32 (*http://www.census.gov/population/ www/documentation/ twps0032/twps0032.html*)

Smith, S. D. (1997). The retirement transition and the later life family unit. *Public Health Nursing, 14,* 207–216.

Sparks, M. J. (1997). Helping a child when a parent has cancer. *Nursing '97, 27*(10), 16–17.

Steinberg, L. (2001). The role of the family in adolescent development: Preventing risk, promoting resilience. Temple University. Available at: *http://www.cyfernet.org/keynote2001.html*

Turnbull A. P., & Turnbull, H. R. III. (1997). *Families, professionals, and exceptionality: Collaborating for empowerment* (3rd ed.). Englewood Cliffs, NJ: Merill/Prentice Hall.

U.S. Bureau of Labor Statistics. (2001). *Labor force statistics from the current population survey.* Washington, D.C.: http://www.bls.gov/news.release/empsit.t01.htm. (Feb. 27, 2002)

U.S. Census Bureau. (1990). *Statistical abstract of the United States: 1990.* Washington, DC: Author.

U.S. Census Bureau. (2000). *Statistical abstract of the United States: 2000.* Washington, DC: Author.

U.S. Census Bureau. (1998). *Current Population Survey (CPS).* Available: *http://www.census.gov/ population/socdemo/ hh-family/98pplb.txt*

Van Riper, M. (2001). Family-provider relationships and well-being in families with preterm infants in the NICU. *Heart & Lung, 30,* 74–84.

BIBLIOGRAPHY

Aroian, K. J., Spitzer, A., & Bell, M. (1996). Family stress and support among former Soviet immigrants. *Western Journal of Nursing Research, 18,* 655–674.

Coyne, I. T. (1997). Chronic illness: The importance of support for families caring for a child with cystic fibrosis. *Journal of Clinical Nursing, 6,* 121–129.

Dorfman, L. T., Holmes, C. A., & Berlin, K. L. (1996). Wife caregivers of frail elderly veterans: Correlates of caregiver satisfaction and caregiver strain. *Family Relations, 45,* 46–55.

Dougherty, C. M. (1997). Family-focused interventions for survivors of sudden cardiac arrest. *Journal of Cardiovascular Nursing, 12,* 45–58.

Douglass, L. G. (1997). Reciprocal support in the context of cancer: Perspectives of the patient and spouse. *Oncology Nursing Forum, 24,* 1529–1536.

Keller, C. S., & Stevens, K. R. (1997). Cultural considerations in promoting wellness. *Journal of Cardiovascular Nursing, 11,* 15–25.

Narayan, M. C., & Rea K. (1997). Nursing across cultures: The South Asian client. *Home Healthcare Nurse, 15,* 460–469.

Odulana, J. A., Camblin, L. D., & White, P. (1996). Cultural roles and health status of contemporary African American young grandmothers. *Journal of Multicultural Nursing and Health, 2*(4), 28–35.

Pinkerton, R., et al. (1995). *Childhood cancer management— A practical handbook* (2nd ed.). Oxford: Chapman & Hall.

Santelli, B., Turnbull, A., Marquis, J., & Lerner, E. (1997). Parent-to-parent programs: A resource for parents and professionals. *Journal of Early Intervention, 21,* 73.

Smith, S. D. (1997). The retirement transition and the later life family unit. *Public Health Nursing, 14,* 207–216.

Stetz, K. M., & Brown, M. A. (1997). Taking care: Caregiving to persons with cancer and AIDS. *Cancer Nursing, 20,* 12–22.

Internet Resources: Family Links

American Association for Marriage and Family Therapy. Professional association link with detailed information about problems facing families. Available at:*http://www.aamft.orgfamilies/ index.htm*

Child Welfare Training Resources Online Network. Network link for educators to locate training materials; focus is on child welfare workers. Available at: *http://www.childwelfare-training.org*

CYFERnet: Children, Youth, and Families Education and Research Network. National network of educators supporting community-based educational programs. Available at http:// *http://www. cyfernet.org*

Minnesota Council on Family Relations. State link to articles that explore family issues; focus is on practice and policy making. Available at: *http://www.mcfr.net*

National Council on Family Relations. National site providing family-oriented web site links. Available at: *http://www. ncfr.com*

Society for Research in Child Development. International multidisciplinary society of researchers and practitioners with news links. Available at: *http://www.srcd.org/news1.html*

University of Delaware Family Resources. University site provides access to multiple family-related resources by topic. Available at: *http://ag.udel.edu/fam/resources/ resbytopic.htm*

48 Loss and Grieving

🔳 Key Terms

anticipatory grief
bereavement
death
dying
dysfunctional grief

grief
hospice
loss
mourning

🔳 Learning Objectives

Upon completion of this chapter, the student will be able to do the following:

1. Define selected terms related to loss, death, dying, and grief.
2. Identify the normal functions of grief.
3. Compare models of grief related to bereavement and grief related to dying.
4. Identify the common signs and symptoms of grief.
5. Evaluate death and grief reactions across the life span.
6. Identify variables that influence normal grieving.
7. Discuss the effects of multiple losses on the grief process.
8. Apply the nursing process to grieving clients.
9. Differentiate between normal and dysfunctional grieving.
10. Identify the principles of hospice care.
11. Recognize physical and emotional signs and symptoms of dying.

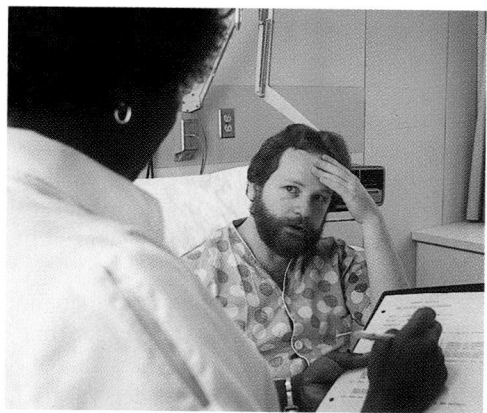

🔳 Critical Thinking Challenge

You are a nurse in an outpatient diagnostic unit. Jim, a middle-aged man, is admitted to your unit for a gastroscopy. As you complete your admission assessment you obtain the following data: (1) Jim has been HIV positive for 14 months; (2) his partner, with whom he lived for 15 years, died from AIDS 6 months ago after numerous hospitalizations. Jim complains of abdominal pain that is "like the pain" his partner had just before his death. Jim lives by himself, has few close friends, and is estranged from his family. During the examination he becomes tearful and states, "I don't know what is wrong with me. I just can't get myself together and do things like I used to."

One of your greatest challenges as a nurse will be to help clients and families deal with loss and grief. As you pursue the profession of nursing, you will meet many people who are experiencing loss. You will need to combine your nursing knowledge and understanding of people to work with those who have suffered a loss and are grieving. Once you have completed this chapter and have incorporated loss and grieving into your knowledge base, review the above scenario and reflect on the following areas of Critical Thinking:

1. From the information provided, consider possible nursing diagnoses for this client.
2. Identify additional information you need to make a thorough assessment of this client and his social support system.
3. Plan actions you should take to assist this client.
4. Examine other resources (professional and nonprofessional) that you think could be mobilized to assist this client.
5. Propose how the client could best use such professional and nonprofessional resources.

Loss and grief are universal experiences that each person experiences from birth until death. Losses vary in importance, from insignificant losses that cause minor and brief sadness to major losses that cause intense and long-lasting distress.

Some losses are the result of normal development, whereas other losses are the result of unexpected events. Regardless of the source of the loss, grief is a necessary and normal reaction to it: grief is the price we pay for becoming attached to people, objects, and beliefs. Through the grief process, the person is able to sever the attachment to the lost person or object and become attached to other people or objects.

NORMAL GRIEVING

Grief has several important functions:

- To make the outer reality of the loss into an internally accepted reality.
- To sever the emotional attachment to the lost person or object.
- To make it possible for the bereaved person to become attached to other people or objects.

Characteristics of Normal Loss and Grieving

Types of Loss

Loss is defined as the experience of parting with an object, person, belief, or relationship that one values; the loss requires a reorganization of one or more aspects of the person's life. Losses range from minor ones, which necessitate only minor adjustments, to major ones, which necessitate major adaptations.

Losses are part of the normal developmental cycle. At birth, the newborn loses the warmth and security of the mother's womb. Later, the infant loses the comfort and gratification of the mother's breast. When a sibling is born, the child loses his or her place as the youngest in the family. Each loss has both negative and positive aspects. For example, by no longer being the youngest in the family, the child gains certain rights and responsibilities, but the child also loses the family's undivided attention and the special benefits attached to being the youngest.

A material loss is a loss of some tangible object or possession; a psychological loss is a loss of something that has no physical form but has some important symbolic meaning. Many losses have both material and psychological components. For example, loss of a job results in the material loss of income, but it also results in numerous psychological losses, such as loss of status, self-esteem, relationships with coworkers, and meaning for living.

An expected loss occurs with forewarning, whereas an unexpected loss occurs without warning. When a loss is expected, as in the case of terminal illness, survivors have time to prepare for it; thus, the distress associated with the loss may be decreased. In contrast, when a loss is unexpected, individ-

uals have no time to prepare and are likely to experience greater distress. When a family member has a terminal illness, the survivors have time to express their love, make amends, and make legal and financial arrangements. This is impossible when an unexpected loss occurs, such as a sudden death from an accident.

Terms Related to Grieving

Grief is the characteristic pattern of psychological and physiologic responses a person experiences after the loss of a significant person, object, belief, or relationship. Grief encompasses the entire range of physical, psychological, cognitive, and behavioral responses to a loss.

Bereavement is a state of desolation that occurs as the result of a loss, particularly the death of a significant other. Bereavement manifestations are the person's total response to a loss and include emotional, physical, social, and cognitive responses.

Mourning encompasses the socially prescribed behaviors after the death of a significant other. Such behaviors vary from culture to culture. Mourning behaviors are socially conventional bereavement behaviors and do not necessarily indicate the presence or absence of grief.

Anticipatory grief is the characteristic pattern of psychological and physiologic responses a person makes to the impending loss (real or imagined) of a significant person, object, belief, or relationship. It is generally believed that anticipatory grief facilitates coping with loss when the loss actually occurs.

Models of Grieving

Many researchers and theorists have attempted to describe the characteristics of the normal grief process. Some have proposed stage models of grief, others task models, and still others models of subconcepts such as bereavement guilt. Although these models are useful in guiding nursing care of clients who are experiencing loss, remember that there are no clear-cut stages of grief, nor are there any exact timetables. Expecting all clients to conform to a specific model is inappropriate. Table 48-1 outlines several models of grief, which are discussed in the following paragraphs.

Two popular stage models of grief are those proposed by Engel and by Parkes. A third model (Fig. 48-1) is the Grief Cycle Model (Demi, 1981), which was derived from Parkes' theory of grief. It can be used to guide practice with bereaved clients and (with minor modifications) with people who have experienced other types of loss.

Engel's Model. Engel (1964), one of the first to study grief, proposed six phases of grief: (a) shock and disbelief, (b) developing awareness, (c) restitution, (d) resolving the loss, (e) idealization, and (f) outcome. In the shock and disbelief stage, the survivor either refuses to accept the loss or shows intellectual acceptance of the loss but denies the emotional impact. Developing awareness occurs as the reality and meaning of the loss penetrate the person's consciousness. The numbness of the first phase is replaced with feelings of

THERAPEUTIC DIALOGUE
Loss and Grieving

Scene for Thought

Maureen O'Hagan, 48 years old, had a simple mastectomy 2 months ago. She is married with two grown children and runs her own business. She is returning to the clinic for a check of her operative site. The nurse notes that she looks pale and tired although she is dressed well and is wearing makeup.

Less Effective

Nurse: Hi, Ms. O'Hagan, I'm Natalie, the clinical specialist. How are you doing?
Client: Okay, I guess.
Nurse: Good! Any pain in the incision or in the muscles underneath? *(Client shakes head no.)* How about your general health? Any problems there? *(Looks at client and chart.)*
Client: Well, I haven't been eating or sleeping too well since the operation. *(Looks down at her hands.)*
Nurse: Really? Your lab works looks good. I wonder what the problem is. Do you have any ideas?
Client: Not really.
Nurse: Well, let me see about getting you some sleep medication to relax you. Getting enough sleep usually makes people feel better right away. Okay? *(Writes in chart and leaves the room. Ms. O'Hagan sighs.)*

More Effective

Nurse: Hi, Ms. O'Hagan. I'm Rosalie, the clinical nurse specialist. I'm going to check your mastectomy site today and see how you're doing in general.
Client: Fine. *(Gives a small smile to be polite.)*
Nurse: So, how are you doing? *(Shows concern, uses good eye contact.)*
Client: I . . . I'm not too sure, actually. I have no pain, the arm feels fine, the scar is okay, but I don't seem to be back to normal yet. My husband is beginning to complain about our not having sex like we used to. I don't get it. *(Looks confused, annoyed, and depressed.)*
Nurse: I'm checking your chart and all your blood work is fine. How have you been eating and sleeping? *(Assessment of the physical signs of grief.)*
Client: Not too well. I can't get to sleep very easily, and then I wake up in the middle of the night with dreams I can't remember. And I have no appetite.
Nurse: It sounds like you've been going through a difficult time. You're having trouble with sleep, disturbing dreams, fatigue, appetite loss, decreased sex drive, and not feeling like yourself. Is there anything else you want to add? *(Summarizes, asks open-ended question.)*
Client: Uh, well, yes, but it's stupid. *(Looks embarrassed.)*
Nurse: Oh? *(Continues with good eye contact and interested posture.)*
Client: I, ah, thought about driving into a wall one day last week. Quickly. I would never do it, but I got worried when I thought about that. Besides, what does it have to do with feeling tired and everything else?
Nurse: I think you haven't finished grieving for the loss of your breast. *(Says gently.)*
Client: *(After a short silence.)* Oh. So, you think I'm depressed? And that I haven't accepted that the breast is gone?
Nurse: Let's talk some more about it. I know some ways to help you feel better. Would that be okay?
Client: Well, maybe. I'm willing to try.

Critical Thinking Challenge
- Compare and contrast the signs that Natalie missed to which Rosalie paid attention.
- Propose the stage of grief Maureen might be in. Give your reason.
- Analyze her potential support systems.
- Specify other assessment factors to consider.
- Select interventions you would use if you were Rosalie.

intense psychological pain, often expressed through crying and anger. The next phase, restitution, consists of the work of mourning and includes the various funeral and religious rituals. The next phase, resolving the loss, occurs intrapsychically as the grieving person focuses energy on thoughts of the deceased. In the phase of idealization, first, all negative feelings toward the deceased are repressed; then, through identification, the survivor incorporates certain characteristics of the deceased into his or her own personality. Gradually, the grieving person's psychological dependence on the

TABLE 48-1

Models of Grief			
Engel's Model	**Parkes' Model**	**Grief Cycle Model**	**Kubler-Ross' Stages of Dying**
1. Shock and disbelief	1. Numbness	1. Shock	1. Denial
2. Developing awareness	2. Yearning	2. Protest	2. Anger
3. Restitution	3. Disorganization	3. Disorganization	3. Bargaining
4. Resolving the loss	4. Reorganization	4. Reorganization	4. Depression
5. Idealization			5. Acceptance
6. Outcome			

deceased diminishes and his or her interest in new relationships returns. According to Engel, the resolution of grief takes 1 year or longer.

Parkes' Model. Parkes (1986) proposed four stages of grief: (a) numbness, (b) yearning, (c) disorganization, and (d) reorganization. In the numbness stage, which is usually brief, trauma so overwhelms the bereaved survivor that he or she must use denial as a psychological defense. The next stage, yearning, usually lasts several months and is characterized by intense psychological distress, with thoughts focusing on the deceased. The disorganization stage is characterized by severe depression, social withdrawal, and lack of interest in people and activities. The last stage, reorganization, usually begins 6 to

9 months after the loss and is characterized by a gradual renewal of interest in people and activities and return of a sense of meaning in life. Parkes proposed that progression through the stages of grief normally takes 2 years or longer.

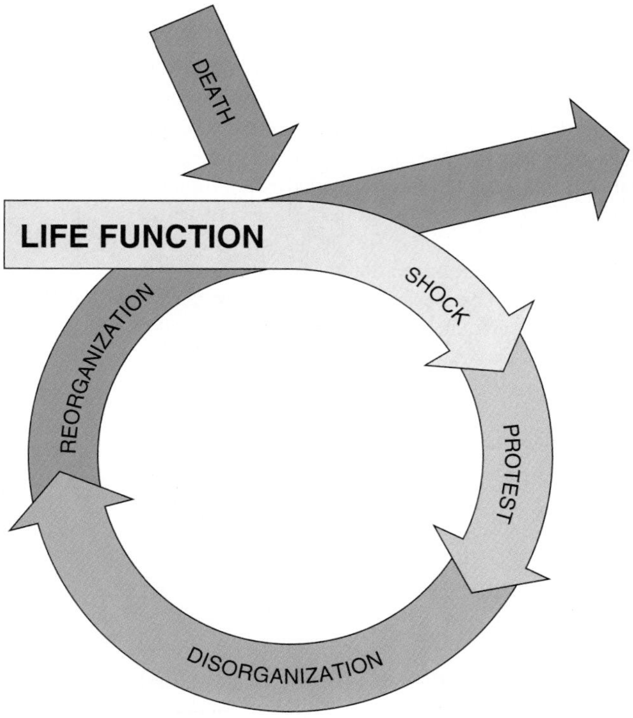

Grief Cycle Model. The grief cycle model assumes that, before a major loss, the person is functioning on a relatively unchanging level. Table 48-2 describes the manifestations of each stage of the grief cycle model: shock, protest, disorganization, and reorganization.

When a loss occurs, the first reaction is shock and a drop to a lower level of functioning. This stage may last several hours to several days.

The second stage of grief, protest, usually starts during the first week after the loss and continues through the third month. The person continues to drop in his or her level of functioning. Intense physical and psychological distress marks this period.

The disorganization stage starts around the third month and continues for 3 to 6 months. The person sinks to the lowest level of functioning. Feelings of depression and social withdrawal characterize this stage.

The reorganization stage starts at approximately the sixth month and usually continues for at least 1 year, but it may continue for a much longer period. People who have sufficient resources during this period are likely to continue to improve their level of functioning and often emerge from the grief cycle at a higher level of functioning than before the loss. Others with more stressors and fewer resources are often unable to recover fully from the grief experience and therefore function at a lower level than before the loss.

In reality, the stages are not as discrete as the grief cycle model indicates. However, it is helpful to use the model as a general guide, while keeping in mind that people may vary greatly in their responses to loss and still fall within the normal response range. Grieving persons may go through the stages at varying rates, go back and forth between stages, or skip stages.

Lifespan Considerations

The person's developmental stage must be considered when assessing reactions to loss and planning interventions. The impact of a traumatic event and the person's reaction to it de-

FIGURE 48-1   Grief wheel. (From Demi, A. [1981]. *Bereavement support group: Leadership manual.* Littleton, CT: Grief Education Institute.)

TABLE 48-2

Major Functional Manifestations During Grief

Stages/Phases of Grief

Realm	Shock	Protest	Disorganization	Reorganization
Cognitive	Slowed and disorganized thinking Blocking of thoughts Wish to join deceased Thoughts of suicide Denial of the loss and its significance	Preoccupation with thoughts of deceased Searching for deceased Dreams/nightmares Hallucinations Concerns about others' health and safety Continued death wishes	Difficulty making decisions Aimlessness Loss of interest in people, work, usual activities Perception of life as meaningless Focus on memories and reminders of deceased	Realistic memory of deceased Comfortable when remembering deceased Return to previous level of ability
Emotional	Blocking of emotions Emotional outbursts May appear unaffected Emotionally numb Feeling of unreality	Sadness Anger Guilt Relief Anxiety Yearning for deceased Feel deceased's presence	Depression Loneliness Meaninglessness Decreased self-esteem Apathy	Feels life has meaning Able to experience pleasure
Physical	Feels physically numb Hyperactive/ underactive, immobile	Pain in heart Sleep or appetite problems Weight loss Neglect of appearance Fatigue Lethargy Poor hygiene	Continued sleep and appetite problems Restlessness Decreased sexual interest/ satisfaction Aimless activity Decreased resistance to illness Accident prone Increased alcohol intake Increased drug use Increased tobacco use	Renewed vigor Restoration to previous level of health Improved health habits Sexual drive renewed
Social	Passive Unaware of others	Dependent on others Seeks help and advice of others	Loss of interest in people and work	New or renewed social relationships New or renewed activities Development of close relationship with at least one person

pend on the individual's developmental stage at the time the traumatic event occurs.

Newborn and Infant

Newborns have no concept of life and death. Growing infants have the ability to sense alterations in existence during cycles of wakefulness and sleep, which can be likened to a beginning understanding of the states of "being" and "nonbeing." The infant's concept of death or loss is related to feelings of separation anxiety when the parent or other caregiver is out of sight. The game of "peek-a-boo" introduces children to the death-related concepts of absence and pres-

ence. The child's delighted reaction to the other person's reappearance in the peek-a-boo game is the result of relief from the terror of separation.

Toddler and Preschooler

Cognitive powers are evidenced by 18 to 24 months and intensify the toddler's experience of separation anxiety. The developmental task of toddlers is to gain a sense of autonomy. Achievement of this task helps toddlers break the tie with their mother or other primary caregiver, who can now be out of sight for some time without the toddler being overly anxious. However, because toddlers vacillate between independence and attachment, such separations still causes them to fear abandonment by the primary caregiver.

Preschoolers perceive death as reversible, avoidable, and occurring in degrees. They develop an increasing awareness of themselves as separate physical and emotional beings. With this deepening awareness of self comes the vague realization that one may cease to exist. Although preschoolers sense their own vulnerability and begin to make the distinction between being alive and being dead, they still cannot grasp death's universality, inevitability, and finality. Preschoolers develop their concept of death from their experiences in real life and the depictions of death in books and the media. On television, animals and people die only to pop up again live in the same program, or on another program, reinforcing the perception that death is reversible. Preschoolers think of death as a long sleep. The death of a pet or a family member plays an important part in a child's development of a concept of death, although the preschooler's cognitive ability does not allow a clear understanding.

School-Age Child and Adolescent

In the early school years, the child perceives death as unnatural, reversible, and avoidable; the child may also personify death (e.g., perceive death to be a person or an animal). At about 9 years of age, the child's concept of death matures, and the child perceives death realistically as irreversible, universal, inevitable, and natural.

Society reinforces concepts of life and death. By school age, children usually have been touched by death in some way (e.g., family member, classmate, friend's family member, pet, news story). Some children live in violent neighborhoods where death is common. The modern school curriculum includes discussions about deaths and traumatic events that are prominent in the news or that occur locally. Religious institutions teach diverse beliefs about death and about life after death. The school-age child gradually realizes that death is an event no one escapes.

As age increases, the child's understanding of death becomes more realistic. A high level of cognitive development allows the adolescent to view life and death with an adult understanding. Adolescents begin to develop a philosophy of life and death. Nevertheless, the thought of one's own death is overwhelming and consequently is suppressed. Adolescents are already in the midst of a developmental crisis during which they experience constant change (Waechter, Phillips, & Holaday, 1985). Adolescents generally have the capacity to mourn fully, but they are at greater risk for poorer outcomes than adults because of the numerous other stressors and developmental changes they are experiencing during this stage of the life cycle (Hogan & DeSantis, 1994).

Adult and Older Adult

In contrast to children, adults tend to grieve more intensely and more continuously, but for a relatively shorter period of time. Furthermore, adults usually do not seek an immediate

replacement for the lost loved person, but rather move toward this after achieving some resolution of their grief.

Young adults often experience many losses within a short period of time, which places them particularly at risk for poor outcomes. They may experience the death of a family member, the ending of their schooling and consequent separation from peers, broken relationships, or failure in their attempt to achieve a satisfying job. These multiple losses, coupled with their inexperience with loss and grief, make them particularly at risk.

Middle-age adults who have a relatively stable lifestyle and adequate support systems usually cope well with loss; however, an untimely loss, such as the death of a child or the death of a spouse, may be extremely stressful, because it is perceived as out of the normal sequence of events.

Older adults often experience numerous losses, sequentially or simultaneously; therefore, they are at higher risk than other adults for poor outcomes after major losses. At a time when their stressors are highest, their resources are often the most meager. Deaths of relatives and friends, retirement, impaired health of self or family members, and decreased economic resources are all common stressors for the older adult. Fewer support networks are available to older adults because of deaths and illnesses of family and friends. Therefore, they may need to rely more heavily on healthcare providers to assist them in coping with their losses.

FACTORS AFFECTING GRIEVING

Many factors influence the grieving process, including the meaning of the loss to the individual, the circumstances of the loss, personal resources and stressors, and sociocultural resources and stressors.

Meaning of the Loss

People have a tendency to ascribe their own values to others, and therefore they incorrectly assume that a specific loss is or is not traumatic to a specific person without first assessing the meaning of the loss to that person. Loss of a finger would have very different meanings to a classical guitarist and a manual laborer. Divorce may be extremely undesired and cause intense grief in one person, whereas it may be welcomed and a cause for rejoicing in another. The age at which a loss occurs has a major impact: the loss of a parent has different meanings to an infant, a child, and an adult (see Lifespan Considerations).

Circumstances of the Loss

Whether a loss is expected or unexpected, violent or peaceful, timely or untimely, natural or unnatural, it affects the grief process. A loss that occurs under violent or frightening conditions is much more difficult to cope with than a loss that occurs under more peaceful conditions. A death that occurs as a result of homicide or suicide is usually more stressful than a death from natural causes. The perception that one in some way caused or contributed to the loss increases the grieving person's distress, such as when loss of function in an auto accident is caused by one's own carelessness. Loss of the ability to conceive a child is stressful if it is untimely (occurs at a young age), but it is timely and therefore not stressful in middle age.

Religious Beliefs and Cultural Practices

An individual's religious beliefs affect the grief process. Some people find strength in dealing with loss through their religious beliefs, whereas others experience greater distress due to their beliefs. Some people believe that death is the end; others believe that death is the beginning of a life in heaven or hell; and still others believe in reincarnation in another form. Some may think that their loss is a punishment for past sins. Nurses should gain knowledge of the specific cultural and religious beliefs of the clients they are serving and help their clients deal with loss in a manner that is congruent with their cultural and religious beliefs and practices.

Personal Resources and Stressors

Each person enters a loss situation with a unique combination of personal resources and stressors. What is a resource for one person may be a stressor for another. For example, health status may be either a resource or a stressor: the person who has good health habits, a variety of coping strategies, and a generally high level of wellness has a major advantage over the person who has poor health habits, limited coping skills, a chronic or acute illness, and a history of emotional instability.

Personal resources and stressors that influence response to a loss include coping skills, previous experiences with loss, emotional stability, spiritual beliefs, physical health, individual developmental stage, family developmental stage, other concurrent stressors, and socioeconomic status. Research indicates that socioeconomic status is one of the major factors related to ability to cope with loss. People with higher levels of education, higher income, and higher job status tend to have better outcomes after a major loss.

Sociocultural Resources and Stressors

Sociocultural resources include the social support that is available from family, friends, coworkers, and formal institutions. Absence of these social supports creates additional stressors for the grieving person. Sometimes the presence of these supports can also be stressors, particularly if the resource people are not able to empathize with the grieving person. Further, if a community is able to deal with loss and has reasonable expectations of the survivors, this reduces stress; however, if the community tends to blame the survivors for their plight (as in the case of AIDS), or if the community has unrealistic expec-

tations, the grieving person will have much more difficulty coping with the loss.

ALTERED GRIEVING

Dysfunctional grief is grief that falls outside the normal response range and may be manifested as exaggerated grief, prolonged grief, or absence of grief. In dysfunctional grief, the grieving person often becomes stuck in one stage of the grief process and is unable to progress to the next stage or stages. Furthermore, the grieving person expends so much energy either repressing the grief or dealing ineffectively with the grief that little time or energy is left to invest in normal growth and development.

Manifestations of Altered Grieving

In a study of bereavement experts' perceptions of "grief that falls outside normal parameters," Demi and Miles (1987) found that more than 30 different terms were commonly used to label dysfunctional grief. The most commonly accepted terms were pathologic grief, unresolved grief, dysfunctional grief, and prolonged grief. Many symptoms that have been considered abnormal or dysfunctional were identified as components of the normal grief process. At 1 year after bereavement, most experts believed that the grief manifestations listed in Display 48-1 were within normal parameters.

Bereavement experts reported that they considered almost all bereavement manifestations to be normal during the early stages of grief but considered most of the manifestations to be abnormal if they continued beyond 3 years after bereavement (Demi and Miles, 1987). Symptoms considered abnormal if present beyond 3 years are also listed in Display 48-1.

Impact on Activities of Daily Living

Dysfunctional grief leads to dysfunction in everyday life activities. This dysfunction may be manifested by individual family members or by the family as a whole. The person may be too tired or too depressed to concentrate on daily household chores or personal hygiene. Loss of appetite or sleep disturbance adds to loss of energy. The adult may no longer be able to maintain a job or provide a safe and healthy home atmosphere, and the child may be unable to keep up with schoolwork. Individual family members may not be able to carry out their family or work roles.

Because family members are unable to carry out their individual roles, the family as a whole is unable to carry out its roles of nurturing and protecting. The family life cycle stage that the family is in at the time it experiences the loss greatly affects family functioning (Demi, 1989). Families are particularly vulnerable when they are gaining or losing family members through normal development. That is, if the family is in the stage of child launching, it is often more difficult to cope with a loss. In addition, if one or both of the parents are deeply

DISPLAY 48-1

 NORMAL AND ABNORMAL GRIEF MANIFESTATIONS

May Be Normal at 1 Year After Bereavement	Abnormal if Present Beyond 3 Years
• Excessive or persistent expression of affect • Inability to experience joy • Clinical symptoms of depression • Inability to form new relationships • Inability to speak of the deceased without intense emotion • Hearing or seeing the deceased • Feelings of emptiness or meaninglessness	• Leaving the deceased's room and belongings intact • Reporting physical symptoms similar to those the deceased had before death • Talking about the loss as if it had just happened • Inability to remember or talk about the deceased • Being preoccupied with thoughts of the deceased • Talking or acting as if the deceased were still alive • Experiencing physical illness that seems to be related to the loss

involved in grieving, they may not be able to carry out their parental roles.

ASSESSMENT

Questions about losses (actual and anticipated) need to be incorporated into the assessment of every client. Frank physical illness may be the result of a loss, actual or anticipated; often the client does not connect the presenting symptom with the loss. On the other hand, physical illness or accident may result in loss, both actual and anticipated. The skillful nurse recognizes the relationship of loss to health status and helps the client recognize and acknowledge this connection.

Subjective Data

Many behaviors previously thought to be dysfunctional are being recognized as normal components of grief. Observation and assessment of a grieving person at a single point in time is not a good way to assess the normality of the grief response. To distinguish between normal and altered grief reactions, one must assess the severity of the symptoms and the pattern of change over time.

Normal Pattern Identification

When interviewing a client, it is helpful to start the interview with some general, nonthreatening questions before moving in to ask questions about the loss. A major factor in understanding the client's loss reaction is assessing the relationship to the lost person or object and the particular circumstances surrounding the loss. Important considerations include the following:

- What was the physical and psychological significance of the lost person or object?
- Was the loss unexpected or expected?
- Did the survivor contribute, or perceive that he or she contributed, to the loss?

Assessment of the client's personal resources and personal stressors is essential. Personal resources are strengths within the person that contribute to a healthy pattern of grieving. Personal stressors are limitations within the person that may inhibit healthy grieving. Personal stressors and resources include personality characteristics, coping skills, communication skills, physical health status, spirituality, and previous experiences with loss. To assess personal stressors and resources, ask the following:

- Do you have a history of emotional illness?
- What coping behaviors do you usually use?
- How well do you communicate with others?
- What previous losses have you experienced?
- How did you cope with the previous losses?
- Are any of those previous losses still unresolved?
- Do you have any physical health problems?
- What are your spiritual beliefs?
- How do your spiritual beliefs influence your reactions to loss?
- What other personal stressors are you experiencing?

Also assess sociocultural resources and stressors. Sociocultural resources are the assets that are available to the client from the interpersonal environment; they include social support, material support (financial assistance, assistance with tasks), and cultural traditions and customs. Sociocultural stressors are strains and tensions that the social and cultural systems exert on the client. Family members, peers, friends, coworkers, and employers can function as either resources or stressors. Cultural traditions also may be either resources or stressors. For example, if the cultural tradition dictates a long mourning period and the bereaved person is ready to move into the reorganization stage of grief, this may create feelings of conflict. However, it is more likely that sociocultural expectations will be that the bereaved person stop grieving and get "back to normal" long before the bereaved person is capable of doing so. To assess sociocultural stressors and resources, ask the following questions:

- What social supports are available to the grieving person?
- Does the grieving person perceive these supports as helpful?
- What are the traditional rituals for dealing with this type of loss?
- To what extent did the grieving person participate in the sociocultural rituals?
- How satisfied is the grieving person with the socio-cultural rituals?
- Do any of the social and cultural traditions conflict with needs of the grieving person?

Risk Identification

The risk for dysfunctional grief can be identified through analysis of the resources and stressors that the client is experiencing. Clients with many stressors and few resources are at greatest risk.

Physical health and psychosocial adjustment are intricately intertwined. The bereaved are known to be at greater risk for mortality and morbidity than are comparable nonbereaved people. This increased risk of mortality is greatest in the first month after bereavement, remains elevated throughout the first year, and then drops to normal range by the end of the second year of bereavement (Biondi & Picardi, 1996).

Dysfunction Identification

People with normal grief may display many diverse and intense signs and symptoms. Nurses must avoid inappropriately placing a label of dysfunctional grief on a normal process. Generally, dysfunction can be identified only after several contacts with the client over an extended period. The frequency and intensity of grief manifestations should decrease over time; prolonged intense grief may be an indicator of dysfunction. Although wishing to die and having brief thoughts of suicide are generally within the normal range, continuing thoughts of suicide, especially when the person has a specific plan in mind, are a sign of dysfunction. Abuse of alcohol or drugs is also a sign of dysfunction.

Objective Data

Grief may manifest itself in many diverse physiologic and psychological signs that are directly observable. Many of these signs are identical to the signs of depression; consequently, it is very difficult to differentiate between normal grieving and depression. Currently, there is no laboratory test to assess the presence of grieving, but there are a few paper-and-pencil tests that are helpful in assessing grief symptomatology, such as the Grief Experience Questionnaire (Sanders & Mauger, 1979), the Bereavement Experience Questionnaire (Demi & Schroeder, 1985), the Impact of Event Scale (Zilberg, Weiss, & Horowitz, 1982), and the Texas Inventory of Grief (Faschingbauer, DeVaul, & Zisook, 1977).

Many of the subjective manifestations of grief have concomitant objective manifestations:

- Dejected physical appearance
- Slowed motor function
- Weeping
- Outbursts of anger
- Emotional blunting
- Unkempt appearance
- Sleep disturbance
- Appetite disturbance (excessive weight loss or gain)

NURSING DIAGNOSES

Anticipatory Grieving and Dysfunctional Grieving are the two approved nursing diagnoses relevant to loss and grief (Johnson, Bulechek, McCloskey-Dochterman, Maas, & Moorland, 2001). A number of nurses believe that another diagnostic category should be added, Normal Grieving (Carpenito, 2000). The rationale for adding this diagnosis is that normal grieving results in numerous physical, emotional, and social consequences that can be ameliorated through nursing interventions.

Diagnostic Statement: Anticipatory Grieving

Definition. Anticipatory Grieving comprises the intellectual and emotional responses and behaviors by which individuals, families, and communities work through the process of modifying self-concept based on the perception of loss (Johnson et al., 2001).

Defining Characteristics. Among the defining characteristics are the following: potential loss of significant object; expression of distress at potential loss; denial of potential loss; guilt, anger, sorrow, or choked feelings; changes in eating habits; alterations in sleep patterns or in activity level; altered libido; and altered communication patterns (Carpenito, 2000).

Diagnostic Statement: Dysfunctional Grieving

Definition. Dysfunctional Grieving is extended, unsuccessful use of intellectual and emotional responses by which individuals, families, and communities attempt to work through the process of modifying self-concept based on the perception of loss (Johnson et al., 2001).

Defining Characteristics. According to Carpenito (2000), the defining characteristics or clinical cues that point to this nursing diagnosis include verbal expression of distress at loss; denial of loss; expression of guilt or expression of unresolved issues; anger, sadness, or crying; difficulty in expressing loss; alterations in eating habits, sleep patterns, dream patterns, activity level, or libido; idealization of the lost object; reliving of past experiences; interference with life functioning; developmental regression; labile affect; and alterations in concentration or pursuit of tasks. These defining characteristics also describe normal grief. Differentiating normal grief from dysfunctional grief requires consideration

ETHICAL/LEGAL ISSUE
Durable Power of Attorney for Healthcare and Advance Directives

You are an RN working in a neurosurgeon's office. Two weeks ago, a 45-year-old physician, Dr. Smithson, had a complete neurologic workup because he was having headaches that were increasing in severity and was having some short-term memory loss. At that time, he was told that he had an operable brain tumor. He was given the choice of (1) having a type of surgery with minimal risk of death, but with the likelihood that he would lose some cortical brain function, or (2) having a type of surgery that had a high risk of death but would not affect his cortical brain function. He chose the latter. Today, he and his wife have come to the office for preoperative preparation and teaching. Mrs. Smithson tells you that she is extremely worried about her husband's prognosis and potential for full recovery.

Reflection
- Consider your own feelings as you encounter this situation. What type of surgery would you have chosen?
- Think about three different ways you could respond to this situation and the consequences of responding in these different ways.
- What additional information would you need to help the couple prepare for the impending surgery?
- What information should you provide to them about advance directives? What information should you provide to them about a durable power of attorney for healthcare? How would you go about discussing these topics?

of the interval between the time of loss and the time of assessment. To be considered dysfunctional, the grief must be unusually prolonged and turbulent (Horowitz et al., 1997).

Related Factors. A variety of etiologic or contributing factors may affect the development of this altered pattern of grieving. The major etiologic factors include perceived object loss ("object loss" is used in the broadest sense). Objects may include people, possessions, a job, status, home, ideals, or parts and processes of the body (NANDA, 2000).

Related Nursing Diagnoses

In addition to the diagnoses of Anticipatory Grieving and Dysfunctional Grieving, clients who have experienced a major loss may also be found to have the nursing diagnoses based on functional health given in Table 48-3.

OUTCOME IDENTIFICATION AND PLANNING

After the nursing diagnoses and related factors have been identified, client goals and nursing interventions are planned. Development of client goals centers on the stage of grief the client is in and whether the grief is normal, anticipatory, or dysfunctional. The client should have input in deciding what his or her personal needs are at the moment. Short-term and long-term goals are needed. The following client goals are samples of what may need to be addressed with such a client.

- The client will move toward resolution of diverse emotions.
- The client will accept the reality of the loss.
- The client will reinvest emotional and physical energy in meaningful people and activities.

Planning evolves around the phase or stage the client is in. It may vary from emotional support, to counseling, to finding a support group. Some interventions used in various phases of grief are listed in the accompanying display.

IMPLEMENTATION

Nurses frequently have contact with people who are anticipating or experiencing a major loss; therefore, they have many opportunities to provide care for grieving people. Because grief can be both devastating and long-lasting, opportunities for intervention occur throughout the grief process.

Health Promotion

Whenever feasible, nursing interventions to promote normal grieving should occur before the loss occurs.

Client Teaching

Loss education should begin in early childhood. Preschoolers should learn about the normality of loss and grief through exposure to naturally occurring events. A visit to a nursing home, the death of a distant relative, the death of a pet, or the loss of a friend—all provide opportunities to discuss the natural life cycle and loss in nonthreatening ways. The parent or other caregiver or relative who can talk about loss honestly and openly, in terms that the child can understand, will help the child establish a healthy attitude toward loss and will serve as a role model (Woodard, 1997).

Loss education should continue throughout childhood and adolescence. Encourage parents to include children in mourning rituals; however, family members should never force children to participate in such rituals. Also, encourage parents to allow children to express their diverse feelings about various losses (Display 48-2). Gradual exposure to loss and death situations concurrent with appropriate preparation and support will prepare the child to cope with losses later in life (Aspinall, 1966).

TABLE 48-3

Sample Nursing Diagnoses Related to Grief and Based on Functional Health	
Functional Health Area	**Nursing Diagnosis**
Health perception and health management	Altered Health Maintenance
	Risk for Injury
	Altered Growth and Development
	Noncompliance
Activity and exercise	Activity Intolerance
	Diversional Activity Deficit
	Impaired Home Maintenance/Management
Nutrition and metabolism	Altered Nutrition: Less Than Body Requirements
Sleep and rest	Sleep Pattern Disturbance
Cognition and perception	Altered Thought Processes
	Knowledge Deficit
	Acute Confusion
	Decisional Conflict
Self-perception	Anxiety
	Fear
	Hopelessness
	Powerlessness
	Body Image Disturbance
	Self-Esteem Disturbance
Roles and relationships	Altered Family Processes
	Risk for Loneliness
	Altered Parenting
	Social Isolation
Coping and stress tolerance	Ineffective Individual Coping
	Impaired Adjustment
	Ineffective Family Coping
	Risk for Suicide
Sexuality and reproduction	Sexual Dysfunction
Values and beliefs	Spiritual Distress

PLANNING: Examples of NIC/NOC Interventions

Accepted Loss and Grieving Nursing Interventions Classification (NIC)
Grief Work Facilitation

Accepted Loss and Grieving Nursing Outcomes Classification (NOC)
Coping
Grief Resolution
Psychological Adjustment Life Change

Refer to the following for specifics regarding NIC/NOC:
  McCloskey, J., & Bulechek, G. (2000). *Iowa Intervention Project: Nursing Interventions Classification (NIC)* (3rd ed.). St. Louis, MO: C. V. Mosby.
  Johnson, M., & Maas, M. (2000). *Iowa Outcomes Project: Nursing Outcomes Classification (NOC)* (2nd ed.). St. Louis, MO: C. V. Mosby.

Nurses should also be directly involved in education of children about grief and loss. Incorporate grief education naturally into your contacts with children in various health-care settings, such as schools, hospitals, physicians' offices, and clinics.

Working through Grief Stages

The following is a discussion of nursing interventions based on the client's present stage of grief. Display 48-3 provides additional information.

During the shock phase, nursing interventions should focus on protecting the client from physical harm and on getting the client to accept the reality of the loss. During this phase, help the client mobilize normal support systems; for example, help the client contact family members and tell them about the loss. Clients may act out impulsively or may have decreased reaction time; therefore, make an effort to protect the client

OUTCOME-BASED TEACHING PLAN

Hugh Sidney, 88 years old, recently died, after a long illness. His daughter, Dottie, has two young grandchildren, Jill (age 9) and Beth (age 6). Candace, the mother of Jill and Beth, wants her children to attend the memorial service for their great-grandfather. Dottie, the grandmother, thinks it would be better to not discuss the death with the children, and to just tell them that Hugh has "gone away." Candace turns to you, the nurse in the children's clinic, for advice.

OUTCOME: Family can verbalize feelings about the death and the memorial service with respect to the children's feelings and understanding.
Strategies
- Encourage Candace to explore her own feelings and beliefs.
- With Candace, evaluate each child's level of understanding of the event.
- Encourage expression of the children's feelings about the event.
- Help the family recognize that children grieve differently than adults.
- Talk openly about death and feelings it generates, expecting children to alternate between grieving and normal functioning.
- Encourage the children and family to discuss their desires about remembrance of the deceased and convey those inclinations to other family members as the basis of their decision making about the upcoming memorial service.

from self-harm (suicide attempts) and from accidents. It usually is helpful to have a family member present when the client is notified of a loss or an anticipated loss and to have this person drive the client home; this is particularly important if the loss was unanticipated. Encourage clients to use coping behaviors that have been helpful to them in the past, such as participation in religious activities or talking with a friend or relative. If the loss was a death, encourage clients to participate in funeral and mourning rituals.

During the protest phase, nursing interventions should focus on getting the client to express thoughts and feelings about the loss and maintaining the client's normal health status.

During the disorganization phase, place emphasis on getting the client to accept the reality of the loss and to begin reorganization of his or her life. Continue interventions instituted during the shock phase.

During the reorganization phase, place emphasis on helping the client to continue changing patterns of behavior so that he or she can find new or renewed meaning in life. Some losses, such as the death of a spouse, a spinal cord injury, or blindness, require a major reorganization of many life activities, whereas other losses, such as reproductive sterility or amputation of a finger, may require reorganization in only a few areas. Clients who experience a greater degree of life reorganization may need additional interventions.

Encouraging Support Groups
To prevent or ameliorate intense emotional distress or lack of social support or prolonged grief, encourage clients to participate in support groups for bereaved persons (Fig. 48-2). The Widow-to-Widow program (Silverman, 1986) and the Reach-to-Recovery program for mastectomy clients provide one-to-one support by nonprofessionals who have experienced a similar loss and have made a satisfactory recovery from the loss. These befriender programs provide role modeling, edu-

DISPLAY 48-2

   PREPARING CHILDREN FOR DEATH

Instruct the parent as follows:

DOs:
- Know your own feelings and beliefs.
- Be honest.
- Begin at the child's level.
- Include the child in family rituals related to death and mourning.
- Encourage expression of feelings.
- Provide security and stability.
- Encourage remembrance of the deceased.
- Recognize that children grieve differently from adults.
- Expect the child to alternate between grieving and normal functioning.

- Talk openly about death and the feelings it generates.
- Introduce death concepts into conversation naturally.

DON'Ts:
- Praise stoicism.
- Encourage forgetting of the deceased.
- Force the child to participate in grief and mourning rituals.
- Emphasize the likeness of the child to the deceased.
- Compare the child to the deceased.
- Use euphemisms.
- Protect the child from exposure to experiences with death.

DISPLAY 48-3

⑤ EXAMPLES OF NURSING INTERVENTIONS USED IN HELPING CLIENTS MOVE THROUGH GRIEF

Interventions During Shock Phase
- Help client mobilize a support system.
- Protect client from physical harm.
- Have a family member present when notifying client of a loss.
- Have someone drive client home.
- Help client establish coping behaviors used in past.
- Encourage client to participate in mourning rituals.

Interventions During Protest Phase
- Encourage expression of diverse feelings (e.g., sadness, loneliness, anger, guilt, resentment, relief).
- Encourage remembering and talking about that which was lost.
- Provide anticipatory guidance regarding the normal grief process.
- Provide role models who have successfully coped with similar loss.

- Encourage client to use existing support systems.
- Identify new support systems.
- Discourage use of alcohol, drugs, and caffeine.
- Promote appropriate sleep habits.
- Promote good nutrition.
- Refer for complete physical examination.
- Encourage participation in religious rituals.
- Encourage use of previous healthy coping behaviors.
- Introduce new coping behaviors.

Interventions During Disorganization Phase
- Continue interventions begun in shock phase.
- Refer client to self-help groups.
- Refer client for individual or group counseling.

Interventions During Reorganization Phase
- Refer client for career counseling.
- Refer client to educational programs.
- Refer client to social activity programs.

---

cation, and emotional support. Self-help support groups serve the same functions as befrienders, but the help is less individualized and is provided primarily in a group setting.

Nursing Interventions for Altered Grieving

Clients experiencing dysfunctional grief need professional help to resolve their problems. This help generally takes one of two forms: individual therapy or professionally led support groups. This type of help may be prescribed in addition to self-help. Professional support is particularly important if the client has inadequate support systems. Many nurse-therapists specialize in grief therapy.

Healthcare Planning and Home or Community-Based Nursing

When a client has experienced a major loss, or is anticipating such a loss, adequate discharge planning and follow-up are essential. Because the grief process extends over a long period, the severity of the client's grief may not be obvious during hospitalization. Nurses may misperceive the client's shock and denial and conclude that the client is "unaffected by the loss." Actually, the client who appears unaffected by a loss is particularly in need of follow-up care, because he or she may have a delayed grief reaction.

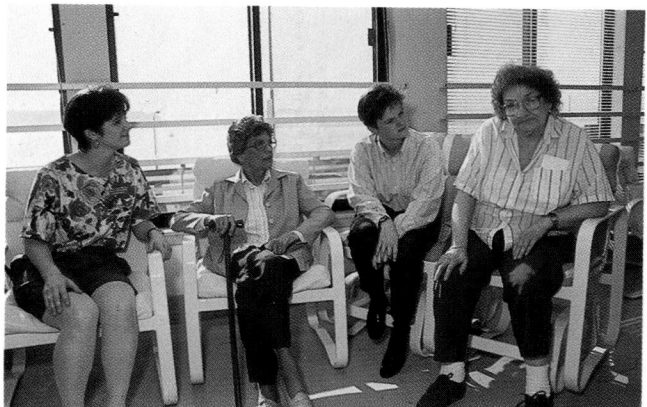

FIGURE 48-2 Support groups can help people work through their feelings with others who share similar experiences.

⑤ APPLY YOUR KNOWLEDGE

You are working in an emergency department when Paulie, 18 years old, is brought in after a terrible accident. His parents are called and arrive less than 1 hour before Paulie dies. They are able to say goodbye, but Paulie never regains consciousness. After Paulie's death, his mother sits crying, saying over and over, "How could this happen? How could this happen?" What phase of grieving is Paulie's mother in? What interventions would be most helpful?

Check your answer in Appendix A.

Referral

Discharge planning should include referral to befriender programs, self-help groups, professionally led support groups, public health nurses, or hospice programs, depending on the client's specific needs and the resources available in the community. Widow and widower groups may help when the client is ready for such a program. Pastoral counselors and other clergy are helpful resources for many people. Encourage clients to continue contact with their primary healthcare provider (physician or nurse) as well, because the grief process often decreases resistance to disease and exacerbates existing illnesses.

EVALUATION

This section lists some general goals and outcome criteria for a grieving client which can be used as a guide for evaluation. Remember, however, that evaluation must be individualized based on the client's specific needs and goals. The items presented here are suggestions, to be amended based on knowledge about the specific client.

Evaluation is an ongoing process that includes assessing the client and comparing the client's status to the outcome criteria. During this process, remember the long-term nature of grief and that progress toward these outcomes may be very slow but nevertheless within the normal range. Use astute clinical judgment to determine whether the client is making satisfactory progress, and revise the nursing care plan as appropriate.

Goal

The client will recognize and express diverse emotions.

Possible Outcome Criteria

- Within 7 days, the client expresses diverse emotions, such as sadness, anger, guilt, loneliness, or relief.
- Within 14 days, the client states that experienced emotions are normal components of the grief process.

Goal

The client will move toward resolution of diverse emotions.

Possible Outcome Criteria

- Within 6 months, the client reports decreased frequency and intensity of painful emotions.
- Within 9 months, the client expresses decreased frequency of preoccupation with thoughts of the lost loved one or object.

Goal

The client will recognize the reality of the loss.

Possible Outcome Criteria

- Within 4 weeks, the client discusses the loss and its meaning.
- Within 4 weeks, the client discusses potential life changes necessary because of the loss.
- Within 6 months, the client disposes of articles no longer needed (e.g., paraplegic gives away skis, widow gives away deceased spouse's clothing).
- Within 12 months, the client plans for major life changes to accommodate the loss (e.g., selling home, taking new job).

Goal

The client will recognize the need for help and seek help appropriately.

Possible Outcome Criteria

- Within 24 hours, the client reaches out to family and friends for emotional and practical help.
- Within 2 months, the client uses family and friends for social support.
- Within 6 months, the client uses community resources for support.
- Within 12 months, the client assumes major responsibility for self.

Goal

The client will retain or regain physical health status.

Possible Outcome Criteria

- The client does not use sleeping pills, alcohol, caffeine, tobacco, or tranquilizers as crutches to ease the pain.
- Within 3 months, the client follows his or her prescribed medical regimen and adheres to healthful behaviors.
- Within 12 months, the client states that he or she has returned to normal eating, sleeping, and exercise habits.

Goal

The client will reinvest emotional and physical energy in meaningful people and activities.

Possible Outcome Criteria

- Within 9 months, the client participates in new activities.
- Within 12 months, the client reports making necessary changes in social, recreational, and occupational spheres.
- Within 12 months, the client identifies renewal of old friendships and development of new friendships.
- Within 24 months, the client expresses a sense of satisfaction with life and a sense of meaning in life.

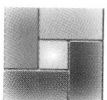

Grief and bereavement are common to families of clients with end-stage Alzheimer's disease. Many clients with end-stage dementia reside in the nursing home setting, where clients with dementia may comprise up to 70% of the client population. Many people do not understand the unique aspects of hospice care in the nursing home and imagine services to duplicate care that is already given. Hospice providers designed this study to determine the prevalence of grief and bereavement services in nursing homes. The researchers performed a telephone survey of 121 nursing homes regarding their on-site grief and bereavement services. A structured telephone survey was administered to nursing home staff, either the social worker or director of nursing. A total of 111 nursing homes responded to the survey, a response rate of 91%. An estimation of proportion and its associated 95% confidence interval (CI) was used, assuming a binomial distribution. The results of the survey found that 55% of the homes sent sympathy cards to family members after the death, 99% did not provide materials to the family or to the primary caregiver on the grieving process or bereavement after death, 99% did not inform family members of avail-

able bereavement support groups, 76% did not offer referral for counseling when bereavement intervention was deemed appropriate, 54% sent a representative from the nursing home to the funeral home or the funeral of a client who died at their facility, 99% had no contact with family members after the death of their clients.

Critical Thinking Considerations. The subjects for this study were limited to nursing homes in one small area of the United States. However, the researchers point out several issues that are important to nurses who provide care for end-stage dementia clients in other settings:

- Nursing home staff and families of clients are unaware of the unique service hospice provides in the nursing home for clients with end-stage Alzheimer's disease and their families.
- Families of dying clients in the nursing home should have an opportunity to receive grief and bereavement programming and support, but these services are often not a part of the care provided at these facilities.

From Murphy, K., Hanrahan, P., & Luchins, D. (1997). A survey of grief and bereavement in nursing homes: The importance of hospice grief and bereavement for the end-stage Alzheimer's disease patient and family. *Journal of the American Geriatrics Society, 45*(9), 1104–1107.

CARING FOR THE DYING PATIENT

Definition of Death

Death is defined in three ways: as cessation of heart-lung function, or of whole-brain function, or of higher-brain function. The heart-lung definition (cessation of heartbeat and respirations) is widely used to define clinical death. Higher-brain death results in a vegetative state in which the patient has no consciousness, speech, or feelings. Lower-brain death results in inability to maintain circulation and respiration; such patients depend on a ventilator for breathing and circulation. The President's Commission for the Study of Ethical Problems in Medical and Biomedical and Behavioral Research (1993) defined death as either irreversible cessation of circulatory and respiratory functions or irreversible cessation of all functions of the entire brain (whole brain), including the brain stem. A determination of death must be made in accordance with accepted medical standards. An organ donor could have an organ harvested while he or she is clinically alive if either higher- or lower-brain death occurs. A death that occurs in a hospital or other healthcare setting needs to be pronounced by a physician. State laws determine who can pronounce a death at home.

Response to Dying and Death

Kubler-Ross' (1969) theory of the stages of grief when an individual is dying has gained wide acceptance in nursing and other disciplines, probably because she was a pioneer in developing sensitive, compassionate care for the dying. Her work provided the impetus for increased attention to the needs of the dying and the bereaved and had an influence on the later development of hospice programs. She proposed five stages of grief: (a) denial, (b) anger, (c) bargaining, (d) depression, and (e) acceptance. Denial may range from complete denial of the illness and impending death to denial of the effect that dying will have on self and others. In the second stage, anger may be directed toward fate, God, family members, healthcare providers, or others. Bargaining occurs as the client seeks to delay the dreaded event; the client bargains with God for more time and, in return, promises to do something to repay God for this favor. Depression occurs when the client acknowledges the reality and inevitability of the impending death. In the final stage, acceptance, the client comes to terms with the loss, begins to detach from supportive people, and loses interest in worldly activities.

Although Kubler-Ross' theory provides a general guideline for understanding responses to dying, many patients do not follow this progression through stages. Many go back and forth from one stage to another; others remain in one stage until their death. Nurses must be aware that there is no one right way for a patient to respond to dying. Nurses must adapt their care based on patients' current responses and needs and not expect them to always progress through defined stages.

Physical Signs of Dying

When a patient is **dying** the lungs become less efficient for gas diffusion and oxygenation, the heart and blood vessels become inadequate to maintain circulation and to perfuse tissues, and the brain ceases to regulate vital centers. Physical signs that often occur are the following: the skin is extremely pale, cyanotic, jaundiced, or mottled; the heartbeat is irregular and the pulse is weak, rapid, and irregular; respirations are changed, shallow, labored, faster or slower, or irregular; urine output is decreased due to system failure and limited intake; fecal retention or impaction occurs due to reduced gastrointestinal motility; incontinence occurs due to relaxation of the sphincter muscles; there is difficulty swallowing, generalized weakness, increased somnolence, decreased responsiveness to external stimuli, decreased pain. As death gets closer, the number of signs increases and they become more pronounced.

Hospice Care

Hospice care is a viable alternative for dying patients and their families (Backer, Hannon, & Russell, 1994). Hospices have become part of our healthcare system. Hospices provide care that focuses on quality of life rather than length of life. The philosophy of hospice is that patients and families are empowered to achieve as much control over their lives as possible (Tarzian, 2000). Hospice-type care can be provided in hospitals, in extended care facilities, in freestanding hospices, and in patients' homes. Hospice programs provide comfort care, such as control of pain and nausea, and also help patients and families to attain a degree of mental and spiritual preparation for death that is in accordance with their wishes. Hospices provide social, psychological, and spiritual support through a team of healthcare professionals and lay volunteers (Wilkes & White, 1995). Research has shown that psychological distress is lower among bereaved spouses who received hospice care than among those who did not (McCorkle, Robinson, Nuamah, Lev, Quint-Benoiel, 1998).

Nursing Diagnoses and Nursing Implementation

The ultimate outcome for dying patients is to achieve good end-of-life care and a good death. A death is defined as "good" if there is an awareness, acceptance, and preparation for death by all those concerned and there is control of physical and emotional pain and distress. Patients often define a "good death" as being pain free, dying with dignity, and dying in their sleep (Payne, Hillier, Langley-Evans, & Roberts, 1996). A "good death" may be defined differently based on patients'

cultural and health beliefs. Seale (1998) described two very different cultural patterns for dying: one was "aware death," which is practiced by Anglo-Americans, and the other was "keeping a secret," which is supported in Japan and some parts of Italy. The nursing care needs of patients vary based on their belief systems.

Nurses need to address the physical, emotional, social, spiritual, and cultural needs of dying patients and their families, and they need to recognize that these needs vary across the stages of dying. Three core competencies are necessary: ability to talk to patients and families about dying, pain control techniques, and comfort care nursing interventions (White, Coyne, & Patel, 2001). A healthcare team is necessary to best meet the complex needs of dying patients and their families. Nurses alone cannot meet these needs. Caring for dying patients can be very stressful to caregivers. Working as a team often provides the support necessary to help the caregivers cope with these stressors.

The following are some of the more common nursing diagnoses for dying patients.

Diagnostic Statement: Pain. Chronic pain is defined as the state in which an individual experiences pain that is persistent or intermittent and lasts for longer than 6 months. Dying patients' pain can be acute or chronic. Most cancer patients have chronic pain near the end of life. The goal of nursing care is to control pain. Strategies to control pain include administration of narcotics, psychosocial interventions, and complementary therapies, such as soothing music, guided imagery, and distraction. Patients and family members should be reassured that giving narcotics to a terminally ill person will not cause addiction, nor will it lead to uncontrollable pain later in the terminal period. Narcotics usually are administered to dying patients orally or rectally. Psychological or social stress and depression can worsen the pain; efforts should be taken to decrease stress and to treat underlying depression. Skin care is essential to prevent decubitus ulcer formation and resultant pain. Frequent oral and eye care can decrease the risk of oral and eye infections, which are also extremely painful.

Diagnostic Statement: Fatigue. Fatigue is defined as the self-recognized state in which an individual experiences an overwhelming, sustained sense of exhaustion and decreased capacity for physical and mental work that is unrelieved by rest. Decreased energy is common for dying patients owing to the disease process, disuse of muscles, and psychological stress. They tire easily and consequently withdraw from many daily activities. Nurses should discuss with the patient what activities he or she wants to do most and schedule those activities at the time of day when the patient is least tired. Strategically schedule treatments and other tasks to conserve the patient's energy and promote a sense of accomplishment.

Diagnostic Statement: Deficient Fluid Volume. Deficient fluid volume is defined as the state in which an individual who is not restricted to nothing by mouth (NPO) experiences, or is at risk of experiencing, vascular, interstitial, or intracellular dehydration. Decreased fluid intake may be related to the disease process, or it may be intentional, to avoid having to urinate. Dehydration can easily be identified by assessment of the client's skin and mucous membranes. Dehydrated clients are uncomfortable owing to a constant thirsty sensation and dry mouth. Nursing interventions include offering ice chips, sips of water, or other liquids frequently; using a bendable straw or unspillable cup; and providing regular mouth care to avoid mouth infection.

Diagnostic Statement: Imbalanced Nutrition (Less Than Body Requirements). Imbalanced nutrition (less than body requirements) is defined as the state in which an individual, who is not NPO, experiences, or is at risk of experiencing, inadequate intake or metabolism of nutrients for metabolic needs with or without visible weight loss. Inadequate nutrition related to the disease process, medical treatments, medications, or nausea and vomiting is common among dying patients. Psychological stress affects appetite and, consequently, nutrition. Dying patients may refuse to take food because of anorexia or a deliberate choice to hasten impending death (Hughes & Neal, 2000). Nursing interventions include providing small servings of favorite foods, serving foods attractively, using a blender to pulverize food so that it can be swallowed easily, and scheduling feeding at times when pain and nausea medications are having the most effect. A feeding tube can be used to supplement nutritional needs, but this should be done only if it is congruent with the patient's wishes.

Diagnostic Statement: Impaired Gas Exchange. Impaired gas exchange is defined as the state in which an individual experiences an actual or potential decreased passage of gasses (oxygen and carbon dioxide) between the alveoli of the lungs and the vascular system. Impaired gas exchange results in a sense of air hunger, suffocation, dyspnea, anxiety, and sometimes panic. Impaired gas exchange is often the most distressing symptom experienced by dying patients, and it is often very difficult to alleviate. Nursing interventions include positioning the patient to promote an open airway and maximum chest expansion; providing oxygen if there is no airway obstruction; giving sufficient narcotic medications to alleviate discomfort; administering a bronchodilator to reduce airway spasm; and setting up a ventilator, provided that this is congruent with the patient's wishes. Patients, in their advance directives, can identify which of these interventions they wish to receive.

Diagnostic Statement: Interrupted Family Process. Interrupted family process is defined as the state in which a normally supportive family experiences, or is at risk of experiencing, a stressor that challenges its previously effective functioning ability. Family members, as well as patients, experience stress related to the patient's impending death. The nurse must attempt to meet the needs of the patient and of family members. In order to be effective in helping the family deal with death and dying, the nurse must first explore his or her own beliefs about death and dying. The nurse should facilitate open communication between the patient and family members, while concurrently recognizing that there is a great deal of variability in personal and cultural beliefs concerning talking about death and dying. Nursing interventions include a number of other strategies: being an active listener; using touch to communicate; mobilizing support systems; promoting reminiscence; encouraging use of a variety of coping behaviors; providing anticipatory guidance about the grief process; and promoting resolution of unresolved business in the family.

Caring for the Deceased

Nursing care continues after the death of the client. Concern for dignity in the care of the body and sensitivity to the needs of the deceased client's family are nurses' responsibilities. Immediately after the client's death has been certified, family members may wish to spend some time alone with the client's body. In an effort to limit exposure to the disturbing sight of equipment and medical supplies, the nurse should remove unneeded items and clean, position, and cover the client. Having time alone with the client is an important step for some families, whereas others appreciate the presence of a nurse, a spiritual leader, or friends. Religious and ethnic beliefs and customs should be observed as much as possible.

KEY CONCEPTS

- Loss is a universal experience, and grieving is a normal response to loss.
- Models of the grief process provide direction for nursing assessment.
- The grief process is similar regardless of the type of loss experienced.
- A major loss results in a long-term life transition.
- Response to loss is influenced by the person's stage of development.
- The characteristics of the loss, personal resources and stressors, and sociocultural resources and stressors affect the grief process.
- The outcome of a loss experience is not predetermined, but rather is determined by the balance of stressors and resources present during the grief period.
- Risk of dysfunctional grieving can be identified through analysis of the stressors and resources that the client is experiencing.
- Physical health and psychosocial adjustment during the grief process are intricately intertwined.
- Nursing interventions should be based on knowledge of the long-term nature of the grief process.
- Many grief manifestations, identified in the literature as dysfunctional, are considered to be components of the normal grief process.
- Caution should be used in labeling a client as having dysfunctional grieving.
- Discharge planning must consider the long-term nature of the grief process.
- End-of-life care should promote quality of life through comfort care measures and open communication.
- Hospice care is a viable option for dying patients and their families.

(text continues on page 1320)

NURSING PLAN OF CARE
THE CLIENT WHO IS GRIEVING

Nursing Diagnosis
Grieving (normal) related to actual loss of significant person manifested by expression of unresolved issues.

SHOCK STAGE
Client Goal
Client will move toward resolution of diverse emotions.

Client Outcome Criteria
- Client cognitively accepts the reality of death within 1 week.
- Client participates in funeral and mourning rituals within 1 week.
- Client expresses emotional affect in discussion, facial expressions, and reactions within 72 hours.
- Client uses family and friends for social support in resolving emotional responses within 1 week.

Nursing Intervention
1. Encourage mourner to see the deceased and allow mourner to touch or hold the deceased, if desired.

2a. Provide anticipatory guidance regarding physical appearance of the deceased.
 b. Encourage mourner to participate in grief and mourning activities that are congruent with his or her sociocultural and spiritual/religious beliefs.
3. Notify family members of the death in person in a private setting whenever possible.
4. Encourage mourner to express diverse feelings (e.g., guilt, sadness, relief, numbness, anger).

5. Encourage mourner to talk about the deceased and to ask questions about the death.

6. Provide anticipatory guidance on the grief process, including common thoughts, feelings, and behaviors; emphasize that there is no one right way to grieve.
7. Assist mourner with making decisions regarding urgent postdeath responsibilities; help mourner contact family members and other support persons.
8. Protect mourner from deliberate or unintentional harm (e.g., inquire about suicidal thoughts, encourage mourner not to drive own car immediately after learning of the death).

Scientific Rationale
1. Cognitive recognition of the reality of death is necessary before beginning to work on acceptance of the emotional significance of the death.
2. Cognitive acceptance of the death is facilitated by participating in funeral and mourning rituals.

3. Trauma of notification of the death can be eased by sensitive attention to family members' needs.
4. Open expression of feelings facilitates gradual resolution of these feelings; some feelings are perceived as socially unacceptable.
5. Preoccupation with thoughts of the deceased is a normal part of the grief process; talking about the deceased's life and death begins breaking emotional bonds with the deceased.
6. Most people have little knowledge about the normal grief process, and it is reassuring for them to know that what they are experiencing is normal.
7. Bereaved person is often in crisis and needs the emotional and practical support from family and other support systems.
8. Bereaved are at greater risk of mortality and morbidity, particularly from accidents and suicide.

NURSING PLAN OF CARE

THE CLIENT WHO IS GRIEVING (*Continued*)

PROTEST STAGE
Client Goal
Client will begin acceptable transition to life without the deceased.

Client Outcome Criteria
- Client recognizes and accepts emotional feelings as acceptable within 2 months.
- Client begins transition to new roles within 2 months.
- Client experiences minimal deterioration of physical health during first 3 months after death of loved one.

Nursing Intervention

1. Encourage mourner to remember and talk about both negative and positive memories of the deceased. Use counseling skills of empathy, warmth, and positive regard. Facilitate reality testing. Assess need for individual or family who have numerous stressors.
2. Teach support people about the emotional needs of the bereaved.

3. Provide appropriate reading materials on the grief process.
4. Reinforce use of healthy coping skills.

5. Assess for suicidal ideation.

6. Encourage client to assume some new roles, to relinquish other roles, and to allow support people to fill some of the deceased's roles. Provide role models for new roles (e.g., Widow-to-Widow befriender). Recommend participation in self-help or mutual help support groups.
7. Teach problem-solving skills related to new roles.
8. Provide appropriate reading materials on practical aspects of role transition (e.g., financial management, automobile maintenance, child care, home maintenance).
9. Encourage complete physical assessment.

10. Promote good health habits (e.g., nutrition, rest, avoidance of alcohol and tobacco).

Scientific Rationale

1. The process of breaking bonds with the deceased continues over an extended period of time. Counseling skills can be used to elicit unrecognized thoughts and feelings. Bereaved people who have numerous stressors and few resources benefit from professional therapy.
2. Adequately prepared support people can augment professional services or may be the only intervention needed.
3. Identification with other bereaved people can be therapeutic.
4. During a crisis, people may be too overwhelmed to use their usual coping skills; therefore, the nurse must help them remember these skills.
5. Transition to new roles is a major stressor for the bereaved; role models and education on the new roles facilitates ease in role transition.
6. The death of a significant other precipitates role changes. Clients often do not know how to function in new roles; role models can show them how to function.

7. New roles require diverse problem-solving skills.
8. Seeing things in written form helps to reinforce ideas and knowledge; books become references.

9. The risk of increased mortality and morbidity is highest during the early bereavement period but continues throughout the first year of bereavement.
10. Good health habits and early identification of health problems may prevent serious illness.

(*continues*)

NURSING PLAN OF CARE

THE CLIENT WHO IS GRIEVING (*Continued*)

DISORGANIZATION STAGE
Client Goal

Client will reinvest emotional and physical energy in meaningful people and activities.

Client Outcome Criteria

- Client emotionally accepts the loss within 9 months, as disclosed by client.
- Client experiences improved functioning in new roles within 9 months.
- Client discusses with nurse a search for new meaning in life within 9 months.
- Client/family verbalizes experiencing increased family cohesiveness within 9 months.

Nursing Intervention	Scientific Rationale
1. Assist client in decision-making regarding disposal of deceased's belongings.	1. During the disorganization state, the client recognizes the emotional significance of the loss and begins to accept the meaning of the loss.
2. Support client's expression of grief (e.g., cemetery visits, memorial services, visiting places of special meaning to the deceased).	2. Activities focusing on the unresolved grief can facilitate resolution of the loss.
3. Normalize thoughts and feelings.	3. Same as above.
4. Use role-play to work through unresolved issues.	4. Same as above.
5. Encourage client to express thoughts and feelings through writing.	5. Same as above.
6. Enhance previous coping skills.	6. New roles continue to cause stress; effort must be directed toward strengthening the bereaved's intrapersonal and interpersonal competence.
7. Introduce additional coping techniques.	7. Same as above.
8. Support independent problem-solving skills.	8. Same as above.
9. Keep support systems mobilized.	9. Same as above.
10. Encourage client to delay major decisions until out of acute grief.	10. Same as above.
11. Support client's reevaluation of the meaning of his or her life.	11. The death of a loved one leads the bereaved to question the meaning of life.
12. Encourage participation in spiritual/religious activities.	12. Same as above.
13. Encourage client to participate in social and recreational activities.	13. Same as above.
14. Teach family members that each person expresses grief differently and resolves his or her grief at a different speed.	14. The family functions as a system; death of a family member affects all parts of the system.
15. Encourage open family communication about the loss and the feelings engendered.	15. Each subsystem affects other subsystems and the system as a whole.
16. Identify and reinforce the strengths of each family member.	16. Strengthening any part of the system has a positive effect on the other subsystems and on the system as a whole.
17. Encourage family members to provide support to each other.	17. Same as above.
18. Mobilize extra family support systems.	18. Friends, coworkers, and others can supplement support received from family members.

NURSING PLAN OF CARE

THE CLIENT WHO IS GRIEVING (Continued)

REORGANIZATION STAGE
Client Goal
Client will increase level of physical, emotional, social, and spiritual functioning (previous level or higher level of functioning)

Client Outcome Criteria
- Client resolves emotional reactions to the loss within 2 years.
- Client reports satisfaction with new roles within 2 years.
- Client reports finding new meaning in life within 2 years.
- Client reports achievement of personal growth within 2 years.
- Client reports improved coping skills within 2 years.

Nursing Intervention

1. Avoid unrealistic expectations for mourner to recover quickly.

2. Remind client that it is normal for grief feelings to be rekindled by trigger events such as holidays and anniversaries.
3. Support renewal of old friendships/interests and development of new friendships/interests.

4. Use gentle confrontation to deal with unresolved feelings toward the deceased.
5. Facilitate recognition of client's own strengths and limitations.
6. Encourage continued participation in support group.

7. Support continued involvement in religious, social, and recreational activities.
8. Praise client for satisfactory achievement of roles.

9. Encourage reevaluation of diverse meanings in life.

10. Support changes in client's behavior and lifestyle.

11. Reinforce use of a variety of coping skills.

Scientific Rationale

1. Resolution of grief after the death of a significant other often takes 2 to 5 years. By the end of the first year, the bereaved should have resolved the major portion of his or her grief but will continue to reexperience grief on anniversaries.
2. Same as above.

3. Meeting with friends and finding new activities eases the emotional loss and gives new meaning to life.
4. It is important to deal with all feelings before the grief period can end.
5. Knowing oneself aids in acceptable functioning.

6. Support is still needed from people with similar problems.
7. By the end of second year, bereaved should have found a satisfactory level of health and functioning.
8. By the end of second year, bereaved should be functioning satisfactorily in roles.
9. The search for meaning continues for a long time after resolution of other aspects of grief.
10. The crisis of bereavement often produces profound personal growth.
11. Bereaved people often report greatly increased coping skills after resolution of grief and also report a sense of confidence that because they managed to handle their grief satisfactorily, they will be able to handle any other stressor satisfactorily.

REFERENCES

Aspinall, S. Y. (1996). Educating children to cope with death: A preventive model. *Psychology in the Schools, 33,* 341–349.

Backer, B. A., Hannon, N. R., & Russell, N. A. (1994). *Death and dying: Understanding and care* (2nd ed.). New York: Delmar Publishers.

Biondi, M., & Picardi, A. (1996). Clinical and biological aspects of bereavement and loss-induced depression: A reappraisal. *Psychotherapy and Psychosomatics, 65*(5), 229–245.

Boss, P. (1999). *Ambiguous loss: learning to live with unresolved grief.* Cambridge, MA: Harvard University Press.

Carpenito, L. (2000). *Nursing diagnosis: Application to clinical practice* (8th ed.). Philadelphia: J. B. Lippincott.

Demi, A. (1981). *Bereavement support group: Leadership manual.* Littleton, CO: Grief Education Institute.

Demi, A. (1989). Death of a spouse. In R. Kalish (Ed.), *Coping with the losses of middle age.* Newbury Park, CA, pp. 218–248.

Demi, A., & Miles, M. (1987). Parameters of normal grief: A Delphi study. *Death Studies, 11,* 397–412.

Demi, A., & Schroeder, M. (1985, June). *Bereavement experience questionnaire.* Presented at Measurement of Clinical and Educational Nursing Outcomes Conference, New Orleans, LA.

Engel, G. (1964). Grief and grieving. *American Journal of Nursing, 64*(9), 88–100.

Faschingbauer, T., DeVaul, R., & Zisook, S. (1977). Development of the Texas Inventory of Grief. *Am J Psychiatry, 134,* 696–698.

Hogan, N. S., & DeSantis, L. (1994). Things that help and hinder adolescent sibling bereavement. *Western Journal of Nursing Research, 16*(2), 132–146; discussion 146–153.

Horowitz, M. J., Siegel, B., Holen, A., Bonanno, G. A., Milbrath, C., & Stinson, C. H. (1997). Diagnostic criteria for complicated grief disorder. *American Journal of Psychiatry, 154,* 904–910.

Hughes, N., & Neal, R. D. (2000). Adults with terminal illness: A literature review of their needs and wishes for food. *Journal of Advanced Nursing, 32*(5), 1101–1107.

Johnson, M., Bulechek, G., McCloskey-Dochterman, J., Maas, M., & Moorhead, S. (2001). *Nursing diagnoses, outcomes and interventions.* St. Louis: Mosby.

Krigger, K. W., McNeely, J. D., & Lippmann, S. B. (1997). Dying, death, and grief. Helping patients and their families through the process. *Postgrad Med, 101*(3), 263–270.

Kubler-Ross, E. (1969). *On death and dying.* New York: Macmillan.

McCorkle, R., Robinson, L., Nuamah, I., Lev, E., & Quint-Benoiel, J. (1998). The effects of home nursing care for patients during terminal illness on the bereaved's psychological distress. *Nursing Research, 47,* 2–10.

North American Nursing Diagnosis Association (NANDA). (2000). *Nursing diagnoses: Definitions and classification 2000–2001.* Philadelphia: Author.

Parkes, C. M. (1986). *Bereavement: Studies of grief in adult life* (2nd ed.). New York: International Universities Press.

Payne, S., Hillier, R., Langley-Evans, A., & Roberts, T. (1996). Impact of witnessing death on hospice patients. *Social Science and Medicine, 43,* 1785–1794.

President's Commission for the Study of Ethical Problems in Medicine and Biomedical and Behavioral Research. (1983). *Deciding to forego life-sustaining treatment: A report on the ethical, medical, and legal issues in treatment decisions.* Washington, DC: U.S. Government Printing Office.

Sanders, C., & Mauger, P. (1979). *A manual for the Grief Experience Inventory.* Tampa, FL: University of Florida.

Seale, C. (1998). Theories in health care and research: Theories and studying the care of dying people. *British Medical Journal, 317,* 1518–1520.

Tarzian, A. J. (2000). Caring for dying patients who have air hunger. *Journal of Nursing Scholarship, 32*(2), 137–143.

Waechter, E. Phillips, J., & Holaday, B. (1985). *Nursing care of children* (10th ed.). Philadelphia: J. B. Lippincott.

White, K., Coyne, P., & Patel, U. (2001). Are nurses adequately prepared for end-of-life care? *Journal of Nursing Scholarship, 33,* 148–152.

Wilkes, L. M., & White, K. (1995). Palliative care nurses' conflict of values. *Journal of Cancer Care, 4*(3), 97–100.

Zilberg, N., Weiss, D., & Horowitz, M. (1982). Impact of event scale: A cross validational study and some empirical evidence supporting a conceptual model of stress response syndromes. *Journal of Consulting and Clinical Psychology, 50*(3), 407–414.

BIBLIOGRAPHY

Aldrich, L. M. (1996). Hospice update: Helping children with the death of someone close. *Caring, 15*(12), 64–66.

Boss, P. (1999). *Ambiguous loss: Learning to live with unresolved grief.* Cambridge, MA: Harvard University. Press.

Cohen, L., Germain, M., Poppel, D., Woods, A., Pekow, P., & Kjellstrand, C. M. (2000). Dying well after discontinuing life-support treatment of dialysis. *Archives of Internal Medicine, 160,* 2513–2518.

Copp, G. (1998). A review of the current theories of death and dying. *Journal of Advanced Nursing, 28,* 382–390.

Curry, L. C., & Stone, J. G. (1992). Moving on: Recovering from the death of a spouse. *Clinical Nurse Specialist, 6*(4), 180–190.

Davis, B. (1993). Sibling bereavement: Research-based guidelines for nurses. *Seminars in Oncology Nursing, 9*(2), 107–113.

Farrar, A. (1992). How much do they want to know? Communicating with dying patients. *Professional Nurse, 7*(9), 606–610.

Gifford, B. J., et al. (1990). Supporting the bereaved. *American Journal of Nursing, 90*(2), 48–55.

Glass, B. C. (1993). The role of the nurse in advanced practice in bereavement care. *Clinical Disease Specialists, 7*(2), 62–76.

Hallal, J. C., & Walsh, M. B. (1992). Loss bereavement and care of the dying patient. In *Gerontological nursing: Care of the frail elderly.* St. Louis: C. V. Mosby, pp. 434–451.

Heiney, S. P., Hasan, L., & Price, K. (1993). Developing and implementing a bereavement program for a children's hospital. *Journal of Pediatric Nursing, 8*(6), 385–391.

Hunt, M. (1992). "Scripts" for dying at home . . . displayed in nurses, "patients," and relatives' talk. *Journal of Advanced Nursing, 17,* 1297–1302.

Hutti, M. H. (1992). Parents' perceptions of the miscarriage experience. *Death Studies, 16*(5), 401–415.

Jones, P. S., & Marinson, I. M. (1992). The experience of bereavement in caregivers of family members with Alzheimer's disease. *Image, 24,* 172–176.

Kriger, K., McNeely, J., & Lippmann, S. B. (1997). Dying, death, and grief. *Postgraduate Medicine, 101,* 263–270.

Lambert, J. W., Delmer, C. M. (1993). Model of family grief assessment and treatment. *Death Studies, 17*(1), 55–67.

Longman, A. J. (1993). Effectiveness of a hospice community bereavement program. *Omega, 27*(2), 165–175.

McCain, N. L., & Gramling, L. F. (1992). Living with dying: Coping with HIV disease. *Issues in Mental Health Nursing, 13*(3), 271–284.

McClelland, M. L. (1993). Our unit has a bereavement program. *American Journal of Nursing, 93*(1), 62.

Mendyka, B. E. (1993). The dying patient in the intensive care unit: Assisting the family in crisis. *AACN Clinical Issues in Critical Care, 4*(3), 550–557.

Moody, L., Becket, T., Long, C., Edmonds, A., & Andrews, S. (2000). Assessing readiness for death in hospice elders and older adults. *The Hospice Journal, 15*(2), 49–65.

Parry, J. K., & Thornwall, J. (1992). Death of a father. *Death Studies, 16*(2), 173–181.

Redding, S. (2000). Control theory in dying: What do we know? *American Journal of Hospice and Palliative Care, 17,* 204–208.

Reynolds, W. (2000). Do nurses and other professional helpers normally display much empathy? *Journal of Advanced Nursing, 31,* 226–234.

Rosen, S. L. (1990). Stillbirth: What the nurse should and should not do. *Imprint, 37*(1), 65–67.

Schoefeld, D. J. (1993). Talking with children about death. *Journal of Pediatric Healthcare, 7*(6), 267–274.

Seymour, J. (1999). Revisiting medicalization and 'natural' death. *Social Sciences and Medicine, 49,* 691–704.

Silverman, P. R., & Cooperband, A. (1984). Widow-to-widow. The elderly widow and mutual help. *Frontiers in Aging Series, 3,* 144–161.

Steele, L. (1992). Risk factor profile for bereaved spouses. *Death Studies, 16*(5), 87–99.

Sweeting, H. N., & Gilhooly, M. L. M. (1990). Anticipatory grief: A review. *Social Sciences and Medicine, 30,* 1073–1080.

Tolle, S., Tilden, V., Rosenfeld, A., & Hickman, S. (2000). Family reports of barriers to optimal care of the dying. *Nursing Research, 49,* 310–317.

Trolley, B. C. (1993). Kaleidoscope of aid for parents whose child died by suicidal and sudden, non-suicidal means. *Omega, 27*(3), 239–250.

Trunnell, E. P., Caserta, M. S., & White, G. L. (1992). Bereavement: Current issues in intervention and prevention. *Journal of Health Education, 23*(5), 275–280.

Walsh, F., & McGoldrick, M. (1991). *Living beyond loss: Death in the family.* New York: W. W. Norton.

Woodard, N. (1997). Helping children cope with death: the role educators can play. *Journal of Health Education, 28*(1), 42–44.

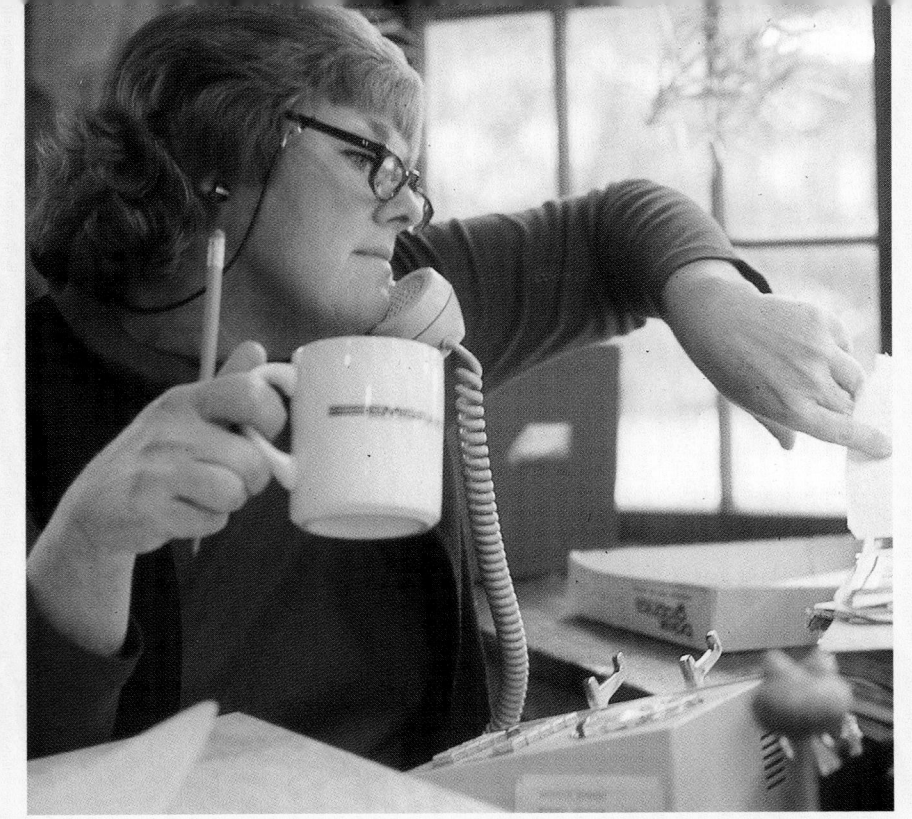

Coping and Stress Management

49 Stress, Coping, and Adaptation

⑤ Learning Objectives

Upon completion of this chapter, the student will be able to do the following:

1. Identify physiologic signs and symptoms of stress.
2. Identify psychological responses to stress.
3. List examples of biophysical and psychosocial stressors.
4. Give examples of variables that affect a person's ability to cope with stress.
5. Describe various types of coping patterns people typically use to handle stress.
6. Identify stress management techniques that nurses can use to help clients adapt to stress.

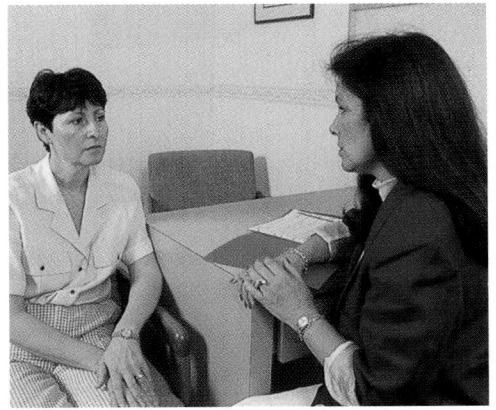

⑤ Critical Thinking Challenge

While caring for an older woman suffering from manic-depression, you interview her 46-year-old daughter. The daughter tells you that her mother has been married for 51 years to a man who has had quadruple cardiac bypass surgery, recurrent kidney and bladder cancer, and a long history of alcoholism, although he is not drinking currently. In assessing the client's home situation, you learn that the client and her husband live in their own home, but the daughter cooks and takes meals to them, drives them to their many healthcare appointments, handles their finances, and provides most of their support. The daughter is married, has three children, and works full-time. She states that she frequently is torn between her responsibilities to her parents and to her husband and children, who feel neglected. Although you began the interview to learn more about your client, you find you are learning more about the daughter's conflicts.

Major nursing responsibilities associated with assisting clients to manage stress include assessing a client's ability to cope with stressors; identifying personal factors that could interfere with coping; promoting effective coping and stress management; and implementing nursing interventions to modify coping as the situation warrants. Once you have completed this chapter and have incorporated stress, coping, and adaptation into your knowledge base, review the above scenario and reflect on the following areas of Critical Thinking:

1. Clarify how you will proceed with this assessment.
2. Identify potential stressors to the people in the situation.
3. Identify factors that may affect the daughter's coping behaviors.
4. Explore factors that place this family at risk for dysfunctional coping.
5. Describe possible manifestations of altered coping in this scenario.
6. Based on the information, plan appropriate nursing interventions.

Stress is a complex phenomenon inherent to life. It is essential, yet sometimes problematic. *Stress* is frequently associated with changes in the physical or social environment that produce tension or distress. It is often considered in the context of a real or an imagined threat. Stress can be the stimulus for constructive change and positive growth, or it can result in illness, disease, and possibly death. *Coping* is a process that a person uses to manage events that he or she encounters, perceives, and interprets as stressful. Successful coping requires adjusting to circumstances, environmental demands, and challenges. The ability to cope is a crucial element that influences well-being. *Adaptation* is generally considered a person's capacity to flourish and survive even with adversity. In the context of stress and coping, adaptation may be considered the outcome of coping. Adaptation depends upon coping processes and ultimately influences long-term health and survival.

NORMAL COPING AND ADAPTATION TO STRESS

Stress is an essential aspect of existence and has always been part of the human experience. Like all organisms, people face environmental demands that necessitate changes to ensure survival. This adaptive process was once assumed to occur as a series of starts and stops. In this framework, constancy and stability were believed to prevail until an organism encountered some threat; faced with danger, the organism changed in some way then entered another period of stability until a new circumstance demanded change. In actuality, both the organism and the environment are involved in a process of continual change. People live in a world full of challenges that require ongoing adjustments. Some adjustments can be made with minimal effort, some are made subconsciously, and others require conscious effort. Stress, coping and adaptation are interrelated. Survival depends upon successful coping responses to ordinary and sometimes extraordinary circumstances and challenges.

Physiologic Function Related to Stress, Coping, and Adaptation

Homeostasis

Homeostasis is a fundamental principle of physiology. Walter B. Cannon (1935), an American physiologist, used the term *homeostasis* to refer to the automatic, coordinated, self-regulating physiologic processes that maintain most steady states in an organism. He coined the notion of the "wisdom of the body" in reference to the beneficial effects of homeostasis. Physiologic homeostasis denotes the relative constancy of the body's internal environment, which is essential for survival and proper functioning. Homeostasis in physiological systems is maintained within a narrow range around a "set point" through continual changes in internal processes. Adjustments in heart rate, blood pressure, body temperature, fluid and electrolyte balance, blood glucose concentration, and blood oxygen level occur automatically to maintain proper system functioning and survival. Homeostatic balance is regulated by numerous interrelated mechanisms that involve all body tissues and organs.

Allostasis

Despite the usefulness of homeostasis to describe the body's self-regulating processes, another term is needed to address the ability of the body's systems to undergo systematic change and adapt appropriately. The concept of *allostasis* was introduced to reflect the capacity of physiologic systems to maintain stability yet alter the set point required for optimum system functioning (Sterling & Eyer, 1988 as cited by McEwen, 2000). Allostasis is a broader concept than homeostasis. Allostasis incorporates homeostatic processes while simultaneously anticipating daily fluctuations and changes. Normal alterations occur in the level at which physiologic systems function throughout the day and also in anticipation of coming events. For example, body temperature is regulated at a higher level during waking hours than during sleep. Allostasis is considered the operating range in which the body's systems increase or decrease to an appropriate level (set point) in response to an actual or anticipated challenge.

Physiologic systems that prepare the body become activated as a person thinks about and anticipates a change. For example, body systems prepare for activity as a person gets ready to exercise, even before the actual exercise begins. This finding is true for stress as well: the body will prepare itself to respond physiologically as a person thinks about or anticipates a threat or challenge even if it never actually happens.

The concept of "allostatic load" was introduced to explain the body's immediate response to actual or anticipated stress as well as the condition of the body once the threat or event has passed (McEwen, 1998, 2000). Allostatic load is described as the "price the body pays" for being forced to adapt repeatedly to psychosocial and environmental circumstances (McEwen, 2000). Allostatic load is increased by (a) frequent exposure to stressors, (b) an inability to habituate to repeated exposures to the same stressor, (c) an inability to mount an adequate physiologic stress response or to turn off the response when it is no longer required (McEwen, 1998). Theorists believe that over time an allostatic load accumulates and adversely affects various body organs, thereby contributing to disease. Allostatic load may be a useful concept to assess the negative impact of the stress response on health.

Neuroendocrine Regulation of Physiologic Functioning

Neuroendocrine integrative functions play a central role in regulating homeostatic and allostatic processes. The neuroendocrine response involves activities of the central nervous system (CNS), autonomic nervous system, and endocrine system.

Central Nervous System. The CNS regulates overt behavior. The brain and spinal cord control the body's rapid muscular movements and motor coordination, perception of sensory inputs, and integration of thoughts, feelings, concerns, and memories. The brain is a remarkable organ, and the cerebral cortex, the highest level of functioning, influences physiologic functioning of the entire body. Thought, memory, and feelings influence a person's response to stress: i.e., how a person perceives or forms beliefs about an event actually shapes subsequent experience and behavior. The way a person perceives a situation is critical to understanding individual responses to potentially stressful encounters. A person's genetic background and experience shape that individual's responses to stress.

Autonomic Nervous System. The autonomic nervous system regulates automatic body functions that involve the dynamic functioning of the smooth muscle of the blood vessels and digestive tract, cardiac muscle, lymph tissue, and the glands of the digestive organs, liver, pancreas, and adrenal medulla. The two divisions of the autonomic nervous system are called parasympathetic and sympathetic. The parasympathetic system innervates peripheral organs in specific, discrete ways. It slows heart rate, stimulates saliva production, and promotes digestion and elimination. The sympathetic system innervates many peripheral organs including the adrenal medulla and organs and cells of the immune system. It responds to sudden demands or threats within seconds. The catecholamines, epinephrine and norepinephrine, are the major hormones secreted in sympathetic responses to stressors. Epinephrine is the main hormone secreted by the adrenal medulla and norepinephrine is the main neurotransmitter secreted from sympathetic nerve endings. Specific peripheral sympathetic responses include increases in heart rate, airway diameter, blood glucose level, and muscle tension. Activation of the autonomic nervous system is a critical component in the immediate or acute physiologic response of the body to an actual or an imagined stressor.

Endocrine System. The functions of five major endocrine glands (pituitary, adrenal, thyroid, parathyroid, and pancreas) secrete chemical substances called hormones, which are specific mediators that alter cellular activity some distance from their source. Figure 49-1 shows the location and function of specific endocrine glands that affect the body's response and coping with stress. The endocrine system is under control of the CNS. The hypothalamus secretes neuropeptides, neurotransmitters, and hormones that regulate the production and release of hormones from the pituitary gland. Hormones secreted by the pituitary (i.e., thyroid-stimulating hormone, corticotropin hormone) are carried in the blood to their peripheral organ targets. Activation of the hypothalamic-pituitary-adrenal (HPA)

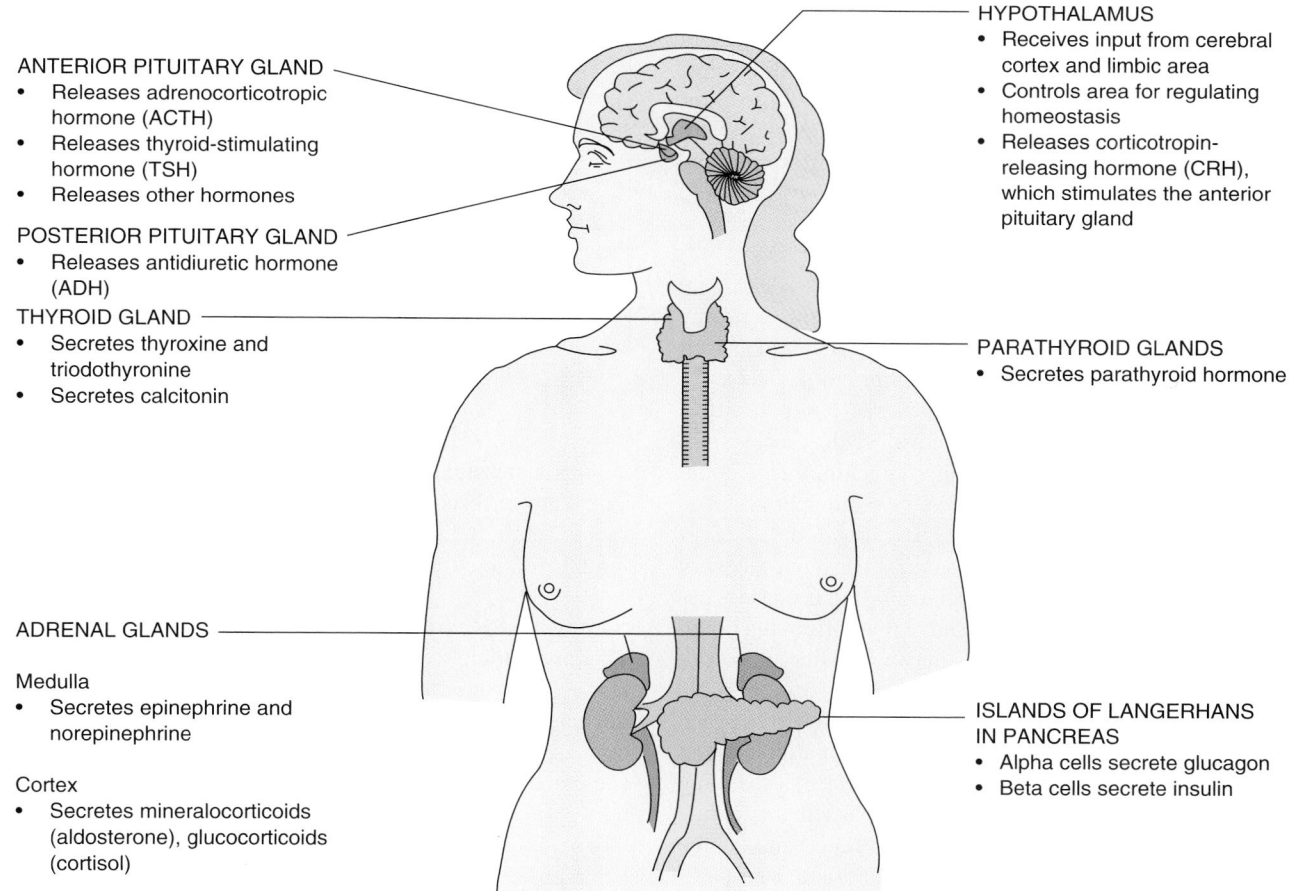

FIGURE 49-1   Location of specific endocrine glands that affect the body's adaptation to stress.

system is an important component of the physiologic response to stress. Cortisol is the main glucocorticoid hormone from the adrenal cortex. Cortisol affects glucose metabolism, which is necessary for increased energy expenditure. The adrenal gland is an important component of the physiologic response to stress because both major parts of this gland, the cortex and the medulla, are activated in a typical stress response.

Characteristics of Stress, Coping, and Adaptation

Although the term *stress* is commonly used, it is difficult to define and very ambiguous. Stress means different things to different people and to the same person at different times. Stress may be considered a stimulus and a stressor, or it may be considered a response. A broader concept of stress encompasses many interacting factors such as stimulus, response, appraisal of the event, and coping processes.

Stress as a Stimulus

When viewed as a stimulus, stress is defined as any event or set of events, a *stressor,* that causes a response (Lazarus, 1992). Everyday triggers associated with work or social relationships, and uncommon events like natural disasters, physical trauma, injuries, illnesses, divorce, death of a loved one, or loss of a job are commonly recognized stressors. Stress is often thought of as negative or "bad" and is associated with events that cause distress. Wolff (1953) described disease states resulting from life stress caused by disruption in lifestyles and relationships, deprivation of human needs, and failure to act in ways to eliminate the cause of the stress. Stressors are also events or behaviors that are considered "good" or are useful to promote well-being. Participating in athletic events, exercising, and soaking in a hot tub will activate physiologic stress responses but these are examples of positive or beneficial stressors.

Lazarus (1981) developed the Everyday Hassles Scale to help identify and rank everyday stressful events (Display 49-1)—events that could be interpreted as distressful as well as those associated with a feeling of exhilaration. The scale contains both "hassles," which create stress, and "uplifts," which promote well-being. People may have different awareness of hassles and uplifts. Knowing the nature of potential stressors, however, provides the means of anticipating problems and their related psychological reactions. The extent of activation of physiologic responses and subsequent recovery to daily hassles is important to a person's health because accumulated allostatic responses may adversely affect the body. Effective coping with daily hassles may help reduce allostatic load and its contribution to disease.

Holmes and Rahe (1967) studied the relationship between specific life changes, such as divorce or death of a spouse, and subsequent onset of illness. They assumed these life-changing events to have negative effects and asked participants to rate such events according to perceived stressfulness and degree of adaptation required. Other researchers advise that variables such as genotype, age, gender, marital status, and ethnic origin can be critical influences on a person's appraisal and evaluation of stressful life events. More recently, researchers have studied the effects or consequences of psychosocial stressors, such as natural disasters or nuclear accidents, on health and immune system functioning (Kaplan, 1991).

Stress as a Response

The physiologic stress response first called a "fight or flight" response (Cannon, 1935) was based largely on research conducted on male subjects (Taylor et al., 2000). This response corresponds to the initial phase of the stress response with acute activation of the sympathetic nervous system with the release of catecholamines by the adrenal medulla and sympathetic nerve endings (see below). This "fight or flight" response is largely considered the prototypic human stress response to real or imagined stressors. The stress response actually involves more than just sympathetic system mediated effects and

DISPLAY 49-1

⑤ LAZARUS'S EVERYDAY HASSLES SCALE

The following scale rank-orders "hassles," which contribute to stress, and "uplifts," which contribute positively to stress management, as evaluated by several middle-aged client groups. Nurses may determine the client's hassles and uplifts for purposes of providing anticipatory guidance. Individual clients may perceive hassles and uplifts differently from the groups studied by Lazarus.

Hassles (Rank Ordered)
1. Feeling concerned about weight.
2. Worrying about health of a family member.
3. Worrying about rising cost of living.
4. Dealing with home maintenance.
5. Having too many things to do.
6. Misplacing or losing things.
7. Doing yard work or outside home maintenance.
8. Worrying about property, investment, or taxes.
9. Worrying about crime.
10. Feeling concern about physical appearance.

Uplifts (Rank Ordered)
1. Relating well to spouse or lover.
2. Relating well with friends.
3. Completing a task.
4. Feeling healthy.
5. Getting enough sleep.
6. Eating out.
7. Meeting responsibilities.
8. Visiting, telephoning, or writing someone.
9. Spending time with family.
10. Taking pleasure in one's home.

(Adapted from Lazarus, R. S. (1981). Little hazards can be hazardous to your health. *Psychology Today, 15*(7), 58–62.)

the neuroendocrine responses may be different in men compared to women (Taylor et al., 2000). Compared to men, women's responses to stress have been described as "tend and befriend" in addition to "flight or fight."

Hans Selye defined stress as "the nonspecific response of the body to any demand upon it" (Selye, 1974, p. 27). Selye used the term *stressor* to differentiate between the stress-producing agent and the body's generalized response to it. The stressor is the stimulus that evokes a generalized stress response in the person; it is anything that places a demand on the person and activates the stress response. Thus if the stress response was not activated, stress was not present.

People may view stressors as positive or negative. Selye (1974) referred to pleasant events as "eustress" from the Greek prefix *eu* meaning good or positive. One example of eustress is going to college, which the person views as positive and desirable, but also stressful because of the changes in routine and adaptation involved. Negative or undesirable events are referred to as "distress." Examples of distress include being fired, having an argument with a close friend, or being hospitalized.

Positive stressors seem to evoke the same physiologic reactions as negative stressors. The distinction between eustress and distress lies in the person's interpretation of the event. Regardless of the type of stressor, Selye (1974) termed the body's response to it as an undifferentiated physiologic reaction. This "nonspecific response" means that the body endures a number of biochemical changes and readjustments regardless of the nature of the stress-producing agent. Because the physiologic response seemed to be universal in all organisms, he referred to this pattern of defense as the general adaptation syndrome. In Selye's model, the hypothalamic-pituitary-adrenal system (HPA) and release of glucocorticoids from the adrenal cortex were critically important in enhancing and mediating the stress response and ultimately lead to exhaustion. Subsequent research has shown that glucocorticoids have enhancing as well as suppressive actions on various target organs (Sapolsky, Romero, & Munck, 2000).

Now it is well accepted that the type of stressor and the extent to which a person appraises the stressor as "stressful" are critical to determining the nature and extent of the physiologic stress response. Responses to stress are influenced by early life experiences that shape a person's "stress reactivity profile" as well as the use of coping strategies or skills learned and modified throughout life. When stressful events are managed through effective coping, the person experiences personal growth and improved problem-solving abilities. A person who is most successful in coping tends to be flexible and to use a variety of strategies to adapt to new situations and stressors.

Physiologic Stress Response. Investigators have shown that corticotropin-releasing hormone (CRH) is increased in hypothalamic neurons involved in coordinating the physiologic stress response (Chappell et al., 1986). CRH administered to animals and to humans has endocrine, physiologic, neurochemical, and behavioral effects that mimic those associated with physiologic arousal responses. Dunn and Berridge (1990) suggest that CRH is the common factor in coordinating the response of the CNS to stress. CRH activates the systems primarily involved in mediating physiologic responses to stress—the autonomic nervous system and the HPA axis. The idea that CRH is the endogenous mediator of the stress response supports Selye's ideas about the body's nonspecific response.

Activation of the physiologic stress response to impending danger is important for survival. In response to actual or perceived danger, muscles are primed, attention is focused, and the body is readied for action. This "fight or flight" response is beneficial in the short term but has detrimental effects in the long term. Cumulative effects increase allostatic load, which contributes to hypertension, heart disease, cancer, and aging.

Events that people perceive and interpret as stressful are processed at multiple levels in the CNS. In the brain, the limbic system and hippocampus are thought to mediate emotional aspects and the memory of perceived events. The limbic system and hippocampus have many neural connections to regulate and inhibit the output of hypothalamic neurons that mediate the physiologic stress response. Neurosecretory cells in the hypothalamus release CRH and other neuropeptides in response to stress to activate the HPA axis. The extent to which this axis is activated is regulated by the extent of inhibitory influences from the limbic system and hippocampus. CRH activates the pituitary gland to secrete corticotropin hormone, which, in turn, stimulates the cortex of the adrenal gland to secrete cortisol and other glucocorticoids associated with the stress response. There are also connections between the hypothalamus and brain stem areas that activate the sympathetic branch of the autonomic nervous system. The sympathetic nervous system releases norepinephrine from peripheral nerve endings and epinephrine from the adrenal medulla. These catecholamines mediate the immediate (within seconds) physiologic manifestations associated with arousal, excitement, or anxiety such as increased heart rate or "palpitations," dilated pupils, increased breathing rate, muscle tension, and "butterflies" in the stomach during the first phase of a stress response. The effects of glucocorticoids constitute the second phase of the stress response that occurs over the course of minutes to hours after the onset of the stressor (Sapolsky, Romero, & Munck, 2000). The neurohormonal components of the stress response are important for mobilizing energy from body stores, making glucose available for metabolism, rapidly delivering this glucose to muscles, stimulating selective components of the immune system, sharpening mental capacities, reducing reproductive behaviors, altering food intake and appetite, and in some cases causing water retention.

The responses of the endocrine and sympathetic nervous systems to stress contribute to altered immune function. A wide variety of neuropeptides and hormones influence lymphocytes and alter their functioning. The acute stress response leads to arousal and sometimes to increased activation of various immune system indicators. On the other hand, chronic stress is associated with immunosuppression. Thus, whether stressors are acute or chronic, the stress response is associated with some form of immune system dysregulation (Dhabhar & McEwen, 1997). Chronic or repeated stressors could lead to an allostatic load that, when combined with continued immune system dysregulation, may contribute to disease. This effect could arise from overexposure to (a) repeated hormone and peptide mediators of the physiologic stress response, (b) failure of components of physiologic arousal response to shut off when the threat is passed, or (c) an inadequate response by one component of the arousal response that in some way triggers another component of the response to become overactive and increase allostatic load (McEwen, 1998, 2000). Although the physiologic stress response is important for survival and unavoidable, the response is modifiable, and how one copes is critical to the response itself.

Cognitive and Psychological Response to Stress. Cognitively, a person encounters an event or stressor, perceives it as a threat (harm/loss) or nonthreat (challenge), and calls on automatic coping responses. Part of the initial physiologic stress response is heightened mental acuity and perception.

The person continues to appraise the stressor to determine if a discrepancy exists between the degree of threat and coping capacity. The person may respond by limiting his or her emotional response, taking direct action to solve a problem, or using defense mechanisms (Lazarus, 1991a; 1991b).

Defense mechanisms are ways to simply withdraw from stress. These self-protective, unconscious processes enable people to cope with stressful encounters, thereby decreasing anxiety (Wineman, Durand & McCulloch, 1994). People use defense mechanisms in several ways; for example, they may use denial or increase time spent sleeping, daydreaming, or fantasizing. Table 49-1 lists and defines common defense mechanisms. If a stressor is more than the person can or wants to deal with, one method of coping is to withdraw to a comforting and nonstressful activity. For example, sleep allows the person to avoid stress temporarily, assuming that the problem does not keep him or her awake. Daydreams and fantasies allow the person to withdraw mentally to a more pleasant, less stressful scene.

Defense mechanisms can become problematic if a person relies on them rather than developing additional coping strategies or perhaps confronting stress and actively problem solving. Although defense mechanisms help to avoid pain, modify strong emotions, and relieve anxiety, overuse can be self-defeating, increase allostatic load, and interfere with productive coping and adapting.

Normal Coping Patterns

Coping successfully with stressful encounters requires ongoing efforts to manage changes, demands, and challenges. Coping is usually described as a process. Various strategies are used to manage daily hassles or life events—the out-of-the-ordinary situations. Although coping may be entirely cognitive, it is more likely to be a psychophysiologic activity that integrates the mind and body. As such, it is a major process crucial to the person's continued growth and adaptation.

TABLE 49-1

Common Defense Mechanisms	
Compensation	The attempt to achieve respect or recognition in one activity as a substitute for inability to achieve in another endeavor
Denial	Refusing to believe or accept something as it is but rather as one wishes it to be
Displacement	Transferring emotion away from the person or situation that incited the emotion to an inappropriate person or object
Introjection	Taking into one's personality the characteristics of another
Projection	Attributing one's own thoughts, emotions, characteristics, or motives to another
Rationalization	Concealing the motive for behavior by giving some socially acceptable reason for the action
Regression	Return to behaviors more appropriate to an earlier stage of development
Repression	Immersing something in the subconscious or unconscious level of thought
Sublimation	Release of libido in socially acceptable behavior rather than using it to obtain sexual gratification
Suppression	Consciously dismissing something from the mind and thoughts

Lazarus (1991a) described two types of cognitive coping processes: problem-oriented (manipulation of the person–environment relationship that is the source of stress) and emotion-focused (regulation of stressful emotions). Display 49-2 gives examples of both. Many common defense mechanisms previously described characterize emotion-focused coping (Lazarus & Folkman, 1984).

Bell (1977) divided *coping mechanisms* (activities or measures for managing stress) into two groups, long term and short term. Long-term coping mechanisms are positive, constructive ways of dealing with stress and can be effective over long periods. Short-term coping methods are temporary measures to reduce stress and tension; however, if used over long periods they may have detrimental effects on the person and may lead to maladaptive behavior. Display 49-2 gives examples.

Lifespan Considerations

An emerging principle in the physiology of brain-behavior interactions is that the interaction of genetic information with early life experiences has a lifelong impact that shapes a person's stress responsiveness (reactivity). There is increasing

DISPLAY 49-2

🔳 EXAMPLES OF COPING STRATEGIES

Examples of Problem-Oriented Coping Mechanisms
- Making a time schedule for studying and sticking to it
- Applying for a job at another company because your current position is too demanding
- Trying to find out more about an illness, such as diabetes, to manage it better

Examples of Emotion-Focused Coping Mechanisms
- Accepting sympathy and understanding from a friend in the loss of a family member
- Releasing tension after a hard day at work by meditating, crying, or taking a walk
- Blaming someone else—for example, a spouse or teacher—for the situation you are in

Examples of Long-Term Coping Mechanisms
- Working out stress through physical exercise
- Talking with others about problems (friend, counselor)
- Relying on belief in a higher power
- Seeking additional information about a situation
- Drawing on past experience
- Developing alternative plans for handling the situation

Examples of Short-Term Coping Mechanisms
- Smoking
- Alcohol use
- Overeating
- "Pill-popping"
- Excessive caffeine intake

evidence that elevated HPA activity enhances the rate of brain aging (Porter, Herman & Landfield, 2001).

Newborn and Infant

Newborns and infants rely largely on reflex responses for coping with the environment and its associated stressors. For example, a hungry newborn will reflexively cry and be physically active to cope with the situation temporarily and to attempt to change it. Parents and other caregivers learn to respond to such communication and to participate in a mutual coping pattern by providing food. With continuing development, infants gradually learn new coping strategies for various situations although they usually are limited to reflex and sensory functions. Responses to stress may be excessive during these stages. Evidence from research in human term neonates suggests that vigorous responses to an adverse stimulus (stressor) during the early neonatal period are associated with decreased psychophysiologic reactions in later infancy (Walker, Anand, & Plotsky, 2001). There is also evidence that a single stressful encounter in a newborn, such as experiencing circumcision without anesthesia, is associated with increased behavioral responses to vaccination injections in later infancy.

Individual differences in the responsivity of the HPA axis is influenced by early experiences and the postnatal environment. Newborns and infants depend totally on their caregivers for physiologic needs, safety, and loving attachment. These needs, if met, help to ameliorate the effects of stress and to provide the basis for future coping.

Toddler and Preschooler

During the toddler and preschool stages, physical development becomes more stable. Children learn strategies for coping with relatively simple stressors such as not getting things exactly when they want them. Learning to handle slight delays in getting wants and having needs met sets a pattern children can apply to other situations later in life.

Parents and family members are a key part of children's frames of reference in terms of handling stress and adapting to situations (Fig. 49-2). Because children are developing

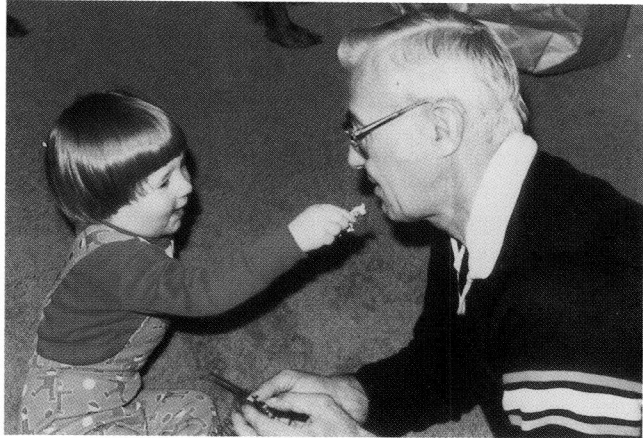

FIGURE 49-2 Children's relationships with family members influence their patterns of coping and adapting to stress.

coping strategies, they may still display excessive responses to minor situations. They depend on their families for safety and limit setting to define the boundaries for handling stress.

School-Age Child and Adolescent

School-age children are expanding their world as they move out of the realm of home into school and interactions with others. Classroom situations, structured play, and interactions with other children and adults present new stresses. For secure children who have experienced only minimal anxiety, attending school for the first time can fill them with real or perceived stress. Children must learn to adapt and to cope with new experiences and rules. At this age, children can identify stressors, begin to reason with parents and others about how to cope with them, and draw from past experience to develop new approaches. Children use a variety of coping strategies that are similar for various stressors including wishful thinking, problem–solving, and trying to regulate emotional reactions. Similar to adults, the way a child appraises a stressful event, such as surgery, determines the coping strategies that a child adopts (LaMontagne, 2000).

Psychological maturation is a primary task of adolescence, requiring behavioral adaptations and development of new coping mechanisms. During adolescence, people move toward achieving emotional independence from parents, developing sexual identity, acquiring values, and exhibiting socially responsible behavior. Such stress-producing tasks require adolescents to use the coping strategies they have learned thus far and to develop additional ones continually (Puskar, Lamb, & Bartolovic, 1993). Adolescents who move to new schools and through various levels of education (i.e., middle school, high school, college) must handle the stresses related to each new situation with increasing maturity (Sorensen, 1994). There are age and gender differences in adolescent responses to stressors. Adolescent girls report more life event-related stress and show higher levels of stress generated from interpersonal conflicts with parents and peers compared to boys (Groer, Thomas, & Shoffner, 1992; Rudolph & Hammen, 1999). Girls are particularly vulnerable to depressive responses in situations in which they feel dependent. Both girls and boys use active (e.g., exercise) and passive (e.g., day dreaming) distraction coping techniques. Although separation from parents is in progress, adolescents still need the security that families can provide.

Adult and Older Adult

The various demands of adulthood (e.g., occupation, lifestyle, relationships, family, transitions) impose daily stress. Adults draw on coping skills developed throughout life and learn new ones. Previous exposures to stressful situations may help people cope with similar situations more constructively than they did in younger years.

As people mature and progress to the developmental tasks of adulthood, transitions related to those events require adequate coping and adaptation. The selection of a mate, marriage, and childbearing are examples of such transitional events. For example, the marriage of two adults is usually a happy occasion. Even so, the involved parties and their families face

stressors relating to decisions about the wedding, new alliances, and possible changes in previous family relationships. When a child is born, new stresses accompany the expansion of the family, even when the baby is anticipated with great delight. There are new demands on both marriage partners in terms of emotions, dependencies, time, and money. Childbearing demands a new set of coping strategies to adapt successfully (Hall, 1994).

In a mobile society such as the United States, many families experience frequent moving and relocation for career purposes. Each move has its own unique stressors related to closure of family life in one community and beginning of family life in a new community. The relocation is not only physical but also emotional, necessitating separation from the family's ties and support systems within the community. Most families can develop these relationships over time in their new community but doing so may be stressful even when all goes well.

As a person ages, stress does not decrease. Among the stresses of aging are retirement, decline in physical energy, decrease in income potential, loss of family and friends, and possibly relocation. Older adults must adapt to these added changes at the same time that their individual reserves and strength are declining. In addition, there is evidence of excess levels of plasma cortisol or altered regulation of glucocorticoid receptors in the brain as important contributors to accelerated aging, memory impairments, and neuronal damage (Porter et al., 2001). There is an age-related increase in the nocturnal level of cortisol and a shortening in the duration of the "quiescent period" or lowest level of the daily cortisol rhythm with age both in men and women (Van Cauter, Leproult, & Kupfer, 1996). These observations have been interpreted as evidence of increased allostatic load.

FACTORS AFFECTING COPING PATTERNS

The extent to which a person considers an event stressful clearly influences subsequent physiologic and behavioral responses. In addition to the previously discussed developmental and age-related considerations, lifestyle factors and prior experience influence coping with daily and "out-of-the-ordinary" events. Factors that create unusual circumstances have the potential to affect coping and adaptation. Examples include such transitions as involuntary relocation, hospitalization, divorce, loss, domestic abuse, fatigue, illness, and death.

Lifestyle Considerations

Choices in nutrition, sleep, exercise, and fitness can influence a person's response to stress. Poor choices in these areas may predispose the person to fatigue, illness, and perhaps death. A person with a lifestyle pattern of poor nutrition, insufficient rest, and irregular exercise is prone to experience inadequate physiologic reserves and increased allostatic load. In these circumstances, the person may overreact psychologically to stress-producing situations, and the neuroendocrine response may be compromised as well.

Diet

Many people are concerned about the quality of their diets not only in terms of total caloric intake but also with food's nutritional value. When the body has adequate nutrients and is neither undernourished nor overfed, nutritional resources provide the body with added reserves for responding to stress. Imbalances in the intake of essential nutrients can enhance or even exaggerate the stress response. A poorly nourished person may be less prepared to handle stressful situations.

Activity and Exercise

When a person combines adequate nutrition with regular exercise, he or she enjoys both physiologic and psychological benefits of fitness. Such benefits include improved cardiovascular conditioning, weight control, enhanced muscle tone, and better sense of well-being. Because many chronic illnesses have some relation to problems in one or more of these areas, exercise programs can be effective in decreasing poor health outcomes. Regular patterns of exercise provide people with a ready outlet for stress before it becomes prolonged or chronic. The exercise routine permits the person to cope with normal, day-to-day hassles so adaptation occurs in smaller increments. This modulated approach prevents the accumulation of many minor stressors to a point where the person can no longer cope.

Sleep and Rest

To feel rested and relaxed, a person needs adequate sleep. When a person is anticipating or experiencing stress, rest and relaxation are particularly important. Many people's busy schedules leave little time for adequate rest and sleep, which compromises their ability to manage stress. People who suffer from inadequate sleep are irritable, tired, and less able to cope effectively with minor and major stressors.

In modern society it has been estimated that adults sleep 1.5 hours less each night compared to adults in the early 1900s. Many adults may accumulate "sleep debt" from chronic insufficient sleep. In a recent study, investigators found that after sleep was restricted to 4 hours a night for a week, subjects had elevated evening cortisol levels, increased sympathetic nervous system activity, and higher blood glucose levels after eating compared to the rested condition (Spiegel, Leproult, Van Cauter, 1999). These results suggest that individuals who restrict their sleep on a chronic basis will increase their allostatic load and their propensity to develop diabetes and cardiovascular diseases.

Safety and Security

The extent to which people perceive situations to be threatening relates directly to their degree of security. This relationship also influences ability to cope and to adapt. For example, if a student is failing a class and feels very insecure about how his or her parents will react, the student will experience greater stress than if he or she felt secure in the parents' support and understanding. Similarly, the effects of other stress-producing situations, such as giving birth, acute illness, or role changes, depend on the person's perception of the event and the presence of adequate support and effective coping mechanisms.

Previous Experience

Prior exposure to and past experience with particular stressors influence the person's response and adaptation to current encounters. A person's responses may be learned from other family members. For instance, a child may develop a fear of heights because his father has this phobia.

Previous exposure to stressful situations may also help the person to cope with present situations. For example, a person who has spoken in public many times may find it much less stressful than the person who has never done so. Clearly the extent to which a person has coped effectively with a stressor will influence subsequent coping with the same or similar stressors.

Involuntary Relocation

Even under the best circumstances, relocation is stressful. When such moves are involuntary, the potential for stress increases greatly. For example, although moving may be necessary for career reasons, it may be disruptive and stressful especially for families that are fragile in some way (e.g., disabled child, unhappy adolescents). Many such families have already developed needed and useful support systems in their present communities. A move may interfere with coping strategies, thereby preventing adaptation.

In another example, an older person may face the realization that living independently is no longer an option but may choose

ETHICAL/LEGAL ISSUE
Transferring a Client

Mrs. Lewis, 85 years old, has lived in your long-term care facility for 5 years. As a result of structural damage to the building, all residents are being moved to a new facility. Because Mrs. Lewis is on public assistance, state representatives have determined that she must move to a different facility than the other residents with whom she is familiar. You are concerned about the stress of relocation and how it will affect Mrs. Lewis, but the state representatives are adamant about their decision.

Reflection
- Identify your concerns about Mrs. Lewis, the move, and her level of stress.
- Describe your feelings in light of the stress and safety concerns in this situation.
- Identify possible approaches to these controversial circumstances.
- Recognizing the client's dependence on state funding, define what you see as your ethically appropriate behavior.

to deny it. Family or other support systems may have to help the older person decide to move to an environment that offers improved safety and more support for daily living activities. This involuntary relocation can produce overwhelming stress and altered coping for the older person (Kammer, 1994).

Another form of involuntary relocation is hospitalization. A person is not admitted to a hospital without a specific health reason, either physical or psychological. Depending on the problem, the person may experience mild or great stress, both of which require coping skills and patterns to manage the problem. The health problem may overwhelm the person's previous patterns of coping, leading to or adding to stress.

Social Interaction

Although families can be great sources of support and social interaction, they can also be sources of distress and altered coping. Many marriages end in separation and divorce that can be amicable or bitter. Divorce, particularly in families with dependent children, can lead to altered coping, which, in turn, requires new adaptation strategies. Research has shown that most children from divorced families function normally, but children and adolescents particularly suffer from the loss of a secure environment and may respond behaviorally or physically with altered coping and adaptation.

Stresses from other sources often have their outlet in the family. When individual coping strategies are inadequate, that outlet may take the form of physical abuse. In the United States, increased public awareness of domestic abuse has led to the growing availability of service agencies and support groups.

Sensory Deficits

Deficits or impairments in the senses can alter a person's ability to cope with and to respond effectively to stress. Sensory deficits in vision and hearing interfere with the ability to interact with the environment and with other people. The person finds it increasingly difficult to make judgments when under stress, to know what coping options exist, and/or to adapt to changes that challenge sensory-perceptual abilities. Inability to see or hear accurately can lead to misperception and the potential for altered coping.

ALTERED COPING PATTERNS

Manifestations of Altered Coping

Altered coping may be manifested in various ways including use of alcohol and drugs, excessive smoking, increased sleeping, overeating, avoidance and withdrawal, daydreaming and fantasizing, and illness. Display 49-3 presents additional examples of expressions of stress.

Addictive Behaviors

Alcohol is a commonly used means of altering reality and awareness. The phrase "crawling into a bottle" illustrates the attempt to withdraw from stress and problems by ingesting

DISPLAY 49-3

🔄 **PSYCHOSOCIAL AND PHYSIOLOGIC EXPRESSIONS OF STRESS**

Psychosocial Expressions	Physiologic Expressions
Behaviors	Back, neck, or shoulder pain
Crying	Breathing irregularities
Decreased motivation	Elevated blood pressure
Decreased self-esteem	Change in appetite
Decreased intellectual processes	Stuttering, trembling
Forgetfulness	Jaw tension
Impulsive behavior	Sexual dysfunction
Inability to make decisions	Constipation or diarrhea
Learning disabilities	Irregular heartbeat
Poor concentration	Muscle cramps, spasms
Emotions	Stomach, digestive disorders
Anger, anxiety	Sweating, skin problems
Nervousness	Tension headaches
Moodiness, depression	Insomnia or fatigue
Emotional instability	
Irritability	
Fears, phobias	
Feeling out of control	
Frustration	
Feelings of worthlessness	

alcohol. Excessive use of legal and illegal drugs is another method for people to escape and cope with stress. The results of excessive alcohol and drug use are addiction, dependency, psychological problems, physiologic consequences, and, probably, more stress and less effective coping. Adolescents are at particular risk for substance abuse because of their need for acceptance and the peer pressure related to this stage of development.

Smoking is also an addictive behavior. People, particularly adolescents, typically begin smoking in an effort to portray a certain image (e.g., older, macho, or more sophisticated). They end up being addicted, relying on the habit as a coping mechanism, and finding it difficult to stop. When stressed, smokers commonly increase their habit. Smoking, although perhaps temporarily relaxing, is ultimately an ineffective coping strategy that causes harmful physiologic alterations including respiratory and cardiovascular disorders.

Eating can become addictive in much the same way as smoking: the person seeks the immediate pleasure of food to avoid discomfort caused by stress. The problem of overeating has no simple cause or explanation. As with sleeping and daydreams, food offers many people a pleasurable escape from difficult situations. The behavior may work in the short term; however, over the long term, overeating leads to obesity with

THERAPEUTIC DIALOGUE
Stress

Scene for Thought
Kathleen O'Brien, an RN and staff member at a clinic, is sitting in the break room alone one morning, looking sad and preoccupied. Jean enters to get a cup of coffee.

Less Effective

Jean: Hi, Kathleen, how are you?

Kathleen: Okay, I guess. *(No eye contact. Looks at the floor.)*

Jean: *(Sits down next to her.)* You don't seem okay. Anything wrong?

Kathleen: *(Smiles embarrassedly.)* I just don't seem to have my usual energy, that's all.

Jean: I've noticed. It's been pretty hectic around here lately. We're all tired, including me! Are you getting enough rest with your busy schedule? *(Concerned tone of voice.)*

Kathleen: Not really. Finals are coming up at school, and I've been working on those. *(No eye contact.)*

Jean: Well, if I can do anything to help, let me know. I've got to get back to my meeting. See you later.

Kathleen: Okay. Thanks. *(Gets up and walks back to her desk to prepare for her next client.)*

More Effective

Jean: Hi, Kathleen, how are you?

Kathleen: Okay, I guess. *(No eye contact. Looks at the floor.)*

Jean: *(Sits down next to her.)* You don't seem okay. Anything wrong?

Kathleen: *(Smiles embarrassedly.)* I just don't seem to have my usual energy, that's all.

Jean: I noticed you've seemed a little tired. What's going on?

Kathleen: Just stressed out, I guess. *(Looks down again.)*

Jean: You mean more stressed than usual? Are the kids and George okay?

Kathleen: Yes, thank goodness.

Jean: How about school? Are you still taking two courses at night?

Kathleen: Yes, I'm doing alright.

Jean: *(Silence.)*

Kathleen: *(Takes a deep breath.)* The only thing that's changed is my brother, Tom. He was diagnosed with a malignant brain tumor last week. The cancer is already in his bowel and liver. *(Tears well in her eyes.)* I feel so helpless. My other brothers expect me to help them and Tom and his family to handle the shock and sorrow. I guess I'm feeling a little overwhelmed.

Jean: I guess so! Who's supporting you? *(Puts her hand on Kathleen's.)*

Kathleen: George has been wonderful and helps all he can. *(Squeezes Jean's hand and sighs.)* It's a matter of finding enough time to keep up my schoolwork and talk on the phone to all the people calling about Tom. I haven't been for a run in weeks. *(Sighs again.)*

Jean: Can I do anything to help?

Kathleen: No, but thanks. Just talking about it to someone who'll listen is comforting.

Jean: Let me know if you need a change in your schedule for anything, including a chance to exercise. Come talk to me anytime.

Kathleen: Thanks. I appreciate that.

Critical Thinking Challenge
- Examine psychosocial expressions of stress that Kathleen exhibited.
- Suggest what you think prevented Kathleen from being able to cope with all the stressors at this time.
- List who and what her resources are, and give reasons.
- Propose what you would do to reduce your stress level if you were Kathleen.

---

significant health consequences. People exhibiting stress and altered coping through substance abuse or overeating require a comprehensive treatment program to address their coping and adaptation problems.

Physical Illness
Prolonged stress increases allostatic load and can lead to physiologic dysfunction. Evidence exists that chronic stress alters health outcomes, reduces susceptibility to the common cold, slows wound healing, and reduces immune responses to vaccines. The physiologic mechanisms that link stress with increased susceptibility to viral infections are not known, but they likely involve alterations in immune system functioning or neuroendocrine regulation of immune system activity. Likewise, evidence exists that stress management, social support, relaxation, and other interventions enhance immune function and can alter disease development or progression (Kiecolt-Glaser & Glaser, 1995).

Anxiety and Depression

Stress can cause anxiety, a subjective reaction to a real or imagined threat. The sense of uneasiness or dread may range from mild to severe. Lack of sleep, poor nutrition, excessive caffeine intake or smoking, or physical illness are possible manifestations.

The extreme response to prolonged stress may be depression and suicide. People with poor coping mechanisms or inadequate support may see suicide as a desirable way to end stress and depression. Adolescents experiencing various kinds of stress have a higher rate of suicide than the general population.

Violent Behavior

People with poor impulse control or inadequate coping mechanisms may respond to stress by acting out violently or abusively. For example, a man experiencing difficulties at work may come home and behave violently with his wife or children as an outlet for stress. Domestic violence and other violent behaviors are related to altered coping.

Impact on Activities of Daily Living

Manifestations of stress and altered coping can interfere with activities of daily living (ADLs). The use of addictive substances, such as alcohol, drugs, and nicotine, ultimately leads to more problems not only with managing stress but also with accomplishing simple activities that are part of daily living. Alcohol and drug use contribute to cognitive impairments, which may compromise personal hygiene, learning, and work performance. The cost of smoking and other substance use diverts income from other personal or household needs.

As stress becomes prolonged or overwhelming, it can dominate a person's awareness or he or she may try to withdraw from it. In either event, activities such as home maintenance, food preparation, cleaning, personal hygiene, and grooming may become less important. If that occurs, stress may actually increase as a result of both changes in ADLs and further compromise of the person's reserves. Thus the family members can experience additional stress.

Stress may interfere with individual employment and family finances if it prevents optimal performance in school or work or the attempt to secure a position. Although some stress may heighten performance, excessive stress may severely impair performance, which adversely affects the person and ultimately the family.

ASSESSMENT

Clients with health problems face many stressors and have various ways of coping with them. Nurses must understand the methods or strategies clients use to individualize care appropriately.

Subjective Data

The focused functional assessment of coping patterns includes obtaining subjective data from clients through a series of purposeful questions and interviews and through observa-

tion and mental notation of nonverbal communication such as body position, facial expressions, gestures, voice, and speech. The nursing history is one of the earliest sources of these data, and in continued interactions nurses may become increasingly focused on specific considerations.

Subjective data help identify normal coping patterns and strategies, determine factors that place clients at risk for ineffective coping, and target any actual dysfunction. The following are possible questions to help gather subjective data:

- Have you experienced any changes or losses in the past year?
- What present situations are causing you stress?
- What does the problem/stressor/loss mean to you?
- Have stressful situations been good or bad for you?
- How have these situations affected you physically and emotionally?
- How do you relieve tension and deal with stress?
- What support systems do you rely on to help you solve problems?
- Do you usually solve your problems?
- Is there something the nurse can do to help you relieve stress? (Fuller & Schaller-Ayres, 1994)

Normal Pattern Identification

To assess coping patterns, obtain information from clients, family members, significant others, and healthcare providers. Because clients may have many stressors with which to cope, it is helpful to assess the variety of potential stressors and typical coping strategies (Fuller & Schaller-Ayers, 1994). To help to clarify stressful feelings and problems, enlist the client's participation in establishing a basis for purposeful nursing interventions.

Physiologic Stress. Because the physiologic response to stress is an activation or arousal response, ask about fatigue, adequacy of sleep, level of physical activity, and bowel elimination patterns. Changes in normal patterns of these or other physiologic activities may be expressions of ineffective coping.

Psychological Stress. Psychological stress is generated from a person's thoughts and feelings about specific events. For a person facing a health problem or hospitalization, stresses may be related to loss of personal control or a sense of powerlessness. Clients may exhibit behavioral responses such as denial, ambivalence, suspicion, hostility, regression, depression, or withdrawal. Asking clients to express their concerns, to identify problems, and to describe feelings associated with specific problems is a beginning approach to obtaining information.

Environmental Stress. Environmental stress may be related to relocation or unfamiliarity with the setting. A change in surroundings with new sounds, smells, and sights may produce stress for clients. In a hospital or long-term care facility, clients also experience changes in privacy, daily activities, and level of sensory stimulation (either more or less). Ask questions that elicit the client's response to the environment, define sources of stress, and disclose areas that both the nurse and the client think may be amenable to mutual planning.

Sociocultural Stress. Sociocultural stress may be related to family, financial, career, and spiritual concerns. For clients experiencing difficulties, elicit information about how the situation is affecting family relationships, whether or not job or career is affected, what kind of financial support or problems are issues, and how current situations affect spiritual beliefs and values. This information highlights the type of planning and collaboration that may be necessary.

Risk Identification

The nursing history includes collecting information that identifies factors placing clients at risk for ineffective coping. Risk assessment areas include transition factors such as moving and relocation, situations involving separation (e.g., divorce, child custody, prison, and hospitalization), and lifestyle factors such as fatigue, malnutrition, and illness.

Many factors that place clients at risk for ineffective coping may actually be positive for long-term outcomes but may add to problems in the short term. For example, a woman leaving an abusive marriage may experience very positive end results, but she may be at risk for ineffective coping while adapting to her new situation and reestablishing herself, and perhaps her children, in a new life.

Some risk factors are directly related to the reason for a client's health problem. If a client has a history of an eating disorder, such as anorexia or bulimia, resulting malnutrition may predispose the client to related health problems. In caring for the client, identify specific risks that may be present.

Dysfunction Identification

To determine the client's coping pattern, assess the client's beliefs about typical levels of stress and usual coping behaviors or strategies. Some people seem to have a high tolerance for stress and are so accustomed to living with an elevated level that they consider ordinary what other people would identify as extremely stressful. Be alert to the fact that these individuals may actually be at greater risk for harmful effects associated with high allostatic loads. Additionally, different people exhibit wide variations in coping behaviors. To gain the most accurate understanding, avoid inserting your personal biases and coping expectations into the assessment. Stay open to learning how clients identify situations.

Altered coping patterns can be identified as significant differences in a client's need to use typical coping behaviors and/or as coping and adaptation patterns outside the range of typical behaviors for that client. For example, the person who usually handles job stress by exercising but reports a current response of fatigue and excessive sleep has identified an altered coping pattern.

Objective Data

Physical Assessment

With activation of the autonomic nervous system and the endocrine system, physiologic responses occur and can be observed in the physical assessment. Because physiologic arousal responses involve general and nonspecific responses, there may be many other causes for some of these same responses.

Do NOT assume that the only cause of some physical findings is stress.

Cardiovascular System. The cardiovascular system is the target system for the effects of epinephrine and norepinephrine, which include increased heart rate, vasoconstriction of peripheral organs, and increased oxygen consumption by the heart. The manifestations of prolonged stimulation by these hormones may include the following:

- An increase in the resting heart rate related to direct stimulation of the myocardium; the client may describe a "pounding in the chest" or palpitations
- An increase in systolic or diastolic blood pressure related to peripheral vasoconstriction
- Dysrhythmias related to ischemia (tissue oxygen deprivation in the face of increased energy demand), noted in an irregular heartbeat or rhythm changes
- Angina, or chest pain, and ischemia-related changes in the electrocardiogram
- Headaches related to vasoconstriction

Respiratory System. Norepinephrine affects the respiratory system, which leads to an increased breathing rate and to bronchiolar dilation. Hyperventilation, a feeling of "air hunger," dizziness, and tingling in the hands and feet are the most common physical manifestations.

Gastrointestinal System. The gastrointestinal system is a common target system in stressful situations. Whereas epinephrine and norepinephrine usually slow gastric motility, people experiencing stress often report loss of appetite, nausea, vomiting, and increased peristaltic activity. Increased peristalsis is manifested by increases in bowel sounds, secretion of hydrochloric acid in the stomach, and number of bowel movements. The increase in hydrochloric acid secretion may also contribute to nausea and vomiting, and, in combination with cortisol, to gastrointestinal ulcerations or gastritis.

Musculoskeletal System. The musculoskeletal system responds to stress by exhibiting increased tension in larger muscles and shakiness and tremor in smaller muscles. The muscle tension is related to the "fight-or-flight" response. Prolonged tension can lead to muscle spasm, particularly in the back, shoulders, and neck.

Integumentary System. The skin, or integumentary system, manifests the peripheral effects of norepinephrine and epinephrine by being diaphoretic (moist) and cool and by exhibiting smooth muscle tension ("making the hairs stand on end").

Diagnostic Tests and Procedures

No simple laboratory tests can determine stress. Although stress-related hormones (epinephrine, norepinephrine, and cortisol) can be detected through laboratory tests and a stress state can be inferred from their existence, these hormones are most often measured in research studies rather than in clinical situations.

Objective data about the client's coping and adaptation are gathered by means of structured interviews and coping and stress assessment tools that attempt to identify and quantify stressors and coping patterns, as described in the section on Subjective Data. Formal assessment tools include instruments such as the Social Readjustment and Rating Scale (SRRS; Holmes & Rahe, 1967); Everyday Hassles Scale (Lazarus, 1981); Interview Guide: Stress and Stress Responses (Fuller & Schaller-Ayers, 1994); and the Stress Audit (Miller, Smith, & Mehler, 1991). These assessment tools are discussed throughout this chapter. Using these instruments helps identify behaviors and feelings that may relate to the amount of stress and the corresponding vulnerability to illness and dysfunction. In some situations nurses may use the scales, which turn subjective factors into objective numbers, or psychosocial clinical nurse specialists, consultants, or psychologists may use the scales. All nurses can employ the interview guide (Display 49-4).

NURSING DIAGNOSES

The North American Nursing Diagnosis Association (NANDA, 2001) has approved several categories of nursing diagnoses related to coping and adaptation. Currently, the diagnoses include Caregiver Role Strain, Risk for Caregiver Role Strain, Ineffective Coping, Impaired Adjustment, Defensive Coping, Disabled Family Coping, Compromised Family Coping, Readiness for Enhanced Family Coping, Readiness for En-

hanced Community Coping, Relocation Stress Syndrome, Risk for Other-directed Violence, Risk for Self-mutilation, Risk for Self-directed Violence, Post-trauma Syndrome, Risk for Post-trauma Syndrome, Rape-trauma Syndrome, Anxiety, Fear, Risk for Relocation Stress Syndrome, and Risk for Suicide. One diagnosis is presented in this text: Ineffective Coping.

Diagnostic Statement: Ineffective Coping

Definition. Inability to form a valid appraisal of the stressors, inadequate choices of practiced responses, and/or inability to use available resources (NANDA, 2001).

Defining Characteristics. Defining characteristics include lack of goal-directed behavior/resolution of problem including inability to attend to and difficulty organizing information; sleep disturbance; abuse of chemical agents; decreased use of social support; use of forms of coping that impede adaptive behavior; poor concentration; fatigue; inadequate problem solving; verbalization of inability to cope or inability to ask for help; inability to meet basic needs; destructive behavior toward self or others; inability to meet role expectations; high illness rate; change in usual communication patterns; risk taking. (NANDA, 2001).

DISPLAY 49-4

🖵 **INTERVIEW GUIDE: STRESS AND STRESS RESPONSES**

Stressors
Major changes/losses in the past year _____
Situations that cause stress: At the present time _____
                    In the past _____

Perception of Stressors/Stress
What does this problem/stressor/loss mean to you? _____
Have stressful situations been good or bad for you? _____
How have stressful situations affected you? (physically and emotionally) _____

Coping Strategies
How do you relieve tension and deal with stress? _____

Talk to others _____	Try to solve the problem _____	Blame someone else for the
Try to forget _____	Try to relieve tension with	problem _____
Do something to get mind off	alcohol _____ drugs _____	Seek help _____
problems _____	overeating _____	Other (describe) _____
Pray _____	Go to sleep _____	_____
Do nothing _____	Accept the situation _____	_____

Is there someone you rely on to help you solve problems? _____
Is there something the nurse can do to make hospitalization (clinic visits, home visits, etc.) less stressful?
_____

Resolution of Stress
Do you usually solve your problems? _____
Do the methods you just described for relieving tension usually help? _____

(From Fuller, J., & Schaller-Ayers, J. (1994). *Health assessment: A nursing approach* (2nd ed.). Philadelphia: J. B. Lippincott.)

Related Factors. Related factors are gender differences in coping strategies, inadequate level of confidence in ability to cope, uncertainty, inadequate social support created by characteristics of relationships, inadequate level of perception of control, inadequate resources available, high degree of threat, situational or maturational crisis, disturbance in pattern of tension release, inadequate opportunity to prepare for stressor, inability to conserve adaptive energies, and disturbance in pattern of appraisal of threat (NANDA, 2001).

Related Nursing Diagnoses

In addition to the previously mentioned nursing diagnoses, there are other diagnoses such as Dysfunctional Grieving and Chronic Sorrow that may also be related to Ineffective Coping. When a person moves beyond normal grieving (see Chapter 48), continued inability to cope with loss leads to Dysfunctional Grieving or Chronic Sorrow in connection with Ineffective Coping.

OUTCOME IDENTIFICATION AND PLANNING

After establishing nursing diagnoses and related factors, nurses work with clients to identify goals and interventions. Goals for clients with ineffective individual coping need to be individualized by considering each client's history, areas of risk, evidence of dysfunction, and related objective data. Examples of client goals include the following:

- The client will identify sources of stress in his or her life.
- The client will identify usual personal coping strategies for stressful situations.
- The client will define the effect of stress and coping strategies on ADLs.

For clients who have related nursing diagnoses or more complex problems with stress, coping, and adaptation, the goals need to be adjusted accordingly along with the time frame in which they can be realized. Examples of some interventions useful in planning are listed in the accompanying display and discussed in the following section.

IMPLEMENTATION

Nurses can intervene independently or collaboratively to help restore function. When working with clients, assist them to recognize signs and symptoms of stress, to identify sources of distress, and to choose appropriate and safe responses. Clients may not recognize that muscle tension or feelings such as depression and anxiety are stress-related. Because the stress response is highly complex and individualized, management of that response must also be individualized. Stress management techniques that are effective for one person may not help another. People may use the same type of intervention differently. For example, people practice meditation as a therapy in many different ways (Orme-Johnson & Walton, 1998). Assist clients to find techniques that are most effective for them.

PLANNING: Examples of NIC/NOC Interventions

Accepted Stress, Coping, and Adaptation Nursing Interventions Classification (NIC)
Coping Enhancement
Self-Awareness Enhancement

Accepted Stress, Coping, and Adaptation Nursing Outcomes Classification (NOC)
Coping
Risk Control: Alcohol Use
Self-Esteem
Social Interaction Skills
Social Support

Refer to the following for specifics regarding NIC/NOC:
McCloskey, J., & Bulechek, G. (2000). *Iowa Intervention Project: Nursing Interventions Classification (NIC)* 2nd ed. St. Louis, MO: C. V. Mosby.
Johnson, M., & Maas, M. (2000). *Iowa Outcomes Project: Nursing Outcomes Classification (NOC)* 2nd ed. St. Louis, MO: C. V. Mosby.

Health Promotion

Helping clients to recognize and to manage stress is an important aspect of health promotion and disease prevention. Learning to cope effectively with stress requires self-awareness and recognition of personal manifestations of stress; this is true for nurses as well as clients (Display 49-5).

Reducing Stressors

Be sensitive to client responses that assist in recognizing stress, its source, and its meaning. By clarifying these parameters, nurses and clients can formulate approaches either to reducing stressors or to removing them entirely. Through health education, which leads to learning the causes of stress, clients can develop strategies for coping and adapting. They can continually appraise their symptoms with respect to significance for well-being and survival and can cope accordingly. For example, the working mother who is tired from putting in overtime and is struggling to spend time with her family may find herself feeling angry, fatigued, and short-tempered with her children. Help her to realize that the mood changes she is experiencing are stress-induced and that coping strategies may include changing jobs to accommodate her own and her family's needs, asking her spouse for help, or hiring part-time help.

Addressing Perfection

Perceptions can contribute to the stress response. Perfectionistic "shoulds, oughts, and musts" may compound a negative response to stress. An example is the person who tells himself or herself, "I must never make a mistake" or "I should always clean the house before going to work." Help such clients realize that a desire for perfection and unrealistic self-expectations are stress-inducing. Encourage clients to be realistic about how much they can and need to accomplish and to remember that relationships are more important than things or tasks.

DISPLAY 49-5

 STRESS MANAGEMENT FOR NURSES

Nursing practice often involves working in stressful environments, caring for clients in noisy or over-crowded spaces, visiting homes or situations that are depressing, adjusting to various work shifts, and being understaffed. Nursing literature describes two conditions that commonly affect nurses: burnout and tedium.

Burnout results from working with people who are demanding and needy, which can produce conflict within the nurse and can lead to depleted energy and low morale. Tedium results from environmental factors that create conflicts or place demands on the nurse. Physical and emotional depletion, negative self-concept, negative attitudes, and feelings of helplessness and hopelessness characterize both burnout and tedium.

Be aware of your own stress levels. Recognize your personal stress and its manifestations. One step is realizing that increased fatigue, anger, disorganization, or other behavior changes may be related to an increased level of stress. Noting changes in lifestyle factors, such as smoking, eating behaviors, or alcohol or other substance use, may provide further evidence of personal stress.

Once you recognize the ways in which you respond to stress, attend to the times when stress is most pronounced and to situations that stimulate a stress response. As you do so, take positive action to institute effective coping strategies by preventing, managing, and alleviating stress.

Suggestions for Stress Management
- Establish a regular program of exercise and activity to focus energy expenditure.
- Eliminate or restrict the amount of alcohol, caffeine, and other mood-altering substances as a means of managing stress.
- Learn to accept failure (your own and others) and turn it into a constructive experience.
- Develop techniques for assertiveness to have more feelings of personal control.
- Develop support systems with colleagues and friends to bolster personal resources.
- Have an optimistic view of the world and believe that most people are doing the best they can.

Using Supportive Internal Messages

An internal dialogue, whereby the person describes and interprets the world, is referred to as "self-talk" or internal messages. Internal messages have definite effects on daily functioning and self-concept. A constant stream of negative self-messages can lead to generalized feelings of inferiority and self-doubt. Instead of being defeated by negative internal messages, clients can learn to control them by substituting

supportive messages to help cope with difficulties. Changing internal messages involves these three steps:

- Identify what one says when the situation occurs (self-talk).
- Evaluate how rational or irrational these messages are.
- Replace the negative messages with supportive coping statements and integrate supportive statements into daily life (Nakagawa-Kogan, 1994).

For example, a person interviews for a job but is not hired. Instead of saying, "I blew it, I'm a failure; I'll never get the job I want," the person learns to restructure the negative thoughts into supportive self-statements such as, "I feel disappointed that I didn't get this job. I know I presented myself well. I have the ability to get the job I want." Encourage clients to examine internal messages and to practice rephrasing those that are negative or irrational.

Another useful behavioral strategy for gaining control over self-defeating thoughts is called "thought stopping." Thought stopping can be accomplished by using the following technique:

- When a negative or self-defeating thought crosses the mind (e.g., "I'll never be able to find a job"), say "stop" inwardly or out loud.
- Substitute a positive, assertive statement for the negative thought (e.g., "I have the skills needed to get the job I want").
- If using the word "stop" is ineffective, place a rubber band around the wrist and snap it whenever negative, unwanted thoughts occur.

Using Assertiveness

Another useful technique for changing behavior in response to stressful encounters is assertiveness. Assertive behavior enables people to act in their best interests, to stand up for themselves, to express their feelings openly and honestly, and to exercise their rights without infringing on the rights of others. Assertiveness is a learned skill that requires practice. When working with clients who have difficulty expressing feelings or meeting their needs, suggest that the client enroll in a class or workshop in assertiveness training.

Making Lifestyle Changes

Adequate rest and nutrition are important components to managing stress and coping effectively. Any person will be more capable of handling daily stressors if the body is not fatigued or malnourished. Encourage clients to get adequate sleep and nutrition, to limit or eliminate smoking, to reduce caffeine consumption, and to avoid dependence on "pill popping" (such as aspirin or tranquilizers). All such measures will promote healthier management of stress.

Exercising

Physical activity or exercise is a technique that helps counter the effects of the stress response. Vigorous physical exertion helps to release tension from the muscles and is a natural out-

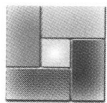

Nursing Research and Critical Thinking
Would Giving Clients a Choice About the Information They Receive Before Day Surgery Help Them to Cope More Effectively?

A nurse's review of the nursing literature led him to believe that an increased element of choice and consideration of the client's locus of control would be crucial in terms of the psychological preparation for day surgery. He designed a correlational study to evaluate the relationship between a high level of information and an internal locus of control, and a low level of information and an external locus of control. The convenience sample (N = 150) was drawn from women who were about to undergo general anesthesia for gynecologic surgery. The subjects were each given the multidimensional health locus of control (MHLC) questionnaire. Three separate scores emerged from this questionnaire: "internal," "external," and "chance" scores. A second questionnaire, the patient information questionnaire (PIQ), was designed to measure the amount of information each subject wished to receive before surgery. The subjects' MHLC score was compared with their PIQ score in order to establish a possible correlation. No correlation was established between the health locus of control and the level of selected preparatory information: in-

ternal LOC and PIQ correlation coefficient 0.02; external LOC and PIQ correlation coefficient 0.12; and chance LOC and PIQ correlation coefficient 0. Only 29.1% of the subjects had a matched coping style.

Critical Thinking Considerations. One of the confounding variables the researcher discussed is that questionnaires given to elicit information need to be completed when anxiety levels are low. However, a large number of subjects were quite anxious during the interview and time of questionnaire completion. Nursing implications of this study are as follows:

- Educational programs should ideally take place a few days or up to a week before admission to the hospital for day surgery.
- The diversity of scores within the PIQ demonstrated a desire for differing levels of preparatory information among clients.
- Each client should be given a choice regarding the level of information he or she requires.

Mitchell, M. (1997). Patients' perceptions of pre-operative preparation for day surgery. *Journal of Advanced Nursing,* 26(2), 356–363.

---

let when the body is in a fight-or-flight state of arousal. Of the broad categories of exercise, aerobic exercise and moderate, low-intensity exercise are recommended. Aerobic exercise involves sustained activity of the large muscle groups and places an increased demand on the cardiopulmonary system. Examples of aerobic exercise include running, bicycling, swimming, cross-country skiing, brisk walking, and rowing. Moderate and low-intensity exercise is less vigorous than aerobic exercise; however, it can increase muscle strength and flexibility. Researchers have recognized that walking for 20 to 30 minutes a day is beneficial and is associated with decreased risk for cardiovascular disease (Haskell, 1994). Low-intensity exercise is particularly good preparation for sedentary persons before they progress to more vigorous aerobic exercise. Additional examples of low-intensity exercise include calisthenics, gardening, and housecleaning.

Regular, moderate-intensity exercise and physical activity have substantial health benefits. Such exercise may take the form of active or passive range of motion either encouraged or performed by nurses. Display 49-6 gives examples of the benefits of exercise.

Using Relaxation Techniques

Another method of decreasing physiologic arousal is through relaxation techniques. The physiologic arousal response activates and can affect all body systems. During this state, muscle tension and heightened awareness begin to compete

with a state of relaxation. The body has the ability to elicit the "relaxation response" that directly opposes the physiologic arousal response. Dr. Herbert Benson (1976) first described the relaxation response. He discovered that meditation brought about an integrated set of physiologic changes in opposition to the fight-or-flight response including decreases in oxygen consumption, heart rate, respiratory rate, and blood lactate. This type of stress management technique is quite useful in reducing the endocrine effects of chronic stress (Orme-Johnson & Walton, 1998).

DISPLAY 49-6

⬒ HEALTH BENEFITS OF EXERCISE

- Improves muscular strength, endurance, and flexibility
- Improves cardiovascular efficiency
- Lowers resting heart rate
- Reduces blood cholesterol levels
- Reduces general anxiety and depression
- Reduces chronic fatigue and insomnia
- Lowers body weight by burning calories and suppressing appetite
- Increases absorption and use of food
- Improves appearance and self-image

Benson is the director of the Mind Body Medical Institute at Harvard. This institute's information is accessible via the Internet at the following address: *http://www.mbmi.org*. This web site contains an overview of stress, stress warning signals, and links to how to carry out the relaxation response. Several techniques have been shown to elicit the relaxation response including deep breathing, progressive relaxation, autogenics, visualization, meditation, yoga, and biofeedback. Table 49-2 presents some selected advanced stress management techniques.

Deep Breathing. Breathing is an important element of the relaxation response. As stress and tension mount during the day, breathing becomes shallow and irregular and the heart rate accelerates. Poorly oxygenated blood contributes to lethargy, tension, and depression. When a person is relaxed, breathing slows and deepens and the heart rate returns to normal. Because breathing is the easiest physiologic system to control, a person can use slow, deep breathing to trigger the relaxation response. In fact, many relaxation techniques begin by having the person slowly inhale and exhale for a few minutes.

As an incentive to practicing deep breathing, a person might associate it with something commonly done during the day such as answering the phone or looking at the clock. Frequently the act of taking a few deep breaths before a stressful situation can decrease fear and anxiety, allowing for a more relaxed frame of mind.

Progressive Relaxation. Progressive relaxation consists of systematically tensing and relaxing various muscle groups from head to toe. Many people do not realize that their muscles are in a state of chronic tension. Progressive relaxation provides a method of identifying particular muscle groups and distinguishing between sensations of tension and tranquility. Display 49-7 shows the steps involved in progressive muscle relaxation. Progressive relaxation has a more generalized systemic response than biofeedback techniques, which affect particular focused muscle responses.

Nursing Interventions for Altered Function

Nurses have a significant role in identifying people at risk for ineffective coping and in initiating appropriate teaching to promote optimal health. Many techniques that promote healthy coping can also be used for altered coping. An advantage of using stress control techniques and promoting effective coping when clients are well is that they then have the skill to use these techniques when altered function exists.

Relaxation Training

Nurses may encounter many stressful situations in all healthcare settings where it is appropriate to teach or to remind clients to use relaxation techniques. Such situations include the following:

TABLE 49-2

Selected Advanced Stress Management and Relaxation Techniques	
Autogenic training	A systematic technique teaching the body and mind to respond to verbal commands, allowing the person to achieve a deep state of relaxation through self-suggestion (or self-hypnosis).
Visualization and imagery	An attempt to affect an unconscious process by using a conscious suggestion or a mental picture of the desired change.
Affirmations	Strong, positive, feeling-rich statements about a desired change to reinforce and increase the effectiveness of visualization; can be done silently, aloud, in writing, or chanted. For example, a person with a strong sense of time urgency might use this affirmation: "I am relaxed and centered. I have plenty of time for everything."
Meditation	A traditional Eastern religious technique to achieve mental and physical relaxation. Four elements include a quiet place; a comfortable position; an object to dwell on such as a word or symbol; and a passive attitude.
Biofeedback	A specialized relaxation technique in which the person learns to monitor physiologic processes, feed back a measure of that function, and exert control over autonomic functions. Information, such as heart rate, muscle tension, and finger temperature, is translated into an auditory or visual signal that the person senses, and through these signals the person learns to discriminate between tension and relaxation.
Therapeutic touch	The use of touch to reduce anxiety and stress, relieve pain, and provide comfort.
Massage	The manipulation of soft tissue, generally with the hands, to provide stimulation and relaxation and to reduce stress and anxiety.
Yoga	A form of exercise (usually combined with meditation) to foster relaxation, mental alacrity, and good health.

DISPLAY 49-7

🔄 **PROGRESSIVE MUSCLE RELAXATION TECHNIQUE**

Progressive relaxation is a self-taught or instructed exercise that involves learning to constrict and relax muscle groups systematically, beginning with the face and finishing with the feet. This exercise may be combined with breathing exercises that focus on inner body processes. Progressive relaxation usually takes 15 to 30 minutes and may be accompanied by a taped instruction that directs the person concerning the sequence of muscles to be relaxed.

1. Wear loose clothing; remove glasses and shoes.
2. Sit or recline in a comfortable position with the neck and knees supported; avoid lying completely flat.
3. Begin with slow, rhythmic breathing.
   a. Close your eyes or stare at a spot and take in a slow, deep breath.
   b. Exhale the breath slowly.
4. Continue rhythmic breathing at a slow, steady pace and feel the tension leave your body with each breath.
5. Begin progressive relaxation of muscle groups.

   a. Breathe in and tense (tighten) your muscles, and then relax the muscles as you breathe out.
   b. Suggested order for tension–relaxation cycle (with tension technique in parentheses).
      Face, jaw, mouth (squint eyes, wrinkle brow)
      Neck (pull chin to neck)
      Right hand (make a fist)
      Right arm (bend elbow in tightly)
      Left hand (make a fist)
      Left arm (bend elbow in tightly)
      Back, shoulders, chest (shrug shoulders up tightly)
      Abdomen (pull stomach in and bear down on chair)
      Right upper leg (push leg down)
      Right lower leg and foot (point toes toward body)
      Left upper leg (push leg down)
      Left lower leg and foot (point toes toward body)
6. Practice technique slowly.
7. End relaxation session when you are ready by counting to three, inhaling deeply, and saying, "I am relaxed."

From Carpenito, L. J. (1995). *Nursing diagnosis: Applications to clinical practice* (6th ed.). Philadelphia: J. B. Lippincott.

- Before and after diagnostic tests or treatments
- During childbirth
- After surgery to help manage postoperative pain
- During recovery from myocardial infarction
- While calming an anxious or agitated person
- Before a painful procedure such as an intramuscular injection or inserting an intravenous line

Having relaxation tapes available for clients to use is becoming a common practice in institutional and community settings. Clients may purchase relaxation tapes or may want to make their own personal recordings. Telling the client to take a few deep breaths before a procedure can decrease a client's anxiety. For example, before a painful procedure or intramuscular injection, ask the client to take two or three slow, deep breaths. Usually clients experience less discomfort physically and emotionally if they are relaxed and calm.

Modifying the Environment

Nurses should be aware of environmental stressors and make adjustments whenever possible to reduce sensory overload and to assist clients with coping and adaptation. For hospitalized clients, that environment, which affords little privacy and is unfamiliar, may be the source of stress. Increased noise levels, constant lights, and unfamiliar procedures all contribute to stress.

Nurses may be instrumental in making modifications in the environment that assist clients to manage the stress of the situation and to cope with the environment. Organizing nursing care to decrease client disturbance, having as few extra lights on as possible, and keeping down the conversational noise in the hallways are a few examples. In the home, encourage families to create a room or space where clients can control the noise level and stimuli (Tyler & Ellison, 1994).

Crisis Intervention

Acute health problems, illness, loss, or trauma may precipitate a crisis in a person's life. A crisis suggests a situation in which usual coping strategies are ineffective, and the person is disorganized or unable to problem solve appropriately. To resolve a crisis, clients need assistance from family, friends, clergy, and healthcare providers including nurses. Adequate support during a crisis and its resolution can help clients realistically perceive the problem or stress and relearn or reinstitute coping strategies.

Healthcare Planning and Home/Community-Based Nursing

People who are convalescing from stress-producing situations are increasingly vulnerable to other stresses and to ineffective coping. Continued support for coping and adaptation is particularly important. Support groups can be especially effective (Fig. 49-3). These groups may be informal, such as family, friends, and spiritual sources, or they can be formal. An

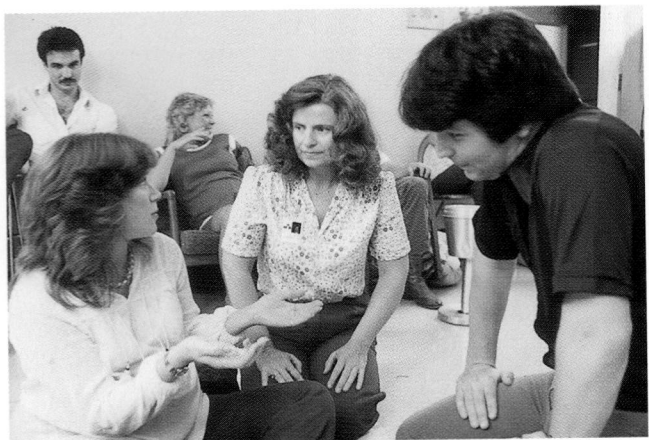

FIGURE 49-3   Support groups are valuable outlets to helping individuals learn to handle stress.

example of a formal support group is the Alzheimer's Disease and Related Disorders Association, which is composed of people who have family members with Alzheimer's disease. A group such as this can be particularly helpful for those experiencing the stress associated with caring for others and can offer many useful ideas for coping strategies and effective adaptation.

Many support groups offer assistance for specialized problems and needs. Be aware of these groups and develop networks with other healthcare professionals to link clients with them appropriately.

EVALUATION

Specific outcome criteria are the tools for measuring the attainment of client goals. Nursing interventions are the means for achieving those goals. Outcome criteria need to be specifically tailored to the individual client so they will uniquely measure the attainment of a client's goals.

Goal

The client will identify sources of stress in his or her life.

Possible Outcome Criteria

- The client defines events that create personal stress by listing them before the next meeting with the nurse.
- The client demonstrates anticipation of stressful situations by discussing them with the nurse before they occur.
- The client identifies the difference between positive and negative sources of stress in the next discussion with the nurse.

Goal

The client will identify usual personal coping strategies for stressful situations.

Possible Outcome Criteria

- The client names at least ten personal coping patterns.
- The client describes techniques that he or she uses to reinforce previous responses or to establish new responses in the next teaching session with the nurse.
- The client consciously initiates effective stress-management techniques during a stressful period, as observed by the nurse.

Goal

The client will define the effect of stress and coping strategies on ADLs.

Possible Outcome Criteria

- At the first home visit, the client identifies specific ADLs that elicit stress effects by describing them to the nurse.
- After the next teaching session with the nurse, the client describes how specific coping strategies interfere with or promote ADLs.
- At the next home visit, the client demonstrates new coping skills effective in managing stress and assisting ADLs to the visiting nurse.

KEY CONCEPTS

- Stress, an inherent part of life, may have positive or negative effects.
- Coping with stress successfully requires ongoing adaptation or change in response to stress.
- Homeostasis consists of coordinated physiologic processes that maintain steady functioning.
- Allostasis reflects the body's capacity to maintain stability in the face of constant change and to adjust to new levels of functioning.
- The hypothalamic-pituitary-adrenal axis and the sympathetic nervous system mediate the physiologic response to stress.
- Coping is a process the person uses to manage stresses or events that he or she encounters.
- Altered coping may be manifested by use of alcohol and drugs, excessive smoking, increased sleeping, withdrawal, and illness.
- Manifestations of altered coping can interfere with the person's effective management of ADLs.
- A focused nursing assessment of coping and adaptation includes the history of the client's previous coping methods, areas of risk for ineffective coping, and identification of coping and adaptation dysfunction.
- Nursing interventions include assisting the client to develop effective coping strategies to promote healthy adaptation to

NURSING PLAN OF CARE
THE CLIENT WITH INEFFECTIVE COPING

Nursing Diagnosis
Ineffective Coping related to situational crises manifested by inability to manage stressors.

Client Goal
Client will identify cause of current problems and usual personal coping strategies for stressful situations.

Client Outcome Criteria
- Client verbalizes feelings related to present emotional state within 24 to 48 hours.
- Client identifies recent stressful life events or sources of stress during first week.
- Client identifies signs and symptoms of current stress.
- Within 1 week, client identifies current coping patterns and consequences of such behavior.

Nursing Intervention	Scientific Rationale
1. Assess causative and contributive factors by discussing with client (i.e., loss, grieving, inadequate support, recent life changes).	1. Assessment of causative factors provides information from which to develop a treatment plan.

2. Assess the person's present coping status:
   Determine onset of symptoms and correlation with recent life changes
   Assess for risk of self-harm.
	2. Identification of current coping skills helps to assess adequacy/inadequacy of coping.

3. Encourage the client to evaluate the effectiveness of current coping skills.	3. Personal understanding of coping skills and outcomes reinforces use of acceptable coping or encourages the client to look for alternatives in coping.

Client Goal
Client will demonstrate appropriate coping strategies.

Client Outcome Criteria
- Client makes environmental changes to reduce stress within 1 to 3 months.
- Client practices several new coping skills (i.e., relaxation techniques, assertiveness, exercise, talking about feelings, thought stopping, affirmations).
- Client assesses effectiveness of social support network and, if inadequate, take steps to correct lack of support within 1 to 3 months.

Nursing Intervention	Scientific Rationale
1. Assist client to problem solve in a constructive manner.	1. Development of healthy coping strategies helps to eliminate or reduce stress and decrease possibility of chronic illness.
2. Help client identify problems in environment that are stressful. Discuss how to change them, if this is possible.	2. Client may need help in knowing how to make necessary changes.
3. When there are problems the client cannot control directly, help him or her identify stress-reducing techniques to use.	3. In addition to identifying techniques, the client needs to understand them and learn proper skills for their usefulness.

4. Assist client in identifying social support network.
   Encourage client to develop this support if it is helpful.
   Assist client in finding support groups to meet his or her needs.
	4. People need external as well as internal resources for coping.

stress and supporting the client in using those strategies in unusually stressful situations.
- Community-based care encompasses the use of support people or groups to maintain effective coping strategies.

REFERENCES

Bell J. M. (1977). Stressful life events and coping methods in mental illness and wellness behaviors. *Nursing Research, 26,* 136–141.

Benson, H. (1976). *The relaxation response.* New York, NY: Avon Books.

Cannon, W. B. (1935). Stressors and strains of homeostasis. *American Journal of the Medical Sciences, 189,* 1.

Chappell, P. B., Smith, M. A., Kilts, C. D., Bissette, G., Ritchie, J., Anderson, C., & Nemeroff, C. B. (1986). Alterations in corticotropin-releasing factor-like immunoreactivity in discrete rat brain regions after acute and chronic stress. *The Journal of Neuroscience, 6*(10), 2908–2914.

Dhabhar, F. S., & McEwen, B. S. (1997). Acute stress enhances while chronic stress suppresses cell-mediated immunity in vivo: A potential role for leukocyte trafficking. *Brain, Behavior, and Immunity, 11,* 286–306.

Dunn, A. J., & Berridge, C. W. (1990). Physiological and behavioral responses to corticotropin-releasing factor administration: is CRF a mediator of anxiety or stress responses? *Brain Research Review, 15*(2), 71–100.

Fuller, J., & Schaller-Ayers, J. (1994). *Health assessment: A nursing approach* (2nd ed.). Philadelphia: J. B. Lippincott.

Groer M. W., Thomas, S. P. & Shoffner, D. (1992). Adolescent stress and coping: a longitudinal study. *Research in Nursing and Health, 15,* 209–217.

Hall, W. A. (1994). New fatherhood: Myths and realities. *Public Health Nursing, 11,* 219–228.

Haskell, W. L. (1994). Health consequences of physical activity: Understanding and challenges regarding dose-response. *Medicine and Science in Sports and Exercise, 26,* 649–660.

Holmes, T. H., & Rahe, R. H. (1967). The social readjustment and rating scale. *Journal of Psychosomatic Research, 11,* 213–218.

Kammer, C. H. (1994). Stress and coping of family members responsible for nursing home placement. *Research in Nursing and Health, 17*(2), 89–98.

Kaplan, H. B. (1991). Social psychology of the immune system: A conceptual framework and review of the literature. *Social Science and Medicine, 33,* 909–923.

Kiecolt-Glaser, J. K., & Glaser, R. (1995). Psychoneuroimmunology and health consequences: Data and shared mechanisms. *Psychosomatic Medicine, 57,* 269–274.

LaMontagne, L. L. (2000). Children's coping with surgery: A process-oriented perspective. *Journal of Pediatric Nursing, 15,* 307–312.

Lazarus, R. S. (1981). Little hazards can be hazardous to your health. *Psychology Today, 15*(7), 58–62.

Lazarus, R. (1991a). Cognition and motivation in emotion. *American Psychologist, 46,* 352–367.

———. (1991b). Progress on a cognitive-motivational-relational theory of emotion. *American Psychologist, 46,* 819–834.

Lazarus, R. S. (1992). Coping with the stress of illness. *WHO Regional Publications European Series, 44,* 11–31.

Lazarus, R. S. & Folkman, S. (1984). *Stress, appraisal, and coping.* New York: Springer.

McEwen, B. S. (1998). Protective and damaging effects of stress mediators. *New England Journal of Medicine, 338*(3), 171–179.

McEwen, B. S. (2000). The neurobiology of stress: From serendipity to clinical relevance. *Brain Research, 886,* 172–189.

Miller, L. H., Smith, A. D., & Mehler, B. L. (1991). *The stress audit.* Brookline, MA: Biobehavioral Association.

Nakagawa-Kogan, H. (1994). Self-management training: Potential for primary care. *Nurse Practitioner Forum, 5*(2), 77–84.

North American Nursing Diagnosis Association (NANDA). (2001). *NANDA nursing diagnoses: Definitions and classification 2000–2001.* Philadelphia: Author.

Orme-Johnson, D. W., & Walton, K. G. (1998). All approaches to preventing or reversing effects of stress are not the same. *American Journal of Health Promotion, 12*(5), 297–299.

Porter, N. M., Herman, J. P., and Landfield, P. W. (2001). Mechanisms of glucocorticoid actions in stress and brain aging. In B. S. McEwen and H. M. Goodman (Eds.), *Handbook of Physiology, Section 7: The Endocrine System* (pp. 293–312). New York: Oxford University Press, Inc.

Puskar, L. R., Lamb, J. M., & Bartolovic, M. (1993). Examining the common stressors and coping methods of rural adolescents. *Nurse Practitioner, 18*(11), 50–53.

Rudolph, K. D. & Hammen C. (1999). Age and gender as determinants of stress exposure, generation, and reactions in youngsters: a transactional perspective. *Child Development, 70,* 660–677.

Sapolsky, R. M., Romero, L. M. & Munck, A. U. (2000). How do glucocorticoids influence stress responses? Integrating permissive, suppressive, stimulatory, and preparative actions. *Endocrine Reviews, 21,* 55–89.

Selye, H. (1974). *Stress without disease.* Philadelphia: J. B. Lippincott.

Sorensen, E. S. (1994). Daily stressors and coping responses: A comparison of rural and suburban children. *Public Health Nursing, 11,* 24–31.

Spiegel, K., Leproult, R., & Van Cauter, E. (1999). Impact of sleep debt on metabolic and endocrine function. *The Lancet, 354,* 1435–1439.

Taylor, S. E., Klein, L. C., Lewis, B. P., Gruenewald, T. L., Gurung, A. R., & Updegraff, J. A. (2000). Biobehavioral responses to stress in females: Tend-and-befriend, not fight-or-flight. *Psychological Review, 107,* 411–429.

Tyler, P. A., & Ellison, R. N. (1994). Sources of stress and psychological well-being in high-dependency nursing. *Journal of Advanced Nursing, 19,* 469–476.

Van Cauter, E., Leproult, R. & Kupfer, D. J. (1996). Effects of gender and age on levels and circadian rhythmicity of plasma cortisol. *Journal of Clinical Endocrinology and Metabolism, 81,* 2468–2473.

Walker, C., Anand, K. J. S., & Plotsky, P. M. (2001). Development of the hypothalamic-pituitary-adrenal axis and the stress response. In B. S. McEwen and H. M. Goodman (Eds.), *Handbook of physiology, section 7: The endocrine system* (pp. 237–270). New York: Oxford University Press, Inc.

Wineman, N. M., Durand, E. J., & McCulloch, B. J. (1994). Examination of the factor structure of the Ways of Coping Questionnaire with clinical populations. *Nursing Research, 43,* 268–273.

Wolff, H. G. (1953). *Stress and disease.* Springfield, IL: Charles C Thomas.

BIBLIOGRAPHY

Beaton, R. D., Egan, K. J., Nakagawa-Kogan, H., & Morrison, K. N. (1991). Self-reported symptoms of stress with temporomandibular disorders: Comparisons to healthy men and women. *Journal of Prosthetic Dentistry, 65,* 289–293.

Brashares, J. J., & Catanzaro, S. J. (1994). Mood regulation expectancies, coping responses, depression, and sense of burden in female caregivers of Alzheimer's patients. *Journal of Nervous and Mental Disease, 182,* 437–442.

Eccles, A. M. (1990). Using humor to relieve stress. *Point of View, 27*(1), 8–9.

Everly, G. S., & Lating, J. M. (1994). *Psychotraumatology: Key papers and core concepts in post-traumatic stress.* New York, NY: Plenum Press.

Gilligan, B. (1993). A positive coping strategy: Humour in the oncology setting. *Professional Nurse, 8,* 231–233.

Hahn, W. K., Brooks, J. A., & Hartsough, D. M. (1993). Self-disclosure and coping styles in men with cardiovascular reactivity. *Research in Nursing and Health, 16,* 275–282.

Humphrey, J. H. (1994). *Human stress: Current selected research, 1986–1993* (Vols. 1–5). New York, NY: AMS Press.

Levine, S., & Scotch, N. (1970). *Social stress.* Chicago, IL: Aldine Publishing.

Maslow, A. (1954). *Motivation and personality.* New York, NY: Harper Brothers.

Mason, J. W. (1975a). A historical view of the stress field, part 1. *Journal of Human Stress, 1,* 6–12.

———. (1975b). A historical view of the stress field, part 2. *Journal of Human Stress, 1*(2), 22–36.

Pelletier, K. (1977). *Mind as healer, mind as slayer.* New York, NY: Dell.

Pepin, J., Ducharme, F., Kerouac, S., Levesque, L., Ricard, N., & Duquette, A. (1994). The development of a research program based on a conceptual model for the discipline of nursing. *Canadian Journal of Nursing Research, 26*(1), 41–53.

Rahe, R. H. (1993). Acute versus chronic post-traumatic stress disorder. *Integrative Physiological and Behavioral Science, 28*(1), 46–56.

Roberts, S. J. (1994). Somatization in primary care: The common presentation of psychosocial problems through physical complaints. *Nurse Practitioner, 19*(5), 47, 50–56.

Ryan-Wenger, N. M. (1994). Coping behavior in children: Methods of measurement for research and clinical practice. *Journal of Pediatric Nursing, 9*(3), 183–195.

Selye, H. (1982). History and present status of the stress concept. In L. Goldberger & S. Breznitz (Eds.), *Handbook of stress.* New York, NY: Free Press.

Smith, J. G. (1990). *Cognitive–behavioral relaxation training.* New York, NY: Springer.

Troop, N. A., Holbrey, A., Trowler, R., & Treasure, J. L. (1994). Ways of coping in women with eating disorders. *Journal of Nervous and Mental Disease, 182,* 535–540.

Vander, A. J., Sherman, J., & Luciano, D. (1997). *Human physiology: The mechanisms of body function* (7th ed.). New York, NY: McGraw-Hill.

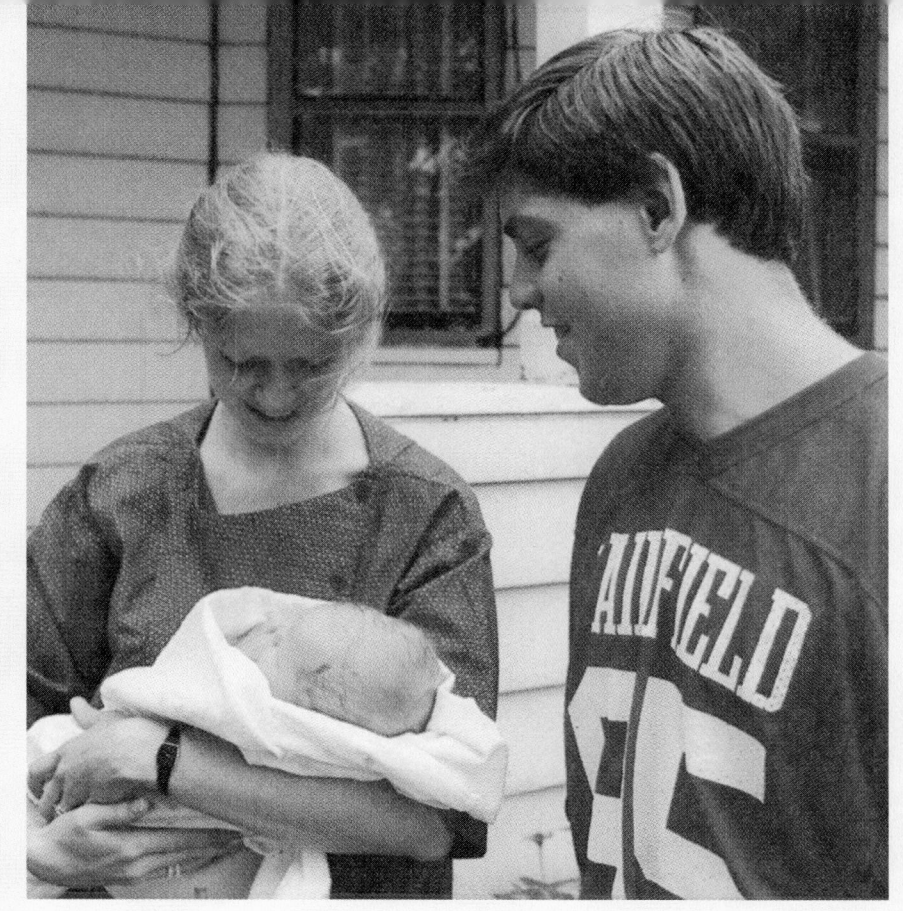

Sexuality and Reproduction

50 Human Sexuality

Key Terms

bisexual
celibacy
climacteric
clitoris
dyspareunia
foreplay
foreskin
heterosexual
homosexual
impotence

masturbation
menarche
menopause
orgasm
premature ejaculation
prepuce
sexuality
transsexual
vaginismus

Learning Objectives

Upon completion of this chapter, the student will be able to do the following:

1. Describe the structures of the male and female reproductive systems.
2. Discuss sexual expression, menstruation, and reproduction as functions of human sexuality.
3. Compare the male and female sexual response cycles.
4. Relate sexuality to all stages of the life cycle.
5. Identify factors that affect sexual functioning.
6. Describe common risks and alterations in sexuality.
7. Understand the nursing process as it relates to sexual functioning.
8. Perform breast self-examination or testicular self-examination.

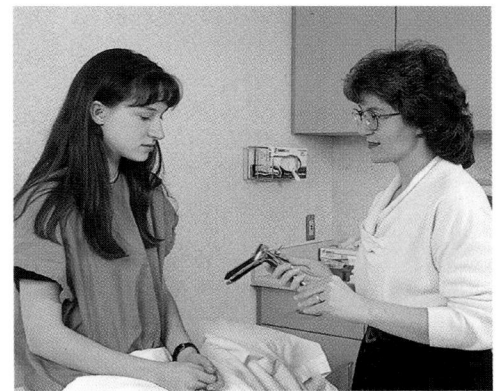

Critical Thinking Challenge

You are a nurse working in a teen clinic. A young woman comes in for an examination because she has noticed a lesion on her labia and she is worried that she might be pregnant. Upon taking a history from her, you learn that she has had sexual intercourse with two different young men and she has not used anything for contraception.

Once you have completed this chapter and added knowledge of human sexuality to your data base, reflect on the following areas of Critical Thinking:

1. Reflect on your feelings and impression about this situation. Distill possible explanations for your reactions.
2. Propose additional information that you would need to elicit from this woman, including your rationale for needing such information.
3. Describe how you would you elicit this information in such a way that this young woman will continue to "trust" you.
4. Describe a plan for follow-up for this patient.

Although marked openness is found in today's media regarding sexual matters, some people are hesitant to discuss personal sexuality and sexual issues especially with strangers. The nurse's challenge relating to such discussions is complex in today's context of more open sexual expression combined with heightened fears of sexually transmitted diseases (STDs).

Most nurses work with clients in settings that are not directly related to sexuality. Clients in any setting, however, may approach nurses with concerns regarding sexuality. Sexual issues, then, should be part of the client history. Although some common problems can be dealt with in the healthcare facility (by healthcare providers with general knowledge of human sexuality), more advanced problems require attention from specially trained personnel. Each nurse must be aware of his or her personal attitudes, expertise, and limitations. These should not, however, interfere with care given.

Recently a thoughtful and provocative document, *The Surgeon General's Call to Action To Promote Sexual Health and Responsible Sexual Behavior* (2001), was released by the U.S. Office of the Surgeon General. Approaching sexuality issues from a public health perspective, this document emphasizes the challenges to promoting responsible sexual behavior with the goal of promoting general health and wellness in our society. In addition, the Surgeon General has deemed responsible sexual behavior as one of the top ten health indicators of the nation (*Healthy People 2010*).

NORMAL HUMAN SEXUALITY

Sexuality includes function of the sexual organs and the person's perceptions of his or her own functioning, sexual expression, and preferences. Human sexual response varies and is influenced by many factors. Such factors include psychological, emotional, and cultural issues; values and moral views;

and comfort with one's body and the quality of any sexual relationships. A person not involved in a sexual relationship is still a sexual being with a sexual identity.

Structure of the Reproductive Systems

Although sexuality is not synonymous with reproduction, the reproductive organs are involved in human sexual response. For purposes of clarity, the male and female reproductive systems are discussed separately.

Male Reproductive System

The male reproductive system (Fig. 50-1) is composed of both external and internal organs. The external organs include the penis and scrotum. The penis is a cylindrical, pendulous, erectile organ composed of the shaft and glans. The shaft contains the urethra, the outlet for urine from the urinary bladder. The glans is the cone-shaped head of the penis; it is covered with loose skin called the **prepuce** or **foreskin.** Uncircumcised men can retract the glans for intercourse and cleaning. In circumcised men, the glans is exposed because the foreskin has been removed surgically. The scrotum is the loose, pouchlike sac containing the testes. The testes are the male gonads, which are the reproductive glands that produce male cells (spermatozoa) and testosterone (male hormone).

The internal organs include the prostate gland and seminal vesicles. These glands produce and store most of the seminal fluid. The combination of seminal fluid and spermatozoa forms semen, the secretion discharged from the urethra during orgasm.

Female Reproductive System

The female reproductive system also includes external and internal organs. External genitalia include the mons pubis, labia majora, labia minora, clitoris, urethral meatus, Skene's

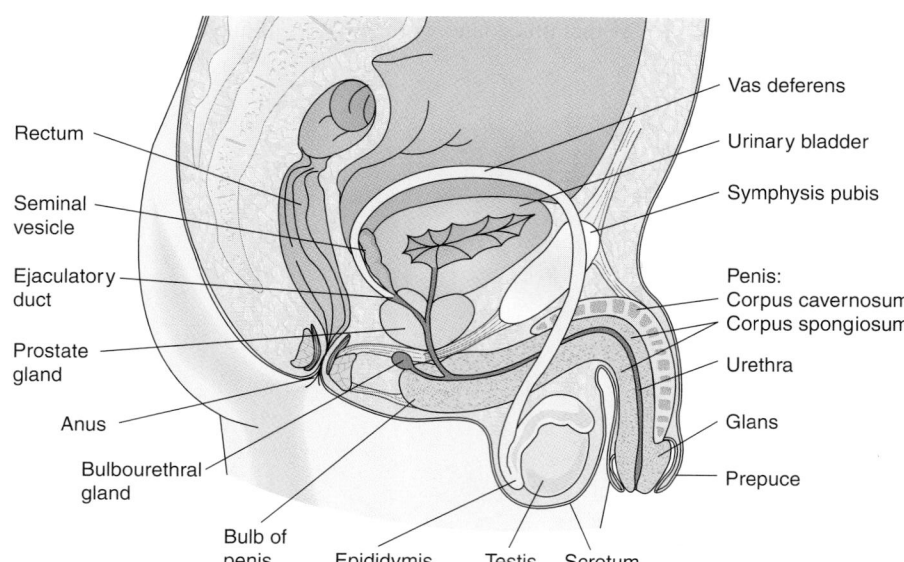

FIGURE 50-1   Internal and external organs of the male reproductive system.

and Bartholin's glands, and the vaginal orifice (Fig. 50-2A). Collectively, these external parts are referred to as the vulva.

The mons pubis is a pad of fatty tissue over the bony prominence called the symphysis pubis. The labia are the fleshy borders of the external genitalia. The labia majora lie on either side of the vaginal opening, forming the lateral borders. The labia minora are thinner folds that lie just inside the labia majora.

The **clitoris** corresponds to the penis in the male in that both organs respond to stimulation that can result in orgasm.

Skene's glands lie inside of and on the posterior of the urethra, and Bartholin's glands are small mucous glands on the lateral wall of the vestibule of the vagina. The Skene's and the Bartholin's glands produce a small amount of lubricant. Although it was once believed that these glands were responsible for producing enough vaginal lubricant during sexual arousal in actuality they only produce a very small amount.

The internal genitalia include the ovaries, fallopian tubes, uterus, and vagina (Fig. 50-2B). The ovaries are two almond-

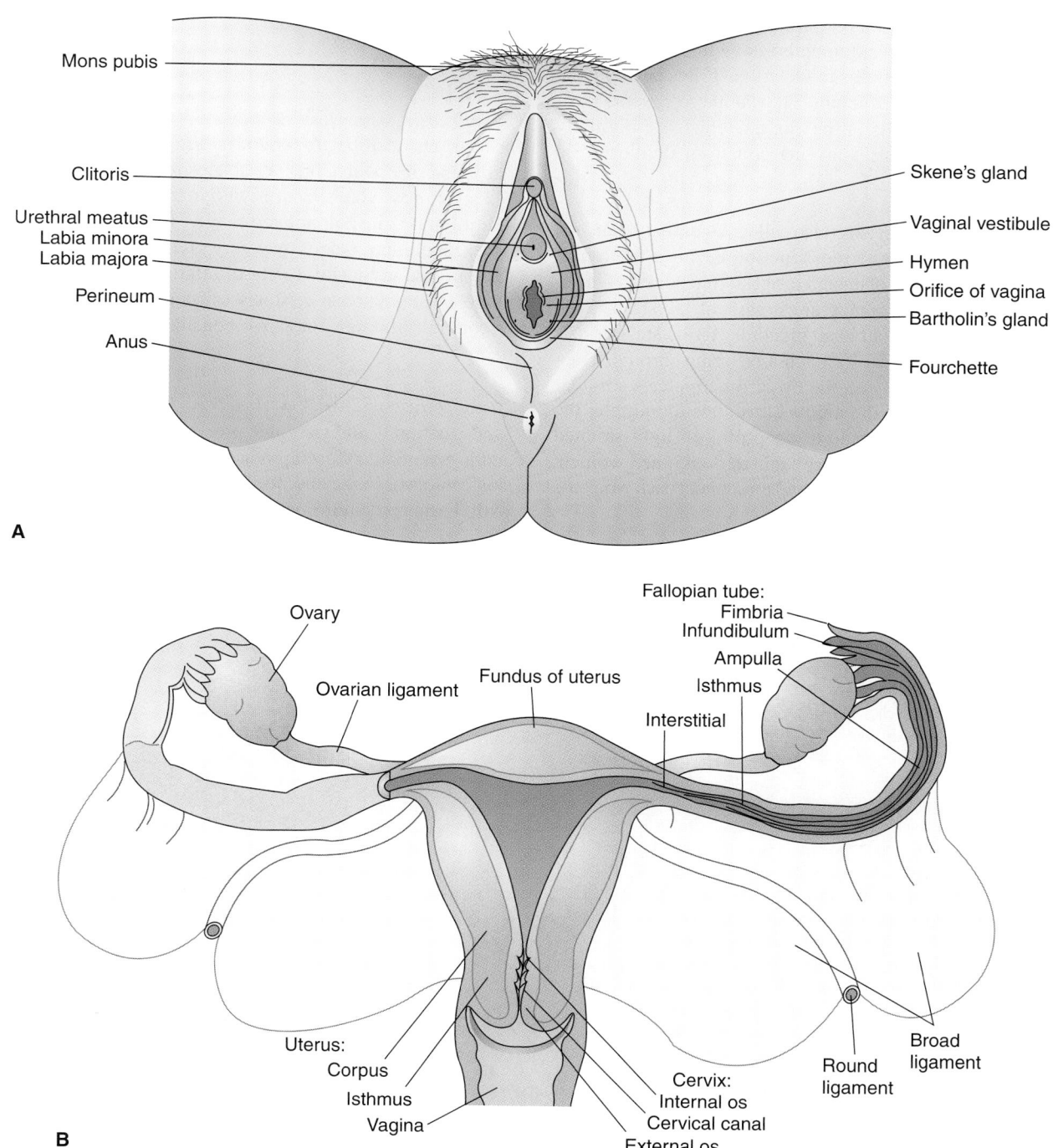

FIGURE 50-2 Female reproductive system. (**A**) External genitalia. (**B**) Internal genitalia.

shaped bodies lying on either side of the pelvic cavity. They contain the ova (female sex cells) and female hormones, specifically estrogen and progesterone. Fallopian tubes are narrow ducts of about 4.5 inches (11.4 cm) in length. They extend laterally on either side of the uterus and terminate in finger-like projections near but not touching the ovaries.

The uterus is a muscular, pear-shaped organ that lies between the sacrum and the symphysis pubis. It consists of three areas: the fundus or upper portion; the cavity, which is hollow; and the lower end, the cervix that connects the uterus to the vagina. The uterus is expandable.

The vagina is a musculomembranous tube that forms a passageway from the uterus to the vulva. It lies between the urinary bladder and the rectum. The vagina represents a potential space—the walls of the vagina, which are normally in contact, stretch for sexual intercourse or delivery of a baby.

Breasts.   The female breasts (also called "mammary glands") are considered organs of reproduction because the reproductive hormones, estrogen and progesterone, directly influence them and because they are organs of lactation. Each breast is composed of fatty and glandular tissue and consists of 15 to 20 lobes (Fig. 50-3). Each lobe drains through a lactiferous duct that opens on the tip of the nipple. A circular pigmented area called the areola surrounds the nipple; the color of the areola is a pale to deep pink in light-skinned women and a light to darker brown in dark-skinned women. Breast size varies among women and throughout each woman's lifespan.

Function of Sexuality and the Reproductive Systems

Reproduction is only one component of sexuality. Human beings can be sexual—engage in sexual relationships and find sexual expression—without reproducing. The male reproductive system is responsible for the generation, maturation, and ejaculation of spermatozoa. The female reproductive system is responsible for cyclic maturation and release of ova and, should fertilization occur, preparation of the uterus for implantation of a fertilized ovum. The experiences of menstruation, ovulation, and lactation are related to the woman's reproductive process.

Sexual Expression

Sexual expression varies among individuals. People may use various positions for coitus and stimulation without any particular one being considered "normal." The frequency of sexual expression also varies with no determined "normal." Additionally, the amount and kind of **foreplay** (activity before sexual intercourse) may vary greatly. Some people engage in **masturbation** (self-stimulation) with a partner or alone. Others choose **celibacy** (abstention from sexual intercourse) although they still consider themselves sexual beings.

Menstruation and Ovulation

Menstruation is a physiologic process that occurs in women and is essential to their reproductive function. Sexual expression can occur in the absence of menstruation (e.g., a woman with Turner's syndrome [a genetic condition in which a

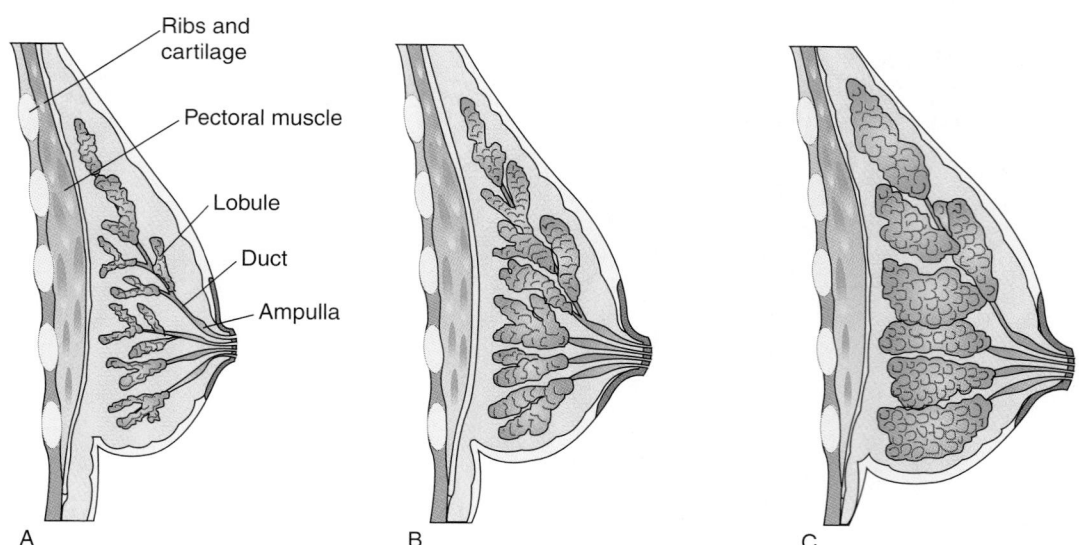

FIGURE 50-3   The structure of the breasts varies among women and during a woman's lifetime. The illustration shows the breast in the **(A)** nonpregnant woman, **(B)** pregnant woman, and **(C)** lactating woman.

woman is born without ovaries and does not menstruate] or a woman who has gone through menopause). Because of its direct connection with reproduction, however, menstruation is appropriate to discuss in this chapter. Menstruation is a cyclic, periodic discharge of bloody fluid from the uterus through the vagina during the woman's reproductive years. The length of a menstrual cycle varies among women and during each woman's lifespan. The cycle repeats itself approximately every 28 days although a normal range could be every 21 to 35 days.

Menstruation depends on the interplay of various hormones (Fig. 50-4). The hypothalamus secretes gonadotropin-releasing hormone, which stimulates the pituitary gland to secrete follicle-stimulating hormone and luteinizing hormone. These hormones stimulate the ovaries to produce estrogen and progesterone, which are necessary for stimulation of the target organs (vagina, breast, uterus) in preparing the body for possible pregnancy. If pregnancy does not occur, levels of estrogen and progesterone fall, menses ensues, and the feedback mechanism begins again with a new menstrual cycle.

The menstrual cycle is discussed in terms of the ovarian cycle and the endometrial or uterine cycle. The ovarian cycle consists of the follicular phase, the ovulatory phase, and the luteal phase. The follicular phase is estrogen-dominant; during this phase, the follicles mature with usually only one follicle reaching full maturity. This follicle, or oocyte, ruptures from the ovary at the time of the ovulatory phase. Progesterone then becomes the dominant hormone during the luteal phase, preparing the uterus for possible implantation and maintenance of a fertilized ovum.

The endometrial or uterine cycle is divided into the proliferative and secretory phases. The proliferative phase refers to the proliferation of the endometrium, or uterine lining. Estrogen is the dominant hormone during the proliferative phase. During the secretory phase, which is progesterone-dominant, the endometrial glands continue to grow, becoming edematous and dense, in preparation for implantation and maintenance of a fertilized ovum.

Hormones also affect the uterus at the cervical level. Under the influence of estrogen, the cervical mucus becomes more watery, alkaline, and stretchy, resembling the quality of egg whites. These qualities are conducive to sperm's survival, thus preparing for the possibility of conception.

Conception, Pregnancy, and Birth

For conception and reproduction to occur, several complicated factors must fully operate. First, the man must produce fully mature spermatozoa in sufficient numbers and with enough motility to penetrate the woman's cervix and to ascend the uterus and fallopian tubes. This transportation occurs by way of cervical mucus, which becomes alkaline and thus receptive to sperm. When the spermatozoa reach the fallopian tubes, they undergo capacitation, a process in which the sperm's surface characteristics change, releasing enzymes that enhance their ability to penetrate the ovum.

The occurrence of ovulation must correspond to the process described earlier because the time period in which the woman can be impregnated is only a few days. In ovulation, the ovary releases a mature follicle into one of the fallopian tubes. The fimbriae or finger-like projections at the end of each fallopian tube assist in extracting the ovum from the ovary and bringing it into the fallopian tube.

Fertilization of one ovum with one spermatozoon normally occurs in the outer third of the fallopian tube (see Fig. 50-2). After fertilization, the fertilized ovum undergoes several cell divisions and moves toward the uterus, where it implants in the uterine wall. The first 2 weeks after fertilization are critical; many pregnancies do not continue beyond this point because of a defective ovum or spermatozoon or because of hormone imbalances. If a pregnancy continues in spite of these complex factors and potential risks, the fertilized ovum, now called an embryo, develops rapidly. The average length of pregnancy, counted from the time of conception, is approximately 267 days or 38 weeks but may vary by about 2 weeks in either direction.

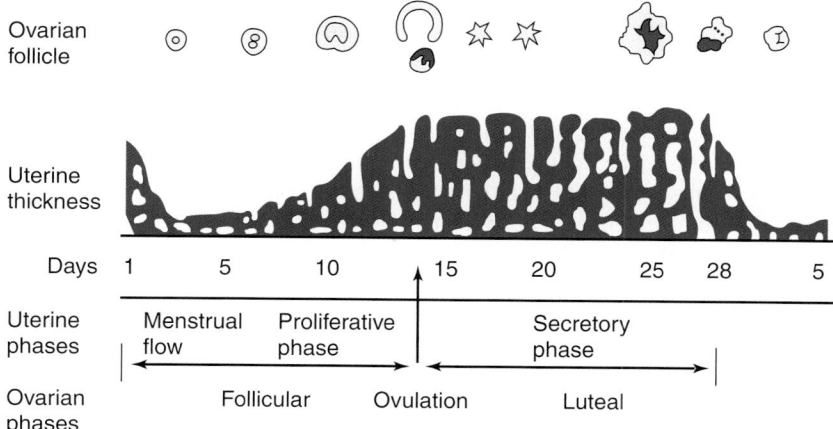

FIGURE 50-4   Schematic representation of one ovarian cycle and the corresponding changes in endometrial thickness. The ovarian cycle includes the changes within the corpus luteum and follicle. The endometrial changes indicate the thickness of the endometrium just before the onset of menstruation and its thinness just as menstruation ends.

Birth is a normal process that occurs in three stages of labor. Although its initiation is not entirely understood, labor involves stimulation by hormones that cause the uterus to contract, thus pushing the fetus through the birth canal after a number of hours.

Milk Production

With pregnancy, the woman's breasts undergo anatomic and physiologic changes (see Fig. 50-3B). They enlarge and become more sensitive. The nipples expand and darken, and the sebaceous glands in the areola hypertrophy. During the second half of pregnancy, the alveolar cells may begin to secrete colostrum. This yellowish fluid, considered a precursor to actual milk, contains important nutrients for the newborn (see Fig. 50-3C).

Milk production occurs under the influence of prolactin, glucocorticoids, insulin, and parathyroid hormone. Estrogen and progesterone actually inhibit milk production; thus with the delivery of the placenta, estrogen and progesterone levels fall dramatically.

Characteristics of Normal Sexuality

Sexual Orientation

Various forms of sexual orientation exist. As mentioned earlier, no one way is "normal" in terms of sexuality and sexual orientation. Some people are **heterosexual,** relating sexually to members of the opposite gender. Others are **bisexual,** relating to both men and women sexually. Others are **homosexual,** relating sexually to members of the same gender. Still others abstain totally from sexual relations either permanently or temporarily.

Gender Identity and Roles

Gender identity and corresponding roles influence sexuality. Nurses must understand each client's perception of his or her gender and the meaning of that gender in terms of identity and roles.

Sometimes a person's biologic gender does not coincide with his or her gender identity, as in the case of people who are transsexual. A **transsexual** man views himself as a woman trapped in a man's body; the reverse is true for a female transsexual. Social roles are usually confusing for transsexuals. Some marry and have families; others do not. Some seek medical intervention in the form of hormones and surgery to change their physical gender. Sometimes, the terms *transsexual* and *transvestite* are used interchangeably although incorrectly. Transsexuals may maintain an appearance consistent with their biologic gender. Transvestites choose to dress like and appear as someone of the opposite sex but may view themselves according to their biologic gender.

Normal Sexual Patterns

Sexual Response

Masters and Johnson (1966) were the first to study scientifically the human sexual response. They found that humans undergo four distinct phases of sexual response: excitement, plateau, orgasm, and resolution. The excitement phase results from various stimuli, both physiologic and psychological. If there are no distracting stimuli, this phase will continue and intensify as the person reaches the plateau phase in which sexual tension increases. If this sexual tension continues without distracting stimuli, orgasm or involuntary climax occurs. During orgasm, the person experiences involuntary contractions and release of vasocongestion that builds in the preceding phases. The resolution phase refers to the period after orgasm in which physiologic changes allow the body to return to its preexcitement state. These phases will be discussed more specifically as experienced by men and women. Note, however, that other researchers have defined the sexual response pattern slightly differently (Lauver & Welch, 1990). Kaplan (1979), for example, defines the sexual response cycle according to three phases: desire, excitement, and orgasm. The American Psychiatric Association (1994) developed a slightly different description of the sexual response consisting of four phases: appetitive, excitement, orgasm, and resolution. Because Masters and Johnson's work is considered "classic" and much subsequent research is based on their work, this chapter presents detailed descriptions based on their model.

Male Sexual Response. Masters and Johnson (1966) found one pattern of sexual response in men, although according to Woods (1984) it is unlikely that male sexual response occurs without variation. The predominant pattern includes a rapid excitement phase, a short plateau phase with orgasm occurring immediately, and a resolution phase that includes an obligatory refractory period.

Excitement. The excitement phase is characterized by rapid erection of the penis with tensing and thickening of the scrotal skin and elevation of the scrotal sac. The spermatic cords shorten, causing partial elevation of both testes toward the perineum. Vasocongestion during this phase is responsible for penile erection, thickening of the scrotal skin, and elevation of the scrotal sac. The testes increase in size. The man may experience nipple erection during the excitement phase. It is not unusual for the man partially to lose his penile erection and regain it. Distractions may interfere with excitement.

Plateau. The plateau phase involves a thickening of the penis circumference at the coronal ridge and an increase in size of the testes by about 50% (Woods, 1984). A few drops of fluid appear at the urethral meatus. This fluid is produced from Cowper's glands and contributes to lubrication. Additionally, this fluid may contain some active spermatozoa. The man may experience nipple erection, and a sex flush, characterized by a maculopapular rash over the epigastric area, may appear during the latter part of this phase. Increases occur in voluntary and involuntary muscle contraction, ventilation, heart rate, and blood pressure.

Orgasm. **Orgasm** is the climax of the plateau phase and consists of expulsive contractions of the entire length of the urethra. The initial three or four contractions are strongest, then they subsequently decrease. Concurrently, the force of ejaculation is greatest with the first several contractions and decreases thereafter. Ejaculation can be viewed as composed of two stages (Woods, 1984). The first stage consists of expulsion of seminal fluid substrate from the seminal vesicles into the prostatic urethra. The second stage consists of expulsion of the seminal fluid from the prostatic urethra to the urethral meatus.

Resolution. Resolution, the fourth and final phase, occurs immediately after orgasm and consists of an initial rapid loss of vasocongestion with an accompanying decrease in penis size. The scrotum becomes less congested, and the testes descend back into the scrotum decreasing to their preexcitement size. Sex flush and nipple erection, if they occurred, disappear. Men experience an obligatory refractory period during which they are unable to be restimulated to erection. The length of this period varies individually.

Female Sexual Response. Although they found only one response pattern in men, Masters and Johnson (1966) found some variability in the patterns of sexual response among women. Some women experience a plateau phase with several peaks without actually experiencing orgasm. Others experience a definite orgasm; still others experience multiple orgasms. Masters and Johnson believe that many other patterns also exist in women's sexual responses.

Excitement. The excitement phase in women consists of clitoral enlargement and vaginal lubrication in response to vasocongestion. The vaginal space expands in the inner one-third portion, and the uterus may become elevated. The vaginal orifice opens as the labia majora and minora either separate or move away slightly. The woman may also experience nipple erection and breast enlargement. She may experience a sex flush similar to that described earlier for men.

Plateau. The plateau phase involves retraction of the clitoris under the clitoral hood. The labia minora increase, and the vagina expands in width and depth. Full elevation of the uterus with concurrent rising of the cervix occurs. Nipple erection may continue, and the sex flush may spread. Both voluntary and involuntary muscle contractions increase, as do ventilation, heart rate, and blood pressure.

Orgasm. The orgasmic platform, or the outer third of the vagina and the labia minora, is the location of primary response during the orgasmic phase. Contractions occur very quickly and strongly in this area. After the initial three to six contractions, intensity and frequency decrease. The woman experiences increased respiratory rate, heart rate, and blood pressure. Controversy exists as to whether women experience fluid expulsion during orgasm. Some research reports that women have described feeling a gushing of fluid along with orgasm (Belzer, 1981). More recently, attention has focused on the differences in women's subjective experiences of orgasm (Bernhard, 1995).

Resolution. The resolution phase includes a return of the clitoris to normal size and position. Vasocongestion dissipates with resulting decrease in size of the orgasmic platform and vaginal relaxation. The woman does not have an obligatory refractory period and may experience multiple orgasms in a short period.

Lifespan Considerations

Rynerson (1990) has outlined the stages of the life cycle with reference to sexuality, incorporating the earlier work of Woods and Stamer (1984), who adapted the work of Mims and Swenson (1980). This section examines sexuality at each developmental stage, emphasizing physiologic, emotional, and social aspects. Figure 50-5 shows couples at two ends of the spectrum of male–female relationships.

Prenatal

The new organism's chromosomal formation is determined when the ovum and spermatozoon unite during fertilization. The sperm carries either an X or a Y chromosome to combine

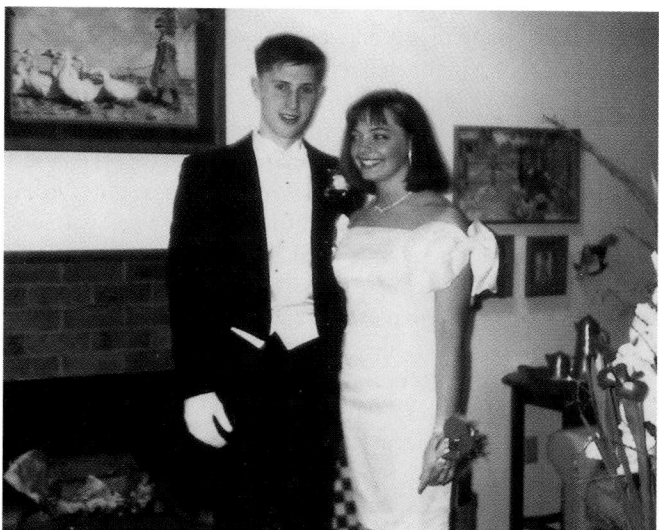
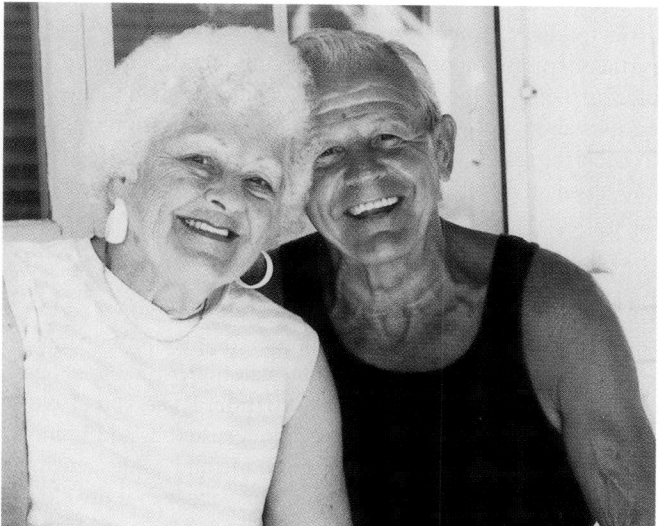

FIGURE 50-5   Expressions of sexuality from two aspects of the lifespan. A key aspect of adolescent development is learning to develop relationships. In older adulthood, warmth, intimacy, and companionship are comfortable aspects of sexuality.

with the X chromosome that the ovum supplies. An XX combination becomes a female and an XY combination becomes a male at about the 5th or 6th week of prenatal life. Hormonal influences also play an important part in determining gonadal sex. In addition to the presence of an XY zygote, androgens must be present and cells must be sensitive to androgens for male genitalia to form. Lack of sensitivity to androgens, even in the presence of an XY genotype, will lead to development of female genitalia.

If genetic errors occur that lead to ambiguous genitalia, parents will have difficulty assigning gender to their newborn. Under normal circumstances, parents automatically interact with their child according to the child's gender. Problems such as ambiguous genitalia or lack of particular sex hormones may create serious problems in relating to a child as male or female and may create serious problems for the child as he or she matures.

Newborn and Infant

Touching and cuddling from parents and other caregivers are of crucial importance to the normal psychosexual development of newborns and infants. Development of trust should occur during these stages, paving the way for future healthy interpersonal relationships. Parents normally relate to their infants as either male or female, which has consequences for later development. Because infants are very sensitive to touch, they commonly explore their own bodies including genitalia. Parents and other caregivers should recognize this developmental process as normal.

Toddler and Preschooler

As children become toddlers, they learn to walk and gain independence. They begin to explore their bodies even more while developing a body image that includes sexual identity. Toddlers may engage in masturbation, and parents should be reassured that this behavior is normal and healthy for development.

As toddlers become preschoolers, they begin to engage in further exploration of the body. Playing with friends and exploring their own bodies are normal. Children at this stage are curious about body parts and may often ask questions related to such things as where babies come from, breast-feeding, and physical differences between men and women and boys and girls.

School-Age Child and Adolescent

During elementary school, children continue to adopt certain sex role behaviors and usually maintain friendships with those of the same sex. Children learn about anatomy, particularly their genitals, and may engage in masturbation. Rynerson (1990) notes that experimentation in both heterosexual and homosexual roles is a normal part of childhood and adolescence.

Adolescence is a turbulent time of psychosexual development. Adolescents not only cope with development of identity and independence from parents; they concurrently experience a surge of hormonal changes leading to the physiologic changes of puberty.

A key point in the development of adolescent girls is the onset of menstruation. The first menstrual period is termed **menarche.** Development of breasts and an adult female shape and proportions coincides with puberty. Adolescent girls become concerned with these physical changes, often equating them with acceptance, confidence, and popularity as well as sexual identity.

Adolescent boys begin to experience nocturnal emissions. They assume a masculine sexual identity and behaviors based on role models and personal expectations. Teen boys are usually competitive in all areas of life, particularly sexual activity.

Sexual experimentation during adolescence is not without consequences. According to the Alan Guttmacher Institute (1994), the previous three decades witnessed major increases in the rate of teenage pregnancies in the United States. Grimes and Wallach (1997) reported that the teenage pregnancy rate has decreased by 19% over the last two decades, but that the proportion of teenagers engaging in intercourse has also increased. Interpersonal relationship conflicts, STDs, as well as pregnancy are common problems during adolescence. Awareness of sexual orientation usually begins during the teen years, and studies have indicated that homosexual teens may be at a higher risk for suicide. Understanding this phenomenon is of critical importance for nurses caring for teenagers.

Adult and Older Adult

The period between the tumultuous changes of adolescence and the climacteric spans about 35 years. Many changes may occur during this time such as becoming involved in adult intimate relationships, raising children, letting children go, and beginning to experience aging. Adults are responsible for educating their children about sexuality and have much influence in shaping their children's attitudes. Adults will continue to grapple with their own issues about sexuality and sexual behavior if they have not developed a high enough comfort level in the past. Many myths and stereotypes persist surrounding sexuality and sexual behavior; and some people fear certain aspects, such as homosexual feelings or behaviors. Adults, therefore, also need guidance from healthcare professionals.

During adulthood, many women experience pregnancy, which poses developmental issues related to sexuality. Additionally, it may lead to sexual difficulties between partners, owing to fear of intercourse during pregnancy or contraindication of sexual intercourse due to high-risk conditions. Couples who desire pregnancy but encounter fertility problems also may face other issues caused by the need to engage in sexual intercourse according to a rigid schedule.

The **climacteric** refers to the period during which significant sexual changes occur in the transition from middle to old age. This term more commonly refers to the transition that women experience as they begin to lose their reproductive function and approach cessation of their menstrual cycles. **Menopause** is the permanent cessation of menstrual activity. It normally occurs between the ages of 40 and 55 but may be surgically induced earlier.

Certain physiologic changes result from decreasing amounts of estrogen in women during the climacteric. Bernhard (1995) describes such physiologic changes as thinning of vaginal tissues and heightened fatigue. Some women require estrogen replacement, which is controversial.

Physiologic changes also occur in older men. Specific effects can be noted in relation to the sexual response cycle, as described by Masters, Johnson, and Kolodny (1988). During the excitement phase, women experience slower onset of and decreased amounts of lubrication, whereas men experience slower and decreased firmness of erection. In women, the clitoris becomes smaller. Men may need more direct genital stimulation during the excitement phase. During the plateau phase, the vaginal canal does not increase as much as it did earlier, and the uterus does not become as elevated as it did previously. Men experience a decrease in the amount of Cowper's gland secretion, are able to maintain an erection longer before ejaculation, and have decreased testicular elevation. The orgasmic phase may become shortened for women and may not occur for men as their need to ejaculate is decreased. Men also experience a decreased force and volume of ejaculate. Men experience longer refractory periods. Both men and women experience more rapid return to nonengorgement of the genitals.

FACTORS AFFECTING SEXUALITY

All people have a basic human need to be loved. Sexuality involves much more. The World Health Organization (1975) has defined sexual well-being as follows:

- A capacity to enjoy and control sexual behavior in accordance with a social and personal ethic
- Freedom from fear, shame, guilt, false beliefs, and other psychological factors inhibiting sexual response and impairing sexual relationships
- Freedom from organic disorder, disease, and deficiencies that interfere with sexual and reproductive functions

As described previously, not all people are involved in sexual relationships but they still regard themselves and are sexual beings. Sexuality or experiences with sex can influence other areas. For example, in the Critical Thinking Challenge at the beginning of this chapter, the woman who is worried about her upcoming pelvic examination may have had sexual difficulties in the past and is now experiencing discomfort relating to a necessary health measure.

Relationships

The quality of a person's relationships can strongly influence the quality of his or her sexual experiences. Love and trust may be key factors in facilitating comfort with sexuality and sexual relations. Again, referring to the Critical Thinking Challenge, the quality of the woman's relationships, particularly sexual relationships, may be important in allowing her to voice any fears or concerns (even perfectly normal concerns).

Cognition and Perception

Psychological factors include aspects leading to sexual arousal such as certain mental images being triggered in the mind. Emotional state may greatly influence sexual response. For example, a person who is depressed may be less concerned with sex than a person who is happy or content. In addition, the degree of knowledge or misperceptions about sexuality will influence sexual functioning.

Culture, Values, and Beliefs

Cultural factors include society's predominant views of sexuality and the social context within which people experience it. Values and morals are additional influences. Religious beliefs and/or personal values may shape views concerning contraception, abortion, sex education, and sex outside marriage. The woman in the Critical Thinking Challenge may be from a culture or ethnic group whose values influence her feelings about a pelvic examination, particularly one done by a male healthcare provider.

Self-Concept

People who are comfortable with themselves as sexual beings are likely to experience pleasure and comfort with sexual relations. A person who feels decreased self-esteem and self-confidence may experience negative effects in sexual functioning. The person may have a decreased sexual drive or conversely may attempt to compensate for this negative self-concept by overemphasizing involvement in sexual relations.

Previous Experience

Previous experience with sexuality or ideas about sexuality influence current sexual functioning. For example, a person who was sexually abused in the past is likely to experience repercussions that will negatively affect current sexual functioning. A more subtle example is that of a man or woman who has grown up with many cultural taboos related to sexuality and finds it difficult later on to engage in a healthy sexual relationship. Fearing another unwanted pregnancy, a woman who has experienced an unwanted pregnancy or possibly an abortion may feel apprehensive about having sexual intercourse.

Pregnancy

Pregnancy clearly influences sexual functioning. Although sexual intercourse is not contraindicated during a normal, low-risk pregnancy, pregnancy may affect sexual drive. Many women find their sexual drive decreased during the first trimester, when they are tired and may feel nauseated. In addition, they may worry about miscarriage during the first trimester so fear having sexual intercourse. During the second trimester, many women experience a surge of energy and a corresponding increase in sexual drive. The third trimester

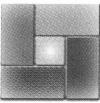

Nursing Research and Critical Thinking
Is the Mother's Relationship With the Father of the Baby Correlated With Maternal–Fetal Attachment?

This nurse was concerned that a lack of acceptance of pregnancy and the child by the mother or significant others may profoundly affect maternal–fetal attachment. She designed an exploratory, longitudinal study to examine the perceived relationship with the baby's father and maternal attachment in pregnant adolescents. A convenience sample of 79 pregnant adolescents attending one of four antepartum clinics for low-income women participated in the study. Data were collected at four different points: before 20 weeks gestation; between 20 and 29 weeks gestation; between 30 and 40 weeks gestation; and within 1 week after delivery. The perceived relationship with the child's father was measured on a five-point Likert-type scale (Father of Baby Scale [FOBS]) using a set of questions the investigator developed. Maternal–fetal attachment (MFA) was measured using Avant's Maternal Attachment Assessment Strategy (MAAS). The adolescents in this sample reported a moderately close prepregnancy relationship with the father of the unborn child (M = 2.88, SD = 0.55). The participants' satisfaction with the relationship, although somewhat high, decreased slightly during the course of the

pregnancy (<20 weeks, M = 3.99, SD 1.34; 20–29 weeks, M = 3.80, SD = 1.44; 30–40 weeks, M = 3.72, SD = 1.45). There was a significantly greater satisfaction expressed after delivery (M = 4.45, SD = 0.93, P = .0015). Analysis of the correlations between scores on the FOBS and the MFA and MAAS showed several statistically significant correlations (P = <.05).

Critical Thinking Considerations. Total attrition resulted in a decreasing group size over time. Chi-square analysis indicated no differences between adolescents who completed the study and those who did not with respect to age, race, gravidity, parity, marital status, or educational level. Implications of this study are as follows:

- A close and satisfying relationship with the baby's father was positively correlated with some aspects of maternal–fetal attachment (r = 0.24 to 0.33, p < 0.05) and maternal–infant attachment (r = 0.38, p < 0.05).
- Fathers of the babies of adolescent mothers should be included, where appropriate, in ongoing care of the mother and infant.

From Bloom, K. C. (1997). Perceived relationship with the father of the baby and maternal attachment in adolescents. *Journal of Obstetric, Gynecologic, and Neonatal Nursing (JOGNN), 27*(4), 420–430.

may again be a time of decreased sexual drive as the woman's abdomen grows, making sexual intercourse uncomfortable. Much variation exists in this pattern, and not all women respond the same way (Bernhard, 1995). Men also may vary in their sexual desires regarding pregnancy. Some men find pregnant women sexually attractive, whereas others are apprehensive about sexual relations during pregnancy for fear of harming the woman or fetus.

Infertility may place stress on a couple's sexual relationship. Couples who are trying to conceive must have sex according to when the woman ovulates. Sex becomes programmed and loses its spontaneity. In addition, couples may feel that they are having sex for a specific purpose rather than for enjoyment and mutual satisfaction. They may believe that they are being judged for how well they have sex in that pregnancy symbolizes "success" and lack of pregnancy symbolizes "failure." Many couples report that normal sexual relations resume after time elapses or they discontinue fertility treatments.

Environment

Environment can largely impact sexual functioning. Hospitalized clients, particularly those undergoing long-term treatments, may find it inhibiting to have sexual relations with a partner or to masturbate within the confines of a hospital room. Lack of privacy becomes a major issue. The same is

true for people in nursing homes. Environment is also a factor for people who are not hospitalized. Living in crowded conditions may preclude privacy. Fears about environmental pollutants affecting fertility may also influence sexuality.

Illness

Illness poses a threat to normal sexual functioning. A person with cardiac problems may fear overexertion from engaging in sexual relations. Although this fear may not be based on physiologic principles, it can still be inhibiting. A person with an STD may fear transmitting the disease to a partner, or conversely a person may fear contracting an STD from a partner. Although the individual may follow safer sex guidelines, this fear can inhibit sexual relations. Pain and joint disorders may make normal sexual intercourse uncomfortable. Motor vehicle accidents have created a sizable population of people with spinal cord injuries (paraplegia and quadriplegia); those affected must develop alternate methods of sexual functioning.

Medication

Some medications affect the ability to perform sexually. Rogers (1990) discusses these medications according to the categories of prescription drugs, over-the-counter drugs,

THERAPEUTIC DIALOGUE
Sexuality

Scene for Thought

Richard Meyers and his wife Aileen are both in their sixties and had been healthy and active until Richard's car accident 3 months ago. At that time, he sustained a comminuted fracture of his right femur that had to be reduced surgically. He still needs crutches to help him ambulate and sometimes has pain in his right leg. Maddie Hines, his clinic health nurse, has been visiting the family since Richard was discharged from the hospital.

Less Effective

Nurse: Hi, Mr. Meyers. How are you today? *(Sits next to him at the kitchen table.)*

Client: Glad to see you, Maddie. Who would have thought a broken leg would give a body such trouble! *(Laughs a little.)*

Nurse: Well, it wasn't just a broken leg, you know. It was pretty severe. What's giving you trouble? *(Good eye contact. Smiles.)*

Client: I'm still having trouble negotiating around the house. The furniture and rugs are still in my way even though you helped us move them. *(Sighs.)* I'm just having trouble with those crutches.

Nurse: *(After assessing client's ability to maneuver and making some suggestions.)* There, that should work better, don't you think?

Client: Yes, that's fine. Could I ask you about something else? *(Looks embarrassed but determined.)*

Nurse: Sure. *(Sits quietly.)*

Client: Um, I seem to be having some trouble in the bedroom.

Nurse: What kind of trouble? *(Looks skeptical about this subject.)*

Client: It's the positioning of this darned leg. It hurts when Aileen and I try to, uh, get close, and then she gets worried and I get annoyed and it all goes to heck! *(Sounds frustrated.)*

Nurse: Oh, I see. Let me tell you about a few things you might try to alleviate the pain that would work for you. *(Settles in for a teaching session.)*

Client: I don't know about trying anything new. We're pretty happy with the way we do it. *(His turn to look skeptical.)*

Nurse: Don't worry, these will work just fine. Other orthopedic clients have told me they were happy with the way things worked out. *(Talks to him about some ways to alleviate pain and pressure on his leg during sex. Says she'll bring pamphlets on the subject next time.)* What do you think? *(Smiles brightly at him.)*

Client: Well, I suppose they're worth a try. I'll let you know. Now, I wonder if you could take my pressure. I've felt it was a little high lately. *(They go on to other subjects, both feeling vaguely unfinished.)*

More Effective

Nurse: Good afternoon, Mr. Meyers. How are you this week? *(Sits down at the kitchen table with him.)*

Client: Glad to see you, Maddie. Who would've thought a broken leg would cause a body such trouble! *(Laughs a little.)*

Nurse: Are you having trouble? *(Good eye contact. Smiles but does not laugh so as to pay attention.)*

Client: Well, I'm still having trouble negotiating around the house. The furniture and rugs and all are still in my way, even though you helped us move them. *(Sighs.)* I'm just having trouble with those crutches.

Nurse: *(After assessing client's ability to maneuver and making some suggestions.)* Is there something else that's causing you trouble?

Client: Uh, *(looks to see where his wife is),* I am having some trouble in the bedroom. *(Looks embarrassed but determined.)*

Nurse: Okay, tell me a little more. *(Sits quietly.)*

Client: It's the positioning of this darned leg. It hurts when Aileen and I try to, uh, get close, and then she gets worried and I get annoyed and it all goes to heck! *(Sounds frustrated.)*

Nurse: Frustrating, huh? *(He nods.)* Let me ask you a few questions so I can find out what you're used to and then we can talk about modifications you might want to try. *(Assesses usual sexual habits and practices, including willingness to experiment with positions and effective use of analgesics. Then suggests two different positions that would afford pleasure without undue pain on the affected leg.)*

Client: That sounds doable, Maddie. I think we'll start out with some dinner and flowers. I'm going to call my son and see if he can help me arrange a dinner here tomorrow night. Aileen's worked hard these last weeks. She deserves it. Then we'll see what we can manage after that. *(Said with a wink. Looks eager to start planning.)*

Nurse: How romantic! Sounds like you two are going to have a great evening. I'm glad we were able to talk about this.

Client: Me too, me too. *(Big smile.)*

Critical Thinking Challenge

- The client in both dialogues received the same information. Discern what was more effective about the second dialogue.
- Distinguish what Maddie did the second time that made it effective for the client's sexual needs.
- Analyze your thoughts about a couple in their sixties, seventies, or eighties having sex.
- List effects pain has on a person's desire to have sex.

and social drugs. Many conventional therapeutic drugs may adversely affect sexual functioning; those drugs include antihypertensives, antipsychotic tranquilizers, antidepressants, neurotransmitters, and hormones. Social drugs that can affect sexuality and sexual response include alcohol, opiates, marijuana, cocaine, sedative-hypnotics, amphetamines, amyl nitrite, LSD, cantharides, and yohimbine. More recently, specific drugs have been developed to enhance sexual functioning, particularly to assist male sexual function (e.g., Viagra).

Surgery

Cesarean births, hysterectomy, and mastectomy are examples of surgical procedures that affect sexuality. Women who undergo cesarean deliveries may experience longer recovery periods than women who deliver vaginally so may feel less desire to resume sexual relations. Women who do not deliver vaginally may believe that they "failed" the labor and birth process even though this thought is irrational. Such thoughts may affect subsequent sexual functioning.

Women who have had hysterectomies may believe their femininity has been adversely affected. Again, this belief is irrational because women with hysterectomies are certainly able to engage in sexual intercourse and have orgasms. The meaning of the hysterectomy may be so negative to some women, however, that it adversely affects sexual functioning.

Women who have had mastectomies may also believe that femininity has been adversely affected, particularly in a society that highly emphasizes breasts as sexual objects. A mastectomy may negatively affect a woman's view of herself, which, in turn, may negatively affect her sexual functioning.

ALTERED HUMAN SEXUALITY

Certain conditions directly related to sexuality influence a person's ability to engage in mutually satisfying sexual relations. Conditions other than those mentioned in this section also may impact sexuality.

Manifestations of Altered Sexuality

Alterations in normal patterns of sexuality can be seen in the following manifestations: sexual abuse, inhibited sexual desire, impotence, ejaculatory dysfunctions, orgasmic dysfunction, dyspareunia, and vaginismus. Nurses can play a key role by assessing alterations in sexuality, assisting in prevention of problems, and helping clients to cope with existing problems.

Sexual Abuse

Some people manifest altered sexual functioning by being sexually abusive to others such as children, spouses, acquaintances, or strangers. Sexual abuse results in sexual problems for abused people as well.

Inhibited Sexual Desire

Lack of or inhibited sexual desire is subjective. Because there is no "normal" frequency of sexual relations, determining the frequency that reflects inhibited sexual desire is difficult. A key feature may be the partner's dissatisfaction with frequency of sexual relations. Thus, relationships play an important role in this issue. Sometimes inhibited sexual desire in one partner accompanies inhibited desire in the other partner. More commonly though, each partner's desires are incongruent and, hence, become a problem. Many factors contribute to inhibited sexual desire. Physical factors include use of certain medications, neurologic problems, and hormonal imbalances. Psychological factors may be depression and inter-

personal difficulties. It may be difficult to determine if depression has resulted from inhibited sexual desire or if it is a cause of inhibited sexual desire and consequent marital problems. Other possible causes are history of sexual abuse, pain with intercourse, or vaginismus.

Impotence

Impotence, the inability to attain or maintain an erection long enough for satisfactory sexual intercourse, is troubling to many men. Most cultures highly value a man's "virility" and view erectile dysfunction as a manifestation of his "failure to perform." Impotence can be primary or secondary. Primary impotence refers to a man who has never been able to achieve an erection necessary for intercourse; secondary impotence refers to a man who was once successful in attaining and maintaining erections but who has subsequently experienced difficulty.

Causes of impotence, whether primary or secondary, can be physiologic, psychological, or both. Certain manifestations may indicate the probability that the problem is secondary to a physiologic or a psychological factor. For example, if a man is able to attain an erection in certain situations but not others, has erections during sleep, or has experienced periods with no erection difficulties, the problem is probably psychological. However, if erection is impossible in any of these situations, the problem is probably physiologic.

Impotence has received much attention recently due to the approval of a new medication, sildenafil citrate (Viagra; The Medical Letter, 1998), to treat erectile dysfunction. This drug is the first oral medication approved by the Food and Drug Administration (FDA) for impotence. It works by causing erection of the penis through release of nitric oxide, which leads to formation of a substance (cyclic guanosine monophosphate) responsible for relaxing smooth muscle, thus allowing engorgement of the corpus cavernosum. One concern with sildenafil is its potential to cause hypotension. It is contraindicated in men who take nitrates or use nitrate patches (The Medical Letter, 1998).

Ejaculatory Dysfunction

Premature Ejaculation. **Premature ejaculation** is a relatively recently acknowledged phenomenon, according to Hogan (1985). This is not because the condition itself has occurred only recently but because many women in today's society are more open and have higher expectations for achieving orgasm than did women in previous eras and cultures. Premature ejaculation is a relative definition depending on the subjective responses of both partners (i.e., whether or not both partners are satisfied). It is a condition in which the man is unable to maintain an erection long enough for satisfactory intercourse to occur. It is believed that premature ejaculation is caused by anxiety on the man's part or fear of failure in the sex act.

Inability to Ejaculate. Inability to ejaculate actually refers to inability to ejaculate in the vagina. This condition is less common than premature ejaculation. The cause of ejaculatory incompetence may be primary or secondary. Primary causes include psychological disturbances; secondary causes may be related to interpersonal problems with one's sexual partner or organic causes such as lumbar sympathectomy or antiadrenergic drugs such as guanethidine or methyldopa (Hogan, 1985).

Orgasmic Dysfunction

Difficulty achieving orgasm is common in women. According to psychoanalytic thought, orgasm was differentiated as vaginal or clitoral with vaginal orgasm considered more mature. Masters and Johnson (1966) found this dichotomy misleading, however, because orgasm occurs through vaginal or clitoral stimulation. In addition, researchers have found that the Graefenberg spot, in the anterior portion of the vagina halfway between the vaginal opening and the cervix, is another area capable of stimulation to orgasm. Lack of information, lack of adequate stimulation, or problems in an intimate relationship may cause difficulty attaining orgasm. Sometimes women feel pressured to have an orgasm to please their partners, and some partners feel pressure to "bring" the woman to orgasm so they will have been "successful" at sex. This kind of pressure may inhibit the woman's ability to attain an orgasm.

Dyspareunia

Dyspareunia, or painful intercourse, is thought to occur regularly in 1% to 2% of adult women (Masters, Johnson, & Kolodny, 1988). These researchers estimate that 15% of adult women occasionally experience pain with intercourse. Parker and Rosenfeld (1997) emphasize the difficulty involved in truly assessing the prevalence of dyspareunia, although they cite a 1990 study by Glatt, Zinner, and McCormack in which 16% of 324 women experienced long-term dyspareunia. Common causes of dyspareunia are organic problems including lack of adequate lubrication at the vaginal opening or within the vaginal walls. Inadequate sexual arousal, drugs (antihistamines, certain tranquilizers, marijuana, alcohol), or estrogen deficiency may inhibit lubrication. Vaginal infections may lead to painful penetration on intercourse. Barrier methods of contraception may irritate the vagina, causing painful intercourse. Pelvic diseases may also cause pain.

Vaginismus

Vaginismus is involuntary contraction of the muscles surrounding the vaginal orifice so that penetration may be impossible and very painful. This condition is uncommon. Heiman (1995) indicated that vaginismus and dyspareunia contribute to about 10% of women's sexual complaints. There usually is no concurrent anatomic abnormality and rarely is there a physiologic abnormality, although these must be ruled out. Vaginismus usually results from psychological problems, namely fear of penetration due to a negative association such as rape, sexual abuse, or fear of sexual intercourse. The woman develops a conditioned reflex in certain situations (e.g., attempted sexual intercourse or a pelvic examination) in which her vaginal muscles involuntarily contract, which precludes penetration.

Impact on Activities of Daily Living

Because sexuality is integral to life, any sexual dysfunction can have a major impact on activities of daily living (ADLs), both for individuals and families. Emotionally, one may suffer from decreases in self-esteem and self-confidence. Consequences are that a person may have less emotional energy to concentrate on important aspects of daily living or may be slow and careless in accomplishing routine tasks. Physically, although a person may function normally, the view of the physical self may be adversely affected.

Sexual difficulties lend themselves to interpersonal difficulties. A person's altered sexual functioning likely does not occur in isolation. Usually such alterations are correlated with interpersonal problems. In fact, some sexual difficulties may be symptoms of underlying problems within a sexual relationship. On the other hand, difficulties may result from sexual dysfunction.

ASSESSMENT

Assessment involves collecting subjective and objective data regarding normal sexual function, risk factors for sexual dysfunction, and any present sexual dysfunction(s). Assessments are made by asking direct questions, observing nonverbal behavior, and evaluating information obtained through physical assessment and diagnostic and laboratory tests.

The historical content is important, although the assessment technique and approach influence the content obtained. Hogan (1985) includes a thorough outline of important content to elicit in a sexual history. This outline is reproduced as an example of necessary information (Table 50-1); however not all clients need to be questioned on all areas. Assess which areas are appropriate for each client.

Subjective Data

Gather subjective data through a careful nursing history. Although the data elicited in a sexual history are crucial, the approach used is equally, if not more, important. Discussing sexual concerns is an excellent opportunity to put a client at ease, encourage expression of any pent-up feelings, and listen actively to any concerns she or he may have. Approaching the sexual history in a humane, open manner can have therapeutic value and provide a source for essential information. Notice nonverbal cues as well.

Nurses should know the slang terms for sexual functions and organs (Hogan, 1985; Poorman, 1988). Some professionals believe that using a client's terminology enhances communication; however others believe that professionals should use formal terminology so clients know that the professional is, indeed, a professional. What is clear is that professionals and clients should understand what each person is saying and that professionals should clarify terminology with the clients if they are not sure they are communicating correctly.

One effective technique in interacting with clients is to ask less sensitive questions initially then gradually progress to

TABLE 50-1

Data to Be Collected by Nursing History for All Clients		
Data	**Significance of Data**	**Nursing History Questions**
Age	Identifies period in life cycle.	In what year were you born; month, day?
Sex	Each sex may react differently to life events; highlights gender identity problems.	Usually is evident by dress; otherwise ask what sex do you consider yourself to be?
Education, occupation	Sexual practices may be related to education–socioeconomic class; change in occupation may contribute to role disturbances.	How far did you go in school? What do you do for a living? What change has there been in your ability to do your job?
Significant others	Other sources of support, stable or otherwise.	What people do you consider most helpful right now? In what way? Are they available?
Quality of relationships with significant others	Relationships may be supportive, negative, or punitive, and these affect ability to cope with sexual problems.	Are there any differences in the way you get along with these people since you have been ill or hospitalized (or recently)?
Interests, hobbies	Indicates other support systems and avocational interests that contribute to self-esteem.	What do you do with your free time? What leisure and work activities are important to you? How are these being affected now?
Spiritual/religious/ philosophical beliefs	Sexual practices may be related to beliefs. Guilt may occur if religious beliefs are compromised. Client may experience conflict and anxiety if nurse suggests different practices.	With what religious denomination are you affiliated? Can you describe any spiritual or other beliefs helpful to you now? Do you have or want the support of a clergyman (minister, priest, rabbi)?
Health problems, medical conditions, surgical procedures in the past and anticipated in the future, medication therapy	Some medical problems, surgical treatment, or medications result in sexual dysfunction (physiologic changes). Anxiety over outcome or change in body image may lead to functional problems.	What illness and/or surgery have you had in the past? Did they affect your usual way of living or work? Did they affect sexual function? Do you expect this illness/hospitalization will have effects on your usual way of living or work? In what ways? What medications do you take?
Changes in role relationships and ability to carry out the usual sexual role	Change in ability to carry out what is perceived as the usual sexual role may cause anxiety, depression, and sexual dysfunction.	What difference has there been in your functioning in the family? Describe. Can you do your usual tasks or jobs? Describe. Have there been any changes in your relationship with the way you get along with others (male, female, significant others)?
Potential changes in ability to carry out usual sexual role	Expectations of problems may cause problems (self-fulfilling prophecy).	What changes do you expect after you get home (or in the future)?
Change in perception of self as male or female due to illness or life events	Anxiety and sexual dysfunction may result from threat to gender identity.	How do you expect this illness (or life event) to affect how you see yourself as a man/woman?
Existing or potential sexual dysfunction	Elicits problems (sexual dysfunction).	Has there been or do you expect to have any changes in sexual functioning (sex life) because of illness, life events? Describe.

Note: Wording of the questions is changed depending on educational level of the client.
From Hogan, R. (1985). *Human sexuality: A nursing perspective* (2nd ed.; pp. 162–163). New York: Appleton-Century-Crofts.

more sensitive areas. For example, an initial question like "When did you begin menstruating?" is much less threatening than such questions as "What is your sexual orientation?" or "How satisfied are you with your sex life?"

Normal Pattern Identification

Specific questions regarding the client's normal functional status will yield information. Approach the client by asking open-ended, nonjudgmental questions. An example is: "How frequently do you masturbate?" instead of "Do you ever masturbate?" The first question grants the client permission to say that he or she masturbates, whereas the second question may imply a more judgmental response to a "yes" answer.

Assessment of the client's psychosocial status is part of the sexual history but should be discussed separately to reinforce the importance of such an assessment. Often, assessing a problem with sexuality is highly subjective because it depends on the client's perspective. For example, an assessment of inadequate frequency of sexual relations is meaningless unless it is placed within the context of what adequate frequency means to the client. Psychosocial assessment includes the client's perception(s) of his or her sexuality. In addition, it includes the healthcare provider's assessment, based on data elicited, of the client's psychosocial functioning. Outlook on life, social support, role relationships, and family functioning are all aspects of a psychosocial assessment.

Risk Identification

Pregnancy, Infertility, and Abortion. Although pregnancy is usually a time of anticipation, that is not always true. Unwanted pregnancies occur and can create many problems for those involved. Be careful not to let personal assumptions influence the assessment. Phrase questions to determine what the pregnancy means to the client, how she feels about it, how her partner feels (if she has a partner), and what her plans are.

When a client loses a pregnancy, either by miscarriage or voluntary termination, assess the effect of the loss on the client. In both voluntary and involuntary abortion, a sense of loss is usually present. Sensitive assessment will assist the client and nurse in planning the type of support from which the client can derive the greatest benefit.

Be particularly sensitive to the stress placed on infertile couples. Assessing the feelings of both partners is essential; there may be guilt, self-blame, or other feelings affecting the situation and the relationship. Inquiring about past illnesses, infections of the reproductive system, and previous nonterm pregnancies may provide useful assessment and counseling information.

Alterations in Gender Identification. For clients experiencing alterations in gender identification, be tactful and discerning. Although the beginning nurse will not have many opportunities to work with these clients, it is useful to be aware of assessment needs including the client's feelings about self, how others regard the client, treatments and medications, and other underlying feelings.

Environment. Lack of privacy, especially in acute and long-term care settings, is a concern related to sexuality. Sensitive assessment of the client's response to the environment is essential. Because acute-care settings involve relatively short stays, long-term care settings are where the nurse will particularly encounter and need to assess the effect of the environment on sexuality. Assessing the client's need for privacy is necessary in nursing homes and other long-term care settings.

Illness. Assessment of present illness, past illnesses, chronic conditions, and medications is integral. Illness may have placed some constraints on sexual relations or sexual performance. Attentive assessment may reveal areas of previously unspoken concern to deal with (Schover, 1988). Careful assessment may reveal misconceptions that some clients (e.g., those with cardiac problems) have about the advisability of sexual relations. Obtaining this information may assist in planning further assessment or counseling.

If the illness a client is concerned about is an STD, diligently assess the person's feelings regarding the diagnosis, fears related to the consequences, and anxiety about future sexual relations. A nonjudgmental approach will support the client in clarifying and focusing on the aspects of greatest concern.

Surgery. Surgical procedures that relate to the reproductive organs create sexual concerns. Procedures such as prostate resection, mastectomy, and hysterectomy may initiate apprehension regarding sexuality, desire, disfigurement, and future sexual relations. Thoughtful questioning and listening as part of assessment may target areas of anxiety and clarify misunderstandings.

ETHICAL/LEGAL ISSUE
Abortion

You are caring for a 35-year-old woman who has come to the primary care clinic for a routine annual exam. You ask her if she has any concerns. She tells you that she has experienced a significant decrease in sexual desire since having a therapeutic abortion 3 years ago. She says her previous health-care provider told her that if she gets pregnant and has another abortion, her pelvic organs will be damaged. She does not want to take birth control pills and does not trust any other form of contraception.

Reflection
- Identify your concerns related to what the woman's previous healthcare provider told her.
- Consider your own feelings about this situation. How might your views influence your assessment?
- Explain how you would approach this woman's concerns.
- Is there any way to address the information given by the previous healthcare provider?

Dysfunction Identification

Dysfunctional patterns can be identified as those that differ significantly from the client's or couple's normal patterns—such as a difference in desire for frequency of sexual intercourse, lack of interest, or anger—which may indicate an underlying problem. Annon (1976) suggests an approach to discovering important data regarding any problem. This technique includes eliciting information in several areas: description of the current problem; onset and course of the problem; client's perception of what has caused the problem and what prevents the problem from being alleviated; any past treatment and treatment outcome; whether treatment was medical, professional, or self-treatment; and client's current expectations and treatment goals.

Objective Data

Physical Assessment

A thorough physical examination includes a complete, systematic, head-to-toe examination with specific focus on the genital organs or any infectious process that might be the result of or might impair sexual activity. Provide privacy and use careful draping. Instruments should be warm. Be sure to wear gloves during physical examination of a client's genitals.

Physical examination includes inspection and palpation, as described in Chapter 24. The nurse's role in examination of the genitals varies according to nursing preparation and type of healthcare facility. Nurses may perform the assessment directly or assist other clinicians.

Examination of Male Genitalia. Help the male client into a position for examination of the penis, scrotum, and testicles. Having the man stand or lie on his back with the knees bent exposes the genitals for examination. Inspect and palpate the genitals. Observe the distribution of hair in the area.

Pay careful attention to any skin masses, skin lesions, discharge from the penis, or anal/rectal abnormalities. Note the absence or atrophy of the testicles and the presence of the foreskin or of circumcision. The urethra's location will indicate whether hypospadias exists. Hypospadias is an abnormal congenital opening of the urethra on the undersurface of the penis rather than at the center of the glans penis. Observe male breasts for deviations from normal. Although rare, breast cancer can occur in men.

Examination of Female Genitalia. Help the female client into the lithotomy position. Ensure that she is comfortable. Inspect her external genitalia for normal and abnormal characteristics including hair distribution and genital development.

A complete pelvic examination is necessary and includes checking for pelvic masses, pelvic tenderness, vaginal discharge, other signs of infection, and vaginal or vulvar lesions. The pelvic examination is conducted in two parts: a speculum examination and bimanual palpation. The speculum examination allows visualization of the vagina and cervix. The speculum is a two-bladed instrument that, after insertion in the vagina, is expanded for viewing. To minimize discomfort,

it is helpful if the client relaxes. The speculum should be warm before insertion. Samples and smears for culture are taken while the speculum is in place. As the speculum is withdrawn, the clinician views the vaginal walls.

 SAFETY ALERT
Use sterile equipment for gynecologic examinations to avoid introducing organisms into the vagina.

In bimanual palpation, the clinician places the index and middle fingers of one hand into the vagina while placing the other hand on the lower abdomen. The cervix, ovaries, and uterus are palpated by this method.

A breast examination is included with the assessment of the reproductive organs. The breast examination is discussed in Chapter 24. The clinician checks for size, symmetry, contour, color, lesions, and nipple discharge. This is also a good time to teach the woman how to do a breast self-examination, which is discussed later in this chapter.

 SAFETY ALERT
Always wash your hands and wear gloves when assessing or performing hygiene in the perineal area. Handle equipment or dressings used in the perineal region appropriately. Limit the spread of contact with body substances.

Diagnostic Tests and Procedures

Certain diagnostic tests may be performed in conjunction with the physical examination. Blood work to detect anemia or infection is routinely ordered. Cultures to detect STDs such as gonorrhea or chlamydia may be indicated. For women, a Pap smear should probably be done if one has not been taken within the past 6 months to 1 year. Depending on the nature of the actual or potential problem, certain other tests may be performed at the healthcare provider's discretion. A summary of various diagnostic tests and procedures is given in Table 50-2.

NURSING DIAGNOSES

The North American Nursing Diagnosis Association (NANDA)-approved nursing diagnoses in the area of sexuality are Sexual Dysfunction and Ineffective Sexuality Patterns. Also included in this pattern is Rape-Trauma Syndrome, although this diagnosis will not be discussed here because it is beyond the scope of information presented in this chapter.

Diagnostic Statement: Sexual Dysfunction

Definition. Sexual Dysfunction is the state in which a person experiences a change in sexual function that is viewed as unsatisfying, unrewarding, or inadequate (NANDA, 2001). The definition of Sexual Dysfunction is subjective in that

TABLE 50-2

Diagnostic Tests and Procedures of the Reproductive Systems	
Test/Procedure	Description
VDRL (Venereal Disease Research Laboratories)	Blood test to detect syphilis ♂ ♀
Chlamydia culture	Cervical culture to detect *Chlamydia*
Gonorrhea culture	Cervical culture to detect gonorrhea
Wet preparation (KOH—potassium hydroxide) (NS—normal saline)	Slide preparation from vaginal secretions to detect *Candida, (Monilia), Gardnerella, Trichomonas* ♀
Pap smear	Slide preparation from endocervical secretions to detect cellular changes in cervix, cervical cancer ♀

how one person perceives the degree of satisfaction in his or her sexual life may differ from how another person perceives such satisfaction. In other words, this diagnosis depends on the person's assessment.

Defining Characteristics. The defining characteristics that contribute to this diagnosis are found mostly in the client's verbalization of the problem. For example, a client may verbalize that he or she is experiencing a change in fulfilling his or her perceived sex role. The client may perceive limitations imposed by disease or therapy, conflicts involving values, alteration in achieving sexual satisfaction, inability to achieve desired satisfaction, or alteration in relationship with significant other. In addition, the client may seek confirmation of his or her desirability and may experience a change of interest in self and others (NANDA, 2001). These defining characteristics reflect the diagnosis's subjective nature. They also reflect the importance of thorough and sensitive history taking on the nurse's part to elicit these perceptions that often are difficult to verbalize.

Related Factors. Several factors may cause or contribute to sexual dysfunction. Any change in sexuality, whether biologic, psychological, or sociologic, may lead to sexual dysfunction. For example, recent surgery, pregnancy, childbirth, drug use, disease process, trauma, radiation, and anomalies can be contributing factors. Ineffectual or absent role models as well as physical and psychosocial abuse may contribute. Such abuse indicates the presence of harmful relationships, which can lead to vulnerability, values conflict, lack of privacy, and lack of a reliable significant other. Misinformation or lack of knowledge also contributes to sexual dysfunction (NANDA, 2001).

Diagnostic Statement: Ineffective Sexuality Patterns

Definition. Ineffective Sexuality Patterns is the state in which a person expresses concern regarding his or her sexuality (NANDA, 2001). Similar to Sexual Dysfunction, this diagnosis is also very subjective depending on the person's own self-

perception. One person's sexual concerns may be very different from another person's sexual concerns, making it difficult to determine objective data to define this pattern. Again, it is essential that the nurse interact sensitively in obtaining a sexual history to elicit Ineffective Sexuality Patterns.

Defining Characteristics. The major point in determining defining characteristics is that these are "reported" difficulties, which emphasizes the subjective nature of the diagnosis. These reports are best elicited through sensitive history taking. These reported difficulties include any limitations or changes in sexual behaviors or activities (NANDA, 2001).

Related Factors. Similar to the diagnosis of Sexual Dysfunction, the related factors for the diagnosis of Ineffective Sexuality Patterns include those that both contribute to and result from the actual diagnosis or pattern. Such factors include lack of knowledge or skills regarding alternative responses to health-related transition; this means that often clients do not have the knowledge or the skill to respond to transitions in their own health in other ways (i.e., in ways that are not necessarily disruptive to their sexual lives). Changes in body function or structure, illness, or certain medical diagnoses can bring on these health-related transitions. Additional contributing factors are lack of privacy, which may lead to disruptions in sexual life; lack of a significant other (or impaired relationship with a significant other), which leads to lack of sexual activity with another person; ineffective or absent role models, which leads to difficulty in making sexual decisions; conflicts with sexual orientation, which leads to conflicts in sexuality; and fear of potential consequences of sexual activity including pregnancy and STDs (NANDA, 2001).

Related Nursing Diagnoses

Other diagnoses may be relevant to clients with sexual difficulties. Such diagnoses are Interrupted Family Processes, Rape-Trauma Syndrome, Ineffective Role Performance, Compromised Family Coping, Ineffective Coping, and Spiritual Distress.

OUTCOME IDENTIFICATION AND PLANNING

After the nursing diagnoses and related factors are identified, client goals and nursing interventions are planned. Common goals for the client or couple with sexual dysfunction should be individualized, depending on assessment findings. General goals for most clients include the following:

- The client/couple will recognize symptoms of sexual dysfunction.
- The client/couple will decrease symptoms of altered sexual functioning.
- The client/couple will express satisfaction with level of sexual functioning.

Planning revolves around the client's motivation to be healthy. Use educational interventions to teach clients about self-care and responsible sex. Examples of nursing interventions commonly used in caring for clients with sexuality needs are listed in the accompanying display and discussed in the next section of this chapter.

IMPLEMENTATION

Nurses play a key role in assisting clients with any of the diagnoses listed earlier. At times, however, they must refer clients to other healthcare providers, for example if a major sexual dysfunction is noted.

Health Promotion

Concerns about sexual issues may or may not be obvious. Clients may enter the healthcare system for a primary problem unrelated to sexuality. Put clients at ease, develop rapport, and allow them to discuss any issues of concern.

Client Teaching

Anticipatory guidance is a major nursing role. Assist clients in anticipating outcomes and consequences; help them to devise plans to cope with or to manage such outcomes and consequences.

Self-Awareness. Assist clients to become more aware of their bodies and body functions. Exploring and understanding the body are essential in assisting men and women to achieve healthy sexual relationships. Women need assistance in understanding their anatomy. The use of a mirror during a pelvic examination is one way to begin this process; a second way is to encourage women to examine themselves with a mirror. Understanding the anatomy of their genitals may help women understand how their bodies respond to sexual stimulation and what helps them to achieve orgasm. Women need to understand what happens to their bodies during menstruation, pregnancy, and menopause.

Men also need assistance in becoming more aware of their bodies. Understanding their anatomy and particularly what kind of stimulation causes them to have an erection will help men to develop healthy sexual relationships.

PLANNING: Examples of NIC/NOC Interventions

Accepted Human Sexuality Nursing Interventions Classification (NIC)
Sexual Counseling

Accepted Human Sexuality Nursing Outcomes Classification (NOC)
Body Image
Physical Aging Status
Self-Esteem

Refer to the following for specifics regarding NIC/NOC:
McCloskey, J., & Bulechek, G. (2000). *Iowa Intervention Project: Nursing Interventions Classification (NIC)* 2nd ed. St. Louis, MO: C. V. Mosby.
Johnson, M., & Maas, M. (2000). *Iowa Outcomes Project: Nursing Outcomes Classification (NOC)* 2nd ed. St. Louis, MO: C. V. Mosby.

Self-Examination. As part of developing awareness of their own bodies, men and women need assistance in learning techniques of self-examination. Men should learn to perform testicular self-examination and women to perform breast self-examination, as illustrated in Displays 50-1 and 50-2.

Kegel Exercises. Self-awareness for women also involves control of the muscle of the pelvic floor. Provide needed instruction in the simple steps necessary during assessment or in a teaching situation. Kegel exercises involve contraction and release of the pubococcygeus muscle, which contracts to prevent urine flow or a bowel movement. Muscles always work better when they are in good shape. Muscle tone can be restored in about 6 weeks of regular practice of Kegel exercises. Benefits of Kegel exercises are increased vaginal lubrication during sexual arousal, enhanced sexual excitement, stronger gripping of the base of the penis, more rapid postpartum recovery of the pelvic floor muscles, increased flexibility of episiotomy scars, and relief of constipation (May & Mahlmeister, 1994). Northrup (1998) notes that if a woman does Kegel exercises consistently and correctly, she will likely experience beneficial changes in about 1 month. Kegel exercises are also used in bladder training. Display 50-3 lists steps of the Kegel exercises.

Sex Education. Parents and caregivers of preschool children need guidance in becoming comfortable answering questions as well as in volunteering information their children may not directly request. During adolescence, both teens and their families need guidance. Adolescents need reassurance that their confusing and conflicting feelings are normal, and adults need to treat teens with patience as they vacillate between wanting to be taken care of and wanting to assert their independence. Assist parents in dealing with adolescent mood swings and unpredictability. Give reassurance and support regarding parents' approach to their children. In addition, parents need help maintaining their own intimate relationships during this turbulent time that often calls attention to their own aging as their children are growing older.

DISPLAY 50-1

🔄 TESTICULAR SELF-EXAMINATION

What Can I Do?

Your best hope for early detection of testicular cancer is a simple 3-minute monthly self-examination. The best time is after a warm bath or shower, when the scrotal skin is most relaxed.

Roll each testicle gently between the thumb and fingers of both hands. If you find any hard lumps or nodules, you should see your doctor promptly. They may not be malignant, but only your doctor can make the diagnosis.

After a thorough physical examination, your doctor may perform certain x-ray studies to make the most accurate diagnosis possible.

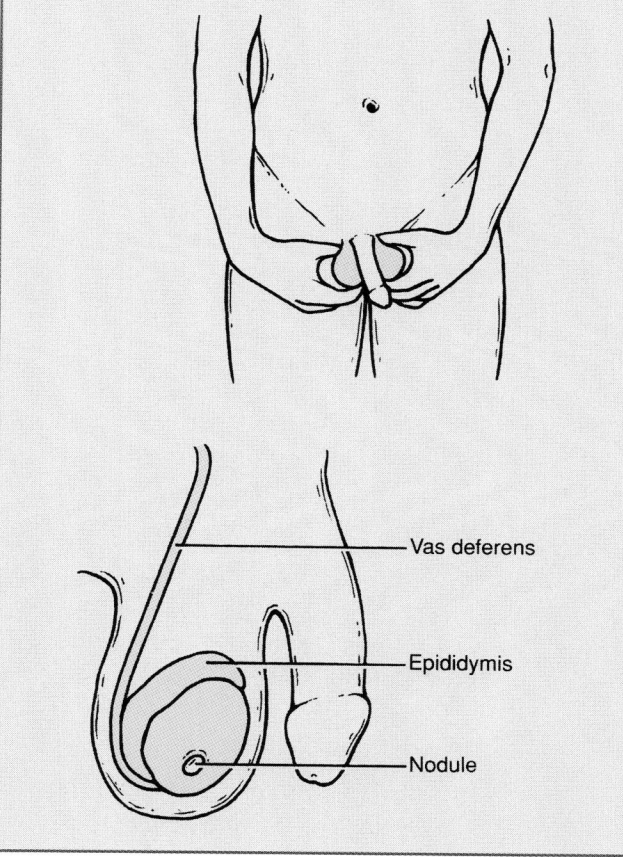

Responsible Sex. Teaching men and women to participate in responsible sex is important. Specifically, limiting the number of sexual partners and using condoms in nonmonogamous relationships are very important. In a nonjudgmental manner, present the importance of limiting sexual contacts. However, if such a discussion might defeat the purpose of the counseling or teaching session, stress the importance of hygiene and condom use. Condoms should always be used in nonmonogamous heterosexual and homosexual relationships

and in other relationships with the potential for AIDS transmission. Much has been said in the media about "safe sex," and nurses should build on this groundwork. Encourage potential sexual partners to talk openly with one another about how to have safer sex and to be honest with one another about any history of STDs.

As part of responsible sex teaching, teach clients about the prevention of STDs. Some STDs are easily treatable, whereas others are not (e.g., herpes). Currently, AIDS is considered incurable and ultimately fatal. The importance of teaching about prevention of STDs cannot be overemphasized.

Contraceptive Use

Decisions regarding family size and spacing are possible largely because of the variety of birth control methods available. Child spacing, limiting family size, and timing the first birth are recognized as preventive health measures (May & Mahlmeister, 1994). Various methods of birth control have improved consistently over the past several decades (Grimes & Wallach, 1997). Health measures must be addressed especially for adolescents because of the significance of teen pregnancy and births.

Men and women need to become aware of the various contraceptive methods available. Nurses are responsible for being familiar with the various contraceptive methods: their advantages and disadvantages, contraindications, effectiveness, safety, and cost. The best method is the one that the client or couple decides is most comfortable to use and will use consistently and correctly (Fig. 50-6).

No perfect contraceptive method exists, but several good methods are available, each with advantages and disadvantages. Although, is beyond the scope of this text to discuss them in detail, they are summarized in Table 50-3 and in the following sections.

Natural Family Planning. Fertility awareness is used in natural family planning. Currently four methods are available; all require some period of abstinence (periodic abstinence). The calendar rhythm method uses calculations of menstrual cycles and fertile and infertile periods. The temperature method uses the rise in basal body temperature to determine ovulation. The cervical mucus method involves teaching the woman to differentiate dryness, moistness, and wetness at the vaginal introitus, and differentiation of types of mucus. The symptothermal method combines the other techniques. These methods are acceptable to couples who follow the tenets of certain religions. Disadvantages are that the methods require motivation, time, consistent daily records, and abstinence for long periods. Miscalculations can occur in any of the methods, and these methods do not allow for spontaneous sex.

Hormonal Methods. Hormonal methods are easy to use and provide the most effective birth control except for surgery. They use estrogen and progestin in various combinations and are introduced by various means into the female body. Oral contraceptives ("the pill") are most commonly used despite years of controversy about them. This controversy has centered on several issues: (1) the pill's potential positive and

DISPLAY 50-2

🖺 BREAST SELF-EXAMINATION

Why Do The Breast Self-Exam?
There are many good reasons for doing the breast self-exam (BSE) each month. One reason is that breast cancer is most easily treated and cured when it is found early. Another is that if you do BSE every month, it will increase your skill and confidence when doing the exam. When you get to know how your breasts normally feel, you will quickly be able to feel any change. Another reason is that it is easy to do.

When To Do BSE
The best time to do BSE is about a week after your period, when breasts are not tender or swollen. If you do not have regular periods or sometimes skip a month, do BSE on the same day every month.

Now, How To Do BSE
1. Lie down and put a pillow under your right shoulder. Place your right arm behind your head.
2. Use the finger pads of your three middle fingers on your left hand to feel for lumps or thickening. Your finger pads are the top third of each finger.
3. Press firmly enough to know how your breast feels. If you're not sure how hard to press, ask your healthcare provider, or try to copy the way your healthcare provider uses the finger pads during a breast exam. Learn what your breast feels like most of the time. A firm ridge in the lower curve of each breast is normal.
4. Move around the breast in a set way. You can choose either the circle (**A**), the up-and-down line (**B**), or the wedge (**C**). Do it the same way every time. It will help you make sure that you've gone over the entire breast area and to remember how your breast feels each month.
5. Now examine your left breast using right hand finger pads.
6. If you find any changes, see your doctor right away.

For Added Safety
You might want to check your breasts while standing in front of a mirror right after you do your BSE each month. See if there are any changes in the way your breasts look: dimpling of the skin, changes in the nipple, or redness or swelling. You might also want to do an extra BSE while you're in the shower. Your soapy hands will glide over the wet skin, making it easy to check how your breasts feel.

Remember: BSE could save your breast—and save your life. Most breast lumps are found by women themselves, but, in fact, most lumps in the breast are not cancer. Be safe, be sure.

Reprinted by permission of the American Cancer Society, Inc.

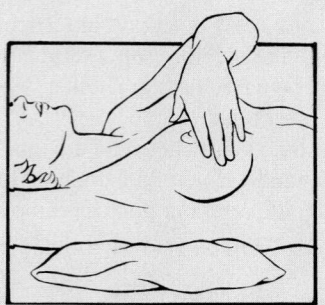

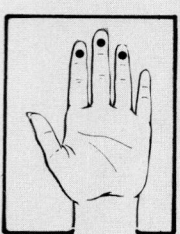

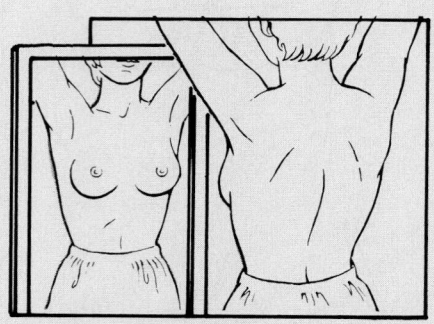

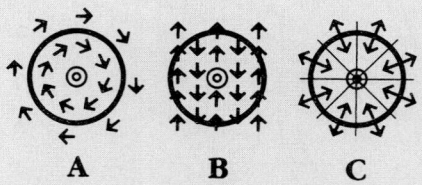

A   B   C

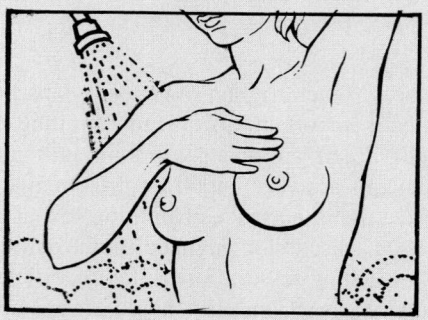

DISPLAY 50-3

🔲 KEGEL EXERCISES

1. Locate the muscles surrounding the vagina by sitting on the toilet and starting and stopping the flow of urine.
2. Test the baseline strength of the muscles by inserting a finger in the opening of the vagina and contracting the muscles.
3. Exercise A–Squeeze the muscles together and hold the squeeze for 3 seconds. Relax the muscles. Repeat.
4. Exercise B–Contract and relax the muscles as rapidly as possible 10 to 25 times. Repeat.
5. Exercise C–Imagine sitting in a pan of water and sucking water into the vagina. Hold for 3 seconds.
6. Exercise D–Push out as during a bowel movement, only with the vagina. Hold for 3 seconds.
7. Repeat exercises A, C, and D 10 times each, and exercise B once. Repeat the entire series three times a day.

From May, K. A., & Mahlmeister, L. R. (1994). *Comprehensive maternity nursing: Nursing process and the childbearing family* (3rd ed.). Philadelphia: J. B. Lippincott.

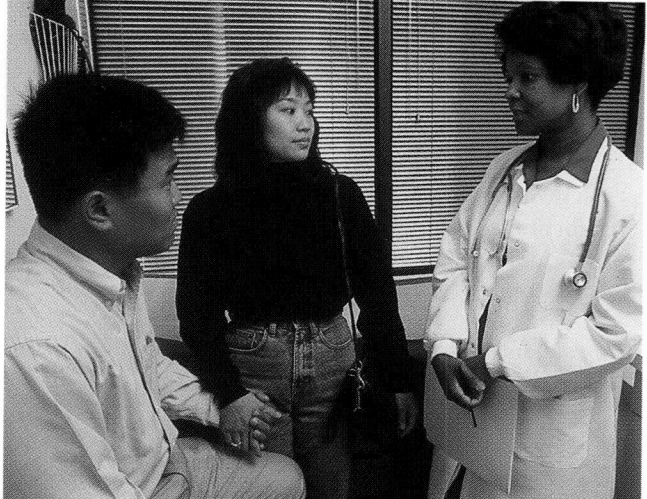

FIGURE 50-6 Providing information about contraceptive methods is an important component of reproductive health for clients.

negative health effects (i.e., possible prevention of ovarian cancer; possible cause of cardiovascular problems); (2) the increased sexual permissiveness resulting from the widespread use of the pill, which contributes to moral dilemmas for some; and (3) the spread of HIV/AIDS because the pill does not provide a barrier to such transmission. Mini-pills and postcoital pills are also used. Oral contraceptives and mini-pills are taken daily. For those women taking daily pills, remembering to take each pill is critical to the method's success. Postcoital pills are used "the day after" coitus.

After use in Europe for years, a progestin implant was introduced to the United States in 1991. Capsules are inserted under the skin of the forearm and are effective for 5 years. Another hormonal method of contraception is depot medroxyprogesterone acetate (DPMA), an injectable form of progesterone that is long-acting and requires injections approximately

🔲 APPLY YOUR KNOWLEDGE

You are a school nurse and two junior high school students drop by the health office to have you settle an argument they have been having. One student thinks you cannot get pregnant if you have sex during your period; the other student thinks it might be possible. How can you answer this question in a way that allows the opening for further discussion about sex?

Check your answer in Appendix A.

every 3 months (Grimes & Wallach, 1997). Hormonal methods allow for spontaneous sex and less stress and anxiety.

There are side effects to these methods, and they can become expensive if used for a lengthy period. Health insurance coverage for contraception is also controversial. Some insurance companies cover such expenses, but much debate and discussion continue over the pros and cons about providing such coverage.

Intrauterine Devices. Intrauterine devices (IUDs) were the subject of much controversy about untoward effects (specifically pelvic inflammatory disease) in the past; consequently some IUDs were taken off the market in the 1970s and 1980s. Two remain: Progestasert and ParaGard (Copper T). Other, newer IUDs are under discussion, and IUDs are experiencing a newfound popularity. Current studies are revealing a very high safety and efficacy (Grimes & Wallach, 1997). In this contraceptive method, a small device is inserted in the uterine cavity, where it remains until removed by a healthcare worker. The exact mechanics for contraception are not clearly understood. Women who use the IUD must be carefully screened because there are a number of contraindications. Women who use the IUD must learn danger signals to report to their healthcare worker. Infection and ectopic pregnancy are the major considerations.

Barrier Methods. Chemical and mechanical barriers are popular with women who cannot or prefer not to use the pill or IUD. Barrier methods are readily available and some can be purchased over the counter. Mechanical barriers include diaphragms, cervical caps, and condoms. Diaphragms and cervical caps are prescribed and fitted over the woman's cervix by a professional. The diaphragm must be used with spermicide. In both cases, the woman has to learn correct insertion methods and must plan ahead for sexual encounters because the devices must be inserted before intercourse. Both seem to be highly effective. Their use may result in discomfort to one

TABLE 50-3

Methods of Fertility Control and Their Relative Effectiveness*

Method	Pregnancy Rate	Drug Contained/ Brand Name	Action	Comments
No protection	85%–90%			
Subcutaneous implant	<1%	Levonorgestrel (Norplant System)	Hormonal	Effective up to 5 years
Injections	<1%	Medroxyprogesterone acetate (Depo-Provera)	Hormonal	Given every 2–3 months
Oral contraceptives	1%–3%	Usually combined— estrogen (such as estradiol, estriol) and progesterone Brand names include the following: *Monophasic* (taken for 20–21 days): Demulen, Levlen, Ovral, Nordette, Ovcon-35, Brevicon, Loestrin *Biphasic* (one color taken for 10 days, next color for 11 days): Nelova 10/11, Ortho-Novum 10/11 *Triphasic* (sequence specified by manufacturer): Tri-Levlen, Triphasil, Tri-Norinyl, Ortho-Novum 7/7/7	Hormonal Simulates pregnancy and depresses ovulation	One pill daily (21 days of medication, 7 days without) in various patterns
"Morning-after" pill	1%	Estrogen/progestin combined (Ovral)	Hormonal	Emergency only
Intrauterine devices	2%–5%	Progestasert Copper-T 380A	Prevents implantation in uterus	Replaced yearly Can remain in place for 4 years
Chemical barriers	5%–25%	Spermicidal douches, suppositories, and so forth	Kills or immobilizes sperm	Most effective if used with mechanical barrier
Mechanical barriers	10%–15%	Male condoms used alone Condoms (male and female), cervical cap, diaphragm	Block sperm from fertilizing egg	Most effective when combined with chemical barrier
	5%–20% 2%–10%	Diaphragm with spermicide Condom with spermicide		Cervical cap and diaphragm must remain in place in female for several hours after intercourse
Rhythm method	11%–30%	None	Planned intercourse to coincide with woman's fertile time	Requires mutual cooperation Woman's cycle must be regular

TABLE 50-3 (Continued)

Methods of Fertility Control and Their Relative Effectiveness*

Method	Pregnancy Rate	Drug Contained/ Brand Name	Action	Comments
Withdrawal (coitus interruptus)	25% when used with extreme care: usual pregnancy rate higher	None	Withdrawal before ejaculation	Requires mutual cooperation Pre-ejaculation fluid may contain sperm
Male sterilization	<0.15%	Vasectomy	Blocks path of sperm	
Female sterilization	<0.5%	Tubal ligation	Blocks path of egg (ovum)	

*Percentages in this table are estimated using a number of sources.
From Rosdahl, C. (1999). *Textbook of basic nursing* (7th ed.). Philadelphia: Lippincott Williams & Wilkins.

or both partners. Infection, including toxic shock syndrome, is among the side effects.

The major form of male birth control is the condom, which ranks in popularity second only to the pill as a contraceptive method. The ability to block STDs is an advantage of this method. With concern about HIV/AIDS transmission, a recently approved contraceptive method is the female condom, which covers the cervix, vaginal walls, and labia (Grimes & Wallach, 1997).

Foams, creams, jellies, and suppositories are chemical barriers. These vaginal spermicides act in two ways: blocking and killing sperm. Chemical barriers are bought without prescription and have few, if any side effects. However, there is some question regarding possible harm to an already implanted embryo.

Elective Abortion. Some people consider elective abortion (therapeutic abortion) to be a contraceptive method although elective abortion remains controversial. There are several methods for performing an abortion. The rate of complications, such as infection, bleeding, and uterine or cervical trauma, may be extremely high in illegal abortions.

Coitus Interruptus. People have used coitus interruptus, withdrawal of the penis just before ejaculation, for centuries. Although no expense is involved in its use and there are no medical side effects, the effectiveness is not high because of difficulty using the method.

Surgical Sterilization. Surgical sterilization may be done for both men and women. Female sterilization includes tubal ligation (cutting and tying the fallopian tubes) and tubal cauterization (cauterizing or burning the tubes) so ova cannot pass through. Vasectomy is the male form of surgical sterilization. Vasectomy involves cutting the vas deferens, thereby preventing sperm from being ejaculated in the semen. Although both male and female sterilizations

are considered permanent, there is a slight chance of reversing each.

Nursing Interventions for Altered Function

A holistic approach addresses both physical and psychological issues related to sexual dysfunction. Each client needs assistance to live as fully as possible, even in the presence of dysfunction. This is accomplished through counseling and education regarding a specific problem area, treating a specific problem if appropriate, promoting ADLs, making referrals to appropriate resources, and assisting with home management.

Levels of Activities of Daily Living

One of the nurse's responsibilities is to assist clients in achieving and maintaining a level of daily living that maximizes their potential. Nurses can be instrumental in suggesting ways to improve clients' levels of ADLs despite sexual dysfunction. For example, nurses play a key role in counseling older adults regarding sexuality and their ability to maintain active sex lives. Give guidance on modifications such as using lubricants to counteract the effect of women's decreased lubrication and engaging in more foreplay to allow more stimulation of men so they can more easily have erections. Also help older adults to discover alternative forms of sexual expression such as physical closeness and caressing in addition to sexual intercourse (see Fig. 50-5).

Counseling

When treating a person with a nursing diagnosis of Sexual Dysfunction, direct interventions toward educating and counseling the client and his or her partner regarding various patterns of human sexual response. Talking with and allowing the client to describe his or her feelings will provide a clearer sense of the client's perspective on the sexual dysfunction.

In this way, you will discover what the dysfunction means to the client and how the client is responding to it; these perspectives will enable the development of individualized interventions.

The PLISSIT Model. One specific technique that nurses can use in working with clients with altered sexual functioning is the PLISSIT model developed by Annon (1976) and based on learning principles. The acronym stands for the following: P 5 permission giving, LI 5 limited information, SS 5 specific suggestions, and IT 5 intensive therapy.

Using this approach, nurses begin with nonthreatening actions: permission giving and limited information. If the client continues to need further therapy or has more serious problems, specific suggestions will be recommended, and, possibly, intensive therapy will be warranted. According to this model, the belief is that many sexual problems stem from lack of education, therefore, applying learning principles may help alleviate many sexual problems. Table 50-4 gives the principles of the PLISSIT model with examples of how it may be used.

Referral

Nurses may refer clients for further counseling if they deem that to be appropriate. In addition, nurses may refer clients to organizations that educate and provide support to people regarding sexuality.

Healthcare Planning and Home/Community-Based Nursing

Many nurses work with clients who are experiencing sexual dysfunction in ambulatory settings or with hospitalized clients preparing for discharge. Because sexual functioning is crucial for all human beings, consider the possibility of sexual dysfunction for all clients regardless of healthcare setting. Many clients are discharged to assisted-living sites or are cared for in day-care facilities. A greater emphasis on case management transcends individual sites of healthcare. Inclusion of sexuality is essential to a comprehensive case management approach.

Discharge Planning

Questions regarding sexual functioning are common as clients prepare to return home. Such questions are common after birth, cesarean section, hysterectomy, or other surgery. Be prepared to give guidance. Refer clients for group therapy in instances that seem appropriate.

Home visits by nurses may be appropriate to assess how well clients are doing. Nurses can reinforce specific treatment protocols prescribed for clients. In addition, they can assess how well clients are after the treatment protocols and can answer any questions that clients may have regarding the treatment. Most importantly, nurses provide support and allow clients to develop a trusting relationship. When clients are

TABLE 50-4

Principles of the PLISSIT Model*		
Acronym	**Definition**	**Example**
P	Permission giving (allows client to speak his/her mind without the nurse communicating value judgments)	The client says, "I need to practice birth control. Too many pregnancies are tiring me out physically and emotionally. But I'm not sure if birth control is right." The nurse may reply, "Some people practice birth control, while others choose not to. It is an individual choice."
LI	Limited Information (gives/provides client with information but not too much to be overwhelming)	After further questions, the nurse says, "A variety of contraceptives exist, each with advantages and disadvantages. People choose contraceptives that are best for their situation."
SS	Specific Suggestions (gives client specific advice in an attempt to solve the client's problems or alleviate concerns/worries)	The nurse gives specific information regarding a variety of contraceptives: advantages, disadvantages, contraindications, side effects, effectiveness, cost, and procedures for each.
IT	Intensive Therapy (provides more in-depth, perhaps long-term treatment if problems are not solved with specific suggestions)	If the client has had several (planned or unplanned) abortions, she may need intensive, professional help related to using a specific contraceptive; dealing with grief, guilt, self-blame, or other emotional results; fitting for a specific method.

* The PLISSIT model provides an organized approach to the client, based on teaching–learning principles.

being treated for sexual problems, many personal issues often arise as well, and the supportive presence of the nurse is important for the client's well-being.

Ambulatory Settings

Education is a prominent nursing role related to sexuality issues. Such teaching can take place in a variety of settings. Schools, walk-in clinics, family planning offices, and malls are examples. Teaching may be as simple as creating wall posters, as informal as a one-to-one counseling session, or as formal as a video presentation.

Nurses may function independently, particularly in the area of anticipatory guidance. Be nonjudgmental, allowing clients to express their feelings, concerns, and fears. Rapport, truth, and respect should be the characteristics of such teaching. Often, nurses can clear up misconceptions and dispel myths that may be interfering with a person's sexual relationship or acceptance of his or her own sexuality.

Clients may approach nurses for information and counseling regarding family planning; therefore, nurses need a working knowledge of family planning and contraceptives. Some nurses may work in family planning clinics, where their major responsibility is assistance in family planning and contraceptive

methods. Adolescents may approach school nurses for counseling. Encourage sex education. It is also appropriate for nurses to become involved at the community level. By supporting and encouraging sex education in the schools, nurses can support educating people about their own bodies and sexuality.

EVALUATION

Specific outcome criteria help to evaluate attainment of client goals related to sexuality. These criteria may differ from criteria related to other physiologic problems where nurses can observe results in many physiologic problems. To evaluate progress toward goals related to sexuality, in most instances the nurse must rely on the client/couple's report of goal achievement in sexuality. Examples of possible outcome criteria for sexuality are listed below. Criteria may be similar because some goals overlap.

Goal

The client/couple will recognize symptoms of sexual dysfunction.

NURSING PLAN OF CARE

THE CLIENT WITH SEXUAL DYSFUNCTION

Nursing Diagnosis

Sexual Dysfunction related to inability to conceive as manifested by altered sexual satisfaction.

Client Goal

The client/couple will restore normal sexual functioning.

Client Outcome Criteria

- Client/couple verbalizes increased satisfaction in sexual relationship within 3 months of treatment, as measured by their self-evaluation.
- Client/couple verbalizes to healthcare provider that they are more relaxed and feeling better within 6 months.

Nursing Intervention	Scientific Rationale
1. Encourage couple to discuss their current patterns of sexual behaviors, with acknowledgment by the nurse that the client's complaints are understandable.	1. If the partners are able to discuss their current patterns of sexual behavior and these patterns are acknowledged by the nurse as normal, the couple may feel more relaxed and less concerned about their new sexual patterns.
2. Suggest possible ways for the couple to attain and maintain a close physical relationship even without sexual intercourse if they are uncomfortable with it.	2. If permission is given to have close physical contact without sexual intercourse, the couple may feel more relaxed and less pressured to have unspontaneous sexual intercourse.
3. Give couple permission to "take a vacation" from infertility at times in an effort to restore their previous sexual relationship.	3. Permission to take a vacation from infertility may help restore some spontaneity into their sexual relationship.

Possible Outcome Criteria

- Client describes male and female reproductive anatomy after next teaching session with the nurse.
- Within 6 months, client/couple describes normal sexual functioning to nurse, as learned in teaching session.
- Client identifies specific symptom experiences, including etiology and treatment, while talking with nurse in next 6 months.

Goal

The client will have decreased symptoms of altered sexual functioning.

Possible Outcome Criteria

- Within 6 months, client verbalizes to nurse that symptoms are decreasing.
- Within 1 year, client and partner report satisfaction with sexual relationship.

Goal

The client/couple will express satisfaction with level of sexual functioning.

Possible Outcome Criteria

- Within 6 months, client states success in using alternate method of sexual functioning.
- Within 6 months, client reports satisfaction with level of sexual functioning.
- Within 1 year, client's partner reports satisfaction with level of sexual relationship.

KEY CONCEPTS

- Nurses must understand the reproductive systems, sexuality, and sexual orientation because sexual health is part of a holistic approach to healthcare.
- Sexuality encompasses function of the sexual organs, individual perceptions of functioning, sexual expression, and preferences.
- Sexual activity is highly individual with wide variations in expression.
- Reproduction depends on the establishment of the menstrual cycle in women and spermatozoa production and motility in men.
- Sexual orientation may be heterosexual, homosexual, or bisexual.
- Factors that affect sexual function include relationships; cognition and perception; culture, values, and beliefs; self-concept; previous experience; pregnancy; gender identification; environment; illness; surgery; and/or medications.
- Altered sexuality may be manifested by sexual abuse, inhibited sexual desire, impotence, ejaculatory dysfunction, orgasmic dysfunction, dyspareunia, and/or vaginismus.

- Assessment includes subjective and objective data regarding normal sexual function, risk factors, and sexual dysfunction.
- Teaching about sexuality includes self-awareness, self-examination, Kegel exercises, sex education, responsible (safer) sex, and contraceptive use.
- Nursing interventions for altered function include guidance in increasing levels of ADLs, ensuring privacy, counseling, and referral as necessary.
- Nurses function independently in areas of teaching and anticipatory guidance and refer clients with major sexual dysfunction to specialists.

REFERENCES

Alan Guttmacher Institute. (1994). *Sex and America's teenagers.* New York: Author.

American Psychiatric Association. (1994). *Diagnostic and statistical manual of mental disorders* (4th ed., text revision). Washington, DC: Author.

Annon, J. S. (1976). *The behavioral treatment of sexual problems, Vol. 1. Brief therapy.* Philadelphia: J. B. Lippincott.

Belzer, E. (1981). Orgasmic expulsions of women: A review and heuristic inquiry. *Journal of Sex Research, 17*(91), 1–12.

Bernhard, L. A. (1995). Sexuality in women's lives. In C. I. Fogel & N. F. Woods (Eds.), *Women's health care: A comprehensive handbook.* Thousand Oaks, CA: Sage Publications.

Glatt, A. E., Zinner, S. H., & McCormack, W. M. (1990). The prevalence of dyspareunia. *Obstetrics and Gynecology, 75,* 433–436.

Grimes, D. A., & Wallach, M. (1997). *Modern contraception: Updates from the contraception report.* Totowa, NJ: Emron.

Heiman, J. R. (1995). Evaluating sexual dysfunction. In D. P. Lemcke, J. Pattison, L. Marshall & D. S. Cowley (Eds.), *Primary care of women.* Norwalk, CT: Appleton & Lange.

Hogan, R. (Ed.). (1985). *Human sexuality: A nursing perspective* (2nd ed.). New York, NY: Appleton-Century-Crofts.

Kaplan, H. S. (1979). *Disorders of sexual desire.* New York, NY: Simon & Schuster.

Lauver, D., & Welch, M. B. (1990). Sexual response cycle. In C. I. Fogel & D. Lauver (Eds.), *Sexual health promotion.* Philadelphia: W. B. Saunders.

Masters, W., & Johnson, V. (1966). *Human sexual response.* Boston, MA: Little, Brown & Co.

Masters, W., Johnson, V., & Kolodny, R. (1988). *Human sexuality* (3rd ed.). Boston, MA: Little, Brown & Co.

May, K. A., & Mahlmeister, L. R. (1994). *Comprehensive maternity nursing: Nursing process and the childbearing family* (3rd ed.). Philadelphia: J. B. Lippincott.

The Medical Letter. (1998, May 8). Sildenafil: An oral drug for impotence. *The Medical Letter on Drugs and Therapeutics, 40*(1026), 51–52.

Mims, F. H., & Swenson, M. (1980). *Sexuality: A nursing perspective.* New York, NY: McGraw-Hill.

North American Nursing Diagnosis Association (NANDA). (2001). *Nursing diagnoses: Definitions and classification 2000–2001.* Philadelphia: Author.

Northrup, C. (1998). *Women's bodies, women's wisdom.* New York, NY: Bantam Books.

Parker, P., & Rosenfeld, J. A. (1997). Dyspareunia and pelvic pain. In J. A. Rosenfeld (Ed.), *Women's health in primary care.* Baltimore, MD: Williams & Wilkins.

Poorman, S. C. (1988). *Human sexuality and the nursing process.* Norwalk, CT: Appleton & Lange.

Rogers, A. (1990). Drugs and disturbed sexual functioning. In C. I. Fogel & D. Lauver (Eds.), *Sexual health promotion.* Philadelphia: W. B. Saunders.

Rynerson, B. (1990). Sexuality through the life cycle. In C. I. Fogel & D. Lauver (Eds.), *Sexual health promotion.* Philadelphia: W. B. Saunders.

Schover, L. R. (1988). *Sexuality and chronic illness.* New York, NY: Guilford Press.

U.S. Department of Health and Human Services. (2000). *Healthy People 2010.* Washington, D.C.: Author.

U.S. Office of the Surgeon General. (2001). *Surgeon General's Call to Action to Promote Sexual Health and Responsible Sexual Behavior.*

Woods, N. F. (1984). Human sexuality: A holistic perspective. In N. F. Woods (Ed.), *Human sexuality in health and illness* (3rd ed.). St. Louis, MO: C. V. Mosby.

Woods, N. F., & Stamer, A. F. (1984). Sexuality throughout the life cycle: Prenatal life through adolescence. In N. F. Woods (Ed.), *Human sexuality in health and illness* (3rd ed.). St. Louis, MO: C. V. Mosby.

World Health Organization. (1975). *Education and treatment in human sexuality: The training of health professionals. Technical Report Series No. 572.* Geneva, Switzerland: Author.

BIBLIOGRAPHY

Johnson, B. K. (1996). Older adults and sexuality: A multidimensional perspective. *Journal of Gerontological Nursing, 22*(2), 6–15.

McLaren, A. (1995). Comprehensive sexual assessment. *Journal of Nurse Midwifery, 40*(2), 104–149.

Internet Resources

http://www.plannedparenthood.org/WOMENSHEALTH/ sexuality.htm

http://www.sxetc.org/

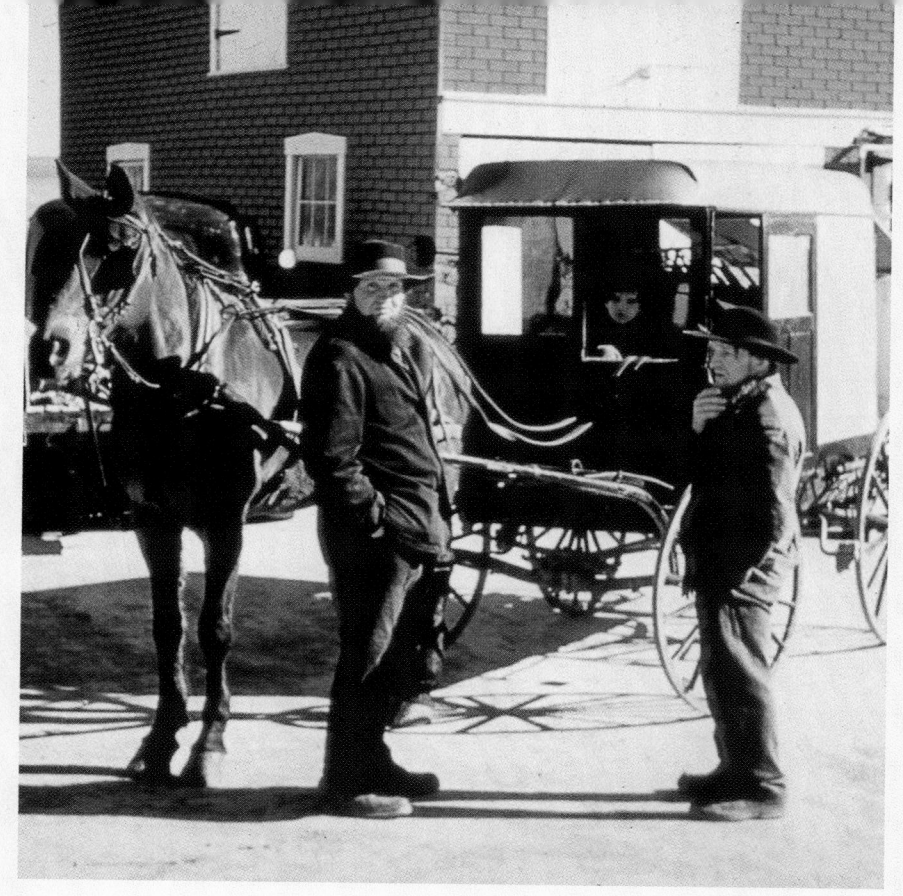

Values and Beliefs

51 Spiritual Health

Key Terms

agnosticism
atheism
faith
holism
spiritual care

spiritual dimension
spiritual need
spiritual well-being
spirituality
theism

Learning Objectives

Upon completion of this chapter, the student will be able to do the following:

1. Explore philosophic questions about life.
2. Discuss his or her personal spiritual journey.
3. Identify spiritual needs in self and others.
4. Identify major local religious faiths and their traditions.
5. Incorporate age-appropriate spiritual assessment questions into nursing assessment.
6. Use appropriate nursing diagnoses in writing plans of care for clients with spiritual problems.
7. Plan how to use self in spiritual support.
8. Develop a resource library of "spiritual" literature.

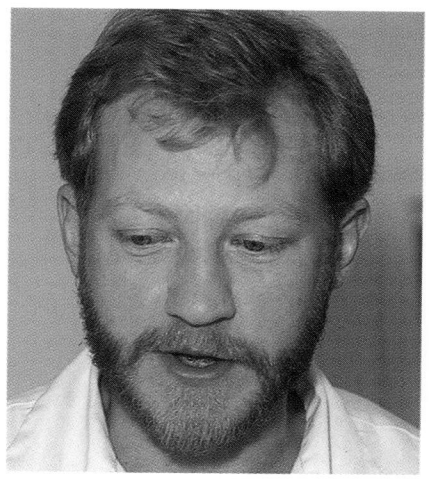

Critical Thinking Challenge

You are a nurse working in a daytime drug rehabilitation program. One of the clients, a cocaine user, tells you that his younger brother attempted suicide by jumping from a building. The client says that the night before the suicide attempt, the brother had called him and asked to go skiing, but the client (on a "high") said "no." The subsequent suicide attempt was unsuccessful, and the brother is now in serious condition, paralyzed from the waist down. The client also learned that this is his brother's second suicide attempt in a month. The client's family had not told him of the previous attempt because he was "stoned" all the time. The client confides that when he visited with his brother last night, "I tried to pray, but nothing would come."

Spiritual health, including the significance of concerns like being unable to pray, plays a crucial role in the function of the "whole" person. Once you have completed this chapter and have incorporated spiritual health into your knowledge base, review the above scenario and reflect on the following areas of Critical Thinking:

1. Consider the potential underlying spiritual issues in the above scenario from the client's point of view, the family's, and the injured brother's.
2. Reflect on your own spiritual perspective. How did you respond to the issues presented above?
3. Construct ideas for how you would respond to this client.

Nurses have the opportunity to contribute to and participate in any client's spiritual health by promoting spiritual well-being and providing the climate for spiritual healing. All people have a spiritual component or dimension that they can develop; however, the ways in which each person expresses spirituality depend on background, family, society, culture, and particular religion.

In terms of spiritual care, your own background, family, culture, and religion are integral parts of interactions with clients. For this reason, taking a step back and examining your own spirituality, values, and beliefs is essential. Often, this examination leads you to reflect on some deep philosophic questions such as: Who am I? Why am I here? What am I doing? Why am I doing it? How can I justify these things? Reflecting on these questions helps to develop a philosophic base for clearer thinking about nursing and health. For example, what one believes about the spiritual dimension is reflected in one's relationship to others.

NORMAL SPIRITUAL FUNCTION

"The **spiritual dimension** is a quality that goes beyond religious affiliation, that strives for inspiration, reverence, awe, meaning and purpose, even for those who do not believe in any god. The spiritual dimension tries to be in harmony with the universe, strives for answers about the infinite, and comes into focus when the person faces emotional stress, physical illness, or death" (Murray & Zentner, 1993, pp. 474–475).

Although all people have the spiritual dimension within their being, not all have the same depth or intensity of it in their lives. **Spirituality** is the quality or essence that pervades, integrates, and transcends one's biopsychosocial nature.

Fromm (1968, p. 68) commented on what it means to be human: "If man were satisfied to spend his life making a living, there would be no problem . . . [however] there is a sphere characteristic of man which one can call the trans-survival or trans-utilitarian sphere . . . He [man] is the only case of life being aware of itself."

Both Assagioli (1971), a psychotherapist, and Tillich (1969), a theologian, describe the human need for synthesis with the Supreme Being or Supreme Other. They describe how all humans have a spiritual dimension, which is the potential to strive toward unity and a higher consciousness to locate meaning and purpose in life.

Characteristics of Spirituality

The major characteristics of spirituality include a sense of wholeness and harmony within one's self, with others, and with God or a higher power as one defines it. People, according to their developmental level, experience and project personal security, strong identity, and a sense of hope. It does not mean that individuals are totally satisfied with life or have all the answers. As each person's life normally unfolds, situations arise that cause anxiety, helplessness, or confusion. Difficult situations generate spiritual questions. Assisting clients with the ensuing spiritual struggle is a valid and important aspect of maintaining health and giving healthcare.

Holism

Holism, the position of viewing the universe as a system of harmonious interconnectedness rather than a sum of isolated parts, integrates the mind and body and emphasizes spirit (Sellers & Haag, 1998). A holistic approach recognizes the spiritual struggle as a valid and important aspect of health and healthcare (Fig. 51-1). It is the integrating factor of "previously compartmentalized constructs of physical body, rational mind, emotional psyche, and intuitive spirit" (Ruffing-Rahal, 1984, p. 12).

Spiritual Need

Definitions of **spiritual need** vary according to each author's belief system. In summarizing the various definitions, spiritual need represents a normal expression of a person's inner being that seeks meaning in all experience and a dynamic relationship with self, others, and to the supreme other as the person defines it. Spiritual needs are derived through affective experiences of faith, hope, love, and positive experiences that serve as catalysts of synthesis and meaning. Spiritual needs include trust, forgiveness, love and relatedness, faith, creativity and hope, meaning and purpose, and grace.

Spiritual Quest

Life may be viewed as a spiritual quest, not only to answer life's philosophic questions but also to seek a higher level of consciousness or a deeper awareness of spiritual life. For example, the Twelve-Step program of Alcoholics Anonymous

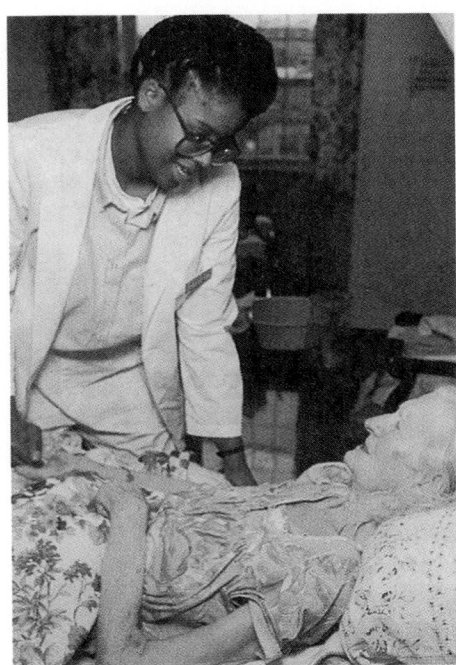

FIGURE 51-1 In spiritual care, the nurse addresses both the physical and spiritual needs of the client.

identifies recovery as a spiritual journey; group members practice a spiritual discipline to live more meaningfully day by day. Recovery begins "through a 'leap of faith' which says that there is no meaning to be found other than that which is beyond one's self; that which transcends man's ability to know—that which is God" (Dyson, Cobb, & Forman, 1997; Kreidler, 1984, p. 175). Chapman (1986, p. 41) also includes the idea of search in defining optimal spiritual health. Spiritual health includes ". . . our ability to discover and articulate our own basic purpose in life, learn how to experience love, joy, peace and fulfillment. . . ."

Spiritual Well-Being

Spiritual well-being is a condition marked by an affirmation of life, peace, harmony, and a sense of interconnectedness with God, self, community, and environment that nurtures and celebrates wholeness (Greer & Moberg, 1998). In the hierarchy of human needs, spiritual well-being appears to connote fulfillment of needs beyond the self-actualization level. For example, Hunglemann and colleagues' (1985) study of older adults found that harmony and interconnectedness were the two major determinants of spiritual well-being with both healthy and terminally ill clients. All the subjects expressed a belief in a Supreme Being, had some means of communication with that entity through prayer and worship, and had an extensive social support system of meaningful personal relationships.

Normal Spiritual Pattern

Part of a person's spiritual pattern relates to his or her values, beliefs, and faith. Beliefs may range from **atheism** (denial of God's existence) to **agnosticism** (belief that God's reality is unknown and unknowable) or to **theism** (belief that God's reality is personal, without a body, perfect in all things, and creator and sustainer of the universe). For example, Christians, Jews, and Muslims are all theists although each group further holds distinct beliefs about God's nature and activity. **Faith,** however, is more than belief; it is the way that a person acts out beliefs in his or her life. It involves "one's dynamic way of making meaning" (Fowler, 1981). It is the personal expression of living out one's spiritual pattern (Fig. 51-2). Thus beliefs, faith, and values are interconnected because what one sets one's heart on, believes in, or lives out comprises one's values. Faith is central to the way the person makes meaning.

The expression of spirituality, often through a specific religious group, usually follows an established order of practices. These practices may range from simple meditation and relaxation to more formal worship such as church services or rituals at shrines. Many observances take place within the home, in private, or with the family. Some traditions involve special foods or ceremonies as part of the celebration of special holy days. These celebrations hold symbolic meaning and a sense of deep mystery or miracle to those who follow the religion.

Some people practice their form of spirituality daily; others formally observe only one or two holy days; still others

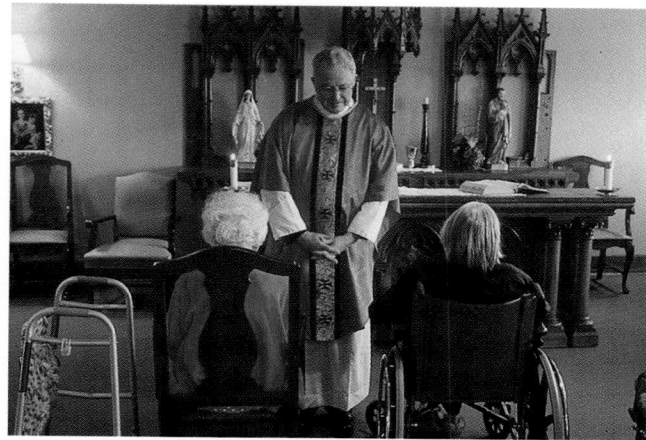

FIGURE 51-2 One's spiritual pattern is lived out in one's belief, faith, and values.

answer a "call" to full-time service in a specific religious group. Whatever the spiritual or religious beliefs the person holds and practices, these beliefs fulfill the following needs:

- Give meaning to life, illness, other crises, and death
- Contribute a sense of security for present and future
- Guide daily living habits
- Drive acceptance or rejection of other people
- Furnish psychosocial support within a group of like-minded people
- Provide strength in meeting life's crises
- Give healing strength and support

The major world religions include Christianity, Judaism, Hinduism, Buddhism, and Islam. All these religions are practiced in the United States and Canada. These groups have many branches that arose from historical events. For example, when the ancient Roman Empire fell, the Catholic Church was divided, becoming the Eastern Orthodox Church and the Roman Catholic Church. Still later, the Roman Catholic Church split again. King Henry VIII of England formed the Anglican Church or the Church of England when he decided to rule the church in place of the Pope. During the Protestant Reformation, more Christian groups formed, including such denominations as Lutheran, Presbyterian, and Methodist. Today, a fourth group, Baptist, is the largest Protestant denomination in the United States. Judaism has three main branches: Reform, Conservative, and Orthodox. Islam also has several branches in the United States. The newest form is the American Muslim Mission (sometimes called the Black Muslims).

Most religious groups have a spiritual leader. That person may be a pastor, priest, or rabbi who is educated in spiritual direction or pastoral counseling, or a shaman or spiritual healer who is trained in ancient cultural traditions. Shamans and spiritual healers are found among Native Americans and many Southeast Asian groups. These leaders are often the center of the spiritual or religious community, leading worship, teaching, and healing.

Lifespan Considerations

A person's level of growth and development influences his or her spiritual expression. Building on the theories of Erikson and Piaget, Fowler (1981) formulated a theory of faith development as the person's integrating center of valuing. Fowler's theory does not address the content of a person's faith, such as a specific religious belief system, but views faith as another way of knowing the world, a spiritual knowing based on a particular phase of psychological and cognitive development. The stages of faith knowing have parallels with Piaget's stages of cognitive development and Erikson's stages of psychosocial development. Table 51-1 is adapted from *Stages of Faith* (Fowler, 1981). The following discussion integrates faith stage concepts with growth and development and identifies spiritual needs arising from these stages.

Newborn and Infant

Trust in caregivers is the basis not only for development of a sense of safety, security of self in the world, and interpersonal relationships but also for faith development. Human beings' initial knowledge of the world is through relationships. If parents who are secure and have a sense of meaning and commitment meet basic trust needs, infants will sense this kinesthetically and incorporate this feeling into their "innermost being." This sense of trust will later broaden and deepen into trust in the world, the universe, and a "higher power."

Toddler and Preschooler

The first stage of faith development, Intuitive-Projective, is characterized by a continuing differentiation of self from others and an awakening of consciousness and memory. The introduction of language and gestures facilitates the child's ability to participate in some faith rituals of the family's religion. Children will respond to routines such as grace before meals, bedtime stories and prayers, special celebrations, and holy days if they are offered as a consistent, natural part of family life. Children also respond positively to those who treat seriously their questions about the world, life, and death. Although children do not know about such matters rationally, they intuitively sense the deeper spiritual questions of existence.

School-Age Child and Adolescent

Children notice the difference between themselves as individuals and others in similar or different groups. Although they are still primarily oriented to the parents' authority, children value belonging and acceptance in their own groups. They continue to be sensitive to good–bad issues, often trying to "make up" for wrongdoing in concrete, literal ways.

Children can now think in a historical perspective and see themselves as part of their family tree. The use of "story" is a major strategy for giving meaning to experience. Childhood is the period when the lore, legends, language, and symbols of a particular religious group are best presented. Wishes, needs, facts, and fantasy may appear somewhat confused, but children are attempting to make sense of the world. This period is the mythic–literal period.

The major change in adolescence is the beginning of the ability to think abstractly, to conceptualize, and to synthesize. Adolescents can ask more sophisticated, philosophic questions, test the truth, evaluate others' behavior, and note incongruities. They develop their own personal style, based on their beliefs, attitudes, and values. Although adolescents are individually involved in this personal synthesis of identity, they carry out this function mainly within the peer group. Mutuality and interpersonal relationships have major effects, making the development process both individualistic and conventional. Although the spiritual need is the same, faith is now centered within the peer group, synthesized differently from the parents. Authority has moved from the parents to the peer group. Thus, the name for this stage is Synthetic–Conventional.

Adult and Older Adult

In the Individuative–Reflective stage, young adults move away from the conforming peer group and clarify boundaries of selfhood and commitment. An encounter with people or groups other than those that provided support in the previous stage often precipitates this shift. Values, beliefs, and attitudes change as a result of interacting in more diverse, pluralistic settings, which can be stressful and frightening. Some situations precipitating this shift include new jobs, international travel, advanced study or education, or new religious affiliations possibly intertwined with achieving intimate re-

TABLE 51-1

Stages of Human Development: Optimal Parallels			
Stages (years)	**Erikson**	**Piaget**	**Fowler**
Infancy (0–1.5)	Trust (hope) Autonomy (will)	Sensorimotor	Undifferentiated–Primal
Early childhood (2–6)	Initiative (purpose)	Intuitive/Preoperational	Intuitive–Projective
Childhood (7–12)	Industry (competence)	Concrete Operational	Mythic–Literal Faith
Adolescence (13–21)	Identity (fidelity)	Formal Operational	Synthetic–Conventional
Young adulthood (21–35)	Intimacy (love)		Individuative–Reflective Faith
Adulthood (35–60)	Generativity (care)		Conjunctive Faith
Maturity (60–)	Integrity (wisdom)		Universalizing Faith

Adapted from Fowler, J. (1981). *Stages of faith* (p. 52). New York: Harper and Row.

THERAPEUTIC DIALOGUE
Afterlife

Scene for Thought

Jeremy Gaston is 17 years old and in the hospital for his third chemotherapy treatment for leukemia. He is lying in bed and seems very quiet when the nurse stops in during morning rounds.

Less Effective

Nurse: Hi, Jeremy. How are you this morning? *(Checks the central venous catheter and the medication's drip rate.)*
Client: I was just thinking about dying. *(Looks off into space.)*
Nurse: *(Stops to look at him in surprise, then continues checking the IV drip.)* What were you thinking?
Client: What it was like, just in case I don't make it through this cancer.
Nurse: I thought we talked about how much better you're getting?
Client: *(Looks sheepish.)* Yeah, I know, but sometimes it gets to me, all the chemo and how long it's taking and the pain. Sorry.
Nurse: You don't have to apologize, Jeremy. I know you get discouraged, but I also know you have Someone *(points up)* watching over you and caring for you. I feel that very strongly. So don't worry about dying just yet. *(Has tears in her eyes that Jeremy doesn't see.)*
Client: Okay. *(Looks off into space again.)*
Nurse: I'll let you rest now. Think good thoughts and this treatment will be over in a jiffy. *(Leaves the room.)*

More Effective

Nurse: Hi, Jeremy. How are you this morning? *(Checks the central venous catheter and the medication's drip rate.)*
Client: I was just thinking about dying. *(Looks off into space.)*
Nurse: *(Stops to look at him in surprise, then continues checking the IV drip.)* What were you thinking?
Client: What it was like, just in case I don't make it through this cancer.
Nurse: What do you think it would be like? *(Sits down next to the bed.)*
Client: My father almost died from a heart attack and said he could see himself on the emergency room table with everyone working on him. He said it wasn't scary, just weird.
Nurse: You've talked about this with your dad?
Client: Yeah. A few years ago. But my family isn't religious at all, so I'm not sure about the bright light or angels or anything like that. *(Sounds worried.)*
Nurse: You sound worried about that.
Client: I am. I'd hate to think there was nothing.
Nurse: So you're worried there might be nothing after death but you're not sure. Is that right?
Client: Yeah.
Nurse: You know, we've talked about pain and chemo and leukemia, but I don't think we've talked about this. What kind of help do you need now?
Client: *(Smiles.)* Maybe a philosophy course! Could we just talk a little about what you think death is?
Nurse: Sure. *(They continue. . . .)*

Critical Thinking Challenge

- From the first nurse's conversation, detect whom she was reassuring and how the client responded.
- Analyze what the second nurse helped the client do.
- Construct your own thoughts about an afterlife and how they affect the way you live.
- Analyze how your thoughts affect the way you care for your clients.

---

lationships, choosing careers, and starting families. The challenge during this stage is to establish one's own sense of faith and commitment based on personal experience and reflection on meaning in life (Fowler, 1981).

The middle years are fulfilled through productive activity—in Erikson's term, generativity. This time is of growth and renewed questioning, in some ways very similar to adolescence. Adults, however, deal with a broader world view rather than with group conformity. Older adults notice the polarities or extremes in life such as young and old, rich and poor, masculine and feminine, war and peace, constructive and destructive, and self-awareness and self-denial. These tensions, enhanced or precipitated by personal and environmental situations, demand integration and resolution. This is referred to as conjunctive faith (Fowler, 1981).

Most people do not achieve the final stage of faith, Universalizing. Usually only great leaders such as Mahatma Gandhi, Martin Luther King, and Mother Theresa appear to have achieved this world view. One's social perspective expands to include everyone as God's children with a more radical living-out of one's vision of the earth community. Terms such as justice, love, and compassion describe the goals of the person in the universalizing stage.

FACTORS AFFECTING SPIRITUAL HEALTH

A number of factors affect expression of spiritual needs. Such things include culture, gender, and previous experience. Individual reactions vary depending on personality and past coping styles. Other factors contributing to spiritual health include appropriate religious education, a firm spiritual identity, a dynamic and adaptable belief system, maintenance of belief systems in times of adversity or under questioning by others, recognition of spiritual assistance when needed, empathy for others' beliefs and values, and a sense of spiritual fulfillment.

Other factors, such as crises, moral issues, and separation, can effect changes in spiritual health and well-being, placing individuals at risk for altered spiritual function. These factors, however, are subjective and mean different things to different people. For example, a job change may challenge one person's sense of meaning whereas a broken relationship may influence another's.

Culture

Attitudes, beliefs, and values arise from one's sociocultural background. Usually, but not always, people follow the spiritual and religious traditions of their families of origin. Children learn the importance of religious practices, including moral values, from family relationships and participation in religious forms. In interfaith marriages, children may follow the practices of one parent over the other. Some parents try to instill the strengths of both religions in their offspring.

Many times, religious preference is tied to ethnic background. For example, many Italians and Irish are Roman Catholics, many Scandinavians and Germans are Lutherans, and many East Indians are Hindus. No matter what religious tradition or belief system a person follows, the inner spiritual experience is uniquely personal.

Gender

Spiritual expression also depends on society's and the religious group's beliefs and teachings about gender or expected behaviors for males and females. For example, in some religions that follow dietary laws, women are responsible to see that their families follow those laws. A person's organized religion may prescribe how each sex dresses and if one wears a head covering. In some cases, the spiritual leader is always male. Some religions encourage women to assume pastoral positions. This change, however, rises from political processes, particularly the equal rights movement.

Previous Experience

Fowler (1981) and others observe that many people direct their lives based on values that have been appropriated more or less uncritically. If something disruptive occurs, the person's "meaning-in-life assumptions" are called into question, which is sometimes termed a test of faith. Thus it would appear that if one's faith and values are confronted, then deeper spiritual needs would arise. During a crisis, past coping styles or learned ways of handling situations are likely to be evident. These coping patterns can be healthy and adaptive or they can be maladaptive. Life experiences in general are influences. Such experiences may or may not be related to age.

Crisis and Change

A crisis may strengthen a person's spirituality (Toth, 1992), which often happens when people face death. One study (Sherman, 1996) has shown that terminally ill clients or those who have life-threatening medical diagnoses demonstrate that spirituality is potentially a very significant variable. When these clients confronted their own mortality, reliance on spiritual assets such as faith and prayer increased when compared with nonterminally ill, hospitalized clients or healthy, nonhospitalized people. The disorienting experience of being near death enabled members of this group to reorient their lives spiritually. In a sense, there was healing.

Just as crisis may strengthen one's faith, it may also weaken it. Many people do not consciously reflect on their personal philosophies of life. They live life as if it were to continue forever. "Often it is not until the crisis, illness, aging, loss, limitation or suffering occurs that the illusion [or security] is shattered. . . . Therefore, illness, suffering, aging, loss, and ultimately death, by their very nature, become spiritual experiences as well as physical and emotional experiences" (Grandstrom, 1985, p. 12).

Crisis may be related to pathophysiologic changes, required treatments, or situations affecting the person. Diagnosis of a debilitating, disfiguring, or terminal illness can lead people to question their belief systems. Sudden trauma, miscarriage, or stillbirth may cause a person to doubt the presence of a Higher Being. Various treatments required for trauma and illness can lead to a sense of isolation or uncertainty. Many treatments generate additional problems such as amputation, surgery, medication administration, dietary restrictions, and other procedures.

Personal changes that result from the death or illness of a loved one, opposition to personal religious beliefs by significant others, or change in personal status can become other sources of spiritual distress. Being hospitalized can interrupt usual religious practices at a time when they are most needed, which can add to spiritual distress.

Separation From Spiritual Ties

Experiences of being hospitalized or becoming a resident in a retirement or nursing home can initially be shattering. To some extent, such individuals are isolated from personal freedom, personal privileges, and social support systems. They may be in private rooms with unfamiliar surroundings and may feel insecure. Daily habits may change. Some people are unable to attend formal services, have the accouterments of faith, or receive support from familiar groups. This separation from spiritual ties places people at risk for altered spiritual function.

Moral Issues Regarding Therapy

Many religions view healers and the healing process as evidence of God at work in the world. Certain religious groups, however, object to some modern medical interventions. For example, Jehovah's Witnesses do not accept blood transfu-

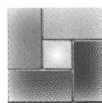

Nursing Research and Critical Thinking
How Can Nurses Assess Spiritual Strategies and the Spiritual Stages Through Which People With Cancer Pass?

Nurses know the necessity of conducting sound assessment before they can implement sound nursing interventions. Physical and psychosocial assessment skills have long been an important and visible part of nursing care, yet the spiritual assessment of human beings has not been well described in the nursing literature. When nurses define professional responsibility as caring for the whole person, they must also find the time, means, and knowledge to incorporate spiritual assessment into nursing care. To explore spiritual assessment strategies and the spiritual stages through which people with cancer pass, a nurse conducted research into the literature of various disciplines: nursing, medicine, theology, and other healthcare professions. She also conducted interviews with people with cancer to explore personal narratives and reflections on their experiences. She found that nursing authors consistently label the human longings to transcend self and circumstances, to discover meaning in suffering, to seek out hope in an unknown future, and to find sustaining relationships with others and God as spiritual. Yet, she found a persistent gap between the needs for spiritual assessment and care expressed by those with cancer and the

nursing care they received. Nurses and clients identified active listening, using words to connect with another, as both spiritual assessment and intervention. Many nurses find it difficult to ask about spiritual concerns. Once a nurse learns to overcome the barriers to asking spiritual assessment questions, the second and more difficult step in assessment is listening. Given the opportunity to reflect aloud, clients may name and begin work on their own spiritual issues.

Critical Thinking Considerations. This study is a beginning search of the literature about spiritual caring and exploration of a few personal narratives of people with cancer. The study points the way for future research into this important area. Implications for nurses from this study are as follows:

- Sound spiritual assessment is a prerequisite for sound spiritual intervention.
- When nurses ask about spiritual concerns, they assume an obligation to attend to the answers.
- Asking question is assessment; listening can become care.

From Highfield, M. F. (1997). Spiritual assessment across the cancer trajectory: methods and reflections. *Seminars in Oncology Nursing, 13*(4), 237–241.

---

sions. Some Christians oppose abortion because of their belief that the soul enters the body at conception. The Amish may refuse expensive treatments for individual members because the cost would impose a severe financial hardship on the entire community. Religious teachings influence attitudes toward many other medical procedures such as right-to-die decisions, organ transplantation, circumcision, birth control, sterilization, autopsies, and handling of the deceased. Some groups, such as Christian Scientists and Amish, have been legally exempted from immunizations; however, many medical decisions are reviewed on a case-by-case basis depending on the client's age and the imminence of death. The choice to treat may be difficult to make if the religious beliefs say "no" and the healthcare system says "yes." Many healthcare agencies have ethics committees to clarify and review such situations so more adequate and informed decisions are made.

Inadequate or Inappropriate Care

When dealing with spiritual care, nurses must be careful neither to avoid assisting clients with such care nor to involve themselves without desire on the client's part (Berggren-Thomas & Griggs, 1995). In general, people receiving healthcare depend on nurses and the healthcare team. Nurses attempt to

overcome this inherent dependency by being advocates for clients and by involving clients as much as possible in mutual goal setting and care planning. However, each client is a captive audience. Thus, doing nothing or jumping in too quickly may result in inadequate or inappropriate care.

Nurses may avoid giving spiritual care for several reasons including insecurity in their own spiritual lives, assigning less value and importance to spiritual care, having little or no educational preparation in spiritual care, or believing that it is the clergy's territory or that spiritual issues are intensely private. Usually too many demands and too little time detract from opportunities to provide spiritual care. Grandstrom (1985) elaborates on these reasons when she identifies five fairly complex values issues between nurses and clients:

- Pluralism: Nurses and clients embrace a wide spectrum of beliefs and creeds
- Fear: Related to not being able to handle situations, intruding on client's privacy, or becoming confused in one's own belief and value system
- Awareness of own spiritual quest: What gives meaning, purpose, hope, and sense of love in one's own life
- Confusion: Confusion over differences between religious and spiritual concepts

- Basic attitudes: Attitudes relative to illness, aging, and suffering

Long (1997) studied spirituality in relation to nurses' own coping strategies when dealing with suffering clients and concluded that nurses who function in a spiritual vacuum feel frustrated, helpless, and anxious when caring for suffering clients. Because relief of suffering is an essential nursing goal, there is a clear need to help nurses face and work effectively with this situation. Kreidler (1984, p. 174) states that "nurses need reassurance that groping for meaning in suffering . . . [is] . . . a sign of strength. . . . Our spiritual distress when facing suffering must be explored and understood if we are to be able to minister to our clients' needs." Kreidler (1984, p. 175) continues, "Spiritual distress is met through the encouragement and preservation of life coupled with the belief that every human life does have meaning; that no one ever lives, suffers, or dies in vain." Thus nurses need opportunities to reflect on their own philosophies and belief systems. Useful questions for this include:

- What do I believe?
- What gives meaning to my life?
- How is my belief system working for me?
- Is my behavior compatible with my belief system?
- How does my belief system relate to my future?
- Is there a relationship between my belief system and my healthcare behavior? (Groer, O'Connor, & Droppleman, 1996)

ALTERED SPIRITUAL FUNCTION

Manifestations of Altered Spiritual Function

Various behaviors and expressions may be warning signs that clients are experiencing spiritual concerns. Table 51-2 is a compilation of categorizations regarding adaptive and maladaptive expressions of spiritual needs that may help examine potential spiritual distress manifested in clients or that may appear in support persons or families.

Verbalization of Distress

Persons suffering spiritual dysfunction may verbalize such distress or express a need for help. The manifestation may be precise: "I feel guilty because I should have realized earlier he was having a heart attack." A person may state that he or she misses Sunday church services and the beautiful music of the choir or may say, "I've never missed a service in 20 years." The manifestation may be more subjective as in the case of the client's rambling speech about life, death, and worth. Clients may ask nurses to pray for them or to notify a spiritual leader of their illness.

Altered Behavior

A change in behavior may be a manifestation of spiritual dysfunction. A client who is nervous about the outcome of a diagnostic test or who shows anger after hearing the re-

sults may be suffering from spiritual distress. Some people become more introspective, attempting to figure out the situation and search for facts in available literature. Some react emotionally, seeking information and support from friends and family. Still others appear not to "hear" and show no outward signs of recognition of the problem; their distress may surface as sleeplessness or lack of concentration. Guilt, fear, depression, and anxiety also may indicate altered spiritual function.

Impact on Activities of Daily Living

All clients need some orientation and understanding of daily structure. The clients' attitudes and moods toward their daily lives influence their acceptance and expectation of care. Clients may go through the motions of daily living but their involvement in living is changed. Their "spirit" level has changed. For example, clients experiencing spiritual distress related to love and relatedness may refuse to cooperate with health regimens or to ask for help. If a client questions pain or the meaning of illness or expresses no reason to live, he or she may be expressing spiritual distress related to loss of meaning and hope. Thus spiritual distress influences the process of daily living rather than the actual tasks.

Clients and families may have divergent spiritual beliefs and practices and not really be aware of these differences on a daily basis (Spiritual Care Work Group, 1990). Thus for example, if family members become involved in home care, there may be unspoken assumptions and expectations regarding life's spiritual dimension. Depending on the ages and maturity of family members, they may or may not be able to articulate needs such as hope, meaning, or forgiveness. Spiritual distress may be experienced as a subtle, "gnawing" feeling of inadequacy. Spiritual distress among family members might be evidenced as anger and blame.

ASSESSMENT

Stoll (1979) cautions that the timing of the spiritual assessment is important and that it should follow the psychosocial assessment. Then if the client has some questions about this portion of the interview, the nurse can explain that spiritual beliefs are also an important part of maintaining health.

Subjective Data

Normal Pattern Identification

Several nurses have developed spiritual assessment tools. Stoll's (1979) Guidelines for Spiritual Assessment is probably most widely recognized. It identifies four areas and suggests questions for each: (1) concept of God or deity, (2) source of hope and strength, (3) religious practices and rituals, and (4) relationship between spiritual beliefs and state of health. Some questions include the following:

- Is religion or God significant to you?
- To whom do you turn when you need help?

TABLE 51-2

Adaptive and Maladaptive Expressions of Spiritual Needs		
Needs	**Adaptive Behavior/Pattern**	**Maladaptive Behavior/Pattern**
Trust	Trusts self and own endurance Accepts that others will be able to meet needs Trusts in life Accepts life's outcomes Is open to God	Shows discomfort with self-awareness Is gullible Feels that only certain people and places are safe Expects people to be unkind and unreliable Is impatient Fears God's intentions
Forgiveness	Accepts fallability of self and others Is nonjudgmental Views illness realistically Experiences self-forgiveness Offers to forgive others Accepts God's forgiveness Has realistic perspective on the past	Views illness as punishment Believes God is judgmental Feels that forgiveness depends on behavior Is unable to accept self Either blames self or projects blame
Love and relatedness	Expresses feelings of being loved by God/others Accepts help Is self-accepting Seeks the good in others	Feels others judge him or her Behaves self-destructively Fears dependence on others Refuses to cooperate with health regimen Worries about separation from loved ones Is self-rejecting or displays false pride and selfishness Lacks love relationship with God Feels distant/separated from God
Faith	Depends on divine wisdom/God Is motivated toward growth Expresses satisfaction with explanation of life after death Expresses need to enter into and/or understand larger drama of human history Expresses need for the symbolic, ritual Expresses need for sense of a shared faith/community	Expresses ambivalent feelings about God Lacks faith in a transcendent power/God Fears death/life after death Senses isolation from faith community Is bitter, frustrated, and/or angry with God Has unclear values, beliefs, and goals Has values conflicts Lacks commitment
Creativity and hope	Asks for information about condition Talks about condition realistically Uses time during illness constructively Seeks ways for self-expression Finds comfort in inner self rather than physical self or worldly criteria Expresses hope in the future Is open to the possibility of peace	Expresses fear of loss of control Expresses boredom Lacks vision of possible alternatives Fears therapy Despairs Cannot help self or accept self Cannot enjoy anything Has put life/major decisions on hold
Meaning and purpose	Expresses contentment with life Lives life in accordance with value system Accepts or uses suffering to understand self Expresses meaning in life/death Expresses commitment and goal orientation Has clear sense of what is important	Expresses no reason to live Finds no meaning in suffering Questions the meaning of suffering Questions the purpose of illness Cannot form goals or has unattainable goals Abuses drugs/alcohol Jokes about life after death

(continues)

TABLE 51-2 (Continued)

	Adaptive and Maladaptive Expressions of Spiritual Needs	
Needs	**Adaptive Behavior/Pattern**	**Maladaptive Behavior/Pattern**
Grace	Is alive in the moment Senses blessing/abundance Senses mercy given beyond self from God Senses harmony/wholeness	Is anxious about the past/future Is oriented toward achievement/production Focuses on regrets/remorse Talks about doing better/trying harder Is perfectionistic

- Do you feel your faith (religion) is helpful to you? If yes, tell me how.
- Has being sick (or what has happened to you) made any difference in your feeling about God or the practice of your faith?

Shelly and Miller (1999) also developed an assessment tool; the questions are similar to Stoll's but the following represent some differences in focus:

- Why are you in the hospital [or healthcare agency]?
- Has being ill affected your outlook in any way?
- Has your illness affected your relationship to the most significant person(s) in your life?
- Has being ill affected the way in which you view yourself?
- What is your greatest need at this time?

Tools also have been modified for various populations. For example, Still (1984) uses different questions to assess children's spiritual needs. Some questions include the following:

- How do you feel when you are in trouble?
- To whom do you turn when you are scared (in addition to your parents)?
- What are the favorite things you like to do when you are happy? When you are sad?
- Do you know who God is? What God is like?

An example of a spiritual assessment tool is given in Display 51-1.

In addition to using assessment tools, the nurse's sensitive observation and listening can elicit other cues. Possible cues regarding children's spiritual needs might include refusal to attend activities, preoccupation with another's situation or illness, reference to Sunday school, statements made in passing by the parents about God's will, and symbolic drawings (Pehler, 1997).

Risk Identification

In one sense, all clients suffering from ill health are at risk for spiritual distress. They may be physically separated from usual sources of spiritual help such as a faith community that maintains relationships and performs rituals of worship. They may be emotionally separated as well, especially if they lack introspection. Even for those who have spiritual strengths, however, the time of illness and accompanying crises in-

crease anxiety. Certainly those clients with critical or terminal illnesses, who are facing death or other profound physical changes, face ultimate, meaning-in-life questions. Shelly and Miller (1999) identify nine situations indicative of a client at spiritual risk:

- One who is lonely and has few, if any visitors
- One who expresses some apprehensions and fears
- One whose illness may have some connection with his or her emotions or religious attitudes
- One who is facing surgery
- One whose surgery or illness forces him or her to change his or her way of living
- One who seems to be doing more than the average amount of thinking about the relationship of his or her religion to his or her health
- One whose pastor is unable to call on him or her or who has no church affiliation and so would receive no pastoral care
- One whose illness has obvious social implications
- One whose illness is terminal

Dysfunction Identification

The discovery of actual spiritual distress depends on the nurse's observation of the client's verbal and nonverbal responses to the nursing history interview. Assist the client in understanding that her or his nursing history is a review of the whole human being and that questions will be wide-ranging, including spiritual health as well as physical and emotional health. A client who appears angry, anxious, depressed, or defensive when asked spiritual questions may need to hear something like, "I can see from your response that you might not have expected these questions; however, they do let you know that we are interested in how you are experiencing your current situation. Do you have a question or concern in this area?" Some clients are relieved to know that the spiritual aspect of their being is worthy of the nurse's concern. Still other clients indicate that they have spiritual concerns but they will deal with them in their own time and way.

Identifying which spiritual need is lacking is related to the nurse's ability to "listen with a third ear." The interview's content or facts combined with nonverbal behavior evolves into a theme or a tone such as distrust, judgment, isolation, or bitterness. Such themes can then be linked with spiritual needs such as trust, forgiveness, love and relatedness, and faith.

DISPLAY 51-1

🖺 SPIRITUAL ASSESSMENT

Client Name _____ Date _____
Days in Treatment _____ Religious Preference _____
Marital Status _____ Children _____ Age _____

Part I. Spiritual Assessment Guide: In the beginning, share with the client that people have several personal aspects, such as physiologic, emotional, and spiritual, and that this is an interview dealing with the spiritual needs. If the client appears to be very uncomfortable, clarify his or her concern and listen.

1. Spiritual Ecology of Childhood
   A. Developmental History: Examples of some questions might be: Describe some early memories of how your family "kept" Sunday (or Saturday) or other Holy Days. How did you feel about yourself? Your family? God? Eternity? Who taught you about spiritual things? Can you remember any religious symbols, hymns, stories that had an impact on you? How did these experiences change as you got older?
   B. Current religious practice: Do you participate in a religious organization? Do you pray, meditate, or participate in some spiritual exercise?
2. Awareness of the Spiritual: Client's awareness of some universal power greater than himself or herself and his or her experience of that power. What do you think or feel about God? Is there an image or a song that expresses how you feel?
3. Meaning and Purpose: Client's concept of the direction that his or her life has taken, the present direction, and who is responsible for life's direction. What meaning does your life have for you right now? When you're feeling down or discouraged, what gives life meaning?

4. Faith and Trust: Client's ability to accept life's uncertainties and his or her willingness to trust and be trustworthy. How do you view the changes in your life? If you were to get a box labeled "Your Next Major Change," what would you do with it?
5. Forgiveness and Grace: Client's acceptance of others and self that allows him or her to confess and admit mistakes. What does the word "sin" mean to you?
6. Hope and Creativity: Client's desire to make changes in life/lifestyle. When you think of the future, how does it make you feel?
7. Love and Relatedness: Client's quality of relationships with family, friends, work associates, community, self, and God. How would you describe your relationship with people?
8. Crises and Peak Experiences: Client's coping abilities and strengths. Have you ever had a time of crisis or suffering when you felt life had no meaning? What happened to you during these times? Did you feel the same or different after these experiences? Did you try to get help from any idea or person? Was there a spiritual thought or expression that was helpful to you during this time? Have you ever had moments of great joy or breakthrough? How has this affected you? Is there any spiritual image, music, or art that expresses your experience?

Part II. Closing: Because this interview will stimulate a lot of thoughts and feelings, be sure to offer some clarification and summary time. Is there anything we haven't discussed that you would like to add? Do you have any questions?

* Adapted from Davis, M. C. (1981). Another look at spiritual assessment: A behavior adaptation model currently in use in a chemical association. *Bulletin of the American Protestant Hospital Association, 45*, 19–26: and Leean, C. (1985). *Faith development in the adult life cycle.* Module 2 (Rev.) Prepared for the Religious Education Association of the United States and Canada.

Objective Data

Objective data can help in assessing spiritual health. Because of the qualities of the spiritual dimension, objective assessment must be verified against subjective information. Sometimes in clients reluctant to verbalize such issues, objective data are the only clues to a difficulty.

Glean as much information about clients from general appearance, facial expression, eye contact, body posture and movement, sleeplessness, anxiety, crying, and inappropriate emotions. Materials such as religious articles, books, cards, and pictures also indicate the spiritual dimension, as do visi-

tors from the church or clergy. Look for physical signs and symptoms of anxiety or distress that may provide additional evidence.

NURSING DIAGNOSES

Spiritual care diagnoses are addressed in the North American Nursing Diagnosis Association (NANDA, 2001) under the domain, Life Principle in Taxonomy II. Life Principle is described as "Principles underlying conduct, thought, and behavior about acts, customs, or institutions viewed as being true or having intrinsic worth." Under this domain are three classes, Values, Beliefs, and Values/Beliefs/Action Congruence. The Beliefs Class has the concept Spiritual Well-being with the diagnosis of Readiness for Enhanced Spiritual Well-being. The third class, Values/Beliefs/Action Congruence, has four nursing diagnoses, Spiritual Distress and Risk for Spiritual Distress, Decisional Conflict (specify), and Noncompliance (specify).

Spiritual Distress (Distress of the Human Spirit)

Definition. Spiritual Distress is disruption in the life principle that pervades a person's entire being and that integrates and transcends one's biologic and psychosocial nature (NANDA, 2001). The distress may be related to the inability to practice spiritual rituals, a conflict between religious or spiritual beliefs and prescribed health regimens, or a crisis of illness, suffering, and death (Carpenito, 1997).

Defining Characteristics. The major defining and present characteristic is that the client is experiencing a disturbance in belief system (Carpenito, 2002). This may involve a particular religious belief or for the nonreligious person a belief in the world, family, or work—whatever gives the person strength, hope, and meaning. Nine minor defining characteristics may be present: client questions credibility of belief system; client demonstrates discouragement or despair; client is unable to practice usual religious rituals; client is ambivalent about beliefs; client expresses no reason to live; client feels a sense of spiritual emptiness; client shows emotional detachment from self and others; client expresses concern, e.g., anger, resentment, fear about the meaning of life or suffering/death; and/or client requests spiritual assistance for disturbance in belief system.

Related Factors. Certain pathophysiologic, treatment-related, or situational factors may precipitate spiritual distress (Carpenito, 1997). For example, loss of a body part or function, terminal illness, debilitating disease, pain, trauma, or miscarriage or stillbirth may be considered pathologic states that raise questions of meaning and purpose. High-risk, treatment-related situations such as abortion, surgery, blood transfusions, dietary restrictions, isolation, amputation, medications, and other medical procedures may precipitate distress as a result of beliefs about health, illness, and healing. Personal or environmental situations such as death or illness of a significant other; childbirth; beliefs opposed by family, peers, or healthcare providers; divorce or separation from a loved one; or embarrassment at practicing spiritual rituals may cause spiritual distress. Hospitals or other healthcare facilities may also present barriers to practicing spiritual rituals. These include restrictions of intensive care, confinement to bed or room, lack of privacy, or lack of availability of special foods or diet.

Readiness for Enhanced Spiritual Well-Being

Definition. Spiritual Well-Being is the process of a person's developing/unfolding of mystery through harmonious interconnectedness that springs from inner strengths (NANDA, 2001). A sense of Spiritual Well-Being affirms life and all its experiences. It also means that people are not alone in life's journey but are spiritually connected with the larger universe.

Defining Characteristics. The major defining characteristics are inner strengths, unfolding mystery, and harmonious interconnectedness. Words used to describe inner strengths include a sense of awareness, self-consciousness, or inner core and a sense of the transcendent, a sacred source, or unifying force. Unfolding mystery connotes the perspective that life experiences of struggles and uncertainty have an ultimate meaning and purpose; however, it may be difficult or impossible to understand them through reason alone. A sense of peace, order, and union with self, others, the environment, and God/Higher Power describes harmonious interconnectedness.

Related Factors. NANDA has not yet established specific related factors, but factors related to spiritual well-being in general have been discussed earlier in this chapter.

Risk for Spiritual Distress

Definition. Risk for Spiritual Distress means that the person is at risk for an altered sense of harmonious connectedness with all of life and the universe in which dimensions that transcend and empower the self may be disrupted (NANDA, 2001).

Defining Characteristics. NANDA has yet to establish defining characteristics.

Related Factors. Related factors include energy-consuming anxiety; low self-esteem; mental or physical illness; blocks to self-love; poor relationships; physical or psychological stress; substance abuse; loss of loved one; natural disasters; situational losses; maturational losses; and inability to forgive (NANDA, 2001).

Decisional Conflict (Specify)

Definition. Decisional Conflict is uncertainty about course of action to take when choice of competing actions involves risks, loss, or challenge to personal life values (NANDA, 2001).

Defining Characteristics. The eight kinds of characteristics are: client verbalizes uncertainty about choices, client verbalizes undesired consequences or alternatives being considered, client vacillates between alternative choices, client delays decision making, client verbalizes feelings of distress while attempting a decision, client focuses on self, client has physical signs of distress or tension, and client questions personal values and beliefs while attempting to make a decision (NANDA, 2001).

Related Factors. Some related factors might be support system deficit, perceived threat to values system, lack of experience of interference with decision making, multiple or divergent sources of information, lack of relevant information, and unclear personal values and beliefs (NANDA, 2001).

Noncompliance (Specify)

Definition. Noncompliance means that the behavior of person or caregiver fails to coincide with health-promoting or therapeutic plan agreed on by the person (and/or family and/or community) and healthcare professional. In the presence of an agreed-on, health-promoting or therapeutic plan, the person's or caregiver's behavior is fully or partially nonadherent and may lead to clinically ineffective or partially ineffective outcomes (NANDA 2001).

Defining Characteristics. The six defining characteristics are behavior indicative of failure to adhere either by direct observation or statement of the patient or significant others, evidence of the development of complications, evidence of exacerbations of symptoms, failure to keep appointments, failure to progress, and failure of objective tests such as laboratory data that demonstrates improvement (NANDA, 2001).

Related Factors. There are three categories of related factors: healthcare plan, individual factors, health system and network. Examples under these categories include cost and complexity of the healthcare plan, person and developmental abilities, health beliefs, cultural influences, spiritual values under individual factors, satisfaction with care, client-provider relationship, and provider reimbursement of teaching and follow-up under health system, and perceived beliefs of significant others (NANDA, 2001).

Related Nursing Diagnoses

Other nursing diagnoses may be evident because of the various causes, manifestations, and results of spiritual distress. Possible diagnoses include Anxiety; Ineffective Denial; Dysfunctional Grieving; Dysfunctional Family Processes; Fatigue; Fear; Hopelessness; Impaired Parenting; Disturbed Personal Identity; Powerlessness; Ineffective Role Perfor-

mance; Self-Esteem; Disturbed Sleep Pattern; and Social Isolation.

OUTCOME IDENTIFICATION AND PLANNING

After nursing diagnoses and related factors are identified, the client and nurse plan outcomes and interventions. Goals for clients with spiritual distress should focus on providing an environment that supports usual religious practices and beliefs. Goals need to be individualized by considering the client's history, areas of risk, evidence of dysfunction, and related objective data. Examples of goals for the client with or at risk for spiritual distress include the following:

- The client will express acceptance of current life situation including satisfaction with the meaning and purpose of illness, suffering, and death.
- The client will participate in spiritual practices that are personally supportive and will express satisfaction with spiritual condition.
- The client will relate feelings of support in decisions regarding health regimens.

Goals for enhancing spiritual well-being can be very similar to those for clients in spiritual distress. The focus is on supporting the client's strengths. The opportunity for spiritual growth may also be present as the client explores creative ways to deal with pain and suffering. Some goals might include the following:

- The client will express a sense of wholeness or integrity during the illness and recovery process.
- The client will relate feelings of intimacy or closeness with others.
- The client will describe feelings for acceptance and respect when working through questions of meaning, purpose, and mystery.

PLANNING: Examples of NIC/NOC Interventions

Accepted Spiritual Health Nursing Interventions Classification (NIC)
Spiritual Support
Spiritual Growth Facilitation

Accepted Spiritual Health Nursing Outcomes Classification (NOC)
Dignified Dying
Hope
Spiritual Well-Being

Refer to the following for specifics regarding NIC/NOC:
McCloskey, J., & Bulechek, G. (2000). *Iowa Intervention Project: Nursing Interventions Classification (NIC)* 2nd ed. St. Louis, MO: C. V. Mosby.
Johnson, M., & Maas, M. (2000). *Iowa Outcomes Project: Nursing Outcomes Classification (NOC)* 2nd ed. St. Louis, MO: C. V. Mosby.

IMPLEMENTATION

Essential in implementing spiritual care are commitment to the nurse–client relationship, good communication skills, trust, empathy, self-awareness, and acceptance of a broad definition of spirituality.

Although qualitative aspects play a large part in performing nursing interventions, implementation also includes continuing data collection, maintaining current documentation, and collaborating with the healthcare team. These steps are important because they ensure consistency and continuity in client care. Spiritual care is not limited to each individual nurse.

The process should affirm the individual. Effective communication helps facilitate the client's use of his or her own spiritual resources or finding someone else to help the client. The timing will not be forced but will demonstrate sensitivity and empathy.

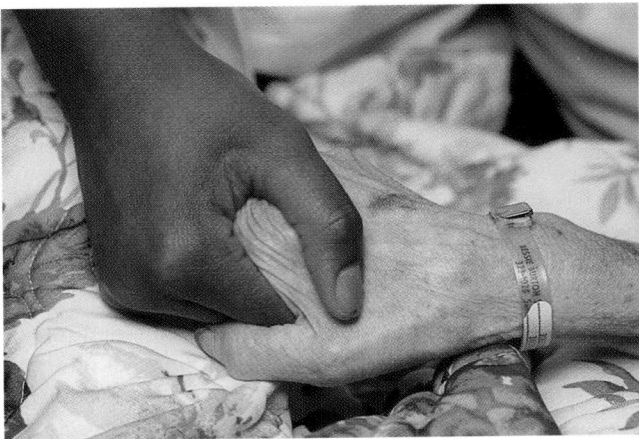

FIGURE 51-3   Being with the client when the client needs someone is an important aspect of spiritual care.

Health Promotion

Spiritual care can be defined as a mutual potentially healing or integrating process in which the client's spiritual needs are met. The word "potential" is inserted here because people of many faiths believe that God (or the Supreme Being as one understands it) ultimately fulfills spiritual needs through people (Wright, 1998).

Use of Self

Spiritual care occurs within the nurse–client relationship. This relationship does not consist only of talking with clients; it is the purposeful use of self to help another person grow in the ability to face reality and to discover potential solutions to problems. Spiritual care is a relationship that the nurse perceives as a valuable part of therapy and to which he or she holds a commitment.

Qualities such as trust and empathy are partially built on good communication skills and an understanding of the processes and phases of the nurse–client relationship. For example, making oneself and one's time available to clients is necessary to build trust in the initial phase of the relationship. Through active listening, nurses can understand the perspectives of clients and be more sensitive to their needs including spiritual needs. Without the establishment of trust and empathy in the relationship's first phase, nurses will be unable to discern deeper concerns such as meaning and purpose.

In discussing spiritual care of older adults, "being" with clients is a much more important aspect of spiritual care than "doing" (Berggren-Thomas & Griggs, 1995; Fig. 51-3). Being able to take part in the lives of clients is a privilege and responsibility. Thus, involvement in the meeting of spiritual needs is very personal for both nurses and clients.

Spiritual Support

Nurses also need to have a broad definition of spirituality to discern the spirituality of others. Relying on their own spiritual traditions and being knowledgeable about other spiritual and religious expressions are helpful. Each client varies in respect to expression of spiritual needs and level or depth of spiritual care. Therefore sensitivity to this variability and offering appropriate care are necessary.

Wright (1998) describes situations in which spiritual faith and belief are beyond the scope of scientific explanation yet appear to be helpful. Nurses should not attempt to change faith that clients already possess. They should support and build on the clients' faith. If faith is removed, clients will lose hope; without the will to live, many people are beyond the help of the most potent medical powers. Conversations regarding faith, however, must not pass judgment or present controversy. The need is to make clients feel accepted in their beliefs and encouraged to remain open in expressing and learning (Boland, 1998).

Piepgras (1984, p. 2613) gives the major principle in dealing with the ethical issue of personal witness in the nurse–client relationship:

Discussion should be confined to the client's ideas, to the client's needs, and to whatever level of religious terminology and frame of reference the client wishes to use. Personal witness by the nurse should be used, if at all, only after the client and the nurse have established a common ground and easy dialogue.

Support of Spiritual Practices

Information regarding the client's spiritual needs and religious preference is obtained during assessment. To facilitate meeting spiritual needs through specific religious practices, become familiar with the various religious groups within the community. Pay attention to special religious considerations such as beliefs about birth, death, sacraments, diet, holy days, and holy objects. For example, dietary practices reflect dietary laws (e.g., no pork or beef) as well as celebration of holy days by fasting or feasting. If the food required is so specialized that the healthcare facility's dietary department cannot accommodate the client's needs, the family may ask to bring in their own food. Table 51-3 gives a brief overview of the major religious groups' practices related to health.

In general, clients have the right to practice personal spiritual expressions in private, such as reading holy scriptures, praying, or meditating while in the hospital. When a client wears special amulets or garments on areas exposed to tests, treatments, or surgery, the circumstances may call for a special consultation with the family and spiritual leader rather than the nurse automatically removing them.

If the spiritual leader or healer plans to visit, prepare the client's room and religious articles appropriately. If the sacraments or other rituals are to be performed, make sure the bedside stand or table is clear.

Nursing Interventions for Altered Spiritual Function

When implementing spiritual care, prioritize emergency client needs. For example, basic survival needs, such as maintaining an airway, take priority over growth needs that have to do with self-actualization. However if the client has found no meaning in suffering, is experiencing hopelessness, or is unable to take part in his or her faith community, the spiritual dimension can become a central need. The client may have regained physical strength, but the spirit remains unfulfilled.

Listening and Supporting

The simplest definition of spiritual care is care given that meets spiritual needs and includes support, comfort, and help. Shelly (1982, p. 15) summarizes spiritual care as follows: Spiritual care is an integrating factor in healthcare. Respecting and encouraging a person's spiritual and religious interest and concerns enhances the healing process. Spiritual support includes communicating love, forgiveness, meaning, purpose, and hope in a time of discouragement and anxiety.

Thus, active listening with empathy and sensitivity becomes one of the most valuable nursing interventions. Through purposeful listening, the client defines personal spiritual questions and directs the most useful type of support. The following situation, adapted from Frye and Long (1985), illustrates the intervention of listening and support as an integral part of spiritual caregiving.

Robert, the son of a practicing physician and the eldest of four children, was a junior medical student. He was a handsome, popular young man with a keen, satirical sense of humor. Robert was scheduled to be at his first family practice clinic, but he didn't make it. Traffic was heavy on the freeway, and Robert found himself between a truck and a semitrailer with cars on either side. He tried to swerve into an adjacent lane and rear-ended a large truck. The impact propelled him off and under his motorcycle, resulting in instant unconsciousness. When he arrived at the emergency room, the outlook was grim.

The next 5 months were a battle. Fluctuating intracranial pressures with complications, pervading depression, and thoughts of suicide haunted him. Having deeply religious parents and a strong background in religious education, Robert seemed to have the spiritual strengths to deal with this crisis . . . until one day when the depth of his loneliness and doubt surfaced.

His nurse approached him, suspecting that he needed permission to doubt previous convictions. As a result, there was an outpouring of questions: Where was God when he needed Him? Why had God let him down?

Many conversations followed with Robert's mother, nurses, doctor, therapists, and chaplain. Family, friends, and staff supported Robert in his questions. Robert identified with the story of Job and began to talk of his hope.

As part of denial of his former convictions, Robert frequently requested pain medication during the day to help him sleep. He stated, "I just don't want to be awake." The nurse confronted him, asking him if he was truly in pain or was trying to escape from the realities of his situation. She recommended that they work together on a different approach.

Referral

Being comfortable listening to a client's spiritual needs and hearing religious requests is important. If the client or family members ask for prayer or scripture reading and you are comfortable doing that, try to identify the special focus or topic before beginning. When the client and family appear to have no religious tradition, ask to assist them in a quiet, reflective moment. Also, respond to any request to see the hospital chaplain, or initiate a referral to see one. One research study done in the Midwest, "Spiritual care in the hospital, who requests it and who needs it" (Fitchett, Meyer, and Burton, 2000), found that 35% of patients requested care in the form of talk with chaplain, prayer with chaplain, or to receive communion. Those who requested these services were likely to be older and nonwhite. Sixty-eight per cent of the patients did list a religious affiliation. However, the conclusion was that in order to have an effective use of time and reach out to patients who did not indicate a religious preference or request care, chaplains need to work with other healthcare colleagues to assess spiritual needs. This is where nurses can be most helpful. For effective referrals, nurses must have some familiarity with the available resources, particularly pastoral care, prayer, Scripture, religious rituals, devotional articles, and sacred music (O'Brien, 1999). Pastoral care departments are also resources for finding representatives of other religious groups.

Age-Specific Interventions

Newborn and Infant. Hospitalization and illness potentially disrupt an infant's basic trust in parents. The nurse can support the spiritual needs of parents by listening, offering support, and promoting stability. Such support of the parents will help, in turn, to meet the infant's needs. Encourage parents to be present and involved in the caring process with infants as much as possible (Pehler, 1997).

Toddler and Preschooler. Carrying out established routines and responding to concrete questions are important consider-

(text continues on page 1398)

TABLE 51-3

Practices of Major Religious Groups Related to Health

Religious Faiths	Dietary Rules	Birth Control and Abortion	Organ Transplants	Death and Dying
Observant Jews	Orthodox Jews observe Kosher dietary laws; Reform Jews usually do not observe dietary restrictions.	Orthodox Jews do not encourage birth control; abortion may be performed only to save mother's life.	Organ transplants generally not permitted by Orthodox or Reform Jews without rabbinical consent.	Advocate use of life support without heroic measures. Believe that family or friends should be with the dying person. Require special procedures for care of the body after death.
Roman Catholics	Observe fasting and abstinence from meat on certain Holy Days; hospitalized patients are excused from dietary obligations.	Birth control is prohibited except for abstinence and natural family planning. Abortion is prohibited.	Organ donation and transplantation are acceptable.	Believe that each Roman Catholic should have the anointing of the sick as well as the Eucharist and penance by a priest before death.
Mainline Protestants (e.g., Baptist, Nazarene, Lutheran, Methodist, Presbyterian, Episcopal)	Use of alcohol and tobacco is forbidden by many denominations. Episcopalians may observe fasting and abstinence from meat on some days.	Birth control is generally left as a matter of personal choice. Abortion is generally discouraged, but there may be some exceptions.	Organ donation and transplantation are acceptable.	Believe that notification of clergy, Scripture reading, and prayer are appropriate.
Islam (Muslims)	Pork and alcohol are forbidden.	Contraception is permitted by Islamic law. Abortion is forbidden.	Donation of body parts or organs is generally not allowed. Vigilant attitude is required to avoid misuse.	Believe family should be with the dying person so they can read the Koran and pray. Believe in special procedures for care of body after death; men wash male bodies and women wash female bodies and perform a variety of other rituals.
Other Western Faiths *Christian Science*	Alcohol and tobacco are prohibited.	Personal choice.	Donations of organs unlikely.	May require that Christian Science practitioner be called.

Special Concerns: Normally do not seek medical care.

TABLE 51-3 (Continued)

Practices of Major Religious Groups Related to Health

Religious Faiths	Dietary Rules	Birth Control and Abortion	Organ Transplants	Death and Dying
Jehovah's Witnesses	Use of alcohol and tobacco are discouraged.	Birth control is personal choice. Abortion is opposed.	Organ transplant is a personal decision but must be cleansed with a nonblood product.	No special practices.
Church of Jesus Christ of Latter Day Saints (Mormons)	Abstinence from tobacco, alcohol, and caffeine-containing beverages such as coffee, tea, and cola.			Notify church elder.
	Special Concerns: A sacred undergarment must be worn at all times.			
Seventh Day Adventists	Alcohol, tobacco, coffee, and tea are prohibited. Most members are vegetarians.	Personal choice.	Personal choice.	No special practices. Notify clergy.
Other Eastern Faiths				
Hinduism represents a 5,000-year tradition. Its many different beliefs and practices depend on the culture and tribal unit. One medical tradition is the Ayurveda system in which illness and wellness are viewed as a state of balance. In this world view, the human being is continuous with the environment.	Wide range from complete vegetarian to restrictions on certain foods such as poultry and milk products. Traditional foods include many legumes, yogurt, and spices. There is also a belief system of "hot" and "cold" food, depending on how the body responds. Balancing tastes is also important (e.g., sour, bitter). In some places, to refuse food means that one is angry or hurt.	All of life is sacred, so generally not practiced; however, there is preference for male children, and female infant sacrifices have been known. There may be some concern that amniocentesis could be used to preference male children. Because India has a population problem, both birth control and abortion are permitted but not generally practiced. Abortion has been legal since 1972.	In the Hindu tradition, ancient myths often are reinterpreted to fit current circumstances. At present, there is no information available as to how this procedure is viewed; however, the wealthy may go to other countries for medical care.	Believe in reincarnation, so life never ends. Regard untimely death with fear and sorrow. The family participates in mourning rituals both before and after mortal death. At death, some place the body on the floor or the earth to facilitate the soul's journey. Cremation is the common practice; fire purifies the body and the family gives the ashes to the holy waters.
Buddhism began in the 6th century BC in northeast India and expanded along trade routes to the	Diet is an issue of balance, similar to Hindu beliefs. Alcohol and other drugs are forbidden because they can lead to moral	There is ambiguity about when life begins so there is no clear-cut view on abortion. They are against killing or injuring humans	At present, there is no stated view about organ transplants. The principles guiding such decisions would include: "all is inter-	Believe life is a temporary state as a combination of body/mental elements, thus death is temporary and is necessary for re-

(continues)

TABLE 51-3   (Continued)

		Practices of Major Religious Groups Related to Health		
Religious Faiths	**Dietary Rules**	**Birth Control and Abortion**	**Organ Transplants**	**Death and Dying**
south, southeast Asia, China, and Japan and in the latter 19th century to the west. The medical system used is the Ayurveda system. The path of health is right living and thinking. There are many different Buddhist groups who follow different leaders.	carelessness. The laity may consume fairly heavily, however, and recent attempts at reform have not been taken seriously.	and animals. Both birth control and abortion have been known and practiced. The practice may not reflect the faith as much as current social and political policies.	dependent (family, donor, healthcare people, society) and suffering." (Personal communication from Ronald Nakasone, Ph.D., Institute of Buddhist Studies, Berkeley, CA)	birth. Family needs to be present; certain prayers need to be said by the priest. The color white means death, so the use of white by healthcare personnel may cause increased anxiety for some patients/families. Priest visits family home every day for prayers until burial. Prayers are said at certain times and up to 1 year after death then every year.

Special Concerns: Most Buddhists have no hesitation about seeking medical advice from non-Buddhist physicians. Thus some see medical interventions, such as organ transplants, as a technologic issue only.

Derived from Anles, P. (1989). Medicine and living tradition of Islam. In L. E. Sullivan (Ed.), *Healing and restoring, health and medicine in the world's religious traditions* (p. 189). New York: Macmillan; Carson, J. B. (1989). *Spiritual dimensions of nursing practice* (pp. 76–112). Philadelphia, W. B. Saunders; Desai, P. N. (1989). *Health and medicine in the Hindu tradition.* New York. Crossroad Publishing Company; Kitagawa, J. M. (1989). Buddhist medical history. In L. E. Sullivan (Ed.), *Healing and restoring, health and medicine in the world's religious traditions* (pp. 9–32). New York: Macmillan.

ations with toddlers and preschoolers. Support families to carry out rituals of faith. If the family is unavailable to do this, carry out these rituals for them. For example, bedtime (often a difficult transition for children at such ages and especially so in hospitals) is a crucial time to offer support (Pehler, 1997).

Young children are very sensitive to good–bad issues. Do not tell them that painful or scary treatments are in any way a punishment. Affirm that the children, although ill or hospitalized, are still loved by their parents, the nurse, God, Jesus, or whoever is appropriate according to the family's faith (Pehler, 1997).

School-Age Child and Adolescent.   Nurses continue to provide major support to families by carrying out familiar religious rituals in the healthcare setting. For children, clarify fact and fantasy when it comes to all medical interventions and procedures. Usually a "story" about a similar situation will aid in this reality-orienting process. Local libraries usually have many books in which children experience going to the health clinic or hospital. Again, children must not associate illness and hospitalization with wrongdoing and punishment, which would increase their anxiety and fear. Ac-

ceptance and clarification of the experiences are the effective modes to offer meaning to children.

For adolescents, development of a personal style and interaction with peers remain priorities even during illness. Involve the adolescent's peers by encouraging them to remain available either through visits, letters, or telephone. If a long-term illness, accident, or some other severe condition is involved, other networks of support might be useful such as the school or church. For example, youth groups might serve as communication links for hospitalized adolescents. Peers also might need the opportunity to explore their own responses to illness to work through their feelings about life. Youth leaders or hospital chaplains are resources for this kind of experience (Fulton & Moore, 1995).

Adolescents are capable of conceptualizing personal relationships with God (Pehler, 1997). In times of illness, they may question the meaning of the experience, trying to integrate it into their lives, much as adults would do under similar circumstances. These issues can often be discerned during a nursing history and assessment. Follow up on the data or involve the hospital chaplain or the adolescent's spiritual counselor.

Adult and Older Adult. Young adults clarify personal beliefs and commitments based on experience and relationships. Their faith challenge is to establish and to reflect on personal faith and life's meaning. Nurses will be unable to act in mentoring relationships with many clients. In some long-term relationships, however, nurses can be available to listen, support, and validate feelings and experiences to facilitate the exploration of meaning-in-life or meaning-in-death. At the very least, all nurses must understand that young adults have the need for spiritual mentoring. Be open to explore with clients the possibilities about whom might fulfill this role. Continue to be supportive of each client's family and social network because these relationships give meaning to the client's life.

During the middle years, adults become more concerned with a broader world view and polarities. Resolution of these polarities lies in being able to see and live with the paradoxes and being open to diversity, not threatened by it. Such people might be described as "wise-hearted." In some ways, they have much to offer others. For example, a young adult nurse might gain personally by spending time with an adult working through a paradox of health and illness. By being available to listen, support, and reflect with the client, the nurse could better understand the client's struggle. By accepting the possibility of mutuality in the relationship, the nurse has the opportunity to give new meaning and hope to the client. Risking mutuality demonstrates true respect and care, which, in turn, enhances both client and nurse (Fowler, 1981).

As with other age groups, listening and support are essential as clients deal with health–illness. Using a life review strategy, in which clients recollect past experiences and come to an understanding of them, is helpful. As infirmity increases, older adults may be less able than in previous years to participate in their faith communities. At this point, facilitate connections with people or groups in the community who can either visit regularly or assist with transportation. Such connections provide meaning and hope for older persons because some faith rituals are satisfactorily performed only in group settings.

For many older adults, other family members and friends have died in the last few years. The older clients not only need to be able to form new relationships with younger generations, they may want to come to terms with their own mortality. Providing answers is not important. Rather the focus is giving clients the opportunity to discuss death and to make their own choices about how arrangements should be handled (Boland, 1998).

Special Populations

The above is a general review of spiritual care needs along the life span continuum, but there are many special groups of patients that may have specialized needs depending upon the type of illness, phase of illness, or setting of care. There are differences in the spiritual concerns of persons with acute illness, persons with chronic illness, persons living with pain, or persons facing surgery (O'Brien, 1999). For example, persons living with a mental illness often have spiritual questions because the mental illness can be in a form expressed in terms of religious delusions or hallucinations. Often, though, healthcare providers including nurses avoid spiritual issues for fear of "supporting" the symptoms of the mental illness. This has led to a lack of assessment of spiritual needs and spiritual care. There are new views of "recovery" for the mentally ill including a key element of recovery as the spiritual need for hope. Hope is the "turning" point in a person's illness. So instead of avoiding spiritual care, several articles suggest ways of incorporating spirituality into care: "Achieving spiritual wellness: Using reflective questions" by Espeland (1999), "Spirituality, meaning, mental health and nursing" by Ameling and Povilonis (2001), and "How people with schizophrenia build their hope" by Kirkpatrick, Landeen, Woodside, and Byrne (2001).

Healthcare Planning and Home/Community-Based Nursing

Assessing and planning for spiritual care comprise an ongoing process. Settings that encourage this process most consistently are usually those in which nurses and clients can establish relationships over time. Examples may be in a clinic with the nurse as case manager, in a long-term care facility with the nurse as team leader, or in a community hospice program with the nurse making regular visits. In acute care settings, nurses most certainly can become aware of clients' spiritual needs and begin to address them. The most important part of that care, however, will be the discharge summary and a plan of care that identifies areas of spiritual distress. In this way, follow-up care can be more holistic.

Some clients want nurses to prearrange visits from pastors, priests, or other members of the religious community after their return home or transfer to another healthcare facility. In some areas of the United States, churches have developed parish nurse programs that assist clients and families to meet spiritual needs (Display 51-2). Clients need not be church members to receive parish nurse visits. They can be referred by geographic area.

Much healing and spiritual growth can occur without professional assistance because some clients find ways to meet their spiritual needs independently. Therefore, a sensitive and nonintrusive attitude on the nurse's part is crucial; nurses cannot force clients to deal with spiritual issues or to assume religious beliefs. "Sometimes [nurses] may set goals for the client and the family which are inflexible and unrealistic; this may inhibit spontaneity and impede the development of a sensitive spiritual relationship" (Spiritual Care Work Group, 1990). Spiritual health is one area that cannot be put onto a specific "road map" or trajectory.

EVALUATION

Specific outcome criteria are the evaluative tools for measuring goal attainment for clients in spiritual distress. Examples of outcome criteria are listed in the following sections and use "Robert" (see the section entitled Listening and Supporting) as an example. Outcome criteria need to be specifically tailored to each client so that the criteria will uniquely measure that client's attainment of goals.

NURSING PLAN OF CARE
THE CLIENT WITH SPIRITUAL DISTRESS*

Nursing Diagnosis
Spiritual Distress related to crisis of illness as evidenced by loss of meaning in life, suicidal thoughts, and overuse of pain medication.

Client Goal
Client will express increased understanding and acceptance of current life situation.

Client Outcome Criteria
- Client verbalizes feelings of despair, anger, and fear after 3 weeks.
- Client identifies support provided by staff, family, and friends during periods of questioning and despair after 5 weeks.
- Client identifies some alternative coping mechanisms other than requesting pain medications after 10 weeks.

Nursing Intervention	Scientific Rationale
1. Offer client opportunity for one-on-one nurse–client relationship. Actively listen to the client. Allow expression of negative feelings.	1. Initiating a one-on-one relationship establishes a climate of acceptance and builds trust and safety.
2. Plan and coordinate a multidisciplinary team conference including the chaplain. Facilitate a care-planning conference involving the social support network including family and friends.	2. Initiating a multidisciplinary social network of conferences facilitates a sense of acceptance, love, and belonging.
3. Explore past coping mechanisms including use of music, scripture, prayer, and relaxation techniques. Help client identify times when he or she can use a variety of these alternative strategies.	3. Building on past positive coping mechanisms enhances a sense of self-control and self-esteem.
4. Use the "life review" technique focusing on faith/spiritual development. Help client explore ways to use this experience in a unique way such as sharing in a group or with medical students or other health-care professional students.	4. By focusing on personal faith/spirit, the client can gain new insights into his or her relationship with God and can sense hope and the potential for creativity or self-actualization.

*Refers to the situation of "Robert."

Goal
The client will express acceptance of current life situation and satisfaction with the meaning and purpose of illness, suffering, and death.

Possible Outcome Criteria
- Client exhibits feelings of despair, anger, and fear during the first few days.
- Client identifies support provided by staff, family, and friends during periods of questioning and despair.

Goal
The client will participate in spiritual practices that are personally supportive and express satisfaction with spiritual condition.

Possible Outcome Criteria
- Within the first month, client asks to speak to a spiritual advisor.
- Client demonstrates spiritual practices such as prayer or reading of religious/spiritual texts within the second month.
- Client expresses satisfaction with being able to maintain relationships with his or her faith community within second month.

KEY CONCEPTS
- Spirituality, like the role of philosophy, is to help people ask the right questions and develop a view of life, rather than answer the questions.
- The spiritual dimension is the essence of a person and is expressed in the need to seek meaning in experiences and to make a spiritual journey through life.

DISPLAY 51-2

🔄 PARISH NURSING

Goal
To promote the health of a faith community and the community by working with the ministry team

Roles
Congregational nurse practitioner and congregational care nurse

Models
(O'Brien, 1999)
- Congregation-based volunteer
- Congregation-based, paid
- Other institutional-based volunteer
- Other institutional-based, paid (e.g., community hospital)

Program Development
(Shelly, 2000)
1. **Assess congregational resources.**
   a. What is the church already doing regarding health and caring ministries?
   b. Who is currently providing the services?
   c. Who are the nurses in the congregation and what is their background?
   d. Who are other health care providers in the congregation?
   e. What are the church library resources?
   f. What resources does the denomination provide? For example, the Presbyterian Church, U.S.A., has a Parish Nurse Task Forces that is a part of the Presbyterian Health Network of the Presbyterian Health, Education and Welfare Association.
   g. What are neighboring churches doing?
   h. What free or collaborative services does the community hospital provide that would support congregational care?

2. **Assess needs of the congregation and community.**
   a. Observe and talk to key members such as pastoral staff, deacons, children and youth leaders
   b. Develop a short survey for key members.
   c. Assess congregational knowledge about spiritual, physical, and emotional health for health promotion and education.
   d. Assess need for consultation and counseling to support individuals and families as they transition between home and hospital or home and long-term care.
   e. Assess the need for systematizing volunteer services such as home visiting, support groups, providing meals, or telephones trees.

3. **Develop a plan.**
   a. Understand the church governance structure.
   b. Depending on the governance structure, develop a support group of interested individuals who may be an ad hoc health care ministries committee or a subcommittee of congregational care or deacons' committees.
   c. With the Health Care Ministries Committee,
      (1) Write a mission statement. For example, one mission statement is "To enhance the church's healing ministry by offering opportunities and activities that include health promotion, social support, health counseling and collaborative care" (Hitchens, E., 2000).
      (2) Develop a proposal with a budget that supports the mission of the parish nurse program and includes space, time, equipment, insurance, record-keeping policies, and linkages to church governance.
      (3) Present plan to church leaders for approval and support.

- Spiritual well-being is the condition in which a person is at peace with God, self, community, and environment.
- Fowler's stages of faith have parallels to Piaget's stages of cognitive development and Erikson's stages of psychosocial development.
- Nurses may provide inadequate or inappropriate care if they have not fully addressed their own spirituality and spiritual well-being and if they hesitate to encourage the client to speak of personal spirituality.
- Altered spiritual function may be expressed verbally or through a variety of altered behaviors.
- Every client has the right to practice his or her spirituality according to personal preference. The nurse should not be judgmental but should assist the client in fulfilling those needs.
- Nursing interventions include use of self, spiritual support, support of religious practices, listening and supporting, and referral.

REFERENCES

Ameling, A & Povilonis, M. (2001). *Journal of Psychosocial Nursing 39*(4), 15–20.

Assagioli, R. (1971). *Psychosynthesis.* New York, NY: Penguin Books.

Berggren-Thomas, P., & Griggs, M. J. (1995). Spirituality in aging: Spiritual need or spiritual journey? *Journal of Gerontologic Nursing, 21*(3), 5–10.

Boland, C. S. (1998). Parish nursing. Addressing the significance of social support and spirituality for sustained health-promoting behaviors in the elderly. *Journal of Holistic Nursing, 16*(3), 355–368.

Carpenito, L. J. (2002). *Nursing diagnosis: Application to clinical practice* (9th ed.). Philadelphia: Lippincott Williams & Wilkins.

Chapman, L. S. (1986). Spiritual health: A component missing from health promotion. *American Journal of Health Promotion, 1*(1), 38–41.

Dyson, J., Cobb, M., & Forman, D. (1997). The meaning of spirituality: A literature review. *Journal of Advanced Nursing, 26*(6), 1183–1188.

Espeland, K. (1999). Achieving spiritual wellness: Using reflective questions. *Journal of Psychosocial Nursing, 37*(7), 36–40.

Fitchett, G., Meyer, P., & Burton, L. (2000). Spiritual care in the hospital: Who requests and who needs it. *The Journal of Pastoral Care, 54*(2), 173–186.

Fowler, J. W. (1981). *Stages of faith.* San Francisco, CA: Harper & Row.

Fromm, E. (1968). *The revolution of hope.* New York, NY: Harper & Row.

Frye, B. & Long, L. (1985). Spiritual counseling approaches following brain injury. *Rehabilitation Nursing, 10,* 14–16.

Fulton, R. A., & Moore, C. M. (1995). Spiritual care of the school-age child with a chronic condition. *Journal of Pediatric Nursing, 10*(4), 224–231.

Grandstrom, S. L. (1985). Spiritual care of oncology clients. *Topics in Clinical Nursing, 7*(1), 39–45.

Greer, J., & Moberg, D. O. (1998). *Research in the social scientific study of religion.* Greenwich, CT: Jai Press.

Groer, M. W., O'Connor, B., & Droppleman, P. G. (1996). A course in health care spirituality. *Journal of Nursing Education, 35*(8), 375–377.

Hunglemann, J., Kenke-Rossi, E., Klassen, L., et al. (1985). Spiritual well-being in older adults: Harmonious inter-connectedness. *Journal of Religion and Health, 24,* 147–153.

Kirkpatrick, H., Landeen, J., Woodside, H. & Byrne, C. (2001). How people with schizophrenia build their hope. *Journal of Psychosocial Nursing 39*(1), 48–52.

Kreidler, M. (1984). Meaning in suffering . . . philosophy for nurses. *International Nursing Review, 31,* 174–176.

Long, A. (1997). Nursing: A spiritual perspective. *Nursing Ethics, 4*(6), 496–510.

Murray, R. B., & Zentner, J. P. (1993). *Nursing concepts for health promotion* (5th ed.). Englewood Cliffs, NJ: Prentice-Hall.

North American Nursing Diagnosis Association (NANDA). (2001). *Nursing diagnoses: Definitions and classification 2001–2002.* Philadelphia: Author.

O'Brien, M. E. (1999). *Spirituality in nursing, standing on holy ground.* Boston: Jones and Bartlett Publishers.

Pehler, S. R. (1997). Children's spiritual response: Validation of the nursing diagnosis spiritual distress. *Nursing Diagnosis, 8*(2), 55–66.

Piepgras, R. (1984). The other dimension: Spiritual help. *American Journal of Nursing, 68,* 2610–2613.

Ruffing-Rahal, M. A. (1984). The spiritual dimension of well-being: Implications for the elderly. *Home Health Nurse, 2,* 12–16.

Sellers, S. C., & Haag, B. A. (1998). Spiritual nursing interventions. *Journal of Holistic Nursing, 16*(3), 338–354.

Shelly, J. A. (1982). Spiritual care . . . planting seeds of hope. *Critical Care Update, 9,* 7–17.

Shelly, J. A., & Miller, A. B. (1999). *Called to care: A Christian theology of nursing.* Downers Grove, IL: InterVarsity Press.

Sherman, D. W. (1996). Nurses' willingness to care for AIDS patients and spirituality, social support, and death anxiety. *Image—The Journal of Nursing Scholarship, 28*(3), 205–213.

Spiritual Care Work Group. (1990). Assumptions and principles of spiritual care. *Death Studies, 14,* 75–81.

Still, J. V. H. (1984). How to assess spiritual needs of children. *Journal of Christian Nursing, 1,* 4–6.

Stoll, R. I. (1979). Guidelines for spiritual assessment. *American Journal of Nursing, 79,* 1574–1577.

Tillich, P. (1969). *What is religion?* New York, NY: Harper & Row.

Toth, J. C. (1992). Faith in recovery: Spiritual support after an acute MI. *Journal of Christian Nursing, 9*(4), 28–31.

Wright, K. B. (1998). Professional, ethical, and legal implications for spiritual care in nursing. *Image—Journal of Nursing Scholarship, 30*(1), 81–83.

BIBLIOGRAPHY

Burkhardt, M. A. (1994). Becoming and connecting: Elements of spirituality for women. *Holistic Nursing Practice, 8*(4), 12–21.

Burkhardt, M. A., & Nagai-Jacobson, M. G. (1994). Reawakening spirit in clinical practice. *Journal of Holistic Nursing, 12*(1), 9–21.

Carson, V. B., & Arnold, N. (1996). *Mental health nursing: The nurse–patient journey.* Philadelphia: W.B. Saunders.

Chang, B. H., Noonan, A. E., & Tennstedt, S. L. (1998). The role of religion/spirituality in coping with caregiving for disabled elders. *Gerontologist, 38*(4), 463–470.

Corcoran, E. (1993). Spirituality: An important aspect of emergency nursing. *Journal of Emergency Nursing, 19,* 183–184.

Freeman, A. (1998). Spirituality, well-being and ministry. *The Journal of Pastoral Care, 52*(1), 7–17.

Hatgidakis, J., Timko, E. R., Plotnikoff, G. A., & Gale, C. (1997). Spirituality and practice: Stories, barriers and opportunities. *Creative Nursing, 3*(4), 7–11, 16.

Hitchens, E. (2000). *Health Ministries Team Mission Statement.* Lake Burien Presbyterian Church, Burien, WA.

Huber, L., & Healy, M. (1992). Grow days: Nurturing spiritually healthy teens. *Journal of Christian Nursing, 9*(3), 18–21.

Kaye, J., & Robinson, K. M. (1994). Spirituality among caregivers. *Image, 26,* 218–221.

Kerfoot, K. (1995). Keeping spirituality in managed care: The nurse manager's challenge. *Nursing Economics, 13*(1), 49–51.

Laukhuf, G., & Werner, H. (1998). Spirituality: The missing link. *Journal of Neuroscience Nursing, 30*(1), 60–67.

Leetun, M. C. (1996). Wellness spirituality in the older adult. Assessment and intervention protocol. *Nurse Practitioner, 21*(8), 60, 65–70.

Macrae, J. (1995). Nightingale's spiritual philosophy and its significance for modern nursing. *Image—Journal of Nursing Scholarship, 27*(1), 8–10.

Mansen, T. G. (1993). The spiritual dimension of individuals: Conceptual development. *Nursing Diagnosis, 4*(4), 140–147.

Martsolf, D. S., & Mickley, J. R. (1998). The concept of spirituality in nursing theories: Differing world-views and extent of focus. *Journal of Advanced Nursing, 27*(2), 294–303.

Mathai, M. K. (1980). *Spirituality in relation to nurses' perception of their own coping strategies when clients are perceived to be suffering.* Ann Arbor, MI: University of Michigan.

Mickley, J. R., Carson, V., & Soeken, K. L. (1995). Religion and adult mental health: State of the science in nursing. *Issues in Mental Health Nursing, 16*(4), 345–360.

Millison, M. B. (1995). A review of the research on spiritual care and hospice. *Hospice Journal, 10*(4), 3–18.

Moberg, D. O. (Ed.). (1979). *Spiritual well-being: Sociological perspectives.* Washington, DC: University Press of America.

O'Brien, M. E. (1999). *Spiritual in nursing: Standing on holy ground.* Sudbury, MA: Jones and Bartlett.

Ozmon, H. A., & Craver, S. M. (1994). *Philosophical foundations of education* (5th ed.). Columbus, OH: Charles E. Merrill.

Pehler, S. (1997). Children's spiritual response: Validation of the nursing diagnosis Spiritual Distress. *Nursing Diagnosis, 8*(2), 55–66.

Shelly, J. A. (2000). *Spiritual care, a guide for caregivers.* Downer's Grove, IL: InterVarsity Press.

Shelley, J. A., & Miller, A. (1999). *Called to care: A Christian theology of nursing.* Downers Grove, IL: InterVarsity Press.

Sumner, C. (1998). Recognizing and responding to Spiritual Distress. *American Journal of Nursing, 98*(1), 26–31.

Tuck, I., Pullen, L., & Lyunn C. (1997). Spiritual interventions provided by mental health nurses. *Western Journal of Nursing Research, 19*(3), 351–363.

Young, C. (1993). Spirituality and chronically ill Christian elderly. *Geriatric Nursing, 14,* 298–303.

Zerwekh, J. (1993). Transcending life: The practice wisdom of nursing hospice experts. *American Journal of Hospice and Palliative Care, 10*(5), 26–31.

Internet Resources

The About.com Death and Dying site is run by a nurse and is semi-commercial. It has some good information on spirituality and spiritual care including a spiritual self-assessment test. Available at: *http:/dying.miningco.com/cs/spiritualcare*

The International Parish Nurse Resource Center web site describes the beginnings of parish nursing, offers classes and symposiums, and has the "approved" parish nurse certificate course curriculum. Available at: *http://www.advocatehealth.com/about/faith/parish/index.html*

The Yahoo! Religion and Spirituality site has information about many religions. Available at *www.yahoo.com* under Society and Culture/Religion and Spirituality

A Answers to "Apply Your Knowledge"

CHAPTER 7—NURSE LEADER AND MANAGER

When an employee calls in sick, other employees usually must increase their productivity to finish the work. As a manager, good listening skills are important. Try to hear and to understand what the new nursing assistant is telling you. Because he is new to the job, his efficiency is still developing. He may feel overwhelmed when asked to add tasks to a workload that he is already having difficulty completing. More important, delegating tasks to an untrained employee is never safe practice. Situations that involve safety and infection control can be especially dangerous.

Acknowledge the nursing assistant's feelings about being unable to complete the extra blood glucose monitoring. Negotiate what additional work he can do safely. For example, tell him "I will have the LPN do the blood glucose monitoring, but then you will have to complete vital signs on her clients." Follow-up should include prompt instruction about glucose monitoring for this employee.

CHAPTER 10— NURSING ASSESSMENT

Primary sources of information are those collected directly from the client: the client's health history (including his complaints and past medical history), physical examination findings, and his perception of ability to cope with life stressors. Secondary sources are laboratory tests, such as CBC and chest x-ray results, description from family members, and the physical therapy report.

CHAPTER 22— CLIENT EDUCATION

Mrs. Babbitt seems motivated to learn, but you must assess her baseline knowledge about medications, attitude about taking medications, daily routine, cognitive abilities, literacy level, ability to hear and see (to read medication labels), and psychomotor ability to remove medications from their containers.

Start teaching as soon as possible. When you give Mrs. Babbitt her medications, say each drug name and explain what each does. A day or two before discharge, sit down with Mrs. Babbitt (and hopefully a close family member) to give written and verbal information regarding each medication.

In consultation with Mrs. Babbitt and her family, develop a medication calendar of when to take medications.

Confusion can occur when the drug regimen is complex. Have both Mrs. Babbitt and her family members restate each medication, dose, purpose, and any special considerations. Provide positive reinforcement for correct answers. Inquire as to the plan for medication administration after discharge (e.g., using a medication administration set, checking off on written schedule). Follow-up by the primary health provider or a home health nurse may be indicated if Mrs. Babbitt does not demonstrate mastery before discharge.

CHAPTER 25—VITAL SIGN ASSESSMENT

Assessing blood pressure in the basal state provides the most accurate data. Stress, increased activity, and anxiety all can elevate blood pressure. The medical assistant should delay blood pressure measurement until Ms. George has a chance to calm down. The assistant should not apply the cuff nor listen with a stethoscope over Ms. George's clothes because hearing will be impaired. Also, blood pressure should not be monitored in the arm that the IV is infusing. The arm should be supported to avoid a falsely high reading, and the assistant should be close enough to the gauge to read it accurately. It appears from the photograph that the cuff is loosely wrapped around the arm and the head of the stethoscope is not placed over the brachial artery.

CHAPTER 26—ASEPSIS AND INFECTION CONTROL

Because influenza is transmitted via the airborne route, it is likely that other family members, including the other children, will contract it. Children are infectious as long as influenza symptoms are present. Instruct the mother to keep the child home from day care/school and isolated from friends during this time. Also stress the need for good handwashing, which is always important. Reinforce hygiene measures including proper disposal of any tissues or secretions. Additionally, encourage the mother not to let the children and other family members share dishes and personal care items to reduce the risk of transmission. Influenza vaccine is now available and should be encouraged, especially for high-risk clients (e.g., elderly, those with respiratory disease).

CHAPTER 27—
MEDICATION ADMINISTRATION

Answer: To calculate the dose to administer, use the formula:

$$\frac{\text{dose on hand}}{\text{quantity on hand}} = \frac{\text{dose desired}}{\text{quantity desired}}$$

$$\frac{10{,}000 \text{ units}}{1 \text{ mL}} = \frac{7{,}500 \text{ units}}{X}$$

$$10{,}000X = 7{,}500$$

$$X = 0.75 \text{ mL}$$

Because the heparin is to be administered subcutaneously, use a short, ½-inch needle. You can use a small gauge (25 to 27) because the medication is not thick and can easily go through a needle with a small diameter. The size of the syringe should be 1 mL so that visualization of 0.75-mL dose will be clear. A tuberculin syringe would be appropriate in this situation.

Many agencies require that heparin be administered in the abdomen away from vascular areas, which might cause more bruising. More research needs to be done to confirm this practice, because some studies show no difference in bruising when arm or thigh sites are used. Additional precautions used for heparin injections to prevent bruising include no aspiration and not rubbing the site after injecting the medication.

CHAPTER 28—
INTRAVENOUS THERAPY

IV controller rate: To calculate the number of cc/hr, divide the total volume by the number of hours for the infusion (3000/24 = 125 cc/hr).

Gravity infusion—macrodrip: Use the formula to obtain the drops/min:

$$\text{Drops/min} = \frac{\text{Total volume infused} \times \text{drop factor}}{\text{Total time for infusion in minutes}}$$

$$\frac{3000 \times 20}{24 \text{ hr} \times 60} = \frac{60{,}000}{1440} = 41.7 \text{ or } 42 \text{ drops/min}$$

An easier method of calculation is to reduce the amount to an hourly rate first (3000/24 hr = 125/60 min). Working with smaller numbers can be less confusing.

$$\frac{125 \text{ cc} \times 20 \text{ drops/cc}}{60 \text{ min}}$$

By reducing to lowest terms, you divide 125 by 3 and arrive at the same answer of 41.7 drops per minute.

Gravity infusion—microdrip: Because the drop factor for a microdrip is 60 and the number of minutes in an hour is 60, you are multiplying and dividing by the same number. When using a microdrip, the number of drops/min is the same as the number of cc/hr, so simply calculate the hourly infusion rate.

CHAPTER 29—
PERIOPERATIVE NURSING

When interpreting postoperative vital signs, evaluate these data in terms of trends, looking for decreasing blood pressure and increasing pulse rate to promptly detect shock. Mr. Johnson's vital signs show some fluctuations, but generally remain close to baseline values. Increased blood pressure and pulse rate may be symptomatic of pain if this upward trend continues.

Other important assessments to regularly monitor include airway patency and quality of respirations, level of consciousness and recovery from anesthetic agent, amount and quality of drainage on dressing or from drains, urinary output, and level of pain.

CHAPTER 30—SAFETY

Restraints are not always the best way to maintain a client's safety. In acute care agencies, restraints may be applied, but a physician's order must be obtained within 24 hours. Protocols should be in place for the appropriate use and monitoring of restraints to prevent injury. Assess circulatory and neurovascular status frequently. Consider other options, such as having a family member sit with the client or using a sitter if a family member is unavailable. Make an effort to detect the cause of Mr. Rau's acute confusion to direct treatment at resolving the underlying cause.

CHAPTER 31—
HEALTH MAINTENANCE

An area for positive feedback is that Patricia introduced low impact exercise into her daily routine. Starting out slowly and focusing on enjoyable things (e.g., walking with a supportive friend) can be successful over a long period. Beginning with very strenuous exercise can result in discouragement if a person does not gradually develop conditioning.

Listen carefully to what Patricia believes are important problems and her understanding of how they will influence health. Help the client develop a realistic plan, providing appropriate information. Try to mention the fat content of her intake calculating the percentage of fat. Provide her with a list of lower fat options (e.g., low fat dressing, substitute roll for muffin, limit desserts to one per day). Ask Patricia to list her favorite fruits and vegetables and encourage her to include at least one more serving of each to her daily diet. Discuss the importance of continuing the Food Diary, stressing the need to also list the amount of food eaten so she can accurately calculate fat and caloric intake.

CHAPTER 32—SELF-CARE

Mrs. Ramirez needs much assistance with bathing due to her mobility and cognitive deficits. A shower using a shower chair seems most appropriate at this point, especially with Mrs. Ramirez's history of falls. First, take Mrs. Ramirez to the toilet, encouraging her to void and defecate. Sometimes, confused clients need prompting for elimination and can be incontinent in the shower when bladder and bowel are full. Verbally keep her informed of what you are doing and encourage as much participation as possible. Give positive feedback for attempts to participate in self-care. Keep Mrs. Ramirez warm by wrapping her in a bath blanket, because older adults can easily become hypothermic. Use mild soap and gently cleanse and inspect all skin surfaces for breakdown or injury. Wash Mrs. Ramirez's hair, using a cream rinse if her hair is tangled or matted. Pat Mrs. Ramirez dry, especially in areas of skinfolds where moisture can accumulate and cause skin maceration and fungal infections. When you return to Mrs. Ramirez's room, dry and comb her hair and provide care for her teeth.

CHAPTER 33—MOBILITY AND BODY MECHANICS

From the data provided, the most important concern before getting Mrs. Jones up is whether she is volume depleted. Data that support this concern are a blood pressure below baseline and a low urine output (less than 30 cc/hr). Fluid volume deficits will cause postural hypotension, which can result in dizziness and possible syncope when arising. The medications she is receiving for pain and nausea could further contribute to hypotension. Before getting Mrs. Jones up, take a postural blood pressure and pulse reading. If Mrs. Jones is orthostatic, her blood pressure will drop and her pulse will rise when she sits on the edge of the bed. She also may complain of dizziness, diaphoresis, and generalized weakness. If the postural drop is significant (a systolic BP drop of 25 mm Hg or greater with a pulse increase), you may need to give her extra fluids. If Mrs. Jones is not orthostatic, get her up slowly, elevating the head of the bed to prevent putting extra pressure on her incision. Make sure she is adequately medicated for pain by using her PCA before ambulation. Mrs. Jones requires standby assistance; a transfer belt is not usually required for postoperative clients with no prior mobility problems. Organize her IV fluids, PCA, and Foley catheter so they are not in the way during ambulation. Assess Mrs. Jones frequently during ambulation to detect signs of activity intolerance quickly.

CHAPTER 34—OXYGENATION: RESPIRATORY FUNCTION

During the first postoperative day of care, Mr. Jacob needs aggressive respiratory interventions to prevent atelectasis. Data that indicate that atelectasis may already be present include elevated temperature; shallow, slow respirations; and diminished breath sounds with crackles. Limited mobility after surgery, pain and the fear of pain when breathing deeply, and diminished respirations from the opiates used to manage pain all contribute to postoperative atelectasis. To reverse atelectasis and promote optimal oxygenation, it is important to

get Mr. Jacob up and moving. Encourage deep breathing, and perhaps see if you can get an order for an incentive spirometer. Supplemental oxygen is usually not given until O_2 saturation falls below 93%.

CHAPTER 35—OXYGENATION: CARDIOVASCULAR FUNCTION

As part of your role as the visiting nurse, you are evaluating the client's recovery from the heart attack. It is normal for the client to experience discomfort from the surgery. Assess the wound for redness, drainage, or swelling that may indicate infection. Take Mr. Brown's vital signs and note any temperature elevation. Encourage Mr. Brown to take his pain medication as needed, and report any increases in pain. Over time, the pain should resolve. The client should report any heart pain that might indicate another heart attack or angina immediately. Risk reduction is another focus of your visit. Provide positive feedback for his attempts at diet revision and walking. Encourage other health promotion activities, such as proper use of medications to reduce the risk of another heart attack and control blood pressure. Reinforce care of incisions to prevent infection. Discuss causes of stress and ways to control it, such as listening to music, talking, or relaxing. In closing the visit, provide praise for all that Mr. and Mrs. Brown have done, review symptoms to report, and leave opportunities for health promotion.

CHAPTER 36—FLUID, ELECTROLYTE, AND ACID-BASE BALANCE

Express your concern for Miss Simpson's discomfort, and explain the rationale for the fluid restriction. Then offer her sugar-free candy or gum. Allow her to rinse her mouth with a sip of water. Tell her to swish it around in her mouth and then spit it out before she swallows the fluid. Also, perform frequent oral care. Miss Simpson may use mouthwashes, but be sure that they are alcohol free because alcohol has a drying effect. Moisten her lips with a water-soluble lubricant to prevent drying and cracking.

CHAPTER 37—NUTRITION

The Isocal has to be diluted with water to obtain a half-strength solution. For a can containing 240 cc, you should add 240 cc of water. Only prepare one can of Isocal at a time. You do not want large volumes of tube feeding hanging for a long time, because warm formula can support microbial growth. Although aspiration is less likely with a gastrostomy tube than with a nasogastric tube, tube placement is important to assess before starting feeding. Quickly inject air into the tube, listening over the gastric area for a swoosh or aspirate gastric contents from the tube. Position Gina in a semi- or high-Fowler's position to prevent gastric reflux and possible aspiration.

CHAPTER 38—SKIN INTEGRITY AND WOUND HEALING

Assess Ms. Nelson's feet, looking for injuries such as blisters, cuts, and abrasions. Examine areas for inflammation, infection, burns, edema, or other problems. Identify what Ms. Nelson understands about foot care and have her explain how she performs it. Caution her about the need for careful foot care in order to maintain skin integrity. Explain that using an emery board on skin will traumatize it, possibly causing breakdown that will then have difficulty healing. Enlisting Ms. Nelson as an active participant in preventing foot trauma or injury is essential—sharing some of the negative consequences of poor foot care may help. Encourage her to seek professional care for her feet if needed and to call the clinic at any time with questions about her feet and skin.

CHAPTER 39—THE BODY'S DEFENSE AGAINST INFECTION

Risk factors that increase the likelihood of infection include abdominal surgery, which breaks skin integrity; abdominal incision and pain level, which promote shallow respirations; reluctance to move, which promotes shallow breathing and increases the likelihood of atelectasis (which can cause a respiratory infection); history of asthma, which indicates a chronic respiratory problem; and age, which decreases the natural defense mechanisms to fight infection.

The most important factor that supports the presence of an infection is a high fever (38°C). Low-grade fevers often occur postoperatively due to stress and inflammation, but when high fevers are present infection should be ruled out, especially in light of Mr. Foscarelli's risk factors for respiratory infection. Elevated respiratory rate, shallow breathing, and a productive cough support this. Pulse rate is elevated due to the increased metabolic rate. Diminished breath sounds might indicate the presence of atelectasis (alveolar collapse), and rhonchi indicate the presence of secretions in the bronchioles, which can occur with respiratory infections such as pneumonia.

Mr. Foscarelli's primary care provider will probably order a WBC with a differential, looking for an elevated leukocyte count and a shift to the left to confirm infection. A sputum culture and sensitivity will be obtained (before giving antibiotics) to identify the organism and determine appropriate antibiotic therapy. Because the culture results are not available for 48 hours, a Gram's stain is usually done to help guide early antibiotic therapy. A chest x-ray will also be ordered.

CHAPTER 40— URINARY ELIMINATION

a. Report Mr. Sanchez's change in status to his physician. Acute confusion has many different causes in older adults, but commonly results from UTI. The presence of an indwelling Foley catheter and the following data also support this tentative diagnosis for Mr. Sanchez: low-grade fever (older adults often do not have a high temperature with infection), low urine output, and cloudy sediment in urine. Some agencies allow you to obtain a urine culture and sensitivity for suspected UTIs, but a physician must then sign this order.

b. One hundred cc's is not an adequate volume for a void. A person usually has the urge to void when 250 to 400 cc are in the bladder. This volume stretches the detrusor muscle, which stimulates the parasympathetic nervous system and alerts the brain that the bladder is full. When an indwelling catheter has been in place for an extended period, the bladder may lose tone, contributing to urinary retention. Because the color of Mr. Phillips's urine is light yellow, he is not volume depleted. If during 6 hours he has only voided 100 cc (less than 20 cc/hr), he is not emptying his bladder completely, which could lead to UTIs. Bladder ultrasound or in and out catheterization can evaluate post void residual volumes.

CHAPTER 41— BOWEL ELIMINATION

Irrigate the NG tube with normal saline as per physician orders. The absence of bowel sounds 2 days postoperatively is normal but indicates that the NG tube should remain in place to prevent abdominal distention. Absence of NG drainage indicates that the tube is probably plugged, especially because the gastric drainage was viscous and contained mucus. Complaints of nausea also support the conclusion that the NG tube is not functioning properly. If, after irrigating, the NG tube still is not draining, reposition the tube by advancing it 1 inch. Know that this action is contraindicated if the client has had gastric surgery. If the NG tube still doesn't drain, notify the physician.

CHAPTER 42—SLEEP AND REST

Although Mrs. Wilson has come to you for help with her sleep difficulties, it is likely that her husband has the most serious problem. Loud snoring is a symptom of sleep apnea, which warrants a full medical evaluation. Suggest to Mrs. Wilson that she ask her husband to come in for an examination and a possible referral to a sleep clinic. Hypnotics can be used as a short-term method to induce sleep, but these pharmacologic agents usually affect sleep quality. Trying nonpharmacologic methods first is a better way to try to improve sleep.

CHAPTER 44— SENSORY PERCEPTION

Discuss with Mr. Myer when he first noticed this blurring of his central vision. Identify whether he has peripheral vision and can move about safely. Do not just assume that he is confused. Mr. Myer may have developed some degenerative changes in the retina's macular area that is distorting his sensory input. Help him to clarify his limited vision versus confusion. Reassurance and reassessment of his vision may be very helpful.

CHAPTER 45— COGNITIVE PROCESS

Assess specifically whether Mr. Moran is oriented to person, place, and time. Complete the neurologic assessment (LOC, reflexes, sensory, and motor function), noting any significant changes from previous readings. Assess Mr. Moran's ability to understand simple directions and willingness to comply with requests (such as staying in bed). You may want to assess his normal alcohol intake, because withdrawal from alcohol can cause delirium.

Try to speak calmly to him, listening to his concerns. Use touch and good communication skills. If he appears disoriented, explain where he is and what happened. Explain why the IV is in place. Keep his call light within reach and hopefully move him to a room close to the nursing station, where he can be constantly observed. Inquire if he has family who might be able to come sit with him. If the confusion continues, and he poses a risk to himself or others, a sitter may need to be employed to stay with him. Medications are contraindicated in this situation because of the head trauma.

CHAPTER 47—FAMILIES AND THEIR RELATIONSHIPS

Young children frequently fall and injure themselves. Your assessment reveals some data, however, that may indicate child abuse (i.e., the child's stoic nature, avoidance of eye contact, multiple bruises). Try to ascertain as much information as possible from the mother, asking her to outline how the incident occurred. Speak with the boyfriend separately for his description of the incident. Compare their individual descriptions for consistency. Closely observe their nonverbal behaviors during the interview. If, after the interviews, you suspect child abuse, you are required by law to report your suspicions to child protective authorities. The law requires *all* healthcare workers to report any incident of suspected abuse so a follow-up investigation may occur.

CHAPTER 48—LOSS AND GRIEVING

Paulie's mother is in shock. Her son's death was completely unexpected and just occurred. Help mobilize support for her and her husband. Do not falsely reassure them that all will be well. Recognize and honor any display of grief. Provide for their physical safety by making sure that they have a ride home from the hospital.

CHAPTER 49—STRESS, COPING, AND ADAPTATION

The symptoms are due to stimulation of the sympathetic nervous system as a response to stress. Stress response is affected by how the individual interprets stimuli. Your concern about the test is heightened by the fact that you did poorly on the first test and probably need to do well now to obtain the grade you desire in the course. Using some relaxation techniques (e.g., slow breathing, focusing) may help decrease your anxiety. Overall, take good care of yourself. Sleeping and eating properly before an exam will help you think clearly as you ponder the correct answers to the test questions. If test anxiety is an ongoing problem, use available resources (such as a learning center or counseling center) to develop strategies that will help ensure your success.

CHAPTER 50— HUMAN SEXUALITY

Start by expressing that the question is good and that you are glad they felt comfortable enough to approach you. Ask each student to discuss why he or she thinks a person can or cannot get pregnant during menstruation. Then give them the correct answer, explaining why it is correct. Assess the need for additional sex information, provide pamphlets, and see if other members of the class might like to participate in an informal discussion about sexuality. If the students seem receptive, you might encourage them to participate in the planning process. Explain when you will be in the health office if they (or their friends) have questions.

B Diagnostic Studies and Interpretation

Test Value Studied

Reference Ranges—Hematology
Reference Ranges—Serum, Plasma, and Whole Blood
    Chemistries
Reference Ranges—Immunodiagnostic Tests
Reference Ranges—Urine Chemistry
Reference Ranges—Cerebrospinal Fluid (CSF)
Miscellaneous Values

Selected Abbreviations Used in Reference Ranges

Conventional Units

kg = kilogram
gm = gram
mg = milligram
μg = microgram
μμg = micromicrogram
ng = nanogram
pg = picogram
dL = 100 milliliters
mL = milliliter
mm^3 = cubic millimeter
fL = femtoliter
mM = millimole
μM = nanomole
mOsm = milliosmole
mm = millimeter
mm = micron or micrometer
mm Hg = millimeters of mercury
U = unit
mU = milliunit
μU = microunit
mEq = milliequivalent
IU = International Unit
mIU = milliInternational Unit

SI Units

g = gram
L = liter
d = day
h = hour
mol = mole
mmol = millimole
mmol = micromole
nmol = nanomole
pmol = picomole

TABLE B-1

Reference Ranges—Hematology*			
Determination	**Reference Range**		**Clinical Significance**
	Conventional Units	*SI Units*	
A_2 hemoglobin	1.5%–3.5% of total hemoglobin	Mass fraction: 0.015–0.035 of total hemoglobin	Increased in certain types of thalassemia
Bleeding time	1–9 min	1–9 min	Prolonged in thrombocytopenia, defective platelet function, and aspirin therapy
Factor V assay (proaccelerin factor)	60%–140%		
Factor VIII assay (anti-hemophiliac factor)	50%–200%		Deficient in classical hemophilia
Factor IX assay (plasma thromboplastin component)	75%–125%		Deficient in Christmas disease (pseudohemophilia)
Factor X (Stuart factor)	60%–140%		Deficient in Stuart clotting defect
Fibrinogen	200–400 mg/dL	2–4 g/dL	Increased in pregnancy, infections accompanied by leukocytosis, nephrosis. Decreased in severe liver disease, abruptio placentae
Fibrin split (degradation) products	Less than 10 mg/L	Less than 10 mg/L	Increased in disseminated intra-vascular coagulation
Fibrinolysins (whole blood clot lysis time)	No lysis in 24 h		Increased activity associated with massive hemorrhage, extensive surgery, transfusion reactions
Partial thromboplastin time (activated)	20–45 sec		Prolonged in deficiency of fibrino-gen, factors II, V, VIII, IX, X, XI, and XII, and in heparin therapy
Prothrombin consumption	Over 20 sec		Impaired in deficiency of factors VIII, IX, and X
Prothrombin time	9.5–12 sec		Prolonged by deficiency of factors I, II, V, VII, and X, far malabsorp-tion, severe liver disease, coumarin anticoagulant therapy.
INR	1.0		
	2–3 for therapy in atrial fibrillation, deep vein throm-bosis, and pul-monary embolism		INR used to standardize the pro-thrombin time and anticoagula-tion therapy
	2.5–3.5 for therapy in prosthetic heart valves		
Erythrocyte count	Males: 4,600,000–6,200,000/cu mm	4.6–6.2×10^{12}/L	Increased in severe diarrhea and de-hydration, polycythemia, acute poisoning, pulmonary fibrosis
	Females: 4,200,000–5,400,000/cu mm	4.2–5.4×10^{12}/L	Decreased in all anemias in leukemia, and after hemorrhage, when blood volume has been restored

TABLE B-1 (Continued)

Reference Ranges—Hematology*

Determination	Reference Range		Clinical Significance
	Conventional Units	*SI Units*	
Erythrocyte indices			
Mean corpuscular volume (MCV)	80–94 (cu μ)	80–94 fL	Increased in macrocytic anemias; decreased in microcytic anemia
Mean corpuscular hemoglobin (MCH)	27–32 μμg/cell	27–32 pg	Increased in macrocytic anemias; decreased in microcytic anemia
Mean corpuscular hemoglobin concentration (MCHC)	33%–38%	Concentration fraction: 0.33–0.38	Decreased in severe hypochromic anemia
Reticulocytes	0.5%–1.5% of red cells	Number fraction: 0.005–0.015	Increased with any condition stimulating increase in bone marrow activity (ie, infection, blood loss [acute and chronically following iron therapy in iron deficiency anemia], polycythemia rubra vera) Decreased with any condition depressing bone marrow activity, acute leukemia, late stage of severe anemias
Erythrocyte sedimentation rate (ESR)—Westergren method	Males under 50 yr: <15 mm/h	<15 mm/h	Increased in tissue destruction, whether inflammatory or degenerative; during menstruation and pregnancy; and in acute febrile diseases
	Males over 50 yr: <20 mm/h	<20 mm/h	
	Females under 50 yr: <20 mm/h	<20 mm/h	
	Females over 50 yr: <30 mm/h	<30 mm/h	
Erythrocyte sedimentation ratio—Zeta centrifuge	41%–54%	Fraction: 0.41–0.54	Significance similar to ESR
Hematocrit	Males: 42%–50%	Volume fraction: 0.42–0.5	Decreased in severe anemias, anemia of pregnancy, acute massive blood loss
	Females: 40%–48%	Volume fraction: 0.4–0.48	Increased in erythrocytosis of any cause, and in dehydration or hemo-concentration associated with shock
Hemoglobin	Males: 13–18 gm/dL Females: 12–16 gm/dL	2.02–2.79 mmol/L 1.86–2.48 mmol/L	Decreased in various anemias, pregnancy, severe or prolonged hemorrhage, and with excessive fluid intake Increased in polycythemia, chronic obstructive pulmonary disease, failure of oxygenation because of congestive heart failure, and normally in people living at high altitudes

(continues)

TABLE B-1 (Continued)

Reference Ranges—Hematology*			

Determination	Reference Range		Clinical Significance
	Conventional Units	*SI Units*	
Hemoglobin F	Less than 2% of total hemoglobin	Mass fraction: <0.02	Increased in infants and children, and in thalassemia and many anemias
Leukocyte alkaline phosphatase	Score of 40–100		Increased in polycythemia vera, myelofibrosis, and infections. Decreased in chronic granulocytic leukemia, paroxysmal nocturnal hemoglobinuria, hypoplastic marrow, and viral infections, particularly infectious mononucleosis
Leukocyte count	Total: 5,000–10,000/cu mm	$5–10 \times 10^9$/L	Elevated in acute infectious diseases, predominantly in the neutrophilic fraction with bacterial diseases, and in the lymphocytic and monocytic fractions in viral diseases
Neutrophils	60%–70%	Number fraction: 0.6–0.7	
Eosinophils	1%–4%	Number fraction: 0.01–0.04	
Basophils	0%–0.5%	Number fraction: 0.00–0.05	Elevated in acute leukemia, following menstruation, and following surgery or trauma
Lymphocytes	20%–30%	Number fraction: 0.2–0.3	Depressed in aplastic anemia, agranulocytosis, and by toxic chemotherapeutic agents used in treating malignancy
Monocytes	2%–6%	Number fraction: 0.02–0.06	
			Eosinophils elevated in collagen disease, allergy, intestinal parasitosis
Platelet count	100,000–400,000/cu mm	$0.1–0.4 \times 10^{12}$/L	Increased in malignancy, myeloproliferative disease, rheumatoid arthritis, and postoperatively; about 50% of patients with unexpected increase of platelet count will be found to have a malignancy Decreased in thrombocytopenic purpura, acute leukemia, aplastic anemia, and during cancer chemotherapy.

*Laboratory values may vary according to the techniques used in different laboratories.

TABLE B-2

Reference Ranges—Serum, Plasma, and Whole Blood Chemistries

Determination	Normal Adult Reference Range		Clinical Significance	
	Conventional Units	*SI Units*	*Increased*	*Decreased*
Acetoacetate	0.2–1.0 mg/dL	19.6–98 µmol/L	Diabetic acidosis Fasting	
Acetone	0.3–2.0 mg/dL	51.6–344.0/µmol/L	Diabetic ketoacidosis Toxemia of pregnancy Carbohydrate-free diet High-fat diet	
Acid, total phosphatase	0–11 UL	0–11 UL	Carcinoma of prostate Advanced Paget's disease Hyperparathyroidism Gaucher's disease	
Acid, phosphatase, prostatic—RLA	0–10 ng/mL Borderline: 2.5–3.3 IU/L	0–10 µg/L	Carcinoma of prostate	
Alkaline phosphatase	Adults: 30–150 mU/mL	30–150 µ/L	Conditions reflecting increased osteoblastic activity of bone Rickets Hyperparathyroidism Hepatic disease Bone disease	
Alkaline phosphatase, thermostable fraction	Thermostable fraction >35%: hepatic disease and combined disease with predominant hepatic component Thermostable fraction between 25% and 35%: combined hepatic and skeletal disease Thermostable fraction <25%: skeletal disease with increased osteoblastic activity			
Adrenocorticotropic hormone (ACTH) (plasma)—RIA*	Less than 50 pg/mL	Less than 50 mg/L	Pituitary-dependent Cushing's syndrome Ectopic ACTH syndrome Primary adrenal atrophy	Adrenocortical tumor Adrenal insufficiency secondary to hypopituitarism
Aldolase	3–8 Sibley-Lehninger U/dL at 37°C	22–59 mU/L at 37°C	Hepatic necrosis Granulocytic leukemia Myocardial infarction Skeletal muscle disease	
Aldosterone (plasma)—RIA	Supine: 3–10 ng/dL Upright: 5–30 ng/dL Adrenal vein 200–800 ng/dL	0.08–0.30 nmol/L 0.14–0.90 nmol/L 5.54–22.16 nmol/L	Primary aldosteronism Secondary aldosteronism	Addison's disease

(continues)

TABLE B-2   (Continued)

Reference Ranges—Serum, Plasma, and Whole Blood Chemistries				
	Normal Adult Reference Range		**Clinical Significance**	
Determination	*Conventional Units*	*SI Units*	*Increased*	*Decreased*
Alpha-1-antitrypsin	200–400 mg/dL	2–4 g/L		Certain forms of chronic lung and liver disease in young adults
Alpha-1-fetoprotein	None detected		Hepatocarcinoma Metastatic carcinoma of liver Germinal cell carcinoma of the testicle or ovary Fetal neural tube defects— elevation in maternal serum	
Alpha-hydroxybutyric dehydrogenase	Up to 140 U/mL	Up to 140 U/L	Myocardial infarction Granulocytic leukemia Hemolytic anemias Muscular dystrophy	
Ammonia (plasma)	40–80 ug/dL (enzymatic method); varies considerably with method	22.2–44.3/μmol/L	Severe liver disease Hepatic decompensation	
Amylase	60–160 Somogyi U/dL	111–296U/L	Acute pancreatitis Mumps Duodenal ulcer Carcinoma of head of pancreas Prolonged elevation with pseudocyst of pancreas Increased by drugs that constrict pancreatic duct sphincters: morphine, codeine, cholinergics	Chronic pancreatitis Pancreatic fibrosis and atrophy Cirrhosis of liver Pregnancy (2nd and 3rd trimesters)
Arsenic	6–20 μg/dL; if 50 μg/dL, suspect toxicity	0.78–2.6 μmol/L	Intentional or unintentional poisoning Excessive occupational exposure	
Ascorbic acid (vitamin C)	0.4–1.5 mg/dL	23–85 μmol/L	Large doses of ascorbic acid as a prophylactic against the common cold	
ALT (alanine aminotransferase), formerly SGPT	10–40 U/mL	5–20 U/L	Same conditions as AST (SGOT), but increase is more marked in liver disease than AST (SGOT)	
AST (aspartate aminotransferase), formerly SGOT	7–40 U/mL	4–20 U/L	Myocardial infarction Skeletal muscle disease Liver disease	

TABLE B-2 (Continued)

Reference Ranges—Serum, Plasma, and Whole Blood Chemistries

Determination	Normal Adult Reference Range		Clinical Significance	
	Conventional Units	*SI Units*	*Increased*	*Decreased*

Bilirubin	Total: 0.1–1.2 mg/dL
	Direct: 0.1–
	  0.2 mg/dL
	Indirect: 0.1–1 mg/dL
		1.7–20.5/µmol/L
		1.7–3.4/µmol/L
		1.7–17.1 µmol/L
			Hemolytic anemia
			  (indirect)
			Biliary obstruction and
			  disease
			Hepatocellular damage
			  (hepatitis)
			Pernicious anemia
			Hemolytic disease of
			  newborn	

Blood gases
  Oxygen, arterial
    (whole blood):
    Partial pressure
    (PaO₂)
	95–100 mm Hg	12.64–13.30kPa	Polycythemia	Anemia
				Cardiac or pul-
				  monary disease

Saturation (SaO₂)	94%–100%	Volume fraction:
		  0.94–1
			Anhydremia	Cardiac
				  decompensation
				Chronic obstructive
				  lung disease

Carbon dioxide,
  arterial (whole
  blood) partial
  pressure (PaCO₂)
	35–45 mm Hg	4.66–5.99 kPa	Respiratory acidosis
			Metabolic alkalosis
				Respiratory alkalosis
				Metabolic acidosis

pH (whole blood, arterial)	7.35–7.45	7.35–7.45	Vomiting Hyperventilation Fever Intestinal obstruction	Uremia Diabetic acidosis Hemorrhage Nephritis

Calcitonin	Basal: nondetectable
	  400 pg/mL
		400 ng/L	Medullary carcinoma of
			  the thyroid
			Some nonthyroid tumors
			Zollinger-Ellison syndrome	

Calcium	8.5–10.5 mg/dL	2.125–
		  2.625 mmol/L
			Tumor or hyperplasia of
			  parathyroid
			Hypervitaminosis D
			Multiple myeloma
			Nephritis with uremia
			Malignant tumors
			Sarcoidosis
			Hyperthyroidism
			Skeletal immobilization
			Excess calcium intake:
			  milk alkali syndrome
				Hypoparathyroidism
				Diarrhea
				Celiac disease
				Vitamin D defi-
				  ciency
				Acute pancreatitis
				Nephrosis
				After parathyroidec-
				  tomy

CO₂, venous	Adults 24–32 mEq/L Infants: 18–24 mEq/L	24–32 mmol/L 18–24 mmol/L	Tetany Respiratory disease Intestinal obstruction Vomiting	Acidosis Nephritis Eclampsia Diarrhea Anesthesia

(continues)

TABLE B-2   (Continued)

Reference Ranges—Serum, Plasma, and Whole Blood Chemistries

Determination	Normal Adult Reference Range		Clinical Significance	
	Conventional Units	*SI Units*	*Increased*	*Decreased*
Catecholamines (plasma)—RIA	Epinephrine random: up to 90 pg/mL Norepinephrine, random 100 550 pg/mL Dopamine, random up to 130 pg/mL	Up to 490 pmol/L 590– 3240 pmol/L Up to 850 pmol/L	Pheochromocytoma	
Ceruloplasmin	30–80 mg/dL	300–800 mg/L		Wilson's disease (hepatolenticular degeneration)
Chloride	95–105 mEq/L	95–105 mmol/L	Nephrosis Nephritis Urinary obstruction Cardiac decompensation Anemia	Diabetes Diarrhea Vomiting Pneumonia Heavy metal poisoning Cushing's syndrome Intestinal obstruction Febrile conditions Pernicious anemia
Cholesterol	150–200 mg/dL	3.9–5.2 mmol/L	Lipemia Obstructive jaundice Diabetes Hypothyroidism	Hemolytic anemia Hyperthyroidism Severe infection Terminal states of debilitating disease
Cholesterol esters	60%–70% of total	Fraction of total cholesterol 0.6–0.7		The esterified fraction decreases in liver diseases
Cholinesterase	Serum: 0.6–1.6 delta pH Red cells—0.6–1 delta pH	0.6–1.6 U 0.6–1 U	Nephrosis Exercise	Nerve gas intoxication (greater effect on red cell activity) Insecticide poisoning
Chorionic gonadotropin, beta subunit	0–5 IU/L	0–5 IU/L	Pregnancy Hydatidiform mole Choriocarcinoma	Threatened abortion Ectopic pregnancy
Complement, human C_3	70–150 mg/dL	880–2520 mg/L	Some inflammatory diseases, acute myocardial infarction, cancer	Acute glomerulonephritis Disseminated lupus erythematosus with renal involvement
Complement C4	16–45 mg/dL	140–510 mg/L	Some inflammatory diseases, acute myocardial infarction, cancer	Often decreased in immunologic disease, especially with active systemic lupus erythematosus

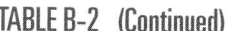

TABLE B-2 (Continued)

Reference Ranges—Serum, Plasma, and Whole Blood Chemistries

Determination	Normal Adult Reference Range		Clinical Significance	
	Conventional Units	*SI Units*	*Increased*	*Decreased*
Complement, total (hemolytic)	90%–94% complement	25–70 U/mL	Some inflammatory diseases	Hereditary angioneurotic edema Acute glomeru-lonephritis Epidemic meningitis Subacute bacterial endocarditis
Copper	70–165 μg/dL	11–25.9 μmol/L	Cirrhosis of liver Pregnancy	Wilson's disease
Cortisol-RIA	8 AM: 7–25/μg/dL 4 PM: 2–9 μg/dL	193–690 nmol/L 55–248 nmol/L	Stress: infectious disease, surgery, burns, etc. Pregnancy Cushing's syndrome Pancreatitis Eclampsia	Addison's disease Anterior pituitary hypofunction
C-peptide reactivity	1.5–10 ng/mL	1.5–10 μg/L	Insulinoma	Diabetes
Creatine	0.2–0.8 mg/mL	15.3–61 μmol/L	Pregnancy Skeletal muscle necrosis or atrophy Starvation Hyperthyroidism	
Creatine phosphoki-nase (CPK)	Males: 50–325 mU/mL Females: 50–250 mU/mL	50–325 U/L 50–250 U/L	Myocardial infarction Skeletal muscle diseases Intramuscular injections Crush syndrome Hypothyroidism Alcohol withdrawal delirium Alcoholic myopathy Cerebrovascular disease	
Creatine phosphoki-nase isoenzymes	MM band present (skeletal muscle)–MB band absent (heart muscle)		MB band increased in myocardial infarction, ischemia	
Creatinine	0.7–1.4 mg/dL	62–124 μmol/L	Nephritis Chronic renal disease	
Creatinine clearance	100–150 mL of blood cleared of creatinine per min	1.67–2.5 mL/s		Kidney diseases
Cryoglobulins, qualitative	Negative		Multiple myeloma Chronic lymphocytic leukemia Lymphosarcoma Systemic lupus erythematosus Rheumatoid arthritis Infective subacute endocarditis	

(continues)

TABLE B-2 (Continued)

Reference Ranges—Serum, Plasma, and Whole Blood Chemistries

Determination	Normal Adult Reference Range		Clinical Significance	
	Conventional Units	*SI Units*	*Increased*	*Decreased*
11-Deoxycortisol	1/µg/dL	<0.029 µmol/L	Some malignancies Scleroderma Hypertensive form of virilizing adrenal hyperplasia due to an 11-β-hydroxylase defect	
Dibucaine number	Normal: 70%–85% inhibition Heterozygote: 50%–65% inhibition Homozygote: 16%–25% inhibition			Important in detecting carriers of abnormal cholinesterase activity who are susceptible to succinylcholine anesthetic shock
Dihydrotestosterone	Males: 50–210 ng/dL Females: none detectable	1.72–7.22 nmol/L		Testicular feminization syndrome
Estradiol—RIA	Females: Follicular: 10–90 pg/mL Midcycle: 100–500 pg/mL Luteal: 50–240 pg/mL Follicular phase: 2–20 ng/dL Midcycle: 12–40 ng/dL Luteal phase: 10–30 ng/dL Postmenopausal: 1–5 ng/dL Males: 0.5–5 ng/dL	37–370 pmol/L 367–1835 pmol/L 184–881 pmol/L	Pregnancy	Depressed or failure to peak—ovarian failure
Estriol—RIA	Nonpregnant females: <0.5 ng/mL Pregnant females: 1st trimester: up to 1 ng/mL 2nd trimester: 0.8–7 ng/mL 3rd trimester: 5–25 ng/mL	<1.75 nmol/L Up to 3.5 nmol/L 2.8–24.3 nmol/L 17.4–86.8 nmol/L	Pregnancy	Depressed or failure to peak—ovarian failure
Estrogens, total—RIA	Females: cycle days: Day 1–10: 61–394 pg/mL Day 11–20: 122–437 pg/mL Day 21–30: 156–350 pg/mL Males: 40–115 pg/mL	61–394 ng/L 122–437 ng/L 156–350 ng/L 40–115 ng/L	Pregnancy Measured on a daily basis, can be used to evaluate response of hypogonadotrophic, hypoestrogenic women to human menopausal or pituitary gonadotropin	Fetal distress Ovarian failure

TABLE B-2 (Continued)

Reference Ranges—Serum, Plasma, and Whole Blood Chemistries				
Determination	**Normal Adult Reference Range**		**Clinical Significance**	
	Conventional Units	*SI Units*	*Increased*	*Decreased*
Estrone—RIA	Females: Day 1–10: 4.3–18 ng/dL Day 11–20: 7.5–19.6 ng/dL Day 21–30: 13–20 ng/dL Males: 2.5–7.5 ng/dL	15.9–66.6 pmol/L 27.8–72.5 pmol/L 48.1–74 pmol/L 9.3–27.8 pmol/L		Depressed or failure to peak—ovarian failure
Ferritin—RIA	Males: 29–438 ng/mL Females: 9–219 ng/mL	29–438 µg/L 9–219 µg/L	Nephritis Hemochromatosis Certain neoplastic diseases Acute myelogenous leukemia Multiple myeloma	Iron deficiency
Folic acid—RIA	2.5–20 ng/mL	6–46 nmol/L		Megaloblastic anemias of infancy and pregnancy Inadequate diet Liver disease Malabsorption syndrome Severe hemolytic anemia
Follicle stimulating hormone (FSH)—RIA	Males: 2–10 mIU/mL Females: Follicular phase: 5–20 mIU/mL Peak of middle cycle: 12–30 mIU/mL Luteinic phase: 5–15 mIU/mL Menopausal females: 40–200 mIU/mL	5–20 IU/L 12–30 IU/L 5–15 IU/L 40–200 IU/L	Menopause and primary ovarian failure	Pituitary failure
Galactose	<5 mg/dL	<0.28 mmol/L		Galactosemia
Gamma glutamyl transpeptidase	Males: <45 IU/L Females: <30 IU/L	45 U/L 30 U/L	Hepatobiliary disease Drug toxicity Myocardial infarction Renal infarction Zollinger-Ellison syndrome	
Gastrin—RIA	Fasting: 50–155 pg/mL Postprandial: 80–170 pg/mL	50–155 ng/L 80–170 ng/L	Peptic ulceration of the duodenum Pernicious anemia	
Glucose	Fasting: 60–110 mg/dL	3.3–6.05 mmol/L	Diabetes Nephritis	Hyperinsulinism Hypothyroidism

(continues)

TABLE B-2 (Continued)

Reference Ranges—Serum, Plasma, and Whole Blood Chemistries

Determination	Normal Adult Reference Range		Clinical Significance	
	Conventional Units	*SI Units*	*Increased*	*Decreased*
	Postprandial (2 h): 65–140 mg/dL	3.58–7.7 mmol/L	Hyperthyroidism Early hyperpituitarism Cerebral lesions Infections Pregnancy Uremia	Late hyperpituitarism Pernicious vomiting Addison's disease Extensive hepatic damage
Glucose tolerance (oral)	Features of a normal response: 1. Normal fasting between 60–110 mg/dL 2. No sugar in urine 3. Upper limits of normal: Fasting = 125 1 hour = 190 2 hours = 140 3 hours = 125	3.3–6.05 mmol/L 6.88 mmol/L 10.45 mmol/L 7.70 mmol/L 6.88 mmol/L	Two-hour value >200 mg/dL (11.1 mmol/L) is diagnostic for diabetes	Decreased 2 and 3 hour values may occur with hypoglycemia
Glucose-6-phosphate dehydrogenase (red cells)	Screening: Decolorization in 20–100 min Quantitative: 1.86–2.5 IU/mL RBC	 1860–2500 U/L		Drug-induced hemolytic anemia Hemolytic disease of newborn
Glycoprotein (alpha-1-acid)	40–110 mg/dL	400–1100 mg/L	Neoplasm Tuberculosis Diabetes complicated by degenerative vascular disease Pregnancy Rheumatoid arthritis Rheumatic fever Infectious liver disease Lupus erythematosus	
Growth hormone— RIA	<10 ng/mL	<10 mg/L	Acromegaly	Failure to stimulate with arginine or insulin— hypopituitarism Hemolytic anemia
Haptoglobin	50–250 mg/dL	0.5–2.5 g/L	Pregnancy Estrogen therapy Chronic infections Various inflammatory conditions	Hemolytic blood transfusion reaction
Hemoglobin (plasma)	0.5–5 mg/dL	5–50 mg/L	Transfusion reactions Paroxysmal nocturnal hemoglobinuria Intravascular hemolysis	Anemia, pregnancy, chronic renal failure

TABLE B-2 (Continued)

Reference Ranges—Serum, Plasma, and Whole Blood Chemistries

| Determination | Normal Adult Reference Range | | Clinical Significance | |
	Conventional Units	*SI Units*	*Increased*	*Decreased*
Glycohemoglobin (GHB, hemoglobin A_{1c}, hemoglobin A1)	Nondiabetics & diabetics with good control: 4.4%–6.4%		Suboptimal glucose control	
Hexosaminidase, total	Controls: 333–375 nM/ mL/h	333–375 µmol/ L/h	Sandhoff's disease	Tay-Sachs disease and heterozygotes
Hexosaminidase A	Controls: 49%–68% of total	Fraction of total: 0.49–0.68		
	Heterozygotes: 26%–45% of total	0.26–0.45		
	Tay-Sachs disease: 0%–4% of total	0–0.04		
	Diabetics: 39%–59% of total	0.39–0.59		
High-density lipoprotein cholesterol (HDL cholesterol)	Males: 35–70 mg/dL	0.91–1.81 mmol/L		HDL cholesterol is lower in patients with increased risk for coronary heart disease
	Females: 35–85 mg/dL	0.91–220 mmol/L		
	Males: 0.4–4 ng/mL	1.2–12 nmol/L	Congenital adrenal hyperplasia	
	Females: 0.1–3.3 ng/mL	0.3–10 nmol/L	Pregnancy	
Homocysteine		4–17 µmol/L	Folic acid deficiency Increased risk for vascular disease Homocystinuria	
17 Hydroxy-progesterone—RIA				
Immunoglobulin A	Children: 0.1–0.5 ng/mL	0.3–1.5 nmol/L	Some cases of adrenal or ovarian adenomas	Ataxia telangiectasis Agammaglobu-linemia
	Adults: 50–300 mg/dL (in children the normals are lower and vary with age)	0.5–3 g/L	Gamma A myeloma Wiskott-Aldrich syndrome Autoimmune disease Hepatic cirrhosis	Hypogammaglobu-linemia, transient Dysgammaglobu-linemia Protein-losing enteropathies
Immunoglobulin D	0–30 mg/dL	0–300 mg/L	IgD multiple myeloma Some patients with chronic infectious diseases	
Immunoglobulin E	20–740 ng/mL	20–740 µg/L	Allergic patients and those with parasitic infections	

(continues)

TABLE B-2 (Continued)

Reference Ranges—Serum, Plasma, and Whole Blood Chemistries

Determination	Normal Adult Reference Range		Clinical Significance	
	Conventional Units	*SI Units*	*Increased*	*Decreased*
Immunoglobulin G	Adults: 565–1765 mg/dL	6.35–14 g/L	IgG myeloma Following hyper-immunization Autoimmune disease states Chronic infections	Congenital and acquired hypogammaglobulinemia IgA myelomas, Waldenström's (IgM) macroglobulinemia Some malabsorption syndromes Extensive protein loss
Immunoglobulin M	Adults: 55–375 mg/dL	0.4–2.8 g/L	Waldenström's macroglobulinemia Parasitic infections Hepatitis	Agammaglobulinemias Some IgG and IgA myelomas Chronic lymphatic leukemia
Insulin—RIA	5–25 µU/mL	0.2–1 µg/L	Insulinoma Acromegaly	Diabetes mellitus
Iron	50–160/µg/dL	9–29 µmol/L	Pernicious anemia Aplastic anemia Hemolytic anemia Hepatitis Hemochromatosis	Iron deficiency anemia
Iron-binding capacity	IBC: 150–235 µg/dL TIBC: 230–410 µg/dL % Saturation: 20–50	26.9–42.1 µmol/L 41–73 µmol/L Fraction of total iron-binding capacity: 0.2–0.5	Iron deficiency anemia Acute and chronic blood loss Hepatitis	Chronic infectious diseases Cirrhosis
Isocitric dehydrogenase	50–180 U	0.83–3 UIL	Hepatitis, cirrhosis Obstructive jaundice Metastatic carcinoma of the liver Megaloblastic anemia	
Lactic acid (whole blood)	Venous: 5–20 mg/dL Arterial: 3–7 mg/dL	0.6–2.2 mmol/L 0.3–0.8 mmol/L	Increased muscular activity Congestive heart failure Hemorrhage Shock Lactic acidosis Some febrile infections May be increased in severe liver disease	
Lactic dehydrogenase (LDH)	100–225 mU/mL	100–225 U/L	Untreated pernicious anemia Myocardial infarction Pulmonary infarction Liver disease	
Lactic dehydrogenase isoenzymes				

TABLE B-2 (Continued)

Reference Ranges—Serum, Plasma, and Whole Blood Chemistries

Determination	Normal Adult Reference Range		Clinical Significance	
	Conventional Units	*SI Units*	*Increased*	*Decreased*
Total lactic dehydrogenase	100–225 mU/mL	100–225 U/L Fraction of total LDH:	LDH-1 and LDH-2 are increased in myocardial infarction, megaloblastic anemia, and hemolytic anemia	
LDH-1	20%–35%	0.2–0.35		
LDH-2	25%–40%	0.25–0.4		
LDH-3	20%–30%	0.2–0.3	LDH-4 and LDH-5 are increased in pulmonary infarction, congestive heart failure, and liver disease	
LDH-4	0–20%	0–0.2		
LDH-5	0–25%	0–0.25		
Lead (whole blood)	Up to 40 µg/dL	Up to 2 µmol/L	Lead poisoning	
Leucine aminopeptidase	80–200 U/mL	19.2–48 U/L	Liver or biliary tract diseases Pancreatic disease Metastatic carcinoma of liver and pancreas Biliary obstruction	
Lipase	0.2–1.5 U/mL	55–417 U/L	Acute and chronic pancreatitis Biliary obstruction Cirrhosis Hepatitis Peptic ulcer	
Lipids, total	400–1000 mg/dL	4–10 g/L	Hypothyroidism Diabetes Nephrosis Glomerulonephritis Hyperlipoproteinemias	Hyperthyroidism
Low-density lipoprotein cholesterol (LDL cholesterol)	mg/dL desirable levels: <160 if no coronary artery disease (CAD) and <2 risk factors <130 if no CAD and 2 or more risk factors <100 if CAD present		LDL cholesterol is higher in patients with increased risk for coronary heart disease	
Luteinizing hormone—RIA	Males: 4.9–15 MIU/mL Females:	4.9–15 mg/L	Pituitary tumor Ovarian failure	Depressed or failure to peak—pituitary failure
	Follicular phase: 2–3 MIU/mL	0.5–6.9 mg/L		
	Ovulatory peak: 40–200 MIU/mL	9.2–46 mg/L		
	Luteal phase: 0–20 MIU/mL	0–5 mg/L		
	Postmenopausal: 35–120 mIU/mL	8–27.5 mg/L		

(*continues*)

TABLE B-2 (Continued)

Reference Ranges—Serum, Plasma, and Whole Blood Chemistries

| Determination | Normal Adult Reference Range | | Clinical Significance | |
	Conventional Units	SI Units	Increased	Decreased
Lysozyme (muramidase)	2.8–8 µg/mL	2.8–8 mg	Certain types of leukemia (acute monocytic leukemia) Inflammatory states and infections	Acute lymphocytic leukemia
Magnesium	1.3–2.4 mEq/L	0.7–1.2 mmol/L	Excess ingestion of magnesium-containing antacids	Chronic alcoholism Severe renal disease Diarrhea Defective growth
Manganese	0.04–1.4 µg/dL	72.9–255 nmol/L		
Mercury	Up to 10 µg/dL	Up to 0.5/µmol/L	Mercury poisoning	
Myoglobin—RIA	Up to 85 ng/mL	Up to 85 µg/mL	Myocardial infarction Muscle necrosis	
5' Nucleotidase	3.2–11.6 IU/L	3.2–11.6 U/L	Hepatobiliary disease	
Osmolality	280–300 mOsm/kg	280–300 mmol/L	Diabetes insipidus Osmotic diuresis	Inappropriate secretion of ADH Addison's disease
Parathyroid hormone	160–350 pg/mL	160–350 ng/L	Hyperparathyroidism	Chronic renal failure Hypoparathyroidism
Phenylalanine	1.2–3.5 mg/dL 1st week 0.7–3.5 mg/dL thereafter	0.07–0.21 mmol/L 0.04–0.21 mmol/L	Phenylketonuria	
Phosphohexose isomerase	20–90 IU/L	20–90 U/L	Malignancy Disease of heart, liver, and skeletal muscles	
Phospholipids	125–300 mg/dL	1.25–3 g/L	Diabetes Nephritis	
Phosphorus, inorganic	2.5–4.5 mg/dL	0.8–1.45 mmol/L	Chronic nephritis Hypoparathyroidism	Hyperparathyroidism Vitamin D deficiency
Potassium	3.8–5 mEq/L	3.8–5 mmol/L	Renal failure Acidosis Cell lysis Tissue breakdown or hemolysis	GI losses Diuretic administration
Progesterone—RIA	Follicular phase: up to 0.8 ng/mL Luteal phase: 10–20 ng/mL End of cycle: <1 ng/mL Pregnant: up to 50 ng/mL in 20th week	2.5 nmol/L 31.8–63.6 nmol/L <3 nmol/L Up to 160 nmol/L	Useful in evaluation of menstrual disorders and infertility and in the evaluation of placental function during pregnancies complicated by toxemia, diabetes mellitus, or threatened miscarriage	

TABLE B-2 (Continued)

Reference Ranges—Serum, Plasma, and Whole Blood Chemistries

Determination	Normal Adult Reference Range		Clinical Significance	
	Conventional Units	*SI Units*	*Increased*	*Decreased*
Prolactin—RIA	6–24 ng/mL	6–24 µg/L	Pregnancy Functional or structural disorders of the hypothalamus Pituitary stalk section Pituitary tumors	
Prostate-specific antigen	<4 ng/mL		Prostatic cancer, benign prostatic hyperplasia, prostatitis	
Protein, total Albumin Globulin	6–8 gm/dL 3.5–5 gm/dL 1.5–3 gm/dL	60–80 g/L 35–50 g/L 15–30 g/L	Hemoconcentration Shock Multiple myeloma (globulin fraction) Chronic infections (globulin function) Liver disease (globulin)	Malnutrition Hemorrhage Loss of plasma from burns Proteinuria

Protein
  Electrophoresis (cellulose acetate)
  Albumin
  Alpha-1 globulin
  Alpha-2 globulin
  Beta globulin
  Gamma globulin
	
	3.5–5 gm/dL
	0.1–0.4 gm/dL
	0.4–1.2 gm/dL
	0.6–1.2 gm/dL
	0.5–1.6 gm/dL
		35–50 g/L
		24 g/L
		6–10 g/L
		1–4 g/L
		4–12 g/L
		5–11 g/L
		5–16 g/L		

Protoporphyrin erythrocyte (whole blood)	15–100 µg/dL	0.27–1.80 µmol/L	Lead toxicity Erythropoietic porphyria	
Pyridoxine	3.6–18 ng/mL			A wide spectrum of clinical conditions, such as mental depression, peripheral neuropathy, anemia, neonatal seizures, and reactions to certain drug therapies
Pyruvic acid (whole blood)	0.3–0.7 mg/dL	34–80 µmol/L	Diabetes Severe thiamine deficiency Acute phase of some infections, possibly secondary to increased -glycogenolysis and glycolysis	

(continues)

TABLE B-2 (Continued)

Reference Ranges—Serum, Plasma, and Whole Blood Chemistries

Determination	Normal Adult Reference Range		Clinical Significance	
	Conventional Units	*SI Units*	*Increased*	*Decreased*
Renin (plasma)—RIA	Normal diet: Supine: 0.3–1.9 ng/mL/h Upright: 0.6–3.6 ng/mL/h	0.08–0.52 ng/L/S 0.16– 1.00 µg/L/S	Renovascular hypertension Malignant hypertension Untreated Addison's disease Primary salt-losing nephropathy Low-salt diet Diuretic therapy	Frank primary aldosteronism Increased salt intake Salt-retaining steroid therapy Antidiuretic hormone therapy
	Low salt diet: Supine: 0.9–4.5 ng/mL/h Upright: 4.1–9.1 ng/mL/h	0.25– 1.25 µg/L/S 1.13– 2.53 µg/L/S	Hemorrhage	Blood transfusion
Sodium	135–145 mEq/L	135– 145 mmol/L	Hemoconcentration Nephritis Pyloric obstruction	Alkali deficit Addison's disease Myxedema
Sulfate (inorganic)	0.5–1.5 mg/dL	0.05– 0.15 mmol/L	Nephritis Nitrogen retention	
Testosterone—RIA	Females: 25–100 ng/dL Males: 300–800 ng/dL	0.9–3.5 nmol/L 10.5–28 nmol/L	Females: Polycystic ovary Virilizing tumors	Males Orchidectomy for neoplastic disease of the prostate or breast Estrogen therapy Klinefelter's syndrome Hypopituitarism Hypogonadism Hepatic cirrhosis
T_3 (triiodothyronine) uptake	25%–35%	Relative uptake fraction: 0.25–0.35	Hyperthyroidism Thyroxine-binding globulin (TBG) deficiency Androgens and anabolic steroids	Hypothyroidism Pregnancy TBG excess Estrogens and anti-ovulatory drugs
T_3 total circulating—RIA	75–200 ng/dL	1.15–3.1 nmol/L	Pregnancy Hyperthyroidism	Hypothyroidism
T_4 (thyroxine)—RIA	4.5–11.5 µg/dL	58.5–150 nmol/L	Hyperthyroidism Thyroiditis Elevated thyroxine-binding proteins caused by oral contraceptives Pregnancy	Primary and pituitary hypothyroidism Idiopathic involvement Cases of diminished thyroxine-binding proteins caused by androgenic and anabolic steroids Hypoproteinemia Nephrotic syndrome

TABLE B-2 (Continued)

Reference Ranges—Serum, Plasma, and Whole Blood Chemistries

Determination	Normal Adult Reference Range		Clinical Significance	
	Conventional Units	*SI Units*	*Increased*	*Decreased*
T_4, free	1–2.2 ng/dL	13–30 pmol/L	Euthyroid patients with normal free thyroxine levels may have abnormal T3 and T4 levels caused by drug preparations	
Thyroid-stimulating hormone (TSH)—RIA		0.3–5 m/IU/L	Hypothyroidism	Hyperthyroidism
Thyroid-binding globulin	10–26 µg/dL	100–260/µg/L	Hypothyroidism Pregnancy Estrogen therapy Oral contraceptives Genetic and idiopathic liver disease	Use of androgens and anabolic steroids Nephrotic syndrome Marked hypoproteinemia
Transferrin	230–320 mg/dL	2.3–3.2 g/L	Pregnancy Iron deficiency anemia due to hemorrhaging Acute hepatitis Polycythemia Oral contraceptives Primary and secondary hyperlipidemias	Pernicious anemia in relapse Thalassemic and sickle cell anemia Chromatosis Neoplastic and hepatic diseases
Triglycerides	10–150 mg/dL	0.10–1.65 nmol/L		Tryptophan-specific malabsorption syndrome
Troponin T and I	Negative	Negative	Myocardial infarction	
Tryptophan	1.4–3 mg/dL	68.6–147 nmol/L	Tyrosinosis	
Tyrosine	0.5–4 mg/dL	27.6–220.8 mmol/L		
Urea nitrogen (BUN)	10–20 mg/dL	3.6–7.2 mmol/L	Acute glomerulonephritis Obstructive uropathy Mercury poisoning Nephrotic syndrome	Severe hepatic failure Pregnancy
Uric acid	2.5–8 mg/dL	0.15–0 mmol/L	Gouty arthritis Acute leukemia Lymphomas treated by chemotherapy Toxemia of pregnancy	Defective tubular reabsorption
Viscosity	1.4–1.8 relative to water at 37°C (98.6°F)		Patients with marked increases of the gamma globulins	

(*continues*)

TABLE B-2 (Continued)

Reference Ranges—Serum, Plasma, and Whole Blood Chemistries

Determination	Normal Adult Reference Range		Clinical Significance	
	Conventional Units	*SI Units*	*Increased*	*Decreased*
Vitamin A	50–220 Hg/dL	1.75–7.7 µmol/L	Hypervitaminosis A	Vitamin A deficiency Celiac disease Sprue Obstructive jaundice Giardiasis Parenchymal hepatic disease
Vitamin B, (thiamine)	1.6–4 µg/dL	47.4– 135.7 nmol/L		Anorexia Beriberi Polyneuropathy Cardiomyopathies
Vitamin B6 (pyridoxal phosphate)	3.6–18 ng/mL	14.6– 72.8 nmol/L		Chronic alcoholism Malnutrition Uremia Neonatal seizures Malabsorption, such as celiac syndrome
Vitamin B12—RIA	130–785 pg/mL	100–580 pmol/L	Hepatic cell damage and in association with the myeloproliferative disorders (the highest levels are encountered in myeloid leukemia)	Strict vegetarianism Alcoholism Pernicious anemia Total or partial gastrectomy Ileal resection Sprue and celiac disease Fish tapeworm infestation
Vitamin E	0.5–2 mg/dL	11.6–46.4 µmol/L		Vitamin E deficiency
Xylose absorption test	2 hr, 30–50 mg/dL	2–3.35 mmol/L		Malabsorption syndrome
Zinc	55–150/µg/dL	7.65– 22.95 µmol/L	Coronary artery disease Arteriosclerosis Industrial exposure	Metastatic liver disease Tuberculosis Sprue

* By radioimmunoassay.

TABLE B-3

Reference Ranges—Immunodiagnostic Tests

Determination	Normal Value	Clinical Significance
Acetylcholine receptor binding antibody	Negative or <0.03 nmol/L	Considered to be diagnostic for myasthenia gravis in patients with symptoms.
Anti-ds-DNA antibody	<70 U by enzyme-linked immunosorbent assay (ELISA)	Valuable in supporting diagnosis or monitoring disease activity and prognosis of systemic lupus erythematosus (SLE).
Antiglomerular basement membrane antibody	<1:20 by indirect fluorescence Negative or less than 10 U	Primarily used in the differential diagnosis of glomerular nephritis induced by antiglomerular basement membrane antibodies from other types of glomerular nephritis.
Anti-insulin antibody	<3% binding of labeled beef and pork insulin by patient's serum; or <9 mIU/L	Helpful in determining the best therapeutic agent in diabetics and the cause of allergic manifestations. Also used to identify insulin resistance.
Antimitochondrial antibody and anti-smooth muscle antibody	<1:5 and <1:20, respectively	Increased in cirrhosis, autoimmune disease, thyroiditis, pernicious anemia.
Antinuclear antibody	Negative, <1:20	Increased in SLE, chronic hepatitis, scleroderma, leukemia, and mononucleosis.
Anti-parietal cell antibody	Negative, <1:20	Helpful in diagnosing chronic gastric disease and differentiating autoimmune pernicious anemia from other megaloblastic anemias.
Antiribonucleoprotein antibody	Negative	Helpful in differential diagnosis of systemic rheumatic disease.
Antiscleroderma antibody	Negative	Highly diagnostic for scleroderma.
Anti-Smith antibody	Negative	Highly diagnostic of SLE.
Anti-SS-A/anti-SS-B antibody	Negative	SS-A antibodies are found in Sjögren's syndrome alone or associated with lupus. SS-B antibodies are associated with primary Sjögren's syndrome.
Antithyroglobulin and anti-microsomal antibodies	<1:100 titer by gelatin or hemaglutination	Presence and concentration is important in evaluation and treatment of various thyroid disorders, such as Hashimoto's thyroiditis and Graves' disease. May indicate previous autoimmune disorders.
CA 15-3 tumor marker	<22 IU/ml	Increased in metastatic breast cancer.
CA 19-9 tumor marker	<37 IU/ml	Increased in pancreatic, hepatobiliary, gastric, and colorectal cancer, gallstones.

EBV Interpretation

	VCA-IgG	VCA-IgM	EA-IgG	EBV-NA
Susceptible	−	−	−	−
Acute infection	+	+	±	−
Convalescent phase	+	±	±	+
Chronic or reactivated	+	−	+	±
Old infection	±	−	−	+

Antibody present: +
Antibody absent: −
VCA, viral capsid antigen; EA, early antigen; EBV-NA, Epstein Barr virus-nuclear antigen

(continues)

TABLE B-3 (Continued)

Reference Ranges—Immunodiagnostic Tests		
Determination	**Normal Value**	**Clinical Significance**
CA 125	0–35 IU/ml	Increased in colon, upper gastrointestinal (GI), ovarian, and other gynecologic cancers: pregnancy, peritonitis.
Carcinoembryonic antigen (CEA)—RLK	0–2.5 11g/L (nonsmoker) 0–5/μg/L (smoker)	The repeatedly high incidence of this antigen in cancers of the colon, rectum, pancreas, and stomach suggests that CEA levels may be useful in the therapeutic monitoring of these conditions, but it is not a screening test
Cold agglutinins	<1:16	Increased in mycoplasma pneumonia, viral illness, mononucleosis, multiple myeloma, scleroderma.
C-reactive protein	<0.8 mg/dL	Increase indicates active inflammation.
Cytomegalovirus antibodies (CMV IgG)	Negative: <0.9 units/mL	Positive >1.0 unit/mL if exposed to CMV at anytime. Acute and convalescent specimens can help identify acute infection.
Cytomegalovirus antibodies (CMV IgM)	Negative: <0.79 Equivocal: 0.80–1.20	Positive >1.20 usually indicates acute infection. Repeat specimen in 1–2 weeks for equivocal result.
Epstein-Barr virus serology (viral capsid antigen IgG and IgM, early antigen IgG, and nuclear antigen IgG)	Negative is <1:20 or <20 for each individual test	Differentiation of acute from chronic or old infection by interpretation of table below.
Hepatitis A virus antibodies, IgM (HAV-Ab/IgM)	Negative	Positive in acute-stage hepatitis A; develops early in disease.
Hepatitis A virus antibodies, IgG (HAV-Ab/IgG)	Negative	Positive if previous exposure and immunity to hepatitis A.
Hepatitis B surface antigen (HBsAg)	Negative	Positive in acute-stage hepatitis B.
Hepatitis B surface antibody (HBsAb)	Negative	Positive if previous exposure and immunity to hepatitis B.
Hepatitis C virus antibodies	Negative	Positive in exposure to hepatitis C virus; may indicate acute, chronic, or cleared infection.
Hepatitis C virus RNA	Negative	Positive in hepatitis C infection, can be quantitative
Infectious mononucleosis tests (monospot, monotest, heterophile antigen test, Epstein-Barr virus (EBV), antiviral capsid antigen IgM and IgG)	Negative, <1:80	Positive monospot and monotest are presumptive, positive EBV IgM and IgG indicate acute and recent or past infection, respectively.
Lyme disease titer	Negative, <1:256 by indirect fluorescent antibody method >0.8 by ELISA	Positive results help diagnose Lyme disease. False positive may occur with high rheumatoid factor titers or syphilis. Positive ELISA confirmed by Western blot test.
Pyroglobulin test	Negative	These abnormal proteins may be associated with myeloma, lymphoma, polycythemia vera, and SLE.
Rheumatoid factor	Negative or less than 60 IU/mL	Elevated in rheumatoid arthritis, lupus endocarditis, tuberculosis, syphilis, sarcoidosis, cancer.

TABLE B-3 (Continued)

Reference Ranges—Immunodiagnostic Tests		
Determination	**Normal Value**	**Clinical Significance**
T and B cell lymphocyte surface markers T-helper/T-suppressor ratio	T and B cell lymphocyte surface markers: Percent T cells (CD2) 60–88% Percent helper cells (CD4) 34–67% Percent suppressor cells (CD8) 10–42% Percent B cells (CD19) 3–21% Absolute counts: Lymphocytes 0.66–4.60 thou/mL T cells 644–2201 cells/mL Helper cells 493–1191 cells/mL Suppressor T cells 182–785 cells/mL B cells 92–392 cells/mL Lymphocyte ratio: T_H/T_S ratio > 1	Done to evaluate immune system by identifying the specific cells involved in the immune response. Valuable in diagnosis of lymphocytic leukemia, lymphoma, and immunodeficiency diseases including acquired immunodeficiency syndrome, and in the assessment of patient response to chemotherapy and radiation.

TABLE B-4

Reference Ranges—Urine Chemistry

Determination	Normal Adult Reference Range		Clinical Significance	
	Conventional Units	*SI Units*	*Increased*	*Decreased*
Acetone and acetoacetate	Zero		Uncontrolled diabetes Starvation	
Aldosterone	With normal salt diet: Normal: 4–20 µg/ 24 h	11.1–55.5 nmol/24h	Primary aldosteronism (adrenocortical tumor) Secondary aldosteronism	
	Renovascular: 10–40 µg/24 h	27.7–111 nmol/24 h	Salt depletion Potassium loading ACTH in large doses	
	Tumor: 20– 100 µg/24 h	55.4–277 nmol/24 h	Cardiac failure Cirrhosis with ascites formation Nephrosis Pregnancy	
Alpha amino nitrogen	50–200 mg/24 h	3.6–14.3 nmol/24 h	Leukemia Phenylketonuria Other metabolic diseases	
Amylase	35–260 units excreted per h	6.5–48.1 U/h	Acute pancreatitis	
Arylsulfatase A	>2.4 U/mL			
Bence-Jones protein	None detected		Myeloma	Metachromatic leukodystrophy
Calcium	<150 mg/24 h	<3.75 mmol/24 h	Hyperparathyroidism Vitamin D intoxication Fanconi's syndrome	Hypoparathyroidism Vitamin D deficiency
Catecholamines	Total: 0–275 µg/24 h Epinephrine; 10%–40% Norepinephrine: 60%–90%	0–275 µg/24 h Fraction total: 0.10–8.4 Fraction total: 0.60–0.90	Pheochromocytoma Neuroblastoma	
Chorionic gonadotrophin, qualitative (pregnancy test)	Negative		Pregnancy Chorionepithelioma Hydatidiform mole	
Copper	20–70 µg/24 h	0.32–1.12 µmol/ 24 h	Wilson's diseases Cirrhosis Nephrosis	
Coproporphyrin	50–300 µg/24 h	0.075–0.45 µmol/24 h	Poliomyelitis Lead poisoning Porphyria	
Cortisol, free	20–90 Hg/24 h	55.2–248.4 mmol/d	Cushing's syndrome	
Creatinine	0–200 mg/24 h	0–1.52 mmol/ 24 h	Muscular dystrophy Fever Carcinoma of liver Pregnancy Hyperthyroidism Myositis	

TABLE B-4   (Continued)

Reference Ranges—Urine Chemistry

Determination	Normal Adult Reference Range		Clinical Significance	
	Conventional Units	*SI Units*	*Increased*	*Decreased*
Creatine	0.8–2 gm/24 h	7–17.6 mmol/24 h	Typhoid fever Salmonella infections Tetanus	Muscular atrophy Anemia Advanced degeneration of kidneys Leukemia
Creatinine clearance	100–150 mL of blood cleared of creatinine per mm	1.67–2.5 mL/s		Measures glomerular filtration rate Renal diseases
Cystine and cysteine	10–100 mg/24 h	0.08–0.83 mmol/24 h	Cystinuria Lead poisoning	
Delta aminole-vulimic acid	0–0.54 mg/dL	0–40/μmol/L	Porphyria hepatica Hepatitis Hepatic carcinoma	
11-Desoxycortisol	20–100 μg/24 h	0.6–2.9/μmol/d	Hypertensive form of virilizing adrenal hyperplasia due to an 11-beta hydroxylase defect	
Estriol (placental)				Decreased values occur with fetal distress of many conditions, including preeclampsia, placental insufficiency, and poorly controlled diabetes mellitus

Weeks of pregnancy	μm/24 h	mmol/24 h
12	<1	<3.5
16	2–7	7–24.5
20	4–9	14–32
24	6–13	21–45.5
28	8–22	28–77
32	12–43	42–150
36	14–45	49–158
40	19–46	66.5–160

Determination	Normal Adult Reference Range		Clinical Significance	
Estrogens, total (fluorometric)	Females: Onset of menstruation: 4–25 μg/24 h	4–25 μg/24 h	Hyperestrogenism due to gonadal or adrenal neoplasm	Primary or secondary amenorrhea
	Ovulation peak: 28 μg/24 h	28 μg/24 h		
	Luteal peak: 22–105 μg/24 h	22–105 μg/24 h		
	Menopausal: 1.4–19.6 μg/24 h	1.4–19.6 μg/24 h		
	Males: 5–18 μg/24 h	5–18 μg/24 h		

(continues)

TABLE B-4   (Continued)

Reference Ranges—Urine Chemistry

Determination	Normal Adult Reference Range		Clinical Significance	
	Conventional Units	SI Units	Increased	Decreased
Etiocholanolone	Males: 1.9–6 mg/24 h Females: 0.5–4 mg/24 h	6.5–20.6 µmol/24 h 1.7–13.8 µmol/24 h	Adrenogenital syndrome Idiopathic hirsutism	
Follicle-stimulating hormone—RIA	Females: Follicular: 5–20 IU/24 h Luteal: 5–15 IU/24 h Midcycle: 15–60 IU/24 h Menopausal: 50–100 IU/24 h Males: 5–25 IU/24 h	5–20 IU/d 5–15 IU/d 15–60 IU/d 50–100 IU/d 5–25 IU/d	Menopause and primary ovarian failure	Pituitary failure
Glucose	Negative		Diabetes mellitus Pituitary disorders Increased ICP Lesion in floor of 4th ventricle	
Hemoglobin and myoglobin	Negative		Extensive burns Transfusion of incompatible blood Myoglobin increased in severe crushing injuries to muscles	
Homogentistic add, qualitative	Negative		Alkaptonuria Ochronosis	
Homovanillic acid	Up to 15 mg/24 h	Up to 82 µmol/d	Neuroblastoma	
17-hydroxycortico-steroids	2–10 mg/24 h	5.5–27.5 µmol/d	Cushing's disease	Addison's disease Anterior pituitary hypofunction
5-Hydroxyin-doleascetic add, qualitative	Negative		Malignant carcinoid tumors	
Hydroxyproline	15–43 mg/24 h	0.11–0.33 µmol/d	Paget disease Fibrous dysplasia Osteomalacia Neoplastic bone diseases Hyperparathyroidism	
17-ketosteroids, total	Males: 10–22 mg/24 h Females: 6–16 mg/24 h	35–76 µmol/d 21–55 µmol/d	Interstitial cell tumor of testes Simple hirsutism, occasionally Adrenal hyperplasia Cushing's syndrome Adrenal cancer, virilism Adrenoblastoma	Thyrotoxicosis Female hypogonadism Diabetes mellitus Hypertension Debilitating disease of mild to moderate severity Eunuchoidism Addison's disease Panhypopituitarism

TABLE B-4 (Continued)

Reference Ranges—Urine Chemistry

Determination	Normal Adult Reference Range		Clinical Significance	
	Conventional Units	*SI Units*	*Increased*	*Decreased*
Lead	Up to 150 μg/24 h	Up to 60 μmol/24 h	Lead poisoning	Myxedema Nephrosis
Luteinizing hormone	Males: 5–18 IU/24 h Females: Follicular phase: 2–25 IU/24 h Ovulatory peak: 30–95 IU/24 h Luteal phase: 2–20 IU/24 h Postmenopausal: 40–110 IU/24 h	2–25 IU/d 30–95 IU/d 2–20 IU/d 40–110 IU/d	Pituitary tumor Ovarian failure	Depressed or failure to peak—pituitary failure
Metanephrines, total	Less than 1.3 mg/24 h	Less than 6.5 μmol/d	Pheochromocytoma, a few patients with pheochromocytoma may have elevated urinary metanephrines but normal catecholamines and vanillylmandelic acid (VMA)	
Osmolality	Males: 390–1090 mM/kg Females: 300–1090 mM/kg	390–1090 mmol/kg 300–1090 mmol/kg	Useful in the study of electrolyte and water balance	
Oxalate	Up to 40 mg/24 h	Up to 456/μmol/d	Primary hyperoxaluria	
Phenylpyruvic acid qualitative	Negative		Phenylketonuria	
Phosphorus, inorganic	0.8–1.3 gm/24 h	26–24 mmol/24 h	Hypoparathyroidism Vitamin D intoxication Paget's disease Metastatic neoplasm to bone	Hypoparathyroidism Vitamin D deficiency
Porphobilinogen, qualitative	Negative		Chronic lead poisoning Acute porphyria Liver disease	
Porphobilinogen quantitative	0–1 mg/24 h	0–4.4 μmol/24 h	Acute porphyria Liver disease	
Porphyrins, qualitative	Negative		See porphyrins, quantitative	
Porphyrins, quantitative (coproporphyrin and uroporphyrin)	Coproporphyrin: 50–160 μg/24 h Uroporphyrin: up to 50 μ/24 h	0.075–0.24 μmol/24h Up to 0.06 μmol/24 h	Porphyria Lead poisoning (only coproporphyrin increased)	

(continues)

TABLE B-4 (Continued)

Reference Ranges—Urine Chemistry

Determination	Normal Adult Reference Range		Clinical Significance	
	Conventional Units	*SI Units*	*Increased*	*Decreased*
Potassium	40–65 mEq/24 h	40–65 mmol/ 24 h	Hemolysis Chronic renal failure Acidosis Cushing's disease	Diarrhea Adrenocortical insufficiency
Pregnanediol	Females: Proliferative phase: 0.5–1.5 mg/24 h Luteal phase: 2–7 mg/ 24 h Menopause: 0.2–1 mg/24 h Pregnancy:	1.6–4.8 µmol/ 24 h 6–22 µmol/24 h 0.6–3.1 µmol/ 24 h	Corpus luteum cysts When placental tissue remains in the uterus following parturition Some cases of adreno-cortical tumors	Placental dysfunction Threatened abortion Intrauterine death
	Weeks of gestation mg/24 h µmol/24 h 10–12 5–15 15.6–47 12–18 5–25 15.6–78.0 18–24 15–33 47.0–103.0 24–28 20–42 62.4–131.0 28–32 27–47 84.2–146.6 Males: 0.1–2 mg/ 24 h	0.3–6.2 µmol/ 24 h		
Pregnanetriol	0.4–2.4 mg/24 h	1.2–7.1 µmol/ 24 h	Congenital adrenal andro-genic hyperplasia	
Protein	Up to 100 mg/24 h	Up to 100 mg/ 24 h	Nephritis Cardiac failure Mercury poisoning Bence-Jones protein in multiple myeloma Febrile states Hematuria	
Sodium	130–200 mEq/24 h	130–200 mmol/ 24 h	Useful in detecting gross changes in water and salt balance	
Titratable acidity	20–40 mEq/24 h	20–40 mmol/ 24 h	Metabolic acidosis	Metabolic alkalosis
Urea nitrogen	9–16 gm/24 h	0.32–0.57 mol/L	Excessive protein catabolism	Impaired kidney function
Uric add	250–750 mg/24 h	1.48–4.43 mmol/ 24 h	Gout	Nephritis
Urobilinogen	Random urine: <0.25 mg/dL 24-hour urine: up to 4 mg/24 h	<0.42 mol/24 h Up to 6.76 µmol/24 h	Liver and biliary tract disease Hemolytic anemias	Complete or nearly complete biliary obstruction Diarrhea Renal insufficiency

TABLE B-4 (Continued)

Reference Ranges—Urine Chemistry

Determination	Normal Adult Reference Range		Clinical Significance	
	Conventional Units	*SI Units*	*Increased*	*Decreased*
Uroporphyrins	Up to 50 µg/24 h	Up to 0.06 µmol/ 24 h	Porphyria	
Vanillylmandelic acid (VMA)	0.7–6.8 mg/24 h	3.5–34.3 µmol/ 24 h	Pheochromocytoma Neuroblastoma Ingestion of coffee, tea, aspirin, bananas, and several different drugs	
Xylose absorption test (5-hour)	16%–33% of ingested xylose	Fraction absorbed: 0.16–0.33		Malabsorption syndromes
Zinc	0.15–1.2 mg/24 h	2.3–18.4 µmol/ 24 h		

TABLE B-5

Reference Ranges—Cerebrospinal Fluid (CSF)

Determination	Normal Adult Reference Range		Clinical Significance	
	Conventional Units	*SI Units*	*Increased*	*Decreased*
Albumin	15–30 mg/dL	150–300 mg/L	Certain neurologic disorders Lesion in the choroid plexus or blockage of the flow of CSF Damage to the blood central nervous system (CNS) barrier	
Cell count	0–5 mononuclear cells per cu mm	$0–5 \times 10^6$/L	Bacterial meningitis Neurosyphilis Anterior poliomyelitis Encephalitis lethargica	
Chloride	100–130 mEq/L	100–300 mmol/L	Uremia	Acute generalized meningitis Tuberculous meningitis
Glucose	50–75 mg/dL	2.75–4.13 mmol/L	Diabetes mellitus Diabetic coma Epidemic encephalitis Uremia	Acute meningitides Tuberculous meningitis Insulin shock
Glutamine	6–15 mg/dL	0.41–1 mmol/L	Hepatic encephalopathies, including Reye's syndrome Hepatic coma Cirrhosis	
IgG	0–6.6 mg/dL	0–66 mg/L	Damage to the blood CNS barrier Multiple sclerosis Neurosyphilis Subacute sclerosing panencephalitis Chronic phases of CNS infections	
Lactic acid	<24 mg/dL	<2.7 mmol/L	Bacterial meningitis Hypocapnia Hydrocephalus Brain abscesses Cerebral ischemia	
Lactic dehydrogenase	$\frac{1}{10}$ that of serum	Activity fraction: 0.1 of serum	CNS disease	
Protein:			Acute meningitides	
Lumbar	15–45 mg/dL	150–450 mg/L	Tubercular meningitis	
Cisternal	15–25 mg/dL	150–250 mg/L	Neurosyphilis	
Ventricular	5–15 mg/dL	50–150 mg/L	Poliomyelitis Guillain-Barré syndrome	

TABLE B-5 (Continued)

Reference Ranges—Cerebrospinal Fluid (CSF)

| Determination | Normal Adult Reference Range | | Clinical Significance | |
	Conventional Units	*SI Units*	*Increased*	*Decreased*
Protein electro- phoresis	% of total:	Fraction:	An increase in the level of albumin alone can be the result of a lesion in the choroid plexus or a blockage of the flow of CSF. An elevated gamma globulin value with a normal albumin level has been reported in multiple sclerosis, neurosyphilis, subacute sclerosing panen-cephalitis, and the chronic phase of CNS infections. If the blood-CNS barrier has been damaged severely during the course of these diseases, the CSF albumin level may also be elevated.	
(cellulose acetate)	3–7	0.03–0.07		
Prealbumin	56–74	0.56–0.74		
Albumin	2–6.5	0.02–0.065		
Alpha, globulin	3–12	0.03–0.12		
Alpha2 globulin	8–18.5	0.08–0.185		
Beta globulin	4–14	0.04–0.14		
Gamma globulin				

TABLE B-6

Miscellaneous Values			
		Clinical Significance	
Determinations	**Normal Value**	*Conventional Units*	*SI Units*
Acetaminophen	Zero	Therapeutic level = 10–20 µg/mL	10–20 mg/L
Aminophylline (theophylline)	Zero	Therapeutic level = 10–20/µg/mL	10–20 mg/L
Bromide	Zero	Therapeutic level = 5–50 mg/dL	50–500 mg/L
Carbamazepine	Zero	Therapeutic level = 8–12 µg/mL	34–51 µmol/L
Carbon monoxide	0%–2%	Symptoms with >20% saturation	
Chlordiazepoxide	Zero	Therapeutic level = 1–3 µg/mL	1–3 mg/L
Diazepam	Zero	Therapeutic level = 0.5–2.5 µg/dL	5–25 µg/L
Digitoxin	Zero	Therapeutic level = 5–30 ng/mL	5–30 µg/L
Digoxin	Zero	Therapeutic level = 0.5–2 ng/mL	0.5–2/µg/L
Ethanol	0%–0.01%	Legal intoxication level = 0.10% or above	
		0.3%–0.4% = marked intoxication	
		0.4%–0.5% = alcoholic stupor	
Gentamicin	Zero	Therapeutic level = 4–10 µg/mL	4–10 mg/L
Lithium	Zero	Therapeutic level = 0.6–1.2 mEq/L	0.6–1.2 mmol/L
Methanol	Zero	May be fatal in concentration as low as 10 mg/dL	100 mg/L
Phenobarbital	Zero	Therapeutic level = 15–40 µg/mL	10–20 mg/L
Phenytoin	Zero	Therapeutic level = 10–20 µg/mL	10–20 mg/L
Primidone	Zero	Therapeutic level = 5–12 µg/mL	5–12 mg/L
Quinidine	Zero	Therapeutic level = 0.2–0.5 mg/dL	2–5 mg/L
Salicylate	Zero	Therapeutic level = 2–25 mg/dL	20–250 mg/L
		Toxic level = >30 mg/dL	300 mg/L
Vancomycin	Zero	Therapeutic peak 18.0–26.0 µg/mL	
		Therapeutic trough 5.0–10.0 µg/mL	
Amitriptyline	Zero	Therapeutic level 120–250 mg/mL	433–903 nmol/L
Doxepin	Zero	Therapeutic level 30–150 ng/mL	107–537 nmol/L
Imipramine	Zero	Therapeutic level 125–250 ng/mL	446–893 nmol/L
Lidocaine	Zero	Therapeutic level 1.5–6.0 µg/mL	6.4–25.6 µmol/L
Methotrexate	Zero	Toxic (48 hr. after high dose) 454 mg/mL	1000 mmol/L
Propranolol	Zero	Therapeutic level 50–100 ng/mL	193–386 nmol/L
Valproic acid	Zero	Therapeutic level 50–100 g/mg	347–693 mmol/L

PEDIATRIC LABORATORY VALUES

Blood Chemistries. These values are compiled from a review of current published literature; however, normal values vary with the analytic method used. If any doubt exists, consult your laboratory for its analytical method and normal range of values.

TABLE B-7

Pediatric Blood Chemistries

Determination	Conventional Units	SI Units	Determination	Conventional Units	SI Units
Acid phosphatase			Aspartate aminotrans- ferase (AST)		
Newborn	7.4–19.4 U/ml	7.4–19.4 U/ml			
2–13 yr	6.4–15.2 U/ml	6.4–15.2 U/ml			
Adult	M: 0.5–11 U/ml	0.5–11.0 U/ml	Newborn/infant	25–65 U/L	25–65 U/L
	F: 0.2–9.5 U/ml	0.2–9.5 U/ml	Child/adult	0–35 U/L	0–35 U/L
Alanine aminotrans- ferase (ALT)			Bicarbonate		
			Premature	18–26 mEq/L	18–26 mmol/L
			Infant	20–25 mEq/L	20–25 mmol/L
Infants	<54 U/L	<54 U/L	>2 yr	22–26 mEq/L	22–26 mmol/L
Children/adults	1–30 U/L	1–30 U/L	Bilirubin (total)		
Aldolase			Cord	<2 mg/dl	<34 µmol/L
Adult	<8 U/L	<8 U/L	24 h		
Children	<16 U/L	<16 U/L	Preterm	≤8 mg/dl	≤137 µmol/L
Newborn	<32 U/L	<32 U/L	Term	≤ 6 mg/dl	≤103 µmol/L
Alkaline phosphatase			48 h		
			Preterm	<12 mg/dl	<205 µmol/L
Infant	150–420 U/L	150–420 U/L	Term	≤ 8 mg/dl	≤137 µmol/L
2–10 yr	100–320 U/L	100–320 U/L	3–5 days		
11–18 yr			Preterm	≤16 mg/dl	≤274 µmol/L
Male	100–390 U/L	50–390 U/L	Term	≤12 mg/dl	<205 µmol/L
Female	100–320 U/L	100–320 U/L	1 mo-Adult	≤ 2 mg/dl	≤34 µmol/L
Adult	30–120 U/L	30–100 U/L	Conjugated	≤ 0.4 mg/dl	≤9 µmol/L
Alpha-1-antitrypsin	93–224 mg/dl		Calcium (total)		
Alpha-fetoprotein	<30 ng/dl	<0.1 g/L	Premature	6–10 mg/dl	1.5–2.5 mmol/L
	<30 mcg/L		<1 week		
Ammonia nitrogen	Newborn:		Full-term	7–12 mg/dl	1.75–3 mmol/L
(venous sample:	90–150 µg/dl	64–107 µmol/L	<1 week		
heparinized	>1 month:		Child	8–10.5 mg/dl	2–2.6 mmol/L
specimen in	29–70 µg/dl	21–50 µmol/L	Adult	8.5–10.5 mg/dl	2.1–2.6 mmol/L
ice water and			Calcium (ionized)	4.4–5.4 mg/dl	0.1–1.35 mmol/L
analyzed within			Carbon dioxide (CO_2 content)		
30 min)					
All ages	0–50 µg/dl	0–35 µmol/L	Cord blood	14–22 mmol/L	14–22 mmol/L
Amylase			Child	20–24 mmol/L	20–24 mmol/L
Newborn	0–44 U/L	5–65 U/L	Adult	24–30 mmol/L	24–30 mmol/L
> 1 yr	0–88 U/L	25–125 U/L			
Arsenic	< 3 µg/dl	<0.4 mmol/L			

(continues)

TABLE B-7 (Continued)

Pediatric Blood Chemistries

Determination	Conventional Units	SI Units	Determination	Conventional Units	SI Units
Carbon monoxide (carboxy-hemoglobin)				Upper Limits, mg/dl (μmol/L)	
			Age (yr)	Males	Females
Nonsmoker	<2% of total hemoglobin		1	0.6 (53)	0.5 (44)
			2–3	0.7 (62)	0.6 (53)
Smoker	<10% of total hemoglobin		4–7	0.8 (71)	0.7 (62)
			8–10	0.9 (80)	0.8 (71)
Lethal	>60% of total hemoglobin		11–12	1.0 (88)	0.9 (80)
			13–17	1.2 (106)	1.1 (97)
Carotenoids (carotenes)			18–20	1.3 (115)	1.1 (97)
			Adult	1.2 (106)	1.4 (124)
Infant	20–70 μg/dl	0.37–1.30 μmol/L			
Child	40–130 μg/dl	0.74–2.42 μmol/L	Ferritin	80–155 μg/dl	μmol/L
			Children		
Adult	50–250 μg/dl	0.95–4.69 μmol/L	Fibrin degradation products	7–140 ng/ml	7–140 μg/L
Ceruloplasmin			Titer		
	23–58 mg/dl	210–530 μmol/L	Fibrinogen	1:50 = positive	
Chloride			Folic acid (folate)	200–400 mg/dl	2–4 g/L
Cholesterol	99–111 mEq/L	99–111 mmol/L	Galactose	3–17.5 ng/L	4–20 nmol/L
Copper	See Lipids		Newborn		
0–6 mo			Thereafter	0–20 mg/dl	0–1.11 mmol/L
6 mo–6 yr	20–70 μg/dl	3.1–11 μmol/L	Gammaglutamyl transferase (GGT)	<5 mg/dl	<0.28 mmol/L
6–17 yr	90–190 μg/dl	14–30 μmol/L			
Adult	80–160 μg/dl	12.6–25 μmol/L 12.6–24.4	Cord		
			Premature	19–270 U/L	19–270 U/L
Creatine Kinase (Creatine Phosphokinase)			0–3 wk	56–233 U/L	56–233 U/L
			3 wk–3 mo	0–130 U/L	0–130 U/L
			>3 mo	4–120 U/L	4–120 U/L
	Upper 95th Percentile (U/L)		M		
			F	5–65 U/L	5–65 U/L
Age	Males	Females	1–15 yr	5–35 U/L	5–35 U/L
1 d	600	500	Gastrin	0–23 U/L	0–23 U/L
2–10 d	440	440	Glucose (serum)	<100 pg/ml	<100 ng/L
<1 yr	170	170	Premature		
1–7 yr	109	100	Full term	45–100 mg/dl	1.1–3.6 mmol/L
7–9 yr	103	85	1 wk–16 yr	45–120 mg/dl	1.1–6.4 mmol/L
9–11 yr	109	88	>16 yr	60–105 mg/dl	3.3–5.8 nmol/L
11–13 yr	108	85	Haptoglobin*	70–115 mg/dl	3.9–6.4 nmol/L
13–15 yr	129	85	Iron	400–1800 mg/L	0.4–1.8 g/L
15–17 yr	247	74			
17–19 yr	190	68			

Creatinine (serum)

TABLE B-7 (Continued)

Pediatric Blood Chemistries

Determination	Conventional Units		SI Units		
	Iron		Iron Binding Capacity		% Saturation
	(μg/dl)	(μmol/L)	(μg/dl)	(μmol/L)	(μg/dl)
Newborn	100–250	18–45	59–175	10.6–31.3	65%
4–10 mo	40–100	7–18	250–400	45–72	25%
3–10 yr	50–120	9–22	250–400	45–72	30%
Adult	50–170	9–30	250–400	45–72	35%

Determination	Conventional Units	SI Units
Ketones		
Qualitative	Negative	
Quantitative	up to 3 mg%	5–30 mg/L
Lactate		
Capillary blood		
Newborn	≤27 mg/dl	<3.0 mmol/L
Child	5–20 mg/dl	0.56–2.25 mmol/L
Venous	5–20 mg/dl	0.5–2.2 mmol/L
Arterial	5–14 mg/dl	0.5–1.6 mmol/L
Lactate dehydrogenase (37°C)		
Newborn	160–1500 U/L	160–1500 U/L
Infant	150–360 U/L	150–360 U/L
Child	150–300 U/L	150–300 U/L
Adult	100–250 U/L	100–250 U/L
Lactate dehydrogenase isoenzymes (% total)		
LD$_1$ Heart		24–34%
LD$_2$ Heart, erythrocytes		35–45%
LD$_3$ Muscle		15–25%
LD$_4$ Liver, trace muscle		4–10%
LD$_5$ Liver, muscle		1–9%
Lipase	4–24 U/dl	20–180 U/L
Lipids		
Cholesterol (mg/dl)		
Desirable: <170		
Borderline: 170–199		
High: ≥200		
HDL: >45 mg/dl		
LDL: (mg/dl)		
Desirable: <110		
Borderline: 110–129		
High: ≥130		
Magnesium	1.3–2 mEq/L	0.65–1 mmol/L

Determination	Conventional Units	SI Units
Manganese (blood)		
Newborn	2.4–9.6 μg/dl	2.44–1.75 μmol/L
2–18 yr	0.8–2.1 μg/dl	0.15–0.38 μmol/L
Methemoglobin	1.3% of total Hb	
5′ Nucleotidase	2.2–15 U/L	2.2–15 U/L
Osmolality	285–295 mOsm/kg	270–285 mOsm/L plasma
Phenylalanine		
Premature	2.0–7.5 mg/dl	0.12–0.45 mmol/L
Newborn	<1.2–3.4 mg/dl	0.07–0.21 mmol/L
Child	<3 mg/dl	<0.18 mmol/L
Phosphorus		
Newborn	4.2–9.0 mg/dl	1.36–2.91 mmol/L
1 yr	3.8–6.2 mg/dl	1.23–2.0 mmol/L
2–5 yr	3.5–6.8 mg/dl	1.13–2.2 mmol/L
Adult	3.0–4.5 mg/dl	0.97–1.45 mmol/L
Porcelain	0.52–1.94 mg/dl	0.32–9.93
Potassium		
<10 days of age	4–6 mEq/L	4–6 mmol/L
>10 days of age	3.5–5 mEq/L	3.5–5 mmol/L
Prolactin		
Newborn	<200 ng/ml	<200 μg/L
Adult	<20 ng/ml	<20 μg/L
Proteins Average (Range) in g/dl		

Age	Total	Albumin	Globulin	Gamma Globulin
Premature	5.5 (4.0–7.0)	3.7 (2.5–4.5)	1.8 (1.2–2.0)	0.7 (0.5–0.9)
FT newborn	6.4 (5.0–7.1)	3.4 (2.5–5.0)	3.1 (1.2–4.0)	0.8 (0.7–0.9)
1-mo	6.6 (4.7–7.4)	3.8 (3.0–4.2)	2.5 (1.0–3.3)	0.3 (0.1–0.5)
3–12 mo	6.8 (5.0–7.5)	3.9 (2.7–5.0)	2.6 (2.0–3.8)	0.6 (0.4–1.2)
1–15 yr	7.4 (6.5–8.6)	4.0 (3.2–5.0)	3.1 (2.0–4.0)	0.9 (0.6–1.2)

Determination	Conventional Units	SI Units
Pyruvate	0.3–0.9 mg/dl	0.03–0.10 mmol/L
Sodium		
Premature	130–140 mEq/L	130–140 mmol/L
Older	135–148 mEq/L	135–148 mmol/L

(continues)

TABLE B-7 (Continued)

Pediatric Blood Chemistries

Determination	Conventional Units	SI Units	Determination	Conventional Units	SI Units
Transaminase (SGOT)	*See Aspartate Aminotransferase (AST)*		5–16 yr	60–100 µg/dl	2.09–3.50 µmol/L
Transaminase (SGPT)	*See Alanine Aminotransferase (AT)*		Adult	20–80 µg/dl	0.70–2.79 µmol/L
Troponin	0.03–0.15 ng/ml		Vitamin B$_1$ (thiamine)	5.3–7.9 µg/dl	0.16–0.23 µmol/L
Urea nitrogen	7–22 mg/dl	2.5–7.9 mmol/L			
Uric acid			Vitamin B$_2$ (riboflavin)	3.7–13.7 µg/dl	98–363 mmol/L
0–2 yr	2.0–6.4 mg/dl	0.14–0.38 mmol/L	Vitamin B$_{12}$ (cobalamin)	130–785 pg/ml	96–579 pmol/L
2–12 yr	2.4–5.9 mg/dl	0.14–0.35 mmol/L	Vitamin C (ascorbic acid)	0.2–2 mg/dl	11.4–113.6 µmol/L
12–14 yr	2.4–6.4 mg/dl	0.14–0.38 mmol/L	Vitamin D (1.25 dihydroxy)		
14–adult					
M	3.5–7.2 mg/dl	2–0.43 mmol/L	Newborn	21 ± 2 pg/ml	50 ± 4.8 nmol/L
F	2.4–6.4 mg/dl	0.14–0.38 mmol/L	Child	43 ± 3 pg/ml	103 ± 7.2 nmol/L
Vitamin A (retinol)			Adult	29 ± 2 pg/ml	69.6 ± 4.8 nmol/L
0–1 yr	20–90 µg/dl	0.7–3.14 µmol/L	Vitamin E	5–20 µg/dl	8.4–23 µmol/L
1–5 yr	30–100 µg/dl	1.05–3.50 µmol/L	Zinc	70–150 µg/dl	10.7–23 µmol/L

* Detectable in only 10%–20% of newborns.
(Adapted from Siberry, G. K. & Iannone, R. [Eds.] [2000]. *The Harriet Lane handbook* [15th ed.]. St. Louis: Mosby.)

TABLE B-8

Normal Values—Hematology

Age	Hgb (gm %) Mean (−2SD)	HCT (%) Mean (−2SD)	MCV (fl.) Mean (−2SD)	MCHC (gm/% RBC) Mean (−2SD)	Retic (%)	WBC/mm³ × 100 Mean (−2SD)	Pits (10³/mm³) Mean (±2SD)
26–30 wk gestation*	13.4 (11)	41.5 (34.9)	118.2 (106.7)	37.9 (30.6)	—	4.4 (2.7)	254 (180–327)
28 wk	14.5	45	120	31	(5–10)	—	275
32 wk	15.0	47	118	32	(3–10)	—	290
Term† (cord)	16.5 (13.5)	51 (42)	108 (98)	33 (30)	(3–7)	18.1 (9–30)‡	290
1–3 days	18.5 (14.5)	56 (45)	108 (95)	33 (29)	(1.8–4.6)	18.9 (9.4–34)	192
2 wk	16.6 (13.4)	53 (41)	105 (88)	31.4 (28.1)		11.4 (5–20)	252
1 mo	13.9 (10.7)	44 (33)	101 (91)	31.8 (28.1)	(0.1–1.7)	10.8 (5–19.5)	
2 mo	11.2 (9.4)	35 (28)	95 (84)	31.8 (28.3)			
6 mo	12.6 (11.1)	36 (31)	76 (68)	35 (32.7)	(0.7–2.3)	11.9 (6–17.5)	
6 mo—2 yr	12 (10.5)	36 (33)	78 (70)	33 (30)		10.6 (6–17)	(150–350)
2–6 yr	12.5 (11.5)	37 (34)	81 (75)	34 (31)	(0.5–1.0)	8.5 (5–15.5)	(150–350)
6–12 yr	13.5 (11.5)	40 (35)	86 (77)	34 (31)	(0.5–1.0)	8.1 (4.5–13.5)	(150–350)
12–18 yr							
Male	14.5 (13)	43 (36)	88 (78)	34 (31)	(0.5–1.0)	7.8 (4.5–13.5)	(150–350)
Female	14 (12)	41 (37)	90 (78)	34 (31)	(0.5–1.0)	7.8 (4.5–13.5)	(150–350)

* Values are from fetal samplings.
† Under 1 month, capillary Hgb exceeds venous: 1 h–3.6 gm difference; 5 days–2.2 gm difference; 3 wks–1.1 gm difference.
‡ Mean (95% confidence limits).
(Adapted from Siberry, G. K. & Iannone, R. [Eds.] [2000]. *The Harriet Lane handbook* [15th ed.]. St. Louis: Mosby.)

TABLE B-9

Normal Serologic Reference Values	
Determination	**Value**
Antinuclear antibody	<1:80
Anti-streptolysin O titer*	
Preschool	<1:85
School ages and adults	<1:170
Older adults	<1:85
Anti-hyaluronidase	<1:256
C-reactive Protein	Negative
C_1 Esterase inhibitor	17.4–24 mg/dl
C_3	
1–6 mo	53–175 mg/dl
7–12 mo	75–180 mg/dl
1–5 yr	77–166 mg/dl
6–10 yr	88–199 mg/dl
Adult	83–177 mg/dl
C_4	
1–6 mo	7–42 mg/dl
7–12 mo	9.5–39 mg/dl
1–5 yr	9–40 mg/dl
6–10 yr	12–40 mg/dl
Adult	15–45 mg/dl
C_{H50}	75–160 U/ml
Rheumatoid factor	<20 negative
	20–40 suggestive
	≥80 positive
Rheumaton titer (modified	Negative
Waaler-Rose slide test)	≥10 may be significant
Total B cells	5%–20% of lymphocytes
Total T cells	50%–80% of lymphocytes
T helper cells	34%–56% of lymphocytes
T suppressor cells	18%–32% of lymphocytes
Helper/suppressor ratio	1.1–2.5

*Significant if rising titer can be demonstrated at weekly intervals.
(Adapted from Siberry, G. K. & Iannone, R. [Eds.] [2000]. *The Harriet Lane handbook* [15th ed.]. St. Louis: Mosby.)

TABLE B-10

Cerebrospinal Fluid Values	
Determination	**Value**
Cell Count	
Preterm mean	9.0 (0–25.4 WBC/mm³) (57% PMNs)
Term mean	8.2 (0.–22.4 WBC/mm³) (61% PMNs)
> 1 mo	0–7 (0% PMNs)
Glucose	
Preterm	24–63 mg/dl (mean 50)
Term	34–119 mg/dl (mean 52)
Child	40–80 mg/dl
CSF Glucose/	
Blood Glucose (%)	
Preterm	55–105
Term	44–128
Child	50%
Lactic acid dehydrogenase	20 U/ml (range 5–30 U/ml)
Myelin basic protein	<4 ng/ml
Pressure (initial lumbar puncture)	
Newborn	80–110 (<110) mm H_2O
Infant	<200 (lateral recumbent
Child	position) mm H_2O
Respiratory movements	5–10 mm H_2O
Protein	
Preterm	65–150 mg/dl (mean 115)
Term	20–170 mg/dl (mean 90)
Children	
Ventricular	5–15 mg/dl
Cisternal	5–25 mg/dl
Lumbar	5–40 mg/dl

(Adapted from Siberry, G. K. & Iannone, R. [Eds.] [2000]. *The Harriet Lane handbook* [15th ed.]. St. Louis: Mosby.)

TABLE B-11

Sample Conversions of Pounds and Ounces to Grams*																
	Ounces															
Pounds	*0*	*1*	*2*	*3*	*4*	*5*	*6*	*7*	*8*	*9*	*10*	*11*	*12*	*13*	*14*	*15*
0	—	28	57	85	113	142	170	198	227	255	283	312	340	369	397	425
1	454	482	510	539	567	595	624	652	680	709	737	765	794	822	850	879
2	907	936	964	992	1021	1049	1077	1106	1134	1162	1191	1219	1247	1276	1304	1332
3	1361	1389	1417	1446	1474	1503	1531	1559	1588	1616	1644	1673	1701	1729	1758	1786
4	1814	1843	1871	1899	1928	1956	1984	2013	2041	2070	2098	2126	2155	2183	2211	2240
5	2268	2296	2325	2353	2381	2410	2438	2466	2495	2532	2551	2580	2608	2637	2665	2693
6	2722	2750	2778	2807	2835	2863	2892	2920	2948	2977	3005	3033	3062	3090	3118	3147

*1 ounce = approximately 30 grams.
(From Avery, GB. [1994]. *Neonatology* [4th ed.]. Philadelphia: J. B. Lippincott.)

CONVERSION TABLES

TABLE B-12

Metric Units and Symbols			
Quantity	**Unit**	**Symbol**	**Equivalent**
Length	millimeter	mm	1000 mm = 1 m
	centimeter	cm	100 cm = 1 m
	decimeter	dm	10 dm = 1 m
	meter	m	1000 m = 1 km
Volume	cubic centimeter	cc or cm^3	1000 cc = 1 cm^3 or liter
	milliliter	ml	1000 mL = 1 liter
	cu decimeter	dm^3	1000 dm^3 = 1 m^3
	liter	L	1000 L = 1 m^3
Mass	microgram	μg	1000 μg = 1 mg
	milligram	mg	1000 mg = 1 g
	gram	g	1000 g = 1 kg
	kilogram	kg	1000 kg = 1 metric ton (t)

To convert from pounds to kilograms, divide by 2.2.
To convert from kilograms to pounds, multiply by 2.2.

TABLE B-13

Celsius (Centigrade) and Fahrenheit Temperatures	
Celsius (Centigrade) 0°	**Fahrenheit 32°**
36.0	96.8
36.5	97.7
37.0	98.6
37.5	99.5
38.0	100.4
38.5	101.3
39.0	102.2
39.5	103.1
40.0	104.0
40.5	104.9
41.0	105.8
41.5	106.7
42.0	107.6

To convert degrees F. to degrees C: Subtract 32, then multiply by ⅝.
To convert degrees C. to degrees F: Multiply by ⅘, then add 32.

TABLE B-14

Table of Metric and Apothecaries' Systems (Approved approximate dose equivalents are enclosed in parentheses. Use exact equivalents in calculations.)			
Metric	**Apothecaries**	**Metric**	**Apothecaries**
1 milligram (mg)	¹⁄₆₄ grain	3.888 cubic centimeters or grams	1 dram (4 cc or grams)
64.79 milligrams	1 grain (65 mg)	31.103 cubic centimeters or grams	1 ounce (30 cc or grams)
1 gram	15.43 grains (15 grains)	473.167 cubic centimeters	1 pint (500 cc)
1 cubic centimeter (cc)*	16 minims		

*Note: A cubic centimeter (cc.) is the approximate equivalent of a milliliter (ml.). The terms are used interchangeably in general medicine.

NOMOGRAM FOR ESTIMATING SURFACE AREA OF INFANTS AND YOUNG CHILDREN

To determine the surface area of the patient, draw a straight line between the point representing the patient's height on the left vertical scale to the point representing the patient's weight on the right vertical scale. The point at which this line intersects the middle vertical scale represents the surface area in square meters. (Courtesy of Abbott Laboratories.

HEIGHT		SURFACE AREA	WEIGHT	
feet	centimeters	in square meters	pounds	kilograms

NOMOGRAM FOR ESTIMATING SURFACE AREA OF OLDER CHILDREN AND ADULTS

See Nomogram for Estimating Surface Area of Infants and Young Children for instructions on use. (Courtesy of Abbott Laboratories.)

HEIGHT		SURFACE AREA	WEIGHT	
feet	centimeters	in square meters	pounds	kilograms

C Medical Terminology: Prefixes, Roots, and Suffixes

Appendix

Medical terms are made up of components that are derived mostly from Latin or Greek. The root is the main part of the word. Prefixes precede the root and suffixes follow the root to modify its meaning. The roots are presented here with combining vowels that are used to ease pronunciation when a suffix is added.

Prefixes

Prefix	Meaning	Example	Definition of Example
a-, an-	without, not	aseptic	Sterile; free of infection
		anoxia	Lack of oxygen
ab-	away from	abduct	To move away from the midline
acro-	extremity	acromegaly	Disease marked by enlargement of the extremities
ad-	to, toward	adduct	To move toward the midline
ambi-	both	ambidextrous	Able to use either hand
ante-	before	antenatal	Occurring before birth; prenatal
anti-	against	antidote	Substance that neutralizes a poison
auto-	self	autoimmunity	An immune response to one's own body tissues
bi-	two, double	binocular	Pertaining to both eyes
brady-	slow	bradycardia	Slow heart rate
circum-	around	circumduction	Circular movement of a limb at a ball-and-socket joint
co-	together	coherent	Sticking together; logical
contra-	against	contraindication	Condition that makes it inadvisable to use a certain form of treatment
de-	without, removal	dehydration	Removal of water
di-	two, twice	diatomic	Having two atoms
dia-	through	dialysis	Separation of substances by passage through a semipermeable membrane
diplo-	double, two	diplopia	Double vision
dis-	removal, separation	disinfect	Remove infectious organisms from
dys-	abnormal, difficult, painful	dysmenorrhea	Painful menstruation
ecto-	outside	ectopic	Outside the normal position
endo-	within	endoscope	Instrument for viewing the inside of a body space
epi-	above	epigastric	Above the stomach
eryth/r/o-	red	erythema	Redness of the skin
		erythrocyte	Red blood cell
eu-	normal, good, true	eupnea	Normal breathing
ex/o-	out, out of	excise	To remove surgically
extra-	outside, in addition to	extracellular	Outside the cell

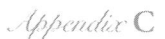

Prefixes (*Continued*)

Prefix	Meaning	Example	Definition of Example
hemi-	half	hemiplegia	Paralysis of one half of the body
hetero-	other, different	heterosexual	Pertaining to the opposite sex
		homograft	Transplant of tissue from same species
homo-, homeo-	same	homeostasis	State of internal constancy
hyper-	high, excessive	hypertension	High blood pressure
hypo-	under, decreased	hypoglycemia	Low blood sugar
in, im-	in, within	inhale	To breathe in
		impacted	Held firmly
in-, im-	not	indigestion	Incomplete digestion
		impermeable	Unable to be penetrated
infra-	below	infrared	Pertaining to heat waves beyond the red spectrum
inter-	between	interstitial	Between cells
intra-	within	intracranial	Within the skull
iso-	equal, same	isotonic	Having the same concentration as cellular fluids
juxta-	near	juxtaglomerular	Near the glomerulus of the kidney
leuk/o-	white, colorless	leukemia	Malignant overgrowth of white blood cells (leukocytes)
macro-	large	macromolecule	Large molecule composed of subunits
mal-	bad, poor	malnutrition	Poor nutrition
melan/o-	black, dark	melanin	Dark pigment found in skin, hair, the brain, and the eye
mega/lo-	large, enlarged	megalocyte	Large red blood cell
mes/o-	middle	mesoderm	Middle germ layer of the embryo
meta-	beyond, over, change	metamorphosis	Change in form or structure; passage from one stage to another
micr/o-	small, one millionth	microscope	Instrument for viewing extremely small objects
mon/o-	one	monocyte	White blood cell with a single large nucleus
multi-	many	multipara	Woman who has borne more than one viable fetus
neo-	new	neoplasm	A new, abnormal growth of tissue; a growth or tumor
noct/i-	night	nocturnal	Occurring at night
non-	not	nontoxic	Not poisonous
olig/o-	little, deficiency	oliguria	Decreased amount of urine formation
ortho-	straight, correct	orthopedics	Medical specialty that deals with prevention and correction of deformities
pan-	all	pandemic	Presence of a disease in most of a large population
para-	beside, near	paramedic	Trained medical assistant
per-	by, through	percutaneous	Through the skin
peri-	around	perioral	Around the mouth
poly-	many	polydactyly	Having more than the normal number of fingers or toes
post-	after, behind	postpartum	Occurring after birth
pre-	before	pre-existing	Present or occurring before a given time
prim/i-	first	primigravida	Woman during her first pregnancy
pro-	before	prognosis	Prediction of the outcome of a disease
pseud/o-	false	pseudostratified	Appearing to be in layers
quad/r/i-	four	quadriplegia	Paralysis of all four limbs
re-	back, again	reflux	Backward flow
retro-	backward, behind	retroperitoneal	Behind the peritoneum
scler/o-	hard, hardening	scerloderma	Disease characterized by hardening of the skin
semi-	half	semilunar	Shaped like a half moon
sub-	below, under	subcutaneous	Under the skin
super-	above, excessive	superinfection	Second infection after an initial infection and caused by a different organism

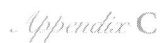

Prefixes (*Continued*)

Prefix	Meaning	Example	Definition of Example
supra-	above	suprapubic	Above the pubis
syn-, sym-	together	synthesis	Union of elements or molecules; a joining of parts
		symmetry	Correspondence in position of parts
tachy-	fast	tachypnea	Rapid respiration rate
trans-	through, across	transfusion	Injection of a substance into the bloodstream
tri-	three	tricuspid	Having three points or cusps
ultra-	beyond	ultrasound	Sound waves beyond the audible range
un-	not	unconscious	Lacking in awareness; insensible
uni-	one	unicellular	Having one cell

Roots

Root	Meaning	Example	Definition of Example
aden/o	gland	adenoma	Neoplasm of glandular epithelium
angi/o	vessel	angioplasty	Surgical repair of a blood vessel
arteri/o	artery	endarteritis	Inflammation of the lining of an artery
arthr/o	joint	arthroscope	Instrument for examining the interior of a joint
audio/o	hearing	audiologist	Specialist in the study and treatment of hearing disorders
bio	life	biopsy	Removal and examination of living tissue
blast/o	immature form, growing form	osteoblast	Growing cell that produces bone tissue
branchi/o	arm	antebrachium	Forearm
bronch/o, bronchi/o	bronchus	bronchogenic	Originating in a bronchus
		bronchiectasis	Chronic dilation of the bronchi
carcin/o	cancer	carcinogen	Agent that causes cancer
cardi/o	heart	cardiomyopathy	Any disease affecting the heart muscle
cerebr/o	brain	cerebrospinal	Pertaining to the brain and spinal cord
cephal/o	head	hydrocephalus	Accumulation of excess cerebrospinal fluid in the brain
cervic/o	neck, cervix	cervical	Pertaining to the neck or cervix
chol/e	bile	cholelithiasis	Presence or formation of gallstones
cholecyst/o	gallbladder	cholecystectomy	Surgical removal of the gallbladder
chondr/o	cartilage	endochondral	Located or occurring within cartilage
cleid/o	clavicle	cleidomastoid	Pertaining to the clavicle and mastoid process
col/o	colon	colostomy	Surgical formation of an opening between the colon and the surface of the body
colp/o	vagina	colpocele	Hernia into the vagina
cost/o	rib	intercostal	Between the ribs
crani/o	skull	craniotomy	Surgery on the cranium
cyst/o	sac, bladder	cystitis	Inflammation of the urinary bladder
cyt/o	cell	cytology	Study of cells
derm, dermat/o	skin	hypodermic	Beneath the skin
		dermatosis	Any skin disease
encephal/o	brain	encephalitis	Inflammation of the brain
enter/o	intestine	enterotoxin	Toxin that acts on the cells lining the intestine

(*continues*)

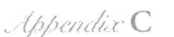
Roots (*Continued*)

Root	Meaning	Example	Definition of Example
gastr/o	stomach	epigastric	Above the stomach
genesis	origin	spermatogenesis	Formation of sperm cells
glomerul/o	glomerulus	glomerulonephritis	Inflammation of the glomeruli of the kidney
gloss/o	tongue	hypoglossal	Under the tongue
hem/o, hemat/o	blood	hemoglobin	Pigment that carries oxygen in red blood cells
		hematoma	Localized collection of clotted blood
hepat/o	liver	hepatomegaly	Enlargement of the liver
hist/o	tissue	histologist	One who studies tissue
hydro/o	water, fluid	hydrophilic	Readily absorbing water
hyster/o	uterus	hysterectomy	Surgical removal of the uterus
ile/o	ileum	ileocecal	Pertaining to the ileum and cecum
ili/o	ilium	iliac	Pertaining to the ilium
kerat/o	cornea, horny layer of the skin	keratoplasty	Plastic surgery of the cornea; corneal grafting
		keratosis	Any horny growth, such as a wart or callus
labi/o	lip, labium	labiodental	Pertaining to the lips and teeth
lact/o	milk	lactogenic	Promoting formation of milk
laryng/o	larynx	laryngospasm	Spasmodic closing of the larynx
lith/o	stone	sialolith	Stone in a salivary gland or duct
lymph/o	lymph	lymphadenopathy	Any disease of a lymph node
mast/o	breast	mastectomy	Surgical removal of a breast
medull/o	central part, medulla oblongata	medullary	Pertaining to the central region of a structure or to the medulla oblongata
men/o	menses	menarche	Beginning of menstrual cycles
mening/o	meninges	meningocele	Hernia of the meninges
metr/o	uterus	endometrium	Lining of the uterus
my/o	muscle	myofiber	Muscle cell
myc/o	fungus	dermatomycosis	Any fungal infection of the skin
myel/o	marrow, spinal cord	myelogenous	Originating in bone marrow
		myelodysplasia	Defective formation of the spinal cord
myring/o	tympanic membrane	myringotomy	Incision of the tympanic membrane
nas/o	nose	paranasal	Near the nose
necr/o	death	necrosis	Death of tissue
nephr/o	kidney	hydronephrosis	Accumulation of fluid in the renal pelvis due to obstruction
neur/o	nerve	neuralgia	Pain along the path of a nerve
ocul/o	eye	oculomotor	Pertaining to eye movements
odont/o	tooth	orthodontics	Branch of dentistry that deals with prevention and correction of irregularities in the teeth
onc/o	tumor, swelling	oncolytic	Destructive of tumor cells
onych/o	nail	paronychia	Infection of the area around a nail
oo	egg, ovum	oocyte	Developing ovum
oophor/o	ovary	oophorectomy	Removal of an ovary
ophthalm/o	eye	exophthalmia	Protrusion of the eyeball
orchi/o, orchid/o	testis	orchiopexy	Surgical fixation of an undescended testis in the scrotum
		orchidoptosis	Dropping of the testis

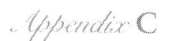

Roots (*Continued*)

Root	Meaning	Example	Definition of Example
os, oste/o	bone	ossification	Formation of bone
		periosteum	Membrane that covers bone
ot/o	ear	otosclerosis	Formation of bone tissue in the inner ear leading to hearing loss
ovari/o	ovary	ovariorrhexis	Rupture of an ovary
path/o	disease	pathophysiology	Study of the physiology of disease
ped/o	child, foot	pediatrics	Branch of medicine that deals with care of children
		pedometer	Instrument for recording numbers of steps
phag/o	eating	phagocyte	Cell that takes in and destroys waste or foreign particles
phak/o, phac/o	lens of the eye	phacolysis	Destruction of the lens
phleb/o	vein	phlebotomist	One who draws blood from a vein
pneum/o, pneumon/o	lung, air, breathing	pneumothorax	Accumulation of air in the pleural space
		pneumonia	Inflammation of the lung
proct/o	rectum	proctoscopy	Endoscopic examination of the rectum
psych/o	mind	psychogenic	Of mental or emotional origin
ptosis	dropping	blepharoptosis	Drooping of the eyelid
py/o	pus	empyema	Accumulation of pus in a body cavity
pyel/o	pelvis, renal pelvis	pyelography	X-ray study of the renal pelvis and ureter
pylor/o	pylorus	pylorospasm	Spasm of the pylorus
rachi/o	spine	rachiocentesis	Lumbar tap
ren/o	kidney	suprarenal	Above the kidney
rhin/o	nose	rhinorrhea	Discharge of thin mucus from the nose
salping/o	tube, oviduct	salpingectomy	Surgical removal of the oviduct
scler/o	hardening	arteriosclerosis	Hardening of the arteries
splen/o	spleen	splenectomy	Removal of the spleen
thorac/o	chest, thorax	thoracotomy	Surgical incision of the chest wall
thromb/o	blood clot	thrombosis	Formation or presence of a blood clot, usually causing obstruction of a vessel
tox/o, toxic/o	poison	toxoid	Modified bacterial toxin used to produce immunity
		toxicology	Study of poisons
trache/o	trachea	tracheostomy	Surgical creation of an opening into the trachea
trich/o	hair	trichology	Study of hair
ureter/o	ureter	ureterectasis	Dilation of the ureter
urethr/o	urethra	urethrostenosis	Narrowing of the urethra
ur/o	urine	anuria	Lack of urine formation
vas/o	vessel, duct	vasomotor	Pertaining to changes in the diameter of a vessel
vesic/o	urinary bladder	vesical	Pertaining to the urinary bladder

Suffixes

Root	Meaning	Example	Definition of Example
-algia	pain	gastralgia	Pain in the stomach
-cele	tumor, hernia, swelling	cystocele	Hernia of the bladder
-centesis	puncture, tap	paracentesis	Surgical puncture of a cavity for removal of fluid
-cide	killing	bactericide	Agent that kills bacteria
-ectasis	dilation, stretching	atelectasis	Incomplete expansion of the lungs
-ectomy	excision	tonsillectomy	Surgical removal of the tonsils
-emia	blood	ischemia	Insufficient blood supply to an area
-esthesia	pertaining to sensation	anesthesia	Loss of sensation
-form	shaped like	cruciform	Shaped like a cross
-gen, -genic	formation, origin, producing	fibrinogen	Substance in the blood that is converted to fibrin during blood clotting
		cardiogenic	Originating in the heart
-gram	record	echocardiogram	Record produced by echocardiography
-graph	recording instrument	pneumograph	Instrument for recording the rate and depth of respiration
-graphy	recording of data	radiography	The taking of x-ray pictures
-iasis	condition	helminthiasis	Infestation with worms
-ism	condition	embolism	Blockage of a blood vessel, usually by a blood clot
-itis	inflammation	pericarditis	Inflammation of the pericardium
-logy	study	etiology	Study of the origin of disease
-lysis	separation, disintegration	hemolysis	Rupture of red blood cells
-malacia	softening	osteomalacia	Softening of the bones
-megaly	enlargement	splenomegaly	Enlargement of the spleen
-meter	measuring instrument	calorimeter	Instruction for measuring heat production
-metry	measurement	pelvimetry	Measurement of the pelvis
-odynia	pain	cephalodynia	Pain in the head; headache
-oid	like, resembling	rheumatoid	Similar to rheumatism
-oma	tumor	sarcoma	Tumor of connective tissue
-osis	condition	narcosis	Unconsciousness due to narcotics
-pathy	disease	myopathy	Any disease of muscle
-penia	lack of	leukopenia	Abnormal decrease in the number of white blood cells
-pexy	surgical fixation	hysteropexy	Surgical fixation of the uterus
-phagia	eating	dysphagia	Difficulty in swallowing
-phil, -philic	attracting	basophil	White blood cell that stains with basic stain
-plasia	formation, molding	hyperplasia	Excessive growth of cells
-plasty	plastic repair	rhinoplasty	Plastic surgery of the nose
-plegia	paralysis	paraplegia	Paralysis of both legs and the lower part of the body
-pnea	breathing	apnea	Absence of breathing
-poiesis	formation, production	erythropoiesis	Formation of red blood cells
-ptosis	dropping	nephroptosis	Dropping of the kidney
-rhage, -rhagia	bursting forth	hemorrhage	Bursting forth of blood
		menorrhagia	Excessive menstrual bleeding
-rhaphy	surgical repair	herniorrhaphy	Surgical repair of a hernia
-rhea	discharge	pyorrhea	Discharge of pus
-rhexis	rupture	amniorrhexis	Rupture of the amnion
-scope	instrument for examining	cystoscope	Instrument for examining the bladder
-scopy	visual examination	bronchoscopy	Examination of the bronchi
-stasis	stoppage of flow	hemostasis	Prevention of blood loss

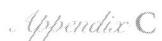

Suffixes (*Continued*)

Root	Meaning	Example	Definition of Example
-stomy	surgical formation of an opening	colostomy	Surgical formation of an opening in the colon
-tomy	incision into	tracheotomy	Incision into the trachea
-trophy	nourishing	atrophy	Wasting or decrease in size of an organ or tissue
-tropic	acting on	gonadotropic	Acting on the gonads
-tripsy	crushing	lithotripsy	Crushing of a stone
-uresis	urination	diuresis	Elimination of large amounts of urine
-uria	urine	hematuria	Presence of blood in the urine

Word Roots According to Body System

Circulatory System
angi/o
arteri/o
cardi/o
hem/o, hemat/o
lymph/o
myel/o
phleb/o
thromb/o
vas/o

Digestive System
chol/e
cholecyst/o
col/o
enter/o
gastr/o
gloss/o
hepat/o
ile/o
lith/o
odont/o
proct/o

Integumentary System
derm, dermat/o
onych/o
trich/o

Musculoskeletal System
arthr/o
brachi/o
cervic/o
chondr/o
cleid/o
cost/o
crani/o
ili/o
my/o
myel/o
os, oste/o
ped/o
rachi/o
sarc/o

Nervous System
audi/o
cerebr/o
encephal/o
kerat/o
medull/o
mening/o
myring/o
neur/o
ocul/o
ophthalm/o
ot/o
phac/o, phak/o
psych/o

Reproductive System
cervic/o
colp/o
hyster/o
labi/o
lact/o
mast/o
men/o
metr/o
oo
oophor/o
orchi/o, orchid/o
ovari/o
salping/o

Respiratory System
bronch/o
laryng/o
nas/o
pneum/o, pneumon/o
rhin/o
thora, thorac/o
trache/o

Urinary System
cyst/o
glomerul/o
nephr/o
pyel/o
ren/o
ureter/o
urethr/o
ur/o
vesic/o

Prepared by Barbara Janson Cohen, MS, Delaware County Community College, Media, PA, and Thomas Jefferson University, Philadelphia, PA.

D Selected Information Resources for Nursing Practice

SELECTED RESOURCES FOR COMMUNITY-BASED CARE

The Academy for Guided Imagery
P.O. Box 2070
Mill Valley, CA 94942
(800) 726-2070
http://www.healthy.net/agi/index-net.html

Academy of Medical-Surgical Nurses
East Holly Avenue
Pitman, NJ 08071-0056
(856) 256-2323
http://www.medsurgnurse.org

Academy of Psychosomatic Medicine
5824 North Magnolia
Chicago, IL 60660
(773) 784-2025
http://www.apm.org

Action on Smoking and Health (ASH)
2013 H Street, NW
Washington, DC 20006
(202) 659-4310
http://www.ash.org

Administration on Aging
Department of Health and Human Services
330 Independence Avenue, SW
Washington, DC 20201
800-677-1116
http://www.aoa.dhhs.gov

Agency for Health Care Research and Policy
Executive Office Center
2101 East Jefferson Street, Suite 501
Rockville, MD 20852
(301) 594-1364
http://www.ahcpr.gov

Al-Anon Family Group Headquarters
1600 Corporate Landing Parkway
Virginia Beach, VA 23454-5617
757-563-1600
http://www.al-anon.org

Alcoholics Anonymous
475 Riverside Drive
New York, NY 10115
http://www.alcoholics-anonymous.org

American Academy of Ambulatory Care Nurses
East Holly Avenue, Box 56
Pitman, NJ 08071-0056
(800) 252-2350
http://www.aaacn.org

American Anorexia Bulimia Association, Inc.
165 West 46th Street, Suite 1108
New York, NY 10036
212-575-6200
http://www.aabainc.org

American Association for the Advancement of Science
1200 New York Ave., NW
Washington, DC 20005
(202) 326-6400
http://www.aaas.org

American Association of Managed Care Nurses, Inc. (AAMCN)
4435 Waterfront Drive, Suite 101
P.O. Box 4975
Glen Allen, VA 23058-4975
(804) 747-9698
FAX: (804) 747-5316
www.aamcn.org

American Association of Retired Persons (AARP)
601 E Street, NW
Washington, DC 20049
1-800-424-3410
http://www.aarp.org

American Burn Association
625 N. Michigan Avenue, Suite 1530
Chicago, IL 60611
http://www.ameriburn.org

American Cancer Society
1599 Clifton Road NE
Atlanta, GA 30329
800-320-3333 or 800-ACS-2345
http://www.cancer.org

American Chronic Pain Association
P.O. Box 850
Rocklin, CA 95677
(916) 632-0922
http://www.theacpa.org

American College of Cardiovascular Nursing
P.O. Box 3345
Riverview, FL 33568-3345
(813) 677-1116
http://www.accn.net

American Diabetes Association
1660 Duke Street
Alexandria, VA 22314
http://www.diabetes.org

American Dietetic Association
216 West Jackson Boulevard
Suite 800
Chicago, IL 60606-6995
312-899-0040
http://www.eatright.org

American Digestive Health Foundation
7910 Woodmont Avenue
7th Floor
Bethesda, MD 20814
(301) 654-2055
http://www.gastro.org

American Foundation for the Blind
11 Penn Plaza, Suite 300
New York, NY 10001
212-502-7661
http://www.afb.org

American Heart Association
National Center, 7272 Greenville Avenue
Dallas, TX 75231
(800) AHA-USA1
http://www.americanheart.org

American Holistic Nurses' Association
P.O. Box 2130
Flagstaff, AZ 86003-2130
(800) 278-2462
http://ahna.org

American Lung Association
1740 Broadway
New York, NY 10019
800-LUNG USA or 212-315-8700
http://www.lungusa.org

American Nurses Association
600 Maryland Avenue, SW
Suite 100 West
Washington, DC 20024
1-800-274-4ANA
http://www.nursingworld.org

American Pain Society
4700 West Lake Avenue
Glenview, IL 60025
http://www.ampainsoc.org

American Psychiatric Association
1400 K Street, NW
Washington, DC 20005
(888) 357-7924
http://www.psych.org

American Psychiatric Nurses Association
1200 19th Street, NW, Suite 300
Washington, DC 20036-2422
202-857-1133
http://www.apna.org

American Psychological Association
750 First Street, NE
Washington, DC 20002-4242
(202) 336-5500
http://www.apa.com

American Public Health Association
800 I Street NW
Washington, DC 20001-3710
202-777-APHA
http://www.apha.org

American Red Cross
430 17th Street, NW
Washington, DC 20006
202-737-8300
http://www.redcross.org

The American Self-Help Clearinghouse
St. Clares-Riverside Medical Center
25 Pocono Road
Denville, NJ 07834
(201) 625-7101
http://mentalhelp/net.selfhelp

American SIDS Institute
2480 Windy Hill Road, Suite 380
Marietta, GA 30067
http://www.sids.org

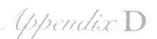

American Speech-Language-Hearing Association
10801 Rockville Pike
Dept. AP
Rockville, MD 20852
301-897-5700
http://www.asha.org

American Spinal Injury Association
345 E. Superior Street, Room 1436
Chicago, IL 60611
312-908-1242
http://www.asia-spinalinjury.org

Americans With Disabilities Act
U.S. Department of Justice
950 Pennsylvania Avenue, NW
Washington, DC 20530-0001
http://www.usdoj.gov/crt/ada/adahoml.htm

The ARC of the United States
(formerly Association for Retarded Citizens of the
   United States)
500 East Border Street, Suite 300
Arlington, TX 76010
817-261-6003
http://TheArc.org

Arthritis Foundation
1330 West Peachtree Street
Atlanta, GA 30309
404-872-7100
http://www.arthritis.org

Asian-Pacific Islander Nurse Association
c/o College of Mount Sinai Vincent
6301 Riverdale Avenue
New York, NY 10471
1-718-405-3354

**Asociacion Nacional por Personas Mayores
   (for Hispanic Seniors)**
3325 Wilshire Boulevard, Suite 800
Los Angeles, CA 90010

Association for Death Education & Counseling
342 North Main Street
West Hartford, CT 06117-2507
860-586-7503
http://www.adec.org

The Association for Integrative Medicine
Box 1
Mont Clare, PA 19453
(610) 933-8145
http://www.integrativemedicine.org

Association of Operating Room Nurses
2170 South Parker Road, Suite 300
Denver, CO 80231-5711
(800) 755-2676
http://www.aorn.org

Asthma and Allergy Foundation of America
1125 Fifteenth Street, NW, Suite 502
Washington, DC 20005
202-466-7643
http://www.aafa.org

Brain Injury Association, Inc.
(formerly National Head Injury Foundation)
105 N. Alfred Street
Alexandria, VA 22314
http://www.biausa.org

The Canadian Federation of Mental Health Nurses
3rd Floor CSB, Nursing
University of Alberta
Edmonton, AB
T6G 2G3
http://www.iciweb.com/cfmhn

Cancer Information Service (CIS)
National Cancer Institute (NCI)
Building 31, Room 10A16
Bethesda, MD 20892
1-800-422-6237
Cancernet: http://cancernet.nci.nih.gov

The Candlelighters Childhood Cancer Foundation
7210 Woodmont Avenue, Suite 460
Bethesda, MD 20814-3015
800-366-2223
http://www.candlelighters.org

Center for Food Safety and Applied Nutrition
200 C Street, SW
Washington, DC 20204
(888) 723-3366
http://vm.cfsan.fda.gov/list.html

Centers for Disease Control and Prevention
Department of Health and Human Services
U.S. Public Health Service
1600 Clifton Road, NE
Atlanta, GA 30333
800-311-3435 or 404-639-3311
http://www.cdc.gov

Children of Aging Parents (CAPs)
1609 Woodbourne Road, Suite 302A
Levitown, PA 19057
(800) 227-7294
http://www.caps4caregivers.org

The Compassionate Friends, Inc.
(Nationwide support group for bereaved parents and siblings)
P.O. Box 3696
Oak Brook, IL 60522-3696
630-990-0010
http://www.compassionatefriends.org

CultureNurse.org
340 Commerce Avenue, SW
Grand Rapids, MI 49503-4129
e-mail: webmaster@culturenurse.org
http://nursing.simplenet.com/main/mainindex.html

Cystic Fibrosis Foundation
6931 Arlington Road
Bethesda, MD 20814
800-FIGHT-CF
http://www.cff.org

Department of Health and Human Services
Health Resources and Services Administration
Office of Minority Health
200 Independence Avenue, SW
Washington, DC 20201
(202) 619-0257
http://www.omhredhhs.gov

Digestive Diseases Clearinghouse
2 Information Way
Bethesda, MD 20892-3570
http://www.mediaconsult.com/mc/mcsite.nsf/conditionnav/
    ibd~educationalmaterial

Eldercare Locator
1112 16th Street, NW
Washington, DC 20036
(800) 677-1116
http://www.aoa.dhhs.gov/elderpage/locator.html

Elderhostel, Inc.
75 Federal Street
Boston, MA 02110-1941
617-426-7788
http://www.elderhostel.org

Emergency Nurses Association
915 Lee Street
Des Plains, IL 60016-6569
(800) 243-8362
http://www.ena.org

Epilepsy Foundation of America
4351 Garden City Drive
Landover, MD 20785
http://www.efa.org

Families USA
1334 G Street, NW
Washington, DC 20005
(202) 628-3030
http://familiesusa.org

The Foundation Fighting Blindness
National Retinitis Pigmentosa Foundation, Inc.
Executive Plaza I, Suite 800
11350 McCormick Road
Hunt Valley, MD 21031-1014
888-394-3937
http://www.libertyresources.org/ffb.html

Grief Recovery Institute
P.O. Box 6061-382
Sherman Oaks, CA 91413
818-907-9600
http://www.grief-recovery.com

Health and Human Services Minority
    HIV/AIDS Initiative
Office of Minority Health Resource Center (OMHRC)
P.O. Box 37337
Washington, DC 20013-7337
(800) 444-6472
http://www.omhrc.gov/OMH/AIDS/aidshome_new.htm

Health Resources and Services Administration
Division of Transplantation
Room 7-29, 5600 Fishers Lane
Rockville, MD 20857
(301) 443-7577
http://www.hrsa.DHHS.gov.bhrd/dot/dotmain.htm

Housecall Medical Resources, Inc.
6501 Deane Hill Drive
Knoxville, TN 37919
(865) 292-6261
www.housecall.com

The International Association of Lion Clubs
300 22nd Street
Oak Brook, IL 60523-8842
630-571-5466
http://www10.lionsclubs.org

Intravenous Nurses Society
220 Norwood Park South
Norwood, MA 02062
(781) 440-9408
http://www.ins1.org

Juvenile Diabetes Foundation International
120 Wall Street
New York, NY 10005-4001
800-JDF-CURE
http://www.jdf.org

Leukemia Society of America
600 Third Avenue
New York, NY 10016
212-573-8484
http://www.leukemia.org

March of Dimes Birth Defects Foundation
1275 Marmaroneck Avenue
White Plains, NY 10605
888-MODIMES
http://www.modimes.org

The Mind/Body Medical Institute
110 Francis Street
Boston, MA 02215
(617) 632-9530
http://mindbody.harvard.edu

Mind-Brain Society
Brown University
http://www.brown.edu/Students/Mind-Brain

Mothers Against Drunk Driving (MADD),
Metroplex Chapter
1341 Mockingbird Lane, #240W
Dallas, TX 75247
(214) 637-0372
http://www.madd.org

Muscular Dystrophy Association
3300 East Sunrise Drive
Tucson, AZ 85718
800-572-1717
http://www.mdausa.org

National Alliance for the Mentally Ill
200 North Glebe Road, Suite 1015
Arlington, VA 22203-3754
(800) 950-6264
http://www.nami.org

National Association for Home Care
228 Seventh Street, SE
Washington, DC 20003
202-547-7424
http://www.nahc.org

National Association of Clinical Nurse Specialists
3969 Green Street
Harrisburg, PA 17110
(717) 234-6799
http://www.nacns.org

National Association of Hispanic Nurses
1501 16th Street, NW
Washington, DC 20036
1-202-387-2477
http://www.thehispanicnurses.org

National Association of Orthopaedic Nurses (NAON)
North Woodbury Road, Box 56
Pitman, NJ 08071-0056
1-609-256-2310
www.inurse.com/~naon

National Black Nurses Association, Inc.
8630 Fenton Street, Suite 330
Silver Spring, MD 20910-3803
301-589-3200
FAX 301-589-3223
http://www.nbna.org

National Cancer Institute
Office of Cancer Communications
Building 31, Room 10A24
National Institutes of Health
Bethesda, MD 20892
800-4-CANCER
http://www.nci.nih.gov

National Center for Cultural Competence
Georgetown University
Child Development Center
3307 M Street NW, Suite 401
Washington, DC 20007-3935
1-800-788-2066
http://www.georgetown.edu/research/gucdc
email: cultural@georgetown.edu

National Center for Environmental Health
Mail Stop F-29
4770 Buford Highway, N.E.
Atlanta, GA 30341-3724
(888) 232-6789
http://www.cdc.gov/nceh

National Clearing House for Alcohol and Drug
Information (NCADI)
P.O. Box 2345
11400 Rockville Pike
Rockville, MD 20847-2345
800-729-6686
http://www.samhsa.gov

National Coalition Against Domestic Violence
P.O. Box 18749
Denver, CO 80218
(303) 839-1852
htto://www.ncadv.org

National Commission for Acupuncture and
Oriental Medicine
11 Canal Center Plaza, Suite 300
Alexandria, VA 22314
(703) 548-9004
http://www.nccaom.org

National Council on Alcoholism and Drug Dependence, Inc.
12 West 21st Street
New York, NY 10010
800-622-2255 or 212-206-6770
http://www.ncadd.org

National Digestive Diseases Information Clearinghouse
2 Information Way
Bethesda, MD 20892-3570
http://www.niddk.nih.gov

National Domestic Violence Hotline
(800) 799-7233
http://www.ndvh.org

National Easter Seal Society
230 West Monroe Street
Suite 1800
Chicago, IL 60606
http://www.easter-seals.org

National Emergency Medical Association
306 W. Joppa Road
Baltimore, MD 21204-4048
http://www.nemahealth.org

National Emergency Number Association
P.O. Box 360960
Columbus, OH 43236
(800) 332-3911
http://nema9-1-1.org

National Hemophilia Foundation
116 West 32nd Street, 11th Floor
New York, NY 10001
212-328-3700
http://www.infohf.org

National Hospice Organization
1901 North Moore Street, Suite 901
Arlington, VA 22209-1714
703-243-5900
http://www.nho.org

National Hydrocephalus Foundation
1670 Green Oak Circle
Lawrenceville, GA 30243

National Indian Council on Aging
10501 Montgomery Boulevard, NE, Suite 210
Albuquerque, NM 87111-3846
505-292-2001
http://www.nicoa.org

National Institute of Allergy and Infectious Diseases
National Institutes of Health
Building 31, Room 7A-50
31 Center Drive
Bethesda, MD 20892-2520
(301) 496-5717
http://www.niaid.nih.gov

National Institute of Arthritis and Musculoskeletal and Skin Diseases
National Institutes of Health
31 Center Drive
Bethesda, MD 20892-2350
301-496-8188
http://www.nih.gov/niams

National Institute of Mental Health (NIMH)
Information Resources and Inquiries Branch
Office of Scientific Information, Room 15C
5600 Fishers Lane
Rockville, MD 20857
(301) 443-4513
http://nimh.nih.gov

National Institute on Aging
P.O. Box 8057
Gaithersburg, MD 20898-8057
(800) 222-2225
http://www/nih.gov/nia

National Institute on Alcohol Abuse and Alcoholism
National Institutes of Health
6000 Executive Boulevard, Willco Building
Bethesda, MD 20892-7003
http://www.niaaa.nih.gov

National Institute on Drug Abuse
5600 Fishers Lane
Rockville, MD 20857
(301) 443-1124
www.nida.nih.gov

National Kidney Foundation
30 East 33rd Street, Suite 1100
New York, NY 10016
212-889-2210
http://www.kidney.org

National League for Nursing
61 Broadway
New York, NY 10006
800-669-9656
http://www.nln.org

National Mental Health Association
1021 Prince Street
Alexandria, VA 22314-2971
800-969-NMHA or 703-684-7722
http://www.nmha.org

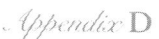

National Mental Health Consumers' Self-Help Clearinghouse
1211 Chestnut Street
Philadelphia, PA 19107
(800) 553-4539
http://www.mhselfhelp.org

Native American Nurses Association
927 Treadale Lane
Cloquet, MN 55720
1-218-879-1227

National Osteoporosis Foundation
1232 22nd Street NW
Washington, DC 20037-1292
202-223-2226
http://www.nof.org

National Psoriasis Foundation
6600 SW 92nd Avenue, Suite 300
Portland, OR 97223
503-244-7404
http://www.psoriasis.org

National Safety Council
1121 Spring Lake Drive
Itasca, IL 60143-3201
630-285-1121
http://www.nsc.org

National Scoliosis Foundation (NSF)
5 Cabot Place
Stoughton, MA 02072
http://laran.waisman.wisc.edu/fv/www/lib_scoliosis.html

National Society to Prevent Blindness
500 East Remington Road
Schaumburg, IL 60173
312-843-2020
http://www.eyeinfo.org/national.html

National Spinal Cord Injury Association
8300 Colesville Road, Suite 551
Silver Spring, MD 20910
301-588-6959
http://www.spinalcord.org

North American Nursing Diagnosis Association
1211 Locust Street
Philadelphia, PA 19107
215-545-8105
FAX: 215-545-8107
www.nanda.org

Office for Handicapped Individuals
Department of Education
Room 3106, Switzer Building
400 Maryland Avenue SW
Washington, DC 20202

Pan American Health Organization
Regional Office of the World Health Organization
525 23rd Street, NW
Washington, DC 20037
202-974-3000
http://www.paho.org

Parkinson's Disease Foundation
Medical Center
William Black Medical Research Building
Columbia-Presbyterian Medical Center
640 West 168th Street
New York, NY 10032
http://www.parkinsons-foundation.org

Philippine Nurses Association of America, Inc.
151 Linda Vista Drive
Daly City, CA 94014
415-468-7995
http://www.pna-america.org

Prevent Blindness America
500 E. Remington Rd.
Schaumburg, IL 60173
http://www.preventblindness.org

Scoliosis Association
PO Box 51353
Raleigh, NC 27609

Sickle Cell Disease Association of America, Inc.
200 Corporate Pointe, Suite 495
Culver City, CA 90230
800-421-8453
http://www.sicklecelldisease.org

Spina Bifida Association of America
4590 MacArthur Boulevard, NW, Suite 250
Washington, DC 20007-4226
800-621-3141
http://www.sbaa.org

Sudden Infant Death Syndrome Clearinghouse
8201 Greensboro Drive
Suite 600
McLean, VA 22102

Transcultural Nursing Society
c/o Madonna University College of Nursing and Health
36600 Schoolcraft Road
Livonia, MI 48150-1173
1-800-TCN-9995
http://www.tcns.org

United Cerebral Palsy Association
1000 Elmwood Avenue
Rochester, NY 14620
http://www.ggw.org/freenet/a/AlSigl/ucpa.html

United Ostomy Association Inc.
19772 MacArthur Boulevard, Suite 200
Irvine, CA 92612-2405
800-826-0826
http://www.uoa.org

U.S. Census Bureau
Washington, DC 20233
Street address: 4700 Silver Hill Road
Suitland, MD 20746
301-457-4608
http://www.uscensusbureau

Visiting Nurse Associations of America (VNAA)
11 Beacon Street, Suite 910
Boston, MA 02108
http://www.vnaa.org/home.htm

World Health Organization
Avenue Appia 20
1211 Geneva 27
Switzerland
(00 41 22) 791 21 11
Fax: (00 41 22) 791 3111
www.who.int

WEB SITES RELATED TO HEALTH

ABC News
http://www.abcnews.go.com/sections/living/index.html

American Academy of Nursing
http://www.nursingworld.org/aan/index.htm

American Association of Colleges of Nursing
http://www.aacn.nche.edu

American Association of Critical-Care Nurses
http://www.aacn.org

American College of Nurse-Midwives
http://www.acnm.org

American Nurses Association
http://www.nursingworld.org

CNN Health News
http://www.cnn.com/HEALTH/index.html

CPR: You CAN do it!
http://www.learncpr.org

Evaluating On-Line Health Information
http://www.healthfinder.gov/smartchoices/onlineinfo/evaluate.htm

Joint Commission on Accreditation of Healthcare Organizations
http://www.jcaho.org

Mayo Clinic Health Oasis
http://www.mayohealth.org/mayo/common/htm/headline.htm

MSNBC Health Front Page
http://www.msnbc.com/news/HEALTH_Front.asp?a

National Center for Complementary and Alternative Medicine
http://www.altmed.od.nih.gov/nccam

National Council of State Boards of Nursing
http://www.ncsbn.org

National Institute for Occupational Safety and Health
http://www.cdc.gov/niosh/homepage.html

NPR Health and Science News
http://www.npr.org/news/healthsci

Sigma Theta Tau, International
http://www.nursingsociety.org

Thinking Critically About World Wide Web Resources
http://www.library.ucla.edu/libraries/college/instruct/web/critical.htm

This Week in JAMA
http://www.ama-assn.org/sci-pubs/journals/most/recent/issues/jama/issue.htm

U.S. Department of Health and Human Services
http://www.hhs.gov

U.S. Public Health Service Nursing
http://www.hhs.gov/progorg/nursing

The Virtual Medical Center
http://www.montana.edu/wwwdhs/vmc.html

"Virtual" Nursing Center
http://www.sci.lib.uci.edu/~martindale/Nursing.html

Wound, Ostomy and Continence Nurses Society
http://www.wocn.org

WEB SITES RELATED TO NURSING RESEARCH

Administration on Aging
www.aoa.dhhs.gov

Agency for Health Care Policy and Research
http://www.ahcpr.gov

American Association for Marriage and Family Therapy
http://www.aamft.org/families/index.htm

American Heart Association
http://www.americanheart.org

American Holistic Nurses Association
http://www.ahna.org

American Journal of Health Promotion
http://www.healthpromotionjournal.com

American Medical Informatics Association, Nursing Informatics Working Group
http://www.amia.org

American Nurses Association
http://www.ana.org

American Nurses Foundation
http://www.nursingworld.org/anf

Australian Health Promotion
http://www.health.usyd.edu.au/achp

Bill Trochim's Center for Social Research Methods
http://trochim.human.cornell.edu

Bioethics Network
www.bioethics.net

Blue Sky Associates (World Wisdom Project)
http://worldwisdomproject.org

Campus-Community Partnerships for Health
http://www.furturehealth.ucsf.edu/ccph/html

Canadian Nursing Association
http://www.cna-nurses.ca

Centers for Disease Control and Prevention
http://www.cdc.gov

Child Welfare Training Resources Online Network
http://www.childwelfaretraining.org

Coalition for Healthier Cities and Communities
http://www.healthycommunities.org

Coalition of Campuses to Support Students and Faulty in Community Partnership Efforts
http://www.compact.org

Cochrane Collaboration and Library
www.cochrane.org

Communicable Disease Prevention and Control
http://www.cdpc.com

Community Formation for Nurses
http://www.nursemanifest.com/manifesto.htm

Computers in Nursing Interactive
http://www.cini.com.org

Continuum Health Partners–Interactive Health Evaluation
http://www.wehealny.com/interactive/evaluation.html

CPRI-HOST (Computer-based Patient Record Institute & Healthcare Open Systems and Trials)
http://www.cpri-host.org

Critical Thinking Foundation
http://www.criticalthinking.org/university

Cultural Diversity in Health Care
http://www.ggalanti.com/index.html

CYFERnet: Children, Youth, and Families Education and Research Network
http://www.cyfernet.org

Disease Prevention and Control Guidelines (Canada)
http://www.hc-sc.gc.ca/pphb-dgspsp/dpg_e.html

Disease Prevention News
http://www.tdh.state.tx.us/phpep/dpn/dpnhome.htm

Environmental Protection Agency
http://www.epa.gov

Evidence-Based Nursing
http://www.bmipg.com/data/ebn.htm

Global Good Services, Inc.
http://www.globalgoodservice.org

Global Health Action
http://www.globalhealthaction.org

A Health Promotion and Wellness Resource for Individuals, Worksites, Communities, and Health Professionals
http://www.siu.edu/departments/bushea

Health Promotion England
http://www.hpe.org.uk

Health Promotion Clearinghouse
http://www.heart-health.ns.ca/hpc

Health Promotion On-Line (Canada)
http://www.hc-sc.gc.ca/hppb/hpo

Healthy Lifestyles and Mental Health
http://www.paho.org/english.hpp

Healthy People 2010
http://www.health.gov/healthypeople

Healthy Mothers, Healthy Babies
http://www.hmhb.org/about/abouthtml

Healthy Schools, Healthy Communities
http://www.bphc.hrsa.dhhs.gov/hshc

Hope Health: A Health Promotion Guide
http://www.hithope.com/corp/main.php3?dir=
    content&file=hpromo.txt

International Food Information Council
http://ificinfo.health.org

International Council of Nurses
www.icn.ch

**The International Healthy Cities/
    Communities Movement**
http://electronicvalley.org/hv2000

International Parish Nurse Resource Center
http://www.advocatehealth.com/about/faith/parishn/
    index.html

Lippincott's Nursing Center
http://www.nursingcenter.com

**Martindales' Health Science Guide–The Virtual
    Nursing Center**
http://www-sci.lib.uci.edu/HSG/Nursing.html

Mental Health Infosearch
http://www.mhsource.com

Mental Health Net
http://www.cmhc.com

Midwest Nursing Research Society
http://www.mnrs.org

Mind Body Medical Institute
http://www.mbmi.org

Minnesota Council on Family Relations
http://www.mcfr.net

Minority Health Project
http://www.minority.unc.edu

**National Center for Complementary and
    Alternative Medicine**
http://www.nccam.nih.gov

**National Center for Chronic Disease Prevention and
    Health Promotion**
http://www.cdc.gov/nccdphp

National Civic League, Healthy Communities Program
http://www.ncl.org

National Council on Family Relations
http://www.ncfr.com/

National Institute of Nursing Research
http://www.nih.gov/ninr

National Wellness Institute
http://www.nationalwellness.org

Native American Viable Village HealthCare Reform
http://globalgoodservices.org

**Nola Pender (Most frequently asked questions
    about the Health Promotion Model)**
http://www.nursing.umich.edu/faculty/
    pender_questions.html

**Nurse Healers-Professional Associates International
    (Therapeutic Touch)**
http://www.therapeutic-touch.org

Nurses Certificate Program in Imagery
http://www.imageryrn.com

Nursing Ethics Network
http://www.nursingethicsnetwork.org

**Nutrition and Your Health: Dietary Guidelines
    for Americans**
http://www.health.gov/dietaryguidelines

Office of Disease Prevention and Health Promotion
http://www.odphp.osophs.ddhs.gov

**Ottawa Charter for Health Promotion
    (First International Conference)**
http://www.who.dk/policy/ottawa.htm

Outcome and Assessment Information Set (OASIS)
www.hcfa.gov/medicare/hhmain.htm#billing

Planned Parenthood
http://www.plannedparenthood.org

PubMed
http://www.ncbi.nlm.nih.gov/PubMed

Relationship-Centered Care
http://www.fetzer.org/rcc

Sex, Etc.
http://www.sxetc.org

Society for Research in Child Development
http://www.srcd.org/news1.html

Southern Nursing Research Society
http://www.snrs.org

Stanford Center for Research in Disease Prevention
http://prevention.stanford.edu

Sustainable Communities Network
http://www.sustainable.org/casestudies/florida

University of Arizona's Health Source Center
http://www.ahsc.arizona.edu/opa/health

University of Delaware Family Resources
http://ag.udel.edu/fam/resources/resbytopic.htm

US Army Center for Health Promotion and Preventive Medicine
http://chppm-www.apgea.army.mil/ento

UW Physicians On Line–Health Risk Assessment
http://www.uwphysicians.org/healthcalc.html

White House Office of Faith and Community-Based Initiatives
http://www.faithbasedcommunityinitiatives.org

You First Health Risk Assessment
http://www.youfirst.com

E Herbal Preparations Used As Health Remedies

Herbal Supplement	Popular Uses	Usual Dose Range	Possible Side Effects	Safety in Pregnancy and Lactation	Possible Medication Interactions	Possible Efficacy *Type of Study*	Probable Safety
Cardiovascular and Circulatory							
CoEnzyme Q10, ubiquinone	Heart problems	100–600 mg daily.	None known	Unknown	None known	+, in vitro and human studies	+
Garlic (*Allium sativa*)	Hyperlipidemia, antiplatelet, hypertension, anti-infective, digestive disorders	3.6–5.4 mg allicin/day (enteric-coated, freeze-dried)	Heartburn, flatulence, increased bleeding risk (with >5 cloves garlic/day), possible allergies	Contraindicated	Antiplatelet agents (aspirin, clopidogrel), anticoagulants, including warfarin	+, human studies	+
Green tea (*Camellia sinensis*)	To prevent heart disease, cancer, lower cholesterol, as an antioxidant, an antimicrobial	3–9 cups/day	Possible increased risk for esophageal cancer due to tannin content, not conclusive; asthma	Contraindicated	May prevent absorption of concomitantly administered medications; separate by several hours	+ in vitro ?, human studies	+
Hawthorn (*Crataegus sp.*)	Mild heart failure (NYHA Stage I or II)	0.3–1.0 g dried fruit, 0.5–1.0 mL 1:1 liquid extract or 1–2 mL 1:5 in 45% alcohol tid (standardized to procyanidin or flavinoid content)	Nausea, fatigue, sweating, hand rashes	Contraindicated	Digoxin	?, human studies	+, human studies
Gastrointestinal							
Aloe (*Aloe barbadensis*)	Juice or latex: laxative	20–30 mg hydroxy-anthrecene derivatives/day as aloin	Cramps, electrolyte depletion with long-term use	Contraindicated	Digoxin, diuretics, other stimulant laxatives	+, human studies	?
	Gel: wound healing	Apply to affected area as needed	None	Unknown	None known	+, human studies	+

	Uses	Dose	Adverse reactions	Contraindicated	Interactions	Evidence	
Chamomile (*Matricaria recutita*)	Gastrointestinal disorders, inflammation of mucous membranes and skin, sedative, anti-inflammatory, anti-infective	2–8 g dried flowers or 1–4 mL 1:1 in 45% alcohol tid	Allergic reactions, #	None known	None known	+, animal studies ?, human studies	+
Flaxseed (*Linium usitatissimum*)	Constipation, irritable bowel syndrome, diverticulitis, estrogenic effects, hyperlipidemia	15–45 g milled seed; contains alpha-linoleic acid	None known Intestinal obstruction, dehydration: contraindicated	Contraindicated	May decrease absorption of concomitantly administered medications	+, human studies	+
Ginger (*Zingiber officinale*)	Nausea, motion sickness, dyspepsia	0.25–1.0 dried ginger root daily	Gallstones: contraindicated	Unknown	Antiplatelet agents (aspirin, clopidogrel), anticoagulants, including warfarin	+, human studies	+
Licorice (*Glycyrrhiza glabra*)	Coughs, colds, gastric ulcers, liver disease	5–15 g root, approximately 200–600 mg glycyrrhizin	Renal insufficiency, high blood pressure, hypokalemia, heart disease, liver disease, diabetes	Contraindicated	Digoxin, diuretics, corticosteroids, insulin, amoliride, spironolactone, stimulant laxatives	+, human studies	?
Milk thistle (*Silybum marianum*)	Dyspepsia, supportive treatment of liver disease, protection from chemical and hepatitis-induced liver damage	12–15 g herb (200–400 mg silymarin as silibinin)	Mild transient gastrointestinal effects Allergic reactions, #	Unknown	None known	+, human studies	+

(continues)

Herbal Supplement	Popular Uses	Usual Dose Range	Possible Side Effects	Safety in Pregnancy and Lactation	Possible Medication Interactions	Possible Efficacy / Type of Study	Probable Safety
Endocrine							
Bilberry (*Vaccinium myrtillus*)	Diarrhea, improving visual acuity, diabetes	20–60 g dried berry	None known	Unknown	None known	?, human studies	?
Bitter melon (*Momordica charantia*)	Diabetes	15 g aqueous extract, 50 mL extract	None reported in humans; seeds are toxic, may cause liver damage (animal data)	Contraindicated	May potentiate the effects of sulfonylureas, insulin, other antidiabetic agents	+, animal studies; +, human studies	? to +
Dehydroepiandrosterone (DHEA)	Multiple uses, including anti-aging agent, in the place of estrogen replacement therapy, memory loss	25–50 mg po qd	High blood pressure, glucose intolerance, increased risk for breast and prostate cancer	Contraindicated	None known	? to +, human studies	? to (–), human studies
Vascular							
Gingko biloba	Decreased circulation (cerebral, intermittent claudication)	40 mg tid (as Egb-761 or LI 1370; 24% flavinoids and 6% terpenes)	Occasional stomach or intestinal upset, headaches, allergy	Unknown	Antiplatelet agents (aspirin, clopidogrel), anticoagulants, including warfarin	+, human studies	+
Grapeseed extract (*Vitis vinifera*)	Vascular insufficiency	50 mg daily	None reported	Unknown	None reported	+, human studies	+
Horse chestnut (*Aesculus hippocastanum*)	Vascular insufficiency	30–150 mg aesculin/day	Gastrointestinal symptoms; Bleeding disorders: contraindicated	Unknown	Antiplatelet agents (aspirin, clopidogrel), anticoagulants, including warfarin	+, human studies	+
Musculoskeletal/Pain							
Indian frankincense tree (*Boswellia serrata*)	Pain reliever, anti-inflammatory, particularly for arthritis	350 mg tid	None reported	Unknown	None reported	?, human studies	+

Devil's claw (*Harpagophytum procumbens*)	To alleviate pain, particularly arthritis and back pain	0.1–0.25 g tid, up to 6 g/day dried root or 50 mg harpagoside	None known	Unknown; may be contraindicated	None reported	?, human studies	? to +
Glucosamine	Arthritis	1500 mg/day	Gastrointestinal side effects	Contraindicated	None known	+	+
Immune System							
Cat's claw, Una de gato (*Uncaria guianensis, U. tomentosa*)	Immunostimulant anticancer agent, anti-inflammatory for arthritis, inflammatory bowel disease, etc.	1–5 g powdered bark or one cup of tea 2–3 times daily	None reported	Unknown	None reported	+, in vitro ?, human studies	?
Echinacea (*Echinacea purpura, E. angustiflora, E. pallida*)	Immune-stimulant, colds, upper respiratory tract, externally for wound healing	6–9 mL freshly pressed plant juice; hydroalcoholic extract, maximum of 6–8 weeks*	Allergic reactions, # Autoimmune diseases (eg, rheumatoid arthritis, lupus), progressive systemic disease (eg, multiple sclerosis), HIV: contraindicated	Unknown	None reported	+, human studies	+, human studies
Goldenseal (*Hydrastis canadensis*)	Anti-infective, digestive disorders, to mask a positive drug screen	Endangered species, banned from international trade.	None reported Contraindicated in ear infection with purulent discharge	Contraindicated	None reported	?, no effect on drug screens.	+
Korean ginseng (*Panax ginseng*)	"Adaptogen" (increases the body's ability to resist stress and resist disease)	1–2 g ginseng or 200–600 mg standardized extract (4–7% ginsenosides)*	Insomnia, diarrhea, skin eruptions	Contraindicated	Monoamine oxidase inhibitors, caffeine, warfarin, insulin (speculative, AS)	?	+

(continues)

Herbal Supplement	Popular Uses	Usual Dose Range	Possible Side Effects	Safety in Pregnancy and Lactation	Possible Medication Interactions	Possible Efficacy	Probable Safety
						Type of Study	
Siberian ginseng, eluthero, ciwujia (*Elutherococcus senticosus*)	"Adaptogen," particularly to improve athletic performance	2–3 g root/day*	None known BP >180/90 mm Hg: possibly contraindicated	Contraindicated	Barbiturates (speculative, AS), monomycin, kanamycin, insulin (speculative, AS)	?	+
Genitourinary							
Cranberry (*Vaccinium macrocarpon*)	Urinary tract infections, particularly in women	5–20 mL cranberry cocktail/day	None reported	Unknown	None known	+, in vitro, ? human studies	+
Uva Ursi (*Arctostaphylos uva ursi*)	Urinary tract inflammatory disorders, diuretic	1.5–4.0 g (100–210 mg hydroquinone) as a tea qid (no longer than 1 week)	Nausea, vomiting Renal disease: contraindicated	Contraindicated	None known	+, animal studies	?
Saw palmetto (*Serenoa repens*)	Benign prostatic hypertrophy	1–2 s berry or 320 mg lipophilic extract (90% v/v hexane or ethanol) daily	Occasional gastrointestinal side effects	Contraindicated	None known	+, human studies, superior to finasteride, comparable to alpha blocker	+
Gynecologic Conditions							
Black cohosh (*Cimicifuga racemosa*)	Menopausal symptoms, premenstrual syndrome, painful menstruation	Alcohol extract (40–60% v/v) equivalent to 40 mg herb	Occasional gastrointestinal discomfort	Contraindicated	None known	?	?

	Use	Dose	Side Effects	Contraindications	Drug Interactions		
Chaste berry (*Vitex agnus castus*)	Premenstrual syndrome, irregularities of the menstrual cycle	Aqueous-alcohol extract (50–70% v/v) equivalent to 30–40 mg berry	Occasional pruritus, urticaria	Contraindicated	May interfere with birth-control pills, may antagonize dopamine antagonists (eg, antipsychotics)	? to +, human studies	+
Dong quai (*Angelica sinensis*)	Menopausal symptoms, premenstrual syndrome, painful menstruation	1000–3390 mg/day dried root	Photosensitivity, particularly with high doses	Contraindicated	None known	?	–
Evening primrose oil (black currant or borage oil, cisgamma linoleic acid-GLA)	Premenstrual syndrome, rheumatoid arthritis, other autoimmune diseases, multiple sclerosis	Dose dependent on reason for taking; most common range is 2–3 g/day of an 8% GLA preparation	Gastrointestinal symptoms Borage oil may cause liver damage, avoid None reported for other forms of GLA	Unknown	None known	?	?
Soy/phytoestrogens (isoflavones)	As a substitute for estrogen replacement therapy	165 mg isoflavones (45 mg soy flour)	Headaches, oily skin	Do not exceed amounts found in foods	None known	?	?
Neurologic							
Feverfew (*Tanacetum parthenium*)	Migraine headaches	2.5 fresh leaves or 50 mg freeze-dried leaves daily	Mouth ulcers, gastrointestinal symptoms Allergic reactions, #	Contraindicated	None known	+, HS	+, HS
Guarana (*Paullinia cupana*)	Stimulant, weight loss	Contains 2.5–5% caffeine	Nervousness, insomnia, rapid or irregular heart beat, heartburn	Contraindicated	Monoamine oxidase inhibitors, ephedrine, adenosine, beta-blockers, phenyl-propanolamine, lithium, theophylline, and fluoroquinolones	?	?

(continues)

Herbal Supplement	Popular Uses	Usual Dose Range	Possible Side Effects	Safety in Pregnancy and Lactation	Possible Medication Interactions	Possible Efficacy	Probable Safety
						Type of Study	
Ma huang (*Ephedra* sp.)	Stimulant, weight loss, asthma	Contains ephedrine, which is a controlled substance in the United States; the status of ma huang is undetermined	Increases blood pressure and heart rate, palpitations, nervousness, headaches, insomnia and dizziness. Contraindicated in heart disease, high blood pressure, diabetes, hyperthyroidism, history of substance abuse	Contraindicated	Theophylline, caffeine, monoamine oxidases, reserpine, amitriptyline	(+) for asthma, ? to (−) for other uses	? to (−)
Psychiatric Kava kava (*Piper methysticum*)	Anxiety	Clinical trials (WS 1490): 90–110 mg dried extract (70 mg kava-pyrones) daily	Yellow discoloration of skin, hair and nails, rare allergic reactions. Depression: contraindicated	Contraindicated	Benzodiazepines (one case report of coma), alcohol, barbiturates	+, human studies	+

Hops	Insomnia, anxiety, restlessness	Single dose: 0.5 g hops (as a tea)	None known	Unknown	Barbiturates (speculative, AS)	+, animal studies	?
Melatonin	Insomnia, jet lag	Jet lag: 5–10 mg/day Insomnia: dose undefined	Headache, may worsen depression	Unknown	None known	+, small human studies	?
Passion flower (*Passiflora incarnata*)	Insomnia	?	None reported	Unknown	Barbiturates (speculative, AS)	+, animal studies	+
St. John's Wort (*Hypericum perforatum*)	Depression	Clinical trials (extract LI 160): 900–1800 mg/day	Photosensitivity, headache, nausea, vomiting, restlessness, dizziness, sedation, gastric symptoms	Contraindicated	Possible monoamine oxidase activity; avoid tyramine in diet, caffeine, decongestants, caffeine, SSRIs, amphetamines	+, human studies, = to 150 mg imipramine	+
Valerian (*Valeriana officinalis*)	Insomnia	2–3 g herb (as tea), up to several times daily, 1–2 mL tincture up to several times daily, 450–900 mg extract at bedtime	Cases of hepatotoxicity reported, may have been secondary to substitution with *Teucrium* species	Unknown	Barbiturates, benzodiazepines (speculative, in vitro, AS)	+, but human study results mixed	+

Key: (+) = possibly effective or safe;? = inconclusive;(−) = ineffective or unsafe;* = prone to adulteration with other plants; # = individuals allergic to ragweed, chrysanthemums, marigolds, daisies, and other members of the Asteraceae/Compositae plant family may also be allergic to this plant. AS = animal studies; HS = human studies.

Glossary

A

Abrasion Wound in which skin or mucous membranes are rubbed or scraped away

Absorption Process by which a medication enters the body

Acid Any substance capable of releasing hydrogen ions in solution

Acronym A word formed from the initial letters of the successive or major parts of a compound term

Active transport Movement of substances across a cell membrane against an electrochemical gradient

Activities of daily living (ADLs) Activities frequently performed on a daily basis, such as bathing, grooming, eating, and toileting

Activity intolerance Physical inability to withstand activity

Actual nursing diagnosis An existing human response to a health problem the nurse identifies that is amenable to nursing intervention

Acute pain Pain that lasts less than 6 months

Adaptation Process by which a person changes to conform to the environment

Advance directive Written document (e.g., living will) that states in advance a client's desires about the types of healthcare he or she wishes to receive should the client become unable to decide

Advanced practice nurse Nurse who has advanced degrees and certification (e.g., nurse practitioner)

Advocacy Communicating and acting on behalf of another person's welfare, especially a client in the healthcare system; keeping the client informed about treatment and nursing care

Aerobic exercise Exercise that requires oxygen for energy and involves elevation of heart rate for an extended period

Affective Refers to emotional reactions or feelings

Agent Any factor (internal or external) that can lead to illness by its presence or absence

Agonist Drug that has affinity for a receptor and is capable of eliciting a pharmacologic response

Agranulocytes Mononuclear cells that lack digestive enzymes

Air embolus Air bubble in the vascular space that may obstruct circulation

Allodynia Enhanced sensation of pain produced by an innocuous stimulus, such as a light touch

Allostasis Capacity of physiologic systems to maintain stability through change

Alopecia Hair loss

Alveoli Spherical, saclike epithelial structures in the lungs through which gas exchange occurs

American Nurses Association Professional nursing organization concerned with all aspects of professional nursing; provides standards and leadership for the profession; comprised of individual state nursing associations and also has nursing specialty bodies representing all nursing practice areas

Anaerobic exercise Exercise in which muscles cannot extract enough oxygen, and anaerobic pathways are used to provide additional energy for a short time; useful in endurance training

Andragogy Adult learning theory

Anesthesiologist Physician who specializes in anesthesia administration

Angina Pain and discomfort about the heart, characteristic of myocardial ischemia; severe pain felt in the anterior chest, shoulder, left arm, neck, and jaw

Anion Negatively charged ion

Anonymity Protection of a research participant in such a way that the participant cannot be linked to the information provided

Anorexia Loss of appetite

Antagonist Pharmacologic agent that binds with a receptor but does not produce a physiologic response or block the effect of an agonist

Antibody Protective substance the body produces to protect itself against an antigen

Anticipatory grief Pattern of psychological and physiologic responses a person makes to the impending loss (real or imagined) of a significant person, object, belief, or relationship

Anticipatory guidance Information given to a client about a situation before it occurs so the client can develop problem-solving and coping strategies

Antigen Substance that provokes irritation or damage to the body tissues and induces the formation of antibodies

Antiseptic Agent that stops or slows the growth of microorganisms on living tissue, commonly used for handwashing, skin preparation, and wound packing or irrigation

Anuria Formation and excretion of less than 100 cc of urine in 24 hours

Aphasia Communication disorder that may affect speech, reading, and writing

Apnea Absence of respiration

Approximated Lightly pulled together

Arthroscopy Direct visualization of a joint by insertion of a scope

Articulation Enunciation of words and sentences

Asepsis Absence of disease-producing microorganisms

Asphyxiation Lack of oxygen, leading to cell death

Assault Threat of touching a person without his or her consent

Assessment First phase of the nursing process in which data are gathered to identify actual or potential health problems

Associate nurse A nurse prepared in an associate degree program

Atelectasis Collapse of alveoli

Atheism Denial of God's existence

Atrophy Wasting away of an organ, muscle, or body tissue

Attention Ability to concentrate on and take in specific sensory stimuli

Attitudes A person's dispositions toward an object or situation; can be a mental or emotional mind-set and positive or negative

Audit Review of records

Auscultation Technique of listening to body sounds with a stethoscope

Auscultatory gap Absence of audible sounds during blood pressure measurement that may cause inaccurate readings

Automaticity Heart's capability of generating its own electrical impulse, which is then conducted through specialized conduction fibers

Autonomy Degree of discretion and independence a practitioner has

B

Bacteremia Presence of bacteria in the blood

Bactericidal Able to kill bacteria

Bacteriostatic Able to inhibit the growth of bacteria

Basal metabolic rate Amount of energy the body uses during absolute rest in an awake state

Base Any substance that can combine with and decrease hydrogen ions in solution; alkali

Battery Unlawful touching of a person's body without his or her consent

Behaviors Observable actions

Beliefs Ideas that a person accepts as true

Beneficence Doing or promoting good, the basis for all healthcare

Bereavement Response to the death of a significant person

Binder Large bandage used to support a body part or to hold a dressing in place

Biofeedback A technique in which the client learns voluntary control over autonomic functions

Bisexual Relating to both men and women sexually

Blended family Two parents with unrelated children who are being raised together

Blood pressure Force the blood exerts against the walls of the blood vessels

Body image Feelings about one's body

Body mechanics Positioning or moving the body to prevent or to correct problems related to activity or immobilization

Borborygmi Loud, rumbling sounds produced by the normal movement of gas through the intestines, referred to as "stomach growling"

Bradycardia Abnormally slow heart rate (usually less than 60 beats per minute in adults)

Bradypnea Abnormally slow respiratory rate (usually less than 10 breaths per minute in adults)

Bronchioles Narrow airways that conduct air into alveolar ducts and alveoli

Bronchospasm Narrowing of the bronchioles caused by tightening of the smooth muscles in the airways

Buccal Pertaining to the inside cheek

Buffer Compound that helps stabilize the pH of a solution by neutralizing added acid or base

Burn Injury cause by exposure to thermal, chemical, electrical, or radioactive energy

C

Calorie (kilocalorie) Unit of heat, commonly used to describe the energy value of food

Carbohydrates Food group containing simple and complex sugars composed of carbon, hydrogen, and oxygen

Care plan conference Meeting to discuss revisions to the plan of care and coordination of care

Caregiver Person (usually a family member) responsible for providing day-to-day care, especially hygiene, nutrition, supervision, and company for someone who has an impairment to ADLs

Caries Cavities in the tooth enamel

Carrier Person from whom a microorganism can be cultured but who shows no sign of a disease

Case management Professional approach to providing care in which one provider coordinates a client's services

Catheter Tube placed into a body cavity or vessel for evacuating or injecting fluid

Cation Positively charged ion

Celibacy Abstention from sexual intercourse

Central venous catheter Catheter whose tip is placed in the superior vena cava or at the entrance of the right atrium

Cerumen Earwax

Change-of-shift report Information passed between nurses at change of shift about client status and plan of care

Charge nurse Nurse responsible for the functioning of a nursing unit for a particular work shift

Charting by exception Charting in which the nurse documents only those findings that fall outside the standard of care and norms the institution has developed

Chronic pain Pain that lasts more than 6 months

Circadian rhythm Regular occurrence of certain phenomena in cycles of about 24 hours

Circle of confidentiality Professionals with whom client information can be shared

Client Person requiring the services of a healthcare provider

Climacteric Menopause

Clinical nurse specialist Registered nurse who holds a master's degree in a nursing specialty and has advanced clinical experience

Clinical pathway Models for ensuring quality of care, providing direction about major interventions to perform for a specific condition

Clitoris Small, erectile organ located just above the urinary meatus in females; plays a key role in female orgasm

Clustering Combining client data into meaningful patterns

Cognition Thinking and awareness; system by which sensory input, past experiences, and emotions are integrated and made meaningful

Cohabitated family People living together without the formal or legal bond of marriage

Collaboration Actions taken in coordination with other professionals

Collaborative health problem Problems based on medical diagnoses, medically ordered treatments, or other related problems that require interdependent standards and activities to be addressed

Colloid Fluids that contain proteins or starch molecules

Colonization State in which a microorganism is present but no immune reaction or tissue destruction occurs

Colostomy Opening of a part of the colon onto the abdominal skin surface

Coma Abnormally deep stupor occurring in illness or as a result of injury; external stimuli fail to arouse the client

Commode Portable chair with a toilet seat and a waste receptacle beneath that can be emptied so a client who cannot walk to the bathroom can manage toileting

Communal family Related and unrelated people with common goals and beliefs who share a household

Communicable disease Disease transmissible between hosts

Communication Interchange of information

Communication channel Medium through which a message is sent (e.g., television, writing, speaking)

Community Social group whose members may or may not share common geographic boundaries but who interact because of common interests or shared values to meet their needs within a larger society

Community-based healthcare Healthcare directed toward a specific group within the community

Community-based nursing care Nursing care directed toward a specific group or population within the community; may be provided for individuals or groups

Complement system Series of proteins found in the bloodstream that enhances phagocytosis of microbes, helps in lysis of bacterial cell walls, and encourages the inflammatory response

Complete protein Protein that contains sufficient amounts of essential amino acids to maintain body tissues and to promote body growth

Compliance (1) Adherence to recommended plan; (2) Measure of the lung's "stretchiness"

Comprehension Capacity for understanding and reasoning

Comprehensive health assessment Assessment that encompasses the physical, psychological, social, and spiritual dimensions of living

Computer-based personal record Record of a client's health saved on and easily accessed by computer system

Conceptual framework Formal explanation that links concepts and emphasizes relationships among them

Condom catheter (external, Texas) Noninvasive urinary collection device for incontinent male clients; consists of a thin, flexible sheath placed over the penis and attached to tubing and a collection bag

Confidentiality Practice of keeping client information private

Consciousness State of awareness and full responsiveness to stimuli

Continuity of care Provision of uninterrupted service as a client moves between settings

Contractility Force of contraction

Contracture Shortening of a muscle and loss of joint mobility from fibrotic changes in the tissues surrounding the joint

Contralateral stimulation Stimulation of the opposite side from pain; common methods including pressure, massage, cold, and heat

Controlled substance Drugs that are considered to have either limited medical use or high potential for abuse or addiction

Coping Problem-solving process a person uses to manage stress

Coping mechanism Effort used to manage stress

Core temperature Internal body temperature

Crime Violation of the law punishable by the state

Critical pathway Standard plan of care used to establish and monitor the extent and timing of care; includes such key elements as diagnostic tests, consultations, treatments, activities, procedures, and discharge planning and teaching

Critical thinking Purposeful process that is disciplined, active, multidimensional, reasonable, rational, and reflective to arrive at insight and draw conclusions

Crystalloid Fluids that are clear

Cue Piece of data, subjective or objective, about a client

Cultural diversity Plurality of ideas and opinions for behavior to which people are exposed, adding to the texture and complexity of a society

Cultural relativity Principle that meaning is created by one's culture and truth is culture-specific; the same experience may carry different meanings to people of different cultures

Cultural value orientation Subset of world view with four general orientations (nature, time, activity, and relationships) and three types of responses (mastery, subjugation, and harmony)

Culture (1) A society's behavior and institutions; (2) Growth of microorganisms in a specialized medium under precise conditions

Culture change Dynamic in which a culture evolves as people come into contact with new beliefs and ideas

Culture shock Failure to comprehend the culture in which one is living

Cycling Interruption of an intravenous infusion for a period of time

Cynosure Emblem of group social identity

D

Dangling Preliminary step to ambulation, especially for clients who may be unable to ambulate initially, which involves sitting on the side of the bed with the legs dependent

Débridement Removal of foreign material or dying tissue from a wound

Decision-making process Method of analyzing a problem, determining alternatives, and selecting the appropriate action

Decoding Process of understanding a message

Deep vein thrombosis A thrombus originating in the large veins of the legs because of the relatively low velocity of blood flow there

Defecation reflex Involuntary response of intestinal contraction and anal sphincter relaxation to rectal distention

Dehiscence Accidental separation of wound edges, especially a surgical wound

Delegation Transferring to a competent person the authority to perform a selected nursing task in a selected situation

Delirium Reversible disorder of cognition; confusion

Delusion Belief that is not based in reality and that reflects an unconscious need or fear

Dementia Cognitive impairment as the result of irreversible organic changes in brain cell function

Dependent variable Variable (or item of interest that varies) that is the outcome; hypothesized to depend on or be caused by another variable

Dermis Layer of skin beneath the epidermis; composed of dense connective fibers, blood vessels, nerves, hair follicles, and glands

Detrusor Smooth muscle of the urinary bladder

Development Process of ongoing change throughout a person's life

Developmental stages Points in life when old responsibilities are discarded and new ones are assumed

Developmental tasks Psychomotor, psychosocial, or cognitive skills attained at certain stages of life that are prerequisites for successive skill development

Diagnosis-related groups (DRGs) Categories or classifications of illnesses, disorders, procedures, or other conditions necessitating hospitalization from which cost of care is predetermined

Diagnostic reasoning process Skills used to make nursing diagnoses

Diarrhea Frequent evacuation of watery stools

Diastole Period of rest in the cardiac cycle, when the ventricles are not contracting and the coronary arteries are filling with blood

Diastolic blood pressure Pressure in the blood vessels during cardiac ventricular relaxation

Diffusion Movement of molecules from an area of higher concentration to one of lower concentration

Digestion Mechanical and chemical processes necessary to convert food to an absorbable state

Directive leadership Leadership style in which the leader makes all the decisions and tells subordinates what to do

Disaccharides Simple sugars

Discharge planning Process of coordinating, planning, and arranging for the transition from one healthcare setting to another

Disease State of disharmony of mind, body, emotions, and spirit

Disease-prevention activities Avoidance behaviors that seek to prevent specific diseases or conditions

Disinfectant Chemical used to kill microorganisms on lifeless objects

Distention Condition of being stretched or inflated

Distribution Process by which a drug passes from the circulation of the blood and lymphatic system across cell membranes to a specified tissue

Diuresis Formation and excretion of large amounts of urine

Documentation Written communication of client information and care

Double effect Action that can produce two outcomes, one helpful and one harmful, at the same time

Drug Substance that alters physiologic function with the potential for affecting health

Dualism Theory that divides concepts into two mutually irreducible elements

Dysarthria Disorders affecting either single or combined motor control of the muscles of speech

Dysfunction Action that does not meet expected norms

Dysfunctional grief Grief that falls outside normal parameters; may manifest as absence of, delayed, exaggerated, or prolonged grief

Dyspareunia Painful sexual intercourse

Dysphagia Inability to swallow

Dyspnea Breathing that requires marked effort

Dysuria Painful voiding

E

Edema Accumulation of fluid in the interstitial tissues

Electrical shock Interruption of body functions due to electrical current

Electrolyte Chemical compound that dissociates into ions when in solution; usually refers to extracellular sodium, potassium, and chloride

Embryo Stage of development from the second week after conception to about 8 weeks, during which time major structures and organs are formed

Empathy Ability to understand how another person sees a situation, while maintaining objectivity

Encoding Process of translating the purpose of a communication into a message that can be sent

Endogenous (autogenous) From a source inside the client

Endurance Ability to withstand physical or other stressors over time

Enema Insertion of fluid into the rectum and colon

Enteral nutrition Delivery of nutrition into the gastrointestinal system, usually in the form of tube feedings

Enuresis Involuntary voiding with underlying pathophysiologic origin after the age that bladder control is usually achieved; nocturnal enuresis is bedwetting

Environment Context in which a person lives; includes social and inanimate characteristics

Epidermis Thin, avascular, outermost skin layer

Eschar Black, leathery crust of dead tissue covering a wound

Ethics Professional standards of behavior related to right and wrong

Ethnicity or **ethnic identity** Shared cultural characteristics that symbolize a common group origin

Ethnocentrism Use of one's own culture to judge the beliefs, behaviors, attitudes, and values of people of another culture

Etiology Cause or origin

Evaluation Judgment of the effectiveness of nursing care in achieving client goals

Evidence-based care Approach to healthcare that emphasizes decision making based on the best available evidence and the use of outcome studies to guide decisions

Evisceration Protrusion of internal organs through an open wound

Excretion Process by which a drug or urine is eliminated from the body

Exogenous From a source other than the client

Extended family Family structure that includes grandparents, aunts, uncles, and cousins

Extracellular fluid (ECF) compartment Body fluid outside the cells; mainly interstitial fluid and plasma

F

Faith Belief held; a relational phenomena

Family Basic human social unit; membership is based on mutual commitment, heredity, or legal arrangements

Family-centered care Caring for the client and family as a unit

Fatigue A subjective state of weariness; lack of energy

Fats Lipid organic substances composed of carbon, hydrogen, and oxygen

Febrile With an elevated temperature

Feedback In communication, the sender and receiver use one another's reactions to produce further messages

Feedback loop Output is rerouted back to the system as input

Fetus Stage of development from 8 weeks after conception to birth

Fiber Component of food that adds bulk to the diet and is not broken down by digestion

Fidelity Being faithful to one's commitments and promises

Filtration Passage of a solution through a semipermeable membrane from a region of higher pressure to a region of lower pressure

Financial resources Allocation and expenditure of money

Fistula Abnormal tubelike passage between organs or between an organ and the body surface, often as the result of poor wound healing

Flaccid Without muscle tone or resistance

Flatus Gas in the gastrointestinal tract

Flowsheet Form for charting routine nursing procedures

Focus system Documentation system that organizes data entry around data (D), action (A), and response (R). The FOCUS can be a problem area but does not need to be. An entry can be positive growth or learning

Focused health assessment Assessment based on the client's problems; components include performing a general survey, taking vital signs, and assessing specific areas that relate to the problem

Foot drop Temporary or permanent plantar flexion due to weakness or paralysis

Foreplay Sexual activity before sexual intercourse

Foreskin Loose skin at the head of the penis, removed during circumcision; prepuce

Functional health assessment Assessment that evaluates the effects of the mind, body, and environment in relation to a person's ability to perform the tasks of daily living

Functional health patterns A framework for collecting and organizing nursing assessment data to ascertain the client's strengths and any actual or potential dysfunctional patterns

Futility Situation in which interventions are unlikely to result in desirable state

Future values Values that people would like to hold but momentarily lack the knowledge or skills necessary to integrate them into their lives

G

Gait Character of one's walk

Gastric lavage Irrigation of the stomach

Gavage Liquid food instilled into the stomach through the nasogastric tube; also called enteral nutrition

General anesthetic Agent used to induce complete loss of sensation and consciousness

General systems theory A systems framework that assumes all systems must be goal directed; a system is more than the sum of its parts; a system is ever-changing and any change in one part affects the whole; boundaries are implicit and in human systems are open and dynamic

Genetics Characteristics determined by the DNA code inherited from biologic mother and father

Gingiva Oral mucosa

Glycogenesis Anabolic process or glycogen storage; formation of glycogen from glucose

Goal Aim or expected end to which the nurse and client work together

Granulation tissue Soft, pink, highly vascularized connective tissue formed during wound repair

Granulocytes Polymorphonuclear white blood cells: neutrophils, eosinophils, and basophils

Grief Psychological and physiologic response after the loss of a significant person, object, belief, or relationship

Ground To connect electricity between an electrical conductor and the ground or earth

Growth Progressive increase in physical size or psychosocial development

Guaiac Test to reveal the presence of blood in feces

H

Hallucination False sensory perception: seeing, hearing, smelling, feeling, or tasting objects that are not there

Health (1) State of well-being and optimal functioning; (2) Interactive process between the person and the internal and external environment

Health maintenance activities Positive health behaviors to preserve a current state of health

Health maintenance organization (HMO) Organization that provides comprehensive health services to members for a set monthly fee

Health promotion activities Health behaviors that enhance a person's level of health

Hematocrit Percentage of red blood cells in a given volume of whole blood

Hematoma Localized accumulation of blood in a body tissue, organ, or space as a result of broken blood vessel

Hematuria Presence of blood in urine

Hemolysis Red blood cell destruction

Hemolytic transfusion reaction When a donor's blood is incompatible with the recipient's blood, hemolysis occurs as the antibodies in the recipient's blood quickly react to the donor's blood cells; symptoms are immediate and include facial flushing, fever, chills, headache, low back pain, tachycardia, dyspnea, hypotension, and blood in the urine

Heterosexual Person who relates sexually to a member of the opposite sex

High-level wellness Way of living in which a person strives toward the highest potential in physical, mental, emotional, and spiritual health

Holism Seeing the universe—and the client—as a system of connected parts rather than a sum of isolated parts

Home healthcare Healthcare services provided at home

Homeostasis State of balance in the body, including the balance of body fluids and their chemical constituents

Homosexual Person who relates sexually to a member of the same sex

Hormonal dyssynchrony Situation in which the circadian rhythms of different hormones adjust to changes in sleeping time at different rates

Hospice Family-focused health service that provides care for terminally ill clients

Host Person or animal who harbors and nourishes a microorganism

Human resources management Maximizing the value of the people who do the work of an organization

Hygiene Observance of health rules as related to self-care activities (bathing, dressing, feeding, and toileting)

Hyperalgesia Enhanced sensation of pain produced by a noxious stimulus

Hyperosmolar One compartment contains a greater concentration of a dissolved substance (hyperosmolar) than the other compartment (hypoosmolar)

Hypertension Abnormally high blood pressure

Hypertonic Of greater concentration than in body fluids

Hyperventilation Breathing in excess of metabolic demands, resulting in removal of too much carbon dioxide from the blood; indicated by decreased $PaCO_2$

Hypnotic Medication that induces or maintains sleep

Hypoosmolar One compartment contains a lesser concentration of a dissolved substance (hypoosmolar) than the other compartment (hyperosmolar)

Hypotension Abnormally low blood pressure

Hypothesis Statement that predicts the relationships between the variables under study

Hypotonic Of lower concentration than in body fluids

Hypoventilation Breathing insufficient to meet metabolic demands and adequately remove carbon dioxide from the blood; indicated by elevated $PaCO_2$

Hypoxemia Below normal amount of oxygen in the blood

Hypoxia Decreased amount of oxygen available to the tissues

I

Identity Awareness of self as separate and distinct from others

Ileostomy Opening of the ileum onto the abdominal skin surface via a stoma

Illiteracy Inability to read or write

Imagery Focusing the mind on a series of images for self-awareness, relaxation, and healing

Imaginal skills Skills that bring imagination and creativity into play

Impaction Accumulation of hardened feces in the rectum

Implementation Action phase of the nursing process in which nursing care is provided

Impotence Inability to attain or maintain an erection long enough to have satisfactory sexual intercourse

Incident Unusual happening to a client or visitor at a healthcare facility

Incomplete protein Protein that does not contain enough amino acids to independently maintain life, build tissue, or promote growth

Independent variable Variable that causes or affects the dependent variable

Infarction Dead tissue resulting from ischemia due to lack of circulation

Infectious disease Process resulting from infection that produces manifestations such as fever, leukocytosis, inflammation, or tissue damage

Infiltration Abnormal or accidental seepage or deposition of a substance into the tissues; accidental administration of IV fluids into subcutaneous tissues that occurs when the needle or catheter becomes dislodged from the vein

Information processing theory Method of organizing information to use cues to make accurate diagnoses

Information resources Sources of all types of data

Informed consent Legal document giving permission for surgical or diagnostic procedure signed by client or legal guardian; before signing, the physician has explained all aspects of the procedure, including risks

Input Information that enters a system

Inquiry Thoughtful questioning and drawing conclusions

Insomnia Difficulty sleeping; may be characterized by trouble falling or staying asleep or by waking too early

Inspection Systematic visual examination of the client

Instrumental skills Skills associated with basic physical and intellectual competencies that enable one to shape ideas and the external environment

Interferon Protein produced by the body cells on exposure to viruses that retards viral replication

Intermittent catheterization In-and-out catheterization performed on a routine, scheduled basis for a particular client

Intermittent claudication Limb pain caused by poor blood flow

International Council of Nurses Nursing organization concerned with health and nursing care throughout the world

Interpersonal skills Skills that determine a person's ability to relate happily and productively with others

Interstitial fluid Fluid between the cells

Interview Goal-directed conversation in which the nurse questions the client

Intracellular fluid (ICF) compartment Portion of body fluid contained within the cells

Intradermal Involving administration of a medication into the dermis located just beneath the skin surface

Intramuscular Involving administration of a medication into the muscle layer beneath the dermis and subcutaneous tissue

Intraoperative period Time that starts when the client is transferred to the operating room bed and ends with transfer to the postanesthetic area

Intravascular fluid Fluid inside the blood and lymphatic vessels

Intravenous (IV) Involving administration of fluid or medication within a vein

Intravenous therapy Infusion of fluid into a vein to treat or to prevent fluid and electrolyte or nutritional imbalances; may be used to deliver medications or blood products

Intuition Use of insight, instincts, and clinical experience to make judgments

Ion Charged particle formed by the dissociation of electrolytes in a solution

Ischemia Insufficient blood supply to a body part due to obstruction of circulation

Isolation Techniques used to prevent or to limit the spread of infection

Isometric exercise Exercise involving muscle contraction without a change in muscle length (often occurs against resistance)

Isotonic Osmotic concentration equal to that of body fluids

Isotonic exercise Dynamic form of exercise in which there is constant muscle tension, muscle contraction, and active movement

J

Judgment Process of reasoning; ability to process incoming stimuli and to determine meanings that encompass many aspects of a situation

Justice Principle of fairness; basis of the obligation to treat all clients equally and fairly

K

Kardex Trade name of a care plan documentation system

Key informant Person who knows and will discuss certain aspects of his or her culture with someone outside that culture

Korotkoff sounds Sounds heard during auscultation that indicate the systolic and diastolic blood pressure

L

Laceration Wound caused by tearing of body tissue

Laws Standards of human conduct established and enforced by the authority of an organized society through its government

Learning Multidimensional process of acquiring knowledge that depends on symbols, language, classifications, concepts, and other concrete operations along with abstract functions

Leukocytosis Increase in production of white blood cells

Liability Responsibility for one's actions; an obligation one is bound to perform

Libel False communication by means of print that results in injury to a person's reputation

Licensed practical nurse Person licensed by a state after completing a state-approved nursing program to provide technical nursing care under the direct supervision of a registered nurse

Literature review Process of selecting published materials about the concepts to be examined in a research study

Local anesthetic Depresses superficial peripheral nerves and blocks conduction of pain impulses from their site of origin

Loss Experience of parting with an object, person, belief, or relationship that one values; the loss requires a reorganization of one or more aspects of the person's life

M

Maceration Softening of tissue due to excessive moisture

Malignant hyperthermia Severe body temperature elevation after administration of certain anesthetics

Malignant pain Pain with recurrent, acute episodes, or persistent, chronic pain, or both acute and chronic pain associated with a progressive, malignant-type process

Malpractice Professional misconduct, causing harm or injury to a person from lack of experience, skill, knowledge, or judgment

Managed care Model of client care delivery in which the person's care from time of contact with the healthcare system to discharge is carefully planned and monitored to ensure that standards are followed and costs are minimized

Management Getting the job done or accomplishing a goal through the functions of planning, organizing, directing, and controlling

Maslow's hierarchy of human needs Theory that states that all humans are born with instinctive needs, grouped into five categories, and arranged in order of importance from those essential to physical survival to those necessary to develop a person's fullest potential

Masturbation Autostimulation of the genitals

Meconium First feces of a newborn

Medicaid Government-funded health insurance plan that provides financial assistance to the disabled or financially needy

Medical asepsis Measures taken to control and to reduce the number of pathogens present; also known as "clean technique"; measures include handwashing, gloving, gowning, and disinfecting to help contain microbial growth

Medical diagnosis Identified disease or pathologic process; treatment focuses on correcting or preventing specific pathology of specific organs or body systems

Medication Drug given for its therapeutic effects

Menarche First menstrual period

Menopause Permanent cessation of menstruation

Metabolism (1) Chemical reactions in the cells that produce heat as a byproduct; (2) Breakdown of a drug (usually in the liver) to an inactive form

Metacognition Thinking about thinking

Metacommunication Meanings beyond the literal level of communication, such as the roles of the communicators and the context in which communication is taking place

Method Procedure a researcher follows to gather and analyze data

Micturition Urination

Milliequivalent (mEq) Unit used to give the concentration of an electrolyte in solution; commonly expressed as mEq/L

Minority Smaller segment of society

Mnemonic A memory tool

Monosaccharides Simple sugars

Moral Involving correct behavior

Moral reasoning Judgments people make about right and wrong behavior within a social context

Moral values Values that involve correct behavior and deal with human interactions that involve the integrity of life or health

Motivation Something that provides drive or incentive

Mourning Behavior after the death of a significant other, which varies among cultures

Movement State of change in which behavior shifts toward a new and more healthful pattern

Myocardium Layer of cardiac muscle that forms the walls of the heart

N

Narcolepsy Sleep disorder characterized by sudden, uncontrollable episodes of sleep

National League of Nursing Organization that serves as the accrediting body for nursing education programs

Negligence Failure to do something that a reasonably prudent person would do, or doing something that a reasonably prudent person would not do

Networking System of meeting and establishing contacts with colleagues who share common interests

Neural plasticity Nervous system adaptation after pain

Neuropathic pain Pain caused by nerve damage

Neutropenia Decrease in the neutrophils in the blood, the white blood cells, responsible for quick response to invasion by infectious organisms

Nociceptors Free nerve endings that sense and respond to potentially noxious thermal, electrical, mechanical, or chemical stimuli

Noncompliance Failure to adhere to a recommended plan

Nonmaleficence Principle of avoidance of doing harm

Nonverbal communication Messages sent without words (e.g., gestures, facial expressions, postures, silence)

Normal flora Microorganisms commonly found in a body location that ordinarily cause no harm

Nosocomial infection Infection acquired during receipt of healthcare

Nurse administrator Nurse who supervises the organization of nursing care to ensure overall safety and quality

Nurse anesthetist (CRNA) Nurse who specializes and is certified in the administration of anesthesia

Nurse educator Nurse responsible for nursing and healthcare education in various settings

Nurse executive Top administrative nursing position in an organization

Nurse midwife Nurse with advanced education and certification in the care of women during pregnancy and childbirth

Nurse practice acts State guidelines that govern the practice of professional nursing

Nurse practitioner Nurse with advanced education and certification who may practice independently in various settings

Nurse researcher Nurse responsible for continued development of nursing knowledge and improvement of practice through research

Nursing Profession that involves diagnosis and treatment of human responses to actual or potential health problems

Nursing diagnosis Actual, potential, or possible health problem identified by the nurse that is amenable to nursing intervention

Nursing informatics Combination of computer science, information science, and nursing science designed to assist in the management and processing of nursing data to support nursing practice and care delivery

Nursing interventions Any treatment the nurse performs to enhance client outcomes based on clinical judgment and knowledge

Nursing monitor Review by a nurse of a client's care or records to determine the extent to which the care or records meet established standards

Nursing process Systematic approach to providing nursing care using assessment, diagnosis, outcome identification, planning, implementation, and evaluation

Nursing research Research that focuses on establishing a scientific base for the practice of nursing

Nursing theory Explanation or description of nursing issues that defines and predicts nursing practice

Nutrients Food containing elements for normal body functioning

O

Obesity Weight more than 20% over ideal body weight

Objective data Observable, measurable information that can be validated or verified

Observation Art of noticing client cues

Oliguria Formation and excretion of less than 500 mL of urine in 24 hours

Ophthalmoscope Instrument for examining the interior of the eye

Opportunistic organisms Organisms that invade the tissues when the body's defenses are suppressed

Orgasm Climax phase of the human sexual response cycle; men experience expulsive contractions of the entire length of the urethra, and women experience contractions in the outer third of the vagina and labia minora, as well as uterine contractions

Orthostatic hypotension Fall in blood pressure associated with a change in position (e.g., from lying to sitting to standing)

Osmolality Concentration of solutes in a solution, expressed as milliosmols per kilogram

Osmolarity Concentration of solutes in a solution expressed as milliosmols per liter

Osmosis Movement of a fluid through a semipermeable membrane from a region of lower to higher solute concentration

Osmotic pressure Pressure exerted by nondiffusible particles in a solution across a semipermeable membrane; tends to hold fluid within its container and is opposed by hydrostatic pressure

Ostomate Client who has a recent ostomy

Otoscope Instrument for examining the ear

Outcome criteria Specific, measurable, realistic statement of goal attainment

Outcome identification Formulation of goals and measurable outcomes that provides the basis for evaluation

Output End-product of a system

Overweight Body mass index (BMI) between 25 and 29.9 kg/m²

P

Pain threshold Lowest intensity at which a certain person perceives a stimulus to be painful

Pain tolerance Highest intensity of pain that the person is willing to tolerate

Palpation Use of the sense of touch to ascertain the size, shape, and configuration of underlying body structures

Paradoxical blood pressure Significant decrease in systolic blood pressure with inspiration

Paralytic ileus Condition in which the bowel is temporarily paralyzed and distention occurs

Parasomnias Group of disorders (e.g., sleepwalking, enuresis) involving autonomic and motor activity associated with partial arousal from sleep

Parenteral nutrition Nutritional elements supplied through an intravenous route, usually into a central vein

Partially complete proteins Proteins that contain sufficient amounts of amino acids to maintain life but do not promote growth

Participative leadership Style of a leader that involves subordinates in setting goals, solving problems, and making decisions

Pathogen Microorganism that can harm humans

Pedagogy Teaching as applied to children or adolescent learners

Pediculosis Infestation with lice

Peer review Evaluation and judgment of performance by other nurses

Perceptions Views of oneself and the world, influenced by culture, religion, family, experiences, expectations, and knowledge

Percussion Examination by tapping the body surface with the fingertips and evaluating the sounds obtained

Perfusion Passing of blood through an area

Peripherally inserted central catheter Long-line catheter made of soft silicone or Silastic material that is placed peripherally but delivers medications and solutions centrally

Peristalsis Motility and movement of the intestines

Person Human being; recipient of nursing care

Pharmacodynamics Study of the physiologic and biochemical effects of a drug on the body

Pharmacokinetics Study of how a medication changes as it passes through the body and undergoes absorption, distribution, metabolism, and excretion

Phlebitis Inflammation or infection of a vein, manifested by redness, swelling, and tenderness along the course of the vein

Phonation Process by which humans create vocal sounds

Physical examination Use of the techniques of inspection, palpation, percussion, and auscultation to obtain information about the structure and function of body parts

PIE charting System of documentation that incorporates the plan of care into the progress notes and structured according to problem (P), intervention (I), and evaluation (E)

Planning Management function of deciding what to do, when, where, how, by whom, and with what resources

Plaque Substance that forms and hardens on the teeth and is composed primarily of bacteria and saliva

Point of care documentation Documentation that takes place as care occurs

Poison Substance or gas that can injure or kill

Pollution Substances in air, water, or land that are potentially harmful to health

Polysaccharides Complex sugars

Polyuria Formation and excretion of large amounts of urine in the absence of a concurrent increase in fluid intake

Positional IV Term used when position changes cause the needle bevel or catheter to rest against a vein wall

Possible nursing diagnosis Health problem amenable to nursing intervention that requires additional data collection and validation before it can be confirmed or deleted as a nursing diagnosis

Postanesthesia care unit Designated area of the hospital or ambulatory care facility where immediate postoperative care is usually given

Postoperative period Phase that begins with transfer to the surgical recovery area and ends with recovery

Premature closure Selecting a diagnosis before analyzing pertinent information

Premature ejaculation Condition in which the man cannot delay ejaculation long enough for the woman to reach orgasm, or for satisfactory sexual intercourse to occur

Preoperative period Phase that begins with the decision to have surgery and ends with transfer to the operating room bed

Prepuce Loose skin at the head of the penis; foreskin

Prescription Directive written by a physician or other person legally permitted to do so (e.g., nurse practitioner)

Primary nursing Model of nursing care in which a professional nurse develops a 24-hour nursing plan of care and integrates that plan with those of other healthcare professionals

Primary source The client

Priority Nursing problem that takes on a position of prominence

Problem solving Systematic process that involves identifying and analyzing the problem, determining and weighing the possible solutions, choosing and implementing a solution, and evaluating the results

Problem statement Key step in the research process that identifies the direction a project will take

Proprioception Awareness of the position and movements of body parts in space, sensed by sensory nerve terminals in muscles, tendons, and the labyrinth of the ear

Protein Organic compound composed of polymers of amino acids connected by peptide bonds

Pruritus Severe itching

Psychomotor Relating to muscle movements resulting from a mental process

Puberty Period of life in which the sex organs mature, secondary sex characteristics appear, and reproduction becomes possible

Pulse deficit Mathematical difference between apical and radial pulse

Pulse oximetry Noninvasive means for approximating oxygenation that uses infrared light and a sensor attached to the client's finger or earlobe to determine the percentage of hemoglobin that has combined with oxygen

Pulse pressure Mathematical difference between systolic and diastolic blood pressure

Purulent Producing or containing pus

Pyuria Presence of pus in urine

Q

Qualifier Description of the parameter for achieving a goal

Qualitative research Involves the systematic collection and analysis of subjective materials, using procedures in which there tends to be a minimum of researcher-imposed control

Quality assurance monitors Mechanisms that ensure that a healthcare facility provides acceptable client care and upholds standards

Quality improvement programs Mechanisms for healthcare organizations to assess and improve care

Quantitative research Involves the systematic collection of numeric information, usually under conditions of considerable control, and analysis of findings using statistical procedures

R

Race Group defined by biologic characteristics

Racism Oppression and exploitation of people of a different skin color or ethnic origin

Range of motion Extent to which a person can move joints and muscles

Reality orientation Nursing technique to help restore the client's awareness of reality

Reflection Identifying the main emotional themes contained in a communication and directing them back to the client for the purpose of verifying and checking feelings that are being heard

Refreezing Long-term solidification of a new behavior pattern

Regional anesthetic Agent used to induce loss of sensation in a selected body area

Registered nurse Person licensed by a state to practice professional nursing; steps toward licensure include completing a state-approved nursing program and passing the state licensure examination

Relativism Theory that knowledge is relative to individuals, groups, and conditions and that there are various approaches to any situation

Reporting Sharing of client information by two or more healthcare professionals

Res ipsa loquitur "The thing speaks for itself"; invoked when it is impossible to prove who was at fault when a client's injury results from negligence

Research design Overall plan for collecting and analyzing data

Resonance Echoing of sound through passages

Resource management Accomplishing the work of a unit within the constraints of available resources

Respiration Exchange of carbon dioxide for oxygen in lungs and in tissues

Respondeat superior "Let the master answer"; doctrine in which a facility is held liable for an employee's negligence

Rest Physical and emotional state of decreased muscle and cognitive activity

Restatement Content portion of communication, in which the nurse, after listening carefully to the client, repeats the content of the message back to the client, to verify understanding

Restraint Device that prevents a client from moving or gaining normal access to a body part

Reticular activating system (RAS) Part of the brain responsible for bringing together information from the cerebellum and other brain parts as well as from the sense organs

Return demonstration Observing a client's performance of a new skill; this tool is valuable for evaluating psychomotor learning

Risk nursing diagnosis State of being at risk for the development of a health problem amenable to nursing intervention

Ritual Common and observable expression of culture

Role Expected function and behavior

Role ambiguity Occurs when the person lacks knowledge of role expectations, which fosters anxiety and confusion

Role conflict Occurs when a person's expectations concerning his or her role differ from the reality

Role strain Occurs when the person perceives himself or herself as inadequate or unsuited for a role

S

Sandwich generation Term used to describe adult children facing the dilemma of meeting their own generativity needs while assisting the older generation (their parents) and the younger generation (their children)

Sanguineous Pertaining to or containing blood

Schizophrenia Serious, persistent brain disease that is characterized by distortion of reality and difficulty processing information

Scientific rationale Reason for a nursing intervention that is supported by clinical research

Scrub person Wears a sterile gown, mask, headgear, gloves, disposable shoe covers, and eye protection, and provides the surgeon with required instruments, sponges, drains, and other equipment, anticipating what will be needed throughout surgery

Seamless care System in which all levels of care are available in an integrated form

Secondary sources Family, significant others, other healthcare professionals, health records, and literature review

Self A person's unique dimensions, potentials, and purposes

Self-actualization Process of developing one's maximum potential and managing one's life confidently

Self-awareness Knowing and caring for oneself; recognizing one's strengths and limitations

Self-care A person's ability to perform primary care functions in the four areas of bathing, feeding, toileting, and dressing without the help of others

Self-concept Mental image of oneself

Self-efficacy A person's belief that he or she is capable of doing something

Self-esteem Evaluation and judgment of one's worth

Self-evaluation Conscious assessment of the self

Self-expectation The self a person wants to be

Self-knowledge Basic understanding of oneself

Self-perception A person's awareness or identification of self; the filtering process of evaluating events and entering them into the subconscious

Sensation information Telling a client what he or she will see, hear, smell, taste, or feel in a particular situation

Sensoristasis State of optimal sensory input, which differs for each person

Sensory deprivation Lack of meaningful sensory stimuli; monotonous input or interference with the processing of information; leads to behavioral changes ranging from boredom to psychosis

Sensory overload State of arousal in which a person cannot manage the intensity or quantity of incoming sensory stimuli

Sepsis Poisoning of body tissues; usually refers to blood-borne organisms or their toxic products

Serosanguineous Containing serum and blood

Serous Thin, watery, serum-like

Sexuality Person's characteristics and perceptions concerning sexual expression

Shock Severe circulatory insufficiency

Sigmoidoscopy Diagnostic examination of the rectum and sigmoid colon

Single-parent family Family consisting of one parent and a child or children

Skin staples Type of wound healing device made of stainless steel that decreases the risk of infection and reduces tissue handling because they allow faster wound closure

Slander False communication by spoken word that results in injury to a person's reputation

Sleep Readily reversible state of altered consciousness in which awareness and responsiveness to the environment are decreased

Sleep apnea Condition in which, at least five times an hour, the client stops breathing for 10 seconds or more during sleep

Sleep deprivation State of having less sleep than needed

Sleep latency Time it takes one to get to sleep after going to bed

SOAP note Method of organizing charting entries so that each entry includes subjective, objective, assessment, and planning information

Social isolation State in which a person's desire for interpersonal relationships is perceived as unattainable; negative feelings of being alone

Social self One's behavior and interaction with others in social situations

Socialization Process in which a person is familiarized with the ways of a specific culture or group

Somnambulism Sleepwalking

Spasticity Sudden, involuntary increase in muscle tone or contractions due to central nervous system lesions

Spinal dorsal horn Site in the spinal cord where complex processing of messages occurs; one of the most important areas for pain modulation

Spiritual care Mutual, potentially healing or integrating process in which the client's spiritual needs are met

Spiritual dimension Quality beyond religious affiliation that strives for inspiration, reverence, awe, meaning and purpose, even for those who do not believe in any god

Spiritual well-being Condition marked by an affirmation of life and a sense of unity with God, self, community, and environment

Standard Precautions The latest CDC isolation system that combines the major features of Universal Precautions (bloodborne transmissions) and Body Substance Isolation (moist body substances transmission), thus protecting against blood and body-fluid transmission of potentially infective agents

Standards Statements of the required quality of nursing care that serve as the model for others to follow

Stereotype Preconceived belief about a person or people

Sterilization (1) Destruction of all bacteria, spores, fungi, and viruses on an item, accomplished by heat, chemicals, or gas; (2) Rendered unable to reproduce biologically

Stethoscope Device that collects and transmits sound, selects frequencies, and screens out extraneous sound

Stoma Artificially created opening of bowel on the abdominal skin surface

Stress State of arousal of mind and body in response to demands made on the person

Stressor Stimulus or event that requires coping or adaptation

Stroke Cerebrovascular accident (CVA); involves a sudden onset of hemorrhage, blood clots, or other vascular lesions, causing damage to the brain

Stroke volume Amount of blood ejected from each cardiac ventricle with each heart contraction

Subculture Beliefs held by a portion (e.g., occupational or age group) of the larger population

Subcutaneous Pertaining to the layer of tissue under the dermis

Subjective data Symptoms or covert cues that include the client's feelings and statements about his or her health problems

Sublingual Under the tongue

Suffering An emotional response to increased pain, associated with events that threaten a person's intactness

Suffocation Oxygen deprivation

Sundown syndrome State of disorientation and agitation that occurs at night in institutionalized clients who are oriented during the day

Suppository Medication inserted into the rectum or vagina

Surgical asepsis Refers to "sterile technique" in which an object is free of all microorganisms to prevent the introduction or spread of pathogens from the environment into the client; employed when a body cavity is entered with an object that may damage the mucous membranes, when surgical procedures are performed, and when the client's immune system is already compromised

Suture Material used to stitch together the edges of traumatic or surgical wounds

Synergism Medication interaction that increases a drug's effects

Systems skills Skills that help a person see the whole picture and the relationships between parts

Systems theory Way of viewing the world or an organization in which the parts are seen in relation to the whole

Systole Period of contraction of the ventricles

Systolic blood pressure Pressure in the blood vessels during cardiac ventricular contraction

T

Tachycardia Abnormally rapid heart rate, usually above 100 beats per minute in an adult

Tachypnea Abnormally rapid respiratory rate, usually more than 20 breaths per minute in an adult

Tangential lighting Light shining from the side to create shadows over the area being examined; accentuates subtle differences in contour and movement

Tartar Plaque that remains and hardens on the teeth, which cannot be removed by simple brushing

Taxonomy Classification system to organize information

Team leader Nurse in the team nursing model who manages the team

Team nursing Model of nursing care in which a team of registered nurses, licensed practical nurses, and nursing assistants are assigned specific functions or procedures to do for a group of clients

Theism Belief in God

Theory Explanation of the relationships among phenomena

Therapeutic communication Interactions that help a person express feelings and work out problems

Therapeutic effect A medication's desired and intentional effects

Therapeutic touch A healing meditation in which the practitioner assesses and treats the client's energy field and attempts to redirect any obstructed, disordered, or depleted areas

Thinking Mental activity in which one forms thoughts or intentions, determines by reflection, or attains clear ideas

Thrombophlebitis Blood clot that accompanies vein inflammation

Thrombus Blood clot in a blood vessel

Throughput Process by which a system transforms, creates, and organizes input, resulting in a reorganization of the input

Tonicity Fluid's effect on cell size

Tort Wrong committed against a person or property; subject to action in a civil court

Total parenteral nutrition (TPN) Administration of hypertonic solutions containing dextrose, proteins, vitamins, and minerals to provide for nutritional deficits

Trace elements Subgroup of minerals found in small amounts in food

Tracheostomy Permanent or temporary opening into the trachea through the neck

Transcultural nursing Synthesis of anthropology and nursing that focuses on the cultural dimension of care and recognizes that a person's cultural background influences and determines both health and illness

Transcutaneous electrical nerve stimulation (TENS) Mild electrical impulse to an area or over the pain zone and controlled by the client

Transdermal medication Topical medication that is released through the epidermis and dermis to the blood

Transfusion Introduction of whole blood or blood components (packed red cells, plasma, platelets) directly into a client's circulatory system

Transient ischemic attack (TIA) Temporary cerebral ischemia due to transient interruption in blood supply

Transsexual Person who psychologically sees himself or herself as a member of the opposite sex

Triage System in which provision of healthcare services is prioritized in order of importance

U

Unfreezing Recognition of the need for change and dissolution of previously held behavioral patterns

Urinal Metal or plastic receptacle into which the penis can be placed to facilitate urinating without spilling

Urinary incontinence Involuntary loss of urine from the bladder

Urinary retention Inability to empty the bladder of urine

V

Vaginismus Involuntary contraction of the muscles around the vaginal orifice, which makes sexual intercourse painful or impossible

Validation Reexamining information to check its accuracy

Values Personal standards for decision making

Values system Enduring set of personal principles and rules

Variable Property that varies from another

Variance Deviation that alters an expected outcome or date of discharge

Venipuncture Insertion of a needle or catheter into a vein

Ventilation Movement of air in and out of the lungs; breathing

Veracity Principle of telling the truth, essential to the integrity of the client-provider relationship

Vision values Future values

Vitamins Organic compounds that do not supply energy but are necessary to the body in small amounts for growth, development, maintenance, and reproduction

W

Wellness Dynamic balance among the physical, psychological, social, and spiritual aspects of a person's life

Wellness nursing diagnosis Diagnostic statement that describes the human response to levels of wellness in an individual, family, or community that have a potential for enhancement to a higher state

World view Unquestioned framework or predominant set of assumptions through which people view life

Index

Note: Page numbers in *italics* indicate illustrations; those followed by t indicate tables; those followed by d indicate display text; and those followed by p indicate procedures.

A

AACN. *See* American Association of Colleges of Nursing
AARP. *See* American Association of Retired Persons
Abbreviations
  in documentation, 234t–236t
  in medication order, 518, 520t
Abdellah, Faye Glenn, 58t–59t, 64t
Abdomen
  organs in, 431t
  physical examination of, 1111t
  quadrants of, 431t
Abdominal assessment, 427–435
  auscultation in, 430–433, 432p–433p, 433
  for bowel function, 427–433
  inspection in, 427–430
  landmarks for, 427
  palpation in, 433
  for urinary function, 433–434
Abdominal distention, 1109–1110
Abdominal girth, measurement of, 1112
Abdominal massage, in bowel training, 1132
Abdominal muscles, decreased tone of, and urinary elimination, 1069–1070
Abdominal thrust (Heimlich maneuver), 855, 856p–857p
Abdominal ultrasound, 1081
Abducens nerve (VI), assessment of, 416t
Abduction, 755t
Abduction pillow, as positioning aid, 784t
ABO blood group, 604
Abortion
  elective, 1373
  ethical/legal issues with, 1365
  in sexual function assessment, 1365
  therapeutic, 1373
Abrasion, 990, 990t
Absorbent antidiarrheals, 1122t
Absorption, 952
  intestinal, 1103
  of medications, 523
Abstinence, periodic, 1369
Abstract thinking, 219, 1224, 1226
Abuse, 1284–1285
  child, 288, 290, 1285, 1293
  client neglect, 1074
  documentation of, 232
  elder, 1285
  by healthcare personnel, 1230
  reporting of, 1293
  sexual, 290, 1285, 1362
  spousal, 312, 1284–1285
Accessibility, of client records, 249–250
Accessory muscle use, 816
Accidental wounds, 990, 990t
Accident-related infections, 1038t
Accidents, 282, 650
Accolate. *See* Zafirlukast
Accommodation, in cognitive development theory, 270
Accountability, 97, 218t
Accreditation, 27, 48
Accuracy, of client records, 231, 232
Acetaminophen
  for fever, 1055

  for pain, 1186, 1187t
Acetasalicylic acid, for pain, 1187t
Acetic acid, as antiseptic, 492t
Ace wraps, 1015–1017
Achilles reflex, 438t
Acid, 916–917
Acid-base balance, 910
  altered, 921–929, 924
    and activities of daily living, 928–929
    evaluation for, 937
    implementation for, 934–937
    manifestations of, 924–928
    nursing diagnoses for, 932–934
    nursing interventions for, 935–936
    outcome-based teaching plan for, 935
    outcome identification and planning for, 934
  assessment of, 929–932
  factors affecting, 918–921
  health promotion for, 934–937
  in home/community-based care, 936–937
  normal, 916–918
  regulation of, 917–918
Acidosis
  metabolic, 924
  respiratory, 924
ACLS. *See* Advanced cardiac life support
Acne vulgaris, 986
Acquired immunodeficiency syndrome (AIDS), 1036t
  culture and, 333–334
  healthcare workers with, 486
Active experimenters, 219
Active immunity, 1031
Active listening, 144, 217, 353–354
Active transport, 914, *914*
Activities of daily living (ADLs)
  altered bowel function and, 1110
  altered cardiovascular function and, 879
  altered cognitive function and, 1232–1233
  altered coping and, 1336
  altered family function and, 1285–1286
  altered grieving and, 1305–1306
  altered health maintenance and, 688
  altered human sexuality and, 1363, 1373
  altered mobility and, 766–771
  altered nutrition and, 963
  altered resistance to infection and, 1044
  altered respiratory function and, 816–818
  altered safety and, 659–660
  altered self-care and, 708–710
  altered self-concept and, 1264
  altered sensory perception and, 1205–1206
  altered skin integrity and, 997
  altered sleep and rest and, 1156
  altered spirituality and, 1388
  altered urinary function and, 1073
  fluid and electrolyte/acid base imbalances and, 928–929
  Index of Independence in, 710, 711t
  pain and, 1176
Activity and exercise, 65, *66*, 147d, 321
  aerobic, 760
  altered mobility and, 766–768
  anaerobic, 760
  assessment of, 161t, 399–400, 413p

  benefits of, 760
  and body temperature, 445
  and bowel elimination, 1105
  and bowel function, 1119–1120
  in cardiac rehabilitation, 902
  cardiovascular function and, 893–894
  and cardiovascular health, 872
  client teaching for, 365t
  and cognitive function, 1241
  in community assessment, 320d
  and coping, 1333, 1340–1341
  in family assessment, 316d
  and grieving, 1309t
  health benefits of, 1341
  and health maintenance, 684d
  in individual assessment, 311d
  isometric, 760
  isotonic, 760
  lifespan considerations, 282–283
  medications to promote normal function of, 515t
  mobility and, 759–760, 767t
  nursing diagnosis and, 180d
  postoperative, 640t
  programs for, 780–781
  and respirations, 459
  and safety, 653, 695
  and sleep and rest, 1151
  surgery and, 613
  types of, 760
  and values, 76
Activity intolerance, 766, 779, 884, 904
Activity orientation, 74t
Activity tolerance, assessment of, 778
Actual nursing diagnosis, 177t, 178, *178*, 179t
Acute care, *versus* home healthcare, 381
Acute care settings, nosocomial infections in, 483
Acute Confusion, 1237–1238
Acute infection, 1041
Acute pain, 1170, 1174, 1181
Acute wound, 990t
Adaptation
  characteristics of, 1328–1330
  in cognitive development theory, 270
  definition of, 1326
  evaluation for, 1344
  in home/community-based nursing, 1343–1344
  implementation for, 1339–1344
  lifespan considerations, 1331–1332
  nursing diagnoses for, 1338–1339
  outcome identification for, 1339
  physiologic functions related to, 1326–1328
  planning for, 1339
  sensory, 1200–1201
Adapted Symptom Distress Scale (ASDS), 1040
Addiction. *See also* Substance abuse
  to opioid analgesics, 1189
Addictive behaviors, as altered coping, 1334–1335
Adduction, 755t
A-delta fibers, 1168, 1173
ADH. *See* Antidiuretic hormone
Adjuvant analgesics, in pain management, 1192
ADLs. *See* Activities of daily living
Administration, 51

Administrative law, 98
Admission
    to healthcare system, 28, 29t
    reporting of, 248
Admission entries, in client record, 243
ADN. *See* Associate degree nursing program
Adolescent. *See also* Child
    activity and exercise in, 283
    bathing of, 719p
    bowel elimination in, 1104–1105
    bowel sounds in, 433p
    breath sounds in, 429p
    cardiovascular function in, 870
    client teaching for, 375–377
    cognition and perception in, 286–287,
        1225–1226
    communication with, 357–358
    coping and stress tolerance in, 289, 1332
    elimination in, 285
    family of, 1279
    feeding assistance for, 970p
    fluid and electrolyte balance in, 916
    grieving in, 1304
    growth and development of, 277
        cognitive, 278
        physical, 277
        psychosocial, 277–278
    hair care of, 731p
    health assessment of, 439
    health maintenance of, 683–684, 692d
    health perception and health management in,
        282
    heart sounds in, 424p
    in home healthcare, 382
    infections in, 1031
        prevention of, 505
    intravenous therapy for, 599
    medication administration for, 571
        inhaled, 542p
    mobility of, 763
    nutrition and metabolism in, 284, 955–956
    pain perception in, 1172
    peak flow monitoring in, 824p
    respiratory function in, 813
    roles and relationships in, 287–288
    safety of, 651–652
    self-care of, 706
    self-perception and self-concept in, 287, 1256t,
        1258, 1258–1259, 1268, 1268t
    sensory perception of, 1201
    sex education for, 1368
    sexuality and reproduction in, 289–290, 1358
    skin of, 986
    sleep and rest in, 285, 1149
    spirituality of, 1384, 1398
    surgery for, 622
    urinary elimination in, 1066t, 1067
    values and beliefs of, 73, 75–76, 76t, 291
    vital signs of, 444t, 475
Adolescent egocentrism, 277
Adolescent Pediatric Pain Tool, *1178*
Adolescent pregnancy, 290, 1358
Adoption, 330, 1277
Adrenal glands, *1327,* 1328
Adrenal medulla, stress and, 1329
Adrenocorticotropic hormone, and sleep-wake
        patterns, 1148
Adult
    activity and exercise in, 283
    antiembolism stockings for, 888p
    blood pressure of, 463
    bowel elimination in, 1105
    cardiopulmonary resuscitation for, 896p–899p
    cardiovascular function in, 870
    client teaching for, 377
    cognition and perception in, 287, 1226

    communication with, 358
    coping and stress tolerance in, 289, 1332
    elimination in, 285
    family of, 1279–1280
    feeding assistance for, 969p–970p
    fluid and electrolyte balance in, 916
    grieving in, 1304
    health assessment of, 439–440
    health maintenance of, 684–685, 692d–693d
    health perception and health management in,
        282
    Heimlich maneuver for, 856p, 857p
    immunizations for, 1054t
    infections in, 1031–1032
        prevention of, 505–509
    intravenous therapy for, 599
    medication administration for, 572
        inhaled, 542p
    medication dosages for, 530
    mobility of, 763
    nutrition and metabolism in, 284, 956–957
    pain perception in, 1172
    pulse rate of, 449
    respiratory function of, 813
    roles and relationships in, 288
    safety of, 652
    self-care of, 706
    self-perception and self-concept in, 287, 1257t,
        1259, 1268, 1268t
    sensory perception in, 1201
    sexuality and reproduction in, 290–291,
        1358–1359
    skin of, 986
    sleep and rest in, 285–286, 1149–1150
    spirituality of, 1384–1385, 1398–1399
    subcutaneous injections for, 555p
    surgery for, 622
    transfer of, 798p
    urinary elimination in, 1067
    values and beliefs of, 76, 76t, 291
    vital signs of, 444t, 475
Advanced beginner, in critical thinking develop-
        ment, 226
Advanced beginner nurse, 46t
Advanced cardiac life support (ACLS), 895
Advanced clinical practice roles, 117
Advance directives, 89, *90,* 102–103, 1308
Advanced practice nursing, 46
    client outcomes and, 187
    private practice, 25
Advanced registered nurse practitioners, 117
Advances in Nursing Science, 124
Adventitious breath sounds, 426–427, *431,* 817t
Adverse effects, of medications, 524
Advice giving, 357
Advisory Committee on Immunization Practices,
        of U.S. Public Health Service, 1052
Advocacy, 348–349, 348t, 387
Advocacy work, 13, 49–50
Aerobic exercise, 760
Aerobic metabolism, 765
Aerobic wound culture, 1049p
AeroBid. *See* Flunisolide
Aerosol therapy, 832–835, 836t
Aesthetic communication, in home healthcare, 388
Affective disorders
    and mobility, 765
    and self-care, 1230
Affective factors, in pain perception, 1174
Affective learning, 363
    teaching methods for, 373–374, 373d
Affective reflectivity, 226t
Affirmations, 1342t
African Americans
    and human immunodeficiency virus, 15
    and religion, 335

    and self-care health promotion, 260
    and sickle cell anemia, 1028
Afterburn, in sensory adaptation, 1200–1201
Afterlife, 1385
Age. *See also* Adolescent; Adult; Child; Infant;
        Lifespan considerations; Newborn;
        Older adult; Preschooler; Toddler
    and blood pressure, 463
    and body fluid variations, 910, 910t
    and body temperature, 445
    and health maintenance, 685, 686
    and respirations, 459
    and wound healing, 995
Agency for Health Care Policy and Research
        (AHCPR), 130–131
    on smoking cessation, 826
    urinary incontinence guidelines of, 1085
Agent, in host-agent-environment model of
        health, 256
Age spots, 986
Aging, and cardiovascular problems, 873
Aging parents, caring for, 1279
Agnosticism, 1383
Agranulocytes, 1028, 1030t
AHA. *See* American Heart Association; American
        Hospital Association
AHCPR. *See* Agency for Health Care Policy and
        Research
AHNA. *See* American Holistic Nurses Association
AIDS. *See* Acquired immunodeficiency syndrome
Air, as physiologic need, 63
Airborne precautions, 495, 496t
Airborne transmission, 482
Air embolism, intravenous therapy and, 597, 597t
Air-fluidized beds, for pressure ulcer prevention,
        1005, *1007*
Air Force Nurse Corps, 45
Air lock injection technique, for intramuscular
        injections, 560p
Air pollution, 655, 659
    and respiratory function, 813
Air vents, clogged, in intravenous therapy, 585
Airway, artificial, 843–847, *846*
Airway hyperreactivity, 815
Airway obstruction, 814–815
    emergency measures for, 851–855
Alarm systems, for safety, 666
Albumin, 603–604
Albuterol (Ventolin, Proventil), 459, 836t
Alcohol
    as antiseptic, 492t
    tolerance of, biocultural variations in, 334
Alcohol abuse
    and cardiovascular problems, 872
    and motor vehicle incidents, 656
    overdose, 656–657
    and respiratory function, 814
    and sleep, 1154
    and sleep apnea, 1155
Alcoholics Anonymous, as spiritual quest,
        1382–1383
Alcohol injections, in pain management, 1193t
Aldosterone, 911, 912
Alginate dressings, 1008, 1009t
Alignment, 755, 776
Alkalosis
    metabolic, 924
    respiratory, 924
Allergens
    reducing, 826
    and respiratory function, 813
Allergy, 1030t
    with blood transfusions, 607
    to medications, 524, 526
    and skin inflammation, 989
Allergy history, 398
    preoperative, 623

Allodynia, 1172–1173
Allostasis, stress and, 1326
Allostatic load, 1326
Aloe latex, 519t
Alopecia, 726
Alternative and complementary medicine, 261–264, 263d
Alternative/complementary therapies, 259
Alternatives, looking at, in therapeutic communication, 354–355
Altitude, and respirations, 459
Alupent. *See* Metaproterenol
Alveoli, 810
Ambien. *See* Zolpidem
Ambiguous genitalia, 1358
Ambulation, 788–794. *See also* Gait; Mobility
   assisting with, 788–793, 791p–792p
   mechanical aids for, 793–794
   muscle strength and, 794
   and respiratory function, 827
Ambulation belts, 793
Ambulatory care facility, 8
   documentation in, 245
   nosocomial infections in, 484
   sexuality and, 1375
Ambulatory surgical center, 613
   discharge from, 641
American Academy of Pediatrics, Committee on Infectious Diseases of, 1052
American Association of Colleges of Nursing (AACN), 45
   values statement of, 70–71, 71t
American Association of Nurse Executives (AONE), 110
American Association of Retired Persons (AARP), 1293
American Heart Association (AHA), 463, 468
American Holistic Nurses Association (AHNA), 261
American Hospital Association (AHA)
   Organizational Ethics Committees of, 97
   Patient's Bill of Rights of, 89, 91d–92d, 362
   on translators, 371
American Hospital Formulary Service, 515
American Journal of Nursing, 42t, 45
American National Red Cross, 41t
American Nurses Association (ANA), 45, 51–52, 310, 362
   Cabinet on Nursing Research, 124
   Code for Nurses of, 70
   Code of Ethics of, 71t, 86, 87d
   Commission on Nursing Research, 124
   definition of nursing, 45–46
   on documentation, 237
   founding of, 41t
   on home healthcare, 383, 384d
   on nursing diagnosis, 164
   on nursing education, 46–47
   on nursing process, 138, 139t
   on nursing research, 123
   on outcome identification, 186
   on pain management, 1186–1189
   quality improvement programs of, 211
   standards of, 51, 52d, 98, 140
   Steering Committee on Data Bases to Support Clinical Nursing Practice, 237
American Psychiatric Association, on sexual response, 1356
American Red Cross, 44
Americans, response to death and dying, 346
American Society of Hypertension, 471
Amino acids, 943
Aminophylline, 836t
Amitriptyline
   in pain management, 1192
   and urine color, 1070

Ammonia, and altered cognitive function, 1236–1237
Ampules, 544, 547p–548p
ANA. *See* American Nurses Association
Anaerobes, 1032
Anaerobic exercise, 760
Anaerobic metabolism, 765
Anaerobic wound culture, 1050p
Anal fissure, 1106
Analgesia. *See also* Pain management
   epidural, 1186–1189
   intrathecal, 1186–1189
Analgesics
   nonopioid, 1186, 1187t
   opioid, 1186
   postoperative, 619
Anaphylactic reaction, 524
Anatomic barriers, to infection, 1028, 1029t
ANCT. *See* Antineoplastic chemotherapy
Andragogy, 362, 363t
Anemia, iron-deficiency, 949
Aneroid manometer, 464
Anesthesia
   age and, 622
   and bowel elimination, 1107
   general, 635
   local, 635–636
   monitoring of, 635
   regional, 635, 636t
   responses to, 636t
   safety, 637
   and thermoregulation, 618
   and urinary elimination, 1070
Anesthesiologist, 635
Anesthetist. *See* Nurse anesthetist
Angina, 878
Angiography, 882t, 883
Angiotensin-converting enzyme inhibitors, and cardiac function, 892t
Angiotensin I, 911
Angiotensin II, 911
Animal fats, 944
Anions, 912, 912t
Ankle joint, 762t
Ankle restraint, 665
Anomia, 1231
Anomic aphasia, 1232, 1232t
Anonymity, in nursing research, 129
Anorexia, 957, 1263
   altered mobility and, 769
Anorexia nervosa, 961
ANP. *See* Atrial natriuretic peptides
ANS. *See* Autonomic nervous system
Antacids, and diarrhea, 1109
Antagonism, 524
Anterior pillar, *418*
Anterior-posterior (AP) diameter, 425
Anthropometric measurements, 964–965
Antiarrhythmics, and cardiac function, 892t
Antiasthmatic agents, 836t
Antibiotics
   for fungal infections, 1039
   preoperative, 618
Antibodies, 1030–1031, 1030t. *See also* Immunoglobulins
Anticholinergics, and urinary elimination, 1070
Anticipatory grief, 1300
Anticipatory Grieving, 1307
Anticipatory guidance, 1292
   and lifespan development, 281–291
   in pain management, 1184
Anticoagulants, and cardiac function, 892t
Antidepressants
   for dementia, 297–298
   in pain management, 1192
   and sleep and rest, 1154, 1160

Antidiarrheal agents, 1121, 1122t
Antidiuretic hormone (ADH), 911–912, 1068
Antiembolism stockings, 885–886, 887p–888p
Antiflatulence agents, 1121
Antigens, 1029
Antihistamines
   in pain management, 1192
   and sleep apnea, 1155
   and urinary elimination, 1070
Antihypertensives
   and blood pressure, 464
   and cardiac function, 892t
Anti-inflammatory agents, 836t
Antilipid agents, and cardiac function, 892t
Antimicrobial therapy, 1056. *See also* Antibiotics
Antineoplastic chemotherapy (ANCT), sensory responses to, 1202
Antipsychotics, for dementia, 297–298
Antipyretics, 1055–1056
Antiseptics, 492, 492t
Antispasmodic antidiarrheals, 1122t
Anus, 1102, 1103, *1352, 1353*
Anxiety
   and altered coping, 1336
   and altered self-concept, 1264
   and altered sensory perception, 1204–1205
   and critical thinking, 217
   and sleep and rest, 1153, 1160
   and urinary elimination, 1068
Anxiolytics, and sleep and rest, 1160
AONE. *See* American Association of Nurse Executives
AORN, 637
Aortic area, 421
AP diameter. *See* Anterior-posterior diameter
Aphasia, 1231–1232, 1232t
   anomic, 1232, 1232t
   assessment of, 1235d
   expressive, 410, 1231, 1232t
   global, 1232, 1232t
   receptive, 410, 1231–1232, 1232t
Apical artery, and pulse assessment, 454, *455,* 456p–457p
Apnea, 459, 812, 818
Apocrine sweat glands, 984
Applied ethics, 72
Applied Nursing Research, 124
Approximated wound, 995
Apresoline, 892t
Aquathermia pads, 1021
Arbovirus, 1034t
Area Agency on Aging, 1293
Areola, 1354
Arizona 2000: Plan for a Healthy Tomorrow, 26
Arizona State University (ASU) EAP and Wellness Program, 23–24, *24*
Arm
   blood pressure measurement in, 464
   circumference measurement of, 964, 965
Army and Navy Nurse Corps, 45
Army Nurse Corps, 44
Army Student Nurse Program, 45
Arousal, altered level of, 1230–1231
Arterial blood gas
   acid-base balance and, 932
   respiratory function and, 820–821
   values of, 821t, 918t
      and fluid and electrolyte/acid-base balance, 932
Arterial dysfunction, 874–878
Arterial oxygen level, and altered cognitive function, 1236
Arterial pulse, assessment of, 435
Arteries, 869
Arterioles, 869
   filtration pressure and, 915

Arthrograms, in mobility assessment, 778
Arthropods z, 1039
Arthroscopy, in mobility assessment, 778
Articles of the Nuremberg Tribunal, 128, 128d
Articulation, 1223
Artificial airways, 843–847, *846*
Artificial eyes, 735
Artificial immunity, 1031
Ascending colon, 1103
Ascending pathways, and pain perception, 1168
Ascorbic acid, and wound healing, 995
Ascribed role, 1255
ASDS. *See* Adapted Symptom Distress Scale
Asepsis, 480, 671. *See also* Infection control
    intraoperative, 637, 637d
    medical (*See* Medical asepsis)
    surgical (*See* Surgical asepsis)
    therapeutic dialogue, 497
Aseptic practices, 486–501
    barriers, 492–494
    cleaning, 491
    disinfection, 491–492
    handwashing, 488–491
    isolation systems in, 494–496
    sterilization, 492
Asian and Pacific Islander Americans, response to
        death and dying, 339, 346
Asphyxiation, 657–658
Aspiration, 814–815, 851–855, 976
Aspirin
    for fever, 1055
    for pain, 1186
Assault, 99
Assertiveness, 1340
Assessment, 139, 149–161. *See also* Evaluation
    activities in, 155–160
    aims of, 151t
    body systems model of, 160
    of bowel function, 1110–1116
    in client record, 230
    in client teaching, 365–368
    of cognitive function, 1233–1237, 1234d
    communication in, 350–359, 352d
    of community, 317, 320d
    confidentiality in, 158
    of coping, 1336–1338
    cues and inferences in, 159d
    cultural, 333, 334–337
    data collection in, 155–157
    emergency, 151, 151t
    of family, 313–314, 315t, 316d, 1286–1287,
        1287d
    focus, 150, 151t
    functional health patterns model of, 160, 161t
    of grieving, 1306–1307
    head-to-toe model of, 160
    of health maintenance, 688–691
    in home healthcare, 384–387, 385d
    of human sexuality, 1363–1366
    of infection resistance, 1044–1051
    initial, 150, 151t
    interviewing in, 152t, 153–154, 153t
    intuition in, 152t, 155
    of mobility, 771–778
    of nutrition, 963–965
    observation in, 152–153, 152t
    of pain, 1176–1181
    physical examination in, 152t, 154–155
    in plan of care, 191
    preparation for, 150–151
    questions in, 350
    and reassessment, 202
    of respiratory function, 818–821
    of safety, 660–663
    of self-care, 710–711
    of self-concept, 1264–1265

of sensory perception, 1206–1207
setting and environment for, 151
skills for, 151–155, 152t
of skin integrity, 997–1001
of sleep and rest, 1156–1157
of spirituality, 1388–1391, 1391d
time frames for, 151t
time-lapsed, 151, 151t
types of, 150–151, 151t
of vital signs, 443–475
Assimilation, in cognitive development theory, 270
Assisted ventilation, 841–843
Assistive devices
    for ambulation, 793–794
    for feeding, 736, *737*
    for older adults, 297
    for positioning, 784t
Assistive range of motion, 784
Associate degree nursing (ADN) program, 48, 130d
Associate nurse, 47
Association for the Care of Children's Health, 1293
Assumed role, 1255
Asthma, 815
    among inner-city children, 23
    medications for, and cardiovascular problems,
        872
    occupational triggers of, 826
Ataxia, 765
Ataxic gait, 766
Atelectasis, 814
Atheism, 1383
Atherosclerosis, 874–878
Athetosis, 765
Athlete's foot, 726t, 990
Ativan. *See* Lorazepam
Atrial natriuretic peptides (ANP), 911
Atrophy
    muscle, 754–755, 766–767
    skin, 993t
Atropine, 449, 1122t
Atrovent. *See* Ipratropium
Attachment, 287
Attapulgite (Kaopectate), 1122t
Attending, in cognition, 1224
Attention
    altered, 1231
    assessment of, 1233
    definition of, 1220
Attention deficit hyperactivity disorder (ADHD),
        286
Attitude
    and critical thinking, 217, 218t
    definition of, 70
Audiometer, 416–417
Audiovisual aids, for client teaching, 370–371
Audit, of client records, 230
Auditory assessment, 416–418, *418*
Auditory learners, 218
Auditory nerve (VIII), assessment of, 416t
Auscultation
    in abdominal assessment, 430–433, 432p–433p,
        433
    in blood pressure assessment, 470
    in bowel function assessment, 1112
    in cardiac assessment, 422, 423p–424p
    in cardiovascular assessment, 881–882
    in physical examination, 155, 409–410
    in pulse assessment, 458
    in respiratory assessment, 425–427,
        428p–429p, 819–820
Auscultatory gap, 470
Authenticity crisis, 1259
Authoritarian nurse-client relationship, 348t
Autoclaving, 492
Autogenics, in pain management, 1185–1186
Autogenic training, 1342t

Autolytic débridement, 1010–1013
Automated medication-dispensing system,
        516–517, *517*
Automaticity, 866–867
Autonomic blockade, postoperative, 639
Autonomic nervous system (ANS)
    and blood pressure, 463
    functions of, 1327
    and orthostatic hypotension, 471
    and pulse rate, 449
Autonomous neurogenic bladder, 1069
Autonomy, 89
Autopsy, 103
Avoidance behaviors, 682
Awakenings, per night, 1147
Axillary temperature, 444, 445t, 447, 452p–453p
Azmacort. *See* Triamcinolone

B

Babinski reflex, 760
Baby. *See* Infant; Newborn
Baccalaureate degree nursing program, 48, 130d
Bachelor of Science in Nursing (BSN), 15
Back massage, 717, 725p
    in pain management, 1183
Bacteremia, 1041
Bacteria, 480, 1032, 1033t–1038t
    in urine, 1080t
Bacterial infections, 989–990. *See also* Infection(s)
Bactericidal, 492
Bacteriostatic, 492
Bag baths, 716
Bailey v. Cooper Green Hospital, et al., 101
Balance, 755, 756
    assessment of, 399–400, 776
Baldness, 726
Bandages, 1015–1017
    application of, *1018*
Baptists, 1396t
Barbiturates, and respiratory function, 814
Bar code medication administration (BCMA),
        517
Bariatric (obese) beds, 1004
Barium enema, 1113–1115
Baroreceptors, 911
Barrel-shaped chest, 425
Barrier methods, of birth control, 1371–1373,
        1372t
Barriers, in aseptic practices, 492–494
Bartholin's gland, 1353, *1353*
Barton, Clara, 41t
Basal ganglia, and motor functions, 755
Basal metabolism, 953
Base(s), 916–917. *See also* Acid-base balance
    in blood, 917
Baseline knowledge, 365
Basophils, 1028, 1030t
Bathing, 704–705, 711t, 715–716
    in bed, 720p–722p
    in fever management, 1056
    in home/community-based care, 742
    methods of, 716
    nursing procedure for, 718p–719p
    types of, 715, 717t
Bathing/Hygiene Self-Care Deficit, 712
Battery, 99
BCMA. *See* Bar code medication administration
B-complex vitamins, 945t–946t, 947
Beans, in Food Guide Pyramid, 951
Beclomethasone (Beclovent, Vanceril), 836t
Beclovent. *See* Beclomethasone
Bed(s)
    bathing in, 720p–722p
    hospital, 739–742
    positioning client in, 785p–787p

positions of, 742d
  for pressure ulcer prevention, 1005, *1007*
Bed cradle, as positioning aid, 784t
Bedmaking, 742, 743p–746p
Bedpans, 738, *739,* 740p–741p
Bed rest, 765
Bedridden clients, infection control for, 1052
Bed scale, 401, 403p
Bedside commode, 738, *738*
Bedsores. *See* Pressure ulcers
Bed-wetting, 285, 1073, 1144, 1156
Behavior
  altered self-concept and, 1263–1264, 1269
  altered spirituality and, 1388
  definition of, 70
  self-destructive, and altered self-concept, 1264
Behavioral factors, in pain perception, 1174
Behavioral observation scales, 1237
Behavioral responses, to pain, 1175–1176, 1176t
The Behavioral System Model for Nursing (Johnson),
  60t
Behavior problems, in children and adolescents,
  291
Being therapies, 261
Beliefs. *See also* Values and beliefs
  definition of, 70
Bell, of stethoscope, 409, *409,* 409t
Belladonna alkaloids, and urinary elimination,
  1070
Bellevue Training School, 41t
Belt restraint, 665
Beneficence, 89
Benzodiazepines, 1160t
  in pain management, 1192
  and sleep and rest, 1160
Bereavement, 1300
Bernard, Claude, 259
Beta-adrenergic blockers, and cardiac function,
  892t
Bethanecol, and urinary elimination, 1070
Bicarbonate, 912, 912t, 917
Biceps reflex, 438t
Bicycle safety, 672
Bilevel positive airway pressure (BiPAP), 841
Bimanual palpation, 1366
Binders, for wound support, 1017
Bingo card, for medication distribution, 516, *516*
Biocultural variation, 334
Biofeedback, 1342t
  in bowel training, 1132
  in pain management, 1186
Biologic vectors, 482
Biotin, 946t
Biot's respirations, 460t
BiPAP. *See* Bilevel positive airway pressure
Bipolar disorder, 300t
Birth, 1355–1356
Birth control, 1369–1373
  during adolescence, 290
Birth control pills, and cardiovascular problems,
  872
Birth weight, average, 274
Bisexual, 1356
Bismuth salicylate (Pepto-Bismol), 1122t
Bladder, 1064–1065
Bladder credé, 1085
Bladder distention, 1071
Bladder function, assessment of, 401
Bladder neck, 1064–1065
Bladder retraining, 1084–1085
Bladder tone
  loss of, 1069–1070, 1071
  optimal, 1083–1084
Bladder training, 1084–1085
Blaylock Risk Assessment Screen (BRASS), 30, 31d
Blended family, 1277, 1284

Blind clients, feeding of, 736
Blink reflex, 760
Blood, 870
  acids and bases in, 917
  alterations in, 874
  components of, 603–604
  and gas transport, 810–811
Blood-borne infections, 1037t
Bloodborne Pathogen Standard, 656
Blood cell counts, 1411
Blood chemistries, 1412–1416
Blood chemistry tests, 882t
Blood compatibility, 604
Blood cultures, 1048
Blood donors, selection of, 604
Blood flow
  altered, 874–878
  and blood pressure, 461
  and cognition, 1226–1227
  through heart, 868
    distribution of, 868
Blood glucose
  levels of, 943
  measurement of, 959p–960p
Blood groups, 604
Blood poisoning, 1041
Blood pressure (BP), 460–473, 868
  abnormalities in, 471–473
  across lifespan, 444t
  age and, 870
  altered cardiovascular function and, 873
  assessment of, 464–473, 466p–468p, 882
    auscultation in, 470
    equipment for, 464–468
    errors in, 465t
    methods of, 468–471
    palpation in, 470–471
    postoperative, 638
    sites for, 464
  factors affecting, 463–464
    physiologic, 461–463
  fluid and electrolyte/acid-base balance and,
    927–928
  high, 871
  normal fluctuations in, 464
  pain and, 1175
  postural, 778
  therapeutic dialogue, 463
Blood products, 576
Blood tests, for kidney disease, 1081
Blood transfusion, 603–607
  allergic reactions with, 607
  complications of, 607
  febrile reactions with, 607
  fluid volume overload in, 607
  hemolytic reactions with, 607
  nursing procedure for, 605p–606p
  septic reactions in, 607
  techniques of, 604–607
  values and beliefs pattern and, 621
Blood typing, 604
Blood urea nitrogen (BUN) test, 1081
Blood vessels, of heart, 868–870, *869*
Blood viscosity, 461
Blue Sky Associates, 25
B lymphocytes, 1029–1035, 1030t
BMI. *See* Body mass index
Body, care of, after death, 103
Body cavity culture, 1048
Body fluid. *See* Fluid(s)
Body fluid culture, 1048
Body image
  altered, 1263
  positive, 1254–1255
  of toddlers and preschoolers, 1257–1258
Body language. *See* Nonverbal communication

Body mass index (BMI), 954, 962
Body mechanics, 756–759
  components of, 756
  and movement of clients, 757p–758p
  principles of, 756–759, 759d
Body-mind connection, 258
Body odor, biocultural variations in, 334
Body positions. *See* Position/positioning
Body-substance isolation, 494
Body system assessment, 160, 394–396, 395t
  in medication assessment, 528
Body temperature, 444–449. *See also* Temperature
  across lifespan, 444t
  assessment of, 446–449, 450p–454p
  factors affecting, 445–446
  measurement of, 446–449
    factors affecting, 446
    instruments for, 447–448
    methods of, 449
    outcome-based teaching plan for, 446
    scales for, 448, *449*
    sites for, 444, 445t, 446–448
  regulation of, 444–445
Body weight. *See* Weight
Bonding, 1278
  parent-child, 1360
Bone(s), and mobility, 754, 763–764
Bone marrow transplantation, 11
Borborygmi, 1112
Bordetella pertussis, 1034t
Boston Training School, 41t
Botanicals, 517–518
Bowel function/elimination, 1101–1138. *See also*
  Elimination
  altered, 1108–1110
    and activities of daily living, 1110
    in home/community-based care, 1137
    implementation for, 1117–1137
    nursing diagnoses for, 1116–1117
    nursing interventions for, 1120–1137
    outcome identification and planning for, 1117
  altered nutrition and, 963
  assessment of, 401, 427–433, 1110–1116
    acid-based balance and, 932
    diagnostic tests/procedures in, 1113–1116
    dysfunction identification in, 1111
    fluid and electrolyte balance and, 932
    normal pattern identification in, 1111
    objective data in, 1111–1113, 1111t
    physical examination in, 1111–1113, 1111t
    risk identification in, 1111
    subjective data in, 1111
  evaluation for, 1137–1138
  factors affecting, 1105–1108
  lifespan considerations, 1103–1105
  normal, 1102–1105
  normal patterns of, 1103
  outcome-based teaching plan for, 1119
  postoperative, 642
  surgery and, 618–619
Bowel habits, 1120
Bowel Incontinence, 1117
Bowel preparation, preoperative, 629–630
Bowel sounds, 432p–433p, 1045, 1112
Bowel training, 1104, *1132,* 1132–1133
Bowman's capsule, 1064
BP. *See* Blood pressure
Brachial artery, and pulse assessment, 454, *455*
Braden Scale, for pressure ulcer risk, 302d–303d,
  998, 999–1000
Bradycardia, 458
Bradypnea, 425, 459, 460t
Brain, 1220, *1222*
Brain damage
  and communication impairment, 1235
  and urinary elimination, 1069

Brain death, 1313
Brain stem, stress and, 1329
Bran, 1118–1119
Brand drug name, 514
BRASS. *See* Blaylock Risk Assessment Screen
Brawny edema, *881*
Breach of duty, 100
Breads, in Food Guide Pyramid, 950
Breakthrough pain, 1170
Breast(s), 1354, *1354*
  examination of, 427, 1366
    self-examination, 696, 1370d
Breast-feeding, 955
  and self-concept, 1257
Breast milk, 283, 284
  and bowel elimination, 1104
Breathing. *See also* Respiratory function; Ventilation
  deep, 828, 829p–830p
  increased work of, 814–815
  muscles of, 810
  normal pattern of, 812, 812t
  pursed-lip, 830
  shallow, 828
Breath sounds, 428p–429p, 819–820
  abnormal, 816, 817t, 819–820
  adventitious, 426–427, *431*
  infections and, 1045
  normal, 425–426, 430t
Brethine. *See* Terbutaline
Brewster, Mary, 41t
Bricanyl. *See* Terbutaline
Brief Pain Inventory, 1180
Brief Symptoms Inventory (BSI), 1040
Broad ligament, *1353*
Broca's aphasia. *See* Expressive aphasia
Broca's area, and cognition, 1220
Bronchial breath sounds, 426, 430t
Bronchial smooth muscle tone, altered, 814–815
Bronchioles, 810
Bronchitis, 816
Bronchodilators, 832–834, 836t
Bronchoscopy, in respiratory function assessment, 821
Bronchospasm, 813, 815
Bronchovesicular breath sounds, 426, 430t
Bronkosol. *See* Isoetharine
Brown, Esther Lucille, 42t, 44
Brown report, 46
Bruits, 418–419
Brushing
  of hair, 723
  of teeth, 729
BSI. *See* Brief Symptoms Inventory
BSN. *See* Bachelor of Science in Nursing
Buccal administration, 537
Buddhism, 1397t–1398t
Buddy system, 652
Budgets, 112
Buffering, in acid-base balance, 917–918
Buffer pair, 917
Building a Healthy Mesa, 25
Bulb, of penis, *1352*
Bulbourethral gland, *1352*
Bulk-forming agents, 1122t
Bulk laxatives, 1121t
Bullae, 991, 992t
BUN test. *See* Blood urea nitrogen test
Burns, 658, 991
  dietary modifications for, 972d
  minor, first aid for, 1007–1008
  prevention of, 670
Burrow, of scabies, 993t
Butorphanol, in pain management, 1188t
Butterflies, 1013

C

Cabinet on Nursing Research, of American Nurses Association, 124
Caffeine
  and cardiovascular problems, 872
  in pain management, 1192
  and sleep, 1154
Calcitonin, and calcium-phosphate balance, 913
Calcium, 912–913, 912t, 947–949, 948t
  as electrolyte source, 937t
  in older adults, 916
Calcium channel blockers, and cardiac function, 892t
Calendar rhythm method, 1369, 1372t
Call light, 739
Calluses, 726t
Calorie count, 965
Calories, 942, 954d
  excessive intake of, 957–958
Canada
  accreditation in, 48
  nursing education in, 48
  nutrient guidelines in, 942
  professional nursing in, 47–48
Canadian Association of University Schools of Nursing, 48
The Canadian Nurse, 42t
Canadian Nurses Association (CNA), 45, 52
  code of ethics of, 86, 87d
  founding of, 41t
  standards of, 51, 52d
Canadian University Nursing Students Association, 42t
Cancer
  and altered health maintenance, 687
  client teaching on, 695–696
  and nutrition, 961
  and spirituality in dealing with, 1387
  treatment of, and nutrition, 961
  and values, 72
  warning signs of, 696d
Candida albicans, 480
Candidal infections, 990
Canes, 793
Cannula, in oxygen therapy, 838p–840p, *841,* 842t
Cantor tube, 1126
Capillaries, 869
  dysfunction of, 878
Capillary refill time, 435, 881, *881*
Caps, 493
Capsule, 516t
Captopril, 892t
Carbohydrates, 943
  metabolism of, 952
Carbon dioxide
  diffusion of, 810
  transport of, 810–811
Cardiac arrest, resuscitation after, outcomes, 461
Cardiac assessment, 421–422
  auscultation in, 422, 423p–424p
  inspection in, 421
  landmarks for, 421, *421*
  palpation in, 421–422
Cardiac catheterization, 882t, 883
Cardiac enzymes, 882
Cardiac failure, fluid and electrolyte balance and, 921
Cardiac glycoside, 892t
Cardiac medications, and blood pressure, 464
Cardiac monitors, 901
Cardiac muscle, 868
  damage to, 874
Cardiac output (CO), 868–869
  decreased, 874
Cardiac rehabilitation, 901–902

Cardiac rhythm, assessment of, postoperative, 638
Cardiac surgery, therapeutic dialogue, 894
Cardiac workload, increased, altered mobility and, 768
Cardiopulmonary resuscitation (CPR), 674, 895–901
  Code Team, 895–900
  initial management, 895
  nursing procedure for, 896p–900p
  procedure following, 900–901
Cardiovascular disease, and infection, 1040
Cardiovascular function, 865–904
  altered, 873–879
    and activities of daily living, 879
    emergency care for, 902
    evaluation for, 902–903
    implementation for, 885–902
    manifestations of, 873–879
    nursing interventions for, 889–901
    outcome identification and planning for, 884–885
    risk factors for, 871
      modification of, 885
    signs and symptoms of, 892d
  assessment of, 879–884, 880d
    diagnostic tests/procedures in, 882–884, 882t
    dysfunction identification in, 880
    normal pattern identification in, 879
    objective data in, 880–884
    physical examination in, 880–882
    risk identification in, 879–880
    subjective data in, 879–880
  factors affecting, 869–873
  health promotion for, 885–889
  in home/community-based care, 901–902
  lifespan considerations, 870
  normal, 866–870, 866–873
  nursing diagnoses for, 884
  outcome-based teaching plan for, 903
Cardiovascular system
  function of, 867–869
  and safety, 653, 661
  stress and, 1337
  structure of, *866,* 866–867
Care. *See also* Nursing care
  coordination of, in home/community-based care, 749
  economic provision of, by family, 1277–1278
  physical provision of, by family, 1277
Care circle, 64t
Career development, 50–51
Career opportunities, 46–49
Caregiver Role Strain, 1287–1288, 1295
Caregivers, nurses as, 49
CareMaps, 194
Care partners, 117
Care plan, 141, 188–198, 237. *See also* Planning
  for Activity Intolerance, 904
  assessment in, 191
  for Caregiver Role Strain, 1295
  client goals in, 190, 192t
  and client record, 230
  in clinical nursing, 191–193, 194d
  collaborative, 193–198
  computerized, 194d
  for Constipation, 1138
  data collection in, 191
  for Disturbed Body Image, 1270
  for Disturbed Sensory/Perception, 1215–1216
  for Disturbed Sleep Pattern, 1162
  for Disturbed Thought Processes, 1248
  evaluation in, 191, 193, 193t
  example of, 191
  for Extracellular Fluid Volume Deficit, 938
  generic, 194d
  for Grieving, 1316–1319

for Health Seeking Behavior, 699
for Imbalanced Nutrition, 979
for Impaired Physical Mobility, 805–806
for Impaired Skin Integrity, 1024–1025
individual, 194d
for Ineffective Airway Clearance, 861
for Ineffective Coping, 1345
instructional, 190
nursing diagnosis in, 190, 191, 192t
nursing interventions in, 190–191, 192t, 193, 193t
outcome criteria in, 190, 192t
outcome identification in, 193
revision of, 210, *210, 211*
for Risk for Infection, 1059
for Risk for Injury, 676
scientific rationale in, 191, 192t, 193
for Self-Care Deficit, 750
for Sexual Dysfunction, 1375
for Spiritual Distress, 1400
standardized, 194d
types of, 190–193
for Urge Incontinence, 1099
writing of, 190
Care plan conferences, reporting of, 248–249
Caries, 704
Carotid artery, and pulse assessment, 454, *455*
Carriers, of infection, 482
Car seats, 651, *651,* 664
Case analysis
client preference in, 95
conducting, 97
contextual features of, 95–96
indications for intervention in, 94–95
model for, 94–96, 94d
quality of life in, 95
Case management, 9, 24–25, 117, 379–389, 1294
Casts, in urine, 1080t
Catabolism, 952
Cataplexy, 1155
Catecholamines, 1327
stress and, 1329
Catheter(s)
central venous, 598
condom, 739, 1085, 1086p–1087p
and decreased bladder tone, 1070
double-lumen, 1088
external urinary, 1085
Foley, 1088, *1094*
indwelling, 1076p, 1088, 1089p–1093p, 1092p, 1094, 1095
and infections, 1039
intermittent, 1088, 1096
multilumen central, 578, *579*
over-the-needle, 577, *579*
peripherally inserted central, 580, *580,* 598
postoperative, 642
silver-impregnated/coated, 1088
straight, 1088, 1089p–1093p
suprapubic, 1095–1096, *1096*
transtracheal, 837, 842t
triple-lumen indwelling, 1088, *1088*
tunneled central venous, 578–580, *580*
urinary, 1088–1097
and urinary tract infections, 1069
Yankauer suction, 847, *855*
Catheter coudé, 1088
Catheterization
cardiac, 882t, 883
urinary, 1088–1097
Catholic University of America, 138
Cations, 912, 912t
CBC. *See* Complete blood count
CBE. *See* Charting by exception
CBI. *See* Continuous bladder irrigation
CCNE. *See* Commission on Collegiate Nursing Education

CDC. *See* Centers for Disease Control and Prevention
Cecum, 1102
Celibacy, 1354
Cellular immunity, 1030
Celsius scale, 448, *449*
Center of gravity, 755, *756*
Centers for Disease Control and Prevention (CDC), 671
and consulting nurse services, 9
on infection control, 484
in isolation, 494
National Nosocomial Infections Surveillance System of, 483
on safety, 664
Central apnea, 1155–1156
Central cyanosis, 419, 816, 873
Central nervous system (CNS)
and central sensitization, 1173
functions of, 1326–1327
infectious processes of, 1228
stress and, 1329
Central sensitization, and pain perception, 1173
Central venous access devices, 578–580
Central venous catheter (CVC), removal of, 598
Central venous pressure, fluid and electrolyte/acid-base balance and, 931–932
Cephalosporin antibiotics, preoperative, 618
Cereal, in Food Guide Pyramid, 950
Cerebellum, and motor functions, 755–756
Cerebral cortex, *1222*
and cognition, 1220
and consciousness, 1222
and motor functions, 755
Cerebrovascular accident (CVA), 879
and cognition, 1227
and urinary elimination, 1069
Certification, 27
Certified registered nurse anesthetist (CRNA), 635
Cerumen, 705
Cervical canal, *1353*
Cervical caps, 1371–1373
Cervical mucus method, 1369
Cervical spine, movements of, 761t
Cervix, *1353,* 1354
Cesarean delivery, and sexuality, 1362
C fibers, 1168, 1173
Chain of infection, *481,* 481–483, 1028
Chair scale, 401, 402p
Change
in growth and development, 268–269
management and, 114, *114*
and spirituality, 1386
Change-of-shift reports, 247
Change theory, 64–65
Changing the subject, 357
Charge nurse, 118
Charting by exception (CBE), 240t, 243
Cheese, in Food Guide Pyramid, 951
Chemical barrier contraceptives, 1372t, 1373
Chemical barriers, to infection, 1028, 1029t
Chemical burns, 991
first aid for, 1007–1008
Chemical name, of medication, 514
Chemicals, and sleep and rest, 1154
Chemical safety, intraoperative, 634
Chemoreceptors, 1168
Chemotherapy
sensory responses to, 1202
and wound healing, 995
Chest, anatomic landmarks of, 422, *426*
Chest drainage, 844p–845p
Chest pain
management of, 893
respiratory function and, 815–816
Chest physiotherapy, 832

Chest tubes, 840–841
Chest x-rays, 820, 883, 1050
Cheyne-Stokes breathing, 425, 460t
CHF. *See* Congestive heart failure
Chickenpox, 1034t
Child. *See also* Adolescent; Infant; Newborn; Preschooler; Toddler
antiembolism stockings for, 888p
bathing of, 719p
bedpan use by, 741p
blood glucose measurement in, 960p
blood pressure of, 463, 467p
blood transfusion for, 606p
body temperature of, 453p–454p
bowel elimination in, 1104–1105
bowel sounds in, 433p
breath sounds in, 429p
cardiopulmonary resuscitation for, 899p
cardiovascular function in, 870
client teaching for, 375–377
cognitive function of, 1225–1226
communication with, 357–358
coping and stress tolerance for, 1332
deep breathing/coughing exercises for, 830p
enemas for, 1125p
falls of, prevention of, 668
family of, 1279
fluid and electrolyte balance in, 916
fluid requirements of, 934
foot and nail care for, 728p
and grieving, 1304, 1308, 1310d
hair care of, 731p
handwashing in, 491
health maintenance of, 683–684
heart sounds in, 424p
Heimlich maneuver for, 856p, 857p
hemoccult test for, 1115p
infection control for, 505
infections in, 1031
intermittent infusion technique for, 570p
intramuscular injections for, 560p
intravenous therapy for, 567p, 590p, 593p–594p, 596p, 599
medication administration for, 571
inhaled, 542p
oral, 536p
medication dosages for, 530
mobility of, 763
nutrition of, 955–956
oral care for, 733p
oxygen therapy for, 840p
pain assessment in, 1178, *1178*
pain perception in, 1172, 1172d
peak flow monitoring for, 824p
pulse oximetry for, 823p
pulse rate of, 449, 457p
respirations of, 462p
respiratory function of, 813
respiratory suctioning for, 854p
safety of, 651–652, 671–672
self-care of, 706
self-concept of, 1256t, 1258–1259, 1267–1268, 1268t
self-esteem of, 1255
sensory perception of, 1201
sex education for, 1368
sexuality of, 1358
skin of, 986
sleep and rest of, 1149
spirituality of, 1384, 1398
subcutaneous injections for, 555p
surgery for, 622
total parenteral nutrition for, 602p
tracheostomy for, 850p
transfer of, 798p
tube feedings for, 976p

Child (*continued*)
  urinary catheterization of, 1093p
  urinary elimination in, 1066t, 1067
  urine specimen collection from, 1077p–1078p, 1079
  values of, 73, 75–76, 76t
  wound cultures from, 1050p
  wound dressings for, 1013p
Child abuse, 288, 290, 1285, 1293
Childbearing, and stress, 1332
Childbirth, and stress incontinence, 1071
Childhood immunization schedule, 1053t
Childhood infections, 1033t–1034t
Chill phase, of febrile episode, 1043, 1055t
Chinese Americans, response to death and dying, 339
Chlamydia, 1036t
Chlamydia trachomatis, 1036t
Chlorhexidine gluconate (Hibiclens), as antiseptic, 492t
Chloride, 911, 912, 912t
Chlorine, as disinfectant, 492t
Chlorothiazide, and urinary elimination, 1070
Choking, 814–815, 851–855
Cholesterol, 871
Cholinergics, and urinary elimination, 1070
Chorea, 765
Christianity, 43
Christian Science, 1396t
Chronic Confusion, 1238
Chronic illness. *See also* Illness
  and altered health maintenance, 687–688
  and fluid and electrolyte/acid-base balance, 920–921
  in older adults, 301
Chronic infection, 1041
Chronic Low Self-Esteem, 1265
Chronic pain, 1170, 1181. *See also* Pain
  management of, 1182–1183
Chronic renal failure, coping strategies for, 280
Chronic wound, 990t
Chronic Wound Management Decision Tree (CWMDT), 203
Church of Jesus Christ of Latter Day Saints, 1397t
Chyme, 1103
Cigarette smoking. *See* Smoking
Circadian rhythm, 1147–1148
  aging and, 1149
  and blood pressure, 464
  and body temperature, 445
  disorders of, 1156
Circle of confidentiality, 349
Circular interaction, 313
Circulating nurse, 632–633
Circulating volume, and blood pressure, 463–464
Circulation. *See also* Blood flow
  coronary, 867
  maintenance of, postoperative, 642
  and mobility, 764–765
  movement, and sensation (CMS), assessment of, 436–437
  and skin integrity, 986, 1003
  and wound healing, 995
Circumcision, 434–435, 1352
Circumduction, 755t
Cirrhosis, dietary modifications for, 972d
Civil law, 98
Civil Rights Act, Title VI of, 337
Clarification, in therapeutic communication, 354
Claudication, management of, 893
Clean-catch urine specimen, 1075
Cleaning, 491
Cleansing, of wounds, 1010
Cleansing baths, 715
Clear liquid diets, 971

Client(s)
  attitude towards pain, 1179–1180
  introduction to, 397
  mistreatment of, 1230
  movement of, 757p–758p, 781–784, 788d
  neglect of, 1074
  preferences of, 95
  preparation of
    for health assessment, 396–397
    preoperative, 627
  value conflicts with, 80
Client advocate, 49–50, 348–349
Client-centered care, 117
Client decision making, 1205
Client discharge. *See also* Discharge planning
  reporting of, 248
Client goals
  barriers to, 209–210
  in evaluation, 208, 209–210, 209t
  facilitators of, 209
  in outcome identification, 188, 188d
  in plan of care, 190, 192t
Client record, 230–245. *See also* Documentation
  access to, 249–250
  accuracy of, 231, 232
  admission entries in, 243
  completeness of, 231–232
  conciseness of entries, 233
  confidentiality of, 249
  as data source, 157
  discharge summary in, 243–245, *244*
  as education tool, 231
  errors in, 232, *233*
  incident reports in, 245
  Kardex, 238, *239*
  as legal document, 231
  medication record in, 245, *246*
  nursing entries on, 237–245
  nursing progress notes and, 238–242
  in nursing research, 231
  objectivity of, 233
  organization of, 233
  plan of care and, 237
  purpose of, 230–231
  timeliness of, 233
  universal computer-based patient record, 236–237
Client resistance, and nosocomial infections, 483
Client response, knowledge of, in evaluation, 207
Client satisfaction, measurement of, 57
Client Satisfaction Tool (CST), 57
Client's rights, and medication administration, 522
Client teaching, 361–377
  about common illnesses, 694–696
  for altered bowel function, 1117–1120
  for altered cardiovascular function, 889
  for altered urinary function, 1083–1084
  amount of information in, 372
  assessment in, 365–368
  communication in, 373
  for coping, 365
  culture and, 337–338
  during discharge, 746
  for disease prevention, 364
  documentation in, 374
  environment for, 372–373
  evaluation of learning in, 374
  for families, 1292
  family/friend involvement in, 372
  for grieving, 1308–1309
  for health restoration, 364–365, 365t
  in home healthcare, 387
  implementation of, 372–374
  individualized teaching sessions in, 373
  for intravenous therapy, 607–608
  learning readiness in, 367–368

  lifespan considerations, 375–377
  methods of, 373–374, 373d
  nursing diagnoses in, 368
  for nutrition, 967, 977
  oral tests in, 374
  outcome identification in, 368
  in parenteral nutrition, 607–608
  planning in, 368–372
  preoperative, 624–626, 628, 628t
  priorities in, 366–367, 372
  purposes of, 364–365, 365t
  realistic approach to, 367
  repetition in, 373
  return demonstration in, 374
  for self-care, *695*
  self-study, 8
  for sensory perception, 1209
  for sexuality, 1368–1369
  simulations in, 374
  for skin integrity, 1003
  teaching-learning process in, 362–364
  teaching-learning relationship in, 364
  teaching methods in, 373–374, 373d
  teaching opportunities in, 366t
  teaching strategies in, 368–372
  therapeutic dialogue, 376
  timing of, 372
  translators in, 371
  for wellness promotion, 364
  written teaching plan in, 372
  written tests in, 374
Client transfer, 711t, 794–801
  from bed to chair, 802p–803p
  equipment for, 801t
  ethical/legal issues of, 1333
  reporting of, 248
  to stretcher, 798p
  to wheelchair, 799p–800p
Client transport
  of client with infectious disease, 494
  to recovery facility, 637–638
  safety of, 665
Climacteric, 1358
Clinical Assessment of Confusion, 1233, 1237
Clinical experience, 220
Clinical judgment, 94
Clinical model, of health, 256
Clinical nurse specialist, 50, 117
Clinical nursing
  nursing research and, 129–132
  plans of care in, 191–193, 194d
Clinical Nursing - A Helping Art (Weidenbach), 59t–60t
Clinical nursing teachers, 223
Clinical practice roles, 114–117
Clinical reasoning, 220
Clinical research, 129–130
  multidisciplinary, 130–131
Clinical study, values in, 73
Clinics
  admission to, 29t
  surgery in, 612–613
Clips, for wound support, 1013–1015
Clitoris, 1353, *1353*
Clonidine, in pain management, 1193t
Closed systems, 313
Closed wound, 990t
Clostridium difficile, and diarrhea, 1109
Clostridium tetani, 1038t
Clove-hitch knot, 666, *667*
Cloze test, 368
Clubbing, 420, *420,* 816
Clusters. *See* Cue clustering
CMS. *See* Circulation, movement, and sensation
CNA. *See* Canadian Nurses Association
CO. *See* Cardiac output

Coagulation-related tests, laboratory values for, 1411
Coalition for Accountable Managed Care, 82–83
Cobalamin, 946t, 947
Cocaine, and cardiovascular problems, 872
Code for Nurses, of American Nurses Association, 70
Codeine, 1122t, 1188t
Code of Ethics for Nurses, of ANA, 86
Codes of ethics, 87d–88d
Coexistent medical problems, and infection, 1040
Cognition and perception, 66, *66,* 147d, 321
    anatomic structures involved in, 1220
    assessment of, 161t, 401–404, 410, 411p–412p
    cardiovascular function and, 878–879
    client teaching for, 365t
    in community assessment, 320d
    definition of, 1220
    in family assessment, 316d
    grieving and, 1309t
    and health maintenance, 684d, 685, 686
    in individual assessment, 311d
    and lifespan development, 286–287
    medications to promote normal function of, 515t
    mobility and, 767t, 770
    nursing diagnosis and, 180d–181d
    postoperative, 640t
    and sexuality, 1359
    surgery and, 619
    and values, 76
Cognitive development
    of adolescent, 278
    of infant, 275
    intrauterine, 274
    of middle adult, 279
    of newborn, 274–275
    of older adult, 280
    of preschooler, 276
    of school-age child, 277
    theories of, 270, 271t, 272t
    of toddler, 276
    of young adult, 278
Cognitive dysfunction, altered sensory perception and, 1205
Cognitive factors, in pain perception, 1174
Cognitive function
    altered, 1230–1233
        and activities of daily living, 1232–1233
        in home/community-based nursing, 1246–1247
        nursing diagnoses for, 1237–1240
        nursing interventions for, 1241–1247
        outcome-based teaching plan for, 1242d
        outcome identification and planning for, 1240
    assessment of, 1233–1237, 1234d
        diagnostic tests/procedures in, 1236–1237
        dysfunction identification in, 1235–1236
        normal pattern identification in, 1233–1235
        objective data in, 1236–1237
        physical examination, 1236
        risk identification in, 1235
        subjective data in, 1233–1236
    cardiovascular function and, 880
    evaluation for, 1247–1248
    factors affecting, 1226–1230
    and home healthcare, 382
    implementation for, 1240–1247
    lifespan considerations, 1225–1226
    normal, 1220–1223
        characteristics of, 1223–1224
        patterns of, 1224
    of older adults, 297–298
    and self-care, 707
    tests of, 1237

Cognitive learning, 363
    teaching methods for, 373, 373d
Cognitive nursing interventions, 204, 205t
Cohabited family, 1277
COI. *See* Concrete objective information
Coitus interruptus, 1373, 1373t
Cold compresses, 1021
Cold medications, and cardiovascular problems, 872
Cold packs, 1019–1021
Cold therapy
    in pain management, 1183
    safety of, 1020t
    uses for, 1020t
    for wound healing, 1018–1021
Collaboration and delegation
    ambulation assistance, 792p, 797p
    antiembolism stockings, 888p
    auscultation of bowel sounds, 433p
    auscultation of breath sounds, 429p
    auscultation of heart sounds, 424p
    bathing, 719p
    bedmaking, 746p, 748p
    bedpan use, 741p
    blood pressure assessment, 468p
    blood transfusion, 606p
    body temperature assessment, 454p
    cardiopulmonary resuscitation, 900p
    chest drainage, 845p
    client transfer, 798p, 803p
    condom catheter application, 1087p
    deep breathing/coughing exercises, 830p
    enemas, 1125p
    fecal ostomy pouch, 1136p
    foot and nail care, 728p
    glove use, 503p, 505p
    gown use, 505p
    hair care, 731p
    handwashing, 490p
    Heimlich maneuver, 857p
    hemoccult test, 1115p
    incentive spirometry, 832p
    inhaled medications, 542p
    intravenous therapy, 590p, 594p, 596p
    movement of clients, 758p
    nasogastric intubation, 1131p
    and neurologic assessment, 414p
    oral administration, 536p
    oral care, 734p
    oxygen therapy, 840p
    peak flow monitoring, 824p
    positioning in bed, 787p
    pulse assessment, 457p
    pulse oximetry, 823p
    range of motion exercises, 790p
    respiratory assessment, 462p
    respiratory suctioning, 855p
    sequential compression device application, 891p
    sterile fields, 508p
    surgical scrub, 501p
    total parenteral nutrition, 602p
    tracheostomy, 851p
    urinary catheterization, 1093p
    urine specimen collection, 1078p
    weight measurement, 403p
    wheelchair transfer, 800p
    wound cultures, 1050p
    wound dressings, 1013p
    wound suction, 1019p
Collaborative care plan, 193–198
    for congestive heart failure, 875–877
    example of, 195–197, 614–617
    for total hip replacement, 772–775
Collaborative health problems, 168, 168t
    interventions for, 203
Collaborative learners, 219

Collecting duct, 1064
Collett-Lester Fear of Death Scale, 346
Colloid oncotic pressure, 914
Colloid solutions, 576–577
Colon, 1102, 1103
Colonization, 1041
Colonoscopy, 1116
Color
    of skin, 985, 998
    as symbol, 326
    of urine, 1080t
Colorectal screening, 1120
Colostomy, 1107, *1107*
    irrigation of, 1136, *1136*
Coma, Glasgow Coma Scale and, 410, 414t
Combing, of hair, 723
Comfort, postoperative, 643
Comfort measures, for altered resistance to infection, 1054–1055
Commission on Collegiate Nursing Education (CCNE), 48, 52
Commission on Nursing Research, of American Nurses Association, 124
Commitment, 219
Committee on Infectious Diseases, of American Academy of Pediatrics, 1052
Commode, bedside, 738, *738*
Common cold, 1033t
Communal family, 1277
Communicable disease, 1041–1043
Communicable period, of infections, 1041
Communication, 1224
    with adults and older adults, 358
    altered, 1226
    alternative methods of, 1242–1243
    and assessment, 350–359, 352d
    assessment of, 410, 1233, 1235d
    with children and adolescents, 357–358
    in client teaching, 373
    cross-cultural, 358–359, 359d
    definition of, 344, 1220
    development of skills, 355, 356t
    and experience, 345–346
    guidelines for, 353d
    in home healthcare, 388
    impaired, 1231–1232
    in implementation, 202
    in intensive care unit, 359
    in interviews, 153, 153t
    and language, 345–346
    language barriers and, 1230
    as management responsibility, 113
    nonverbal, 113, 344, 344d, 359, 396, 397, 1224
    in nurse-client relationship, 343–359
    and nursing process, 350–359
    in nursing process, 144
    of older adults, 297–298
    oral (*See* Reporting)
    process of, *344,* 344–346
    self-concept and, 1227
    skin and, 985
    special situations in, 357–359
    therapeutic, 349–350, 353t, 1244
    through client record, 230
    with tracheostomy, 846–847
    translators for, 359, 359d
    types of, 344–345, 344d
    verbal, 113, 344, 344d, 1224
    written (*See* Documentation)
Communication channel, 345
Communicators, nurses as, 50
Community, 314–320
    advanced concepts of, 318–320
    assessment of, 317, 320d
    definition of, 315–316
    and functional health patterns, 317, 320d

Community (*continued*)
    functional health patterns of, 320–322
    and health promotion, 682
    and home healthcare, 381, 387
    nursing interventions for, 318t–319t
    and safety, 653
    types of, 316–317, 317t, 318t–319t
    and values, 74
Community-based healthcare, 21
    bowel function in, 1137
    cognitive function in, 1246
    complementary and alternative services in,
        27–28
    continuity of, 28–33
    discharge planning in, 29–33
    entrance and exit within, 28–33
    for families, 1293–1294
    fragmentation of service in, 27
    grieving in, 1311–1312
    health maintenance in, 697
    infections in, 1057–1058
    intravenous therapy in, 607–608
    medication administration in, 562–564
    nutrition in, 977
    pain management in, 1194
    parenteral nutrition in, 607–608
    quality of care in, 27
    resources for, 1425–1432
    safety in, 673, 674–675
    self-care and, 28
    self-concept in, 1269–1270
    sensory perception in, 1211–1214
    sexuality in, 1374–1375
    shift to, 8
    skin integrity in, 1021–1022
    sleep and rest in, 1160
    spirituality in, 1399
    stress, coping, and adaptation in, 1343–1344
    trends in, 20–21, *21*
    and urinary dysfunction, 1097–1098
Community-based no code order, 103
Community-based nursing, 22–26
    cardiovascular function in, 901–902
    competencies needed for, 26, 27d
    definition of, 22
    fluid, electrolyte, and acid-base balance in,
        936–937
    focus of care in, 22
    global initiatives for, 25–26
        discipline specific, 25–26
        interdisciplinary, 25
    mobility in, 801–804
    postoperative, 643
    respiratory function in, 858–860
    in schools, 23
    self-care in, 742–749
    settings for, 22–25
    therapeutic dialogue for, 322
    transition of, 22
    web sites regarding, 26d
Community coalitions, 25
Community healthcare agencies, 8–9
Community health nursing, 22
Community nursing centers, 22–25, 23d
Community resources, in home healthcare, 383,
    388–389
Compensation
    in acid-base balance, 918
    renal, 918
    respiratory, 918
Competence
    in critical thinking development, 226
    and self-esteem, 1255
Competent nurse, 46t
Competitive learners, 219

Complementary and alternative healthcare ser-
    vices, in community-based care, 27–28
Complementary and alternative medicine (CAM),
    261–262
    ethics and, 264
    modalities of, 263–264, 263d
Complement system, 1031
Complete blood count (CBC), 882, 882t
Completeness, of client record, 231–232
Complete proteins, 943
Compliance
    in client teaching, 367
    with medication routine, 528–529, 563
Comprehension, 1223
Comprehensive Drug Abuse Prevention and
    Control Act, 102, 521
Comprehensive health assessment, 394
Compromised Family Coping, 1289
Compromised host, 1039–1041
Computed axial tomography (CT) scan
    in infection detection, 1050–1051
    of urinary system, 1081
Computer-based personal record, 236–237
Computerized plan of care, 194d
Computers, and documentation, 233–237
Conception, 1355–1356
Conceptual framework, 56
Conceptual reflectivity, 226t
Conciseness, of client record, 233
Concluding phase, of interview process, 154
Concrete objective information (COI), 8
Concrete thinkers, 219
Concrete thinking, 1224
Condom catheter, 739
    application of, nursing procedure for,
        1086p–1087p
    for urinary elimination, 1085
Condoms, 1369, 1373
Conduct disorders, in children and adolescents,
    291
Conduction, and heat loss, 445
Conduction system, of heart, 866–867, *867*
    problems with, 874
Conerly v. State, 100
Confidence, 218t
Confidentiality, 230, 249
    of assessment findings, 158
    in health assessment, 396
    of nurse-client relationship, 349
    in nursing research, 129
    in professional-patient relationship, 93–94
Confusion, 1228, 1228t, 1230, 1246
    in older adults, 1154
    postoperative, 619, 1154
Congenital disorders, and mobility, 765
Congestive heart failure (CHF)
    collaborative care plan for, 875–877
    dietary modifications for, 972d
Conjunctivitis, and work restriction, 487t
Connected knowledge, 219
Connecticut Training School, 41t
Consciousness, 1222
    assessment of, 1233
    definition of, 1220
    level of, 410
Conscious sedation, 636–637
Conservation Model (Levin), 60t
Conservative thinkers, 219
Constipation, 1106, 1108, 1116, 1118
    altered mobility and, 770
    medications for, 1120–1121, 1121t
    nursing plan of care for, 1138
    in older adults, 1105
    postoperative, 642
    during pregnancy, 1106
    treatment for, 1120

Consulting nurse services unit, 9
Consumerism, 10–11
Contact lenses, 734–735
    removing, nursing procedure for, 1212p
Contact precautions, 495, 496t
Contact transmission, 482
Continence, 711t
Continent fecal diversion, 1107–1108
    management of, 1136–1137
Continent ileostomy, 1107–1108
Continuous bladder irrigation (CBI), *1095*
Continuous breath sounds, 817t
Continuous enteral tube feedings, 973,
    975p–976p
Continuous infusion technique, in intravenous
    administration, 556–560
Continuous positive airway pressure (CPAP), 841
Continuous quality improvement, 210–212, 230
Contraception, 1369–1373, 1372t–1373t
Contract, in nurse-client relationship, 347–348,
    348d
Contractility, of cardiac muscle, 868
Contraction, of muscles, 754
Contractures, 766, 767–768
Contralateral stimulation, in pain management,
    1183–1184
Controlled substances, 521t
    administration of, 521–522
    laws concerning, 102
Controlled Substances Act, 521, 521t
Contusion, 990t
Convalescent period, of infections, 1041
Convection, and heat loss, 445
Cool-water bath, 717t
Coordinated movement, 755–756
Coordinating nursing interventions, 204–205
Coordination
    assessment of, 776
    in discharge planning, 30, *32*
    lack of, and altered mobility, 765
Coordination of care, in home/community-based
    care, 388, 749
Coping and stress tolerance, 66, *66*, 147d, 321
    altered, 1334–1336
        and activities of daily living, 1336
        evaluation for, 1344
        implementation for, 1339–1344
        nursing diagnoses for, 181d, 1338–1339
        nursing interventions for, 1342–1343
        outcome identification and planning for, 1339
    altered mobility and, 770–771
    assessment of, 161t, 405, 1336–1338
        dysfunction identification in, 1337
        normal pattern identification in, 1336–1337
        objective data in, 1337–1338
        risk identification in, 1337
        subjective data in, 1336–1337
    characteristics of, 1328–1330
    with chronic renal failure, 280
    client teaching for, 365, 365t
    in community assessment, 320d
    definition of, 1326
    emotion-focused, 1331d
    factors affecting, 1332–1334
    and family, 1281
    in family assessment, 316d
    grieving and, 1309t
    and health maintenance, 684d, 687
    in home/community-based nursing, 1343–1344
    in individual assessment, 311d
    lifespan considerations, 1331–1332
    and lifespan development, 288–289
    long-term, 1331d
    medications to promote normal function of,
        515t
    mobility and, 767t

normal, 1326–1332
  patterns of, 1330–1331, 1331d
of older adults, 305
with pain, 1175d
physiologic functions related to, 1326–1328
postoperative, 640t
preoperative, 1341
problem-oriented, 1331d
and safety, 653
and self-concept, 1261
short-term, 1331d
surgery and, 619–620
values and, 79
Cordotomy, in pain management, 1193t
Core circle, 64t
Core temperature, 444
Corns, 726t
Coronary artery disease, dietary modifications for, 972d
Coronary circulation, 867
Coronary heart disease, risk factors for, 871d
Corpus cavernosum, *1352*
Corpuscular values, of erythrocytes, 1411–1412
Corpus spongiosum, *1352*
Corticosteroids
  inhaled, 824
  in pain management, 1187t, 1192
Corticotropin-releasing hormone (CRH), stress and, 1329
Cortisol, 1328
  nocturnal level of, 1332
  and sleep-wake patterns, 1148
Cost savings, 131, 131d
  critical pathways and, 193–194
Cough, 815, 818, 828–830, 829p–830p
  deep, 828
  low-flow, 830
  quad, 830
  stacked, 828–830
Cough reflex, 812
Coumadin, 892t
Counseling, for altered sexuality, 1373–1374
Courage, intellectual, 227t
Course rales, 817t, 819
CPAP. *See* Continuous positive airway pressure
CPR. *See* Cardiopulmonary resuscitation
Crackles, *431*, 817t, 819
Cranial nerves, assessment of, 415, 416t, 419
Craven, Ruth, 6
Cream, 516t
Creams, administration of, 537
Creatinine clearance, 1081
Creatinine excretion, in nutritional assessment, 965
Creativity, 218t, 1389t
Crepitus, 776
Cretinism, 949
CRH. *See* Corticotropin-releasing hormone
Crimes, 99, 99d, 101–102
Criminal law, 98
Crisis, and spirituality, 1386
Crisis intervention, 1343
Crisis phase, of febrile episode, 1044
Critical care hospitalization, impact on family roles, 1284
Critical pathways, 193–198, 243
  for congestive heart failure, 875–877
  documentation in, 194–198
  example of, 195–197, 614–617
  for total hip replacement, 772–775
  variances in, 194, 243
Critical periods, in development, 269
Critical thinking, 215–227
  anxiety and, 217
  application to learning activities, 227
  attitude and, 217, 218t

conceptual development of, 216–217
definitions of, 216–217, 216d
development of, 220–222, 226–227
diagnostic reasoning in, 222–224
factors affecting, 217–219
gender issues in, 219
importance of, 216
learning styles and, 218–219
level of preparation and, 217–218
nursing judgment in, 224
nurturing of skills, 225d
parts of, 221, 221d
reflection in, 224–226, 226t
CRNA. *See* Certified registered nurse anesthetist
Cromolyn (Intal), 824
Cromolyn sodium (Intal), 836t
Crushing, of medications, 537
Crust, 992t
Crutches, 793–794, 795p–797p
Cryoprecipitate, 604
Crystalloid solutions, 576
CST. *See* Client Satisfaction Tool
CT scan. *See* Computed axial tomography scan
Cue clusters, in nursing diagnosis, 175–177
Cues
  in assessment, 151, 159d
  in nursing diagnosis, 175–176
Cuff size, in blood pressure assessment, 468–469, 469t
Cultural assessment, 333, 334–337
Cultural diversity, 328–329
Culturally sensitive nursing care, 333–334
Cultural relativity, 329
Cultural value orientation, 73, 74t
Culture, 325–339
  and body image, 1254–1255
  characteristics of, 327–330, 327d
  and client teaching, 337–338, 366
  and cognitive function, 1229–1230
  and communication, 345–346, 358–359, 359d
  concepts related to, 330–332
  definitions of, 326
  descriptions of, 329
  dynamic nature of, 328
  ethnocentrism of, 329
  and family, 1279, 1280
  and grieving, 1305, 1306
  habituated assumptions of, 329
  and health assessment, 396
  and health maintenance, 687
  and infection resistance, 1028
  and language differences, 337, 338d
  as learned, 327
  and nurses' use of touch, 153
  and nursing, 332–338
  and nutrition, 961
  pervasiveness of, 329–330
  reasonableness of, 329
  recognizability of, 330
  rituals of, 330
  and self-care, 706
  and self-concept, 1259
  and sexuality, 1359
  and spirituality, 1386
  therapeutic dialogue for, 336
  and transcultural nursing, 332–333, *333*
  unequal sharing among members, 327–328
  and values, 73, 74t
  views of health and, 76–77
Culture change, 328
Cultures
  blood, 1048
  body cavity, 1048
  for infection detection, 1047–1049
  sputum, 820, 1048
  stool, 1048, 1113

throat, 1048
  wound, 1048, 1049p–1050p
Culture shock, 327
Curative surgery, 612t
Cure circle, 64t
Curiosity, 218t
Current Procedural Terminology, 165
Cutaneous stimulation, in pain management, 1183
Cutaneous warts, 989
CVA. *See* Cerebrovascular accident
CWMDT. *See* Chronic Wound Management Decision Tree
Cyanoacrylate glue, 1015
Cyanocobalamin, 947
Cyanosis, 419, 816, 819, 873
Cyclic infusions, in total parenteral nutrition, 600
Cynosure, 330
Cystectomy, 1070
Cystitis, 1069
Cystoscopy, 1081

D

Daily living assessment, 400
Dalmane. *See* Flurazepam
Damages (legal), 101
Dandruff, 724–726
Dangling, of legs, before ambulation, 788
DAT. *See* Diet as tolerated
Data
  collection of, 155–157
    in evaluation, 208–209
    in plan of care, 191
  in health assessment, 394, 396–410
  management of, 127, 231–233
  objective, 156, 157t, 208
  organization of, 160
  primary sources of, 396
  recording of, 157
  secondary sources of, 396
  sources of, 156–157
  subjective, 156, 157t, 208–209
  types of, 156, 157t
  validation of, 158–160, *159*
Data entry, 231–233
Day after pill, 1371, 1372t
Day care, 281, 1246
Daytime naps, 1147, 1150
Death and dying, 14. *See also* Grief; Grieving; Loss
  caring for deceased patient, 1315
  caring for dying patient, 1313–1315
  definitions of, 1313
  legal issues concerning, 102–103
  nursing diagnoses for, 1314–1315
  physical signs of, 1314
  precipitous, with opioid analgesics, 1191
  responses to, 1313–1314
    cultural variations in, 339
    in older adults, 306
  value conflicts and, 80
  wills and, 89, *90*, 102–103, 1308
Death certificate, 103
Débridement, of wounds, 1010–1013
Deceased patient, caring for, 103, 1315
Decisional Conflict (Specify), 1392–1393
Decision making
  by client, 1205
  decision trees and, 203
  ethical/legal issues of, 928
  in implementation, 202
  in nursing process, 49, 142–143
Decision trees, 203
Decoding, in communication process, 345
Decreased Cardiac Output, 884
Decubitus ulcers. *See* Pressure ulcers
Deduction, in information-processing theory, 143

Deep breathing, 828, 829p–830p, 1342
Deep cough, 828
Deep palpation, 407, 408, 1112
Deep tendon reflexes, assessment of, 437, 438t
Deep vein thrombosis (DVT), 768
Defamation of character, 99
Defecation, 1103, 1106. *See also* Bowel
     function/elimination
Defecation reflex, 1103
Defense mechanisms, 1330, 1331t
Defensive self-esteem, 1261
Deficient Fluid Volume, 1314–1315
Deficient Knowledge, 368
Defining characteristics, in nursing diagnosis, 175
Definition, in nursing diagnosis, 175
Degenerative processes, and cognition, 1228
Degermation, 497
Dehiscence, and wound healing, 996–997, *997*
Dehydration. *See also* Fluid balance, altered
     hypertonic, 923
     isotonic, 921
Delayed primary closure of wounds, 995
Delayed sleep phase syndrome, 1156
Delegation of care. *See also* Collaboration and
     delegation
     ethical/legal issues of, 723
     as management responsibility, 113–114, 113d
Delirium, 297, 1230, 1231
Deltoid site, for intramuscular injections, 552,
     556t, *562*
Delusional disorder, 300t
Delusions, 1205, 1230
Dementia, 1228, 1228t, 1230
     behavioral symptoms of, 297d
     nursing interventions for, 298
     in older adults, 297
Demonstrations, in client teaching, 369
Dental hygiene, 704, 729–731, 732p–734p
Dentures, care of, 729–731, *734*
Denuded skin, treatment of, 1008
Deontologic framework, of ethics, 88–89
Dependence
     on opioid analgesics, 1189
     on pain medication, 1191
Dependent variables, 127
Depot medroxyprogesterone acetate (DPMA),
     1371
Depression, 300t
     and altered coping, 1336
     and altered self-concept, 1264
     and altered sensory perception, 1205
     and cognitive function, 1229
     and nutrition, 961
     in older adults, 298
         postoperative, 146
     and self-care, 707
     and sleep and rest, 1154, 1160
Deprived environment, 1203–1204
Depth, of respirations, 460
Dermatitis, 989
Dermatologic illness, and altered health mainte-
     nance, 687–688
Dermatomes, 436, *436*
Dermis, 984, *984*
Descending colon, 1103
Descending pathways, and pain perception, 1169
Descriptors, of nursing diagnosis, 169–175
Desquamation, 984
Detrusor muscle, 1064, 1065
Development. *See also* Growth and development
     change and, 268–269
     cognitive (*See* Cognitive development)
     concepts of, 269–272
     critical periods in, 269
     definition of, 268
     integration and, 269

patterns of, 268
     physical (*See* Physical development)
     psychosocial (*See* Psychosocial development)
     reorganization and, 269
Developmental framework, of family, 310–312, 312t
Developmental healthcare requisites, 64t
Developmental level
     and health maintenance, 685
     and self-concept, 1262
Developmental problems
     and altered family function, 1285
     and altered health maintenance, 688
Developmental role transitions, 1262
Developmental stages
     of families, 311–312
     and home healthcare, 382
Developmental tasks, incomplete, and self-concept,
     1262
Developmental task theory, 271, 273t
     of self-concept, 1256t–1257t
The Development Cycle in Domestic Groups
     (Fortes), 311
Dexamethasone, in pain management, 1187t
Dezocine, in pain management, 1188t
Diabetes mellitus
     and cardiovascular problems, 872
     and foot care, 723
     and nutrition, 958
Diabetic ketoacidosis, 924
Diagnosis. *See also* Nursing diagnosis(es)
     medical, 167–168, 168t
*Diagnostic and Statistical Manual of Mental
     Disorders* (APA), 165
Diagnostic imaging, in infection detection,
     1050–1051
Diagnostic label, of nursing diagnosis, 169
Diagnostic reasoning, 222–224
     in nursing process, 144
     steps in, 223d
Diagnostic statement
     accurate *versus* inaccurate, 179t
     of nursing diagnosis, 177–179, 177t
     types of, 177t, *178*
Diagnostic surgery, 612t
Diagnostic tests/procedures
     for altered sensory perception, 1207
     in bowel function assessment, 1107,
         1113–1116
     in cardiovascular assessment, 882
     in cognitive function assessment, 1236–1237
     in coping assessment, 1337–1338
     in fluid and electrolyte/acid-base balance assess-
         ment, 932
     in health maintenance assessment, 691
     in human sexuality assessment, 1366, 1367t
     in infection resistance assessment, 1046–1051
     in mobility assessment, 778
     in nutrition assessment, 965
     in pain assessment, 1181
     in respiratory function assessment, 820–821
     in safety assessment, 663
     in skin integrity assessment, 1001
     in sleep and rest assessment, 1157
     in urinary function assessment, 1075–1081
Dialysis, renal, 1097, *1098*
Diaper rash, 986
Diaphoresis, 920
Diaphragm, of stethoscope, 409, *409,* 409t
Diaphragm (anatomical), 810
Diaphragm (contraceptive), 1371–1373
Diarrhea, 920, 1109, 1116–1117
     healthcare personnel with, work restrictions for,
         487t
     medications for, 1121, 1122t
     traveler's, 1109
     treatment for, 1120

Diastole, 422, 868
Diastolic blood pressure, 461. *See also* Blood
     pressure
Diastolic murmur, 422, *425*
Dickens, Charles, 44
Diet, 971–972. *See also* Feeding; Food; Nutrition
     and metabolism
     biocultural variations in, 334
     clear liquid, 971
     and coping, 1333
     full liquid, 971
     mechanical soft, 971
     and medication administration, 527
     restrictive, 971–972
     soft, 971
Dietary fiber, 943
Dietary Guidelines for Americans, 953, 953d
Dietary Reference Intakes (RDIs), 942, 944
Diet as tolerated (DAT), 642, 971
Dieting, safety, 690
Diet teaching, 889–892, 936
Diffusion, 810, 811, 913
Digestion
     chemical process of, 952
     mechanical process of, 952
Digestive system, 951–953
     functions of, 952–953
     structure of, 951
Digoxin, 449, 892t
Dilantin. *See* Phenytoin
Diphenoxylate/atropine (Lomotil), 1122t
Diphtheria-tetanus vaccine, 1054t
Diploma nursing programs, 48
Directive leadership, 110, *111*
Disabled Family Coping, 1289
Disaccharides, 943, 952
Disaster plans, 673
Discharge planning
     in ambulatory surgical center, 641
     basic plan, 32, 32t
     Blaylock Risk Assessment Screen in, 30
     and client teaching, 746
     in community-based care, 29–33
     complex referrals, 32–33, 32t
     coordination in, 30, *32*
     elements of
         for client, 30
         for nurse, 30–32
     facilitation in, 30–32
     goal setting in, 30
     and grieving, 1312
     levels of, 32–33
     negotiation in, 32
     postoperative, 643
     in preoperative nursing, 623
     referrals in, 32–33, 32t, 33t
     sexuality and, 1374–1375
     simple referrals, 32, 32t
     transitions in, 30
Discharge summary, in client record, 243–245,
     244
Discipline, 218t
Discontinuous breath sounds, 817t, 819
Discriminant reflectivity, 226t
Discussions, in client teaching, 369
Disease
     classification of, 165
     definition of, in holistic healthcare, 259
     effects on safety, 655–656
     prevention of, 364, 399, 680, 683t
         activities in, 682, 683
Disinfection, 491–492
     agents for, 492, 492t
     of wounds, 1010
Disorganized thinking, 1230
Disposable paper thermometer, 448, *448*

Distal tubule, 1064
Distention, abdominal, 1109–1110
Distraction, in pain management, 1184
Distress, 1329
    verbalization of, 1388
Distress of the Human Spirit, 1392
Distribution, of medications, 523
Distribution systems, for medications, 515–517
Disturbed Body Image, 1265, 1270
Disturbed Sensory Perception, 1207–1208, 1215–1216
Disturbed Sleep Pattern, 1157–1158, 1162
Disturbed Thought Processes, 1239, 1248
Disuse osteoporosis, altered mobility and, 769
Diuresis, 1068
Diuretics, 920, 936, 1070
    and blood pressure, 464
    and cardiovascular function, 872, 892t
    and fluid and electrolyte balance, 916
    and pulse rate, 449
Divorce, 1283–1284
Dix, Dorothea, 41t, 44
DNR orders, 103
Doctoral degree nursing program, 49, 130d
Documentation, 230. *See also* Client record
    abbreviated forms of, 242–243
    abbreviations in, 234t–236t
    of abuse, 232
    in critical pathway, 194–198
    data entry and, 231–233
    data management and, 231–233
    errors in, 236d
    ethics and, 249–250
    of evaluation, 210
    of health assessment, 397
    in implementation, 203
    of intravenous therapy, 588
    of learning, 374
    legal, 231
    legal need for, 105
    legibility of, 233
    of medication administration, 532
    point of care, 237
    and reimbursement, 231
    settings and, 245
    standardized vocabulary in, 237
    technology and, 233–237
    timeliness of, 233
    of vital signs, 473, *474*
Doing therapies, 261
Domains of knowledge, 363–364
Domestic violence, 1284–1285
Dong Quai, 519t
Doppler devices
    for blood pressure assessment, 464–465
    for pulse assessment, 455, *455*
Doppler examination, 883
Dorsalis pedis pulse, 455, *455*
Dorsogluteal site, for intramuscular injections, 556, 556t, *563*
Double-gloving, 494
Double-lumen catheters, 1088
Double-lumen gastric sump tube, 1126, *1127*
DPMA. *See* Depot medroxyprogesterone acetate
Drainage systems, *843,* 1001
Draping, during physical examination, 407
Draw sheet, 759
Dressing, 705, 711t, 739
    altered respiratory function and, 816
    in home/community-based care, 742–746
    in intravenous therapy, 588
Dressing/Grooming Self-Care Deficit, 713
Dreyfuss model, of socialization, 45, 46t
Drip rate, in intravenous therapy, calculation of, 582

Drop factor, in intravenous therapy, calculation of, 582
Droplet precautions, 495, 496t
Droplet transmission, 482
Drowning, 657–658, 669
Drowsiness, with opioid analgesics, 1191
Drug(s). *See also* Medication(s)
    actions of, 523–526
    classifications of, 514
    definition of, 514
    preparations of, 514, 516t
    and respiratory function, 814
Drug abuse. *See* Substance abuse
Drug incompatibility, 526
Drug monographs, 515
Drug-nutrient interactions, 961
Drug overdose, 656–657, 1229, 1237
Drug-resistant microbial strains, 481
Dry shampoo, 724
Dual-career families, 1278, 1280, 1281, 1284
Dualism, in critical thinking, 219
Dull tones, 408, 408t
Duodenocolic reflex, 1120
Duodenum, 1102
Durable power of attorney, 89, 1308
Duration, of sound, 410
Duty, 100
    breach of, 100
DVT. *See* Deep vein thrombosis
The Dynamic Nurse-Patient Relationship (Orlando), 59t
Dysarthria, 1232, 1242–1243
Dysfunction, definition of, in holistic healthcare, 260–261
Dysfunctional Family Processes: Alcoholism, 1288–1289
Dysfunctional Grieving, 1307–1308
Dyspareunia, 1363
Dysphagia, 737, 1236
Dyspnea, 460, 815, 815d, 818
    causes of, 858
    comfort measures for, 858
    management of, 858
    measurement of, 859
Dysrhythmias, 874, 882
Dystonia, 765
Dysuria, 1070

E

EAPs. *See* Employee assistance programs
Ear(s)
    assessment of, 416–418, *417*
    care of, 704–705, 735
    temperature assessment via, 444, 445t, 447, 453p
Eardrops, 538, 539d
Early-awakening insomnia, 1155
Earwear, protective, 1209
Eating
    as altered coping behavior, 1334–1335
    discomfort during, 957
Eating disorders, 961
Eccrine sweat glands, 984
ECF. *See* Extracellular fluid
ECG. *See* Electrocardiography
Echinacea, 519t
Echocardiography, 882t, 883
Economic factors
    in family function, 1277–1278, 1280–1281, 1280t
    in healthcare, 12–13
    in health maintenance, 681–682, 686
    in home healthcare, 383, 388–389
    in nutrition, 961
Eczema, 986

Edema, 435, 873, 916, 931
    grading of, *881*
    palpating for, 881
    in pregnancy, 922
    reduction of, 889–893
Education. *See also* Client teaching; Nursing education
    as function of family, 1278
Educational nursing interventions, 204
Educators, nurses as, 50
Eggs, in Food Guide Pyramid, 951
Ego, 269
Ego theory, of self-concept, 1256t–1257t
EID. *See* Electronic infusion devices
Ejaculation, 1356–1357
    inability, 1362–1363
    premature, 1362
Ejaculatory dysfunction, 1362–1363
Ejaculatory gland, *1352*
Elaborating, in therapeutic communication, 354
Elbow joint, 761t
Elbow protector, as positioning aid, 784t
El Camino Hospital, 233
Elder abuse, 1285
Elderly. *See* Older adult
Elective abortion, 1373
Elective surgery, 612t
Electrical burns, 991
    first aid for, 1008
Electrical hazards, 655
Electrical neutrality, 913
Electrical safety, 658, 670
    intraoperative, 634
Electrical shock, 658–659
Electrocardiography (ECG), 882–883, 882t, *883*
Electroencephalogram, of sleep stages, *1146*
Electrolyte(s), 912. *See also under* Fluid
    and cardiovascular function, 882
    and cognitive function, 1227, 1236
    dietary sources for, 937t
    distribution of, 913–916
    movement of, 913–914
        pressures affecting, 914–916
    normal serum values, 912t
    output, 920
    replacement of, 936
Electrolyte balance, 910
    altered, 921–929, 925t–927t
        and activities of daily living, 928–929
        evaluation for, 937
        health promotion for, 934–937
        in home/community-based care, 936–937
        implementation for, 934–937
        manifestations of, 924–928
        nursing diagnoses for, 932–934
        nursing interventions for, 935–936
        outcome-based teaching plan for, 935
        outcome identification and planning for, 934
    assessment of, 929–932
    factors affecting, 918–921
    lifespan considerations, 916
    normal, 910–916
Electrolyte supplements, 936
Electronic blood pressure devices, 465–468, *469*
Electronic infusion devices (EID), 582, 585–586
Electronic thermometer, 447, *448,* 451p–452p, 452p–453p
Electrophysiology, 882t, 883–884
    of sleep, 1144–1145, *1146*
Elimination, 66, *66,* 147d, 321. *See also* Bowel function/elimination; Urinary elimination
    altered, and home healthcare, 383
    altered mobility and, 769–770
    altered respiratory function and, 816
    assessment of, 161t, 401

Elimination (*continued*)
  client teaching for, 365t
  in community assessment, 320d
  in family assessment, 316d
  and health maintenance, 684d
  in individual assessment, 311d
  and lifespan development, 284–285
  medications to promote normal function of, 515t
  mobility and, 767t
  nursing diagnosis for, 180d
  in older adults, 299–300
  as physiologic need, 63
  postoperative, 640t, 642
  and sleep and rest, 1151
  surgery and, 618–619
  and values, 76
Elixir, 516t
Embolism, 878
  air, 597, 597t
  altered mobility and, 768
  pulmonary, 878
Embryo, 272
Emergency assessment, 151, 151t
Emergency care
  for airway obstruction, 851–855
  for cardiovascular problems, 902
  for poisoning, 673–674
Emergency medical services (EMS), and consulting nurse services, 9
Emergency room, admission to, 29t
Emergent surgery, 612t
Emesis. *See* Vomiting
Emollient laxatives, 1121t
Emotional problems
  and altered family function, 1285
  and self-care, 707
Emotional support
  intraoperative, 633–634
  for wound healing, 1021
Emotion-focused coping mechanisms, 1331d
Emotions
  and illness, 260
  and listening, 353
  and pain response, 1174
  and self-concept, 1263–1264
  validation of, 96–97
Empathy, 349–350
  intellectual, 227t
  and spirituality, 1394
Emphysema, 815
  dietary modifications for, 972d
Employee assistance programs (EAPs), 23–24
Employee health, infection control and, 484–486
EMS. *See* Emergency medical services
Emulsification, 952
Emulsion, 516t
Encephalitis, 1034t
Encoding, in communication process, 345
Endemic goiter, 949
Endocardium, 866
Endocrine system, *1327,* 1327–1328
Endogenous opioids, and pain modulation, 1169
Endometrial cycle, 1355, *1355*
Endoscopic examination
  in bowel function assessment, 1116
  in infection detection, 1050
Endotoxins, 1032
Endotracheal tubes, 843, *846*
Enema, 1113–1115, 1121–1125
  administration of, 539, 1123p–1125p
  barium, 1113–1115
  large-volume, 1122, 1123p–1124p
  oil retention, 1121
  return-flow, 1125
  small-volume, 1121–1122, 1124p

Energy. *See also* Nutrition and metabolism
  decreased, 963
  measurement of, 942
  and mobility, 765
  and respiratory function, 859–860
  and self-care, 707
Energy balance, 953–954, 954d
Energy conservation, for altered cardiovascular function, 894–895
Enteral nutrition, 972–977, 1126. *See also* Nasogastric intubation
  continuous *versus* intermittent, 973
  formulas in, 973
  hazards and complications of, 973–977
  nursing procedure for, 974p–976p
  types of, 972–973, 972t
Enteric-coated tablets, 516t, 537
Enterostomal therapist (ET), 1133, 1136p
Enterovirus, 1034t
Enuresis, 1073, 1144, 1156
  nocturnal, 285, 1073
Environment
  for assessment, 151
  and body temperature, 445
  care of, 739–742
  and circadian rhythms, 1148
  for client teaching, 372–373
  and cognitive function, 1229, 1243
  concept of, 57, 58t–62t
  definition of, 268
  and growth and development, 268–269
  for health assessment, 396–397
  and health maintenance, 685–686
  in home healthcare, 381, 385d, 386–387
  in host-agent-environment model of health, 256
  and nosocomial infections, 483
  and respiratory function, 813
  safety of, 652, 653–655, 654d
  and self-care, 706–707
  and sensory deprivation, 1203–1204
  and sensory overload, 1203
  and sensory perception, 1201
  and sexuality, 1360, 1365
  and sleep and rest, 1150, 1158
  and stress management, 1343
Environmental Protection Agency (EPA), 655
Environmental stress, 1336
Enzymatic débridement, 1010
Eosinophils, 1028, 1030t
EPA. *See* Environmental Protection Agency
Ephedra, 519t
Epicardium, 866
Epidermis, 984, *984, 989*
Epididymis, *1352*
Epidural analgesia, 1186–1189
Epinephrine, 1327
  and body temperature, 446
  stress and, 1329
Episcopalians, 1396t
Equilibrium, 755
Equipment
  handling of, asepsis and, 494
  practice on, for client teaching, 371
Equipment safety, intraoperative, 634
Erikson, Erik, 269, 270t, 1256t–1257t
Erosion, 992t
Errors, in documentation, 232, *233,* 236d
Erythrocyte sedimentation rate (ESR), 1047, 1412
Eschar, 987
Escherichia coli
  and diarrhea, 1109
  and urinary tract infections, 1069
Esophagogastroduodenoscopy, 1116
Esophagostomy, 972t
Esophagus, 951, 1102

ESR. *See* Erythrocyte sedimentation rate
Essentials of Baccalaureate Education for Professional Nursing Practice (AACN), 70–71
Esteem needs, 63
Estrogen
  and milk production, 1356
  and stress incontinence, 1071
ET. *See* Enterostomal therapist
Ethical/legal issues
  abortion, 1365
  accuracy of client records, 232
  advance directives, 1308
  alternative therapies, 264
  anorexia, 1263
  caregiver involvement in home healthcare, 386
  child abuse, 288
  client decision making, 1205
  client transfer, 1333
  confidentiality, 158, 349
  delegation of care, 723
  dependence on pain medication, 1191
  durable power of attorney, 1308
  ending tube feeding, 957
  family conflict over healthcare, 1117
  following orders, 766
  health assessment, 397
  independence of older adults, 660
  informed consent, 630
  IV hydration in terminally ill patients, 599
  literacy, 368
  medication refusal, 523
  mistreatment of client by staff, 1230
  needlestick injuries, 487
  nursing homes, 1294
  possible neglect of a client, 1074
  poverty, 81
  prejudice, 332
  refusal of treatment, 687, 895
  research studies on human subjects, 129
  self-care, 1004
  shift work, 1153
  spousal abuse, 312
  substance abuse by healthcare worker, 523
  treatment decisions, 928
  vital signs assessment, 469
  withdrawal of ventilator support, 846
Ethics
  applied, 72
  dilemmas in, resolutions of, 96–98
  and documentation, 249–250
  in nursing, 86–98
  and nursing research, 128–129, 128d
  principles of, 89–92
  professional, 86
  in professional-patient relationship, 93–94
  and reporting, 249–250
  theoretical frameworks for, 88–89
  therapeutic dialogue, 104
Ethics committees, 97
Ethnic group, 331
Ethnic identity, 330–331
Ethnicity, 330–331. *See also* Culture
  of older adult, 296, *296*
Ethnocentrism, 329
Ethnographic interview, in cultural assessment, 335
Eustress, 1329
Euthanasia, 102
Evaluation, 206–210. *See also* Assessment
  activities in, 208–210
  documentation of, 210
  of family, 1294–1296
  and functional health patterns, 210
  in nursing process, 141
  outcome, 208
  in plan of care, 191, 193, 193t

process, 208
purposes of, 207
of safety, 675
skills for, 207–208
structure, 208
types of, 208
Evaporation, and heat loss, 445
Evening people, 1150
Eversion, 755t
Everyday Hassles Scale, 1328, 1328d, 1338
Evidence-based care, 122
Evisceration, and wound healing, 997, *997*
Excitatory signals, 1168
Excitement phase, of sexual response, 1356
female, 1357
male, 1356
Excoriation, 993t
Excretion
digestive waste, 953 (*See also* Bowel function/
elimination)
of medications, 523
Exercise. *See* Activity and exercise
Exercises
Kegel, 737, 1368, 1371d
range of motion, 788, 789p–790p
Exercise testing, 883
Exhalation, 810
Exogenous opioids, and pain modulation, 1169
Exotoxins, 1032
Expectancy, 1261
Experiments. *See* Nursing research
Expert, in critical thinking development, 227
Expert nurse, 46t
Explorative surgery, 612t
Exploring, in therapeutic communication,
354–355
Expressive aphasia, 410, 1231, 1232t
Extended care facilities. *See* Long-term care
facilities
Extended family, 1277
Extension, 755t
External anal sphincter, 1103
External disaster, 673
External eye, assessment of, 415
External locus of control, 1261
External os, *1353*
External rotation, 755t
External urinary catheters, 1085
External urinary sphincter, 1065, 1066
Exteroceptors, 1220–1222
Extracellular fluid (ECF), 910
and urinary elimination, 1068
volume of, 911
deficit, 921–923
excess, 923
Extracellular Fluid Volume Deficit, 932–933, 938
Extracellular Fluid Volume Excess, 933
Extraocular movement, assessment of, 415
Extrapyramidal tracts, and motor function, 755
Extravasation, with intravenous administration,
565t
Extremities
assessment of, 435–437
inspection in, 435
palpation in, 435–437
blood pressure assessment at, 464
Eye(s)
artificial, 735
assessment of, 415
care of, 704–705, 734–735
in unconscious client, 735
and cognition, 1220, *1221*
structures of, 415
Eyeglasses, 734–735
Eye medications, 538, 539d
Eyewear, protective, 1209

F

Face, assessment of, 410–419
Facial mask of pain, 1180
Facial muscles, assessment of motor control of,
1236
Facial nerve (VII), assessment of, 416t
Facilitator, in discharge planning, 30–32
Facilitator, nurse as, in home healthcare, 383
Fahrenheit scale, 448, *449*
Fairmindedness, 227t
Fairness, 218t
Faith, 1383, 1384, 1384t, 1389t. *See also* Religion;
Spirituality
Faith Health Network, 25
Faith in reason, 227t
Fallopian tubes, *1353*, 1354
Falls, 656
altered mobility and, 766
in older adults
causes of, 764
prevention of, 301
prevention of, 301, 664–668
risks for, 776, 778
False imprisonment, 100
False reassurance, 355–357
Family, 310–314, 1275–1296
altered relationships in, 1282–1286
evaluation of, 1294–1296
health promotion for, 682
implementation for, 1292–1294
nursing diagnoses for, 1287–1291
nursing interventions for, 1292–1293
outcome identification and planning for,
1291–1292
altered safety and, 660
assessment of, 313–314, 315t, 316d,
1286–1287, 1287d
dysfunction identification in, 1286
normal pattern identification in, 1286
objective data in, 1286–1287
risk identification in, 1286
subjective data in, 1286
blended, 1277, 1284
and client goals, 209, 210
of clients with acute confusion, 1246
cohabitated, 1277
communal, 1277
conceptual frameworks of, 310–313
conflicts in, 80, 1117, 1280, 1280t
as data source, 157
developmental framework of, 310–312, 312t
developmental stages of, 311–312
extended, 1277
factors affecting, 1280–1282
and functional health patterns, 314, 316d,
320–322, 1278
functions of, 1277–1278
home/community-based care for, 381, 383,
385, 1293–1294
infection transmission in, 1044
involvement in client teaching, 372
lifespan considerations, 1278–1280
normal relationships in, 1276–1280
nuclear, 1276–1277
roles and relationships pattern in, 405
single-parent, *1276*, 1277
structure of, 1276–1277
systems framework of, 312–313, *313*
therapeutic dialogue, 1046, 1283
Family-centered care, 1276
Family counseling, 1293
Family health history, 398, 872
Family Medical Leave Act, 1278
Family nursing, factors affecting, 314
Family planning, 1369

Family rules, 313
Family themes, 313
Fat, 943–944
digestion of, 952
excessive intake of, 957–958
in Food Guide Pyramid, 951
metabolism of, 952
and wound healing, 995
Father of Baby Scale (FOBS), 1360
Fatigue, 1146
with dying, 1314
pain and, 1174, 1176
and safety, 653
Fat-soluble vitamins, 944–947, 945t
Fax orders, for medications, 519–520
F-COPES, 280
FDA. *See* U.S. Food and Drug Administration
Febrile episodes
with blood transfusions, 607
phases of, 1043–1044, 1055t
Fecal diversion, *1107*, 1107–1108, 1136–1137
Fecal impaction, *1108*, 1108–1109
removal of, 1131–1132
Fecal incontinence, 1109
fecal collection during, 1133
treatment for, 1120
Feces, characteristics of, 1103, 1104t
Feedback, in communication process, 345
Feedback loops, 312–313
Feedback mechanism, 210, *210*
Feeding, 705, 711t, 735–737. *See also* Enteral
nutrition; Nutrition and metabolism;
Parenteral nutrition
assisting adults with, 969p–970p
assistive devices for, 736, *737*
in home/community-based care, 749
needs for, 736d
Feeding Self-Care Deficit, 712
Feelings. *See* Emotions
Feet. *See under* Foot
Felony, 99d
Female genitalia, assessment of, 434, 1366
Female reproductive system, 1352–1354, *1353*
Female sexual response, 1357
Female sterilization, 1373, 1373t
Femoral pulse, 454, *455*
Fentanyl, 1188t. *See also* Opioid analgesics
Fertilization, 1355
Festinating gait, 766
Fetal development. *See* Intrauterine development
Fetus, 272, 273, 281
Fever
and infection, 1043–1044
and infection resistance, 1028–1029
management of, 1055–1056, 1055t
and respirations, 459
Feverfew, 519t
Fever phase, of febrile episode, 1043–1044, 1055t
FFP. *See* Fresh frozen plasma
Fiber, dietary, 943
and bowel elimination, 1105, 1117–1119
Fidelity, in professional-patient relationship, 93
Fight or flight response, 1328–1330
Filipino Americans, response to death and dying,
339
Filter needles, 543
Filtration, 914, *914*, 1065
Filtration pressure, *915*, 915–916
Financial factors
in family function, 1280–1281, 1280t
in healthcare, 12–13
in health maintenance, 681–682, 686
in home healthcare, 383, 388–389
in nutrition, 961
Financial resources management, 112
Fine rales, 817t, 819

Fingers
  clubbing of, 420, *420*
  joints of, 761t
Finland, family nursing in, 314
Firearm safety, 658, 670
Fire evacuation plans, 673
Fire extinguishers, 670t
Fire safety, 651, 658, 669
First aid
  for minor burns, 1007–1008
  for minor wounds, 1005–1006
First degree burns, 991
First-line managers, 118, *118*
First trimester, growth and development in, 272, *274*
Fish, in Food Guide Pyramid, 951
Fissure, 992t
Fistula, 997
Five rights of medication administration, 530–532, 531d
Flaccidity, of muscles, 765
Flat tones, 408, 408t
Flatulence, 1109
  medications for, 1121
  treatment for, 1120
Flatus, 1109
Flatworms, 1039
Fleas, 1039
Flexion, 755t
Flexion contractures, 767–768
Flora, normal, 1028
Flossing, 729
Flowsheets, 242–243
Fluent aphasia, 410, 1231–1232, 1232t
Fluid(s)
  distribution of, 913–916
  24-hour intake and output, 919t
  loss of, and urinary elimination, 1068
  movement of, 913–914
    pressures affecting, 914–916
  stasis of, and infections, 1039
  variations in, by age and sex, 910, 910t
  water concentration of, 911–912
Fluid balance, 910. *See also* Acid-base balance; Electrolyte balance
  altered, 921–929
    and activities of daily living, 928–929
    evaluation for, 937
    health promotion for, 934–937
    implementation for, 934–937
    manifestations of, 924–928
    nursing diagnoses for, 932–934
    nursing interventions for, 935–936
    outcome identification and planning for, 934
  assessment of, 929–932
  factors affecting, 918–921
  in home/community-based care, 936–937
  lifespan considerations, 916
  normal, 910–916
  outcome-based teaching plan for, 935
Fluid compartments, 910–912
Fluid intake, 918–920, 919t
  in bladder training, 1084
  and bowel elimination, 1105, 1119
  and cognitive function, 1227, 1243
  monitoring of, 929–932, *930*
  and urinary elimination, 1068, 1083
Fluid orders, medication administration and, 527
Fluid output, 920
  monitoring of, 929–932, *930*
Fluid overload, 874
  intravenous therapy and, 594–597, 597t
  total parenteral nutrition and, 603
Fluid replacement, 934, 935–936
Fluid restriction, for edema reduction, 892–893
Fluid volume deficit, and blood pressure, 463–464

Fluid volume overload, with blood transfusions, 607
Flunisolide (AeroBid), 836t
Fluoride, 704, 950
Flushing, in intravenous therapy, 588, 595p–596p
Flush phase, of febrile episode, 1044, 1055t
Fly larvae, 1039
FOBS. *See* Father of Baby Scale
Focus assessment, 150, 151t, 394. *See also* Health assessment
Focusing, in therapeutic communication, 354
FOCUS notes, 240t, 241–242, *242*
Focus on Critical Care, 132
Focus value, 75, *75*
Folacin, 946t, 947
Foley catheters, 1088, *1094*
Folic acid, 946t, 947
Follicle-stimulating hormone, and menstruation, 1355
Follicular phase, of ovarian cycle, 1355, *1355*
Follow through, 97
Food. *See also* Diet; Feeding; Nutrient(s); Nutrition and metabolism
  optimal intake, 968
  preparation of, 957
    in home/community-based care, 749
  withholding of, 968–971
Food and Nutrition Board, of the Institute of Medicine/National Academy of Sciences, 942
Food-borne infections, 1037t–1038t
Food-drug interactions, 526
Food Guide Pyramid, *950,* 950–951
Food labels, 967, *968*
Footboard, as positioning aid, 784t
Footboards, 741–742
Foot care, 704, 706, 723, 726t, 727p–728p
Foot drop, 768
Foot joints, 762t
Foot odor, 726t
Foot strength, assessment of, 435
Foot ulceration, 986, *987. See also* Pressure ulcers
Forearm, joints of, 761t
Foreplay, 1354
Foreskin, 1352
Forgiveness
  and spirituality, 1389t
  and terminal illness, 72
Formaldehyde, as disinfectant, 492t
Formal thinking, 277
Formula (newborn nutrition), 283, 284, 955, 1104
Fortes, Meyer, 311
Foster children, 1277
Foundation value, 75, *75*
Fourchette, *1353*
Fowler's position, 742d, *782*
Fraud, 99
Fremitus, 819
Frequency
  of pulse, 449
  of sound, 409–410
  of urination, 1071
Fresh frozen plasma (FFP), 603
Freud, Sigmund, 269, 269t, 1256t–1257t
Friction, and pressure ulcers, 988
Fruits, in Food Guide Pyramid, 950
Full liquid diets, 971
Full-thickness burns, 991
Functional health patterns, *66. See also specific functional health pattern*
  assessment of, 160, 161t, 394, 395t
  of community, 317, 320–322, 320d
  and evaluation, 208, 210
  of family, 314, 316d, 320–322
  health maintenance and, 684d

and implementation, 206
  of individual, 311d, 320–322
  and lifespan development, 281–291
  nursing diagnosis by, 180d–181d, 182
  as nursing framework, 65–66
  and nursing process, 145–146, *147,* 147d
  in older adults, following elective surgery, 146
  planning and, 198
  postoperative, 640t
  surgery and, 613–621
  typology of, 147d
  values and, 76–79, 78d–79d
Functional incontinence, 299, 1072–1073
Functional Urinary Incontinence, 1082
Function restoration, client teaching for, 364–365, 365t
Fundus, of uterus, *1353,* 1354
Fungal infections, 989–990. *See also* Infection(s)
Fungi, 480, 1032–1039
Furosemide, and urinary elimination, 1070
Futility, medical, 95
The Future of Public Health, 26
Future value, 75, *75*

G

Gag reflex, 760
  in assessment of motor control, 1236
  safety and, 661
Gait
  altered, 766
  assessment of, 399–400, 776
  normal, 760
Gallbladder, 951
Gamma benzene hexachloride (Kwell), for pediculosis, 724
Garlic, 519t
Gas exchange, 810, 811
  impaired, 824
    dying and, 1315
Gas sterilization, 492
Gas transport, 810–811
Gastric decompression, 1126
Gastric feeding, 1126. *See also* Enteral nutrition
Gastric gavage, 1126. *See also* Enteral nutrition
Gastric lavage, 1126
Gastroenteritis, manifestations of, 1043d
Gastrointestinal illness
  altered health maintenance and, 687
  infections and, 1044
  stress and, 1110, 1337
Gastrointestinal infections, manifestations of, 1043d
Gastrointestinal motility, and medication administration, 527
Gastrointestinal tract
  assessment of, 401, 427–435
  digestion and, 951
  fluid loss through, 920
  inflammation of, 958
  obstruction of, 958
  stress and, 1337
  structures of, *1102,* 1102–1103
Gastrostomy, 972t, 973, 974p–976p
Gate control theory of pain, 1169
Gauze dressings, 1008, 1009t
Gavage feeding, 1126. *See also* Enteral nutrition
G-CSF. *See* Granulocyte colony-stimulating factors
Gel, 516t
Gender
  and critical thinking, 219
  and nutrition, 961
  and respirations, 459
  and spirituality, 1386
  and stress, 1329, 1332

Gender identity, 289, 1356, 1358, 1365
Gender roles, 1356
General anesthesia, 635
Generalized anxiety disorder, 300t
General systems theory, 57–62
Generativity, 279
Generic drug name, 514
Generic plan of care, 194d
Genetics, 268–269
Genital herpes, 1035t
Genitalia
  assessment of, 434–435
  female, 434, 1366
  male, 434–435, 1366
Genitourinary tract, *1065*
Geriatric client. *See* Older adult
German measles (rubella), 1033t
Gill v. Foster, 100
Ginger, 519t
Gingiva, care of, 704
Ginkgo biloba, 519t
Ginseng, 519t
Glans penis, 1352, *1352*
Glasgow Coma Scale, 410, 414t
Glass mercury thermometer, 447, *447*
Global aphasia, 1232, 1232t
Global Good Services, Inc., 25
Global initiatives, for community-based nursing, 25–26
Global Nursing Exchange, 25
Glomerular filtrate, 1065
Glomerulus, 1064
Glossopharyngeal nerve (IX), assessment of, 416t
Gloves, 493–494
  closed method with, 499, 504p–505p
  for infection control, 485
  and latex allergy, 656
  nursing procedure for use, 502p–503p
  open method with, 499
  in surgical asepsis, 499
Glucocorticoids
  and milk production, 1356
  stress and, 1329
Glucose
  metabolism of, 952
  and osmolarity, 923
  in urine, 1080t
Glutaraldehyde, as disinfectant, 492t
Gluten intolerance, 1105
Glycerol, 952
Glycogenesis, 952
Glycolysis, 765
Goals. *See also* Client goals
  in discharge planning, 30
  identification of, 97
Goiter, endemic, 949
Goldenseal, 519t
Goldmark report, 42t, 45, 46
Gonadotropin-releasing hormone, and menstruation, 1355
Gonorrhea, 1035t
Good Samaritan Law, 103–104
Gordon, Marjory, 65
Gowns, in asepsis, 493, 504p–505p
Grab bars, 665
Grace, and spirituality, 1390t
Grade-oriented students, 219
Graduate school, 15–16, 48–49
Graefenberg spot, 1363
Gram-negative bacteria, 1032, 1034t
Gram-positive bacteria, 1032
Gram stains, 1047
Grandparents, 1280
Granulation tissue, 995
Granulocyte(s). *See* White blood cell(s)

Granulocyte colony-stimulating factors (G-CSF), 1056
Gravity line, 755, *756*
Grenade drain, 1001
Grief, definition of, 1300
Grieving. *See also* Death and dying; Loss
  altered, 1305–1306
    and activities of daily living, 1305–1306
    evaluation for, 1312
    health promotion for, 1308–1311
    home/community-based nursing for, 1311–1312
    implementation for, 1308–1312
    manifestations of, 1305, 1306d
    nursing diagnoses for, 1307–1308, 1309t
    nursing interventions for, 1311, 1311d
    outcome identification and planning for, 1308
  among older adults, 304
  anticipatory, 1300, 1307
  assessment of, 1306–1307
    dysfunction identification in, 1307
    normal pattern identification in, 1306–1307
    objective data in, 1307
    risk identification in, 1307
    subjective data in, 1306–1307
  characteristics of, 1300–1302
  factors affecting, 1304–1305
  lifespan considerations, 1302–1303, 1302–1304
  models of, 1300–1302, 1302t
    Engel's, 1300–1302, 1302t
    grief cycle, 1302, *1302*, 1302t, 1303t
    Kubler-Ross', 1302t, 1313–1314
    Parkes', 1302, 1302t
  normal, 1300–1304
    manifestations of, 1306d
  nursing plan of care for, 1316–1319
  outcome-based teaching plan for, 1310
  referrals for, 1312
  stages of, 1309–1310, 1311d
  terms related to, 1300
  therapeutic dialogue, 1301
Grooming, 705. *See also* Hygiene; Self-care
  in home/community-based care, 742–746
  poor, 708
Ground, electrical, 659
Group therapy, 205–206
Growth, definition of, 268
Growth and development
  of adolescent, 277
  biocultural variations in, 334
  environment and, 268–269
  genetics and, 268–269
  of infant, 275
  intrauterine, 272–274
  of middle adult, 279
  of newborn, 274–275
  of older adult, 279
  of preschooler, 276
  principles of, 269
  of school-age child, 276–277
  theories of, 269–272
    cognitive development theory, 270, 271t, 272t
    developmental task theory, 271, 273t
    psychodynamic theory, 269, 269t, 270t
  of toddler, 275–276
  of young adult, 278
Growth hormone, and sleep-wake patterns, 1148
Guaiac test, 1113
Guided imagery, in pain management, 1184
Guidelines for Preventing the Transmission of Mycobacterium tuberculosis in Health-Care Facilities (CDC), 671
Guidelines for Spiritual Assessment, 1388
Guilt inducement, in nurse-client relationship, 348t

Gums, care of, 704
Gun safety, 658, 670
Gurgles, 817t, 819

H

Habit retraining, 1085
Habits
  and health maintenance, 685
  and mobility, 763
  and nutrition, 958–961
  and respiratory function, 813–814
  and sensory perception, 1201
  and skin integrity, 989
  and sleep and rest, 1151–1152
Hair, 984
  altered nutrition and, 963
  assessment of, 419–420
  care of, 704, 723–726, 730p–731p
  examination of, 998
  loss of, 726
Haitian Americans, and religion, 335
Half-bow knot, 666
Half-hitch knot, 666, *667*
Hall, Lydia E., 59t, 64t, 138, 139t
Hallucinations, 1205, 1230
Hallux valgus, 726t
Hand-held nebulizers, 825, *837*
Hand restraint, 665
Hand roll, as positioning aid, 784t
Hand strength, assessment of, 435
Handwashing, 488–491
  in children, 491
  in infection transmission prevention, 1057
  for medical asepsis, 488, 489p–490p
  for surgical asepsis, 488, 499, 500p–501p
Hand-wrist splint, as positioning aid, 784t
Hard palate, *418*
Harris tube, 1126
Hat, for urine collection, 1074
Havighurst, Robert, 271, 273t, 1256t–1257t
Hayes, Anna Mae, 45
Hay fever, 813
Hazardous waste. *See* Waste disposal
HCl. *See* Hydrochloric acid
HCO$_3$, 918t
HDL cholesterol, 871
Head
  assessment of, 410–419
  trauma to, and cognitive function, 1229
Head-to-toe framework
  for health assessment, 160, 394, 395d, 395t
  for physical examination, 410–437
Health, 255
  concept of, 57, 58t–62t
  definitions of, 256
  determinants of, 20–21
  models of, 256–258
    clinical, 256
    health belief, 256–257, *257*
    high-level wellness, 257–258
    holistic, 258
    host-agent-environment, 256, *256*
  web sites related to, 1432
Health assessment, 393–440. *See also* Assessment; Physical examination
  comprehensive, 394
  conclusion of, 437
  conducting, 396–397
  cultural sensitivity in, 396
  data in, 394, 396
  documentation of, 397
  ethical/legal issues in, 397
  focused, 394
  frameworks for, 394–396, 395t
    body systems, 394–396, 395t
    head-to-toe, 394, 395d, 395t

Health assessment (*continued*)
  functional, 394, 395t
  interview phase of, 397–406
  lifespan considerations in, 437–440
  objective data in, 406–410
  physical examination phase of, 406–410
  preparation for, 396–397
  purpose of, 394
  subjective data in, 397–406
  therapeutic dialogue, 439
Health assessment forms, 397
Health belief model, 256–257, *257*
Healthcare
  access to, 12–13
  community-based (*See* Community-based care)
  delivery of, 116–117
  at home (*See* Home healthcare)
  levels of, 20–26
  reasons for seeking, 398
  as a right, 10
Healthcare ethics, principles of, 89–92
Healthcare personnel
  abuse by, 1230
  with AIDS, 486
  attitude towards pain, 1178–1179
  as barriers to client goals, 210
  certification of, 27
  and infection control, 485
  licensure of, 27, 48, 98
  safety of, 654, 655–656, 671
  substance abuse by, 523
Health Care Professionals' Experiences With and
    Attitudes Toward Death and Dying,
    346
Healthcare reform, 42t
Healthcare settings, 8–10
  documentation and, 245
  and nosocomial infections, 483–484
  safety in, 654
Healthcare system
  admission to, 28, 29t
  attitude towards pain, 1179
  discharge from (*See* Discharge planning)
Health curriculum, 260
Health deviations, 64t
The Health Hazard Appraisal, 690
Health history, 397, 398. *See also* Health
    assessment
  and cardiovascular problems, 872
  in medication assessment, 526
  in preoperative nursing, 622–623
  and respiratory function, 818
Healthier People, 690
Health Insurance Portability and Accountability
    Act (HIPAA), 100
Health interview information, 1047
Health maintenance
  altered, 687–688
  assessment of, 688–691
    dysfunction identification in, 690
    normal pattern identification in, 688
    objective data in, 690
    risk identification in, 690
    subjective data in, 688–690
  characteristics of, 680–682
  in community-based care, 697
  evaluation in, 698
  factors affecting, 685–687
  functional health patterns and, 684d
  in home healthcare, 697
  implementation in, 694–697
  lifespan considerations and, 683–685,
    692d–693d
  normal, 680–685, *681*
  nursing diagnoses for, 691–694
  nursing interventions in, 694–697

  in older adults, 300–301
  outcome-based teaching plan for, 697
  outcome identification and planning in, 694
  patterns of, 682–683
  therapeutic dialogue, 689
Health-maintenance activities, 680
Health maintenance organizations (HMOs), ac-
    creditation of, 27
Health management. *See* Health perception and
    health management
Health Patterning Clinic, 25
Health perception and health management, 65,
    66, 147d, 321
  assessment of, 161t, 398–399
  client teaching for, 365t
  in community assessment, 320d
  in family assessment, 316d
  grieving and, 1309t
  and health maintenance, 684d
  in individual assessment, 311d
  and lifespan development, 281–282
  mobility and, 767t
  nursing diagnosis and, 180d
  postoperative, 640t
  surgery and, 613
  and values, 76
Health Predict: Personal Health Analysis, 690
Health-Promoting Lifestyle Profile (HPLP), 962
Health promotion, 260, 680, 694–697
  for altered grieving, 1308–1311
  for bowel function, 1117–1120
  for cardiovascular function, 885–889
  client teaching and, 364
  for cognitive function, 1240–1241
  for family, 1292
  for fluid and electrolyte/acid-base balance,
    934–935
  in home healthcare, 382
  for infection control, 1052–1054
  for mobility, 780–781
  for nutrition, 967–968
  for pain management, 1182–1183
  for respiratory function, 824–828
  for safety, 664–673
  for self-care, 713–714
  for self-concept, 1266–1268
  for sensory perception, 1209–1210
  for sexuality, 1368–1373
  for skin integrity, 1003–1005
  for sleep and rest, 1158–1159
  for spirituality, 1394–1395
  for stress, coping, and adaptation, 1339–1342
  for urinary function, 1083–1084
Health-promotion activities, 682, 683, 686
Health-protection activities, 682
Health records. *See* Client records
Health restoration, client teaching for, 364–365,
    365t
Health screenings, 696
Health-Seeking Behaviors, 693, 699
Health Style: A Self-Test, 690
Healthy Chico Kids 2000, 318–319
Healthy People 2010, 26, 259, 310
Hearing
  assessment of, 1208t
  normal, 1200
  in observation, 152–153
  and perception of information, 1220–1222
  and safety, 661
  sensory aids for, 1211d
Hearing aids
  care of, 735
  inserting, 1213p
  types of, 736d
Hearing impairments. *See also* Sensory perception,
    altered

  and surgery, 622
Hearing loss, 416
Hearing tests, 416–418, *418*
Heart
  blood flow through, 868
    distribution of, 868
  blood vessels of, 868–870, *869*
  conduction system of, 866–867, *867*
    problems with, 874
  function of, 867–869, *868*
  impulse conduction in, 868
  layers of, 866
  muscle of, 868
    damage to, 874
  structure of, 866, *866,* 866–867
  valves of, 867
    dysfunction of, 874
Heart attack, 874
  in older adults, 1172
  symptoms of, 696d
Heart catheterization, 882t, 883
Heart disease, client teaching on, 695
Heart-lung death, 1313
Heart murmurs, 422, *425*
Heart rate (HR). *See also* Pulse rate
  altered cardiovascular function and, 873
  assessment of, postoperative, 638
  and cardiac output, 868–869
  fluid and electrolyte/acid-base balance and, 927
  pain and, 1175
Heart rhythm, fluid and electrolyte/acid-base bal-
    ance and, 927
Heart sounds, 421, *421,* 423p–424p
  abnormal, 422, *425*
  assessment of, 882
  extra, 422
  normal, 422
Heat lamps, 1021
Heat loss, 445
Heat production, 444–445
Heat therapy
  in pain management, 1183
  safety of, 1020t
  uses for, 1020t
  for wound healing, 1018–1021
Heel protector, as positioning aid, 784t
Height
  measurement of, 401, 964
  weight and, standardized tables of, 964
Heimlich maneuver, 855, 856p–857p
Helminths, 481, 1039
Helpers, 262, 262t
Hematocrit, 1412
  in nutritional assessment, 965
Hematologic studies, in mobility assessment, 778
Hematology, 1411–1412
Hematomas, and wound healing, 996
Hematuria, 1071
Hemiplegic gait, 766
Hemoccult test, 1113, 1114p–1115p
Hemoglobin
  concentration of, 1412
  in nutritional assessment, 965
Hemolysis, 604
Hemolytic transfusion reaction, 607
Hemorrhage, and wound healing, 996
Hemorrhoids, 1106, *1106*
Hemovac drain, 1001, *1001*
Henderson, Virginia, 58t, 64t
Henry Street Settlement, 41t
Heparin, 550, 892t
Hepatitis A, 487t, 1037t
Hepatitis B, 487t, 1037t, 1054t
Hepatitis C, 1037t
Herbal preparations, 517–518, 519t
  effects on surgery, 622–623

Herbal remedies, and cardiovascular problems, 872
Herpes, genital, 1035t
Herpes simplex virus
type 2, 1035t
and work restriction, 487t
Herpesvirus, 989
Herpes zoster virus, 487t
Heterosexual, 289, 1356
Hexachlorophene, antiseptic use of, 492t
HHPPS. *See* Home health prospective payment system
Hierarchy of human needs, 62–64, *63, 64*
Hierarchy of skills, 79–80
High-density lipoprotein (HDL) cholesterol, 871
High-grade fever, 1043
High-level wellness model, of health, 257–258
Hinduism, 1397t
HIPAA. *See* Health Insurance Portability and Accountability Act
Hippocampus
and memory, 1223
stress and, 1329
Hippocrates, 43
Hip replacement, collaborative care plan for, 772–775
Hip surgery, positioning after, 784
Hirnle, Connie, 6–7
Hives, 991
Holism, 258, 1382
Holism and Evolution (Smuts), 258
Holistic healthcare, 258–261
disease definition in, 259
dysfunction definition in, 260–261
illness definition in, 259–260
informed choices in, 259
modalities of, 263–264
nursing in, 261–264
practice of, 258–259
self-responsibility in, 259
self-worth and, 259
stress definition in, 261
Holistic health model, 258
Holistic perspective, 313
Holistic practice, 65
Homan sign, 881
Home environment
safety of, 652, 653, 654d, 673
toxins in, 657d
Home health aide, referrals to, 33t
Home healthcare, 9, 11, 380–389
versus acute care, 381
admission to, 29t
ambulation assistance in, 792p, 797p
antiembolism stockings in, 888p
assessment in, 384–387, 385d
of community resources, 387
of family, 385
of home environment, 386–387
of individual, 385
of risks, 385–386
bathing in, 719p, 722p
blood glucose measurement in, 960p
blood pressure assessment in, 468p
blood transfusion in, 606p
body temperature assessment in, 454p
bowel function in, 1137
cardiopulmonary resuscitation in, 899p–900p
cardiovascular function in, 901–902
cognitive function in, 1246
community resources for, 383
condom catheter application in, 1087p
coping and stress tolerance in, 1343–1344
documentation in, 245
enemas in, 1125p
environment of, 381, 385d, 386–387

ethical/legal issues in, 386
factors affecting, 381–383
for families, 1293–1294
family roles in, 381, 383
fecal ostomy pouch use in, 1136p
feeding in, 970p
fluid, electrolyte, and acid-base balance in, 936–937
focus of, 22
functional abilities and, 382–383
glove use in, 503p
grieving in, 1311–1312
hair care in, 731p
handwashing in, 490p
health maintenance in, 697
hemoccult test in, 1115p
infections in, 1057–1058
intramuscular injections in, 560p
intravenous therapy in, 590p, 594p, 596p, 607–608
medication administration in, 533, 562–564
inhaled, 542p
oral, 536p
parenteral, 550p
medication records in, 245
mobility in, 801–804
movement of clients in, 757p
nosocomial infections in, 484
nurses in, 383–389
nursing progress notes in, 238
nursing visit in, 383–384
nutrition in, 977
oral care in, 734p
oxygen therapy in, 840p
pain management in, 1194
parenteral nutrition in, 607–608, *608*
for peak flow monitoring, 824p
positioning in bed in, 787p
pulse assessment in, 457p
pulse oximetry in, 823p
range of motion exercises in, 790p
respiratory assessment in, 462p, 858–860
respiratory suctioning in, 854p–855p
responsibilities in, 387–389
Rice model of, 383, *384*
safety in, 674–675
self-care in, 742–749
self-concept in, 1269–1270
sensory perception in, 1211–1214
sexuality in, 1374–1375
skin integrity in, 1021–1022
sleep and rest in, 1160
social supports in, 383
spirituality in, 1399
standards of, 383, 384d
sterile field in, 508p
subcutaneous injections in, 555p
systems view of, 381
telenursing and, 381
total hip replacement and, 772–775
total parenteral nutrition in, 602p
tracheostomy in, 851p
trends affecting, 380–381, 380t
tube feedings in, 976p
urinary catheterization in, 1093p
urinary function in, 1097–1098
weight measurement in, 403p
wheelchairs in, 800p
wound cultures in, 1050p
wound dressings in, 1013p
Home health nurse
referrals to, 33t
and self-care promotion, 714t
Home health prospective payment system (HHPPS), 382
Homeostasis, 259, 1326

Homicide, firearms and, 658
Homosexuality, 289, 1356, 1358
Hope, and spirituality, 1389t
Hormonal dysynchrony, and sleep-wake patterns, 1148
Hormone(s), 1327–1328
and birth control, 1369–1371
and body temperature, 445–446
and sleep and rest, 1153
Hormone replacement therapy, and cardiovascular problems, 872
Hospice, 389, 1313, 1314. *See also* Home healthcare
admission to, 29t
ethical/legal issues in, 96
Hospice nurses, 22
Hospital, admission to, 29t
Hospital-acquired infections, 483–484, 655, 659, 1032, 1041
Hospital beds, 739–742
Hospitals
accreditation of, 27
and cognitive function, 1229
infection control in, 485
and sleep and rest, 1153, *1153*
surgery in, 613
Hospital waste. *See* Waste disposal
Host
compromised, 1039–1041
in host-agent-environment model of health, 256
of infection, 482–483
Host-agent-environment model, of health, 256, *256*
Hot packs, 1021
Hot-water bath, 717t
HPA axis, 1327–1328, 1329
HPLP. *See* Health-Promoting Lifestyle Profile
HR. *See* Heart rate
Huff coughing, 830
Human immunodeficiency virus (HIV), 1036t. *See also* Acquired immunodeficiency virus
in African American community, 15
transmission of, through blood transfusions, 604
Human needs theory, 62–64, *63, 64*, 271–272
Human resource management, 112
Human sexuality. *See* Sexuality and reproduction
Humility, 218t
intellectual, 227t
Humor, 205
Humoral immunity, 1030–1031
Hydration. *See also* Fluid balance
in infection control, 1052
postoperative, 642
and respiratory function, 827
of skin, 1003
of tissues, abnormal, 928
Hydraulic lift, 801, 801t, 802p–803p
Hydrochloric acid (HCl), 917
Hydrochlorothiazide, and urinary elimination, 1070
Hydrocolloid dressings, 1008, 1009t
Hydrocortisone, in pain management, 1187t
Hydrogels, 1008, 1009t
Hydrogen peroxide, as antiseptic, 492t
Hydrolysis, 952
Hydromorphine, 1188t
Hydronephrosis, 1069, 1071
Hydrostatic pressure, 915
Hygiene, 704–705. *See also* Self-care
in children and adolescents, 282
and infection control, 1052
mobility and, 771
in pain management, 1183
poor, 708

Hygiene (*continued*)
  postoperative, 643
  respiratory function and, 816
  and safety, 655
  scheduled care for, 714–715, 716d
  and skin integrity, 1003
Hymen, *1353*
Hyperactive bowel sounds, 1112
Hyperalgesia, 1172–1173
Hypercalcemia, 926t
Hypercoagulability, altered mobility and, 768
Hyperemia, reactive, altered mobility and, 769
Hyperextension, 755t
Hyperglycemia, 943, 977
Hyperkalemia, 925t
Hypermagnesemia, 926t
Hypernatremia, 923
Hyperosmolar, 913
Hyperosmolarity, 923
Hyperphosphatemia, 926t
Hyperpigmentation, of skin, 985
Hyperpyrexia, 1043
Hyperresonant tones, 408, 408t
Hypersensitivity reactions, to medications, 524
Hypertension, 871, 872. *See also* Blood pressure
  client teaching about, 695
  dietary modifications for, 972d
Hyperthermia, malignant, 618
Hypertonic dehydration, 923
Hypertonic fluids, 576, *577, 578t*
Hypertonicity, 923
Hypertonic solution, 914–915
Hyperventilation, 425, 821, 858, 924
Hypervigilance, 1230–1231
Hypnosis, in pain management, 1184
Hypnotics, 1154, 1159–1160, 1160t
  and sleep apnea, 1155
Hypoactive bowel sounds, 1112
Hypocalcemia, 926t
Hypoglossal nerve (XII), assessment of, 416t
Hypoglycemia, 943
Hypokalemia, 925t
Hypomagnesemia, 926t
Hyponatremia, 924
Hypoosmolarity, 913, 924
Hypophosphatemia, 927t
Hypopnea, 1155
Hypospadias, 1366
Hypotension, 471. *See also* Blood pressure
  orthostatic, 471–473
    altered mobility and, 768
    assessment for, 472p–473p
  and urinary elimination, 1069
Hypothalamic osmoreceptors, 911
Hypothalamic-pituitary-adrenal (HPA) axis, 1327–1328
  stress and, 1329
Hypothalamus, 1327, *1327*
  stress and, 1329
  and thermoregulation, 444
Hypothermia, during surgery, 618
Hypothermia blankets, in fever management, 1056
Hypotheses, in nursing research, 122, 127
Hypotonic disorder, 924
Hypotonic fluids, 576, *577, 578t*
Hypotonicity, 924
  of muscles, 765
Hypotonic solution, 914–915
Hypoventilation, 425, 821
Hypovolemia, 921
  orthostatic hypotension and, 471
Hypoxemia, 819, 820, 820d
Hypoxia, 874. *See also* Oxygenation
  and clubbing, 816
Hysterectomy, and sexuality, 1362

I
Iacano v. St. Peter's Medical Center, 100, 101
IBS. *See* Irritable bowel syndrome
Ibuprofen, in pain management, 1187t
IBW. *See* Ideal body weight
ICD-10-CM. *See International Classification of Diseases*
Ice bags, 1019–1021
ICF. *See* Intracellular fluid
ICNP. *See* International Classification of Nursing Practice
ICU. *See* Intensive care unit
Id, 269
Ideal body weight (IBW), 954
Idealized body image, 1254
Identification bracelet, 28
Identified client, lack of, 313
Identity, 1255
IIFS. *See* Iowa ICU Family Scale
Ileoanal reservoir, 1107, *1108*
Ileocecal valve, 1103
Ileostomy, 1107, *1107*
Ileum, 1102
Illicit drugs, and cardiovascular problems, 872
Illiteracy, 367–368
Illness. *See also* Disease
  acute phase of, 1041
  chronic
    and altered health maintenance, 687–688
    and family function, 1282
    fluid and electrolyte balance and, 920–921
  and cognition, 1226
  coping with, 1335
  definition of, in holistic healthcare, 259–260
  dietary modifications for, 972d
  and family function, 1281–1282
  and self-care, 707
  and self-concept, 1263
  and sensory perception, 1201–1202
  and sexuality, 1360, 1365
  and sleep and rest, 1152–1153
  and spirituality, 1387
Imagery, 264, 1342t
Imaginal skills, 79–80
Imbalanced Nutrition, 979
Imbalanced Nutrition: Less Than Body Requirements, 965, 1315
Imbalanced Nutrition: More Than Body Requirements, 965
Imbalanced Nutrition: Risk for More Than Body Requirements, 965
Immediate memories, 1223
Immobility. *See* Mobility, altered
Immune system
  dysfunction of, 1040
  immobility and, 769
  in older adults, 303, 1032
  stress and, 1040, 1329–1330
  and wound healing, 995
Immunity, 1029–1031
  active, 1031
  cellular, 1030
  humoral, 1030–1031
  passive, 1031
Immunization programs, 1052–1054
Immunizations, 697, 1031, 1052–1054
  adult, 1054t
  childhood, 1053t
  for infection control, 671
  refusal of, 687
Immunocompetence testing, nutrition and, 965
Immunocompromised patient, 1039–1041
Immunoglobulins, 1030–1031, 1030t. *See also* Antibodies
Imovane. *See* Zopiclone

Impaired Bed Mobility, 779
Impaired Gas Exchange, 824, 1315
Impaired Memory, 1239
Impaired Parenting, 1290
Impaired Physical Mobility, 778, 805–806
Impaired Skin Integrity, 1001–1002, 1024–1025
Impaired Swallowing, 156, 965
Impaired thought processes, 1230–1232
Impaired Tissue Integrity, 1002
Impaired Transfer Ability, 779
Impaired Verbal Communication, 1239
Impaired Walking, 779
Impaired Wheelchair Mobility, 779
Impetigo, 989
Implantable venous access devices, *582*
Implanted vascular access devices, 580
Implementation, 202–206
  activities in, 202–203
  of client teaching, 372–374
  documentation in, 203
  in health maintenance, 694–697
  nursing interventions in
    performance of, 203
    types of, 203–206
  in nursing process, 141
  priority setting in, 202–203, *204*
  reassessment in, 202
  skills in, 202
Implementing Community-Based Education in the Undergraduate Nursing Curriculum, 26
Impotence, 1362
Impulse conduction, in heart, 868
Incentive spirometry, 828, 831p–832p
Incident pain, 1170
Incident reports
  in client record, 245
  filing, 674
Incomplete proteins, 943
Incontinence
  fecal (*See* Fecal incontinence)
  urinary (*See* Urinary incontinence)
Incontinent briefs, 1087
Incubation period, of infections, 1041
Incubator, in oxygen therapy, 842t
Independence, of older adults, 660, 1294
Independent nurse practitioners, 25
Independent thinking, 218t
Independent variables, 127
Inderal, 892t
Index of Independence in Activities of Daily Living, 710, 711t
Indirect percussion, 408–409, *409*
Individual, 310
  functional health patterns of, 320–322
Individual peer review, 212
Individual plan of care, 194d
Individual therapy, 205–206
Indomethacin, 1187t
Induction, in information-processing theory, 143
Indwelling catheters, 1088
  care of, 1094
  insertion of, 1089p–1093p
  removal of, 1092p, 1095
  urine specimen collection from, 1076p
Ineffective Airway Clearance, 824, 861
Ineffective Breathing Pattern, 821–824
Ineffective Coping, 1338–1339, 1345
Ineffective Family Therapeutic Regiment Management, 1290
Ineffective Health Maintenance, 691–693
Ineffective Role Performance, 1266
Ineffective Sexuality Patterns, 1367
Ineffective Tissue Perfusion (Renal, Cerebral, Cardiopulmonary, Gastrointestinal, Peripheral), 884

Infant. *See also* Child; Newborn
  activity and exercise in, 282–283
  bathing of, 719p
  blood glucose measurement in, 960p
  blood pressure of, 467p
  blood transfusion for, 606p
  body temperature of, 453p–454p
  bowel elimination in, 1103–1104
  bowel sounds in, 432p
  breath sounds in, 429p
  cardiovascular function in, 870
  client teaching for, 375
  cognition and perception in, 286, 1225
  coping and stress tolerance in, 288, 1331
  deep breathing/coughing exercises for, 830p
  elimination in, 284
  enemas for, 1125p
  family of, 1278
  feeding of, 736
  fluid and electrolyte balance in, 916
  foot and nail care for, 728p
  grieving in, 1303
  growth and development of, 275
    cognitive, 275
    physical, 275
    psychosocial, 275
  hair care of, 731p
  health assessment of, 437
  health maintenance of, 683, 692d
  health perception and health management in, 281
  heart sounds in, 423p–424p
  hemoccult test for, 1115p
  in home healthcare, 382
  infections in, 1031
    prevention of, 501–505
  intramuscular injections for, 560p
  intravenous therapy for, 567p, 570p, 590p, 593p–594p, 596p, 598, *598*
  medication administration for, 564–570
    inhaled, 542p
    oral, 536p
  mobility of, 760–762
  nasogastric intubation of, 1131p
  neurologic assessment of, 414p
  nutrition and metabolism in, 283–284, 955
  oral care for, 733p
  oxygen therapy for, 840p
  pain perception in, 1171
  pulse oximetry for, 823p
  pulse rate of, 449, 457p
  respiratory function of, 462p, 812
  respiratory suctioning for, 854p
  roles and relationships of, 287
  safety of, 651
  self-care of, 705
  self-perception and self-concept of, 287, 1255–1257, 1256t, 1267, 1268t
  sensory perception of, 1201
  sexuality and reproduction in, 289, 1358
  skin of, 985–986
  sleep and rest in, 285, 1148–1149
  spirituality of, 1384, 1395
  subcutaneous injections for, 555p
  surgery for, 621
  total parenteral nutrition for, 602p
  tracheostomy for, 850p
  transfer of, 798p
  tube feedings for, 976p
  urinary elimination in, 1066–1067, 1066t
  values and beliefs of, 75, 76t, 291
  vital signs of, 444t, 474
  weight measurement of, 403p
  wound cultures from, 1050p
Infant-parent attachment, 1278
Infant scales, 401

Infection(s), 1027–1059. *See also* Disease; Illness
  causes of, 480–481
  chain of, *481*, 481–483
  in childhood, 1033t–1034t
  and cognition, 1228
  defenses against
    acquired, 1029–1031, 1029t
    nonspecific natural, 1028–1029, 1029t
  in home/community-based care, 1057–1058
  host for, 482–483
  intravenous therapy and, 565t, 594, 597t
  lifespan considerations, 1031–1032
  manifestations of, 1043–1044, 1043d
  microorganisms in, 480–484
  modes of transmission, 482
  nosocomial, 483–484, 655, 659, 1032, 1041
  in older adults, 303
  outcome-based teaching plan for, 1057
  portal of entry of, 482
  portal of exit of, 482
  predispositions for, 1042d
  progress of, 1041–1043
  resistance to
    altered, 1041–1044
      and activities of daily living, 1044
      evaluation of, 1058
      implementation for, 1052–1058
      nursing diagnoses for, 1051
      nursing interventions for, 1054–1057
      outcome identification and planning for, 1051–1052
    assessment of, 1044–1051
      diagnostic tests and procedures in, 1046–1051
      dysfunction identification in, 1045
      normal pattern identification in, 1044–1045, 1047d
      objective data in, 1045–1051
      physical examination in, 1045–1046
      risk identification in, 1045
      subjective data in, 1044–1045
    normal, 1028–1031, 1029t
      factors affecting, 1032–1041
  and safety, 655, 659
  and skin integrity, 989–990
  source of, 482
  spread of, prevention of, 1057
  surgery and, 618
  total parenteral nutrition and, 600–603
  transmission of, 482
  types of, 1041
  urinary catheterization and, 1093p
  wounds and, 996, 1001
Infection control, 484–486, 671. *See also* Asepsis
  and employee health, 484–486
  in home/community-based nursing, 858
  lifespan considerations, 501–509
  regulatory agencies for, 484
  waste disposal in, 486
  in workplace, 484–486
    for healthcare personnel, 485
    work restrictions and, 485–486, 487t
Infectious agents, 480–481, 482, 1032–1039
Infectious disease, definition of, 480
Infectious waste, disposal of, 486, *488*
Inferences, in assessment, 159d
Infertility, 1360, 1365
Infiltration, intravenous fluid, 594, 597t
Inflammation
  of airways, 814
  in wound healing, 994
Inflammatory disorders, and infection, 1040
Inflammatory response
  and infection resistance, 1028
  infections and, 1044

Influenza, 1033t
  immunization for, 1054t
Information, perception of, 1220–1222
Information giving, in therapeutic communication, 354
Information-processing theory
  client teaching and, 362–363
  nursing research and, 143, *143*
Information resource management, 112
Informed choices, and holistic healthcare, 259
Informed consent, 95, 98–99, 626–627, 630
Informed consent form, *629*
Ingrown nails, 726t
Inhaled medications, 540, 541p–542p
Inhibited sexual desire, 1362
Inhibitory signals, 1168
In-home phase, of home healthcare visit, 384
Initial assessment, 150, 151t
Initiation phase, of home healthcare visit, 383–384
Injectable contraceptives, 1372t
Injuries. *See also* Safety
  and altered health maintenance, 688
  prevention of, 781
  unintentional, 650
Inner ear, assessment of, 416, *417*
Input, in systems theory, 142
Insensible water loss, 920
Insight, 1223
Insomnia, 286, 1155
Inspection
  in abdominal assessment, 427–430
  in bowel function assessment, 1112
  in breast assessment, 427
  in cardiovascular assessment, 421, 880
  of extremities, 435
  in physical examination, 154–155, 407
  in respiratory assessment, 422–425, 819
  of skin, 998
  in urinary elimination assessment, 433, 1075, 1075t
  of wound, 998–1001
Inspiration (respiratory), 810
Institute of Medicine (IOM), 532
Institute of Medicine/National Academy of Sciences, Food and Nutrition Board of, 942
Institutional medication policies, 522
Institutional policies, 86
Institutional review board (IRB), 128
Institutional waste
  categories of, 487d
  disposal of, 486
Instructional nursing plan of care, 190
Instrumental skills, 79
Insulin
  and milk production, 1356
  and potassium, 912
  subcutaneous injections of, 548–550
Insulin pens, 548
Insulin syringes, 543, *543*
Insurance
  and home healthcare, 382
  professional liability, 105
Intal. *See* Cromolyn
Integration, in growth and development, 269
Integrity, 218t
  intellectual, 227t
Integumentary function. *See* Skin integrity
Intellectual courage, 227t
Intellectual development, 219. *See also* Cognition
Intellectual empathy, 227t
Intellectual humility, 227t
Intellectual integrity, 227t
Intellectual perseverance, 227t
Intelligence, 1223
Intelligence tests, 1237

Intensity, of sound, 410
Intensive care unit (ICU), client in, communication with, 359
Intentional torts, 99–100, 99d
Intercostal muscles, 810
Interdepartmental reporting, 248
Interdisciplinary team, reporting to, 248–249
Interferons, 1028
Intermediate memory, 410, 1223
Intermittent catheters, 1088, 1096
Intermittent claudication, 878
Intermittent enteral tube feedings, 973, 975p
Intermittent infusion devices, 556, 577–578, *579*
    converting to, 595p–596p
    flushing of, 595p–596p
    tunneled, 579–580
Intermittent infusion technique, 556, 568p–570p
Intermittent pneumatic compression devices, 888
Intermittent positive pressure breathing (IPPB), 841
Internal anal sphincter, 1103
Internal dialogue, 1340
Internal disaster, 673
Internal eye, assessment of, 415
Internal locus of control, 1261
Internal os, *1353*
Internal rotation, 755t
Internal urinary sphincter, 1064–1065
International Classification of Diseases (ICD-10-CM), 165
International Classification of Nursing Practice (ICNP), 165
International Council of Nurses (ICN), 45, 51, 53
    code of ethics of, 86, 87d–88d
    founding of, 42t
    International Classification of Nursing Practice of, 165
Interoceptors, 1222
Interpersonal Aspects of Nursing (Travelbee), 61t
Interpersonal nursing interventions, 204–206, 205t
Interpersonal Relations in Nursing (Peplau), 58t
Interpersonal role conflict, 1262–1263
Interpersonal theory, of self-concept, 1256t–1257t
Interpreters, for language differences, 338d
Interrole conflict, 1263
Interrupted Family Process, 1315
Interrupted Family Processes, 1288
Interstitial fluid, 910
    loss of, and wound healing, 996
    volume of, 923
Intertrigo, 986
Interventions. *See* Nursing interventions
Interview Guide: Stress and Stress Response, 1338, 1338d
Interviewing, 208
    in assessment, 152t, 153–154, 153t
    concluding phase of, 154
    in cultural assessment, 335
    ethnographic, 335
    introductory phase of, 154
    key informants for, 328, 335–337
    maintenance phase of, 154
    open-ended, 335
    phases of, 153–154
    preparatory phase of, 154
Interview phase, of health assessment, 397–406
Intestinal diversions, *1107*, 1107–1108
Intestines, 1103
Intimacy, and sleep and rest, 1158–1159
Intolerances, to medications, 526
Intracellular fluid (ICF), 910
Intradermal injections, 546–548, 551p
Intramuscular injections, 550–556, *556, 558p–560p, 564*

complications with, 561t
sites for
    deltoid, 552, 556t, *562*
    dorsogluteal, 556, 556t, *563*
    rectus femoris, 552–555, 556t, *562*
    vastus lateralis, 552–555, 556t, *562, 563*
    ventrogluteal, 555–556, 556t, *563*
    Z-track technique for, 560p, *564*
Intraoperative nursing, 612, 632–638
    assessment in, 632
    evaluation in, 638
    nursing diagnoses in, 632, 633t
    nursing interventions in, 632–638
    outcome identification in, 632, 633t
Intrapersonal role conflict, 1262
Intrathecal analgesia, 1186–1189
Intrauterine development, 272–274, *274*
    cognitive, 274
    physical, 272–274
    psychosocial, 274
Intrauterine device (IUDs), 1371, 1372t
Intravascular fluid, 910
Intravascular lines, and infections, 1039
Intravenous administration set, 581–582, *583, 584*
Intravenous flow rates, 582–586
    calculation of, 582
    factors affecting, 583–586
    regulation of, 583, 585–586
Intravenous flowsheets, 245
Intravenous lock, flushing of, 588
Intravenous medications
    administration of, 556–560
        advantages and disadvantages of, 556
        complications with, 565t
        continuous infusion technique in, 556–560
        of electrolyte supplements, 936
        intermittent infusion technique in, 556, 568p–570p
        intravenous push technique in, 556, 566p–567p
        patient-controlled analgesia in, 560
    and cardiovascular problems, 872
Intravenous pyelogram (IVP), 1081
Intravenous (IV) therapy, 575–608
    and air embolism, 597, 597t
    for blood transfusions, 603–607
    bottle changes in, 588
    catheter breakage in, 598
    client preparation for, 586
    client teaching for, 607–608
    clogged air vents in, 585
    complications with, 588–598, 597t
    definition of, 576
    discontinuing, 598
    documentation of, 588
    dressing changes in, 588
    equipment for, 577–582
    and fluid overload, 594–597, 597t
    in home/community-based care, 607–608
    and infection, 594, 597t
    infiltration in, 594, 597t
    initiation of, 586–588
    intermittent flushing in, 588
    lifespan considerations, 590p, 598–599
    maintenance of, 588
    monitoring of, 588, 589p–590p, 608
    needleless system accessories for, 582, *584*
    nurse's role in, 586–599
    obstruction of tubing in, 584
    outcome-based teaching plan for, 581
    patency of, 584–585
    and phlebitis, 594, 597t
    and pneumothorax, 597–598
    positional, 584
    positioning of access in, 584
    positioning of extremity in, 583–584

preoperative, 628–629, 642
    site preparation in, 586
    site selection in, 586
        for infants, *598*
    solutions in, 576–577, *577*, 578t
        changing, 591p–594p
        containers for, 580, *582*, 583
    for terminally ill patients, 599
    therapeutic dialogue, 587
    tubing changes in, 588, 591p–594p
    venipuncture in
        securing of device, 587–588
        technique for, 586
Introductory phase, of interview process, 154
Intuition, in assessment, 152t, 155
Invasion of privacy, 99–100
Invasive devices, and infections, 1039
Invasive medical techniques, in pain management, 1193–1194, 1193t
Invasiveness, of infectious agent, 482
Inversion, 755t
Involuntary relocation, coping with, 1333–1334
Iodine, 948t, 949
IOM. *See* Institute of Medicine
Ions, 912
Iowa ICU Family Scale (IIFS), 1284
IPPB. *See* Intermittent positive pressure breathing
Ipratropium (Atrovent), 836t
IQ tests, 1237
IRB. *See* Institutional review board
Iron, 948t, 949
Iron-deficiency anemia, 949
Irregularly irregular pulse, 458
Irrigation
    colostomy, 1136, *1136*
    continuous bladder, *1095*
    stomal, 1136, *1136*
    of urinary catheters, 1094–1095, *1095*
    of wounds, 1016p–1017p
Irritable bowel syndrome (IBS), 1110
Ischemia, 878
Ischemic pain, management of, 893
Islam, 1396t
Islands of Langerhans, *1327*
Isoetharine (Bronkosol), 836t
Isolation
    protective, 495
        psychological effects of, 496
Isolation systems, 494–496
Isometric exercise, 760
Isotonic dehydration, 921
Isotonic exercise, 760
Isotonic fluids, 576, *577, 578t*
I statements, 1269
Itching. *See* Pruritus
IUDs. *See* Intrauterine device
IVP. *See* Intravenous pyelogram
IV therapy. *See* Intravenous therapy

J

Jacket restraint, 665
Jackson-Pratt drain, 1001, *1001*
Japanese Americans, response to death and dying, 339
JCAHO. *See* Joint Commission on Accreditation of Healthcare Organizations
Jehovah's Witnesses, 1397t
Jejunostomy, 972t, 973
Jejunum, 1102
Jelly, as drug preparation, 516t
Jet lag, 1156
Jews, 1396t
Job satisfaction, 116
Jock itch, 990
Johnson, Dorothy E., 60t, 138, 139t

Joint(s)
  assessment of, 776–777
  flexibility of, decreased, 766
  mobility of, 755, 755t, 761t–762t, 763–764
    assessment of, 435
    maintenance, 784–788
    pain with, 767–768
Joint Commission on Accreditation of Healthcare
    Organizations (JCAHO), 27
  on assessment, 150
  on audits of client records, 230
  on client teaching, 362
  on confidentiality, 249
  on infection control, 484
  on nursing diagnosis, 164
  Organizational Ethics Committees of, 97
  on plans of care, 141, 190
  quality improvement programs of, 211
  standards of care of, 98
  on translators, 371
  on use of restraints, 665
Journals. *See* Nursing journals
J pouch, 1107
Judgment, 1223, 1226
Judgmental reflectivity, 226t
Jugular venous distention, fluid and electrolyte/
    acid-base balance and, 931, *931*
Jugular venous pressure, assessment of, 419, *420*
Justice, 89–92

K

Kalamazoo Community Indicators, 26
*Kalamazoo County Healthier Community
    Assessment,* 26
Kaolin/pectin (Donnagel), 1122t
Kardex, 238, *239,* 247
Kava-kava, 519t
Kegel exercises, 737, 1368, 1371d
Keratoses, 986
Ketoacidosis, diabetic, 924
Ketonuria, 1080t
Key informants, 328, 335–337
Kidney(s), 1064. *See also* under Renal
  acid-base balance and, 918
  fluid and electrolyte balance and, 920
  magnesium and, 913
  potassium and, 912
  and urine formation, 1065
Kidney function studies, 882
Kidneys, ureters, and bladder (KUB), 1081
Kidney stones, altered mobility and, 769–770
Kilocalorie, 942
Kinesthetic learners, 218
Kinetic therapy beds, 1004
King, Imogene M., 61t, 64t
Klebsiella, and urinary tract infections, 1069
Knee joint, 762t
Knots, for restraints, 666, *667*
Knowledge
  baseline, 365
  domains of, 363–364
  for nursing process, 144
  types of, 219
Knowledge base, 220
Knowles, Lois, 138, 139t
Kock's pouch, 1107–1108
Kohlberg, Lawrence, 270, 272t
Krieger, Dolores, 264
KUB film, 1081
Kubler-Ross grief model, 1302t, 1313–1314
Kunz, Dora, 264
Kussmaul respirations, 460t
Kwell. *See* Gamma benzene hexachloride
Kyphosis, 399

L

Labia majora, 1353, *1353*
Labia minora, 1353, *1353*
Labor, 1356
Laboratory tests. *See also* Diagnostic tests/procedures
  as data source, 157
  interpretation of, 208
Laboratory values, 954, 1411–1416
Lacerations, 990, 990t
Lack of coordination, and altered mobility, 765
Lactation, 1354, *1354,* 1356
  iodine and, 949
  medication assessment and, 526–527
  nutrition and, 954–955
Lactose intolerance, 334, 1105
Lamellar bone, 754
Landmarks
  for abdominal assessment, 427
  for cardiac assessment, 421, *421*
  for respiratory assessment, 422, *426*
Language, 345–346, 1224. *See also* Communica-
    tion; Speech
  assessment of, 410
  in client teaching, 366, 371
  cultural differences and, 337, 338d
  in sexual function assessment, 1363
Language barriers, 1230
Language Line Service, 371
Lanugo, 985
Large intestine, 951, 1102
Large-volume enemas, 1122, 1123p–1124p
Large volume pneumatic nebulizer, 842t
Larynx, impairment in use of, 1236
Lasix, 892t
Latch-key children, 1281
Latent infection, 1043
Latex allergy, 493–494, 623, *625,* 656
Latex gloves, 493–494
Latex Risk Tool, 623, *625*
Lavage
  gastric, 1126
  saline, 851
Laws
  administrative, 98
  civil, 98
  criminal, 98
  Good Samaritan, 103–104
  sources of, 98
Laxatives, 1109, 1120–1121, 1121t
  abuse of, 1105
  and fluid and electrolyte balance, 916
Lay health workers, 24
LDL cholesterol, 871
Leadership, 110–111
  application to nursing roles, 114–119
  directive, 110, *111*
  participative, 110, *111*
  styles of, 110–111, *111*
  therapeutic dialogue for, 115
Lead time, in sensory adaptation, 1200–1201
Learning, 362, 1224. *See also* Client teaching
  approaches to, 362, 363t
  definition of, 1220
  documentation of, 374
  evaluation of, 374
  maintenance of skills for, 1241
  readiness for, 367–368
Learning needs
  assessment of, 365–367
  in preoperative nursing, 623
Learning-oriented students, 219
Learning styles, 218–219
Lectures, in client teaching, 369
Leftward shift, 1047
Legal documentation, 231

Legal guidelines, 86
Legal issues, 98–105. *See also* Ethical/legal issues
  in medication administration, 521–523
  and nursing research, 128–129, 128d
Leg bags, 1097, *1097*
Legibility, of documentation, 233
Legs
  blood pressure measurement in, 464
  dangling of, before ambulation, 788
  elevation of, for edema reduction, 889
  exercises for, to improve circulation, 885, *886*
  ulceration of, 986, *987*
Lesions, 991, 992t–993t
Leukocytes. *See* White blood cells
Leukocytosis, 1046
Leukotriene inhibitors, 836t
Level of consciousness, 410
Levin, Myra Estrin, 60t
Liability, 101, 102t
Liability insurance, 105
Libel, 99
Liberal thinkers, 219
Lice, 724, 1039
Licensed practical nurses (LPNs), 9, 48
Licensed vocational nurses, 48
Licensure, 27, 98
  routes to, 48
Lichenification, 993t
Licorice, 519t
Life cycle, of family, 311–312
Life experience, and values, 74–75
Lifespan considerations
  for ambulation assistance, 797p
  for antiembolism stockings, 888p
  for bathing, 719p
  for bedpan use, 741p
  for blood transfusion, 606p
  for bowel elimination, 1103–1105
  for cardiovascular function, 870
  for client transfer, 798p, 803p
  for cognitive function, 1225–1226
  for condom catheter application, 1087p
  for deep breathing/coughing exercises, 830p
  for enemas, 1125p
  family, 1278–1280
  for fecal ostomy pouch use, 1136p
  for fluid and electrolyte balance, 916
  for foot and nail care, 728p
  for hair care, 731p
  for health assessment, 437–440
  for health maintenance, 683–685, 692d–693d
  for hemoccult test, 1115p
  for incentive spirometry, 832p
  for infection control, 501–509, 1031–1032
  for inhaled medications, 542p
  for intermittent infusion technique, 570p
  for intramuscular injections, 560p
  for intravenous therapy, 567p, 590p,
      593p–594p, 596p, 598–599
  for medication administration, 564–572
  for mobility, 760–763
  for nasogastric intubation, 1131p
  for nutrition, 954–957
  for oral administration, 536p
  for oral care, 733p
  for oxygen therapy, 840p
  for pain perception, 1171–1172
  for peak flow monitoring, 824p
  for pulse oximetry, 823p
  for respiratory function, 812–813
  for respiratory suctioning, 854p
  for safety, 650–652
  for self care, 705–706
  for self-concept, 1255–1259, 1256t–1257t
  for sensory perception, 1201
  for skin integrity, 985–986

Lifespan considerations (*continued*)
for sleep and rest, 1148–1150, *1149*
for spirituality, 1384–1385, 1384t, 1395–1398
for stress, coping, and adaptation, 1331–1332
for subcutaneous injections, 555p
for surgery, 621–622
for total parenteral nutrition, 602p
for tracheostomy, 850p
for urinary catheterization, 1093p
for urinary elimination, 1066–1067.6t
for values, 75–76, 76t
for vital signs, 473–475
for wound cultures, 1050p
for wound dressings, 1013p
Lifespan development, 267–291. *See also* Growth and development
functional health patterns and, 281–291
therapeutic dialogue for, 290
Lifestyle
and bowel elimination, 1106
and cognitive function, 1240–1241
and coping, 1332, 1340
of families, 1281
and health maintenance, 685
and mobility, 763
and nutrition, 958–961
and respiratory function, 813–814
and safety, 656
and sensory perception, 1201
and skin integrity, 989
and sleep and rest, 1151–1152
Lifestyle Assessment Questionnaire, 690
Lifestyle modification, 263
Lifting
hydraulic devices for, 801
injury prevention during, 665
mechanical, 759
stand-up assist, 801, *803*
two- or three-person, 794
Lift sheet, 759
Ligaments, 755
Light, and sleep and rest, 1150
Lighting, tangential, in physical examination, 407
Light palpation, 407–408, *408*
Limbic system, stress and, 1329
Limbs, elevation of, for edema reduction, 889
Liniment, 516t
Lipids. *See also* Fat
and cardiovascular function, 882
Lips. *See also* Mouth
color of, 419
Liquid diets, 971
Listening, 113, 144, 217, 349, 353–354, 1395
Literacy, and client teaching, 217, 367–368
Literature review
as data source, 157
in nursing research, 126
Liver, 951
Liver disease, dietary modifications for, 972d
Liver spots, 986
Living wills, 89, *90,* 102–103, 1308
Local anesthesia, 635–636, 1193t
Local health department, and consulting nurse services, 9
Local infections, 1041
Local tissue barriers, to infection, 1029t
Lockjaw, 1038t
Locus of control, 1261
Logotherapy, 305
Logrolling, 783
Loneliness, in older adults, 304–305
Long bones, 754
Long-term care, 1246–1247
Long-term care facilities
medication distribution in, 516, *516*
nosocomial infections in, 483–484

Long-term coping mechanisms, 1331d
Long-term memory, 410, 1223
Loop of Henle, 1064
Loperamide (Imodium), 1122t
Lorazepam (Ativan), 1160
Lordosis, 399
Loss. *See also* Death and dying; Grieving
among older adults, 304
circumstances and meaning of, effect on grieving, 1304–1305
therapeutic dialogue for, 1301
types of, 1300
Loss education, 1308–1309
Lotions, 516t
administration of, 537
Lovastatin, 892t
Love, 63, 1389t
Low-air-loss beds, for pressure ulcer prevention, 1005
Low-density lipoprotein (LDL) cholesterol, 871
Lower extremities. *See* Legs
Low-flow cough, 830
Low-grade fever, 1043
Lozenge (troche), 516t
LPNs. *See* Licensed practical nurses
L-Tryptophan, 1151
Lumpers, 218
Lung(s), 810
anatomic landmarks of, 422
auscultation of, 425–427, 428p–429p, 819–820
capacity of, age and, 459
decreased expansion of, altered mobility and, 768
defenses of, 812
fluid loss through, 920
percussion of, 425, 819
restricted movement of, 814
Luteal phase, of ovarian cycle, 1355, *1355*
Luteinizing hormone, and menstruation, 1355
Lutherans, 1396t
Lymphatic vessels, filtration pressure and, 915
Lymph nodes
assessment of, 419
infections and, 1044, 1045–1046
Lysaught report, 45

M

MAAS. *See* Maternal Attachment Assessment Strategy
Macrodrip tubing, 581–582, *583*
Macrophages, 1030t
Macule, 992t
Magnesium, 912, 912t, 913, 937t, 948t
Magnetic resonance imaging (MRI), in infection detection, 1051
Ma-Huang, 519t
Mainline Protestants, 1396t
Maintenance insomnia, 1155
Maintenance nursing interventions, 206
Maintenance phase, of interview process, 154
Major depression, 300t
Malabsorption, of nutrients, 958
Male genitalia, assessment of, 434–435, 1366
Male-pattern baldness, 726
Male reproductive system, 1352, *1352*
Male sexual response, 1356–1357
Male sterilization, 1373, 1373t
Malignant hyperthermia, 618
Malignant pain, 1170
Malnutrition, and infections, 1039
Malpractice, 100, 101, 102t
Mammary glands. *See* Breast(s)
Managed care delivery model, 117
Managed care organizations (MCOs), 10, 81–83
Management, *111,* 111–114

application to nursing roles, 114–119
change and, 114, *114*
communication in, 113
delegation in, 113–114, 113d
effective, skills for, 112–114
of financial resources, 112
of health maintenance, 681
of human resources, 112
of information resources, 112
planning and, 112
problem solving in, 113
of resources, 111–112
roles of, *118,* 118–119
of safety, 650
supervision in, 113d
therapeutic dialogue and, 115
Managers, nurses as, 50
Man-Living-Health: Theory of Nursing (Parse), 62t
Manning v. Twin Falls Clinic and Hospital, 101
Mantoux test, 546–548
Manual resuscitation bag and mask, 841–843
Martin Chuzzlewit (Dickens), 44
Mask(s)
in asepsis, 493, *493*
manual resuscitation bag and, 841–843
in oxygen therapy, 838p–840p, *841,* 842t, 842t
Maslow, Abraham, 271–272
Maslow's hierarchy of human needs, 62–64, *63, 64*
Massage, 1342t
abdominal, in bowel training, 1132
back, 717, 725p
in pain management, 1183
Mastectomy, and sexuality, 1362
Master's degree nursing program, 48–49, 130d
Mastication, 951
Masturbation, 1354
Maternal Attachment Assessment Strategy (MAAS), 1360
Maternal-child nursing, in ancient Egypt, 43
Maternal-fetal attachment (MFA), mother-father relationship and, 1360
Mattresses
in hospitals, 739
for pressure ulcer prevention, 1005
Mattress overlays, for pressure ulcer prevention, 1005, *1007*
Maturation, in wound healing, 994
McGill-Melzack Pain Questionnaire, 1178, *1179,* 1180
MCOs. *See* Managed care organizations
MDI. *See* Metered-dose inhaler
Meaning
and self-esteem, 1255
and spirituality, 1389t
Measles, 1033t
healthcare personnel with, work restrictions for, 487t
Measles-mumps-rubella (MMR) vaccine, 1054t
Meat, in Food Guide Pyramid, 951
Mechanical barrier contraceptives, 1372t
Mechanical barriers, to infection, 1028, 1029t
Mechanical lifts, 759
Mechanical receptors, 1168
Mechanical soft diets, 971
Mechanical vectors, 482
Mechanical ventilator, for inhaled medications, 540
Meconium, 1103–1104
Medicaid
and Civil Rights Act, 337
and client records, 231
and plans of care, 190
Medical asepsis, 488, 489p–490p. *See also* Asepsis
Medical diagnosis, 167–168, 168t
Medical futility, 95
Medical history. *See* Health history
Medical model, of assessment, 160

Medical records. *See* Client records
Medical Symptoms Reduction Programs, 263
Medical terminology, 1417–1424
Medical treatment
  indications for, 94–95
  moral issues regarding, 1386–1387
Medicare
  and Civil Rights Act, 337
  and client records, 231
  and home healthcare, 381
  hospice nursing home benefit of, 1313
  and plans of care, 190
Medication(s)
  administration of, 513–572
    diet and fluid orders and, 527
    documentation of, 532
    five rights of, 530–532, 531d
    in home/community-based care, 533,
      562–564
    legal aspects of, 521–523
    lifespan considerations, 564–572
    medication assessment prior to, 527–528
    outcome-based teaching plan for, 528
    safety of, 529–564
    teaching of, 529
    therapeutic dialogue, 571
    timing of, 532
    topical medications, 537–539
  adverse effects of, 524
  allergic reactions to, 524
  and blood pressure, 464
  and bowel elimination, 1106, 1120–1121
  and cardiovascular function, 872, 880, 889, 892t
  classifications of, 514, 515t
  client response to, evaluation of, 564
  and cognition, 1228–1229, 1235, 1247
  crushing, 537
  definition of, 514
  and diarrhea, 1109
  distribution systems for, 515–517
    automated medication-dispensing system,
      516–517, 517
    bar code medication administration, 517
    self-administered medication system, 517
    stock supply system, 515–516
    unit-dose system, 516
  dosages of, 531
    calculation of, 530
    in medication order, 518
  hypersensitivity reactions to, 524
  and infection, 1040–1041
  interactions of, 524–526
  mixing, 546, 549p–550p
  names of, 518
  nonprescription, 517
  overdose of, 656–657
  over-the-counter, 517
  pharmacodynamics of, 524–526
  pharmacokinetics of, 523
  preoperative administration, 630
  prescription, 517
  and pulse rate, 449
  reconstituting, 544–546
  refusal of, 523
  and respiratory function, 459, 836t
  route of administration, 531
    aerosol, 832–834
    inhaled, 540
    nasogastric, 1128–1131
    oral, 533–537
    topical, 537–539
  and sensory perception, 1202
  and sexuality, 1360–1361
  side effects of, 524
  for sleep and rest, 1154, 1159–1160
  sources of information about, 514–515

and surgery, 622–623
therapeutic effects of, 524
tolerance to, 524
in total parenteral nutrition, 600
toxicity of, 524
and urinary elimination, 1070
and wound healing, 996
Medication assessment, 526–529
  allergies in, 526
  client knowledge and compliance in, 528–529
  diet and fluid orders in, 527
  intolerances in, 526
  laboratory values in, 527
  medical history in, 526
  medication history in, 526
  medication record in, 527
  physical examination in, 527–528
  pregnancy and lactation status in, 526–527
  prior to medication administration, 527–528
Medication errors, 532–533
Medication history, 526
Medication order, 518–520
  abbreviations in, 518, 520t
  components of, 518
  fax, 519–520
  interpretation of, 530
  medication dosage in, 518
  medication name in, 518
  one-time, 519
  PRN, 518
  route of administration in, 518
  routine, 518
  signature in, 518
  standing, 518
  standing protocols, 518–519
  stat, 519
  telephone, 519–520
  types of, 518–520
  verbal, 519–520
Medication record, 245, 246, 527
Medication standards, 514
Meditation, 263–264, 1342t
  in pain management, 1185–1186
MedWatch, 524, 525
Melanin, 334
Melatonin, and sleep-wake patterns, 1147, 1160
Memorial Pain Assessment Card, 1180
Memory, 1223, 1224
  assessment of, 410
  in children, 288–289
  definition of, 1220
  impaired, 1231
  improving, 1241
  in older adults, 377
  therapeutic dialogue, 1245
Men. *See also* Gender; Male
  adolescent, 277
  bladder of, 1064
  body temperature of, 445
  moral development of, 291
  respirations of, 459
  stress response in, 1329, 1332
  urinary catheterization for, 1091p–1092p, 1093p
  urinary hesitancy in, 1067
  urinary tract infections in, 1069
Menarche, 277, 1358
Meningitis, 1034t
Menopause, 1358
Menstruation, 1354–1355
Mental illness, and spirituality, 1399
Mental status
  fluid imbalance and, 927
  pressure ulcers and, 988
Mental status questionnaire, 1233
Menthol products, in pain management, 1183
Meperidine, 1188t

Mercury manometer, 464
Mercury thermometer, 447, 447
Metabolic acidosis, 924
Metabolic alkalosis, 924
Metabolic demand, 958
Metabolic rate, decreased, altered mobility and,
  769
Metabolic response, pain and, 1175
Metabolism, 952–953. *See also* Nutrition and
  metabolism
  aerobic, 765
  age and, 956
  anaerobic, 765
  basal, 953
  of carbohydrates, 952
  definition of, 942
  of fats, 952
  of medications, 523
  and pressure ulcers, 989
  of proteins, 952–953
  skin in, 985
  and sleep and rest, 1151
Metacommunication, 344–345
Metaproterenol (Alupent), 836t
Metered-dose inhaler (MDI), 540, 541p–542p,
  824, 837
Methadone, 1188t
Methodists, 1396t
Mexican Americans, and religion, 335–336
MFA. *See* Maternal-fetal attachment
MHC. *See* Minimum inhibitory concentration
MHLC questionnaire. *See* Multidimensional
  health locus of control questionnaire
MI. *See* Myocardial infarction
Microdrip tubing, 582, 583
Microorganisms. *See also specific organism*
  drug-resistant, 481
  and infection, 480–484
  as normal flora, 1028
  sensitivity testing of, 1047
Micturition, 1065–1066, 1084. *See also* Urinary
  elimination
Middle adult. *See also* Adult
  growth and development of, 279
    cognitive, 279
    physical, 279
    psychosocial, 279
  health maintenance of, 693d
  values development in, 76t
Middle managers, 118, 118
Midstream urine specimen, 1075, 1077p
Midwife. *See* Nurse midwife
Milia, 985
Military nursing, 44–45
Milk, in Food Guide Pyramid, 951
Milk production, 1356
Miller-Abbot tube, 1126–1127
Milliequivalent, 912
Mind-body connection, 258
Mind Body Medical Institute, 1342
Minerals, 947–950, 948t, 995. *See also specific*
  minerals
Mini-Mental Status Examination (MMSE), 1233,
  1237, 1238d, 1247
Minimum inhibitory concentration (MHC), for
  infection detection, 1047
Mini-pills, 1371
Minorities, 331
Mirrored body image, 1254
Misdemeanor, 99d
Mites, 1039
Mitral (apical) area, 421
Mitt restraint, 665
Mixed apnea, 1156
MMR vaccine. *See* Measles-mumps-rubella vaccine
MMSE. *See* Mini-Mental Status Examination

Mobility
  altered, 765–771
    and activities of daily living, 771
    and functional activities, 766–771, 767t
    health promotion for, 780–781
    in home/community-based nursing,
        382–383, 801–804
    implementation for, 780–804
    manifestations of, 765–766
    nursing diagnoses for, 778–780
    nursing interventions for, 781–801
    outcome identification and planning for, 780
  altered respiratory function and, 816
  assessment of, 400, 413p, 771–778
    diagnostic tests/procedures in, 778
    dysfunction identification in, 776
    normal pattern identification in, 771
    objective data in, 776–778
    physical examination in, 776–778
    risk identification in, 776
    subjective data in, 771–776
  and cognitive function, 1243–1244
  evaluation, 804
  factors affecting, 763–765
  lifespan considerations, 760–763
  normal, 754–763
    characteristics of, 760
  and normal physiologic function, 755–760
  of older adults, 298–299
  outcome-based teaching plan for, 804
  postoperative, 642–643
  and safety, 663
  surgery and, 621d
  therapeutic dialogue, 777
Models, in client teaching, 371
Modular nursing, 117
Moisture, of skin, 985
  and pressure ulcers, 988
Mongolian spots, 334
Monocytes, 1028, 1030t
Monosaccharides, 943, 952
Mons pubis, 1353, *1353*
Montgomery straps/ties, for wound dressings,
    1008, *1010*
Mood
  assessment of, 410
  and sleep and rest, 1154
Mood disorders, in older adults, 298
Moral development, 270, 272t
Moralism, 357
Moral issues, regarding medical treatment,
    1386–1387
Morality, personal, 86
Moral judgment, 291
Moral reasoning, 291
  in cognitive development theory, 270
Moral values, 70
Mormons, 1397t
Morning after pill, 1371, 1372t
Morning people, 1150
Moro reflex, 414p, 760
Morphine
  in pain management, 1186, 1188t
  and sleep, 1154
  withdrawal from, 1189
MOSES. *See* Multidimensional Observation Scale
    for Elderly Subjects
Motility, intestinal, 1103
Motivation
  client teaching and, 367
  and health maintenance, 680–681
  and self-care, 707
Motor aphasia, 410, 1231, 1232t
Motor vehicle incidents, 652, 656, 664
Mourning, 1300. *See also* Grieving
Mouth, 951, 1102

  assessment of, 418
  inspection of, 965
  structures of, *418*
Movement. *See also* Mobility
  in change theory, 65
MRI. *See* Magnetic resonance imaging
Mucous membranes
  altered nutrition and, 963
  assessment of, 418
  breaks in, infections and, 1039
  protection of, in infection control, 1052
Multidimensional health locus of control
    (MHLC) questionnaire, 1341
Multidimensional Observation Scale for Elderly
    Subjects (MOSES), 182
Multidisciplinary clinical research, 130–131
Multilumen central catheters, 578, *579*
Multiplicity, 219
Mummy restraint, 665
Mumps, 1033t
  healthcare personnel with, work restrictions for,
    487t
Muscle(s)
  of breathing, 810
  contraction of, 754
  injections into (*See* Intramuscular injections)
  and mobility, 754–755, 763–764
Muscle atrophy, 754–755, 766–767
Muscle mass
  assessment of, 777–778
  and medication administration, 527
Muscle relaxants, intraoperative, 635
Muscle relaxation, 1342, 1343d
Muscle sensation, abnormal, 928
Muscle strength
  and ambulation, 794
  assessment of, 435, 436d, 777–778
  decreased, and altered mobility, 765
Muscle tone
  abnormal, 928
  assessment of, 777–778
  decreased
    and altered mobility, 765
    and urinary elimination, 1069–1070
  promotion of optimal, for urinary function,
    1083–1084
Muscle weakness, 766–767
Muscular dysfunction, and cognition, 1226
Musculoskeletal system
  and altered health maintenance, 687–688
  and mobility, 763–764
  and safety, 652
  stress and, 1337
  structure of, 754–755
Music therapy, 1246
Muslims, 1396t
Myelograms, in mobility assessment, 778
Myocardial infarction (MI), 874
  in older adults, 1172
  symptoms of, 696d
Myocardium, 866

N
Nails, 984
  assessment of, 419–420
  care of, 704, 723, 727p–728p
  clubbing of, 420, *420*
  color of, 419
  examination of, 998
Nalbuphine, 1188t
Naloxone, 1186, 1188t
NANDA. *See* North American Nursing Diagnosis
    Association
NANDA Taxonomy II, 167, 170d–174d
Naproxen, 1187t

Naps, 1147, 1150
Narcolepsy, 1155
Narcotics
  and blood pressure, 464
  and respiratory function, 459, 814
  and urinary elimination, 1070
Narrative nursing progress notes, 238, 240t, *241*
Nasal cannula, in oxygen therapy, 838p–840p,
    841, 842t
Nasal medications, administration of, 538–539
Nasal pharyngeal airway, 843, *846*
Nasal prongs, in oxygen therapy, 842t
Nasogastric decompression, preoperative, 629
Nasogastric intubation, 972–973, 972t, *1126,*
    1126–1131
  equipment for, 1126–1127
  intake and output monitoring with, 1128
  medication administration with, 1128–1131
  nasal and oral care with, 1128
  nursing considerations in, 1127–1131
  nursing procedure for, 974p–976p,
    1129p–1131p
  placement of, 1127–1128
  suction in, 1127, 1128
  tube patency, 1128
Nasointestinal intubation, 1126–1127
National Center for Complementary and Alterna-
    tive Medicine (NCCAM), 28, 259,
    263, 263d
National Center for Nursing Research, 42t, 124
National Commission on Nursing and Nursing
    Education, 45
National Committee for Quality Assurance
    (NCQA), 27
National Formulary, 514
National Institute for Nursing Research, 51, 124
National League for Nursing (NLN), 21, 23, 45,
    48, 52, 221, *221,* 222t
National Nosocomial Infections Surveillance
    (NNIS), 483
National Student Nurses' Association (NSNA),
    42t, 53
Native Americans, 330–331, 336
Natural Death Act, 102
Natural family planning, 1369
Natural immunity, 1031
Nature and nurture, 1259. *See also* Environment;
    Genetics
The Nature of Nursing (Henderson), 58t
Nausea
  and nutrition, 957
  with opioid analgesics, 1191
Navy Nurse Corps, 44
Nazarenes, 1396t
NCCAM. *See* National Center for Complemen-
    tary and Alternative Medicine
NCQA. *See* National Committee for Quality
    Assurance
NDEC. *See* Nursing Diagnosis Extension and
    Classification
Nebulizers, 540, 825, 832, *837,* 842t
Neck
  assessment of, 410–419, 418–419
  movements of, 761t
  veins in, distention of, 931, *931*
Nedocromil (Tilade), 824, 836t
NEECHAM Confusion Scale, 1233, 1237
Needle(s), 543, *543*
Needle-housing systems, 485, *486*
Needleless access adapters, in intravenous therapy,
    582, *584*
Needleless systems, 485, *486,* 543–544, *544*
Needle sharing, 655
Needlestick injuries, 485, *485, 486,* 487, 587, 671
Needs, 62–64
Negative-airflow rooms, 494

Negative feedback, 313
Negative stressors, 1329
Neglect, of client, 1074
Negligence, 100, 102t
Negotiation, in discharge planning, 32
Neisseria gonorrhoeae, 1035t
Neonate. *See* Newborn
Neoplasms, and skin integrity, 990
Nephron, 1064
Nerve blocks, in pain management, 1193t
Nerve sprouts, 1173–1174
Nervous system
    and cognition, 1220
    and mobility, 764
    and safety, 652–653
Networking, 128
Neuman, Betty, 61t
The Neuman Systems Model (Neuman), 61t
Neural plasticity, and pain perception, 1172–1174
Neurectomy, in pain management, 1193t
Neuroendocrine regulation, of physiologic func-
    tioning, 1326–1328
Neuroendocrine response, pain and, 1175
Neurologic assessment, 410, 411p–414p
    postoperative, 639
    for safety concerns, 661
Neurologic infections, 1034t–1035t
Neurologic injury, and urinary elimination, 1069
Neuromas, 1173–1174
Neuromuscular function, and self-care, 708
Neuropathic pain, 1192
Neuropeptides, stress and, 1329
Neurotransmitters, and sleep, 1145
Neutropenia, precautions against, 1056
Neutrophils, 1028, 1030t, 1046–1047
Newborn. *See also* Child; Infant
    activity and exercise in, 282–283
    bathing of, 719p
    body temperature of, 445, 453p–454p
    bowel elimination in, 1103–1104
    bowel sounds in, 432p
    breath sounds in, 429p
    cardiovascular function in, 870
    client teaching for, 375
    cognition and perception in, 286, 1225
    coping and stress tolerance in, 288, 1331
    elimination in, 284
    family of, 1278
    fluid and electrolyte balance in, 916
    grieving in, 1303
    growth and development of, 274–275
        cognitive, 274–275
        physical, 274
        psychosocial, 274
    health assessment of, 437
    health maintenance of, 683
    health perception and health management in,
        281
    heart sounds in, 423p–424p
    infection control for, 501–505
    infections in, 1031
    intravenous therapy for, 598, *598*
    medication administration for, 564–570
    mobility of, 760–762
    neurologic assessment of, 414p
    nutrition and metabolism in, 283–284, 955
    pain perception in, 1171
    respiratory function of, 812
    roles and relationships of, 287
    safety of, 651
    self-care of, 705
    self-perception and self-concept in, 287,
        1255–1257, 1256t, 1267, 1268t
    sensory perception of, 1201
    sexuality and reproduction in, 289, 1358
    skin of, 985–986

    sleep and rest of, 285, 1148–1149
    spirituality of, 1384, 1395
    surgery for, 621
    urinary elimination in, 1066–1067, 1066t
    values and beliefs in, 75, 291
    vital signs of, 444t, 474
New England Medical Center Hospital, 194
NF. *See National Formulary*
Niacin, 946t, 947
NIC. *See* Nursing Intervention Classification
Nicotine, and sleep, 1154
Nifedipine, 892t
Nightingale, Florence, 41t, 44, 45, 56, 58t, 64t,
        70, 123, 261
Nightingale Pledge, 70, 71d
Nightmares, 285
Night terrors, 1156
Nitrates, and cardiac function, 892t
Nitrogen balance, 769, 943
Nitroglycerin, 892t
    in emergency cardiovascular care, 902
    transdermal administration of, 538
NLN. *See* National League for Nursing
NNIS. *See* National Nosocomial Infections
        Surveillance
NOC. *See* Nursing-Sensitive Outcomes
        Classification
Nociceptors, 1168
Nocturia, 1071
Nocturnal enuresis, 285, 1073
Nodule, 992t
Noise, and sleep and rest, 1150
Noise pollution, 655
Noncompliance, 367, 1393
Nonfluent aphasia, 410, 1231, 1232t
Noninvasive urine volume monitoring,
        1074–1075
Nonmaleficence, 89
Nonopioid analgesics, 1186, 1187t
Nonprescription medications, 517
Nonprofessional relationships, 357
Nonproprietary drug name, 514
Non-rapid eye movement sleep, 1144, 1149
Nonsteroidal antiinflammatory drugs (NSAIDs),
        in pain management, 1186, 1187t
Nontherapeutic responses, to therapeutic commu-
        nication, 355–357
Nonverbal behavior, observation of, 152
Nonverbal communication, 113, 344, 344d, 359,
        396, 397, 1176t, 1224
Norepinephrine, 892t, 1327
    and body temperature, 446
    stress and, 1329
Normal flora, 1028
North American Nursing Diagnosis Association
        (NANDA), 140, 147, 222–223
    definition of nursing diagnosis, 164
    goal of, 165
    and International Classification of Nursing
        Practice, 165
    and Nursing Diagnosis Extension and Classifi-
        cation project, 167
    review and staging process of, 165–167
    Taxonomy II of, 167, 170d–174d
Norton Scale, for pressure ulcer risk, 998
Nose, care of, 704–705
Nosocomial infections, 483–484, 655, 659, 1032,
        1041
Notes on Nursing (Nightingale), 56, 58t
Novice, in critical thinking development, 226
Novice nurse, 46t
NPO orders, 968–971
NPO status, 627–628
NSNA. *See* National Student Nurses' Association
Nuclear family, 1276–1277
Nuremberg Tribunal, 128, 128d

Nurse(s)
    as barriers to client goals, 210
    as caregivers, 49
    as client advocate, 49–50
    as communicators, 50
    as decision makers, 49
    as educators, 50 (*See also* Client teaching)
    in home healthcare, 383–389
    leadership roles of, 110–111
    legal protection for, 104–105
    as managers and coordinators, 50
    participation in nursing research, 129–132
    self-concept of, 47
    stress management for, 1340d
    subculture of, 331–332
    values of
        challenges to, 81–83
        manifestations of, 79–80
Nurse administrator, 51
Nurse anesthetist, 50–51, 117
Nurse anthropologists, 326
Nurse-client interaction, and sensory perception,
        1209–1210
Nurse-client relationship, 343–359
    advocacy in, 348–349, 348t
    authoritarian, 348t
    confidentiality in, 349
    contract setting in, 347–348, 348d
    guilt inducement in, 348t
    phases of, 347
    and spirituality, 1394
    vs. social relationships, 347t
Nurse Corps of the United States Army, 44
Nurse educator, 51
Nurse executive, 112, *118*, 119
Nurse Healers-Professional Associates Interna-
        tional, 264
Nurse midwife, 50, 117
Nurse practice acts, 51, 522
Nurse practitioners, 25, 50, 117
Nurse researcher, 51
Nursing
    administrative, 9
    advanced clinical practice roles, 117
    career opportunities in, 46–49
    clinical practice roles, 114–117
    community-based, 22–26 (*See also* Community-
        based nursing)
    concept of, 57, 58t–62t
    culturally sensitive, 333–334
    culture and, 332–338
    current issues and trends in, 8–16, 53
    current status of, 13–16
    definitions of, 40, 45–46, 47t
    ethics in, 86–98
    future of, 45, 53
    history of, 40–45, 41t–42t
        during American Civil War, 44
        in ancient Greece, 43
        in ancient history, 43
        in early Christian era, 43
        in Middle Ages, 43
        during the Reformation, 43
        during the Renaissance, 43
        in 18th century, 44
        in 19th century, 44
        in 20th century, 44–45
        in 21st century, 45
    in holistic healthcare, 261–264
    leadership and, 114–119
    legal issues in, 98–105
    management roles of, *111*, 111–114, 114–119,
        118–119
    personal accounts of, 6–16
    as practice, 56
    professional practice, 51–53

Nursing (*continued*)
    professional values in, 70–73, 71t
    responsibilities in, 49–50
    roles of, 50–51, 110
    as science, 56
    as therapeutic partnership, 262
    transcultural, 332–333, *333*
Nursing: A Social Policy Statement (ANA), 138, 164
Nursing: Concepts of Practice (Orem), 60t
Nursing: Human Science and Human Care
        (Watson), 62t
Nursing: What Is It? (Hall), 59t
Nursing Care Management Exchange, 25
Nursing care plan. *See* Care plan
Nursing diagnoses
    for altered bowel function, 1116–1117
    for cardiovascular function, 884
    for client teaching, 368
    for cognitive function, 1237–1240
    for dying, 1314–1315
    for family, 1287–1291
    for fluid and electrolyte/acid-base balance,
        932–934
    for grieving, 1307–1308, 1309t
    for health maintenance, 691–694
    for human sexuality, 1366–1367
    for infection, 1051
    in intraoperative nursing, 632, 633t
    for mobility, 778–780
    for nutrition, 965–967
    for pain, 1181
    in postoperative nursing, 639, 641t
    in preoperative nursing, 623, 626t
    for respiratory function, 821–824
    for safety, 663
    for self-care, 711–713
    for self-concept, 1265–1266
    for sensory perception, 1207–1208
    for skin integrity, 1001–1002
    for sleep and rest, 1157–1158
    for spirituality, 1391–1393
    for stress, coping, and adaptation, 1338–1339
    for urinary elimination, 1081–1083
    for wellness, 262–263
Nursing diagnosis(es), 139–140, 140, 163–183,
        164
    activities in, 175–179
    actual, 177t, 178, *178*, 179t
    components of, 169–175
    defining characteristics in, 175
    definition in, 175
    descriptors of, 169–175
    diagnostic label of, 169
    diagnostic statement of, 177–179, 177t
    by functional health patterns, 180d–181d, 182
    high-priority, 187
    historical development of, 164
    low-priority, 187
    medium-priority, 187
    NANDA review and staging process of, 165–167
    and nursing practice, 179–182
    and other healthcare problems, 167–169, 168t,
        169
    pattern identification in, 175–177
    in plan of care, 190, 191, 192t
    possible, 177t, 179, 179t
    priority of, 187
    related factors in, 175
    risk, 177t, 178, *178*, 179t
    risk factors in, 175
    significance of, 179–182
    taxonomy of, 164–169
        development of, 165, 166t–167t
    validation of, 177
    wellness, 177t, *178*, 178–179, 179t
Nursing Diagnosis: Reference Manual, 177

Nursing Diagnosis Extension and Classification
        (NDEC), 146–147, 167
Nursing education, 12, 15–16, 46–49. *See also*
        Critical thinking
    accreditation in, 27, 48
    advanced degrees, 48–49
    client records in, 231
    military influences on, 44–45
    in 19th century, 44
    types of programs, 48–49
Nursing framework, functional health patterns as,
        65–66
Nursing history, data in, 1364t
Nursing homes, 10–11, 29t, 1294, 1313
Nursing informatics, 237
Nursing Intervention Classification (NIC), 147,
        189, 189d, 203–204
Nursing interventions. *See also* Implementation
    cognitive, 204, 205t
    by community type, 318t–319t
    coordinating, 204–205
    educational, 204
    effectiveness of, monitoring of, 208
    for family, 1292–1293
    interpersonal, 204–206, 205t
    maintenance, 206
    performance of, 203
    planning of, 189
    in plan of care, 190–191, 192t, 193, 193t
    psychomotor, 206
    psychosocial, 205–206
    supervisory, 204
    supportive, 205
    surveillance, 206
    taxonomy of, 189
    technical, 205t, 206
    types of, 203–206, 205t
Nursing journals, 45, 124
Nursing judgment, 220, *220,* 224
Nursing Manifesto, 26
Nursing monitors, 211–212
Nursing organizations, 51–53, 53d
Nursing Outcome Classification (NOC). *See*
        Nursing-Sensitive Outcome
        Classification
Nursing plan of care. *See* Care plan
Nursing practice
    application of research to, 131–132
    nursing diagnosis and, 179–182
    nursing process and, 144–147
Nursing process
    assessment in, 139 (*See also* Assessment)
    characteristics of, 138
    communication in, 144, 350–359
    components of, 138–142
    decision-making in, 142–143
    definitions of, 138, 140d
    diagnostic reasoning process in, 144
    evaluation in, 141 (*See also* Evaluation)
    functional health patterns and, 145–146, *147,*
        147d
    historical development of, 138, 139t
    implementation in, 141 (*See also* Implementation)
    knowledge base for, 144
    listening in, 144
    nursing diagnosis in, 139–140 (*See also* Nursing
        diagnosis)
    nursing practice and, 144–147
    outcome identification in, 140 (*See also* Out-
        come identification)
    phases of, 139–141, *140*
        interactive nature of, *141,* 141–142
    planning in, 140–141 (*See also* Planning)
    problem-solving in, 142, 143t
    professional relevance of, 144–145
    respirations assessment, 462p

skill requirements for, 144
    theoretical foundations of, 142–144
    therapeutic dialogue for, 145
    trends in, 146–147
Nursing progress notes, 238–242
    FOCUS, 240t, 241–242, *242*
    narrative, 238, 240t, *241*
    PIE, 240–241, 240t, *242*
    SOAP, 238–240, 240t, *241*
Nursing research, 51, 121–132
    application to practice, 131–132
    awareness of, 208
    characteristics of, 124–125
    client records in, 231
    clinical, 129–130
    data management in, 127
    design of, 127
    ethical and legal issues in, 128–129, 128d
    history of, 123–124
    hypotheses in, 127
    information-processing theory in, 143, *143*
    literature review in, 126
    methods of, 125
    multidisciplinary clinical research, 130–131
    priorities of, 124d
    problem area identification in, 125–126
    problem statement in, 126–127
    process of, 125–128
    professional nurses and, 129–132
    qualitative, 125, 125t
    quantitative, 125, 125t
    in relation to other forms of research, 132
    results in
        analysis of, 127
        dissemination of, 127–128
    scientific process in, 123
    subject rights in, 129
    theoretical frameworks of, 126
    web sites related to, 1433–1435
Nursing Research, 123
Nursing rounds, 247
Nursing's Agenda for Health Care Reform (ANA),
        21, 26
Nursing schools, history of, 41t–42t
Nursing-sensitive client outcomes, 186
Nursing-Sensitive Outcomes Classification
        (NOC), 147, 186, 187d
Nursing theory(ies), 56–57, 58t–62t, 64t
    concepts in, 57
    development of, 56–57
    and evaluation, 207
    non-nursing theories in, 57–65
    and nursing process, 142–144
    and nursing research, 126
Nurturing, as function of family, 1278
Nutrient(s), 942–951. *See also specific nutrients*
    absorption of, 1103
    deficiency of, 963t
    definition of, 942
    guidelines for, 942
    intake of, 957–958
    malabsorption of, 958
    use of, 958
Nutrient density, 953
Nutritional status, 954
Nutritional supplements, 972
    effects on surgery, 622–623
Nutrition and metabolism, 65, *66,* 147d, 321,
        941–980. *See also* Parenteral nutrition
    altered, 962–963
        and activities of daily living, 963
        evaluation of, 977–980
        in home/community-based care, 383, 977
        implementation for, 967–977
        nursing diagnoses for, 180d, 965–967
        nursing interventions for, 968–977

outcome identification and planning for, 967
signs of, 963t
assessment of, 161t, 400–401, 963–965
diagnostic tests/procedures in, 965
dysfunction identification in, 964
normal pattern identification in, 963–964
objective data in, 964–965
physical examination in, 964–965
risk identification in, 964
subjective data in, 963–964
biocultural variations in, 334
and bowel function, 1105, 1117–1119
and cardiovascular function, 871–872, 879
characteristics of, 953–957, 964d
client teaching and, 365t
and cognitive function, 1227, 1241, 1243
in community assessment, 320d
and edema reduction, 889–892
factors affecting, 957–961
in family assessment, 316d
grieving and, 1309t
and health maintenance, 684d
in individual assessment, 311d
infections and, 1039, 1052
knowledge of, 957
lifespan considerations, 283–284, 954–957
medications to promote normal function of, 515t
mobility and, 767t, 769
normal, 942
in older adults, 300–301
as physiologic need, 63
postoperative, 640t, 642
and pressure ulcers, 989
religion and, 1394–1395
and respiratory function, 814, 816
and safety, 659–660
and skin integrity, 989, 1003
and sleep and rest, 1151
special diets, 971–972
surgery and, 613–618
therapeutic dialogue, 978
and urinary elimination, 1068
and values, 76
and wound healing, 995
Nutritionist, referrals to, 33t
Nuts, in Food Guide Pyramid, 951

O

OASIS. *See* Outcome and Assessment Information Set
Obesity, 962
antiembolism stockings and, 888p
and cardiovascular problems, 872
and health promotion, 962
Heimlich maneuver and, 857p
in older adults, 301
and respiratory function, 814
and stress incontinence, 1071
and subcutaneous injections, 555p
and wound healing, 995
Objective data, 156, 157t, 208
in health assessment, 394, 406–410 (*See also* Physical examination)
Objectivity, of client record, 233
Observant Jews, 1396t
Observation, in assessment, 152–153, 152t, 1236
Obstructive sleep apnea, 1155
Occupational hazards, and infection control, 485
Occupational health and safety, 672–673
Occupational health nurses, 22
and safety, 674
Occupational Safety and Health Administration (OSHA), 653
on infection control, 484
on safety, 664

Occupational therapist, 33t, 714t
Oculomotor nerve (III), assessment of, 416t
Odor
body, 334
foot, 726t
skin, 985
urine, 1066
Office of Alternative Medicine, 28, 259
Official drug name, 514
Oil retention enemas, 1121
Oils, in Food Guide Pyramid, 951
Ointments, 516t, 537
Older adult, 295–306
abuse of, 1285
activity and exercise of, 283
ambulation assistance for, 797p
assistive devices for, 297
bathing of, 719p
bedpan use by, 741p
blood pressure of, 468p
blood transfusion in, 606p
body temperature of, 445, 454p
bowel elimination in, 1105
bowel sounds in, 433p
breath sounds in, 429p
cardiovascular function in, 870
chronic conditions in, 296d, 301
client teaching for, 377, 377d
cognition and perception in, 287, 297–298, 1226, 1247
communication with, 297–298, 358
confusion in, postoperative, 1154
coping and stress tolerance in, 289, 305, 1332
demographics of, *296*, 296–297
depression in, postoperative, 146
elimination in, 285, 299–300
enemas for, 1125p
ethnicities of, 296, *296*
falls and, 764
family of, 1279–1280
feeding assistance for, 970p
fluid and electrolyte balance in, 916
fluid requirements of, 935
foot and nail care for, 728p
grieving in, 1304
growth and development of, 279
cognitive, 280
physical, 279
psychosocial, 279–280
hair care of, 731p
health assessment in, 439–440
health maintenance in, 300–301, 684–685, 686, 693d
health perception and health management in, 282
heart sounds in, 424p
home healthcare for, 382
immunity in, 303
independence of, 660, 1294
infections and, 303, 505–509, 1031–1032
intravenous therapy for, 567p, 599
involuntary relocation of, 1333–1334
loneliness in, 304–305
loss and grieving, and, 304
medication administration in, 572
inhaled, 542p
oral, 536p
mobility of, 298–299, 400, 763
mood disorders in, 298
neurologic assessment of, 414p
noise disturbance and, 1150
nutrition and metabolism in, 284, 300–301, 956–957
opioid analgesics and, 1191
oral care in, 733p
pain management for, 304, 304d

pain perception in, 1172
pulse oximetry for, 823p
pulse rate of, 457p
relocation stress syndrome in, 182
respiratory function of, 813
roles and relationships of, 288, 305–306
safety of, 652
self-care and, 298, 706
self-perception and self-concept of, 287, 306, 1257t, 1259, 1262, 1268, 1268t
sensory perception of, 1201
sexuality and reproduction in, 290–291, 305, 1358–1359
skin of, 300, 986
sleep and rest of, 285–286, 1149–1150, 1160
spirituality of, 306, 1384–1385, 1398–1399
surgery for, 622
urinary catheterization of, 1093p
urinary elimination in, 1067
values and beliefs of, 76, 76t, 291, 306
vital signs of, 444t, 475
wound dressings for, 1013p
Olfactory nerve (I), assessment of, 416t
Oliguria, 1070–1071
One-time order, 519
Onset insomnia, 1155
Open-ended interviewing, in cultural assessment, 335
Open-ended questions, in assessment, 350
Opening remarks, in assessment, 350–353
Open systems, 313
Open Systems Model (King), 61t
Open wound, 990t
Operating room. *See* Surgery
Ophthalmic medications, administration of, 538, 539d
Ophthalmoscope, 415, *417*
Opiates
cardiovascular problems and, 872
for diarrhea, 1122t
Opioid agonist-antagonists, in pain management, 1186, 1188t
Opioid agonists, in pain management, 1186, 1188t
Opioid analgesics, 1186
addiction to, 1189
adverse effects of, 1190–1191
dependence on, 1189
patient-controlled, 1191
precipitous death with, 1191
and respiratory depression, 1189
tolerance to, 1189–1190
Opioid antagonists, in pain management, 1186, 1188t, 1193t
Opium alkaloids, in pain management, 1188t
Opportunistic organisms, 1032
Opposition (joint), 755t
Optic nerve (II), assessment of, 416t
Oral administration, 533–537
nursing procedure for, 534p–536p
Oral airways, 843, *846*
Oral care, 704, 729–731, 732p–734p
for unconscious client, 729
Oral communication. *See* Reporting
Oral contraceptives, 1369–1371, 1372t
Oral fluids, 935–936
Oral medications
buccal administration of, 537
oral administration of, 534–537
preparations of, 516t
routes of administration, 533–537
sublingual administration of, 537
tube administration of, 537
Oral temperature, 444, 445t, 446
Oral tests, in client teaching, 374
Orem, Dorothea E., 60t, 64t
Organ donation, 103, *103*

Organ dysfunction, 878
Organ failure, 878
Organization, in cognitive development theory, 270
Organizational Ethics Committees, 97
Orgasm, in sexual response, 1356
    female, 1357
    male, 1356–1357
Orgasmic dysfunction, 1363
Orientation, 1223
    assessment of, 410, 1233
    reality, 1223, 1233, 1234–1235, 1244
    to surroundings, 1242
    time, 74t
Orientation phase
    of interview process, 154
    of nurse-client relationship, 347
Orlando, Ida Jean, 59t, 64t, 138, 139t
Orthostatic hypotension, 471–473
    altered mobility and, 768
    assessment for, 472p–473p
    and falls, 665
OSHA. *See* Occupational Safety and Health Administration
Osmolality, 911
Osmolar imbalance, 923–924
Osmolarity
    of body fluids, 911–912
    of solutions, 576
Osmosis, 913, *915*
Osmotic pressure, 914–915
Osteoporosis, 949
    and altered health maintenance, 687–688
    client teaching on, 696
    disuse, 769
    prevention of, 781
Ostomy pouch, 1133, *1133,* 1134p–1136p
OTC medications. *See* Over-the-counter medications
Otic medications, administration of, 538, 539d
Otoscope, 416
Outcome and Assessment Information Set (OASIS), 381, 382
Outcome criteria
    in evaluation, 208
    in outcome identification, 188
    in plan of care, 190, 192t
Outcome evaluation, 208, 209–210
Outcome identification, 140, 186
    activities in, 186–188
    advanced practice nursing and, 187
    client goals in, 188, 188d
    in client teaching, 368
    for family, 1291–1292
    nursing-sensitive client outcomes, 186
    outcome criteria in, 188
    in plan of care, 193
    priorities in, 186–188
Output, in systems theory, 142
Ovarian cycle, 1355, *1355*
Ovarian ligament, *1353*
Ovaries, *1353,* 1353–1354
Overeating, 957–958
Overflow incontinence, in older adults, 299
Overstimulation, 1243–1244
Over-the-counter medications, 517
Over-the-needle IV catheters, 577, *579*
Overweight, 962
Ovulation, 445–446, 1354–1355
Ovulatory phase, of ovarian cycle, 1355, *1355*
Oximetry, in respiratory function assessment, 821
Oxybutynin, 1070
Oxycodone, 1188t
Oxygenation
    and cardiovascular function, 865–904
    and mobility, 764–765

and respiratory function, 809–862
    and wound healing, 995
Oxygen diffusion, 810
Oxygen mask, *841,* 842t
Oxygen perfusion, and cognitive function, 1241
Oxygen saturation, 821
Oxygen tent, in oxygen therapy, 842t
Oxygen therapy, 825–840, 838p–840p
    equipment in, 842t
    in home healthcare, 859, *860*
    principles of, 836–837
    safety of, 837–840
    system selection for, 837, *841*
Oxygen transport, 810–811
Oxyhood, in oxygen therapy, 842t
Oxymorphone, 1188t

P
PaC$_2$, 918t
Packed red blood cells, 603
Packing, of wounds, 1008–1010
PaCO$_2$, 918t
PACU. *See* Postanesthesia care unit
Pain
    and activities of daily living, 1176
    acute, 1170, 1174, 1181
    altered function resulting in, 1174–1176
    with altered skin integrity, 991
    assessment of, 398, 1176–1181
        diagnostic tests/procedures in, 1181
        dysfunction identification in, 1180
        normal pattern identification in, 1176–1178
        objective data in, 1180–1181
        and pain management, 1177
        physical assessment in, 1180–1181
        risk identification in, 1178–1180
        subjective data in, 1176–1180
    associated characteristics of, 1180
    behavioral responses to, 1175–1176, 1176t
    with cardiovascular problems, 878
    characteristics of, 1169–1170
    chest, 815–816, 893
    and cognitive function, 1229
    coping with, 1175d
    descriptions of, 1170d
    with dying, 1314
    gate control theory of, 1169
    implementation for, 1182–1194
    infections and, 1044
    intensity of, 1170
        assessment of, 1177–1178, *1178*
    location of, 1169
        assessment of, 1177, *1178*
    manifestations of, 1174–1176
    modulation of, 1169
        peripheral, 1169
        spinal cord and, 1169
        spinal reflexes and, 1169
    on movement, 766
    nonverbal responses to, 1176t
    nursing diagnoses for, 1181
    nursing interventions for, 1183–1194
    outcome identification and planning for, 1182
    perception of, 1168–1172
        affective factors in, 1174
        behavioral factors in, 1174
        cognitive factors in, 1174
        factors affecting, 1172–1174, *1173*
        lifespan considerations, 1171–1172
        physiologic factors in, 1172–1174
        structures related to, *1168,* 1168–1169
            central, 1168–1169
            peripheral, 1168
    physical expressions of, 1180–1181
    physiologic responses to, 1174–1175

postoperative, 619
    management of, 1191–1192, *1192*
    therapeutic dialogue, 620
quality of, 1170
    assessment of, 1178, *1180*
referred, 1169, *1171*
responses to, 1172–1176, *1173*
and self-care, 707–708
and sleep and rest, 1152–1153
temporal pattern of, 1170
    assessment of, 1178
theories of, 1169
verbal responses to, 1175–1176, 1176t, 1181
Pain management
    adjuvant analgesics in, 1192
    alcohol injections in, 1193t
    for altered cardiovascular function, 893
    anticipatory guidance in, 1184
    behavioral techniques in, 1184–1186
    biofeedback in, 1186
    cognitive techniques in, 1184
    contralateral stimulation in, 1183–1184
    cutaneous stimulation in, 1183
    distraction in, 1184
    epidural analgesia in, 1186–1189
    evaluation of, 1194
    guided imagery in, 1184
    heat and cold therapy in, 1183
    in home/community-based care, 1194
    hygiene in, 1183
    hypnosis in, 1184
    invasive techniques in, 1193–1194, 1193t
    massage in, 1183
    meditation in, 1185–1186
    nerve blocks in, 1193t
    for older adults, 304, 304d
    outcome-based teaching plan for, 1185
    and pain assessment, 1177
    patient-controlled analgesia in, 560, 1191, *1192*
    pharmacologic, 1186–1193, 1187t–1188t
    physical techniques in, 1183–1184
    placebos in, 1192–1193
    positioning in, 1183
    postoperative, 643, 1191–1192, *1192*
    relaxation in, 1184–1185
    therapeutic dialogue, 1190
    transcutaneous electrical nerve stimulation in, 1184
Pain medication, dependence on, 1191
Pain threshold, 1170
Pain tolerance, 1170
Palliative surgery, 612t
Palpation
    in abdominal assessment, 433
    in blood pressure assessment, 470–471
    in bowel function assessment, 1112
    in breast assessment, 427
    in cardiovascular assessment, 421–422, 880–881
    deep, 407, 408
    of extremities, 435–437
    in genital assessment, 435
    light, 407–408, *408*
    in physical examination, 155, 407–408
    in pulse assessment, 455
    in respiratory assessment, 425, *427,* 819
    superficial, 407
    in urinary elimination assessment, 434, 1075, 1075t
    of wounds, 1001
Pamphlets, in client teaching, 369–370
Pancreas, 951, *1327,* 1327–1328
Pantothenic acid, 946t
Paper thermometer, 448, *448*
Papillomavirus, 989
Papule, 992t
Paradoxical blood pressure, 469

ParaGard, 1371
Paralytic ileus, 618–619, 1112
Paraplegia, 764
Parasitic infections, 480–481, 1039, 1048. *See also* Infection(s)
Parasomnias, 1156
Parasympathetic nervous system, functions of, 1327
Parathyroid glands, *1327,* 1327–1328
Parathyroid hormone (PTH)
    and calcium-phosphate balance, 913
    and milk production, 1356
Paregoric, 1122t
Parental Role Conflict, 1291
Parenteral medications, administration of, 540–560
    drawing up medications in, 544–546, 545p–546p
    equipment for, 543–544
        disposal of, 546
    intradermal, 546–548, 551p
    intramuscular, 550–556, *556,* 558p–560p, 561t, *562, 563, 564*
    intravenous, 556–560, 565t
    mixing medications in, 546, 549p–550p
    reconstituting medications in, 544–546
    subcutaneous, 548–550, *552,* 553p–555p
Parenteral nutrition, 576–577, 599–603
    client teaching in, 607–608
    in home/community-based care, 607–608, *608*
Parenting, and sleep and rest, 1151
Parish nursing, 24, 1399
Parse, Rosemarie Rizzo, 62t
Partially complete proteins, 943
Partial-thickness burns, 991
Participative leadership, 110, *111*
Particulate respirator, 493, *493*
Passive immunity, 1031
Passive range of motion (PROM), 784
Pasta, in Food Guide Pyramid, 950
Paste, 516t
Patch, 992t
Patellar reflex, 438t
Patency, in intravenous therapy, 584–585
Pathogenicity, of infectious agent, 482
Pathogens, 480
Pathways, 10
Patient-Centered Approaches to Nursing (Abdellah), 58t–59t
Patient-controlled analgesia (PCA), 560, 1191, *1192*
Patient information questionnaire (PIQ), 1341
Patient's Bill of Rights, 89, 91d–92d, 362
Patient Self-Determination Act, 102
Pattern identification, in nursing diagnosis, 175–177
PCA. *See* Patient-controlled analgesia
Peak flow monitoring, 823p–824p, 828
Peak level, of drug concentration, 1050
Pedagogy, 362, 363t
Pedal pulse, 455, *455*
Pediatrics, 10, 11–12, 116
Pediculosis, 724
Peer culture, and values, 74
Peer pressure, 683
Peer relationships, among adolescents, 287–288
Peer review, 211–212
PEG. *See* Percutaneous endoscopic gastrostomy
Pelvic examination, 1366
Pelvic floor exercises, in bowel training, 1132
Penis, 1352, *1352*
Penrose drain, 1001
Pentazocine, 1188t
People-oriented learners, 218
Peplau, Hildegard E., 58t, 344
Perceived Constipation, 1116

Perceiving, in cognition, 1224
Perception. *See also* Cognition and perception
    definition of, 268
    and health maintenance, 680, 685, 686
    of information, 1220–1222
    of reality, 1223, 1233, 1234–1235
    of safety, 650
Percocet (oxycodone with acetaminophen), 1186
Percodan (oxycodone with aspirin), 1186
Percussion
    in bowel function assessment, 1112
    in chest physiotherapy, 832
    indirect, 408–409, *409*
    in physical examination, 155, 408–409, 408t
    in respiratory assessment, 425, 819
    in urinary elimination assessment, 434, 1075, 1075t
Percutaneous endoscopic gastrostomy (PEG), 973, *973*
Perfectionism, stress and, 1339
Performance appraisals, 112
Perfusion. *See* Tissue perfusion
Perineal care, 716–717, *724*
Perineal muscles, decreased tone of, and urinary elimination, 1069–1070
Perineum, *1353*
Periodic abstinence, 1369
Periodic limb movements disorder, 1156
Perioperative nursing, 611–644
    lifespan considerations and, 621–622
    phases of, 612
        intraoperative (*See* Intraoperative nursing)
        postoperative (*See* Postoperative nursing)
        preoperative (*See* Preoperative nursing)
Peripheral cyanosis, 419, 873
Peripheral insertion devices, 577
Peripheral ischemic pain, management of, 893
Peripherally inserted central catheters (PICCs), 580, *580,* 598
Peripheral nervous system, and peripheral sensitization, 1173
Peripheral parenteral nutrition (PPN), 599
Peripheral sensitization, and pain perception, 1173
Peripheral vision, assessment of, 415
Perirectal area, examination of, 433, 1111t, 1113
Peristalsis, 1103
PERRLA, 415
Perseverance, 218t
    intellectual, 227t
Person, concept of, 57, 58t–62t
Personal factors, in cognition, 1226
Personality type, and cardiovascular problems, 872–873
Personal morality, 86
Personal resources and stressors, and grieving, 1305, 1306
Personal values, 86. *See also* Values and beliefs
Person-nature orientation, 74t
Perspiration, 920
Pertussis (whooping cough), 1034t
Pfeiffer Short Portable Mental Status Questionnaire, 1237, 1237d
pH. *See also* Acid-base balance
    arterial blood, 918t
    of urine, 1080t
Phagocytes, 1030t
Pharmacodynamics, 524–526
Pharmacokinetics, 523
Pharyngostomy, 972t
Pharynx, *418,* 951, 1102
Phenazopyridine (Pyridium), 1070
Phenothiazines, 1070
Phenytoin (Dilantin), 1154
Phlebitis, intravenous therapy and, 594, 597t
Phonation, 1223

Phosphate, 912, 912t
Phosphorus, 913, 937t, 948t
pH scale, 917, *917*
Physical appearance, surgery and, 621d
Physical development
    of adolescent, 277
    of infant, 275
    intrauterine, 272–274
    of middle adult, 279
    of newborn, 274
    of older adult, 279
    of preschooler, 276
    of school-age child, 276–277
    of toddler, 276
    of young adult, 278
Physical examination, 152t
    of abdomen, 427–435
    auscultation in, 155, 409–410
    in bowel function assessment, 1111–1113, 1111t
    of breasts, 427
    in cardiovascular assessment, 421–422, 880–882
    in cognitive function assessment, 1236
    draping during, 407
    and evaluation, 208
    of extremities, 435–437
    in fluid and electrolyte/acid-base balance assessment, 929–932
    of genitalia, 434–435
    of hair, 419–420
    of head, face, and neck, 410–419
    head-to-toe framework for, 410–437
    in health assessment, 406–410
    in health maintenance assessment, 690
    in human sexuality assessment, 1366
    in infection resistance assessment, 1045–1046
    inspection in, 154–155, 407
    in medication assessment, 527–528
    in mobility assessment, 776–778
    of mouth, 418
    of nails, 419–420
    of neck, 418–419
    in nutrition assessment, 964–965
    in pain assessment, 1180–1181
    palpation in, 155, 407–408
    percussion in, 155, 408–409, 408t
    positioning during, 407
    in preoperative nursing, 622–623
    in respiratory assessment, 422–427, 819–820
    in safety assessment, 661–663
    in sensory assessment, 1207, 1208t
    in skin assessment, 419–420
    in skin integrity assessment, 998–1001
    in sleep and rest assessment, 1157
    techniques in, 154–155
    in urinary elimination assessment, 1075, 1075t
Physical expression of pain, 1180–1181
Physical fitness, promotion of, 780–781
Physical health, assessment of, 394
Physical provision of care, by family, 1277
Physical restraints, 665–666, *667*
Physical state
    and client teaching, 367
    nutrition and, 954
Physical therapist
    referrals to, 33t
    and self-care promotion, 714t
Physician-assisted suicide, 102
Physician's office
    admission to, 29t
    surgery in, 612–613
Physiologic functioning, neuroendocrine regulation of, 1326–1328
Physiologic needs, 62–63
Physiologic stress, 1336

Physiologic tests, in cognitive function assessment, 1236–1237
Piaget, Jean, 270, 271t
PICCs. *See* Peripherally inserted central catheters
PIE notes, 240–241, 240t, *242*
The Pill, 1369–1371
Pillow, as positioning aid, 784t
Pinworms, 1039
PIQ. *See* Patient information questionnaire
Pitch, of phonation, 1223
Pitting edema, *881,* 931
Pituitary gland, *1327,* 1327–1328
Placebos, in pain management, 1192–1193
Planning, 188–198. *See also* Care plan; Outcome identification
    activities in, 189–198
    in client teaching, 368–372
    disaster, 673
    discharge (*See* Discharge planning)
    health maintenance and, 694
    in management, 112
    nursing interventions in, 189
    in nursing process, 140–141
Plantar warts, 726t
Plaque, 992t, 993t
    dental, 704
Plasma, 870
Plateau phase, of sexual response
    female, 1357
    male, 1356
Platelet-derived growth factors, in wound dressings, 1008
Platelets, 603
Play
    and self-concept, 1257
    and socialization, 1279
Pleural friction rub, *431,* 817t, 820
PLISSIT model, 1374, 1374t
PMI. *See* Point of maximal impulse
Pneumatic compression devices, 888–889, 890p–891p
Pneumatic nebulizer, 842t
Pneumococcal vaccination, 1054t
Pneumocystosis, 1039
Pneumonia, 816
Pneumothorax, intravenous therapy and, 597–598
Point of care documentation, 237
Point of maximal impulse (PMI), 421–422
Poisoning, 656–657, *657,* 657d
    emergency care for, 673–674
    prevention of, 668–669
Polio, 1035t
Pollen, and respiratory function, 813
Pollution, 655, 659, 813
Polycythemia, 874
Polygraph, of REM sleep, *1147*
Polysaccharides, 943, 952
Polyurethane film dressings, 1008
Polyurethane foam dressings, 1008, 1010t
Polyuria, 1070
Popliteal pulse, 454–455, *455*
Portal of entry, of infectious agent, 482
Portal of exit, of infectious agent, 482
Positional IV, 584
Position/positioning
    aids for, 784t
    in bed, 785p–787p
    of bed, 742d
    for blood pressure measurement, 469
    for cardiac auscultation, 422
    and cardiovascular function, 893
    for defecation, 1105–1106
    in intravenous therapy, 583–584
    in pain management, 1183
    during physical examination, 407
    and respiratory function, 459, 813, 827

during sleep, 1146
during surgery, 622, 634–635
therapeutic, 781–784, *782–783*
for urinary catheterization, 1088
for urinary elimination, 1068
Positive body image, 1254–1255
Positive feedback, 313
Positive pressure breathing, 841–843
Positive-pressure ventilators, 843
Positive regard, 350
Positive stressors, 1329
Possible nursing diagnosis, 177t, 179, 179t. *See also* Nursing diagnosis(es)
Postanesthesia care unit (PACU), 612
Posterior pillar, *418*
Posterior tibial pulse, 455, *455*
Postoperative nursing, 612, 638–644
    assessment in, 638–639, 639t
    community-based, 643
    evaluation in, 643–644
    functional health patterns and, 640t
    nursing diagnoses in, 639, 641t
    nursing interventions in, 639–641, 641–643
    outcome identification in, 639, 641t
Postoperative pain, management of, 1191–1192, *1192*
Postoperative protocols, 626, 628t
Postural blood pressure, 778
Postural drainage, in chest physiotherapy, *825,* 832
Postural hypotension. *See* Orthostatic hypotension
Posture, 399, 755, *756*
Postvisit phase, of home healthcare visit, 384
Potassium, 912, 912t, 949
    as electrolyte source, 937t
    preoperative levels of, 919
    supplements, 936
Poultry, in Food Guide Pyramid, 951
Poverty. *See also* Financial factors
    as ethical/legal issue, 81
    and health maintenance, 686
Povidone-iodine, as antiseptic, 492t
Powder, 516t
Power, and self-esteem, 1255
Power of attorney, 89, 1308
PPN. *See* Peripheral parenteral nutrition
Practical nursing programs, 48
Practice. *See* Nursing practice
Practice standards. *See* Standards of practice
Preanesthetic assessment form, *624*
Precipitous death, with opioid analgesics, 1191
Precordium, 421
Prednisone, 1187t
Prefilled syringes, 543, *544*
Pregnancy, 1355–1356
    abuse during, 232
    acid-base balance in, 921
    adolescent, 290
    and bowel elimination, 1106
    breasts in, *1354*
    edema in, 922
    fluid and electrolyte balance in, 921
    health maintenance and, 688, 692d–693d
    Heimlich maneuver in, 857p
    iodine and, 949
    medication assessment and, 526–527
    nutrition and, 954–955
    in sexual function assessment, 1365
    and sexuality, 1359–1360
    and stress incontinence, 1071
    unwanted, 688
    and urinary elimination, 1070
Preinteraction phase, of interview process, 154
Prejudice, 332
Premature closure, in nursing diagnosis, 176
Premature ejaculation, 1362
Prenatal care, abuse documentation during, 232

Prenatal sexuality, 1357–1358
Preoperative care unit, 630–631
Preoperative checklist, 630–631, *631*
Preoperative evaluation, 632
Preoperative nursing, 612, 622–632
    allergy assessment in, 623
    assessment in, 622–623, 623t
    discharge needs in, 623
    health history in, 622–623
    learning needs in, 623
    nursing diagnoses in, 623, 626t
    nursing interventions in, 624–631
    outcome-based teaching plan for, 627
    outcome identification and planning in, 623, 626t
    physical examination in, 622–623
Preoperative protocols, 626
Preparatory phase, of interview process, 154
Prepuce, 1352, *1352*
Presbyterians, 1396t
Preschooler. *See also* Child
    activity and exercise in, 283
    bowel elimination in, 1104
    bowel sounds in, 433p
    breath sounds in, 429p
    cardiovascular function in, 870
    client teaching for, 375
    cognition and perception in, 286, 1225
    coping and stress tolerance in, 288–289, 1331–1332
    elimination in, 285
    family of, 1278–1279
    fluid and electrolyte balance in, 916
    grieving in, 1303–1304
    growth and development of, 276
        cognitive, 276
        physical, 276
        psychosocial, 276
    health assessment in, 437
    health maintenance in, 683, 692d
    health perception and health management in, 281–282
    heart sounds in, 424p
    infections in, 1031
        prevention of, 505
    intravenous therapy for, 598–599
    medication administration for, 570–571
    mobility of, 763
    neurologic assessment of, 414p
    nutrition and metabolism in, 284, 955
    pain perception in, 1171–1172
    respiratory function of, 812
    roles and relationships of, 287
    safety of, 651
    self-care of, 705–706
    self-perception and self-concept of, 287, 1256t, 1257–1258, 1267, 1268t
    sensory perception of, 1201
    sexuality and reproduction in, 289, 1358
    skin of, 986
    sleep and rest in, 285, 1149
    spirituality of, 1384, 1395–1398
    surgery in, 621–622
    urinary elimination in, 1066t, 1067
    values and beliefs of, 75, 76t, 291
    vital signs of, 444t, 474
Prescription medications, 517
President's Commission for the Study of Ethical Problems in Medical and Biomedical and Behavioral Research, 1313
Pressure devices, for safety, 666
Pressure receptors, 911
Pressure ulcers, 986–989
    altered mobility and, 769
    Braden Scale of, 302d–303d, 998, 999–1000
    friction and, 988

locations of, *988*
mental status and, 988
metabolism and, 989
moisture of skin and, 988
nutrition and, 989
in older adults, 300
prediction of, 1004d
prevention of, 1003–1005, 1004d
risk factors for, 988
shearing force and, 988, *989*
staging of, 987d
Prevention. *See* Disease, prevention of
Previous experience
and communication, 345–346
and coping, 1333
and family, 1281
and health maintenance, 685
and self-concept, 1261
and sensory perception, 1201
and sexuality, 1359
and spirituality, 1386
Previsit phase, of home healthcare visit, 384
Primary care provider, reporting to, 247–248
Primary data, in health assessment, 396
Primary disease prevention, 682, 683t
Primary intention wound healing, *994*, 994–995
Primary nursing, 9, 116–117
Primary sources, 139, 156
Privacy
for bowel elimination, 1104
draping for, 407
in health assessment, 396
in professional-patient relationship, 93
for urinary elimination, 1069
Private rooms, for asepsis, 494
PRN orders, 518
Problem-oriented coping mechanisms, 1331d
Problem solving
for families, 1292–1293
as management responsibility, 113
methods of, 143t
in nursing process, 142, 143t
Problem statement, in nursing research, 126–127
Procedural knowledge, 219
Process evaluation, 208
Process recording, in communication skills development, 356t
Proctoscopy, 1116
Prodromal period, of infections, 1041
Professional development, 45, 47t
Professional ethics, 86
Professionalism, 45–49
definitions of, 45–46, 47t
and self-concept, 47
Professional liability insurance, 105
Professional nurse, 47
Professional nursing practice, 51–53
Professional-patient relationship, ethics of, 93–94
Professional practice, legal protection in, 105
Professional Self-Concept of Nurses Instrument (PSCNI), 47
Professional values, 70–73, 71t
Proficiency, in critical thinking development, 226
Proficient nurse, 46t
Progestasert, 1371
Progesterone
and body temperature, 445
and milk production, 1356
Progestin implant, 1371
Program for Reversing Heart Disease, 263
Progressive relaxation, 1185, 1342, 1343d
Progress notes. *See* Nursing progress notes
Projection cells, 1168
Prolactin
and milk production, 1356
and sleep-wake patterns, 1148

Proliferation, in wound healing, 994
Proliferative phase, of uterine cycle, 1355, *1355*
PROM. *See* Passive range of motion
Prompted voiding, 1085
Pronation, 755t
Prone position, *782*
Propranolol, and pulse rate, 449
Proprioceptors, 1222
Prostate gland, 1352, *1352*
Prosthetic eyes, 735
Protective clothing, 493–494, 633, *634,* 655–656, 1209
Protective function, of skin, 985
Protective isolation, 495
Protective pants, for incontinence, 1085, 1087–1088
Protective reflexes, 760
Protein, 943
digestion of, 952
metabolism of, 952–953
in urine, 1080t
Protestants, 1396t
Proteus, 1069
Protozoal infections, 1039
Proventil. *See* Albuterol
Proximal convoluted tubules, 1064
Proximate cause, 100–101
Proxy directive, 89
Pruritus, 986, 991
relief for, 1005
PSCNI. *See* Professional Self-Concept of Nurses Instrument
Psoriasis, 990
Psychiatric facility, admission to, 29t
Psychic reflectivity, 226t
Psychodynamic theories
of growth and development, 269, 269t, 270t
of self-concept, 1256t–1257t
Psychological disorders, 298, 300t
and cognitive function, 1229
and urinary elimination, 1068–1069
Psychological health
assessment of, 394
isolation and, 496
Psychological state, and nutrition, 961
Psychological stress, 1336
Psychomotor learning, 363–364
teaching methods for, 373d, 374
Psychomotor nursing interventions, 206
Psychophysiologic insomnia, 1155
Psychosexual theory, of growth and development, 269, 269t
Psychosocial development
of adolescent, 277–278
of infant, 275
intrauterine, 274
of middle adult, 279
of newborn, 274
of older adult, 279–280
of preschooler, 276
of school-age child, 277
of toddler, 275–276
of young adult, 278
Psychosocial nursing interventions, 205–206
Psychosocial problems, and altered health maintenance, 688
Psychosocial stress, 261
Psychosocial theory, of growth and development, 269, 270t
Psychosomatic, 258
Psychostimulants, in pain management, 1192
Psyllium (Metamucil, Effer-syllium), 1122t
PTH. *See* Parathyroid hormone
Puberty, 277, 289, 1358
Puerto Ricans, and religion, 336–337
Pulmonary artery pressure, 932

Pulmonary embolism, 878
Pulmonary function tests, in respiratory function assessment, 820
Pulmonary toilet, 1055
Pulmonic area, 421
Pulse, 449–459
across lifespan, 444t
altered cardiovascular function and, 873
assessment of, 435, 435d, 449–459, 456p–457p
auscultation in, 458
equipment for, 455
methods of, 455–458
palpation in, 455
postoperative, 638
sites for, 449–455, *455*
characteristics of, 449, 458
infections and, 1044
Pulse deficits, 458–459
Pulse oximetry, 821, 822p–823p
Pulse pressure, 461
Pulse quality, 449, 458, 458t
Pulse rate, 449
assessment of, 458
factors affecting, 449
fluid and electrolyte/acid-base balance and, 927–928
Pulse rhythm, 449, 458
Pulsus bigeminus, 458
Puncture wound, 990, 990t
Pupillary reflex, assessment of, 415
Pupils, assessment of, 415, *415*
Purified protein derivative (PPD) test, 546–548
Purpose, and spirituality, 1389t
Pursed-lip breathing, 830
Purulent drainage, 1001, 1044
Pustules, 991, 992t
Pyramidal tract, and motor functions, 755
Pyridoxine, 946t
Pyuria, 1071

Q

Quad canes, 793
Quad cough, 830
Quadriplegia, 764
Qualifiers, of client goals, 188
Qualitative research, 125, 125t
Quality
of phonation, 1223
of pulse, 449, 458, 458t
of respirations, 460
of sound, 410
Quality assurance memos, 245
Quality assurance monitors, 210–212
Quality control, 27
Quality improvement programs, 210–212, 230
Quality of care, 27
Quality of life, 20–21, 95
Quantitative research, 125, 125t
Questions, open-ended, in assessment, 350
Quiescent period, 1332
Quinidine sulfate, 892t

R

Race, 331, 962
Racism, 331
Radial pulse, 454, *455,* 456p
Radiation
and heat loss, 445
symbol for, *671*
and wound healing, 995
Radiation injury, 659, 991
Radiation safety, 634, 655, 670–671
Radiography
in bowel assessment, 1113–1115

Radiography (*continued*)
  chest, 883
  in mobility assessment, 778
  in urinary assessment, 1081
Radon, 655
Rales, 817t, 819
Random collection, of urine specimen, 1075
Random thinkers, 219
Range of motion (ROM), 760
  exercises for, 789p–790p
    automatic equipment for, 788
    general principles of, 788
  types of, 784
Rapid Estimate at Adult Literacy in Medicine
    (REALM), 368
Rapid eye movement (REM) sleep, 1144, *1146,
    1147*
  deprivation of, 1151, 1155
  in newborns and infants, 1149
  in older adults, 1149
RAS. *See* Reticular activating system
Rash, 991
  infections and, 1044
RBCs. *See* Red blood cells
RDAs. *See* Recommended Dietary Allowances
RDIs. *See* Dietary Reference Intakes
Reabsorption, in urine formation, 1065
Reacher, for altered mobility, 803, *803*
Reach-to-Recovery program, 1310
Reactive hyperemia, 769
Readiness for Enhanced Family Coping, 1290
Readiness for Enhanced Spiritual Well-Being, 1392
Reading ability, assessment of, 368, 410
Reagent strips, in urine tests, 1079–1080
Reality orientation, 1223, 1233, 1234–1235, 1244
REALM. *See* Rapid Estimate at Adult Literacy in
    Medicine
Reasoning, 1223
Reassessment, 202
Recall, 1224
Received knowledge, 219
Receptive aphasia, 410, 1231–1232, 1232t
Recognition, 1224
Recommended Dietary Allowances (RDAs), 942,
    944
Reconstituting, of medications, 544–546
Reconstructive surgery, 612t
Records. *See* Client records; Documentation;
    Reporting
Recovery facility
  assessment in, 638–639, 639t
  client transport to, 637–638
  nursing interventions in, 639–641
Recreating Professional Practice for a New Century,
    26
Recreation therapy, 1246
Rectal examination, 433, *434*
Rectal medications, administration of, 539, *540*
Rectal suppository, 1120–1121
Rectal temperature, 444, 445t, 446, 447,
    451p–452p
Rectal tubes, 1125–1126
Rectum, 1102, 1103, *1352*
Rectus femoris site, for intramuscular injections,
    552–555, 556t, *562*
Red blood cells (RBCs), 870
  packed, 603
  in urine, 1080t
Re-epithelialization, in wound healing, 994
Referrals
  for altered sexuality, 1374
  in discharge planning, 32–33, 32t, 33t
  for family problems, 1293
  for grieving, 1312
  in spiritual care, 1395
Referred pain, 1169, *1171*

Reflection
  in critical thinking, 224–226, 226t
  in therapeutic communication, 354
Reflective observers, 219
Reflex(es). *See also specific reflexes*
  assessment of, 414p
  protective, 760
  survival, 760
Reflex arcs, and safety, 661
Reflex incontinence, 1072, 1082
Reflex voiding, 1069
Refreezing, in change theory, 65
Refugee behaviors, 337–338
Refusal
  of medication, 523
  of treatment, 332, 895
Regeneration, in wound healing, 994
Regenerative neuronal growth, and pain percep-
    tion, 1173–1174
Regional anesthesia, 635, 636t
Registered nurses (RNs), 9
  in primary nursing, 116–117
  and self-care promotion, 714t
Regression, as coping mechanism, 706
Rehabilitation, cardiac, 901–902
Rehabilitation physician, and self-care promotion,
    714t
Reimbursement, documentation for, 231
Reinen v. Northern Arizona Orthopedics, LTD, 105
Related factors, in nursing diagnosis, 175
Relatedness, and spirituality, 1389t
Relational orientation, 74t
Relationships. *See also* Family; Roles and
    relationships
  and sexuality, 1359
  and sleep and rest, 1151
Relativism, 219
Relaxation
  in infection control, 1052
  in pain management, 1184–1185
  techniques for, 1341–1342, 1342t
Relaxation response, 1341
Relaxation tapes, 1343
Relaxation training, 1342–1343
Religion, 1396t–1398t. *See also* Spirituality
  and client teaching, 366
  and cultural diversity, 335–336
  and family, 1280
  and grieving, 1305
  and nursing, 43, 44
Relocation, involuntary, coping with, 1333–1334
Relocation stress syndrome (RSS), 182
Remembering, 1224
Reminiscence therapy, 280, 1246
REM sleep. *See* Rapid eye movement sleep
Renal calculi, altered mobility and, 769–770
Renal compensation, acid-base balance and, 918
Renal dialysis, 1097, *1098*
Renal disease, dietary modifications for, 972d
Renal failure, fluid and electrolyte balance and, 921
Renal scan, 1081
Renin, 911
Reorganization, in growth and development, 269
Replacement mattresses, for pressure ulcer preven-
    tion, 1005
Reporting, 230, 245–249
  change-of-shift, 247
  of child abuse, 1293
  ethics and, 249–250
  interdepartmental, 248
  to interdisciplinary team, 248–249
  nurse to nurse, 247
  to primary care provider, 247–248
  by telephone, 247–248
Reproduction. *See also* Sexuality and reproduction
  as family function, 1278

Reproductive system
  female, 1352–1354, *1353*
  function of, 1354–1356
  male, 1352, *1352*
  structure of, 1352–1354
Required surgery, 612t
Rescue feelings, 355
Rescuers, 262, 262t
Research. *See* Nursing research
Research design, 127
Research in Nursing and Health, 124
Reservoir mask, in oxygen therapy, *841,* 842t
Reservoirs, of infection, 482
Res ipsa loquitur, 100
Resistance, and blood pressure, 461–463
Resolution, of value conflicts, 80–81
Resolution phase, of sexual response, 1356
  female, 1357
  male, 1357
Resonance, 408
Resonant tones, 408, 408t
Resource management, 111–112
Respiration(s), 459–460
  abnormal, 460t
  acid-base balance and, 927
  across lifespan, 444t
  altered cardiovascular function and, 873
  assessment of, 459–460, 460, 462p, 638 (*See
    also* Respiratory function, assessment of)
  Biot's, 460t
  Cheyne-Stokes, 425, 460t
  depth and, 927
  depth of, 460
  factors affecting, 459
  Kussmaul, 460t
  quality of, 460
  rhythm of, 460
Respiratory acidosis, 924
Respiratory alkalosis, 924
Respiratory compensation, acid-base balance and,
    918
Respiratory cycle, blood pressure and, 469–470
Respiratory depression, opioid analgesics and, 1189
Respiratory failure, fluid and electrolyte balance
    and, 921
Respiratory function, 809–862
  altered, 815–818
    and activities of daily living, 816–818
    diet and, 972d
    evaluation for, 860–862
    health promotion for, 824–828
    in home/community-based nursing,
      858–860
    implementation for, 824–860
    manifestations of, 815–816
    nursing diagnoses for, 821–824
    nursing interventions for, 828–858
    outcome identification and planning for, 824
  assessment of, 422–427, 818–821
    auscultation in, 425–427, 428p–429p
    diagnostic tests/procedures in, 820–821
    dysfunction identification in, 818–819
    inspection in, 422–425
    landmarks for, 422, *426*
    normal pattern identification in, 818
    objective data in, 819–821
    palpation in, 425, *427*
    percussion in, 425
    physical examination in, 819–820
    risk identification in, 818
    subjective data in, 818–819
  factors affecting, 813–815
  lifespan considerations, 812–813
  normal, 810–813
  outcome-based teaching plan for, 827
  therapeutic dialogue, 825

Respiratory infections, 659
  in children, 1031
    manifestations of, 1043d
    predispositions for, 1042d
    prevention of, 824–825
Respiratory maintenance, postoperative, 641–642
Respiratory medications, 836t, 858–859
Respiratory rate, 459, 812, 812t
    fluid and electrolyte/acid-base balance and, 927
    infections and, 1044
    pain and, 1175
Respiratory system
    defenses of, 811–812
    function of, 810–812
    and safety, 653, 661
    stress and, 1337
    structure of, 810, *811*
Respiratory therapist, referrals to, 33t
Respite care, 1246
Respondeat superior, 101
Responsibility, 218t
Responsible sex, 1369
Rest. *See also* Sleep and rest
    definition of, 1144
    in infection control, 1052
    nursing interventions for, 1159
    in older adults, 303–304
    as physiologic need, 63
    postoperative, 643
Restatement, in therapeutic communication, 353–354
Restless leg syndrome, 1156
Restoril. *See* Temazepam
Restraints, 301, 665–666, *667*, 1244
    alternatives to, 668d
Restrictive diets, 971–972
Resuscitation, 103
Reticular activating system (RAS)
    and cognition, 1220
    and consciousness, 1222
    and sensory perception, 1200
Retirement, 279, 1259, 1285
Return demonstration, in client teaching, 364, 374
Return-flow enemas, 1125
Reverse Trendelenburg position, 742d
Review of systems, 160
Reward structure, in employment, 112
Reye's syndrome, 1055
Rh factor, 604
Rhinovirus, 1033t
Rhizotomy, in pain management, 1193t
Rhonchi, 817t, 819
Rhythm
    of pulse, 449, 458
    of respirations, 460
    of sleep, 1144–1145
Rhythm method of contraception, 1371, 1372t
Riboflavin, 946t, 947
Rice, in Food Guide Pyramid, 950
Rice model, of home healthcare, 383, *384*
Richards, Linda, 44
Right hemisphere syndrome, 1232
Ringworm, 726t
Rinne test, 417–418, *418*
Risk assessment, in home healthcare, 385–386
Risk factors, in nursing diagnosis, 175
Risk for Caregiver Role Strain, 1288
Risk for Disuse Syndrome, 779
Risk for Impaired Parent/Infant/Child Attachment, 1291
Risk for Impaired Parenting, 1290–1291
Risk for Impaired Skin Integrity, 1002
Risk for Infection, 1051, 1059
Risk for Injury, 663, 676
Risk for Spiritual Distress, 1392

Risk nursing diagnosis, 177t, 178, *178,* 179t. *See also* Nursing diagnosis(es)
Risk taking, 218t
Rituals, cultural, 330
RNs. *See* Registered nurses
Rogers, Martha E., 60t, 64t
Role(s)
    definition of, 1255
    gender, 1356
Role ambiguity, 1262
Role conflict, 1262
Role modeling
    and pain perception, 1172d
    and values, 74
Role performance, 1255
Role playing, in client teaching, 369
Roles and relationships, 66, *66,* 147d, 321
    altered mobility and, 770
    assessment of, 161t, 404–405
    client teaching and, 365t
    in community assessment, 320d
    in family assessment, 316d
    grieving and, 1309t
    health maintenance and, 684d, 687
    in individual assessment, 311d
    lifespan development and, 287–288
    mobility and, 767t
    nursing diagnosis and, 181d
    of older adults, 305–306
    postoperative, 640t
    surgery and, 619
    values and, 79
Role strain, 1262, 1284
Role transition, and self-concept, 1262–1263
Roller board, 801t
ROM. *See* Range of motion
Roman Catholics, 1396t
Room temperature, and sleep and rest, 1150
Rooting reflex, 414p
Rotation (joint), 755t
Round ligament, *1353*
Roundworms, 1039
Route of administration, in medication order, 518
Routine healthcare, 696–697
Routine orders, 518
Roy, Sister Callista, 61t, 64t, 128
Roy Adaptation Model of Nursing, 207
RSS. *See* Relocation stress syndrome
Rubella, 1033t
    healthcare personnel with, work restrictions for, 487t
Rubeola, 1033t
Rubor, 873

S

S₁, 422
S₂, 422
S₃, 422
S₄, 422
Safe sex, 1369
Safety, 649–676
    altered, 656–660
        and activities of daily living, 659–660
        evaluation of, 675
        in home/community-based care, 382, 674–675
        implementation for, 664–675
        nursing diagnoses for, 663
        nursing interventions for, 673–674
        outcome-based teaching plan for, 669
        outcome identification and planning for, 663–664
    altered mobility and, 801
    altered sensory perception and, 1210–1211
    assessment of, 660–663

    dysfunction identification in, 661
    normal pattern identification in, 660
    objective data in, 661–663
    physical examination in, 661–663
    risk identification in, 661
    subjective data in, 660–661
  characteristics of, 650
  of children and adolescents, 282
  cognitive function and, 1244
  coping and, 1333
  disregard for, 656
  factors affecting, 652–656
  of infants, 281
  intraoperative, 633, *634,* 634–635
  lifespan considerations, 650–652
  management of, 650
  of medication administration, 529–564
  nonrestraint devices for, 666–668
  normal, 650–652
  with oxygen therapy, 837–840
  perception of, 650
  pervasiveness of, 650
  physiologic factors of, 652–653
  restraints for, 665–666
  therapeutic dialogue, 662
  of toddlers and preschoolers, 281–282
Safety belts, 652
  as ambulation aid, 793
Safety needs, 63
Saline deficit, 921
Saline lavage, 851
Saline laxatives, 1121t
Salivary glands, 951
Salmonella, 1038t
Salmonella, 1038t
Salt. *See* Sodium
SAM. *See* Suitability Assessment of Materials
Sanguineous drainage, 1001
Sanitation, 653
SA node. *See* Sinoatrial node
Saturated fats, *943*–944
Saw palmetto, 519t
Scabies, 993t
  healthcare personnel with, work restrictions for, 487t
Scale, 992t
Scales
  for temperature measurement, 448, *449*
  in weight measurement, 401, 402p–403p
Scalp, assessment of, 419
Scar, 993t
Scarlet fever, 1034t
Scavenger cells, synthesis of, 1030t
SCDs. *See* Sequential compression devices
Schizophrenia, 300t, 1230, 1231
School, nosocomial infections in, 484
School-age child. *See also* Child
  activity and exercise in, 283
  cognition and perception in, 286–287
  coping and stress tolerance in, 289
  elimination in, 285
  growth and development of, 276–277
    cognitive, 277
    physical, 276–277
    psychosocial, 277
  health assessment of, 439
  health maintenance of, 692d
  health perception and health management in, 282
  nutrition and metabolism in, 284
  roles and relationships of, 287–288
  self-perception and self-concept of, 287, 1256t, 1267–1268, 1268t
  sexuality and reproduction in, 289–290
  sleep and rest in, 285
  values and beliefs of, 291
  vital signs of, 444t, 475

School lunch programs, 956
School nurses, 22, 23, 934
    and physical education, 780
    and safety, 674
Science, of nursing, 56
The Science of Unitary Man (Rogers), 60t
Scientific process, in nursing research, 123
Scientific rationale, in plan of care, 191, 192t, 193
SCN. *See* Superchiasmatic nucleus
Scoliosis, 399
Scrotum, 1352, *1352*
Scrub person, 632
Search for meaning, 219
Sebaceous glands, 984
Secondary data sources, in health assessment, 396
Secondary disease prevention, 682, 683t
Secondary intention wound healing, *994, 995*
Secondary sources
    in assessment, 139
    of data, 156–157
Second degree burns, 991
Second trimester, growth and development in,
        273, *274*
Secretion, in urine formation, 1065
Secretory phase, of uterine cycle, 1355, *1355*
Security
    and coping, 1333
    and sleep and rest, 1158–1159
Sedation, with opioid analgesics, 1191
Sedatives, and respiratory function, 814
Segmentation, 1103
Seizures, and sleep and rest, 1153
Self
    definition of, 1254
    normal function of, 1254–1259
    sense of, 350, 1266
    and spirituality, 1394
Self-actualization needs, 63–64
Self-administered medication system, 517. *See also*
        Patient-controlled analgesia
Self-awareness, 259, 1368
Self-care, 310, 400d, 1004
    altered, 708–710
        and activities of daily living, 708–710
        evaluation for, 749–750
        in home/community-based care, 742–749
        manifestations of, 708
        nursing diagnoses for, 711–713
        nursing interventions for, 714–749
        outcome-based teaching plan for, 715
        outcome identification and planning for, 713
    assessment of, 400, 710–711
        dysfunction identification in, 710–711
        normal pattern identification in, 710
        objective data in, 711, 712d
        risk identification in, 710
        subjective data in, 710–711
    community-based care and, 28
    definition of, 704
    factors affecting, 706–708
    health promotion for, 260
    internal and external resources for, 711, 712d
    levels of, 710, 710t
    lifespan considerations, 705–706
    mobility and, 771
    normal, 704–706
        characteristics of, 704–705
        patterns of, 705
    in older adults, 298
    postoperative, 642–643
    reluctance to perform, verbalization of, 708
    scheduled, 714–715
    therapeutic dialogue, 709
Self-care deficit, 750, 1263
Self-care education, 694–696, *695*

Self-concept, 1253–1271. *See also* Self-perception
    altered, 1263–1264
        and activities of daily living, 1264
        evaluation of, 1270–1271
        in home/community-based care, 1269–1270
        implementation for, 1266–1270
        nursing diagnoses for, 1265–1266
        nursing interventions for, 1268–1269
        outcome-based teaching plan for, 1269
        outcome identification and planning for,
                1266
    assessment of, 1264–1265
        dysfunction identification in, 1265
        normal pattern identification in, 1264
        objective data in, 1265
        risk identification in, 1264–1265
        subjective data in, 1264–1265
    characteristics of, 1254
    client teaching and, 365t
    cognition and, 1227
    communication and, 1227
    definition of, 1254
    development of, 1266–1268
    factors affecting, 1259–1263
    and health maintenance, 685
    lifespan considerations, 1255–1259,
            1256t–1257t
    of nurses, 47
    postoperative, 640t
    safety and, 660
    sexuality and, 1359
    surgery and, 619
    therapeutic dialogue, 1260
Self-destructive behavior, self-concept and, 1264
Self-disclosure, 357
Self-efficacy
    in older adults, postoperative, 146
    and self-concept, 1261, 1262
Self-esteem, 63, 71, 1255
    defensive, 1261
    respiratory disorders and, 860
Self-evaluation, 350, 1254, 1269
Self-examination
    breast, 427, 696, 1370d
    and sexuality, 1368
    skin, 696
    testicular, 696, 1369d
Self-expectation, 1254
Self-help groups, 1294
Self-knowledge, 1254
Self-perception, 66, *66*, 147d, 321. *See also* Self-
        concept
    assessment of, 161t, 404
    in community assessment, 320d
    definition of, 1254
    in family assessment, 316d
    grieving and, 1309t
    health maintenance and, 684d
    in individual assessment, 311d
    lifespan development and, 287
    mobility and, 767t, 770
    nursing diagnosis and, 181d
    of older adults, 306
    and values, 76
Self-reported health, 399
Self-responsibility, in holistic healthcare, 259
Self-talk, 1340
Self-worth, in holistic healthcare, 259
Semi-Fowler's position, *782*
Seminal vesicles, 1352, *1352*
Sender, in communication process, 345
Senile lentigines, 986
Senility, 1228
Senior Citizen's Service Act, 13
Sensation (sensory) information, 1209
Sensitivity testing, for infection detection, 1047

Sensorimotor deficits, and self-care, 708
Sensoristasis, 1200
Sensory adaptation, 1200–1201
Sensory aids, 415, 1210, 1211d
Sensory aphasia, 410, 1231–1232, 1232t
Sensory awareness, 1200
Sensory deficits, 1205, 1334
Sensory deprivation, 1202, 1203–1204
    in healthcare environment, 1207d
    risk factors for, 1207d
Sensory overload, 1202–1203
    environment and, 1203, 1207d
    imparting of information and, 1203
    internal factors in, 1202
    prevention of, 1209
    risk factors for, 1207d
Sensory perception, 1199–1216
    altered, 1204–1206
        and activities of daily living, 1205–1206
        cognitive function and, 1241
        evaluation for, 1214–1216
        in healthcare environment, 1207d
        in home/community-based care, 382,
                1211–1214
        implementation for, 1209–1214
        nursing diagnoses for, 1207–1208
        nursing interventions for, 1210
        outcome identification and planning for,
                1208
        and safety, 1210–1211
        therapeutic dialogue, 1204
    assessment of, 410–418, 411p–412p, 436, *436*,
            1206–1207
        diagnostic tests/procedures in, 1207
        dysfunction identification in, 1207
        normal pattern identification in, 1206, 1206t
        objective data in, 1207
        physical assessment in, 1207, 1208t
        risk identification in, 1206–1207, 1207d
        subjective data in, 1206–1207
    factors affecting, 1201–1204
    input in, 1200
    lifespan considerations in, 1201
    normal, 1200–1201
        characteristics of, 1200
    safety and, 661
    skin and, 985
Sensory reception, altered, 1203
Sensory retraining, 1133
Sensory status
    assessment of, 404
    and client teaching, 367
Sensory stimulation
    in dementia, 297
    provision of, 1210
    reduction of, 1210
    variations in, 1202
Separation
    coping with, 1334
    of families, 1283–1284
Separation anxiety, 287
Sepsis, 480
Septicemia, 480, 1041
Septic reactions, with blood transfusions, 607
Sequential compression devices (SCDs), 888–889,
        890p–891p
Sequential thinkers, 219
Serology tests, for infection detection, 1047
Serosanguineous drainage, 1001
Serous drainage, 1001
Serum albumin, in nutritional assessment, 965
Serum creatinine test, 1081
Serum electrolytes, 932. *See also* Electrolyte(s)
Serum enzymes, 882t
Serum glucose, and altered cognitive function,
        1236

Serum osmolarity, 932
Serum prealbumin, in nutritional assessment, 965
Serum transferrin, in nutritional assessment, 965
Settings
    for assessment, 151
    for community-based nursing, 22–25
Seventh Day Adventists, 1397t
Sex
    and body fluid variations, 910, 910t
    as physiologic need, 63
    responsible/safe, 1369
Sex education, 1368
Sexual abuse, 290, 1285, 1362
Sexual desire, inhibited, 1362
Sexual development, in adolescents, 277
Sexual Dysfunction, 1366–1367, 1375
Sexual expression, 1354
Sexual function, cardiovascular problems and, 902
Sexual history, 406
Sexual intimacy, as function of family, 1278
Sexuality and reproduction, 66, 66, 147d, 321
    altered, 1362–1363
        and activities of daily living, 1363, 1373
        evaluation for, 1375–1376
        implementation for, 1368–1375
        nursing diagnoses for, 181d, 1366–1367
        nursing interventions for, 1373–1374
        outcome identification and planning for,
            1368
    assessment of, 161t, 405–406, 1363–1366
        diagnostic tests/procedures in, 1366, 1367t
        dysfunction identification in, 1366
        normal pattern identification in, 1365
        objective data in, 1366
        physical examination in, 1366
        risk identification in, 1365–1366
        subjective data in, 1363–1366
    characteristics of, 1356
    client teaching for, 365t
    in community assessment, 320d
    factors affecting, 1359–1362
    in family assessment, 316d
    function of, 1354–1356
    grieving and, 1309t
    and health maintenance, 684d
    in home/community-based care, 1374–1375
    in individual assessment, 311d
    lifespan considerations, 289–291, 1357–1359
    medications to promote normal function of,
        515t
    mobility and, 767t, 771
    normal, 1352–1359, 1356–1357
    of older adults, 305
    postoperative, 640t
    respiratory function and, 860
    surgery and, 620–621
    therapeutic dialogue, 1361
    values and, 79
Sexually transmitted diseases (STDs), 655, 1028,
        1035t–1036t
    and altered health maintenance, 688
    among adolescents, 282
    prevention of, 671
    and sexuality, 1365
Sexual misconduct, 357
Sexual orientation, 1356, 1358
Sexual response, 1356–1357
    age and, 1359
    female, 1357
    male, 1356–1357
Shaft, of penis, 1352
Shallow breathing, 828
Shampooing, of hair, 723–724, 730p–731p
Shaving, 726–729, *731*
Shearing force, and pressure ulcers, 988, *989*
Shift to the left, 1047

Shift work
    ethics and, 1153
    and sleep and rest, 1151
Shigellosis, 1038t
Shock, 874
    electrical, 658–659
Shoe coverings, 493
Shortness of breath, 815, 818
Short-term coping mechanisms, 1331d
Short-term memory, 410
Shoulder joint, 761t
Showering. *See* Bathing
Sibilant wheeze, 817t
Sibling rivalry, 288, 1278
Sickle cell anemia, 1028
Side effects, of medications, 524
Side-lying position, *782*
Side rails, 665–666, 668d, 741, 784t
Sighs, 460
Sigmoid colon, 1103
Sigmoid colostomy, *1107*
Sigmoidoscopy, 1116
Signature, in medication order, 518
Significant others. *See* Family
Sildenafil citrate (Viagra), 1362
Silence, 219, 355
Silver-impregnated/coated catheter, 1088
Sims' position, *782*
Simulations, in client teaching, 374
Single-parent family, *1276, 1277*
Singleton v. AAA Home Health, Inc., 101
Sinoatrial (SA) node, and pulse, 449
Sinus dysrhythmia, 458
Sitting position, 788, *793*
Situational Low Self-Esteem, 1265–1266
Situational role transitions, 1262
Sitz baths, 717t, 1021
Skene's gland, 1353, *1353*
Skilled nursing facilities, documentation in, 245
Skin
    abdominal, 430
    abnormal growth rate of, 990
    allergies and, 989
    altered, nutrition and, 963
    assessment of, 419–420
        altered cardiovascular function and, 873–874
        fluid imbalance and, 931
        postoperative, 638
    breaks in, and infections, 1039
    characteristics of, 985
    color of, 419, 873, 880, 985, 998
    denuded, treatment of, 1008
    functions of, 985
    habits and, 989
    infections and, 989–990, 1032, 1052
    inspection of, 998
    layers of, 984, *984*
    lifestyle and, 989
    moisture of, 985, 988
    nutrition and, 989
    odor of, 985
    self-examination of, 696
    stress and, 1337
    structure of, 984, *984*
    temperature of, 419, 873, 985
    texture of, 419, 985, 998
    thickness of, 985
Skin appendages, 984
Skin care, 715–716, 1003, 1003d
Skin color, biocultural variations in, 334
Skin diseases, and sleep and rest, 1153
Skinfold measurements, 964–965
Skin integrity
    altered, 991–997
        and activities of daily living, 997
        evaluation for, 1022–1023

    in home/community-based care, 1021–1022
    implementation for, 1003–1022
    nursing diagnoses for, 1001–1002
    nursing interventions for, 1005–1021
    outcome-based teaching plan for, 1023
    outcome identification and planning for,
        1002–1003
    assessment of, 997–1001
        diagnostic tests/procedures in, 1001
        dysfunction identification in, 998
        objective data in, 998–1001
        physical examination in, 998–1001
        risk identification in, 998
        subjective data in, 997–998
    circulation and, 986
    factors affecting, 986–991
    lifespan considerations, 985–986
    normal, 984–986
    in older adults, 300
    and safety, 662
    systemic diseases and, 990
    therapeutic dialogue, 1022
    trauma and, 990–991
Skin lesions
    altered cardiovascular function and, 874
    assessment of, 420
Skin preparation
    preoperative, 630
    in surgical asepsis, 497–499
Skin tags, 986
Skin tests, in respiratory function assessment, 821
Skin turgor, assessment of, 420
Slander, 99
Sleep and rest, 66, 147d, 321, 1143–1162
    altered, 1154–1156
        and activities of daily living, 1156
        evaluation of, 1160–1161
        implementation for, 1158–1160
        nursing diagnoses for, 180d, 1157–1158
        nursing interventions for, 1159–1160
        outcome-based teaching plan for, 1161
        outcome identification and planning for, 1158
        safety and, 660
    assessment of, 161t, 401, 1156–1157
        diagnostic tests in, 1157
        dysfunction identification in, 1157
        normal pattern identification in, 1157
        objective data in, 1157
        physical examination in, 1157
        risk identification in, 1157
        subjective data in, 1156–1157
    characteristics of, 1146
    client teaching for, 365t
    cognitive function and, 1227, 1241
    in community assessment, 320d
    coping and, 1333
    definition of, 1144
    deprivation of, 1154, 1155
    factors affecting, 1150–1154
    in family assessment, 316d
    good habits for, 303d
    grieving and, 1309t
    health maintenance and, 684d
    in home/community-based care, 1160
    in individual assessment, 311d
    lifespan considerations, 285–286, 1148–1150,
        1149
    medications to promote normal function of,
        515t
    mobility and, 767t, 770
    need for, 1146, 1150, 1159
    normal, 1144–1150
    in older adults, 303–304
    patterns of, 1146–1148
    physiologic functions of, 1144–1145
    as physiologic need, 63

Sleep and rest (*continued*)
  physiology of, 1144–1145
  postoperative, 640t
  psychological functions of, 1145–1146
  stages of, 1145t, *1146*
  surgery and, 619
  therapeutic dialogue, 1152
  values and, 76
Sleep apnea, 286, 818, 1155–1156
  central, 1155–1156
  mixed, 1156
  obstructive, 1155
Sleep debt, 1333
Sleep Deprivation, 1158
Sleepiness, 1146, 1150
Sleeping pills, 1154
Sleep latency, 1146
Sleep rhythm, 1144–1145
Sleep rituals, 1159
Sleep routine, 1160
Sleep talking, 1156
Sleepwalking, 1156
Slo-bid. *See* Theophylline
Small intestine, 951, 1102
Small-volume enemas, 1121–1122, 1124p
Smegma, 435, 1075
Smell
  assessment of, 1208t
  decreased sense of, safety and, 1211
  normal, 1200
  in observation, 152
  and perception of information, 1222
  and safety, 661
  sensory aids for, 1211d
SMOG Readability Formula, 370, 370d
Smokeless tobacco, 813
Smoking
  in adolescence, 282, 813
  as altered coping behavior, 1334
  cardiovascular problems and, 871
  cessation of, 825–826
  respiratory function and, 813–814, 818
  risks of, 1241
  wound healing and, 995–996
Smuts, Jan Christian, 258
Sneeze reflex, 812
Snellen test, 415
SNO MED. *See Systemized Nomenclature of Medicine*
Soaks, 717t
SOAP notes, 238–240, 240t, *241*
Social health, assessment of, 394
Social interaction
  and cognitive function, 1241
  and coping, 1334
  Dreyfuss model of, 45, 46t
  as function of family, 1278
  in home healthcare, 383
  and professional nursing, 45–49
  safety of, 651
  and values, 71, 73–75
Social isolation, 1285
Socialization therapies, 1244–1246
Social Readjustment and Rating Scale (SRRS), 1338
Social resources, for health maintenance, 681–682
Social self, 1254
Social worker
  referrals to, 33t
  and self-care promotion, 714t
Sociocultural resources and stressors, and grieving, 1305, 1306–1307
Sociocultural stress, 1337
Sodium, 912, 912t, 949
  and blood pressure, 871
  and cardiovascular problems, 871–872
  as electrolyte source, 937t

Sodium chloride, 911
Sodium hypochlorite (Dakin's), antiseptic use of, 492t
Sodium-potassium pump, 914, *914*
Sodium restriction, 936–937
Soft diets, 971
Soft palate, *418*
Somatic senses, 1200
  assessment of, 1208t
Somnambulism, 1144, 1156
Sonorous wheeze, 817t
Sound
  properties of, 409–410
  transmission of, 1220
Spansule, 516t
Spastic gait, 766
Spasticity, 765
Special senses, 1200
Specialty beds, for pressure ulcer prevention, 1005, *1007*
Specific gravity, of urine, 1079, *1079*, 1080t
Specificity, of infectious agent, 482
Speculum examination, 1366
Speech, 1223. *See also* Communication
Speech deficits, assessment of, 410
Speech therapist
  referrals to, 33t
  and self-care promotion, 714t
Speed shock, with intravenous administration, 565t
Spermicides, 1373
Sphygmomanometer, 464, *468*
  cuff inflation and deflation, 470
  cuff size of, 468–469, 469t
Spinal accessory nerve (XI), assessment of, 416t, 419
Spinal cord, and pain modulation, 1169
Spinal cord injury, and urinary elimination, 1069
Spinal dorsal horn, and pain modulation, 1169
Spinal reflexes, and pain modulation, 1169
Spinothalamic tract, and pain perception, 1168
Spiritual care
  in home healthcare, 388
  inadequate/inappropriate, 1387–1388
Spiritual dimension, definition of, 1382
Spiritual Distress, 1392, 1400. *See also* Spirituality, altered
Spirituality, 291, 1381–1401
  altered, 1388, 1389t–1390t
    and activities of daily living, 1388
    evaluation for, 1399–1400
    in home/community-based care, 1399
    implementation for, 1394–1399
    nursing diagnoses for, 1391–1393
    nursing interventions for, 1395–1399
    outcome identification and planning for, 1393
  among special populations, 1399
  assessment of, 394, 406, 1388–1391, 1391d
    dysfunction identification in, 1390
    normal pattern identification in, 1388–1390
    objective data in, 1391
    risk identification in, 1390
    subjective data in, 1388–1390
  characteristics of, 1382–1383
  definition of, 1382
  factors affecting, 1385–1388
  and family, 1280
  lifespan considerations, 1384–1385, 1384t, 1395–1398
  normal, 1382–1385, 1383
  of older adults, 306
  religious practices, 1396t–1398t
Spiritual leader, 1383
Spiritual need, 1382, 1389t–1390t
Spiritual practices, support of, 1394–1395
Spiritual quest, 1382–1383
Spiritual support, 1394

Spiritual ties, separation from, 1386
Spiritual well-being, 1383
Spirochetes, 1035t
Spironolactone, and urinary elimination, 1070
Splitters, 218–219
Sports drinks, 934
Spousal abuse, 312, 1284–1285
Sputum assessment, 820
Sputum culture, 820, 1048
Sputum production, 815
SRRS. *See* Social Readjustment and Rating Scale
St. John's wort, 519t
Stacked cough, 828–830
Staff nurse, 112, 114–117
Stages of change model, of health promotion, 364, 366t
Standardized plan of care, 194d
Standardized tests of intelligence, 1237
Standard Precautions, 494, 495d
Standards: Nursing Practice (ANA), 310
Standards of care, 51, 52d, 98, 207
Standards of Clinical Nursing Practice (ANA), 51, 138, 140, 186, 211, 212, 362
Standards of Holistic Nursing Practice, 261
Standards of Home Health Nursing Practice, 383, 384d
Standards of Nursing Practice (ANA), 138, 164, 211
Standards of practice, 51, 52d
Standards of professional performance, 51, 52d
Standard syringes, 543
Standing orders, 518
Standing protocols, 518–519
Standing scale, 402p
Stand-up assist lifts, 801, *803*
Staphylococcus aureus, infection with, work restrictions for, 487t
Staples, in wound closure, 637, 1013–1015, *1017*
Startle reflex, 760
Stasis dermatitis, 986, *987*
Stat order, 519
STDs. *See* Sexually transmitted diseases
Steam sterilization, 492, *493*
Steering Committee on Data Bases to Support Clinical Nursing Practice, of American Nurses Association, 237
Stepfamily, 1277
Stepping response, 760
Stereotypes, 332
Sterile field, 499, 506p–508p
Sterile gloves
  nursing procedure for, 502p–503p
  in surgical asepsis, 499
Sterile technique, 488, 1057
Sterilization, 492, *493*
  female, 1373, 1373t
  male, 1373, 1373t
Steristrips, 1013
Stethoscope, 409, *409*, 409t, 455, 464
Stimulant laxatives, 1121t
Stock supply system, of medication distribution, 515–516
Stoma, 1107
Stomach, 951, 1102
Stoma management, 1133–1137
  assessment in, 1133
  continent fecal diversion management, 1136–1137
  fecal collection in, 1133–1136
  irrigation in, 1136, *1136*
Stool culture, 1048, 1113
Stool softeners, 1121t
Stool specimens
  collection of, 1113, 1133–1136
  for parasitic infection detection, 1048
Straight catheters, 1088, 1089p–1093p

Strengths
  identification of, 1266
  reinforcement of, in families, 1292
Streptococcal bacteria, 1034t
Streptococcal infections, and work restriction, 487t
Stress. *See also* Coping and stress tolerance
  and body temperature, 445
  and cardiovascular function, 872–873
  characteristics of, 1328–1330
  and cognitive function, 1229, 1241
  cognitive response to, 1330
  definition of, 1326
  and diarrhea, 1109
  effects of, 261
  environmental, 1336
  evaluation for, 1344
  and fluid and electrolyte balance, 920
  and immune function, 1040
  implementation for, 1339–1344
  and infections, 1039–1040
  and irritable bowel syndrome, 1110
  lifespan considerations, 1331–1332
  nursing diagnoses for, 1338–1339
  outcome identification and planning for, 1339
  physiologic functions related to, 1326–1328
  physiologic response to, 1329–1330, 1334d, 1336
  psychological response to, 1330, 1336
  psychosocial expressions of, 261, 1334d
  and respirations, 459
  as response, 1328–1330
  and sleep and rest, 1154
  sociocultural, 1337
  as stimulus, 1328
  therapeutic dialogue, 1335
  and urinary elimination, 1068
  and wound healing, 996
Stress Audit, 1338
Stress ECG, 882t, 883
Stress incontinence, 299, 1071–1072
Stress management
  in home/community-based nursing, 1343–1344
  for nurses, 1340d
  techniques for, 1342t
Stressors, 1328, 1329
  chronic, 1329–1330
  reducing, 1339
Stress Reduction and Relaxation Program, 263
Stress-related illness, effects on safety, 659
Stress tolerance, of older adults, 305
Stress Urinary Incontinence, 1082
Stretcher, client transfer to, 798p
Stretch receptors, 911
Striae, 430
Stridor, 460, 820
Stroke, 879
  and cognition, 1227
  and urinary elimination, 1069
Stroke volume (SV), and cardiac output, 868–869
Structure evaluation, 208
Study skills, 218
Subcultures, 331–332
Subcutaneous injections, 548–550, 552, 553p–555p
Subcutaneous tissue, 984, 984
Subjective data, 156, 157t, 208–209
Subject rights, in nursing research, 129
Sublingual administration, 537
Substance abuse
  as altered coping behavior, 1334–1335
  family function and, 1282
  by healthcare professional, 523
  and nutrition, 961
  and overdoses, 656–657
Sucking reflex, 414p

Suctioning, in respiratory care, 847–851, 852p–855p
  hazards of, 847–851
Suffering, 1174
Suffocation, 657–658
  prevention of, 669
Suicide, 1358
  firearms and, 658
  physician-assisted, 102
Suitability Assessment of Materials (SAM), 8
Sulfate, 912
Summarizing, in therapeutic communication, 355
Sunburns, 670
Sundowner's syndrome, 1149, 1231
Sun protection, 670, 1003
Superchiasmatic nucleus (SCN), and sleep-wake patterns, 1147–1148
Superego, 269
Superficial palpation, 407
Superinfection, 1040, 1056
Supervisory nursing interventions, 204
Supination, 755t
Supine position, 782
Support
  for families, 1292
  in spiritual care, 1395
Support groups, 1294, 1343–1344
  as function of family, 1278
  for grieving, 1310–1311
  postoperative, 619
Supportive nursing interventions, 205
Support surfaces, for pressure ulcer prevention, 1005, 1006
Suppository, 516t, 540
  rectal, 1120–1121
Suprapubic catheters, 1095–1096, 1096
Surfactant, 812
The Surgeon General's Call to Action To Promote Sexual Health and Responsible Sexual Behavior, 1352
Surgery, 612–622
  and bowel elimination, 1107
  classification of, 612, 612t
  client preparation for, 369
  coping with, 1341
  fever following, 1043
  and fluid and electrolyte balance, 921
  and functional health patterns, 613–621
  intraoperative nursing, 632–638
  lifespan considerations and, 621–622
  and nutrition, 961
  postoperative nursing, 638–644
  preoperative nursing, 622–632
  and self-care, 707
  and self-concept, 1263
  and sexuality, 1362, 1365
  skin preparation for, 499
  and urinary elimination, 1070
Surgical asepsis, 488, 496–502
  handwashing in, 488, 499, 500p–501p
  principles of, 496, 498t–499t
  skin preparation in, 497–499
  sterile field in, 499
  sterile gloves in, 499
Surgical débridement, 1010
Surgical drains, and infections, 1039
Surgical facilities, 612–613, 641–643
Surgical scrub, 497, 499, 500p–501p
Surgical sterilization, 1373
Surgical wounds, 990–991, 990t. *See also* Wound(s)
Surroundings, orientation to, 1242
Surveillance nursing interventions, 206
Survival reflexes, 760
Survivor, role of, 1282
Susceptible host, 482–483

Suspension, 516t
Sustained-release medications, 537
Sutures, 637, 1013–1015
SV. *See* Stroke volume
Swallowing
  assessment of, 156, 1236
  evaluation of, 965
  impaired, 156, 737, 957
  and medication administration, 527
Sweat glands, 984
Sweating, 920
Sweets, in Food Guide Pyramid, 951
Symbolic meaning, 326
Sympathectomy, in pain management, 1193t
Sympathetic nervous system
  and blood pressure, 463
  functions of, 1327
  and pulse rate, 449
  stress and, 1329
Sympathomimetics, and respirations, 459
Symphysis pubis, *1352*
Symptothermal contraceptive method, 1369
Syndrome X, 872
Synergism, 524
Synovial joints, 755
Syphilis, 1035t
Syringes, 543, *543, 544*
Syrup, 516t
Syrup of ipecac, 673d
Systemic circulation, 869, *869*
Systemic disease, and skin abnormalities, 990
Systemic infections, 1041
Systemized Nomenclature of Medicine (SNO MED), 165
Systems framework. *See also* General systems theory
  of family, 312–313, *313*
Systems skills, 80
Systems theory, and nursing process, 142, *142*
Systole, 422, 868
Systolic blood pressure, 461
Systolic murmur, 422, *425*

T

Tablet, as drug preparation, 516t
Tachycardia, 458
Tachypnea, 425, 459, 460t
TAH. *See* Total abdominal hysterectomy
Tangential lighting, in physical examination, 407
Tape, for wound dressings, 1008, 1010t
Tartar, oral care and, 704
Task Force on Nursing Information Systems, 237
Task-oriented learners, 218
Taste
  assessment of, 1208t
  normal, 1200
  and perception of information, 1222
  and safety, 661
  sensory aids for, 1211d
Taxonomy
  definition of, 165
  of nursing diagnosis, 164–169
    development of, 165, 166t–167t
  of nursing interventions, 189
Teaching. *See* Client teaching
Teaching aids, in client teaching, 369–371
Teaching-learning process
  approaches to learning in, 362, 363t
  in client teaching, 362–364
  domains of knowledge in, 363–364
  information processing in, 362–363
Teaching-learning relationship, 364
Team leader, 116
Team nursing, 9, 115–116
Team rounds, reporting of, 248–249

Technical nursing interventions, 205t, 206
Technology
    advances in, 11–12
    and confidentiality, 249
    and documentation, 233–237
    and evaluation, 208
    and home healthcare, 381
    and information resource management, 112
    and nursing process, 146
    in risk identification, 690
Teenager. *See* Adolescent
Teeth, 951
    altered nutrition and, 963, 1111
    care of, 704, 729–731, 732p–734p
Tele-home health, 381
Telephone orders, 519–520
Telephone reporting, 247–248
Temazepam (Restoril), 1160t
Temperature. *See also* Body temperature
    environmental, safety and, 654–655
    of skin, 985
Temperature method of contraception, 1369
Temperature-sensitive strips, 448
Temporal pulse, 454, *455*
Tendons, 755
TENS. *See* Transcutaneous electrical nerve
    stimulation
Tepid baths, in fever management, 1056
Terbutaline (Brethine, Bricanyl), 836t
Terminal illness
    forgiveness and, 72
    intravenous therapy in, 599
Termination phase
    of home healthcare visit, 384
    of interview process, 154
    of nurse-client relationship, 347
Terminology, medical, 1417–1424
Tertiary disease prevention, 682, 683t
Tertiary intention wound healing, *994,* 995
Testes, 1352, *1352*
Testicular self-examination, 696, 1369d
Tetanus, 1038t
Texture, of skin, 985, 998
Theism, 1383
Theo-Dur. *See* Theophylline
Theophylline (Theo-Dur, Slo-bid), 836t
Theoretical reflectivity, 226t
Theory. *See* Nursing theory
Therapeutic abortion, 1373
Therapeutic baths, 715, 717t
Therapeutic communication, 344, 349–350,
    1244. *See also* Communication
    nontherapeutic responses to, 355–357
    techniques in, 353t
Therapeutic drug monitoring, for infections,
    1048–1050
Therapeutic effects, of medications, 524
Therapeutic modalities, and mobility, 765
Therapeutic partnership, nursing as, 262
Therapeutic regimen, and nosocomial infections,
    483
Therapeutic Regimen Management: Effective and
    Ineffective — Focus: Individual, Fam-
    ily, and Community, 694
Therapeutic relationships, self-concept and,
    1268–1269
Therapeutic touch, 264, 1342t
Therapy
    group, 205–206
    individual, 205–206
Thermal burns, 991, 1007
Thermometers
    electronic, 447, *448,* 451p–452p, 452p–453p
    glass mercury, 447, *447*
    paper, 448, *448*
    tympanic membrane, 447–448, *448*

Thermoreceptors, 1168
Thermoregulation, 444
    as physiologic need, 63
    skin and, 985
    sleep and rest and, 1151
    during surgery, 618
Thiamine, 946t, 947
Thickness, of skin, 985
Thinking, 1224. *See also* Critical thinking
Third degree burns, 991
Third party reimbursers
    and client records, 231
    and plans of care, 190
Third spacing, 921
Third trimester, growth and development in, 273,
    274
Thoughts, 1222–1223
Three-person lift, 794
Throat culture, 1048
Thrombophlebitis, 594
    intravenous therapy and, 565t
Thrombus, 768, 873, 878
Throughput, in systems theory, 142
Thumb joint, 762t
Thyroid gland, *1327,* 1327–1328
    assessment of, 419, *420*
    enlarged, 949
Thyroxine, and body temperature, 446
TIA. *See* Transient ischemic attack
Ticks, 1039
Tilade. *See* Nedocromil
Timbre, of phonation, 1223
Time, 24-hour time conversions, 236t
Timed voiding, 1085
Time-lapsed assessment, 151, 151t
Timeliness, of documentation, 233
Time of day, and body temperature, 445
Time orientation, 74t
Time tape, in intravenous therapy, 583, *585*
Timing, of medication administration, 532
Tincture, 516t
Tincture of belladonna, 1122t
Tinea capitis, 990
Tinea corporis, 990
Tinea cruris, 990
Tinea pedis, 726t, 990
Tinea unguium, 990
Tissue hydration, abnormal, 928. *See also* Edema
Tissue perfusion, 870, 878
Titration, 1190
T lymphocytes, 1029–1035, 1030t
Toddler
    activity and exercise in, 283
    bowel elimination in, 1104
    bowel sounds in, 433p
    breath sounds in, 429p
    cardiovascular function in, 870
    client teaching for, 375
    cognition and perception in, 286, 1225
    coping and stress tolerance in, 288–289,
        1331–1332
    elimination in, 285
    family of, 1278–1279
    fluid and electrolyte balance in, 916
    grieving in, 1303–1304
    growth and development of, 275–276
        cognitive, 276
        physical, 275
        psychosocial, 275–276
    health assessment of, 437
    health maintenance of, 683, 692d
    health perception and health management in,
        281–282
    heart sounds in, 424p
    infection control for, 505
    infections in, 1031

inhaled medications for, 542p
    intravenous therapy for, 598–599
    medication administration for, 570–571
    mobility of, 763
    neurologic assessment of, 414p
    nutrition and metabolism in, 284, 955
    pain perception in, 1171–1172
    respiratory function of, 812
    roles and relationships of, 287
    safety of, 651
    self-care of, 705–706
    self-perception and self-concept of, 287, 1256t,
        1257–1258, 1267, 1268t
    sensory perception of, 1201
    sexuality of, 289, 1358
    skin of, 986
    sleep and rest of, 285, 1149
    spirituality of, 1384, 1395–1398
    surgery for, 621–622
    urinary elimination in, 1066t, 1067
    values and beliefs of, 75, 76t, 291
    vital signs of, 444t, 474
Toe joints, 762t
Toilet, 737–738, *738*
Toileting, 705, 711t, 737–739
    in home/community-based care, 749
    and safety, 663
Toileting Self-Care Deficit, 713
Tolerance
    to medications, 524
    to opioid analgesics, 1189–1190
Tolmetin, 1187t
Tongue, *418,* 951
    and airway obstruction, 851
    assessment of motor control of, 1236
    color of, 419
Tonicity, 914–915
Tonic neck reflex, 414p, 760
Tonsils, 418, *418*
Tonsil-tip (Yankauer) suction tube, 847, *855*
Topical drug preparations, 516t
    administration of, 537–539
Torts, 99–101, 99d
    intentional, 99–100, 99d
    unintentional, 99d, 100–101
Total abdominal hysterectomy (TAH), collaborative
    care plan for, 614–617
Total client care, 116
Total hip replacement, collaborative care plan for,
    772–775
Total incontinence, 1073. *See also* Urinary
    incontinence
Total parenteral nutrition (TPN), 576, 599,
    600–603
    administration of, 600
    complications of, 600–603
    cyclic infusions of, 600
    and fluid overload, 603
    and infections, 600–603
    metabolic complications with, 603
    nursing procedure for, 601p–602p
Total quality improvement. *See* Quality improve-
    ment programs
Total quality management. *See* Quality improve-
    ment programs
Total Urinary Incontinence, 1082
Touch
    in observation, 153
    and perception of information, 1222
    sensory aids for, 1211d
    therapeutic, 264
Towel baths, 716, 720p–722p
Toxicity. *See also* Poisoning
    of medications, 524
Toxins, common household, 657d
Toy safety, 651, 672

TPN. *See* Total parenteral nutrition
Trace elements, 942, 948t
Trachea, assessment of, 419
Tracheostomy, 843–847
  care of, 847, 848p–851p
  equipment for, 845–846, *847*
  indications for, 845
  risks of, 846–847
Trade name of medications, 514
Traditional bladder retraining, 1085
Transcendental meditation, in pain management, 1185
Transcultural nursing, 332–333, *333. See also under* Cultural; Culture
Transcutaneous electrical nerve stimulation (TENS), in pain management, 1184
Transdermal medications, administration of, 538, *538*
Transdermal patch, 516t
Transfer, of clients. *See* Client transfer
Transfer belts, 793, 801t
Transfer board/sled, 801t
Transfusions. *See* Blood transfusion
Transient ischemic attack (TIA), 879
Translators, 359, 359d
  in client teaching, 371
  in health assessments, 396
Transmission, of infection, 482
Transmission-Based Precautions, 494–495, 496t
Transplant surgery, 612t
Transsexual, 1356
Transtheoretical model, of health promotion, 364
Transtracheal catheters, 837, 842t
Transverse colon, 1103
Transverse (loop) colostomy, *1107*
Transvestite, 1356
Trapeze bar, as positioning aid, 784t
Trauma
  effect on family, 1282
  to head, and cognitive function, 1229
  and self-concept, 1263
  and skin integrity, 990–991
Travel, and infection exposure, 1032
Travelbee, Joyce, 61t
Traveler's diarrhea, 1109
Treatment
  alternative/complementary, 259
  ethical/legal issues in, 928
  mobility restriction due to, 765
  refusal of, 895
Tremor, 765
Trendelenburg position, 742d
Treponema pallidum, 1035t
Triage, 9
Triamcinolone (Azmacort), 836t
Triamterene, and urinary elimination, 1070
Triceps reflex, 438t
Trichomoniasis, 1039
Tricuspid area, 421
Tricyclic antidepressants, and urinary elimination, 1070
Trigeminal nerve (V), assessment of, 416t
Triple-lumen indwelling catheters, 1088, *1088*
Trochanter roll, as positioning aid, 784t
Trochlear nerve (IV), assessment of, 416t
Trough level, of drug concentration, 1050
Trust, and spirituality, 1389t, 1394
TST. *See* Tuberculin skin testing
Tubal ligation/cauterization, 1373
Tube(s)
  endotracheal, 843, *846*
  for intravenous therapy, 581–582, *583*
  medication administration through, 537
  nasogastric, 972–973, 972t, 1126, *1126*
  nasointestinal, 1126–1127
  for total parenteral nutrition, 576, 599, 600–603
  tracheostomy, 845–846, *847*
Tube feedings. *See also* Nasogastric intubation
  ending, ethical/legal issues of, 957
  enteral, 972–977
  fluid replacement in, 935
Tuberculin skin testing (TST), 546–548
Tuberculin syringes, 543, *543*
Tuberculosis, dietary modifications for, 972d
Tumor, 992t
Tunneled central venous catheters, 578–580, *580*
Turbidity, of urine, 1080t
Turning, of clients, schedule for, 782–783
Turn sheet, 759, 784t
Tuskegee project, 331
24-hour time conversions, 236t
24-hour urine specimen, 1075–1078
Two-person lift, 794
Tympanic membrane, assessment of, 416, *417*
Tympanic membrane thermometer, 447–448, *448,* 453p
Tympanic temperature, 444, 445t, 447, 453p
Tympanic tones, 408, 408t
Tympany, 1112
Typhoid fever, 1038t

U

Ulcers, 992t
  of leg and foot, 986, *987*
  pressure (*See* Pressure ulcers)
Ultrasound
  abdominal, 1081
  Doppler, 883
    for blood pressure assessment, 464–465
    for pulse assessment, 455, *455*
  echocardiographic, 882t, 883
Unconscious client
  coma assessment and, 410, 414t
  eye care for, 735
  Heimlich maneuver for, 857p
  oral care for, 729
Under-axilla lift technique, 794
Underweight, 962. *See also* Weight
Unfreezing, in change theory, 65
Uniform Anatomical Gift Act, 103
Unintentional injuries, 650
Unintentional torts, 99d, 100–101
Unit-dose system, for medication distribution, 516, *516*
United Nations Food and Agriculture Organization, nutrient guidelines of, 942
United States Pharmacopeia, 514
Unit environment, care of, 739–742
Unit level managers, 118, *118*
Universal computer-based patient record, 236–237
Universal donors, 604
Universal healthcare requisites, 64t
Universal intellectual standards, 224, 224t
Universal Precautions, 494
Unlicensed personnel. *See also* Collaboration and delegation
  delegation of care to, 723
Unsaturated fats, 944
Upper extremity. *See* Arm
Upper respiratory tract infections, healthcare personnel with, work restrictions for, 487t
Upright scale, 401
Urea levels, and altered cognitive function, 1236–1237
Ureteritis, 1069
Ureters, 1064
Urethra, 1065, *1352*
Urethral meatus, *1353*

Urethritis, 1069
Urge incontinence, 1072, 1082, 1099
  in older adults, 299
Urgency, urinary, 1071
Urgent surgery, 612t
Urge Urinary Incontinence, 1082
Urinal, 738
Urinalysis, 1048, 1080, 1080t
Urinary bladder, *1352*
Urinary catheters/catheterization, 1088–1097
  care of, 1094
  condom, 1085
  Foley, 1088, *1094*
  indications for, 1088
  infections and, 1039
  insertion of, 1088, 1089p–1093p
  intermittent, 1096
  irrigation of, 1094–1095, *1095*
  leg bags for, 1097, *1097*
  removal of, 1095
  risks of, 1088–1094
  suprapubic, 1095–1096, *1096*
  surgery and, 618
  triple-lumen, 1088, *1088*
  types of, 1088
Urinary diversion, 1070
Urinary drainage bags, 1093p, 1094
Urinary elimination, 1063–1099. *See also* Elimination
  altered, 1070–1073
    and activities of daily living, 1073
    evaluation for, 1098
    in home/community-based care, 1097–1098
    implementation for, 1083–1098
    nursing interventions for, 1084–1098
    outcome identification and planning for, 1083
  assessment of, 433–434, 1073–1081
    diagnostic tests and procedures in, 1075–1081
    dysfunction identification in, 1074
    normal pattern identification in, 1073
    objective data in, 1074–1081
    physical examination in, 1075, 1075t
    risk identification in, 1073–1074
    subjective data in, 1073–1074
  factors affecting, 1068–1070, 1068d
  lifespan considerations, 1066–1067.6t
  normal, 1064–1067
  nursing diagnoses for, 1081–1083
  outcome-based teaching plan for, 1084
  surgery and, 618
Urinary frequency, 1071
Urinary incontinence, 1067, 1071–1073
  bladder training for, 1084–1085
  functional, 1072–1073
  in older adults, 299–300
  reflex, 1072
  stress, 1071–1072
  therapeutic dialogue, 1072
  total, 1073
  urge, 1072
Urinary meatus, inspection of, 1075
Urinary retention, 1071, 1082–1083
Urinary stasis, 769
Urinary system, 1069
  function of, 1065–1066
  structures of, *1064,* 1064–1065
Urinary tract infections (UTIs)
  altered mobility and, 769
  manifestations of, 1043d
  predispositions for, 1042d
  during pregnancy, 1070
  prevention of, 1083
Urinary tract obstruction, 1069
Urinary urgency, 1071
Urination. *See* Micturition

Urine
    assessment of, 1074
    bacteria in, 1080t
    casts in, 1080t
    clarity of, 1066
    color of, 1066, 1070, 1080t
    excretion of, 1065–1066
    fluid intake and, 1074–1075
    formation of, 1065
    glucose in, 1080t
    ketones in, 1080t
    normal, characteristics of, 1066
    odor of, 1066
    osmolarity of, 932
    output of, 920
        monitoring, 930, *931*, 1074–1075
    protein in, 1080t
    red blood cells in, 1080t
    specific gravity of, 932, 1079, *1079,* 1080t
    turbidity of, 1080t
    volume of, 1066
    white blood cells in, 1080t
    yeast in, 1080t
Urine culture and sensitivity, 1080–1081
Urine specimen, collection of, 1074, 1075–1079
    from catheter, 1076p, 1078–1079
    from child, 1077p–1078p, 1079
    clean-catch, 1075
    midstream, 1075, 1077p
    nursing procedure for, 1076p–1078p
    random, 1075
    24-Hour, 1075–1078
Urine tests, 1079–1081
Urinometer, 1079, *1079*
Urodynamic studies, 1081
Urticaria, 991
U.S. Department of Agriculture
    Dietary Guidelines for Americans of, 953
    Food Guide Pyramid of, *950,* 950–951
U.S. Department of Health and Human Services,
        Dietary Guidelines for Americans of,
        953
U.S. Department of Labor, on infection control,
        484
U.S. Food and Drug Administration
    on herbal preparations, 518
    on medication administration, 521
    on use of restraints, 665, 666d
U.S. Preventive Services Task Force, 26
U.S. Public Health Service, Advisory Committee
        on Immunization Practices of, 1052
USP. *See United States Pharmacopeia*
Utah, family nursing in, 314
Uterine cycle, 1355, *1355*
Uterus, *1353,* 1354
Utilitarian framework, of ethics, 88
UTIs. *See* Urinary tract infections
Uvula, 418, *418*

V

Vaccinations. *See* Immunizations
Vagina, *1353,* 1354
    perineal care and, 716–717, *724*
Vaginal medications, 539, *540*
Vaginal speculum, 1366
Vaginal spermicides, 1373
Vaginal vestibule, *1353*
Vaginismus, 1363
Vagus nerve (X), assessment of, 416t
Valerian, 519t
Validation
    of data, 158–160, *159*
    of nursing diagnosis, 177
Validation therapy, 297, 297d
Valsalva maneuver, 1103

Values and beliefs, 70–73
    assessment of, 161t, 406
        postoperative, 640t
    challenges to, 81–83
    in classroom study, 71–72
    client teaching and, 365t
    cognition and, 1229–1230
    community and, 74, 320d
    conflicting, 80–83
    cultural influences on, 73, 74t
    definition of, 70
    developmental stage and, 291
    family and, 316d, 1280
    and functional health patterns, 66, *66,* 76–79,
        78d–79d, 147d
    grieving and, 1309t
    health maintenance and, 684d, 687
    individual, family and community focus for,
        321–322
    in individual assessment, 311d
    life experience and, 74–75
    lifespan considerations and, 75–76, 76t
    of nurses, 79–80
    nursing diagnoses and, 181d
    nutrition and, 961
    of older adults, 306
    peer culture and, 74
    personal, 86
    role models and, 74
    self-care and, 706
    self-concept and, 1259
    sexuality and, 1359
    socialization and, 73–75
    sources of, 73–76
    surgery and, 621
    terminal illness and, 72
    therapeutic dialogue and, 82
    validation of, 96–97
Values clarification, 71, 72d
Values inquiry, 71–72
Value system, 70
Valuing, as human response pattern, 74–75, *75*
Valves, heart, 867
    dysfunction of, 874
Vanceril. *See* Beclomethasone
Variables, in nursing research, 127
Variances, in critical pathways, 194, 243
Varicella, healthcare personnel with, work restric-
        tions for, 487t
Varicella-zoster virus, 1034t
Varicose veins, prevention of, 885
Vascular access devices. *See also* Venous access
        devices
    implanted, 580
Vascular fluid, 910
    volume of, 921–923
Vasculature, *869,* 869–870
Vas deferens, *1352*
Vasectomy, 1373
Vasoconstriction, orthostatic hypotension and, 471
Vasodilators, and cardiac function, 892t
Vasopressors, 892t
Vastus lateralis site, for intramuscular injections,
        552–555, 556t, *562, 563*
Vectorborne transmission of infections, 482
Vegetables, in Food Guide Pyramid, 950
Vehicle transmission of infections, 482
Veins, 869–870
    dysfunction of, 878
    neck, distention of, 931, *931*
Venipuncture, 576
    in intravenous therapy, 586–588
Venous access devices, 577–580. *See also*
        Catheter(s)
    implantable, *582*
    for medication administration, 527

Venous stasis
    immobility and, 768
    postoperative, 642
    prevention of, 885–889, 887p–888p, 890p–891p
Venous thrombosis, 768, 873, 878
Ventilation, 810. *See also* Breathing;
        Respiration(s)
    assisted, 841–843
    control of, 811
Ventilators, 843
    in home healthcare, 859
    withdrawal of, 846
Ventolin. *See* Albuterol
Ventrogluteal site, for intramuscular injections,
        555–556, 556t, *563*
Venturi mask, *841, 842t*
Venules, 869
Veracity, in professional-patient relationship, 93
Verbal communication, 113, 344, 344d, 1224
Verbalization
    of distress, 1388
    in pain response, 1175–1176, 1176t, 1181
Verbal orders, 519–520
Vertical gravity line, 755, *756*
Vesicles, 991, 992t
Vesicular breath sounds, 426, 430t
Vestibular apparatus, and balance, 755
Vest restraint, 665
Viable Village model, of community-based
        nursing, 25
Viagra. *See* Sildenafil citrate
Vials, parenteral medications in, 544, 545p–546p
Vibration, in chest physiotherapy, 832
Vicarious liability, 101
Victim-rescuer-persecutor triangle, 262, *262*
Vietnamese Americans, response to death and
        dying, 339
Vigilance, in sleep and rest, 1151
Vinyl gloves, 494
Violence. *See also* Abuse
    altered coping and, 1336
    among adolescents, 282, 289
    domestic, 1284–1285
    firearms and, 658
    against healthcare workers, 654
Viral infections. *See also* Infection(s)
    skin effects of, 989–990
Virtue, and self-esteem, 1255
Virulence, of infectious agent, 482
Viruses, 480, 655, 1032, 1033t–1038t. *See also*
        Infection(s); *specific virus*
Vision
    assessment of, 1208t
    normal, 1200
    in observation, 152
    and perception of information, 1220–1222
Vision impairments
    and safety, 661
    sensory aids for, 370–371, 1211d
    and surgery, 622
Visual acuity, assessment of, 415
Visual aids, 370–371, 1211d
Visual fields, assessment of, 415
Visualization, 264, 1342t
Visual learners, 218
Vital signs, 443–475. *See also specific vital signs*
    acid-base balance and, 927–928
    altered cardiovascular function and, 873
    documentation of, 473, *474*
    fluid and electrolyte balance and, 927–928, 931
    infections and, 1045
    lifespan considerations, 473–475
    medication administration and, 527–528
    normal, 392, 444t
    pain and, 1180
    postoperative, 638–639, 639t

Vitamin(s), 944–947, 945t–946t
  fat-soluble, 944–947, 945t
  water-soluble, 945t–946t, 947
  in wound healing, 995
Vitamin A, 944, 945t, 995
Vitamin B, 995
Vitamin B₁, 946t, 947
Vitamin B₂, 946t, 947
Vitamin B₃, 946t, 947
Vitamin B₆, 946t
Vitamin B₁₂, 946t, 947
Vitamin C, 945t, 947, 995
Vitamin D, 913, 944, 945t
Vitamin E, 944, 945t
Vitamin K, 944–947, 945t, 995
Vocabulary, standardized, in documentation, 237
Vocalization, 1223
Voiding. *See* Micturition; Urinary elimination
Volume, of phonation, 1223
Volume-controlled intravenous administration
    set, 582, *583*
Volunteer Nurse Corps, 44
Vomiting
  enteral feeding and, 973
  fluid and electrolyte balance and, 920
  induction of, 673d
    for poisoning, 924
  and metabolic alkalosis, 924
  nutrition and, 957
  opioid analgesics and, 1191
Vulva, 1353

W
Waddling gait, 766
Waist measurement, 964
Wald, Lillian, 41t
Walkers, 793, *794*
Walking, 760, 788–794. *See also* Mobility
  assistance with, 788–793, 791p–792p
  dangling legs prior to, 788
  gait and
    altered, 766
    assessment of, 399–400, 776
    normal, 760
  impaired, 766
  mechanical aids for, 793–794
  muscle strengthening for, 794
  respiratory function and, 827
Walking rounds, 247
Walsh, Mary, 138, 139t
Warm compresses, 1021
Warm soaks, 1021
Warm-water bath, 717t
Warts, plantar, 726t
Waste disposal, *488*
  for asepsis, 494
  infection control and, 486
  parenteral medications and, 546
  for sharps, *486*
Water. *See also* Fluid(s)
  concentration of, in body fluids, 911–912
  fluoride in, 950
  in nutrition, 950
  as physiologic need, 63
Water-borne infections, 1037t–1038t
Water deficit, 923, 933
Water excess, 924, 933
Water imbalance, 923–924
Water intake, 919–920
  assessment of, 929–931, *930*
    in nasogastric intubation, 1128
  and body weight, 927, 931
  and bowel elimination, 1105, 1119
  and cognitive function, 1243

  monitoring of, 929–932, *930*
  and urinary elimination, 1068, 1083
Water pollution, 655
Water safety, 652
Water-soluble vitamins, 945t–946t, 947
Watson, Jean, 62t, 64t
WBCs. *See* White blood cells
Weakness, muscle atrophy and, 754–755, 766–767
Weather conditions, respiratory function and, 813
Weber test, 417, *418*
Web sites
  related to health, 1432
  related to nursing research, 1433–1435
Wedge cushion, 668d
Weidenbach, Ernestine, 59t–60t, 138
Weight. *See also* Obesity
  birth, average, 274
  extracellular fluid volume excess and, 923
  in fluid balance assessment, 931
  fluid intake and output and, 927, 931
  height and, standardized tables of, 964
  ideal, 954
  measurement of, 400–401, 402p–403p, 964
  of older adults, 300–301
  overweight, 962
  significant changes in, altered nutrition and,
    962–963
  underweight, 962
Weir report, 42t
Wellness, 255. *See also* Health
  definitions of, 256
  high-level, 257–258
  holistic healthcare and, 258–261
  nursing and, 261–264
  self-responsibility for, 259
Wellness-illness continuum, 257, *258*
Wellness nursing diagnoses, 177t, *178,* 178–179,
    179t, 262–263. *See also* Nursing
    diagnosis(es)
Wellness programs, 23–24
  client teaching and, 364
Wernicke's aphasia, 410, 1231–1232, 1232t
Wernicke's area, 1220
Western Interstate Commission for Higher
    Education (WICHE), 138, 139t
Western Journal of Nursing Research, 124
Wheals, 991, 992t, 993t
Wheelchairs
  mobility in, impaired, 779
  safety in, 665
  self-care and, 707
  transfer of client to, 799p–800p
Wheezing, *431,* 460, 817t, 819–820
White blood cell(s) (WBCs), 603
  and infection resistance, 1028, 1029t, 1030t
  in urine, 1080t
White blood cell count, 1046–1047
White House Office of Faith-Based and Commu-
    nity Initiatives, 24
WHO. *See* World Health Organization
Whole blood, 603
Wholeness, 313
Whole person concept, 65
Whooping cough, 1034t
WICHE. *See* Western Interstate Commission for
    Higher Education
Wide Range Achievement Test (WRAT), 368
Widows/widowers, support groups for, 1310
Wills, living, 89, *90,* 102–103, 1308
Winged infusion needles, 577
Withdrawal
  altered sensory perception and, 1205
  from morphine, 1189
Withdrawal method, of contraception, 1373, 1373t
Withdrawal reflex, 760
Withholding food, 968–971

Women. *See also under* Female; Gender
  adolescent, 277
  aging of, 279
  bladder of, 1064
  body temperature of, 445–446
  genitalia of, 434
  genitourinary tract of, *1065*
  health promotion for, 962
  moral development of, 291
  noise disturbance and, 1150
  pregnant, health maintenance of, 692d–693d
  reproductive system of, 1352–1354, *1353*
  respirations of, 459
  sexual response in, 1357
  sterilization of, 1373, 1373t
  stress response in, 1329, 1332
  urinary catheterization of, 1089p–1091p,
    1093p
  urinary elimination in, 1069
  urinary incontinence in, 1067
  urinary tract infections in, 1069
  urine specimen collection from, 1077p
Workers' compensation insurance, 231
Working phase
  of interview process, 154
  of nurse-client relationship, 347
Workplace/working conditions
  and asthma, 826
  and hydration, 934
  infection control in, 484–486
    in hospitals, 485
    personnel monitoring and counseling in, 485
  nosocomial infections in, 484
  and respiratory function, 813
  roles and relationships pattern in, 405
  safety of, 653, 672–673
  and sleep and rest, 1151
Work restriction, for infection control, 485–486
World Health Organization (WHO)
  definition of health of, 255
  on health promotion, 680
  nutrient guidelines of, 942
World Nutrient Guidelines, 942
World view, 73
Wound(s)
  accidental, 990, 990t
  appearance of, 998–1001
  assessment of, 420
  cleaning and disinfection of, 1010
  closure of, 637
  débridement of, 1010–1013
  drainage of, 1001
    management of, 1017–1018
    postoperative assessment of, 638–639
    systems for, 1001, *1001*
  dressings for
    application of, 1014p–1015p
    changing of, 1008, 1011p–1013p
    securing, 1008
    types of, 1008, 1009t–1010t
  infection of, 1001
    manifestations of, 1043d
    predispositions for, 1042d
  inspection of, 998–1001
  irrigation of, 1016p–1017p
  minor, first aid for, 1005–1006
  palpation of, 1001
  suction of, 1019p
  surgical, 990–991, 990t
  types of, 990t
Wound culture, 1048, 1049p–1050p
Wound healing, 991–997
  adjunctive therapies for, 1021
  complications of, 996–997
  decision-making and, 203
  emotional support for, 1021

Wound healing (*continued*)
  factors affecting, 995–996
    individual, 995–996
    local, 996
    systemic, 995
  heat and cold application for, 1018–1021
  phases of, 994
  postoperative, 642
  therapeutic dialogue, 1022
  topical therapy for, 1008–1013
  types of, *994,* 994–995
Wound packing, 1008–1010
Wound support, 1013–1017
Woven bone, 754
WRAT reading test, 368
Wrist, movement of, 761t
Wrist restraints, 665
Writing, 217
  assessment of, 410
  communication through, 144

Written communication. *See* Documentation
Written materials, in client teaching, 369–370
Written teaching plan, in client teaching, 372
Written tests, in client teaching, 374

X
X-ray examination
  in bowel assessment, 1113–1115
  in cardiovascular assessment, 883
  in mobility assessment, 778
  in respiratory assessment, 820
  safety of, 655, 671
  in urinary tract assessment, 1081

Y
Yankauer suction catheter, 847, *855*
Yeast, in urine, 1080t
Yeast infections, 1032–1039
Yesavage Geriatric Depression Scale, 298, 299d

Yin-yang symbol, 261, *261*
Yoga, 1185, 1342t
Yogurt, in Food Guide Pyramid, 951
Young adult. *See also* Adolescent; Adult
  growth and development of, 278
    cognitive, 278
    physical, 278
    psychosocial, 278
  health maintenance of, 692d
  values and beliefs of, 73, 76t
Yura, Helen, 138, 139t

Z
Zafirlukast (Accolate), 836t
Zileuton (Zyflo), 836t
Zinc, 948t
Zolpidem (Ambien), 1160t
Zopiclone (Imovane), 1160t
Z-track injection, 560p, *564*
Zyflo. *See* Zileuton

NURSING PROCEDURES

Procedure	Page	Procedure	Page
24-1, Measuring Weight	402	33-3, Providing Range-of-Motion Exercises	789
24-2, Assessing the Neurologic System	411	33-4, Assisting with Ambulation	791
24-3, Auscultating Heart Sounds	423	33-5, Helping Clients with Crutchwalking	795
24-4, Auscultating Breath Sounds	428	33-6, Transferring a Client to a Stretcher	798
24-5, Auscultating Bowel Sounds	432	33-7, Transferring a Client to a Wheelchair	799
25-1, Assessing Body Temperature	450	33-8, Transferring a Client from Bed to a Chair Using a Hydraulic Lift	802
25-2, Obtaining a Pulse	456	34-1, Monitoring with Pulse Oximetry	822
25-3, Assessing Respirations	462	34-2, Teaching Coughing and Deep-Breathing Exercises	829
25-4, Obtaining Blood Pressure	466		
25-5, Assessing for Orthostatic Hypotension	472	34-3, Promoting Breathing with the Incentive Spirometer	831
26-1, Handwashing	489		
26-2, Surgical Hand Scrub	500	34-4, Monitoring Peak Flow	833
26-3, Applying and Removing Sterile Gloves	502	34-5, Administering Oxygen by Nasal Cannula or Mask	838
26-4, Donning a Sterile Gown and Closed Gloving	504		
26-5, Preparing and Maintaining a Sterile Field	506	34-6, Monitoring a Client with a Chest Drainage System	844
27-1, Administering Oral Medications	534		
27-2, Administering Medication by Metered-Dose Inhaler	541	34-7, Providing Tracheostomy Care	848
		34-8, Suctioning Secretions from Airways	852
27-3, Withdrawing Medication from a Vial	545	34-9, Managing an Obstructed Airway (Heimlich Maneuver)	856
27-4, Withdrawing Medication from an Ampule	547		
27-5, Drawing Up Two Medications in a Syringe	549	35-1, Applying Antiembolic Stockings	887
27-6, Administering Intradermal Injections	551	35-2, Applying a Sequential Compression Device (SCD)	890
27-7, Administering Subcutaneous Injections	553		
27-8, Administering Intramuscular Injections	558	35-3, Administering Cardiopulmonary Resuscitation	896
27-9, Administering Medications by Intravenous Push	566	37-1, Measuring Blood Glucose By Skin Puncture	959
		37-2, Assisting an Adult with Feeding	969
27-10, Administering Intravenous Medications Using Intermittent Infusion Technique	568	37-3, Administering Nutrition Via Nasogastric or Gastrostomy Tube	974
28-1, Monitoring an Intravenous Infusion	589		
28-2, Changing Intravenous Solution and Tubing	591	38-1, Changing a Dry Sterile Dressing	1011
28-3, Converting to an Intermittent Infusion Device (IID) and Flushing	595	38-2, Applying a Saline-Moistened Dressing	1014
		38-3, Irrigating a Wound	1016
28-4, Administering Total Parenteral Nutrition	601	38-4, Maintaining a Portable (Hemovac) Wound Suction	1019
28-5, Administering a Blood Transfusion	605		
32-1, Assisting with the Bath or Shower	718	39-1, Obtaining a Wound Culture	1049
32-2, Bathing a Client in Bed	720	40-1, Collecting Urine Specimens	1079
32-3, Massaging the Back	725	40-2, Applying a Condom Catheter	1086
32-4, Performing Foot and Nail Care	727	40-3, Inserting a Straight or Indwelling Urinary Catheter	1089
32-5, Shampooing Hair of a Bedridden Client	730		
32-6, Providing Oral Care	732	41-1, Assessing Stool for Occult Blood	1114
32-7, Using a Bedpan	740	41-2, Administering an Enema	1123
32-8, Making an Unoccupied Bed	743	41-3, Inserting a Nasogastric Tube	1129
32-9, Making an Occupied Bed	747	41-4, Applying a Fecal Ostomy Pouch	1134
33-1, Using Body Mechanics to Move Clients	757	44-1, Removing Contact Lenses	1212
33-2, Positioning a Client in Bed	785	44-2, Assisting an Adult with Inserting a Hearing Aid	1213

NANDA-APPROVED NURSING DIAGNOSES

This list represents the NANDA-approved nursing diagnoses for clinical use and testing.

Activity Intolerance
Activity Intolerance, Risk for
Adjustment, Impaired
Airway Clearance, Ineffective
Allergy Response, Latex
Allergy Response, Risk for Latex
Anxiety
Anxiety, Death
Aspiration, Risk for
Attachment, Risk for Impaired
    Parent/Infant/Child
Autonomic Dysreflexia
Autonomic Dysreflexia, Risk for
Body Image, Disturbed
Body Temperature, Risk for Imbalanced
Bowel Incontinence
Breastfeeding, Effective
Breastfeeding, Ineffective
Breastfeeding, Interrupted
Breathing Pattern, Ineffective
Cardiac Output, Decreased
Caregiver Role Strain
Caregiver Role Strain, Risk for
Comfort, Impaired
Communication, Impaired Verbal
Conflict, Decisional
Conflict, Parental Role
Confusion, Acute
Confusion, Chronic
Constipation
Constipation, Perceived
Constipation, Risk for
Coping, Ineffective
Coping, Ineffective Community
Coping, Readiness for Enhanced
    Community
Coping, Defensive
Coping, Compromised Family
Coping, Disabled Family
Coping, Readiness for Enhanced Family
Denial, Ineffective
Dentition, Impaired
Development, Risk for Delayed
Diarrhea
Disuse Syndrome, Risk for

Diversional Activity, Deficient
Energy Field, Disturbed
Environmental Interpretation
    Syndrome, Impaired
Failure to Thrive, Adult
Falls, Risk for
Family Processes: Alcoholism,
    Dysfunctional
Family Processes: Interrupted
Fatigue
Fear
Fluid Volume, Deficient
Fluid Volume, Excess
Fluid Volume, Risk for Deficient
Fluid Volume, Risk for Imbalanced
Gas Exchange, Impaired
Grieving
Grieving, Anticipatory
Grieving, Dysfunctional
Growth and Development, Delayed
Growth, Risk for Disproportionate
Health Maintenance, Risk for Ineffective
Health-Seeking Behaviors
Home Maintenance, Impaired
Hopelessness
Hyperthermia
Hypothermia
Identity, Disturbed Personal
Incontinence, Functional Urinary
Incontinence, Reflex Urinary
Incontinence, Risk for Urge Urinary
Incontinence, Stress Urinary
Incontinence, Total Urinary
Incontinence, Urge Urinary
Infant Behavior, Disorganized
Infant Behavior, Readiness
    for Enhanced Organized
Infant Behavior, Risk for Disorganized
Infant Feeding Pattern, Ineffective
Infection, Risk for
Injury, Risk for
Injury, Risk for Perioperative-Positioning
Intracranial, Adaptive Capacity,
    Decreased
Knowledge, Deficient
Loneliness, Risk for
Memory, Impaired
Mobility, Impaired Bed
Mobility, Impaired Physical

Mobility, Impaired Wheelchair
Nausea
Neglect, Unilateral
Noncompliance
Nutrition: Less Than Body
    Requirements, Imbalanced
Nutrition: More Than Body
    Requirements, Imbalanced
Oral Mucous Membrane, Impaired
Pain, Acute
Pain, Chronic
Parenting, Impaired
Parenting, Risk for Impaired
Peripheral Neurovascular Dysfunction,
    Risk for
Poisoning, Risk for
Post-Trauma Syndrome
Post-Trauma Syndrome, Risk for
Powerlessness
Powerlessness, Risk for
Protection, Ineffective
Rape-Trauma Syndrome
Rape-Trauma Syndrome: Compound
    Reaction
Rape-Trauma Syndrome, Silent Reaction
Relocation Stress Syndrome
Relocation Stress Syndrome, Risk for
Role Performance, Ineffective
Self-Care Deficit
Self-Care Deficit, Bathing/Hygiene
Self-Care Deficit, Feeding
Self-Care Deficit, Toileting
Self-Esteem, Chronic Low
Self-Esteem, Situational Low
Self-Esteem, Risk for Situational Low
Self-Mutilation
Self-Mutilation, Risk for
Sensory Perception, Disturbed
Sexual Dysfunction
Sexuality Patterns, Ineffective
Skin Integrity, Impaired
Skin Integrity, Risk for Impaired
Sleep Deprivation
Sleep Pattern, Disturbed
Social Interaction, Impaired
Social Isolation
Sorrow, Chronic
Spiritual Distress
Spiritual Distress, Risk for